Dietary Reference Intakes (DRIs): Recommended Intakes for Individuals, Minerals

Life-Stage Group	Calcium (mg/day)	Chromium (mcg/day)	Copper (mcg/day)	Fluoride (mg/day)	Iodine (mcg/day)	Iron (mg/day)	Magnesium (mg/day)	Manganese (mg/day)	Molybdenum (mcg/day)	Phosphorus (mg/day)	Selenium (mcg/day)	Zinc (mg/day)	Potassium (g/day)	Sodium (g/day)	Chloride (g/day)
Infants															
0-6 mo	210*	0.2*	200*	0.01*	110*	0.27	30*	0.003*	2*	100*	15*	2*	0.4	0.12	0.18
7-12 mo	270*	5.5*	220*	0.5*	130*	11	75*	0.6*	3*	275*	20*	3*	0.7	0.37	0.57
Children															
1-3 yr	500*	11*	340	0.7*	90	7	80	1.2*	17	460	20	3	3.0	1.0	1.5
4-8 yr	800*	15*	440	1*	90	10	130	1.5*	22	500	30	5	3.8	1.2	1.9
Males															
9-13 yr	1300*	25*	700	2*	120	8	240	1.9*	34	1250	40	8	4.5	1.5	2.3
14-18 yr	1300*	35*	890	3*	150	11	410	2.2*	43	1250	55	11	4.7	1.5	2.3
19-30 yr	1000*	35*	900	4*	150	8	400	2.3*	45	700	55	11	4.7	1.5	2.3
31-50 yr	1000*	35*	900	4*	150	8	420	2.3*	45	700	55	11	4.7	1.5	2.3
50-70 yr	1200*	30*	900	4*	150	8	420	2.3*	45	700	55	11	4.7	1.3	2.0
>70 yr	1200*	30*	900	4*	150	8	420	2.3*	45	700	55	11	4.7	1.2	1.8
Females															
9-13 yr	1300*	21*	700	2*	120	8	240	1.6*	34	1250	40	8	4.5	1.5	2.3
14-18 yr	1300*	24*	890	3*	150	15	360	1.6*	43	1250	55	9	4.7	1.5	2.3
19-30 yr	1000*	25*	900	3*	150	18	310	1.8*	45	700	55	8	4.7	1.5	2.3
31-50 yr	1000*	25*	900	3*	150	18	320	1.8*	45	700	55	8	4.7	1.5	2.3
50-70 yr	1200*	20*	900	3*	150	8	320	1.8*	45	700	55	8	4.7	1.3	2.0
>70 yr	1200*	20*	900	3*	150	8	320	1.8*	45	700	55	8	4.7	1.2	1.8
Pregnant															
≤18 yr	1300*	29*	1000	3*	220	27	400	2.0*	50	1250	60	12	4.7	1.5	2.3
19-30 yr	1000*	30*	1000	3*	220	27	350	2.0*	50	700	60	11	4.7	1.5	2.3
31-50 yr	1000*	30*	1000	3*	220	27	360	2.0*	50	700	60	11	4.7	1.5	2.3
Lactating															
≤18 yr	1300*	44*	1300	3*	290	10	360	2.6*	50	1250	70	13	5.1	1.5	2.3
19-30 yr	1000*	45*	1300	3*	290	9	310	2.6*	50	700	70	12	5.1	1.5	2.3
31-50 yr	1000*	45*	1300	3*	290	9	320	2.6*	50	700	70	12	5.1	1.5	2.3

Data from Food and Nutrition Board, Institute of Medicine: Dietary reference intakes for calcium, phosphorus, magnesium, vitamin D, and fluoride (1997); *Dietary reference intakes for thiamin, riboflavin, niacin, vitamin B₆, folate, vitamin B₁₂, pantothenic acid, biotin, and choline* (1998); *Dietary reference intakes for vitamin C, vitamin E, selenium, and carotenoids* (2000); and *Dietary reference intakes for vitamin A, vitamin K, arsenic, boron, chromium, copper, iodine; manganese, molybdenum, nickel, silicon, vanadium, and zinc* (2001), Washington, DC, National Academies Press (www.nap.edu).

NOTE: * This table presents Recommended Dietary Allowances (RDAs) in **bold type** and Adequate Intakes (AIs) in regular type followed by an asterisk (*). RDAs and AIs may both be used as goals for individual intake. RDAs are set to meet the needs of almost all (97%-98%) individuals in a group. For healthy breast-fed infants, the AI is the mean intake. The AI for other life-stage and gender groups is believed to cover needs of all individuals in the group, but lack of data or uncertainty in the data prevent being able to specify with confidence the percentage of individuals covered by this intake.

Dietary Reference Intakes (DRIs): Tolerable Upper Intake Levels (UL[a]), Minerals

Life-Stage Group	Arsenic[b]	Boron (mg/day)	Calcium (g/day)	Chromium	Copper (mcg/day)	Fluoride (mg/day)	Iodine (mcg/day)	Iron (mg/day)	Magnesium (mg/day)[c]	Manganese (mg/day)	Molybdenum (mcg/day)	Nickel (mg/day)	Phosphorus (g/day)	Selenium (mcg/day)	Silicon[d]	Vanadium (mg/day)[e]	Zinc (mg/day)	Potassium	Sulfate	Sodium (g/day)	Chloride (g/day)
Infants																					
0-6 mo	ND[f]	ND	ND	ND	ND	0.7	ND	40	ND	ND	ND	ND	ND	45	ND	ND	4	ND	ND	ND	ND
7-12 mo	ND	ND	ND	ND	ND	0.9	ND	40	ND	ND	ND	ND	ND	60	ND	ND	5	ND	ND	ND	ND
Children																					
1-3 yr	ND	3	2.5	ND	1000	1.3	200	40	65	2	300	0.2	3	90	ND	ND	7	ND	ND	1.5	2.3
4-8 yr	ND	6	2.5	ND	3000	2.2	300	40	110	3	600	0.3	3	150	ND	ND	12	ND	ND	1.9	2.9
Males, Females																					
9-13 yr	ND	11	2.5	ND	5000	10	600	40	350	6	1100	0.6	4	280	ND	ND	23	ND	ND	2.2	3.4
14-18 yr	ND	17	2.5	ND	8000	10	900	45	350	9	1700	1.0	4	400	ND	ND	34	ND	ND	2.3	3.6
19-70 yr	ND	20	2.5	ND	10,000	10	1100	45	350	11	2000	1.0	4	400	ND	1.8	40	ND	ND	2.3	3.6
>70 yr	ND	20	2.5	ND	10,000	10	1100	45	350	11	2000	1.0	3	400	ND	1.8	40	ND	ND	2.3	3.6
Pregnant																					
≤18 yr	ND	17	2.5	ND	8000	10	900	45	350	9	1700	1.0	3.5	400	ND	ND	34	ND	ND	2.3	3.6
19-50 yr	ND	20	2.5	ND	10,000	10	1100	45	350	11	2000	1.0	3.5	400	ND	ND	40	ND	ND	2.3	3.6
Lactating																					
≤18 yr	ND	17	2.5	ND	8000	10	900	45	350	9	1700	1.0	4	400	ND	ND	34	ND	ND	2.3	3.6
19-50 yr	ND	20	2.5	ND	10,000	10	1100	45	350	11	2000	1.0	4	400	ND	ND	40	ND	ND	2.3	3.6

Data from Food and Nutrition Board, Institute of Medicine: *Dietary reference intakes for calcium, phosphorus, magnesium, vitamin D, and fluoride* (1997); *Dietary reference intakes for thiamine, riboflavin, niacin, vitamin B₆, folate, vitamin B₁₂, pantothenic acid, biotin, and choline* (1998); *Dietary reference intakes for vitamin C, vitamin E, selenium, and carotenoids* (2000); and *Dietary reference intakes for vitamin A, vitamin K, arsenic, boron, chromium, copper, iodine, manganese, molybdenum, nickel, silicon, vanadium, and zinc* (2001), Washington, DC, National Academies Press (www.nap.edu).

[a] UL = The maximum level of daily nutrient intake that is likely to pose no risk of adverse effects. Unless otherwise specified, the UL represents total intake from food, water, and supplements. Due to lack of suitable data, ULs could not be established for arsenic, chromium, and silicon. In the absence of ULs, extra caution may be warranted in consuming levels above recommended intakes.

[b] Although the UL was not determined for arsenic, there is no justification for adding arsenic to food or supplements.

[c] The ULs for magnesium represent intake from a pharmacologic agent only and do not include intake from food or water.

[d] Although silicon has not been shown to cause adverse effects in humans, there is no justification for adding silicon to supplements.

[e] Although vanadium in food has not been shown to cause adverse effects in humans, there is no justification for adding vanadium to food, and vanadium supplements should be used with caution. The UL is based on adverse effects in laboratory animals, and this data could be used to set a UL for adults but not children and adolescents.

[f] ND = Not determinable due to lack of data of adverse effects in this age group and concern with regard to lack of ability to handle excess amounts. Source of intake should be from food only to prevent high levels of intake.

Dietary Reference Intakes (DRIs): Values for Energy for Active Individuals*

Life-Stage Group	Criterion	Active Pal EER (kcal/day)† Male	Female
Infants			
0-6 mo	Energy expenditure + Energy deposition	570	520 (3 mo)
7-12 mo	Energy expenditure + Energy deposition	743	676 (9 mo)
Children			
1-2 yr	Energy expenditure + Energy deposition	1046	992 (24 mo)
3-8 yr	Energy expenditure + Energy deposition	1742	1642 (6 yr)
9-12 yr	Energy expenditure + Energy deposition	2279	2071 (11 yr)
14-18 yr	Energy expenditure + Energy deposition	3152	2368 (16 yr)
Adults			
>18 yr	Energy expenditure	3067‡	2403‡ (19 yr)
Pregnant Women			
14-18 yr	Adolescent female EER + Change in TEE + Pregnancy energy deposition		
First Trimester			2368 (16 yr)
Second Trimester			2708 (16 yr)
Third Trimester			2820 (16 yr)
19-50 yr	Adult female EER + Change in TEE + Pregnancy energy deposition		
First Trimester			2403‡ (19 yr)
Second Trimester			2743‡ (19 yr)
Third Trimester			2855‡ (19 yr)
Lactating Women			
14-18 yr	Adolescent female EER + Milk energy output - Weight loss		
First 6 mo			2698 (16 yr)
Second 6 mo			2768 (16 yr)
19-50 yr	Adult female EER + Milk energy output - Weight loss		
First 6 mo			2733‡ (19 yr)
Second 6 mo			2803‡ (19 yr)

From Institute of Medicine of The National Academies: *Dietary reference intakes for energy, carbohydrate, fiber, fat, fatty acids, cholesterol, protein, and amino acids,* Washington, DC, 2002, The National Academies Press.

*For healthy active Americans and Canadians at the reference height and weight.

†*PAL,* Physical activity level; *EER,* estimated energy requirement; *TEE,* total energy expenditure.

‡Subtract 10 kcal/day for men and 7 kcal/day for women for each year of age above 19 years.

Dietary Reference Intakes (DRIs): Recommended Intakes for Individuals, Macronutrients

Life-Stage Group	Protein RDA/AI g/day[a]	AMDR[b]	Carbohydrate RDA/AI g/day	AMDR	Fiber RDA/AI g/day	AMDR	Fat RDA/AI g/day	AMDR	n-6 Polyunsaturated Fatty Acids (Linoleic Acid) RDA/AI g/day	AMDR	n-3 Polyunsaturated Fatty Acids (α-Linolenic Acid) RDA/AI g/day	AMDR[d]	Saturated and trans Fatty Acids and Cholesterol RDA/AI g/day	AMDR
Infants														
0-6 mo	9.1	ND[c]	60	ND	ND		31		4.4	ND	0.5	ND		
7-12 mo	11	ND	95	ND	ND		30		4.6	ND	0.5	ND		
Children														
1-3 yr	13	5-20	130	45-65	19			30-40	7	5-10	0.7	0.6-1.2		
4-8 yr	19	10-30	130	45-65	25			25-35	10	5-10	0.9	0.6-1.2		
Males														
9-13 yr	34	10-30	130	45-65	31			25-35	12	5-10	1.2	0.6-1.2		
14-18 yr	52	10-30	130	45-65	38			25-35	16	5-10	1.6	0.6-1.2		
19-30 yr	56	10-35	130	45-65	38			20-35	17	5-10	1.6	0.6-1.2		
31-50 yr	56	10-35	130	45-65	38			20-35	17	5-10	1.6	0.6-1.2		
50-70 yr	56	10-35	130	45-65	30			20-35	14	5-10	1.6	0.6-1.2		
>70 yr	56	10-35	130	45-65	30			20-35	14	5-10	1.6	0.6-1.2		
Females														
9-13 yr	34	10-30	130	45-65	26			25-35	10	5-10	1.0	0.6-1.2		
14-18 yr	46	10-30	130	45-65	26			25-35	11	5-10	1.1	0.6-1.2		
19-30 yr	46	10-35	130	45-65	25			20-35	12	5-10	1.1	0.6-1.2		
31-50 yr	46	10-35	130	45-65	25			20-35	12	5-10	1.1	0.6-1.2		
50-70 yr	46	10-35	130	45-65	21			20-35	11	5-10	1.1	0.6-1.2		
>70 yr	46	10-35	130	45-65	21			20-35	11	5-10	1.1	0.6-1.2		
Pregnant														
≤18 yr	71	10-35	175	45-65	28			20-35	13	5-10	1.4	0.6-1.2		
19-30 yr	71	10-35	175	45-65	28			20-35	13	5-10	1.4	0.6-1.2		
31-50 yr	71	10-35		45-65	28			20-35	13	5-10	1.4	0.6-1.2		
Lactating														
≤18 yr	71	10-35	210	45-65	29			20-35	13	5-10	1.3	0.6-1.2		
19-30 yr	71	10-35	210	45-65	29			20-35	13	5-10	1.3	0.6-1.2		
31-50 yr	71	10-35	210	45-65	29			20-35	13	5-10	1.3	0.6-1.2		

Data from *Dietary reference intakes for energy, carbohydrate, fiber, fat, fatty acids, cholesterol, protein, and amino acids,* Washington, DC, 2002, The National Academies Press.

NOTE:* This table presents Recommended Dietary Allowances (RDAs) in **bold type** and Adequate Intakes (AIs) in regular type. RDAs and AIs may both be used as goals for individual intake. RDAs are set to meet the needs of almost all (97%-98%) individuals in a group. For healthy breast-fed infants, the AI is the mean intake. The AI for other life stage and gender groups is believed to cover the needs of all individuals in the group, but lack of data prevents being able to specify with confidence the percentage of individuals covered by this intake.

[a]Based on 1.5 g/kg/day for infants, 1.1 g/kg/day for 1-3 yr, 0.95 g/kg/day for 4-13 yr, 0.85 g/kg/day for 14-18 yr, 0.8 g/kg/day for adults, and 1.1 g/kg/day for pregnant (using pre-pregnancy weight) and lactating women.

[b]Acceptable Macronutrient Distribution Range (AMDR) is the range of intake for a particular energy source that is associated with reduced risk of chronic disease while providing intakes of essential nutrients. If an individual has consumed in excess of the AMDR, there is a potential of increasing the risk of chronic diseases and insufficient intakes of essential nutrients.

[c]ND = Not determinable due to lack of data of adverse effects in this age group and concern with regard to lack of ability to handle excess amounts. Source of intake should be from food only to prevent high levels of intake.

[d]Approximately 10% of the total can come from longer-chain, n-3 fatty acids.

Krause's *Food & Nutrition Therapy*

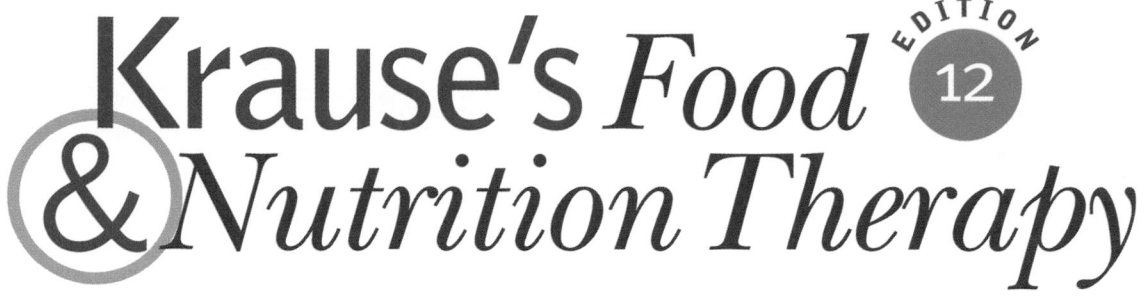

Krause's *Food* & *Nutrition Therapy*

EDITION 12

L. Kathleen Mahan, MS, RD, CDE

Clinical Associate
Department of Pediatrics
School of Medicine
University of Washington
Seattle, Washington

Nutrition Counselor
Nutrition by Design
Seattle, Washington

Sylvia Escott-Stump, MA, RD, LDN

Dietetic Programs Director
Department of Nutrition and Dietetics
East Carolina University
Greenville, North Carolina

Consulting Nutritionist
Nutritional Balance
Winterville, North Carolina

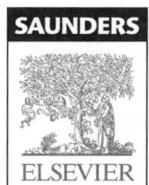

SAUNDERS

ELSEVIER

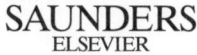

SAUNDERS
ELSEVIER

11830 Westline Industrial Drive
St. Louis, Missouri 63146

Notice

Knowledge and best practice in this field are constantly changing. As new research and experience broaden our knowledge, changes in practice, treatment, and drug therapy may become necessary or appropriate. Readers are advised to check the most current information provided (i) on procedures featured or (ii) by the manufacturer of each product to be administered, to verify the recommended dose or formula, the method and duration of administration, and contraindications. It is the responsibility of the practitioners, relying on their own experience and knowledge of the patient, to make diagnoses, to determine dosages and the best treatment for each individual patient, and to take all appropriate safety precautions. To the fullest extent of the law, neither the Publisher nor the Editors assumes any liability for any injury and/or damage to persons or property arising out of or related to any use of the material contained in this book.

The Publisher

Acquisitions Editor: Yvonne Alexopoulos
Managing Editor: Kristin Hebberd
Associate Developmental Editor: Heather Bays
Publishing Services Manager: John Rogers
Senior Project Manager: Cheryl Abbott
Design Direction: Amy Buxton
Cover Art: Dennis Kunkel Microscopy, Inc.
Cover Image: Copyright Dennis Kunkel Microscopy, Inc.

Working together to grow
libraries in developing countries

www.elsevier.com | www.bookaid.org | www.sabre.org

ELSEVIER   BOOK AID International   Sabre Foundation

Printed in Canada

Last digit is the print number: 9 8 7 6 5 4 3 2 1

The authors dedicate this edition to all of the wonderful dietitians and students who have used this text and continue to consider it as their "nutrition bible." We are most grateful to them for their insights and devotion to the field.

—The Authors, 12th Edition

Contributors

Diane M. Anderson, PhD, RD, CSP, FADA
Associate Professor
Department of Pediatrics
Baylor College of Medicine
Houston, Texas

John J. B. Anderson, PhD
Professor of Nutrition
University of North Carolina
Chapel Hill, NC

Cynthia Taft Bayerl, MS, RD, LDN
Nutrition Coordinator
Coordinator, Massachusetts Fruit & Vegetable
   Nutrition Coordinator
Nutrition and Physical Activity Unit
Division of Health Promotion and Disease Prevention
Massachusetts Department of Public Health
Boston, Massachusetts

Peter L. Beyer, MS, RD
Associate Professor
Dietetics & Nutrition
University of Kansas Medical Center
Kansas City, Kansas

Abby S. Bloch, PhD, RD, FADA
Executive Director
The Dr. Robert C. Atkins Foundation
Jenkintown, Pennsylvania

Pamela Charney, PhD, RD, CNSD
Consultant, Dietetic Internship, Nutrition Sciences
Affiliate Clinical Associate Professor
College of Pharmacy
University of Washington
Seattle, Washington;
Adjunct Assistant Professor
College of Human Ecology
SUNY Oneonta
Oneonta, New York

Harriet Cloud, MS, RD, FADA
Nutrition Matters, Owner
Professor Emeritus, Department of Nutrition Sciences
School of Health Related Professions
University of Alabama at Birmingham
Birmingham, Alabama

Sarah C. Couch, PhD, RD, LD
Associate Professor
Department of Nutritional Sciences
University of Cincinnati
Cincinnati, Ohio

Sr. Jeanne P. Crowe, PharmD, RPH
Director of Pharmacy
Camilla Hall Nursing Home
Immaculata, Pennsylvania

Ruth DeBusk, PhD, RD
Geneticist and Clinical Dietician
Private Practice
Tallahassee, Florida

Judith L. Dodd, MS, RD, FADA
Adjunct Assistant Professor
Department of Sports Medicine and Nutrition
School of Health and Rehabilitation Sciences
University of Pittsburgh
Pittsburgh, Pennsylvania

Lisa Dorfman, MS, RD, CSSD, LMHC
Adjunct Professor
Department of Exercise Science
University of Miami
Miami, Florida

Kristine Duncan, MS, RD, CDE
Lead Educator
Life Quest Department
St. Joseph Hospital
Bellingham, Washington;
Adjunct Instructor
Skagit Valley College
Mt. Vernon, Washington

Robert Earl, DrPh, RD
Senior Director for Nutrition Policy
Food Products Association
Washington, DC

Miriam Erick, MS, RD, CDE, LDN
Senior Clinical Dietitian
Department of Nutrition
Brigham and Women's Hospital
Boston, Massachusetts

Marcy Fenton, MS, RD
Office of AIDS Programs and Policy
Los Angeles County Department of Public Health
Los Angeles, California

Sharon A. Feucht, MA, RD, CD
Nutritionist
Center on Human Development and Disability
University of Washington
Seattle, Washington

Marion J. Franz, MS, RD, LD, CDE
Nutrition Concepts by Franz, Inc.
Minneapolis, Minnesota

Carol D. Frary, MS, RD
Public Health Nutrition Specialist
Vermont State WIC Program
Burlington, Vermont

Margie Lee Gallagher, PhD, RD
Acting Dean
Human Ecology
East Carolina University
Greenville, North Carolina

Molly Gee, MEd, RD
Project Leader
Behavioral Medicine Research Center
Baylor College of Medicine
Houston, Texas

Barbara Grant, MS, RD
Oncology Clinical Dietitian
Saint Alphonsus Cancer Care Center
Boise, Idaho

Kathy Hammond, MS, RN, RD, LD, CNSD
Coordinator, Continuing Education
Clinical Nutrition Specialist
Chartwell Diversified Services, Inc.
Atlanta, Georgia;
Adjunct Assistant Professor
Department of Food and Nutrition
University of Georgia
Athens, Georgia

Jeanette M. Hasse, PhD, RD, LD, CNSD, FADA
Manager, Transplant Nutrition
Baylor Regional Transplant Institute
Baylor University Medical Center
Dallas, Texas

Sherry K. Hubbard, RD, LD
Clinical Dietitian
Medical Nutrition Department
Oklahoma Allergy and Asthma Clinic
Oklahoma City, Oklahoma

Rachel K. Johnson, PhD, RD
Dean and Professor of Nutrition
College of Agriculture and Life Sciences
University of Vermont
Burlington, Vermont

Veena Juneja, MSc, RD
Senior Renal Dietitian
Nutrition Services
St. Joseph's Healthcare
Hamilton, Ontario, Canada

Barbara J. Kamp, MS, RD
Project Coordinator
National Resource Center on Nutrition, Physical
    Activity, and Aging
Florida International University
Miami, Florida

Debra A. Krummel, PhD, RD
Endowed Professor
Nutritional Sciences
University of Cincinnati
Cincinnati, Ohio

Mary Demarest Litchford, PhD, RD, LDN
President
CASE Software & Books
Greensboro, North Carolina

Betty L. Lucas, MPH, RD, CD
Nutritionist
Center on Human Development and Disability
University of Washington
Seattle, Washington

Ainsley M. Malone, MS, RD, CNSD
Nutrition Support Team
Mt. Carmel West Hospital
Columbus, Ohio

Laura E. Matarese, MS, RD, LDN, CNSD, FADA
Director of Nutrition
Intestinal Rehabilitation and Transplantation Center
Thomas E. Starzl Transplantation Institute
University of Pittsburgh Medical Center
Pittsburgh, Pennsylvania

Kelly N. McKean, MS, RD, CD
Clinical Pediatric Dietitian
Children's Hospital and Regional Medical Center
Seattle, Washington

Charles Mueller, PhD, RD, CNSD, CDN
Nutrition Research Manager
Weill Medical College
Cornell University
New York, New York

Donna H. Mueller, PhD, RD, FADA, LDN
Associate Professor
Department of Bioscience and Biotechnology
Drexel University
Philadelphia, Pennsylvania

Beth N. Ogata, MS, RD, CD
Nutritionist
Center on Human Development and Disability
University of Washington
Seattle, Washington

Zaneta M. Pronsky, MS, RD, LDN, FADA
Author/Consultant
Food Medication Interactions

Diane Rigassio Radler, PhD, RD
Assistant Professor
Department of Primary Care
University of Medicine and Dentistry of New Jersey
School of Health Related Professions
Newark, New Jersey

Valentina M. Remig, PhD, RD, LD, FADA
Consultant/Author
Nutrition & Healthy Aging
Manhattan, Kansas

Janet E. Schebendach, MA, RD
Nutritionist
Eating Disorders Research
New York State Psychiatric Institute
New York, New York

Ellyn C. Silverman, RD, MPH
President
ECS Nutrition Services
Director of Nutritional Services
Long Beach, California

Linda G. Snetselaar, RD, LD, PhD
Professor
Department of Epidemiology
College of Public Health
University of Iowa
Iowa City, Iowa

Jamie Stang, PhD, MPH, RD
Assistant Professor and Director
Leadership Education and Training Program
    in MCH Nutrition
School of Public Health, Division of Epidemiology
    and Community Health
University of Minnesota
Minneapolis, Minnesota

Tracy Stopler, MS, RD
President
Nutrition ETC (Exercise, Training, and Counseling) Inc.
Plainview, New York;
Associate Professor
Nutrition and Human Performance
Adelphi University
Garden City, New York

Cynthia A. Thomson, PhD, RD
Associate Professor
Nutritional Sciences, Public Health, and Medicine
University of Arizona
Tucson, Arizona

Riva Touger-Decker, PhD, RD, FADA
Professor and Director
Graduate Programs in Clinical Nutrition
School of Health Related Professions
University of Medicine and Dentistry of New Jersey
Newark, New Jersey

Cristine M. Trahms, MS, RD, CD, FADA
Senior Lecturer
Division of Genetics and Development
Department of Pediatrics;
Head, Nutrition
Center on Human Development and Disability
University of Washington
Seattle, Washington

Nancy S. Wellman, PhD, RD, FADA
Professor and Director
National Resource Center on Nutrition, Physical
    Activity, and Aging
Florida International University
Miami, Florida

Katy G. Wilkens, MS, RD
Manager
Nutrition & Fitness Services
Northwest Kidney Centers
Seattle, Washington

Marion F. Winkler, MS, RD, LDN, CNSD
Surgical Nutrition Specialist and Senior Teaching Associate
  of Surgery
Rhode Island Hospital and Brown Medical School
Providence, Rhode Island

Monika M. Woolsey, MS, RD
Owner
After the Diet Network
Glendale, Arizona

Reviewers

Thelma B. Baker, PhD
Associate Professor
Department of Nutritional Sciences
College of Pharmacy
Nursing and Allied Health Sciences
Howard University
Washington, DC

Bonita E. Broyles, RN, BSN, PhD
ADN Faculty
Piedmont Community College
Roxboro, North Carolina

Melany Tracy Burns, PhD, RD
Associate Professor and DPD Coordinator
School of Family and Consumer Sciences
Eastern Illinois University
Charleston, Illinois

Kathryn Camp, MS, RD, CSP
Pediatric Nutritionist
Walter Reed Army Medical Center
Department of Pediatrics
Washington DC;
Assistant Professor
Pediatrics
Uniformed Services University
Bethesda, Maryland

Malinda D. Cecil, MS, RD, LDN
Dietetics Program Director and Lecturer
University of Maryland Eastern Shore
Department of Human Ecology
Princess Ann, Maryland

Dorice M. Czajka-Narions, PhD
Former Professor and Chair
Department of Nutrition and Food Science
Texas Women's University
Denton, Texas

Judith L. Dodd, MS, RD, FADA
Adjunct Assistant Professor
Department of Sports Medicine and Nutrition
School of Health and Rehabilitation Sciences
University of Pittsburgh
Pittsburgh, Pennsylvania

Rebecca L. Dunn, MA, RD, LD, CNSD
Instructor
Department of Health Science/Nutrition
Keene State College
Keene, New Hampshire

Christine Filipowski, MS, RD, LDN
Clinical Dietitian
Rush University Medical Center
Chicago, Illinois

Margie Lee Gallagher, PhD, RD
Acting Dean
College of Human Ecology
East Carolina University
Greenville, North Carolina

Andrea Goyshor, MPH, RD, LDN
Clinical Dietitian
Department of Food and Nutrition Services
Rush University Medical Center
Chicago, Illinois

Debra Hodge, RN, BSN, MSN
Clinical and Theory Instructor
Academy of Careers and Technology
School of Nursing
Beckley, West Virginia

Sharon Kaye Hunt, MS, RD
Associate Professor
Fort Valley State University
Fort Valley, Georgia

Judith M. Lukaszuk, PhD, RD, LDN
Assistant Professor
School of Family, Consumer, and Nutrition Services
Director
Didactic Program in Dietetics
Northern Illinois University
Dekalb, Illinois

Alisa Montgomery, RN, MSN
Associate Degree Nursing Faculty
Level Coordinator
Piedmont Community College
Roxboro, North Carolina

Sharon M. Nickols-Richardson, PhD, RD
Associate Professor
Department of Human Nutrition, Foods, and Exercise
Virginia Polytechnic Institute and State University
Blacksburg, Virginia

Ruth Novitt-Schumacher, RN, BSN, MSN
Instructor
University of Illinois at Chicago
College of Nursing
Department of Maternal Child Nursing
Chicago, Illinois

Emily J. Porterfield, RD, LDN
Consulting Dietitian
Private Practice
Kalispell, Montana;
Freelance Copyeditor and Proofreader

Cynthia A. Stegeman, RDH, MeD, RD, LD, CDE
Assistant Professor
Dental Hygiene Department
University of Cincinnati
Cincinnati, Ohio

Foreword

"Be willing to change to remain the same" is a favorite quote of mine and exemplifies the quality of the 12th edition of the *Krause's Food & Nutrition Therapy* textbook. Fifty-five years ago, the vision of Marie Krause Mendelson was to publish a "universally recognized, authoritative, and popular nutrition textbook," a vision that remains in the forefront for the authors today. As the world of dietetics and nutrition changes over the years, the Krause textbook continues to evolve and remain a valuable resource guide for practitioners, as well as remain the textbook for medical nutrition therapy in higher education. As a practitioner, I always have the latest edition on my bookshelf to serve as a ready reference in communicating the message of nutrition to industry and consumers.

The current edition is not the same as the textbook I used at the University of Kentucky in the 1970s, but neither is the practice of dietetics. Today we face a multitude of challenges and opportunities that will shape the future practice of dietetics not only in our society but also globally. The American Dietetic Association's 2006 report, "The Profession of Dietetics at a Critical Juncture," defines the challenges and opportunities that will change the nature of professional practice, not just for the dietitian but for all health and medical professionals. Trends that will have the greatest impact on the future of dietetics include the aging of the U.S. population and the associated rise in chronic diseases and Alzheimer's disease; the continuation of obesity as a public and global issue; a growing economic gap between the haves and have-nots in American society; the global explosion in the communication and how the consumer obtains nutrition knowledge; and the increasing multiculturalism of the U.S. society with its differing attitudes, languages, and food choices.

The 12th edition of *Krause's Food & Nutrition Therapy* addresses the future trends as evidenced by the inclusion of two new chapters—"Medical Nutrition Therapy for Psychiatric Conditions" and "Medical Nutrition Therapy for Developmental Disabilities," as well as the newest information on the Dietary Guidelines for Americans 2005. This edition also expands on the nutrition care process and provides "real-life" sample diagnoses in a case study format vital in promoting learning for students and practitioners. In keeping with the global explosion, the inclusion of Canada's 2007 Food Guide is a new feature. This edition remains true to its vision of being a " universally recognized and authoritative reference" as it continues to provide its audience with the latest information on some of the nutritional hot topics: *trans*-fatty acids; childhood obesity; the prevalence of celiac disease; and the rising incidence of type 2 diabetes and prediabetes, especially in children.

Opportunities for the profession of dietetics abound along with the challenges. As health professionals, we must create the new avenues of communication and counseling for the consumer, develop a practice that meets the needs of an aging but "forever young" generation, and understand the role that genetics and nutrigenomics will play in medical nutrition therapy. The 12th edition of *Krause's Food & Nutrition Therapy* opens the door for students and practitioners to find the knowledge and assistance to navigate the challenges and opportunities of the future.

Marianne Smith Edge, MS, RD, LD, FADA
President
MSE & Associates, LLC
Owensboro, Kentucky;
2003-2004 President
American Dietetic Association

Preface

The 12th edition of this classic text supports the nutrition care process as the standard for dietetics. This process plays a major role in the empowerment of dietitians to manage and solve nutrition problems independently. Not only will students be able to grasp this concept, but also practitioners will continue to evolve and embrace the standardized language for their own settings, whether for individuals, families, groups, or communities.

AUDIENCE

The text furnishes theoretical knowledge and clinical information in a form that is useful to students in dietetics, nursing, and other allied health professions in an interdisciplinary format. It is valuable as an ancillary text for use in other disciplines such as medicine, dentistry, child development, health education, and lifestyle counseling. **Nutrient and assessment appendixes, tables, illustrations,** and **Clinical Insight boxes** provide practical hands-on procedures and clinical tools for students and practitioners alike.

This textbook accompanies the graduating student into clinical practice as a treasured reference. All of the popular features such as **Key Terms, Focus On** and **New Directions boxes, Useful Websites,** and **Pathophysiology and Clinical Management Algorithms** have been retained in this edition. New features are **nutrition diagnoses for all Clinical Scenarios and Focal Points** summarizing each chapter. All material has been updated and referenced extensively to reflect the most current information, especially for evidence-based practice.

A few new guest authors join those who are back by popular demand. Many new reviewers also joined the preparation process. The contributions of these reputable authors and reviewers, all experts in their fields, reflect the effort of this text to cover the increasing sophistication of nutrition care and education.

Our goal with each new edition has always been to maintain this book as a premier text in the field of dietetics that students and educators will turn to and that clinicians will continue to use with ease and confidence when providing nutrition care.

ORGANIZATION

The premise of this edition follows the Conceptual Framework for Steps of the Nutrition Care Process (see inside of back cover). All nutrition care components (assessment, nutrition diagnosis, intervention, monitoring and evaluation) are addressed to enhance or improve the nutritional well-being of individuals, their families, or populations. The role of the educated nutrition practitioner is to identify nutrition problems and to help solve them within the scope of practice.

With this in mind, the 12th edition is organized into five parts and includes information about all key elements related to nutrition care. The first two parts, "Nutrition Basics" and "Nutrition in the Life Cycle," are appropriate for understanding the basics of nutrition related to nutrient requirements and life stages. The third part, "Nutrition Care Process," addresses new standardized language to promote more predictable outcomes from nutritional care. The fourth part, "Nutrition in Health and Fitness," emphasizes how nutritional interventions can make a difference in retaining health or recovering from a decline in nutritional status. The fifth part, "Medical Nutrition Therapy," provides in-depth discussion of nutritional therapies and their rationale for successful clinical practice.

Part 1, Nutrition Basics, continues to furnish practical information with many tables and clinical applications such as calculation of energy requirements and expenditure. The macronutrient chapters have been merged into one chapter; discussion of vitamins and minerals is included here and remains essential reading for background to medical nutrition therapy.

Part 2, Nutrition in the Life Cycle, presents in-depth information on the nutrition for life stages from pregnancy throughout aging.

Part 3, Nutrition Care Process, describes the process from nutrition genomics to individual eating habits, pharmacological and nutritional treatments, and the nutrition resources in the community. Understanding the nutrition care process allows practice to reflect critical thinking skills regardless of the setting or environment. The process is used for individuals but can also be applied when helping families, teaching groups, or when evaluating the nutrition weaknesses in a community or population.

Part 4, Nutrition for Health and Fitness, brings together nutrition concepts that have particular meaning in the achievement and maintenance of health and fitness and the prevention of chronic disease. Weight management, eating disorders, dental health, bone health, and sports nutrition focus on the role of nutrition in promoting long-term health.

Part 5, Medical Nutrition Therapy, reflects evidence-based knowledge and current trends in nutrition therapies. All of the chapters are written and reviewed by specialists in the nutritional aspects of conditions such as cardiovascular disorders, diabetes, liver disease, renal disease, and pulmonary disease.

NEW TO THIS EDITION

- **New title:** The updated title reflects the profession's change in focus from "diet therapy" to "nutrition therapy" while still providing the most current information upon which instructor's and students alike have come to rely.
- **Newest Recommendations:** Throughout the text we have incorporated all of the Dietary Reference Intakes (DRI), including Recommended Dietary Allowances (RDA), Adequate Intakes (AI), and Tolerable Upper Levels of Intake (UL).
- **Clinical Scenarios:** Each chapter, where relevant, includes "Clinical Scenarios" with a new sample **Nutrition Diagnosis** (Problem, Etiology, Signs & Symptoms) statement to promote thinking of how to intervene, what other assessment and monitoring factors are needed, and how to evaluate the outcomes.
- **Medical Nutrition Therapy:** Two new chapters have been added to the section on "Medical Nutrition Therapy": *Medical Nutrition Therapy for Psychiatric Conditions* and *Medical Nutrition Therapy for Developmental Disabilities.* They are written by specialists in the fields and are timely for the scope of practice today. We think they will be useful for the student and practitioner staying current in nutritional care.
- **Nutrition Care Process Tools:** In the extensive appendixes, the reader will find updated clinical references and tools that have always been a valued feature of this text. There are several new appendixes, including more nutrient tables as useful guides for specific foods in the dietary management of various conditions.

PEDAGOGY

UNIQUE Pathophysiology and Care Management Algorithms: Pathophysiology, related to nutrition care, continues to be a basic part of the text. Newly drawn algorithms illustrate pathophysiology and appropriate medical and nutritional management. These algorithms equip the reader with an understanding of the illness as background for providing optimal nutritional care.

Clinical Insight boxes expand on clinical information in the text and highlight areas that may go unnoticed. These boxes contain information on studies and clinical resources for the student and practitioner.

Focus On boxes provide thought-provoking information on key concepts for well-rounded study and to promote further discussion within the classroom.

New Directions boxes suggests areas for further research by spotlighting emerging areas of interest within the field.

- **Key Terms** are defined at the beginning of each chapter and are highlighted within the text where they are discussed in more detail.
- **Useful Websites** direct the reader to online resources that relate to the chapter topics.

ANCILLARIES

Accompanying this edition are the Instructor's Electronic Resource on CD-ROM and the Evolve site online. These valuable resources have been completely updated for this edition. All Instructor materials can be found on CD-ROM and online, and students can access resources for further study through the Evolve site by going to http://evolve.elsevier.com/Mahan/nutrition/.

INSTRUCTOR RESOURCES

- **PowerPoint Presentations:** Over 900 slides to help guide classroom lectures.
- **NEW Image Collection:** Approximately 200 images are included that contain the illustrations from the PowerPoint Presentations, as well as more illustrations that can be downloaded and used to develop other teaching resources.
- **NEW Audience Response System Questions (for use with iClicker and other systems):** 2 to 4 questions per chapter to help the instructor incorporate this new technology into the classroom.
- **Testbank:** Each chapter includes NCLEX-formatted questions with page references specific to that chapter's content to offer over 900 multiple-choice questions.
- **NEW Animations:** Approximately 50 animations have been developed to visually complement the text and the processes discussed.
- **NEW Nutrition Care Process Tools:** Consisting of Assessment/Monitoring Tools and Intervention Tools, this information can be used by the student and by the practitioner in teaching and guiding the client in his or her specific nutrition care.

STUDENT RESOURCES

WebLinks: Online resources consisting of the sites needed for further study within the nutrition field.

Study Exercises With Answers: With over 20 questions per chapter, these exercises give instant feedback on questions related to the chapter's content.

Acknowledgements

We heartily thank the contributors of this edition who devoted hours of committed time to the accuracy and reliability of this book. We could not do this without them!

The contributors would like to thank Sanford C. Garner, PhD, for his help in the preparation the Nutrition and Bone Health chapter; Marijane Staniec, MS RD, CNSD, Department of Nutrition, Boston University, Claire Cotes, RN, BA, IBCLC, Lactation Specialist, and Gina Abbascia, RN, ADNm IBCLC, Brigham & Women's Hospital, Lactation Support Services, for their help on the Pregnancy and Lactation chapter; Jan King, MD, MPH, Medical Director, Office of AIDS Programs and Policy, Los Angeles County Department of Public Health, for her help on the Medical Nutrition Therapy for HIV Disease chapter; University of Houston's Dietetic Internship students, especially Rebecca J. Mitchell, RD, and Angie Sutphin, RD, NSCA-CPT, for their help on the Weight Management chapter; Amy Pflum M ED, RD, Research Dietitian and Coordinator, University of Cincinnati, and Sara King Tamsukhin, RD, Clinical Research Coordinator, Cincinnati Children's Hospital Medical Center, for their help on the Cardiovascular, Hypertension, and Heart Failure and Transplant chapters; Nicole Bergier, BS, Research Assistant, Department of Nutritional Sciences, University of Arizona, for her help on the Dietary Supplementation and Integrative Nutrition Therapy chapter; Lori S. Brizee, MS, RD, CSP, of Children's Hospital & Medical Center, Seattle, Washington, for her expertise in writing the section on renal failure in children; Alysun Deckert, MS, RD, CD, and Elizabeth Mullins, RD, CD, of the University of Washington Medical Center, Seattle, Washington, for their expertise in writing the section on renal transplantation; and Fiona Wolf, RD, for her work in reviewing the chapter on Renal Disorders.

We also wish to acknowledge the hard work and support of Yvonne Alexopoulos, Acquisitions Editor; Kristen Hebberd, Managing Editor; Heather Bays, Associate Developmental Editor; Cheryl Abbott, Senior Project Manager; Pam Charney, who assisted with the Clinical Scenarios and Nutrition Diagnosis statements; Maria Montesano, who helped update the Appendixes and Evolve sites; Gill Robertson and Joseph Bonilla for Instructor and Student ancillaries; and all of our wonderful reviewers.

Most important is the continuing encouragement and support from our families, without whom this work would not be possible. Kathleen thanks Robert, Carly, and Ana Raab and Jim Mahan and his family. Sylvia thanks Russ, Matthew, and Lindsay Stump; Clara Escott; Florianne Stump; and Joyce Stanley and her family. Their never-ending support is incredible, and so important.

L. Kathleen Mahan

L. Kathleen Mahan, MS, RD, CDE

Sylvia Escott-Stump

Sylvia Escott-Stump, MA, RD, LDN

Contents

PART 5
MEDICAL NUTRITION THERAPY

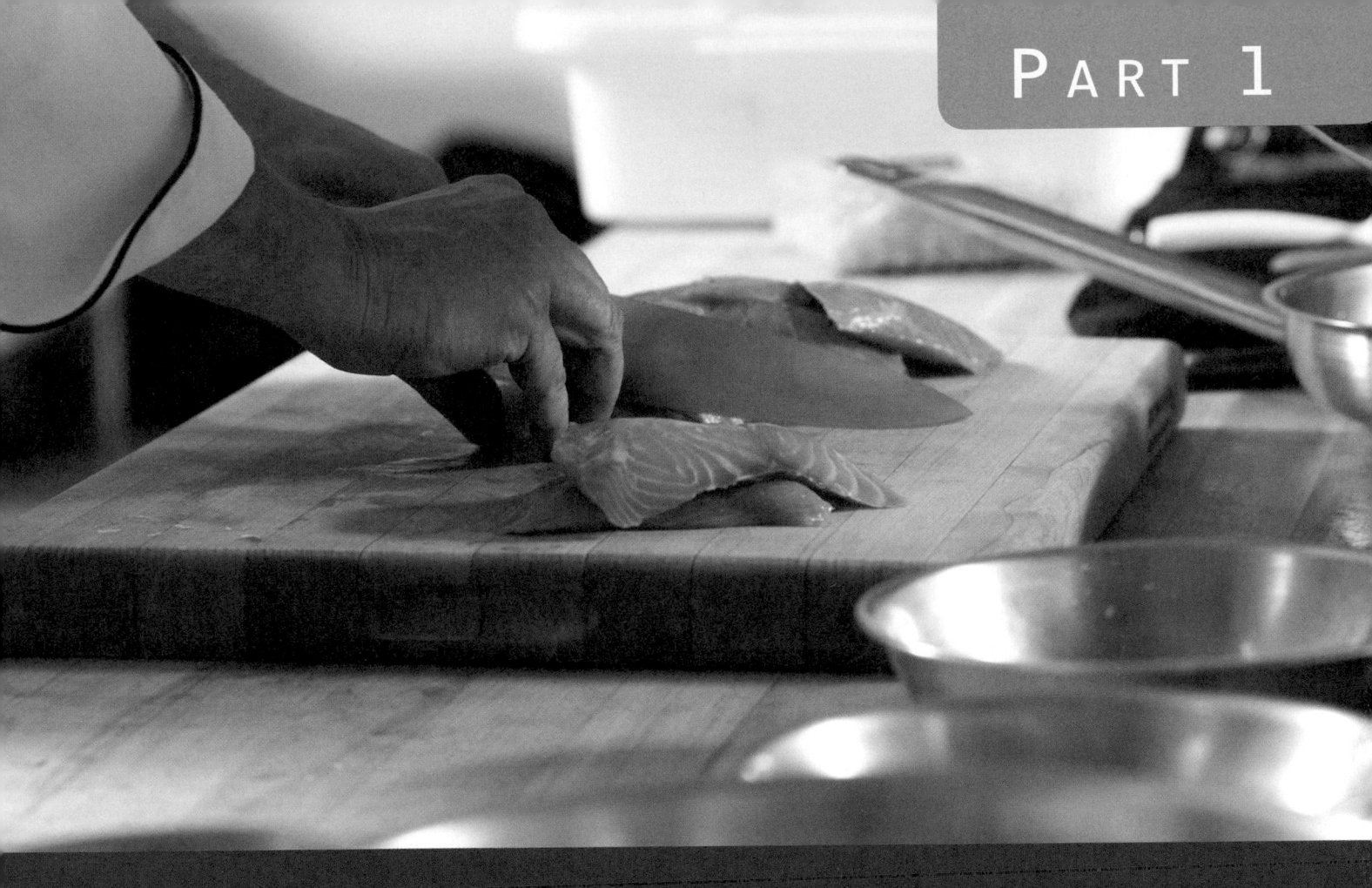

PART 1

Nutrition Basics

FOOD provides the energy and building materials for the countless substances that are essential for the growth and survival of living things. The way nutrients become integral parts of the body and contribute to its function depends on the physiologic and biochemical processes that govern their actions.

This section opens with a brief overview of digestion, absorption, transportation, and excretion. These steps describe the remarkable processes involved in converting myriads of complex foodstuffs into individual nutrients ready to be used in metabolism. Different characteristics of foods, including color, form, texture, and flavor, and a host of psychosocial factors, invite consumption. However, once inside the alimentary tract, their appeal is no longer important. The process of digestion reduces them to a size and form capable of absorption and transportation to individual cells.

Proteins, fats, and carbohydrates all contribute to the total energy pool, but ultimately the energy they yield is all in the same form. Release of the energy for use in synthesis, movement, and other functions requires the involvement of vitamins and minerals, which function as coenzymes, co-catalysts, and buffers in the miraculous, watery arena of metabolism.

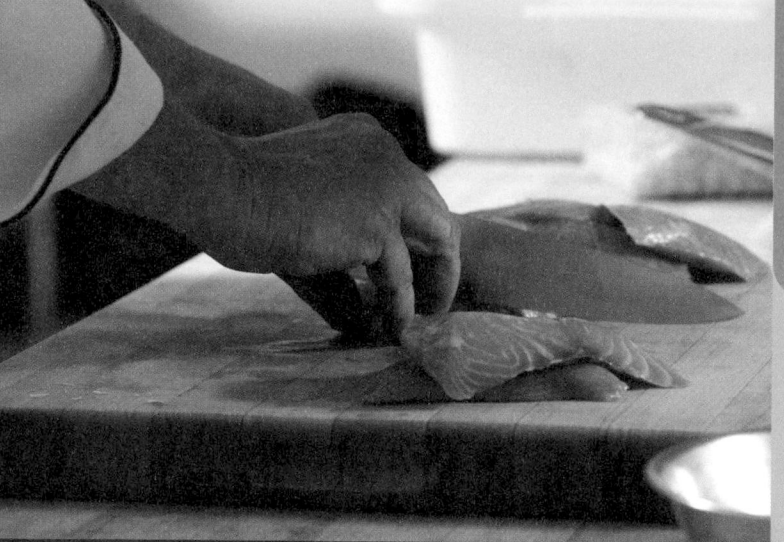

CHAPTER 1

Peter L. Beyer, MS, RD

Digestion, Absorption, Transport, and Excretion of Nutrients

KEY TERMS

active transport the movement of particles via a carrier protein across cell membranes and epithelial layers; requires expenditure of energy

amylase an enzyme that is secreted in saliva and from the pancreas and catalyzes the hydrolysis of starch

brush border the microvilli that greatly increase the surface area of intestinal mucosal cells

chelation the process by which a mineral is bound to a ligand—usually an acid, an organic acid, or a sugar—so that it is in a form capable of being absorbed into intestinal cells

cholecystokinin (CCK) a hormone that is secreted by the proximal small bowel and stimulates the pancreas to secrete enzymes (and, to a lesser extent, bicarbonate and water), stimulates gallbladder contraction, slows gastric emptying, stimulates colonic activity, and may regulate appetite

chyme the semifluid, gruel-like material produced by the gastric digestion of food

colonic salvage the process of fermenting and absorbing end products of dietary carbohydrates, fiber, and amino acids in the large intestine

enterogastrone a hormone secreted by the duodenal mucosa in response to the presence of fat in the duodenum; inhibits gastric secretion and motility, slowing the delivery of additional lipids into the duodenum

facilitated diffusion the movement of particles across a membrane via a transporter or carrier protein

gastrin a hormone that is produced by the antral mucosa of the stomach and stimulates gastric secretions and motility

glucagon-like peptide 1 (GLP-1) a hormone released from the intestinal mucosa that decreases gastric emptying, lowers glucagon secretion, stimulates insulin secretion, and increases insulin sensitivity and satiety

glucose-dependent insulinotropic polypeptide (GIP) a hormone that is released from the intestinal mucosa in the presence of glucose, fat, and/or protein and increases insulin release by pancreatic islet cells

lactase an intestinal enzyme that hydrolyzes lactose into glucose and galactose

maltase an intestinal enzyme that hydrolyzes maltose into glucose

micelle a complex of primarily free fatty acids, monoglycerides, and bile salts that allows lipids to be absorbed into intestinal mucosal cells

microvilli minute cylindrical processes that are found on the surface of the intestinal cells and greatly increase their absorptive surface area

motilin a polypeptide gastrointestinal hormone that promotes gastric emptying and intestinal motility

pancreatic lipase an enzyme in pancreatic juice that hydrolyzes the ester linkages between fatty acids and glycerol

parietal cells large cells that are scattered along the walls of the stomach and secrete hydrochloric acid in gastric juice

passive diffusion the random movement of particles through openings in cellular membranes according to electrochemical and concentration gradients

pepsin a protease active only in the acid environment of the stomach; serves to change the shape and size of some proteins in a meal

peristalsis the movement by which the alimentary canal propels its contents

prebiotic food, usually carbohydrates or specific oligosaccharides (fructooligosaccharides, inulin) from vegetables, grains, and legumes; may also include resistant starch, soluble dietary fiber, and malabsorbed sugars that are the preferred energy substrates of "friendly" microbes in the gastrointestinal tract

probiotic food or concentrate of live organisms that contribute to a healthy microbial environment and suppress potential harmful microbes

2

proteolytic enzymes the enzymes trypsin, chymotrypsin, and carboxypeptidase, all of which break down protein into proteoses, peptones, peptides, and amino acids

secretin a hormone released from the duodenal wall into the bloodstream that stimulates the pancreas to secrete water and bicarbonate and inhibits gastrin secretion

somatostatin a polypeptide hormone secreted from the stomach, small intestine, and pancreas that tends to inhibit other gastrointestinal secretions and motility

sucrase the intestinal enzyme that hydrolyzes sucrose into glucose and fructose

synbiotic a combination of probiotics and prebiotics of a long-chain inulin-type fructans

villi the numerous fingerlike projections that cover the surface of the small intestine mucosa

Most of the major nutrients in foods must be made smaller, unbound, or more soluble before they can be absorbed from the intestine. The digestive system is responsible for reducing these large particles and molecules into smaller, more readily absorbed units and converting the insoluble molecules into soluble forms. Proper functioning of the absorptive and transport mechanisms is crucial in the delivery of the products of digestion to individual cells. Malfunctions in any of these systems can result in malnutrition, even when an adequate diet is being consumed.

THE GASTROINTESTINAL TRACT

The primary roles of the gastrointestinal (GI) tract are to (1) extract macronutrients, protein, carbohydrates, lipids, water, and ethanol from ingested foods and beverages; (2) absorb necessary micronutrients and trace elements; and (3) serve as a physical and immunologic barrier to microorganisms, foreign material, and potential antigens consumed with food or formed during the passage of food through the GI tract. In addition to its primary roles, the GI tract also participates in many other regulatory, metabolic, and immunologic functions that affect the entire body.

The human GI tract is well suited for digesting and absorbing nutrients from a tremendous variety of foods, including meats, dairy products, fruits, vegetables, grains, complex starches, sugars, fats, and oils. Depending on the nature of the diet consumed, about 90% to 97% of food is digested and absorbed; most of the unabsorbed material is of plant origin. Compared with ruminants and animals with a very large cecum, humans are considerably less efficient at extracting energy from grasses, stems, seeds, and other coarse fibrous materials because they lack the enzymes to hydrolyze the chemical bonds that link the molecules of sugars that make up plant fibers. Fibrous foods and any undigested carbohydrates are fermented to varying degrees by bacteria in the human colon, but only 5% to 10% of the energy needed by humans can be derived from this process (Engylst and Engylst, 2005). The GI tract extends from the mouth to the anus and includes the oropharyngeal structures, esophagus, stomach, liver and gallbladder, pancreas, and small and large intestine. It is one of the largest organs in the body (Figure 1-1). In addition to having the largest surface area, the GI tract is extremely active in carrying out the physiologic and metabolic functions of secretion, digestion, absorption, and cellular replication. The human intestine is about 7 m long and configured in a pattern of folds, pits, and fingerlike projections called **villi.** The villi are lined with epithelial cells and even smaller, cylindrical extensions called **microvilli.** The result is a tremendous increase in surface area compared with that expected from a smooth, hollow cylinder. The cells lining the intestinal tract have a life span of approximately 3 to 5 days, and then they are sloughed into the lumen and "recycled," adding to the pool of nutrients available. The cells are fully functional only for the last 2 to 3 days as they migrate from the crypts to the distal third of the villi.

It is becoming increasingly apparent that the health of the body depends on a healthy and functional GI tract. Because of the unusually high metabolic activity and requirements of the GI tract, the cells lining it are more susceptible than most tissues to micronutrient deficiencies; protein calorie malnutrition; and damage resulting from toxins, drugs, irradiation, or interruption of its blood supply. Approximately 45% of the energy requirement of the small intestine and 70% of the energy requirement of cells lining the colon are supplied by nutrients passing through its lumen. After only a few days of starvation, the GI tract atrophies (i.e., the surface area decreases; and secretions, synthetic functions, blood flow, and absorptive capacity are all reduced). Resumption of food intake, even with less than adequate calories, results in cellular proliferation and return of normal GI function after only a few days. Optimum function of the human GI tract seems to depend on a more constant supply of foods rather than consumption of large amounts of foods interrupted by prolonged fasts.

BRIEF OVERVIEW OF DIGESTIVE AND ABSORPTIVE PROCESSES

In the mouth, chewing reduces the size of food particles, which are mixed with salivary secretions that prepare them for swallowing. A small amount of starch is degraded by salivary amylase, but its contribution to overall carbohydrate digestion is small. The esophagus transports food and liquid from the oral cavity and pharynx to the stomach. In the stomach, food is mixed with acidic fluid and proteolytic and lipolytic enzymes. Small amounts of lipid digestion take place, and some proteins are changed in structure or partially digested to large peptides (Soybel, 2005). When food reaches the appropriate consistency and concentration, the stomach allows its contents to pass into the small intestine, where most digestion takes

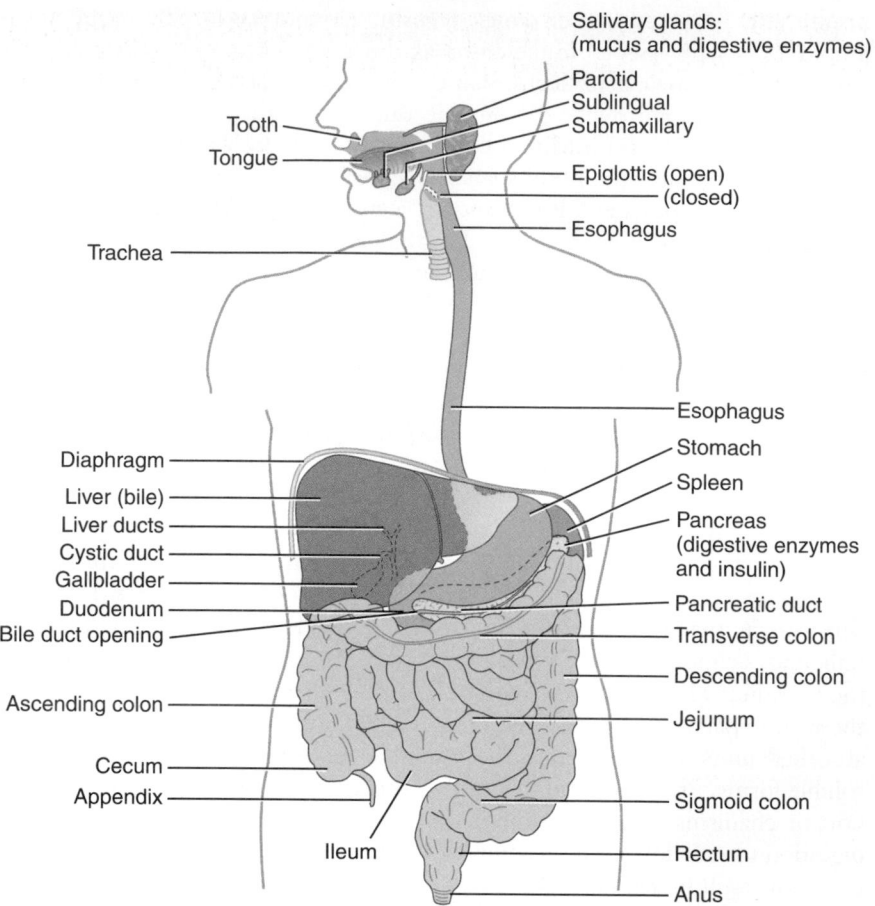

FIGURE 1-1 The digestive system.

place. In the first 100 cm of small intestine, a flurry of activity occurs, resulting in the digestion and absorption of most of the food ingested. The presence of food in the small intestine stimulates the release of hormones that in turn stimulate the production and release of powerful enzymes from the pancreas and small intestine and bile from the liver and gallbladder. The result is the reduction of starches and proteins to smaller-molecular-weight carbohydrates and small- to medium-size peptides. Dietary fats are reduced from visible globules of fat, first to microscopic droplets of triglycerides and then to free fatty acids and monoglycerides. Enzymes from the brush border of the small intestine further reduce the remaining carbohydrates to monosaccharides and peptides to single amino acids, dipeptides, and tripeptides (Keller and Layer, 2005; Thompson, 2003). Together with salivary and gastric secretions, secretions from the pancreas, small intestine, and gallbladder contribute about 7 to 9 L of fluid in a day, about three to four times more fluid than is normally consumed orally. All but about 100 to 150 ml of the total fluid entering the lumen is reabsorbed.

The movement of ingested and secreted material in the GI tract is regulated primarily by peptide hormones, nerves, and enteric muscles (Rehfeld, 2004). Along the remaining length of the small intestine, almost all the macronutrients, minerals, vitamins, trace elements, and fluid are absorbed before reaching the colon, or large intestine.

The colon and rectum absorb most of the remaining liters of fluid delivered from the small intestine; the colon absorbs electrolytes and only a small amount of remaining nutrients. Most of the nutrients absorbed from the GI tract make their way to the liver by way of the portal vein, where they may be stored, transformed into other substances, or released into circulation. End products of most dietary fats are transported ultimately to the bloodstream by lymphatic circulation. The colonic flora play an essential role in fermentation of part of the remaining fiber, resistant starch, sugar, and amino acids. Fermentation of the remaining carbohydrates results in the production of short-chain fatty acids (SCFAs) and gas. SCFAs help maintain normal mucosal function, salvage a small amount of energy from some of the residual substrates, and facilitate the absorption of the remaining salt and water (Englyst and Englyst, 2005). The remaining substrates, especially fermentable fibers, also serve as "prebiotic" material by producing SCFAs, decreasing the colonic pH, and increasing the mass of "helpful" bacteria (Delzenne, 2003). The large intestine also provides temporary storage for waste products; and the distal colon, rectum, and anus control defecation (see *Clinical Insight:* The Gastrointestinal Tract: The Ultimate Food Processor).

Enzymes in Digestion

Digestion of food is accomplished by hydrolysis under the direction of enzymes. Cofactors such as hydrochloric acid, bile, and sodium bicarbonate support the digestive and absorptive processes. Digestive enzymes are synthesized in

The Gastrointestinal Tract: The Ultimate Food Processor

Each day a varying mixture of foods enters the gastrointestinal (GI) tract, and with remarkable efficiency the GI tract goes about its tasks.

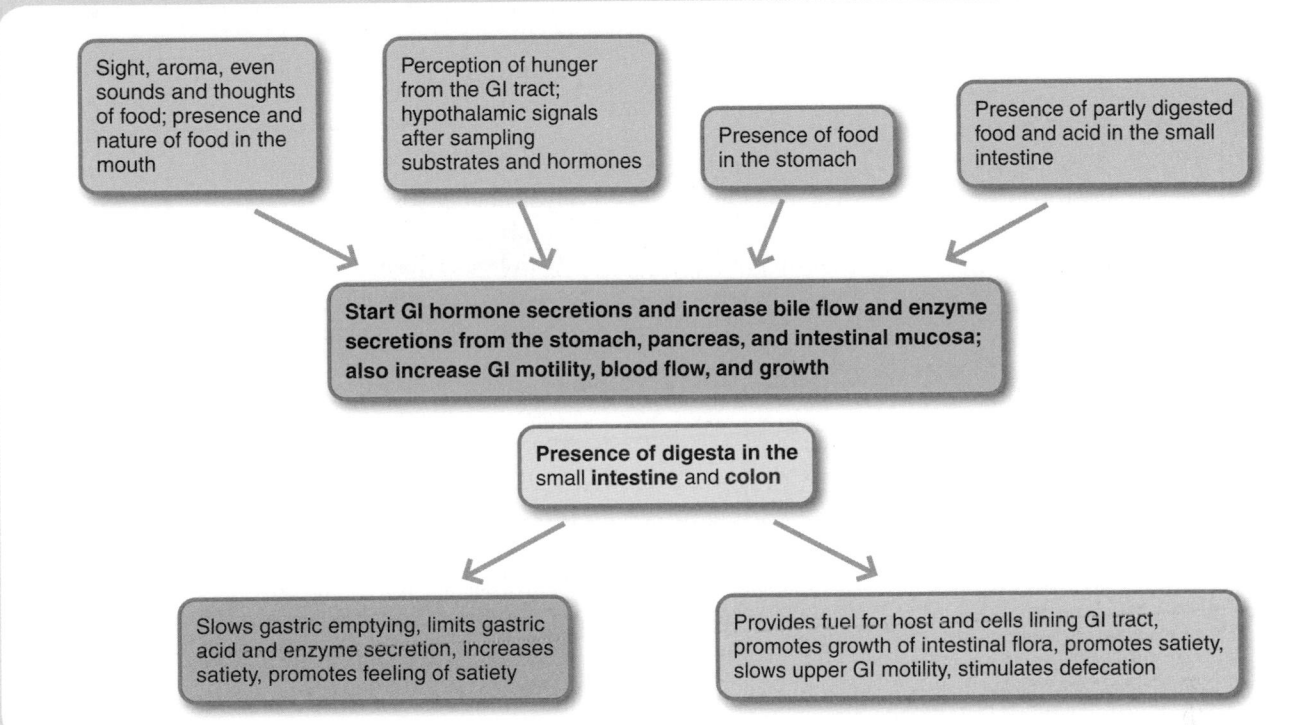

The GI tract is also remarkable because of the following:

- The extent and type of hormonal, motor, and secretory response are appropriate for the amount and type of foods consumed.
- It is remarkably efficient in digestion and absorption of foods and fluids, despite tremendous variations in types and mixtures of foods.
- It has the largest surface area, greatest number of immune cells, and most hormones produced of all organs.
- It protects host tissues from strong acids and potent digestive enzymes, a host of antigens, potenially toxic compounds, and high concentrations of microbes that coexist in the colon just millimeters from sterile tissues.

specialized cells in the mouth, stomach, pancreas, and small intestine and released into the lumen. Some enzymes are localized in the lipoprotein membranes of the mucosal cells and attach to their substrates as they enter the cell. Table 1-1 summarizes the GI enzymes and their functions in the small intestine. No additional digestive enzymes are secreted from the large intestine. Except for fiber and some carbohydrates, digestion and absorption are essentially completed in the small intestine. Water, monosaccharides, vitamins, minerals, and alcohol are usually absorbed in their basic form but in many cases must be unbound from other molecules or attached to carriers before being absorbed. For the most part, the carbohydrates, lipids, and proteins must be converted to their simple constituents by digestive enzymes before they are absorbed (see Chapter 3).

Regulators of Gastrointestinal Activity: Nerves, Neurotransmitters, and Neuropeptide Hormones

Neural Mechanisms

GI movement, including contraction, mixing, and propulsion of luminal contents, is the result of the coordinated activity of enteric nerves, extrinsic nerves, endocrine cells, and smooth muscle. The neural mechanisms include (1) an intrinsic system consisting of two layers of nerves embedded in the gut wall, and (2) an external system of nerve fibers running to and from the central and autonomic nervous systems. Mucosal receptors in the gut wall are appropriately sensitive to the composition of the **chyme** (a semiliquid substance of acid, fatty acids, and amino acids) and lumen distention (i.e., fullness)

TABLE 1-1

Summary of Enzymatic Digestion and Absorption

Secretion and Source	Enzymes	Substrate	Action and Resulting Products	Final Products Absorbed
Saliva from salivary glands in mouth	Ptyalin (salivary amylase)	Starch	Hydrolysis to form dextrins and branched oligosaccharides	—
Gastric juice from gastric glands in stomach mucosa	Pepsin	Protein (in presence of hydrochloric acid)	Hydrolysis of peptide bonds to form polypeptides and amino acids	—
	Gastric lipase	Fat, especially shorter chain	Hydrolysis to form free fatty acids	—
Exocrine secretions from pancreas	Lipase	Fat (in presence of bile salts)	Hydrolysis to form monoglycerides and fatty acids; incorporated into micelles	Fatty acids into mucosal cells; reesterified as triglycerides
	Cholesterol esterase	Cholesterol	Hydrolysis to form esters of cholesterol and fatty acids; incorporated into micelles	Cholesterol into mucosal cells; transferred to chylomicrons
	α-Amylase	Starch and dextrins	Hydrolysis to form dextrins and maltose	—
	Trypsin (activated trypsinogen)	Proteins and polypeptides	Hydrolysis of interior peptide bonds to form polypeptides	—
	Chymotrypsin (activated chymotrypsinogen)	Proteins and peptides	Hydrolysis of interior peptide bonds to form polypeptides	
	Carboxypeptidase	Polypeptides	Hydrolysis of terminal peptide bonds (carboxyl end) to form amino acids	Amino acids
	Ribonuclease and deoxyribonuclease	Ribonucleic acids and deoxyribonucleic acids	Hydrolysis to form mononucleotides	Mononucleotides
	Elastase	Fibrous protein	Hydrolysis to form peptides and amino acids	—
Small intestine enzymes (primarily in brush border)	Carboxypeptidase, aminopeptidase, and dipeptidase	Polypeptides	Hydrolysis of carboxyl terminus, amino terminus, or internal peptide bonds	Amino acids
	Enterokinase	Trypsinogen	Activates trypsin	Dipeptides and tripeptides
	Sucrase	Sucrose	Hydrolysis to form glucose and fructose	Glucose and fructose
	α-Dextrinase (isomaltase)	Dextrin (isomaltose)	Hydrolysis to form glucose	Glucose
	Maltase	Maltose	Hydrolysis to form glucose	Glucose
	Lactase	Lactose	Hydrolysis to from glucose and galactose	Glucose and galactose
	Nucleotidases	Nucleic acids	Hydrolysis to form nucleotides and phosphates	Nucleotides
	Nucleosidase and phosphorylase	Nucleosides	Hydrolysis to form purines, pyrimidines, and pentose phosphate	Purine and pyrimidine bases

TABLE 1-2		
Examples of Neurotransmitters and Their Actions		
Neutotransmitter	**Site of Release**	**Primary Actions**
α-Aminobutyric acid (GABA)	Central nervous system	Relaxes lower esophageal sphincter
Norepinephrine	Central nervous system, spinal cord, sympathetic nerves	Decreases motility, increases contraction of sphincters, inhibits secretions
Acetylcholine	Central nervous system, autonomic system, other tissues	Increases motility, relaxes sphincters, stimulates secretions
Neurotensin	Gastrointestinal (GI) tract, central nervous system	Inhibits release of gastric emptying and acid secretion
Serotonin (5-HT)	GI tract, spinal cord	Facilitates secretion and peristalsis
Nitric oxide	Central nervous system, GI tract	Regulates blood flow, maintains muscle tone, maintains gastric motor activity
Substance P	Gut, central nervous system, skin	Increases sensory awareness (mainly pain), and peristalsis

and send impulses through submucosal and mysenteric nerves. Neurotransmitters and neuropeptides with small molecular weights signal nerves to contract or relax muscles, increase or decrease fluid secretions, or change blood flow. The GI tract then largely regulates its own motility and secretory activity. However, signals from the central nervous system can override the enteric system and affect GI function (Furness and Clerc, 2000). Numerous hormones, neuropeptides, and neurotransmitters in the GI tract not only affect GI function but also have an impact on other nerves and tissues in many parts of the body. Some examples of neurotransmitters released from enteric nerve endings and their actions are listed in Table 1-2. In people with GI disease (e.g., infections, inflammatory bowel disease, irritable bowel syndrome), the enteric nervous system may be overstimulated, resulting in abnormal secretion, altered blood flow, increased permeability, and altered immune function.

Autonomic innervation is supplied by the sympathetic fibers that run along blood vessels and by the parasympathetic fibers in the vagal and pelvic nerves. In general, sympathetic neurons, which are activated by fear, anger, and stress, tend to slow transit of GI contents by inhibiting neurons affecting muscle contraction and inhibiting secretions. The parasympathetic nerves innervate specific areas of the alimentary tract. For example, the sight or smell of food stimulates vagal activity and subsequent secretion of acid from **parietal cells** scattered along the walls of the stomach. The GI tract also sends signals that are perceived as colicky pain, sharp pain, nausea, urgency or gastric fullness, or gastric emptiness by way of the vagal and spinal nerves. Inflammation, dysmotility, and various types of intestinal damage may intensify these perceptions.

Neuropeptide Hormones

Regulation of the GI system also involves numerous peptide hormones that can act locally or distally. These regulators can act locally in an autocrine or a paracrine role or as endocrine hormones by traveling through the blood to their target organs. More than 100 peptide hormones and hormonelike growth factors secreted by more than 30 different types of neuroendocrine cells have been identified. Their actions are often complex and extend well beyond the GI tract. Some of the hormones (e.g., of the cholecystokinin and somatostatin family) also serve as neurotransmitters between neurons (see *Focus On:* Roles of Gastrointestinal Neuropeptide Hormones and Neurotransmitters). The digestive and secretory functions of several GI hormones have been well described, but the complete actions of these and many other peptide hormones that affect GI cell growth, DNA synthesis, proliferation, secretion, movement, or metabolism have not been fully evaluated (Rehfeld, 2004). Some of the classic hormones involved in digestive and absorptive processes are reviewed in the following paragraphs and summarized in Table 1-3. Knowledge of major hormone functions becomes especially important when the sites of their secretion or action are diseased or removed in surgical procedures or when hormones and their analogs are used to suppress or enhance some aspect of GI function.

Gastrin, a hormone that stimulates gastric secretions and motility, is secreted primarily from endocrine "G" cells in the antral mucosa of the stomach. Secretion is initiated by (1) distention of the antrum after a meal, (2) impulses from the vagus nerve such as those triggered by the smell or sight of food, and (3) the presence in the antrum of secretagogues such as partially digested proteins, fermented alcoholic beverages (e.g., wine), caffeine, or food extracts (e.g., bouillon). When the lumen gets more acidic, feedback involving other hormones inhibits gastrin release. The receptors for gastrin and cholecystokinin are related and constitute the gastrin/cholecystokinin receptor family, although their affinity for binding gastrin and cholecystokinin depends on their subtypes (Wank, 1998).

◎ **FOCUS ON**

Role of Gastrointestinal Neuropeptide Hormones and Neurotransmitters

Scientists continue to discover more gastrointestinal (GI) neuropeptide hormones that not only affect digestive activity but participate in many other regulatory functions within and beyond the GI tract. The GI tract secretes more than 30 families of neuropeptide hormones, which makes it the largest endocrine organ in the body (Ahlman and Nilsson, 2001; Rehfeld, 2004). GI hormones are involved in initiating and terminating feeding, bringing on sensations of hunger and satiety, increasing or decreasing movements of the GI tract, enhancing or retarding esophageal and gastric emptying, regulating blood flow and permeability, regulating immune functions, and stimulating the growth of cells (within and beyond the GI tract). *Ghrelin*, a relatively newly identified neuropeptide that is secreted from the stomach, sends a "hungry" message to the brain, whereas *PYY 3-36*, another recently identified hormone that is produced by the digestive tract, seems to signal appetite suppression. Cholecystokinin, glucagon-like polypeptide-1 (GLP-1), oxyntomodulin, pancreatic polypeptide, and gastrin-releasing polypeptide (bombesin) also tend to decrease hunger and increase satiety (Stanley et al., 2005).

Some of the GI hormones, including some of those that affect satiety, seem to slow gastric emptying and decrease secretions (e.g., somatostatin). Other GI hormones (e.g., motilin) increase motility. These signaling agents of the GI tract are also involved in several metabolic functions. The neuropeptides glucose-dependent insulinotropic polypeptide and GLP-1 are called *incretin hormones* because they help lower blood sugar by facilitating insulin secretion, decreasing gastric emptying, and increasing satiety.

Several of these neuropeptide hormones and analogs are already being used in clinical practice or being tested in the management of clinical problems such as obesity, anorexia, cachexia, delayed or rapid gastrointestinal transit, inflammatory bowel disease, irritable bowel syndrome, diarrhea and constipation, diabetes, GI malignancies, and a host of others.

Gastrin binds to receptors on parietal cells and histamine-releasing cells to stimulate gastric acid, to receptors on chief cells to release pepsinogen, and to receptors on smooth muscle to increase gastric motility.

Secretin, the first hormone to be discovered and named, is released from "S" cells in the wall of the proximal small intestine into the bloodstream. It essentially opposes the action and secretion of gastrin. It is secreted in response to gastric acid and digestive end products in the duodenum, it stimulates the pancreas to secrete water and bicarbonate into the duodenum, and it inhibits gastric acid secretion and emptying. Neutralization of the acidity protects the duodenal mucosa from prolonged exposure to acid and provides the appropriate environment for the activity of intestinal and pancreatic enzymes. The receptor is a 7-transmembrane G protein-coupled receptor and is found in the stomach and ductal and acinar cells of the pancreas. In different species other organs may express secretin, including the liver, colon, heart, kidney, and brain (Chey and Chang, 2003).

Other cells of the small bowel mucosa ("I" cells) secrete **cholecystokinin (CCK),** an important multifunctional hormone released primarily in response to the presence of protein and fat. Receptors for CCK are in pancreatic acinar cells, pancreatic islet cells, gastric somatostatin-releasing D cells, smooth muscle cells of the GI tract, and the central nervous system. The major GI functions of CCK are to (1) stimulate the pancreas to secrete enzymes (and to a lesser extent bicarbonate and water), (2) stimulate gallbladder contraction, (3) increase colonic and rectal motility, (4) slow gastric emptying, and (5) increase satiety, at least to a limited degree (Keller and Layer, 2005; Thompson et al., 2003; Wank, 1998).

Glucagon-like peptide 1 (GLP-1) and **glucose-dependent insulinotropic polypeptide (GIP),** released from the intestinal mucosa in the presence of meals rich in glucose and fat, stimulate insulin synthesis and release. GLP-1 also decreases glucagon secretion, delays gastric emptying, and may help promote satiety. GLP-1 and GIP are examples of incretin hormones, which help keep blood glucose from rising excessively after a meal (Efendic and Portwood, 2004). This may explain why a glucose load received enterally results in less of an increase in blood glucose than when an equal amount of glucose is received intravenously.

Motilin, which is released by the cells of the upper small intestine in response to bile and pancreatic secretions into the duodenum, increases the rate of gastric emptying and stimulates gut motility. Motilin acts on G protein-coupled receptors on enteric neurons in the duodenum and colon and stimulates contraction of smooth muscle in the stomach. Erythromycin, an antibiotic, has been shown to bind to motilin receptors; thus analogs of erythromycin and motilin have been used as therapeutic agents to treat delayed gastric emptying (Feighner et al., 1999; Sarna et al., 2000).

Somatostatin, released by D cells in the antrum and pylorus, is a hormone with far-reaching actions. Its general roles seem to be inhibitory and antisecretory. It decreases motility of the stomach and intestine and inhibits or regulates the release of several GI hormones. Somatostatin and its analog octreotide are being used to treat certain malignant diseases (Low, 2004), as well as numerous GI disorders such as diarrhea, short bowel syndrome, pancreatitis, dumping syndrome, and gastric hypersecretion.

TABLE 1-3

Functions of Major Gastrointestinal Hormones

Hormone	Site of Release	Stimulants for Release	Organ Affected	Effect on Organ
Gastrin	Gastric mucosa duodenum	Peptides, amino acids, caffeine Distention of the antrum Some alcoholic beverages, vagus nerve	Stomach, esophagus, gastrointestinal (GI) tract, in general	Stimulates secretion of hydrochloric acid (HCl) and pepsinogen Increases gastric antral motility Increases lower esophageal sphincter tone
			Gallbladder	Weakly stimulates contraction of gallbladder
			Pancreas	Weakly stimulates pancreatic secretion of bicarbonate
Secretin	Duodenal mucosa	Acid in small intestine	Pancreas	Increases output of H_2O and bicarbonate Increases some enzyme secretion from the pancreas and insulin release
			Duodenum	Decreases motility Increases mucus output
Cholecystokinin (CCK)	Proximal small bowel	Peptides, amino acids, fats, HCl	Pancreas	Stimulates secretion of pancreatic enzymes
			Gallbladder	Causes contraction of gallbladder
			Stomach	Slows gastric emptying
			Colon	Increases motility May mediate feeding behavior
Glucose-dependent insulinotropic polypeptide (GIP)	Small intestine	Glucose, fat	Stomach, pancreas	Stimulates insulin release
Glucagon-like peptide (GLP-1)	Small intestine	Glucose, fat	Stomach, pancreas	Prolongs gastric emptying Inhibits glucagon release Stimulates insulin release
Motilin	Stomach, small and large bowel	Biliary and pancreatic Secretions	Stomach, small bowel, colon	Promotes gastric emptying and GI motility

Digestion in the Mouth

In the mouth the teeth grind and crush food into small particles. The food mass is simultaneously moistened and lubricated by saliva. Three pairs of salivary glands—the parotid, submaxillary, and sublingual glands—produce about 1.5 L of saliva daily. A serous secretion containing **amylase** (ptyalin) begins the digestion of starch. The starch digestion is minimal, and the amylase becomes inactive when it reaches the acidic contents of the stomach. Another type of saliva contains mucus, a protein that causes particles of food to stick together and lubricates the mass for swallowing. The oropharyngeal secretions also contain a lipase that is capable of digesting some fats. Because fatty materials are still mixed with whole foods, not extensively processed, and not retained in the mouth or esophagus for any length of time, the contribution of this lipase to overall fat digestion is usually minimal.

The masticated food mass, or bolus, is passed back to the pharynx under voluntary control, but throughout the esophagus the process of swallowing (deglutition) is involuntary. **Peristalsis** then moves the food rapidly into the stomach (see Chapter 41 for a more detailed discussion of swallowing).

Digestion in the Stomach

Food particles are propelled forward and mixed with gastric secretions by wavelike contractions that progress forward from the upper portion of the stomach (fundus), to the midportion (corpus), and then the antrum and pylorus. In the stomach gastric secretions are mixed with food and beverages. An average of 2000 to 2500 ml of gastric juice is secreted daily. The gastric secretions contain hydrochloric acid (secreted by the parietal cells in the walls of the fundus and corpus), a protease, gastric lipase, mucus, intrinsic factor (a glycoprotein that facilitates vitamin B_{12} absorption in the ileum), and the GI hormone gastrin. The protease is **pepsin,** which is also secreted from glands in the fundus and corpus. It is first secreted in an inactive form, pepsinogen, which is converted by hydrochloric acid to its active form. Pepsin is active only in the acid environment of the stomach and serves primarily to change the shape and size of some of the proteins in a normal meal.

An acid-stable lipase is secreted into the stomach by chief cells. Although this lipase is considerably less active than pancreatic lipase, it contributes to the overall processing of dietary triglycerides. Gastric lipase is more specific for triglycerides composed of medium- and short-chain fatty acids, but the normal diet contains few of these fats. Lipases secreted in the upper portions of the GI tract may have a relatively important role in the liquid diet of infants, but, when pancreatic insufficiency occurs, it becomes apparent that lingual and gastric lipases are not sufficient to prevent lipid malabsorption (Keller and Layer, 2005). In the process of gastric digestion, most of the food becomes semiliquid chyme, containing approximately 50% water. Gastric secretions are also important in increasing the availability and downstream absorption of vitamin B_{12} and several metals and trace elements, including calcium, iron, and zinc (Soybel, 2005).

When food is consumed, significant numbers of microorganisms are also consumed. The acid in the stomach is quite strong, with a pH ranging from about 1.0 to 4.0. The combined actions of hydrochloric acid and proteolytic enzymes from the stomach result in a significant reduction in the concentration of microorganisms ingested. Some microbes may escape and enter the intestine if consumed in sufficient concentrations. Achlorhydria, gastrectomy, GI dysfunction or disease, poor nutrition, or drugs that suppress acid secretions may increase the risk of bacterial overgrowth in the intestine.

The stomach continuously mixes and churns food and normally releases the mixture in small quantities into the small intestine. The amount emptied with each contraction of the antrum and pylorus varies with the volume and type of food consumed, but only a few milliliters are released at a time. Most of a liquid meal empties in 1 to 2 hours, and most of a solid meal empties within 2 to 3 hours. When eaten alone, carbohydrates leave the stomach the most rapidly, followed by protein, fat, and fibrous food. In a meal with mixed types of foods, emptying of the stomach depends on the overall volume and characteristics of the foods. Liquids empty more rapidly than solids, large particles empty more slowly than small particles, and concentrated food tends to empty more slowly than low-calorie meals. These factors are important considerations for practitioners who counsel patients with nausea, vomiting, diabetic gastroparesis, or partial obstruction, or practitioners monitoring patients after GI surgery or those who are malnourished.

The lower esophageal sphincter above the entrance to the stomach prevents reflux of gastric contents into the esophagus, and the pyloric sphincter in the distal portion of the stomach helps regulate exit of gastric contents and prevents backflow of chyme from the duodenum into the stomach. Emotional changes, food, and GI regulators can affect the activity of these sphincters. Irritation from nearby ulcers may also alter the performance of strictures. Certain foods and beverages may alter the lower esophageal sphincter pressure, permitting reflux of the GI contents into the esophagus. The presence of food in the intestine and regulatory hormones provide feedback to slow gastric emptying (see Chapter 26).

Digestion in the Small Intestine

The small intestine is the primary site for digestion of foods and nutrients. The small intestine is divided into the duodenum, the jejunum, and the ileum (Figure 1-2). The duodenum is about 0.5 m long, the jejunum is 2 to 3 m, and the ileum is 3 to 4 m. Most of the digestive process is completed in the duodenum and upper jejunum, and the absorption of most nutrients is largely complete by the time the material reaches the middle of the jejunum. The acidic chyme from the stomach enters the duodenum, where it is mixed with duodenal juices and the secretions from the pancreas and biliary tract. As a result of the secretion of bicarbonate-containing fluid from the pancreas and dilution from other secretions, acid chyme is neutralized. Enzymes of the small intestine and pancreas operate more effectively in a more neutral pH.

The entry of partially digested foods, primarily fats and protein, stimulates the release of several hormones that in turn stimulate the secretion of enzymes and fluids and affect GI motility and satiety. Bile, which is predominantly a mixture of water, bile salts, and small amounts of pigments and cholesterol, is secreted from the liver and gallbladder. Through their surfactant properties, the bile salts facilitate the digestion and absorption of lipids. The pancreas secretes potent enzymes capable of digesting all of the major nutrients, and enzymes from the small intestine help complete the process. The primary lipid-digesting enzymes secreted by the pancreas are **pancreatic lipase** and colipase (Lowe, 2002). **Proteolytic enzymes** include trypsin and chymotrypsin, carboxypeptidase, aminopeptidase, ribonuclease, and deoxyribonuclease. Trypsin and chymotrypsin are secreted in their inactive forms and are activated by enterokinase (also known as enteropeptidase), which is secreted when chyme contacts the intestinal mucosa. Pancreatic amylase serves to hydrolyze large starch molecules eventually into units of approximately two to six sugars. Enzymes lining the brush border of the villi further break down the carbohydrate molecules into monosaccharides before absorption. Varying amounts of resistant starches and most ingested dietary fiber escape digestion in the small intestine and may add to fibrous material available for fermentation by colonic microbes (Englyst and Englyst, 2005).

Intestinal contents move along the small intestine at a rate of 1 cm per minute, taking from 3 to 8 hours to travel through the entire intestine to the ileocecal valve, while along the way remaining substrates continue to be digested and absorbed. The ileocecal valve, like the pyloric valve, serves to limit the amount of intestinal material passed back and forth from the small intestine to the colon. A damaged or nonfunctional ileocecal valve results in the entry of significant amounts of fluid and substrate into the colon and increased chance for microbial overgrowth in the small intestine (see Chapter 27).

THE SMALL INTESTINE: PRIMARY SITE OF NUTRIENT ABSORPTION

Structure and Function

The primary organ of nutrient and water absorption is the small intestine, which is characterized by its expansive absorptive area. The surface area is attributable to its extensive length, as well as to the organization of the mucosal lining. The small intestine has characteristic folds in its surface called *valvulae conniventes*. These convolutions are covered with fingerlike projections called villi (Figure 1-3), which in turn are covered by microvilli, or the **brush border.** The combination of folds, villous projections, and microvillous border creates an enormous absorptive surface of about 200 to 300 m^2. The villi rest on a supporting structure called the lamina propria. Within the lamina propria, which is composed of connective tissue, the blood and lymph vessels receive the products of digestion. Each day, on average, the small intestine absorbs 150 to 300 g of monosaccharides, 60 to 100 g of fatty acids, 60 to 120 g of amino acids and peptides, and 50 to 100 g of ions. The capacity for absorption in the healthy individual far exceeds the normal macronutrient and caloric requirements. In

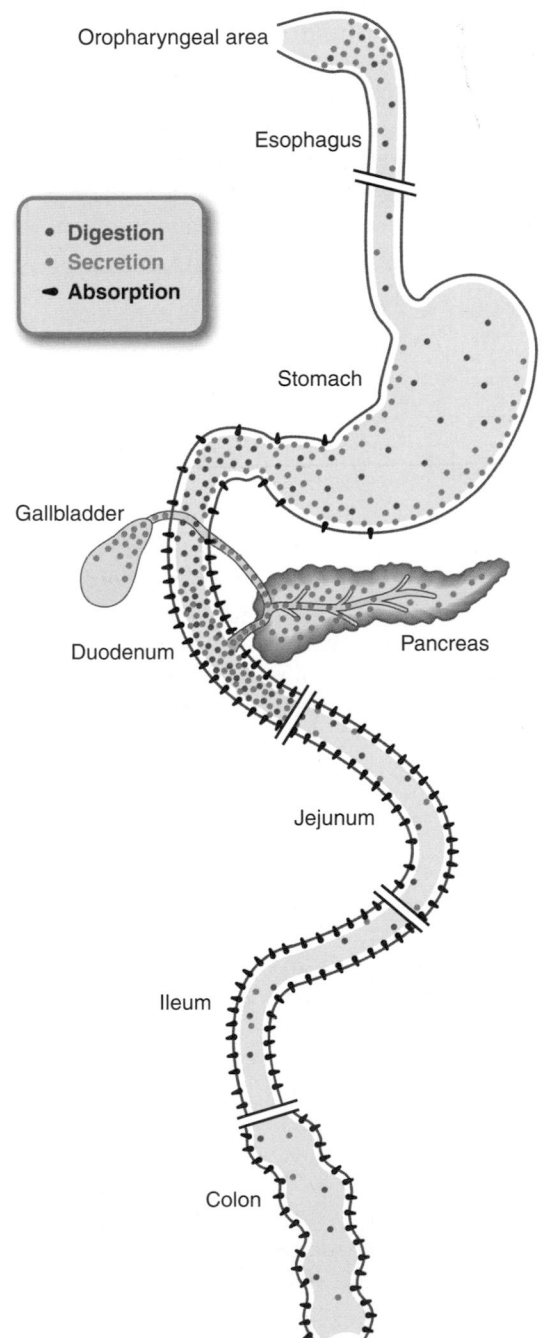

- Digestion
- Secretion
- Absorption

Oropharyngeal area

Esophagus

Stomach

Gallbladder

Duodenum

Pancreas

Jejunum

Ileum

Colon

FIGURE 1-2 Sites of secretion, digestion, and absorption.

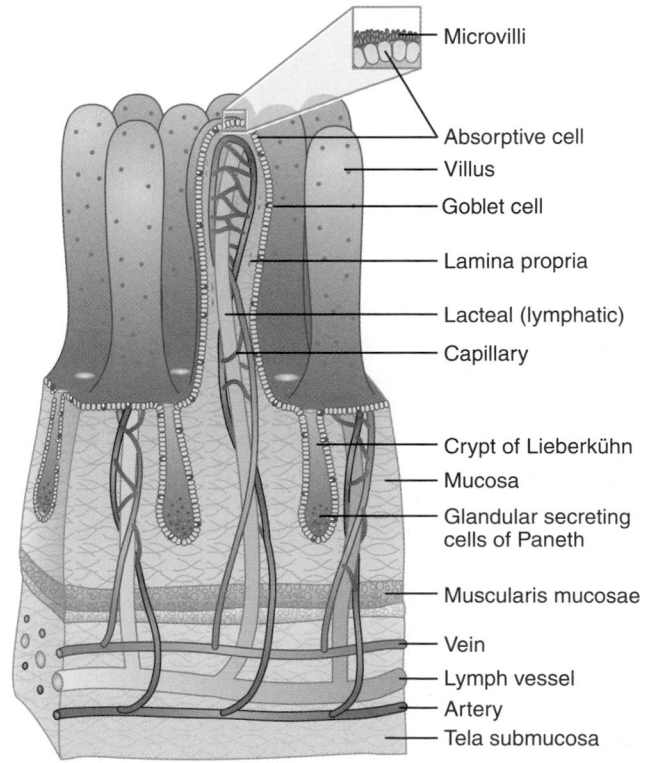

Microvilli

Absorptive cell

Villus

Goblet cell

Lamina propria

Lacteal (lymphatic)

Capillary

Crypt of Lieberkühn

Mucosa

Glandular secreting cells of Paneth

Muscularis mucosae

Vein

Lymph vessel

Artery

Tela submucosa

FIGURE 1-3 Structure of the villi of the human intestine showing blood and lymph vessels.

the small intestine, all but 1 to 1.5 L of the 7 or 8 L of fluid secreted from the upper portions of the GI tract, in addition to 1.5 to 3 L of dietary fluids, is absorbed by the time the contents reach the end of the small intestine. About 95% of the bile salts secreted from the liver and gallbladder are reabsorbed as bile acids in the distal ileum. Without this recycling of bile acids from the GI tract (enterohepatic circulation), de novo synthesis of bile acids in the liver would not keep pace with needs for adequate lipid digestion. Bile salt insufficiency becomes clinically important in patients who have resections of the distal small bowel and diseases affecting the small intestine such as Crohn's disease, radiation enteritis, and cystic fibrosis. The distal ileum is also the site for vitamin B_{12} (with intrinsic factor) absorption.

Emulsification of fats in the small intestine is followed by their digestion, primarily by pancreatic lipase, into free fatty acids and β-monoglycerides. Pancreatic lipase typically cleaves the first and third fatty acid, leaving one attached to the middle glycerol carbon. When the concentration of bile salts reaches a certain level, they form **micelles** (i.e., complexes of free fatty acids, monoglycerides, and bile salts), which are organized with the polar ends of the molecules oriented toward the watery lumen of the intestine. The products of lipid digestion are rapidly solubilized in the central portion of the micelles and carried to the area of the brush border (Figure 1-4).

At the surface of the unstirred water layer (UWL) (i.e., the slightly acidic and watery plate that forms a boundary

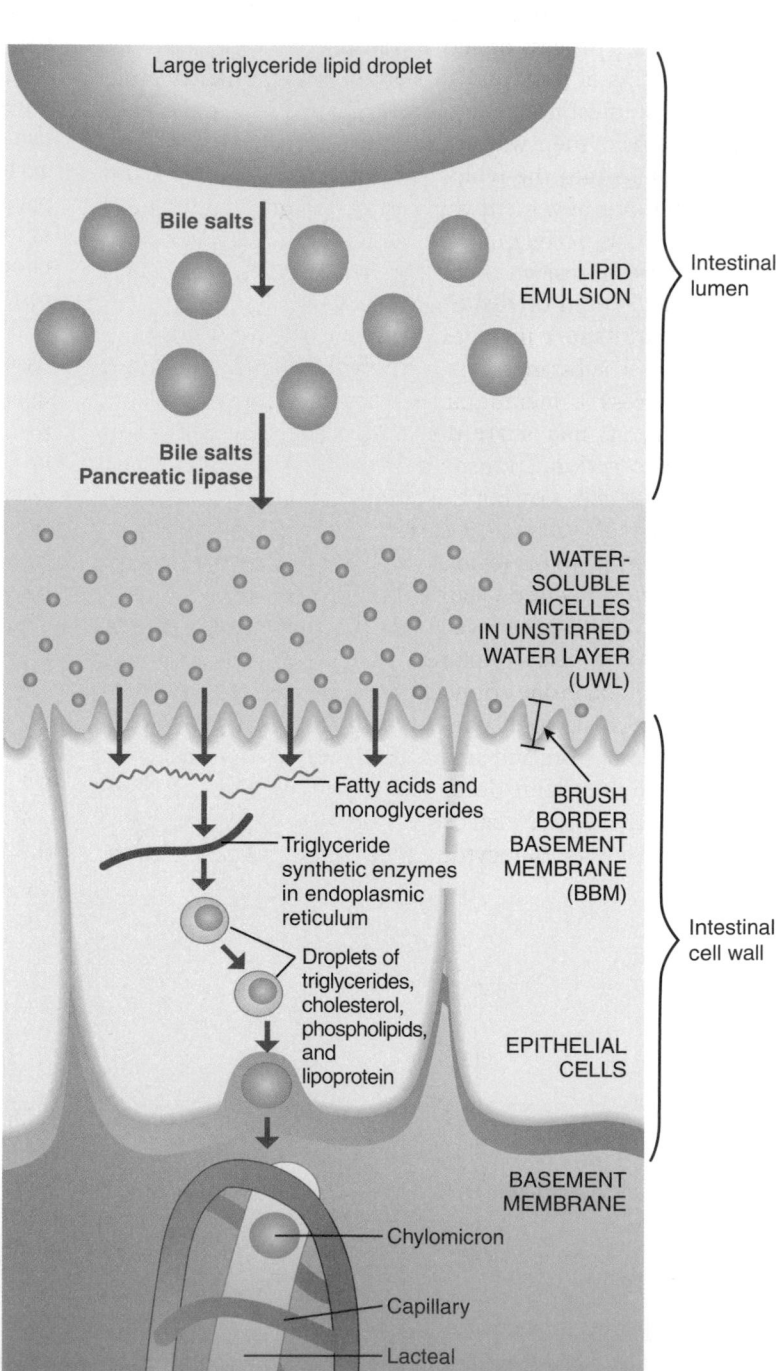

FIGURE 1-4 Summary of fat absorption.

between the intestinal lumen and the brush border membranes) the lipids detach from the micelles, and the remnants of the micelles return to the lumen for further transport. The monoglycerides and fatty acids are thus left to make their way across the lipophobic UWL to the more lipid-friendly membrane cells of the brush border. When they arrive, they are rapidly taken up for processing and entry into the transport system. Cholesterol absorption may be accomplished through both passive and facilitated transfer that involves a protein transport system specific to cholesterol and not to other sterols (Lammert and Wang, 2005; Thompson et al., 2003).

Absorptive Mechanisms

Absorption is an extremely complex process, combining the more intricate process of active transport and the relatively simple process of **passive diffusion,** in which nutrients pass through the intestinal mucosal cells (enterocytes or colonocytes) and make their way eventually into the venous system to the liver or into the lymphatic circulation. Diffusion involves random movement through openings in or between the membranes of the mucosal cell walls using channel proteins (simple diffusion) or carrier (transport) proteins as a form of **facilitated diffusion** (Figure 1-5).

Active transport involves the input of energy to move ions or other substances, in combination with a transport protein, across a membrane against an energy gradient. Some nutrients may share the same carrier and thus compete for absorption. Transport or carrier systems can also become saturated, slowing the absorption of the nutrient. A notable example of such a carrier is the previously mentioned intrinsic factor, which is responsible for the absorption of vitamin B_{12} (see Chapters 3 and 31).

Some molecules are moved from the intestinal lumen into mucosal cells by means of pumps, which require a carrier and energy from adenosine triphosphate. The absorption of glucose, sodium, galactose, potassium, magnesium, phosphate, iodide, calcium, iron, and amino acids occurs in this manner.

Pinocytosis has been described as the "drinking in," or engulfing, by the epithelial cell membrane of a small drop of intestinal contents. Pinocytosis allows large particles such as whole proteins to be absorbed in small quantities. The movement of foreign proteins across the GI tract into the bloodstream, where they cause allergic reactions, may be the result of pinocytosis. The immunoglobulins from breast milk are probably absorbed through pinocytosis.

THE LARGE INTESTINE

The large intestine is the site of absorption of the remaining water and salts, bacterial fermentation, synthesis of a small amount of vitamins, storage, and excretion. The large intestine is approximately 1.5 m long and consists of the cecum, colon, and rectum. Mucus secreted by the mucosa of the large intestine protects the intestinal wall from excoriation and bacterial activity and provides the medium for binding the feces together. Bicarbonate ions secreted in exchange for absorbed chloride ions help to neutralize the acidic end products produced from bacterial action.

Most of the water contained in the 500 to 1000 ml of chyme entering the colon each day is absorbed, leaving 50 to 200 ml to be excreted in the feces. Colonic contents move forward slowly at a rate of 5 cm/hr, and some remaining nutrients may be absorbed.

Defecation, or expulsion of feces through the rectum and anus, occurs with varying frequency, ranging from three times daily to once every 3 days or more. Average stool weight is in the range of 100 to 200 g, and mouth-to-anus transit time may vary from 18 to 72 hours. The feces generally consist of 75% water and 25% solids, but the proportions vary greatly. About two thirds of the contents of the wet weight of the stool is bacteria, with the remainder coming from GI secretions, mucus, sloughed cells, and undigested foods. A diet that includes abundant fruits, vegetables, and whole grains typically results in a shorter overall GI transit time, more frequent defecation, and larger and softer stools.

Bacterial Action

The gut microflora make up a complex community that is estimated to involve 400 species of microorganisms (Hao and Lee, 2004; Bourlioux et al., 2003). At birth the GI

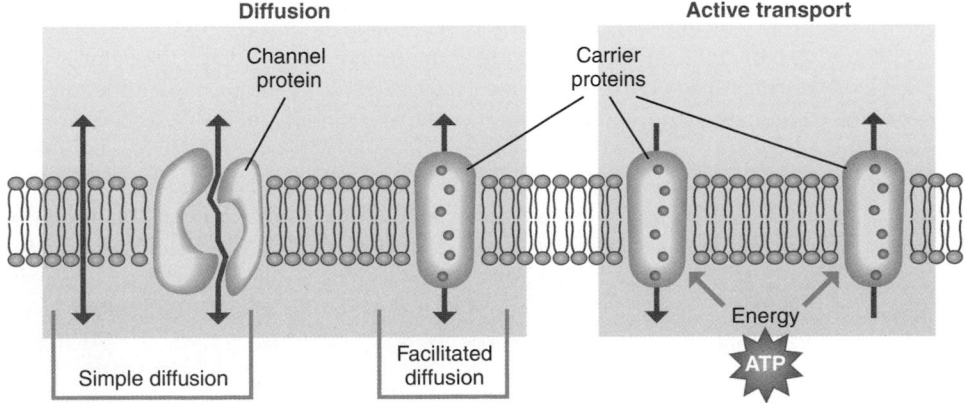

FIGURE 1-5 Transport pathways through the cell membrane, as well as basic transport mechanisms. *ATP,* Adenosine triphosphate.

tract is essentially sterile, but accumulation of various microorganisms soon takes place. *Lactobacillus* organisms are the chief component of the GI tract flora until an infant begins to eat solid foods. *Escherichia coli* then become predominant in the distal ileum, and the primary colonic flora are anaerobic, with species of the genus *Bacteroides* occurring most frequently. Lactobacilli are also present in the stools of most people who consume an ordinary mixed diet; but dietary intake differences in the host's genome, dietary intake, hygiene, and medical and surgical history may affect the kind of flora in the GI tract.

Normally relatively few bacteria remain in the stomach or small intestine after meals because the actions of hydrochloric acid, pepsin, and bile serve as a germicidal agent. However, decreased gastric secretions may allow increased survival of microbes. Decreased gastric secretions can increase the risk of inflammation of the gastric mucosa (*gastritis*), increase the risk of bacterial overgrowth in the small intestine, or increase the numbers of microbes

reaching the colon. An acid-tolerant bacterium is known to infect the stomach (*Helicobacter pylori*) and may cause gastritis and ulceration in the host (see Chapter 26).

Bacterial action is most intense in the large intestine. Following a meal, dietary fiber, resistant starches, remaining bits of amino acids, and mucus sloughed from the intestine are fermented in the colon. Colonic bacteria contribute to the formation of gases (e.g., hydrogen, carbon dioxide, nitrogen, and in some individuals methane) and SCFAs (e.g., acetic, propionic, butyric, and to a lesser degree lactic acids). Colonic bacteria continue the digestion of some materials that have resisted previous digestive activity. During the process, several nutrients are formed by bacterial synthesis (Hill, 1997). These nutrients are used to varying degrees by GI mucosal cells but usually contribute little to meeting the nutrient requirements of the human host. Examples of nutrients produced include vitamin K, vitamin B_{12}, thiamin, and riboflavin.

◉ FOCUS ON

Microbes in the Gastrointestinal Tract: Friend, Foe, or Passive-Aggressive Resident?

In addition to the important roles of secretion, digestion, and absorption, the gastrointestinal (GI) tract also serves as a physical, chemical, and immunologic barrier. The immunologic functions of the GI tract are receiving renewed interest, and it is now considered that the gut-associated lymphatic tissue that lines the GI tract is the largest immune tissue in the body. The GI tract protects the host against pathogenic microorganisms and prevents penetration of immunogenic components of the luminal contents (e.g., foods, bacteria, medications, and contaminants) beyond the mucosal surfaces (Tlaskalova-Hogenova et al., 2004; Bourlioux et al., 2003). Each individual's innate and acquired GI immune system has a formidable task: It is charged with having to: (1) mount and subsequently turn off an attack against transient invading pathogens that make their way into the GI tract; (2) prevent antigenic components of foodstuffs (e.g., peptides) from interacting or being absorbed and producing allergic responses locally and systemically; and (3) tolerate the mixture of approximately 400 species of "normal" bacteria that reside in the GI tract, their secretions, and degradation products (e.g., cell wall components, DNA, proteins).

The innate and acquired immune systems and the interactions that occur evolve based on one's genetic heritage and exposure to the myriad of environmental substances consumed over one's lifetime. Malnutrition, exposure to toxic agents, and disease may all affect the relationships among the physical and immunologic components of the GI tract and the tremendous number of substances that reside or pass through its lumen. Several diseases may be exacerbated by or even causally linked with disruption of the tenuous har-

mony between the GI tract and the contents of its lumen, especially in those who are genetically predisposed to the specific disorder. Mounting evidence supports that impaired interactions between the host and GI antigens may be linked with several infectious and inflammatory bowel diseases, allergies, autoimmune disorders, and neoplasms. In addition to the therapeutic use of antibiotics and anti-inflammatory and immunosuppressive agents, new attention is being given to the consumption of:

- **Probiotics:** foods or concentrates of live organisms that contribute to a healthy microbial environment and suppress potential harmful microbes
- **Prebiotics:** oligosaccharide components of the diet (e.g., fructo-oligosaccharides, inulin) that are the preferred energy substrates of "friendly" microbes in the GI tract.

When prebiotics, other sources of soluble dietary fiber, and other carbohydrates resistant to digestion are fermented by bacteria in the distal ileum and colon, they also produce short-chain fatty acids (SCFAs) that serve as fuel for the cells lining the GI tract. SCFAs also serve as regulatory agents for several GI and host functions (Gill and Guarner, 2004). **Synbiotics** are a combination of probiotics and prebiotics that are being tested in clinical settings. Beneficial effects are achieved by synbiotics, which are long-chain inulin-type fructans compared to short-chain derivatives; these fructans, extracted from chicory roots, are prebiotic food ingredients that are fermented to lactic acid and SCFAs in the gut lumen and may protect against conditions such as colon cancer (Pool-Zobel, 2005.)

Increased consumption of prebiotic material may lead to an increase in SCFAs and in the microbial mass—in particular, indigenous bifidobacteria and lactobacilli species thought to be beneficial. Prebiotic carbohydrates typically refer to specific oligosaccharides from vegetables, grains, and legumes but may also include resistant starch, soluble dietary fiber, and malabsorbed sugars (Gibson et al., 2005; Guarner, 2005; Englyst and Englyst, 2005). A low-fiber diet based primarily on meat, fat, and highly digestible carbohydrates is said to result in a higher ratio of "putrefactive" or potentially harmful bacteria such as *Pseudomonas*, *Clostridia*, *E. coli*, and *Proteus* organisms (Bourlioux et al., 2003; Roberfroid, 2001). Probiotic foods are foods or concentrates containing very high quantities of live bacteria considered to be healthy or protective against pathogenic organisms and disease. Recently, research into their role in preventing and treating a host of GI and systemic disorders has expanded tremendously (Gill and Guarner, 2004; Snelling, 2005) (see Chapter 27 and *Focus On: Microbes in the Gastrointestinal Tract: Friend, Foe, or Passive-Aggressive Resident?*).

Bacterial action also may result in the formation of potentially toxic substances such as ammonia, indoles, amines, and phenolic compounds such as indolacetate, tyramine, histamine, and cresol (MacFarlane and MacFarlane, 1997). Some of the gases and organic acids contribute to the odor of feces.

Colonic Salvage of Malabsorbed Energy Sources and SCFA

Normally, varying amounts of some small-molecular-weight carbohydrates and amino acids remain in the chyme after leaving the small intestine. Accumulation of these small molecules could become osmotically important if it weren't for the action of bacteria in the colon. The disposal of residual substrates through production of SCFAs is called **colonic salvage** (Figure 1-6). SCFAs produced in fermentation are rapidly absorbed and take water with them. They also serve as fuel for the colonocytes and gut microbes, stimulate colonocyte proliferation and differentiation, enhance the absorption of electrolytes and water, and reduce the osmotic load of malabsorbed sugars. SCFAs may also help slow the movement of GI contents and participate in several other regulatory functions.

The ability to salvage carbohydrates is limited in humans, and colonic fermentation normally disposes of about 20 to 25 g of carbohydrate in 24 hours. Excess amounts of carbohydrate and fermentable fiber in the colon can cause increased gas production, abdominal (colonic) distention, bloating, pain, increased flatulence, and decreased colonic pH. If large amounts of poorly digested sugars or carbohydrates are consumed at once, diarrhea may also occur. Adaptation seems to occur in individuals consuming diets high in carbohydrates and fiber that are resistant to human digestive enzymes. Current recommendations are for the consumption of about 24 to 38 g of dietary fiber per day from fruits, vegetables, legumes, seeds, and whole grains for (1) maintaining the health of the cells lining the colon, (2) preventing excessive intra-colonic pressure, and (3) preventing constipation and maintaining a stable and healthful microbial population.

Digestion and Absorption of Specific Types of Nutrients

Carbohydrates and Fiber

Most dietary carbohydrates are consumed in the form of starches, disaccharides, and monosaccharides. Starches, or polysaccharides, usually make up the greatest proportion of carbohydrates. Starches are large molecules composed of straight or branched chains of sugar molecules that are joined together, primarily in $\alpha1$-4 and $\alpha1$-6 linkages. Most

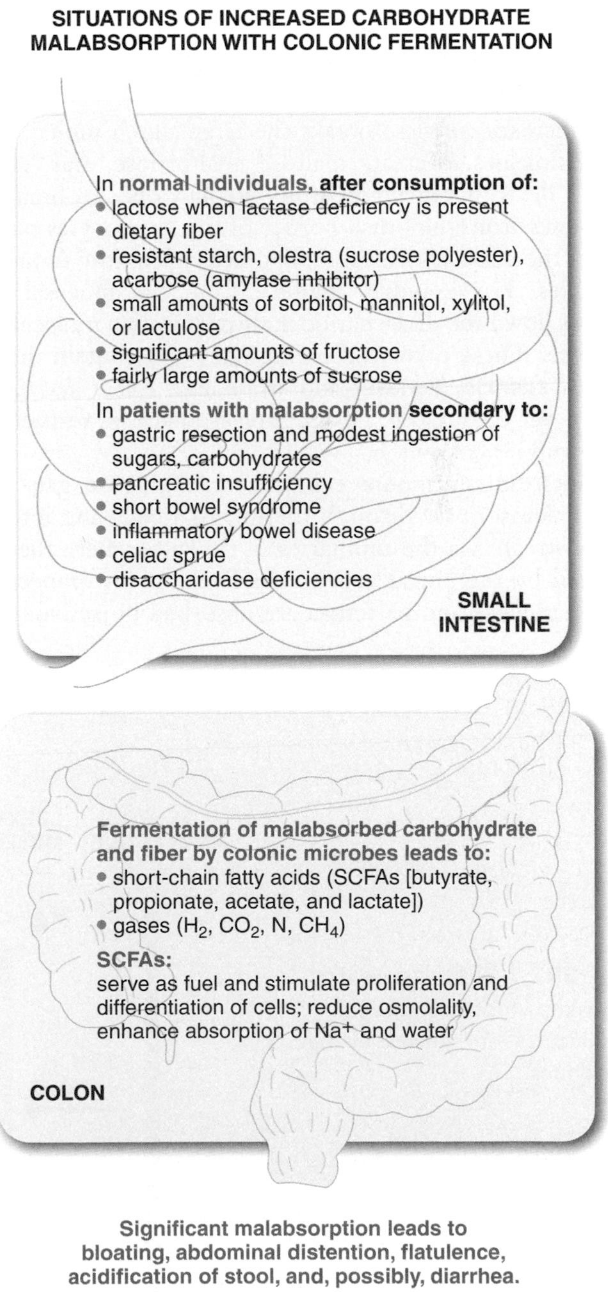

SITUATIONS OF INCREASED CARBOHYDRATE MALABSORPTION WITH COLONIC FERMENTATION

In normal individuals, **after consumption of:**
- lactose when lactase deficiency is present
- dietary fiber
- resistant starch, olestra (sucrose polyester), acarbose (amylase inhibitor)
- small amounts of sorbitol, mannitol, xylitol, or lactulose
- significant amounts of fructose
- fairly large amounts of sucrose

In patients with malabsorption **secondary to:**
- gastric resection and modest ingestion of sugars, carbohydrates
- pancreatic insufficiency
- short bowel syndrome
- inflammatory bowel disease
- celiac sprue
- disaccharidase deficiencies

SMALL INTESTINE

Fermentation of malabsorbed carbohydrate and fiber by colonic microbes leads to:
- short-chain fatty acids (SCFAs [butyrate, propionate, acetate, and lactate])
- gases (H_2, CO_2, N, CH_4)

SCFAs: serve as fuel and stimulate proliferation and differentiation of cells; reduce osmolality, enhance absorption of Na^+ and water

COLON

Significant malabsorption leads to bloating, abdominal distention, flatulence, acidification of stool, and, possibly, diarrhea.

FIGURE 1-6 Colonic fermentation of malabsorbed carbohydrates and fiber.

of the dietary starches are *amylopectins*, the branching poly-saccharides, and *amylose*, the straight chain–type polymers.

Dietary fiber is also largely made of chains and branches of sugar molecules, but in this case the hydrogens are positioned on the beta (opposite) side of the oxygen in the link instead of the alpha side. That humans have significant ability to digest starch, and not most forms of fiber, is an example of the stereospecificity of enzymes.

In the mouth the enzyme salivary amylase (ptyalin), which operates at a neutral or slightly alkaline pH, starts the digestive action by hydrolyzing a small amount of the starch molecules into smaller fragments (Figure 1-7). Amylase deactivates after contact with hydrochloric acid. If digestible carbohydrates remained in the stomach long enough, acid hydrolysis could eventually reduce most of them into monosaccharides. However, the stomach usually empties before significant digestion can take place. By far, most carbohydrate digestion occurs in the proximal small intestine.

Pancreatic amylase breaks the large starch molecules at α1-4 linkages to create maltose, maltotriose, and "alpha-limit" dextrins remaining from the amylopectin branches. Enzymes from the brush border of the enterocytes further break the disaccharides and oligosaccharides into monosac-charides. For example, **maltase** from the mucosal cells breaks down the disaccharide maltose into two molecules of glucose. These outer cell membranes also contain the enzymes **sucrase, lactase,** and isomaltase (or α-*dextrinase*), which act on sucrose, lactose, and isomaltose, respectively (Figure 1-8).

The resultant monosaccharides (i.e., glucose, galactose, and fructose) pass through the mucosal cells and into the bloodstream via the capillaries of the villi, where they are carried by the portal vein to the liver. At low concentrations, glucose and galactose are absorbed by active trans-port, primarily by a sodium-dependent transporter, glu-cose (galactose) cotransporter (SGLT1). At higher luminal concentrations of glucose, GLUT 2 becomes a primary facilitative transporter into the intestinal cell. Fructose is more slowly absorbed and uses GLUT 5 and the facilita-tive transporter from the lumen. GLUT 2 is used to trans-port both glucose and fructose across the intestinal cell membranes into the blood (Wright et al., 2003; Kellett and Brot-Laroche, 2005).

The sodium-dependent transport of monosaccharides is the reason why sodium-glucose drinks are used to rehydrate infants with diarrhea or athletes who have lost too much fluid. Glucose is transported from the liver to the tissues, although some glucose is stored in the liver and muscles as glycogen. Most of the fructose, as in the case of galactose, is transported to the liver, where it is converted to glucose. Consumption of large amounts of lactose (especially in in-dividuals with a lactase deficiency), fructose, stachyose, raf-finose, or alcohol sugars (e.g., sorbitol, mannitol, or xylitol) can result in considerable amounts of these sugars passing unabsorbed into the colon (Beyer et al., 2005; Thompson et al., 2003) and may cause increased gas and loose stools. Fructose is found naturally in many fruits (e.g., in sucrose and high-fructose corn syrup) but is likely only to produce symptoms if consumed as the single monosaccharide or if the food has an abundance of fructose compared to glucose (as in the case of apple juice).

Some forms of carbohydrates (i.e., cellulose, hemicellu-lose, pectin, gum, and other forms of fiber) cannot be di-gested by humans because neither their salivary nor pancre-atic amylase has the ability to split the β1-2 and β1-4 linkages connecting the constituent sugars. These carbohy-drates pass relatively unchanged into the colon, where they are partially fermented by bacteria in the colon. However, unlike humans, cows and other ruminants can subsist on

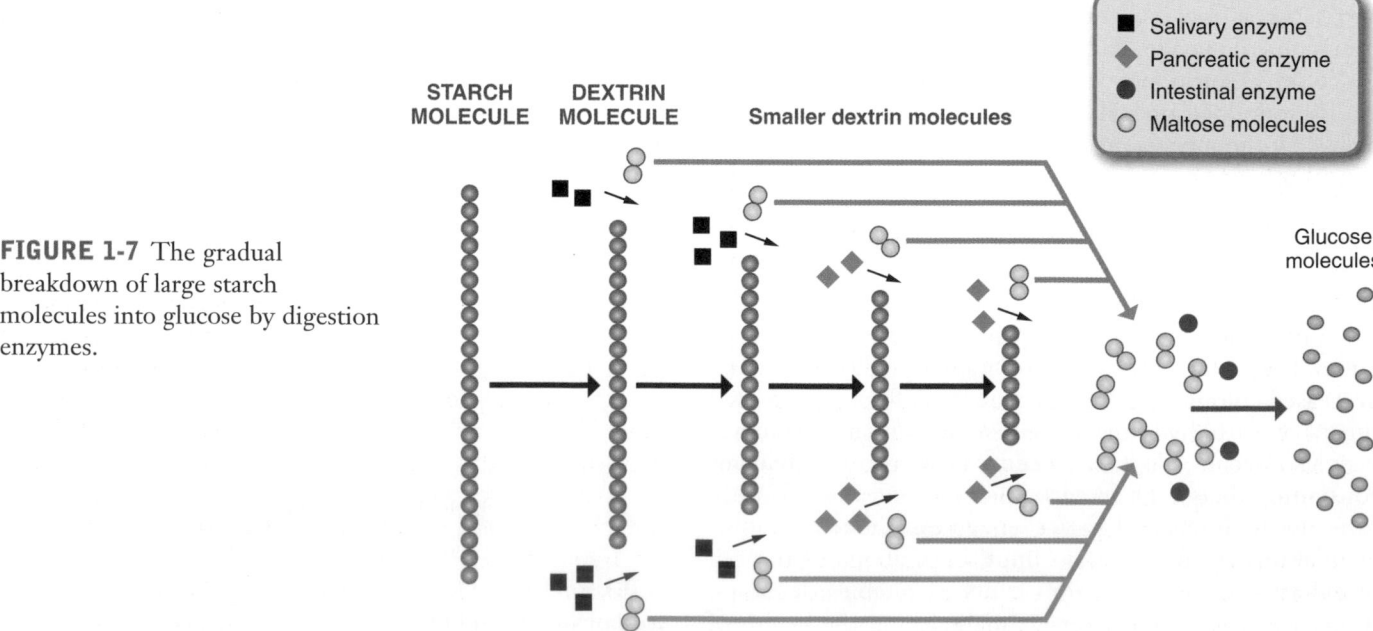

FIGURE 1-7 The gradual breakdown of large starch molecules into glucose by digestion enzymes.

high-fiber food because of the bacterial digestion of these carbohydrates that takes place in the rumen. Other resistant starches and sugars are also less well-digested or absorbed by humans; thus their consumption may result in significant amounts of starch and sugar in the colon. The resistant starches and some types of dietary fiber are fermented into SCFAs and gases. Starches resistant to digestion tend to include plant foods with a high protein and fiber content such as those from legumes and whole grains. One form of dietary fiber, lignin, is made of cyclopentane units and is not readily soluble or fermentable.

Proteins

Protein intake in the Western world ranges from about 50 to 100 g daily, and a good deal of the protein consumed is from animal sources. Additional protein is added all along the GI tract from GI secretions and cells sloughed from GI tissues. The GI tract is one of the most active synthetic tissues in the body, and the life span of enterocytes migrating from the crypts of the villi until they are shed is only 3 to 4 days. The number of cells shed daily is in the range of 10 to 20 billion cells. The latter accounts for an additional 50 to 60 g of protein that is digested and "recycled" and contributes to the daily supply. In general, animal proteins are more efficiently digested than plant proteins, but human GI physiology allows for very effective digestion and absorption of large amounts of ingested protein sources.

Protein digestion begins in the stomach, where some of the proteins are split into proteoses, peptones, and large polypeptides. Inactive pepsinogen is converted into the enzyme pepsin when it contacts hydrochloric acid and other pepsin molecules. Unlike any of the other proteolytic enzymes, pepsin digests collagen, the major protein of connective tissue. Most protein digestion takes place in the upper portion of the small intestine, but it continues throughout the GI tract (Soybel, 2005; Thompson et al., 2003). Any residual protein fractions are fermented by colonic microbes.

Contact between chyme and the intestinal mucosa stimulates release of enterokinase, an enzyme that transforms inactive pancreatic trypsinogen into active trypsin, the major pancreatic protein digesting enzyme. Trypsin in turn activates the other pancreatic proteolytic enzymes. Pancreatic trypsin, chymotrypsin, and carboxypeptidase break down intact protein and continue the breakdown started in the stomach until small polypeptides and amino acids are formed.

Proteolytic peptidases located on the brush border also act on polypeptides, breaking them down into amino acids, dipeptides, and tripeptides. The final phase of protein digestion takes place in the brush border, where some of the dipeptides and tripeptides are hydrolyzed into their constituent amino acids by peptide hydrolases.

End products of protein digestion are absorbed as both amino acids and small peptides. Several transport molecules are required for the different amino acids, probably because of the wide differences in the size, polarity, and configuration of the different amino acids. Some of the transporters are sodium- and/or chloride-dependent, and some are not. Considerable amounts of dipeptides and tripeptides are also absorbed into intestinal cells using a peptide transporter (PEPT1), a form of active transport (Daniel, 2004). Absorbed peptides and amino acids are transported to the liver via the portal vein for metabolism by the liver and are released into the general circulation.

The presence of antibodies to many food proteins in the circulation of healthy individuals indicates that immunologically significant amounts of large intact peptides escape hydrolysis and can enter the portal circulation. The exact mechanisms that cause a food to become an allergen are not entirely clear, but these foods tend to be high in protein, be relatively resistant to complete digestion, and produce an immunoglobulin E (IgE) response (Bannon, 2004) (see Chapter 29).

Almost all protein is absorbed by the time it reaches the end of the jejunum, and only 1% of ingested protein is found in the feces. Small amounts of amino acids may remain in the epithelial cells and are used for synthesis of new proteins, including intestinal enzymes and new cells.

Lipids

About 97% of dietary lipids are in the form of triglycerides, and the rest are in the form of phospholipids and cholesterol. Only small amounts of fat are digested in the mouth with lingual lipase and in the stomach from the action of gastric lipase (*tributyrinase*). Gastric lipase hydrolyzes some triglycerides, especially short-chain triglycerides (such as those found in butter), into fatty acids and glycerol. However, most fat digestion takes place in the small intestine through pancreatic lipase. As in the case of carbohydrates and protein, the capacity for digestion and absorption of dietary fat is in excess of ordinary needs.

Entrance of fat and protein into the small intestine stimulates the release of CCK and **enterogastrone,** which

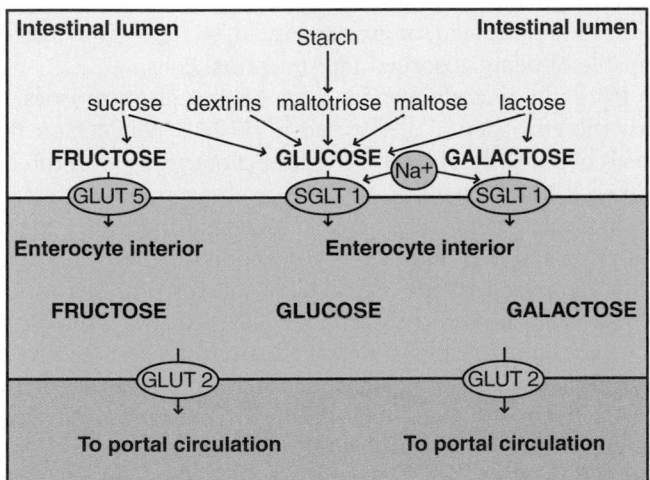

FIGURE 1-8 Starch, sucrose, maltotriose, and galactose are digested to their constituent sugars. Glucose and galactose are transported through the apical brush border membrane of the enterocyte by a sodium-dependent transporter, SGLT1; and fructose is transported by GLUT 5. Glucose, fructose, and galactose are transported across the serosal membrane by the sodium-independent transporter, GLUT 2.

inhibit gastric secretions and motility, thus slowing the delivery of lipids. As a result, a portion of a large, fatty meal may remain in the stomach for 4 hours or longer. In addition to its many other functions, CCK stimulates biliary and pancreatic secretions. The combination of the peristaltic action of the small intestine and the surfactant and emulsification action provided by bile reduces the fat globules into tiny droplets, thus making them more accessible to digestion by the most potent lipid-digesting enzyme, pancreatic lipase (Keller and Layer, 2005).

Bile is a liver secretion composed of bile acids (primarily conjugates of cholic and chenodeoxycholic acids with glycine or taurine), bile pigments (which color the feces), inorganic salts, some protein, cholesterol, lecithin, and many compounds such as detoxified drugs that are metabolized and secreted by the liver. From its storage organ, the gallbladder, about 1 L of bile is secreted daily in response to the stimulus of food in the duodenum and stomach.

The free fatty acids and monoglycerides produced by digestion form complexes with bile salts called *micelles.* The micelles facilitate passage of the lipids through the watery environment of the intestinal lumen to the brush border (see Figure 1-4). The micelles release the lipid components and are returned to the gut lumen. Most of the bile salts are actively reabsorbed in the terminal ileum and returned to the liver to reenter the gut in bile secretions. This efficient recycling process is known as the *enterohepatic circulation.* The pool of bile acids may circulate from three to fifteen times per day, depending on the amount of food ingested.

In the mucosal cells the fatty acids and monoglycerides are reassembled into new triglycerides. A few are further digested into free fatty acids and glycerol and then reassembled to form triglycerides. These triglycerides, along with cholesterol, fat-soluble vitamins, and phospholipids, are surrounded by a β-lipoprotein coat, forming chylomicrons (see Figure 1-4). The lipoprotein globules pass into the lymphatic system instead of entering portal blood and are transported to the thoracic duct and emptied into the systemic circulation at the junction of the left internal jugular and left subclavian veins. The chylomicrons are then carried through the bloodstream to several tissues, including liver, adipose tissue, and muscle. In the liver triglycerides from the chylomicrons are repackaged into very low–density lipoproteins and transported primarily to the adipose tissue for metabolism and storage.

The fat-soluble vitamins A, D, E, and K are also absorbed in a micellar fashion, although water-soluble forms of vitamins A, E, and K supplements and carotene can be absorbed in the absence of bile acids.

Under normal conditions approximately 95% to 97% of ingested fat is absorbed into lymph vessels. Because of their shorter length and thus increased solubility, fatty acids of 8 to 12 carbons (i.e., medium-chain fatty acids) can be absorbed directly into colonic mucosal cells without the presence of bile and micelle formation (Thompson et al., 2003). After entering mucosal cells, they are able to go directly without esterification into the portal vein, which carries them to the liver.

Use of medium-chain triglycerides (which have fatty acids of 8 to 12 carbons) is clinically valuable for individuals who lack necessary bile salts for emulsification and micellar formation required for long-chain fatty acid transport (see Chapter 27) or lack the ability to transport triglycerides from the intestinal epithelial cells into the lymphatics, as occurs in abetalipoproteinemia. Supplements for clinical use are normally provided in the form of oil or a dietary beverage with other macronutrients and micronutrients.

Increased motility, intestinal mucosal changes, pancreatic insufficiency, or the absence of bile can decrease absorption of fat. When undigested fat appears in the feces, the condition is known as *steatorrhea* (see Chapter 27).

Vitamins and Minerals

Vitamins and minerals from foods are made available as macronutrients are digested and absorbed across the mucosal layer, primarily in the small intestine (Figure 1-9). Besides adequate passive and transporter mechanisms, various factors affect the bioavailability of vitamins and minerals, including the presence or absence of other specific nutrients, acid or alkali, phytates, and oxalates. Each day about 8 to 9 L of fluid is secreted from the GI tract and serves as a solvent, a vehicle for chemical reactions, and a medium for transfer of several nutrients.

At least some of most vitamins and water pass unchanged from the small intestine into the blood by passive diffusion, but several different mechanisms might be used to transport individual vitamins across the GI mucosa. Drugs are absorbed by a number of mechanisms and may share or compete with mechanisms for the absorption nutrients into intestinal cells (see Chapter 16).

Mineral absorption is more complex, especially the absorption of the cation minerals. These cations, such as selenium, are made available for absorption by the process of **chelation,** where a mineral is bound to a ligand—usually an acid, an organic acid, or an amino acid, so that it is in a form capable of being absorbed into intestinal cells.

Iron and zinc absorption share several characteristics in that the efficiency of absorption is partly dependent on the needs of the host. They also use at least one transport protein, and each has mechanisms to increase absorption when stores are inadequate. Phytates and oxalates impair the absorption of both iron and zinc, and their reabsorption is better when consumed from animal rather than plant sources. The absorption of zinc is impaired with disproportionately increased amounts of magnesium, calcium, and iron. Calcium absorption into the enterocyte occurs through channels in the brush border membrane, where it is bound to a specific protein carrier for transportation across the basolateral membrane. The process is regulated by the presence of vitamin D. Phosphorus is absorbed by a sodium phosphorus cotransporter, which is also regulated by vitamin D or low phosphate intake.

The GI tract is the site of important interactions among minerals. Supplementation with large amounts of iron or zinc may decrease the absorption of copper. In turn, the presence of copper may lower iron and molybdenum absorption. Cobalt absorption is increased in pa-

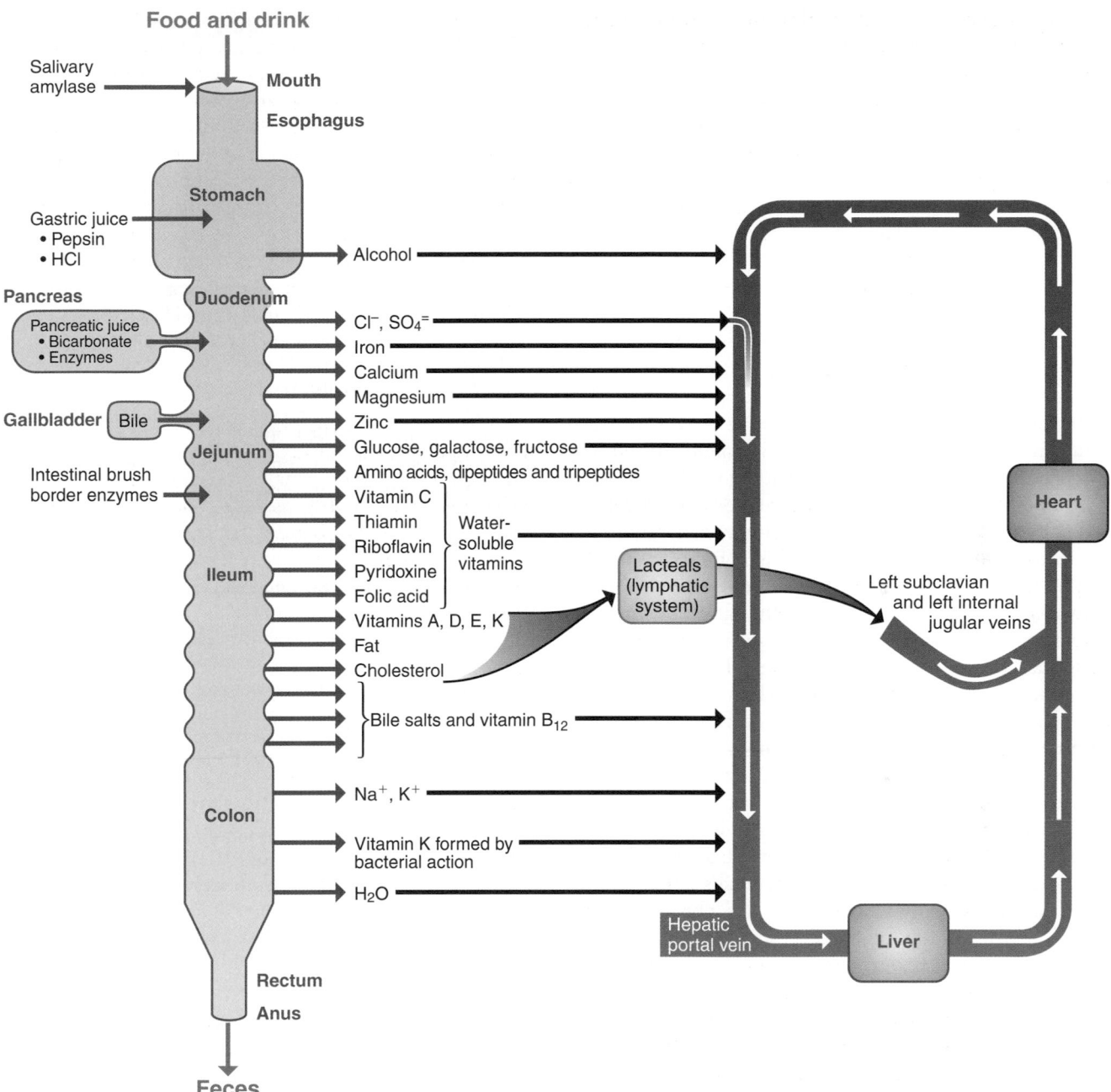

FIGURE 1-9 Sites of secretion and absorption in the gastrointestinal tract.

tients with iron deficiency, but cobalt and iron compete and inhibit one another's absorption. These interactions are probably the result of an overlap of mineral absorption mechanisms.

Minerals are transported in blood bound to protein carriers. The protein binding is either specific (e.g., transferrin, which binds with iron) or general (e.g., albumin, which binds with a variety of minerals). A fraction of each mineral is also carried in the serum in the form of amino acid or peptide complexes. Specific protein carriers are usually not completely saturated; the reserve capacity may serve as a buffer against excessive exposure. Toxicity from minerals usually results only after this buffering capacity is exceeded.

Factors Affecting Digestion

Psychologic Factors

The appearance, smell, and taste of food, in addition to emotional states, have an impact on digestion. The sight, smell, taste, and even the thought of food increase secretion of GI hormones, fluids, and enzymes and increase the muscular activity of the GI tract (Keller and Layer, 2005; Furness and Clerc, 2000). After ingestion of food, digestive products then trigger feedback mechanisms to inhibit GI activity and limit food intake. Fear, anger, and worry stimulate the hypothalamus to activate the autonomic nervous system, which then depresses secretions, inhibits peristalsis, and slows propulsion of food by increasing sphincter tone

(Bray, 2000; Katschinski, 2000). Strong odors, noxious stimuli, and very strong emotions may induce nausea and vomiting. Strong signals from the GI tract as a result of disease, inflammation, distention, or dysmotility may send signals to the central nervous system, resulting in the perception of nausea or abdominal comfort. Aging affects digestion through impaired protein turnover rate, reduced anabolic hormone production, and inadequate intake (Walrand and Boirie, 2005).

Food Processing

The processes of freezing, preserving, microwaving, baking, and frying foods can, to varying degrees, alter the solubility, microbial counts, structure, and digestibility of foods and even increase the formation of potentially harmful foods (Friedman, 2003; Meade et al., 2005). Several nutrients such as ascorbic acid and folate can be destroyed with prolonged cooking. In general, however, when foods are properly prepared, stored, and cooked, many tend to be safe and more digestible than raw food. For example, cooking meat loosens its connective tissue, facilitates chewing, and makes the meat more accessible to digestive juices. Cooking softens dietary fiber, makes certain fiber more fermentable, and may make the digestible nutrients attached to fiber more available. Claims have been made that fruits and vegetables should be consumed raw because their inherent carbohydrate- or protein-digesting enzymes facilitate digestion of foods and are destroyed with cooking. Enzymes from a few raw fruits and vegetables may still have some activity in the GI tract, but their contribution to the digestion of foods is miniscule and pales compared with the powerful human digestive enzymes. During grain refinement for breads and cereals, many of the nutrients, phytochemicals, and fibrous materials are lost. Enrichment replaces several of the lost nutrients but not the dietary fiber or phytochemicals.

⊙ FOCAL POINTS

- With few exceptions the human GI tract is remarkably efficient: humans can consume a wide variety of foods in random combinations without significantly affecting digestion.
- The nature of secretions changes in amount and type to accommodate foods consumed.
- The GI tract has self-regulating mechanisms for coordinating digestive, immunologic, secretory, and absorptive functions.
- A transient disruption of these homeostatic mechanisms may occur as a result of dietary extremes; more long-term dysfunction can result from malnutrition, disease, surgery or trauma.

USEFUL WEBSITES

American Gastroenterological Association
www.gastro.org/public/digestinfo.html

NIH Digestive Diseases
www.niddk.nih.gov/health/digest/digest.htm

References

Ahlman H, Nilsson O: The gut as the largest endocrine organ in the body, *Ann Oncol* 12(suppl 2):63, 2001.

Bannon GA: What makes a food protein an allergen? *Curr Allergy Asthma Rep* 4:43, 2004.

Beyer P et al: Fructose intake at current level, in the United States may cause gastrointestinal distress in normal adults. *J Am Diet Assoc* 105:1559, 2005.

Bourlioux P et al: The intestine and its microflora are partners for the protection of the host: report on the Danone symposium, *Am J Clin Nutr* 78:675, 2003.

Bray GA: Afferent signals regulating food intake, *Proc Nutr Soc* 59:373, 2000.

Chey WY, Chang TM: Secretin, 100 years later, *J Gastroenterol* 38:1025, 2003.

Daniel H: Molecular and integrative physiology of intestinal peptide transport, *Annu Rev Physiol* 66:361 2004.

Delzenne NM: Oligosaccharides: state of the art, *Proc Nutr Soc* 62:177, 2003.

Efendic S, Portwood N: Overview of incretin hormones, *Hormone Metab Res* 36:742, 2004.

Englyst KN, Englyst HN: Carbohydrate bioavailability, *Br J Nutr* 94:1, 2005.

Feighner SD et al: Receptor for motilin identified in the human gastrointestinal system, *Science* 284:2184, 1999.

Friedman M: Nutritional consequences of food processing, *Forum Nutr* 56:350 2003.

Furness JB, Clerc N: Responses of afferent neurons to the contents of the digestive tract and their relation to endocrine and immune responses, *Prog Brain Res* 122:159, 2000.

Gibson GR et al: Prebiotics and resistance to gastrointestinal infections, *Br J Nutr* Suppl 1(93):S31, 2005.

Gill HS, Guarner F: Probiotics and human health: a perspective, *Postgrad Med* 80:516, 2004.

Guarner F: Inulin and oligofructose: impact on intestinal diseases and disorders, *Br J Nutr* Suppl 1(93):S61, 2005.

Hao WL, Lee YK: Microflora of the gastrointestinal tract: a review, *Methods Mol Biol* 268:491, 2004.

Hill MJ: Intestinal flora and endogenous vitamin synthesis, *Eur J Cancer Prev* 6(Suppl 1):43 1997.

Katschinski M: Nutritional implications of cephalic phase gastrointestinal responses, *Appetite* 34:189, 2000.

Keller J, Layer P: Human pancreatic endocrine response to nutrients in health and disease, *Gut* 54:1, 2005.

Kellett G, Brot-Laroche E: Apical GLUT 2: a major pathway of intestinal sugar absorption, *Diabetes* 54:3056, 2005.

Lammert F, Wang DO: New insights into the genetic regulation of intestinal cholesterol absorption, *Gastroentorology* 128:718, 2005.

Low MJ: Clinical endocrinology and metabolism: the somatostatin neuroendocrine system: physiology and clinical relevance in gastrointestinal and pancreatic disorders, *Best Pract Res Clin Endocrinol Metabol* 18:607, 2004.

Lowe ME: The triglyceride lipases of the pancreas, *J Lipid Res* 43:2007, 2002.

MacFarlane GT, MacFarlane S: Human colonic microbiota: ecology physiology and metabolic potential of intestinal bacteria, *Scand J Gastroenterol* 222(suppl):3, 1997.

Meade SJ et al: The impact of processing on the nutritional quality of food proteins, *J AOAC Int* 88(3):904, 2005.

Pool-Zobel BL: Inulin-type fructans and reduction in colon cancer risk: review of experimental and human data. *Br J Nutr* 93:S73, 2005.

Rehfeld JF: A centenary of gastrointestinal endocrinology, *Horm Metab Res* 36:735, 2004.

Roberfroid MB: Prebiotics: preferential substrates for specific germs? *Am J Clin Nutr* 73(suppl):406, 2001.

Sarna SK et al: Enteric locus of prokinetics: ABT-229, motilin, and erythromycin, *Am J Physiol Gastrointest Liver Physiol* 278: G744, 2000.

Snelling AM: Effects of probiotics on the gastrointestinal tract, *Curr Opin Infect Dis* 18:420, 2005.

Soybel DI: Anatomy and physiology of the stomach, *Surg Clin North Am* 85:875, 2005.

Stanley S et al: Hormonal regulation of food intake, *Physiol Rev* 85:1131 2005.

Thompson ABR et al: Small bowel review. Normal physiology, Part 1, *Dig Dis Sci* 48:1546, 2003.

Tlaskalova-Hogenova H et al: Commensal bacteria (normal microflora), mucosal immunity and chronic inflammatory and autoimmune diseases, *Immunol Let* 93:97, 2004.

Walrand S, Boirie Y: Optimizing protein intake in aging, *Curr Opin Clin Nutr Metabol Care* 8:89, 2005.

Wank SA: G Protein-coupled receptors in gastrointestinal physiology. I. CCK receptors: an exemplary family, *Am J Physiol Gastrointest Liver Physiol* 274:G607, 1998.

Wright EM et al: Intestinal absorption in health and disease, *Best Pract Res Clin Gastroenterol* 17:943, 2003.

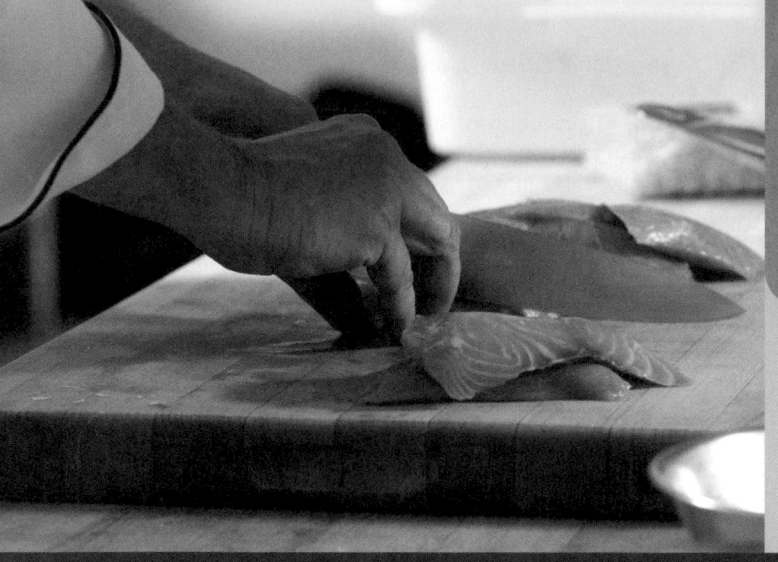

CHAPTER 2

Carol D. Frary, MS, RD
Rachel K. Johnson, PhD, RD

Energy

KEY TERMS

activity thermogenesis (AT) the energy expended during active exercise such as fitness and sports exercise and the energy expended during activities of daily living, referred to as nonexercise activity thermogenesis

basal energy expenditure (BEE) the measurement of the basal metabolic rate extrapolated to 24 hours; usually expressed as kilocalories per 24 hours (kcal/24 hr)

basal metabolic rate (BMR) the energy needed to sustain the metabolic activities of cells and tissues and to maintain circulatory, respiratory, gastrointestinal, and renal processes; expressed as kilocalories per kilogram of body weight per hour; measured in the morning 10 to 12 hours after ingestion of food, drink, alcohol, or nicotine

calorie the amount of energy required to raise the temperature of 1 ml of water at 15° C by 1° C

direct calorimetry a method for measuring the amount of energy expended by monitoring the rate at which a person loses heat from the body to the environment when placed inside a structure large enough to permit moderate amounts of activity

doubly labeled water (DLW) used to measure total energy expenditure in free-living people using two stable isotopes of water (deuterium [^2H_2O] and oxygen-18 [$H_2{}^{18}O$]); the difference in the turnover rates of the two isotopes measures the carbon dioxide production rate, from which total energy expenditure can be calculated

estimated energy requirement (EER) the average dietary energy intake that is predicted to maintain energy balance in a healthy adult of a defined age, gender, weight, height, and level of physical activity consistent with good health; in children and pregnant and lactating women, the EER is taken to include the energy needs associated with the deposition of tissues or the secretion of milk at rates consistent with good health

excess postexercise oxygen consumption (EPOC) 8% to 14% increase in metabolic rate for a period after exercise has ceased

facultative thermogenesis a portion of the thermic effect of food; "excess" energy expended in addition to the obligatory thermogenesis—thought to be partially mediated by sympathetic nervous system activity

indirect calorimetry a method for estimating energy production by measuring oxygen consumption and carbon dioxide production rather than by directly measuring heat transfer; typically takes 30 minutes to 1 hour to complete

joule (J) the measure of energy in terms of mechanical work; the amount of energy required to accelerate 1 Newton (N) a distance of 1 m; 1 kcal = 4.184 kJ

kilocalorie (kcal or Cal) 1000 calories; sometimes written as Calorie

metabolic equivalents (METs) the measure of caloric expenditure by the amount of oxygen consumed per minute per kilogram of body weight; 1 MET = ~3.5 ml oxygen consumed per kilogram of body weight per minute in adults

nonexercise activity thermogenesis (NEAT) the energy expended during activities of daily living

obligatory thermogenesis a portion of the thermic effect of food; the energy required to digest, absorb, and metabolize nutrients

physical activity level (PAL) the ratio of total energy expenditure (TEE) to basal energy expenditure (BEE); PAL = TEE/BEE

resting energy expenditure (REE) a measurement of the resting metabolic rate extrapolated to 24 hours; usually expressed as kilocalories per 24 hours (kcal/24 hr)

resting metabolic rate (RMR) the energy expended for the maintenance of normal body functions and homeostasis; represents the largest portion of total energy expenditure; expressed as kilocalories per kilogram of body weight per hour; may be as much as 10% to 20% higher than the basal metabolic rate, allowing for the energy spent as a result of the thermic effect of food or excess postexercise oxygen consumption

respiratory quotient (RQ) the ratio of moles of carbon dioxide produced to the moles of oxygen consumed

thermic effect of food (TEF) the increase in energy expenditure associated with the processes of digestion, absorption, and metabolism of food; represents approximately 10% of the sum of the resting metabolic expenditure and the energy expended in physical activity and includes facultative thermogenesis and obligatory thermogenesis; often called diet-induced thermogenesis, specific dynamic action, or the specific effect of food

total energy expenditure (TEE) the sum of basal energy expenditure, activity thermogenesis, and the thermic effect of food; the daily total energy expended by a person in 24 hours

Energy is defined as "the capacity to do work." The ultimate source of all energy in living organisms is the sun. Through the process of photosynthesis, green plants intercept a portion of the sunlight reaching their leaves and capture it within the chemical bonds of glucose. Proteins, fats, and other carbohydrates are synthesized from this basic carbohydrate to meet the needs of the plant. Animals and humans obtain these nutrients and the energy they contain by consuming plants and the flesh of other animals. The body makes use of the energy from carbohydrates, proteins, fats, and alcohol in the diet. Energy provided from the macronutrients is locked in chemical bonds within food and is released when food is metabolized. Energy must be supplied regularly to meet the energy needs for the body's survival. Although all energy eventually takes the form of heat, which dissipates into the atmosphere, unique cellular processes first make possible its use for all of the tasks required to maintain life. Among these processes are chemical reactions that accomplish synthesis and maintenance of body tissues, electrical conduction of nerve activity, the mechanical work of muscles, and heat production to maintain body temperature.

Energy requirements are defined as the dietary energy intake that is required to maintain energy balance in a healthy person of a defined age, gender, weight, height, and level of physical activity consistent with good health. In children and pregnant or lactating women, energy requirements include the needs associated with the deposition of tissues or the secretion of milk at rates consistent with good health (Institute of Medicine, 2002; 2005).

Body weight is an indicator of energy adequacy or inadequacy. The body has the unique ability to shift the fuel mixture of carbohydrates, proteins, and fats to accommodate energy needs. However, consuming too much or too little energy over time results in body weight changes. Thus body weight reflects adequacy of energy intake, but it is not a reliable indicator of macronutrient or micronutrient adequacy (see *New Directions:* Will Eating Less Make You Live Longer?).

⇄ NEW DIRECTIONS

Will Eating Less Make You Live Longer?

Calorie restriction (CR), otherwise referred to as dietary restriction of energy intake but with adequate intakes of essential nutrients and vitamins, has been found to extend the aging process in species with limited life spans (Hursting et al., 2003), yet findings are inconsistent (Masoro, 2006). Some of the proposed hypotheses linking CR to the slowing of aging relate to reduced body fat, reduced metabolic rate, less oxidative damage, and lower plasma glucose and insulin levels (Masoro, 2005).

Ongoing research that began in 1987 in cohorts of rhesus monkeys consuming a 30% CR diet revealed improved regulation of glucose, decreased blood pressure and blood lipids, reduced body weight and abdominal fat, and reduced body temperature (a possible factor associated with anti-aging) over their age-matched controls (Mattison et al., 2003). Male monkeys presented with slower rates of decline in age-related hormones (Mattison et al., 2003). Allowing for the maximum 40-year life expectancy of the rhesus monkey, findings will be uncertain for another two to three decades.

CR research in humans is limited. The Comprehensive Assessment of the Long-Term Effects of Reducing Intake of Energy (CALERIE) study conducted between 2002 and 2004 examined the effects of CR in overweight (BMI 25 to <30) people during a 6-month intervention (Heilbronn et al., 2006). Forty-eight adults were randomly assigned to either a control group or one of three intervention groups: (1) 25% CR (about 1500 kcal/day for a man requiring 2000 kcal/day), (2) 12.5% CR plus 12.5% increase in energy expenditure with exercise, and (3) very low–calorie diet (850 kcal/day until 15% weight reduction, followed by weight maintenance diet). After 6 months all three intervention groups experienced decreased fasting serum insulin levels, reduced metabolic rate beyond what would be expected from reduced metabolic mass, and less DNA damage; groups 1 and 2 also had lowered core body temperatures (biomarkers of longevity) (Heilbronn et al., 2006).

Although studies have linked lower energy intakes to a reduction in risk factors for some diseases associated with aging (Weindruch, 2006), CR in humans has also been associated with health risks. Some of the negative effects include hypotension, slower wound healing, depression, and excessive loss of fat and muscle mass, which in turn can trigger a host of additional health concerns such as loss of strength, sensitivity to cold, bone loss, loss of libido, menstrual irregularities, and infertility (Dirks and Leeuwenburgh, 2006). Preliminary CR research in humans is inconclusive, and the effects of long-term CR and longevity may not be known for several decades.

COMPONENTS OF ENERGY EXPENDITURE

Energy is expended by the human body in the form of basal metabolic rate, thermic effect of food, and activity thermogenesis (Levine and Kotz, 2005). These three components make up a person's daily **total energy expenditure (TEE)** (Figure 2-1).

Basal and Resting Energy Expenditure

Definition

Basal energy expenditure (BEE) can be simply defined as the minimum amount of energy expended that is compatible with life. A person's BEE reflects the amount of energy used over 24 hours while physically (i.e., lying down) and mentally resting in a thermoneutral environment that prevents the activation of heat-generating processes such as shivering. **Basal metabolic rate (BMR)** measurements are made early in the morning, before the person has engaged in any physical activity and 10 to 12 hours after the ingestion of any food, drink, or nicotine. The BMR remains remarkably constant on a daily basis (Durnin, 1996) and typically represents approximately 60% to 70% of the total energy expenditure (Shetty et al., 1996). If any of the conditions for the BMR are not met, energy expenditure should be referred to as the **resting metabolic rate (RMR).** For practical reasons the BMR is now rarely measured. RMR measurements are used in its place, which in most cases are higher than the BMR by 10% to 20% (Institute of Medicine, 2002; 2005).

Resting energy expenditure (REE) is the energy expended in the activities necessary to sustain normal body functions and homeostasis. These activities include respiration and circulation, the synthesis of organic compounds, the pumping of ions across membranes, the energy required by the central nervous system, and the maintenance of body temperature. Organs in the body contribute to heat production (Figure 2-2). Nearly 60% of REE can be accounted for by the heat produced by the liver, brain, heart, and kidneys (Gallagher et al., 1998).

Factors Affecting Resting Energy Expenditure

Numerous factors cause the REE to vary among individuals. Major variables include body size and composition; but age, sex, and hormonal status also affect REE.

Body Size. Larger people generally have higher metabolic rates than smaller people; but tall, thin people have higher metabolic rates than short, wide people. For example, if two people weigh the same but one person is taller, the taller person with the larger body surface area has the higher metabolic rate (Whitney and Rolfes, 2002). Thus those with the greater surface area have the higher metabolic rate.

The amount of lean body mass is highly correlated with total body size. For example, obese children have higher RMRs than nonobese children; but, when RMR is adjusted for body composition, fat free mass, and fat mass, no RMR differences are found (Molnar and Schutz, 1997).

Body Composition. *Fat-free mass (FFM)*, the metabolically active tissue in the body, is a predictor of REE. FFM contributes to approximately 80% of the variance in REE (Illner et al., 2000; Bosy-Westphal et al., 2004). Because of their greater FFM, athletes with greater muscular development have approximately a 5% higher resting metabolism than nonathletic individuals.

FFM can be measured most accurately by using reference body composition methods. These methods include underwater weighing *(hydrodensitometry)*, dual x-ray absorptiometry *(DEXA or DXA)*, and air-displacement plethysmography (e.g., the BOD POD). Underwater weighing determines body fat by measuring a person's body density and is considered the gold standard for measuring body composition. Body density is the difference between the dry weight before underwater weighing and the underwater weight. Be-

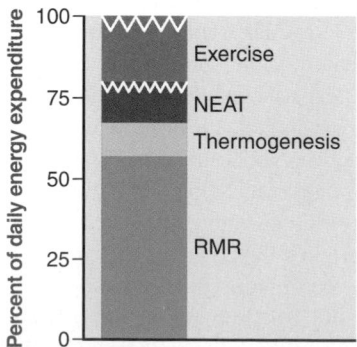

FIGURE 2-1 The components of total energy expenditure (TEE): Activity thermogenesis (active exercise and nonexercise activity thermogenesis [NEAT]), diet-induced thermogenesis, and resting metabolic rate (RMR). *(From Ravussin E: Physiology: a NEAT way to control weight? Science 307(5709):530, 2005 (the percent of daily energy expenditure portion only).*

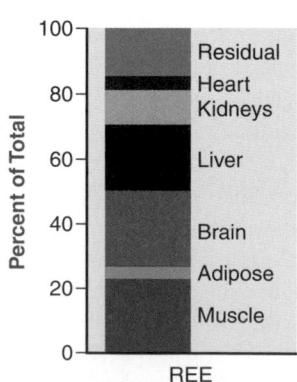

FIGURE 2-2 Proportional contribution of organs and tissues to calculated resting energy expenditure (REE). *(Modified and used with permission from Gallagher D et al: Organ-tissue mass measurement allows modeling of REE and metabolically active tissue mass, Am J Physiol Endocrinol Metabol 275:E249, 1998. Copyright American Physiological Society.)*

cause fat is less dense and more buoyant in water than FFM, the less a person weighs underwater, the higher the body fat. (The underwater procedure can be viewed at http://nutrition.uvm.edu/bodycomp [Pintauro and Buzzell, 2006]). The BOD POD (Figure 2-3) is based on the same principle as underwater weighing, except that it uses air displacement technology (Callahan, 2002). DXA is a novel scanning technique that accurately estimates bone mineral, fat, and fat-free soft tissue. Radiation exposure is minimal—approximately a single day's background radiation—for a whole-body composition analysis (Figure 2-4).

However, because of the expense and impractical nature of some of these reference methods, less accurate but more practical methods such as skinfold anthropometry (SFA) and bioelectrical impedance analysis (BIA) are often used to estimate body composition (see Appendixes 24 and 27). SFA is used to determine the percentage of body fat by measuring subcutaneous fat tissue with a skinfold caliper (see Chapter 14 and Figures 14-10 and 14-11). A highly trained person should perform and read skinfold thickness measurements to obtain the most accurate data. The BIA technique can be used to determine FFM in the extremities and involves placing electrodes on the wrist and ankle. BIA electrical measurements are used to estimate a person's total body water (TBW). From TBW measurements, FFM can be estimated because FFM is primarily composed of water. Subsequently an approximation of fat mass can be calculated as the difference between body weight and FFM (Pintauro and Buzzell, 2006).

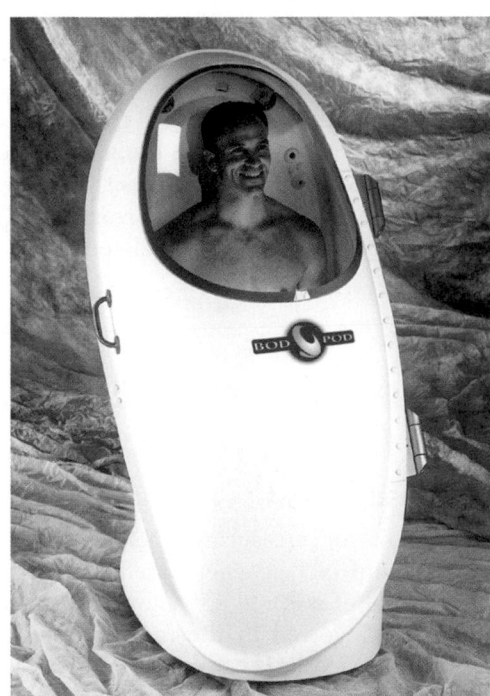

FIGURE 2-3 The BOD POD uses air displacement technology to measure body composition. *(Courtesy Life Measurement, Inc., Concord, Calif.)*

Age. Because it is determined by the FFM, RMR is highest during periods of rapid growth, chiefly during the first and second years of life (Butte et al., 2000). The additional energy required for synthesizing and depositing body tissue is about 5 kcal/g of tissue gained (Roberts and Young, 1988). Growing infants may store as much as 12% to 15% of the energy value of their food in the form of new tissue. As a child becomes older, the caloric requirement for growth is reduced to about 1% of the total energy requirement.

After early adulthood there is a decline in RMR of 1% to 2% per kilogram of FFM per decade (Keys et al., 1973). Exercise can help maintain a higher lean body mass and thus a higher RMR (Dolezal and Potteiger, 1998).

Sex. Sex differences in metabolic rates are primarily attributable to differences in body size and composition. Women, who generally have more fat in proportion to muscle than men, have metabolic rates that are approximately 5% to 10% lower than men of the same weight and height.

Hormonal Status. Hormonal status can affect metabolic rate, particularly in those with endocrine disorders such as hyperthyroidism and hypothyroidism, which increase or decrease energy expenditure, respectively. Stimulation of the sympathetic nervous system (e.g., during periods of emotional excitement or stress) causes the release of epinephrine, which directly promotes glycogenolysis and increases cellular activity. Endogenous growth hormone levels among healthy adults were determined to have no association with RMR (Jorgensen et al., 1998).

The metabolic rate of women fluctuates with the menstrual cycle. Some studies show that during the luteal phase (i.e., the time period between ovulation and the onset of menstruation) metabolic rate increases slightly (Institute of Medicine, 2005). During pregnancy, growth in uterine,

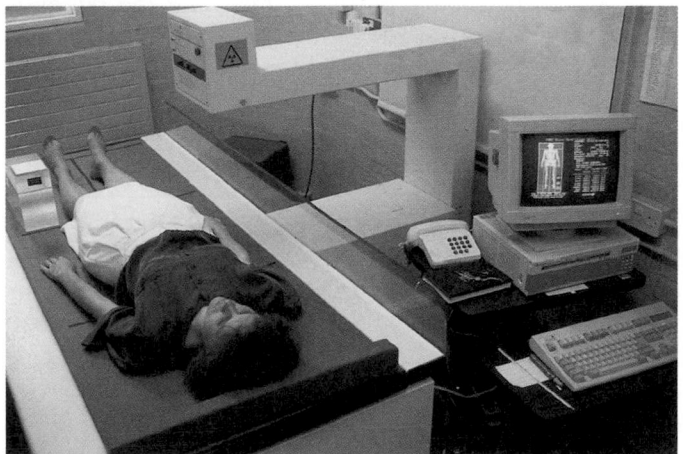

FIGURE 2-4 Dual-energy x-ray absorptiometry (DXA) is a scanning technique that accurately estimates bone mineral, fat, and fat-free soft tissue. Radiation exposure for a whole-body analysis is minimal, being approximately equivalent to the x-ray associated with a dental x-ray. *(Courtesy The Dunn Nutrition Centre, University of Cambridge, Cambridge, England.)*

placental, and fetal tissues along with the mother's increased cardiac workload contributes to gradual increases in BMR. On average, BMR increases 11 calories per week during gestation (Butte et al., 2004).

Other Factors. Caffeine, nicotine, and alcohol use stimulate metabolic rate. Caffeine intakes of 200 to 350 mg in men and approximately 240 mg in women increased mean RMR by 7% to 11% and 8% to 15%, respectively (Compher et al., 2006). Nicotine use increased mean RMR by 3% to 4% among men and by 6% among women (Compher et al., 2006). Alcohol consumption among women increased mean RMR by 9% (Compher et al., 2006). Fevers increased the metabolic rate by about 7% for each degree of increase in body temperature above 98.6° F (13% for each degree above 37° C).

RMR is also affected by extremes in environmental temperature. People living in tropical climates usually have RMRs that are 5% to 20% higher than those living in temperate areas. Exercise in temperatures greater than 86° F also imposes a small additional metabolic load of about 5% from increased sweat gland activity. The extent to which energy metabolism increases in extremely cold environments depends on the insulation available from body fat and protective clothing.

Thermic Effect of Food

Definition

The **thermic effect of food (TEF)** is the increase in energy expenditure associated with the consumption of food. The TEF accounts for approximately 10% of TEE (Institute of Medicine, 2002; 2005). The TEF is also referred to as *diet-induced thermogenesis (DIT)*, *specific dynamic action (SDA)*, and the *specific effect of food (SEF)*. TEF can be separated into obligatory and facultative (or adaptive) subcomponents. **Obligatory thermogenesis** is the energy required to digest, absorb, and metabolize nutrients, including the synthesis and storage of protein, fat, and carbohydrates. Adaptive or **facultative thermogenesis** is the "excess" energy expended in addition to the obligatory thermogenesis and is thought to be attributable to the metabolic inefficiency of the system stimulated by sympathetic nervous activity.

Factors Affecting the Thermic Effect of Food

The TEF varies with the composition of the diet and is greater after consumption of carbohydrates and proteins than after fat. Fat is metabolized efficiently, with only 4% wastage, compared with 25% wastage when carbohydrate is converted to fat for storage. These factors are thought to contribute to the obesity-promoting characteristics of fat (Prentice, 1995). Women who follow a regular eating schedule have a higher TEF response than women who eat irregularly (Farshchi et al., 2004). The role of TEF in weight management is discussed in more detail in Chapter 21.

Spicy foods enhance and prolong the effect of the TEF. Meals with chili and mustard may increase the metabolic rate as much as 33% more than unspiced meals, and this effect may last for more than 3 hours (McCrory et al., 1994).

Activity Thermogenesis

Definition

Activity thermogenesis (AT) is the energy expended during sports or fitness exercise; the energy expended during activities of daily living is referred to as **nonexercise activity thermogenesis (NEAT)** (Levine and Kotz, 2005). The contribution of physical activity is the most variable component of TEE, which may be as low as 100 kilocalories (kcal)/day in sedentary people or as high as 3000 kcal/day in very active people. NEAT is the energy expended during activities of daily living such as the energy expended during the work day and that expended during leisure-type activities (e.g., shopping, fidgeting, and even gum chewing), which may account for vast differences in energy costs among people (Levine and Kotz, 2005).

Factors Affecting Activity Thermogenesis

AT varies considerably, depending on body size and the efficiency of individual habits of motion. The level of fitness also affects the energy expenditure of voluntary activity, probably because of variations in muscle mass.

AT tends to decrease with age, a trend that is associated with a decline in FFM and an increase in fat mass (Roubenoff et al., 2000). Most men generally have a greater skeletal muscle than women, which may account for higher AT (Janssen et al., 2000). **Excess postexercise oxygen consumption (EPOC)** affects energy expenditure. The duration (Bahr et al., 1987) and magnitude (Bahr et al., 1992) of physical activity have been shown to increase EPOC, resulting in an elevated metabolic rate even after exercise has ceased. Habitual exercise does not cause a significantly prolonged increase in metabolic rate per unit of active tissue, but it does cause an 8% to 14% higher metabolic rate in men who are moderately and highly active, respectively, because of their increased FFM (Horton and Geissler, 1994). These differences seem to be related to the person, not to the activity.

MEASUREMENT OF ENERGY EXPENDITURE

Units of Measurement

The standard unit for measuring energy is the **calorie,** which is the amount of heat energy required to raise the temperature of 1 ml of water at 15° C by 1° C. Because the amount of energy involved in the metabolism of food is fairly large, the **kilocalorie (kcal or Cal)** (1000 calories) is commonly used to measure it. A popular convention is to designate kilocalorie by *Calorie* (with a capital "C"). In this text, *kilocalorie* is abbreviated *kcal*.

The **joule (J)** measures energy in terms of mechanical work and is the amount of energy required to accelerate with a force of 1 Newton (N) for a distance of 1 m; this measurement is widely used in countries other than the United States. One kcal is equivalent to 4.184 kilojoules (kJ).

Measuring Human Energy Expenditure

Various methods are available to measure human energy expenditure. It is important to gain an understanding of the differences in these methods and how they can be applied in practical and research settings.

Direct Calorimetry

Direct calorimetry monitors the amount of heat produced by a person placed inside a structure large enough to permit moderate amounts of activity. These structures are referred to as *whole-room calorimeters*. Direct calorimetry provides a measure of energy expended in the form of heat but provides no information on the kind of fuel being oxidized. The method is also limited by the confined nature of the testing conditions. Hence the measurement of TEE using this method is not representative of a free-living (i.e., engaged in normal daily activities) individual in a normal environment because physical activity within the chamber is limited. Its high cost and complex engineering and the scarcity of appropriate facilities around the world also limit the use of this method.

Indirect Calorimetry

Indirect calorimetry estimates energy expenditure by determining the oxygen consumption and carbon dioxide production of the body over a given period. The equipment varies, but the person usually breathes into a mouthpiece or ventilated hood through which his or her expired gases are collected. Indirect calorimetry has the advantage of mobility and low equipment cost. The most widely used form of indirect calorimetry is the measurement of RMR through a respirator gas-exchange canopy (Figure 2-5). These ventilated hoods are useful for short- and long-term measurements. Although less advantageous in measuring AT, indirect calorimetry can be used to measure AT during various activities in a laboratory setting. Handheld indirect calorimeters are less cumbersome and typically more cost-effective to operate. The MedGem indirect calorimeter by HealtheTech is a handheld portable device that determines measured RMR.* Comparison studies among healthy people measuring RMR using the Deltatrac metabolic cart (Datex-Ohmeda, Inc.) and the MedGem handheld monitor (HealtheTech Inc, Golden, Col) found no significant differences (St-Onge et al., 2004; Stewart et al., 2005). In the clinical setting metabolic carts are often used at the hospital bedside to assess patients' energy requirements.

Food, caffeine, alcohol, and nicotine increase RMR and should be limited before indirect calorimetry measurements. Among healthy people a minimum of a 5-hour fast after meals and snacks is recommended. Caffeine should be avoided for at least 4 hours, and alcohol and smoking for at least 2 hours. Testing should occur no sooner than 2 hours after moderate exercise; following vigorous resistance exercise, a 14-hour time period is advised (Compher et al.,

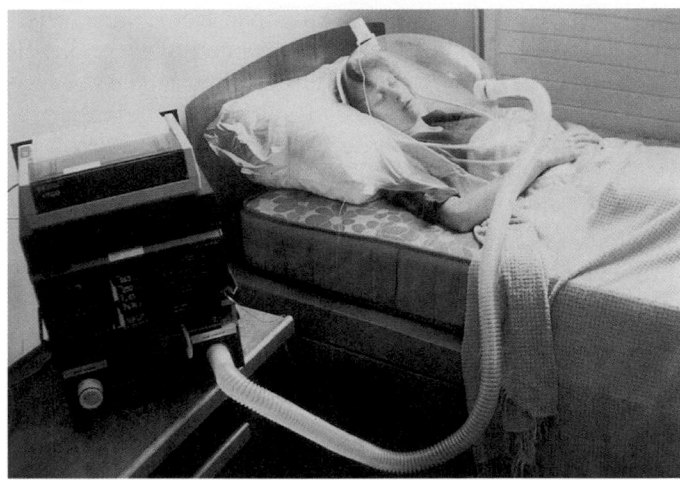

FIGURE 2-5 Measuring resting metabolic rate (RMR) using a ventilated hood system. *(Courtesy The Dunn Nutrition Centre, University of Cambridge, Cambridge, England.)*

2006). On the test day there should be a rest period of 10 to 20 minutes before measurements are taken. The accuracy of RMR can be determined after the first 5 minutes of testing have been completed.

Data are obtained from indirect calorimetry in a form that permits calculation of the **respiratory quotient (RQ):**

$$RQ = \text{Moles } CO_2 \text{ expired/Moles } O_2 \text{ consumed}$$

This determination is converted into kilocalories of heat produced per square meter of body surface per hour and is extrapolated to energy expenditure in 24 hours.

The RQ depends on the fuel mixture being metabolized. The RQ for carbohydrate is 1 because the number of carbon dioxide molecules produced is equal to the number of oxygen molecules consumed.

$$RQ = 1 \text{ for carbohydrate, } 0.85 \text{ for a mixed diet,}$$
$$0.82 \text{ for protein, and } 0.7 \text{ for fat}$$

Doubly Labeled Water

The **doubly labeled water (DLW)** technique for measuring TEE revolutionized the understanding of energy requirements and energy balance in humans. The method was first applied to humans in 1982, and since that time scientists developed a database that is used to develop recommendations for energy intake (Institute of Medicine, 2002; 2005). The DLW method is based on the principle that carbon dioxide production can be estimated from the difference in the elimination rates of body hydrogen and oxygen. After administering an oral loading dose of water labeled with deuterium oxide (^2H_2O) and oxygen-18 ($H_2^{18}O$)—hence the term *doubly labeled water*—the deuterium is eliminated from the body as water, and the oxygen-18 is eliminated as water and carbon dioxide. The elimination rates of the two isotopes are measured for 10 to 14 days by periodic sampling of body water from urine, saliva, or plasma. The difference between the two elimination rates is a measure of carbon dioxide production. Carbon dioxide production can then be

---

*RMR is calculated using the Weir equation. The Weir equation and a constant RQ value of 0.85 (RMR = $6.931 \times VO_2$) are used to convert VO_2 to RMR (Weir, 1949).

equated to TEE using standard indirect calorimetric techniques for the calculation of energy expenditure.

The DLW technique has numerous advantages, which make it the ideal method for measuring TEE in various populations (Friedman and Johnson, 2002). First, it provides a measure of energy expenditure that incorporates all the components of TEE, REE, TEF, and AT. The administration is easy, and the person is able to engage in typical activities of daily living throughout the measurement period. Therefore the technique provides a measure of the person's usual daily TEE, which is beneficial for those such as infants, young children, older adults, and disabled individuals, who cannot easily withstand the rigorous testing involved in the measurement of oxygen consumption during various activities. DLW also provides a method by which more subjective estimates of energy intakes (e.g., diet recalls and records) and energy expenditure (e.g., physical activity logs) can be validated (Schoeller, 1990). Most important, the method is accurate and has a precision of 2% to 8% (Schoeller, 1988).

However, the DLW technique also has drawbacks (i.e., the expense of the stable isotopes and the expertise required to operate the highly sophisticated and costly mass spectrometer for the analysis of the isotope enrichments). These disadvantages make the DLW technique impractical for daily use by clinicians. However, DLW research studies have provided the data used to develop prediction equations to estimate total energy requirements (Institute of Medicine, 2002; 2005). These equations should be used only as a guide or starting point, after which the person must be monitored closely, and interventions developed to promote optimal nutrition status.

Thermic Effect of Food

Actual measurement of the TEF is appropriate only for research purposes. For practical purposes it is calculated as 10% of the sum of the RMR and the AT. The TEF is the energy expended in excess of BMR after a meal. Thus to measure the TEF it is necessary to determine a baseline BMR and the energy expended in excess of BMR every 30 minutes for at least 5 hours after a meal.

Activity-Related Energy Expenditure

Doubly Labeled Water

The caloric value of AT can be estimated using the DLW method in conjunction with indirect calorimetry. After the postprandial RMR (which includes a measure of the TEF) has been measured using indirect calorimetry, an estimated AT can be determined by subtracting the postprandial RMR from the TEE that was measured using DLW (Goran et al., 1995). This method is generally only used in research settings but can be used to validate other, more practical and easily administered methods of measuring physical activity.

Caltrac Monitor

Uniaxial monitors measure the degree and intensity of movement in a vertical plane. Resembling a pager worn on the hip, the uniaxial monitor is a portable device designed for children

and adults to use to estimate activity-related energy expenditure. The accuracy of the Caltrac accelerometer (Muscle Dynamic Fitness Network, Torrance, Calif) was found to be effective in measuring activity-related energy expenditure among school-age children within a supervised setting (Sallis et al., 1989). However, the Caltrac was not useful in assessing activity-related energy expenditure in free-living children (Johnson et al., 1998). Among adults the Caltrac accelerometer was found to be an effective tool for measuring energy expenditure when compared with the DLW technique (Gretebeck et al., 1991, 1992). It may be acceptable for estimates of activity-related energy expenditure in groups of people, but it has limited use with individuals.

Tracmor Monitor

Because human movement is multidirectional, studies that measure movements on three different planes may be superior to those relying on one-plane measurements. A triaxial accelerometer monitor has three uniaxial accelerometers. The Tracmor (Philips Research, Eindhoven, The Netherlands) is a triaxial monitor with a data unit. Determined by DLW, the measurement of activity-related energy expenditure was found to be more accurate using the triaxial monitors than the uniaxial monitors (Bouten et al., 1996).

Heart Rate Monitor

A heart rate monitor is a simple-to-use and inexpensive device that estimates energy expenditure. In the past the validity of the equipment for monitoring sedentary intervals was questionable because of the uncertain relationship between heart rate and oxygen consumption. However, the use of a minute-by-minute heart rate monitor has been found to be a reliable method for estimating habitual TEE and physical activity level in groups of free-living, healthy children but not for individuals (Livingstone et al., 1992).

Physical Activity Questionnaire

Physical activity questionnaires are easily used, inexpensive tools for gaining information about a person's activity level (Winters-Hart et al., 2004; Philippaerts et al., 1999). DLW allows researchers to determine the validity of questionnaires. The Seven-Day Recall and the Yale Physical Activity Survey are two questionnaires that have been shown to be valid (Bonnefoy et al., 2001). The Baecke questionnaire and an adapted version of the Tecumseh Community Health Study questionnaire have been shown to be useful for determining whether a group or an individual is active or inactive (Philippaerts et al., 1999).

ESTIMATING ENERGY REQUIREMENTS

Knowledge of energy requirements throughout the life cycle to meet various physiologic conditions such as pregnancy and lactation and for those with various diseases is essential for the promotion of optimal health. In the past the measurement of energy *intake* served as an important tool from which recommendations for energy requirements for all age-groups were derived (World Health Organization [WHO], 1985). However, since the advent of the DLW technique, scientists have established energy requirements based on the actual measurement of TEE in free-living individuals.

Measuring Energy Intake

Traditionally recommendations for energy requirements were based on self-recorded estimates (e.g., diet records) or self-reported estimates (e.g., 24-hour recalls) of food intake. However, it is now well accepted that these methods do not provide accurate or unbiased estimates of a person's energy intake and that underestimation of food intake is pervasive (Johnson, 2000). The percentage of people who underestimate or underreport their food intake ranges from 10% to 45%, depending on the person's age, sex, and body composition. Underestimating tends to increase as children age, is worse among women than men, and is more prevalent and severe among the obese in comparison with the lean (Johnson, 2000) (see Chapter 14). This conclusion is confirmed by studies using the DLW technique, which measures TEE to assess the accuracy of estimates of energy intake (Schoeller, 1990).

Determining who is likely to underestimate energy intake is important. It is also necessary to identify the foods and food groups that are frequently underreported such as beer, chips, popcorn, pizza, pretzels, cookies and brownies, pancakes and waffles, cakes and pies, frozen dairy desserts, ready-to-eat cereals (and milk on cereal), meat mixtures, and condiments. Diet soft drinks are more likely to be recorded than nondiet (Krebs-Smith et al., 2000).

Until methods of determining energy intake are developed that minimize the problem of underreporting, it is no longer acceptable to base recommendations for energy requirements on estimates of energy intake (Black and Cole, 2000; Johnson, 2002; Livingstone, 1995). The World Health Organization (WHO, 1985) stated that "as a matter of principle, we believe the estimates of energy requirements should, as far as possible, be based on estimates of energy expenditure."

Estimations for Basal and Resting Metabolic Rate

Over the years several equations have been developed to measure the RMR. The Harris-Benedict equations, developed in 1919, are some of the most widely used equations in the United States (Harris and Benedict, 1919). The Harris-Benedict formulas have been found to overestimate REE by 7% to 24% (Daly et al., 1985; Owen et al., 1986; 1987). Newer BEE predictive equations have been formulated (Henry, 2000; Schofield, 1985).

Estimations of Energy Expenditure

The National Academy of Sciences, Institute of Medicine, and Food and Nutrition Board in partnership with Health Canada, developed the estimated energy requirements for men, women, children, and infants and for pregnant and lactating women (Institute of Medicine, 2002; 2005). The **estimated energy requirement (EER)** is the average dietary energy intake that is predicted to maintain energy balance in a healthy adult of a defined age, gender, weight, height, and level of physical activity consistent with good health. In children and pregnant and lactating women, the EER is taken to include the energy needs associated with the deposition of tissues or the secretion of milk at rates consistent with good health. Table 2-1 lists average dietary reference intake values for energy in healthy, active people of reference height, weight, and age for each life-

---

TABLE 2-1

Dietary Reference Intake Values for Energy for Active Individuals*

Life-Stage Group	Criterion	Active PAL EER (kcal/day) Male	Female
Infants			
0-6 mo	Energy expenditure + Energy deposition	570	520 (3 mo)
7-12 mo	Energy expenditure + Energy deposition	743	676 (9 mo)
Children			
1-2 yr	Energy expenditure + Energy deposition	1046	992 (24 mo)
3-8 yr	Energy expenditure + Energy deposition	1742	1642 (6 yr)
9-13 yr	Energy expenditure + Energy deposition	2279	2071 (11 yr)
14-18 yr	Energy expenditure + Energy deposition	3152	2368 (16 yr)

From Institute of Medicine of The National Academies: *Dietary reference intakes for energy, carbohydrate, fiber, fat, fatty acids, cholesterol, protein, and amino acids,* Washington, DC, 2002/2005, The National Academies Press.

EER, Estimated energy requirement; *PAL*, physical activity level; *TEE*, total energy expenditure.

*For healthy active Americans and Canadians at the reference height and weight.

†Subtract 10 kcal/day for men and 7 kcal/day for women for each year of age above 19 years.

Continued

TABLE 2-1

Dietary Reference Intake Values for Energy for Active Individuals*—cont'd

Life-Stage Group	Criterion	Active PAL EER (kcal/day)	
		Male	**Female**
Adults			
>18 yr	Energy expenditure	3067[†]	2403[†] (19 yr)
Pregnant Women			
14-18 yr	Adolescent female EER + Change in TEE + Pregnancy energy deposition		
First trimester			2368 (16 yr)
Second trimester			2708 (16 yr)
Third trimester			2820 (16 yr)
19-50 yr	Adult female EER + Change in TEE + Pregnancy energy deposition		
First trimester			2403[†] (19 yr)
Second trimester			2743[†] (19 yr)
Third trimester			2855[†] (19 yr)
Lactating Women			
14-18 yr	Adolescent female EER + Milk energy output −Weight loss		
First 6 mo			2698 (16 yr)
Second 6 mo			2768 (16 yr)
19-50 yr	Adult female EER + Milk energy output −Weight loss		
First 6 mo			2733[†] (19 yr)
Second 6 mo			2803[†] (19 yr)

From Institute of Medicine of The National Academies: *Dietary reference intakes for energy, carbohydrate, fiber, fat, fatty acids, cholesterol, protein, and amino acids,* Washington, DC, 2002/2005, The National Academies Press.

EER, Estimated energy requirement; *PAL,* physical activity level; *TEE,* total energy expenditure.

*For healthy active Americans and Canadians at the reference height and weight.

[†]Subtract 10 kcal/day for men and 7 kcal/day for women for each year of age above 19 years.

stage group (Institute of Medicine, 2002; 2005). Supported by DLW studies, prediction equations have been developed to estimate energy requirements for people according to their life-stage group. Box 2-1 lists the EER prediction equations for people of normal weight. TEE prediction equations are also listed for various overweight and obese groups, as well as for weight maintenance in obese girls and boys. All equations have been developed to maintain current body weight (and promote growth when appropriate) and current levels of physical activity for all subsets of the population; they are not intended to promote weight loss (Institute of Medicine, 2002; 2005).

The EER incorporates age, weight, height, gender, and level of physical activity for people ages 3 years and older. Although variables such as age, gender, and feeding type (i.e., breast milk, formula) can impact TEE among infants and young children, weight has been determined as the sole predictor of TEE needs (Institute of Medicine, 2002; 2005). Beyond TEE requirements, additional calories to support the deposition of tissues needed for growth are required for infants and young children, children ages 3 through 18, and pregnant and lactating females; thus the EER among these subsets of the population is the sum of TEE plus the caloric requirements for energy deposition. The prediction equations include a physical activity (PA) coefficient for all groups except infants and young children (see Box 2-1). PA coefficients correspond to four **physical activity levels (PAL)** lifestyle categories: *sedentary, low active, active, and very active.* Because PAL is the ratio of TEE to BEE, the energy spent during activities of daily living, the *sedentary* lifestyle category has a PAL range of 1 to 1.39. PAL categories beyond *sedentary* are determined according to the energy spent by an adult walking at a set pace. The walking equivalents that correspond to each PAL category (i.e., *low-active, active,* and *very active*) for an average-weight adult walking at 3 to 4 mph are 2, 7, and 17 miles per day, respectively (Institute of Medicine, 2002; 2005).

BOX 2-1

Estimated Energy Expenditure* Prediction Equations at Four Physical Activity Levels†

EER for Infants and Young Children 0-2 Years (Within the 3rd-97th Percentile for Weight-for-Height)

EER = TEE‡ + Energy deposition

0-3 months	(89 × Weight of infant [kg] − 100) + 175 (kcal for energy deposition)
4-6 months	(89 × Weight of infant [kg] − 100) + 56 (kcal for energy deposition)
7-12 months	(89 × Weight of infant [kg] − 100) + 22 (kcal for energy deposition)
13-35 months	(89 × Weight of child [kg] − 100) + 20 (kcal for energy deposition)

EER for Boys 3-8 Years (Within the 5th-85th Percentile for BMI§)

EER = TEE + Energy deposition

EER = 88.5 − 61.9 × Age (yr) + PA × (26.7 × Weight [kg] + 903 × Height [m]) + 20 (kcal for energy deposition)

EER for Boys 9-18 Years (Within the 5th-85th Percentile for BMI)

EER = TEE + Energy deposition

EER = 88.5 − 61.9 × Age (yr) + PA × (26.7 × Weight [kg] + 903 × Height [m]) + 25 (kcal for energy deposition)

where

PA = Physical activity coefficient for boys 3-18 years:

PA = 1.0 if PAL is estimated to be ≥ 1.0 < 1.4 (Sedentary)

PA = 1.13 if PAL is estimated to be ≥ 1.4 < 1.6 (Low active)

PA = 1.26 if PAL is estimated to be ≥ 1.6 < 1.9 (Active)

PA = 1.42 if PAL is estimated to be ≥ 1.9 < 2.5 (Very active)

EER for Girls 3-8 Years (Within the 5th-85th Percentile for BMI)

EER = TEE + Energy deposition

EER = 135.3 − 30.8 × Age (yr) + PA × (10 × Weight [kg] + 934 × Height [m]) + 20 (kcal for energy deposition)

EER for Girls 9-18 Years (Within the 5th-85th Percentile for BMI)

EER = TEE + Energy deposition

EER = 135.3 − 30.8 × Age (yr) + PA × (10 × Weight [kg] + 934 × Height [m]) + 25 (kcal for energy deposition)

where

PA = Physical activity coefficient for girls 3-18 years:

PA = 1.0 if PAL is estimated to be ≥ 1.0 < 1.4 (Sedentary)

PA = 1.16 if PAL is estimated to be ≥ 1.4 < 1.6 (Low active)

PA = 1.31 if PAL is estimated to be ≥ 1.6 < 1.9 (Active)

PA = 1.56 if PAL is estimated to be ≥ 1.9 < 2.5 (Very active)

EER for Men 19 Years and Older (BMI 18.5-25 kg/m²)

EER = TEE

EER = 662 − 9.53 × Age (yr) + PA × (15.91 × Weight [kg] + 539.6 × Height [m])

where

PA = Physical activity coefficient:

PA = 1.0 if PAL is estimated to be ≥ 1.0 < 1.4 (Sedentary)

PA = 1.11 if PAL is estimated to be ≥ 1.4 < 1.6 (Low active)

PA = 1.25 if PAL is estimated to be ≥ 1.6 < 1.9 (Active)

PA = 1.48 if PAL is estimated to be ≥ 1.9 < 2.5 (Very active)

From Institute of Medicine, Food and Nutrition Board: *Dietary reference intakes for energy, carbohydrate, fiber, fat, fatty acids, cholesterol, protein, and amino acids,* Washington, DC, 2002, The National Academies Press, www.nap.edu.

*Estimated energy expenditure (EER) is the average dietary energy intake that is predicted to maintain energy balance in a healthy adult of a defined age, gender, weight, height, and level of physical activity consistent with good health. In children and pregnant and lactating women, the EER includes the needs associated with the deposition of tissues or the secretion of milk at rates consistent with good health.

†Physical activity level (PAL) is the physical activity level that is the ratio of the total energy expenditure to the basal energy expenditure.

‡Total energy expenditure (TEE) is the sum of the resting energy expenditure, energy expended in physical activity, and the thermic effect of food.

§Body mass index (BMI) is determined by dividing the weight (in kilograms) by the square of the height (in meters).

Continued

BOX 2-1

Estimated Energy Expenditure* Prediction Equations
at Four Physical Activity Levels†—cont'd

EER for Women 19 Years and Older (BMI 18.5-25 kg/m²)

EER = TEE

EER = $354 - 6.91 \times$ Age (yr) + PA $\times$ ($9.36 \times$ Weight [kg] + $726 \times$ Height [m])

where

  PA = Physical activity coefficient:

  PA = 1.0 if PAL is estimated to be $\geq 1.0 < 1.4$ (Sedentary)

  PA = 1.12 if PAL is estimated to be $\geq 1.4 < 1.6$ (Low active)

  PA = 1.27 if PAL is estimated to be $\geq 1.6 < 1.9$ (Active)

  PA = 1.45 if PAL is estimated to be $\geq 1.9 < 2.5$ (Very active)

EER for Pregnant Women

14-18 years: EER = Adolescent EER + Pregnancy energy deposition

First trimester = Adolescent EER + 0 (Pregnancy energy deposition)

Second trimester = Adolescent EER + 160 kcal (8 kcal/wk 1 $\times$ 20 wk) + 180 kcal

Third trimester = Adolescent EER + 272 kcal (8 kcal/wk $\times$ 34 wk) + 180 kcal

19-50 years: EER = Adult EER + Pregnancy energy deposition

First trimester = Adult EER + 0 (Pregnancy energy deposition)

Second trimester = Adult EER + 160 kcal (8 kcal/wk $\times$ 20 wk) + 180 kcal

Third trimester = Adult EER + 272 kcal (8 kcal/wk $\times$ 34 wk) + 180 kcal

EER for Lactating Women

14-18 years: EER = Adolescent EER + Milk energy output − Weight loss

First 6 months = EER + 500 − 170 (Milk energy output − Weight loss)

Second 6 months = Adolescent EER+ 400 − 0 (Milk energy output − Weight loss)

19-50 years: EAR = Adult EER + Milk energy output − Weight loss

First 6 months = Adult EER + 500 − 170 (Milk energy output − Weight loss)

Second 6 months = Adult EER + 400 − 0 (Milk energy output − Weight loss)

Weight Maintenance TEE for Overweight and At-Risk for Overweight Boys 3-18 Years (BMI >85th Percentile for Overweight)

TEE = $114 - 50.9 \times$ Age (yr) + PA $\times$ ($19.5 \times$ Weight [kg] + $1161.4 \times$ Height [m])

where

  PA = Physical activity coefficient:

  PA = 1.0 if PAL is estimated to be $\geq 1.0 < 1.4$ (Sedentary)

  PA = 1.12 if PAL is estimated to be $\geq 1.4 < 1.6$ (Low active)

  PA = 1.24 if PAL is estimated to be $\geq 1.6 < 1.9$ (Active)

  PA = 1.45 if PAL is estimated to be $\geq 1.9 < 2.5$ (Very active)

Weight Maintenance TEE for Overweight and At-Risk for Overweight Girls 3-18 years (BMI >85th Percentile for Overweight)

TEE = $389 - 41.2 \times$ Age (yr) + PA $\times$ ($15 \times$ Weight [kg] + $701.6 \times$ Height [m])

where

  PA = Physical activity coefficient:

  PA = 1.0 if PAL is estimated to be $\geq 1.0 < 1.4$ (Sedentary)

  PA = 1.18 if PAL is estimated to be $\geq 1.4 < 1.6$ (Low active)

  PA = 1.35 if PAL is estimated to be $\geq 1.6 < 1.9$ (Active)

  PA = 1.60 if PAL is estimated to be $\geq 1.9 < 2.5$ (Very active)

BOX 2-1

Estimated Energy Expenditure* Prediction Equations at Four Physical Activity Levels†—cont'd

Overweight and Obese Men 19 Years and Older (BMI ≥25 kg/m²)

TEE = 1086 − 10.1 × Age (yr) + PA × (13.7 × Weight [kg] + 416 × Height [m])
where
PA = Physical activity coefficient:
PA = 1.0 if PAL is estimated to be ≥ 1.0 < 1.4 (Sedentary)
PA = 1.12 if PAL is estimated to be ≥ 1.4 < 1.6 (Low active)
PA = 1.29 if PAL is estimated to be ≥ 1.6 < 1.9 (Active)
PA = 1.59 if PAL is estimated to be ≥ 1.9 < 2.5 (Very active)

Overweight and Obese Women 19 Years and Older (BMI ≥25 kg/m²)

TEE = 448 − 7.95 × Age (yr) + PA × (11.4 × Weight [kg] + 619 × Height [m])
where
PA = Physical activity coefficient:
PA = 1.0 if PAL is estimated to be ≥ 1.0 < 1.4 (Sedentary)
PA = 1.16 if PAL is estimated to be ≥ 1.4 < 1.6 (Low active)
PA = 1.27 if PAL is estimated to be ≥ 1.6 < 1.9 (Active)
PA = 1.44 if PAL is estimated to be ≥ 1.9 < 2.5 (Very active)

Normal and Overweight or Obese Men 19 Years and Older (BMI ≥18.5 kg/m²)

TEE = 864 − 9.72 × Age (yr) + PA × (14.2 × Weight [kg] + 503 × Height [m])
where
PA = Physical activity coefficient:
PA = 1.0 if PAL is estimated to be ≥ 1.0 > 1.4 (Sedentary)
PA = 1.12 if PAL is estimated to be ≥ 1.4 > 1.6 (Low active)
PA = 1.27 if PAL is estimated to be ≥ 1.6 > 1.9 (Active)
PA = 1.54 if PAL is estimated to be ≥ 1.9 > 2.5 (Very active)

Normal and Overweight or Obese Women 19 years and Older (BMI ≥18.5 kg/m²)

TEE = 387 − 7.31 × Age (yr) + PA × (10.9 × Weight [kg] + 660.7 × Height [m])
where
PA = Physical activity coefficient:
PA = 1.0 if PAL is estimated to be ≥ 1.0 < 1.4 (Sedentary)
PA = 1.14 if PAL is estimated to be ≥ 1.4 < 1.6 (Low active)
PA = 1.27 if PAL is estimated to be ≥ 1.6 < 1.9 (Active)
PA = 1.45 if PAL is estimated to be ≥ 1.9 < 2.5 (Very active)

From Institute of Medicine, Food and Nutrition Board: *Dietary reference intakes for energy, carbohydrate, fiber, fat, fatty acids, cholesterol, protein, and amino acids,* Washington, DC, 2002, The National Academies Press, www.nap.edu.

*Estimated energy expenditure (EER) is the average dietary energy intake that is predicted to maintain energy balance in a healthy adult of a defined age, gender, weight, height, and level of physical activity consistent with good health. In children and pregnant and lactating women, the EER includes the needs associated with the deposition of tissues or the secretion of milk at rates consistent with good health.

†Physical activity level (PAL) is the physical activity level that is the ratio of the total energy expenditure to the basal energy expenditure.

‡Total energy expenditure (TEE) is the sum of the resting energy expenditure, energy expended in physical activity, and the thermic effect of food.

§Body mass index (BMI) is determined by dividing the weight (in kilograms) by the square of the height (in meters).

Estimated Energy Expended in Physical Activity

Energy expenditure in physical activity can be estimated using two methods: (1) the method shown in Appendix 28, which represents energy spent during common activities and incorporates body weight and the duration of time for each activity as variables, and (2) using information in Table 2-2, which represents energy spent by adults during various *intensities* of physical activity—energy that is expressed as metabolic equivalents (Institute of Medicine, 2002; 2005).

Estimating Energy Expenditure of Selected Activities Using Metabolic Equivalents (METs)

Energy expenditure is determined by the amount of oxygen metabolized by the body. **Metabolic equivalents (METs)** are units of measure that correspond to a person's

TABLE 2-2

Intensity and Impact of Various Activities on Physical Activity Level in Adults*

Physical Activity	METs[†]	Δ PAL/10 min[‡]	Δ PAL/hr[‡]
Daily Activities			
Lying quietly	1	0	0
Riding in a car	1	0	0
Light activity while sitting	1.5	0.005	0.03
Watering plants	2.5	0.014	0.09
Walking the dog	3	0.019	0.11
Vacuuming	3.5	0.024	0.14
Doing household tasks (moderate effort)	3.5	0.024	0.14
Gardening (no lifting)	4.4	0.032	0.19
Mowing lawn (power mower)	4.5	0.033	0.20
Leisure Activities: Mild			
Walking (2 mph)	2.5	0.014	0.09
Canoeing (leisurely)	2.5	0.014	0.09
Golfing (with cart)	2.5	0.014	0.09
Dancing (ballroom)	2.9	0.018	0.11
Leisure Activities: Moderate			
Walking (3 mph)	3.3	0.022	0.13
Cycling (leisurely)	3.5	0.024	0.14
Performing calisthenics (no weight)	4	0.029	0.17
Walking (4 mph)	4.5	0.033	0.20
Leisure Activities: Vigorous			
Chopping wood	4.9	0.037	0.22
Playing tennis (doubles)	5	0.038	0.23
Ice skating	5.5	0.043	0.26
Cycling (moderate)	5.7	0.045	0.27
Skiing (downhill or water)	6.8	0.055	0.33
Swimming	7	0.057	0.34
Climbing hills (5-kg load)	7.4	0.061	0.37
Walking (5 mph)	8	0.067	0.40
Jogging (10-minute mile)	10.2	0.088	0.53
Skipping rope	12	0.105	0.63

Modified from Institute of Medicine of The National Academies: *Dietary reference intakes for energy, carbohydrate, fiber, fat, fatty acids, protein, and amino acids,* Washington, DC, 2002, The National Academies Press.

*Physical activity level (PAL) is the physical activity level that is the ratio of the total energy expenditure (TEE) to the basal energy expenditure (BEE).

[†]*METs,* Metabolic equivalents. METs are multiples of an individual's resting oxygen uptakes, defined as the rate of oxygen (O_2) consumption of 3.5 ml of O_2/min/kg body weight in adults.

[‡]The Δ PAL is the allowance made to include the delayed effect of physical activity in causing excess postexercise oxygen consumption (EPOC) and the dissipation of some of the food energy consumed through the thermic effect of food (TEF).

metabolic rate during selected physical activities of varying intensities and are expressed as multiples of RMR (see Table 2-2) (Institute of Medicine, 2002; 2005). A MET value of 1 is the oxygen metabolized at rest (3.5 ml of oxygen per kilogram of body weight per minute in adults) and can be expressed as 1 kcal per kilogram of body weight per hour (Ainsworth et al., 1993). Thus the energy expenditure of adults can be estimated using MET values (1 MET = 1 kcal/kg/hour). For example, an adult who weighs 65 kg and is walking moderately at a pace of 4 mph (which is a MET value of 4.5) for 1 hour would expend 293 calories (4.5 kcal × 65 kg × 1 = 293).

To estimate a person's energy requirements using the Institute of Medicine EER equations, it is necessary to

TABLE 2-3

Physical Activity Level Categories and Walking Equivalence

PAL Category	PAL Values	Walking Equivalence (miles/day at 3-4 mph)
Sedentary	1-1.39	
Low active	1.4-1.59	1.5, 2.2, 2.9 for PAL = 1.5
Active	1.6-1.89	3, 4.4, 5.8 for PAL = 1.6
		5.3, 7.3, 9.9 for PAL = 1.75
Very active	1.9-2.5	7.5, 10.3, 14 for PAL = 1.9
		12.3, 16.7, 22.5 for PAL = 2.2
		17, 23, 31 for PAL = 2.5

From Institute of Medicine, The National Academies: Dietary reference intakes for energy, carbohydrate, fiber, fat, fatty acids, cholesterol, protein, and amino acids, Washington, DC, 2002/2005, The National Academies Press.

PAL, Physical activity level.

*In addition to energy spent for the generally unscheduled activities that are part of a normal daily life. The low, middle, and high miles/day values apply to relatively heavyweight (120-kg), midweight (70-kg), and lightweight (44-kg) individuals, respectively.

identify a PAL value for that person. A person's PAL value can be *affected* by various activities performed throughout the day and is referred to as the *change in physical activity level* (Δ PAL). To determine (Δ PAL), take the sum of the Δ PALs for each activity performed for 1 day from Table 2-2 (Institute of Medicine, 2002; 2005). To calculate the PAL value for 1 day, take the sum of activities and add the BEE (1) plus 10% to account for the TEF (1 + 0.1 = 1.1). For example, take the sum of the Δ PAL values for activities of daily living such as walking the dog (0.11) and vacuuming (0.14) for 1 hour each, sitting for 4 hours doing light activity (0.12), and then performing moderate to vigorous activities such as walking for 1 hour at 4 mph (0.20) and ice skating for 30 minutes (0.13) for a total of (0.7). To that value include the BEE adjusted for the 10% TEF (1.1) for the final calculation (0.7 + 1.1 = 1.8). To calculate the EER for an adult woman, use the EER equation for women 19 years and older (BMI 18.5-25 kg/m²) (see Box 2-1) (Institute of Medicine, 2002; 2005). For this woman the PAL value (1.8) falls within an *active* range. The *PA coefficient* (PA) that correlates with an *active* lifestyle for this woman is 1.27. The following equation estimates the EER for this 30-year-old active woman who weighs 65 kg, is 1.77 m tall, with a PA coefficient (1.27).

$$EER = 354 - 6.91 \times Age \text{ (yr)} + PA \times$$
$$(9.36 \times Weight \text{ [kg]} + 726 \times Height \text{ [m]})$$

$$EER = 354 - (6.91 \times 30) +$$
$$1.27 \times ([9.36 \times 65] + [726 \times 1.77])$$

$$EER = 2551 \text{ kcal}$$

Physical Activity in Children

Energy spent during various activities and the intensity and impact of selected activities can also be determined for children and teens (see Box 2-1) (Institute of Medicine, 2002; 2005).

CALCULATING FOOD ENERGY

The total energy available from a food is measured with a bomb calorimeter. This device consists of a closed container in which a weighed food sample, ignited with an electric spark, is burned in an oxygenated atmosphere. The container is immersed in a known volume of water, and the rise in the temperature of the water after igniting the food is used to calculate the heat energy generated.

Not all of the energy in foods and alcohol is available to the body's cells. The processes of digestion and absorption are not completely efficient, and the nitrogenous portion of amino acids is not oxidized but is excreted in the form of urea. Therefore the biologically available energy from foods and alcohol is expressed in values rounded off slightly below those obtained using the calorimeter. These values for protein, fat, carbohydrate, and alcohol (Figure 2-6) are 4, 9, 4, and 7 kcal/g, respectively. The figure of 2 kcal/g has been proposed for fiber because of the "unavailable carbohydrate" that resists digestion and absorption (Guenther and Jensen, 2000).

Although the energy value of each nutrient is known precisely, only a few foods such as oils and sugars are made up of a single nutrient. More commonly, foods contain a mixture of protein, fat, and carbohydrate. For example, the energy value of one medium-size (50-g) egg calculated in terms of weight is derived from protein (13%), fat (12%), and carbohydrate (1%) as follows:

Protein: 13 % × 50g = 6.5g × 4 kcal/g = 26 kcal

Fat: 12% × 50g = 6g × 9 kcal/g = 54 kcal

Carbohydrate: 1% × 50g = 0.05g × 4 kcal/g = 2 kcal

Total = 82 kcal

Energy values of foods based on chemical analyses may be obtained from the U.S. Department of Agriculture (USDA) Nutrient Data Laboratory website: http://www.nal.usda.gov/fnic/foodcomp. Another source of nutrient values for common serving sizes of foods is Bowes and Church's *Food Values of Portions Commonly Used* (Pennington and Douglass, 2004). Many computer software programs that use the USDA nutrient database as the standard reference are also available. In addition, the diet analysis program of the Department of Nutrition and Food Sciences at the University of Vermont is available at the website: http://nutrition.uvm.edu/htm/fs_inter.htm.

Kilocalories in alcoholic beverages may be calculated as shown in the *Clinical Insight* box: Calculation of Energy Value of Alcoholic Beverages and Mixes; see also Appendix 44.

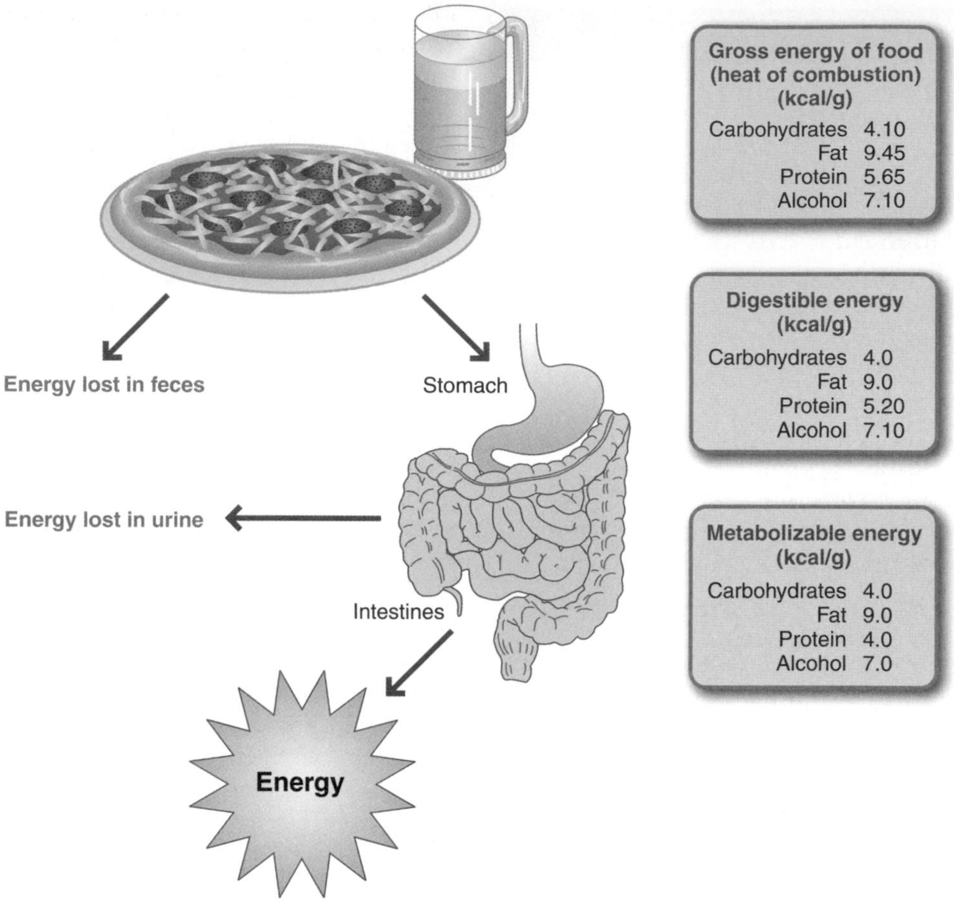
Gross energy of food
(heat of combustion)
(kcal/g)
Carbohydrates 4.10
Fat 9.45
Protein 5.65
Alcohol 7.10
Digestible energy
(kcal/g)
Carbohydrates 4.0
Fat 9.0
Protein 5.20
Alcohol 7.10
Metabolizable energy
(kcal/g)
Carbohydrates 4.0
Fat 9.0
Protein 4.0
Alcohol 7.0
Energy lost in feces
Stomach
Energy lost in urine
Intestines
Energy

FIGURE 2-6 Energy value of food.

CLINICAL INSIGHT

Calculation of Energy Value of Alcoholic Beverages and Mixes

The energy value of alcoholic beverages, which is expressed in kilocalories, can be determined by the following equation (Gastineau, 1976):

Kilocalories = Amount of beverage (oz) × Proof × 0.8kcal/proof/1 oz

where

Proof = The proportion of alcohol to water or other liquids in an alcoholic beverage. (The standard in the United States defines 100-proof as being equal to 50% of ethyl alcohol by volume.)

To determine the percentage of ethyl alcohol in a beverage, divide the proof value by 2. For example, 86-proof whiskey contains 43% ethyl alcohol.

The latter part of the equation—0.8 kcal/proof/1 oz—is the factor that accounts for the caloric density of alcohol (7 kcal/g) and the fact that not all of the alcohol in liquor is available for energy. For example, the number of kilocalories in 1½ oz of 86-proof whiskey would be determined as follows:

1½ oz × 86-proof × 0.8 kcal/proof/1 oz = 103 kcal

See Appendix 38.

FOCAL POINTS

- Metabolic rate in the human body is affected by several variables, including daily TEE, 60% to 70% of which is the BEE.
- The energy cost of physical activity is the most variable of factors related to an individual's TEE, and can be altered by the individual.
- Physical activity has the most impact on a person's energy balance, usually due to the energy expended during activities of daily living.
- Estimates of energy expenditure (EER) at various levels of physical activity can be determined using the EER prediction equations; application of these prediction equations is a valuable tool for assessing energy needs.
- With the obesity epidemic facing many individuals, encouragement to expend energy through activity should be recommended.

USEFUL WEBSITES

American Dietetic Association
http://adaevidencelibrary.com

Centers for Disease Control
www.cdc.gov/needphp/dnpa

National Academy Press—Publisher of Institute of Medicine DRIs for Energy
www.nal.usda.gov/fnic/foodcomp/

National Institutes of Health—Bioelectrical Impedance Analysis
http://consensus.nih.gov/ta/015/015_statement.htm

U.S. Department of Agriculture Food Composition Tables
www.nal.usda.gov/fnic/foodcomp/www.nap.edu/books/0309085373/html/

University of Vermont Body Composition and Diet Analysis
http://nutrition.uvm.edu/bodycomp
http://nutrition.uvm.edu/htm/fs_inter.htm

References

Ainsworth BE et al: Compendium of physical activities: classification of energy costs of human physical activities, *Med Sci Sports Exerc* 25:71, 1993.

Bahr R et al: Effect of duration of exercise on excess postexercise O₂ consumption, *J Appl Physiol* 62:485, 1987.

Bahr R et al: Effect of supramaximal exercise on excess postexercise O₂ consumption, *Med Sci Sports Exerc* 24:66, 1992.

Black AE, Cole TJ: Within- and between-subject variation in energy expenditure measured by the doubly labeled water technique: implications for validating reported dietary energy intake, *Eur J Clin Nutr* 54:386, 2000.

Bonnefoy M et al: Simultaneous validation of ten physical activity questionnaires in older men: a doubly labeled water study, *J Am Gerontolical Society* 49:28, 2001.

Bosy-Westphal A et al: Effect of organ and tissue masses on resting energy expenditure in underweight, normal weight and obese adults, *Int J Obes Related Metabol Disord* 28(1):72, 2004.

Bouten C et al: Daily physical activity assessment: comparison between movement registration and doubly labeled water, *J Appl Physiol* 81:1019, 1996.

Butte NF et al: Energy requirements derived from total energy expenditure and energy deposition during the first 2 years of life, *Am J Clin Nutr* 72:1558, 2000.

Butte NF et al: Energy requirements during pregnancy based on total energy expenditure and energy deposition, *Am J Clin Nutr* 79(6):1078, 2004.

Callahan T: Personal communication, May 29, 2002.

Compher C et al: Best practice methods to apply to measurement of resting metabolic rate in adults: a systematic review, *J Am Diet Assoc* 106:881, 2006.

Daly JM et al: Human energy requirements: overestimation by widely used prediction equation, *Am J Clin Nutr* 42:1170, 1985.

Dirks AJ, Leeuwenburgh C: Caloric restriction in humans: potential pitfalls and health concerns, *Mech Aging Dev* 127:1, 2006.

Dolezal BA, Potteiger JA: Concurrent resistance and endurance training influence basal metabolic rate in nondieting individuals, *J Appl Physiol* 85(2):695, 1998.

Durnin JVGA: Energy requirements: general principles, *Eur J Clin Nutr* 50(suppl 1):2, 1996.

Farshchi HR et al: Decreased thermic effect of food after an irregular compared with a regular meal pattern in healthy lean women, *Int J Obes Relat Metabol Disord* 28:653, 2004.

Friedman A, Johnson RK: Doubly labeled water: new advances and applications for the practitioner, *Nutr Today* 27:243, 2002.

Gallagher D et al: Organ-tissue mass measurement allows modeling of REE and metabolically active tissue mass, *Am J Physiol Endocrinol Metabol* 275:E249, 1998.

Gastineau CF: Alcohol and calories, *Mayo Clin Proc* 51(2):88, 1976.

Goran MI et al: Energy requirements across the life span: new findings based on measurement of total energy expenditure with doubly labeled water, *Nutr Res* 15:115, 1995.

Gretebeck R et al: Comparison of the doubly labeled water method for measuring energy expenditure with Caltrac accelerometer recordings, *Med Sci Sports Exerc* 23 (suppl):60, 1991.

Gretebeck R et al: Assessment of energy expenditure in active older women using doubly labeled water and Caltrac recordings, *Med Sci Sports Exerc* 23(suppl):68, 1992.

Guenther PM, Jensen HH: Estimating energy contributed by fiber using a general factor of 2 vs. 4 kcal/g, *J Am Diet Assoc* 100:944, 2000.

Harris JA, Benedict FG: A biometric study of basal metabolism in man, Pub No. 279, Washington, DC, 1919, Carnegie Institute of Washington.

Heilbronn LK et al: Effect of 6-month calorie restriction on biomarkers of longevity, metabolic adaptation, and oxidative stress in overweight individuals: a randomized controlled trial, *JAMA* 295:1539, 2006.

Henry CJ: Mechanisms of changes in basal metabolism during aging, *Eur J Clin Nutr* 54(suppl 3):77, 2000.

Horton T, Geissler C: Effect of habitual exercise on daily energy expenditure and metabolic rate during standardized activity, *Am J Clin Nutr* 59:13, 1994.

Hursting SD et al: Calorie restriction, aging, and cancer prevention: mechanisms of action and applicability to humans, *Ann Rev Med* 54:131, 2003.

Illner K et al: Metabolically active components of fat free mass and resting energy expenditure in nonobese adults, *Am J Physiol Endocrinol Metabol* 278(2):E308, 2000.

Institute of Medicine, Food and Nutrition Board: Dietary reference intakes: for energy, carbohydrate, fiber, fat, fatty acids, cholesterol, protein, and amino acids, Washington, DC, 2002/2005, The National Academies Press.

Janssen I et al: Skeletal muscle mass and distribution in 468 men and women aged 18-88 yr, *J Appl Physiol* 89(1):81, 2000.

Johnson RK: What are people really eating, and why does it matter? *Nutr Today* 35:40, 2000.

Johnson RK: Dietary intake—how do we measure what people are really eating? *Obes Res* 10(suppl 1):63, 2002.

Johnson RK et al: Physical activity related energy expenditure in children by doubly labeled water as compared with the Caltrac accelerometer, *Int J Obes Related Metabol Disord* 22:1046, 1998.

Jorgensen J et al: Resting metabolic rate in healthy adults: relation to growth hormone status and leptin levels, *Metabolism* 47:1134, 1998.

Keys A et al: Basal metabolism and age of adult man, *Metabolism* 22(4):579, 1973.

Krebs-Smith SM et al: Low energy reporters vs. others: a comparison of reported food intakes, *Eur J Clin Nutr* 54:281, 2000.

Levine JA, Kotz CM: NEAT—non-exercise activity thermogenesis—egocentric & geocentric environmental factors vs. biological regulation, *Acta Physiol Scand* 184(4):309, 2005.

Livingstone MBE: Assessment of food intake: are we measuring what people eat? *Br J Biomed Sci* 52:58, 1995.

Livingstone MBE et al: Daily energy expenditure in free-living children: comparison of heart-rate monitoring with the doubly labeled water method, *Am J Clin Nutr* 56:343, 1992.

Masoro EJ: Overview of caloric restriction and aging, *Mech Aging Dev* 126:913, 2005.

Masoro EJ: Caloric restriction and aging: controversial issues, *J Gerontol Series A: Biol Sci Med Sci* 61:14, 2006.

Mattison JA et al: Calorie restriction in rhesus monkeys, *Esp Gerontol* 38:35, 2003.

McCrory P et al: Energy balance, food intake and obesity. In Hills AP, Wahlqvist ML, editors: *Exercise and obesity*, London, 1994, Smith-Gordon.

Molnar D, Schutz Y: The effect of obesity, age, puberty and gender on resting metabolic rate in children and adolescents, *Eur J Pediatr* 156:376, 1997.

Owen OE et al: A reappraisal of caloric requirements in healthy women, *Am J Clin Nutr* 44:1, 1986.

Owen OE et al: A reappraisal of the caloric requirements of men, *Am J Clin Nutr* 46:875, 1987.

Pennington JA, Douglass JS: *Bowes and Church's food values of portions commonly used*, ed 18, Philadelphia, Lippincott Williams and Wilkins, 2004.

Philippaerts RM et al: Doubly labeled water validation of three physical activity questionnaires, *Int J Sports Med* 20:284, 1999.

Pintauro S, Buzzell P: Methods of body composition analysis tutorials, accessed 6/15/06 from http://nutrition.uvm.edu/bodycomp.

Prentice AM: All calories are not equal, *International dialogue on carbohydrates* 5(4):1, 1995.

Roberts SB, Young VR: Energy costs of fat and protein deposition in the human infant, *Am J Clin Nutr* 48:951, 1988.

Roubenoff R et al: The effect of gender and body composition method on the apparent decline in lean mass–adjusted resting metabolic rate with age, *J Gerontol Series A: Biol Sci Med Sci* 55: M757, 2000.

St-Onge MP et al: A new hand-held indirect calorimeter to measure postprandial energy expenditure, *Obes Res* 12:704, 2004.

Sallis JF et al: The Caltrac accelerometer as a physical activity monitor for school-age children, *Med Sci Sports Exerc* 22:698, 1989.

Schoeller DA: Measurement of energy expenditure in free-living humans by using doubly labeled water, *J Nutr* 118:1278, 1988.

Schoeller DA: How accurate is self-reported dietary energy intake? *Nutr Rev* 48:373, 1990.

Schofield WN: Predicting basal metabolic rate, new standards and review of previous work, *Hum Nutr Clin Nutr* 39(suppl 1): 5, 1985.

Shetty PS et al: Energy requirements of adults: an update on basal metabolic rates (BMRs) and physical activity levels (PALs), *Eur J Clin Nutr* 50 (suppl 1):11, 1996.

Stewart CL et al: Comparison of two systems of measuring energy expenditure, *JPEN J Parenter Enteral Nutr* 29(3): 212, 2005.

Weindruch R: Will dietary restriction work in primates? *Biogerontology*, May 6, 2006.

Weir JB: New methods of calculating metabolic rate with special reference to protein metabolism, *J Physiol* 109:1, 1949.

Whitney EN, Rolfes SR: *Understanding nutrition*, ed 9, Belmont, Calif, 2002, Wadsworth-Thomson Learning.

Winters-Hart CS et al: Validity of a questionnaire to assess historical physical activity in older women, *Med Sci Sports Exerc* 36:2082, 2004.

World Health Organization: Energy and protein requirements. Report of a Joint Food and Agriculture Organization/World Health Organization/United Nations University (FAO/WHO/UNU) Expert Consultation, Technical Report Series 724, Geneva, 1985, WHO.

CHAPTER 3

Margie Lee Gallagher, PhD, RD

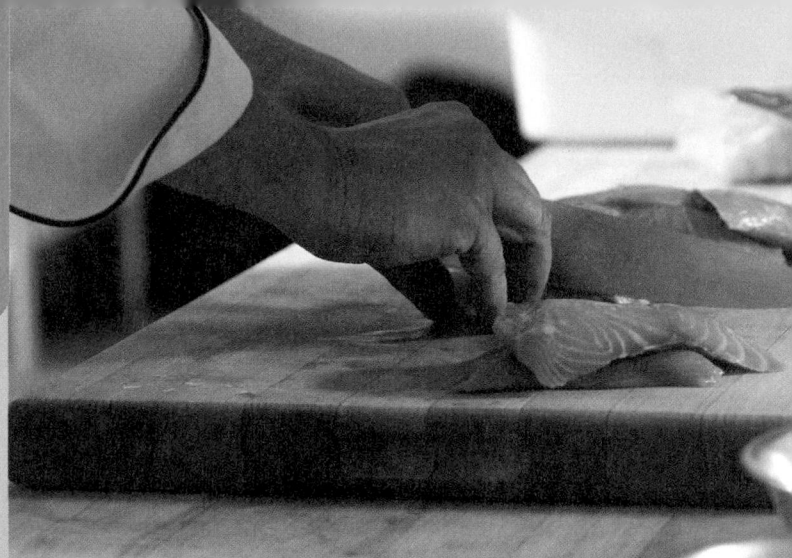

The Nutrients and Their Metabolism

KEY TERMS

acetyl coenzyme a (acetyl CoA) a molecule produced by fatty acid oxidation

amino acid an organic compound containing an amino (NH_2) group and a carboxyl (COOH) group; links with other amino acids to form proteins

amino acid score a method of protein evaluation in which the milligrams of the limiting essential amino acid in the test protein are divided by the milligrams of the same essential amino acid in the reference protein

amylopectin a form of starch made up of highly branched glucose polymers

amylose a form of starch composed of smaller, linear molecules (10^5 to 10^6 daltons) that is less than 1% branched

antioxidant a substance that can inhibit reactions of free radicals such as reactive species of oxygen; used to describe vitamins C and E, some carotenoids, ubiquinones, and bioflavonoids

ascorbic acid vitamin C, a water-soluble vitamin that plays essential roles in mineral metabolism and intracellular antioxidant functions; biosynthesized from glucose by most nonprimate species

beta-glucans (glucopyranose) polysaccharides that occur with branching, which make them less linear than cellulose and therefore more soluble; found in oats and barley

beriberi neuropathy caused by thiamin deficiency

bioavailability the availability of a mineral within the small intestine for absorption and the actual absorption (efficiency) of the mineral; implies retention of the mineral in the body and its use in cellular or tissue functions

bioflavonoids group of vitamin-like substances found in plants with antioxidant activities

biotin a sulfur-containing vitamin synthesized by microorganisms in the lower gastrointestinal tract

calbindins calcium-binding proteins found in intestinal absorbing cells and other cells of the body

calcitriol hormonally active form of vitamin D produced by the kidney; 1,25-dihydroxycholecalciferol (1,25-$[OH]_2D_3$)

carnitine a required cofactor derived from the essential amino acids methionine and lysine that facilitates transfer of long-chain fatty acids across the mitochondrial membranes and is essential for the oxidation of fatty acids

carotenoids yellow or red pigments found in carrots, sweet potatoes, leafy vegetables, milk fat, and egg yolk, which can be converted into vitamin A (retinol) in the body

ceruloplasmin a plasma protein that transports copper and acts as an oxidase (enzyme)

cellulose a carbohydrate made of long, straight glucose polymers in β linkage that resists hydrolysis in the human digestive tract; a dietary fiber

chiral carbon a carbon atom with four different atoms or groups attached, can form isomers

chitin a homopolymer of *N*-acetylglucosamine in the exoskeleton of invertebrates; sometimes included in food products as chitosan, a fiber component; possibly has a hypercholesterolemic effect in humans

cholecalciferol the form of the fat-soluble vitamin D_3, produced when 7-dehydrocholesterol in the skin is photolysed by ultraviolet irradiation

cholesterol a sterol found in cell membranes of all animal tissues that is also necessary for production of bile and steroid hormones

choline a metabolic precursor of the key structural element of membranes, phosphatidylcholine, and the neurotransmitter acetylcholine

chylomicrons lipoprotein particles formed in the intestine after lipid absorption to transport dietary triglycerides and cholesterol through the lymph and into the systemic circulation

Sections of this Chapter were written by Susan Ettinger, PhD, RD, and John J.B. Anderson, PhD, for the previous edition of this text.

cobalamin—vitamin B$_{12}$ a B-complex vitamin with porphyrin-like, cobalt-centered corrin nucleus; plays important roles in the metabolism of propionate, amino acids, and single carbons; absorption requires presence of intrinsic factor (IF)

coenzyme Q$_{10}$ (CoQ$_{10}$) a ubiquinone that exists naturally in the body and is an essential component of the mitochondrial electron transport system; vitamin-like metabolite with redox properties

cretinism a congenital condition typically caused by severe iodine deficiency during gestation; characterized by arrested physical and mental development and subnormal intelligence

deamination removal of nitrogen groups from organic molecules

denaturation dissociation of the tertiary structure of proteins by mechanical agitation, heat, cold, acidity, or alkalinity

dextrins intermediate products of starch hydrolysis

dextrose glucose produced by the hydrolysis of cornstarch

dietary fiber intact and intrinsic plant material that is not digestible by human gastrointestinal tract enzymes; may be soluble or insoluble

diacylglycerols (diglycerides) lipids with only two fatty acids attached to the glycerol molecule

disaccharides sugars capable of being hydrolyzed into two monosaccharide molecules

essential amino acids amino acids for which bodily synthesis is inadequate to meet metabolic needs and that must be supplied in the diet: threonine, tryptophan, histidine, lysine, leucine, isoleucine, methionine, valine, and phenylalanine; formerly called "indispensable amino acids"

essential fatty acids fatty acids that the body needs but cannot synthesize; the primary essential fatty acids are linoleic and α-linolenic acids

ferritin an iron-apoferritin complex that is the major storage form of iron in the liver and other tissues

folic acid (folate) a specific folate vitamer also called pteroylglutamic acid, a deficiency of which results in macrocytic anemia

free radicals atomic or molecular species with unpaired electrons that are highly reactive, take part in chemical reactions, and can cause cell destruction; one example is highly reactive oxygen

fructans nonabsorbed polymers of fructose; support the growth of beneficial colonic bacteria; examples are fructooligosaccharides and inulin

fructose a monosaccharide in fruit, honey, and some vegetables; the sweetest of the monosaccharides

functional fiber nondigestible carbohydrates that have been extracted or manufactured from plants that have a beneficial physiologic effect in humans

galactose a monosaccharide produced by the hydrolysis of lactose by digestive enzymes

glucose the main monosaccharide in blood and an important source of energy for living organisms; usually found as a disaccharide linked to fructose (sucrose), galactose (lactose), or glucose (maltose)

glucose tolerance factor (GTF) a biologically active chromium complex found in foods; unknown structure

glutathione peroxidase (GSH-Px) a selenium-containing enzyme that is the major active form of selenium in cells

glycemic index the ranking of different dietary carbohydrates on their ability to raise blood glucose levels as compared with a reference food

glycogen a branched-chain glucose polymer used for glucose storage in animals

glycolipids membrane lipids with one or more sugar molecules attached to the polar head group; high concentrations in the brain

goiter a chronic enlargement of the thyroid gland, visible as a swelling at the front of the neck; commonly associated with iodine deficiency

goitrogens compounds that block the uptake and use of iodine by thyroid cells and contribute to iodine deficiency and goiter; some are cabbage, turnips, rapeseeds (from rape plants), peanuts, cassava, sweet potatoes, kelp, and soybeans; inactivated by cooking

heme iron the nonprotein, insoluble, iron-containing protoporphyrin that is a constituent of hemoglobin, myoglobin, and a few other proteins

hemoglobin a conjugated protein containing four heme groups and globin, with the property of reversible oxygenation

hemosiderin a complex insoluble form of storage iron

hepcidin a small regulatory peptide hormone that acts on the mucosa cell and inhibits iron absorption and iron release; amount produced by the liver is related to the amount of iron stored in the liver

hydrogenation the process of adding hydrogen across the unsaturated fatty acid double bond; commercial hydrogenation of oils increases saturation and makes the oil more solid at room temperature

hydroxyapatite a crystalline structure in bone consisting of calcium phosphate and calcium carbonate

hypercarotenodermia an accumulation of carotenoids in the skin, causing skin yellowing

isoprenoids members of a large family of lipids with a carbon skeleton based on five-carbon isoprene units with alternating single- and double-bond structure (conjugated double bonds); long isoprenoid structures function as antioxidants by quenching free radicals; examples include fat-soluble vitamins, carotenoids, and other phytochemicals—lycopene and limonene—as well as steroid hormones

ketone bodies three compounds (acetoacetic acid, acetone and β-hydroxybutyric acid) formed by linking two acetyl coenzyme A (acetyl coA) groups

lactose the principal sugar in mammalian milk; a disaccharide composed of glucose and galactose

lecithin (phosphatidylcholine) a phospholipid containing choline; found in the membranes of biologic organisms; is part of bile, where it emulsifies fats, and is part of lipoproteins, where it transports triglyceride and cholesterol

lignin a woody fiber found in the stems and seeds of fruits and vegetables and in the bran layer of cereals; because of conjugated double bonds, is an excellent antioxidant; some, such as that found in flaxseed, have phytoestrogen activity

limiting amino acid an amino acid in short supply as a precursor for protein synthesis; lack of a specific limiting amino acid restricts the level of protein synthesis in the body

macrominerals minerals required by humans in amounts of 100 mg/day or more (i.e., in large quantities)

macronutrients macromolecules in plant and animal structures that can be digested, absorbed, and used by another organism as energy sources and as substrates for synthesis of the carbohydrates, fats, and proteins required to maintain cell and system integrity

maltose (malt sugar); formed from two glucose molecules, is seldom found naturally in the food supply but is formed by hydrolysis of starch polymers

medium-chain triglycerides (MCTs) a fat with fatty acid chain lengths of between 6 and 12 carbons, which are short enough to be water soluble; requires less bile salt for solubilization, is not reesterified in the enterocyte, and is transported as free fatty acid bound to albumin through the portal system

menadione a fat-soluble synthetic form of vitamin K_3

menaquinones vitamin K_2 form produced by bacteria and found in animal tissue

metallothionein a nonenzymatic, zinc-binding protein found in intestinal absorbing cells and other tissues of the body, especially the liver

microminerals (trace elements) minerals required by humans in amounts of less than 100 mg/day (i.e., in quantities of a few milligrams or even micrograms)

monoglycerols (monoacylglycerides) lipids with only one fatty acid attached to the glycerol molecule

monosaccharides the simplest sugar units with the formula $(CH_2O)n$

monounsaturated fatty acids (MFAs) fatty acids containing one double bond

myoglobin an oxygen-storing iron protoporphyrin-globin complex in striated muscle

myo-inositol a vitamin-like factor synthesized from glucose that plays important metabolic roles as a constituent of phospholipids and mediator of cellular responses to external stimuli

niacin vitamin B_3; the general term for the antipellagra vitamers nicotinamide (also niacinamide) and nicotinic acid, which play essential roles as cofactors for numerous enzymes involved in the metabolism of carbohydrates, protein, and energy

night blindness impaired dark adaptation caused by loss of visual pigments from vitamin A deficiency; also called nyctalopia

nonessential amino acids amino acids with a carbon skeleton made in the body; if needed, the body can add an amino group to endogenous intermediates to form the nonessential amino acids

nonheme iron the form of iron found in plants; less well absorbed than heme iron

oligosaccharides low–molecular-weight polymers containing 2 to 20 sugar molecules that are small, readily water soluble and often sweet

omega-3 fatty acid a fatty acid with the first double bond located at the third carbon from the methyl end (e.g., eicosapentaenoic acid [C20:5 ω-3])

omega-6 fatty acid a fatty acid with the first double bond located at the sixth carbon from the methyl end (e.g., linoleic acid [C18:2 ω-6])

pantothenic acid a B-complex vitamin that plays essential roles in the synthesis and oxidation of fatty acids

pellagra a dermatitis caused by niacin deficiency in humans

peptide bond a chemical bond between two amino acids; links amino acids into proteins

phospholipids a lipid molecule used to construct biologic membranes; composed of two fatty acids and one of several polar groups linked to glycerol phosphate

phytic acid (phytate) a phosphorus-containing compound that is found in the outer husks of cereal grains; binds with minerals and inhibits absorption

polysaccharides a carbohydrate polymer with more than 10 monosaccharide units

polyunsaturated fatty acids (PUFAs) fatty acids containing at least two double bonds

proteins complex nitrogenous compounds made up of amino acids in peptide linkages

protein digestibility corrected amino acid score (PDCAAS) the official assay for evaluating protein quality in humans

pyridoxine (PN) a B-complex vitamin (B_6) that plays essential roles in the metabolism of amino acids

resistant starch starch that resists digestive enzyme action and reaches the colon; a starch encased in a nondigestible plant seed coat or modified by cooking or processing can be resistant

retinol a form of vitamin A that is essential to the visual process and cell differentiation

retinol activity equivalents (RAEs) the measure of the vitamin A activity in foods

riboflavin a B-complex vitamin, vitamin B_2, that plays essential roles as a cofactor of enzymes involved in many cell oxidation-reduction reactions

rickets a disease of infants and young animals characterized by impaired mineralization of growing bone caused by deficiencies of vitamin D, calcium, or phosphorus

S-containing amino acids sulfur-containing amino acids, methionine and cysteine, which provide the bulk of the sulfur used in organic reactions

saturated fatty acids (SFAs) fatty acids in which all available carbon binding sites are saturated with hydrogen

short-chain fatty acids (SCFAs) fatty acids with 4 to 6 carbons; the fatty acids acetate (2 carbons), butyrate (4 carbons), and proprionate (3 carbons), which account for 85% of all SCFAs produced in the human colon; are readily absorbed by the intestinal and colonic mucosa

scurvy a disease characterized by impaired maturation of connective tissues caused by a vitamin C deficiency

structured lipids a synthetic triglyceride with medium- and long-chain fatty acids esterified to glycerol; used in parenteral nutrition formulas

sucrose a disaccharide composed of one glucose unit and one fructose unit; the major form in which glucose is transported between plant cells; ordinary table sugar

tetany muscle twitching, spasms, and (eventually) convulsions caused by low blood levels of calcium or magnesium

thiamin a B-complex vitamin (B_1) that plays an essential role as a cofactor of enzymes involved in dehydrogenase and transketolase reactions

thyroxine (T_4) an iodine-containing hormone secreted by the thyroid gland to regulate the rate of cell metabolism

tocopherol biologically active form of the fat-soluble vitamin E

transamination reversible transfer of an amino group between an amino acid and a keto acid

***trans*-fatty acids** stereoisomers of the naturally occurring cis-fatty acid in which hydrogen is added back across the double bond; result from a hydrogenation process and are naturally occurring to a limited extent in milk and in meat from ruminants, where microflora convert *cis*- to *trans*-fatty acids; present to a much greater extent in processed foods

triglycerides (triacylglycerols) lipids consisting of three fatty acid chains esterified to a glycerol phosphate molecule

triiodothyronine (T_3) an iodine-containing thyroid hormone with several times more biologic activity than thyroxine

tryptophan an amino acid that serves as the metabolic precursor of niacin

ubiquinones vitamin-like metabolites such as coenzyme Q_{10} that play essential roles in processes such as respiratory energy metabolism and have antioxidant functions that may spare vitamin E in cells

ultratrace elements minerals in the body, each of which exists in small quantities and is typically measured in micrograms

urea product of the urea cycle containing two nitrogen atoms and carbon dioxide; the chief form in which nitrogenous end products are excreted in terrestrial animals

vitamer one of multiple forms (all isomers and active analogs) of a vitamin

vitamin an organic compound, essential in very small amounts in supporting normal physiologic function, that generally cannot be biosynthesized quickly enough to meet the needs of the body

vitamin K a fat-soluble vitamin that plays essential roles in the biosynthesis of several proteins involved in blood clotting and bone mineralization

xerophthalmia a disease caused by vitamin A deficiency; characterized by dryness and eventual ulceration of the cornea

The major nutrients and their roles in the human body that will be discussed are the macronutrients (i.e., carbohydrates, lipids, protein, and alcohol) and the micronutrients (i.e., vitamins and minerals). In addition, an important indigestible dietary component, fiber, is included, as well as a review of the basis concepts regarding the structure, function, and use of nutrients in the body.

MACRONUTRIENTS

CARBOHYDRATES

Carbohydrates are manufactured by plants and are a major source of energy in the diet comprising around half the total calories. Carbohydrates are composed of carbon, hydrogen, and oxygen in a ratio of $C:O:H_2$. Important dietary carbohydrates can be categorized as (1) monosaccharides, (2) disaccharides and oligosaccharides, and (3) polysaccharides.

Monosaccharides

Monosaccharides do not normally occur as free molecules in nature but as basic components of disaccharides and polysaccharides. Only a small number of the many monosaccharides found in nature can be absorbed and used by humans. Monosaccharides can have three, four, five, six, or seven carbons, but the most important monosaccharides in the human diet are the three six-carbon hexoses: glucose, galactose, and fructose.

These hexoses all have the same chemical formula but differ importantly from one another. These differences result from small but significant differences in their chemical structure, some resulting from the presence of chiral carbons. A **chiral carbon** is one with four different atoms or groups attached. These groups can occur in different positions, resulting in isomers. For example, as illustrated in Figure 3-1, glucose and galactose are both aldehydes (C-1)

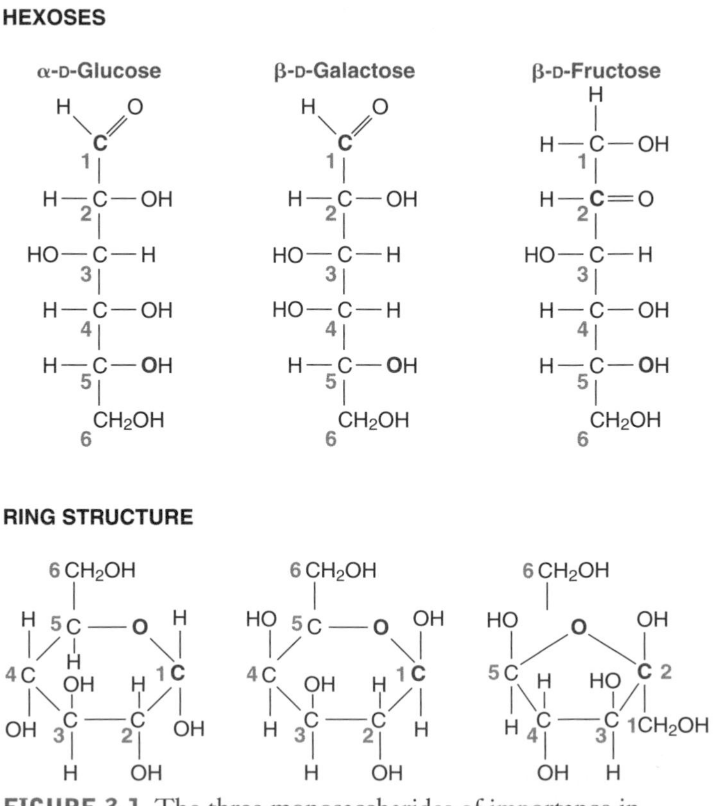

HEXOSES

RING STRUCTURE

FIGURE 3-1 The three monosaccharides of importance in humans differ from each other in how they are handled metabolically even though they have very similar structures. They are isomers of one another.

and have exactly the same chemical structure, except that the position of the –OH group on the number four carbon (C-4) on glucose is in the opposite position compared to the same –OH group, in the same position on galactose. This small difference results in a completely different compound with completely different absorption and metabolism in the body.

In addition to forming isomers, monosaccharides (both those with aldehyde groups such as glucose and galactose and those with ketone groups such as fructose) also cyclize, forming ring structures that give rise to further isomers. Isomerism has important implications for use of sugars (as well other nutrients such as amino acids and lipids) since enzymes in the body are stereospecific and can only act on specific isomers. Thus only three monosaccharide isomers are of major significance in human metabolism. They are α-D-glucose, β-D-fructose and α-D-galactose. All other carbohydrates must be effectively digested to these component monosaccharides for absorption.

The most important of the monosaccharides is the 6-carbon sugar α-D-**glucose**. Glucose is the most widely distributed sugar in nature, usually as a component of disaccharides or polysaccharides. **Dextrose** is glucose that is produced after the hydrolysis of cornstarch. "Blood sugar" refers to glucose, and the brain is highly dependent on a regular, predictable supply. The body has highly adapted physiologic mechanisms to maintain adequate blood glucose levels.

Fructose (also known as *levulose* and *fruit sugar*) is the sweetest of all monosaccharides (Table 3-1). Most fruits contain from 1% to 7% fructose, with some containing considerably greater concentrations. Fructose makes up about 3% of the dry weight in vegetables and about 40% of

honey. As fruit ripens, enzymes cleave sucrose into glucose and fructose (invert sugar, see "Disaccharides and Oligosaccharides"), resulting in a sweeter taste. *High-fructose corn syrup* is intensely sweet and inexpensive. It is manufactured enzymatically by changing the glucose in cornstarch to fructose. The overall 23% increase in sugar consumption in recent years is largely a result of an increase in corn sweetener intake, 45% in beverages, 18% in cereal and bakery products, and 11% in confectionary products. Kantor (1998) and Guthrie and Morton (2000) reported that regular soft drinks accounted for about one third of the approximately 82 g of added sweeteners per day consumed by Americans 2 years and older.

Last, dietary **galactose** is produced from lactose (milk sugar) by hydrolysis during the digestive process. Some infants are born with an inability to metabolize galactose, a condition called galactosemia (see Chapter 44). Both galactose and fructose are metabolized in the liver by incorporation into metabolic pathways for glucose. Fructose is incorporated into the glycolytic pathway but bypasses a major control enzyme in the pathway (Figure 3-2).

In view of the recent increase of high fructose corn syrup in the American diet, the metabolism of fructose may have important health implications. Recent epidemiologic evidence and experimental data (Gross et al., 2004) have provided evidence that high-fructose diets (in conjunction with other factors) may contribute to the development of type 2 diabetes and syndrome X (see Chapters 9, 30, and 32).

Disaccharides and Oligosaccharides

Although a wide variety of disaccharides and oligosaccharides exist in nature, the three most important **disaccharides** in human nutrition are sucrose, lactose, and maltose. These sugars are formed from monosaccharides joined by a glycosidic linkage between the active aldehyde or ketone carbon and a specific hydroxyl on another sugar (Figure 3-3). **Sucrose** (e.g., table sugar, cane sugar, beet sugar, grape sugar) is formed when glucose and fructose are linked together. Sucrose occurs naturally in many foods and is also an additive in commercially processed items; it is consumed in large amounts by most Americans. *Invert sugar* is also a natural form of sugar (unlinked glucose and fructose in a 1:1 ratio) used commercially because it is sweeter than equal concentrations of sucrose. Invert sugar forms smaller crystals than sucrose; thus invert sugar is preferred to sucrose in the preparation of delicate candies and icings. *Honey* is an invert sugar. Honey is made up of glucose and fructose produced by the action of honeybee *sucrase* and *amylase* enzymes on sucrose in nectar. **Lactose**, or milk sugar, is formed by glucose and galactose and made almost exclusively in the mammary glands of lactating animals; it accounts for 7.5% and 4.5% of the composition of human and cow's milk, respectively. **Maltose** (malt sugar) formed from two glucose molecules is seldom found naturally in the food supply but is formed by hydrolysis of starch polymers during digestion and is also consumed as an additive in numerous food products.

Enzymes found in the brush border of the intestine (see Chapter 1) break (digest) bonds between molecules in

TABLE 3-1	
Sweetness of Sugars and Artificial Sweeteners	
Substance	**Sweetness Value**
Sugar or Sugar Product	
Levulose, fructose	173
Invert sugar	130
Sucrose	100
Glucose	74
Sorbitol	60
Mannitol	50
Galactose	32
Maltose	32
Lactose	16
Artificial Sweeteners	
Cyclamate (banned in United States)	30
Aspartame (NutraSweet)*	180
Acesulfame-K (Sunette)	200
Saccharin (Sweet 'n Low)	300
Sucralose (Splenda)	600
Alitame (approval pending)	2000

*Nutritive (has calories).

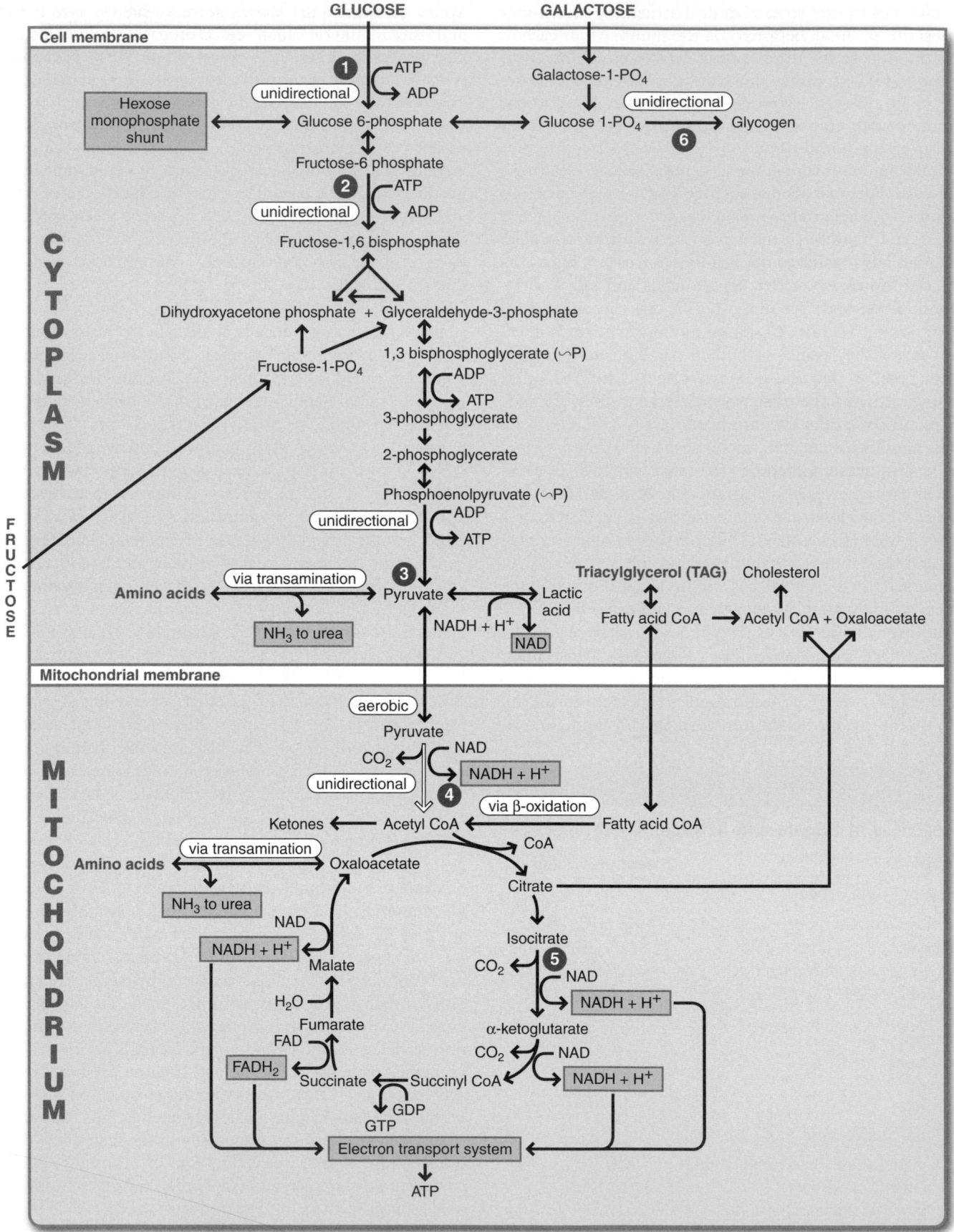

FIGURE 3-2 Overview of macronutrient metabolism. Legend on opposite page.

disaccharides and are specific to the particular bond. *Sucrase* cleaves the α bond between glucose (C-1) and fructose (C-2), *lactase* cleaves the β bond between galactose (C-1) and glucose (C-4), *maltase* cleaves the α bond between glucose (C-1) and glucose (C-4), and *isomaltase* cleaves the α bond between glucose (C-1) and glucose (C-6). There are the only four glycosidic bonds hydrolyzed in the brush border. Carbohydrates containing any other linkages cannot be digested and are classified as **dietary fiber**.

Oligosaccharides are low-molecular-weight polymers containing 2 to 20 sugar molecules. Because they are small, they are readily water soluble and often sweet (Roberfroid et al., 2005). Larger molecules are not digestible and are classified as dietary fiber.

Polysaccharides

Polysaccharides are carbohydrates with more than 10 monosaccharide units. Plants store these carbohydrates as *starch* granules formed by linking glucose in α-1,4 straight chains and branching the straight chains with α-1,6 linkages into a complex granular structure. Plants make two types of starch: amylose and amylopectin. **Amylose** is a smaller, linear molecule (10^5 to 10^6 daltons) that is less than 1% branched. **Amylopectin** is highly branched, containing up to 5% α-1,6 branches, with a very high molecular weight (10^7 to 10^8 daltons). Because of its larger size, amylopectin is more abundant in the food supply and makes up a greater fraction of the starch in grains and starchy tubers. Raw starch (i.e., raw potato and grains) is poorly digested. Moist cooking causes the granules to swell, gelatinizes the starch, softens and ruptures the cell wall, and makes the starch much more digestible, primarily by pancreatic amylase. However, some starch remains intact throughout the cooking process or recrystalizes after cooling and resists enzyme breakdown. This **resistant starch** yields limited amounts of glucose for absorption.

Starches from different plant sources such as corn, arrowroot, rice, potatos, tapioca, and other plants are all glucose polymers with the same chemical composition. Their unique character, including their taste, texture, and absorbability, is determined by the relative numbers of glucose units in straight (amylase) and branched configurations (amylopection) and the degree of accessibility to digestive enzymes.

Waxy starch is obtained from corn and rice strains bred to contain a greater percentage of branched amylopectin chains. When dissolved in water, waxy starch forms a smooth paste that does not gel until the concentration becomes very high. Once a gel forms, the product remains thick during freezing and thawing, making it an ideal thickener for commercially frozen fruit pies, sauces, and gravies. *Modified food starch* is chemically or physically modified to change its viscosity, ability to gel, and other texture properties. Pregelatinized starch, dried on hot rolls or drums and made into powder, is porous and rapidly rehydrated with cold liquid. This starch rapidly thickens, making it useful for instant puddings, salad dressings, pie fillings, gravies, and baby food.

Dextrins result from the digestive process and are large, linear glucose polysaccharides of intermediate lengths cleaved from high amylose starch by α-amylase. *Limit dextrins* are

FIGURE 3-2 Overview of macronutrient metabolism.
1, Hexokinase/glucokinase (liver) reaction; uses ATP, is reversed by glucose 6-phosphotase in gluconeogenesis.
2, Phosphofructokinase reaction: modulated by ATP, positively modified by AMP and ADP, uses ATP; is reversed by specific phosphatase in gluconeogenesis.
3, Pyruvate kinase reaction: second example of substrate level phosphorylation of ADP → ATP, is not reversible and must be bypassed for gluconeogenesis.
4, Pyruvate dehydrogenase enzyme complex reaction: unidirectional and cannot be reversed.
5, Dehydrogenase reaction: similar to pyruvate dehydrogenase, characterizes the removal of hydrogens in the Kreb cycle.
6, Glycogenesis uses a glycogenin primer reaction and then glycogen synthetase and branching enzymes to synthesize glycogen. The reactions are not reversible. Glycogen is catabolized by a highly controlled phosphorylase.
ADP, adenosine diphosphate; *cAMP,* cyclic adenosine monophosphate (cAMP); *ATP,* adenosine triphosphate. (*Courtesy of Margie Gallagher, PhD, RD, East Carolina University.*)

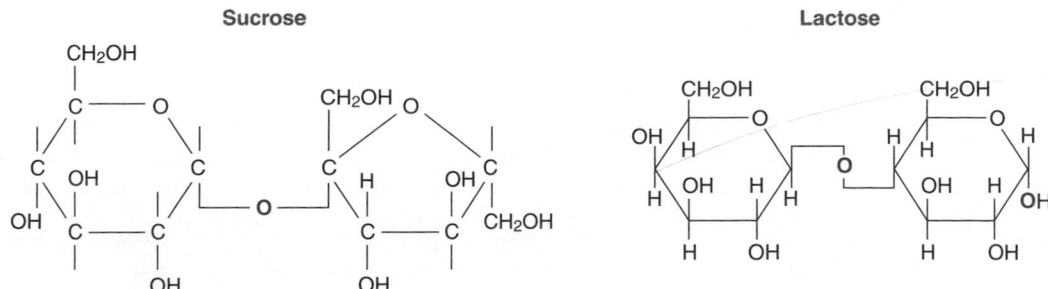

FIGURE 3-3 Disaccharides of importance in humans: sucrose (glucose and fructose) and lactose (glucose and galactose).

cleaved from amylopectin containing branch points not cleaved by amylase; they can subsequently be digested into glucose by the mucosal enzyme isomaltase.

In contrast to plants, animals use carbohydrates primarily to maintain blood glucose concentrations between feedings. To ensure a readily available supply, all cells (primarily the liver and muscles) store carbohydrate in the easily mobilized **glycogen** polymer (Figure 3-4). As with

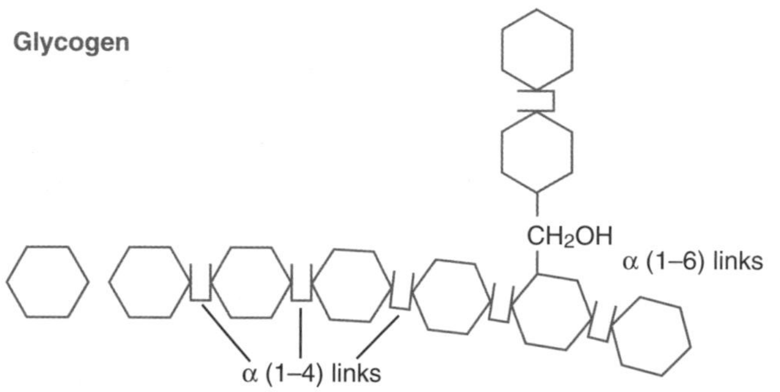

all carbohydrates, glycogen is stored hydrated with water. The adsorbed water makes glycogen a large and cumbersome molecule, unsuitable for long-term energy storage. The 70-kg "average man" stores only an 18-hour fuel supply as glycogen, compared with a 2-month supply stored as fat. It has been estimated that if all human energy stores were glycogen, humans would need to weigh 60 additional pounds (Alberts et al., 2002). About 150 g of glycogen is stored in muscle; this amount can be increased fivefold with physical training (see Chapter 23) but is not available to maintain blood glucose directly. It is the glycogen store in the human liver (about 90 g) that is involved in the hormonal control of blood sugar (see *Clinical Insight:* Hormonal Control of Blood Sugar).

The recommended amount of digestible carbohydrate required in the diet ranges between 45% and 65% of total calories (Institute of Medicine, Food and Nutrition Board, 2002). The carbohydrate content of selected foods is given in Table 3-2. The dietary guidelines recommend that consumers select foods with less added sugar and consume carbohydrates as fiber-rich fruits, vegetables, and whole grains, thus linking digestible carbohydrate consumption with fiber intake (USDA, 2005).

FIGURE 3-4 Glycogen is a branched glucose polymer similar to amylopectin, but the branches in glycogen are shorter and more numerous.

✶ CLINICAL INSIGHT

Hormonal Control of Blood Sugar

In the body blood glucose must be maintained at a minimum level (70 to 100 mg/100 ml) to provide fuel for the brain, central nervous system, and other obligate consumers of glucose. If blood glucose is chronically higher than this range, damage to cells and systems takes place, as it does in patients with diabetes. Glucose homeostasis (equilibrium) is controlled in the fed and fasted states through actions of hormones that store, release, or oxidize glucose as needed.

In the fed state insulin is the principal anabolic hormone and is responsible for fuel storage and use. It is produced by the β cells of the islets of Langerhans in the pancreas and released into the bloodstream in response to the postprandial increase in blood glucose. Insulin release can also be stimulated, although to a lesser extent, by the ingestion of protein or infusion of amino acids or **ketone bodies**. Insulin release is also stimulated by gastrointestinal hormones, vagus nerve activity, and certain drugs (e.g., glucotrol, an oral hypoglycemic agent). Insulin binds to receptors on muscle and adipose cells and facilitates glucose entry through specialized GLUT 4 transporters. In the liver insulin facilitates glucose oxidation and glycogen synthesis. If food intake is excessive, insulin also facilitates fatty acid synthesis and storage in the adipose cells, thereby reducing the glucose concentration in the bloodstream.

In the fasted state, glucagon is secreted by the α cells of the islets of Langerhans. This hormone acts primarily on the liver to stimulate glycogen breakdown to maintain blood glucose

levels. In the absence of insulin, glucagon inhibits hepatic glucose oxidation and enhances gluconeogenesis. The net result of these activities is return of blood glucose levels to the normal range. Fasting also stimulates the release of epinephrine from the adrenal medulla and norepinephrine from peripheral nerve endings. These catabolic hormones act primarily on the muscle to mobilize glycogen and on adipocytes to release triglycerides.

Epinephrine and norepinephrine levels increase when a person is angry or afraid, resulting in the "fight-or-flight" response. Under these conditions glucose is needed to provide extra energy for crisis response. Glucocorticoids such as cortisol are steroid hormones elaborated by the adrenal cortex in the fasting or stressed state. As the name suggests, glucocorticoids increase blood glucose levels, largely by stimulating gluconeogenesis. Cortisol also enhances the release of fat and amino acids from adipose and muscle tissue, thereby providing a substrate for adenosine triphosphate synthesis and gluconeogenesis. Growth hormone, produced by the anterior pituitary gland, increases the blood glucose level by antagonizing insulin action and diminishing cellular uptake of glucose. It also increases amino acid uptake and protein synthesis by all cells and increases the mobilization of fat for energy. Finally, in the absence of insulin binding, muscle and adipose tissues cannot take up glucose. The net actions of these counter-regulatory hormones maintain the blood glucose concentration within the range required for optimal cell function.

Dietary Fiber and Functional Fiber

Dietary fiber refers to intact plant components that are not digestible by gastrointestinal (GI) enzymes, whereas **functional fiber** refers to nondigestible carbohydrates that have been extracted or manufactured from plants. Both of these types of fiber have been shown to have beneficial physiologic functions in the GI tract and in reducing risk of certain disease states. These fibers and their functions are summarized in Table 3-3.

TABLE 3-2	
Carbohydrate Content of Foods	
Food	**Carbohydrate (Percentage of Weight)**
Sugar	
Concentrated Sweets	
Sugar: Cane, beet, powdered,	99.5
brown, maple	90-96
Candies	70-95
Honey (extracted)	82
Syrup: Table blends, molasses	55-75
Jams, jellies, marmalades	70
Carbonated, sweetened beverages	10-12
Fruits	
Prunes, apricots, figs (cooked, unsweet)	12-31
Bananas, grapes, cherries, apples, pears	15-23
Fresh: Pineapples, grapefruits, oranges, apricots, strawberries	8-14
Milk	
Skim	6
Whole	5
Starch	
Grain Products	
Starches: Corn, tapioca, arrowroot	86-88
Cereals (dry): Corn, wheat, oat, bran	68-85
Flour: Corn, wheat (sifted)	70-80
Popcorn (popped)	77
Cookies: Plain, assorted	71
Crackers, saltines	72
Cakes: Plain, without icing	
Bread: White, rye, whole wheat	48-52
Macaroni, spaghetti, noodles, rice (cooked)	23-30
Cereals (cooked): Oat, wheat, grits	10-16
Vegetables	
Boiled: Corn, white and sweet potatoes, lima and dried beans, peas	15-26
Beets, carrots, onions, tomatoes	5-7
Leafy: Lettuce, asparagus, cabbage, greens, spinach	3-4

Homopolysaccharides contain repeating units of the same molecule. The most abundant fiber is **cellulose**, a homopolysaccharide made up of glucose molecules linked by β-1-4 linkages that cannot be hydrolyzed by amylase enzymes. Cellulose is the most abundant organic compound in the world, constituting 50% or more of all the carbon in vegetation. The long cellulose molecule folds back on itself and is held in place by hydrogen bonding, thus giving cellulose fibrils great mechanical strength but limited flexibility. Cellulose is found in carrots, celery, broccoli, and many other vegetables.

Other homopolymers called **beta-glucans (glucopyranose)** occur with branching, which makes them less linear than cellulose and therefore more soluble. Soluble fiber sources such as oats and barley are rich in beta-glucans.

Chitin and chitosan are also homopolymers of glucosamine and are widely distributed among various organisms, including algae, fungi, and yeasts. **Chitin** is best known as the major component in the exoskeleton of arthropods, mollusks, and marine invertebrates, including lobster and shrimp, and is usually consumed as an isolated supplement. Chitin forms a matrix on which minerals are deposited, much as collagen forms a matrix for vertebrate bone mineralization. *Chitosan* is obtained by the deacetylation of acetylglucosamine of chitin (Shiau and Yu, 1998). Chitin and chitosan have been studied for their hypocholesterolemic effect. The strong positive charge on chitosan binds negatively charged lipids, blocking their absorption. Hypercholesterolemic mice given chitosan for 20 weeks had significantly lower blood cholesterol levels (64% of controls) and highly significant inhibition of athcrogenesis in the aorta (Ormrod et al., 1998). In contrast, chitosan feeding resulted in severe malabsorption of fat-soluble vitamins and bone minerals in rats (Deuchi et al., 1995). More research is needed to assess the safety of this substance for long-term human consumption.

Heteropolysaccharides are made by modifying the basic cellulose structure to form compounds with different water solubilities. *Hemicellulose* is a glucose polymer substituted with other sugars; different sugar molecules have different water solubilities. The predominant sugar is used to name the hemicellulose (e.g., xylan, galactan, mannan, arabinose, galactose). *Pectins* and *gums* contain sugars and sugar alcohols that make these molecules even more water soluble than hemicellulose. The galacturonic acid structure of pectin absorbs water and forms a gel; thus it is widely used for making jams and jellies. The galacturonic acid backbone has rhamnose units inserted at intervals and side chains of arabinose and galactose. Pectin is found in apples, citrus fruit, strawberries, and other fruits. *Gums and mucilages* (e.g., guar gum) are similar in structure to pectin, except that their galactose units are combined with other sugars (e.g., glucose) and polysaccharides. Gums are found in plant secretions and seeds. The specific textural qualities of gums and mucilages are commercially useful when added to processed foods such as ice cream.

Fructans include *fructooligosaccharides (FOSs), inulin, inulin-type fructans* and *oligofructose* and are composed of fructose

TABLE 3-3

Types, Composition, Sources, and Functions of Fibers

Type of Fiber	Major Chemical Components	Sources	Major functions
Less Soluble Fiber			
Cellulose	Glucose (β-1-4 linkages)	Whole wheat, bran, vegetables	Increase water-holding capacity, thus increasing fecal volume and decreasing gut transit time
Hemicellulose	Xylose, mannose, galactose	Bran, whole grains	
Lignin	Phenols	Fruits and edible seeds, mature vegetables	Fermentation produces short-chain fatty acids associated with decreased risk of tumor formation
More Soluble Fibers			
Gums	Galactose and glucuronic acid	Oats, legumes, guar, barley	Cause gel formation, thus decrease gastric emptying, slow digestion, gut transit time, and glucose absorption
Pectins	Polygalacturonic acid	Apples, strawberries, carrots, citrus	Also binds minerals, lipids, and bile acids increasing excretion of each, thus decreasing serum cholesterol
Functional Fibers*			
Chitin	Glucopyranose	Supplement from crab or lobster shells	Reduces serum cholesterol
Fructans (including inulin)	Fructose polymers	Extracted from natural sources: chicory, onions etc	Prebiotic which stimulates growth of beneficial bacteria in gut, used as fat replacer
Beta-glucans	Glucopyronoase	Oat and barley bran	Reduces serum cholesterol
Algal polysaccharides (carrageenan)		Isolated from algae and seaweed	Gel forming—used as thickeners, stablizers (can be toxic)
Polydextrose, polyols	Glucose and sorbitol etc.	Synthesized	Bulking agent or sugar substitute
Psyllium		Extracted from psyllium seeds	High water binding capacity (choking hazard)

*Isolated or extracted.

polymers, often linked with an initial glucose. Inulin comprises a diverse group of fructose polymers widely distributed in plants as a storage carbohydrate. Oligofructose is a subgroup of inulin, containing less than 10 fructose units. All are poorly digested in the upper GI tract and thus supply only about 1 kcal/g (Roberfroid, 2005). Because they contain fructose, fructans have a sweet, clean flavor and are half as sweet as sucrose. Major sources of fructans include wheat, onions, garlic, bananas, and chicory; other sources include tomatoes, barley, rye, asparagus, and Jerusalem artichokes. Inulin and related compounds are used widely in the commercial formulation of innovative food products to improve the flavor (added sweetness) of low-calorie foods and to improve the stability and acceptability of fat-reduced foods. Because they are not absorbed in the proximal intestine, fructans have been used as a sugar replacement for diabetic patients.

In addition, fructans (synthesized or extracted), as well as other fibers, may have prebiotic properties and are likely to be considered functional fiber in the future. *Prebiotics* are nondigestible food substances that selectively stimulate the growth or activity of beneficial bacterial species already resident in the colon (*probiotics*) and are beneficial to the host. Various prebiotics, especially FOSs, variably stimulate the growth of intestinal bacteria, principally *bifidobacteria*. In a healthy person 80% to 90% of nonabsorbable carbohydrate is fermented by colonic bacteria into carbon dioxide, hydrogen, methane, and short-chain fatty acids (SCFAs) (Cummings et al., 2001).

Algal polysaccharides (e.g., carrageenan) are extracted from seaweed and algae and used as thickening and stabilizing agents in many processed foods such as infant formulas, ice cream, milk pudding, and sour cream products.

Algal polysaccharides are used commercially because they form weak gels with proteins and stabilize food mixtures, preventing suspended ingredients from settling. Tobacman (2001) demonstrated that carrageenan damages human cells in culture and destroys human mammary myoepithelial cells at concentrations as low as 0.00014%. With its wide use in commercial food preparation and uncertainty about the extent of human sensitivity, further investigation of carrageenan is needed.

Polydextrose and other polyols are synthetic polymers of sugar alcohols that are used as sugar substitutes in foods. They are not digestible, contribute to increased fecal bulk, and may be fermented in the small intestine. More data are needed before they can be classified as functional fibers (Institute of Medicine, Food and Nutrition Board, 2002).

Lignin is a woody fiber found in the stems and seeds of fruits and vegetables and the bran layer of cereals. It is not a carbohydrate but is a polymer composed of phenylpropyl alcohols and acids. The phenyl groups contain conjugated double bonds, which make them excellent antioxidants. Flaxseed lignin also has phytoestrogen activity and can mimic estrogen at its receptors on reproductive organs and bone; the role of flaxseed in the prevention of cancer and other chronic diseases is under investigation (Stark and Madar, 2002).

Role of Fiber in Digestion and Absorption

The role of fiber in the GI tract is complex and varies based on the solubility of the fiber. A growing body of evidence suggests that nonabsorbable oligosaccharides and fibers have a significant impact on human physiology. Generally insoluble fibers such as cellulose increase the water-holding capacity of undigested material and lead to increased fecal volume (bulk) and decreased GI transit time (increases the frequencies of defecation). On the other hand, soluble fibers can form gels, resulting in slowed GI transit time and slowed or decreased nutrient absorption. Soluble fibers also bind other nutrients such as cholesterol and minerals and decrease absorption of these. However, certain nondigestible oligosaccharides (NDOs), which are fermented by intestinal bacteria, stimulate the intestinal absorption and retention of some minerals, including calcium, magnesium, zinc, and iron (Scholz-Ahrens et al., 2001).

Serum lipid concentrations can be modified by insoluble fibers such as cellulose, lignin, chitin, and more soluble fibers because (1) fibers bind fecal bile acids and increase excretion of bile acid–derived cholesterol, (2) fibers prevent dietary fat and cholesterol absorption by binding bile acids or fat and lipids, and (3) fermentable oligosaccharides and dietary fiber are converted by intestinal bacteria to short-chain fatty acids, which lower blood lipids by mechanisms that are currently unclear. However, evidence for the hypocholesterolemic effect of soluble fibers, including FOSs, synthetic polydextrose and polyols, viscous pectin, guar gum, oat bran, psyllium husk, beans, legumes, and fruits and vegetables, is conflicting. Cholesterol-lowering effects have been reported, but the effect varies with the type and amount of fiber.

A possible mechanism for prebiotic modulation of metabolic pathways by fiber is by their fermentation into the **short-chain fatty acids (SCFAs),** (acetate, butyrate, and proprionate), which account for 85% of all SCFAs produced in the human colon. SCFAs are readily absorbed by the intestinal and colonic mucosa; and they (1) enhance sodium and water absorption, (2) increase colonocyte proliferation, (3) increase metabolic energy production, (4) enhance colonic blood flow, (5) stimulate the autonomic nervous system, and (6) increase GI hormone production (Compher et al, 1997).

More than 70% of the fuel for colonocytes is the SCFA butyrate (4C), which is actually produced more from starch than from fat. Proprionate (3C) is absorbed and cleared by the liver and may be important in hepatic lipid or glucose metabolism. Acetate (2C) is produced in the greatest quantities from undigested carbohydrate, is rapidly metabolized into carbon dioxide by peripheral tissues, and can serve as substrate for lipid and cholesterol synthesis (Cummings et al., 2001).

The roles of fiber in the physiology of the GI tract are complex, and our understanding is evolving. The adequate intake (AI) of total fiber is set at 38 g/day for men and 25 g/day for women (Institute of Medicine, Food and Nutrition Board, 2002). Mean intake of Americans is currently less than half this.

In addition to fiber, other nonnutrient components of plants, including tannins, saponins, lectins, and phytates, interact with dietary macronutrients, vitamins, and minerals and can reduce macronutrient and micronutrient absorption. **Phytic acid** or **phytate,** a six-carbon ring with phosphate bound to each carbon, is found in the seed coat of grains and legumes and has the ability to bind metal ions, especially calcium, copper, iron, and zinc. Because calcium catalyzes the action of amylase, which hydrolyzes starch, excess phytate also reduces starch hydrolysis.

Glucose Absorption and the Glycemic Index

Dietary carbohydrates are digested into glucose, fructose, and galactose through the actions of α-amylase and brush border digestive enzymes in the upper GI tract. The ability to digest carbohydrates is modified by (1) the relative availability (or resistance) of the starch to enzyme action; (2) the activity of digestive enzymes, especially lactase, at the mucosal brush border; and (3) the presence of other dietary factors such as fat that slow stomach emptying, nonabsorbable oligosaccharides, and viscous dietary fibers such as pectins, β-glucans, and gums that dilute enzyme concentration. Thus a diet rich in whole foods such as fruits, vegetables, legumes, nuts, and minimally processed grains tends to slow down the pace of glucose absorption.

Once digested, glucose is actively absorbed across the intestinal cell and transferred to the portal blood for transport to the liver as described in Chapter 1. The liver removes about 50% of absorbed glucose for oxidation and storage as glycogen. Galactose (absorbed actively) and fructose (absorbed by facilitated diffusion) are also taken up by the liver and incorporated into glucose metabolic pathways (see Figure 3-2). Glucose exits the liver and enters the systemic circulation. Only then is it available for insulin-dependent uptake by peripheral tissues. Thus the major regulators of blood glucose concentration after a meal are (1) the amount and digestibility of ingested carbohydrate, (2) the absorption and degree of liver uptake, and (3) insulin secretion and the sensitivity of peripheral tissues to insulin action.

In 1981 Jenkins defined a **glycemic index** to rank different dietary carbohydrates on their ability to raise blood glucose levels as compared with a reference food (Jenkins, 1981). Studies suggest that the glycemic index of a diet has a predictable effect on blood glucose levels and may have use in the dietary management of diabetes and hyperlipidemia (Brand-Miller et al., 2002). There are significant data indicating that slowly absorbed starchy foods (i.e., those with a low glycemic index) may have health advantages over those with a high glycemic index. However, the Institute of Medicine (IOM) declined to set an upper limit (UL) for the glycemic index in its 2002 recommendations. Compelling reasons were that data from healthy individuals were not adequate and that it is difficult to separate other factors that may contribute to blood glucose levels from the effect of the glycemic index. For example, the beneficial effects of dietary fiber on blood glucose levels are well established. Certainly fiber is known to decrease the glycemic index; yet, as noted in a previous paragraph, the median fiber intake of Americans is only half of the AI recommendations for healthy individuals. The question is: Does a low glycemic index diet have any effect on healthy individuals receiving adequate amounts of dietary fiber? Published data on the glycemic indexes of individual foods, using white bread and glucose as reference foods, have been consolidated for the convenience of users. Use of the glycemic index to modify diets and prevent and control chronic disease is under intense investigation (see Chapters 9 and 30).

In addition, it is possible that some high-risk individuals have subtle genetic changes that impair their ability to tolerate dietary carbohydrates (Salas et al., 1998). Observations from the Third National Health and Nutrition Examination Survey (NANES III) clearly demonstrate that prevalence of this condition manifests as the metabolic syndrome in various age-groups (Ford et al., 2002). Prevalence rises from less than 10% for individuals in the 20- to 29-year-age-group to 45% in the 60- to 69-year-age-group, suggesting possible interactions between the process of aging and the cumulative effect of increased sugar (or perhaps other carbohydrates) consumption. For more details about the metabolic syndrome (which is also called *insulin resistance* and *syndrome X*), see Chapters 9, 30, 32, and 33.

Regulation of Blood Lipids

Carbohydrate-induced hypertriglyceridemia can result from consuming a high-carbohydrate diet. It is important to remember that fat intake does not translate directly into blood lipid changes because the body regulates macronutrient levels to provide adequate supplies of fuel to body tissues. For example, the brain uses the major por-

tion of the approximately 200 g of glucose required per day. If the blood glucose level falls below 40 mg/dl, counter-regulatory hormones release macronutrients from stores; if the blood glucose level rises above 180 mg/dl, glucose is spilled into the urine. High intakes of carbohydrate can trigger large releases of insulin. This anabolic hormone stimulates compensatory responses, including insulin-dependent glucose uptake by muscle and fat and active glycogen and fat synthesis, thereby lowering the blood glucose level to a normal range. About 2 hours after a meal, intestinal absorption is complete, but insulin effects persist, and the blood glucose level falls, sometimes below the normal range. The body interprets this hypoglycemic state as starvation and secretes counter-regulatory hormones that release free fatty acids from fat cells (Ludwig, 2002). Fatty acids are packed into transport lipoproteins (very low–density lipoproteins [VLDLs]) in the liver, thereby elevating serum triglycerides.

Parks and Hellerstein (2000) reviewed evidence for the paradoxic rise in serum lipid levels and fall in high-density lipoprotein (HDL) levels after consumption of a diet higher than usual in carbohydrates. Although conclusive human studies have not yet been done, researchers are focusing on the increase in Americans' obesity coupled with their higher sugar (especially fructose) consumption as the cause and are calling for additional studies to clearly define the way the macronutrient composition of the diet can influence health.

FATS AND LIPIDS

Lipid Structures and Functions

Fats and lipids constitute approximately 34% of the energy in the human diet. Because fat is energy rich and provides 9 kcal/g of energy, humans are able to obtain adequate energy with a reasonable daily consumption of fat-containing foods. Dietary fat is stored in *adipose* (fat) cells located in depots on the human frame. The ability to store and use large amounts of fat enables humans to survive without food for weeks and sometimes months.

Some fat deposits are not used effectively during a fast and are classified as *structural fat*. Structural fat pads hold the body organs and nerves in position and protect them against traumatic injury and shock. Fat pads on the palms and buttocks protect the bones from mechanical pressure. Humans also have a subcutaneous layer of fat that insulates the body, preserving body heat and maintaining body temperature. Dietary fat is also essential for the digestion, absorption, and transport of the fat-soluble vitamins and phytochemicals such as carotenoids and lycopenes. As described in Chapter 1, dietary fat depresses gastric secretions, slows gastric emptying, and stimulates biliary and pancreatic flow, thereby facilitating the digestive process. Fat also conveys important textural properties to foods such as ice creams (smoothness) and baked goods (tenderness—due to "shortening" of strands of gluten). Box 3-1 shows the fat content of some common foods.

BOX 3-1

Fat Content of Some Common Foods

0 g

Most fruits and vegetables
Nonfat milk
Nonfat yogurt
Plain pasta and rice
Angel food cake
Popcorn, air popped, unbuttered
Soft drinks
Jam or jelly

1 to 3 g

Popcorn, oil popped, unbuttered, 1 cup
Low-calorie salad dressing, 1 tbsp
Baked beans, ½ cup
Soup, chicken noodle, canned, 1 cup
Whole wheat bread, 1 slice
Dinner roll, 1
Waffle, frozen, 4 inch, 1
Coleslaw, ½ cup
Flounder or sole, baked, 3 oz
Chicken, without skin, baked or roasted, 3 oz
Tuna, canned in water, 3 oz
Cheese, cottage, 2% fat, ½ cup
Ice milk, soft serve, ½ cup

4 to 6 g

Low-fat yogurt, 1 cup
Cheese, mozarella, part skim, 1 oz
Chicken, baked or roasted with skin, 3 oz
Egg, scrambled, 1
Turkey, roasted, 3 oz
Granola, 1 oz
Muffin, bran, 1 small
Pizza, cheese, ¼ of 12 inch
Burrito, bean, 1
Brownie, with nuts, 1 small
Margarine or butter, 1 tsp
Popcorn, oil popped, buttered, 1 cup
French dressing, regular, 1 tbsp

7 to 10 g

Cheese, cheddar, 1 oz
Milk, whole, 1 cup
Bologna, beef, 1 slice
Sausage, 1 patty
Steak, sirloin, broiled, 3 oz
Potatoes, French fried, 10
Chow mein, chicken, 1 cup
Chocolate candy bar, 1 oz
Corn chips, 1 oz
Doughnut, cake type, plain, 1
Mayonnaise, 1 tbsp

15 g

Hot dog, beef, 2 oz
McDonald's Chicken McNuggets, 6 pieces
Peanut butter, 2 tbsp
Pork chop, broiled, 3 oz
Sunflower seeds, dry roasted, ¼ cup
Avocado, ½ medium
Chop suey, beef and pork, 1 cup
Cinnamon roll, 1

20 g

Cheesecake, ½ cake
Lasagna with meat, 1 medium piece
Macaroni and cheese, homemade, 1 cup
Peanuts, dry roasted, ¼ cup
Ground beef, broiled, 3 oz

25+ g

Polish sausage, 3 oz
Cheeseburger, large
Pie, pecan, ⅛ of 9 inch
Chicken pot pie, frozen, baked, 1 pie
Quiche, bacon, ⅛ pie

Unlike carbohydrates, lipids are not polymers; they are small molecules extracted from animal and plant tissues. Lipids comprise a heterogeneous group of compounds characterized by their insolubility in water, and they can be classified into three major groups (Box 3-2). Figure 3-5 shows some of the more important lipid structures.

Fatty Acids

Fatty acids are rarely free in nature and almost always are linked to other molecules by their *hydrophilic* carboxylic acid head group (see Figure 3-5, *1*). Fatty acids occur primarily as unbranched hydrocarbon chains with an even number of carbons and are classified according to the number of carbons, the number of double bonds, and the position of the double bonds in the chain. Chain length and extent of saturation contribute to the melting temperature of a fat. In general, fats with shorter fatty acid chains or more double bonds are liquid at room temperature. Saturated fats, especially those with long chains (e.g., beef tallow), are solid at room temperature; but a fat such as coconut oil, which is also highly saturated, is semiliquid at room temperature because the predominant fatty acids are short (8 to 14 carbons). Some manufacturers cool oil and filter out solidified lipid particles before sale; the resultant "winterized" oil remains clear when refrigerated. In general, SCFAs are considered to have 4 to 6 carbons, medium-chain fatty acids

Classification of Lipids

Simple Lipids

Fatty Acids

Neutral fats: Esters of fatty acids with glycerol
  Monoglycerides, diglycerides, triglycerides
Waxes: Esters of fatty acids with high-molecular-weight
  alcohols
  Sterol esters (e.g., cholesterol ester)
  Nonsterol esters (e.g., retinyl palmitate [vitamin A esters])

Compound Lipids

Phospholipids: Compounds of phosphoric acid, fatty acids,
  and a nitrogenous base
  Glycerophospholipids (e.g., lecithins, cephalins,
    plasmologens)
  Glycosphingolipids (e.g., sphingomyelins)
Glycolipids: Compounds of fatty acids, monosaccharides, and
  a nitrogenous base (e.g., cerebrosides, gangliosides,
  ceramide)
Lipoproteins: Particles of lipid and protein

Miscellaneous Lipids

Sterols (e.g., cholesterol, vitamin D, bile salts)
Vitamins A, E, K

From Examples of current and proposed ingredients for fats, *J Am Diet Assoc* 92:472, 1992.

(MCFAs) to have 8 to 14, and long-chain fatty acids (LCFAs) to have 16 to 20 or more.

In a **saturated fatty acid (SFA),** all carbon binding sites not linked to another carbon are linked to hydrogen and are therefore saturated. There are no double bonds between carbons. **Monounsaturated fatty acids (MFAs)** contain only one double bond, and **polyunsaturated fatty acids (PUFAs)** contain two or more double bonds. In MFAs and PUFAs one or more pairs of hydrogen have been removed, and double bonds form between adjacent carbons. Because fatty acids with double bonds are vulnerable to oxidative damage, humans and other warm-blooded organisms store fat predominantly as saturated palmitic fatty acid (C16:0) and stearic fatty acid (C18:0). On the other hand, cell membranes must be stable and flexible for optimum function. To achieve this requirement, membrane phospholipids contain one SFA and one highly PUFA, the most abundant of which is arachidonic acid (C20:4). Some commonly occurring fatty acids are listed in Table 3-4 with a typical food source. Fatty acids are also characterized by the location of their double bonds. Two notation conventions are used to describe the location of the double bonds Table 3-5. Omega notation is used in this chapter. In omega notation a lower case omega (ω) or *n* is used to refer to the placement of the first double bond counting from the methyl end (referred to as the fatty acid's omega number). Thus arachidonic acid (20:4 ω-6 or 20:4 *n*-6), the major highly polyunsaturated fat in mem-

branes of land animals, is an **omega-6 fatty acid.** It has twenty carbons and four double bonds, the first of which is six carbons from the terminal methyl group. Eicosapentaenoic acid (EPA) (20:5 ω-3 or 20:5 *n*-3) is found in marine organisms and is an **omega-3 fatty acid.** It has five double bonds, the first of which is three carbons from the terminal methyl group. Only plants (including marine phytoplankton) can synthesize omega-6 and omega-3 fatty acids. Animals including humans can only place double bonds as low as the omega-9 carbon and therefore cannot synthesize omega-6 and omega-3 fatty acids.

Sources of omega-3 fatty acids from selected marine sources are listed in Table 3-6. However, the fatty acid content in the diet of an organism determines the proportion of that fatty acid in the animal product (Farrell, 1998); thus values given in Table 3-6 and other nutrient databases should be used as an estimate of the fatty acid content.

Essential Fatty Acids and the Omega-6/Omega-3 Ratio

As mentioned previously, neither omega-3 nor omega-6 fatty acids can be synthesized by humans, although humans can desaturate and elongate linoleic acid (18:2 *n*-6) to arachidonic acid (20:4 *n*-6) and alpha-linolenic acid (ALA) (C18:3 ω-3) to EPA (C20:5 ω-3) and docosahexaenoic acid (DHA) (C22:6 ω-3). Because of this ability, Cunnane (2003) suggested that the term ***essential fatty acid,*** especially as it refers to linoleic and linolenic acids, be replaced by referring to omega-3 and omega-6 fatty acids more generally. It is the longer-chain fatty acids that are required (essential), but if sufficient amounts of shorter-chain precursors occur in the diet they need not be supplied directly. The longer-chain fatty acids are important components of the cell membranes and as precursors of eicosanoids such as prostaglandins, thromboxanes, and leukotrienes. Eicosanoids act as localized (paracrine) hormones and have multiple local functions. They can alter the size and permeability of the blood vessels, alter the activity of platelets and contribute to blood clotting, and modify the processes of inflammation (see Figure 3-6). McCowen and Bistrian (2005) recently concluded that derivatives of *n*-3 fatty acids from dietary sources or fish oil can have beneficial effects in a number of disease states. Roles for omega-3 fatty acids related to paracrine hormones and cardiovascular disease are discussed in Chapter 32, arthritis and inflammatory conditions are discussed in Chapter 40, and their role in brain function is discussed in Chapter 42.

Although both omega-6 and omega-3 fatty acids are essential in the diet, excess omega-6 fatty acids in the diet saturate the enzymes that desaturate and elongate both *n*-3 and *n*-6 fatty acids and prevent conversion of ALA into longer EPA and DHA forms (Kris-Etherton, 2000). Haag (2003) concluded that the omega-6/omega-3 ratio in the diet influences neurotransmission and thus brain function. The optimal omega-6/omega-3 ratio has been estimated to be 2:1 to 3:1, four times lower than the current intake; therefore it is recommended that humans consume more

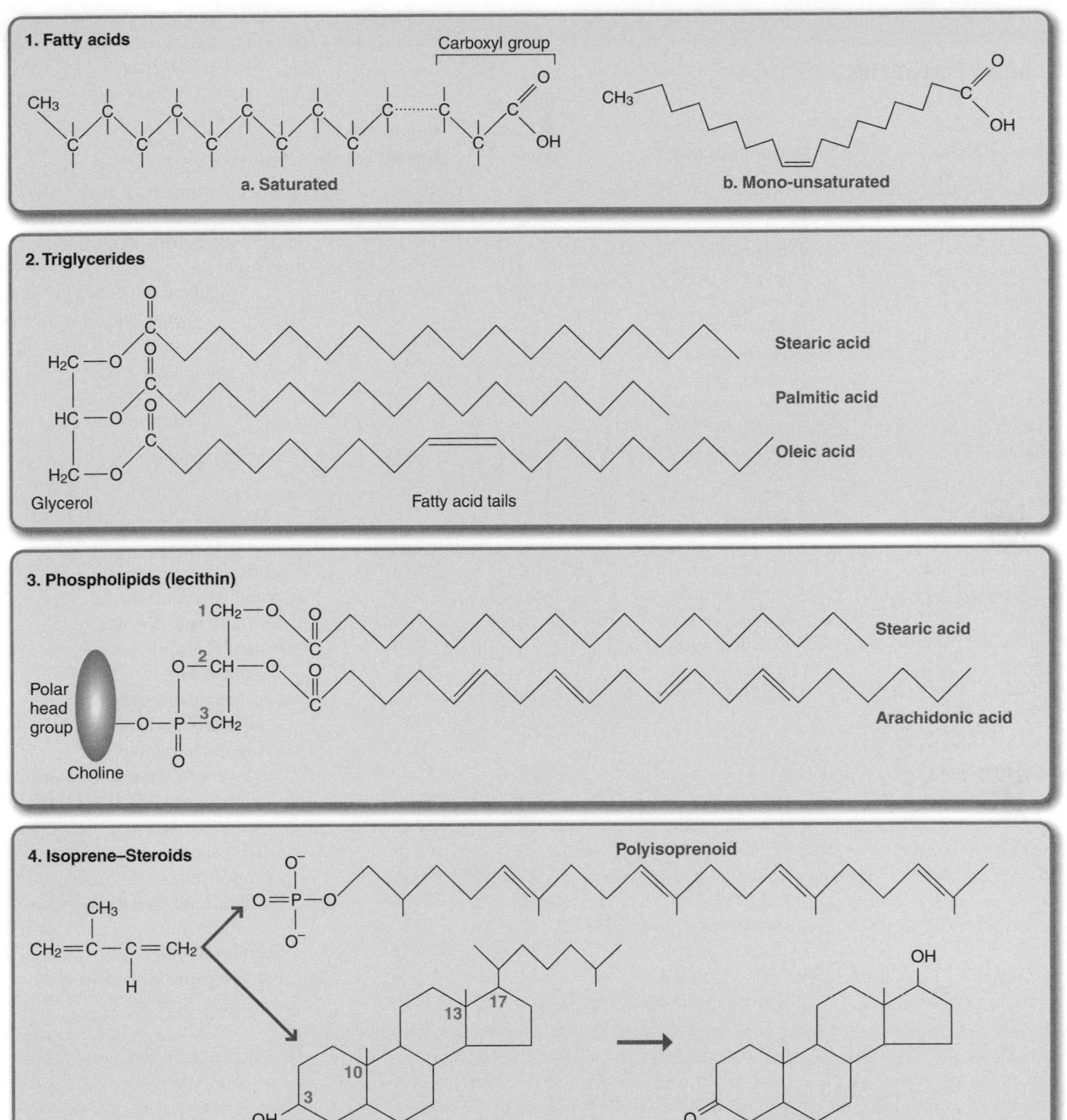

FIGURE 3-5 Structures of physiologically important fats and lipids.

omega-3 fatty acids from vegetable and marine sources. ALA can be obtained from flaxseed (57%), canola (8%), and soybean (7%) oils and green leaves in a few plants such as purslane. Sources of the longer EPA and DHA omega-3 fatty acids are primarily marine: cod liver oil, mackerel, salmon, and sardines, as well as crab, shrimp, and oysters (see Table 3-6).

Trans-Fatty Acids

In natural unsaturated fatty acids, the two carbons participating in a double bond each bind a hydrogen on the *same* side of the bond (the *cis*-isomer form), causing the fatty acid to bend (see Figure 3-5, *1*). The more double bonds per fatty acid, the more bends in the molecule. **Hydrogenation** of unsaturated fatty acids adds hydrogen to liquid oils to

TABLE 3-4

Common Fatty Acids

Common Name	Systematic Name	Number of Carbon Atoms*	Number of Double Bonds	Typical Fat Source
Saturated Fatty Acids				
Butyric	Butanoic	4	0	Butterfat
Caproic	Hexanoic	6	0	Butterfat
Caprylic	Octanolic	8	0	Coconut oil
Capric	Decanoic	10	0	Coconut oil
Lauric	Dodecanoic	12	0	Coconut oil, palm kernel oil
Myristic	Tetradecanoic	14	0	Butterfat, coconut oil
Palmitic	Hexadecanoic	16	0	Palm oil, animal fat
Stearic	Octadecanoic	18	0	Cocoa butter, animal fat
Arachidic	Elcosanoic	20	0	Peanut oil
Behenic	Docosanoic	22	0	Peanut oil
Unsaturated Fatty Acids				
Caproleic	9-Decenoic	10	1	Butterfat
Lauroleic	9-Dodecenoic	12	1	Butterfat
Myristoleic	9-Tetradecenoic	14	1	Butterfat
Palmitoleic	9-Hexadecenoic	16	1	Some fish oils, beef fat
Oleic	9-Octadecenoic	18	1	Olive oil, canola oil
Elaidic	9-Octadecenoic	18	1	Butterfat
Vacceric	11-Octadecenoic	18	1	Butterfat
Linoleic	9, 12-Octadecadienoic	18	2	Most vegetable oils, especially safflower, corn, soybean, cottonseed
Linolenic	9, 12, 15-Octadecatrienoic	18	3	Soybean oil, canola oil, walnuts, wheat germ oil, flaxseed oil
Gadoleic	9-Eicosenoic	20	1	Some fish oils
Arachidonic	5, 8, 11, 14-Eicosatetraenoic	20	4	Lard, meats
—	5, 8, 11, 14, 17-Eicosapentaenoic (EPA)	20	5	Some fish oils, shellfish
Erucic	13-Docosenoic	22	1	Canola oil
—	4, 7, 10, 13, 16, 19-Docosahexaenoic (DHA)	22	6	Some fish oils, shellfish

Modified from Institute of Shortening and Edible Oils: *Food fats and oils*, ed 6, Washington, DC, 1988, The Institute.

*All double bonds are in the *cis* configuration except for elaidic acid and vaccenic acid, which are *trans*.

form a stable, solid fat such as margarine. Hydrogen can be added both in the natural *cis* position (with two hydrogens on the same side of the double bond) and in the *trans* position (with one hydrogen on opposite sides of the double bond). Major sources of ***trans*-fatty acids** in the U.S. diet are chemically hydrogenated margarine, shortening, commercial frying fats, high-fat baked goods, and salty snacks containing these fats (see Table 32-8). Butter and animal fat can also contain *trans*-fatty acids from bacterial fermentation in the rumen of cows and sheep. It has been postulated that *trans*-fatty acids have a negative effect on human health due to their influence on membrane function.

Membrane function depends on the three-dimensional configuration of membrane fatty acids found in phospholip-ids. The *cis* double bonds in the membrane bend, allowing the fatty acids to pack loosely, thus making the membrane fluid. Because proteins embedded in a membrane float or sink, depending on the membrane's fluidity, membrane viscosity is important for membrane protein function. *Trans*-fatty acids do not bend; they pack into the membrane as tightly as if they were fully saturated. Clinical and epidemiologic studies suggest that higher intakes of *trans*-fatty acids are associated with increased risk for coronary heart disease, cancer, and other chronic diseases (including type 2 diabetes and allergies [Stender and Dyerberg, 2004]), possibly because of their potential to influence membrane fluidity (see Chapter 32). *Trans*-fatty acids have also been shown to inhibit the desaturation and elongation of linoleic and

TABLE 3-5

Fatty Acid Families

α-Linolenic Family (Omega-3)	Linoleic Family (Omega-6)	Oleic Family (Omega-9)
18:3 n-3 →18:4 n-3 linolenic ↓	18:2 n-6 →18:3 n-6 linoleic ↓	18:1 n-9 → 18:2 n-9 oleic ↓
20:4 n-3→20:5 n-3 eicosapentaenoic ↓	20:3 n-6→20:4 n-6 arachidonic ↓	20:2 n-9→20:3 n-9 eicosatrienoic* ↓
22:5 n-3→22:6 n-3 docosahexanoic	22:4 n-6→22:5 n-6 docosapentaenoic	

Elongation, ↓; desaturation, →
*Increases in essential fatty acid deficiency.

TABLE 3-6

Sources of Omega-3 Fatty Acids

Food Source (100 g Edible Portion, Raw)	Total Fat (g)	Omega-3 Fat DHA (22:6 ω-3) EPA (20:5 ω-3)
Sardines, in sardine oil	15.5	3.3
Mackerel, Atlantic	13.9	2.5
Herring, Atlantic	9	1.6
Salmon, Chinook	10.4	1.4
Anchovy	4.8	1.4
Salmon, Atlantic	5.4	1.2
Bluefish	6.5	1.2
Salmon, pink	3.4	1
Pompano, Florida	9.5	0.6
Tuna	2.5	0.5
Trout, brook	2.7	0.4
Shrimp	1.1	0.3
Catfish, channel	4.3	0.3
Lobster, northern	0.9	0.2
Haddock	0.7	0.2
Flounder	1	0.2

Modified from Conner SL, Conner WE: Are fish oils beneficial in the prevention and treatment of coronary artery disease? *Am J Clin Nutr* (suppl 4):1020-1031, 1997.

DHA, Docosahexenoic acid; *EPA,* eicosapentaenoic acid.

ALA to form long-chain essential fatty acids, as discussed previously. Long-chain PUFAs are critical for fetal brain and organ development (see Chapters 5 through 8). Until more is known about the extent of their risk, it is recommended that dietary consumption of hydrogenated and saturated fatty acids be reduced. The U.S. Department of Agriculture Dietary Guidelines for Americans (2005) recommends limiting intake of *trans*-fatty acids and saturated fatty acids to as little as possible (see *Clinical Insight:* Essential Fatty Acid Deficiency).

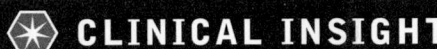

✳ CLINICAL INSIGHT

Essential Fatty Acid Deficiency

The consequences of reduced availability of omega-3 fatty acids are just now beginning to be understood. The human brain, central nervous system, and membranes throughout the body require omega-3 fatty acids, especially eicosapentaenoic acid (EPA) and docosahexaenoic acid (DHA), for optimum function. Connor et al. (1992) proposed that greater availability of long-chain omega-3 fatty acids allowed humans to develop their complex brain and neural system. An animal deficient in omega-3 fatty acids grows and reproduces normally but is at risk for developing learning problems, impaired vision, and polydipsia.

The impact of omega-3 fatty acids on cardiovascular disease, arthritis, cancer, and other chronic diseases, as well as on altered immune and mental states, including attention deficit hyperactivity disorder and depression, is under intense study. Abnormal omega-6/omega-3 ratios have been linked to changes in vascular membrane lipid composition and increased incidence of atherosclerosis and inflammatory disorders (see Chapters 32, 40, and 42). Deficiencies of omega-6 essential fatty acids also have clinical implications, including growth retardation, skin lesions, reproductive failure, fatty liver, and polydipsia. Fat-free diets may lead to essential fatty acid deficiencies and eventually death if the missing nutrient is not provided.

Triglycerides

The body forms **triglycerides (triacylglycerols)** (TAG) by joining three fatty acids to a glycerol side chain (see Figure 3-5, *2*), thereby neutralizing reactive fatty acids and making triglycerides water insoluble (hydrophobic). Neutral fats can be safely transported in the blood and stored in fat cells (adipocytes) as an energy reserve. More than 95% of lipids in the food supply are in the triglyceride storage form. As indicated in Figure 3-5, 2, the hydroxyl group on each fatty acid is bound to a hydroxyl group on glycerol, releasing water and forming an ester linkage. Different fatty acids can comprise a single triglyceride and are dependent on the dietary fatty acids and the amount of synthesis taking place. SFAs are relatively inert and not susceptible to oxidative damage during storage. Thus storage triglycerides from land animals are predominately saturated. Cold-water creatures must maintain their fatty acids in liquid form even at low temperatures; therefore triglycerides in fish oils and marine-derived fats contain even longer (C20 and C22) and highly unsaturated fatty acids.

Phospholipids

Phospholipids are derivatives of phosphatidic acid, a triglyceride modified to contain a phosphate group at the third position (see Figure 3-5, 3). Phosphatidic acid is esterified into a nitrogen-containing molecule, usually a choline, serine, inositol, or ethanolamine, and named for its nitrogenous base (e.g., phosphatidylcholine, phosphatidylserine). Membrane phospholipids usually contain one SFA (C16 to C18) at C-1 and a highly PUFA (C16 to C20) at C-2, usually one of the essential fatty acids. ALA (C18:3 ω-3), arachidonic acid (C20:4 ω-6), and omega-3 substitutes can be cleaved from the lipid bilayer

and provide substrate for synthesis of prostaglandins and other local mediators of cell activity, as noted previously. Because it is polar at physiologic pH, the phosphate-containing portion of the molecule forms hydrogen bonds with water, whereas the two fatty acids have hydrophobic interactions with other fatty acids (Figure 3-6). The polar head groups face outward into the aqueous external and cytoplasmic fluids, whereas the centrally placed fatty acid tails participate in hydrophobic interactions at the membrane center. The barrier formed by this lipid bilayer can only be crossed by very small lipid soluble molecules (e.g., oxygen, carbon dioxide, and nitrogen) and to a limited extent by small, uncharged polar molecules such as water and urea.

Lecithin (phosphatidylcholine) is a major phospholipid, and it is the primary component of lipid in the membrane lipid bilayer. Lecithin is also a major component of lipoproteins (i.e., VLDLs, low-density lipoproteins [LDLs], HDLs) used to transport fats and cholesterol. Lecithin is made by the body de novo (but with the essential fatty acid, arachidonic acid) and is widely distributed in the food supply. Because all cells contain lecithin as a lipid bilayer component, animal products, especially liver and egg yolks, are rich sources of lecithin. Plant products such as soybeans, peanuts, legumes, spinach, and wheat germ are also rich sources. Lecithin is added to food products such as margarine, ice cream, snack crackers, and confections as a stabilizer.

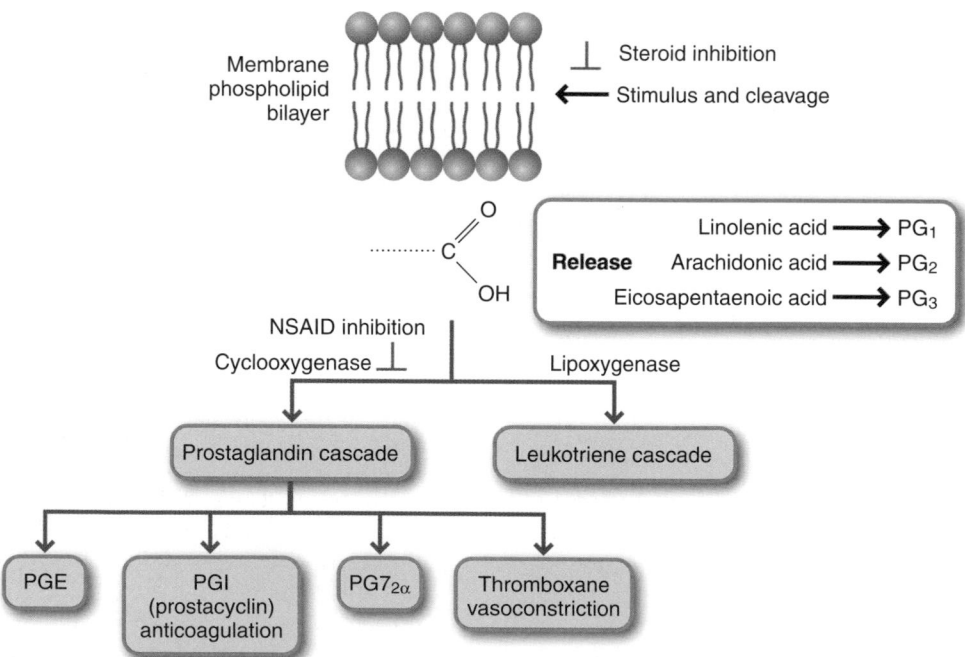

FIGURE 3-6 Eicosanoid synthesis after phospholipid cleavage in the biomembrane. Injury, inflammation, and other stimuli cleave the highly unsaturated fatty acid at the C-2 position of the membrane phospholipid. Arachidonic acid (AA) or eicosapentaenoic acid (EPA) is the major fatty acid released; the pathway entered depends on the degree to which the target tissue expresses the enzyme. The cyclooxygenase pathway leads to prostaglandin (PG), thromboxane, and prostacyclin synthesis. The lipoxygenase pathway, which is common in the lungs and bronchi, leads to leukotriene synthesis and subsequent bronchoconstriction. Note the point at which steroidal and nonsteroidal antiinflammatory drugs (NSAIDs) act.

Sphingolipids, Alcohols, Waxes, Isoprenoids, and Steroids

All organisms produce small amounts of complex lipids with specialized, critical functions. Many of these lipids do not contain glycerol and are built from two-carbon **acetyl coenzyme A (acetyl CoA)** units. *Sphingolipids* are lipid esters attached to a sphingosine base rather than a glycerol. They are widely distributed in the nervous systems of animals and the membranes of plants and lower eukaryotes such as yeast. Sphingomyelin includes the nitrogenous base choline and makes up more than 25% of the myelin sheath, the lipid-rich structure that protects and insulates cells of the central nervous system. In addition to phosphatidylcholine, sphingomyelin is found in all membranes. Sphingolipidoses comprise a group of genetic lipid storage diseases in which normal sphingolipid degradation is blocked. Tay-Sachs disease is an example of such a lipid storage disease.

Long-chain alcohols are metabolic by-products of lipids. The feces contain cetyl alcohol, a by-product of palmitic acid. Beeswax is rich in the alcohol myricyl palmitate. Waxes consist of LCFAs bound to long-chain alcohols. These molecules are almost completely water insoluble and often used as water repellants, as they are in the feathers of birds and on the leaves of plants.

Isoprenoids, activated derivatives of isoprene, are an extraordinarily large and diverse group of lipids built from one or more five-carbon units. Isoprene contains alternating single and double (conjugated) bonds, an arrangement that can quench free radicals by accepting or donating electrons. Terpene is a generic term for all compounds synthesized from isoprene precursors and includes essential oils of plants (e.g., turpentine from trees and limonene from lemons). Plant pigments that transfer electrons in photosynthesis are also isoprenoids and include lycopene (the red pigment in tomatoes), carotenoids (the yellow and orange pigments in squash and carrots), and the yellow/green chlorophyll group. Fat-soluble vitamins A, D, E, and K and the electron transducer coenzyme Q have isoprenoid structures. Vitamin E, lycopene, and β-carotene are effective antioxidants (see Table 9-1 and Appendix 47). Nonnutritive phytochemicals with antioxidant function usually have an isoprenoid structure (see Chapter 9).

Steroids constitute a class of lipids derived from a four-membered saturated ring (see Figure 3-5, *4*). **Cholesterol** is the basis for all steroid derivatives made in the body, including glucocorticoids (cortisone) and mineralocorticoids (aldosterone), which are made in the adrenal gland, androgens (testosterone) and estrogens (estradiol) made in the testes and ovaries, respectively, and bile acids made in the liver. Vitamin D hormone is made when ultraviolet rays from the sun cleave cholesterol in subcutaneous fat to form cholecalciferol (D_3). Synthetic vitamin D is made by irradiating the plant steroid ergosterol to form ergocalciferol (D_2).

Cholesterol also plays an important role in membrane function. The rigid, four-ringed cholesterol molecule is bound into the hydrophobic membrane by its hydroxyl group. The stiff, planar rings spread apart and partially immobilize the fatty acid chains near the polar region. At the same time, the nonpolar hydrocarbon tail contributes to greater fluidity in the interior of the membrane. Plasma membranes contain large amounts of cholesterol—up to one molecule for every phospholipid molecule.

Glycolipids include the cerebrosides and gangliosides, which are composed of a sphingosine base and very long–chain (22C) fatty acids. Cerebrosides contain galactose; gangliosides also contain glucose and a complex compound containing an amino sugar. Structurally both compounds are components of nerve tissue and certain cell membranes, where they play a role in lipid transport.

Synthetic Lipids

Medium-chain triglycerides (MCTs) are SFAs with a chain length of between 6 and 12 carbons. Although MCTs occur naturally in milk fat, coconut oil, and palm kernel oil, they are also produced commercially (MCT oil) as a by-product of margarine production. MCT oils provide 8.25 kcal/g and are of value in a number of clinical situations (see discussions in Chapters 27 and 41) because they are short enough to be water soluble, require less bile salt for solubilization, are not reesterified in the enterocyte, and are transported as free fatty acids, bound to albumin, through the portal system. Because the portal blood flow rate is about 250 times faster than the lymph flow, MCTs are digested quickly and not likely to be affected by intestinal factors that inhibit fat absorption. They are not stored in adipose tissue but are oxidized to acetic acid.

Structured lipids include MCT oil esterified with a desired fatty acid such as linoleic acid or an omega-3 lipid. The combined product is absorbed faster than the long-chain triglyceride alone. Clinically, structured lipids are being studied for their role in parenteral and enteral formulas in specific situations (e.g., to enhance immune function or athletic performance).

Fat replacers (Table 3-7) are structurally different from fats and do not provide readily absorbable nutrients. Their commercial importance is that they imitate the texture and other sensations of fat, especially in the mouth. Fat replacers differ in their macronutrient base and the extent to which they mimic the characteristics of fat. The caloric value of these substitutes varies between 5 kcal/g (e.g., caprenin) and 0 kcal/g (e.g., olestra, carrageenan).

The largest group of fat replacers is derived from plant polysaccharides such as gums, cellulose, dextrins, fiber, maltodextrins, starches, and polydextrose Olestra is a sucrose polyester in which sucrose is esterified with six to eight fatty acids to form esters. The fatty acid chains range in length from 12 to 24 carbons and are derived from edible oils such as soybean, cottonseed, and corn oils. The product has the physical properties of natural dietary fats. Because they are nonabsorbable, sucrose polyesters do not contribute calories to the diet.

Protein-based fat replacers alter the texture of a product in various ways. Microparticulated proteins can act like small ball bearings, providing a fatlike feeling in the mouth. These replacers contribute between 1.3 and 4 kcal/g and augment the protein content of the food. Note that some of

TABLE 3-7

Examples of Fat Replacers and Their Functions and Properties

Class of Fat Replacers	Trade Names	Applications	Functional Properties
Carbohydrate Based			
Polydextrose	Litesse,[a] Sta-Lite[b]	Dairy products, sauces, frozen desserts, salad dressings, baked goods, confections, gelatins, puddings, meat products, chewing gum, dry cake and cookie mixes, frostings and icings	Moisture retention, bulking agent, texturizer
Starch (modified food starch)	Amalean I & II,[c] N-Lite,[d] Instant Stellar,[e] Sta-Slim,[b] OptaGrade,[e] Pure-gel[f]	Processed meats, salad dressings, baked goods, fillings and frostings, condiments, frozen desserts, dairy products	Gelling, thickening, stabilizing, texturizer
Maltodextrins	CrystaLean,[e] Maltrin,[f] Lycadex,[g] Star-Dri,[b] Paselli Excell,[h] Rice-Trim[i]	Baked goods, dairy products, salad dressings, spreads, sauces, fillings and frostings, processed meat, frozen desserts, extruded products	Gelling, thickening, stabilizing, texturizer
Grain based (fiber)	Betatrim,[j] Opta[e] Oat Fibere,[k] Snowite[k] TrimChoice,[b] Fibrim[l]	Baked goods, meats, extruded products, spreads	Gelling, thickening, stabilizing, texturizer
Dextrins	N-Oil,[d] Stadex[b]	Salad dressings, puddings, spreads, dairy products, frozen desserts, chips, baked goods, meat products, frostings, soups	Gelling, thickening, stabilizing, texturizer
Gums (xanthan, guar, locust bean carrageenan, alginates)	Kelcogel,[m] Keltrol,[n] Viscarin,[o] Gel-carin,[o] Fibrex,[p] Novagel,[q] Rohodi-gel,[j] Jaguar[r]	Salad dressings, processed meats, formulated foods (e.g., desserts, processed meats)	Water retention, texturizer, thickener, mouth texture, stabilizer
Pectin	Grindsted,[s] Slendid,[t] Splendid[t]	Baked goods, soups, sauces, dressings	Gelling, thickening, mouth texture
Cellulose (carboxymethyl cellulose, microcrystalline cellulose)	Avicel,[q] cellulose gel, Methocel,[u] Solka-Floc,[v] Just Fiber[w]	Dairy products, sauces, frozen desserts, salad dressings	Water retention, texturizer, stabilizer, mouth texture
Fruit Based (fiber)	Prune paste, dried plum paste, Lighter Bake,[x] WonderSlim[y] fruit powder	Baked goods, candy, dairy products	Moisturizer, mouth texture
Protein Based	Simplesse,[z] K-Blazer[aa] Dairy-lo,[bb] Veri-lo,[bb] Ultra-Bake,[b] Powerpro,[cc] Proplus,[dd] Supro[dd]	Cheese, mayonnaise, butter, salad dressing, sour cream, spreads, bakery products	Mouth texture
Fat Based	Caprenin,[ee] Olean,[ee] Benefat,[bb] Dur-Em[w] Dur-Lo[w]	Chocolate, confections, bakery products, savory snacks	Mouth texture
Combinations	Prolestra,[ff] Nutrifat,[ff] Finesse[ff]	Ice cream, salad oils, mayonnaise, spreads, sauces, bakery products	Mouth texture

From American Dietetic Association: Position of the American Dietetic Association: fat replacers, *J Am Diet Assoc* 98:463, 1998.

[a]Cultor Food Science, Inc, Ardsley, N.Y.
[b]AE Staley manufacturing Co, Decatur, Ill.
[c]Cerestar USA, Inc, Hammond, Ind.
[d]National Starch and Chemical Co. Bridgewater, N.J.
[e]Opta Food Ingredients, Bedford, Mass.
[f]Grain Processing Corp, Muscatine, Iowa.
[g]Roquette America, Inc, Keokuk, Iowa.
[h]AVEBE America Inc, Princeton, N.J.
[i]Zumbro, Inc, Hayfield, Minn.
[j]Rhone-Poulenc, Inc, Cranbury, N.J.
[k]Canadian Harvest USA, Cambridge, Minn.
[l]Protein Technologies International, Pryor, Okla.
[m]Monsanto, Chicago, Ill.
[n]Kelco, Division of Merck, Clark, N.J.
[o]FMC Corp, Rockland, Me.
[p]Purity Foods, Okemos, Mich.

[q]FMC Corp, Philadelphia, Pa.
[r]Aston Chemicals, Aylesbury, Buckinghamshire, England.
[s]Danisco, New Century, Ky.
[t]Hercules Inc, Wilmington, Del.
[u]Dow Chemical, Midland, Mich.
[v]Fiber Sales and Development Corp, Green Brook, N.J.
[w]Loders Croklaan, Glen Ellyn, Ill.
[x]Sunsweet Growers, Yuba City, Calif.
[y]The Heart Garden Corporation, Los Angeles, Calif.
[z]Nutrasweet, San Diego, Calif.
[aa]Kraft Food Ingredients, Memphis, Ind.
[bb]Cultor Food Science, Ardsley, N.Y.
[cc]Land O'Lakes Food Division, Arden Hill, Minn.
[dd]Protein Technologies International, St Louis, Mo.
[ee]Procter and Gamble, Cincinnati, Ohio.
[ff]Reach Associates, South Orange, N.J.

these proteins can stimulate an allergic or antigenic response in susceptible individuals (see Chapter 29).

Fat sources can be modified to reduce GI absorption, thereby reducing caloric availability. **Monoacylglycerides (monoglycerols)** and **diacylglycerols (diglycerides)** are used as emulsifiers and contribute to the sensory properties of fat but have fewer calories (approximately 5 kcal/g). Salatrim (an SFA and an LCFA triglyceride molecule) also contains approximately 5 kcal/g because of reduced absorbability.

Concerns about the long-term effects of fat substitutes center on their ability to bind essential fatty acids and fat-soluble vitamins and contribute to their malabsorption. However, under most circumstances they appear to be safe, effective, and feasible alternatives for controlling fat and energy in diets (The American Dietetic Association, 2005).

Recommendations for Lipid Intake

Recommendations for lipid intake must take into account the documented physiologic and health effects of various lipid components, as well as the growing obesity epidemic in the United States and the world. For example, saturated fatty acids are known to increase LDLs and HDLs, whereas PUFAs decrease the "bad" and "good" lipoproteins. The 2005 Dietary Guidelines for Americans (USDA) recommended the consumption of less than 10% of calories as SFA. On the other hand, too much PUFA can be dangerous. Double bonds are highly reactive and bind oxygen to form peroxides when exposed to air or heat. When subjected to routine frying or cooking, PUFAs can generate high levels of toxic aldehyde products that promote cardiovascular disease and cancer. SFAs and MFAs, especially those in olive oil, that are similarly thermally stressed do not produce these toxic products. Saturated fat and partially hydrogenated oils have fewer oxygen-binding sites and thereby have increased stability and a longer shelf life; however, their intake is associated with greater risk of cardiovascular disease. The association between high serum cholesterol concentrations and risk for heart disease is well documented, and current guidelines recommend a dietary cholesterol intake of less than 300 mg/day (see Chapter 32). In addition, the guidelines recommend that the consumption of *trans*-fatty acids from partially hydrogenated oils be kept to a minimum and that total fat intake be kept between 20% to 35% of total calories with most of the fat coming from PUFA and MFAs.

Alcohol (Ethyl Alcohol)

Although moderate amounts of ethyl alcohol have been reported to have positive effects on such diseases as cardiovascular disease (Corder et al., 2006), it is still a toxic substance that contains approximately 7 kcal/g and no other nutrients. It is able to permeate all membranes and is absorbed quickly and easily. It is metabolized primarily by the liver enzyme alcohol dehydrogenase (ADH) to acetaldehyde and then to acetyl-CoA, where it can be used to synthesize fat or enter the tricarboxylic acid (TCA) cycle. ADH requires both thiamin and niacin to function. When the amount of alcohol in the cell exceeds the capacity of alcohol dehydrogenase to metabolize it or when niacin (as NAD^+) is depleted, the microsomal ethanol oxidizing system (MEOS) will also metabolize alcohol to acetaldehyde. Chronic alcohol consumption induces both ADH and certain enzymes in the MEOS system. Since the MEOS system is also responsible for the metabolism of many drugs, chronic ingestion of large amounts of alcohol (alcoholism) can alter drug responses in unpredictable ways. For example, overall alcoholism leading to induction of the MEOS causes a person to be tolerant not only of alcohol but other drugs as well. But, if at any given time the MEOS is saturated with alcohol, drugs are not metabolized at the expected rate, and a drug overdose can occur. In addition the production of acetaldehyde in these pathways may be toxic in itself leading to cirrhosis of the liver.

AMINO ACIDS AND PROTEIN

Whereas plant structures are primarily composed of carbohydrates, the body structure of humans and animals is built on protein. **Proteins** differ molecularly from carbohydrates and lipids in that they contain nitrogen. Primary roles for proteins in the body include structural protein, enzymes, hormones, transport, and immunoproteins. Proteins are comprised of amino acids (Figure 3-7) linked by **peptide bonds** (Figure 3-8). The sequence of the amino acids determines the ultimate structure and function of the protein and is determined by the genetic code stored in the cell nucleus as deoxyribonucleic acid (DNA) (see Chapter 13). As illustrated in Figure 3-9, protein synthesis is a complex process through which the protein pattern is copied from DNA to ribonucleic acid (RNA). The pattern for protein synthesis is carried to the rough endoplasmic reticulum via messenger RNA (mRNA). New proteins are built by attaching amino acids as dictated by the mRNA in a precise linear sequence. When the protein has been built, it detaches from the message and is ready to be used or further processed for use (see *Focus On*: DNA Transcription and RNA Translation).

Proper folding of the completed linear amino acid chain is essential for a protein to perform its unique functions. The linear sequence of individual amino acids dictates the configuration of the mature protein. As indicated in Figure 3-9, R groups protrude from the newly synthesized peptide chain and are in position to react with each other. Folding is accomplished through hydrogen bonding, ionic bonding, and hydrophobic and other interactions between individual R groups on each amino acid. For example, a negative charge on one amino acid R group forms an attraction with a positive charge on another. This allows the protein to form a precise, three-dimensional structure. Proteins have four levels of structure, as indicated here:

1. *Primary structure:* Peptide bonds are formed between sequential amino acids according to directions on mRNA. The completed protein is a linear chain of amino acids.
2. *Secondary structure:* Attractions between R groups of amino acids create helices and pleated sheet structures.

All amino acids have the same general structure (structure shown: $O=C(OH)-C^{\alpha}(NH_2)(H)-R$) in which R is different for each.

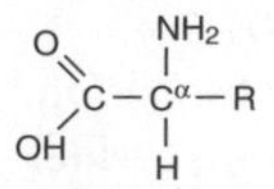

FUNCTIONAL TYPE	AMINO ACID (abbr.)	R GROUP	CHARACTERISTICS OF THE AMINO ACID
Aliphatic	Glycine (Gly) G	H	Tiny R group (H), which allows hairpin bends in the peptide chains
	Alanine (Ala) A	CH_3	Can be deaminated to pyruvate and used for glucose synthesis
	Valine (Val) V*	$-CH(CH_3)_2$	Branched-chain amino acids; metabolized in muscle
	Leucine (Leu) L*	$-CH_2-CH(CH_3)_2$	Branched-chain amino acids more hydophobic; muscle metabolism
	Isoleucine (Ile) I*	$-CH(CH_3)-CH_2-CH_3$	Branched-chain amino acids most hydophobic; muscle metabolism
Sulfur	Cysteine (Cys) C**	$-CH_2-SH$	Essential for glutatione synthesis; synthesis limited in chronic diseases
	Methionine (Met) M*	$-CH_2-CH_2-S-CH_2$	Converted to S-adenosylmethionine (SAM), the universal methyl donor, and cysteine
Hydroxyl	Serine (Ser) S	$-CH_2-OH$	Hydroxyl group phosphorylated to activate and inactivate protein
	Threonine (Thr) T	$-CH_2-OH-CH_3$	Also site for regulatory phosphorylation
Aromatic	Phenylalanine (Phe) F*	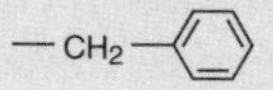 $-CH_2-$ (benzene ring)	Converted to tyrosine for synthesis of norepinephrine, epinephrine, and dopamine
	Tyrosine (Tyr) Y	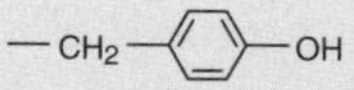 $-CH_2-$ (phenol ring, OH)	Converted to neurotransmitters norepinephrine, epinephrine, and dopamine
	Tryptophan (Trp) W*	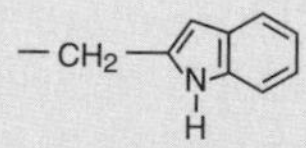 $-CH_2-$ (indole ring)	Converted to neurotransmitter serotonin and to niacin
Cyclic	Proline (Pro) P*	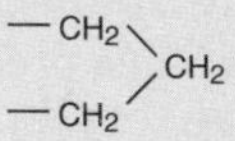 $-CH_2-CH_2-CH_2$ (ring)	Allows triple helix; proline in collagen to be hydroxylated for cross-linkage
Basic	Lysine (Lys) K	$-CH_2-CH_2-CH_2-CH_2-\overset{+}{N}H_3$	Site for hydroxylation in proteins; hydrophylic; used in signaling
	Histidine (His) H**	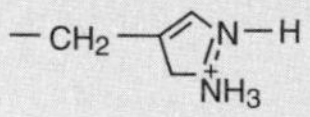 $-CH_2-$ (imidazole ring, N-H, $\overset{+}{N}H_3$)	Hydrophilic, binds zinc in signaling proteins
	Arginine (Arg) R	$-CH_2-CH_2-CH_2-NH-C(=\overset{+}{N}H_2)-NH_2$	Formed in the urea cycle; essential for synthesis of nitric oxide signaling pathway
Acidic	Aspartic acid (Asp) D	$-CH_2-C(=O)-O^-$	Takes a second nitrogen to form asparagine (Asn) N $-CH_2-C(=O)-NH_2$
	Glutamic acid (Glu) E	$-CH_2-CH_2-C(=O)-O^-$	Takes a second nitrogen to form glutamine (Gln) Q $-CH_2-CH_2-C(=O)-NH_2$

FIGURE 3-7 Structures and functions of the 20 amino acids required by humans. All amino acids have the same general structure, but the R group is different for each. Amino acids are abbreviated using a three-letter and single-letter code. Amino acids marked with an asterisk (*) are essential; those marked with double asterisks (**) are essential for infants and those with certain chronic diseases.

3. *Tertiary structure:* Helices and pleated sheets are folded into compact domains. Small proteins have one domain, and large proteins have multiple domains.

4. *Quaternary structure:* Individual polypeptides can serve as subunits in the formation of larger assemblies, or complexes. Subunits are bound together by numerous weak, noncovalent interactions; sometimes they are stabilized by disulfide bonds. For example, four hemoglobin monomers are joined to form the tetramer hemoglobin molecule.

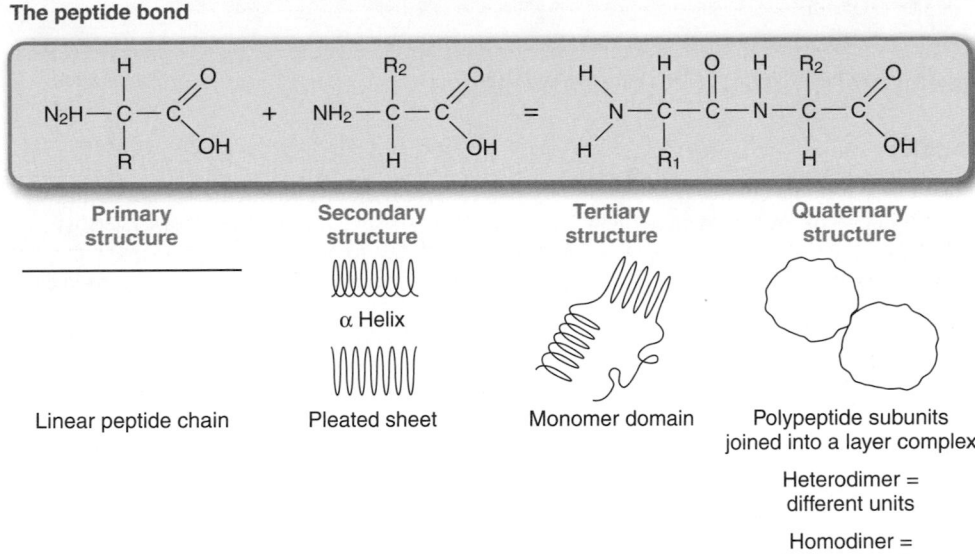

FIGURE 3-8 The peptide bond and protein folding.

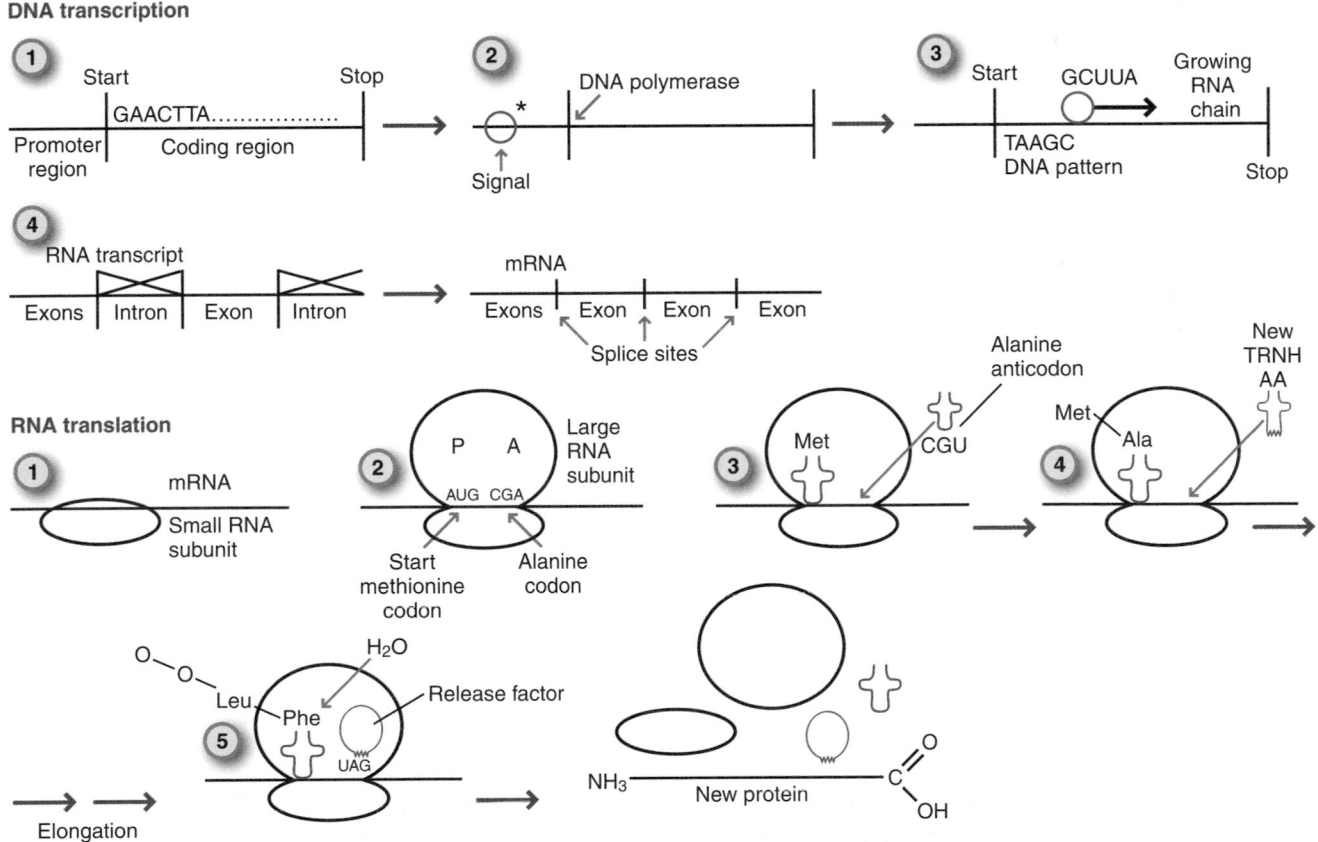

FIGURE 3-9 Summary of DNA transcription and RNA translation in the eukaryotic cell.

Protein structure is a critical component of protein function. The active and catalytic sites at which protein action occurs are formed by juxtaposing functional groups from nearby but occasionally distant R groups. If the linear protein sequence is altered, as it is in those with certain genetic diseases, the protein is unable to form active sites, and its activity may be reduced or eliminated entirely.

Essential Amino Acids

Synthesis of proteins requires the presence of all necessary amino acids during the process. Chemically **amino acids** are carboxylic acids with an amino group attached to the α-carbon (see Figure 3-7). All amino acids have this same general structure; it is the side chain also attached to the α-carbon (the R group), which dictates the identity and function of

◎ FOCUS ON

DNA Transcription and RNA Translation

DNA Transcription*

1. All cells have the ability to make all proteins needed by the body. The linear sequence of each protein is dictated by the linear sequence of nucleotide bases: thymine, adenine, guanine, and cytosine. A linear sequence of three bases, or codon, codes for each of the 20 amino acids. Because the four bases can be combined in 64 ways, more than one three-base codon can code for a single amino acid.
2. As they differentiate, cells inactivate various regions of the DNA that codes for specific proteins. For example, only the precursor to the red blood cell makes hemoglobin. The gene for hemoglobin is inactivated in all other differentiated cells.
3. In front of each coding region is a promoter region. The promoter region receives a signal that the protein is needed. Nutrients, including vitamins A and D and minerals such as zinc, play major roles in regulating gene expression in the promoter region.
4. When nutrients and other molecules bind to the promoter region, RNA polymerase binds to the start code in the coding region, opens the DNA double helix, and builds a new RNA chain complementary to the DNA coding region.
5. When the RNA polymerase reaches the stop code at the end of the protein coding region, polymerase detaches, releasing the completed RNA transcript. The DNA helix re-forms, and the RNA transcript is modified to remove introns, which are intervening, noncoding sequences that are not part of the final protein pattern. The modified RNA transcript is called messenger RNA (mRNA).

6. At the same time, in another region of the DNA, RNA polymerase molecules make copies of ribosomal RNA (rRNA) and transfer RNA (tRNA).
7. The mRNA, rRNA, and tRNA leave the nucleus and enter the cytoplasm (see Figure 3-9).

RNA Translation*

1. Small rRNA subunits are activated and bind mRNA. Large rRNA subunits bind and hold the mRNA firmly. The mRNA is sandwiched between the two rRNA subunits, and two three-base codons are available for binding tRNA.
2. Each of 20 tRNA types binds the amino acid that matches its anticodon region. The tRNA, with its attached amino acid and matching anticodon, recognizes its mRNA codon. This process ensures that the linear amino acid sequence is an exact representation of the original DNA code.
3. After each tRNA binds the A site, its amino acid is linked to the growing peptide chain by an enzyme, peptidyl transferase, which forms a peptide bond between the end carboxyl and the amino group of the incoming amino acid.
4. The ribosome moves forward. The tRNA is now attached to the peptide chain in the P (peptide) site, and another tRNA enters.
5. The stop codon, UAG, signals the end of the protein. A release factor binds at the A site and attaches a water molecule to the peptide chain, creating the carboxyl (COOH) terminus. The newly formed peptide chain detaches, and the tRNA and rRNA units separate.

*See Figure 3-9.

DNA, Deoxyribonucleic acid; *RNA*, ribonucleic acid.

---

each amino acid. Note that the α-carbon is a chiral carbon, and isomers can be formed. It is the L-isomer that is functional in the human body. Many amino acids can be synthesized from carbon skeletons produced as intermediates in the major metabolic pathways by a process called **transamination,** which adds an amino group from another amino acid without actually producing a free amino group. Transamination is an important process because it allows for the production of **nonessential amino acids** from metabolic intermediates while using free amino groups, so that they are not left to produce toxic ammonia. For example, pyruvate formed during glycolysis is easily converted to the amino acid alanine by adding an amino group via the enzyme alanine aminotransaminase. On the other hand, **essential amino acids** have carbon skeletons that humans cannot make (or cannot make enough) and can obtain only from the diet (Table 3-8).

Protein can also be an energy source. Proteins contain over 5 kcal/g. However, using protein for energy necessi-

tates the removal of the amino group and the formation and excretion of urea in a process involving **deamination,** which has a metabolic cost of over 1 kcal/g. Therefore the resulting carbon skeleton product can be used for energy at the rate of 4 kcal/g. These carbon skeletons can also be used to produce glucose; in fact, when the diet is low in carbohydrate or an individual is starving, protein is the only good source of de novo synthesis of glucose available. The process of de novo synthesis of glucose is called gluconeogenesis. Oxaloacetate is moved out of the mitochondria and converted to phospho*enol*pyruvate (PEP) (see Figure 3-2). From PEP the glycolytic pathway can be reversed because all the enzymes with the exception of phosphofructokinase and glucokinase are reversible. Both of these enzymes can be reversed by specific phosphatase enzyme when there is a need for blood glucose. Since glucokinase is found primarily in the liver, it is only reversed there, making the liver the primary site for de novo synthesis of blood glucose. Amino acids that produce carbon skeletons that can be converted to

TABLE 3-8

Estimates of Amino Acid Requirements

| Amino Acid | Requirements (mg/kg/day) by Age-Group | | | |
	Infants, Age 3-4 mo*	Children, Age ~2 yr†	Children, Age 10-12 yr‡	Adults§
Histidine	28	Not determined	Not determined	8-12
Isoleucine	70	31	28	10
Leucine	161	73	44	14
Lysine	103	64	44	12
Methionine plus cystine	58	27	22	13
Phenylalanine plus tyrosine	125	69	22	14
Threonine	87	37	28	7
Tryptophan	17	12.5	3.3	3.5
Valine	93	38	25	10
Total without histidine	714	352	216	84

Modified from World Health Organization: *Energy and protein requirements report of a joint FAO/WHO/UNU expert consultation*, Technical Report Series 724, p. 65, Geneva, 1985, WHO.

*Based on amounts of amino acids in human milk or cow's milk formulas fed at levels that supported good growth.

†Based on achievement of nitrogen balance sufficient to support adequate lean tissue gain (16 mg nitrogen/kg/day).

‡Based on upper range of requirement for positive nitrogen balance.

§Based on highest estimate of requirement to achieve nitrogen balance.

glucose are called glucogenic amino acids. Only two of the 20 amino acids cannot be used to produce at least some glucose. These amino acids are lysine and threonine. They produce products that are converted to ketones and used for energy, thus they are known as ketogenic amino acids.

According to current recommendations, a healthy adult human requires 0.8 g of protein per kilogram of healthy body weight (Institute of Medicine, Food and Nutrition Board, 2002). To obtain this quantity of protein, humans benefit when dietary protein makes up approximately 10% to 15% of total energy intake. Protein requirements increase during times of stress and disease (see Chapter 39). Protein-rich foods are obtained primarily from animal flesh or animal products such as eggs and milk. Most plant foods are relatively poor sources of protein, with the exception of legumes and beans.

Dietary Protein Quality

As noted previously, the ability to synthesize all of the proper proteins for the body depends on the availability of all necessary amino acids. Therefore the quality of a dietary protein is dependent on its amino acid makeup and the bioavailablity of these amino acids. A number of methods have been used to measure the quality of proteins based on one or both of these properties. More than 50 years ago, Block and Mitchel (1946) determined that a protein's biologic value could be determined by the essential amino acid profile compared with human requirements. The essential amino acid which occurred in the least concentration compared to human requirement was the **limiting amino acid,** from which a "chemical score" of protein quality could be calculated.

Protein quality is also determined by measuring the amount of protein actually used by an organism; *net protein utilization (NPU)* is the one method of doing so. Dietary protein is equated with its metabolic products by measuring nitrogen in the diet and biologic samples and converting it to the amount of protein on the basis of the formula (nitrogen [grams] $\times$ 6.25 = protein [grams]). The nitrogen content in the bodies of protein test animals is compared with the nitrogen in the carcasses of an experimental group fed a protein-free diet for the same length of time. The gain in nitrogen is compared with the nitrogen intake, and the proportion of nitrogen retained in the body is computed to obtain the NPU. The NPU ranges from approximately 40 to 94, with protein from animal products scoring higher and protein from vegetables scoring lower.

Care must be taken when using animals in trials for determining the quality of a protein for humans. For example, soy protein originally received a low NPU score when tested with rats until it was recognized that methionine, which is low in soy protein, is a limiting amino acid for rats. Rats require approximately 50% more methionine than humans (Sarwar et al., 1985). The World Health Organization (WHO) and the U.S. Food and Drug Administration (FDA) adopted a **protein digestibility corrected amino acid score (PDCAAS)** as the official assay for evaluating protein quality in the human. The PDCAAS is based on amino acid requirements of children ages 2 to 5 years and represents the **amino acid score** after correcting for digestibility (Messina, 1995). After being corrected for digestibility, proteins that provide amino acids equal to or in excess of requirements receive a PDCAAS of 1. Soy protein has a PDCAAS of 1 and meets protein needs of human adults when consumed as a sole source of protein at the rate of at least 0.6 g/kg of body weight (Young, 1991).

Digestibility is a major factor affecting protein quality, and the digestibility of protein sources is affected by multiple factors. Meat preparation procedures often involve wine or vinegar marinades and moist heat to tenderize tough cuts of meat through **denaturation.** Proteins are kept in their functional three-dimensional structure by hydrogen and ionic interactions; these bonds loosen in the presence of acid, salt, and heat. Because they denature proteins, these methods also soften gristle, or connective tissue proteins, and release muscle proteins from their attachments, thereby making all proteins more available to digestive enzymes.

Vegetable protein is less well digested than animal protein, partly because it is encased in carbohydrate cell walls and is less available to digestive enzymes. Some plants also contain enzymes that interfere with protein digestion; thus the enzymes must be heat inactivated before consumption. For example, soybeans contain a trypsinase that inactivates trypsin, the major protein-digesting enzyme in the intestine.

Food processing can also damage amino acids and reduce their digestive availability in several ways (Crim and Munro, 1994). Mild heat treatment in the presence of reducing sugars (e.g., glucose and galactose), a procedure used in milk processing, causes a loss of available lysine. Lactose reacts with lysine side chains and renders them unavailable. This reaction, which is called *browning*, or the *Maillard reaction*, can cause significant lysine loss at high temperatures. Under severe heating conditions in the presence (or even absence) of sugars or oxidized lipids, all amino acids in food proteins become resistant to digestion. When protein is exposed to severe treatment with alkali, the amino acids lysine and cysteine can react together and form a potentially toxic lysinoalanine. Exposure to sulfur dioxide and other oxidative conditions can result in loss of methionine. Thermal processing and low-moisture storage of proteins can also result in reductive binding of vitamin B_6 to lysine residues, thereby inactivating the vitamin. Therefore proper handling of protein foods is necessary to maintain their integrity and usefulness.

As noted previously, if the amino acid profile of a food does not match human needs, the amino acids that are in short supply are considered limiting. The quality of dietary protein can be improved by combining protein sources with different limiting amino acids. Diets based on a single plant food staple do not foster optimal growth because the diet does not have enough of the limiting amino acid to provide substrates for protein synthesis. If another plant protein that contains an excess of the limiting amino acid is added to the diet, the protein combination is *complemented*. In other words, the plant combination provides adequate amounts of essential amino acids to adequately support human protein synthesis. The concept of protein complementarity is primarily important for populations at risk for consuming insufficiently diverse mixed foods that contain various amino acids. Certain foods, when eaten together, provide all of the essential amino acids (Table 3-9).

TABLE 3-9

Food Combinations Providing All Essential Amino Acids

Excellent Combinations*	Examples
Grains and legumes	Rice and beans, pea soup and toast, lentil curry and rice
Grains and dairy	Pasta and cheese, rice pudding, cheese sandwich
Legumes and seeds	Garbanzo beans and sesame seeds; hummus as dip, falafel, or soup

*Other combinations, such as dairy and seeds, dairy and legumes, grains and seeds, are less effective because the chemical scores are similar and not effectively complementary.

It is now considered unnecessary to eat complementary amino acids during a single meal, but they should be eaten within the same day (American Dietetic Association, 1997). Children, pregnant women, and nursing mothers who have vegetarian diets need to plan their diets carefully to include a mixture of amino acid–containing foods.

Nitrogen Balance

Homeostatic regulations control the concentrations of specific amino acids in the amino acid pool and the rate at which muscle and plasma proteins are synthesized and broken down. Body protein synthesis and breakdown, or turnover, is regulated. Nitrogen balance studies have demonstrated that in healthy individuals the amount of protein taken in is exactly balanced by protein used for body maintenance and excreted in feces, in urine, and from skin, resulting in a zero protein balance (Figure 3-10). This balance reflects homeostatic regulations within tissues. For example, muscle mass, often described as *somatic protein*, is equilibrated with the circulating amino acid pool such that similar quantities of muscle protein are destroyed and rebuilt daily. Muscle mass can be estimated using the creatinine/height index and the midarm muscle circumference (see Chapter 14). Amino acids are also required for synthesis of visceral proteins by the liver and other tissues (see Chapter 15). On the other hand, a person with an infection or a traumatic injury excretes more nitrogen than is ingested. Inflammatory cytokines and other mediators are thought to cause nitrogen loss and negative nitrogen balance under these conditions (see Chapter 39). The pregnant woman and her growing child use ingested protein for growth and maintain a positive nitrogen balance (i.e., retain more protein than is lost daily).

Nitrogen in the form of ammonia (NH_3) is highly toxic, easily crosses membranes, and cannot be allowed to travel unbound throughout the body. In the fed state, pyruvate and other carbon skeletons take up nitrogen (via transamination) and transport it to the liver as nonessential amino acids, usually alanine and glutamic acid (from α-ketoglutarate). When these amino acids reach the liver, they are deaminated or

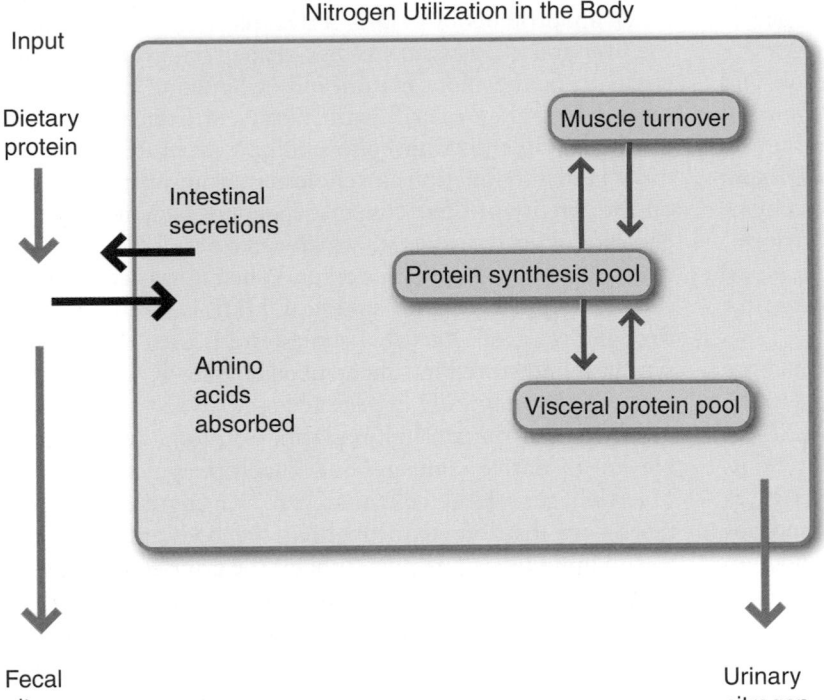

Nitrogen Utilization in the Body

Input

Dietary protein

Intestinal secretions

Amino acids absorbed

Muscle turnover

Protein synthesis pool

Visceral protein pool

Fecal nitrogen

Urinary nitrogen

FIGURE 3-10 Nitrogen use in the body. Protein supplies nitrogen in the form of amino acids, according to the formula (Nitrogen [grams] = Protein [grams] ÷ 6.25). Dietary protein and protein from endogenous secretions are available for absorption across the GI tract. More than 95% of protein is normally absorbed and enters the synthetic pool. Muscle proteins and visceral (i.e., plasma) proteins are broken down and built up daily. Nitrogen is converted to urea and excreted in the urine. Minor amounts of nitrogen are lost in the menstrual flow and the normal secretions and turnover of skin and its appendages. In a healthy individual, nitrogen intake equals nitrogen losses; the person is in zero protein balance. (*Modified from Crim MC, Munro HN: Proteins and amino acids. In Shils ME et al, editors:* Modern nutrition in health and disease, *Philadelphia, 1994, Lea & Febiger.*)

transaminated back into the carbon skeleton. A deaminated ammonia ion is combined with carbon dioxide in the presence of high-energy phosphate and magnesium by the enzyme *carbamoyl phosphate synthase* to form carbamoyl phosphate, the first intermediate of the urea cycle. A second amino group enters the urea cycle via aspartic acid. Thus with each urea molecule formed, two excess amino groups can be excreted. **Urea** makes up 90% of urinary nitrogen in the fed state. Arginine, one of the basic amino acids (see Figure 3-7), is also a product of the urea cycle and is a nonessential amino acid because it is produced in the urea cycle. Recent research has found that arginine is required for formation of nitric oxide and other mediators of the inflammatory response (Abcouwer and Souba, 1998). Although classified as a nonessential amino acid, arginine may be essential for critically ill individuals (see Chapter 39). Details of the urea cycle are in Chapter 44, Figure 44-7.

MACRONUTRIENT USE AND STORAGE IN THE FED STATE

As discussed in Chapter 1, absorbed carbohydrates are transported as plasma glucose in the portal vein. An increase in the glucose level in the portal vein stimulates preformed insulin secretion from the pancreas. One of the most dramatic effects of insulin is it effects on the glucose transporters (GLUT 4) in insulin-dependent tissues (adipose and muscle). However, the liver is the first organ to receive portal blood glucose. The liver takes up approximately 50% of absorbed glucose via noninsulin-dependent transporters (GLUT 2) and immediately phosphorylates glucose into

glucose-6-phosphate using the high-capacity enzyme glucokinase, thereby retaining glucose in the liver cells (see Figure 3-2). Insulin also enhances the oxidation of glucose in the glycolytic pathway by increasing the activity of glucokinase. *Pyruvate dehydrogenase* is also stimulated, increasing glycolysis and acetyl CoA production in both the liver and the muscle, which generates adenosine triphosphate (ATP). In addition, insulin increases glycogen synthase activity in the liver and muscle, maximizing glucose storage as glycogen storage under fed conditions (see *Clinical Insight:* Hormonal Control of Blood Sugar). Muscle glycogen is used within the muscle cell to provide ATP for muscle contraction. Its concentration in the muscle depends on the physical activity of the individual and can be greatly increased by physical training. Liver glycogen serves as a reservoir, providing a readily available supply of glucose to maintain blood glucose levels during the fasting state.

If carbohydrate intake exceeds the body's oxidative and storage capacities, the cells can convert carbohydrate into fat. Carbohydrate-induced lipogenesis in the rat model has been well described (Kibir et al., 1998). Elevated insulin levels increase the activity of fatty acid and triglyceride synthesis enzymes such as acetyl CoA carboxylase in the liver, lipoprotein lipase in the adipose tissue, and fatty acid synthetase. The increase in synthetase has been confirmed in human subjects maintained on moderate carbohydrate (fat at 30% kcal) and high carbohydrate (fat at 10% kcal) diets (Hudgins, 2000).

Because they are fat soluble, lipids cannot be transported unbound through the aqueous media of the body. Absorbed fatty acids and monoglycerides (monoacylglycerols) are re-esterified into triglycerides within mucosal cells, and the fat-soluble center is surrounded with a thin layer of protein and phospholipid for transport. The protein component includes apoproteins ([Apo] B, A, C, and E) with specific functions. The resulting **chylomicrons** contain only 2% protein; the rest is triglycerides (84%), cholesterol, and phospholipids. The lipid-rich particles leave the mucosal cells and travel through lymphatic channels to the thoracic duct that empties into the right side of the heart. Rapid blood flow in the heart prevents the large, lipid-rich chylomicrons from forming clumps and fat emboli. Chylomicrons transport dietary fat and are usually found in blood only after meals and can make the plasma appear milky after a high-fat meal.

Chylomicrons leave the heart through the aorta and are dispersed into the general circulation and transported to the adipocytes (fat cells). An enzyme, *lipoprotein lipase (LPL),* is expressed on the membrane of endothelial cells lining capillaries in the region of the adipocytes and elsewhere. LPL is activated by lipoprotein-bound Apo C to bind chylomicrons and cleave triglycerides, releasing fatty acids and monoglycerides that cross the fatty lipid membrane, enter the adipocytes, and become reesterified into triglyceride for safe and hydrophobic storage. Note that insulin, the predominant hormone in the fed state, activates LDL and facilitates fat storage. The chylomicron remnant, relieved of some of its triglyceride content, is bound to liver receptors through its surface markers Apo B and Apo E and recycled.

The liver receives fat from numerous sources: (1) chylomicron remnants, (2) circulating fatty acids, (3) uptake of intermediate lipoproteins and other lipoproteins, and (4) its own endogenous synthesis. The liver reesterifies fat from all sources and forms VLDLs. These lipoproteins are richer in cholesterol compared with chylomicrons but still contain a large proportion of triglycerides. See Figure 32-1 for characteristics of lipoproteins. VLDLs also contain apoproteins B, E, and C and adsorb Apo A as they circulate. In the fed state numerous VLDLs are formed and transported to the adipocytes, where triglycerides are again hydrolyzed, reesterified, and stored. Even in the fasted state, VLDLs can be formed to carry endogenous lipids.

Dietary cholesterol is transported via chylomicrons and VLDLs but is not removed by LPL activity. After LPL has cleaved the maximum triglyceride from VLDLs, the remnant remaining is called an intermediate-density lipoprotein (IDL). Once the maximum triglyceride is removed, the lipoprotein is known as an LDL and primarily carries cholesterol. Although LDLs can be taken up by the liver on receptors for Apo B and Apo E, they are first taken up by specific LDL receptors that bind these cholesterol-rich particles. After uptake, endocytic vesicles containing LDL fuse with a lysosome. The digestive enzymes in the lysosome break down the protein and phospholipids, leaving free cholesterol. Free cholesterol regulates cholesterol synthesis and LDL uptake within the cell by inhibiting HMG CoA reductase, the rate-limiting enzyme for cholesterol synthesis from acetyl CoA. It downregulates cellular synthesis of the LDL receptor and reduces receptor expression on the membrane. Free cholesterol also increases the esterification of cholesterol for storage.

Cholesterol is removed from the cell membrane and other lipoproteins by HDLs. HDL particles are formed in the liver and other tissues as disk-shaped lipoproteins. They circulate in the bloodstream and accumulate free cholesterol, which they esterify with fatty acid from their phosphatidylcholine (lecithin) phospholipid structure. The ability of HDLs to function as a cholesterol transporter depends on the activity of their copper-dependent enzyme lecithin-cholesterol acyltransferase, which esterifies cholesterol and stores it in its hydrophobic center. When it has accumulated sufficient lipid to become spherical, HDL is taken up by the liver and recycled. Recycled cholesterol is used for bile acid synthesis and stored in subcutaneous tissue, where it can be formed into vitamin D or secreted as VLDL.

LDLs that remain in circulation too long are susceptible to oxidative damage and macrophage scavenging. Macrophages—large cells that "eat," or engulf, other particles—are distributed throughout the body, play a major role in immune defense, and inhabit the arteries, where they serve as a surveillance mechanism against foreign and microbial agents in the blood. Although macrophages do not recognize and ingest normal lipoproteins, they do recognize as foreign those lipoproteins that have undergone oxidation. Macrophages ingest oxidized LDLs and accumulate ingested fat within their cytoplasm, giving them a foamy appearance (thus the name *foam cells*). LDL ingestion activates macrophages and stimulates them to secrete mediators that trigger multiple inflammatory and proliferative cascades, some of which lead to atherosclerosis. Evidence now supports the proposal that the macrophage plays a role in the pathogenesis of atherosclerosis (Chisolm and Penn, 1996) (see Chapter 32).

MACRONUTRIENT CATABOLISM IN THE FASTED STATE

The body has a remarkable ability to withstand food deprivation, allowing humans to survive cycles of feast and famine. Adaptive changes allow the body to access stored macronutrients to provide for routine activities.

Individuals with protein energy, or protein-calorie, malnutrition can have varying symptoms, determined by the cause of the malnutrition. Simple starvation (the absolute deprivation of food) leads to marasmus and represents one end of the protein-energy malnutrition continuum. At the opposite end of the continuum is protein deprivation that occurs in individuals who are consuming carbohydrates almost entirely. This condition is called kwashiorkor, the Ghanaian word for the disease that develops when a mother's first child is weaned from protein-rich breast milk to a protein-poor carbohydrate food source. Although recently Ciliberto et al. (2005) have proposed that some symptoms in kwashiorkor patients are caused by an imbalance between free radical production and their safe disposal, the disease is generally thought to be caused by severe protein deficiency and hypoalbuminemia.

Glucose is an obligate nutrient for the brain and nervous system, red blood cells, white blood cells, and other glucose-requiring tissues. To maintain function, the blood glucose level must be maintained within a normal range at all times. During early fasting, glucose is obtained from glycogen by the action of the hormones glucagon and epinephrine, but these stores are depleted within 24 hours. At this point, glucose must be synthesized de novo using protein as a substrate. The catabolic hormones epinephrine, thyroxine, and glucagon stimulate the release of muscle protein and other available substrates for gluconeogenesis. The most common amino acid substrate for gluconeogenesis is alanine because, when its nitrogen is removed, alanine becomes pyruvate. Note that glycogen is never totally depleted, even during long-term starvation. A small amount of preformed glycogen is carefully guarded as a primer for glycogen resynthesis.

As fasting is prolonged and the body adapts to starvation conditions (marasmus or adapted stravation), liver gluconeogenesis decreases from producing 90% of the glucose to less than 50%, with the remainder being supplied by the kidney. Although the muscle and brain are unable to release free glucose, the muscle can release pyruvate and lactate for gluconeogenesis in a process called the Cori cycle. Muscles also release glutamine and alanine. These amino acids can be deaminated or transaminated into α-ketoglutarate or pyruvate, respectively, and converted into oxaloacetate and then to glucose. During prolonged fasting the kidney requires ammonia to excrete acidic metabolic products. Muscle-derived glutamine is used for this purpose, and the deaminated glutaminc (α-ketoglutarate) can then be used to produce glucose. Thus during starvation glucose production by the kidney increases, and production by the liver decreases.

In addition to glucose, a reliable energy source is required during fasting. The best source is fat that is stored in adipocytes and used primarily by muscles, including the heart muscle, to make ATP. Fatty acid release and use requires low insulin levels and an increase of the anti-insulin hormones glucagon, cortisone, epinephrine, and growth hormone. Anti-insulin hormones activate the hormone-sensitive lipase enzyme on the adipocyte membrane. This enzyme cleaves stored triglycerides, releasing fatty acids and glycerol from fat cells. Fatty acids travel to the liver bound to serum albumin and easily enter the liver cells. Once inside the cell, fatty acids enter the liver mitochondria via the carnitine acyltransferase transport system, which carries fatty acid **carnitine** esters cross the mitochondrial membrane. Once inside the mitochondria, acetyl CoA is formed from fatty acid CoA via the process of β-oxidation. During starvation excess acetyl CoA molecules accumulate in the liver, since the liver is able to obtain all necessary energy from the process of β-oxidation and form ketones, which then enter the bloodstream and are able to act as a source of energy for the muscles, thus sparing protein.

Adaptation to starvation depends on ketone production. As the blood ketone level rises during fasting, the brain and nervous system, although obligate glucose consumers, begin to use ketones as an energy source. Because the brain is using a fuel other than glucose, the demand on muscle protein for gluconeogenesis declines, thereby reducing the rate of muscle catabolism. Reduced muscle catabolism reduces the amount of ammonia received by the liver. Liver synthesis of urea decreases precipitously, reflecting the slower rate of muscle protein deamination. If the fast extends for weeks, the rate of urea synthesis and excretion is minimized. As discussed previously, in an individual who has adapted to starvation, urea is excreted at approximately the same rate as uric acid produced by the kidney.

Thus, in an individual who is adapting to starvation, protein losses are minimized, and lean body mass spared. Although fat cannot be converted into glucose, it does provide fuel for the muscle and brain in the form of ketones. As long as water is available, a normal-weight individual can fast for a month. Relatively normal nutritional indices, immune function, and other system function are maintained. However, when fat stores are exhausted, protein is used, and death is the ultimate concequence.

In certain cases of trauma and sepsis, the individual is not able to adapt to fasting or starvation. If an individual who is fasting develops an infection, inflammatory mediators such as interleukin-1 and tumor necrosis factor stimulate insulin secretion and prevent the development of mild ketosis. Without ketones the brain and other tissues continue to depend on glucose, thereby limiting the person's ability to adapt to starvation. Muscle mass erodes to provide glucose substrates. A fasting person with an infection rapidly develops a negative nitrogen balance (see Chapter 15). When 50% of the protein stores is exhausted, the person's ability to recover from the infection is poor; the person may die if the respiratory muscles cannot support breathing.

Adaptation to starvation is also not possible for those with protein-calorie malnutrition (kwashiorkor) because the carbohydrate intake stimulates insulin production. Insulin is a storage hormone that prevents fat stores from being accessed for fuel. It also inhibits fat from being formed into ketones, thereby limiting adaptation to starvation. Insulin secretion inhibits muscle breakdown. Protein cannot be used to make albumin and other visceral proteins. Edema results because albumin exerts osmotic pressure in the vessels. If the albumin concentration is low, fluid remains in the extracellular spaces and causes edema. Compromised neural function and GI absorption, decreased cardiac output, immune function, fatigue, and other symptoms of protein-calorie malnutrition result from inadequate protein synthesis, inadequate ATP production, and fluid accumulation in the tissues.

Nonadapted protein-calorie malnutrition is dangerous. Not only can unremitting protein loss become life threatening by compromising the muscles of the heart and respiratory system, it can compromise the immune system. By limiting a person's immune defenses, it makes the individual susceptible to a vicious cycle of infections, diarrhea, additional nutrient loss, an even weaker immune system, and, finally, opportunistic infections and death. Iatrogenic, or "physician-induced," malnutrition was recognized long ago as a danger for hospitalized patients and remains so to this day (Kruizenga et al., 2005).

MICRONUTRIENTS: VITAMINS

The discovery of vitamins gave birth to the field of nutrition. The elucidation of these compounds is an exciting and convoluted story (see *Focus On:* Pellagra, Politics, and the Poor). Eventually the term **vitamin** came to describe a group of essential micronutrients that generally satisfy the following criteria: (1) organic compounds (or class of compounds) distinct from fats, carbohydrates, and proteins, (2) natural components of foods; usually present in minute amounts, (3) not synthesized by the body in amounts adequate to meet normal physiologic needs, (4) essential, also usually in minute amounts, for normal physiologic function (i.e., maintenance, growth, development, and reproduction), and (5) cause a specific deficiency syndrome by their absence or insufficiency.

Vitamers are the multiple forms (all isomers and active analogs) of vitamins. Although the vitamins have few close chemical similarities, their metabolic functions have classically been described in one of four general categories: (1) membrane stabilizers, (2) hydrogen (H^+) and electron donors and acceptors, (3) hormones, and (4) coenzymes. Their functions in human health are much broader and often include roles in gene expression. Studies indicate that subclinical or even less than optimum levels of some vitamins can contribute to disease states that are not normally associated with vitamin status (see *Clinical Insight:* Vitamins and Minerals in Prevention of Chronic Disease).

The vitamins can be classified based on their solubilities: the fat-soluble vitamins (A, D, E, and K) and the water-soluble vitamins (ascorbic acid, thiamin, riboflavin, niacin, pyridoxine, biotin, pantothenic acid, folate, and cobalamin). The fat-soluble vitamins are absorbed passively and must be transported with dietary lipid. They tend to be found in the lipid portions of the cell such as membranes and lipid droplets. The water-soluble vitamins are absorbed by passive and active mechanisms, transported by carriers, and not stored in appreciable amounts in the body. Fat-soluble vitamins are generally excreted with the feces via enterohepatic circulation, whereas water-soluble vitamins or their metabolites are excreted in the urine.

THE FAT-SOLUBLE VITAMINS

Vitamin A

Vitamin A (retinoids) refers to three preformed compounds that exhibit metabolic activity: the alcohol (retinol), the aldehyde (retinal or retinaldehyde), and the acid (retinoic

◎ FOCUS ON

Pellagra, Politics, and the Poor

The history of niacin and pellagra is an example of the long and often convoluted search for the vitamins. Even though oranges and lemons were used as early as 1601 on the ships of the East India Company to prevent scurvy, the idea that a chemical in the diet could prevent certain diseases eluded the scientific and medical communities for hundreds of years. Pellagra was among these diseases. In 1915, 11,000 deaths from pellagra were reported in the southern United States. By 1917 more than 170,000 cases developed in the southern United States. The situation was so grave that the Public Health Service sent Joseph Goldberger to the South to investigate the deaths. He determined a nutrient deficiency to be the cause of the disease and that it could be cured by a diet containing high-quality protein. In fact, he showed that he could eliminate the disease simply by improving the diet. In 1918 Goldberger published these findings (Goldberger, 1918). Considering these facts, why in 1927 were 120,000 cases reported in the South? Between 1927 and 1930, 27,103 deaths were recorded. Why were there so many deaths from a disease that was entirely preventable?

Several factors contributed to the situation. First, Pasteur's germ theory of disease was sweeping the scientific community. In fact, it was accepted that scurvy, beriberi, and rickets were each caused by a microbe rather than by the lack of a nutrient. The antiberiberi actions of whole grain rice were thought to be caused by a pharmacologic substance that acted against an unknown bacterium, rather than a substance that served as a nutrient (thiamin). Even after Goldberger showed that pellagra was not contagious, doubts persisted. The problem was further complicated, as is now known, because (1) high-quality protein does not contain niacin—it contains the **tryptophan** precursor, and (2) the isolation of individual vitamins from the B-complex isolate took many years of painstaking laboratory research. Many more years passed before tryptophan was recognized as an important precursor of niacin, the missing B vitamin leading to pellagra.

Perhaps the most significant factors contributing to the numerous deaths from pellagra—factors that affected the southern United States into the 1940s (with more than 2000 deaths per year) and early 1950s (with more than 500 deaths per year)—were economic and social. All of those who died from pellagra were poor and became poorer as the Great Depression of the late 1920s and 1930s deepened. The deaths primarily affected black Americans. In the South, people died from a lack of food, whereas in other parts of the country, farmers burned or threw away food because they could not sell the excess.

acid) (Table 3-10). Stored retinol is often esterified to a fatty acid (usually palmitate) and is called retinyl-palmitate. These retinyl esters are also usually found complexed with proteins in foods. These active forms of vitamin A exist in only animal products.

In addition to preformed vitamin A found in animal products, plants contain a group of compounds known collectively as **carotenoids**, which can yield retinoids when metabolized in the body. Although several hundred carotenoids exist in foods naturally as antioxidants, only a few have significant vitamin A activity. The most important of these is β-carotene. The amount of vitamin A available from dietary carotenoids depends on how well they are absorbed and how efficiently they are converted to retinol. Absorption varies greatly (from 5% to 50%) and is affected by other dietary factors such as the digestibility of the proteins complexed with the carotenoids and the level and type of fat in the diet. (Fat-soluble vitamins need fat for proper absorption.)

Absorption, Transport, and Storage

Before either vitamin A or its carotenoid provitamins can be absorbed, proteases in the stomach and small intestine must hydrolyze proteins that are usually complexed with these compounds. In addition, retinyl esters must be hydrolyzed in the small intestine by lipases to retinol and free fatty acids (Figure 3-11, *A*). Retinoids and carotenoids are incorporated into micelles along with other lipids for passive absorption into the mucosal cells of the small intestine. Once in the intestinal mucosal cells, retinol is bound to a cellular retinol-binding protein (CRBP) and reesterified (primarily by lecithin retinol acyl transferase [LRAT]) into retinyl esters. Carotenoids and retinyl esters are incorporated into chylomicrons for transport into the lymph and eventually the bloodstream or may be cleaved into retinal, which is then reduced to retinol and reesterified into retinyl esters. These retinyl esters, like those produced from absorbed retinol, are also incorporated into chylomicrons (Figure 3-11, *B*).

The liver plays an important role in vitamin A transport and storage (Figure 3-11, *C*). Chylomicron remnants deliver retinyl esters to the liver. These esters are immediately hydrolyzed into retinol and free fatty acids. **Retinol** in the liver has three major metabolic fates. First, retinol may be bound to CRBP, which controls free retinol concentrations that can be toxic in the cell. Second, retinol may be reesterfied to form retinyl esters, mostly retinyl palmitate, for storage. Approximately 50% to 80% of the

---

⬢ **CLINICAL INSIGHT**

Vitamins and Minerals in Prevention of Chronic Disease

Recent studies have demonstrated that (1) a number of vitamins and minerals may have roles beyond those functions normally given to them in prevention of symptoms of deficiency diseases, and (2) subclinical deficiencies may have important impacts on development of chronic disease. For example, it is known that folate and B₁₂ are critical for both deoxyribonucleic acid (DNA) synthesis and repair and that low intake levels are common in the general population and in particular the elderly. Duthie et al. (2004) reported evidence that folate also has a role in maintaining the stability of DNA. Individuals who are homozygous for the gene that controls key folate-metabolizing enzymes have decreased risk of colorectal cancer. Similarly Kirkland (2003) concluded that there was strong evidence that niacin status also impacts cancer risk by playing an important role in response to DNA damage, including repair and maintenance of genomic stability. Riboflavin deficiency has also been suggested as a risk factor for cancer (Powers, 2003), although more studies are needed. More substantial evidence supports the role of riboflavin in iron metabolism and anemia. Likewise, it is known that vitamin D is essential for healthy bones and is protective against bone diseases, but there is now evidence that vitamin D also protects against certain types of cancers, multiple sclerosis, and type 1 diabetes (Grant and Holick, 2005).

Peterlik and Cross (2005) suggest that there is clear evidence that vitamin D and calcium deficits predisposed individuals to certain types of cancers, chronic inflammatory and autoimmune diseases, and metabolic disorders such as metabolic syndrome and hypertension. They noted the widespread deficit of these nutrients in the American population as a major challenge for preventive medicine. However, Guerrero-Romero and Rodriguez-Moran (2005) in a review of the beneficial role of chromium, magnesium, and antioxidants in the treatment of diabetes, warn against focusing on micronutritent supplementation and emphasize the need for an adequate diet that would prevent deficiencies noting that most adults in the United States do not get the dietary recommended intake [DRI] for many nutrients. Multiple nutrients have been implicated in the development of osteoporosis (Nieves, 2005) and lung disease (Romieu, 2005). As the roles of vitamins and minerals in preventing secondary disease responses become clear, DRIs may need to be revised, especially for some populations. In the assessment statement from the National Institutes of Health State-of-the-Science Conference on Multivitamin/Mineral Supplement and Chronic Disease Prevention, the panel noted in experimental trials that examined cancer end points that supplements resulted in a reduction of cancer incidence and mortality. However, they also noted that supplements might increase cancer risk in some groups (retrieved from www. concensus.nih.gov, May 22, 2006).

vitamin A in the body is stored in the liver, although other tissues such as the adipose tissue, lungs, and kidneys also store retinyl esters in specialized cells called stellate cells. This storage capacity buffers the effects of highly variable patterns of vitamin A intake and is particularly important during periods of low intake when a person is at risk for developing a deficiency.

Finally, retinol may be bound to retinol-binding protein (RBP). Retinol bound to RBP leaves the liver and enters the blood, where another protein—transthyretin (TTR)—attaches, forming a complex that is used to transport retinol in the blood to the peripheral tissues. Hepatic RBP synthesis depends on adequate protein. Therefore blood levels of retinol can be affected by protein deficiency as well as by chronic vitamin A deficiency. Thus children with protein-calorie malnutrition typically have low circulating retinol levels that may not respond to vitamin A supplementation unless the protein deficiency is also corrected (see Chapter 15).

The retinol-RBP-TTR complex delivers retinol to other tissues via cell surface receptors. Retinol is transferred from RBP to CRBP with the subsequent release of Apo retinol-binding protein (Apo RBP) into binding protein and TTR to the blood. Apo RBP is eventually metabolized and excreted by the kidney. In addition to CRBP, cellular retinoic acid–binding proteins (CRABPs) bind retinoic acid in the cell and serve to control retinoic acid concentrations similar to the way CRBP controls retinol concentrations.

Metabolism

In addition to being esterified for storage, the transport form of retinol can also be oxidized into retinal and then into retinoic acid or conjugated into retinyl glucuronide or retinyl phosphate. After retinoic acid is formed, it is converted to forms that are readily excreted. Chain-shortened and oxidized forms of vitamin A are excreted in the urine; intact forms are excreted in the bile and feces.

TABLE 3-10

Vitamins, Vitamers, and Their Functions

Group	Vitamers	Provitamins	Physiologic Functions
Vitamin A	Retinol Retinal Retinoic acid	β-carotene Cryptoxanthin	Visual pigments; cell differentiation; gene regulation
Vitamin D	Cholecalciferol (D_3) Ergocalciferol (D_2)		Ca homeostasis; bone metabolism
Vitamin E	α-tocopherol γ-tocopherol Tocotrienols		Membrane antioxidant
Vitamin K	Phylloquinones (K_1) Menaquinones (K_2) Menadione (K_3)		Blood clotting; Ca metabolism
Vitamin C	Ascorbic acid		Reductant in hydroxylations in biosynthesis of collagen and carnitine and in the metabolism of drugs and steroids
	Dehydroascorbic acid		
Vitamin B_1	Thiamin		Coenzyme for decarboxylations of 2-keto acids and transketolations
Vitamin B_2	Riboflavin		Coenzyme in redox reactions of fatty acids and the TCA cycle
Niacin	Nicotinic acid Nicotinamide		Coenzymes for several dehydrogenases
Vitamin B_6	Pyridoxol Pyridoxal Pyridoxamine		Coenzymes in amino acid metabolism
Folate	Folic acid Pteroylmonoglutamate		Coenzymes in single-carbon metabolism
	Polyglutamyl folacins		
Biotin	Biotin		Coenzyme for carboxylations
Pantothenic acid	Pantothenic acid		Coenzyme in fatty acid metabolism
Vitamin B_{12}	Cobalamin		Coenzyme in metabolism of propionate, amino acids, and single carbon fragments

TCA, Tricarboxylic acid.

Functions

Vitamin A has essential but separate roles in vision and various systemic functions, including normal cell differentiation and cell surface function (e.g., cell recognition), growth and development, immune functions, and reproduction.

Retinal is a structural component of the visual pigments of the rod and cone cells of the retina and is essential to photoreception. The 11-*cis* isomer, 11-*cis*-retinal, constitutes the photosensitive group of various visual pigment proteins (i.e., the opsins—rhodopsin in the rods and iodopsin in the cones). Photoreception results from light-induced isomerization of 11-*cis*-retinal to the completely all-*trans* form. For example, in the rod, rhodopsin progresses through a series of reactions leading to the dissociation of "bleached" rhodopsin into all-*trans*-retinal and opsin, a reaction that is coupled to nervous stimulation of the visual centers of the brain. All-*trans*-retinal can then be converted back enzymatically to 11-*cis*-retinal for subsequent binding to opsin (Figure 3-12). The movement of retinal into designated sites in the retina is controlled by the proteins and interphotoreceptor retinal-binding protein (IRBP), which, although distinct from other retinal–retinal-binding proteins, serves a similar function.

Although the systemic functions of vitamin A are not completely understood, they can be separated into two major categories. First, vitamin A (specifically, retinoic acid) acts as a hormone to affect gene expression (see Chapter 13). Within the cell, CRABP transports retinoic acid to the nucleus. In the nucleus, retinoic acid and 9-*cis*-retinoic acid bind to retinoic acid receptors (RARs) or retinoid receptors (RXRs) on the gene (Figure 3-13). Subsequent interactions allow stimulation or inhibition of transcription of specific genes, thus affecting protein synthesis and many body processes. Only a few of these processes are known, and they include morphogenesis in embryonic development and epithelial cell function (including differentiation and production of keratin proteins). The second major role of vitamin A in systemic functions involves glycoprotein synthesis. In a series of reactions, retinol forms retinyl-phosphomannose and then transfers the mannose to the glycoprotein. Glycoproteins are important for normal cell surface functions such as cell aggregation and cell recognition. This role in glycoprotein synthesis may also account for the importance of vitamin A in cell growth because it may increase glycoprotein synthesis for cell receptors that respond to growth factors.

Vitamin A (retinol) is also essential for normal reproduction, bone development and function, and immune system function, although its actions in these roles are currently unclear.

Although a consistent body of epidemiologic evidence indicates that higher blood levels of carotenoids reduce the risk of several chronic diseases, the only clear function of the carotenoids is as provitamin A (Institute of Medicine, Food and Nutrition Board, 2001). β-Carotene can act as an antioxidant, but its other properties that are unrelated to antioxidant actions, such as retinoid-dependent signaling, gap junction communications, regulation of cell growth, and induction of enzymes, may be more important properties (Stahl et al., 2002).

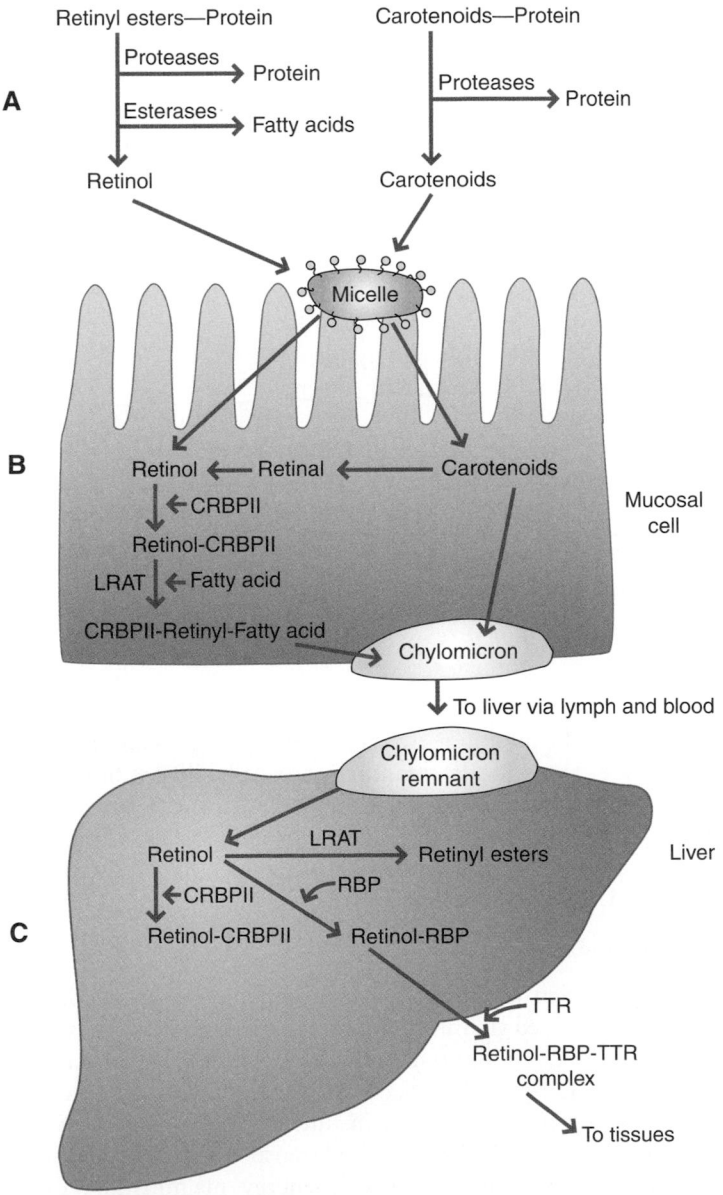

FIGURE 3-11 Retinol and carotenoids. **A,** Digestion. **B,** Absorption. **C,** Transport. *CRBPII,* Cellular retinol-binding protein II; *RBP,* retinol-binding protein; *TRR,* transthyretin.

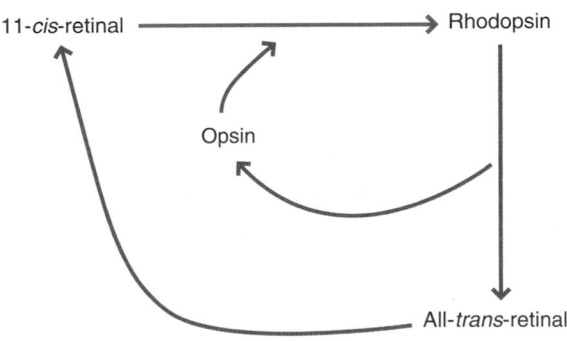

FIGURE 3-12 The visual cycle.

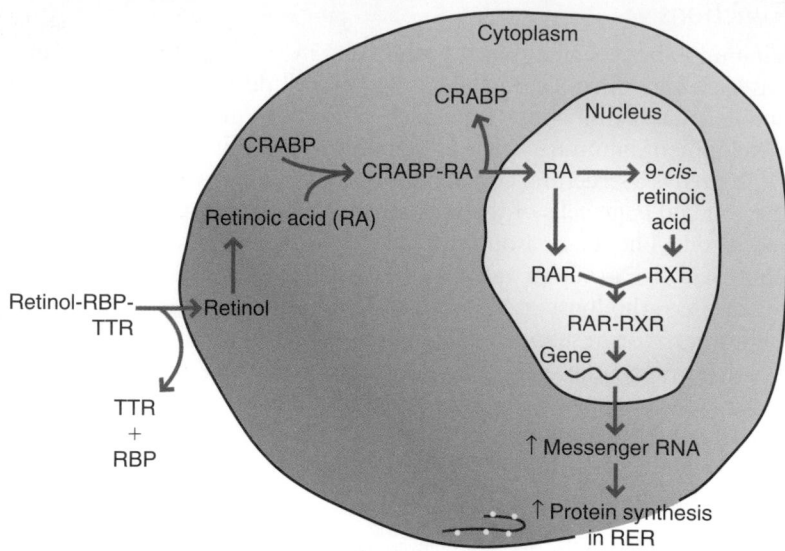

FIGURE 3-13 Role of vitamin A in gene expression. *CRABP*, Cellular retinoic acid-binding protein; *RAR*, retinoic acid receptor; *RBP*, retinol-binding protein; *RXR*, retinoid X receptor; *TTR*, transthyretin.

Dietary Reference Intakes Measurement

The vitamin A content of foods is measured as **retinol activity equivalents (RAEs).** One RAE equals the activity of 1 mcg of retinol (1 mcg of retinol is equal to 3.33 international units [IU]) (Box 3-3). Because new data show that the efficiency of β-carotene absorption is much less (14%) than that previously believed (33%), 12 mcg of β-carotene is equal to 1 RAE, and 24 mcg of other carotenoids equal 1 RAE. In other words, approximately twice as much carotenoid is needed in the diet as was previously believed.

Dietary reference intakes (DRIs) have been determined for vitamin A and are expressed in micrograms per day (mcg/day). The AI for infants is based on the amount of retinol in human milk. The DRIs for adults are based on levels that provide adequate blood levels and liver stores and are adjusted for differences in average body size. Increased amounts of the vitamin during pregnancy and lactation allow for fetal storage and the vitamin A in breast milk.

No DRIs have been established for the carotenoids. Indeed, supplementation has not been shown to be beneficial and may be harmful. However, increased consumption of fruits and vegetables with carotenoids is clearly beneficial (Institute of Medicine, Food and Nutrition Board, 2001). (For a complete explanation of the DRIs, see Chapter 12.)

Sources

Preformed vitamin A exists only in foods of animal origin, either in storage areas such as the liver or in the fat of milk and eggs. Very high concentrations of vitamin A are found in cod and halibut liver oils. Nonfat milk in the United States, which by U.S. law can contain 0.1% fat, is routinely fortified with retinol. Provitamin A carotenoids are found in dark green leafy and yellow-orange vegetables and fruit; deeper colors are associated with higher carotenoid levels. In much of the world, carotenoids supply most of the dietary vitamin A. The American food supply provides roughly equal amounts of preformed vitamin A and provitamin A carotenoids. Carrots, greens, spinach, orange juice, sweet

> ### BOX 3-3
> ## Vitamin A Activity
>
> 1 retinol activity equivalent (RAE) =
>   1 mcg of retinol
>   12 mcg of β-carotene (from food)
>   3.33 IU of vitamin A activity (on a label)*
> For example: 5000 IU vitamin A (supplement or food label) =
>   1500 RAE = 1500 mcg of retinol
>
> Data from Institute of Medicine, Food and Nutrition Board: *Dietary reference intakes for vitamin A, vitamin K, arsenic, boron, chromium, copper, iodine, iron, manganese, molybdenum, nickel, silicon, vanadium, and zinc,* Washington, DC, 2001, National Academies Press.
>
> *The vitamin A activity on a food or supplement label is stated in international units (IU), a term outdated scientifically but still required legally on labels.

potatoes, and cantaloupe are rich sources of provitamin A. In many of these foods, vitamin A bioavailability is limited by binding of carotenoids to proteins, but this can be overcome by cooking, which disrupts the protein association and frees the carotenoid. Table 3-11 and Appendix 47 list the vitamin A content of selected foods.

Deficiency

Primary deficiencies of vitamin A result from inadequate intakes of preformed vitamin A or provitamin A carotenoids (see *New Directions:* Biophotonic Measurement of Antioxidant Capacity in Chapter 15). Secondary deficiencies can result from malabsorption caused by insufficient dietary fat, biliary or pancreatic insufficiency, impaired transport from abetalipoproteinemia, liver disease, protein-energy malnutrition, or zinc deficiency.

Vitamin A deficiency is the most significant cause of blindness in the developing world, and an estimated 250 million children are at risk. Between 250,000 and 500,000

TABLE 3-11

Vitamin A Content of Selected Foods

Food	RAE*
Turkey, 1 cup	15,534
Sweet potato, baked, 1 small	7,374
Carrots, raw, 1 cup	5,553
Spinach, cooked, 1 cup	6,882
Squash, butternut, 1 cup	2,406
Mixed vegetables, frozen, 1 cup	2,337
Apricots, canned, 1 cup	1,329
Cantaloupe, 1 cup	1,625
Broccoli, cooked, 1 cup	725
Brussel sprouts, 1 cup	430
Tomatoes, 1 cup	450
Peaches, canned, 1 cup	283

DRIs

Infants and young children, AI = 400-500 RAE/day, depending on age

Older children and adolescents, RDA = 600-900 RAE/day, depending on age

Adults, RDA = 700-900 RAE/day, depending on gender

Pregnant, RDA = 750-770 RAE/day, depending on age

Lactating, RDA = 1200-1300 RAE/day, depending on age

From U.S. Department of Agriculture, Agricultural Research Service: Nutrient Database for Standard Reference, Release 18, retrieved 2005, Data Laboratory home page, http://www.nal.usda.gov/fnic/foodcomp/Data/SR18/sr18.html.

*RAE, Retinol activity equivalents, 1 RAE = 1 mcg of retinol; RAE from plant sources calculated based on 12 mcg β-carotene = 1 RAE.

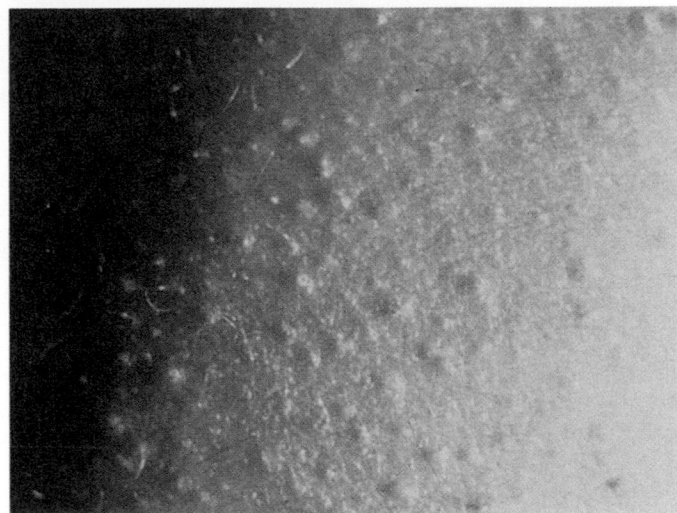

FIGURE 3-14 Follicular hyperkeratosis. Dry, bumpy skin associated with vitamin A or linoleic acid (essential fatty acid) deficiency. Linoleic acid deficiency may also result in eczematous skin, especially in infants. *(From Taylor KB, Anthony LE:* Clinical nutrition, *New York, 1983, McGraw-Hill.)*

tence (reduced numbers and mitogenic responsiveness of circulating T lymphocytes), and fewer osteoclasts, with subsequent excessive deposition of periosteal bone. Vitamin A deficiency also leads to the keratinization of the mucous membranes that line the respiratory tract, alimentary canal, urinary tract, skin, and epithelium of the eye. Clinically these conditions manifest as poor growth, blindness caused by xerophthalmia, corneal ulceration, or occlusion of the optic foramina from periosteal overgrowth of the cranium. **Xerophthalmia** involves atrophy of the periocular glands, hyperkeratosis of the conjunctiva, and, finally, involvement of the cornea, leading to softening (keratomalacia) and blindness. Although the condition is now rare in the United States (where it is usually associated with malabsorption), it is more common in developing countries.

Vitamin A deficiency produces characteristic changes in skin texture involving follicular hyperkeratosis (phrynoderma). Blockage of the hair follicles with plugs of keratin causes the distinctive "goose flesh" or "toad skin"; and the skin becomes dry, scaly, and rough. At first the forearms and thighs are affected, but in advanced stages the whole body is affected (Figure 3-14). Loss of mucous membrane integrity as a result of vitamin A deficiency increases host susceptibility to bacterial, viral, or parasitic infections. The deficiency also leads to impairments in certain aspects of cell-mediated immunity, ultimately increasing the risk for infection, particularly for respiratory infections.

Acute vitamin A deficiency is treated with large doses of vitamin A given orally. When the deficiency is part of concomitant protein-energy malnutrition, the malnutrition must be treated for the patient to benefit from vitamin A treatment. The signs and symptoms of deficiency respond to vitamin A supplementation in about the same order as they appear; night blindness responds very quickly, whereas the skin abnormalities may take several weeks to resolve. Massive, intermittent dosing with large doses of vitamin A has

cases of blindness from vitamin A deficiency occur annually. Research shows that, 4.4 million preschool children, most from South Asia, had clinical eye disease (xerophthalmia) caused by vitamin A deficiency (West, 2003). Two thirds of those newly diagnosed die within months of going blind because of enhanced susceptibility to infections. Even subclinical vitamin A deficiency increases childhood morbidity and mortality.

One of the first signs of vitamin A deficiency is impaired vision from the loss of visual pigments. This manifests clinically as **night blindness,** or nyctalopia. This impairment of dark adaptation (the ability to adapt from being in a bright light or glare to being in darkness [e.g., while driving at night or moving from a brightly lighted to a dark room]), results from the failure of the retina to regenerate rhodopsin. Individuals with night blindness have poor visual discriminatory abilities and may not be able to see in dim light or at twilight. In addition to measuring plasma retinol levels, dark adaptation testing is one of the recommended methods for testing for vitamin A adequacy (Institute of Medicine, Food and Nutrition Board, 2001).

Subsequently vitamin A deficiency leads to failures in its systemic functions, which are characterized by impaired embryonic development, impaired spermatogenesis or spontaneous abortion, anemia, impaired immunocompe-

been used in developing countries. Treatments with single doses of 60,000 RAE of vitamin A have reduced child mortality by 35% to 70% (Institute of Medicine, Food and Nutrition Board, 2001).

Toxicity

Persistent, large doses of vitamin A (more than 100 times the required amount) overcome the capacity of the liver to store the vitamin and can produce intoxication and eventually lead to liver disease. This intoxication is marked by high plasma levels of retinyl esters associated with lipoproteins. Hypervitaminosis A in humans is characterized by changes in the skin and mucous membranes (Box 3-4). Dry lips (cheilitis) are a common initial sign, followed by dryness of the nasal mucosa and eyes; more advanced signs include dryness, erythema, scaling and peeling of the skin, hair loss, and nail fragility. Headache, nausea, and vomiting have also been reported. Animals with hypervitaminosis A frequently have bone abnormalities involving overgrowth of periosteal bone; an increased incidence of hip fractures was found in women with high vitamin A intakes (Feskanick et al., 2002).

Acute hypervitaminosis A can be induced by single doses of retinol greater than 200 mg (200,000 RAEs) in adults or greater than 100 mg (100,000 RAEs) in children. Chronic hypervitaminosis A can result from chronic intakes (usually from misuse of supplements) greater than at least 10 times the AI (i.e., 4000 RAEs/day for an infant or 7000 RAEs/day for an adult). Dramatic stories in the literature describe reddening and exfoliation of the skin of Arctic explorers and fishermen who feasted on polar bear or halibut liver, both extremely high in vitamin A.

Retinoids can be toxic to embryos exposed in the womb. This is particularly true for 13-*cis*-retinoic acid (Accutane), a form very effective in treating severe cystic acne but which can cause craniofacial, central nervous system, cardiovascular, and thymic malformations in the fetus. Fetal malformations have also been linked to daily exposures of 6000 to 7500 RAEs of vitamin A from supplements, and pregnant women are advised against exceeding 3000 RAEs/day of vitamin A.

BOX 3-4

Signs of Vitamin A Toxicity

Serum vitamin A of 75-2000 RAE/100 ml
Bone pain and fragility
Hydrocephalus and vomiting (infants and children)
Dry, fissured skin
Brittle nails
Hair loss (alopecia)
Gingivitis
Cheilosis
Anorexia
Irritability
Fatigue
Hepatomegaly nud abnormal liver function
Ascites and portal hypertension

The toxicities of carotenoids are low, and daily intakes of as much as 30 mg of β-carotene have no side effects other than the accumulation of the carotenoid in the skin and consequent yellowing. **Hypercarotenodermia** can be differentiated from jaundice in that the former affects only the skin, leaving the sclera (white) of the eye clear. Hypercarotenodermia is reversible if excessive carotene intake is decreased. However, high doses of β-carotene have been implicated as playing a role in some types of lung cancer, especially in smokers (see Chapter 37).

Vitamin D (Calciferol)

Vitamin D is known as the sunshine vitamin because modest exposure to sunlight is usually sufficient for most people to produce their own vitamin D using ultraviolet light and cholesterol in the skin. Because the vitamin can be produced in the body, has specific target tissues, and does not have to be supplied in the diet, it better meets the definition of a hormone rather than a vitamin and usually acts as a steroid hormone.

Two sterols—one in the lipids of animals (7-dehydrocholesterol) and one in plants (ergosterol)—can serve as precursors of vitamin D. Each of these can undergo photolytic ring opening when exposed to ultraviolet irradiation. Ring opening of 7-dehydrocholesterol yields a provitamin form of 7-dehydrocholesterol, which yields **cholecalciferol,** or vitamin D_3 (see Table 3-24). Ergosterol ring opening yields ergocalciferol, or vitamin D_2. Vitamins D_2 and D_3 require further metabolism to yield the metabolically active form of 1,25-dihydroxyvitamin D **(calcitriol)** (Figure 3-15). In this way, vitamin D plays an important role, in addition to calcium and phosphorus, in the maintenance of calcium homeostasis and healthy bones and teeth. Are vitamin D_2 and D_3 equally metabolically active?

Absorption, Transport, and Storage

Dietary vitamin D is incorporated with other lipids into micelles and absorbed with lipids into the intestine by passive diffusion. Inside the absorptive cells the vitamin is incorporated into chylomicrons, enters the lymphatic system, and subsequently enters the plasma, where it is delivered to the liver by chylomicron remnants or to the specific carrier vitamin D–binding protein (DBP), or transcalciferin. The efficiency of this absorption process seems to be about 50%. Vitamin D synthesized in the skin from cholesterol enters the capillary system and is transported by DBP. Vitamin D attached to DBP is delivered to the peripheral tissues. Little vitamin D is stored in the liver.

Metabolism

Vitamin D must be activated by two sequential hydroxylations. The first occurs in the liver and yields 25-hydroxyvitamin D_3 (25-hydroxycholecalciferol). This metabolite is the predominant circulating form of the vitamin. The second hydroxylation is carried out by the enzyme α-1-hydroxylase in the kidney and yields 1,25-dihydroxyvitamin D_3 (1,25(OH)$_2$D$_3$), the most active form of the vitamin. The activity of α-1-hydroxylase is increased by parathyroid hormone (PTH) in the presence of low plasma concentrations of calcium, yielding increased production of $1,25(OH)_2D_3$ (calcitriol). The activity of the enzyme decreases when calcitriol levels are increasing (see Figure 3-15).

Functions

Calcitriol (1,25-dihydroxyvitamin D_3) functions primarily like a steroid hormone. Its major actions involve interaction with cell membrane receptors and nuclear vitamin D receptor (VDR) proteins to affect gene transcription in a wide variety of tissues (see Chapter 13). When calcitriol binds to VDR proteins in the nucleus, the affinity of the VDR proteins for specific promoter regions of the genes—vitamin D response elements (VDRE)—increases, allowing the VDR-

calcitriol complex to bind to the VDRE. Once the VDR-calcitriol complex is attached to the VDRE region, transcription for specific mRNAs for specific proteins is enhanced (promoted) or inhibited (Figure 3-16). More than 50 genes are known to be regulated by vitamin D (Omdahl et al., 2002), including the gene for the calcium-binding protein calbindin; however, most of the genes regulated by vitamin D are not involved in mineral metabolism.

The most well understood functions of vitamin D are in the maintenance of calcium and phosphorus homeostasis, which it can affect in three major ways. First, through gene expression, calcitriol in the small intestine enhances the active transport of calcium across the gut, which stimulates synthesis of calcium-binding proteins (including calbindin)

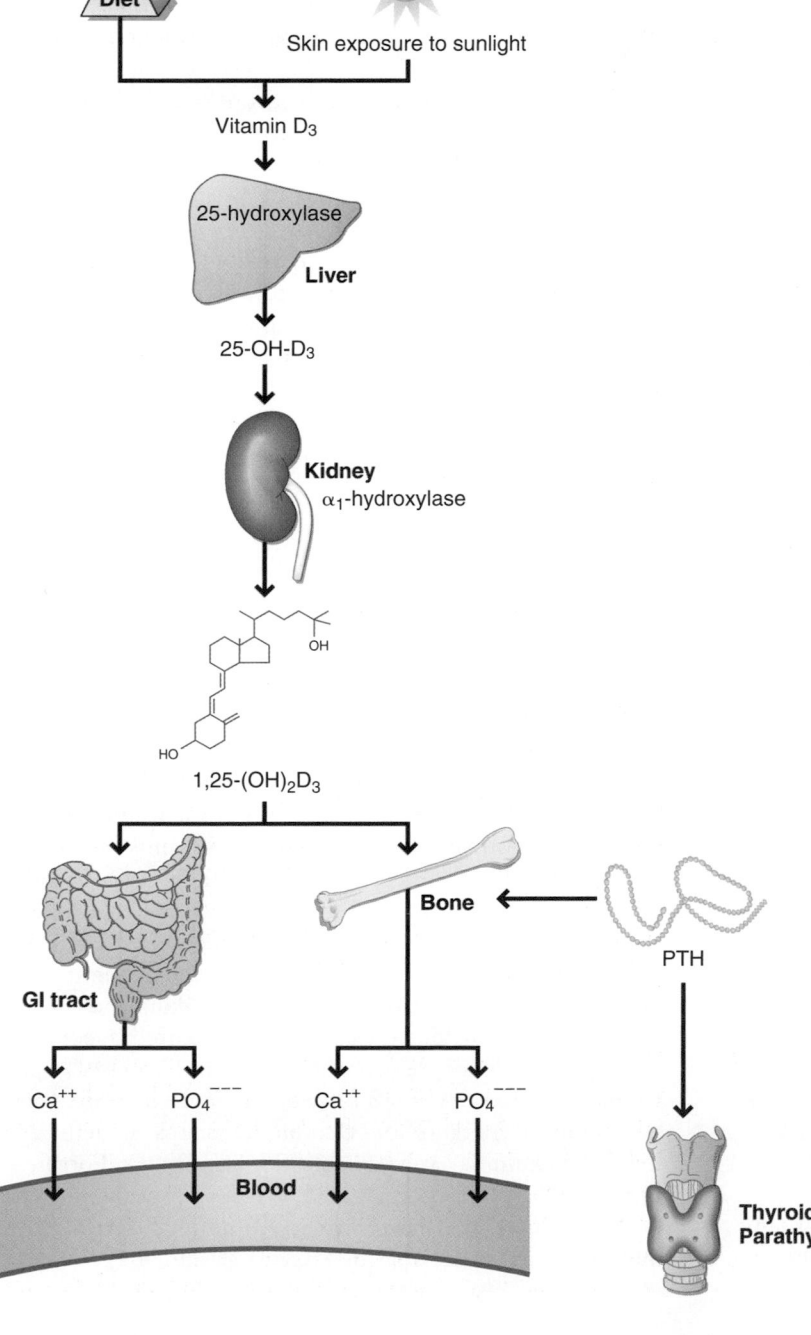

FIGURE 3-15 Metabolism and function of vitamin D. Vitamin D_3 (cholecalciferol) changes into its biologically active forms: $25-(OH)D_3$ and $1,25-(OH)_2D_3$ (calcitriol). Calcitriol increases calcium and phosphate absorption in the intestine, increases calcium and phosphate resorption in bone, and acts on the kidney to decrease calcium loss in urine.

in the mucosal brush border. These proteins then increase calcium absorption. (Vitamin D may also increase calcium absorption in a separate mechanism unrelated to gene expression. This mechanism apparently operates by opening voltage-gated calcium channels [Brown et al., 2002].) Phosphate absorption is also increased by enhancing acid phosphatase activity, which cleaves phosphate esters and allows increased phosphorus absorption. Second, in the bone PTH alone or with calcitriol, estrogen, or both, moves calcium and phosphorus from the bone to maintain normal blood levels. The process most probably involves increased osteoclast activity, increased numbers of new osteoclasts through cell differentiation, or both. Finally, in the kidney calcitriol increases renal tubular reabsorption of calcium and phosphate. These activities are coordinated with the purpose of maintaining plasma calcium concentrations within a narrow range. Calcitonin secreted by the thyroid counters the activity of calcitriol and PTH by suppression of bone mobilization and increases the renal excretion of calcium and phosphate (see Chapter 24).

Calcitriol plays roles that are not well understood in cell differentiation, proliferation, and growth in many tissues, including skin, muscles, pancreas, nerves, parathyroid gland, and immune system. For example, as mentioned previously, it stimulates differentiation of intestinal epithelial cells and osteoblasts; however, it seems to inhibit cell proliferation and growth.

Dietary Reference Intakes

The preferred units for quantification of vitamin D are micrograms (mcg) of vitamin D_3. For nonavian species, vitamins D_2 and D_3 have equivalent biologic activities; thus both are used to quantify total vitamin D. IUs are still used on some labels. One IU of vitamin D_3 equals 0.025 mcg of vitamin D_3, and 1 mcg of vitamin D_3 equals 40 IU of vitamin D_3.

DRIs for vitamin D are AIs set to meet the body's needs when a person has inadequate exposure to sunlight, and the

tolerable upper intake levels (ULs) are set at those considered to pose no risk of adverse effects. Although 2.5 mcg (100 IU) of vitamin D daily is sufficient to prevent vitamin D–deficiency rickets, higher levels (AI of 5 mcg/day) are recommended for infants and children throughout the period of skeletal development. Continued intake of the vitamin at this level during adulthood is necessary to support the normal process of continual bone remodeling and adequate calcium and phosphorus homeostasis. The AI increases to 10 mcg/day (400 IU) for adults age 51 years and older and increases even more to 15 mcg/day (600 IU) for adults 71 years and older. The UL for vitamin D for infants is 25 mcg/day (1000 IU) and for children and adults, 50 mcg/day (2000 IU).

The normal adult is presumed to obtain sufficient vitamin D from exposure to sunlight and incidental ingestion through small amounts in foods (see *Focus On: Sunshine,*

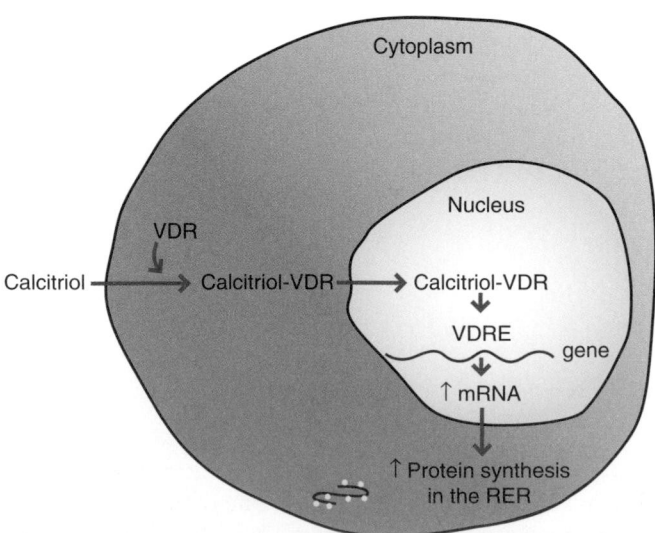

FIGURE 3-16 Role of vitamin D in gene expression. *VDR*, Vitamin D receptor protein; *VDRE*, vitamin D response elements; *RER*, rough endoplasmic reticulum.

◎ FOCUS ON

Sunshine, Vitamin D, and Fortification

Brief and casual exposure of the face, arms, and hands to sunlight is thought to equal about 5 mcg (200 IU) of vitamin D, and prolonged exposure with erythema raises plasma 25-(OH)D_3 concentrations as much as long-term ingestion of 250 mcg (10,000 IU) of vitamin D daily (Haddad, 1992). Ultraviolet light penetration depends on the amount of melanin in the skin, clothing type, blockage of effective rays by window glass, and use of sunscreens. Holick (2004) describes sensible sun exposure as 5 to 10 minutes of exposure of the arms and legs or the hands, arms, and face, 2 or 3 times per week. This type of casual exposure seems to provide sufficient vitamin D to last through the winter months except in those unable or unwilling to go outside. For these individuals who get sun exposure in the summer and who live in the United States, the present level of fortification of foods with vitamin D seems to be adequate. However, there may be a growing number of individuals for whom this is not adequate.

Milk continues to be a food of choice for vitamin D fortification because of its calcium content. Soy milks and other nondairy milks are now often fortified with the same amount of vitamin D and calcium found in cow's milk. However, milk and infant formulas may not always contain the amount of vitamin D stated on the label (Holick, 2006). Eight cases of hypervitaminosis D resulting from drinking incorrectly and excessively fortified milk have been reported (Jacobus et al., 1992), but there are probably many more cases of hypovitaminosis D as new roles for vitamin D are identified and new clinical markers of vitamin D status (serum 25-hydroxyvitamin D) are available (Holick, 2006). Fortification must be carefully regulated. Overfortification and underfortification are dangerous, so a unified fortification monitoring program is needed (Calvo et al., 2004).

Vitamin D, and Fortification). However, increasing evidence suggests that vitamin D status in the United States (Parks and Johnson, 2005) and worldwide (Reginster, 2005; Pettifor, 2005) is low, and increasing vitamin D in the diet has been recommended (Reginster, 2005; Grant and Holick, 2005). Supplemental vitamin D is appropriate for individuals consistently shielded from sunlight, such as those who are housebound, live in northern latitudes or areas with high atmospheric pollution, wear clothing that completely covers the body, or work at night and stay indoors during the day. Grant and Holick (2005) have noted that the current requirements are set based on protection against bone disease, but because of evidence of the protective effect of vitamin D against cancer, multiple sclerosis, and type I diabetes mellitus, these requirements may be revised upward (Hathcock et al., 2007).

Sources

Vitamin D_3 exists naturally in animal products, and the richest sources are fish liver oils. It is found in only small and highly variable amounts in butter, cream, egg yolk, and liver. Human milk and unfortified cow's milk tend to be poor sources of vitamin D_3, providing only 0.4 to 1 mcg/L. However, approximately 98% of all fluid milk sold in the United States is fortified with vitamin D_2 (usually 10 mcg [400 IU]/qt), as is most dried whole milk, evaporated milk, some margarines, butters, soy milks, certain cereals, and all infant formula products. Vitamin D is very stable and does not deteriorate when foods are heated or stored for long periods (Table 3-12; see also Appendix 51).

TABLE 3-12	
Vitamin D Content of Selected Foods	
Food	**Content (mcg)***
Herring, fresh, raw, 1 oz	6.6
Salmon, cooked, 1 oz	3.5
Milk, cow's, fortified, 1 cup	2.5
Sardines, canned, 1 oz	2.1
Liver, chicken, cooked, 3 oz	1.1
Shrimp, canned, 1 oz	0.7
Egg yolk	0.6
Milk, human, 1 cup	0-0.6
Liver, calf, cooked, 3 oz	0.4
DRIs	
Infants and young children	5 mcg/day
Older children and adolescents	5 mcg/day
Adults	5-15 mcg/day, depending on age and gender
Pregnant	5 mcg/day
Lactating	5 mcg/day

From U.S. Department of Agriculture: Composition of foods, Handbook No. 8 Series, Washington, DC, 1976-1986, Agricultural Research Service, USDA.

*Recalculated in micrograms of D_3; IU = 0.025 mcg; 1mcg = 40 IU.

Deficiency

Vitamin D deficiency manifests as rickets in children and growing animals and as osteomalacia in adults. Reginster (2005) noted the high prevalence of inadequate vitamin D intake on a global basis, regardless of age or health status. It is recommended that a level of 30 ng/ml be considered as the minimum level of serum 25-hydroxy vitamin D indicating deficiency (see Chapter 15).

Rickets

Rickets is a disease involving impaired mineralization of growing bones. It is the result not only of deprivation of vitamin D, but of deficiencies of calcium and phosphorus. Rickets is characterized by structural abnormalities of the weight-bearing bones (e.g., tibia, ribs, humerus, radius, ulna) (Figure 3-17) and is associated with accompanying bone pain, muscular tenderness, and hypocalcemic tetany. Soft, pliable, rachitic bones cannot withstand ordinary stresses and strains, resulting in bowed legs, "knock knees," beaded ribs (the rachitic rosary), pigeon breast, and frontal bossing of the skull. Radiography reveals enlarged epiphyseal growth plates manifested as enlarged wrists and ankles resulting from their failure to mineralize and continue growth. Patients have increased plasma and serum levels of alkaline phosphatase, which is released by the affected osteoblasts.

Historically those with rickets have been poor children in industrialized cities where exposure to sunlight is limited. In North America the vitamin D supplementation of foods has

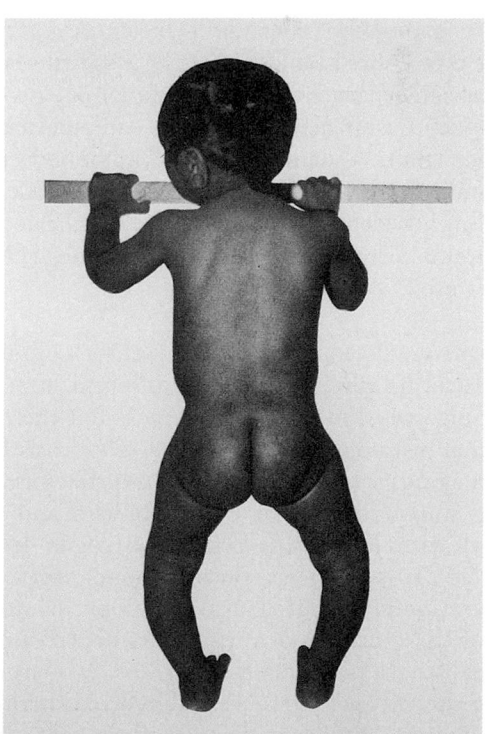

FIGURE 3-17 Severely bowed legs caused by rickets, an indication of vitamin D and calcium deficiencies in children. (Rickets is a disorder of cartilage cell growth and enlargement of epiphyseal growth plates). (*From Latham MC et al: Scope manual on nutrition, Kalamazoo, Mich, 1980, The Upjohn Company. Copyright by Rose Lee Nemir, MD.*)

virtually eliminated the disease. However, the incidence of vitamin D–dependent rickets is increasing in American children. The children most at risk have dark skin and breast-feed for long periods without exposure to sunlight or vitamin D supplements (Holick, 2006). Rickets can also develop in children with chronic problems of lipid malabsorption and in those undergoing long-term anticonvulsant therapy (which reduces the circulating levels of 1,25-dihydroxyvitamin D_3) (see Chapter 16).

Rickets caused strictly by vitamin D deprivation can be treated effectively with oral preparations of the vitamin or natural sources rich in the vitamin. For example, vitamin D concentrates of fish-liver oil have been prescribed; 1 teaspoon (4 ml) of cod-liver oil contains 9 mcg (360 IU) of vitamin D. For those with calcium deficiency–related or hypophosphatemic vitamin D–refractory rickets, vitamin D treatment alone may not be effective, and active vitamin D metabolites such as 25-(OH)D_3 or 1,25(OH)2D_3, or a synthetic analog become necessary.

Osteomalacia. Osteomalacia develops in adults whose epiphyseal closures make that portion of the bone resistant to vitamin D deficiency. Therefore the disease involves generalized reductions in bone density and the presence of pseudofractures, especially of the spine, femur, and humerus. Patients experience muscular weakness and bone tenderness and have a greater risk of fractures, particularly of the wrist and pelvis.

Prevention of osteomalacia is usually possible with an adequate consumption of vitamin D, calcium, and phosphorus in the diet. It has been estimated that as little as 10 to 15 minutes of sun exposure on a clear summer day two or three times a week is sufficient to prevent osteomalacia among most older adults. Osteomalacia can be treated effectively with vitamin D_3 in doses of 25 to 125 mcg (1000 to 1250 IU/day); in those whose conditions are complicated by lipid malabsorption, daily doses as large as 1250 mcg (12,500 IU) have been used.

Osteoporosis. Osteoporosis is frequently confused with osteomalacia; however, it is a very different bone disease, one that involves diminished bone mass but the retention of a normal histologic appearance. Osteoporosis is associated with aging; it is thought to be a multifactorial disease involving impaired vitamin D metabolism and function associated with low or decreasing estrogen levels (see Chapter 24). It is the most common bone disease of post-menopausal women, but it also develops in older men. Studies of the efficacies of various vitamers D in treating osteoporosis have been inconsistent, but two large studies involving the chronic use of 1,25-dihydroxyvitamin D_3 by women showed significant delay of the onset (and some reversal) of the signs and symptoms of osteoporosis. However, another study concluded that neither calcium nor vitamin D supplements alone are sufficient treatment for individuals with osteoporosis but are useful in conjunction with hormone replacement therapy in early postmenopausal women (Delmas, 2002).

Toxicity

Excessive intake of vitamin D can produce intoxication characterized by elevated serum calcium (hypercalcemia) and phosphorus (hyperphosphatemia) levels and ultimately the calcification of soft tissues (calcinosis), including the kidney, lungs, heart, and even the tympanic membrane of the ear, which can result in deafness. Patients often complain of headache and nausea (Box 3-5). Infants given excessive amounts of vitamin D may have GI upset, bone fragility, and retarded growth.

Hypervitaminosis D is a progressive intoxication, and individuals seem to vary in their susceptibility to the condition. The UL for vitamin D is 25 mcg (1000 IU)/day for infants and 50 mcg (2000 IU)/day for children and adults. It is clear that infants and small children are most susceptible to hypervitaminosis D.

Vitamin E

Vitamin E has a fundamental role in protecting the body against the damaging effects of reactive oxygen species that are formed metabolically or encountered in the environment. Vitamin E includes two classes of biologically active substances: (1) the **tocopherols** and (2) the related but much less biologically active compounds, the tocotrienols. The vitamers of each series are named according to the position and number of methyl groups on their ring systems. The most important of these is α-tocopherol (see Table 3-24) in the natural D-isomer form.

Absorption, Transport, and Storage

Vitamin E is absorbed in the upper small intestine by micelle-dependent diffusion, and, like the other fat-soluble vitamins, its use depends on the presence of dietary fat and adequate biliary and pancreatic function. The esterified forms of vitamin E found in supplements (which are more stable) can only be absorbed after hydrolysis by esterases at the duodenal mucosa. However, esters of natural and synthetic α-tocopherol are digested equally well (Institute of Medicine, Food and Nutrition Board, 2000b). The absorption of vitamin E is highly variable, and efficiencies range

---

BOX 3-5

Signs of Vitamin D Toxicity

Excessive calcification of bone
Kidney stones
Metastatic calcification of soft tissues (kidney, heart, lung, and tympanic membrane)
Hypercalcemia
Headache
Weakness
Nausea and vomiting
Constipation
Polyuria
Polydipsia

from 20% to 70%. Absorbed vitamin E is incorporated into chylomicrons and transported into the general circulation via lymph. Vitamin E delivered to the liver is incorporated into VLDLs using a transport protein specific for vitamin E. In the plasma, tocopherol is also partitioned into LDLs and high-density lipoproteins HDLs, where it may protect the lipoproteins from oxidation.

The cellular uptake of vitamin E can occur either as a receptor-mediated process (in which LDLs deliver the vitamin into the cell), or as a process mediated by LP as vitamin E is released from chylomicrons and VLDLs by the action of LP. Within the cell, intracellular transport of the tocopherol requires an intracellular tocopherol-binding protein (TBP). In most nonadipose cells vitamin E is located almost exclusively in membranes from which it can be mobilized; in adipose tissues it is partitioned primarily in the bulk lipid phase, from which it is not readily mobilized.

Metabolism

The metabolism of vitamin E is limited. It is primarily oxidized into the biologically inactive tocopheryl quinone, which can be reduced to tocopheryl hydroquinone. Glucuronic acid conjugates of the hydroquinone are secreted in the bile, making excretion in the feces the major route of elimination of the vitamin. With usual intakes of vitamin E, a very small portion is excreted in the urine as water-soluble, side-chain metabolites (tocopheronic acid and tocopheronolactone).

Functions

Vitamin E is the most important lipid-soluble **antioxidant** in the cell. Located in the lipid portion of cell membranes, it protects unsaturated phospholipids of the membrane from oxidative degradation from highly reactive oxygen species and other **free radicals**. Vitamin E performs this function through its ability to reduce such radicals into harmless metabolites by donating a hydrogen to them (Figure 3-18). This process is called free radical scavenging.

As a membrane free radical scavenger, vitamin E is now understood to be an important component of the cellular antioxidant defense system, which involves other enzymes (e.g., superoxide dismutases [SODs], glutathione peroxidases [GSH-Pxs], glutathione reductase [GR], catalase, thioredoxin reductase [TR]) and nonenzymatic factors (e.g., glutathione, uric acid), many of which depend on other essential nutrients. For example, the expressions of the GSH-Px and TR depend on adequate selenium status; the expressions of the SODs depend on adequate copper, zinc, and manganese statuses; and the activity of GR depends on adequate riboflavin status. Therefore the antioxidant function of vitamin E can be affected by the levels of many other nutrients.

This antioxidant function suggests that vitamin E and related nutrients may collectively be important in protecting the body against and treating conditions related to oxidative stress such as aging, arthritis (Can et al., 2002), cancer (Malmberg et al., 2002), cardiovascular disease (Fairfield and Fletcher, 2002), cataracts, diabetes, infection, and some cases of Alzheimer's disease (Morris et al., 2000). However,

care must be taken in making broad statements regarding these antioxidant effects. For example, although vitamin E is known to inhibit processes related to the development of atherosclerosis, clinical trials have given variable results, mostly negative (Weinberg, 2005). Recent evidence has indicated that vitamin E also functions in regulation of cell signaling processes and gene expression, particularly of drug metabolizing enzymes (Brigelius-Flohe, 2005).

Dietary Reference Intakes

Vitamin E is quantified in terms of α-tocopherol equivalents (α-TEs); 1 mg of R,R,R-α-tocopherol is defined as 1 α-TE, and 1 mg of the synthetic all-rac-α-tocopherol is defined as 0.5 α-TE. Although outdated, IUs of vitamin E are still found on food labels. An IU of vitamin E is equal to 0.67 mg of RRR-α-tocopherol and 1 mg of all-rac-α-tocopherol (Institute of Medicine, Food and Nutrition Board, 2000b). The DRIs for vitamin E have been established (Institute of Medicine, 2000b) with AIs for infants and recommended dietary allowances (RDAs) for children and adults based solely on the α-tocopherol form of the vitamin because other forms are not converted to α-tocopherol in humans. The present DRIs are generally higher than the previous RDAs (Institute of Medicine, Food and Nutrition Board, 1997). The need for vitamin E depends in part on the amount of PUFAs consumed. For Americans typical intakes are about 0.4 mg α-TE/mg of PUFAs; because the United

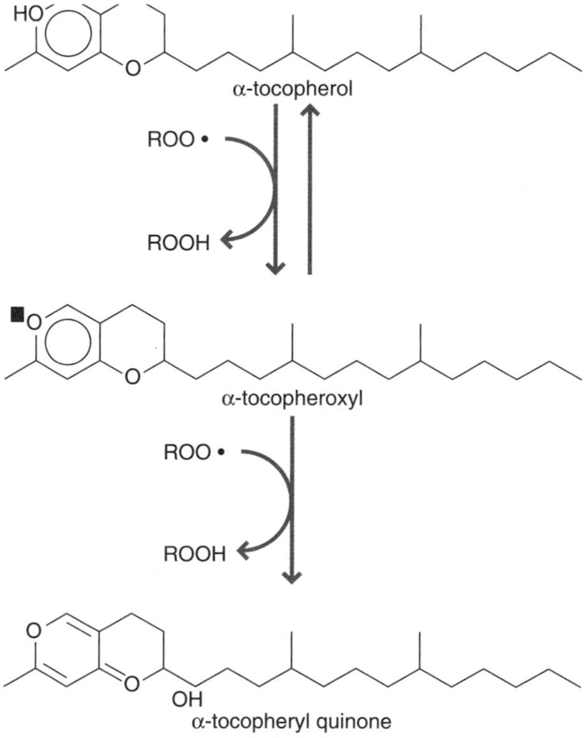

FIGURE 3-18 Mechanism of vitamin E scavenging oxygen-centered free radicals (ROO). *(From Combs GF: The vitamins: fundamental aspects in nutrition and health, ed 2, Orlando, 1998, Academic Press.)*

States does not have significant vitamin E deficiency problems, this ratio is thought to be adequate.

Sources

Because tocopherols and tocotrienols are synthesized only by plants, plant products—especially the oils—are the best sources of them, with α- and γ-tocopherols being the predominant forms in most common foods. Nearly two thirds of the vitamin E in the typical American diet is supplied by salad oils, margarines, and shortenings; about 11% by fruits and vegetables; and about 7% by grains and grain products. Table 3-13 and Appendix 49 list the vitamin E content of selected foods (Institute of Medicine, Food and Nutrition Board, 2000b).

The free alcohol forms of vitamin E (e.g., tocopherols) are fairly stable but can be destroyed by oxidation. Vitamin E esters (e.g., tocopheryl acetate) are very stable, even in oxidizing conditions. Because the vitamers E are insoluble in water, they are not lost by cooking in water but can be destroyed by deep-fat frying.

Deficiency

The clinical manifestations of vitamin E deficiency vary considerably among species. In general, the targets of deficiency are the neuromuscular, vascular, and reproductive systems. In the neuromuscular system, vitamin E deficiency, which may take 5 to 10 years to develop, manifests clinically as loss of deep tendon reflexes, impaired vibratory and position sensation, changes in balance and coordination, muscle weakness, and visual disturbances (Sokol, 2001). Symptoms in humans are uncommon and have occurred only in those with lipid malabsorption (e.g., biliary atresia, exocrine pancreatic insufficiency) or lipid transport abnormalities (e.g., abetalipoproteinemia).

At the cellular level, a deficiency of vitamin E is accompanied by an increase in lipid peroxidation of the cell membrane. Because of this, vitamin E–deficient cells exposed to an oxidant stress experience more rapid injury and necrosis.

The limited transplacental movement of vitamin E results in newborn infants having low tissue concentrations of vitamin E. Therefore premature infants may be at risk for vitamin E deficiency because they typically have a limited lipid absorptive capacity for some time (see Chapter 43).

Toxicity

Vitamin E is one of the least toxic of the vitamins. Humans and animals seem to be able to tolerate relatively high intakes—at least 100 times the nutritional requirement. The UL for vitamin E in adults is 1000 mg/day. However, in very high dose, vitamin E can decrease the body's ability to use other fat-soluble vitamins. For example, animals fed excessive amounts of vitamin E have developed impaired bone mineralization, impaired hepatic vitamin A storage, and prolonged blood coagulation. This may show up as nosebleeds. The latter effect on vitamin K status may be a concern for patients receiving anticoagulant therapy because a regular daily intake of 800 TE of vitamin E was found to exacerbate the effect of a coumarin drug.

Vitamin K

In addition to playing an essential role in blood clotting, scientists now know that **vitamin K** plays a role in bone formation and regulation of multiple enzyme systems (Denisova and Booth, 2005). Naturally occurring forms of vitamin K are the phylloquinones (the vitamin K_1 series), which are synthesized by green plants, and the **menaquinones** (the vitamin K_2 series), which are synthesized by bacteria. Both of these natural forms have a 2-methyl-1,4-napthoquinone ring and alkylated side chains (see Table 3-24). The synthetic compound **menadione** (vitamin K_3) has no side chain but can be alkylated in the liver to produce menaquinones. Menadione is twice as potent biologically as the naturally occurring forms vitamins K_1 and K_2.

TABLE 3-13

Vitamin E Content of Selected Foods

Food	α-TE (mg)
Raisin bran, 1 cup	13.50
Almonds, 1 oz	7.33
Sunflower oil, 1 tbsp	5.59
Mixed nuts 1 oz	3.10
Canola oil, 1 tbsp	2.39
Asparagus, 1 cup	2.16
Peanut oil, 1 tbsp	2.12
Corn oil, 1 tbsp	1.94
Olive oil, 1 tbsp	1.94
Apricots, canned, sweetened, ½ cup	1.55
Margarine, 1 tbsp	1.27
Flounder, 3 oz	0.56
Cashews, 1 oz	0.26
Baked beans, canned with pork, 1 cup	0.25

DRIs	
Infants	4-5 α-TE (mg)/day, depending on age
Young children	6-7 α-TE (mg)/day, depending on age
Older children and adolescents	11-15 α-TE (mg)/day, depending on age
Adults	15 α-TE (mg)/day
Pregnant	15 α-TE (mg)/day
Lactating	19 α-TE (mg)/day

From U.S. Department of Agriculture, Agricultural Research Service: Nutrient Database for Standard Reference, Release 18, retrieved 2005, Data Laboratory home page: http://www.nal.usda.gov/fnic/foodcomp/Data/SR18/sr18.html.

α-TE, α-Tocopherol equivalents.

Absorption, Transport, and Storage

The phylloquinones (K_1) are absorbed by an energy-dependent process in the small intestine. However, the menaquinones (K_2) and menadione (K_3) are absorbed in the small intestine and colon by passive diffusion. Like the other fat-soluble vitamins, absorption depends on a minimum amount of dietary fat and on bile salts and pancreatic juices. The absorbed vitamers K are incorporated into chylomicrons in the lymph and taken to the liver, where they are incorporated into VLDLs and subsequently delivered to the peripheral tissues by LDLs.

Vitamin K is found in low concentrations in many tissues, where it is localized in cellular membranes. Because of the metabolism of the vitamin, tissues show mixtures of vitamers K even when a single form is consumed. Most tissues contain phylloquinones and menaquinones.

Metabolism

Phylloquinones can be converted to menaquinones by successive bacterial dealkylation and realkylation before absorption. Side-chain shortening and oxidation produce metabolites that are excreted in the feces via the bile, frequently as glucuronic acid conjugates, and catabolize phylloquinones and menaquinones. Menadione is metabolized more rapidly; it is excreted primarily in the urine as a phosphate, sulfate, or glucuronide derivative.

Functions

Vitamin K is essential for the posttranslational carboxylation of glutamic acid residues in proteins to form carboxyglutamate ([GLA] residues); the residues bind calcium. In the process of generating residues, vitamin K is oxidized (i.e., donates a hydrogen) to an epoxide. It is restored to its hydroquinone form by the enzyme expoxide reductase (Figure 3-19). This process is known as the vitamin K cycle. The vitamin K cycle can be disrupted by inhibitors of the regeneration of reduced vitamin K, including coumarin-type drugs such as warfarin and dicumarol (which is the basis for their anticoagulant activities).

Four plasma-clotting GLA proteins have been identified, including thrombin, which is necessary for the conversion of fibrinogen to fibrin in blood clotting. In addition, at least three proteins found in calcified tissues (including osteocalcin; see Chapter 24) and at least one protein found in calcified atherosclerotic tissue (atherocalcin; see Chapter 32) have been identified.

Denisova and Booth (2005) concluded that vitamin K may play a role in the regulation of multiple enzymes involved in sphingolipid metabolism in the brain as well as other enzyme systems. The mechanisms of action may be related to a vitamin K role in carboxylation of glutamic acid residues, but other mechanisms may be involved.

Dietary Reference Intakes

Although the various vitamers K vary widely in their biopotencies, no standardization of means exists for accommodating these differences when quantifying the amounts of the vitamin K in foods or diets. Each vitamer is expressed in terms of its mass in micrograms of vitamin K.

The DRIs for vitamin K are given as AIs, and no UL has been determined. However, it should not be assumed that high vitamin K consumption has adverse effects because data on such effects are very limited.

Sources

Vitamin K is found in large amounts in green leafy vegetables, especially broccoli, cabbage, turnip greens, and dark lettuces, usually at levels greater than 100 mcg/100 g. The amounts of the vitamin in dairy products, meats, and eggs tend to vary, ranging from 0 to 50 mcg/g, and fruits and cereals usually contain about 15 mcg/g. Breast milk tends to be low in vitamin K and does not provide enough of the vitamin for infants less than 6 months of age (see Chapters 5 and 6). Table 3-14 and Appendix 50 show the vitamin K contents of some selected foods. Vitamin K content of foods is currently under revision, with the U.S. Department of Agriculture (USDA, 2000) recently publishing data on the contents of grains, cereals, fast-food breakfasts and baked goods. Researchers report that products that contain plant oils can be a good source of phylloquinone and that meat, dairy, and fast foods, which are not particularly good sources of vitamin K, do contain menaquinone, which could be physiologically significant (Elder et al., 2006).

The analytic task of determining the vitamers K in foods is formidable; therefore it is understandable that tabulated vitamin K values for food are often inaccurate.

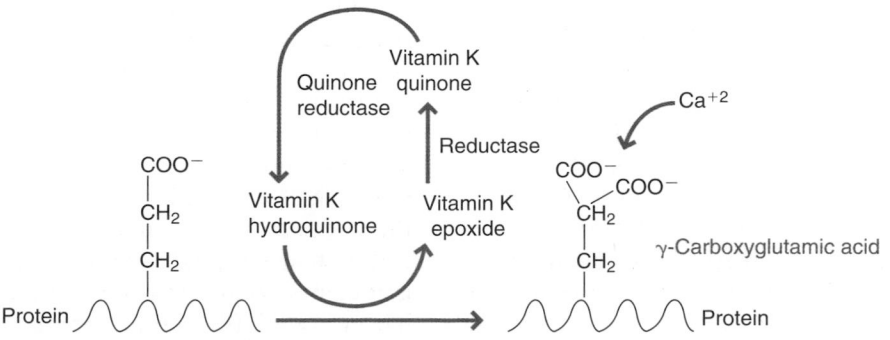

FIGURE 3-19 Function and regeneration of vitamin K in the production of γ-carboxyglutamic acid.

TABLE 3-14

Vitamin K Content of Selected Foods

Food	Content (mcg)
Spinach, frozen, cooked 1 cup	1027
Broccoli, cooked, 1 cup	220
Asparagus, cooked, 1 cup	144
Cabbage, cooked, 1 cup	73
Green beans, raw, 1 cup	47
Carrot, raw, 1 cup	14
Lettuce, iceberg, 1 cup	13
Avocado, raw, 1 oz	6
Turkey, cooked, 3 oz	0.03
Potato, baked, 1 medium	0.5
Ground beef, cooked, 3 oz	1.0
Orange, raw, 1 medium	0

DRIs

Infants	2.0-2.5 mcg/day, depending on age
Young children	30-55 mcg/day, depending on age
Older children and adolescents	60-75 mcg/day, depending on age
Adults	90-120 mcg/day, depending on gender
Pregnant	75-90 mcg/day, depending on age
Lactating	75-90 mcg/day, depending on age

From U.S. Department of Agriculture, Agricultural Research Service: Nutrient Database for Standard Reference, Release 18, retrieved 2005, Data Laboratory home page: http://www.nal.usda.gov/fnic/foodcomp/Data/SR18/sr18.html.

Nevertheless, the absence of evidence of a significant vitamin K deficiency in the general population indicates that adequate amounts of the vitamin can normally be obtained by foods or produced by enteric microflora. Vitamin K is fairly stable; it is not destroyed by ordinary cooking methods, nor is it lost in cooking water. However, it is sensitive to light and alkalis.

Deficiency

The predominant sign of vitamin K deficiency is hemorrhage, which in severe cases can cause fatal anemia. The underlying condition is hypoprothrombinemia, which is characterized by prolonged clotting time. Vitamin K deficiencies are rare among humans but have been associated with lipid malabsorption, destruction of intestinal flora in those receiving chronic antibiotic therapy, and liver disease. Newborn infants, particularly those who are premature or exclusively breast-fed, are susceptible to hypoprothrombinemia during the first few days of life as the result of poor placental transfer of vitamin K and failure to establish a vitamin K–producing intestinal microflora. Hem-

orrhagic disease in the newborn is treated prophylactically by administering menadione intramuscularly at birth. Low intakes of vitamin K have been associated with increased incidence of hip fractures in older adults (U.S. Department of Agriculture, 2000).

Toxicity

Neither the phylloquinones nor the menaquinones have shown any adverse effects by any route of administration. However, menadione can be toxic; excessive doses have produced hemolytic anemia in rats and severe jaundice in infants.

THE WATER-SOLUBLE VITAMINS

Thiamin, riboflavin, niacin, vitamin B_6, pantothenic acid, biotin, folic acid, vitamin B_{12}, and vitamin C are usually referred to as the water-soluble vitamins; and solubility in water is one of the only characteristics that they share. Because they are water soluble, these vitamins tend to be absorbed by simple diffusion when ingested in large amounts and by carrier-mediated processes when ingested in smaller amounts. They are distributed in the aqueous phases of the cell (i.e., the cytoplasm and mitochondrial matrix space) and are essential cofactors or cosubstrates of enzymes involved in various aspects of metabolism). Most are not stored in appreciable amounts, making their regular consumption a necessity.

Thiamin

Thiamin (see Table 3-24) plays essential roles in carbohydrate metabolism and neural function. The vitamin must be activated by phosphorylation into thiamin triphosphate (TTP), or cocarboxylase, which serves as a coenzyme in energy metabolism and the synthesis of pentoses. Thiamin's role in neural function is unclear, but it probably does not act as a coenzyme (Gropper et al., 2005).

Absorption, Transport, and Storage

Thiamin is absorbed from the proximal small intestine by active transport (in low doses) and passive diffusion (in high doses—i.e., >5 mg/day). Active transport is inhibited by alcohol consumption, which interferes with transport of the vitamin, and by folate deficiency, which interferes with the replication of enterocytes. The mucosal uptake of thiamin is coupled to its phosphorylation into thiamin pyrophosphate (TPP). The activated TPP is carried to the liver by the portal circulation.

Most (approximately 90%) of circulating thiamin is carried as TPP by erythrocytes, although small amounts exist primarily as free thiamin and thiamin monophosphate (TMP) bound chiefly to albumin. Uptake by cells of peripheral tissues occurs by passive diffusion and active transport. Tissues retain thiamin as phosphate esters, most of which are bound to proteins. Tissue levels of thiamin vary, with no appreciable storage of the vitamin.

Metabolism

Thiamin is phosphorylated in many tissues by specific kinases into the diphosphate and triphosphate esters. Each of these esters can be catabolized by a phosphorylase to yield TMP. Small amounts of some 20 other excretory metabolites are also produced and excreted in the urine.

Functions

The functional form of thiamin is TPP, which is a coenzyme for several dehydrogenase enzyme complexes essential in the metabolism of pyruvate and other α-keto acids. Thiamin is essential for the oxidative decarboxylation of α-keto acids, including the oxidative conversion of pyruvate to acetyl coenzyme A (acetyl CoA), which enters the tricarboxylic acid (TCA), or Krebs, cycle to generate energy. It is also required for the conversion of α-ketoglutarate and the 2-ketocarboxylates derived from the amino acids methionine, threonine, leucine, isoleucine, and valine. TPP also serves as the coenzyme for transketolase, which catalyzes 2-carbon fragment exchange reactions in the oxidation of glucose by the hexose monophosphate shunt.

Dietary Reference Intakes

Thiamin is expressed quantitatively in terms of its mass, usually in milligrams. The DRIs for thiamin include AIs for infants and the newly defined RDAs. In general, the RDAs are based on levels of energy intake because of the direct role of thiamin in energy metabolism, whereas the AIs for infants are based on the thiamin levels typically found in human milk.

Sources

Thiamin is widely distributed in many foods, most of which contain only low concentrations. The richest sources are yeasts and liver; however, cereal grains comprise the most important source of the vitamin in most human diets. Although whole grains are typically rich in thiamin, most of it is removed during milling and refining. However, in the United States most refined grain products are supplemented with thiamin and other B vitamins. Plant foods contain thiamin predominantly in the free form, whereas almost all of the thiamin in animal products exists as the more efficiently used TPP (Table 3-15).

Thiamin can be destroyed by heat, oxidation, and ionizing radiation, but it is stable when frozen. Cooking losses of the vitamin tend to vary widely, depending on cooking time, pH, temperature, quantity of water used and discarded, and whether the water is chlorinated. Thiamin can be destroyed by several sulfites added in processing; by thiamin-degrading enzymes (thiaminases) in raw fish, shellfish, and some bacteria; and by certain heat-stable factors in several plants (e.g., ferns, tea, betel nuts).

Deficiency

Thiamin deficiency is characterized by anorexia and weight loss, as well as cardiac and neurologic signs (Table 3-16). In humans thiamin deficiency eventually results in **beriberi**, the

TABLE 3-15

Thiamin Content of Selected Foods

Food	Content (mg)
Fortified ready to eat cereal, 1 cup	Up to 9.90
Pork chop, lean, 3 oz	1.06
Ham, lean, 3 oz	0.82
Sunflower seeds, shelled, 1 oz	0.59
Bagel, plain, 4 inch	0.53
Tuna sushi, 6-inch roll	0.46
Green peas, 1 cup	0.45
Beans, baked, 1 cup	0.13
Pasta, spaghetti, cooked, 1 cup	0.29
Rice, white, enriched, cooked, 1 cup	0.26
Potato, mashed, 1 cup	0.23
Doughnut, yeast, 1	0.22
Orange juice, from frozen concentrate, 6 fl oz	0.2

DRI Range

.2-1.4 mg/day, depending on age and gender

From U.S. Department of Agriculture, Agricultural Research Service: Nutrient Database for Standard Reference, Release 18, retrieved 2005, Data Laboratory home page: http://www.nal.usda.gov/fnic/foodcomp/Data/SR18/sr18.html.

symptoms of which include mental confusion, muscular wasting, edema (in those with wet beriberi), peripheral neuropathy, tachycardia, and cardiomegaly. The nonedematous (or dry) form of the disease is usually associated with energy deprivation and inactivity, whereas the wet form is usually associated with a high carbohydrate intake along with strenuous physical exertion. The latter is characterized by edema caused by biventricular heart failure with pulmonary congestion.

Without TPP, pyruvate cannot be converted to acetyl CoA and enter the TCA cycle, and energy deprivation of the heart muscle results in heart failure. Beriberi has been reported in infants (infantile beriberi) who were fed formulated diets that were not supplemented with thiamin; deterioration was sudden and characterized by cardiac failure and cyanosis. Beriberi responds to thiamin treatment, particularly if neural damage and cardiac involvement are not great.

Historically, beriberi has been endemic among the poor in areas of the world where polished white rice is the major staple food and particularly where people also consume raw fish or other sources of thiaminase. Such conditions usually produce not only beriberi but also multiple nutritional deficiencies.

Frank thiamin deficiency is not common in the United States because of the thiamin supplementation of rice and other refined cereal products. Subclinical thiamin deficiency develops in those with alcoholism who tend to have inadequate thiamin intake and impaired absorption of the

TABLE 3-16

Clinical Features of Thiamin Deficiency

Deficiency Type	Features
Early stage of deficiency	Anorexia
	Indigestion
	Constipation
	Malaise
	Heaviness and weakness of legs
	Tender calf muscles
	"Pins and needles" and numbness in legs
	Anesthesia of skin, particularly at the tibia
	Increased pulse rate and palpitations
Wet beriberi	Edema of legs, face, trunk, and serouscavities
	Tense calf muscles
	Fast pulse
	Distended neck veins
	High blood pressure
	Decreased urine volume
Dry beriberi	Worsening of early-stage polyneuritis
	Difficulty walking
	Wernicke-Korsakoff syndrome: possible
	Encephalopathy
	• Loss of immediate memory
	• Disorientation
	• Nystagmus (jerky movements of eyes)
	• Ataxia (staggering gait)
Infantile beriberi (2-5 mo of age)	Acute:
	• Decreased urine output
	• Excessive crying; thin and plaintive whining
	• Cardiac failure
	Chronic:
	• Constipation and vomiting
	• Fretfulness
	• Soft, toneless muscles
	• Pallor of skin with cyanosis

vitamin. In addition thiamin is required for the metabolism and detoxification of alcohol, so those with alcoholism need more. Some older Americans are at risk for thiamin deficiency because of their poor diets and long-term use of diuretics. Affected individuals have a type of encephalopathy called Wernicke-Korsakoff syndrome, the signs of which range from mild confusion to coma (see Chapter 28). Many have an apparently inherited abnormal transketolase incapable of normal TPP binding. Biochemical changes that reflect thiamin status occur well before the appearance of overt symptoms. Thus thiamin status can be assessed by determining erythrocyte transketolase activity, measuring blood or serum levels of thiamin, or measuring urinary thiamin excretion levels (see Appendix 30).

Toxicity

Little information exists about the toxic potential of thiamin, although massive doses (i.e., 1000 times greater than nutritional needs) of the commercial form, thiamin hydrochloride, have suppressed the respiratory center, causing death (Institute of Medicine, Food and Nutrition Board, 2000a). Parenteral doses of thiamin at 100 times the recommended levels have produced headache, convulsions, muscular weakness, cardiac arrhythmia, and allergic reactions.

Riboflavin

Riboflavin (see Table 3-24) is essential for the metabolism of carbohydrates, amino acids, and lipids and supports antioxidant protection. It carries out these functions as the coenzymes flavin adenine dinucleotide (FAD) and flavin adenine mononucleotide (FMN). Because of its fundamental roles in metabolism, riboflavin deficiencies are first evident in tissues that have rapid cellular turnover such as the skin and epithelia.

Absorption, Transport, and Storage

Riboflavin is absorbed in the free form by a carrier-mediated process in the proximal small intestine. Because most foods contain the vitamin in its coenzyme forms, FMN and FAD, absorption occurs only after the hydrolytic cleavage of free riboflavin from its various flavoprotein complexes by various phosphatases. Riboflavin absorption is a carrier-mediated process that requires ATP. The mucosal uptake of free riboflavin depends on its phosphorylation into FMN.

Riboflavin is transported in the plasma as free riboflavin and FMN, both of which are mainly bound to plasma proteins, primarily albumin. A specific riboflavin-binding protein (RfBP) has also been identified and is thought to function in the transplacental movement of the vitamin. Riboflavin is transported in its free form into cells by a carrier-mediated process. It is then converted to FMN or FAD; because both are primarily protein bound, it prevents their diffusion out of the cell and makes them resistant to catabolism. Although small amounts of the vitamin are found in the liver and kidney, it is not stored in any useful amount and therefore must be supplied in the diet regularly.

Metabolism

Riboflavin is converted to its coenzyme forms by ATP-dependent phosphorylation to yield riboflavin-5′-phosphate, or FMN, by the enzyme flavokinase. Most FMN is then converted to FAD by FAD-pyrophosphorylase. Both steps are regulated by the thyroid hormones adrenocorticotropic hormone (ACTH) and aldosterone.

Most excess riboflavin is excreted as such in the urine. However, free riboflavin can be glycosylated in the liver, and the glycosylated metabolite excreted. Riboflavin may also have a direct metabolic function. It can also be catabolized by oxidation, demethylation, and hydroxylation of its ring system to yield products that are excreted in the urine with free riboflavin.

Functions

The flavin coenzymes FMN and FAD accept pairs of hydrogen atoms forming $FMNH_2$ or $FADH_2$. As such they can participate in either one- or two-electron redox reactions. FMN and FAD serve as prosthetic groups of several flavoprotein enzymes that catalyze oxidation-reduction reactions in the cells and function as hydrogen carriers in the mitochondrial electron transport system. FMN and FAD are also coenzymes of dehydrogenases (such as in the TCA cycle, Figure 3-2) that catalyze the initial oxidations of fatty acids and several intermediates in glucose metabolism. FMN is also required for the conversion of pyridoxine (vitamin B_6) to its functional form, pyridoxal phosphate. FAD is also required for the biosynthesis of the vitamin niacin from the amino acid tryptophan.

In other cellular roles, mechanisms dependent on riboflavin and nicotinamide adenine dinucleotide phosphate (NADPH) seem to combat oxidative damage to the cell. A cataract study suggests that nutritional supplements (including riboflavin) help to improve cataracts (Jacques et al., 2005). Powers (2003) reviewed the implications of riboflavin in human health and concluded that it was implicated in a number of disease states (see *Clinical Insight:* Vitamins and Minerals in Prevention of Chronic Disease).

Dietary Reference Intakes

The DRIs for riboflavin include AIs for infants and newly defined RDAs. In general, the RDAs are based on the amount required to maintain normal tissue reserves based on urinary excretion, red blood cell riboflavin contents, and erythrocyte glutathione reductase activity. Riboflavin requirements are higher during pregnancy and lactation so that they can meet the needs of increased tissue synthesis and the losses of riboflavin secreted in breast milk.

Sources

Riboflavin, measured in milligrams in foods, is widely distributed in foods in a form bound to proteins as FMN and FAD. Rapidly growing, green leafy vegetables are rich in the vitamin; however, meats and dairy products are the most important contributors to the American diet (Table 3-17). More than half of the vitamin is lost when flour is milled; however, most breads and cereals are enriched with riboflavin and contribute appreciably to the total daily intake.

Riboflavin is stable when heated but can be readily destroyed by alkali and exposure to ultraviolet irradiation. Very little of the vitamin is destroyed during the cooking and processing of foods; however, because of its sensitivity to alkali, the practice of adding baking soda to soften dried peas or beans destroys much of their riboflavin content. Wax-lined paper containers protect milk against riboflavin loss from exposure to sunlight.

TABLE 3-17

Riboflavin Content of Selected Foods

Food	Content (mg)
Liver, beef, 3 oz	2.91
Fortified ready to eat cereal, 1 cup	Up to 1.70
Milk, 2% fat, 1 cup	0.45
Yogurt, fruit flavored, low fat, 1 cup	0.40
Clams, canned, 3 oz	0.36
Cheese, cottage, 1 cup	0.37
Egg, 1	0.25
Custard, baked, ½ cup	0.25
Pork, roast loin, 3 oz	0.27
Bagel, plain, 1	0.22
Hamburger, lean, broiled medium, 3.5 oz	0.21
Spinach, fresh, cooked, ½ cup	0.21
Chicken, dark meat, 3 oz	0.21
Broccoli, 1 cup	0.19
Cheese, American, 1 oz	0.10
Banana, 1	0.09
DRI Range	

.3-1.6 mg/day, depending on age and gender

From U.S. Department of Agriculture, Agricultural Research Service: Nutrient Database for Standard Reference, Release 18, retrieved 2005, Data Laboratory home page: http://www.nal.usda.gov/fnic/foodcomp/Data/SR18/sr18.html.

Deficiency

Riboflavin deficiency becomes manifest after several months of deprivation of the vitamin. The initial symptoms include photophobia; tearing; burning and itching of the eyes; loss of visual acuity; and soreness and burning of lips, mouth, and tongue. More advanced symptoms include cheilosis (fissuring of the lips); angular stomatitis (cracks in the skin at the corners of the mouth); a greasy eruption of the skin in the nasolabial folds, scrotum, or vulva; a purple, swollen tongue (Figure 3-20); capillary overgrowth around the cornea of the eye; and peripheral neuropathy (Box 3-6). Riboflavin has also been implicated in cataract formation when multiple vitamin deficiencies are present (Jacques et al., 2005).

Phototherapy for infants with hyperbilirubinemia often leads to riboflavin deficiency (by photodestruction of the vitamin) if the therapy does not also include riboflavin supplementation. Otherwise riboflavin deficiencies usually occur in combination with deficiencies of other water-soluble vitamins such as thiamin and niacin in those who are malnourished. Riboflavin status is measured by assessment of the activity of erythrocyte glutathione reductase. This enzyme requires FAD and converts oxidized glutathione to reduced glutathione (see Appendix 30).

Toxicity

Riboflavin is not known to be toxic; high oral doses are considered essentially nontoxic. However, high doses are not beneficial.

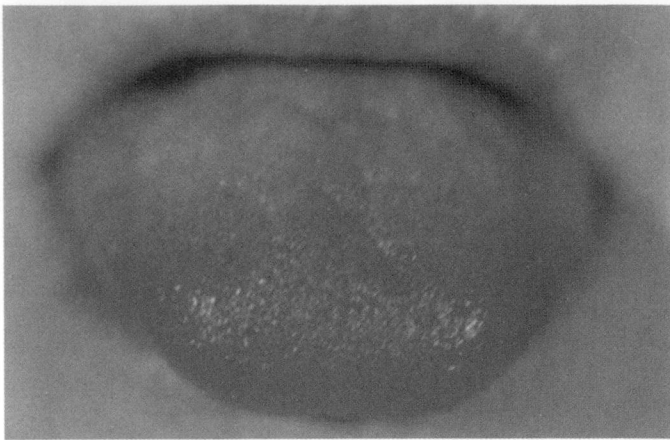

FIGURE 3-20 Magenta tongue, a sign of riboflavin deficiency. In contrast, a person with an iron deficiency often has a pale tongue; and vitamin B–complex deficiency results in a beefy, red-colored tongue. *(From McLaren DS:* Colour atlas of nutritional diseases, *England, 1981, Yearbook Medical Publishers.)*

BOX 3-6
Signs of Possible Riboflavin Deficiency

Soreness and burning of lips, mouth, and tongue*
Cheilosis*
Angular stomatitis*
Glossitis*
Purplish or magenta tongue*
Hypertrophy or atrophy of tongue papillae*
Seborrheic dermatitis of nasolabial folds, vestibule of nose, and sometimes the ears and eyelids, scrotum, and vulva
Ocular pathologic conditions (sometimes)
  • Inflammation of conjunctiva
  • Superficial vascularization of cornea
  • Ulcerations of cornea
  • Photophobia
Anemia—normocytic and normochromic
Neuropathy

Modified from Goldsmith GA: Riboflavin deficiency. In Rivlin RS, editor: *Riboflavin,* New York, 1975, Plenum Press.

*Tongue and mouth changes are difficult to differentiate from those caused by niacin, folic acid, thiamin, vitamin B_6, or vitamin B_{12} deficiency.

Niacin

Niacin is the generic term for nicotinamide and nicotinic acid (see Table 3-24). It functions as a component of the pyridine nucleotide coenzymes nicotinamide adenine dinucleotide (NAD) and NADPH, which are essential in all cells for energy production and metabolism. Recall that NAD and NADPH are the reduced forms of NAD and NADP (i.e., they carry a hydrogen ion).

Niacin was identified as a result of the search for the cause and cure of pellagra, a disease common in Spain and Italy in the eighteenth century and which devastated the

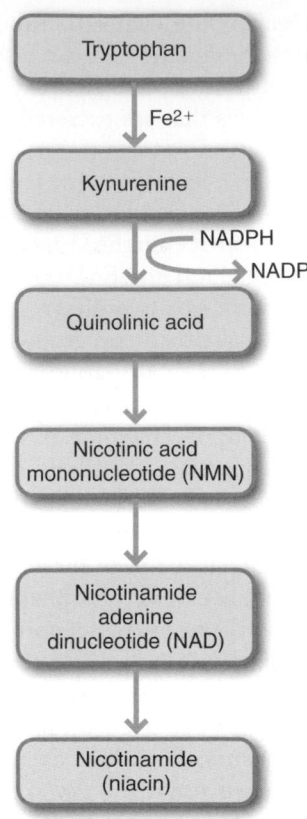

FIGURE 3-21 Synthesis of niacin from tryptophan. *NADPH,* Nicotinamide adenine dinucleotide phosphate in the reduced form.

southern United States in the early twentieth century (see *Focus On: Pellagra, Politics, and the Poor*).

Biosynthesis, Absorption, Transport, and Storage

Niacin can be synthesized from the essential amino acid tryptophan. Even though this process is not efficient, dietary tryptophan intake is important to the overall niacin status of the body (Figure 3-21).

Niacin in many foods, particularly those from animal sources, consists mostly of the coenzyme forms NAD and NADPH, each of which must be digested to release the absorbed forms, nicotinamide (Nam) and nicotinic acid (NA). Many foods derived from plants, particularly grains, contain niacin in covalently bound complexes with small peptides and carbohydrates that are not released during digestion. These forms, collectively referred to as niacytin, are not biologically available but can become bioavailable through alkaline hydrolysis. Thus the Central American tradition of soaking maize in lime water before preparing tortillas effectively increases the bioavailability of niacin in what otherwise would be considered a low-niacin food.

Ultimately Nam and NA are absorbed in the stomach and small intestine by carrier-mediated facilitated diffusion. Both are transported in the plasma in free solution, and each is taken up by most tissues through passive diffusion, although some tissues (e.g., erythrocytes, kidney, brain) also have a transport system for NA. Niacin is retained in tissues by being converted primarily to NAD but is also converted to NADPH.

Metabolism

The de novo synthesis of NAD and NADPH occurs from quinolinic acid, a metabolite of the indispensable amino acid tryptophan (see Figure 3-21). The conversion of tryptophan to niacin depends on such factors as the amount of tryptophan and niacin ingested and pyridoxine status (B₆); therefore the body must have adequate levels of riboflavin and to a lesser extent vitamin B₆. Humans are moderately efficient at this conversion; and 60 mg of tryptophan is considered equal to 1 mg of niacin.

NAD and NADPH can be produced from NA and Nam obtained from the diet. Nam is deaminated to yield NA. Then two ribose phosphates are attached to the nitrogen in the pyridine ring. Next, adenosine is attached to the ribose. Finally, an amino group is added to the acid group, forming an amide, yielding NAD. NAD can be phosphorylated in the hexose monophosphate shunt to yield NADPH.

NAD and NADPH are catabolized by hydrolysis to yield Nam, which can be deaminated into NA or methylated to yield 1-methylnicotinamide (mNAm). Dietary protein deficiency changes the profile of urinary metabolites, presumably because of changes in the amount of tryptophan converted to niacin.

Functions

The coenzymes NAD and NADPH are the most central electron carriers of cells, playing essential roles as cosubstrates of more than 200 enzymes involved in the metabolism of carbohydrates, fatty acids, and amino acids. In general, NAD and NADPH facilitate hydrogen transport by two-electron transfers, which use the hydride ion (H⁺) as the carrier, but play very different roles in metabolism. The NAD-dependent reactions are involved in intracellular respiration (e.g., beta-oxidation, TCA cycle function [see Figure 3-2], and the electron transport system). NADPH, on the other hand, is important for biosynthetic (e.g., fatty acid, sterol) pathways. Because of its fundamental role in metabolism, niacin may play an important role in mechanisms for DNA repair and gene stability and, therefore influence cancer risk (Kirkland, 2003) (see *Clinical Insight*: Vitamins and Minerals in Prevention of Chronic Disease).

Dietary Reference Intakes

Niacin is expressed in total milligrams of niacin or niacin equivalents (NEs), which are calculated from the preformed niacin content plus 1/60 of the tryptophan content. The DRIs established for niacin include AIs for infants, RDAs, and the tolerable UL. Requirements are directly related to energy intake because of niacin's role in energy-producing reactions in metabolism. They are expressed as NEs from preformed niacin and tryptophan.

Sources

Significant amounts of niacin are found in many foods; lean meats, poultry, fish, peanuts, and yeasts are particularly rich

TABLE 3-18

Preformed Niacin Content of Selected Foods*

Food	Content (mg)
Ready-to-eat cereals	Up to 26.43
Chicken, ½ breast	14.73
Tuna, canned in water, 3 oz	11.29
Rice, white, 1 cup	7.75
Mushrooms, cooked, 1 cup	6.96
Beef, ground regular, cooked	4.55
Ham, canned, 3 oz	4.28
Peanuts, dry roasted, 1 oz	3.83
Coffee, 2 fl oz	3.12
Egg bagel, 4 inch	3.06
Pizza with pepperoni	3.05
Noodles, 1 cup	2.68

DRI Range

2-18 mg/day, depending on age and gender

From U.S. Department of Agriculture, Agricultural Research Service: Nutrient Database for Standard Reference, Release 18, retrieved 2005, Data Laboratory home page: http://www.nal.usda.gov/fnic/foodcomp/Data/SR18/sr18.html.

*These data do not take into account niacin available from food via synthesis from tryptophan.

sources. Niacin exists predominantly as protein-bound NA in plant tissues and as Nam, NAD, and NADPH in animal tissues. Milk and eggs contain small amounts of niacin, but they are excellent sources of tryptophan, giving them significant niacin equivalent contents. The amount of niacin in foods depends on the total milligrams of niacin (NA and Nam) plus 1/60 of the tryptophan content. Table 3-18 lists the preformed niacin content of various foods. Many tables of food nutrient composition list only preformed niacin, thus underestimating the total niacin equivalencies of many foods.

Deficiency

Niacin deficiency symptoms initially include muscular weakness, anorexia, indigestion, and skin eruptions. Severe deficiency of niacin leads to **pellagra**, which is characterized by dermatitis, dementia, and diarrhea ("the 3 Ds"); tremors; and sore tongue (or "beef tongue"). The dermatologic changes are usually the most prominent. Skin that has been exposed to the sun develops cracked, pigmented, scaly dermatitis (Figure 3-22). Central nervous system involvement symptoms include confusion, disorientation, and neuritis. Digestive abnormalities cause irritation and inflammation of the mucous membranes of the mouth and the GI tract. Untreated pellagra can cause death (which is often referred to as "the fourth D").

Patients with pellagra can also show clinical signs of riboflavin deficiency, highlighting the metabolic interrelationships of these vitamins. Patients with pellagra are likely to have very poor diets that not only provide very little niacin but also lack protein and other nutrients. The most reliable

TABLE 3-21

Folate Content of Selected Foods

Food	Content (mcg)
Fortified dry cereal, 1 cup	100-672
Black-eyed peas, boiled, 1 cup	358
Lentils, boiled, 1 cup	358
Beans, white, boiled, 1 cup	263
Spinach, cooked, ½ cup	131
Asparagus, cooked, 1 cup	243
Broccoli, cooked, 1 cup	168
Spagetti, cooked, enriched, 1 cup	167
Cabbage, Chinese, 1 cup	70
Fresh orange juice, 1 cup	75
Cabbage, raw, 1 cup	30
Egg yolk, 1	27
Banana, 1	24

DRI Range

65-600 mcg, depending on age and gender

From U.S. Department of Agriculture, Agricultural Research Service: Nutrient Database for Standard Reference, Release 18, retrieved 2005, Data Laboratory home page: http://www.nal.usda.gov/fnic/foodcomp/Data/SR18/sr18.html.

the presence or absence of conjugase inhibitors and folate binders, and the nutritional status of the host (e.g., deficiencies of iron and vitamin C can impair folate use). Thus the bioavailabilities of folates in foods vary widely—from 25% to 50%.

Deficiency

Deficiencies of folate result in impaired biosynthesis of DNA and RNA, thus reducing cell division, which is most apparent in rapidly multiplying cells such as red blood cells; leukocytes; and epithelial cells of the stomach, intestine, vagina, and uterine cervix. In blood this is characterized by megaloblastic, macrocytic anemia with large, immature erythrocytes that have excessive amounts of hemoglobin (see Chapter 31). Initial signs of deficiency in humans include nuclear hypersegmentation of circulating polymorphonuclear leukocytes followed by megaloblastic anemia and then general weakness, depression, and polyneuropathy. Dermatologic lesions and poor growth are also symptoms.

Folate-responsive homocysteinemia (which is related to the role of folate in regeneration of methionine from homocysteine) is a condition associated with elevated risk for occlusive vascular disease and is prevalent among apparently healthy Americans, suggesting that subclinical folate deficiencies may be common. The role of folate in normal cell division makes it particularly important in embryogenesis (see Chapter 5). Thus the finding that periconceptual folate supplementation can reduce the risk of serious birth defects (including neural tube defects) by as much as half, combined with the findings regarding subclinical folate deficiencies, stimulated the U.S. govern-

ment to regulate the addition of folate to wheat flour (see Chapter 11). However, increased dietary methionine is also associated with decreased risk of neural tube defects (Shoob et al., 2001). Low levels of folate are associated with development of epithelial cell tumors (Duthie et al., 2004). Folate status is assessed by measuring the erythrocyte folate concentration, sometimes in conjunction with plasma homocysteine concentrations (see Appendix 33).

Toxicity

No adverse effects of high oral doses of folate have been reported in animals, although parenteral administration of amounts some 1000 times the dietary requirement produce epileptiform seizures in the rat. It has been suggested that high levels of folate may render zinc unavailable through the formation of nonabsorbable complexes in the gut, and studies have shown that folate treatment can exacerbate the teratogenic effects of nutritional zinc deficiency in animals.

Vitamin B$_{12}$

The term **vitamin B$_{12}$** (see Table 3-22) refers to a family of **cobalamin** compounds containing the porphyrin-like, cobalt-centered corrin nucleus. This family includes analogs containing cobalt-bound methyl groups (methylcobalamin), 5'-deoxyadenosyl groups (adenosylcobalamin), hydroxl (OH−) groups (hydroxocobalamin), nitrito groups (nitritocobalamin), or water (aquacobalamin). Of the several cobalamin compounds that exhibit vitamin B$_{12}$ activity, cyanocobalamin and hydroxycobalamin are the most active.

Absorption, Transport, and Storage

Vitamin B$_{12}$ is bound to protein in food and must be released from it by pepsin digestion in the stomach. The vitamin then combines with R proteins (cobalophilins) in the stomach and moves into the small intestine, where the R proteins are hydrolyzed and intrinsic factor (IF), a specific binding protein for B$_{12}$ produced in the stomach, binds the cobalamin. The majority of vitamin B$_{12}$ is absorbed by this active transport, and IF is essential to the process. Only about 1% can be absorbed by simple diffusion even in high amounts. IF can bind any of the four cobalamins in an IF–vitamin B$_{12}$ complex by which the vitamin is taken into the enterocyte by a process involving binding to a specific membrane receptor on the ileal brush border (Figure 3-24) (see Chapter 31).

After absorption cobalamin binds to the plasma R proteins known as transcobalamins (TCs: TCI, TCII, and TC III). TCII is the main transporter protein for newly absorbed cobalamins as they circulate to peripheral tissues (Gropper et al., 2005).

Cellular uptake of vitamin B$_{12}$ seems to be mediated by a specific TC receptor that internalizes the TC-vitamin complex. After lysosomal degradation of TC, the free vitamin is released for binding to vitamin B$_{12}$–dependent enzymes.

In adequately nourished individuals, vitamin B$_{12}$ is stored in appreciable amounts (≈2000 mcg) mainly in the liver, which typically accumulates a substantial store—some 5 to

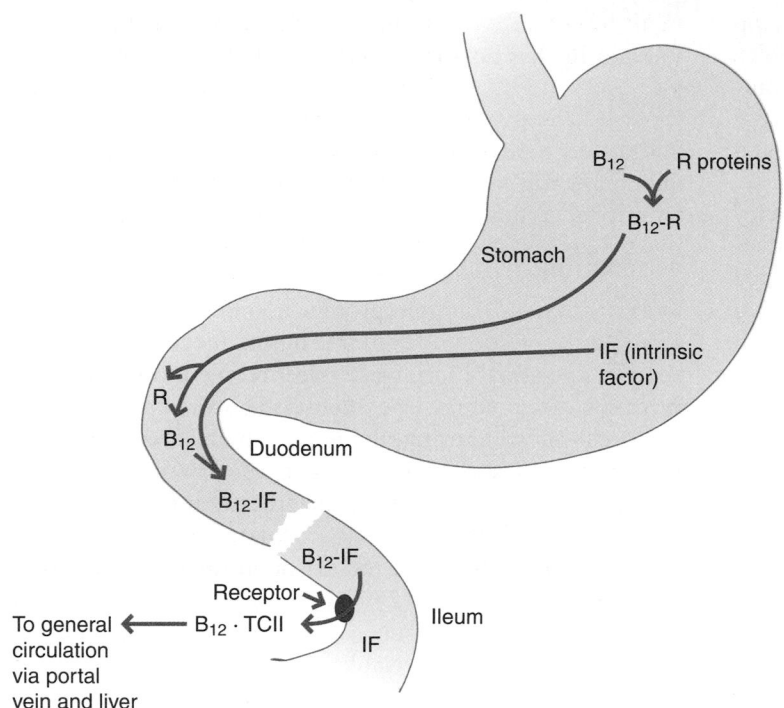

FIGURE 3-24 Digestion and absorption of B_{12}. B_{12}-R: B_{12}, R Protein complex; B_{12}-IF: B_{12}, intrinsic factor complex; B_{12}-TCII: B_{12}, transcobalamin II complex

7 years worth—most of which is in the form of adenosylcobalamin. Enterohepatic circulation of the vitamin also contributes to these stores.

Metabolism

Vitamin B_{12} is metabolically active only as derivatives that have either a 5′-deoxyadenosine or a methyl group attached covalently to the corrin ring cobalt atom. These conversions are accomplished by vitamin B_{12} coenzyme synthetase and 5-methyl-FH_4:homocysteine methyltransferase, respectively. Little if any metabolism of the corrinoid ring system occurs, and the vitamin is excreted intact by renal and biliary routes. Apparently only the free cobalamins (not the adenosylated or methylated forms) in plasma are available for excretion.

Functions

Vitamin B_{12} functions in two coenzyme forms: adenosylcobalamin (with methylcalonyl-CoA mutase and leucine mutase) and methylcobalamin (with methionine synthetase). In these reactions these forms of the vitamin play important roles in the metabolism of propionate, amino acids, and single carbons, respectively. These steps are essential for normal metabolism of all cells, especially for those of the GI tract, bone marrow, and nervous tissue. Therefore a deficiency of the vitamin is marked by increases in plasma and urinary levels of methylmalonic acid, aminoisocaproate, and homocysteine and losses of FH_4 (via the methyl folate trap).

Dietary Reference Intakes

Vitamin B_{12} is expressed in micrograms. The DRIs for vitamin B_{12} include AIs for infants and defined RDAs. The adult RDA provides for substantial body stores because of the prevalences of achlorhydria and atrophic gastritis associated with losses of IF production and of pernicious anemia in those older than 60 years of age.

Sources

Vitamin B_{12} is synthesized by bacteria, but the vitamin produced from the microflora in the colon is not absorbed. The richest sources of the vitamin are liver and kidney, milk, eggs, fish, cheese, and muscle meats (Table 3-22; see also Appendix 46).

Foods of plant origin contain the vitamin only through contamination or bacterial synthesis. Many people believe that fermented foods contain sufficient vitamin B_{12} to meet their needs; however, this theory is not supported by analysis. Individuals consuming strictly vegetarian diets, particularly after 5 to 6 years, typically have lower circulating levels of vitamin B_{12} unless they supplement with the vitamin. This is not true for ovolactovegetarians whose diets include food sources of vitamin B_{12}.

Because the vitamin is found in food bound to protein, approximately 70% of its activity is retained during the cooking of most foods; however, appreciable amounts of the vitamin can be lost when milk is pasteurized or evaporated.

Deficiency

Vitamin B_{12} deficiency causes impaired cell division, particularly in the rapidly dividing cells of the bone marrow and intestinal mucosa, through arrested synthesis of DNA. The ensuing reduction in mitotic rate results in abnormally large cells and a characteristic megaloblastic anemia (see Chapter 31). The anemia of B_{12} deficiency is related to the fact that inadequate B_{12} leads to a secondary folate deficiency because of the methyl folate trap (see previous discussion). Folate supplementation alleviates the anemia caused by B_{12} deficiency; however, other symptoms progress. Cobalamin deficiency also produces neurologic abnormalities that develop much later than the anemia. These abnormalities involve progressive neuropathy, with nerve demyelination commencing peripherally and proceeding centrally. Symptoms include numbness, tingling and burning of the feet, and stiffness and generalized weakness of the legs.

Perhaps the most common cause of vitamin B_{12} deficiency is malabsorption of the vitamin because of inadequate production and secretion of IF. Clinically this condition is called pernicious anemia, which can result from aging associated with atrophy of gastric parietal cells, hereditary deficiencies in IF synthesis, or autoimmune incapacitation of IF. The long-term (i.e., for several years) consumption of strict vegan diets without supplemental vitamin B_{12} typically leads to very low circulating levels of the vitamin (Stabler and Allen, 2004).

Wolters et al. (2004) reported that vitamin B_{12} deficiency is a common disorder in elderly adults (up to 43%), largely due to atrophic gastritis, although Andres et al. (2004) noted that food cobalamin malabsorption was also a significant cause. Food cobalamin malabsorption is caused by the inability to release cobalamin from food or a deficiency of intestinal transport proteins. Its symptoms often include (1) a lemon-yellow tint to the skin and eyes resulting from concurrent anemia and jaundice from ineffective erythropoeisis; (2) a smooth, beefy, red tongue; and (3) neurologic disorders. Psychiatric manifestations such as impaired mentation and depression may be present. Although the methods are expensive, vitamin B_{12} status is best assessed by measuring blood levels of the metabolites methylmalonic acid and homocysteine, which are B_{12} dependent, serum B_{12} level is not a good indicator of status (see Chapters 15 and 31).

TABLE 3-22

Vitamin B_{12} Content of Selected Foods

Food	Content (mcg)
Liver, beef, 3.5 oz	70.66
Clams, canned, 3 oz	84.06
Oysters, raw, eastrn, 6 medium	16.35
Crab, Alaskan king, raw, 3 oz	9.78
Tuna, light, canned, in water, 3 oz	2.54
Beef, hamburger, lean, broiled, 3 oz	2.39
Halibut, baked, ½ filet	2.18
Cottage cheese, 1 cup	1.60
Yogurt with fruit, 8 oz	1.07
Pork chop, boiled, 3.5 oz	0.93
Skim milk, 1 cup	1.30
Bologna, beef and pork, 2 slices	1.03
Ready to eat cereals	0.5-6.00

DRI Range

.4-2.8 mcg/day, depending on age and gender

From U.S. Department of Agriculture, Agricultural Research Service: Nutrient Database for Standard Reference, Release 18, retrieved 2005, Data Laboratory home page: http://www.nal.usda.gov/fnic/foodcomp/Data/SR18/sr18.html.

Toxicity

Vitamin B_{12} has no appreciable toxicity.

Biotin

Biotin (see Table 3-24) consists of a ureido ring joined to a thiophene ring with a valeric acid side chain and is necessary for critical carboxylations in metabolism.

Absorption, Transport, and Storage

Biotin in foods is largely protein bound. It is released by proteolytic digestion to yield free biotin, biocytin, or biotin-peptide. Intestinal biotinidase releases free biotin from the latter two compounds. Free biotin is absorbed in the proximal small intestine primarily by carrier-mediated diffusion. Smaller amounts of biotin can also be absorbed from the colon, which facilitates the use of the vitamin produced by hind gut microflora.

Biotin is transported in the plasma primarily as free biotin, but approximately 12% is also bound to protein and biotinidase. Biotin is taken into cells by a specific carrier-mediated process. Appreciable amounts of the vitamin are stored in the liver; however, these stores do not seem to be mobilized well when the body is deprived of the vitamin.

Metabolism

Little catabolism of biotin occurs, but some of the vitamin is oxidized to biotin sulfoxides. The vitamin is rapidly excreted in the urine (95% of an oral dose is excreted within 24 hours)—half as free biotin and the balance as bisnorbiotin, biotin sulfoxides, and various side-chain metabolites.

Functions

Biotin is a carboxyl carrier covalently bound to the carboxylase enzymes pyruvate carboxylase (which converts pyruvate to oxaloacetate in gluconeogenesis), acetyl CoA carboxylase (which synthesizes malonyl CoA for fatty acid formation), propionyl CoA carboxylase (which allows the use of odd-chain fatty acids by converting propionate to succinate), and 3-methylcrotonyl-CoA carboxylase (which catabolizes leucine). These roles of biotin link it to the metabolic roles of folic acid, pantothenic acid, and vitamin B_{12}. In recent years noncarboxylase roles for biotin have been elucidated, including a direct effect of biotin at the transcription level on glucokinase and phosphoenogyl pyruvate carboxykinase, as well as other enzymes (Dakshinamurti, 2005).

Dietary Reference Intakes

AIs for biotin have been established. However, because of uncertainty about the amount of biotin provided by intestinal flora and differences in bioavailability of biotin from foods, the establishment of EARs and RDAs is problematic.

Sources

Biotin is widely distributed in foods, but its content varies significantly, it has been determined for relatively few foods, and it may not be accurate for many. Peanuts, almonds, soy protein, eggs, yogurt, nonfat milk, and sweet potatoes are sources. Biotin content is not usually reported in food composition tables (Institute of Medicine, Food and Nutrition Board, 2000a). In addition to foods, intestinal bacteria can also contribute appreciable amounts. Fecal and urinary excretion are considerably higher than dietary intake, reflecting the magnitude of the microfloral synthesis of biotin.

The bioavailability of biotin varies considerably among different foods because of differences in the digestibility of various biotin-protein complexes. Biotin is unstable in oxidizing conditions and is destroyed by heat, especially in the presence of lipid peroxidation.

Deficiency

Because biotin can be obtained from many foods and gut microbial metabolism, simple biotin deficiency in animals is rare. Biotin deficiency has been induced by feeding raw egg white or its active component—the heat-labile, biotin-binding protein avidin. Avidin impairs biotin absorption, causing such symptoms as seborrheic dermatitis, alopecia, and paralysis. Impaired biotin absorption can also occur in such GI tract disorders as inflammatory bowel diseases or achlorhydria.

The few cases of biotin deficiency that have been described in humans have involved patients receiving incomplete parenteral nutrition and nursing infants whose mothers' milk contained very low amounts of the vitamin. In each case the signs included dermatitis, glossitis, anorexia, nausea, depression, hepatic steatosis, and hypercholesterolemia. Inherited defects in all of the known biotin enzymes have been identified in humans, but they are rare and usually have serious neurologic consequences. Blood levels of biotin are most often used to assess biotin status.

Toxicity

Biotin has no known toxic effects, even in very large doses.

Ascorbic Acid

Vitamin C, or **ascorbic acid** (see Table 3-24), functions in oxidation-reduction reactions and is synthesized from glucose and galactose by plants and most animals. However, humans, other primates, guinea pigs, some bats, and a few species of birds, lack the enzyme l-gulonolactone oxidase and thus cannot biosynthesize the factor, which for them consequently is a vitamin.

Absorption, Transport, and Storage

Species that cannot biosynthesize ascorbic acid absorb it from the diet by active transport and passive diffusion. The oxidized form of the vitamin, dehydroascorbic acid, is better absorbed than the reduced form, ascorbate, or ascorbic acid. The efficiency of enteric absorption of the vitamin is high (80% to 90%) at low intakes but declines markedly at intakes greater than about 1 g/day.

Vitamin C is transported in the plasma in the reduced form (ascorbic acid) in free solution. It is taken up by cells through a glucose transporter and a specific active transport system. Each system moves dehydroascorbic acid into cells, where it is readily reduced to ascorbate. The glucose transporter-based system of uptake is not as fast as the specific system, but it is stimulated by insulin and inhibited by glucose. Thus diabetic patients with high glucose levels typically have high plasma levels and low cellular levels of dehydroascorbic acid. The vitamin is concentrated primarily as dehydroascorbic acid in many vital organs, particularly the adrenals, brain, and eye. It has been suggested that hyperglycemia-induced cellular vitamin C deficiency may lead to oxidative stress in cells and contribute to an increased risk of atherosclerotic disease (Price et al., 2001).

Metabolism

Ascorbic acid is oxidized in vivo by two successive losses of single electrons forming the free radical (monodehydroascorbic acid). This intermediate can be further oxidized to dehydroascorbic acid (Figure 3-25). Subsequently the oxidized product undergoes irreversible hydrolysis to yield 2,3-diketo-l-gulonic acid, which can be decarboxylated to yield carbon dioxide and several five-carbon fragments (e.g., xylose, xylonic acid) or oxidized to yield oxalic acid and several four-carbon fragments (e.g., threonic acid). In addition, the vitamin can be converted to ascorbic acid 2-sulfate.

Functions

Because ascorbic acid easily loses electrons and is reversibly converted to dehydroascorbic acid, it serves as a biochemical redox system involved in many electron transport reactions, including those involved in the synthesis of collagen and carnitine and other metabolic reactions. During collagen

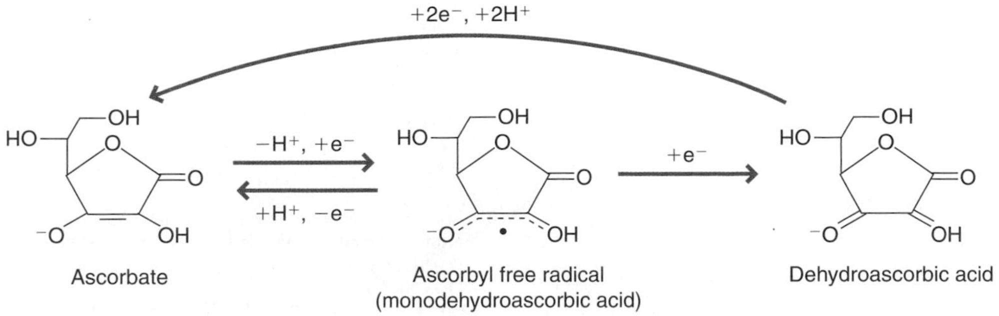

FIGURE 3-25 Oxidation-reduction reaction of vitamin C. *(From Combs GF: The vitamins: fundamental aspects in nutrition and health, ed 2, Orlando, 1998, Academic Press.)*

and carnitine synthesis, vitamin C acts as a reducing agent to keep iron in its ferrous state, thus enabling hydroxylation enzymes to function. For example, collagen, the major protein of fibrous tissues (connective tissue, cartilage, bone matrix, tooth dentin, skin, and tendons) depends on the posttranslational hydroxylation of proline residues in procollagen to form hydroxyproline, resulting in collagen. Ascorbic acid also participates in the hydroxylation of certain steroids synthesized in adrenal tissue. Vitamin C concentration decreases in periods of stress when adrenal cortical hormone activity is high. During periods of emotional, psychological, or physiologic stress, the urinary excretion of ascorbic acid increases.

Ascorbic acid also acts as an antioxidant as it undergoes single-electron oxidation to the ascorbyl radical and dehydroascorbate (see Figure 3-25). By reacting with potentially toxic reactive oxygen species such as the superoxide or hydroxyl radical, the vitamin can prevent oxidative damage. Vitamin C is essential for the oxidation of phenylalanine and tyrosine, the conversion of folate to tetrahydrofolic acid, the conversion of tryptophan to 5-hydroxytryptophan and the neurotransmitter serotonin, and the formation of norepinephrine from dopamine. It also reduces ferric to ferrous iron in the intestinal tract to facilitate iron absorption and is involved in the transfer of iron from plasma transferrin to liver ferritin.

Vitamin C promotes resistance to infection through its involvement with the immunologic activity of leukocytes, the production of interferon, the process of inflammatory reaction, and the integrity of the mucous membranes. The value of large amounts of ascorbic acid to prevent and cure the common cold has been reported, but conclusions from these studies are controversial. It is generally accepted that taking high doses of vitamin C for colds reduces the severity of the symptoms, but does not prevent them. Vitamin C maintains proper lung function (Romieu and Trenga, 2001).

Dietary Reference Intakes

The DRIs for vitamin C are expressed quantitatively in milligrams. Although as little as 10 mg of vitamin C can prevent scurvy, this level does not provide acceptable reserves of the vitamin. Because of the lower concentrations of ascorbic acid in the serum of cigarette smokers, it has been recommended that smokers increase their intake to at least 100 mg/day (Lykkesfeldt et al., 2000).

Sources

Vitamin C is found in plants and animal tissues as ascorbic acid and dehydroascorbic acid. The best sources are fruits, vegetables, and organ meats, but the actual ascorbic acid contents of foods can vary with the conditions of growth and degree of ripeness when harvested. Refrigeration and quick freezing help retain the vitamin. Most commercially frozen foods are processed so close to the source of supply that their ascorbic acid content is often higher than that of fresh foods that have been shipped across the country and spent time in storage and on supermarket shelves. Table 3-23 and Appendix 48 list the vitamin C content of selected fruits and vegetables. Citrus fruits and juices are very important sources of the vitamin for many Americans, who tend not to eat many servings of other fruits and vegetables.

Ascorbic acid is easily destroyed by oxidation, and, because it is soluble in water, it is often extracted and discarded in cooking water. Sodium bicarbonate, added to preserve and improve the color of cooked vegetables, destroys vitamin C. The cumulative losses of the vitamin from prepared vegetables refrigerated for 24 hours can be as high as 45% in fresh products and 52% in frozen products. Because consumers are eating out more frequently and more foods are being supplied to restaurants or institutions partially prepared (e.g., shredded lettuce, peeled and diced vegetables) or served from open salad bars, this vitamin loss must be considered when evaluating dietary intake.

Deficiency

Acute vitamin C deficiency results in **scurvy** in individuals unable to synthesize the vitamin. In human adults signs are manifest after 45 to 80 days of vitamin C deprivation. In children the syndrome is called Moeller-Barlow disease; it can also develop in infants fed formulas not enriched with

TABLE 3-23

Vitamin C Content of Selected Foods

Food	Amount	Content (mg)
Pepper, sweet, yellow	1 cup	283
Orange juice		
Fresh	1 cup	124
Frozen, diluted, canned	1 cup	97
Canned	1 cup	86
Broccoli		
Fresh, boiled	1 cup	116
Frozen, chopped, boiled	1 cup	74
Brussels sprouts, cooked	1 cup	97
Strawberries	1 cup	106
Grapefruit juice, from frozen concentrate, unsweetened	1 cup	83
Cantaloupe	1 cup	68
Mango	1	57
Kale, from raw, cooked	1 cup	53
Tomato juice	1 cup	45

DRI Range

15-120 mg/day, depending on age and gender

From U.S. Department of Agriculture, Agricultural Research Service: Nutrient Database for Standard Reference, Release 18, retrieved 2005, Data Laboratory home page: http://www.nal.usda.gov/fnic/foodcomp/Data/SR18/sr18.html.

vitamin C. In both cases lesions occur in mesenchymal tissues and result in impaired wound healing; edema; hemorrhages; and weakness in bone, cartilage, teeth, and connective tissues (Figure 3-26). Adults with scurvy may have swollen, bleeding gums and eventual tooth loss, lethargy, fatigue, rheumatic pains in the legs, muscular atrophy, skin lesions, and various psychological changes (e.g., hysteria, hypochondria, depression).

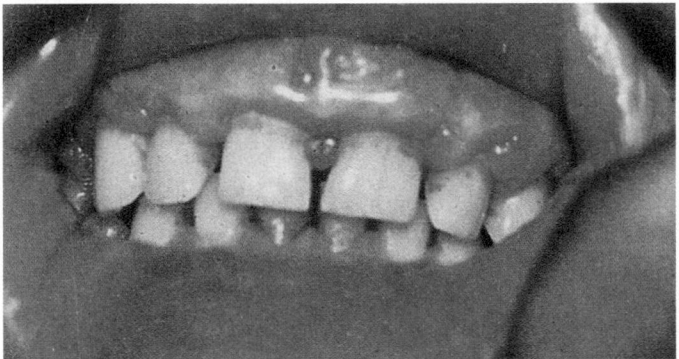

FIGURE 3-26 Scorbutic gums in vitamin C deficiency. Gums are swollen, ulcerated, and bleeding because of vitamin C–induced defects in oral epithelial basement membrane and periodontal collagen fiber synthesis. *(From Taylor KB, Anthony LE:* Clinical nutrition, *New York, 1983, McGraw-Hill.)*

Toxicity

Vitamin C is one of the most commonly used supplements in the United States. The adverse effects of high doses of vitamin C in humans include GI disturbances and diarrhea. In spite of the fact that there is considerable evidence that vitamin C may protect against gastric cancer, in a recent review Zhang and Farthing (2005) have suggested that, in conjunction with *Helicobacter pylori*, vitamin C may increase the risk of gastric carcinogenesis. The authors also note that some studies show that high levels of vitamin C may increase the general risk of cancer through its prooxidant activity. The relationship of vitamin C to cancer is discussed in Chapter 37.

Because the catabolism of vitamin C yields oxalate (among other metabolites), it is also reasonable to be concerned about the possibility of high doses of the vitamin increasing the risk of forming renal oxalate stones (see Chapter 36). However, clinical studies have shown that subjects given multiple daily doses of the vitamin developed only slight oxaluria (Sauberlich, 1994). Nevertheless, prudence dictates that individuals with histories of forming renal stones should avoid consuming too much vitamin C. Excess ascorbic acid excreted in the urine can give a false-positive urinary glucose test. Table 3-24 summarizes the preceding information on the known vitamins.

Text continued on p. 100

TABLE 3-24

Summary of Vitamins

	RDA for Adults	Sources	Stability	Comments
Fat-Soluble Vitamins				
Vitamin A (retinol; α-, β-, γ-carotene)	M: 900 RAE F: 700 RAE	Liver, kidney, milk fat, fortified margarine, egg yolk, yellow and dark-green leafy vegetables, apricots, cantaloupe, peaches.	Stable in presence of light, heat, and usual cooking methods. Destroyed by oxidation, drying, very high temperature, ultraviolet light.	Essential for normal growth, development, and maintenance of epithelial tissue. Essential for the integrity of night vision. Helps promote normal bone development and influences normal tooth formation. Functions as antioxidant. Toxic in large quantities.

All-*trans*-retinal

β-carotene

M, Male; *F,* female; *RAE,* retinol activity equivalents.

Continued

TABLE 3-24

Summary of Vitamins—cont'd

	RDA for Adults	Sources	Stability	Comments
Fat-Soluble Vitamins				
Vitamin D (calciferol)	M: 5-15 mcg F: 5-15 mcg AI	Vitamin D–fortified mild, irradiated foods, some in milk fat, liver, egg yolk, salmon, tuna fish, sardines. Sunlight converts 7-dehydro-cholesterol to cholecalciferol.	Stable in presence of heat and oxidation.	Is a prohormone. Essential for normal growth and development; important for formation and maintenance of normal bones and teeth. Influences absorption and metabolism of phosphorus and calcium. Toxic in large quantities.

Vitamin D (cholecalciferol)

	RDA for Adults	Sources	Stability	Comments
Vitamin E (tocopherols and tocotrienols)	M: 15 α-TE F: 15 α-TE	Wheat germ, vegetable oils, green leafy vegetables, milk fat, egg yolk, nuts.	Stable in presence of heat and acids. Destroyed by rancid fats, alkali, oxygen, lead, iron salts, and ultraviolet irradiation.	Is a strong antioxidant. May help prevent oxidation of unsaturated fatty acids and vitamin A in intestinal tract and body tissues. Protects red blood cells from hemolysis. Role in reproduction (in animals). Role in epithelial tissue maintenance and prostaglandin synthesis.

α-tocopheral

	RDA for Adults	Sources	Stability	Comments
Vitamin K (phylloquinone and menaquinone)	M: 120 mcg F: 120 mcg AI	Liver, soybean oil, other vegetable oils, green leafy vegetables, wheat bran. Synthesized by intestinal tract bacteria.	Resistant to heat, oxygen, and moisture. Destroyed by alkali and ultraviolet light.	Aids in production of prothrombin, a compound required for normal clotting of blood. Involved in bone metabolism. Toxic in large amounts.

Phylloquinone (vitamin K_1)

	RDA for Adults	Sources	Stability	Comments
Water-Soluble Vitamins				
Thiamin	M: 1.2 mg F: 1.1 mg	Pork liver, organ meats, legumes, whole-grain and enriched cereals and breads, wheat germ, potatoes.	Unstable in presence of heat, alkali, or oxygen. Heat stable in acid solution.	As part of cocarboxylase, aids in removal of CO_2 from α-keto acids during oxidation of carbohydrates. Essential for growth, normal appetite, digestion, and healthy nerves.

Thiamin

AI, Adequate intake; α-*TE*, α-tocopherol equivalents.

TABLE 3-24

Summary of Vitamins—cont'd

	RDA for Adults	Sources	Stability	Comments
Water-Soluble Vitamins—cont'd				
Riboflavin Flavin	M: 1.3 mg F: 1.1 mg	Milk and dairy foods, organ meats, green leafy vegetables, enriched cereals and breads, eggs.	Stable in presence of heat, oxygen, and acid. Unstable in presence of light (especially ultraviolet) or alkali.	Essential for growth. Plays enzymatic role in tissue respiration and acts as a transporter of hydrogen ions. Coenzyme forms FMN and FAD.
Niacin (nicotinic acid and nicotinamide) Nicotinic acid (niacin)	M: 16 mg NE F: 14 mg NE	Fish, liver, meat, poultry, many grains, eggs, peanuts, milk, legumes, enriched grains.	Stable in presence of heat, light, oxidation, acid, and alkali.	As part of enzyme system, aids in transfer of hydrogen and acts in metabolism of carbohydrates and amino acids. Involved in glycolysis, fat synthesis, and tissue respiration.
Pantothenic acid Pantothenic acid	5 mg AI	All plant and animal foods. Eggs, kidney, liver, salmon, and yeast are best sources. Possibly synthesized by intestinal bacteria.	Unstable in presence of acid, alkali, heat, and certain salts.	As part of coenzyme A, functions in the synthesis and breakdown of many vital body compounds. Essential in the intermediary metabolism of carbohydrate, fat, and protein.
Vitamin B$_6$ (pyridoxine, pyridoxal, and pyridoxamine) Pyridoxine (PN)	M: 1.3-1.7 mg F: 1.3-1.5 mg	Pork, glandular meats, cereal bran and germ, milk, egg yolk, oatmeal, legumes.	Stable in presence of heat, light, and oxidation.	As a coenzyme, aids in the synthesis and breakdown of amino acids and of unsaturated fatty acids from essential fatty acids. Essential for conversion of tryptophan to niacin. Essential for normal growth.

NE, Niacin equivalents; *FMN*, flavin adenine mononucleotide; *FAD*, flavin adenine dinucleotide.

Continued

TABLE 3-24

Summary of Vitamins—cont'd

	RDA for Adults	Sources	Stability	Comments
Water-Soluble Vitamins—cont'd				
Folate (folic acid, folacins)	400 mcg	Green leafy vegetables, organ meats (liver), lean beef, wheat, eggs, fish, dry beans, lentils, cowpeas, asparagus, broccoli, collards, yeast.	Stable in presence of sunlight when in solution. Unstable in presence of heat in acid media.	Essential for biosynthesis of nucleic acids—especially important in early fetal development. Essential for normal maturation of red blood cells. Functions as a coenzyme—tetrahydrofolic acid.
Biotin	30 mcg AI	Liver, mushrooms, peanuts, yeast, milk, meat, egg yolk, most vegetables, banana, grapefruit, tomato, watermelon, strawberries. Synthesized by intestinal bacteria.	Stable under most conditions.	Essential component of enzymes. Involve din synthesis and breakdown of fatty acids and amino acids through aiding the addition and removal of CO_2 to or from active compounds and the removal of NH_2 from amino acids.
Vitamin C (ascorbic acid)	M: 90 mg F: 75 mg	Acerola (West Indian cherry-like fruit), citrus fruit, tomato, melon, peppers, greens, raw cabbage, guava, strawberries, pineapple, potato, kiwi.	Unstable in presence of heat, alkali, and oxidation, except in acids. Destroyed by storage.	Maintains intracellular cement substance with preservation of capillary integrity. Cosubstrate in hydroxylations requiring molecular oxygen. Important in immune responses, wound healing, and allergic reactions. Increases absorption of nonheme iron.

Folate (structural diagram)

Biotin (structural diagram)

Ascorbate (structural diagram)

OTHER VITAMIN-LIKE FACTORS

Other food factors have vitamin characteristics but do not meet the criteria of vitamin status. These quasi-vitamins include those that can be biosynthesized but may be beneficial as supplements (e.g., choline, carnitine) and those yet to be proven to be essential (e.g., myo-inositol, the ubiquinones, the bioflavonoids). Some, such as choline, may need to be provided in the diet only at certain stages of life.

Choline

Choline (2-hydroxy-N,N,N-trimethylenthanolamine) is a methyl-rich essential component of animal tissues, where it is a structural component of **lecithin (phosphatidylcholine)** in membrane phospholipids and the neurotransmitter acetylcholine. Choline can be biosynthesized from ethanolamine by sequential methylations using S-adenosylmethionine, but most humans obtain it from dietary phosphatides. Choline is widely distributed in fat, existing predominantly

TABLE 3-24

Summary of Vitamins—cont'd

	RDA for Adults	Sources	Stability	Comments
Water-Soluble Vitamins—cont'd				
Vitamin B$_{12}$ (Cobalamin) 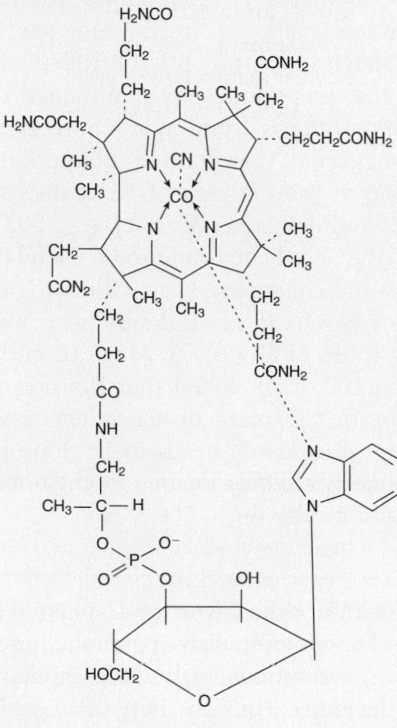	2.4 mcg	Liver, kidney, milk and dairy foods, meat, eggs. Vegans require supplement.	Slowly destroyed by acid, alkali, light, and oxidation.	Involved in the metabolism of single-carbon fragments. Essential for biosynthesis of nucleic acids and nucleoproteins. Role in metabolism of nervous tissue. Involved with folate metabolism. Related to growth.

Cobalamin

in the form of lecithin in eggs, liver, soybeans, beef, milk, and peanuts. Free choline is present in liver, oatmeal, soybeans, iceberg lettuce, cauliflower, kale, and cabbage. Choline is released by the hydrolysis of lecithin by pancreatic and intestinal lipases and is absorbed by a carrier-mediated process and passive diffusion. Absorbed choline is transported via chylomicrons in the lymphatic circulation primarily in the form of lecithin; it is transferred to lipoproteins in this form for distribution to peripheral tissues.

Choline has several functions as a methyl donor in metabolism. As phosphatidylcholine it is a structural element of membranes, a precursor to the sphingolipids, and a promoter of lipid transport. As acetylcholine it is a neurotransmitter and a component of platelet-activating factor. It functions as an emulsifier in bile, thus helping with the absorption of fat, and is also a component of pulmonary surfactant.

Meck and Williams (2003) reported that choline deficiency during the perinatal period results in "metabolic imprinting," a permanent alteration in the cholinergic organization of brain function. In adults supplemental choline has been used to diminish the short-term memory loss associated with Alzheimer's disease, and very high doses (up to 20 g/day) have been reported to alleviate symptoms of tardive dyskinesia and Huntington's disease (Canty and Zeisel, 1994). Certain kinds of cancer may induce choline deficiency (Lehman-McKeeman et al., 2002). AIs were established for choline as part of the 1998 DRIs. The UL has been set at 3.5 g/day.

Carnitine

Carnitine (β-hydroxy-γ-N-trimethylaminobutyrate) helps transport LCFAs into the mitochondria for oxidation as sources of energy, a process called the carnitine transport shuttle. Mammals and birds can synthesize carnitine from the amino acid lysine using a process that requires vitamin C. Little data exist on the carnitine biosynthetic capacities of humans, but the low tissue levels typical in neonates fed diets low in carnitine (e.g., nonsupplemented, soy-based formulas) suggest that they may have limited capacities for synthesizing the factor (Atkins and Clandinin, 1990). In some instances carnitine may be a conditionally essential nutrient. Stanley (2004) described disorders in children in which lack of carnitine limits fatty acid oxidation, but notes that efficacy of supplementation has not been documented.

Foods of plant origin are generally low in carnitine, but meats and dairy products in particular are good sources. Carnitine is efficiently absorbed across the gut by active transport and simple diffusion. About half of carnitine is acetylated during absorption; free and acetylated forms are found in circulation in plasma and erythrocytes. Carnitine is taken up primarily by skeletal peripheral tissues, which contain approximately 90% of the body stores.

Tissue depletion of carnitine has been reported in adults undergoing hemodialysis, adults with liver disease, and preterm infants. Carnitine may also be effective in certain disease states such as cardiovascular disease and type 2 diabetes (Mingrone, 2004), in which supplementation improves fatty acid oxidation. It's deficiency is also apparent in some genetic metabolic disorders (see Chapter 44).

Myo-inositol

Myo-inositol (*cis*-1,2,3,5-*trans*-4,6-cyclohexanehexol) functions in metabolism as phosphatidylinositol (PI), which provides structural support in membranes and serves as an anchor for membrane proteins by covalent bonding. It is a source of arachidonic acid for the biosynthesis of eicosanoids (see Table 3-5). In addition, PI is the source of important intracellular signals and secondary cell messengers in response to hormonal stimuli. For example, hormone-sensitive phospholipase C can act on phosphorylated PI, producing free inositol triphosphate (IP3) and a diacylglycerol (DAG). IP3 activates the release of calcium ions, which in turn stimulate calcium-dependent enzymes. DAG initiates a process that results in the alteration of some cellular enzyme activities (Gropper et al., 2001). IP is concentrated in the brain and cerebrospinal fluid but also exists in other tissues. Myo-inositol may be useful in the treatment of bipolar disorder due to abnormalities in the role of PI as a cell messenger but has not yet been found relevant to other psychiatric disorders (Kim, 2005).

Mammals synthesize myo-inositol from glucose; but it is also obtained from fruits, grains, vegetables, nuts, legumes, and organ meats such as liver and heart. Dietary sources include various inositol phospholipids in animal products and phytic acid (inositol hexaphosphate) in plant materials. Because humans and most other mammals lack an intestinal phytase, phytic acid is not a useful source of myo-inositol.

Myo-inositol is efficiently absorbed in its free form by an active transport process. It is transported in the blood primarily in its free form, with some as PI associated with lipoproteins. Free myo-inositol is converted in the tissue to PI, which is metabolized by sequential phosphorylations to the monophosphate and diphosphate forms. Only female gerbils and certain fish have been shown to have a clear dietary need for preformed myo-inositol. In these animals deprivation of the factor produced anorexia, dermatologic lesions, and intestinal lipdystrophy. A requirement for humans has yet to be defined.

Ubiquinones

The **ubiquinones** are a group of substituted 1,4-benzoquinone derivatives with varying lengths of isopentyl side chains. The principal species has 10 such side-chain units and is referred to as **coenzyme Q_{10} (CoQ_{10}),** which was first isolated in 1957. The ubiquinones are essential components of the mitochondrial electron transport chain, in which they undergo reversible reduction-oxidation reactions to pass electrons from flavoproteins (NAD or succinic dehydrogenases) to the cytochromes via cytochrome b5. In addition, the redox properties of CoQ_{10} enable it to function as a fat-soluble antioxidant, much like α-tocopherol. Relatively high concentrations of the ubiquinones are maintained in tissues, apparently by biosynthesis from endogenous precursors. It has been suggested that limited ubiquinone synthesis may play a role in the etiology of heart disease (Rosenfeldt et al., 2002) and diabetes (Watts et al., 2002). Indeed, supplemental CoQ_{10} has been found to be useful in treating cardiomyopathy and congestive heart failure (Tran et al., 2001). The use of CoQ_{10} in clinical situations was extensively reviewed by Jones et al. (2002). More recently Bonakdar and Guarneri (2005) concluded that the use of CoQ_{10} is most promising in treatment of neurodegenerative disorders but that more research needs to be done in other areas. CoQ_{10} is concentrated in various foods, notably fish oils, nuts, fish, and meats.

Bioflavonoids

The **bioflavonoids** (phenolic derivatives of 2-phenyl-1, 4-benzopyrone) have no known immediate metabolic function; however, they have been shown to reduce capillary fragility and potentiate the antiscorbutic activity of ascorbic acid, both of which may involve their chelation of divalent metal ions (Cu^{++}, Fe^{++}) and their intrinsic antioxidant properties (Manach et al., 1996). Epidemiologic studies have shown an association between diets high in bioflavonoids and reduced risks for cardiovascular disease and several cancers. The bioflavonoids are ubiquitous in foods of plant origin; more than 800 different bioflavonoids such as quercetin, rutin, and hesperidin have been isolated from plants in which they are the major sources of noncarotenoid red, blue, and yellow pigments (see Chapter 9).

MICRONUTRIENTS: MINERALS

The mineral nutrients most are traditionally divided into **macrominerals** ($\geq$100 mg/day required) and **microminerals** or trace elements (<15 mg/day required). More recently studies of patients receiving long-term total parenteral nutrition (TPN) have helped to determine the essentiality of **ultratrace elements** that are necessary in microgram (mcg) quantities each day. Mineral nutrients are recognized as essential for human function, even though specific requirements have not been established for a few of them.

MINERAL COMPOSITION OF THE BODY

Minerals represent about 4% to 5% of body weight, or 2.8 to 3.5 kg in adult women and men, respectively. Approximately 50% of this weight is calcium, and another 25% is phosphorus, existing as phosphates; almost 99% of the calcium and 70% of the phosphates are found in bones and teeth. The five other essential macrominerals (magnesium, sodium, potassium, chloride, and sulfur) and the eleven established microminerals (iron, zinc, iodide, selenium, manganese, fluoride, molybdenum, copper, chromium, cobalt, and boron) constitute the remaining 25%. The ultratrace elements without established essentiality for humans, such as arsenic, aluminum, tin, nickel, vanadium, and silicon, provide a negligible amount of weight.

Macrominerals exist in the body and food chiefly in the ionic state. For example, sodium, potassium, and calcium form positive ions (cations), whereas other minerals exist as negative ions (anions). The latter include chlorine (as chloride), sulfur (as sulfate), and phosphorus (as phosphates). Minerals also exist as components of organic compounds such as phosphoproteins, phospholipids, metalloenzymes, and other metalloproteins such as hemoglobin. (See Chapter 4 for a discussion of the electrolytes sodium, potassium, and chloride.)

With the exception of heme iron, minerals are usually absorbed in the ionic state. Therefore minerals that remain bound to organic molecules (chelated) or remain as inorganic complexes after the digestion usually cannot be absorbed and are not considered to be bioavailable. However, a few minerals may be absorbed better in a chelated form when they are properly bound to an amino acid in a covalent bond (e.g., selenomethionine). Unabsorbed minerals are excreted in the feces. Once a mineral is absorbed at the brush border of the intestinal epithelial cells, each must transfer through the cytosol and be transported across the basolateral membrane into the blood, usually by an active transport mechanism, at least for the mineral cations. If the mineral is not transported across the basolateral membrane, it remains in the intestinal cell bound to proteins. For example, calcium ions bind to calbindins, iron to intestinal ferritin, and zinc to metallothionein; if not transported into the blood, they are excreted when the intestinal cells die and slough off into the intestinal lumen. Such mechanisms may have evolved to protect the body against the potential toxicity of excessive absorption.

Bioavailability also is equated with absorption of a mineral element after its digestion from food and before its use in tissue and cells. Several factors can affect bioavailability of ingested minerals. Low bioavailability may also result from the formation of soaps, from calcium and magnesium binding to free fatty acids in the lumen in fat malabsorption, or from precipitation when one of a pair of ions (e.g., calcium, which combines with phosphates) is present in the lumen in a very high concentration. Mineral-mineral interactions also can result in depressed absorption of elements or reduce their bioavailability. For example, the absorption of zinc is typically reduced by nonheme iron supplementation; excessive intake of zinc reduces the absorption of copper; and excessive intake of calcium may reduce the absorption of manganese, zinc, and iron. However, interaction studies are difficult to conduct, and definitive conclusions about the cited interactions await additional investigation.

Many organic molecules in foods influence bioavailability, either by enhancing absorption or inhibiting absorption. Examples of inhibitors include the binding by phytates and oxalates of calcium and other divalent cations. Enhancers include ascorbate for nonheme iron or the hemoglobin protein for iron. These chelation states often enhance absorption. Vegetarians tend to consume foods with higher quantities of many of the inhibiting factors, but they typically also ingest more ascorbic acid, an enhancer. In addition, the bioavailability of elements may be influenced by many physiologic factors such as gastric acidity, homeostatic adaptations, and stress (that affect GI function). As noted previously, nondigestible oligosaccharides (NDOs), which are fermented by intestinal bacteria, stimulate the intestinal absorption and retention of calcium, magnesium, zinc, and iron (Scholz-Ahrens et al., 2001).

Certain minerals generally have a low bioavailability from foods (e.g., iron, chromium, manganese), whereas others have a high bioavailability (e.g., sodium, potassium, chloride, iodide, fluoride). Other minerals, including calcium and magnesium, have a medium bioavailability. (See following discussion and Chapter 24 for additional information on calcium bioavailability.)

Problem Minerals in the U.S. Diet

A few minerals such as calcium and iron continue to be consumed in less than optimal amounts by a large percentage of people in the United States. The intakes of magnesium, zinc, and possibly a couple of other trace minerals are also generally insufficient in the population. In the last decade fortification of foods, especially of ready-to-eat cereals, has improved intakes of iron and zinc but not calcium (Berner et al., 2001); the mean intakes still do not meet DRI levels.

Calcium

Calcium, the most abundant mineral in the body, makes up about 1.5% to 2% of the body weight and 39% of total body minerals. Approximately 99% of the calcium exists in the bones and teeth. (NOTE: The calcium in teeth cannot be mobilized back to the blood because the minerals of erupted teeth are fixed for life.) The remaining 1% of calcium is in the blood and extracellular fluids and within the cells of all tissues, where it regulates many important metabolic functions. Figure 3-27 illustrates the pathways of calcium metabolism. Bone is a dynamic tissue that returns calcium and other minerals to the extracellular fluids and blood on demand. Bone also takes up calcium and other minerals from the blood when they are consumed (i.e., during the postprandial period). However, late in life bone retention of

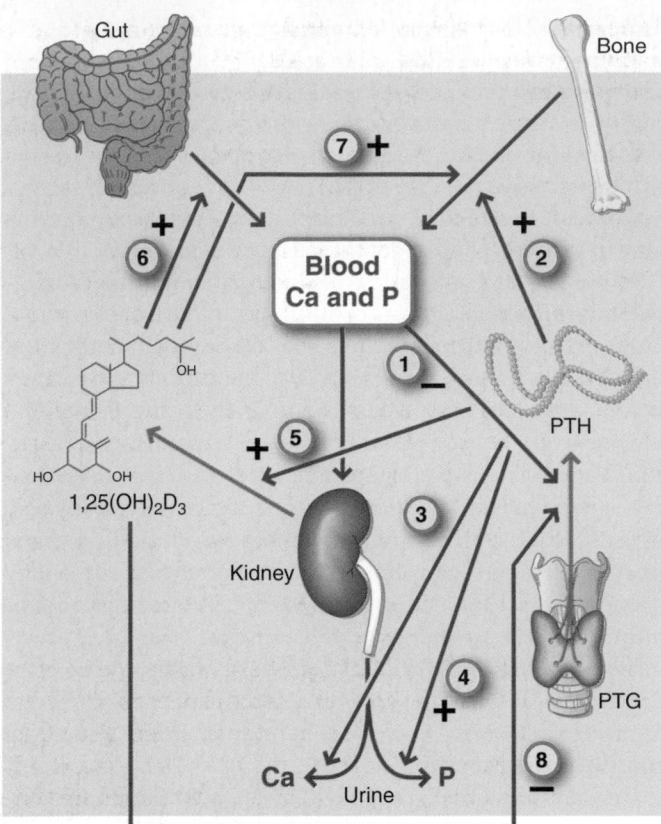

FIGURE 3-27 Pathways of calcium metabolism. The regulation of calcium metabolism involves intestinal absorption (gut), blood calcium (*Ca*) and phosphate (*P*) concentrations, bone, the kidneys—which produce the hormonal form of vitamin D (1,25[OH]₂D₃)—and the parathyroid glands (*PTG*), which secrete parathyroid hormone (*PTH*). Steps 1 through 8 are specific regulation points. A low serum calcium or high serum phosphate level stimulates PTH secretion *(Step 1)* through negative feedback.

calcium derived from food and supplements is limited unless the calcium is consumed along with sufficient vitamin D or a bone-conserving drug. (The roles of calcium in bone metabolism are discussed in Chapter 24.)

Absorption, Transport, Storage, and Excretion

Calcium is absorbed by all parts of the small intestine, but the most rapid absorption after a meal occurs in the more acidic (pH <7.0) duodenum. Absorption is slower in the remainder of the small bowel because of the alkaline pH, but the amount of calcium absorbed is actually greater in the lower segments of the small intestine, including the ileum. Calcium can also be absorbed in the colon, but only in small amounts. Only about 30% of ingested calcium is absorbed by adults, but a few individuals may absorb as little as 10% and some (rarely) as much as 60% of ingested calcium.

Calcium is absorbed by two mechanisms: (1) active transport, which operates predominantly at low luminal concentrations of calcium ions, and (2) passive transport, or paracellular transfer, which operates at high luminal concentrations of calcium ions. The active transport mechanism, mainly in the duodenum and proximal jejunum, has limited capacity, and it is controlled through the action of 1,25-dihydroxyvitamin D (1,25[OH]₂D₃). This vitamin/hormone increases calcium uptake at the brush border of the intestinal mucosal cell by also stimulating the production of calcium-binding proteins **(calbindins)** and other mechanisms. The role of calbindins in the actions of the intestinal absorbing cells is to store calcium ions temporarily after a meal and ferry them to the basolateral membrane for the final step of absorption. The calcium-binding proteins bind two or more calcium ions per protein molecule within the cytosol.

The second absorption mechanism, which is passive, nonsaturable (with no limit), and independent of vitamin D, occurs along the entire length of the small intestine. When large amounts of calcium are consumed in a single meal (e.g., from a dairy food or a supplement), much of the calcium that is absorbed occurs by this passive route. The active transport mechanism is more important when calcium intakes are well below recommended intakes and body requirements are not being met.

Numerous factors influence (favorably and unfavorably) the bioavailability and hence the absorption of calcium within the gut lumen. In general, the greater the need and/or the smaller the dietary supply, the more efficient the absorption of calcium is. Increased needs encountered during growth, pregnancy, lactation, and calcium-deficient states, as well as during levels of exercise resulting in high bone density, enhance calcium absorption. Low vitamin D intake or inadequate exposure to sunlight reduces calcium absorption, especially among older adults. In addition, the efficiency of skin production of vitamin D by older adults is considerably lower than that of younger people. Aging is also characterized by achlorhydria (a lack of gastric acid secretion), which results in less gastric acidity and reduced calcium absorption (see Chapter 10).

Calcium is absorbed only if it is present in an ionic form. Thus calcium is best absorbed in an acidic medium; the hydrochloric acid secreted in the stomach, such as that secreted during a meal, increases calcium absorption by lowering the pH in the proximal duodenum. This also applies to calcium supplements; therefore taking a calcium supplement with a meal improves absorption, especially in older adults. Lactose enhances calcium absorption. Even in adults with lactose intolerance, lactose probably improves calcium absorption (see Chapter 24).

Calcium is not absorbed if it is precipitated by another dietary constituent such as oxalate or if it forms soaps with free fatty acids. Oxalic acid (oxalate) in rhubarb, spinach, chard, and beet greens forms insoluble calcium oxalate in the digestive tract (see Box 36-4). For example, only 5% of the calcium in spinach is absorbed. Phytic acid (phytate), a phosphorus-containing compound found principally in the outer husks of cereal grains, combines with calcium to form calcium phytate, which is also insoluble and cannot be absorbed. These unabsorbed forms of calcium are excreted in the feces as calcium oxalates and calcium soaps.

Dietary fiber may decrease calcium absorption, but this may only be a problem for those who consume large amounts of fiber (i.e., more than 30 g/day). Less fiber has little effect on calcium availability in the gut lumen and hence on absorption. Medications can affect bioavailability or increase calcium excretion, both of which may contribute to bone loss (see Chapter 16). In individuals with fat malabsorption, calcium absorption is decreased because of the formation of calcium–fatty acid soaps. Calcium absorption does not seem to be affected by the amount of phosphate in the diet unless the intake of phosphate is excessively high or by the calcium/phosphorus ratio (see following discussion on phosphorus).

Renal Excretion. About 50% of the ingested calcium is excreted in the urine each day, but an almost equivalent amount is also secreted into the intestine (and joins unabsorbed calcium in the feces). Calcium resorption from the renal tubules occurs by transport mechanisms similar to those in the small intestine. Urinary calcium excretion varies throughout the life cycle, but it is typically low during periods of rapid skeletal growth. At menopause calcium excretion increases greatly, but in postmenopausal women treated with estrogen, less calcium is excreted. After approximately 65 years of age, calcium excretion decreases, most likely because of decreased intestinal absorption of calcium. In general, urinary calcium levels correlate well with calcium intake.

High urinary calcium excretion (hypercalciuria) can be induced experimentally by a diet high in animal protein due to the generation of inorganic acids such as sulfuric acid from the sulfur-containing amino acids. However, this effect has not been established in long-term studies of populations with diets high in meat. Consumption of several cups of caffeinated coffee daily increases urinary calcium loss, but results from studies have not been consistent. A high sodium intake also contributes to lower renal resorption of calcium and higher urinary calcium losses.

Skin Losses. Dermal losses of calcium occur in the form of skin exfoliation and sweat. The amount of calcium lost in sweat is about 15 mg/day. Strenuous physical activity with sweating increases the loss, even in persons with a low calcium intake.

Serum Calcium. Total serum calcium consists of three distinct fractions: (1) free, or ionized, calcium (47.6%); (2) complexes between calcium and anions such as phosphate, citrate, or other organic anions (6.4%); and (3) calcium that is protein bound, primarily with albumin (46%). Serum albumin binds between 70% and 90% of the calcium that is protein bound.

Ionized calcium (Ca^{++++}) is regulated and equilibrates rapidly with protein-bound calcium in blood. The serum ionized calcium concentration is controlled primarily by PTH, although other hormones have minor roles in its regulation. These other hormones include calcitonin, vitamin D, estrogens, and others (see the following section). The total serum

calcium level is maintained within a narrow range of 8.8 to 10.8 mg/dl, of which the ionized calcium concentrations range from 4.4 to 5.2 mg/dl because hypocalcemia (serum calcium values below the lower limit) and hypercalcemia (serum calcium level values higher than the upper limit) have significant physiologic effects. Serum levels of calcium are highest early in life, gradually decreasing throughout life and reaching the lowest levels during the older years.

Several factors affect the relative distribution of calcium in blood serum or plasma. One of these is pH; the ionized calcium fraction is higher in acidosis and lower in alkalosis (see Chapter 4). Total calcium changes concurrently with changes in plasma protein levels; however, the ionized fraction usually remains within normal limits. The strict regulation of ionized calcium makes it a useful diagnostic tool in assessing parathyroid gland function, monitoring kidney disease, and monitoring sick neonates for whom hypocalcemia could be life threatening.

Regulation of Serum Calcium. Calcium in bones is in equilibrium with calcium in the blood. PTH plays the major role in maintaining serum calcium as noted previously. When the blood calcium concentration falls below this level, PTH stimulates the transfer of exchangeable calcium from the bone into the blood. At the same time, PTH promotes renal tubular resorption of calcium, and it indirectly stimulates increased intestinal absorption of calcium by increasing kidney production of vitamin D ($1,25[OH]_2D_3$) (see Figure 3-27).

Other hormones such as glucocorticoids, thyroid hormones, and sex hormones also have important roles in calcium homeostasis. Glucocorticoid excess leads to bone loss, particularly of trabecular bone, due to impaired calcium absorption through both active and passive mechanisms. Thyroid hormones (T_4 and T_3) may stimulate bone resorption; chronic hyperthyroid conditions result in loss of compact and trabecular bone. In women normal bone balance requires serum estrogen concentrations to be within normal limits. The rapid decrease of the serum estrogen concentration during menopause is a major factor contributing to bone resorption. Treating postmenopausal women with estrogen slows the rate of bone resorption (see Chapter 24). Bone reabsorption is also inhibited by testosterone.

Functions

Adequate dietary calcium is needed to permit optimal gains in bone mass and density in the prepubertal and adolescent years. These gains are especially critical for girls because the accumulated bone may provide additional protection against osteoporosis in the years after menopause. Peak calcium retention by girls has been shown to occur in the prepubertal and early pubertal periods and is influenced by race with black girls having significantly higher retention rates (Wigertz et al., 2005) (see Chapter 24).

Postmenopausal women need to obtain sufficient amounts of calcium to maintain bone health and suppress PTH, which increases later in life in most individuals, perhaps as a result of inadequate calcium in the diet (see Chapters 10 and 24).

Additional amounts of calcium are recommended to meet the needs of pregnancy and lactation. Calcium requirements during pregnancy, infancy, childhood, and adolescence are discussed in detail in Chapters 5 through 8. In addition to its function in building and maintaining bones and teeth, calcium also has numerous critical metabolic roles in cells in all other tissues. However, compared with the significant needs of the skeleton, only small amounts of calcium are required for all other cellular and extracellular functions.

The transport functions of cell membranes are influenced by calcium, which affects membrane stability in poorly understood ways. Calcium also influences the transmission of ions across membranes of cell organelles, the release of neurotransmitters at synaptic junctions, the function of hormones, and the release or activation of intracellular and extracellular enzymes.

Calcium is required for nerve transmission and regulation of heart muscle function. The proper balance of calcium, sodium, potassium, and magnesium ions maintains skeletal muscle tone and controls nerve irritability. A significant increase in the serum calcium level can cause cardiac or respiratory failure, whereas a decrease results in **tetany** of skeletal muscles. In addition, calcium ions play a critical role in smooth muscle contractility.

Ionized calcium initiates the formation of a blood clot by stimulating the release of thromboplastin from blood platelets. Calcium ions also serve as required cofactors for several enzymatic reactions, including the conversion of prothrombin to thrombin, which aids in the polymerization of fibrinogen to fibrin and the final step in blood clot formation.

High dietary calcium intakes are associated with decreased prevalence of overweight and obesity. The mechanism for this affect appears to be related to (1) depression of the PTH and 1,25 hydroxy vitamin D, which leads to inhibition of lipogenesis and increased lipolysis, and (2) increased excretion of fecal fat due to soaps formation (Schrager, 2005) (see Table 3-36).

Dietary Reference Intakes

The AI for calcium is based on estimates of requirements of both genders throughout the life cycle. The tolerable UL has also been established for this nutrient for the first time. During several periods of the female life cycle, calcium intake is critical: prepuberty and adolescence, postmenopause, and during pregnancy and lactation (Kovacs, 2005). In a study of adolescent girls, calcium intakes of 1300 mg or more each day were necessary for maximum calcium retention by the body's skeleton. Abrams (2005) noted that calcium supplementation was helpful to children and adolescents and that catch-up mineralization was possible later in puberty if intakes were adequate. Men also need adequate amounts of calcium throughout the life cycle, but less is known about their requirements.

Food Sources and Intakes

Cow's milk and dairy products are the most concentrated sources of calcium. Dark green leafy vegetables such as kale, collards, turnip greens, mustard greens, and broccoli; al-

monds; blackstrap molasses; the small bones of sardines and canned salmon; and clams and oysters are good sources of calcium. Soybeans also contain ample amounts of calcium. Oxalic acid limits the availability of calcium in rhubarb, spinach, chard, and beet greens. Fortified orange juice and other juices and most fortified soy, nut, grain and rice milks contain as much calcium as cow's milk. Many bottled waters and energy bars have calcium and sometimes vitamin D added. Tofu prepared by calcium precipitation is also a source of calcium. Table 3-25 and Appendix 51 show the calcium content of selected foods.

Calcium supplements are now commonly used to increase calcium intakes. The most common form is calcium

TABLE 3-25

Calcium Content of Selected Foods

Food	Content (mg)
Milkshake, vanilla, 11 oz	457
Yogurt, low fat, with fruit, 1 cup	345
Fast-food enchilada, 1	324
Rhubarb, cooked, ½ cup	318
Spinach, frozen, cooked, 1 cup	291
Milk, 2% milkfat, 1 cup	285
Cheese, cheddar, 1 oz	204
Waffle, frozen, 4-inch diameter, 1	191
Salmon, canned, with bones, 3½ oz	181
Tofu, regular, ¼ block	163
Cheese, cottage, 2% fat, 1 cup	155
Ice cream, vanilla, softserve, ½ cup	113
Almonds, 1oz	70
Baked beans, white, ½ cup	64
Broccoli, cooked from fresh, 1 cup	62
Frankfurter, turkey, 1	58
Orange, 1 medium	52
Halibut, baked, 3 oz	51
Kale, fresh, cooked, ½ cup	47
Bread, whole wheat, 1 slice	20
Banana, 1 medium	7
Ground beef, lean, 3 oz	4

DRIs = AIs

Infants and young children	210-800 mg/day, depending on age
Older children and adolescents	1300 mg/day
Adults	1000-1200 mg/day, depending on age and gender
Pregnant	1000-1300 mg/day, depending on age
Lactating	1000-1300 mg/day, depending on age

From U.S. Department of Agriculture, Agricultural Research Service: Nutrient Database for Standard Reference, Release 18, retrieved 2005, Data Laboratory home page: http://www.nal.usda.gov/fnic/foodcomp/Data/SR18/sr18.html.

carbonate, which is relatively insoluble, particularly at a neutral pH. Although it has less calcium than calcium carbonate by weight, calcium citrate is much more soluble. Therefore calcium citrate would be suitable for patients with achlorhydria (lack of hydrochloric acid in the stomach). In patients with achlorhydria, the efficiency of calcium absorption is greatly decreased because of the higher pH of the stomach contents; however, calcium absorption is increased by the consumption of a meal, which improves the solubility of calcium ions because of the increased gastric acidity. The selection of the most appropriate calcium supplement depends on several factors, including physical and chemical properties, interactions with other medications being taken concurrently, current medical conditions, and age. Beginning at the age of 11 years, median dietary calcium intakes in the United States are considerably less than the AIs (Figure 3-28). Therefore calcium intakes of Americans are insufficient for the critical ages of bone deposition in both genders, as well as being inadequate at other critical stages.

Deficiency

The development of peak bone mass requires adequate amounts of calcium and phosphorus, vitamin D, and other nutrients. Compared with adulthood, greater amounts of calcium and phosphate are required for skeletal development; therefore adequate intakes of these minerals and others have a significant impact on peak bone mass development until the time of puberty and throughout adolescence. After adolescence, bone gains may still occur, but the amounts of calcium required decrease. Vitamin D status may or may not be a problem, depending on the intakes of calcium and phosphorus. Almost any time during the life cycle when the calcium intake is well below the recommended amount, PTH concentrations in the blood increase. A persistent elevation may contribute to low bone mass (see "Phosphorus" in the following paragraphs and Chapter 24). Calcium and vitamin D intakes of many older women are inadequate.

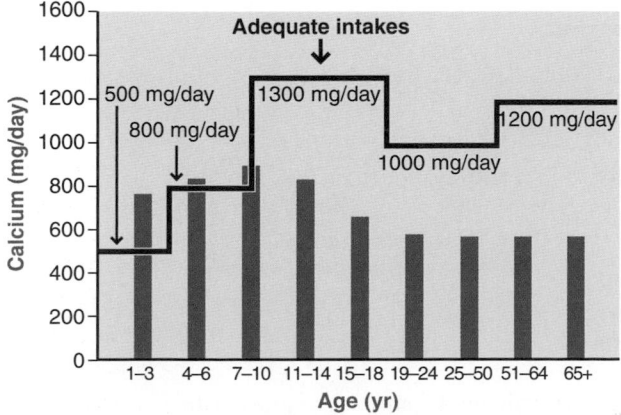

FIGURE 3-28 Comparison of the median daily calcium intake for females in the United States and the adequate intakes established in 1998.

An inadequate intake of calcium, in addition to an inadequate intake of vitamin D, has also been demonstrated to contribute to osteomalacia (see Chapter 24). A low calcium intake may be an important factor in several chronic diseases, such as colon cancer (see Chapter 37) and hypertension (see Chapter 33), that commonly occur in Western societies. Data from the Dietary Approaches to Stop Hypertension (DASH) study show that adequate dietary intakes of calcium, magnesium, potassium, and other micronutrients from low-fat dairy foods, fruits, and vegetables can both substantially reduce blood pressure in those with hypertension and prevent the development of hypertension (see Chapter 33). Hogan (2005) suggested that epidemic obesity and subsequent dieting may have a detrimental affect on bone status, leading to osterporosis. But, as pointed out previously (Schrager, 2005), calcium, especially from dairy products, is associated with decreased body fat, and these foods work well in weight loss diets.

Toxicity

A very high intake of calcium (i.e., 2000 mg or more per day), especially in a person with a high level of vitamin D (e.g., from ingestion of combined supplements of calcium and vitamin D), is a potential cause of hypercalcemia. Such toxicity may lead to excessive calcification in soft tissues, especially the kidneys, and may be life threatening (the tolerable ULs for calcium are found on the inside front cover). In addition, Klompmaker (2005) proposed that long-term high intakes of calcium may lead to increased bone fractures in the elderly, perhaps due to high bone remodeling rates that lead to exhaustion of osteoblast.

High intakes of calcium may also interfere with the absorption of other divalent cations such as iron, zinc, and manganese. Therefore supplements of certain minerals should be taken at different times. Another potential adverse, although not toxic per se, effect of excessive calcium intake is constipation. Constipation is common among older women who take calcium supplements.

Physical Immobility

Prolonged bed rest or periods of weightlessness during space travel promote significant calcium losses in response to a lack of tension or gravity on the bones. Older individuals who require a prolonged recovery with limited activity, such as those with hip fractures or other illnesses, also have increased calcium losses. Many studies have shown that physical activity promotes bone health (see Chapter 24).

Phosphorus

Phosphorus, another essential element, ranks second to calcium in abundance in human tissues; approximately 700 g of phosphorus exists in adult tissues, and about 85% is present in the skeleton and teeth as calcium phosphate crystals. The remaining 15% exists in the metabolically active pool in every cell in the body and in the extracellular fluid compartment. Almost 50% of the inorganic phosphate is present in serum as free ions (i.e., $H_2PO_4^-$ and $H_2PO_4^{2-}$). Smaller percentages are bound to protein ($\approx 10\%$) or complexed ($\approx 40\%$).

The serum inorganic phosphorus level is closely maintained by PTH at 3 to 4 mg/100 ml in adults, but it is not as closely regulated as the serum calcium level. Normal blood concentrations in infants are higher. In older adults serum phosphate concentrations are typically lower; hypophosphatemia (<2.5 mg/dl) may be more common among older adults than previously thought. Phosphorus balance is illustrated in Figure 3-29 (see Chapter 24).

Absorption, Transport, Storage, and Excretion

The relative amounts of inorganic and organic phosphates in the diet vary with the food or supplement consumed. Regardless of the form, most phosphates are absorbed in the inorganic state. Organically bound phosphate is hydrolyzed in the lumen of the intestine and released as inorganic phosphate, primarily through the action of pancreatic or intestinal phosphatases. Bioavailability depends on the form of the phosphate and the pH. The acidic milieu of the most proximal portion of the duodenum is important in maintaining phosphorus solubility and therefore bioavailability. In vegetarian diets the major portion of the phosphorus exists as phytate, which is poorly digested by humans. Humans do not have the phytase enzyme to cleave the phosphorus from the phytate; however, intestinal bacteria have the enzyme needed to hydrolyze phosphates. The yeast used in making bread contains a phytase, which releases phosphate.

In general, the efficiency of phosphate absorption is 60% to 70% in adults, almost twice as high as for calcium; phosphate absorption is also much more rapid than that of calcium. For example, the peak of absorption of phosphates occurs approximately 1 hour after ingestion of a meal, whereas the peak for calcium entry into the blood occurs 3 to 4 hours after a meal (Anderson et al., 1998).

The primary route of phosphorus excretion is renal, which also is the primary site of phosphate regulation. Major determinants of urinary phosphorus loss are an increased intake of phosphate, an increase in phosphate absorption, and the plasma phosphorus concentration. Other factors contributing to increased urinary phosphate loss are hyperparathyroidism, acute respiratory or metabolic acidosis, the intake of diuretics, and the expansion of extracellular volume. If PTH levels are high, the urinary route excretes additional phosphate. Starvation or chronic undernutrition typically contributes to most of the alterations in metabolism that result in hypophosphatemia and renal losses of phosphate. Regulation of serum phosphate and hence urinary phosphate losses is not as precise as it is for calcium, but endogenous fecal phosphate excretion may be better regulated and provide a way to eliminate some of the excessive phosphate when PTH levels are elevated. The latter route of excretion may increase when the phosphate load in the blood and tissues is excessively high. Reduced phosphate excretion is associated with dietary phosphorus restriction; increases in plasma insulin, thyroid hormone, growth hormone, glucagon, or glucocorticoids; metabolic or respiratory alkalosis; and extracellular volume contraction.

Functions

As phosphates, phosphorus participates in numerous essential functions of the body. DNA and RNA are based on phosphate. The major cellular form of energy, ATP, contains high-energy phosphate bonds, as do creatinine phosphate and phosphoenolpyruvate (see Chapter 23). Cyclic adenosine monophosphate (cAMP) acts as a secondary signal within cells following peptide hormone activation of

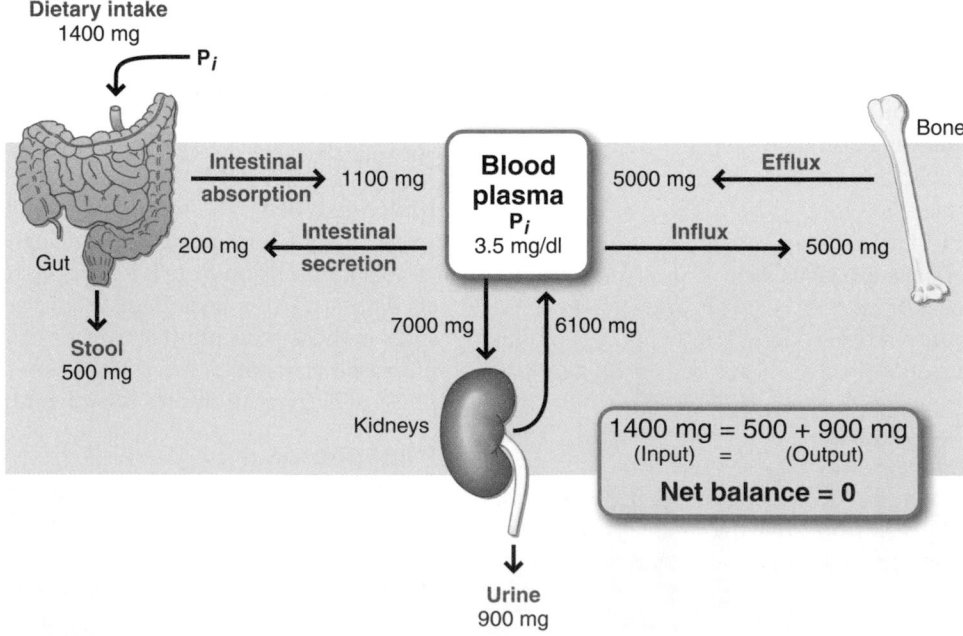

FIGURE 3-29 Phosphorus balance is maintained primarily by the amount of phosphate absorbed versus the amount excreted by the kidneys and intestine. Bone is the major storage site for phosphate, as it is for calcium. The metabolic pathways share many similarities with the calcium pathways

many membrane receptors. As part of phospholipids, phosphorus is present in every cell membrane in the body. Numerous phospholipid molecules also act as secondary messengers within the cytosol. Phosphorylation-dephosphorylation reactions control various steps in the activation or deactivation of cytosolic enzymes by kinases or phosphatases. Total intracellular concentrations of phosphate (but not ionic concentrations) are much higher than extracellular concentrations because phosphorylated compounds do not cross cell membranes easily and are trapped within the cell. The phosphate buffer system is important in intracellular fluid and the kidney tubules, where phosphate functions in the excretion of hydrogen ion. Filtered phosphate reacts with secreted hydrogen ions, releasing sodium in the process. In turn, the sodium can be resorbed under the influence of aldosterone (see Chapter 4) (see Table 3-36).

Finally, phosphate ions combine with calcium ions to form **hydroxyapatite,** the major inorganic molecule in teeth and bones. The bone mineral, not the tooth mineral, provides phosphate ions via homeostatic regulation of serum calcium by PTH.

Dietary Reference Intakes

DRIs for phosphorus are somewhat lower than those for calcium for all age-groups. Tolerable ULs are also established (see inside front cover).

Food Sources and Intakes

In general, good sources of protein are also good sources of phosphorus. Meat, poultry, fish, and eggs are excellent sources. Milk and milk products are good sources, as are nuts and legumes, cereals, and grains. (Phosphorus is bound to a few amino acids, especially serine, threonine, and tyrosine, in food proteins.) In the outer coating of cereal grains, particularly wheat, phosphorus exists in the form of phytic acid, which can form a complex with some minerals to create insoluble compounds. In conventional breads phytic acid is converted to the soluble form of orthophosphate during the leavening process. However, in the unleavened breads commonly eaten in the Middle East, the availability of practically all minerals is much lower. Table 3-26 lists the phosphorus content of selected foods.

The average intakes of phosphorus by adults in the United States are approximately 1300 mg/day for men and 1000 mg/day for women. Most phosphorus (about 60%) comes from milk, meat, poultry, fish, and eggs. Cereals and legumes provide another 20%, and less than 10% is derived from fruits and their juices. Other dietary sources such as tea, coffee, vegetable oils, and spices supply only small amounts of phosphorus. The estimated amount provided by food additives to such products as meats, cheeses, dressings, beverages, and bakery products can be significant.

Deficiency

Phosphate deficiency is rare, but it could possibly develop in individuals who are taking drugs known as phosphate binders (see Chapter 36). However, among older adults,

phosphorus deficiencies may be more common than previously thought because of poor intakes in general. The widespread and ultimately fatal consequences of severe phosphorus depletion reflect its ubiquitous roles in body functions. Symptoms result primarily from decreased synthesis of ATP and other organic phosphate molecules. Neural, muscular, skeletal, hematologic, renal, and other abnormalities occur.

Because phosphorus is so widely available from foods, including processed foods and soda types of soft drinks, little likelihood of a dietary inadequacy exists. Clinical phosphate depletion and hypophosphatemia can result from long-term administration of glucose or TPN without sufficient phosphate, excessive use of phosphate-binding antacids, hyperparathyroidism, or treatment of diabetic acidosis, and it may

TABLE 3-26

Phosphorus Content of Selected Foods

Food	Content (mg)
Fast food pancakes, 2	476
Sole (½ fillet)	246
Fast food hamburger (1)	284
Macaroni and cheese, 1 cup	322
Milk, 2% fat, 1 cup	232
Cheddar cheese, 1oz	146
Ham, 3 oz	210
Ice milk, soft serve, 1 cup	202
Mixed nuts, 1 oz	123
Cheese, cottage, 2% fat, 1 cup	341
Cheese, cheddar, 1 oz	146
Shrimp, boiled, 2 large	137
Baked beans, 1 cup	293
Ground beef, cooked, 3 oz	165
Tofu, regular, ½ cup	120
Potato, baked, with skin, 1	115
Egg, 1	96
Bread, whole wheat, 1 slice	65
Cola beverage, 1 can, 12 oz	46
Potato chips, 14	43
Bread, white, 1 slice	23
Cauliflower, fresh, ½ cup	23
Orange, 1	18

DRIs

Infants and young children	100-500 mg/day, depending on age
Older children and adolescents	1250 mg/day
Adults	700 mg/day
Pregnant	700-1250 mg/day, depending on age
Lactating	700-1250 mg/day, depending on age

From U.S. Department of Agriculture, Agricultural Research Service: Nutrient Database for Standard Reference, Release 18, retrieved 2005, Data Laboratory home page: http://www.nal.usda.gov/fnic/foodcomp/Data/SR18/sr18.html.

develop in those who have alcoholism with or without decompensated liver disease. Premature infants who are fed unfortified human milk may also develop hypophosphatemia.

Toxicity

A persistently high concentration of PTH may result because of the chronic consumption of a low-calcium, high-phosphorus diet. This condition was often previously referred to as "nutritional secondary hyperparathyroidism." In humans the PTH levels in blood that result from a low dietary calcium/phosphorous ratio typically remain within the normal range but usually at the high end. A persistently high PTH, even within the normal range, contributes to increased bone turnover that potentially can result in a reduction of bone mass and density. If this condition is chronic, it could contribute to fragility fractures because of excessive resorption and thinning of trabecular plates at bone sites throughout the skeleton. Individuals with a low calcium/phosphorous ratio would benefit from increasing their calcium intake from foods or supplements. Adequate calcium intakes, whether provided by food or supplements, have been shown to reduce the serum PTH concentration and presumably help inhibit bone loss. The effects of a low dietary calcium/phosphorous ratio on the PTH concentration is illustrated in Figure 3-30. The persistently high

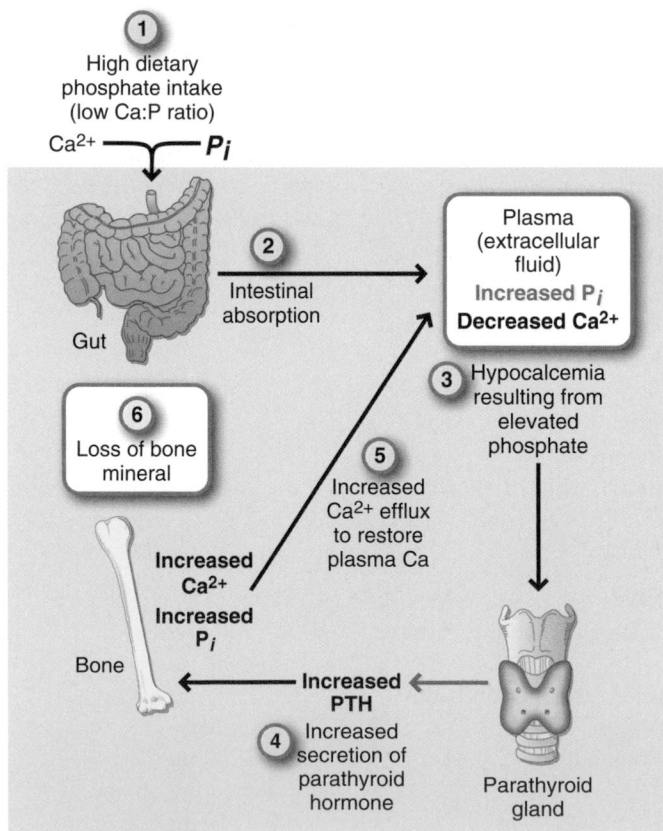

FIGURE 3-30 Mechanism through which a low dietary calcium/phosphorus (*Ca:P*) ratio contributes to the development of a persistently high parathyroid hormone (*PTH*) concentration.

PTH level contributes to the limited bone mineralization during growth (i.e., the inadequate peak bone mass accumulation in adolescents and young adults and the loss of bone mass in adults) (Anderson et al., 1998).

Magnesium

Magnesium is the second-most abundant (after potassium) intracellular cation in the body. The adult human body contains approximately 20 to 28 g of magnesium, of which approximately 60% is found in bone, 26% in muscle, and the remainder in soft tissues and body fluids. Gender differences in the body content of magnesium begin before puberty. Magnesium in bone is present in exchangeable and nonexchangeable pools. Magnesium ions in the bone fluid compartment are much more exchangeable than magnesium ions that have become part of the crystal lattice. Normal serum levels are usually in the range of 1.5 to 2.1 mEq/L (0.75 to 1.1 mmol/L). About half the magnesium in plasma is free, approximately one third is bound to albumin, and the remainder is complexed with citrate, phosphate, or other anions. Magnesium homeostasis is governed by intestinal absorption and renal excretion. No hormone is known to have a major role in the control of serum magnesium.

Absorption, Transport, Storage, and Excretion

The efficiency of absorption of magnesium varies widely from 35% to 45%. Magnesium may be absorbed along the length of the small intestine, but most absorption occurs in the jejunum. Like other divalent cation minerals, the entry of magnesium from the gut lumen occurs by two mechanisms: a carrier-facilitated process and simple diffusion. A saturable facilitated mechanism operates at low intraluminal concentrations, whereas paracellular movement across the mucosa predominates throughout the length of the small bowel when intraluminal concentrations are high. The efficiency of absorption varies with the magnesium status of the individual, the amount of magnesium in the diet, and the composition of the diet as a whole. Vitamin D has little or no effect on magnesium absorption.

No homeostatic system for serum magnesium regulation has been identified, but the serum magnesium concentration is remarkably constant. Maintenance of these constant values depends on absorption, excretion, and transmembranous cation flux rather than on hormonal regulation. Once in the cells, magnesium is bound mainly to protein and energy-rich phosphates. The magnesium balance is illustrated in Figure 3-31.

Primarily the kidneys control magnesium balance by conserving magnesium efficiently, particularly when intake is low. Supplementing a normal intake increases urinary excretion, and the serum magnesium level remains normal. Low dietary intake of magnesium results in reduced urinary excretion of magnesium. To allow nursing mothers to meet the increased needs for magnesium, urinary excretion of the mineral tends to decrease during lactation. Renal resorption varies inversely with that of calcium.

Functions

The major function of magnesium is to stabilize the structure of ATP in ATP-dependent enzyme reactions. Magnesium is a cofactor for more than 300 enzymes involved in the metabolism of food components and the synthesis of many metabolic products. Among the reactions requiring magnesium are the synthesis of fatty acids and proteins, phosphorylation of glucose and its derivatives in the glycolytic pathway, and transketolase reactions. Magnesium is important in the formation of cAMP, which was the first cytosolic second messenger to be identified as a mechanism for transmitting messages from outside the cells in response to hormones, local hormonelike factors, or other molecules.

Magnesium plays a role in neuromuscular transmission and activity, working in concert with and against the effects of calcium, depending on the system involved. In a normal muscle contraction, calcium acts as a stimulator, and magnesium acts as a relaxant. Magnesium acts as a physiologic calcium-channel blocker. High magnesium intakes are associated with greater bone density (Rude and Gruber, 2004). The reactivity of vascular and other smooth muscle cells depends on the ratio of calcium to magnesium in the blood. Large doses of magnesium can result in central nervous system depression, anesthesia, and even paralysis, especially in patients with renal insufficiency. Thus patients with renal problems should not be given magnesium supplements (see Chapter 36) (see Table 3-36).

Dietary Reference Intakes

The RDA for magnesium was increased in 1997, and for the first time different recommendations were made for females and males beginning at puberty. ULs were also established (see inside front cover), as were AIs for infants (Institute of Medicine, Food and Nutrition Board, 1997).

Food Sources and Intakes

Magnesium is abundant in many foods, and the ordinary diet usually provides adequate amounts. Good sources are seeds, nuts, legumes, and milled cereal grains, as well as dark green vegetables, because magnesium is an essential constituent of chlorophyll. Milk is a moderately good source of magnesium, especially because milk and other dairy products are so widely consumed. Fish, meat, and the most commonly eaten fruits (i.e., oranges, apples, and bananas) are poor sources of magnesium. Tofu prepared by magnesium precipitation (e.g., check the label) is a good source. Diets high in refined foods, meat, and dairy products are usually lower in magnesium than diets rich in vegetables and unrefined grains (Table 3-27; see also Appendix 55). Magnesium is lost during the refining of wheat cereals and the processing of foods such as sugar, and it is not generally replaced as part of the enrichment of cereals.

The most commonly consumed food sources of magnesium in the U.S. diet include milk, bread, coffee, ready-to-eat cereals, beef, potatoes, and dried beans and lentils. Recent data (Lopez et al., 2004) have indicated that a decrease in pH of bread dough during preparation (as with sourdough) reduces phytate content of flour and increases the availability of magnesium and other minerals from bread.

Over 10 years ago Alamio et al., (1994) showed that Americans' median intakes of magnesium were well below the RDAs, with older adults having the lowest intakes of any adult group Figure 3-32. More recent studies (Rude and Gruber, 2004; He et al., 2006) suggest that this trend continues and is implicated in development of diseases such as osteoporsis and diabetes. High intakes of calcium, protein, vitamin D, and alcohol all increase the requirements for magnesium; physical or psychological stress may also increase magnesium needs.

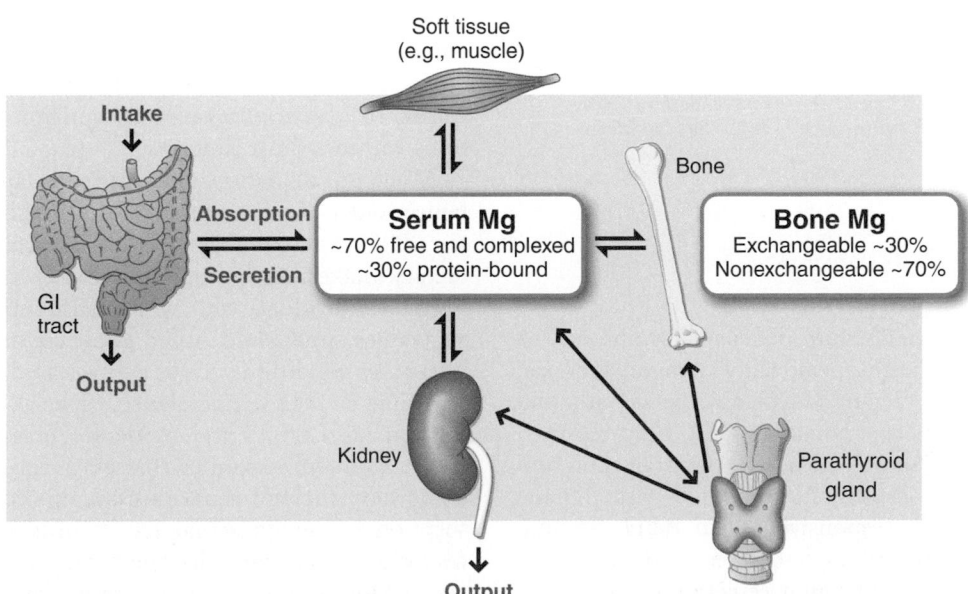

FIGURE 3-31 Magnesium *(Mg)* balance is maintained largely by gastrointestinal *(GI)* absorption and renal excretion.

TABLE 3-27

Magnesium Content of Selected Foods

Food	Content (mg)
Halibut, baked, ½ fillet	170
Spinach, canned, 1 cup	163
Cow peas, cooked, 1cup	91
Muffin, oat bran 1	89
Rice, brown, cooked, 1 cup	84
Refried beans, 1 cup	83
Cashews, roasted, 1 oz	77
Orange juice, 6 oz	72
Mixed nuts, roasted, 1 oz	67
Baked potato with skin, 1	57
Raisins, 1 cup	46
Tofu, firm, ¼ block	30
Bread, whole wheat, 1 slice	29
Milk, 2% fat, 1 cup	27
Spinach, fresh, 1 cup	24
Ground beef, lean, cooked, 3 oz	18
Fruits	10-25

DRIs

Infants, AIs	30-75 mg/day, depending on age
Young children, RDAs	80-130 mg/day, depending on age
Older children and adolescents, RDAs	240-410 mg/day, depending on age and gender
Adults	310-400 mg/day, depending on age and gender
Pregnant	350-400 mg/day, depending on age
Lactating	310-360 mg/day, depending on age

From U.S. Department of Agriculture, Agricultural Research Service: Nutrient Database for Standard Reference, Release 18, retrieved 2005, Data Laboratory home page: http://www.nal.usda.gov/fnic/foodcomp/Data/SR18/sr18.html.

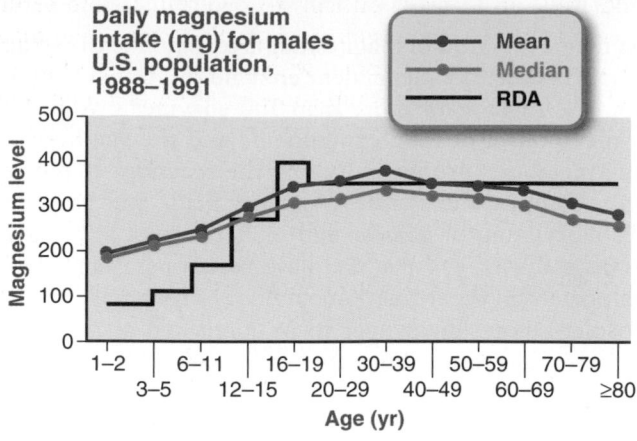

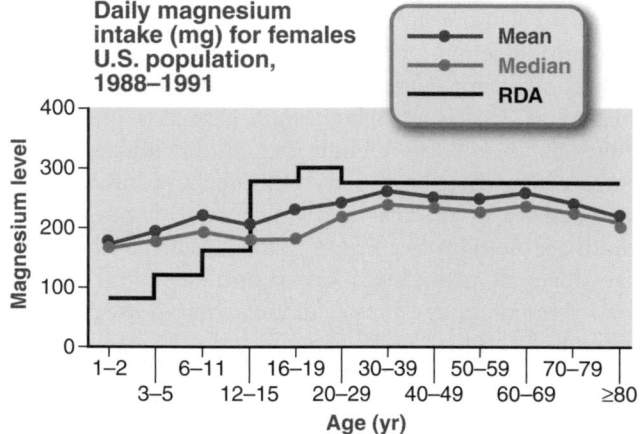

FIGURE 3-32 Comparison of the median daily magnesium intake for Americans and the DRIs.

serum $1,25(OH)_2D_3$, vitamin D resistance, altered hydroxyapatite crystal formation, and impaired bone growth in young patients or the development of osteoporosis in older patients). With continued depletion of magnesium, PTH concentrations decrease even further. Intravenous administration of magnesium reverses the clinical signs and symptoms within a short time.

Moderate depletion of magnesium apparently is prevalent in older populations in Western nations (Leenhardt et al., 2005). Such deficiencies are typically precipitated by dietary intakes that are persistently low in magnesium, especially in individuals who avoid consuming dark green leafy vegetables, milk, and other good sources of magnesium. Any other condition such as an increased loss of electrolytes or a shift in electrolyte balance, especially a decrease in potassium, also triggers a moderate magnesium deficiency. Conditions and situations that may cause acute deficiencies to develop include renal disease, diuretic therapy, malabsorption, hyperthyroidism, pancreatitis, kwashiorkor, diabetes, parathyroid gland disorders, postsurgical stress, and vitamin D–resistant rickets. Magnesium deficiency has also been linked to insulin resistance and metabolic syndrome because magnesium is required for carbohydrate metabolism (He et al., 2006).

Deficiency

Although rare, severe magnesium deficiency symptoms include tremors, muscle spasms, personality changes, anorexia, nausea, and vomiting. Tetany, myoclonic jerks, athetoid movements, convulsions, and coma have also been reported in those with a magnesium deficiency. Hypocalcemia and hypokalemia typically occur first, combined with impairment of the individual's responsiveness to PTH. Sodium retention may also occur.

The effects of severe magnesium depletion on bone metabolism include decreased PTH secretion by the parathyroid glands, very low concentrations of serum PTH, impaired responsiveness of bone and kidneys to PTH, decreased

Magnesium status is difficult to determine from serum measurements of magnesium because the total serum magnesium level remains constant within a wide range of intake levels. Leukocyte magnesium contents are much more sensitive to nutritional status, which makes them a superior marker. Urinary excretion of magnesium (and often of potassium) is less in those with a magnesium deficiency than in those with sufficient magnesium, suggesting that those with magnesium deficiencies have greater retention of magnesium and improved tissue magnesium status throughout the body. Attention has been focused on the interrelationships of magnesium and other electrolytes, particularly potassium, and the effects of these relationships on the development of various tissue abnormalities. For example, a low magnesium intake is now considered to be a potential risk factor for hypertension, as are inadequate intakes of potassium, calcium, and other micronutrients (see Chapter 33).

Oral magnesium supplementation in middle-age and older women with mild-to-moderate hypertension was found to reduce systolic and diastolic blood pressure significantly (see Chapter 33). Low magnesium intakes have been associated with coronary heart disease. Studies of magnesium use by patients who had experienced acute myocardial infarction (MI) suggest that rapid post-MI magnesium treatment reduces mortality. Magnesium deficits may also be a factor in osteoporosis, although the mechanism has not been established. Researchers in Israel who administered magnesium supplements for 2 years to postmenopausal women with established osteoporosis demonstrated improved trabecular but not cortical bone mass (Stendig-Lindenberg et al., 1993).

Toxicity

Although excess magnesium can inhibit bone calcification, magnesium excesses from dietary sources, including supplements, are very unlikely to result in toxicity. However, the ULs for magnesium from supplements or pharmacologic agents were established for the first time in 1998. The only cases of toxicity that have been reported involve smelter workers who inhale or otherwise ingest toxic levels of magnesium dust.

Sulfur

Although sulfur has long been studied as a mineral, it functions almost entirely as a component of organic molecules (see *Focus On:* Sulfur: It's Not a Mineral; It's an Organic Molecule). Sulfur exists in the body as a constituent of three amino acids—cystine, cysteine, and methionine—and of many other organic molecules. As such, it exists as part of these organic molecules in all cells and extracelluar compartments such as connective tissue. The tertiary structure of proteins is attributable in part to covalent bonding between cysteine residues in which the $-SH$ groups are oxidized to form disulfide ($-S$-$S-$) bridges. These bridges also provide the three-dimensional structural modifications necessary for the activity of some enzymes, insulin, and other proteins.

Sulfhydryl groups of proteins also participate in diverse cellular reactions. For example, the poisonous effects of ar-

◎ FOCUS ON

Sulfur: It's Not a Mineral; It's an Organic Molecule

The sulfur-containing amino acids **(S-containing amino acids)** methionine and cysteine provide almost 100% of the sulfur in the human diet. (A small percentage of the methionine molecules have selenium as a substitute for the sulfur.) The transmethylation pathway within cells, especially in the liver, converts methionine to homocysteine while transferring the methyl group to other molecules. This pathway is linked to the metabolism of other important molecules such as cysteine, adenine (a nucleoside), and polyamines. S-adenosylmethionine is a critical intermediate in these pathways. The sulfur atoms remain part of the organic structures until hepatic degradation (oxidation) of the cysteine and the formation of inorganic sulfate groups that are excreted by the kidneys.

Several nonhepatic cells use sulfate (bound to an organic donor) for the synthesis of iron-sulfur proteins. In addition, structural molecules within cells (i.e., proteoglycans) contain sulfated monosaccharide (glucose and galactose) residues. Taurine, a sulfur-containing amino acid made by liver cells, is used to conjugate bile acids before secretion.

In summary, sulfur acts primarily as a component of organic molecules in cells rather than as an inorganic element.

senic are caused by its ability to bind sulfhydryl groups of enzymes. The sulfur of cysteine binds to iron-sulfur clusters in electron transfer proteins involved in basic, life-sustaining processes, such as photosynthesis, nitrogen fixation, and oxidative phosphorylation.

Glutathione, a tripeptide-containing cysteine, acts as a donor of reducing equivalents for the reduction of hydrogen peroxide and organic peroxides by GSH-Px. In the broadest sense, sulfur can be considered an antioxidant. Sulfur exists as a component of heparin, an anticoagulant found in liver and some other tissues and as chondroitin sulfate in bone and cartilage. Sulfur is also an essential component of three vitamins—thiamin, biotin, and pantothenic acid. Other important molecules such as *S*-adenosylmethionine also contain sulfur.

Excess inorganic sulfur generated as a result of hepatic or renal metabolism is excreted in the urine as sulfates. The metabolism of sulfur-containing amino acids generates inorganic acids, especially sulfate anions, in substantial amounts. These sulfates are thought to combine with calcium ions in the glomerular ultrafiltrate, thereby reducing the renal tubular resorption of calcium. This mechanism may explain as much as 50% of the calcium loss associated with protein-induced hypercalciuria, which develops after consumption of meals rich in animal proteins—proteins that are rich in sulfur. Food sources of sulfur include meat, poultry, fish, eggs, dried beans, broccoli, and cauliflower. Sulfur deficiency or toxicity is highly unlikely. There are no DRIs for sulfur.

MICROMINERALS (TRACE ELEMENTS)

Numerous elements that are present in minute amounts in body tissues are essential for optimum human growth, health, and development. These **microminerals (trace elements)** are defined as those that have been shown through appropriately designed and corroborated experiments to be required for optimum performance of a particular function.

Deficiency of a nutrient has historically been identified and defined based on investigations using animal models. Increasing amounts of a nutrient (beginning with intake of almost zero) evokes a biologic response that increases until a plateau is reached, beyond which larger intakes can produce pharmacologic effects and eventually toxicity. Low intakes produce signs and symptoms of deficiency.

The spectrum of effects produced by trace element deficiencies is more subtle and difficult to identify, partly because many of these effects occur at the cellular or subcellular level. For example, iron deficiency eventually results in a type of anemia that is easy to identify. The cellular effects cannot be identified as easily but may actually be more harmful to the individual (see Chapter 31). The knowledge of the various functions of trace and ultratrace minerals continues to grow.

DRIs and ULs have been established for nine essential trace elements—chromium, copper, iodine, iron, manganese, molybdenum, selenium, zinc, and fluoride. DRIs for five potentially essential trace elements—arsenic, boron, nickel, silicon, and vanadium—have not yet been published (Trumbo et al., 2001). No DRI exists for cobalt, just for cobalt-containing vitamin B_{12} (cobalamin).

General Characteristics

Trace elements exist typically in two forms: (1) as charged ions, or (2) bound to proteins or complexed in molecules (e.g., metalloenzymes). Each element has different chemical properties that become critical in its functional role in cells or extracellular compartments. In blood and other tissue and cellular fluids, the trace elements do not exist in the free ionic state; they are typically bound to transporting or holding proteins. Fluoride ions become bound in the hydroxyapatite crystals of bones and teeth.

Functions

Many enzymes require small amounts of one or more trace metals for full activity. Metals function in enzyme systems by (1) participating directly in the catalyzed reaction, (2) combining with substrates to form complexes on which enzymes act, (3) forming metalloenzymes that bind substrates, (4) combining with reaction end products, or (5) maintaining quaternary structures.

Minute concentrations of trace minerals affect the whole body through interactions with the enzymes or hormones that regulate masses of substrate. This ability is amplified if, in turn, the substrate has some regulatory function. Trace minerals may also interact with DNA to control the transcription of proteins important for the metabolism of that particular trace mineral.

Food Sources

Compared with other sources, foods of animal origin are generally superior sources of trace elements because concentrations of the elements tend to be higher and the metals more available for absorption. Seafood in particular is usually rich in nearly all micronutrients except manganese, which is more readily available from plant sources. Trace elements are not distributed evenly in wheat grains, and the germ and outer layers that contain major amounts of most minerals are removed to a large extent by the milling process. However, the small quantities of minerals that remain in white flour are more biologically available than those in whole wheat flour, which are in complexes with or bound by molecules in the inner layer such as phytate and fiber. Unless the pH is lowered during product production as noted previously in sourdough bread, these minerals remain unavailable.

Iron

Iron has been recognized as an essential nutrient for more than a century. Nutritional iron deficiency and iron deficiency anemia remain far too common in the 21st century given the wide availability of iron-rich foods (see Chapter 31). Indeed, iron deficiency anemia is the world's most common nutritional deficiency disease. Many advances have been made in the study of iron metabolism and iron defi-

TABLE 3-28

Relative Proportions of Iron in Young, Healthy Adults

Iron Type	Men: Iron Content (mg)	Men: Iron Content (%)	Women: Iron Content (mg)	Women: Iron Content (%)
Functional				
Hemoglobin	2300	64	1700	73
Myoglobin	320	9	180	8
Heme enzymes	80	2	60	3
Nonheme enzymes	100	3	80	3+
Storage				
Ferritin	540	15	200	9
Hemosiderin	230	6	100	4
Transferrin	5	<1	4	<1
TOTAL	3575	100	2314	100

ciency, but questions about the mechanisms regulating the intestinal absorption of iron and iron balance persist. The adult human body contains iron in two major pools: (1) functional iron in hemoglobin, myoglobin, and enzymes; and (2) storage iron in ferritin, hemosiderin, and transferrin (a transport protein in blood). Healthy adult men have about 3.6 g of total body iron, whereas women have about 2.4 g. Table 3-28 lists the relative proportions of the major categories of iron in men and women. Adult women have much lower amounts of iron in storage than do men. Iron is highly conserved by the body; approximately 90% is recovered and reused every day. The rest is excreted, primarily in the bile. Dietary iron must be available to maintain iron balance to meet this 10% gap, or iron deficiency results.

Two concerns about iron nutritional status predominate: the incidence of iron deficiency anemia and the role of excessive iron intake in coronary heart disease and cancer. Because of food fortification and the use of iron supplements by so many individuals, high iron intakes by men and postmenopausal women may be contributing to the risk of these chronic diseases. In fact, a study of older adults replete with iron in the Framingham Heart Study cohort concluded that increased iron stores were a liability (Fleming et al., 2001).

Absorption, Transport, Storage, and Excretion

Dietary iron exists in two chemical forms: (1) **heme iron,** which is found in hemoglobin, myoglobin, and some enzymes; and (2) **nonheme iron,** which is found predominantly in plant foods but also in some animal foods, as are non-

heme enzymes and ferritin. Heme iron (i.e., the intact ferroporphyrin ring) is absorbed across the brush border (mucosa) of intestinal absorbing cells (enterocytes) after it is digested from animal sources. After heme enters the cytosol, the ferrous iron is enzymatically removed from the ferroporphyrin complex. The free iron ions combine immediately with apoferritin to form ferritin in the same way that free nonheme iron combines with apoferritin.

Ferritin is an intracellular store and a ferry that carries bound iron from the brush border to the basolateral membrane of the absorbing cell. The final step of absorption by which iron ions are moved into the blood occurs at the basolateral membrane of the absorbing cell and involves an active transport mechanism. At this point, it is the same for heme and nonheme iron, and a diagram of these steps is presented in Figure 3-33. The absorption of heme iron is affected only minimally by the composition of meals and GI secretions. Heme iron represents only 5% to 10% of the dietary iron of individuals who consume a mixed diet, but absorption may be as high as 25%, compared with only 5% or so for nonheme iron. Because vegans consume only plant foods, sufficient amounts of nonheme iron must be ingested and absorbed to meet body requirements.

Three steps of absorption also precede the entry of nonheme iron into the blood circulation. Nonheme iron must be digested free from plant sources and enter the duodenum and upper jejunum in a soluble (and ionized) form if it is to be transferred across the brush border (mucosa). The acid of gastric secretions enhances the solubility and the change of

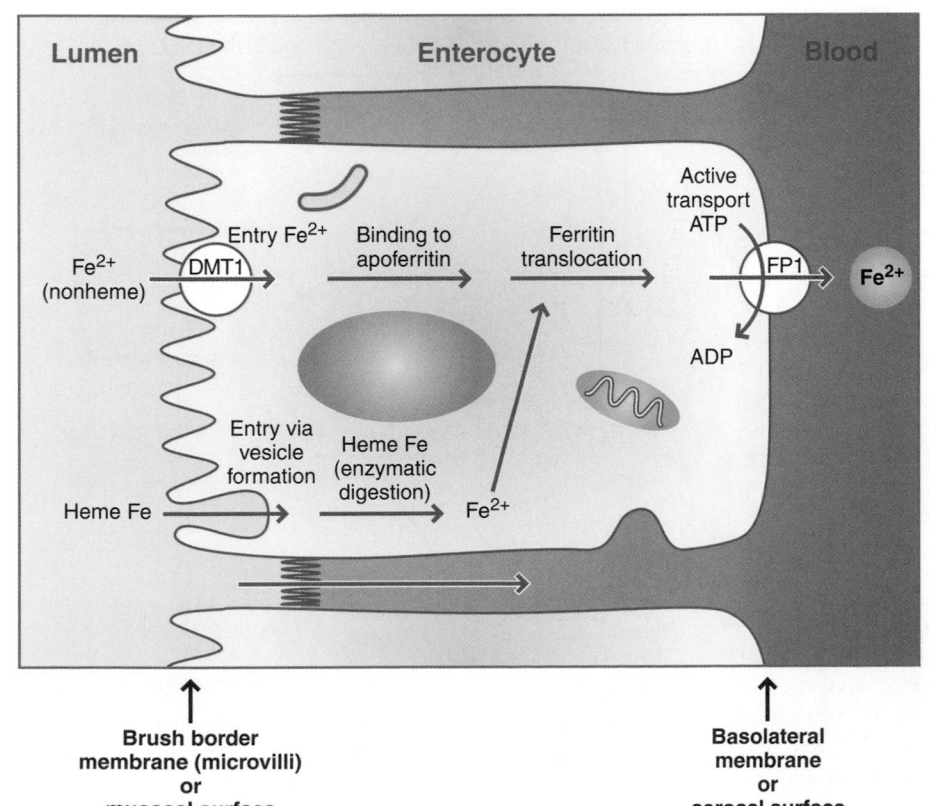

FIGURE 3-33 Intestinal absorption of iron from heme and nonheme sources by an intestinal absorbing cell, or enterocyte. Enerocytes contain two membranes: the brush border membrane and the basolateral membrane. The entry step of nonheme iron at the brush border membrane is different from that of heme iron. Heme iron enters by vesicle formation around the heme, whereas nonheme iron (ionic iron) enters by facilitated diffusion down a concentration gradient. Absorbed ions combine with apoferritin to form ferritin complexes that move across the cell by diffusion to the basolateral membrane for the exit step of absorption by active transport. The iron of heme iron is enzymatically removed, and these ions exit at the basolateral membrane by an unknown mechanism. *ATP,* Adenosine triphosphate; *ADP,* adenosine disphosphate.

iron to the ionic state—either as ferric (+3 oxidation state) or ferrous (+2 oxidation state) iron—within the gut luminal contents. Iron in the reduced or ferrous state is preferred for the entry step of absorption, but some ferric iron is also transferred across the brush border. The brush border iron transporter, divalent metal transporter 1 (DMT1) transports ferrous iron. Ferric iron may be reduced by a brush border enzyme, ferric reductase, for absorption (Frazer and Anderson, 2005). In addition, as chyme moves down the duodenum, the addition of pancreatic and duodenal secretions increases the pH of the contents to 7.0, at which point most ferric iron is precipitated unless it has been chelated. However, ferrous iron is significantly more soluble at a pH of 7, so these ions remain available for absorption in the remainder of the small intestine.

The efficiency of nonheme (but not heme) iron absorption seems to be controlled by the intestinal mucosa, which allows certain amounts of iron to enter the blood from the cytosolic ferritin pool according to the body's needs. A small peptide hormone known as **hepcidin** produced by the liver acts on the mucosa cell and inhibits iron absorption. The amount of hepcidin produced by the liver is related to the amount of iron stored in the liver (Frazer and Anderson, 2005).

Other signals from the body to the absorbing cells may be transferrin saturation, or the percentage of iron bound to transferrin (Figure 3-34). Normally transferrin saturation is 30% to 35% in healthy, iron-consuming individuals. The percentage can vary greatly, depending on iron intake and bioavailability. A low percentage (e.g., 15%) of the total iron-binding capacity (TIBC) of transferrin would stimulate the absorbing cells to transport iron by the exit step at the basolateral membrane to the blood. Conversely, if the iron concentration in the body is excessive, the absorbing cells would be downregulated, and less iron would be absorbed. The latter situation occurs during iron overloads to protect the body against toxicity.

The life span of an intestinal absorbing cell is approximately 5 to 6 days. During this time the cell emerges from the crypt after cell division, passes up the villus to the tip, and eventually sloughs off as a dead cell. During the early life of the individual cell, signals resulting from the saturation percentage of circulating transferrin are sent to the young cells to adjust their number of receptors for transferrin (e.g., to increase iron absorption in a state of iron deficiency). Other cells formed before or after may have different numbers of receptors, depending on the nutritional supply of iron. In individuals who persistently con-

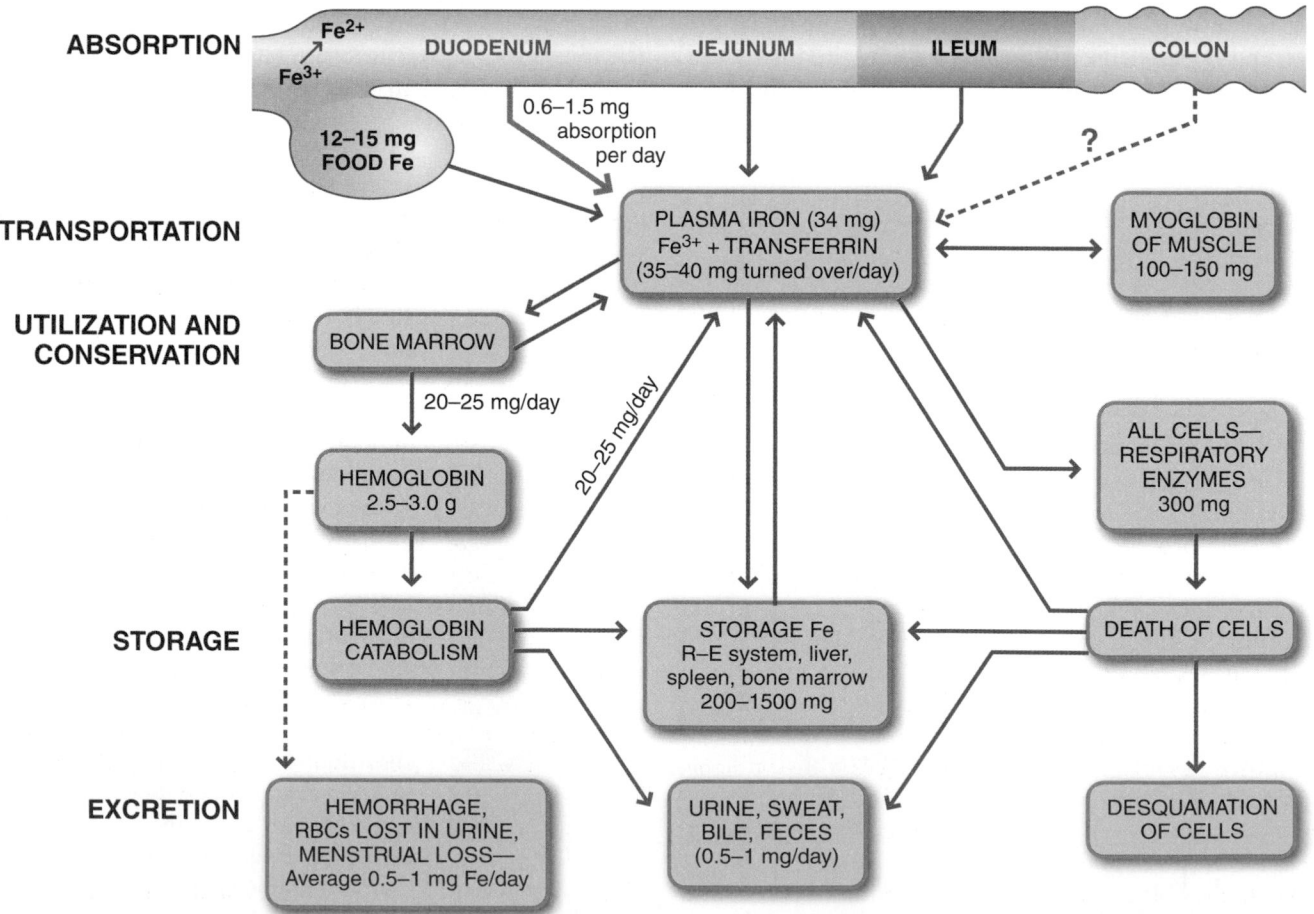

FIGURE 3-34 Iron metabolism in adults. Most iron is absorbed from the duodenum and jejunum, after which it is transported as plasma iron or bound to transferrin. *RBCs,* Red blood cells; *R-E system,* reticuloendothelial system.

sume inadequate levels of iron, especially women in their childbearing years, the number of receptors may consistently be upregulated to maximize the efficiency of iron absorption.

The efficiency of iron absorption (from gut lumen to blood) by adults with normal hemoglobin values averages 5% to 15% of the iron (heme and nonheme combined) contained in food and supplements. Although absorption may be as high as 50% in those with iron deficiency anemia, this level of absorption is not common. Most women with an iron deficiency, but no anemia, probably have absorption efficiencies of 20% to 30%. From 2% to 10% of nonheme iron in vegetables is absorbed, and from 10% to 30% of iron (heme and nonheme) in animal sources is typically absorbed.

Several factors affect the intestinal absorption of iron, especially nonheme iron. The efficiency of iron absorption is determined to some extent by the foods from which it is derived or with which it is consumed. For example, both ascorbic acid and sodium ethylenediaminetetraacetic acid (EDTA) improved iron absorption from a school breakfast meal (Davidsson et al., 2001). Ascorbic acid, the most potent enhancer of iron absorption, reduces ferric to ferrous iron and forms a chelate with iron that remains soluble at the alkaline pH of the lower small intestine. However, the effect of prolonged daily dietary increases in ascorbic acid on iron absorption from a complete diet does not seem to be strong enough to improve iron status over time without additional iron supplementation (Cook and Reddy, 2001). Other food molecules such as sugars and sulfur-containing amino acids may also enhance iron entry by forming chelates with ionic iron. In addition, animal proteins from beef, pork, veal, lamb, liver, fish, and chicken enhance absorption. The substance responsible for this improved absorption—which is called the meat factor—remains unknown, but specific amino acids or dipeptide digestion products may enhance iron absorption.

Although the iron content of human milk is very low, it is highly bioavailable because of the presence of milk lactoferrin, which enhances iron absorption. Infants retain more iron from human milk than from cow's milk or infant formulas because of the presence of lactoferrin in breast milk. Whey protein (lactalbumin), which constitutes a greater percentage of the total protein in human milk than in cow's milk, may also improve iron absorption.

The degree of gastric acidity enhances solubility and therefore bioavailability of iron derived from foods. Therefore achlorhydria (lack of gastric acid secretion), hypochlorhydria (inadequate acid secretion), or administration of alkaline substances such as antacids can interfere with nonheme iron absorption by not permitting the solubilization of iron in gastric and duodenal fluids. Gastric secretions also seem to increase the absorption of heme iron.

Certain physiologic states such as pregnancy and growth that involve increased blood formation stimulate iron absorption. In addition, more iron is absorbed during iron deficiency states because of adaptive mechanisms that enhance nonheme iron absorption.

Foods with high phytate content have low iron bioavailability, but whether phytate is the cause is not clear. Oxalates can inhibit absorption. Tannins, which are polyphenols, in tea also reduce nonheme iron absorption. On the other hand, the presence of an adequate amount of calcium helps to remove phosphate, oxalate, and phytate that would otherwise combine with iron and inhibit its absorption.

The availability of iron from various compounds used for food enrichment or as supplements varies widely according to their chemical composition. Although iron in the ferrous form is most readily absorbed, not all ferrous compounds are equally available. Ferrous pyrophosphate is used frequently in products such as breakfast cereals because it does not add a gray color to the food; however, this compound and others such as ferrous citrate and ferrous tartrate are poorly absorbed. Iron is usually added to baby foods in an elemental form, the absorbability of which depends on the iron particle size. Increased intestinal motility decreases iron absorption by decreasing contact time and rapidly removing the chyme from the area of highest intestinal acidity. Poor fat digestion leading to steatorrhea also decreases iron absorption and the absorption of other cations.

Transport. Iron (nonheme) is transported, bound to transferrin (see Figure 3-34), from the intestinal absorbing cells to various tissues to meet their needs. It rarely exists in the free ionic state in serum.

Storage. Between 200 and 1500 mg of iron is stored in the body as ferritin and hemosiderin; 30% of the body's iron store is in the liver, 30% is in the bone marrow, and the rest is found in the spleen and muscles. Up to 50 mg/day can be mobilized from storage iron, 20 mg of which is used in hemoglobin synthesis. (Estimates of these amounts are listed in Table 3-28.) The amounts of circulating **ferritin** in blood correlate closely with total body iron stores, which make this measurement an invaluable tool for clinical evaluation of iron status (see Chapters 15 and 31).

Intestinal Excretion. Iron is only lost from the body through bleeding and in very small amounts through defecation, sweat, and the normal exfoliation of hair and skin. Most of the iron lost in the feces could not be absorbed from food. The remainder comes from bile and the cells exfoliated from the GI epithelium. Almost no iron is excreted in the urine. Daily iron loss is approximately 1 mg for men and slightly less for nonmenstruating women. The loss of iron accompanying menstruation averages about 0.5 mg/day. However, wide variations exist among individuals, and menstrual losses of more than 1.4 mg of iron daily have been reported in approximately 5% of normal women.

Functions

The functions of iron relate to its ability to participate in oxidation and reduction reactions (Beard, 2001). Chemically iron is a highly reactive element that can interact with oxygen to form intermediates with the potential of damaging cell membranes or degrading DNA. Iron must be tightly bound to proteins to prevent these potentially destructive oxidative effects.

Iron metabolism is complex because this element is involved in so many aspects of life, including red blood cell function, myoglobin activity, and the roles of numerous heme and nonheme enzymes. Because of its oxidation-reduction (redox) properties, iron has a role in the blood and respiratory transport of oxygen and carbon dioxide, and it is an active component of the cytochromes (enzymes) involved in the processes of cellular respiration and energy (ATP) generation. Iron also seems to be involved in immune function and cognitive performance. Although these latter relationships have not been clearly identified, they underscore the importance of preventing iron deficiency anemia in the world population. Table 3-29 lists the major iron molecules in the body and their functions.

Hemoglobin, present in red blood cells, is synthesized in immature cells in bone marrow. Hemoglobin works in two ways: (1) the iron-containing heme combines with oxygen in the lungs; and (2) the heme releases the oxygen in tissues, where it picks up carbon dioxide and then releases it in the lungs after its return from the tissues. **Myoglobin,** also a heme-containing protein, serves as an oxygen reservoir within muscle.

Oxidative production of ATP within the mitochondria involves many heme and nonheme iron-containing enzymes. The cytochromes, present in nearly all cells, function in the mitochondrial respiratory chain in the transfer of electrons and the storage of energy through the alternate oxidation and reduction (redox) of iron ($Fe^{2++} = Fe^{3+++}$). Numerous water-insoluble drugs and endogenous organic molecules are transformed by the iron-containing cytochrome P-450 system in the liver into more water-soluble molecules that can be secreted in the bile and eliminated. Ribonucleotide reductase, the rate-limiting enzyme involved in DNA synthesis, is also an iron enzyme. Although these vital enzymes represent only a small portion of the total iron in the body (see Table 3-29), a severe decrease in their concentrations can have long-term consequences. Other enzymes, including several in the brain, also require iron.

An adequate iron intake is essential for the normal function of the immune system. Iron overloads and deficiencies result in changes in the immune response. Iron is required by bacteria; therefore an iron overload (especially intravenously) may result in an increased risk of infection. Iron deficiency affects humoral and cellular immunity. Concentrations of circulating T-lymphocytes decrease in individuals with an iron deficiency, and the mitogenic response is typically impaired. Natural killer (NK) cell activity also decreases. Production of interleukin-1 has been shown to be reduced in iron-deficient animals, and depressed interleukin-2 production has been reported in humans and animals.

Two iron-binding proteins—transferrin (in blood) and lactoferrin (in breast milk)—seem to protect the body against infection by withholding iron from microorganisms that need it for proliferation. Iron is used by brain cells for normal function in people of all ages. Iron is involved in the function and synthesis of neurotransmitters and possibly myelin. The detrimental effects of early iron deficiency anemia in children persist for many years (Beard, 2001). For example, declines have been found between the scholastic performance, sensorimotor competence, attention, learning, and memory of children with anemia. Iron supplementation in children with iron deficiency anemia has been found to improve learning, as indicated by achievement test scores (Beard, 2001). Changes occur in iron metabolism in those with certain diseases such as Alzheimer's disease. Iron distribution in the brain has also been reported to change during normal aging (Johnson et al., 1994).

Dietary Reference Intakes

DRIs have been established for iron. The RDA for men and postmenopausal women is 8 mg/day. The RDA for women of childbearing age (to replace iron loss from menstruation and provide for iron stores sufficient to support a pregnancy) is 18 mg/day. For teenage boys (ages 14 to 18) the iron RDA is 11 mg/day. Full-term infants are born with a reserve supply of iron from placental transfer during gestation, but normal-term infants still require adequate iron from food sources and fortified milk products during the first year of life. Premature infants have limited iron stores because they lack most of the iron and other trace minerals that are normally transferred during the last trimester of pregnancy. The need for iron to support rapid growth in premature infants becomes apparent at approximately 2 to 3 months of age (see Chapter 43). The

TABLE 3-29

Iron Molecules in the Body

Molecule	Function
Metabolic Proteins	
Heme proteins	
Hemoglobin	Oxygen transport from lungs to tissues
Myoglobin	Transport and storage of oxygen in muscle
Enzymes: Heme	
Cytochromes	Electron transport
Cytochrome P-450	Oxidative degradation of drugs
Catalase	Conversion of hydrogen peroxide to oxygen and water
Enzymes: Nonheme	
Iron-sulfur and metalloproteins	Oxidative metabolism
Enzymes: Iron-Dependent	
Tryptophan pyrolase	Oxidation of tryptophan
Transport and Storage Proteins	
Transferrin	Transport of iron and other minerals
Ferritin	Storage
Hemosiderin	Storage

RDAs for ages 1 year and older are (variably) 7, 8, or 10 mg/day until adolescence (age 14) begins. Figure 3-35 shows the physiologic requirements for iron in relation to age. Requirements are highest during infancy and adolescence. Iron needs among males decrease after the adolescent growth spurt, whereas the iron needs of their female counterparts continue to be high until the menopausal transition. Iron allowances increase during pregnancy (from 15 to 30 mg/day) but not during lactation, although many lactating women are told to continue taking supplements.

Food Sources and Intakes

By far the best source of dietary ion is liver, followed by seafood (oysters and fish), kidney, heart, lean meat, and poultry. Dried beans and vegetables are the best plant sources. Some other foods that provide iron are egg yolks, dried fruits, dark molasses, whole grain and enriched breads, wine, and cereal. Milk and milk products are practically devoid of iron. Corn is a notoriously poor source of iron, so it is not surprising that cultures with diets based primarily on corn have high rates of anemia. Old-fashioned iron skillets used for cooking add to the total iron intake.

The median iron intakes of most women are lower than the RDA, whereas the median intakes of men generally exceed the RDA, as reported from NHANES III (Alaimo et al., 1994). An adequate diet containing meats and other animal sources typically has high iron content, containing approximately 6 mg of iron per 1000 kcal. Therefore the average omnivorous woman of childbearing age consuming 2000 kcal takes in only 12 mg of iron, or approximately 67% of the RDA of 18 mg/day. This intake level meets the needs of almost no menstruating woman. However, iron intakes totaling much less than 12 mg/day place women at more serious risk for developing deficiency anemia. Women with

high daily iron losses compensate with an increased rate of absorption, but even with this adaptation, insufficient stores of iron typically exist, and the risk of anemia remains high.

The availability of iron derived from food is important in the consideration of dietary sources. For example, only 50% or less of the iron in whole grain cereals and in some green vegetables is available in a usable form. Table 3-30 and Appendix 54 present the iron content of selected foods. Vegetarian or vegan women can obtain enough iron from their plant-based diet, but they must consume suffi-

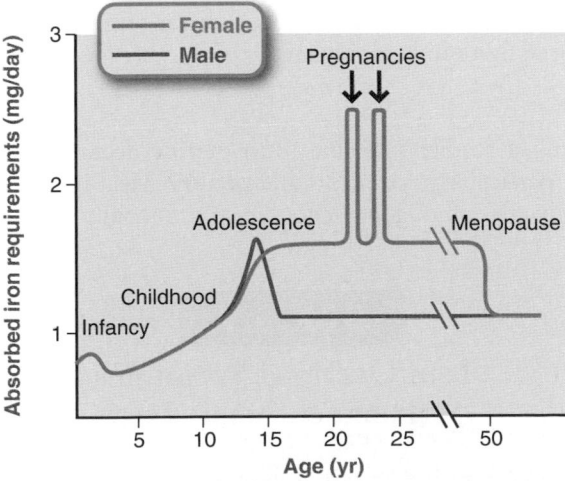

FIGURE 3-35 The absorbed iron requirement for various ages. The greatest requirements for iron occur during infancy. During childhood, requirements are the same for boys and girls. During the adolescent growth spurt, iron needs increase and are greater for boys than girls. However, because of menstruation, the requirements after adolescence remain high for females but decrease for males.

TABLE 3-30

Iron Content of Selected Foods

Food	Content (mg)
Cereal, ready-to-eat, fortified, 1 cup	1-22
Clams, canned, 3 oz	23.7
Rice, white, enriched, 1 cup	9.73
Baked beans, 1 cup	8.2
Braunschweiger, 2 slices	6.35
Oysters, cooked, 3 oz	5.9
Bagel, enriched, 1, 4-inch	5.38
Beef liver, fried, 3 oz	5.24
Fast food roast beef sandwich, 1	4.23
Refried beans, 1 cup	4.18
Potato skin, 1	4.08
Burrito, bean, 1	1.13
Ground beef, lean, 3 oz	1.8
Oatmeal, unfortified, 1 cup	1.6
Spinach, cooked, 1 cup	6.43
Corn dog, 1	6.18
Macaroni and cheese, 1 cup	1.86
Egg, 1	0.92
Peanuts, dry roasted, 3 oz	0.8
Blueberries, frozen, ½ cup	4.5
Chicken, breast, roasted, ½	0.64
Broccoli, fresh, cooked, ½ cup	0.64
Wine, red, ½ cup	0.5
Cheese, cheddar, 1 oz	0.2
Milk, 2% fat, 1 cup	0.07
RDA	
Infants and young children	7-11 mg/day, depending on age
Older children and adolescents	8-15 mg/day, depending on age
Adults	8-18 mg/day, depending on age and gender
Pregnant	27 mg/day
Lactating	9-10 mg/day, depending on age

From U.S. Department of Agriculture, Agricultural Research Service: Nutrient Database for Standard Reference, Release 18, retrieved 2005, Data Laboratory home page: http://www.nal.usda.gov/fnic/foodcomp/Data/SR18/sr18.html.

cient amounts of moderately iron-rich foods, such as legumes and dried fruits. Soy products are typically good sources of iron and zinc.

Iron fortification of cereals, flours, and bread has added significantly to the total iron intake of the U.S. population. Fortified cereals have become a substantial source of iron for infants and children, as well as for adolescents and adults. Concern about potential iron overloading from fortified breakfast foods was raised because analyzed values of iron content were considerably greater than labeled values (Whittaker et al., 2001).

The foods that supply the greatest amount of iron in the U.S. diet include ready-to-eat cereals fortified with iron; bread, cakes, cookies, doughnuts, and pasta (all fortified with iron); beef; dried beans and lentils; and poultry (Subar et al., 1998).

Deficiency

Iron deficiency, the precursor of iron deficiency anemia, is the most common of all nutritional deficiency diseases (see Chapter 31). In the United States and worldwide, iron deficiency anemia is prevalent among children and women of childbearing age. The groups considered to be at greatest risk for iron deficiency anemia are infants younger than 2 years of age, adolescent girls, pregnant women, and older adults. Pregnant teenagers are frequently at high risk because of poor eating habits and continuing growth (see Chapters 5 and 8). Women in their childbearing years who are iron deficient benefit from either a diet rich in iron-containing foods or supplements (Patterson et al., 2001).

The final stages of iron deficiency include hypochromic, microcytic anemia. Anemia may be corrected by providing high-dose supplements in the form of ferrous sulfate or ferrous gluconate until blood parameters return to normal. To prevent worsening of the iron deficiency, individuals should be counseled regarding a diet that is appropriately rich in iron.

Iron deficiency can be caused by injury, hemorrhage, or illness (e.g., blood loss from hookworms, GI diseases that interfere with iron absorption). Iron deficiency may also be aggravated by an unbalanced diet containing insufficient iron, protein, folate, and vitamin C. Anemia typically develops because of an inadequate amount of dietary iron or faulty iron absorption. (Iron deficiency anemia is discussed in detail in Chapter 31.)

Female athletes, especially cross-country runners and others involved in endurance sports, often have an iron deficiency at some point in their training if they are not taking iron supplements or do not have diets high in iron. The source of the additional iron losses in those with athletic amenorrhea has not been determined, but it is thought that iron losses occurring through the gut may increase during the stressful conditions of training. One cross-country runner became so anemic that she developed hairline fractures in her proximal femur (hip), which illustrates the potential severity of the consequences of inadequate iron consumption (Anderson et al., 1998). It seems that without supple-

mentation, the greater the intensity of training, the worse the iron levels become in women (see Chapter 23).

Toxicity

The major cause of iron overload is hereditary hemochromatosis, whereas transfusion iron overload is rare. The latter may be seen in individuals with sickle cell disease or thalassemia major who require transfusions for their anemia. Iron overload is linked to a distinct gene that favors excessive iron absorption if the iron is available in the diet. Genetic testing may eventually become a routine, readily available method for detecting this gene and reducing the risk of overload. The characteristic chemical parameters of iron overload are listed in Box 3-7 and described in more detail in Chapter 31.

Frequent blood transfusions or long-term ingestion of large amounts of iron can lead to abnormal accumulation of iron in the liver. Saturation of tissue apoferritin with iron is followed by the appearance of **hemosiderin,** which is similar to ferritin but contains more iron and is very insoluble. Hemosiderosis is an iron storage condition that develops in individuals who consume abnormally large amounts of iron or in those with a genetic defect resulting in excessive iron absorption. If the hemosiderosis is associated with tissue damage, it is called hemochromatosis (see Chapter 31).

Iron supplements may not be beneficial for either older (postmenopausal) women or older men because of the associated increased risks for heart disease and cancer. A dietary intake of iron in excess of the RDA for adult men and postmenopausal women may contribute to an enriched oxidative environment in the body that favors oxidation of LDL cholesterol, arterial vessel damage, and other adverse effects involving the cardiovascular system. In addition, excessive iron may help generate excessive amounts of free radicals that attack cellular molecules, thereby increasing the number of potentially carcinogenic molecules within cells. These potential adverse iron-disease linkages must be explored more to be confirmed.

Zinc

The most readily available form of zinc occurs in animal flesh, particularly red meats and poultry. Meat intake is frequently low among preschoolers, occasionally because of

---

BOX 3-7

Iron Overload Symptoms (Hemochromatosis)

Abnormal accumulation of iron in the liver
Excessive tissue ferritin levels
Elevated serum transferrin levels
Oxidation of LDL cholesterol
Cardiovascular complications

LDL, Low-density lipoprotein.

personal preferences or socioeconomic reasons, but usually because meats are displaced by cereal foods, milk, and milk products that children tend to prefer. Observation led to the fortification of infant and children's foods, especially cereals, with zinc. Milk is a good source of zinc, but high intakes of calcium from milk may interfere with the absorption of iron and zinc (see Mineral Interactions section). The phytates from whole grains in unleavened breads may limit zinc absorption in some populations.

The WHO highlighted zinc deficiency as one the the 10 major factors contributing to disease in developing countries (Shrimpton et al., 2005). Deficiencies are less likely to be a problem in Western nations, where breads, breakfast foods, and other cereal-based foods are made primarily from refined grains and are typically fortified (see *Clinical Insight: The Role of Zinc in Children's Health*).

Zinc is abundantly distributed throughout the human body and is second only to iron among trace elements. The human body has aproximately 2 to 3 g of zinc, with the highest concentrations in the liver, pancreas, kidney, bone, and muscles. Other tissues with high concentrations include various parts of the eye, prostate gland, spermatozoa, skin, hair, fingernails, and toenails. Zinc is primarily an intracellular ion, functioning in association with more than 300 different enzymes of various classes. Even though zinc is abundant in the cytosol, virtually all of it is bound to proteins, but it is in equilibrium with a small ionic fraction.

Absorption, Transport, Storage, and Excretion

Zinc absorption and excretion are controlled by poorly understood homeostatic mechanisms. The mechanism of absorption involves two pathways similar to those of calcium: (1) a saturable carrier mechanism operating most efficiently at low zinc intakes when luminal zinc concentrations are low, and (2) a passive mechanism involving paracellular movement when zinc intakes and luminal concentrations are high. Solubility of zinc in the gut lumen is critical, but zinc ions are generally bound to amino acids or short peptides in the lumen, and the ions are released at the brush border for absorption via the carrier mechanism (hZIPI family). The entry step of absorption across the brush border is followed by the binding of zinc ions to metallothionein and other proteins within the cytosol of the absorbing cell. Metallothionein carries the zinc (via transcellular movement) to the basolateral border for the exit step from the absorbing cell to the blood. The exit step occurs by active transport because the blood concentration of zinc is significantly greater than the cytosolic ion concentration. The process of zinc absorption is illustrated in Figure 3-36.

Zinc absorption is affected not only by the level of zinc in the diet but also by the presence of interfering substances, especially phytates. After the consumption of zinc in a meal, the serum zinc level rises and then decreases in a dose-response pattern. A protein-rich diet promotes zinc absorption by forming zinc–amino acid chelates that present zinc in a more absorbable form. Zinc absorption is slightly higher during pregnancy and lactation. Absorbed zinc is taken up from the portal circulation initially by the liver, but most of the zinc is subsequently redistributed to other tissues. Impaired absorption is associated with a variety of intestinal diseases such as Crohn's disease or pancreatic insufficiency.

Several dietary factors affect zinc absorption. Phytate decreases zinc absorption, but other complexing agents

---

✴ CLINICAL INSIGHT

The Role of Zinc in Children's Health

The first studies linking zinc and growth were carried out in Iran and Egypt almost three decades ago. "Nutritionally dwarfed" boys, characterized by short stature, iron deficiency anemia, and delayed sexual maturity, showed remarkable improvements with zinc supplementation. Some grew as much as 5 inches in 1 year and had parallel progression in gonadal development. The primary cause of zinc deficiency in these boys was identified as an impoverished diet consisting mainly of fibrous, unleavened bread. Although the whole grains used to make the bread were relatively high in zinc, they also contained phytates, which are known to form insoluble complexes with zinc and iron.

At the time, the circumstances leading to growth impairment secondary to zinc deficiency were believed to be unique to less developed countries. However, studies of preschool children from apparently well-nourished families in Denver and other cities demonstrated a correlation between short stature and low zinc levels in hair.

In addition to inhibited growth, mild zinc deficiency is probably associated with reduced resistance to infection in children, but it has been difficult to establish this link (Prentice, 1993). However, children with severe zinc deficiency, as measured by plasma zinc concentrations, have been found to be at increased risk for diarrhea and respiratory diseases (Bahl et al., 1998). Therefore adequate zinc status plays a central role not only in growth and health promotion but also in disease prevention.

Zinc and iron deficiencies remain a global problem, especially in developing countries. Fischer Walker et al. (2005) recently reviewed studies where zinc and iron were given as dual micronutrient supplements. Although in some of the studies supplementation with zinc and iron were less effective than each nutrient alone, the authors concluded that there was not strong evidence against dual supplementation.

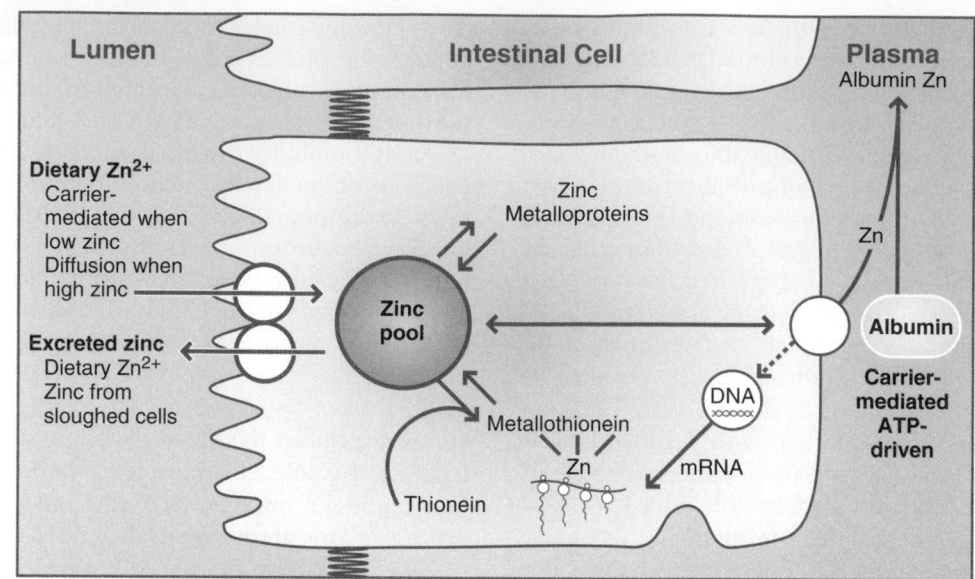

FIGURE 3-36 Model for zinc absorption showing the relationship between metallothionein and cysteine-rich intestinal protein. *DNA*, Deoxyribonucleic acid; *mRNA*, messenger ribonucleic acid; *ATP*, adenosine triphosphate.

(e.g., tannins) do not. Copper and cadmium compete for the same carrier protein; thus they reduce zinc absorption. Concern exists that high intakes of iron may reduce the amounts of zinc absorbed. High calcium intakes reduce zinc absorption and balance. Folic acid may also reduce zinc absorption when zinc intake is low. On the other hand, high doses of zinc can impair absorption of iron from ferrous sulfate, the form usually found in vitamin and mineral supplements. Dietary fiber may also interfere with zinc absorption, but the significance of this interaction within the gut lumen is unclear. Zinc absorption may be enhanced by glucose or lactose and by soy protein consumed alone or mixed with beef. Red table wine also increases zinc absorption, probably because of its congeners. Like iron, zinc is better absorbed from human milk than from cow's milk.

Transport in Blood. Albumin is the major plasma carrier of zinc, and the amount of zinc transported in the blood depends not on zinc but also on the availability of albumin, a transport protein for many mineral cations. Some zinc is transported by transferrin and by α_2-macroglobulin. Most of the zinc in blood is localized in erythrocytes and leukocytes. Plasma zinc is metabolically active and fluctuates in response to dietary intake and physiologic factors such as injury or inflammation. Plasma zinc levels drop by 50% in the acute phase of a response to an injury, probably because of the sequestering of zinc by the liver.

Intestinal Excretion. Excretion of zinc in normal individuals is almost entirely via the feces. When zinc is administered intravenously, about 10% of the dose appears in the intestine within 30 minutes. However, increased urinary excretion has been reported in those who are starving and those with nephrosis, diabetes, alcoholism, hepatic cirrhosis, and porphyria. Plasma and urine concentrations of amino acids, specifically the zinc-binding cysteine and histidine,

and other urinary metabolites may have a role in increasing zinc losses in these patients.

Functions

Zinc, primarily an intracellular ion, functions in association with more than 300 different enzymes. It participates in reactions involving either synthesis or degradation of major metabolites—carbohydrates, lipids, proteins—and nucleic acids. This trace mineral also plays important structural role as a component of several proteins and functions as an intracellular signal in brain cells. Zinc is also involved in the stabilization of protein and nucleic acid structure and the integrity of subcellular organelles, as well as in transport processes, immune function, and expression of genetic information.

Metallothionein is the most abundant, nonenzymatic zinc-containing protein known today. This low–molecular-weight protein is rich in cysteine and exceptionally high in metals, among which are zinc and lesser amounts of copper, iron, cadmium, and mercury. The biologic role of metallothionein has not been defined conclusively, but it does have a function in zinc absorption. Metallothionein may function as an intracellular reservoir that can donate zinc ions to other proteins, or it may have a redox role that reduces oxidative stress, especially in cells with high stress. Thus metallothionein may have a role in the detoxification of metals as well as in their absorption.

Zinc is abundant in the nucleus, where it stabilizes RNA and DNA structure, and is required for the activity of RNA polymerases important in cell division. Zinc also functions in chromatin proteins involved in transcription and replication.

A relationship between zinc intake and age-related macular degenerative (AMD) disease was suggested by previous reports, and a recent publication suggests that zinc supplementation (200 mg/day for 24 months) reduces AMD (Group, 2001).

Although widely touted to cure or prevent common colds, zinc gluconate lozenges were not proved to do so in a randomized, controlled trial with children and adolescents (Macknin et al., 1998) or in a study with adults (Turner and Cetnarowski, 2000). Nasal zinc sprays do not seem to be effective either (Belongia et al., 2001).

Zinc appears in the crystalline structure of bone, in bone enzymes, and at the zone of demarcation. It is thought to be needed for adequate osteoblastic activity, formation of bone enzymes such as alkaline phosphatase, and calcification. Unless bone resorption is occurring, the zinc in bone is not available (see Chapter 24 and Table 3-36).

Dietary Reference Intakes

The zinc DRIs established for adolescent and adult males are 11 mg/day. Because of the lower body weight of adolescent and adult women, their DRI is 8 mg/day. The DRIs for preadolescents are estimated to be 8 mg/day. The DRIs for infants are 2 mg/day for the first 6 months and 3 mg/day for the second 6 months of life.

Food Sources and Intakes

For most Americans almost 80% of the daily intake of zinc is provided by meat, fish, poultry, ready-to-eat breakfast cereals fortified with zinc, and milk and milk products (Subar et al., 1998). Oysters (which are especially high in zinc) and other shellfish, liver, whole grain cereals, dry beans, and nuts are all good sources (Table 3-31; see also Appendix 58). Soy products may also be fairly good sources of zinc. In general, zinc intake correlates well with protein intake.

The zinc content of typical diets of adults in Western countries ranges between 10 and 15 mg/day, but women consume less than men because of their lower caloric intakes. The zinc density of the American adult's diet is about 5.6 mg/1000 kcal (Subar et al., 1998).

Deficiency

The clinical signs of zinc deficiency in humans that were first described involved young boys and included short stature, hypogonadism, mild anemia, and low plasma zinc level (Prasad et al., 1963) (see *Clinical Insight: The Role of Zinc in Children's Health*). This deficiency is caused by a diet high in unrefined cereals and unleavened breads, which contain high levels of fiber and phytate, both of which chelate with zinc in the intestine and prevent absorption. The anemia in the youths may have reflected a coexisting iron deficiency from the same cause. Additional symptoms of zinc deficiency include hypogeusia (decreased taste acuity), delayed wound healing, alopecia, and diverse forms of skin lesions. Acquired zinc deficiency may occur as the result of malabsorption, starvation, or increased losses via urinary, pancreatic, or other exocrine secretions.

Patients with alcoholism may have altered zinc metabolism. Pregnant women and older adults are also at increased risk for deficiency. Low-dose zinc supplementation may improve measures of poor zinc status.

Acrodermatitis enteropathica, an autosomal-recessive disease characterized by zinc malabsorption, results in ecze-

TABLE 3-31

Zinc Content of Selected Foods

Food	Content (mg)
Baked beans, with pork, ½ cup	6.93
Liver, beef, fried, 3 oz	4.45
Ground beef, lean, 3 oz	5.31
Oysters, Eastern, 3 oz	3.94
Turkey, dark meat, baked, 3 oz	3.8
Pork, cooked, 3 oz	3.5
Ham, cooked, 3 oz	2.18
Wild rice, cooked, ½ cup	2.2
Lobster, 3 oz	1.65
Peas, green, cooked, 1 cup	1.21
Yogurt plain, 8 oz	1.30
Pecans, 1 oz	1.28
Peanuts, dry roasted, 1 oz	0.94
Spinach, frozen cooked, 1 cup	0.93
Bread, whole wheat, 1 slice	0.54
Gingerbread, 1 piece	0.39

DRIs

Infants and young children	2-5 mg/day, depending on age
Older children and adolescents	8-11 mg/day, depending on age and gender
Adults	8-11 mg/day, depending on gender
Pregnant	11-13 mg/day, depending on age
Lactating	12-14 mg/day, depending on age

From U.S. Department of Agriculture, Agricultural Research Service: Nutrient Database for Standard Reference, Release 18, retrieved 2005, Data Laboratory home page: http://www.nal.usda.gov/fnic/foodcomp/Data/SR18/sr18.html.

matoid skin lesions (Figure 3-37), alopecia, diarrhea, intercurrent bacterial and yeast infections, and eventually death if left untreated. Symptoms generally first develop during weaning from human milk to cow's milk. A potential adverse interaction between iron and zinc may contribute to acrodermatitis enteropathica.

Zinc deficiency results in various immunologic defects. Severe deficiency is accompanied by thymic atrophy, lymphopenia, reduced lymphocyte proliferative response to mitogens, a selective decrease in T_4-helper cells, decreased NK cell activity, anergy, and deficient thymic hormone activity. Even mild zinc deficiency can reduce immune function (e.g., by producing impaired interleukin-2 production). Supplementation with zinc may improve immune status, but more studies are needed to confirm this. Moderate zinc deficiency is associated with anergy and diminished NK cell activity but not with thymic atrophy or lymphopenia. Box 3-8 summarizes the clinical manifestations of human zinc deficiency. Similarities between patients with sickle cell anemia and zinc

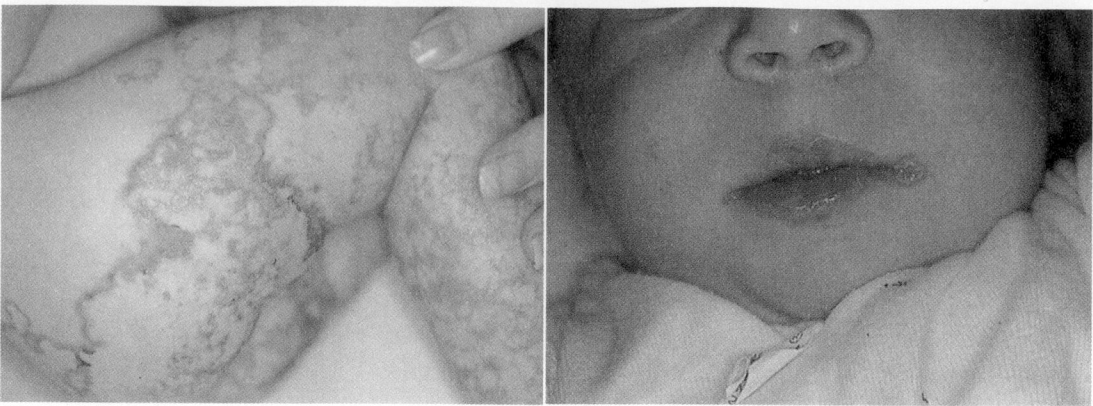

FIGURE 3-37 Cutaneous manifestations of zinc deficiency. *(From Callen WBS et al:* Color atlas of dermatology, *Philadelphia, 1993, Saunders.)*

deficiency suggest the possibility of a secondary zinc deficiency in those with the anemia (see Chapter 31).

Low zinc intakes are associated with low concentrations of insulin-like growth factor 1 (IGF-l) in postmenopausal women, but the meaning of this finding is unclear (Devine et al., 1998). If calcium supplements are taken by postmenopausal women, it is possible that zinc absorption becomes suppressed, reducing IGF-l, which normally supports tissue growth. Problems caused by low zinc intakes seem to be increasing, partly because of the low bioavailability of zinc (Salgueiro and Boccio, 2002). Athletes may also have an increased risk for developing zinc deficiency. Physical activity may increase mobilization of zinc from bone stores for cellular needs (e.g., for the synthesis of zinc-metalloenzymes) (see Chapter 23).

Toxicity

Oral ingestion of toxic amounts of zinc (100 to 300 mg/day) is rare, but the UL for zinc in adults is 40 mg/day. Excessive zinc supplementation has long been known to interfere with copper absorption. A major form of zinc toxicity develops in patients receiving hemodialysis for renal failure (see Chapter 36). Contamination of dialysis fluids from the adhesive plastic used on the dialysis coils or from galvanized pipes has been reported. The toxic syndrome in these patients is characterized by anemia, fever, and central nervous system disturbances. Zinc sulfate in amounts of 2 g/day or more may cause GI irritation and vomiting. Inhalation of zinc fumes during welding may be toxic, but exposure to fumes can be prevented with proper precautions.

Fluoride

Fluoride is a natural element found in nearly all drinking water and soil, although the fluoride content varies greatly throughout the world (Palmer and Anderson, 2000). For example, some well water has much more fluoride than other water, so families who use well water need to monitor fluoride levels periodically to make sure that levels are not in the toxic range. Although fluoride is not considered an essential element, this anion is known to be important for

---

BOX 3-8

Zinc Deficiency Symptoms

Growth retardation
Delayed sexual maturation
Hypogonadism and hypospermia
Alopecia
Delayed wound healing
Skin lesions
Impaired appetite
Immune deficiencies
Behavioral disturbances
Eye lesions, including photophobia and night blindness
Impaired taste (hypogeusia)

---

the health of bones and teeth (see Chapters 24 and 25). The average skeleton contains 2.5 mg of fluoride.

Functions

Fluoride is considered important, if not essential, because of its benefits for tooth enamel. Fluoride incorporation into enamel produces more stable apatite crystals (Robinson et al., 2004). Fluoride also acts as an antibacterial agent in the oral cavity, serving as an enzyme inhibitor. Fluoride has no known requirement in human metabolic pathways.

The prevalence of dental caries has decreased by 50% in recent decades because of fluoridation of drinking water and the use of topical fluorides. The prevalence of dental caries has also decreased in communities without fluoridated water. The cause of this decrease probably results from the use of fluoridated toothpaste, topical fluoride applications, and increased use of fluorides in food, especially in fluoridated water used in food processing, all of which provide fluoride for incorporation into teeth. Soft drinks typically are prepared with fluoridated waters at bottling plants in urban areas (see Chapter 25 for fluoride supplementation recommendations).

Fluoride substitutes for the hydroxyl group on the lattice structure of calcium phosphate salts (i.e., hydroxyapatites) of the bones and teeth to form fluoroapatite, which is harder and less readily resorbed than hydroxyapatite. However, after fluoridation bone tissue formed at high flouride blood levels is not as healthy because it is subject to greater numbers of fractures from too tight binding of the flouroapatite (crystals) compared with the hydroxyapatite unfluoridated bone (see Chapter 24 and Table 3-36).

Dietary Reference Intakes

The AIs for fluoride were established for the first time in 1997. AIs for adult men and women are 4 and 3 mg/day, respectively. Depending on age, the AIs range from 2 to 3 mg/day for children and adolescents and from 0.7 to 1 mg/day for young children between the ages of 1 and 8 years. For comparison, an 8-oz glass of fluoridated water (1 ppm or 1 mg/L) provides about 0.2 mg of fluoride. ULs have also been established for fluoride.

Food Sources and Intakes

The major dietary sources of fluoride are drinking water and processed foods that have been prepared or reconstituted with fluoridated water. Seafood also is high in fluoride, but the flouride content of freshwater fish is lower than that of saltwater fish. The standard recommendation is 1 ppm in fluoridated community water supplies. Children who consume fluoridated water typically consume more fluoride than children who consume unfluoridated water. Intakes higher than 2 mg begin to raise concerns about mild fluorosis, which has been reported in a few U.S. communities.

Although fluorides exist in fruits and vegetables, the amounts in most foods other than seafood and tea are not significant. The amount in tea leaves can be quite substantial, depending on the brewing strength. One cup of tea may contain as much as 1 mg of fluoride. Soups and stews made with fish and meat bones also provide substantial fluoride. Beef liver and mechanically deboned meat and fowl are also high in fluoride. Cooking foods in Teflon pans (a fluoride-containing polymer) may increase fluoride intake, although solid scientific data are not available to support this fact. Fluoridated toothpastes are also a souce of fluoride. Lynch and Cate (2005) reported that calcium carbonate–based fluoride toothpastes are effective in reducing caries and provide oral calcium.

Deficiency

Because no known metabolic function exists for fluoride, fluoride cannot have a true deficiency that results in disease. Fortuitous binding in hydroxyapatite crystals, especially from fluoridated water supplies, reduces dental caries, but it does not seem to have any effect on reducing osteoporotic fractures (Palmer and Anderson, 2000).

Toxicity

A mild fluorosis can develop from daily doses of 0.1 mg/kg (i.e., greater than approximately 2 to 3 ppm of fluoride in the drinking water) (see Chapter 25). The resulting discoloration of the teeth, or mottling, is not usually visible and has no adverse effect except cosmetically. However, higher intakes lead to tooth flaking and more serious dental effects.

Some evidence suggests that fluoride intakes are increasing among toddlers and young children because of the proliferating sources of fluoride. When drinking water contained less fluoride, the average intake was lower. Even the highest values did not exceed the recommendation of 0.08 mg/kg daily. Intakes of fluoride by young children may vary greatly because of the widespread availability of foods prepared with fluoridated water, the use of dentifrices, and other sources. Therefore some are concerned that some children may ingest total amounts of fluoride that exceed the optimum intake level (0.05 to 0.07 mg/kg daily), possibly causing dental fluorosis.

Copper

Copper, a normal constituent of blood, is another established essential micronutrient. Recent interest in copper and several other trace elements has increased because of the many tissue-related functions and the potential (though unlikely) risk of deficiency (Uauy et al., 1998). Concentrations of copper are highest in the liver, brain, heart, and kidney. Muscle contains a low level of copper, but, because of its large mass, skeletal muscle contains almost 40% of all the copper in the body. Recent investigations have increased the understanding of the physiologic roles of copper, copper homeostasis, and copper needs throughout the life cycle (Bonham et al., 2002).

Absorption, Transport, Storage, and Excretion

Copper absorption occurs in the small intestine. Entry at the mucosal surface is by facilitated diffusion, and exit across the basolateral membrane is primarily by active transport, but facilitated transfer may also occur. Competition between copper ions and other divalent cations exists at each step. Within the intestinal absorbing cells, copper ions are bound to metallothionein with greater affinity than zinc or other ions. Some evidence suggests that the amount of copper absorbed is regulated by the amount of metallothionein in the mucosal cells. Net absorption of copper varies from 25% to 60%. Low absorption efficiencies help to regulate the retention of copper in the body; therefore the percentage of absorption decreases with increased intake. Fiber and phytate, known to affect bioavailability of several minerals, may slightly inhibit copper absorption, as shown by a study comparing a vegetarian diet with an omnivorous diet. However, because the total content of copper in the study's vegetarian diet was higher, the total amount of copper absorbed was also higher than from the nonvegetarian diet (Hunt and Vanderpool, 2001).

Approximately 90% of the copper in serum is incorporated into **ceruloplasmin;** the rest is bound loosely to albumin, transcuprein, and other proteins; free amino acids; and possibly histidine. Copper is transported in the blood to other tissues, primarily bound to albumin. It also exists in blood as ceruloplasmin, a functional protein that acts as an enzyme at the erythrocyte-forming cells of the bone marrow. Serum copper and immunoreactive ceruloplasmin levels tend to be higher in women than in men. The serum copper concentration is greatest in the neonate and decreases gradually during the first year of life.

Copper bound to albumin in the blood may serve as a temporary storage site for copper. In the liver copper binds to metallothionein, which serves as a storage form, and is incorporated into ceruloplasmin and secreted into the plasma for the transport of copper to cells. Copper is also secreted from the liver as a component of bile, the major route of excretion of copper. Once in the GI tract, copper becomes part of the pool that may be resorbed or excreted, depending on the body's need for copper. Biliary excretion increases in response to excessive intakes of copper but may not be able to keep up with intake, sometimes allowing it to reach toxic levels.

Small amounts of copper are found in urine, sweat, and menstrual blood. Copper can be conserved by the kidney if necessary when substantial amounts are filtered through the glomeruli and resorbed in the tubules.

The interaction of copper with other nutrients negates the fallacy that taking excessive amounts of vitamin and mineral supplements above the recommended levels of consumption is good. In amounts of 150 mg/day, zinc has been shown to induce copper deficiency by overwhelming the capacity of metallothionein in intestinal absorbing cells to bind copper (even though metallothionein has a greater affinity for copper than for zinc). High ascorbic acid intake (1500 mg/day) also reduces blood concentrations of copper, which may decrease the role of ceruloplasmin in red cell formation.

Functions

Copper is a component of many enzymes, and symptoms of copper deficiency are attributable to enzyme failures. Copper in ceruloplasmin has a well-documented role in oxidizing iron before it is transported in the plasma. Lysyl oxidase, a copper-containing enzyme, is essential in the lysine-derived cross-linking of collagen and elastin, connective tissue proteins with great tensile strength. Through the involvement of copper-containing electron transport proteins, copper also has roles in mitochondrial energy production. As part of copper-containing enzymes such as superoxide dismutase, copper protects against oxidants and free radicals and promotes the synthesis of melanin and catecholamines. Other functions of copper-containing enzymes have not yet been completely defined (see Table 3-36).

Dietary Reference Intakes

RDAs of 900 mcg/day (0.9 mg/day) for adolescents and adults of both genders have been established for copper (Institute of Medicine, Food and Nutrition Board, 2001; Trumbo et al., 2001). Copper intakes should range between 200 and 220 mcg/day for infants and between 340 and 440 mcg for young children. Premature infants are born with low copper reserves and may require additional dietary copper during their first few months of life (see Chapter 43).

Food Sources and Intakes

Copper is distributed widely in foods, including animal products (except for milk), and most diets provide between 0.6 and 2 mg/day. Foods high in copper are shellfish (oysters), organ meats (liver, kidney), muscle meats, chocolate, nuts, cereal grains, dried legumes, and dried fruits (Table 3-32).

In general, fruits and vegetables contain little copper. Cow's milk, a poor source of copper, contains 0.015 to 0.18 mg/L, whereas the copper in human milk is well absorbed and ranges from 0.15 to 1.05 mg/L. Infants fed cow's milk may be at risk for copper deficiency because of its low copper content.

Copper intakes of individuals in several age categories in the United States have been consistently below recommended amounts, with adolescent girls consuming only about 50% of the recommended intakes, according to estimated median intakes reported in the Total Diet Study of the FDA (Pennington and Schoen, 1996). Typically the copper content of drinking water is not considered in diet surveys, but the amount of copper in water from copper pipes is considered to be very low, perhaps insignificant.

Copper intakes may be low in U.S. diets because until recently, ready-to-eat cereals typically were not fortified with copper as they were for several other trace minerals such as iron and zinc. Another reason for the potential existence of low copper intakes is the inaccuracy associated with short-term assessments of dietary copper (Pang et al., 2001).

Deficiency

Copper deficiency has historically been assessed by a decrease in serum copper and ceruloplasmin levels, but more

TABLE 3-32

Copper Content of Selected Foods

Food	Content (mg)
Beef liver, fried, 3 oz	12.4
Oysters, 3 oz	3.63
Orange juice, 1 cup	0.11
Cashews, dry roasted, ¼ cup	0.61
Sunflower seeds, ¼ cup	0.59
Baking chocolate, 1 square	0.92
Mushrooms, cooked, 1 cup	0.79
Tropical trail mix, 1 cup	0.74
Beans, white, canned, 1 cup	0.61
Yogurt, 8 oz	0.03
Broccoli, raw, 1 cup	0.04
Peaches, canned, 1 cup	0.05
Milk chocolate, 1 oz	0.16
Milk, 2% fat, 1 cup	0.03
DRI Range	
0.2-1.3 mg/day, depending on age and gender	

From U.S. Department of Agriculture, Agricultural Research Service: Nutrient Database for Standard Reference, Release 18, retrieved 2005, Data Laboratory home page: http://www.nal.usda.gov/fnic/foodcomp/Data/SR18/sr18.html.

sensitive indicators of copper status—copper-containing enzymes in blood cells—have now been identified. Copper deficiency is characterized by anemia, neutropenia, and skeletal abnormalities, especially demineralization. Other changes may also develop, including subperiosteal hemorrhages, hair and skin depigmentation, and defective elastin formation. The failure of erythropoiesis, as well as cerebral and cerebellar degeneration, may lead to death. Neutropenia and leukopenia are the best early indications of copper deficiency in children. Copper deficiency anemia is discussed in Chapter 31.

Classical cases of copper deficiency were reported in the 1960s among Peruvian infants who were poorly nourished, had diarrhea, and were fed diluted cow's milk (Cordano, 1998). Other cases of deficiency have been reported since then. Premature infants are likely to have copper deficiency unless given a copper supplement, because most of the copper is normally transferred across the placenta during the last few months of a full-term pregnancy (see Chapter 43). Pathak and Kapil (2004) reported that diets in developing countries continue to be low in trace minerals, including copper. They emphasize the importance of zinc, copper, and magnesium in successful pregnancy outcomes and note that further study is needed.

Copper is stored in the liver; therefore deficiency develops slowly as copper stores become depleted. Deficiencies have not been reported in otherwise healthy humans consuming a varied diet. Low serum copper, ceruloplasmin, and superoxide dismutase levels provide supportive evidence of copper deficiency, but these markers are not sensitive to marginal copper status. Bone changes, including osteoporosis, metaphyseal spur formation, and soft tissue calcification in infants receiving prolonged TPN may resolve with copper supplementation. The only signs of copper deficiency found in adults are neutropenia and microcytic anemia, but deficiency is very rare in adults, probably because copper accumulates in the liver throughout life in most individuals.

Menkes syndrome, also known as kinky-hair syndrome, is a sex-linked recessive defect that results in copper malabsorption, increased urinary copper loss, and abnormal intracellular copper transport, all of which cause an abnormal distribution of copper among organs and within cells. Affected infants have retarded growth, defective keratinization and pigmentation of the hair, hypothermia, degenerative changes in aortic elastin, abnormalities of the metaphyses of long bones, and progressive mental deterioration. These infants typically do not survive the first few months of life. Many of the features of this disorder result from interference with the cross-linking of collagen and elastin, steps that require one or more copper enzymes. Brain tissue is practically devoid of cytochrome C oxidase, and a marked accumulation of copper occurs in the intestinal mucosa, although serum copper and ceruloplasmin levels remain very low. Many defects exist in connective tissue in patients with Menkes syndrome.

One copper deficiency manifests as a demyelinating neuropathy with chronic intestinal pseudoobstruction, osteoporosis, testicular failure, retinal degeneration, and cardiomyopathy. The underlying defect seems to involve hepatic incorporation of copper into ceruloplasmin (Buchman et al., 1994). Decreased plasma copper levels develop in patients with malabsorption diseases such as celiac sprue, tropical sprue, protein-losing enteropathies, and nephrotic syndrome. Like zinc, low copper intakes may also contribute to reduced immune responses in otherwise healthy individuals.

Toxicity

Copper toxicity from food consumption is considered impossible, but toxicity from excessive supplementation or copper salts used in agriculture has been reported. Liver cirrhosis typically develops from toxic intake levels, and abnormalities in red blood cell formation also occur.

Ceruloplasmin concentrations increase during pregnancy and with the use of oral contraceptives. Serum copper concentrations in pregnant women are approximately twice those in women who are not pregnant. Serum copper concentrations are also elevated in patients with acute and chronic infections, liver disease, and pellagra. The physiologic significance of these elevations is not known, but bile also contains substantial amounts of copper in these patients. Any chronic liver disease that interferes with the excretion of bile may contribute to the retention of copper. Primary biliary cirrhosis, as well as mechanical obstruction of the bile ducts, contributes to a progressive rise in liver copper content.

Wilson's disease (hepatolenticular degeneration) is characterized by excessive accumulation of copper in body tissues such as the eyes as a result of a genetic deficiency in the liver synthesis of ceruloplasmin (see Chapter 28). A strict vegetarian diet may benefit patients with Wilson's disease because of the low copper content of fruits and vegetables.

ULTRATRACE MINERALS

Ultratrace minerals such as iodine, selenium, manganese, molybdenum, chromium, and a few other nonessential minerals are found in the body in small quantities; their amounts are typically measured in micrograms. Each of these elements has one or more essential roles. Because of their small quantities in human tissues, special analytic instrumentation and ultra-clean laboratories are necessary for the routine analysis or experimental work relating to the ultratrace minerals.

Iodine

Iodine deficiency in the United States and many Western nations has practically been eliminated with the iodinization of salt. However, people living in many mountainous areas of the world and a few low-lying delta regions still have low iodine intakes because of the low iodine content of the soil used in cultivating crops. Others living in lowlands may have high goitrogen consumption that reduces iodine use by the thyroid gland. The body normally contains 20 to 30 mg of iodine, with more than 75% in the thyroid gland and the rest distributed throughout the body, particularly in the lactating mammary gland, gastric mucosa, and blood. Dietary iodine is needed for the synthesis of thyroid hormones.

Absorption, Transport, Storage, and Excretion

Iodine is absorbed easily as iodide. In the circulation iodine exists freely and protein bound, but the bound iodide predominates. Excretion is primarily via urine, but small amounts are found in the feces as a result of biliary secretion.

Functions

Iodine is stored in the thyroid gland, where it is used in the synthesis of **triiodothyronine (T_3)** and **thyroxine (T_4)**. Uptake of iodide ions by the thyroid cells may be inhibited by goitrogens (substances that exist naturally in foods). Thyroid hormone is degraded in target cells and the liver, and the iodine is highly conserved under normal conditions. Selenium is important in iodine metabolism because of its presence in one enzyme responsible for forming active T_3 from thyroglobulin stored in the thyroid gland (see Table 3-36).

Dietary Reference Intakes

An iodine intake of 150 mcg/day has been suggested as sufficient for all adults and adolescents. The RDA for pregnant and lactating women increases to 220 mcg and 290 mcg, respectively. The RDA is 110 mcg for infants up to 6 months of age and 130 mcg for older infants. The RDA for children is between 90 and 120 mcg and increases with age (or body size).

Food Sources and Intakes

Iodine exists in variable amounts in food and drinking water. Seafood such as clams, lobsters, oysters, sardines, and other saltwater fish is the richest source of iodine. Saltwater fish contain 300 to 3000 mcg/kg of flesh; freshwater fish contain 20 to 40 mcg/kg, but they are still good sources. The iodine content of cow's milk and eggs is determined by the iodides available in the diet of the animal; the iodide content of vegetables varies according to the iodine content of the soil in which they grow. Iodine also enters the food chain through iodophors, which are used as disinfectants in dairy processing, coloring agents, and dough conditioners. These sources add significant amounts of iodine to the food supply. Table 3-33 and Appendix 53 list the iodine content of various foods.

The use of iodized salt should still be advocated in certain areas to prevent goiter. The best way to obtain an adequate intake of iodine is to use iodized salt (which has about 60 mcg of iodine per gram of salt in the United States and Canada) in food preparation (Kuhajek, 2000). Sea salt naturally contains variable amounts of iodine, and only about 1/10 the level of iodized salt. More than 50% of the table salt sold in the United States is iodized; however, iodized salt is not used in processed foods. Mandatory iodinization has been adopted by many nations, including Canada, but is not legally required in the United States, where iodine deficiency is now very rare. The Total Diet

Study of the FDA showed that median adult iodine intakes from 1982 to 1991 ranged from 130 to 140 mcg/day for women and 182 to 204 mcg/day for men. The median iodine intake for male and female teenagers was even higher, with adolescent boys consuming almost twice the RDA (Pennington and Schoen, 1996). Intakes of iodine in the United States seem adequate for most people because of iodinization of salt and the use of iodofors.

A small subset of vegans who eat only uncooked, lactobacilli-rich food were tested for thyroid function and found to be within normal limits (Rauma et al., 1994). These vegans consumed iodine in seaweed or kelp tablets. Some of the individuals in this study had iodine intakes high enough to cause potential problems, but symptoms of toxicity were not observed.

Deficiency

An estimated 2 billion people worldwide living in less developed nations remain at risk for iodine deficiency. These individuals may have a moderate iodine deficiency, even when obvious goiter, a severe condition, is not evident. In schoolchildren iodine deficiency is associated with poor cognition. Iodine deficiency is the most common preventable cause of mental retardation in the world (Lee et al., 1999). Use of

TABLE 3-33

Iodine Content of Selected Foods

Food	Content (mcg)
Salt, iodized, 1 tsp	400
Bread, made with iodate dough conditioner and continuous mix process, 1 slice	142
Haddock, 3 oz	104-145
Bread, made with regular process, 1 slice	35
Cheese, cottage, 2% fat, ½ cup	26-71
Shrimp, 3 oz	21-37
Egg, 1	18-26
Cheese, cheddar, 1 oz	5-23
Ground beef, 3 oz	8

DRIs

Infants and young children	90-130 mcg/day, depending on age
Older children and adolescents	120-150 mcg/day, depending on age
Adults	150 mcg/day
Pregnant	220 mcg/day
Lactating	290 mcg/day

From U.S. Department of Agriculture: Composition of foods, USDA Handbook No. 8 Series, Washington, DC, 1976-1986, Agricultural Research Service, The Department.

iodized salt or the oral administration of a single dose of iodized oil, and weekly iodine supplements are effective. Use of iodized salt should be encouraged during pregnancy, especially through the end of the second trimester (Xue-Yi et al., 1994). Very low iodine intakes are associated with the development of endemic or simple **goiter,** which is an enlargement of the thyroid gland (Figure 3-38). The deficiency may be nearly total, especially in mountainous areas and regions of high goitrogen intakes, or relative, subsequent to an increased need for thyroid hormones (e.g., by females during adolescence, pregnancy, and lactation).

Although many countries have worked to eliminate iodine deficiency (Kusic and Jukic, 2005), goiter may affect as many as 200 to 300 million people worldwide. In some countries goiter is so common that it is regarded as a normal physical feature. In the United States the prevalence rate of goiter for all ages is 1.9/1000 persons. The rate is higher in women than in men and in older individuals than in younger ones.

Goitrogens, which exist naturally in foods, can also cause goiter by blocking uptake of iodine from the blood by thyroid cells. Foods containing goitrogens include cabbage, turnips, rapeseeds (from rape plants), peanuts, cassava, sweet potatoes, kelp, and soybeans. Goitrogens are inactivated by heating or cooking. Severe iodine deficiency during gestation and early postnatal growth results in **cretinism** in infants, a syndrome characterized by mental deficiency, spastic diplegia or quadriplegia, deaf mutism, dysarthria, a characteristic shuffling gait, shortened stature, and hypothyroidism. Less severe variations of this syndrome also exist, manifesting as moderate retardation in intellectual or neuromotor maturation.

Toxicity

Even though iodine intakes have a wide margin of safety, tolerable ULs have been established (Institute of Medicine, Food and Nutrition Board, 2001). Adults have a UL of 1100

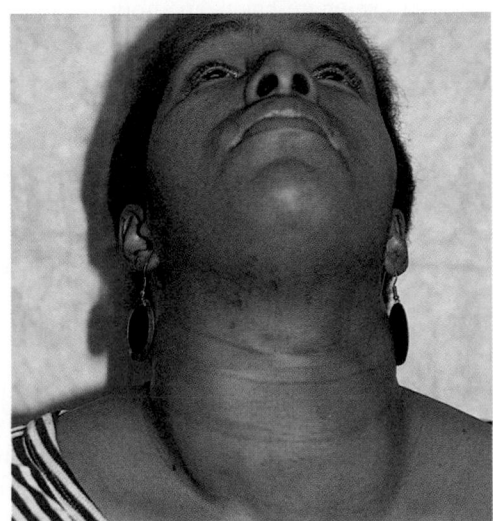

FIGURE 3-38 Goiter caused by iodine deficiency. *(From Swartz MH:* Textbook of physical diagnosis history and examination, *ed 3, Philadelphia, 1998, Saunders.)*

mcg/day, and young children have a UL of 200 to 300 mcg/day. In some cases goiter develops slowly as a consequence of long-term iodine intakes that are much higher than physiologic requirements. The role of excessive iodine in thyroid disease or disorder is not clear. Today the level of iodine in foods is not considered a significant public health problem in the United States or Canada. However, two different studies, one in Canada and the other in the United States, reported iodine intakes that were either greater than or approximately equal to recommended intake levels throughout the life cycle (Pennington and Schoen, 1996). The level of iodine in most American diets is appropriate for good health, but for small groups of people with underlying thyroid pathologic conditions, excessive iodine in the diet may result in hypothyroidism, goiter formation, or hyperthyroidism (Mussig et al., 2006).

Selenium

A rather narrow dietary intake range exists for selenium, below which deficiency occurs and above which toxicity develops. Only in China have these extremes been shown to relate to the selenium content of the soil. A dietary intake of approximately 40 mcg of selenium per day seems to be necessary to maintain **glutathione peroxidase (GSH-Px),** an enzyme containing selenium. The diets of practically all nations other than China supply selenium in sufficient amounts to maintain adequate levels of GSH-Px; thus selenium deficiency is extremely rare. GSH-Px, discovered to be a selenoenzyme in the early 1970s, is considered the major active form of selenium in tissues, although other selenium proteins have since been discovered.

Tissue levels are influenced by dietary intake and reflect the geochemical environment. Regions of North America identified as low in selenium content are the Northeast, Pacific, Southwest, and coastal plain of the southeastern region of the United States, as well as north central and eastern Canada. The lowest selenium content of soil exists in a few regions of China, especially in Keshan, where severe selenium deficiency was first reported in a human population in 1979. Other areas with low selenium content include parts of Finland and New Zealand.

Absorption, Transport, Storage, and Excretion

Absorption of selenium, which occurs in the upper segment of the small intestine, is more efficient under conditions of deficiency. Increased intake frequently results in increased excretion of selenium in the urine. Selenium status is assessed by measuring selenium or GSH-Px in serum, platelets, and erythrocytes or in whole blood. Erythrocyte selenium measurement is an indicator of long-term intake (Neve, 2000). Selenium is transported bound to albumin initially and subsequently to α_2-globulin.

Functions

Many but not all of the pathologic changes caused by selenium deficiency can be explained on the basis of inadequate levels of GSH-Px enzymes. Because GSH-Px acts together with other antioxidants and free radical scavengers, these molecules reduce cellular peroxides and free radicals in general into water and other harmless molecules.

Selenium, as selenomethionine or selenocysteine, exists in several proteins that are widely distributed in the body. Cellular GSH-Px (cGSH-Px) has been found in almost all cells and extracellularly in serum and milk. This family of enzymes may help provide a reserve of selenium in proteins that can be drawn on when needed. Phospholipid hydroperoxide GSH-Px (phGSH-Px), which has a distribution in lipid-soluble fractions of the cell, may have other roles in lipid and eicosanoid metabolism.

Type 1 iodothyronine 5'-deiodinase, an enzyme capable of converting T_4 to T_3, is a selenoprotein. Moderate selenium intakes (40 mcg/day) seem adequate to maintain activities of these deiodinases. However, high intakes (350 mcg/day) are associated with depressed T_3 levels, suggesting less activity of iodothyronine deiodinase (Neve, 2000). GSH-Px enzymes have also been shown to be critical in several endocrine systems (Beckett and Arthur, 2005).

Selenoprotein P, another selenium-containing molecule, may act as a free radical scavenger or a transporter of selenium. Selenium is used in the synthesis of these molecules in the anionic form, but in the molecules selenium is covalently bound, as is sulfur, which it typically replaces in some of these molecules.

The antioxidant effects of selenium and vitamin E may reinforce each other by the overlap of their protective actions against oxidative damage. These two antioxidant nutrients may participate in other cooperative activities that help maintain healthy cells. GSH-Px acts in the cytosol and the mitochondrial matrix, whereas vitamin E exerts its antioxidative actions within cell membranes (see Table 3-36).

The GSH-Px reaction step is illustrated in Figure 3-39. Other selenium-dependent enzymes exist in mammalian systems, but less is known about the requirements of these enzymes for selenium. The antioxidative roles of cellular selenium-containing enzymes may have a role in preventing cancer. For example, modest doses of selenium supplements given to adults resulted in a great reduction in prostate cancer, as well as lesser decreases in several other cancers after a period of several years (Clark et al., 1996; Patrick, 2004). Many other selenoproteins have been identified, but their functions have not yet been eludicated (Burk et al., 2001).

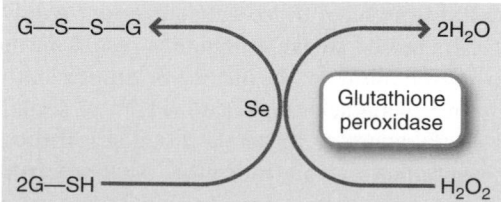

FIGURE 3-39 Enzymatic reaction catalyzed by the selenium-containing enzyme, glutathione peroxidase *(GSH-Px)*. Selenium is a prosthetic form of the enzyme that removes highly reactive hydrogen peroxide *(H₂O₂)* from within cells by converting it to water *(H₂O)* while simultaneously converting two molecules of reduced glutathione *(GUSH)* to oxidized glutathione *(G-S-S-G)*.

Dietary Reference Intakes

The RDAs for selenium 55mc mcg/day for women, men, and adolescents (ages 14 to 18), whereas the RDAs for children range from 20 to 30 mcg/day. The AIs for infants is 15 to 20 mcg/day (Trumbo et al., 2001). The RDA during pregnancy is 60 mcg, and the RDA during lactation is 70 mcg/day. Requirements for selenium may increase with a high consumption of SFAs because of the need for the antioxidant activity of selenium.

Food Sources and Intakes

No comprehensive table of the selenium content of foods has been published. The selenium concentration in foods depends on the selenium content of the soil and water where the food was grown. Improvements in analytic techniques have resulted in changes being made to many previously published data of the selenium content of foods during the last few decades. Table 3-34 and Appendix 57 list the selenium contents of some foods.

Major food sources of selenium are Brazil nuts, seafood, kidney, liver, meat, and poultry. Fruits and vegetables are low in selenium content. The major food source of selenium identified by the Total Diet Study of the FDA is animal flesh foods. Grains vary in selenium content, depending on where they are grown.

Selenium content and GSH-Px activity in human breast milk are influenced directly by maternal selenium intake and by the form of selenium consumed. Plasma selenium concentrations of infants fed unsupplemented formula are lower than those of infants fed supplemented formula or human milk.

Data summarized for the Total Diet Study of the FDA (1982 to 1991) showed that the estimated median selenium intakes of adults and children were greater than the age-specific RDAs (Pennington and Schoen, 1996). Typical diets consumed by Americans provide sufficient amounts of selenium daily to prevent any selenium deficiency and promote health (Levander et al., 1995). Selenium fortification of infant formulas with selenate has been shown to improve the selenium status of preterm infants (Tyrala et al., 1996).

Deficiency

Despite a wide range of selenium intakes from food, selenium deficiency is rare in populations throughout the world. Selenium deficiency takes years to develop when food intake is adequate. Severe selenium deficiency in a population has only been reported for regions in China, including Keshan. Keshan disease, a form of cardiomyopathy that mainly affects children and women, was first observed in the Keshan province of China. A viral infection combined with selenium deficiency has been suggested as the etiology of Keshan disease (Beck et al., 1995). Since its discovery, supplementation programs in Keshan have totally eradicated the disease. However, in individuals with established disease the response to supplementation is poor, probably because of other factors contributing to myopathy.

The second selenium deficiency disease, discovered in Mongolia, is known as Kashan-Beck disease and is common in preadolescent and adolescent children. These two human diseases occur in areas where the content of selenium in the soil is very low. This disease may also have a viral component combined with the selenium deficiency in the diet, but very little is known of its etiology. Illness initially involves symmetric stiffness, swelling, and often pain in the interphalangeal joints of the fingers, followed by generalized osteroarthritis. Kashan-Beck disease may also have iodine deficiency as a risk factor.

Selenium deficiency has previously been reported in malnourished patients receiving long-term TPN. Supplementation resulted in improved serum selenium levels, platelet GSH-Px activity, and reduced clinical symptoms. Selenium deficiency should no longer be a problem in patients receiving long-term TPN or enteral nutrition because the preparation of these solutions now includes a trace element supplement (see Chapter 20).

Deficient selenium intakes may also contribute to carcinogenesis. Patients with some cancers have been shown to have low serum selenium levels, although the underlying mechanisms for this correlation have not been established. One possible explanation lies in the possible failure of GSH-Px to scavenge free radicals efficiently in dividing cells. In addition, patients with cirrhosis have low plasma selenium concentrations, which may predispose them to cancer (Latavayova et al., 2006).

Toxicity

Indicators of selenium toxicity have been reported in China and Australia. Signs of toxicity, referred to as selenosis, include skin and nail changes, tooth decay, and nonspecific GI and neurologic abnormalities.

Manganese

Manganese deficiency in humans was first reported in 1972, and its essentiality in humans is well established. Symptoms of deficiency are weight loss, transient dermatitis, and occasionally nausea and vomiting, a change in hair color, and slow hair growth. Manganese deficiency in animals also affects reproductive capacity, pancreatic function, and several aspects of carbohydrate metabolism.

Absorption, Transport, Storage, and Excretion

Manganese is absorbed throughout the small intestine. Iron and cobalt compete for common binding sites for absorption. Men absorb less manganese than women, a difference that may be related to iron status, according to a study by Finley et al. (1994). In this study, manganese absorption was significantly associated with plasma ferritin.

Heme iron has no influence on manganese status, but diets high in nonheme iron were associated with lower serum manganese values, higher urinary manganese losses, and somewhat lower activity of a manganese-dependent enzyme called superoxide dismutase. Manganese is transported bound to a macroglobin, transferrin, and transmanganin. Excretion of manganese occurs mainly in the feces after secretion into the intestine via the bile.

Functions

The 10 to 20 mg of manganese contained in the adult human body tends to be concentrated predominantly in tissues rich in mitochondria. Manganese is a component of many enzymes, including glutamine synthetase, pyruvate carboxylase, and mitochondrial superoxide dismutase. In addition, manganese activates many other enzymes, most of which can also be activated by magnesium. Manganese is associated with the formation of connective and skeletal tissues, growth and reproduction, and carbohydrate and lipid metabolism (see Table 3-36).

Dietary Reference Intakes

The AIs for manganese are 2.3 mg/day for men and 1.8 mg/day for women. For children 9 years of age and older the AIs are 1.9 to 2.2 mg/day for boys and 1.6 mg/day for girls. For children the AIs are 1.2 to 1.5 mg/day, depending on their age.

TABLE 3-34

Selenium Content of Selected Foods

Food	Content (mcg)
Brazil nuts, 1 oz	543
Fast food fish sandwich, 1	89
Halibut, baked, ½ fillet	74
Tuna , canned, 3oz	68
Oysters, raw, 3 oz	56
Rice, white, long grain, 1 cup	44
Chicken, breast, baked, 3 oz	39
Pie crust, 1	38
Egg noodles, cooked, 1 cup	38
Lobster, 3 oz	36
Wheat germ, toasted, ¼ cup	28
Bagel, 1, 4-inch	27
Sunflower seeds, ¼ cup	25
Egg, 1	16
Bread, whole wheat, 1 slice	10
Asparagus, cooked, 1 cup	7
Milk, 2% fat, 1 cup	6

DRIs

Infants	15-20 mcg/day, depending on age
Young children	20-30 mcg/day, depending on age
Older children and adolescents	40-55 mcg/day, depending on age
Adults	55 mcg/day
Pregnant	60 mcg/day
Lactating	70 mcg/day

From U.S. Department of Agriculture, Agricultural Research Service: Nutrient Database for Standard Reference, Release 18, retrieved 2005, Data Laboratory home page: http://www.nal.usda.gov/fnic/foodcomp/Data/SR18/sr18.html.

Food Sources and Intakes

The manganese content of foods varies greatly. The richest sources are whole grains, legumes, nuts, and tea. Fruits and vegetables are moderately good sources. Animal tissues, seafood, and dairy products are poor sources. Relatively high amounts exist in instant coffee and tea. Human milk is relatively low in manganese. The Total Diet Study of the FDA (1982 to 1991) revealed that the median manganese intakes approximated the recommended intake for men and women but were too low for adolescent girls (Pennington and Schoen, 1996).

Deficiency

Even though the Total Diet Study of the FDA reported that manganese intakes were below recommended levels for adolescent girls (Pennington and Schoen, 1996), no physiologic evidence of insufficiency has been reported. Data on the physiologic effects resulting from manganese deficiency are confined to the results of animal studies. These studies have established the essentiality of manganese for reproduction. Sterility develops in both sexes; striking skeletal abnormalities and ataxia characterize the offspring of mothers who are manganese deficient.

Toxicity

Manganese toxicity has developed in miners as a result of absorption of manganese through the respiratory tract. The excess, which accumulates in the liver and central nervous system, produces Parkinson-like symptoms. Toxicity has also been reported in patients receiving TPN including manganese. Symptoms include headaches, dizziness, and abnormal magnetic resonance imaging (MRI) results and hepatic dysfunction (Masumoto et al., 2001). ULs of manganese have been difficult to establish (Greger and Malecki, 1997).

Chromium

A biologic role for chromium was first proposed in 1954. However, chromium was not accepted as an essential nutrient until 1977, when patients receiving TPN exhibited abnormalities of glucose metabolism that were reversed with chromium supplementation. The low concentrations of chromium in food, body tissues, and body fluids have required careful and appropriate analytic techniques and new standard reference materials for accurate measurements.

Absorption, Transport, Storage, and Excretion

As with other minerals, organic and inorganic forms of chromium are absorbed differently. Organic chromium is readily absorbed but quickly passes out of the body. Less than 2% of the trivalent chromium consumed is absorbed. Chromium absorption is increased by oxalate and is higher in iron-deficient animals than in animals with adequate iron, suggesting it shares some similarities with the iron absorption pathway. With dietary intakes of 40 mcg or more per day, chromium absorption reaches and remains at a plateau; at such high intakes, urinary excretion increases to maintain balance. The type of dietary carbohydrate consumed modifies absorption from chromium chloride; starch, rather than sugar, increases absorption. The absorption of chromium ions from chromium picolinate is greater than that from chromium chloride, the absorption efficiency of which is 2% or less.

Chromium and iron are carried by transferrin; however, albumin is also capable of assuming this role if iron transferrin saturation is high. In addition, α- and β-globulins and lipoproteins can also bind chromium.

Primarily the kidney excretes inorganic chromium, with small amounts being excreted through hair, sweat, and bile. Organic chromium is excreted through bile. Strenuous exercise, physical trauma, or an increased intake of simple sugar results in increased chromium excretion.

Functions

Chromium potentiates insulin action and as such influences carbohydrate, lipid, and protein metabolism. Although the chemical nature of the relationship between chromium and insulin activity has not been clearly identified, chromium may have a beneficial effect on serum triglyceride levels in patients with noninsulin-dependent diabetes mellitus (Lee and Reasner, 1994).

The proposed role of chromium with a so-called **glucose tolerance factor (GTF)** is controversial. A possible chromium-nicotinic acid (chromium polynicotinate) complex has been identified, but its structure has not been established by modern chemical techniques. Chromium may regulate the synthesis of a molecule that potentiates insulin action. Another possible role for chromium, similar to that of zinc, is in the regulation of gene expression (see Table 3-36).

Dietary Reference Intakes

The AIs recommended for chromium range from 25 to 35 mcg/day for males 9 years of age and older and 21 to 25 mcg/day for females of the same age. Depending on the age of the child, 11 to 15 mcg/day has been established for children 1 to 8 years of age (Trumbo et al., 2001).

Food Sources and Intakes

Precise assessment of chromium in foods is difficult; biologically available chromium and inorganic chromium cannot be distinguished from each other. Analyses done before 1980 must be considered with caution because determinations were flawed by contamination and analytic problems.

Brewer's yeast, oysters, liver, and potatoes have high chromium concentrations; seafood, whole grains, cheeses, chicken, meats, and bran have medium chromium concentrations. The refining of wheat removes chromium with the wheat germ and the bran; refining sugar fractionates the chromium into the molasses portion. Dairy products, fruits, and vegetables are low in chromium. Table 3-35 and Appendix 52 present the chromium content of selected foods.

Usual chromium intakes range between 25 and 35 mcg/day for women and men, respectively. Chromium intakes are not assessed in the USDA, NHANES, or Total Diet Study surveys because of inadequate methodology. Human breast milk contains 3 to 8 nmol/L of chromium, which is lower than the recommended intake for infants.

TABLE 3-35

Chromium Content of Selected Foods

Food	Content (mcg)
Broccoli, 1 cup	22.0
Turkey, leg, 3 oz	10.4
Juice, grape, 1 cup	7.5
Waffle, egg, 1	6.7
Ham, 3 oz	3.6
English muffin, 1	3.6
Cookies, chocolate chip, 1 large	3.4
Potatoes, mashed, 1 cup	2.7
Bagel, egg, 1	2.5
Juice, orange, 1 cup	2.2
Green beans, 1 cup	2.2
Beef cubes, 3 oz	2.0
Lettuce, 1 wedge	1.8
Barbecue sauce, 1 tbsp	1.7
Ketchup, 1 tbsp	1.0
American cheese, 1 oz	0.56
Maple syrup, 1 tbsp	0.5

DRIs = AIs	
Infants	.2 • -5.5 mcg/day, depending on age
Young children	11-15 mcg/day, depending on age
Older children and adolescents	21-35 mcg/day, depending on age and gender
Adults	20-35 mcg/day, depending on age and gender
Pregnant	29-30 mcg/day, depending on age
Lactating	44-45 mg/day, depending on age

From Anderson RA, Bryden NA, Polansky MM: Dietary chromium intake, *Biol Trace Elem Res* 32:117, 1992.

Deficiency

Chromium deficiency results in insulin resistance and a few lipid abnormalities, which can be ameliorated by chromium supplementation. Insufficient chromium may be consumed by some Americans, but true deficiency is more likely to be significant in populations with very low chromium intakes. Some epidemiologic studies suggest low tissue levels of chromium in patients with diabetes. However, they recommended long-term clinical trials to assess safety of chronic chromium supplementation before it is used in these patients.

Recent claims that the ingestion of high doses of chromium (as chromium picolinate) improves strength, body composition, endurance, or other characteristics of physical fitness are controversial, with some studies supporting these claims and others not. Lukaski et al. (1996) found that chromium supplements did not improve body composition or

strength in healthy men. However, both acute and chronic resistive exercise did increase urinary chromium losses in men who consumed the American Heart Association Phase I diet (with no supplements) (Rubin et al., 1998). The investigators concluded that these losses indicated increased absorption of chromium during the 16-week study. A period of 12 weeks of chromium picolinate supplementation was not shown to have any effects on plasma glucose concentrations, glucose-regulating hormones, or any other measure in moderately obese women who had completed an exercise program (Volpe et al., 2001).

Toxicity

Chromium toxicity from food has not been reported, but chromium picolinate taken as a supplement in high doses by athletes and power lifters has resulted in some adverse effects, primarily skin lesions.

Molybdenum

Molybdenum has been established as an essential micronutrient, particularly because of its requirement in the enzyme xanthine oxidase (see Table 3-36). Interrelationships among molybdenum, copper, and sulfate absorption in livestock and between molybdenum intake and copper excretion in humans and animals have been demonstrated. Individuals receiving long-term TPN have displayed symptoms of molybdenum deficiency, including mental changes and abnormalities of sulfur and purine metabolism.

Absorption, Transport, Storage, and Excretion

Molybdenum, which is found in minute amounts in the body, is readily absorbed from the stomach and small intestine, with the rate of absorption being higher in the proximal small intestine than in the distal small intestine. As with other minerals, molybdenum is absorbed by two mechanisms: carrier-mediated and passive diffusion. Molybdenum is excreted primarily in the urine. Excretion rather than absorption is the homeostatic mechanism. Some molybdenum is also excreted in the bile.

Functions

Xanthine oxidase, aldehyde oxidase, and sulfite oxidase, all enzymes that catalyze oxidation-reduction reactions, require a prosthetic group containing molybdenum. Sulfite oxidase is important to the degradation of cysteine and methionine and catalyzes the formation of sulfate from sulfite. Genetic sulfite oxidase deficiency is a fatal disorder of cysteine metabolism. Clinical symptoms include severe brain damage with mental retardation, dislocation of the lens, and increased urinary output of sulfate. Whether molybdenum is involved in the response of some asthmatics to sulfites is not known (see Table 3-36).

Dietary Reference Intakes

The RDAs for molybdenum throughout the life cycle range from 43 to 45 mcg/day for adolescent and adult males and females. Depending on age, RDAs range from 17 to 34 mcg/day for children.

Food Sources and Intakes

Molybdenum is distributed widely in commonly consumed foods such as legumes, whole grain cereals, milk and milk products, and dark green leafy vegetables. Estimated intakes, as determined by the Total Diet Study of the FDA, ranged from 50 mcg/day in infants to 80 and 126 mcg/day for 14- to 16-year-old girls and boys, respectively. These intakes were found to decrease slowly over the lifetime.

Deficiency

Molybdenum deficiency has not been established in humans other than patients treated with TPN. Symptoms of molybdenum deficiency include mental changes and abnormalities of sulfur and purine metabolism.

Toxicity

An excessive molybdenum intake of 10 to 15 mg/day is associated with a goutlike syndrome (Nielsen, 2001). However, no good biomarkers are available to accurately assess the presence of molybdenum excess. However, plasma molybdenum does seem to reflect molybdenum intake (Turnlund and Keyes, 2004).

Boron

The essentiality of boron for humans has not yet been established, but its essentiality for plants and animals is widely accepted. Boron, an ultratrace element, is obtained from foods such as sodium borate, and it is rapidly and almost completely (90%) absorbed. The highest concentrations of boron are found in bone, spleen, and thyroid, although it is present in all other tissues of the body. Boron influences the activity of many metabolic enzymes and the metabolism of such nutrients as calcium, magnesium, and vitamin D (Devirian and Volpe, 2003). However, the roles of boron in humans have not been well studied, and symptoms of severe boron deficiency have not been established (Nielsen, 2001). Additional studies of this ultratrace element, especially its relationship to bone metabolism, are being conducted.

Functions

Boron is associated with cell membranes and in plants is involved with the functional efficiency of cell membranes. Response to boron deprivation is enhanced when other nutrients that alter membrane functions are also deficient. Boron apparently binds to the active site of some enzymes, reducing their ability to function. Boron is also thought to compete with some enzymes for the coenzyme NAD.

Evidence from animal studies shows that boron deprivation affects two major organs: the brain and bone. Boron deficiency alters brain composition and function and reduces bone composition, structure, and strength. Because of the role of boron in bone, studies in humans have focused on its potential role in the development of osteoporosis. Some evidence suggests that boron may have actions similar to estrogens on bone (Nielsen, 2001) (see Chapter 24).

Dietary Reference Intakes

No DRIs have been established for boron.

Food Sources and Intakes

Foods that are good sources of boron include plant foods, especially noncitrus fruits, vegetables, nuts, and legumes. Wine, cider, and beer are other good sources of boron.

Deficiency and Toxicity

Boron deficiency has not been reported in humans, and no toxicity level has been established.

Cobalt

Most of the cobalt in the body exists with vitamin B_{12} stores in the liver, but one enzyme has an established specific requirement for cobalt. Blood plasma contains approximately 1 mcg of cobalt per 100 ml.

Absorption, Transport, Storage, and Excretion

Cobalt may share at least part of the same intestinal transport mechanism as iron. Absorption is higher in patients with deficient iron intake, portal cirrhosis with iron overload, and idiopathic hemochromatosis. The major route of cobalt excretion is the urine; small amounts are excreted via feces, sweat, and hair.

Functions

The well-known essential role of cobalt is as a component of vitamin B_{12} (cobalamin). This vitamin is essential for the maturation of red blood cells and the normal function of all cells (see previous section on vitamin B_{12} and Chapter 31). In addition, methionine aminopeptidase, an enzyme involved in the regulation of translation (i.e., of DNA to RNA), is the only enzyme in humans known to have an established requirement of this trace element (see Table 3-36).

Dietary Reference Intakes

The dietary requirement for cobalt is expressed in terms of vitamin B_{12}. Approximately 2 to 3 mcg of vitamin B_{12} is needed daily.

Food Sources and Intakes

Cobalt exists in foods; however, only microorganisms are able to synthesize vitamin B_{12}. Ruminant animals obtain cobalamin as the result of a symbiotic relationship with the microorganisms of their GI tract. The microorganisms of monogastric species such as humans have an extremely limited capacity for synthesis in areas where the vitamin can be absorbed; therefore humans must obtain vitamin B_{12}—and thus cobalt—from animal foods such as organ and muscle meats. In some circumstances ordinary bacterial contamination of foods of vegetable origin may supply the minute amounts of this vitamin required for normal function

Strict vegetarians who avoid all animal products may develop vitamin B_{12} deficiency. However, the deficiency may develop only after 3 to 6 years or not at all.

Deficiency

A cobalt deficiency develops only in relation to a vitamin B_{12} deficiency. Insufficient vitamin B_{12} causes a macrocytic anemia. A genetic defect limiting vitamin B_{12} absorption results in pernicious anemia, which is treated appropriately with massive doses of the vitamin. These forms of anemia are discussed in detail in Chapter 31.

Toxicity

A high intake of inorganic cobalt (existing freely from cobalamin) in animal diets produces polycythemia (an overproduction of red blood cells), hyperplasia of bone marrow, reticulocytosis, and increased blood volume.

The information on the microminerals (trace elements) known to be required by humans is summarized in Table 3-36.

OTHER TRACE ELEMENTS

Several other trace elements of uncertain essentiality exist, including aluminum, lithium, nickel, silicon, tin, and vanadium. A few other ultratrace elements, including arsenic, may be added to this list in the future. They are classified as ultratrace elements because of their very low quantities in human tissues. Requirements remain undefined for all of these elements because of their uncertain essentiality. The ultratrace elements continue to be enigmas because of their uncertain roles in human function. It has long been established that these elements exist in human tissues, especially in the skeleton, because of their abundance on the earth's surface, but the essentiality of any of these in humans remains questionable. These ultratrace elements have been reviewed by Nielsen (2001).

TABLE 3-36

Minerals in Human Nutrition

	Body Location and Selected Biologic Functions	DRIs	Food Sources	Likelihood of Deficiency
Macronutrients Essential at Daily Levels of 100 mg or More				
Calcium	99% is found in bones and teeth. Ionic calcium in body fluids is essential for ion transport across cell membranes. Calcium may also be bound to protein, citrate, or inorganic acids.	1000 mg for adults 19-50 yr; 1200 mg for adults 51+ yr (AI)	Milk and milk products, sardines, clams, oysters, kale, turnip greens, mustard greens, tofu	Dietary surveys indicate that many people do not meet AIs for calcium. Because bone serves as a homeostatic mechanism to maintain calcium levels in the blood, many essential functions are maintained, regardless of dietary intake. Long-term dietary deficiency is probably one of the factors responsible for development of osteroporosis later in life.

From The Food and Nutrition Board, National Academy of Sciences, Institute of Medicine: *Dietary reference intakes for vitamin A, vitamin K, arsenic, boron, chromium, copper, iodine, iron, manganese, molybdenum, nickel, silicon, vanadium, and zinc*, Washington, DC, 2001, National Academies Press; and the Food and Nutrition Board, National Academy of Sciences, Institute of Medicine: *Dietary reference intakes for vitamin C, vitamin E, selenium, and carotenoids*, Washington, DC, 2000, National Academy Press.

DRI, Dietary reference intake; *RDA*, recommended dietary allowance; *AI*, adequate intake.

Continued

TABLE 3-36

Minerals in Human Nutrition—cont'd

	Body Location and Selected Biologic Functions	DRIs	Food Sources	Likelihood of Deficiency
Macronutrients Essential at Daily Levels of 100 mg or More—cont'd				
Phosphorus	About 80% is found in inorganic portion of bones and teeth. Phosphorus is a component of every cell, as well as of important metabolites, including DNA, RNA, ATP, and phospholipids. Phosphorus I is also important for pH regulation.	700 mg for adults (RDA)	Cheese, egg yolk, milk, meat, fish, poultry, whole-grain cereals, and almost all other foods	Dietary inadequacy is not likely if protein and calcium intake are adequate.
Micronutrients Essential at Daily Levels of a Few Milligrams or Less				
Magnesium	About 50% is in bone; the remaining 50% is almost entirely inside body cells, with only about 1% located in extracellular fluid.	400-420 mg for men, 310-320 mg for women 14-70+ yr (RDA)	Whole-grain cereals, tofu nuts, meat, milk, green vegetables, legumes, chocolate	Dietary inadequacy is considered unlikely, but conditioned deficiency often develops and is usually associated with surgery, alcoholism, malabsorption, loss of body fluids, and certain hormonal and renal diseases.
Sulfur	Bulk of dietary sulfur is present in sulfur-containing amino acids needed for synthesis of essential metabolites. Sulfur functions in oxidation-reduction reactions, as part of thiamin and biotin.	No DRI; the need for sulfur is satisfied by essential sulfur-containing amino acids.	Protein foods such as meat, fish, poultry, eggs, milk, cheese, legumes, nuts	Dietary intake is chiefly from sulfur-containing amino acids, and adequacy is related to protein intake.
Iron	About 70% is found in hemoglobin; about 25% is stored in liver, spleen, and bone. Iron is a component of hemoglobin and myoglobin and is important in oxygen transfer. It is also present in serum transferring and certain enzymes. Almost none exists in ionic form.	8 mg for men, 18 mg for women (after menopause, 8 mg) (RDA)	Liver, meat, egg yolk, legumes, whole or enriched grains, dark green vegetables, dark molasses, shrimp, oysters	Iron deficiency anemia occurs in women of reproductive age and infants and preschool children. Deficiency may be associated with unusual blood loss, parasites, or malabsorption. Anemia is the last state of deficiency.

TABLE 3-36

Minerals in Human Nutrition—cont'd

	Body Location and Selected Biologic Functions	DRIs	Food Sources	Likelihood of Deficiency
Micronutrients Essential at Daily Levels of a Few Milligrams or Less—cont'd				
Zinc	Zinc is present in most tissues, with greatest amounts in the liver, voluntary muscle, and bone. A constituent of many enzymes and of insulin, zinc is important for nucleic acid metabolism.	11 mg for men, 8 mg for women (RDA)	Oysters, shellfish, herring, liver, legumes, milk, wheat bran	The extent of dietary zinc inadequacy in the United States is not known. Conditioned deficiency may develop with systemic childhood illnesses and in patients who are nutritionally depleted or have been subjected to severe stress such as surgery.
Copper	Copper is found in all body tissues, with the bulk in the liver, brain, heart, and kidney. Copper is a constituent of enzymes and ceruloplasmin and erythrocuprein in blood. It may be an integral part of DNA or RNA.	900 mcg for men and women (RDA)	Liver, shellfish, whole grains, cherries, legumes, kidney, poultry, oysters, chocolate, nuts	No evidence shows that specific deficiencies of copper occur in humans. Menkes' disease is a genetic disorder resulting in copper deficiency.
Iodine	Iodine is a constituent of T_4 and related compounds synthesized by the thyroid gland. T_4 functions in the control of reactions involving cellular energy.	150 mcg for men and women (RDA)	Iodized table salt, seafood, water and vegetables in regions without goiter	Iodization of table salt is recommended, especially in areas where food is low in iodine.
Manganese	The highest concentration of manganese is in bone; relatively high concentrations also exist in pituitary, liver, pancreas, and gastrointestinal tissue. Manganese is a constituent of essential enzyme systems and is rich in mitochondria of liver cells.	2.3 mg for men, 1.8 mg for women (AI)	Beet greens, blueberries, whole grains, nuts, legumes frit, tea	Deficiency is unlikely to occur in humans.
Fluoride	Fluoride exists in bones and teeth. In optimal amounts from water and diet, fluoride reduces dental caries and may minimize bone loss.	4 mg for men, 3 mg for women (AI)	Drinking water (1 ppm), tea, coffee, rice, soybeans, spinach, gelatin, onions, lettuce	In areas where the fluoride content of water is low, fluoridation of water (at 1 ppm) has reduced the incidence of dental caries.

Continued

TABLE 3-36

Minerals in Human Nutrition—cont'd

	Body Location and Selected Biologic Functions	DRIs	Food Sources	Likelihood of Deficiency
Micronutrients Essential at Daily Levels of a Few Milligrams or Less—cont'd				
Molybdenum	Molybdenum is a constituent of an essential enzyme (xanthine oxidase) and flavoproteins.	45 mcg for men and women (RDA)	Legumes, cereal, grains, dark green leafy vegetables, organ meats	No available information.
Cobalt	Cobalt is a constituent of cyanocobalamin (vitamin B_{12}), existing bound to protein in foods of animal origin. Cobalt is essential for the normal function of all cells, particularly cells of bone marrow and nervous and gastrointestinal systems.	2.4 mg vitamin B_{12}	Liver, kidney, oysters clams, poultry, milk	Primary dietary inadequacy is rare except in those who consume no animal products. Deficiency may be associated with lack of gastric intrinsic factor, gastrectomy, or malabsorption syndromes.
Selenium	Selenium is involved in fat metabolism, cooperates with vitamin E, and acts as an antioxidant.	55 mcg for men and women (RDA)	Grains, onions, meats, milk; varied amounts in vegetables depending on selenium content of soil	Keshan disease is a selenium-deficient state. Deficiency has occurred in patients receiving long-term TPN without selenium supplementation.
Chromium	Chromium is associated with glucose metabolism.	35 mcg for men, 25 mcg for women (AI)	Corn oil, clams, whole-grain cereals, brewer's yeast, meats, drinking water (amount varies)	Deficiency is found in those with severe malnutrition and may be a factor in diabetes in older adults and cardiovascular disease.

 FOCAL POINTS

The major nutrients with roles in the human body include energy-containing macronutrients (carbohydrates, lipids, protein and alcohol) as well as the micronutrients (vitamins and minerals.)

- The indigestible food component, fiber is essential for health, especially related to the gastrointestinal tract and cardiovascular system, but 80% of Americans do not get enough fiber.
- Alcohol contains calories for heat but not for muscular work, and it impacts health positively in moderation and negatively in excess.

- Changing concepts regarding the structure, function, and utilization of nutrients in the body are important to keep in mind as they determine the impact of nutrient deficiencies or excesses on health and disease management.
- Miscellaneous trace elements exist in human tissues, especially in the skeleton, because of their abundance on the earth's surface; their essentiality in humans is not totally clear.

Useful Websites

Institute of Medicine, Dietary Reference Intakes
http://www.iom.edu/CMS/3788/21370.aspx

Use of Dietary Reference Intakes
http://www.nap.edu/books/0309072794/html/554.html

American Society for Bone and Mineral Research
www.asbmr.org/

Dietary Reference Intakes for Energy, Carbohydrate, Fiber, Fat, Fatty Acids, Cholesterol, Protein, and Amino Acids (Macronutrients) (2005)
http://www.nap.edu/books/0309085373/html/R1.html

Food and Drug Administration
http://www.fda.gov/

National Dairy Council
www.nationaldairycouncil.org/

National Institutes of Health State of the Science Conference

Multivitamin/Mineral Supplements and Chronic Disease Prevention
www.consensus.nih.gov

National Institute of Medicine
http://www.iom.edu/

National Academy of Sciences: DRI Tables for Macronutrients
http://www.newtexts.com/newtexts/nutrition%20tables.pdf

Tufts University Nutrition Navigator
http://www.navigator.tufts.edu/

USDA Dietary Guidelines 2005
http://www.health.gov/dietaryguidelines/dga2005/document/

USDA Nutrient Database Laboratory (food composition tables)
http://www.nal.usda.gov/fnic/foodcomp/

References

Abcouwer SF, Souba WW: Glutamine and arginine. In Shils ME et al, editors: *Modern nutrition in health and disease*, ed 9, Baltimore, 1998, Williams & Wilkins.

Abrams SA: Calcium supplementation during childhood: long-term effects on bone mineralization, *Nutr Rev* 63:251, 2005.

Alaimo K et al: *Dietary intake of vitamins, minerals, and fiber of persons aged 2 and over in the United States: third health and nutrition examination survey, phase 1, 1988-1991, advance data from Vital and Health Statistics*, No. 258, Hyattsville, Md, 1994, National Center for Health Statistics.

Alberts B et al: Cell chemistry and biosynthesis (Chapter 2); Membrane structure (Chapter 11); Energy conversion, mitochondria and chloroplasts (Chapter 14). In *Molecular biology of the cell*, ed 4, New York, 2002, Garland Science; Taylor and Francis Group.

American Dietetic Association: Position of the American Dietetic Association: vegetarian diets, *J Am Diet Assoc* 97:1317, 1997.

American Dietetic Association: Position of the American Dietetic Association: fat replacers, *J Am Diet Assoc* 105:266, 2005.

Anderson JJB et al: Nutrition and bone in physical activity and sport. In Wolinsky I, editor: *Nutrition in exercise and sport*, p 219, ed 3, Boca Raton, Fla, 1998, CRC Press.

Andres E et al: Vitamin B_{12} (cobalamin) deficiency in elderly patients, *Can Med Assoc J* 171:251, 2004.

Atkins J, Clandinin MT: Nutritional significance of factors affecting carnitine-dependent transport of fatty acids in neonates: a review, *Nutr Res* 10:117, 1990.

Bahl R et al: Plasma zinc as a predictor of diarrheal and respiratory morbidity in children in an urban slum setting, *Am J Clin Nutr* 68:414, 1998.

Beard JL: Iron biology in immune function, muscle metabolism, and neuronal functioning, *J Nutr* 131:568, 2001.

Beck M et al: Rapid genomic evolution of a non-virulent coxsackievirus B_3—in selenium-deficient mice results in selection of identical virulent isolates, *Nature Med* 1:433, 1995.

Beckett GJ, Arthur JR: Selenium and endocrine systems, *J Endocrinol* 184:455, 2005.

Belongia EA et al: A randomized trial of zinc spray for treatment of upper respiratory illness in adults, *Am J Med* 111:103, 2001.

Berner LA et al: Fortification contributed greatly to vitamin and mineral intakes in the United States, 1989-1991, *J Nutr* 131:2177-2183, 2001.

Block RJ, Mitchel HH: The correlation of the amino acid composition of proteins with their nutritive value, *Nutr Abstr Rev* 16:249, 1946.

Bonakdar RA, Guarneri E: Coenzyme Q_{10}. *Am Fam Physician* 72:1065, 2005.

Bonham, M et al: The immune system as a physiological indicator of marginal copper status? *Br J Nutr* 87(5):393, 2002.

Brand-Miller JC et al: Glycemic index and obesity, *Am J Clin Nutr* 76:281S-285S, 2002.

Brigelius-Flohe R: Induction of drug metabolizing enzymes by vitamin E, *J Plant Physiol* 162:797, 2005.

Brown AJ et al: Differential effects of 19-nor-1,25-dihydroxyvitamin D(2) and 1,25-dihydroxyvitamin D(3) on intestinal calcium and phosphate transport, *J Lab Clin Med* 139:279, 2002.

Buchman AL et al: Copper deficiency secondary to a copper transport defect: a new copper metabolic disturbance, *Metabolism* 12:1462, 1994.

Burk RF et al: Plasma selenium in specific and non-specific forms, *Biofactors* 14:107, 2001.

Calvo MS et al: Vitamin D fortification in the United States and Canada: current stats and data needs, *Am J Clin Nutr* 80 (6 Suppl):1710S, 2004.

Can C et al: Vascular endothelial dysfunction associated with elevated serum homocysteine levels in rat adjuvant arthritis: effect of vitamin E administration, *Life Sci* 71:401, 2002.

Canty DJ, Zeisel SJ: Lecithin and choline in human health and disease, Nutr Rev 52:327, 1994.

Chisolm GM III, Penn MS: Oxidized lipoproteins and atherosclerosis. In Fuster V et al, editors: *Atherosclerosis and coronary artery disease*, Philadelphia, 1996, Lippincott-Raven.

Ciliberto H et al: Antioxidant supplementation for the prevention of kwashiorkor in Malawian children: randomized, double blind, placebo-controlled trial, *Br Med J* 330:1109, 2005.

Clark LC et al: Effects of selenium supplementation for cancer prevention in patients with carcinoma of the skin: a randomized controlled trial, *JAMA* 276:1957, 1996.

Compher C et al: Dietary fiber and its clinical applications to enteral nutrition. In Rombeau JL, Rolandelli RH, editors: *Enteral and tube feeding*, ed 3, Philadelphia, 1997, Saunders.

Connor WE et al: Essential fatty acids: the importance of n-3 fatty acids in the retina and brain, *Nutr Rev* 50:21, 1992.

Cook JD, Reddy MB: Effect of ascorbic acid intake on non-heme-iron absorption from a complete diet, *Am J Clin Nutr* 73:93, 2001.

Corder R et al: Oenology: red wine procyanidins and vascular health. *Nature* 444:566, 2006.

Cordano A: Clinical manifestations of nutritional copper deficiency in infants and children, *Am J Clin Nutr* 67(suppl):1012, 1998.

Coursin DB: Convulsive seizures in infants with pyridoxine deficient diet. *JAMA* 154:406, 1954.

Crawford MA: The role of dietary fatty acids in biology: their place in the evolution of the human brain, *Nutr Rev* 50:3, 1992.

Crim MC, Munro HN: Proteins and amino acids. In Shils ME et al, editors: *Modern nutrition in health and disease*, Philadelphia, 1994, Lea & Febiger.

Cummings JH et al: Prebiotic digestion and fermentation, *Am J Clin Nutr* 73:415S, 2001.

Cunnane SC: Problem with essential fatty acids: time for a new paradigm? *Prog Lipid Res* 42:544, 2003.

Dakshinamurti K: Biotin–a regulator of gene expression, *J Nutr Biochem* 16:419, 2005.

Davidsson L et al: Improving iron absorption from a Peruvian school breakfast meal by adding ascorbic acid or Na$_2$EDTA, *Am J Clin Nutr* 73:283, 2001.

Delmas PD: Treatment of postmenopausal osteoporosis, *Lancet* 359:2018, 2002.

Dengel JL et al: Magnesium homeostasis: conversion mechanism in lactating women consuming a controlled-magnesium diet, *Am J Clin Nutr* 59:990, 1994.

Denisova NA, Booth SL: Vitamin K and sphingolipid metabolism: evidence to date, *Nutr Rev* 63:111, 2005.

Deuchi K et al: Continuous and massive intake of chitosan affects mineral and fat-soluble vitamin status in rats fed on a high-fat diet, *Biosci Biotechnol Biochem* 59:1211, 1995.

Devine A et al: Effects of zinc and other nutritional factors on insulin-like growth factor I and insulin-like growth factor binding proteins in postmenopausal women, *Am J Clin Nutr* 68:200, 1998.

Devirian TA, Volpe SL: The physiological effects of dietary boron, *Crit Rev Food Sci Nut* 43:219, 2003.

Duthie SJ et al: Folate, DNA stability, and colo-rectal neoplasia, *Proc Nutr Soc* 63:571, 2004.

Elder SJ et al: Vitamin K contents of meat, dairy, and fast foods in the U.S. Diet, *J Agric Food Chem* 54:463, 2006.

Fairfield KM, Fletcher RH: Vitamins for chronic disease prevention in adults: scientific review, *JAMA* 287: 3116, 2002.

Farrell DJ: Enrichment of hen eggs with *n*-3 long-chain fatty acids and evaluation of enriched eggs in humans, *Am J Clin Nutr* 68:538, 1998.

Ferland G: The vitamin K–dependent proteins: an update, *Nutr Rev* 56:223, 1998.

Feskanick et al: Vitamin A intake and hip fracture among postmenopausal women, *JAMA* 287:47, 2002.

Finley JW et al: Sex affects manganese absorption and retention by humans from a diet adequate in manganese, *Am J Clin Nutr* 60:949, 1994.

Fisher Walker et al: Interactive effects of iron and zinc on biochemical and function outcome in supplementation trials, *Am J Clin Nutr* 82:5, 2005.

Fleming DJ et al: Iron status of the free-living, elderly Framingham Heart Study cohort: an iron-replete population with a high prevalence of elevated iron stores, *Am J Clin Nutr* 73:638, 2001.

Ford ES et al: Prevalence of the metabolic syndrome among US adults: findings from the Third National Health and Nutrition Examination Survey, *JAMA* 287:356, 2002.

Frazer DM, Anderson GJ: Iron Imports. I. Intestinal iron absorption and its regulation, *Am J Physiol Gastrointest Liver Physiol* 289:G631, 2005.

Goldberger J et al: A study of the diet of nonpellagrous and pellagrous households, *JAMA* 71:944, 1918.

Grant WB, Holick MF: Benefits and requirement of vitamin D for optimal health: a review, *Altern Med Rev* 10:94, 2005.

Greger JL, Malecki EA: Manganese: how do we know our limits? *Nutr Today* 32:116, 1997.

Gregory, J III: Case study: folate bioavailability, *J Nutr* 131(suppl 4):1376, 2001.

Gropper SS et al: Advanced nutrition and human metabolism, ed 4, Stamford, Conn, 2005, Wadsworth, p 584.

Gross LS et al: Increased consumption of refined carbohydrates and the epidemic of type 2 diabetes in the United States: an ecologic assessment, *Am J Clin Nutr* 79(5):774, 2004.

Group (Age-Related Eye Disease Study Research): A randomized, placebo-controlled, clinical trial of high-dose supplementation with vitamins C and E, beta-carotene, and zinc for age-related macular degeneration and vision loss: AREDS report no. 8, *Arch Ophthalmol* 119(10):1417, 2001.

Guerrero-Romero F Rodriguez-Moran M: Complementary therapies for diabetes: the case of chromium, magnesium and antioxidants, *Arch Med Res* 36:250, 2005.

Guthrie JF, Morton JF: Food sources of added sweeteners in the diets of Americans, *J Am Diet Assoc* 100:43-51, 2000.

Haag M: Essential fatty acids and the brain, *Can J Psychiatry* 48:195, 2003.

Haddad J: Vitamin D: solar rays, the Milky Way, or both? *N Engl J Med* 326:1213, 1992.

Hathcock JN et al: Risk assessment for vitamin D, *Am J Clin Nutr*, 85:6, 2007.

He K et al: Magnesium intake and incidence of metabolic syndrome among young adults, *Circulation* 113:1675, 2006.

Hogan SL: The effects of weight loss on calcium and bone, *Crit Care Nurs Q* 28:269, 2005.

Holick M et al: The vitamin D content of fortified mik and infant formula, *N Engl J Med* 326:1178, 1992.

Holick MF: Resurrection of vitamin D deficiency and rickets, *J Clin Invest* 116:2062, 2006.

Holick MF: Sunlight and vitamin D for bone health and prevention of autommune diseases, cancers and cardiovascular disease, *Am J Clin Nutr*, 80(Suppl 6):1678S, 2004.

Hudgins LC: Effect of high-carbohydrate feeding on triglyceride and saturated fatty acid synthesis. *Proc Soc Exp Biol Med* 225:178, 2000.

Hunt JR, Vanderpool RA: Apparent copper absorption from a vegetarian diet, *Am J Clin Nutr* 74:803, 2001.

Institute of Medicine, Food and Nutrition Board: *Dietary reference intakes for calcium, phosphorus, magnesium, vitamin D, and fluoride*, Washington, DC, 1997, National Academies Press.

Institute of Medicine, Food and Nutrition Board: *Dietary reference intakes for vitamin A, vitamin K, arsenic, boron, chromium, copper, iodine, iron, manganese, molybdenum, nickel, silicon, vanadium, and zinc*, Washington, DC, 2001, National Academies Press.

Institute of Medicine, Food and Nutrition Board: *Dietary reference intakes for vitamin C, vitamin E, selenium, and carotenoids*, Washington, DC, 2000a, National Academies Press.

Institute of Medicine, Food and Nutrition Board: *Dietary reference intakes for thiamin, riboflavin, niacin, vitamin B6, folate, vitamin B12, pantothenic acid, biotin, and choline*, Washington, DC, 2000b, National Academies Press.

Institute of Medicine, Food and Nutrition Board: *Dietary reference intakes for energy, carbohydrates, fiber, fat, protein and amino acids (macronutrients)*, Washington, DC, 2002, National Academies Press.

Jacobus C et al: Hypervitaminosis D associated with drinking milk, *N Engl J Med* 326:1173, 1992.

Jacques PF et al: Long-term nutrient intake and 5-year change in nuclear lens opacities, *Arch Opthalmol* 123:517, 2005.

Johnson MA et al: Iron nutriture in elderly individuals, *Fed Am Soc Exp Biol J* 8:609, 1994.

Jones K et al: Coenzyme Q10: efficacy, safety, and use, *Int J Integrative Med* 4:28, 2002.

Kantor LS: *A dietary assessment of the U.S. food supply: comparing per capita food consumption with Food Guide Pyramid serving recommendations*, Food and Rural Economics Division, Economics Research Service, U.S. Department of Agriculture Agricultural Economic Report No 772, 1998.

Kibir M et al: A high glycemic index starch diet affects lipid storage–related enzymes in normal, and to a lesser extent in diabetic rats, *J Nutr* 128:1878, 1998.

Kim H: A review of the possible relevance of inositol and the phosphatidylinositol second messenger system (PI-cycle) to psychiatric disorder—focus on magnetic resonance spectroscopy (MRS) studies, *Hum Psychopharmacol* 20:309, 2005.

Kirkland JB: Niacin and carcinogenesis, *Nutr Cancer* 46:110, 2003.

Klompmaker TR: Lifetime high calcium intake increases osterporotic fracture risk in old age, *Med Hypotheses* 65:552, 2005.

Kovacs CS: Calcium and bone metabolism during pregnancy and lactation, *J Mammary Gland Biol Neoplasia* 10:105, 2005.

Kris-Etherton PM et al: Polyunsaturated fatty acids in the food chain in the United States, *Am J Clin Nutr* 71:179, 2000.

Kruizenga HM et al: Effectiveness and cost-effectiveness of early screening and treatment of malnourished patients, *Am J Clin Nutr* 82:1082, 2005.

Kuhajek EJ: Letter to the editor: iodized salt, *Nutr Rev* 58:250, 2000.

Kusic Z, Jukic T: History of endemic goiter in Croatia: from severe iodine deficiency to iodine sufficiency, *Coll Antropol* 29:9, 2005.

Latavayova L et al: Selenium: From cancer prevention to DNA Damage, *Toxicology* 227(1-2):1-14, 2006.

Lee K et al: Too much versus too little: the implications of current iodine intake in the United States, *Nutr Rev* 57:177, 1999.

Lee N, Reasner C: Beneficial effect of chromium supplementation on serum triglyceride levels in NIDDM, *Diabetes Care* 17:1449, 1994.

Leenhardt F et al: Moderate decrease of pH by sourdough fermentation is sufficient to reduce phytate content of whole wheat flour through endogenous phytase activity, *J Agric Food Chem* 53:98, 2005.

Lehman-McKeeman LD et al: Diethanolamine induces hepatic choline deficiency in mice, *Toxicol Sci* 67:38, 2002.

Levander GA et al: Vitamin E and selenium, *Proc Nutr Soc* 54:475, 1995.

Lopez HW et al: New data on the bioavailability of bread magnesium, *Magnes Res* 17:335, 2004.

Ludwig DS: The glycemic index: physiological mechanisms relating to obesity, diabetes and cardiovascular disease, *JAMA* 287:2414-2423, 2002.

Lukaski HC et al: Chromium supplementation and resistance training: effects on body composition, strength, and trace element status of men, *Am J Clin Nutr* 63:954, 1996.

Lykkesfeldt J et al: Ascorbate is depleted by smoking and repleted by moderate supplementation: a study in male smokers and nonsmokers with matched dietary antioxidant intakes, *Am J Clin Nutr* 71:530, 2000.

Lynch RJ, Cate JM: The anti-caries efficacy of calcium carbonate-based fluoride toothpastes, *Int Dent J* 55:175, 2005.

Macknin ML et al: Zinc gluconate lozenges for treating the common cold in children, *JAMA* 279:1962, 1998.

Malik S, Kashyap ML: Niacin, lipids, and heart disease, *Curr Cardiol Rep* 5:470, 2003.

Malmberg KJ et al: A short-term dietary supplementation of high doses of vitamin E increases T helper 1 cytokine production in patients with advanced colorectal cancer, *Clin Cancer Res* 8:1772, 2002.

Manach C et al: Bioavailability, metabolism and physiological impact of 4-oxo-flavonoids, *Nutr Res* 16:517, 1996.

Masumoto K et al: Manganese intoxication during intermittent parenteral nutrition: report of two cases, *J Parenter Enter Nutr* 25:95, 2001.

McCowen KC Bistrian BR: Essential fatty acids and their derivatives, *Curr Opin Gastroenterol* 21: 207, 2005.

McNulty H, Pentieva K: Folate bioavailablity, *Proc Nutr Soc* 63:529, 2004.

Meck WH, Williams CL: Metabolic imprinting of choline by its availability during gestation: implications for memory and attentional processing across the lifespan, *Neurosci Biobehav Rev* 27:385, 2003.

Messina M: Modern applications for an ancient bean: soybeans and the prevention and treatment of chronic disease, *J Nutr* 125:567S, 1995.

Meydani SN et al: Vitamin E supplementation and in vivo immune response in healthy elderly subjects: a randomized controlled trial, *JAMA* 277:1380, 1997.

Mingrone G: Carnitine in type 2 diabetes, *Ann NY Acad Sci* 1033:99, 2004.

Morris MC et al: Dietary intake of antioxidant nutrients and the risk of incident Alzheimer disease in a biracial community of older persons, *J Gerontol a Bio Sci Med* 55:30, 2000.

Mussig K et al: Iodine-induced thyrotoxicosis after ingestion of kelp-containing tea, *J Gen Intern Med* 21:666, 2006.

Neve J: New approaches to assess selenium status and requirement, *Nutr Rev* 58:363, 2000.

Nielsen FH: Boron, manganese, molybdenum, and other trace elements. In Bowman BA, Russell RM, editors: *Present knowledge in nutrition*, ed 8, Washington, DC, 2001, ILSI Press.

Nieves JW: Osteoporosis: the role of micronutrients, *Am J Clin Nutr* 81:1232S, 2005.

Omdahl JL et al: Hydroxylase enzymes of the vitamin D pathway: expression, function, and regulation, *Annu Rev Nutr* 22:139, 2002.

Ormrod DJ et al: Dietary chitosan inhibits hypercholesterolemia and atherogenesis in the apolipoprotein E-deficient mouse model of atherosclerosis, *Atherosclerosis* 138:329, 1998.

Palmer C, Anderson JJB: Position of the American Dietetic Association: the impact of fluoride on health, *J Am Diet Assoc* 200:1208, 2000.

Pang Y et al: A longitudinal investigation of aggregate oral intake of copper, *J Nutr* 131:2171, 2001.

Parks EJ, Hellerstein MK: Carbohydrate-induced hypertriacylglycerolemia: historical perspective and review of biological mechanisms, *Am J Clin Nutr* 71:41, 2000.

Parks S, Johnson MA: Living in low-latitude regions in the United States does not prevent poor vitamin D status, *Nutr Rev* 63:203, 2005.

Pathak P, Kapil U: Role of trace elements zinc, copper and magnesium during pregnancy and it outcome, *Indian J Pediatr* 71:1003, 2004.

Patrick L: Selenium biochemistry and cancer: a review of the literature, *Altern Med Rev* 9:239, 2004.

Patterson AJ et al: Dietary treatment of iron deficiency in women of child-bearing age, *Am J Clin Nutr* 74: 650, 2001.

Pennington JAT, Schoen SA: Total diet study: estimated dietary intakes of nutritional elements, 1982-1991, *Int J Vitam Nutr Res* 66:350, 1996.

Penniston KL, Tanumihardjo SA: The acute and chronic toxic effect of vitamin A, *Am J Clin Nutr* 83: 191, 2006.

Peterlik, M Cross HS: Vitamin D and calcium deficits predispose for multiple chronic diseases, *Eur J Clin Invest* 35: 290, 2005.

Pettifor JM: Rickets and vitamin D deficiency in children and adolescents, *Endocrinol Metab Clin North Am* 34:537, 2005.

Powers HJ: Riboflavin (vitamin B₂) and health, *Am J Clin Nutr* 77:1352, 2003.

Prasad AS et al: Zinc metabolism in patients with the syndrome of iron deficiency anemia, hepatosplenomegaly, dwarfism and hypogonadism, *J Lab Clin Med* 61:537, 1963.

Price KD et al: Hyperglycemia-induced ascorbic acid deficiency promotes endothelial dysfunction and the development of atherosclerosis, *Atherosclerosis* 158:1, 2001.

Prentice A: Does mild zinc deficiency contribute to poor growth performance? *Nutr Rev* 51:268, 1993.

Rauma AL et al: Iodine status in vegans consuming a living food diet, *Nutr Res* 14:1789, 1994.

Reginster JY: The high prevalence of inadequate serum vitamin D levels and implication for bone health, *Curr Med Res Opin* 21:579, 2005.

Roberfroid MB: Introducing inulin-type fructans, *Br J Nutr* 93 Suppl 1:S13, 2005.

Robinson C et al: The effect of fluoride on the developing tooth, *Caries Res* 38:268, 2004.

Romieu I: Nutrition and lung health, *Int J Tuberc Lung Dis* 9:362, 2005.

Romieu I, Trenga G: Diet and obstructive lung diseases, *Epidemiol Rev* 23:268, 2001.

Rosenfeldt et al: Coenzyme Q₁₀ protects the aging heart against stress: studies in rats, human tissues, and patients, *Ann NY Acad Sci* 959:355, 2002.

Rubin MA et al: Acute and chronic resistive exercises increase urinary chromium excretion in men as measured with an enriched chromium stable isotope, *J Nutr* 128:73, 1998.

Rude RK, Gruber HE: Magnesium deficiency and osteoporosis: animal and human observation, *J Nutr Biochem* 15:710, 2004.

Salas J et al: The SstI polymorphism of the apolipoprotein C-III gene determines the insulin response to an oral-glucose-tolerance test after consumption of a diet rich in saturated fats, *Am J Clin Nutr* 68:396, 1998.

Salgueiro MJ, Boccio J: Zinc intake versus zinc absorption: a bioavailability factor, *Nutrition* 18:354, 2002.

Sarwar G et al: Corrected relative net protein ratio (CRNPR) method based on differences in rats and human requirements for sulfur amino acids, *J Am Oil Chem Soc* 68:689, 1985

Sauberlich HE: Pharmacology of vitamin C, *Annu Rev Nutr* 14:371, 1994.

Schaumberg HJ et al: Sensory neuropathy from pyridoxine abuse, *N Engl J Med* 309:445, 1983.

Scholz-Ahrens KE et al: Effects of prebiotics on mineral metabolism, *Am J Clin Nutr* 73:459S, 2001.

Schrager S: Dietary calcium intake and obesity, *J Am Board Fam Pract* 18:205, 2005.

Shiau SY, Yu YP: Chitin but not chitosan supplementation enhances growth of grass shrimp, Penaeus monodon, *J Nutr* 128:908, 1998.

Shoob et al: Dietary methionine is involved in the etiology of neural tube defect–affected pregnancies in humans, *J Nutr* 131:2653, 2001.

Shrimpton R et al: Zinc deficiency: what are the most appropriate interventions? *BMJ* 330:347, 2005.

Sokol, RJ: Antioxidant defenses in metal-induced liver damage, *Semin Liver Dis* 16:39, 2001.

Stahl W et al: Non-antioxidant properties of carotenoids, *Biol Chem* 383:553, 2002.

Stanley CA: Carnitine deficiency disorder in children, *Ann NY Acad Sci* 1033:42, 2004.

Stark A, Madar Z: Phytoestrogens: a review of recent findings, *J Pediatr Endocrinol Metab* 15:561, 2002.

Stender S, Dyerberg J: Influence of transfatty acids on health, *Ann Nutr Metab* 48:61, 2004.

Stendig-Lindenberg G et al: Trabecular bone density in a two-year controlled trial of peroral magnesium in osteoporosis, *Magnes Res* 6:155, 1993.

Subar AF et al: Dietary sources of nutrients among US adults, 1989 to 1991, *J Am Diet Assoc* 98:537, 1998.

Tobacman JK: Review of harmful gastrointestinal effects of carrageenan in animal experiments, *Environ Health Perspect* 109:983, 2001.

Tran MT et al: Role of coenzyme Q_{10} in chronic heart failure, angina, and hypertension, *Pharmacotherapy* 21:797, 2001.

Trumbo P et al: Dietary reference intakes: vitamin A, vitamin K, arsenic, boron, chromium, copper, iodine, manganese, molybdenum, nickel, silicon, vanadium, and zinc, *J Am Diet Assoc* 101:294, 2001.

Turner RB, Cetnarowski WE: Effect of treatment with zinc gluconate or zinc acetate on experimental and natural colds, *Clin Infect Dis* 31:1202, 2000.

Turnlund JR, Keyes WR: Plasma molybdenum reflects dietary molybdenum intake, *J Nutr Biochem* 15:90, 2004.

Tyrala EE et al: Selenate fortification of infant formulas improves the selenium status of preterm infants, *Am J Clin Nutr* 64:860, 1996.

Uauy R et al: Essentiality of copper in humans, *Am J Clin Nutr* 67(suppl):952, 1998.

U.S. Department of Agriculture: Agriculture Research Service Quarterly Report, Human nutrition, 2000, website: www.ars.usda.gov/is/qtr.

United States Department of Agriculture. Dietary Guidelines for Americans 2005, website:. http://www.health.gov/dietaryguidelines/dga2005/document/.

Volpe SL et al: Effect of chromium supplementation and exercise on body composition, resting metabolic rate and selected biochemical parameters in moderately obese women following an exercise program, *J Am Coll Nutr* 20:293, 2001.

Watts et al: Coenzyme Q_{10} improves endothelial dysfunction of the brachial artery in type II diabetes mellitus, *Diabetologia* 45:420, 2002.

Weinberg PD: Analysis of the variable effect of dietary vitamin E supplements on experimental atherosclerosis, *Plant Physiol* 162:823, 2005.

West KP: Vitamin A deficiency disorders in children and women, *Food Nutr Bull* 24(4 Suppl):S78, 2003.

Whittaker P et al: Iron and folate in fortified cereals, *J Am Coll Nutr* 20:247, 2001.

Wigertz K et al: Racial differences in calcium retention in response to dietary salt in adolescent girls, *Am J Clin Nutr* 81:895, 2005.

Wolters M et al: Cobalamin: a critical vitamin in the elderly, *Prev Med* 39:1256, 2004.

Young VR: Soy protein in relation to human protein and amino acid nutrition, *J Am Diet Assoc* 91:828, 1991.

Zhang ZW Farthing MJ: The roles of vitamin C in *Helicobacter pylori*–associated gastric carcinogenesis, *Chin J Dig Dis* 6:53, 2005.

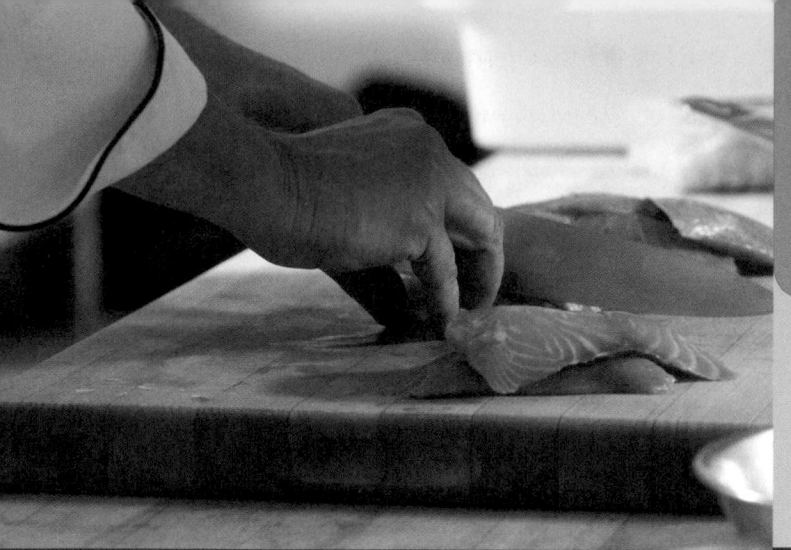

CHAPTER 4

Pamela Charney, PhD, RD, CNSD

Water, Electrolytes, and Acid-Base Balance

KEY TERMS

acid-base balance a dynamic equilibrium state of hydrogen ion concentration in the body

acidemia a state in which the pH of arterial blood decreases below the normal range of 7.35 to 7.45 because of an increase in circulating acids or a reduction in bicarbonate levels

acidosis a physiologic process or disease state that, if left untreated, results in acidemia

alkalemia a state in which the pH of arterial blood exceeds the normal range of 7.35 to 7.45 because of an increase in bicarbonate levels or a reduction in circulating acids

alkalosis a physiologic process or disease state that, if left untreated, results in alkalemia

anion gap the difference between measured cations and measured anions

buffer a proton donor and acceptor system that helps preserve homeostasis of the hydrogen ion concentration

contraction alkalosis metabolic alkalosis resulting from hypovolemia; occurs when decreased blood flow to the kidneys stimulates resorption of water and sodium; bicarbonate is resorbed with the sodium, causing alkalosis

dehydration excessive loss of body water

edema an abnormal accumulation of fluid in the intercellular tissue spaces or body cavities

electrolytes substances that dissociate into positively and negatively charged ions when dissolved in water

extracellular fluid the water and dissolved substances in the plasma, lymph, spinal fluid, and secretions; includes the intercellular (interstitial) water between and around the cells

extracellular water water in plasma, lymph, spinal fluid, and secretions; includes the intercellular (interstitial) water between and around the cell

insensible water loss unmeasured water loss (e.g., when water exits with air expired from the lungs or water vapor evaporates from the skin's surface)

intercellular (interstitial) water water between and around the cells

intracellular fluid the water and dissolved substances contained within cells

intracellular water (ICW) water contained within the cell

metabolic acidosis acidosis caused by an increase in circulating noncarbonic acids, an excessive loss of bicarbonate, or both

metabolic alkalosis alkalosis caused by an increase in circulating bicarbonate, an excessive loss of acid, or both

metabolic water abolism of carbohydrate, protein, or fat

oncotic pressure (colloidal osmotic pressure) pressure at the capillary membrane that is caused by dissolved proteins in the plasma and interstitial fluids

osmolality a measure of the osmotically active particles per kilogram of solvent in which the particles are dispersed

osmolarity a measure of the osmotically active particles per liter of solution

osmotic pressure the pressure of a solution directly related to its solute osmolar concentration

respiratory acidosis acidosis caused by acute or chronic retention of carbon dioxide by the lungs

respiratory alkalosis alkalosis caused by increased ventilation and elimination of carbon dioxide

sensible water loss water that is lost from urine, feces, emesis and gastric suctioning

"third space" fluid fluid that is extracellular and extravascular (in the body cavities), accumulation of which results in edema

water intoxication a state in which excess water increases intracellular volume and dilutes body fluids

---

Sections of this chapter were written by Susan J. Whitmore, RD, LDN, CNSD, for the previous edition of this text.

The volume, composition, and distribution of body fluids have profound effects on cell function. A stable internal environment is maintained through a sophisticated network of homeostatic mechanisms. Protein-energy malnutrition, disease, trauma, and surgery can disrupt fluid, electrolyte, and acid-base balance, causing alterations in the composition, distribution, and amount of body fluids. Even small changes in pH, electrolyte concentrations, and fluid status can have adverse effects on cell function. If these derangements are not corrected, severe consequences, including death, can ensue.

BODY WATER

Water is the largest single component of the body. At birth, water accounts for approximately 75% to 85% of total body weight; this proportion decreases with age and level of adiposity. Water accounts for 60% to 70% of total body weight in the lean adult and 45% to 55% of total body weight in the obese adult. Metabolically active cells of the muscle and viscera have the highest concentration of water, whereas calcified tissue cells have the lowest. Total body water is higher in athletes than in nonathletes and decreases significantly with age because of diminished muscle mass (Figure 4-1). Although the proportion of body weight accounted for by water varies with age and body fat, there is little day-to-day variation in the percentage of body water.

Functions

Water is an essential component of all body tissues as it makes many solutes available for cell function and is the medium needed for all reactions. Water also participates as a substrate in metabolic reactions and as a structural component providing form to cells. Water is essential for the physiologic processes of digestion, absorption, and excretion. It plays a key role in the structure and function of the circulatory system and acts as a transport medium for nutrients and all body substances.

Water maintains the physical and chemical constancy of intracellular and extracellular fluids and has a direct role in maintaining body temperature. Evaporation of perspiration cools the body during warm weather, preventing or delaying hyperthermia. Loss of 20% of body water **(dehydration)** may cause death; loss of only 10% causes severe disorders (Figure 4-2). In moderate weather, healthy adults can live up to 10 days without water, and children can live up to 5 days. In contrast, it is possible to survive for several weeks without food.

Distribution

Intracellular water (ICW) is the water contained within cells and accounts for two thirds of total body water. **Extracellular water** is commonly estimated to account for one third of total body water or 20% of body weight, and includes the water in plasma, lymph, spinal fluid, and secretions. **Extracellular fluid** is the water and dissolved substances in the plasma, lymph, spinal fluid, and secretions and also includes the **intercellular (interstitial) water** between and around the cells. Most interstitial water is part of intracellular fluid and is held in a gel in the intercellular spaces and is continuous with the plasma through pores in the capillaries. Abnormal accumulation of fluid in the intercellular tissue spaces or body cavities is called **edema.**

The distribution of body water varies under different circumstances, but the total amount in the body remains relatively constant. The understanding of the role of body water in health and disease has improved through the use of bioelectrical impedance analysis (BIA), a measurement of electrical conduction used to estimate the amount of

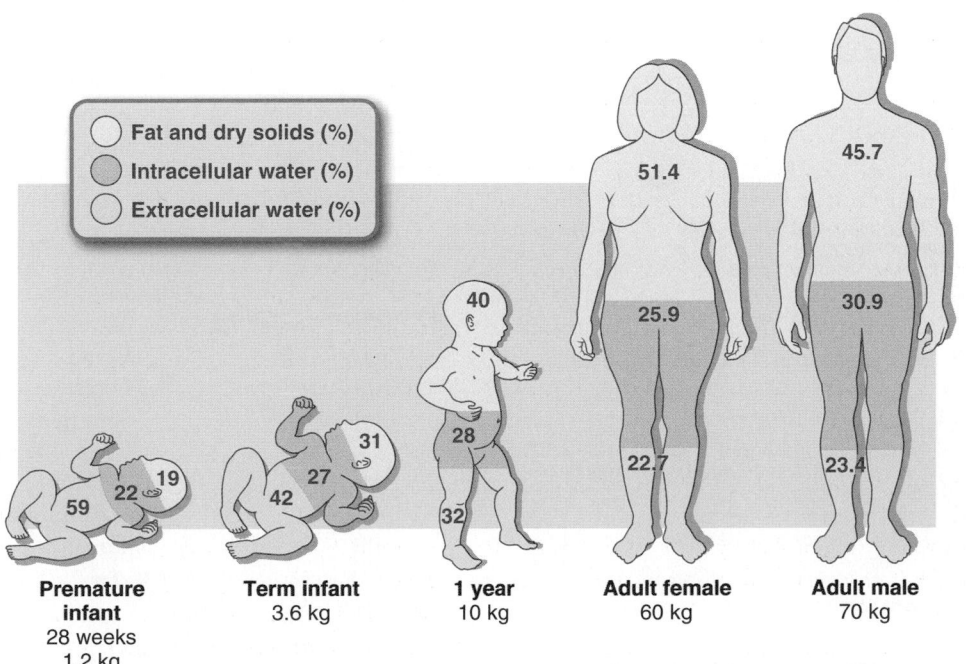

FIGURE 4-1 Distribution of body water as a percentage of body weight.

body water (Kyle et al., 2004) (see Chapter 14 and Appendix 27).

Balance

Shifts in water balance can have adverse consequences. For this reason, homeostatic regulation by the gastrointestinal (GI) tract, kidneys, and brain keeps body water content fairly constant. The amount of water taken in daily is approximately equivalent to the amount lost (Table 4-1).

Water Intake

In healthy individuals water intake is controlled primarily by thirst. Both cellular dehydration and decreased extracellular fluid volume play a role in stimulating thirst. Changes in cellular water content are sensed by baroreceptors in the central nervous system that provide feedback to the hypothalamus, which is close to the centers that regulate antidiuretic hormone (ADH), also known as vasopressin. ADH signals the kidneys to conserve water. Baroreceptors in the vascular system are stimulated by decreased extracellular fluid volume (Kenney, 2001). These sensors stimulate the renin-angiotensin system. Renin is an enzyme that is released by the kidney and acts as a catalyst in the production of angiotensin II, and one of the actions of angiotensin II is stimulation of thirst centers. The sensation of thirst is a signal to consume fluids.

Water is ingested as fluid and part of food (Table 4-2). The oxidation of foods in the body also produces **metabolic water** as an end product. The oxidation of 100 g of fat, carbohydrate, or protein yields 107, 55, or 41 g of water, respectively, for a total of approximately 200 to 300 ml/day. When water cannot be ingested orally or by a feeding tube, it may be administered intravenously in the form of salt (saline) solutions, which closely resemble the electrolyte content of body fluids; dextrose solutions; parenteral nutrition; or in blood or plasma as transfusions.

Water is absorbed rapidly because it moves freely through some membranes by diffusion. This movement is controlled mainly by osmotic forces generated by inorganic ions in solution in the body (see *Clinical Insight:* Osmotic Forces).

Water intoxication occurs as a result of water intake in excess of the body's ability to excrete water. Ensuing increased **intracellular fluid** volume is accompanied by osmolar dilution. The increased volume of intracellular fluid causes the cells, particularly the brain cells, to swell, leading to headache, nausea, blindness, vomiting, muscle twitching, and convulsions with impending stupor. If left untreated, water intoxication can be fatal.

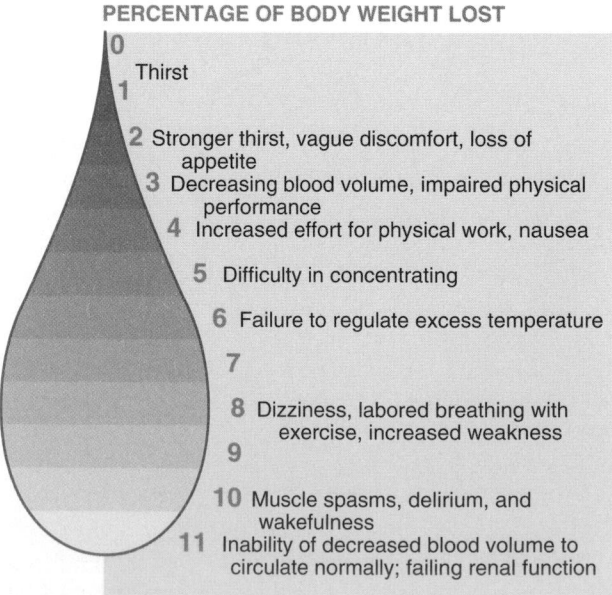

PERCENTAGE OF BODY WEIGHT LOST

0

1 — Thirst

2 — Stronger thirst, vague discomfort, loss of appetite

3 — Decreasing blood volume, impaired physical performance

4 — Increased effort for physical work, nausea

5 — Difficulty in concentrating

6 — Failure to regulate excess temperature

7

8 — Dizziness, labored breathing with exercise, increased weakness

9

10 — Muscle spasms, delirium, and wakefulness

11 — Inability of decreased blood volume to circulate normally; failing renal function

FIGURE 4-2 Adverse effects of dehydration.

TABLE 4-1

Water Balance

Water Intake and Output (ml)*	Water Source
Water intake	
1400	Fluids
700	Food
200	Cellular oxidation of food
2300	TOTAL
Water Output	
Normal Temperature	
1400	Urine
100	Feces
100	Skin (perspiration)
	Insensible loss
350	Skin
350	Respiratory tract
2300	TOTAL
Hot Weather	
1200	Urine
100	Feces
1400	Skin (perspiration)
	Insensible loss
350	Skin
250	Respiratory tract
3300	TOTAL
Prolonged Exercise	
500	Urine
100	Feces
5000	Skin (perspiration)
	Insensible loss
350	Skin
650	Respiratory tract
6600	TOTAL

Modified from Guyton AC: *Textbook of medical physiology,* ed 9, Philadelphia, 1996, Saunders.

*Average values.

Water Elimination

Water loss normally occurs through the kidneys as urine and through the GI tract in the feces (measurable or **sensible water loss**), as well as through air expired from the lungs and water vapor lost through the skin (nonmeasurable or **insensible water loss**) (see Table 4-1). The kidney is the primary regulator of sensible water loss. Natural diuretics are substances in the diet that increase urinary excretion; they include alcohol and caffeine.

Insensible water loss is continuous and usually unconscious. High altitude, low humidity, and high temperatures can increase insensible fluid loss through the lungs and through sweat. Athletes can lose 3 to 4 lb from fluid loss when exercising in a temperature of 80° F and low humidity and even more at higher temperatures (see Chapter 23).

TABLE 4-2

Percentage of Water in Common Foods

Food	Percentage
Lettuce, iceberg	96
Celery	95
Cucumbers	95
Cabbage, raw	92
Watermelon	92
Broccoli, boiled	91
Milk, nonfat	91
Spinach	91
Green beans, boiled	89
Carrots, raw	88
Oranges	87
Cereals, cooked	85
Apples, raw, without skin	84
Grapes	81
Potatoes, boiled	77
Eggs	75
Bananas	74
Fish, haddock, baked	74
Chicken, roasted, white meat	70
Corn, boiled	65
Beef, sirloin	59
Cheese, Swiss	38
Bread, white	37
Cake, angel food	34
Butter	16
Almonds, blanched	5
Saltines	3
Sugar, white	1
Oils	0

From U.S. Department of Agriculture, Agricultural Research Service: *Nutrient Database for Standard Reference*, Release 16, retrieved May, 2006. Data Laboratory home page: http://www.nal.usda.gov/fnic/foodcomp/Data/SR18/sr18.html.

The GI tract can be a major source of water loss. Under normal conditions the water contained in the 7 to 9 L of digestive juices and other extracellular fluids secreted daily into the GI tract is almost entirely resorbed in the ileum and colon, except for about 100 ml that is excreted in the feces. Because this volume of resorbed fluid is about twice that of the blood plasma, excessive GI fluid losses through diarrhea may have serious consequences, particularly for very young and very old individuals.

Fluid loss through diarrhea has been responsible for thousands of children's deaths in developing countries. Oral rehydration therapy with a simple mixture of water, sugar, and salt has been highly effective in reducing the number of deaths (Victora et al., 2000) (see Chapter 27). Other abnormal fluid losses may occur as a result of emesis, hemorrhage, fistula drainage, burn and wound exudates, gastric and surgical tube drainage, and the use of diuretics.

When water intake is insufficient or water loss is excessive, healthy kidneys compensate by conserving water and excreting more concentrated urine. The renal tubules increase water resorption in response to the hormonal action of ADH. However, the concentration of the urine made by the kidneys has a limit: approximately 1400 mOsm/L. Once this limit has been reached, the body loses its ability to excrete solutes. The ability of the kidneys in older individuals to concentrate the urine may be compromised, resulting in increased risk of developing dehydration and hypernatremia, especially during illness.

Signs of dehydration include headache, fatigue, decreased appetite, light-headedness, poor skin turgor (although this may be present in well-hydrated older persons), skin tenting on the forehead, concentrated urine, decreased urine output, sunken eyes, dry mucous membranes of the mouth and nose, orthostatic blood pressure changes, and tachycardia (Armstrong, 2005). In a dehydrated person the specific gravity, a measure of the dissolved solutes in urine, increases above the normal levels of 1.008 to 1.030, and the urine becomes remarkably darker (Shirreffs, 2003).

Requirements

The body has no provision for water storage; therefore the amount of water lost every 24 hours must be replaced to maintain health and body efficiency. Under ordinary circumstances a reasonable allowance based on recommended caloric intake is 1 ml/kcal for adults and 1.5 ml/kcal for infants. This translates into approximately 35 ml/kg of usual body weight in adults, 50 to 60 ml/kg in children, and 150 ml/kg in infants. In most cases a suitable daily allowance for water from all sources, including foods in adults, is approximately 3.7 L (125 oz) for males and 2.7 L (91 oz) for females, depending on body size (see *Focus On: Drink Up! Why Eight Glasses per Day?*) (Sawka, 2005).

Infants need more water because of the limited capacity of their kidneys to handle the renal solute load, their higher percentage of body water, and their large surface area per unit of body weight. A lactating woman's need for water also

✦ CLINICAL INSIGHT

Osmotic Forces

Osmotic Pressure

Osmotic pressure is directly proportional to the number of particles in solution and usually refers to the pressure at the cell membrane. It is convenient (although not entirely accurate) to consider the osmotic pressure of the intracellular fluid as a function of its potassium content because potassium is the predominant cation in the intracellular fluid. In contrast, the osmotic pressure of extracellular fluid may be considered relative to its sodium content because sodium is the major cation present in extracellular fluid. Although variations in the distribution of sodium and potassium ions are the principal causes of water shifts between the various fluid compartments, chloride and phosphate also influence water balance. Proteins, which cannot diffuse because of their size, also play a key role in maintaining osmotic equilibrium.

Oncotic Pressure

Oncotic pressure, or **colloidal osmotic pressure**, is the pressure at the capillary membrane and is maintained by dissolved proteins in the plasma and interstitial fluids. Oncotic pressure helps to retain water within blood vessels, preventing its leakage from plasma into the interstitial spaces. In patients with an exceptionally low plasma protein content, such as those who are under physiologic stress or have certain diseases, water leaks into the interstitial spaces, causing edema. This process is referred to as third spacing, and the fluid is called **"third space" fluid**.

Osmoles and Milliosmoles

Concentrations of individual ionic constituents of extracellular or intracellular fluids are expressed in terms of milliosmoles per liter (mOsm/L). One mole equals the gram molecular weight of a substance; dissolved in 1 L of water, it becomes 1 osmole (osm). One milliosmole (mOsm) equals 1/1000th of an osmole. The number of milliosmoles per liter equals the number of millimoles per liter times the number of particles into which the dissolved substance dissociates. Thus 1 mmol of a nonelectrolyte (e.g., glucose) equals 1 mOsm; similarly, 1 mmol of an electrolyte containing only monovalent ions (e.g., sodium chloride [NaCl]) equals 2 mOsm. One mOsm dissolved in 1 L of water has an osmotic pressure of 17 mm Hg.

Osmolality and Osmolarity

Osmolality is a measure of the osmotically active particles per kilogram of the solvent in which the particles are dispersed. It is expressed as milliosmoles of solute per kilogram of solvent (mOsm/kg). **Osmolarity** is the term formerly used to describe concentration—milliosmoles per liter of the entire solution; but osmolality is now expressed in this form for most clinical work. However, in reference to certain conditions such as hyperlipidemia, it makes a difference whether osmolality is stated as milliosmoles per kilogram of solvent or per liter of solution.

The average sum of the concentration of all the cations in serum is about 150 mEq/L. The cation concentration is balanced by 150 mEq/L of anions, yielding a total serum osmolality of about 300 mOsm/L. Serum osmolality can be estimated as follows:

$$\text{Serum osmolality} = (\text{Serum sodium [mEq/L]} \times 2) + \text{Glucose (mg/dl)}/18 + \text{Blood urea nitrogen (mg/dl)}/2.8$$

An osmolar imbalance is caused by a gain or loss of water relative to a solute or a gain or loss of solute relative to water. An osmolality of less than 285 mOsm/L generally indicates a water excess; an osmolality of greater than 300 mOsm/L indicates a water deficit.

---

increases—theoretically by an additional 600 to 700 ml/day—because of the large amount required for milk production (see Chapter 5).

Thirst is usually an adequate signal for the need to consume water, except in infants, heavily exercising athletes, those who are ill, and sometimes older adults, who may have a diminished thirst sensation (see Chapter 10). Anyone sick enough to be hospitalized, regardless of the diagnosis, is at risk for water and electrolyte imbalance. Older adults are particularly susceptible because of other factors such as impaired renal concentrating ability, fever, diarrhea, vomiting, and a decreased ability to care for themselves. In situations involving extreme heat or excessive sweating, thirst may not keep pace with the actual water requirements of the body (see Chapter 23).

ELECTROLYTES

Electrolytes are substances that dissociate into positively and negatively charged ions (cations and anions) when dissolved in water. Electrolytes can be simple inorganic salts of sodium, potassium, or magnesium or complex organic molecules; they play a key role in a host of normal metabolic functions (Table 4-3). One milliequivalent (mEq) of any substance has the capacity to combine chemically with 1 mEq of a substance with an opposite charge. For univalent ions (e.g., Na^+) 1 millimole (mmol) equals 1 mEq; for divalent ions (e.g., Ca^{++}) 1 mmol equals 2 mEq (see Appendix 3 for milligram-to-milliequivalent conversion guidelines).

The major extracellular electrolytes are sodium, calcium, chloride, and bicarbonate. Potassium, magnesium, and

◎ FOCUS ON

Drink Up! Why Eight Glasses per Day?

The primary determinants of maintenance water requirements are metabolic. Ultimately the water intake of the body must be sufficient to meet metabolic demands and balance sensible and insensible water losses. Sound easy? Metabolic demand is influenced by body size, composition, physical activity, and fever. Nonrenal water loss such as perspiration varies greatly according to activity, altitude, humidity, and temperature, as does insensible water loss via the lungs. Considering these and other variables that affect water requirements, it is obvious that estimating water requirements for individuals is anything but easy and individual requirements are highly variable.

The well-known recommendation for 8 glasses of water per day arose from the need to have a guideline that stresses the importance of adequate water intake that would be easily understood by the public. For practical purposes, the National Research Council recommends 1 ml of water/kcal of energy expenditure for adults under "average conditions of energy expenditure and environmental conditions." To calculate fluid needs, clinical models are typically based on an "average" 70-kg (154-lb) male. Baseline adequate intakes for fluid (water plus other beverages) have been set by the Institute of Medicine at 3 L and 2.2 L for sedentary men and women, respectively, with higher intakes needed to account for physical activity and exposure to extreme environments (Manore, 2005).

Solid food typically contributes about 750 ml (approximately 3 cups) of water daily, and oxidative metabolism contributes another 250 ml (approximately 1 cup), leaving a minimum of 1200 to 2000 ml (5 to 8 cups) of noncaffeinated, nonalcoholic fluids to be consumed daily. For example, the water requirement for a huge 40-year-old, 170-kg man is calculated as follows:

(First 10 kg = 1000 ml) + (Second 10 kg = 500 ml) +
(Remaining 150 kg = 3000 ml) = 4500 ml

An individual of this size may receive more water from solid food and oxidative metabolism because of his overall increased dietary intake. Even so, his fluid intake requirement could be as high as 14 cups per day. The daily water requirement using this method for the reference 70-kg man is 2500

ml, and if 1000 ml is provided by water in food and from metabolic water, he would still need to drink 1500 ml of water—about 5 cups. Roughly translated, every 25 pounds that a person (who is less than 50 years old) is above the ideal 70-kg weight increases the water requirement by about another 1 cup (i.e., 240 ml):

$$(25 \text{ lb}) \times (1 \text{ kg}/2.2 \text{ lb}) \times (20 \text{ ml/kg}) = 227 \text{ ml (about 1 cup)}$$

Healthy individuals are seldom at risk for water intoxication when their intake exceeds their water requirements. In terms of health and performance, people are more at risk for chronic underhydration. Dehydration causing as little as a 2% loss of body weight results in impaired physiologic and performance responses (Kleiner, 1999). Chronic mild dehydration is also associated with diminished salivary gland function (see Figure 4-2), an increased risk of kidney stones in susceptible individuals (Borghi et al., 1996), an increased risk of colon cancer (Shannon et al., 1996), an increased risk of breast cancer (Stookey et al., 1997), an increased risk of childhood obesity (Levine, 1996), and an increased risk of mitral valve prolapse in susceptible individuals (Lax et al., 1992). Therefore drink plenty of noncaffeinated, nonalcoholic beverages . . . to your health!

For many individuals, bottled water appears to be a safe, easy way to meet water requirements. Sales of bottled water are increasing exponentially. Consumers might think that bottled waters, particularly the more expensive brands, are somehow safer or purer than tap water. Because there are no labeling standards for bottled water, there is no guarantee that bottled water is anything but tap water. In most cases, tap water might actually be a safer water source, as tap water safety is regulated by the Environmental Protection Agency (EPA), whereas bottled waters are regulated by the Food and Drug Administration only if they cross state lines. Those who make the choice to drink bottled water should consider the environmental impact of the packaging. According to the UC Berkeley Wellness Letter (2005), more than a million tons of nonbiodegradable plastic are required to produce bottles for bottled water purchased in the United States. Finally, infants and children should not be given bottled water because fluoridated tap water may be their only source of that mineral.

---

phosphate are the major intracellular electrolytes. These elements, which exist as ions in body fluids, are distributed throughout all body fluids and involved in maintaining physiologic body functions, including osmotic equilibrium, acid-base balance, and intracellular and extracellular concentration differentials. Changes in either intracellular or extracellular electrolyte concentrations can have a major impact on body functions. The Na/K ATPase pump func-

tions to closely regulate cellular electrolyte contents by actively pumping sodium out of cells in exchange for potassium. Other electrolytes follow ion gradients.

Calcium

Although approximately 99% of the body's calcium (Ca^{++}) is stored in the bone, the remaining 1% has important physiologic functions. The ionized calcium content of the blood

✳ CLINICAL INSIGHT

Anion Gap

The number of positively charged ions (cations) in the body equals the number of negatively charged ions (anions). However, not all cations and anions are measured routinely. Sodium is the principal measured cation, whereas chloride and bicarbonate are the principal measured anions. The term **anion gap** refers to the difference between measured cations and measured anions (and is normally 12 to 14 mEq/L):

$$\text{Anion gap (AG)} = \text{Serum sodium} - (\text{Serum chloride} + \text{bicarbonate})$$

Nongap Metabolic Acidosis

Nongap metabolic acidosis occurs when a decrease in bicarbonate concentration is balanced by an increase in chloride concentration, resulting in a normal anion gap. This type of acidosis, which is also referred to as hyperchloremic metabolic acidosis, may develop in association with the following (which are represented by the acronym USED CARP) (Wilson, 1992):

Ureterosigmoidostomy *Carbonic anhydrase inhibitor*
Small bowel fistula *Adrenal insufficiency*
Extra chloride ingestion *Renal tubular acidosis*
Diarrhea *Pancreatic fistula*

Anion Gap Metabolic Acidosis

Anion gap metabolic acidosis occurs when a decrease in bicarbonate concentration is balanced by increased acid anions other than chloride. This causes the calculated anion gap to exceed the normal range of 12 to 14 mEq/L. This type of acidosis, which is also referred to as normochloremic metabolic acidosis, may develop in association with the following conditions (which are represented by the acronym MUD PILES) (Wilson, 1992):

Methanol ingestion *Paraldehyde ingestion*
Uremia *Iatrogenic*
Diabetic ketoacidosis *Lactic acidosis*
  Ethylene glycol or ethanol ingestion
  Salicylate intoxication

(decreased pH) compensate by increasing bicarbonate resorption, thereby creating a metabolic alkalosis. This response helps to increase the pH. Similarly, in response to a primary metabolic acidosis (decreased pH), the lungs compensate by increasing ventilation and carbon dioxide elimination, thereby creating a respiratory alkalosis. This compensatory respiratory alkalosis helps to increase pH.

Respiratory compensation for metabolic acid-base disturbances occurs quickly—within minutes. In contrast, renal compensation for respiratory acid-base imbalances may take 3 to 5 days to be maximally effective. Compensation does not always occur; when it does, it is not completely successful (i.e., does not result in a pH of 7.4). The pH level still reflects the underlying primary disorder. It is imperative to distinguish between primary disturbances and compensatory responses because treatment is always directed toward the primary acid-base disturbance and its underlying cause. As the primary disturbance is treated, the compensatory response corrects itself.

Predictive values for compensatory responses are available and may aid the clinician in differentiating between primary acid-base imbalances and compensatory responses (Whitmire, 2002). Alternatively, clinicians can also use acid-base maps or clinical algorithms (DuBose et al., 1996).

◉ FOCAL POINTS

- Acid-base patterns often serve as a common diagnostic tool within medical specialties. (Whittier and Rutecki, 2004).
- Despite wide daily variations in intake of water and minerals that function as electrolytes, the body strives to maintain a stable internal environment to maintain physiologic functioning.
- When normal homeostatic mechanisms are rendered ineffective by disease or injury, or when intakes exceed the body's normal regulatory capacities, the internal environment and ultimately cell function are disrupted.
- All changes in blood pH, in health and in disease, occur in carbon dioxide, electrolyte concentrations, and total weak acid concentrations. (Kellum, 2005).
- Knowledge of fluid, electrolyte, and acid-base balance is important for understanding many aspects of nutrition in health and disease.

USEFUL WEBSITES

Acid-Base Tutorial
http://www.acid-base.com/

Harrison's Online
www.harrisons.accessmedicine.com/

The Merck Manual of Diagnosis and Therapy
www.merck.com/pubs/mmanual/section2/chapter12/
12a.htm

References

Armstrong LE: Hydration assessment techniques, *Nutr Rev* 63 (6 Pt 2):S40, 2005.

Borghi L et al: Urinary volume, water, and recurrences in idiopathic calcium nephrolithiasis: a 5-year randomized prospective study, *Urology* 155:839, 1996.

Burger H et al: Osteoporosis and salt intake, *Nutr Metab Cardiovasc Dis* 10(1):46-53, 2000.

Centers for Disease Control and Prevention: Lactic acidosis traced to thiamine deficiency related to nationwide shortage of multivitamins for total parenteral nutrition—United States, 1997, *MMWR Morb Wkly Rep* 46:523, 1997.

Clemens LH et al: The effect of eating out on the quality of diet in premenopausal women, *J Am Dietetic Assoc* 99:442, 1999.

Cohn JN et al: New guidelines for potassium replacement in clinical practice: a contemporary review by the National Council on Potassium in Clinical Practice, *Arch Intern Med* 160:2429, 2000.

DuBose TD et al: Acid-base disorders. In Brenner BM, Rector FC, editors: *The kidney*, ed 5, Philadelphia, 1996, Saunders, pp 929-998.

Institute of Medicine, Food and Nutrition Board: *Dietary reference intakes for water, potassium, sodium, chloride, and sulfate*, Washington, DC, 2004, National Academies Press.

Kellum JA: Determinants of plasma acid-base balance, *Crit Care Clin* 21:329, 2005.

Kenney WL, Chiu P: Influence of age on thirst and fluid intake, *Med Sci Sports Exerc* 33(9):1524-1532, 2001.

Kleiner SM: Water: an essential but overlooked nutrient, *J Am Diet Assoc* 99:200, 1999.

Kyle UG et al: Bioelectrical impedance analysis. Part I: Review of principles and methods, *Clin Nutr* 23:1430, 2004.

Lax D et al: Mild dehydration induces echocardiographic signs of mitral valve prolapse in healthy females with prior normal cardiac findings, *Am Heart J* 124:1533, 1992.

Levine B: Role of liquid intake in childhood obesity and related diseases, *Curr Concepts Persp Nutr* 8:2, 1996.

Manore MM: Exercise and the Institute of Medicine recommendations for nutrition, *Curr Sports Med Rep* 4(4):193, 2005.

Romanski SA, McMahon MM: Metabolic acidosis and thiamine deficiency, *Mayo Clinic Proc* 74:259, 1999.

Rude RK: Magnesium. In Stipanuk MH, editor: *Biochemical and physiological aspects of human nutrition*, Philadelphia, 2000, Saunders.

Sawka MN et al: Human water needs, *Nutr Rev* 63 (6 Pt 2): S30-S39, 2005.

Shannon J et al: Relationship of food groups and water intake to colon cancer risk, *Cancer Epidemiol Biomarkers Prev* 5:495, 1996.

Shirreffs SM: Markers of hydration status, *Eur J Clin Nutr* 57(Suppl 2):S6-S9, 2003.

Stookey JD et al: Correspondence: relationship of food groups and water intake to colon cancer risk, *Cancer Epidemiol Biomarkers Prev* 6:657, 1997.

Teucher B, Fairweather-Tait S: Dietary sodium as a risk factor for osteoporosis: where is the evidence? *Proc Nutr Soc* 62:859, 2003.

The Seventh Report of the Joint National Committee on Prevention, Detection, Evaluation, and Treatment of High Blood Pressure: NIH Pub No 03-5233, 2003.

Victora CG et al: Reducing deaths from diarrhea through oral rehydration therapy, *Bull WHO* 78:1246, 2000.

Whitmire SJ: Fluids, electrolytes, and acid-base balance. In Matarese LE, Gottschlich MM, editors: *Contemporary nutrition support practice: a clinical guide*, ed 2, Philadelphia, 2002, Saunders.

Wilson RF: Acid-base problems. In Tintinalli JE, Krome RL, Ruiz E, editors: *Emergency medicine: a comprehensive study guide*, ed 3, New York, 1992, McGraw-Hill.

Wood RJ: Calcium and phosphorus. In Stipanuk MH, editor: *Biochemical and physiologic aspects of human nutrition*, Philadelphia, 2000, Saunders.

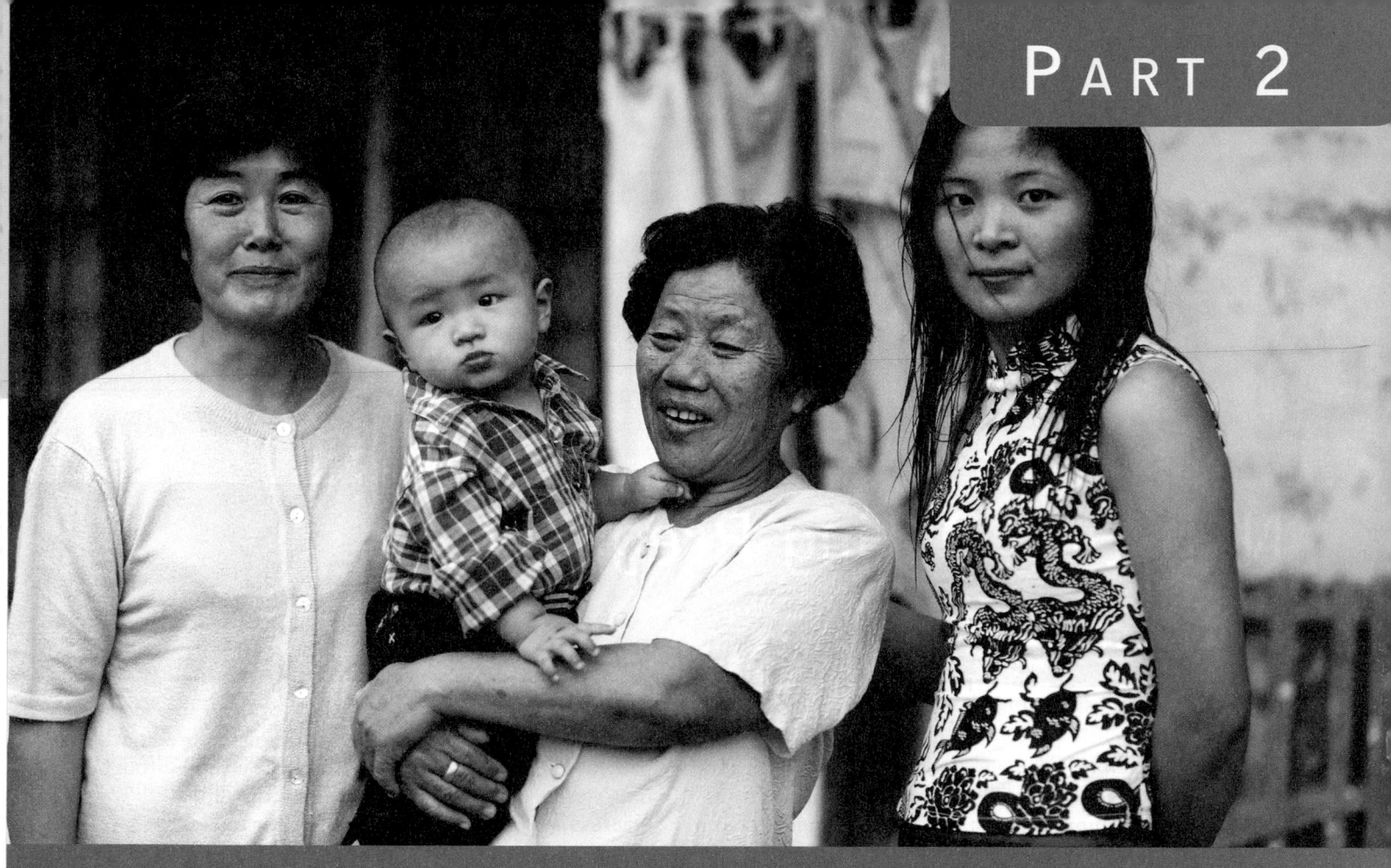

PART 2

Nutrition in the Life Cycle

THE importance of nutrition throughout the life cycle cannot be refuted. However, the significance of nutrition during specific times of growth, development, and aging is becoming increasingly appreciated.

Health professionals have recognized for quite some time the effects of proper nutrition during pregnancy on the health of the infant and mother, even after her childbearing years. Maternal nutrition and possibly even paternal nutrition before conception affect the health of the newborn. "Fetal origin" has far more lifelong effects than originally thought.

Establishing good dietary habits during childhood lessens the possibility of inappropriate eating behavior later in life. Although the influence of proper nutrition on morbidity and mortality usually remains unacknowledged until adulthood, dietary practices aimed at preventing the degenerative diseases that develop later in life should be instituted in childhood.

During early adulthood many changes begin that lead to the development of diseases of aging years later. Many of these changes can be accelerated or slowed over the years, depending on the quality of the individual's nutritional intake, the health of the gut, and the function of the immune system.

With the rapid growth of the oldest adult population has evolved a need to expand the limited nutrition data currently available for these individuals. Although it is known that energy needs decrease with aging, little is known about whether requirements for specific nutrients increase or decrease. Identifying the unique nutritional differences among the various stages of aging is becoming even more important.

A woman with a BMI of 22 would be considered normal weight and counseled to gain 25 to 35 lb during her pregnancy. Pregnancy weight gain curves currently in use reflect the prepregnancy weight, height, and age of the mother (Figure 5-2). Several studies suggest that 50% of overweight women gain more than the target weight recommendations (Scotland et al., 2005). It is important that providers assess weight gain against caloric intake. If a weight gain is excessive and not supported by an overconsumption of calories, it is likely that the woman is accumulating fluid in the form of edema or amniotic fluid excess (i.e., polyhydramnios). Older women with multiple gestations are more prone to cardiac compromise and may have more overall fluid retention.

One way to appreciate the complexity of the combination of maternal weight status and pregnancy gain is depicted in

Table 5-1. The pregnancy weight matrix is a model to follow weight categories throughout pregnancy by looking at the two aspects of pregnancy: maternal prepregnancy body status, which is a constant variable, and the variable factor (weight gained during the 9 months of pregnancy). Looking at the matrix, a woman was overweight before pregnancy and who is gaining too rapidly would be a #9 or a OW-EG. If she slows her rate of weight gain (see Table 5-2) she could become an OW-AG by the end of her pregnancy.

Weight gain charts created by U.S. Department of Health, Education, and Welfare suggest the "pattern of normal prenatal gain in weight." These weight grids are standard assessment tools used by maternity centers and the Women, Infants, and Children (WIC) program. The ideal weight situation is "appropriate gain" for all BMIs; however, clinical reality demonstrates that excessive and inadequate weight performances occur. An example of evaluating weight gain using the matrix model at midgestation (20 weeks) and term (40 weeks) delivery is illustrated in Table 5-2.

Obesity

Trends among U.S. women reveal an increasing prevalence of obesity. For example, the prevalence of overweight as defined in one study as a BMI 27.8, increased among women ages 20 to 29 years from 12.6% in 1971-1974 to 20.2% in 1988-1991 (Flegal, 2005). The risk of gestational diabetes, pregnancy-induced hypertension, (PIH) and cesarean section increases in women who are obese (ACOG, 2005).

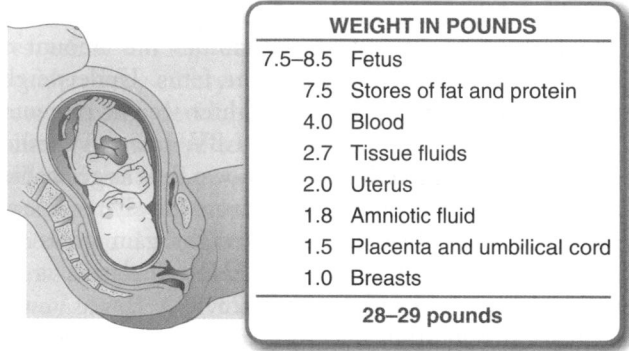

WEIGHT IN POUNDS

7.5–8.5	Fetus
7.5	Stores of fat and protein
4.0	Blood
2.7	Tissue fluids
2.0	Uterus
1.8	Amniotic fluid
1.5	Placenta and umbilical cord
1.0	Breasts

28–29 pounds

FIGURE 5-1 Distribution of weight gain during pregnancy.

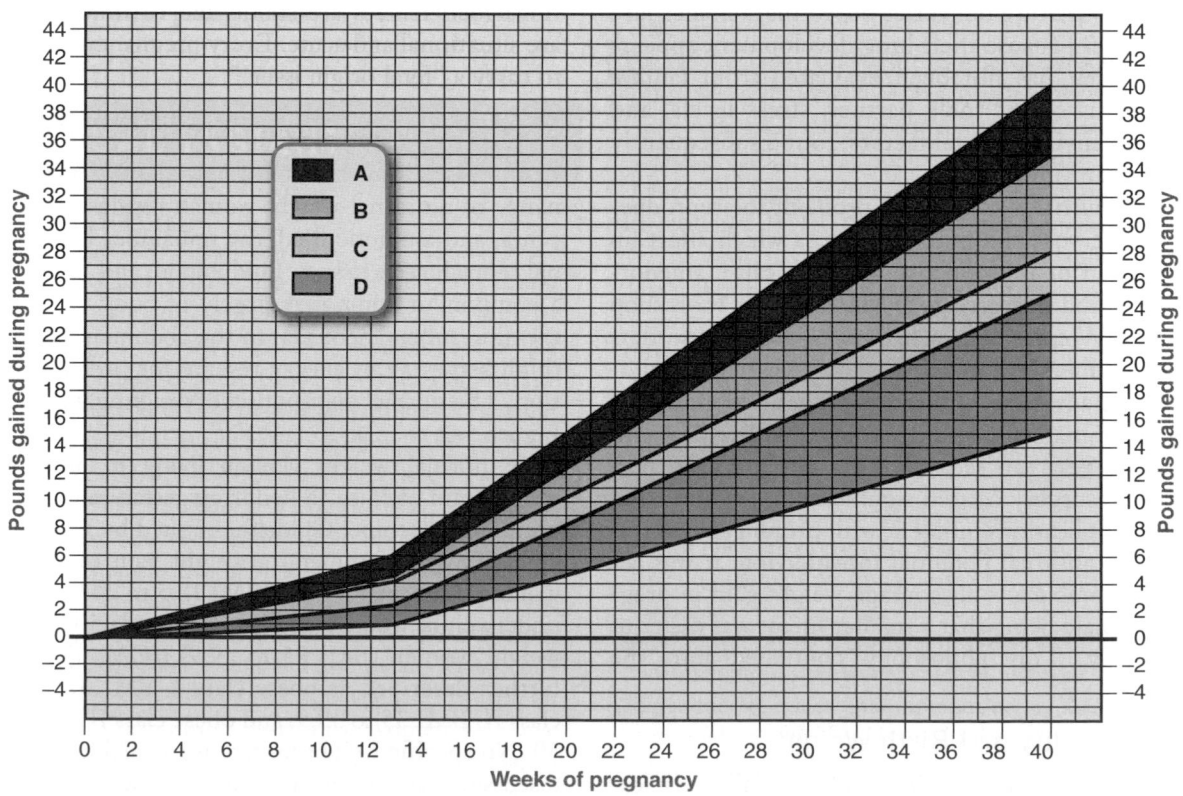

FIGURE 5-2 Desirable weight gain during pregnancy. Females who are of normal weight before their pregnancy should aim for a weight gain in the *B* to *C* range (25 to 35 lb) during pregnancy. Underweight females should gain in the *A* to *B* range (28-40 lb). Females who are overweight before pregnancy should gain in the *D* range (15 to 25 lb).

Overweight and obese women are also at increased risk for late pregnancy (>28 weeks' gestation) and term **intrauterine fetal demise (IUFD)** or miscarriage (Stephansson et al., 2001). The risk for delivery of a very preterm ($\leq$32 weeks) infant or an infant with a cardiac defect, NTD, and **macrosomia** (birthweight greater than 4000 gm), increases in women who are obese (Watkins et al., 2003).

Obese pregnant women (BMI >30) have a twofold increased risk of delivering an infant with **neural tube defects (NTDs),** anomalies resulting in anencephaly or spina bifida, compared to normal weight women. The associa-

tion of maternal obesity and increased incidence of NTDs is puzzling. An adequate folate intake at 600 mcg/day seems to provide less protection against NTDs in obese women than it does in normal-weight pregnant women (Watkins et al., 2003; Scialli and Public Affairs Committee, 2006). There is speculation that the increased body size may require additional supplementation. Since vitamin B_{12} (methyl cobalamin) is a cofactor for methionine synthase, an enzyme that plays a key role in folate metabolism, it may also be required in larger amounts to prevent NTDs. In addition, there is a suggestion that nutrients such as

TABLE 5-1

Pregnancy Weight Matrix

The woman's current gestational weight status as determined by BMI is compared with the recommended weight gain goal by pregravid body size (see Table 5-2 and Figure 5-2).

Prepregnancy Body Size Based on BMI	Inadequate Gain IG	Appropriate Gain AG	Excessive Gain EG
	During Pregnancy		
BMI <18.5 or IBW <85%	1	2	3
Underweight (UW)	UW-IG	UW-AG	UW-EG
BMI 18.5-24.9 or IBW 100%	4	5	6
	AW-IG	AW-AG	AW-EG
BMI 25-29.9 or IBW 120%	7	8	9
	OW-IG	OW-AG	OW-EG
BMI >30 or IBW 150%+	10	11	12
	Obese-IG	Obese-AG	Obese-EG

Modified from Pregnancy Weight Combination Matrix 1990. Used with permission of the author (Erick, 1991).

TABLE 5-2

Pregnancy Weight Matrices

Pregnancy Weight Matrix at Midgestation (20 weeks)

Current gestational weight status (in pounds) compared with BMI specific reference weight goal

Prepregnancy Body Size Based on BMI	Inadequate Gain	Appropriate Gain	Excessive Gain
BMI <18.5 or IBW <85%	<11	11-16	>16
BMI 18.5-24.9 or IBW 100%	<12	12-16	>16
BMI 25-29.9 or IBW 120%	<5	5-8	>8
BMI >30 or IBW 150%+	Weight loss or no gain	Not determined	Not determined

Pregnancy Weight Matrix at Term (40 weeks)

Current gestational weight status (in pounds) compared to BMI specific reference weight goal

Prepregnancy Body Size Based on BMI	Inadequate Gain	Appropriate Gain	Excessive Gain
BMI <18.5 or IBW <85%	<28	28-40	>40
BMI 18.5-24.9 or IBW 100%	<25	25-35	>35
BMI 25-29.9 or IBW 120%	<15	15-25	>25
BMI >30 or IBW 150%+	Weight loss or no gain	15	Not determined

Modified from Pregnancy Weight Combination Matrix 1990. Used with permission of the author (Erick, 1991).

iron, magnesium, and niacin, may play a role in NTDs (Groenen et al, 2004). One study analyzing intakes of 206 mothers using a food frequency questionnaire 14 months after delivery indicated that periconceptual intakes of thiamin, niacin, and vitamin B_6 (pyridoxine) might reduce the incidence in orofacial clefts (OFC) in conjunction with folate, whereas riboflavin and vitamin B_{12} showed no association (Krapels et al., 2004). Inadequate choline may be implicated in NTDs since, like folate, it functions as a methyl donor (Zeisel and Niculescu, 2006).

The 1990 IOM guideline of 15 to 25 pounds for the overweight woman presumably was made to allow for adequate fetal growth without increasing maternal adipose tissue; however, the average term baby is about 7.5 to 8.5 pounds. A recent study evaluated 2910 pregnant women, including 597 obese women for the risk of spontaneous preterm birth, and interestingly found a lower incidence among the obese cohort (Hendler et al., 2005). Another study found that prepregnancy obesity was associated with an increasing risk of fetal death with advancing gestation and speculated that placental dysfunction may be a contributing factor (Nohr et al., 2005). Obesity is considered by some to be a low-grade systemic inflammation with higher levels of C-reactive protein (CRP), interleukin-6, and leptin (Ghezzi et al., 2002).

At this time obese women should be counseled that pregnancy is not a time for weight loss. A proactive nutritional goal would be to choose foods of high antioxidant quality, which are known to help mitigate free radicals. It is known that adipose tissue is a depot for lipid-soluble toxins; unfortunately no research has been done to date evaluating serum levels of these toxins with weight loss (Lordo et al., 1996). There is a theoretic concern that mobilized lipid-soluble toxins may have a detrimental impact on fetal neurologic development. Because obese women have an increased incidence of obstetric complications, the pattern of weight gain during pregnancy should be monitored carefully by the nutrition professional, with appropriate dietary interventions as necessary. Optimum weight gain for the obese woman still is being debated.

Postgastric Bypass Surgery. The prevalence of prepregnancy obesity has resulted in more gastric bypass operations for weight reduction, which has tremendous implications for pregnancy. Although prepregnant weight loss may increase the rate of pregnancy, it has the potential to provide a suboptimum uterine environment for the developing fetus. One study suggests that the fetus will develop adequately if the pregnancy occurs no sooner than 1 year after surgery with adequate nutrient supplementation (Sheiner et al., 2004). After gastric bypass surgery, some women fail to use appropriate methods to prevent pregnancy or fail to be refitted for a diaphragm, and experience an unintended pregnancy because weight loss has corrected underlying endocrine imbalances.

Complications from gastric bypass do occur in pregnancy. For example, internal hernia formation can develop as the growing fetus displaces viscera, which can migrate or rotate more easily as abdominal adipose is reduced. This complication can be life threatening (Kakarla et al., 2005). The optimum nutrient prescription and caloric requirement for pregnant women following gastric bypass surgery has not been determined. The theoretic requirements need to be assessed against the real problems of diminished gastric space and frequent complaints of nausea and heartburn. Depending on length of time from procedure, it is advised to assess iron, thiamin, vitamin B_{12}, 25-hydroxy vitamin D, vitamin A, zinc, and folate to establish a baseline. Women found to have low levels of any nutrient need repletion. An evaluation of 279 morbidly obese patients seeking gastric bypass (mean age 43 ± 9 years, 87% women and 72% white women) showed that 60% of them had vitamin D levels considered deficient (<20ng/ml) and that was *before* their surgeries (Carlin et al., 2006).

The postdelivery nutritional status of the woman with a gastric bypass who plans to breast-feed needs reevaluation. Her breast milk, like that of any other postpartum woman, will reflect her nutritional status; however, it may be more compromised because food volume is less. Obese postpartum women may have higher rates of anemia than normal-weight women. The reason suggested is that more obese women have emergency cesarean deliveries with more blood loss as a result.

Adolescence

Approximately 1 million U.S. adolescents become pregnant every year, which accounts for roughly 25% of U.S. pregnancies. Teens have a higher incidence of delivering a LBW infant (Menacker et al., 2004). Risk factors for poor outcome in pregnant adolescents are listed in Box 5-2.

Public health initiatives have helped reduce the incidence of teen pregnancies (Martin et al., 2002); however, teenage pregnancy continues as a major public health problem in the United States and is associated with significant medical and

---

BOX 5-2

Risk Factors for Poor Pregnancy Outcome in Teenagers

Maternal age, especially younger than age 16
Pregnancy less than 2 years after onset of menarche
Poor nutrition and low prepregnancy weight
Poor weight gain
Infection
Sexually transmitted disease infection
Preexisting anemia
Substance abuse: Smoking, drinking, and drugs
Poverty
Lack of social support
Lack of education
Rapid repeat pregnancies
Lack of access to age-appropriate prenatal care
Late entry into the health system
Unmarried status

nutritional risks (see *Pathophysiology and Care Management Algorithm: Pregnancy in Adolescence*). Many teens enter pregnancy with suboptimal nutritional status; low iron, calcium, and folic acid intakes are common. Improved dietary practices can be one of the most important and controllable factors for both the teen and her baby (Story and Stang, 2000). In counseling teen mothers, the nutrition professional must be aware of the teen's psychosocial, cultural, and literacy level; economic status and dependencies; and any educational frameworks that influence her food choices.

Arranged marriages of adolescent girls are common in some parts of the world. These women and their families may present to Western providers if complications in pregnancy develop and humanitarian care is needed. Pregnancy care in some cultures is limited to female providers because of societal restrictions about intimate exposure. Knowledge of ethnic foods is critical, and comments about unusual foods and preparation must not be negative if a client is referred for nutritional evaluation. Regardless of origin, it is recommended that normal-weight adolescents as a group

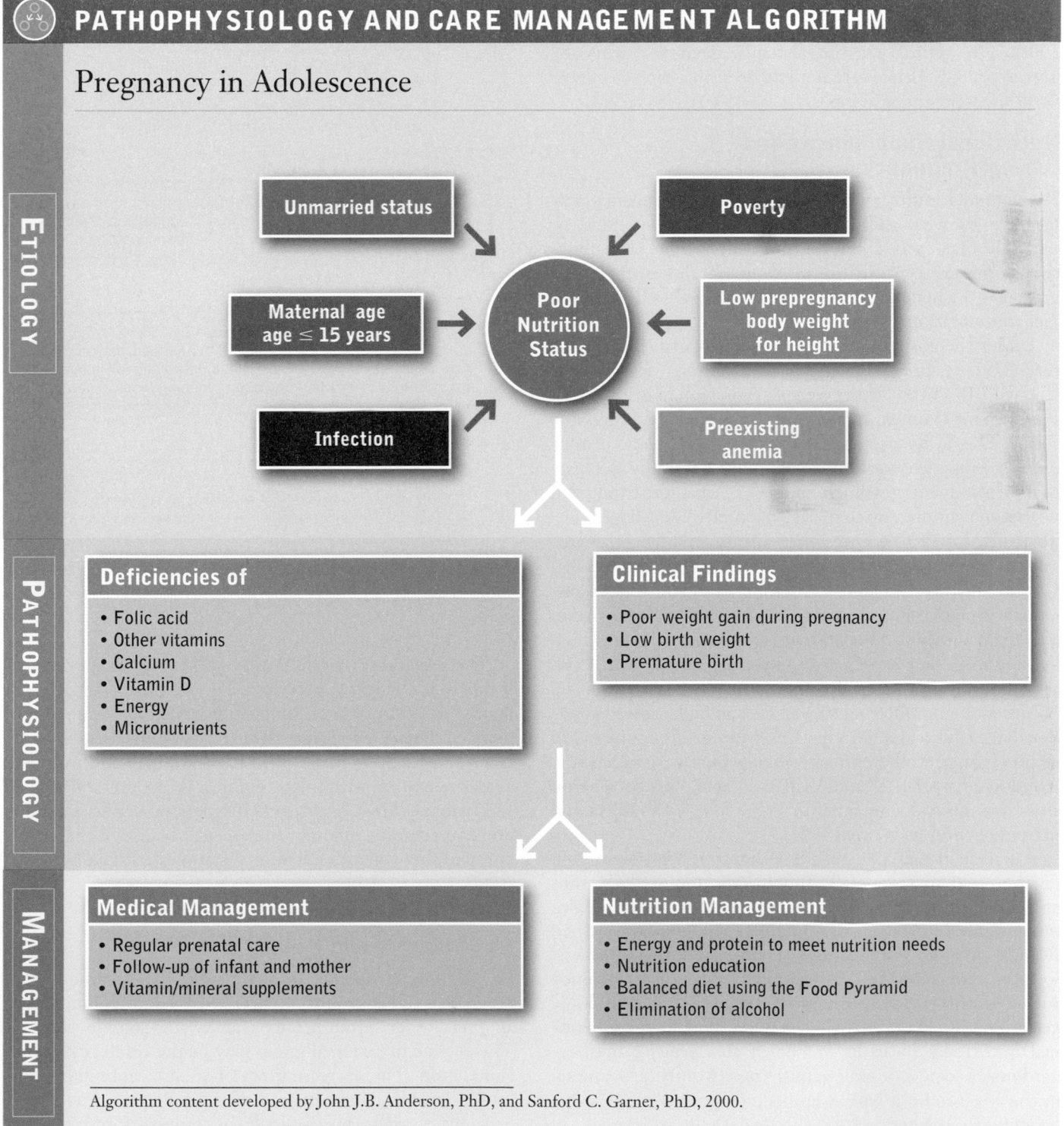

PATHOPHYSIOLOGY AND CARE MANAGEMENT ALGORITHM

Pregnancy in Adolescence

ETIOLOGY

Unmarried status → Poor Nutrition Status

Poverty → Poor Nutrition Status

Maternal age age ≤ 15 years → Poor Nutrition Status

Low prepregnancy body weight for height → Poor Nutrition Status

Infection → Poor Nutrition Status

Preexisting anemia → Poor Nutrition Status

PATHOPHYSIOLOGY

Deficiencies of

- Folic acid
- Other vitamins
- Calcium
- Vitamin D
- Energy
- Micronutrients

Clinical Findings

- Poor weight gain during pregnancy
- Low birth weight
- Premature birth

MANAGEMENT

Medical Management

- Regular prenatal care
- Follow-up of infant and mother
- Vitamin/mineral supplements

Nutrition Management

- Energy and protein to meet nutrition needs
- Nutrition education
- Balanced diet using the Food Pyramid
- Elimination of alcohol

Algorithm content developed by John J.B. Anderson, PhD, and Sanford C. Garner, PhD, 2000.

gain 28 to 40 lb during pregnancy. The benefits of prenatal counseling for teens are noted in Figure 5-3.

Multiple Births

The incidence of multiple births in the United States is rising in part because of the increased use of fertility drugs, embryo transfer, and the increased incidence of pregnancy in older women. Infants of multiple-birth pregnancies have a much greater risk of being born prematurely with IUGR or LBW than do singletons. Adequate maternal weight gain has been shown to be particularly important in these higher-risk pregnancies. Optimal weight gain and infant gestational ages for this population are presented in Table 5–3 (Luke, 2005). The optimal nutritional requirements for twins and higher-order multiples are not known at this time (see *Focus On:* Development of Twins).

Nutritional Supplementation During Pregnancy

Supplementation of a mother's diet during pregnancy may take the form of additional energy, protein, vitamins, or minerals that exceed her routine daily intake. The more compromised the nutritional status of the woman, the greater is the benefit for pregnancy outcome with improved diet and nutritional supplementation.

Under the auspices of the U.S. Department of Agriculture (USDA), pregnant women at nutritional risk are encouraged to enroll in the Special Supplemental Nutrition Program for Women, Infants and Children, better known as WIC. The WIC program serves pregnant women, non-breast-feeding postpartum women until 6 months' postpartum, breast-feeding women up until 1 year postpartum, and infants and children up to the age of 5 years (see Chapter 11). To qualify for WIC services, participants must live in an area served by WIC, be at nutritional risk, and have a low income. Criteria for "nutritional risk" may include anemia, poor gestational weight gain, inadequate diet, or failure to thrive in the infant or child. WIC provides vouchers for foods high in vitamin A, vitamin C, iron, protein, and calcium. WIC actively promotes breast-feeding. Outcome studies of WIC document higher mean birth weights and higher mean gestational ages in infants born to WIC participants compared to infants born to women who are eligible but not participating. A reduction of LBW and VLBW infants, and better iron status has been documented in WIC-enrolled toddlers and preschool children (Owen, 1997).

A balanced diet that results in appropriate weight gain during pregnancy generally supplies the required vitamins and minerals needed for pregnancy. Routine use of supplements is needed in high-risk pregnancies in undernourished women, women with substance abuse, teenage mothers, women with short interval between pregnancies, women with a history of delivering an LBW infant, and multiple gestations (IOM, 1990). Many studies have found suboptimal nutritional status in women of childbearing ages, regardless of socioeconomic status. Some women growing up in the fast-food era have a limited comprehension of what constitutes "balance."

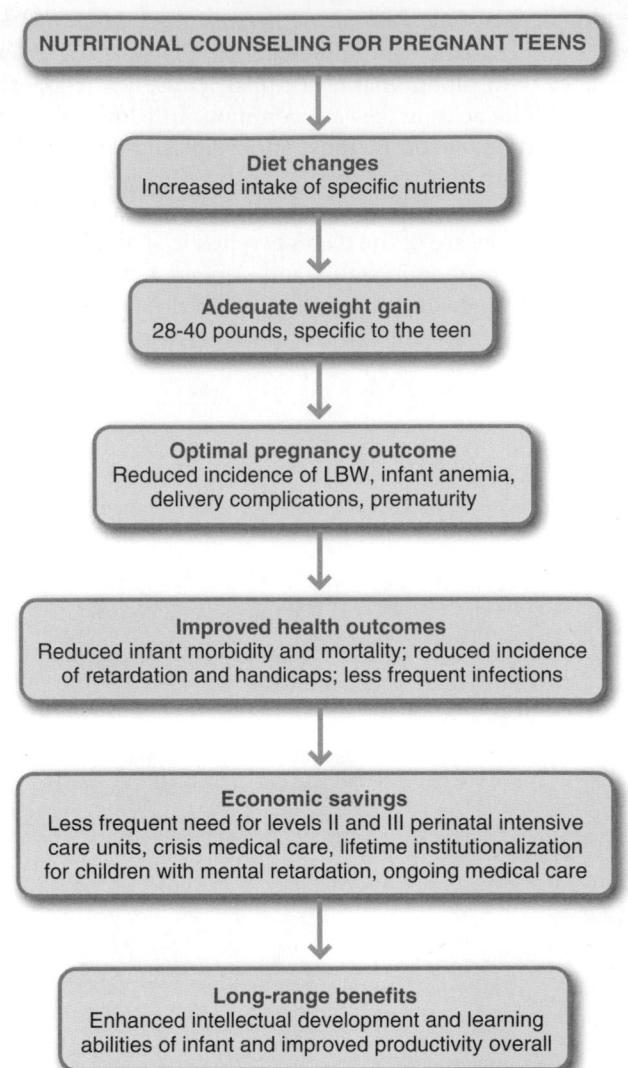

FIGURE 5-3 Benefits of nutritional counseling for pregnant adolescents.

The variability in the composition of prenatal supplements is not widely appreciated. For example, slightly more than 60% of prenatal supplements include the recommended dietary allowance (RDA) for iodine (Pearce et al., 2004). Fortunately they are all high in folate and iron, and supplementation with folate and iron is recommended in all pregnancies. Most health practitioners prescribe a general prenatal vitamin-mineral supplement because of the uncertainty of the woman's nutritional status and intake.

Physiologic Changes of Pregnancy

Blood Volume and Composition

Blood volume expands approximately 50% by the end of pregnancy. This results in decreased hemoglobin, serum albumin, other serum proteins, and water-soluble vitamins. The decline in serum albumin may be the result of fluid accumulation. The decrease in water-soluble vitamin concentrations makes determination of an inadequate intake or a deficient nutrient state difficult. In contrast, serum concen-

TABLE 5-3

Weight Gains of Mothers and Multiple-Birth Babies*

Plurality	Live-Born Infants†	LBW (%) * (<2500 g)	VLBW (%)* (<1500 g)	Maternal Weight by 24 Wk	Weight Gain Total (lb)	Weeks' Gestation	Mean Birth Weight (g)
Singletons	3,899,627	6	1	12	25-35	38-41	3700-4000
Twins	96,445	50	10	24	40-45	36-37	2500-2800
Triplets‡	4168	90	32	36	50-60	34-35	1900-2200

From Luke B: Managing maternal nutrition: prenatal and postpartum, *Perinat Nutr Rep* 3:2, 1997.

*LBW, Low birth weight; *VLBW*, very low birth weight.

†Based on 1994 U.S. vital statistics.

‡Those pregnant with quadruplets should have gained at least 50 lb by 24 weeks.

trations of fat-soluble vitamins and other lipid fractions such as triglycerides, cholesterol, and free fatty acids increase. Unfortunately normative data for early and late gestational vitamin and mineral ranges are not available; therefore it is difficult to make a diagnosis of suboptimal intake by assessing single laboratory data.

Cardiovascular and Pulmonary Function

Increased cardiac output accompanies pregnancy, and cardiac size increases by 12%. Diastolic blood pressure decreases during the first two trimesters because of peripheral vasodilation, but returns to prepregnancy values in the third trimester. Mild lower extremity edema is a normal condition of pregnancy resulting from the pressure of the expanding uterus on the inferior vena cava. Blood return to the heart decreases, leading to decreased cardiac output, a fall in blood pressure, and lower extremity edema. Mild physiologic lower extremity edema is associated with slightly larger babies and a lower rate of prematurity.

Maternal oxygen requirements increase, and the threshold for CO_2 lowers, making the pregnant woman feel dyspneic. Adding to this feeling of dyspnea is the growing uterus pushing the diaphragm upward. Compensation results from more efficient pulmonary gas exchange.

Gastrointestinal Function

During pregnancy the function of the gastrointestinal (GI) system changes in several ways that affect nutritional status. In the first trimester nausea and vomiting may occur, followed by a return of appetite that may be ravenous (see "Nausea and Vomiting" later in the chapter). Cravings for and aversions to foods are common. Increased progesterone concentrations relax the uterine muscle to allow for fetal growth while also decreasing GI motility with increased reabsorption of water. This often results in constipation. In addition, a relaxed lower esophageal sphincter and pressure on the stomach from the growing uterus can cause regurgitation and gastric reflux (see "Heartburn" later in the chapter).

Gallbladder disease represents one of the most common medical problems in pregnancy, affecting approximately 3.5% of pregnant women. Not only does gallbladder emp-

◎ FOCUS ON

Development of Twins

The developmental process of twins is not all the same. The most common development is the dichorionic/diamniotic twins, meaning that each fetus has its own membranes, inner and outer. These are often referred to as *di/di twins*. Sometimes each twin has its own internal sac but shares one outer sac—dichorionic/monoamnionic—or referred to as *di/mono twins*. When both fetuses share one common set of membranes, both the chorion and amnion, they are referred to as *mono-mono twins* and have a very high rate of fetal loss. Cord entanglement is common because there are no separating barriers.

tying becomes less efficient due to the effect of progesterone on muscle contractility, but there is an increase in lysogenicity of bile as well. During the second and third trimester the volume of the gallbladder increases almost twofold, and its ability to empty efficiently is reduced. Constipation and dehydration are also known risk factors for gallstone development, as is a low-calorie diet or poor intake, whatever the etiology.

Celiac disease affects at least one in 100 people in Western Europe and adversely affects the reproductive career of a woman (Hernandez and Green, 2006) (see Chapter 27). Women with celiac disease are at higher risk of spontaneous abortion, LBW infants, and reduced duration of lactation. Celiac disease induces malabsorption and deficiencies of factors essential for organogenesis (e.g., iron, folic acid and vitamin K) (Stazi and Mantovani, 2000). Although gluten-free products are available to replace foods made with wheat and other grains known also to have gliadin inherent in them, not all gluten-free products are enriched with thiamin, riboflavin, and niacin. A survey of 368 gluten-free flours, breads, pastas and cereals demonstrated that only 35 assessed for enrichment were enriched (Thompson, 1999).

The woman with celiac disease planning a pregnancy should be assessed for deficiencies of B vitamins.

Renal Function

The glomerular filtration rate (GFR) increases by 50% during pregnancy, although the volume of urine excreted each day is not increased. Increased blood volume results in an increased GFR with lower serum creatinine and blood urea nitrogen (BUN). Renal tubular resorption is less efficient than in the nonpregnant state, and glucosuria may occur, along with increased excretion of water-soluble vitamins. Small amounts of glycosuria increase the risk for urinary tract infections. Pregnant women with acute pyelonephritis are hospitalized for aggressive antibiotic treatment as there is a high correlation of adult respiratory distress syndrome (ARDS) if left untreated.

TABLE 5-4

Dietary Reference Intakes: Recommended Dietary Allowances and Adequate Intakes for Women

	14-18 Yr of Age	19-50 Yr of Age	Pregnant	Lactating
Energy (kcal)	2368	2403	+10 1st trimester +340 2nd trimester +452 3rd trimester	+330 1st 6 mo +400 2nd 6 mo
Protein (g)	46	46	71	71
Vitamin A (mcg RE)	700	700	770 (>18 yr) 750 (≤18 yr)	1300 (>18 yr) 1200 (≤18 yr)
Vitamin D (mcg) AI	5	5	5	5
Vitamin E (mg α-TE)	8	15	15	19
Vitamin K (mcg)	55	90	90 (>18 yr) 75 (≤18 yr)	90 (>18 yr) 75 (≤18 yr)
Vitamin C (mg)	60	75	85 (>18 yr) 80 (≤18 yr)	20 (>18 yr) 115 (≤18 yr)
Thiamin (mg)	1	1.1	1.4	1.4
Riboflavin (mg)	1	1.1	1.4	1.6
Niacin (mg NE)	14	14	18	17
Vitamin B_6 (mcg)	1.2	1.3	1.9	2
Folate (mcg)*	400	400	600	500
Vitamin B_{12} (mcg)	2.4	2.4	2.6	2.8
Biotin (mcg) AI	25	30	30	35
Pantothenic acid (mg) AI	5	5	6	7
Choline (mg) AI	400	425	450	550
Calcium (mg) AI	1300	1000	1000 (>18 yr) 1300 (≤18 yr)	1000 (>18 yr) 1300 (≤18 yr)
Phosphorus (mg)	1250	700	700 (>18 yr) 1250 (≤18 yr)	700 (>18 yr) 1250 (≤18 yr)
Magnesium (mg)	360	310	350 (>18 yr) 400 (≤18 yr)	310 (>18 yr) 360 (≤18 yr)
Fluoride (mg) AI	3	3	3	3
Iron (mg)	15	18	27	9 (>18 yr) 10 (≤18 yr)
Zinc (mg)	9	8	11 (>18 yr) 12 (≤18 yr)	12 (>18 yr) 13 (≤18 yr)
Iodine (mcg)	150	150	220	290
Selenium (mcg)	55	55	60	70

Modified from Institute of Medicine, Food and Nutrition Board, National Academy of Sciences: *Dietary reference intakes for energy, carbohydrate, fiber, fat, fatty acids, cholesterol, protein, and amino acids,* Washington, DC, 2002, National Academies Press; *Dietary reference intakes for calcium, phosphorus, magnesium, vitamin D, and fluoride,* Washington, DC, 1997, National Academies Press; *Dietary reference intakes for thiamin, riboflavin, niacin, vitamin B_6, folate, vitamin B_{12}, pantothenic acid, biotin and choline,* Washington, DC, 1998, National Academies Press; *Dietary reference intakes for vitamin C, vitamin E, selenium, and carotenoids,* Washington, DC, 2000, National Academies Press; *Dietary reference intakes for vitamin A, vitamin K, boron, chromium, copper, iodine, iron, manganese, molybdenum, nickel, silicon, vanadium, and zinc,* Washington, DC, 2001, National Academies Press.

*This is synthetic folic acid from fortified foods or supplements.

RE, retinol equivalents; *AI,* adequate intake; α-*TE,* alpha-tocopherol; *NE,* niacin equivalents.

Placenta

The placenta is the principal site of production for several hormones responsible for regulating fetal growth and development of maternal support tissues and it is the conduit for exchange of nutrients, oxygen, and waste products. Placental insults compromise the ability to nourish the fetus, regardless of how well nourished the mother. Placental insults can be the result of poor placentation from early pregnancy or small infarcts associated with preeclampsia or hypertension disorders. Placental size can be 15% to 20% below normal in fetuses with IUGR. A small placenta has a smaller surface area of placental villi, with a reduced functional capacity. Sometimes twins share the same placenta, and issues of placental perfusion arise where one fetus transfuses the other, to the detriment of both. This is called *twin-to-twin transfusion syndrome (TTTS)* and has a high rate of mortality.

Nutritional Requirements

Fetal growth and pregnancy demand additional nutrients, and these requirements are defined in the new dietary reference intakes (DRIs), which include adequate intakes (AIs) and RDAs (see inside front cover and Table 5-4).

Energy

Additional energy is required during pregnancy to support the metabolic demands of pregnancy and fetal growth. Metabolism increases by 15% in pregnancy. The 2002 DRIs for energy for the pregnant female are the same as for the nonpregnant female in the first trimester but then increase an additional 340 to 360 kcal/day during the second trimester and another 112 kcal/day in the third trimester (IOM, 2002).

If maternal weight gain is within the desirable limits, the range of acceptable energy intakes varies widely, given individual differences in energy output and basal metabolic rate.

At the origination of the IOM guidelines there was no established "kcal/kilograms of body weight" formula based on BMI to achieve IOM target weight goals (Erick, 2005). In pregnancy there can be many measured weights or "kilograms." There is the "actual pregravid weight in kilograms," or the "desirable pregravid body weight in kilograms," as well the "actual kilograms of body weight at a set time in the gestation" and the "adjusted pregravid body weight in kilograms." The lack of definition has created problems of assigning appropriate calories based on "kcal/kg body weight" and BMI (see *Clinical Insight:* Calculating Pregnancy Energy Requirements).

Exercise. Energy expended in voluntary physical activity is the largest variable in overall energy expenditure. Physical activity increases energy expenditure proportional to body weight. However, most pregnant women compensate for increased weight gain by slowing work pace; thus total daily energy expenditure may not be substantially greater than before pregnancy.

Excessive exercise, combined with inadequate energy intake, may lead to suboptimal maternal weight gain and poor fetal growth; therefore a pregnant woman should always discuss exercise with her primary health practitioner. Acute insults at early gestation, resulting in rapid drop in oxygen delivery to the fetal brain at a time when neurogenesis and neural migration are at their peak, can result in the death of neurons, including Purkinje cells in the cerebellum,

---

✺ CLINICAL INSIGHT

Calculating Pregnancy Energy Requirements

A 5'5" woman with a pregravid weight of 250 lb or 113.6 kg has a BMI of 33.5. She arrives for care at 12 weeks' gestation with a 20-lb (9-kg) weight loss due to hyperemesis gravidarum. She is now 230 lb (104.5 kg). According to the Institute of Medicine, an acceptable weight gain at this time is zero pounds; however, at term she is expected to gain at least 15 lb. Currently she has an 8% loss. Her ideal pregravid body weight range is 124 to 139 lb (56 to 63 kg), assuming the 2-inch heel rule. Using a 30 kcal/kg recommendation for first-trimester needs:

Scenario No. 1: 30 kcal/kg × Upper range IBW =
30 kcal/kg × 63 kg = 1890 kcal

Scenario No. 2: 30 kcal/kg ×
Current real time obese with weight loss =
30 kcal/kg x 104.5 kg × 230 lb) = 3136 kcal

Scenario No. 3: 30 kcal/kg × actual pregravid body weight =
30 kcal/kg × 113.6 kg (250 lb) = 3409 kcal

Note that the definition of kilogram changes the amount of calories in the answer—there is a range of 1890 to 3409 kcal!

Which of these formulas is appropriate at this point in gestation (i.e., 12 weeks), and which of them can be expected to generate a 15-lb weight gain at term? To achieve a gain of 15 lb over pregravid body weight, a total 25-lb gain is necessary to bring this woman to the desired level. Which number for calorie requirements is correct? This clinical reality needs to be appreciated for the complexity it generates: overprescribing calorie requirements adds real weight to a mother and fetus. Underprescribing calories results in weight loss and the mobilization of adipose stores and subsequent ketone production, which may adversely impact neonatal IQ. What is your answer?

pyramidal cells in the hippocampus and cortical neurons, and a slowing of neural mitigation, at least in the hippocampus (Rees and Inder, 2005).

Exercising during pregnancy at high altitudes may compromise fetal oxygen delivery. Resting uterine blood flow is lower in residents residing at 3100 m than at 1600 m, and blood flow is likely to decrease further during exercise in proportion to the intensity and duration. A more conservative stance regarding exercise at elevations over 1600 m during pregnancy may need consideration (Entin and Coffin, 2004) (see *Focus On: Exercise in Pregnancy*).

Consequences of Energy Restriction.

A once popular concept held that the fetus develops at the expense of the mother during nutritional deprivation. However, evidence from famines in Holland and Germany during World War II (see p. 163) clearly contradicts this assumption. It is now accepted that an inadequately nourished mother is proportionately less affected than her fetus. One consequence of severe energy restriction is increased ketone production. Although the fetus has a limited ability to metabolize ketone bodies, the short- and long-term effects of maternal ketonemia are unclear. Both animal and human data indicate that ketone bodies are normally presented to the fetal brain at various times during pregnancy. After an overnight fast, maternal blood ketone body concentrations are greater in pregnant than in nonpregnant women, and even ketonuria can be detected. Ketones are the result of fat metabolism and are suspected of being more detrimental to the fetus in a pregnancy complicated by insulin-dependent diabetes mellitus.

Protein

There is an additional protein requirement for a pregnant woman to support the synthesis of maternal and fetal tissues, but the magnitude of this increase is uncertain. Protein requirement increases throughout gestation and is maximum during the third trimester. The current RDA of 0.66 g/kg/day of protein for pregnant women is the same as that for the nonpregnant women in the first half of pregnancy and increases for the second half to 71 g/day (IOM, 2002) (see Table 5-5). For each additional fetus another 25 g/day of protein is recommended.

Protein deficiency during pregnancy has adverse consequences, but limited intakes of protein and energy usually occur together, making it difficult to separate the effects of energy deficiency from those of protein deficiency. Providing extra energy to a pregnant woman influences pregnancy outcome equal to that of providing both energy and protein. Thus it appears that an energy deficit rather than a protein deficit determines an unfavorable pregnancy outcome.

Carbohydrates

For the first time, DRIs for carbohydrates in pregnancy are presented. The estimated average requirement (EAR) is 135 g/day, and the AI is 175 g/day (IOM, 2002) (see Chapter 12). This 135 to 175 g/day is the recommended amount to provide enough calories in the diet to prevent ketosis and maintain appropriate blood glucose during pregnancy. This 175 grams translates to 700 calories and is 35% of an average 2000 calorie/day regime. Careful choices are needed to include all the nutrients for pregnancy in the daily diet.

◎ FOCUS ON

Exercise in Pregnancy

Exercise programs have become increasingly popular with the heightened concern about weight control, particularly during the reproductive years when some women have a tendency to gain weight as a result of overeating, labor-saving devices, and transportation. Health care providers need to espouse the benefits of activity for many while discussing the risks of exercise for a few during pregnancy.

Research shows that continuing a regular exercise regimen throughout pregnancy reduces subcutaneous fat deposition in midpregnancy and subcutaneous fat retention in late pregnancy. Rate of weight gain is diminished after the 15th week, and the overall weight gain is reduced but remains well within the normal range. Additional outcome data confirm that the incidence of obstetric complications in women who continue a regular exercise regimen throughout pregnancy is either unchanged or reduced.

The potential benefits of prenatal exercise include improved fitness, prevention of gestational diabetes, facilitation of labor, and reduced stress. A healthy fetus is generally able to compensate for periods of transitory stress that occur during maternal exercise. However, a pregnant women should follow particular guidelines to avoid extreme stress to either herself or the fetus. Guidelines for exercise during pregnancy have been developed by the American College of Obstetricians and Gynecologists (ACOG, 2002). Some women have unidentified preexisting health problems; thus it is advised that women wanting to embark on an exercise routine in pregnancy be sure to talk to their health providers before initiation. Most providers will encourage the effort.

A woman who is just beginning an exercise program during pregnancy should exercise at a level that keeps her heart rate below 140 beats/min. A good fitness program would be 1 hour of physical activity 3 days per week, with an intensity that keeps the maternal heart between 120 and 130 beats/min. The types of exercise that provide the best cardiovascular and psychologic benefits with the least pregnancy risks are brisk walking, stationary cycling, and swimming.

Fiber

Daily consumption of whole-grain breads and cereals, leafy green and yellow vegetables, and fresh and dried fruits should be encouraged to provide additional minerals, vitamins, and fiber. The DRI for fiber during pregnancy is 28 g/day (IOM, 2002). Careful attention to the selection of foods that are also good sources of iron and folic acid is important (see Chapters 3 and 31).

Lipids

There is no DRI for lipids during pregnancy. The amount of fat in the diet should depend on energy requirements for proper weight gain. However, for the first time there is a recommendation (an AI of 13 g/day) for the amount of n-6 polyunsaturated fatty acids (linoleic acid) and an AI of 1.4 g/day for the amount of n-3 polyunsaturated fatty acids (α-linolenic acid) in the diet (IOM, 2002).

Vitamins

Certain vitamins have particular significance for optimal pregnancy outcome. In some instances the provision of these specific vitamins may be met through diet, and for others a vitamin-mineral supplement is necessary. Periconceptional multivitamin supplementation has been documented to reduce the risk of heart defects in infants by 43% if started very early in pregnancy (Bailey and Berry, 2005).

Folic Acid. Folic acid requirements increase during pregnancy in response to the demands of maternal erythropoiesis and fetal and placental growth and, most important, for the prevention of NTDs. The RDA for folic acid in pregnancy is 600 mcg, a 200 mcg increase over that for nonpregnant females. The IOM recommends that 400 mcg of the 600 mcg/day be provided by folate-fortified foods or supplements because it is better absorbed, with 200 mcg from food and beverages (IOM, 1998). A tolerable upper intake level (UL) is 800 to 1000 mcg/day from fortified foods or supplements (IOM, 1998).

Folic acid deficiency is marked by a reduced rate of deoxyribonucleic acid (DNA) synthesis and mitotic activity in individual cells. Megaloblastic anemia is the latest stage of folate deficiency, and it may not present until the third trimester; however, white cell morphologic and biochemical changes signaling deficiency may precede overt anemia (see Chapter 31). In experimental animals maternal folate deficiency is associated with an increased incidence of congenital malformations. Malformations can also occur in infants of women using folate antagonist drugs such as the anticonvulsant medications phenytoin (dilantin), carbamazepine, and diphenylhydantoin. Oral contraceptives and some antibiotics (trimethoprim, triamterene, and carbamazepine) may also cause folate insufficiency (see Chapter 16). Approximately 2500 new cases of NTDs occur in the United States each year. Moreover, NTDs have a fairly high recurrence rate in future pregnancies (i.e., approximately 2% to 10%).

Two randomized trials in Europe in the early 1990s strengthened the association between periconceptional supplementation with folic acid and the prevention of NTDs. In the Medical Research Council (MRC) Vitamin Study, 1817 women who had previously delivered an infant with an NTD were randomized to receive a folic acid supplement, a multivitamin supplement, folic acid plus the multivitamin supplement, or placebo. The group that received the folic acid supplement demonstrated a 72% reduction in the risk of recurrence of an NTD. So striking were the results that the trial was halted early (MRC, 1991). The second study of 5520 European women demonstrated that periconceptual supplementation with a multivitamin containing 800 mcg of folic acid reduced the incidence of NTDs (Czeizel, 1994).

Red blood cell (RBC) folate concentrations exceeding 906 mmol/L (400 ng/ml) are associated with the fewest NTDs. In a study of 189 healthy women attempting to become pregnant, only one in four women had RBC folate levels greater than 906 mmol/L. Women who consumed only food sources of folate had the lowest folate intake and the lowest RBC folate concentrations. Only those women who consumed folic acid supplements in addition to dietary folate achieved RBC folate concentrations considered to be optimal for protection against NTDs.

The Centers for Disease Control and Prevention (CDC) have recommended that all women of childbearing age increase their intake of folic acid because 50% of all U.S. pregnancies are unplanned and the neural tube closes by 28 days of gestation (before most women realize they are pregnant). Therefore supplementation with folic acid should begin before conception—hence the CDC's general recommendation to increase folate intake throughout the childbearing years. The Food and Drug Administration (FDA) has mandated that grain products such as bread, rice, and pasta be enriched with folic acid. All women of childbearing age should be encouraged to take a folic acid supplement and to include generous amounts of folic acid food sources in their diets.

Women who smoke, consume moderate-to-heavy alcohol, or use recreational drugs are at risk for marginal folate status, as are those using oral contraceptives, antiseizure medications (such as phenytoin), and those with malabsorption syndromes. Women using antiseizure medications must be closely monitored when starting folic acid because folic acid supplementation can reduce seizure threshold.

Fewer than 40% of U.S. women are taking folic acid supplements periconceptually as evidenced from a telephone survey through the California Teratogen Information Service between 2003 and 2004. Three hundred twenty seven women were called to assess attitudes and compliance toward advice to continue vitamin use following pregnancy to be protected in a future pregnancy (Goldberg et al., 2006).

Not all countries have a folate food fortification program in place. Currently only the United States, Canada, and Chile have programs and have documented the reduction of NTDs by 31% to 78% (Eichholzer et al., 2006).

Choline. Choline is considered an essential nutrient because it cannot be synthesized in sufficient quantities to meet metabolic demands. It is needed for structural integrity of cell membranes, cell signaling, and nerve impulse transmission and is a major source of methyl groups, as is folate (Williams, 2005). IOM recommends choline at 450 mg/day during pregnancy, 25 mg more than for the nonpregnant woman. Choline has been shown to alter brain structure and function in rats whose mothers were supplemented in the last trimester (Zeisel and Niculescu, 2006). Choline has also been shown to protect against memory loss after grand mal seizures and prevents the development of memory impairment in offspring of alcoholic mothers. Foods containing high amounts of choline are beef liver, pork, chicken, turkey, fish, egg yolks, soy lecithin, and wheat germ. Supplementation may be needed to meet DRIs since the mean intake for females in the United States is 314 mg/day (Cho et al., 2006).

Vitamin B₆. The RDA for vitamin B_6 during pregnancy is 1.9 mg/day. The additional 0.6 mg above that recommended for nonpregnant adult women provides for increased needs associated with synthesis of nonessential amino acids in growth and vitamin B–dependent niacin synthesis from tryptophan. The UL for vitamin B_6 is 80 to 100 mg/day (IOM, 1998).

Vitamin B_6 has also been used to manage severe nausea and vomiting in pregnancy. Although this vitamin catalyzes a number of reactions involving neurotransmitter production, it is not known whether this function is involved in the relief of symptoms. Megadoses of vitamin B_6 (25 mg three times per day) are presumed to achieve antiemetic effects; therefore its administration should be closely monitored (Jewel and Young, 2002). The mechanism by which vitamin B_6 functions to reportedly decrease emesis has not been elucidated, but the vitamin functions as a cofactor in approximately 50 decarboxylase and transaminase enzymes.

Ascorbic Acid. An additional 10 mg/day of vitamin C is recommended for pregnant women. The total recommendation of 80 to 85 mg/day is met by the diet (IOM, 2000) if five servings of fruit are selected a day. Although ascorbic acid deficiency has not been associated with adverse pregnancy outcome in large population studies, a few studies have suggested an association between low plasma levels of vitamin C and preeclampsia, as well as premature rupture of the membranes (PROM) (Woods, 2001). The concept that excessive vitamin C in pregnancy can result in "rebound scurvy" in the neonate was articulated in only one paper and is not thought to be of concern.

Vitamin A. The RDA for vitamin A is 770 mcg of retinol equivalents (RAEs) or 2564 international units (IU) for pregnant and nonpregnant women. Maternal stores of vitamin A easily meet fetal accretion rate. Vitamin A deficiency is teratogenic in experimental animals, but confirmatory evidence in humans is lacking (see *Clinical Insight:* Nutritional Deficiency in a Pregnancy Postbariatric Surgery).

Recently it has been shown that vitamin A plays a role in gene expression for acrosin and plasminogen activators, which are important for spermatogenesis in rams (Zervos et al., 2005). In human cord blood vitamin A concentrations correlated with birth weight, head circumference, length, and gestation duration.

In contrast to a number of earlier reports that 10,000 IU or more of vitamin A increased the risk for a **neural crest defect,** the National Institutes of Health (NIH) issued an alert announcing that moderate doses of vitamin A (8,000 to 10,000 IU do not pose a risk for birth defects (NICHD, 2001). However, the alert cautions against the use of large doses of vitamin A such as unintentional intakes greater than 30,000 IU. Women who are taking the vitamin A analog, Accutane, for acne and become pregnant are at extremely high risk for fetal anomalies. Women who have high vitamin A in their diets, such as from large proportions of animal liver on a regular basis, need to be closely evaluated.

Vitamin D. The AI for vitamin D is 5 mcg (200 international units (IU)/day in pregnant and nonpregnant women. The DRIs also suggest a UL of 50 mcg (2000 IU)/day during pregnancy (IOM, 1997). Vitamin D has long been appreciated for its positive effects on calcium balance during pregnancy. This vitamin and its metabolites cross the placenta and appear in fetal blood in the same concentration as in maternal circulation. Emerging data suggest additional roles for vitamin D, including enhanced immune function and brain development (Feron et al, 2005). Vitamin D may

✦ CLINICAL INSIGHT

Nutritional Deficiency in a Pregnancy After Bariatric Surgery

This woman had a biliopancreatic diversion for morbid obesity in 1987. Eight years later in 1995, she became pregnant for the first time, and she bore a healthy infant. Her second pregnancy in 1999 resulted in a spontaneous abortion at 10 weeks' gestation. The male infant from her third pregnancy in 2000 was born at almost 35 weeks' gestation and weighed 1935 g (25th percentile) and had a head circumference of 45 cm (30th percentile). His plasma vitamin A concentration was <0.1 mg/L (normal range 0.3 to 0.9 mg/L) and he was vitamin A deficient. Mom reported that during her pregnancy she was taking a children's multivitamin containing 2500 IU of vitamin A, which is 100% of the usual recommended for a pregnant woman. She said that she experienced night-blindness during her pregnancy (Huerta et al., 2002).

Because of changes in digestive and absorptive capacities after gastric or intestinal bypass, women who have had these surgeries and who are pregnant require extra attention to their diets and their use of appropriate nutritional supplements (Mason et al., 2005). They may require more than pregnant women who have not had these surgeries.

have a role in cytokine (Th_1 and Th_2) regulation and is implicated in multiple sclerosis and recurrent pregnancy loss. Evidence suggests that low vitamin D levels during pregnancy predispose to preeclampsia, a hypertensive condition of pregnancy affecting up to 8% of pregnant women (Hypponen, 2005).

Maternal vitamin D deficiency is associated with neonatal hypocalcemia and hypoplasia of tooth enamel. Fetal bone mineralization may be affected by maternal vitamin D deficiency. Vitamin D blood concentrations are often low in infants born to vitamin D–deficient mothers, and vitamin D deficiency is increasingly recognized in dark-skinned and veiled women in the United States and northern European countries where sun exposure is low (van der Meer et al., 2006).

Excessive amounts of vitamin D may be harmful during gestation. One case of severe infantile hypercalcemia has been reported in a newborn when maternal ingestion was excessive.

Vitamin E. Vitamin E requirements are increased during pregnancy, but vitamin E deficiency in humans is rare and has not been linked with reduced fertility or fetal malformations as it has in animals. However, the 2000 RDA of 15 mg of α-tocopherol for nonpregnant women is the same as for the pregnant woman (IOM, 2000). The UL is set at 800 mg/day for pregnant women 18 years of age or younger and 1000 mg/day for pregnant women 19 to 50 years old (IOM, 2000).

Vitamin K. The RDA for vitamin K during pregnancy (90 mcg/day for adult women ages 19 to 50) applies to nonpregnant women as well (IOM, 2002). Usual diets provide adequate amounts of vitamin K; no ULs are defined for vitamin K during pregnancy. Vitamin K also has a role in bone health, so adequate amounts during pregnancy are important. Vitamin K deficiency in pregnancy has been reported (Robinson et al., 1998).

Minerals

Calcium. Hormonal factors strongly influence calcium metabolism in pregnant women. Human chorionic somatomammotropin from the placenta increases the rate of maternal bone turnover. Estrogen, also largely derived from the placenta, inhibits bone resorption, provoking a compensatory release of parathyroid hormone, which maintains maternal serum calcium while enhancing maternal absorption of calcium across the gut. The net effect of these changes, which predates fetal skeletal mineralization, is the promotion of progressive calcium retention to meet progressively increasing fetal skeletal demands for mineralization. Fetal hypercalcemia and subsequent endocrine adjustments ultimately stimulate the mineralization process.

Approximately 30 g of calcium is accumulated during pregnancy, almost all of it in the fetal skeleton (25 g). The remainder is stored in the maternal skeleton, presumably held in reserve for the calcium demands of lactation. Most fetal accretion occurs during the last trimester of pregnancy, an average of 300 mg/day.

The latest AI for calcium during pregnancy is 1300 mg/day for women 18 years old or younger and 1000 mg/day for women 19 years old or older with a singleton pregnancy. This recommendation is the same as that for nonpregnant females because the hormonal changes of pregnancy increase the absorption and use of calcium. Daily intakes less than the AI may cause increased calcium loss from the maternal skeleton. Multiparous women with poor calcium intake can develop osteomalacia.

The UL for calcium during pregnancy is 2500 mg/day. Overconsumption of calcium in food form is not common; however, elevated serum level of calcium can be the result of excess antacid ingestion for heartburn of pregnancy or gastroesophageal reflux disease (GERD), and dangerous levels of calcium from "milk-alkali syndrome" have been reported (Gordon et al, 2005).

Phosphorus. The RDA for phosphorus is the same for pregnant and nonpregnant women: 1250 mg/day for women younger than 19 years of age and 700 mg/day for those 19 years of age and older. The UL during pregnancy is 3500 mg/day.

Phosphorus is found in such a wide variety of foods that deficiency is rare when one is eating. Low phosphorous levels can be found in women experiencing hyperemesis gravidarum. Hypophosphatemia can be life threatening because phosphorous is important in energy metabolism as a component of adenosine triphosphate (ATP) (Marinella, 2005).

Iron. A marked increase in the maternal blood supply during pregnancy greatly increases the demand for iron. Normal erythrocyte volume increases by 20% to 30% in pregnancy. A pregnant woman must consume an additional 700 to 800 mg of iron throughout her pregnancy: 500 mg for hematopoiesis and 250 to 300 mg for fetal and placental tissues. Most accretion occurs after the 20th week of gestation when maternal and fetal demands are greatest. Iron requirements are increased; therefore the 2001 RDA for iron during pregnancy is 27 mg/day, an increase of 9 mg/day over that for the nonpregnant woman, and 12 mg/day over that for the nonpregnant teen. The UL is 45 mg/day (IOM, 2001).

Rarely do women become pregnant with sufficient iron stores to cover the physiologic needs of pregnancy. Therefore iron supplementation, usually in the form of ferrous salts, is often necessary to prevent iron deficiency anemia. Maternal anemia, defined by a hematocrit less than 32% and a hemoglobin level less than 11 g/dl, occurs in some pregnant women who do not use iron supplements or who are anemic when they enter pregnancy. An anemic woman poorly tolerates hemorrhage with delivery, which subsequently increases cardiac stress. An anemic woman is also more prone to develop puerperal infection.

The fetal effects of maternal anemia are poorly understood. Some data suggest that fetal effects are relatively mild, but several reports suggest that pregnancy outcome may be compromised. It might be hypothesized that poor iron consumption leads to poor hemoglobin production, followed by compromised delivery of oxygen to the uterus, placenta, and developing fetus. The added workload of the heart from maternal anemia with increased cardiac output could compromise the pregnancy.

It is recommended that all pregnant women, even those eating a well-balanced diet, take 30 mg of ferrous iron supplement daily in divided doses during the second and third trimesters as fetal iron needs are increasing (IOM, 1990). Further, for optimal absorption, the iron supplement should ideally be taken between meals and not with milk, tea, or coffee, because they interfere with absorption. Beverages containing ascorbic acid enhance absorption.

If iron deficiency anemia is diagnosed, therapy consists of 60 to 120 mg of ferrous iron in divided doses throughout the day. Iron supplements greater than 56 mg per dose interfere with zinc absorption and should be avoided. When hemoglobin returns to a level appropriate for the women's stage of pregnancy, 30 mg/day in divided doses may be resumed (IOM, 1990) (see Chapter 31). Iron in divided doses may be better tolerated but, on a practical level, divided doses are often forgotten.

Excessive amounts of iron should be avoided because it has been implicated in the pathogenesis of preeclampsia and gestational diabetes (Erick, 2005). Elevated maternal hemoglobin concentrations (>13.2 g/dl) are associated with increased fetal risk and maternal hypertension and are often observed in the pregnant woman who smokes. Elevated hemoglobin may reflect a failure in plasma volume expansion that negatively influences the uteroplacental circulation.

Zinc. The 2001 RDA for zinc is 11 to 13 mg during pregnancy, 3 to 5 mg more than for the nongravid woman (IOM, 2001). Data from NHANES III suggest that the average total zinc intake is approximately 11.1 mg and 13 mg in adults, owing to zinc included in supplements. A zinc-deficient diet does not result in the effective mobilization of zinc stored in the maternal skeleton; therefore a compromised zinc status develops rapidly.

Animal studies of zinc status in gestation have shown that zinc deficiency is highly teratogenic in rats and leads to the development of a variety of congenital malformations. Non-human primates are also affected by zinc deficiency, which results in abnormal brain development in the fetus and abnormal behavior in the newborn. Women in developing countries with low plasma zinc concentrations are 2.5 times more at risk for delivering an infant weighing less than 2000 g, with women younger than 19 years old being even more at risk; plasma zinc level in the mother correlates with plasma zinc level in the offspring (Rwebembera et al., 2005; Scheplyagina, 2005).

Maternal zinc status may be inversely related to the degree of prenatal iron supplementation since excess iron ingestion inhibits zinc absorption (IOM, 1990). The UL for zinc intake during pregnancy is 34 mg/day for the pregnant teen and 40 mg/day for the pregnant woman ages 19 to 50 years old.

Copper. Diets of pregnant women are often marginal in copper; however, it has not been determined if moderate dietary copper deficiency affects the developing human fetus. Copper deficiency is teratogenic in animals. The RDA for copper during pregnancy is 1000 mcg/day, 100 mcg/day more than for the nonpregnant female (IOM, 2001). Excessive iron supplementation inhibits copper absorption. The UL for copper is 8000 mcg/day for the woman 18 years and younger and 10,000 mcg/day for the 19- to 50-year-old pregnant woman, the same as for a nonpregnant individual.

Sodium. The hormonal milieu of pregnancy affects sodium metabolism. Increased maternal blood volume leads to increased glomerular filtration of sodium of 5,000 to 10,000 mEq/day. Compensatory mechanisms maintain fluid and electrolyte balance.

Restriction of dietary sodium or the use of diuretics in pregnant women with edema is not recommended. Rigorous sodium restriction in pregnant animals stresses the renin-angiotensin-aldosterone system and results in water intoxication and renal and adrenal tissue necrosis.

Although moderation in the use of salt and other sodium-rich foods is appropriate for everyone, aggressive restriction is usually unwarranted in pregnancy, and consumption of sodium should remain above 2 to 3 g/day. The salt selected should be iodized salt.

Magnesium. The RDA of 350 to 400 mg of magnesium in pregnancy is an increase of 40 mg over that for the nonpregnant women. The term fetus accumulates 1 g of magnesium during gestation. The IOM reports that magnesium supplementation during pregnancy reduces the incidence of preeclampsia and IUGR. However, the IOM has also set an UL for magnesium from supplements or pharmacologic agents (outside of food and beverages) during pregnancy at 350 mg/day (IOM, 1997). (See "Edema and Leg Cramps" later in the chapter for a further discussion of the role of magnesium.)

Fluoride. The role of fluoride in prenatal development is controversial. Development of primary dentition begins at 10 to 12 weeks' gestation; from the sixth to the ninth month, the first four permanent molars and eight of the permanent incisors are forming. Thus 32 teeth are developing during gestation. Controversy involves the extent to which fluoride is transported across the placenta and its value *in utero* in the development of caries-resistant permanent teeth (see Chapter 25). The AI for fluoride in pregnancy is 3 mg/day, and the UL is 10 mg/day (IOM, 1997).

Iodine. An additional increment of 70 mcg of iodine has been added to the RDA of 150 mcg for females to make the RDA for iodine during pregnancy 220 mcg/day. The UL in pregnancy is set at 900 to 1100 mcg/day (IOM, 2001). The only known role of iodine is in the thyroxine molecule. The thyroxine hormone has critical roles in metabolism of macronutrients. Maternal iodine deficiency has long been recognized as a cause of neonatal cretinism. Suboptimal iodine intake without overt deficiency in the pregnant women may compromise fetal development, even in the absence of cretinism, leading to developmental delays in the infant (Ohara et al., 2004). Previous studies established that preconception iodine supplementation prevents endemic cretinism. In instances in which preconception iodine intake cannot be ensured, supplementation before the end of the second trimester can also protect the fetal brain from the effects of iodine deficiency (see Chapter 3).

Approximately 2.2 billion, or 38% worldwide, are at risk for iodine deficiency, and the etiologies vary widely. Low intake of sea products and fish (because of cost, dislike, or allergy); intakes of produce grown in iodine-deficient soils; food industry use of noniodized salt; exposure to cigarette smoke, which contains cyanate, which prevents iodine uptake; and variable iodization of salt, can all contribute to low iodine levels (Erick, 2005).

In a study of iodine in bread products in the Boston area, three samples were found with over 313 mcg/slice, and the remaining 15 samples with 2.2 to 54 mcg/slice (Pearce et al., 2004). A study of 230 infants in New Zealand found that formula-fed babies had an average urinary iodine excretion (UIE) of 99 mcg/L, whereas breast-fed babies averaged only 44 mcg/L (Skeaff et al., 2005). Clearly the maternal diet needs higher iodine supplementation, and the prenatal supplements need careful review.

The Philippines is considered to be an iodine-deficient country. In a study evaluating 44 infant-mother pairs 24 hours after delivery, 18% of the neonates had a UIE of less than 10 mcg/dl (deficient), whereas 71% had values between 10 and 30 mcg/dl (normal) and 11% of the neonates had high values >30 mcg/dl (Chan-Cua et al., 2003). The results of this small study require further attention by public health officials, and the iodine intake of pregnant women appears to vary widely. Other factors such as the potential presence of perchlorates in the environment may also play a role.

Since pregnant women seeking health care come with their own personal history of nutrition and dietary issues, it is critical that providers appreciate agricultural issues of the country of origin. As an example, the iodine levels in the Pakistani general diet have been deemed below the intakes recommended by the IOM in the U.S. (Akhter et al., 2004). An evaluation of the diets of university students in East Germany pointed out that canteen (dormitory) meals contained approximately 50% of the daily recommended iodine intake (Brauer et al., 2005). One hundred and twenty three pregnant Turkish women were evaluated for urinary iodine excretion and were found to be mildly iodine deficient in the first and third trimesters and moderately so in the second trimester according to WHO Criteria (Gultepe et al., 2005).

There are few reliable databases for iodine, making it difficult to ascertain dietary intake. The etiology of these reported low levels of iodine intake are not fully elucidated. Recent findings in the United States of an industrial pollutant, perchlorate, that is generated from rocket fuel and firework production, show that it inhibits iodine uptake and may impair thyroid and neurodevelopment in infants (Kirk et al., 2005). Most important, insufficient iodine intake has been associated with increased miscarriage rates and spontaneous abortion (Redmond, 2004).

Guide for Eating During Pregnancy

Recommended Food Intake

The increased requirements of pregnancy can be met by following the Daily Food Guide presented in Table 5-5.

TABLE 5-5

Daily Food Guide for Females

Food Group	Minimum Number of Servings		
	Nonpregnant 11- to 24-Year-Olds	Nonpregnant 25- to 50-Year-Olds	Pregnant or Lactating 11- to 50-Year-Olds
Protein, foods	5*	5*	7†
Milk products	3	2	3
Breads, grains	7	6	7
Whole-grain	4	4	4
Enriched	3	3	3
Fruits, vegetables	5	5	5
Vitamin C rich	1	1	1
β-carotene rich	1	1	1
Folate rich	1	1	1
Other	2	2	2
Unsaturated fats	3	3	3

Modified from *Nutrition during pregnancy and the postpartum period: a manual for health care professionals,* 1990, California Department of Health Services, Maternal Child Health Branch.

*Equivalent in protein to 5 oz of animal protein; at least three servings per week should be from the vegetable proteins.

†Equivalent in protein to 7 oz of animal protein; at least one of these servings should be a vegetable protein.

Calcium Intake

A number of milk choices are available: whole milk, low-fat milk, skim milk, nonfat powdered milk, buttermilk, acidophilus milk, Lactaid-treated milk, evaporated milk, enriched soy milk, enriched rice milk, enriched nut milks, and yogurt. Goat milk is also available but historically has had low folate content. Approximately ⅓ cup of dried skim milk is equivalent to 1 cup of fluid milk. Milk can be made richer in calcium, protein, and calories by adding 2 tablespoons of dried nonfat milk to a glass of fluid milk.

Not all milk products are fortified with vitamin D_3, a derivative from an animal source. Some soymilks are fortified with vitamin D_2; as a nonanimal source, this may be preferred by vegans (Armas et al, 2004). Vitamin D_2 potency is less than one third of that of vitamin D_3. However, some non-dairy milks have no vitamin D added at all. If fluid milk is used in limited amounts, a vitamin D supplement is necessary, especially if exposure to sunlight is also limited and the diet lacks other sources.

Many women, primarily non–white and black women, are unable to digest the lactose in milk unless it is taken in small amounts at a time or cooked. If necessary, calcium supplements such as calcium lactate or calcium carbonate may be prescribed (see Chapter 24).

Fluids

Drinking eight to ten glasses of quality fluid daily, mainly water, is encouraged. Although the 2004 report by the National Academies set the AI at 1.5 L/day with a UL of 2.3 L/day, one needs to evaluate a woman's body size as well as climatic conditions. The importance of adequate hydration cannot be overemphasized; however, the caloric contribution of beverages other than water needs to be appreciated. Suboptimal hydration predisposes women in midtrimester and beyond to premature contractions and reduced amniotic fluid volume (Stan et al., 2002; Fait et al., 2003; Margann et al., 2003). Frequent urination is often a complaint from pregnant women; however, the benefits of optimal hydration include reduced risks of urinary tract infections, kidney stones, and constipation.

Pregnant women are usually highly motivated and very receptive to well-presented nutritional advice. A full discussion of individual needs and involvement of the mother (and perhaps her partner or other siblings) in planning dietary changes is usually an effective strategy (Figure 5-4). See Box 5-3 for a suggested menu and Box 5-4 for a summary of nutritional care for the pregnant woman.

Alcohol

Abundant evidence from both animal studies and human experience associates maternal alcohol consumption with **teratogenicity** and a specific pattern of abnormalities in the neonate. It is known as **fetal alcohol syndrome.** Features of this syndrome include prenatal and postnatal growth failure, developmental delay, microcephaly, eye changes (including

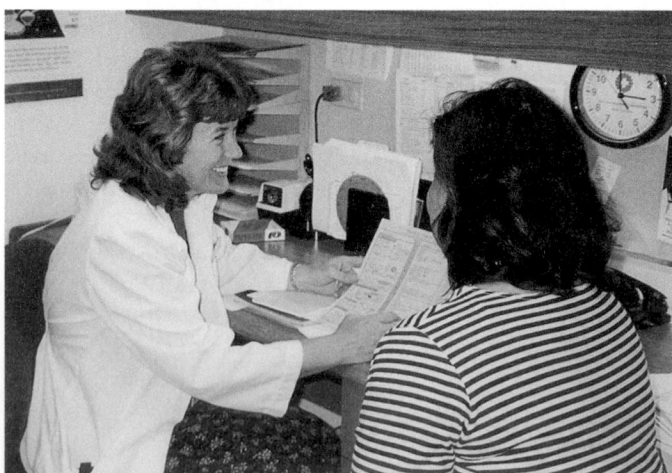

FIGURE 5-4 Nutritionist with client. A prospective mother learns about nutrition during pregnancy.

BOX 5-3
Suggested Menu During Pregnancy*

Breakfast

Orange juice, ½ cup
Oatmeal, ½ cup
Whole-grain or enriched toast, 1 slice
Peanut butter, 2 tsp
Decaffeinated coffee or tea

Midmorning snack

Apple
High-bran cereal, ¼ cup
Nonfat or reduced-fat milk, ½ cup

Lunch

Turkey (2 oz) sandwich on rye or whole-grain bread with lettuce and tomato and 1 tsp mayonnaise
Green salad
Salad dressing, 2 tsp
Fresh peach
Nonfat or low-fat milk, 1 cup

Midafternoon Snack

Nonfat or low-fat milk, 1 cup
Graham crackers, 4 squares

Dinner

Baked chicken breast, 3 oz
Baked potato with 2 tbsp sour cream
Peas and carrots, ½ cup
Green salad
Salad dressing, 2 tsp

Evening snack

Nonfat, yogurt, ½ cup
Fresh strawberries

*Quantities of food should be adjusted to meet individual energy needs to promote appropriate weight gain. Pregnant adolescents and very active or underweight pregnant women require greater quantities.

involvement of the epicanthal fold), facial abnormalities, and skeletal joint abnormalities (Figure 5-5). It is termed *fetal alcohol effects* when a limited number of these features are present.

Use of alcohol during pregnancy has been associated with an increased rate of spontaneous abortion, abruptio placentae, and LBW delivery. The American College of Obstetricians and Gynecologists (ACOG), as well as the March of Dimes and other professional organizations, recommend no alcohol in pregnancy. Because reduced-alcohol wines and beers contain small amounts of alcohol, they are also contraindicated in pregnancy. Despite the multiple

---

BOX 5-4

Summary of Nutritional Care During Pregnancy

1. Energy intake to meet nutritional needs and allow for about a 0.4-kg (14-oz) weight gain per week during the last 30 weeks of pregnancy
2. Protein intake to meet nutritional needs, about an additional 25 g/day; additional 25 g/day/fetus if more than one fetus
3. Sodium intake that is not excessive but is no less than 2-3 g/day
4. Mineral and vitamin intakes to meet the recommended daily allowances (folic acid and possibly iron supplementation is required)
5. Alcohol omitted
6. Caffeine in moderation: less than 200 mg/day—equivalent of 2 cups of coffee

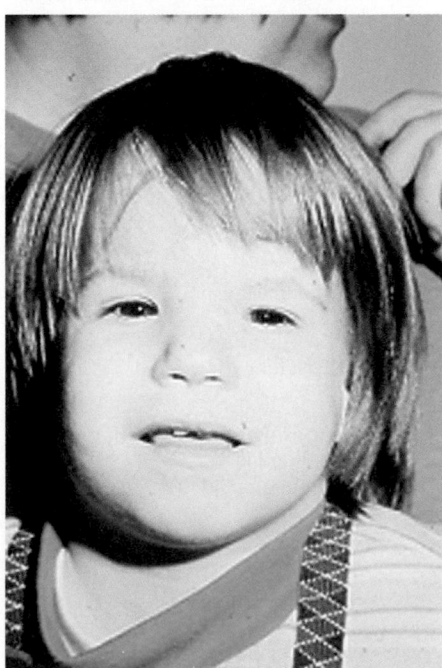

FIGURE 5-5 One-year-old child with fetal alcohol syndrome. *(From Streissguth AP et al: Teratogenic effects of alcohol in humans and laboratory animals, Science 209:353, 1980.)*

warnings of fetal injury caused by alcohol, it has been shown that some women continue to consume alcohol in pregnancy (Houet et al., 2005; Smuts et al., 2003).

The mechanisms by which alcohol affects the fetus are not completely understood. Alcohol may be toxic during blastogenesis and cell differentiation, or fetal damage could be the result of dietary deficiencies or altered metabolism of key nutrients. The nutrients likely to be affected are folic acid, vitamin B_6, niacin, thiamin, magnesium, and zinc; but alcohol affects protein metabolism as well. Alcohol also contains congeners, which are pharmacologically active molecules other than ethanol. In addition to the adverse impact on the developing nervous system, in utero alcohol exposure may have a detrimental impact on metabolism (Yao et al., 2005).

The role of alcohol exposure in rat offspring during pregnancy has been shown to increase insulin resistance. A subset of adult alcohol-exposed rats had fasting hyperglycemia and an exaggerated glycemic response to pyruvate compared with controls. The data suggest that, after prenatal alcohol exposure, the expression of gluconeogenic genes is exaggerated in adult rats and increases gluconeogenesis. In rats these alterations persist through adulthood and may contribute to the pathogenesis of type 2 diabetes.

Nonnutritive Substances in Foods

Caffeine. The effect of caffeine on pregnancy has been extensively researched. Caffeine intake appears to increase the risk of first-trimester spontaneous abortions. Caffeine may not contribute to IUGR or other major complications after the first trimester; however, it appears sensible to limit coffee and caffeine intake during pregnancy, although there are insufficient data for making a specific recommendation (Grosso et al., 2006).

Artificial Sweeteners. There are four types of artificial sweeteners sold in the United States; their chemical names are saccharin, acesulfame-K, sucralose, and aspartame; and their brand names are Sweet 'n' Low, Sunette (or Sweet One), Splenda, Equal, or NutraSweet, respectively.

Saccharin is not classified as a teratogen; however it is weakly, carcinogenic in rats in very high doses. Its consumption in pregnancy has not been restricted. Acesulfame-K consumption by pregnant women is classified as safe; however, there are few or no long-term studies during human pregnancy. Both saccharin and acesulfame-K cross the placenta and appear in breast milk but have no known adverse effect on the fetus or infant.

Sucralose was approved for general use in all foods by the FDA in 1998. It is a carbohydrate derived from sucrose, but it is 600 times sweeter. A 93% to 97% amount of radiolabeled sucralose is eliminated unchanged through the urine and feces within 5 days of ingestion. Approximately 3% is eliminated as glucuronide conjugates of sucralose (Roberts et al., 2000). It has not been found to be mutagenic or teratogenic in high doses in animals. No studies of sucralose in breast milk or during lactation have been reported in the medical literature.

The use of aspartame is unsafe for women with phenylketonuria (PKU) whether or not they are pregnant. Aspartame is metabolized to phenylalanine and aspartic acid. In people without PKU, phenylalanine is rapidly broken down into a relatively harmless substance; persons with PKU lack the enzyme necessary for its conversion. In these individuals brain damage is a consequence of high blood phenylalanine concentrations. High circulating concentrations of phenylalanine are known to damage the fetal brain (see Chapter 44).

Because artificially sweetened soft drinks may substitute for other beverages, including water and beverages that have greater nutritional value such as milk or juice, artificially sweetened beverage use in pregnancy should be discouraged.

Contaminants

Contaminants in food are the exception rather than the rule in the United States, but they do occur. However, dishware with poor glazing and lead crystal decanters for wine or spirits have been found to contain high amounts of lead. Insecticides, pesticides, lawn chemicals, new house out-gassing, and old Teflon pans are all sources of contamination and need to be avoided. In high concentrations, they can pass across the placenta to the fetus (Figure 5-6). Pregnant women should be advised against using dolomite as a calcium supplement because it comes from seashells or sea coral and often contains lead, the result of industrialization.

Methyl Mercury. In January 2001 the USDA and the FDA issued a warning for pregnant and lactating women and women of childbearing age to limit consumption of shark, mackerel, tilefish, tuna, and swordfish to no more than two times a week in 4-oz portions. Traces of methyl mercury are found in most fish, but concentrations may be higher in fish from waters close to areas of industrial mercury pollution. The usual concentration of methyl mercury in most fish ranges from less than 0.01 ppm to 0.5 ppm. Few species of fish reach the FDA limit for human consumption of 1 ppm except shark, swordfish, large tuna (the type used to make sushi or fresh steaks), tilefish, and king mackerel. Fresh-water predatory species such as pike and walleye sometimes have methyl mercury levels in the 1-ppm range (CFSAN, 2006). The rest of the fish advisory states to reduce the total fish meals consumed by pregnant women to approximately 1.4 servings per month (Oken et al., 2003).

Seafood that makes up 80% of the market (i.e., canned tuna, shrimp, pollock, salmon, cod, catfish, clams, flatfish, crabs and scallop) all have methyl mercury levels of <0.2 ppm, and restrictions do not apply unless people eat more than 2.2 pounds of these types of seafood per week. Farm-raised fish are subject to pollution via acid rain; thus they are not totally immune.

In addition to restricting specific types of fish, the U.S. agencies advise that fresh and frozen tuna also be restricted in the diet of pregnant and lactating women and women of childbearing age. Since pollution is not a predictable activity, care providers need to continually monitor ocean products.

Polychlorinated Biphenyls (PCBs). Over 1.2 billion pounds of polychlorinated biphenyls (PCBs) were produced in the United States before 1976, and half still remain in the environment, where they have primarily been taken up through water systems. They concentrate in the fatty flesh of larger fish such as salmon, lake trout, and carp. Although PCBs can be absorbed through the skin and lungs, they primarily enter the body from ingestion of contaminated fatty fish. They readily pass through the placenta and breast milk; thus pregnant and nursing women and women of

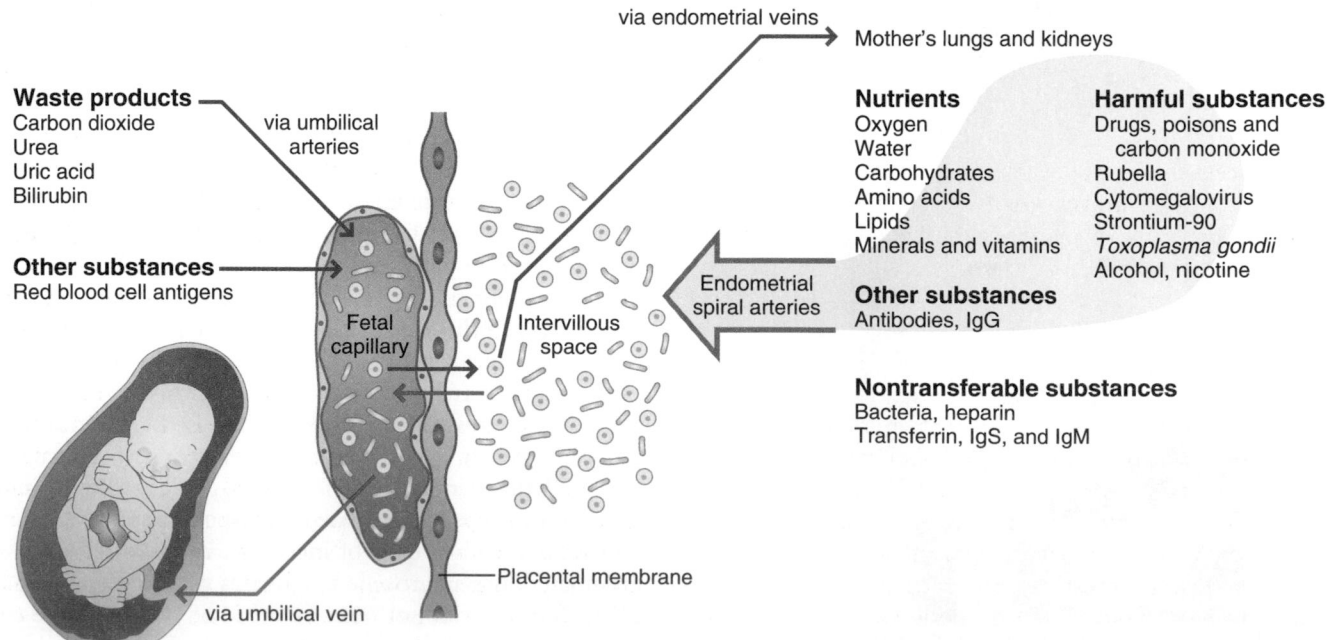

FIGURE 5-6 Transfer of substances across the placental membrane. *Ig,* Immunoglobulin.

childbearing age should avoid eating fish from water known to be contaminated with PCBs. State Land and Natural Resource departments usually regulate fresh-water fish; thus questions regarding methyl mercury, PCBs, and other contamination can be directed to them.

Listeria Monocytogenes. *Listeria monocytogenes* infects 2500 Americans each year; 500 of those infected die. Pregnant women are 20 times more likely than other healthy adults to become infected with *Listeria*. It is a known cause of spontaneous abortion and meningitis of the fetus and newborn. *Listeria* is a soil-borne organism; infection results from eating contaminated foods of animal origin and raw vegetables. Raw milk, smoked seafood, frankfurters, pâté, soft cheeses, cold cuts from the deli counter, and uncooked meats are likely sources. Produce irrigated with wastewater needs to be carefully washed with potable water before ingestion.

Beliefs, Avoidances, Cravings, and Aversions

Most women change their diets during their pregnancies. Change may be due to medical advice, folk medicine beliefs, or a change in food preference and appetite. Food avoidances may not reflect a mother's conscious choice to eliminate certain foods during her pregnancy. Some reasons include smell adversity due to enhanced perception of aroma, altered gag response, getting ill while eating or smelling a particular food, or altered gastric comfort.

Cravings and aversions are powerful urges toward or away from foods, including foods about which women experience no unusual attitudes when not pregnant. The most commonly craved foods are sweets and dairy products or foods quick to eat. The most common aversions reported are to alcohol, coffee, other caffeinated drinks, and meats. However, cravings and aversions are not limited to any particular food or food groups. Cravings and aversions can be deleterious and need exploration.

Pica. **Pica** of pregnancy most often involves **geophagia** (consumption of dirt or clay) or **amylophagia** (consumption of starch such as laundry starch). However, nonfood substances subject to pica of pregnancy include ice, paper, burnt matches, stones or gravel, charcoal, soot, cigarette ashes, antacid tablets, milk of magnesia, baking soda, and coffee grounds. The incidence of pica is not limited to any one geographic area, race, sex, culture, or social status; nor is it limited to pregnancy.

Malnutrition can be a consequence of pica because nonfood substances displace essential nutrients in the diet. Starch in excessive amounts can contribute to obesity, and it can be deleterious in women with diabetes mellitus. Some substances contain toxic compounds such as heavy metals; others can interfere with the absorption of minerals such as iron. Excessive intake of nonfood substances such as starch and clay can lead to intestinal obstruction.

The etiology of pica is poorly understood. One theory suggests that the ingestion of nonfood substances relieves nausea and vomiting. It has also been hypothesized that a deficiency of an essential nutrient such as calcium or iron results in the eating of nonfood substances that contain these nutrients. Some research suggests that there is a higher incidence of pica in Latino cultures (Lopez et al., 2004). In addition, the nutritionist needs to be aware of a religious connection of pica in the form of molded religious icons known as *panito del senor* from the Shrine of the Black Christ or *el Christo Negro* located in Esquipas, Guatemala (Erick, 2004).

Complications of Pregnancy With Dietary Implications

Nausea and Vomiting

Morning sickness or **nausea and vomiting in pregnancy (NVP)** affects 50% to 90% of all pregnant women during the first trimester of pregnancy, and it usually resolves around the 17th week of gestation. There are no clear distinctions of when "morning sickness" becomes "hyperemesis gravidarum." Usually women with "morning sickness" are functional and able to work and are not losing weight. This common form of morning sickness may be helped by simple dietary measures. Small, frequent, dry meals of easily digested carbohydrate-containing foods may be tolerated by some women, whereas protein foods may reduce nausea for others.

Although it has historically been suggested that liquids are best taken between meals, there has been no study to validate this recommendation. In a small study of 14 nauseated women, it was shown that protein-dominated meals reduced nausea and arrhythmic activity to greater degrees than equicaloric carbohydrate and fat meals and calorie-free meals; meal consistency did not affect symptom responses, but liquid meals decreased arrhythmias more than solids did (Jednak et al., 1999). More research is needed.

Although some women often do not tolerate fats because of the olfactory aspect of hot foods, room temperature foods containing fat such as potato chips and snack foods may be preferred by a sick woman. Unfortunately there is no cure-all. It is suggested that the woman suffering with nausea eat whatever reduces the sensation of nausea and avoid odors that trigger nausea. Other elements that can increase nausea include motion, noise (including gum snapping and "boom boxes"), bright lights, and adverse climate conditions (Erick, 2004).

Most pregnant women are aware of the importance of nourishing their fetus and are often confused by comments that weight loss in early pregnancy is acceptable. Although dry crackers and ginger ale are often prescribed for nausea, they do not constitute a high-quality diet. Overhydrating a starving woman reduces ketones but does not indicate that adequate nutrition has been achieved (Erick, 2004). Vitamin B_6 has been reported to relieve symptoms in mild cases only (Jewel and Young, 2002). Smelling lemons has been found by many women to help block noxious background odors (Erick, 2001). Other therapies used include eating crackers or potato chips, elastic sea bands, electronic wrist bands ("Relief Band"), special lollipops ("Reggie Pops"), vitamin B_6, red raspberry leaf, folic-acid enriched ginger elixir

("Morning sickness magic"), vitamin B_6 coupled with Unisom (a sleep aid), noise reduction, acupuncture, long showers, and hypnosis. However 5% to 10% of women can be ill until delivery (Erick, 2001).

When early pregnancy is characterized by excessive vomiting and weight loss, the client likely has **hyperemesis gravidarum,** and her nutritional status is greatly compromised. Fluid and electrolyte imbalances can require hospitalization for rehydration and nutritional support. Historically hyperemesis was considered by some to be psychiatric in nature because women became apathetic regarding their pregnancies and often requested care by their own mothers.

Cognitive alterations accompany starvation, and physical brain changes can be found on a magnetic resonance image (MRI). In addition, consider that some of the medically administered therapies have included injections of husband's blood (Hughes and Robinson, 1942) and application of leeches (Munch, 2002). One of the most common complications of hyperemesis gravidarum is Wernicke's encephalopathy. Wernicke's has commonly been associated with alcoholism but has many other etiologies, mainly starvation (see Chapter 28). Other physical deleterious outcomes noted in the medical literature include ruptured esophagus, acute renal failure, visual deterioration, and splenic avulsion (Hill et al., 2002; Henry and Vadas, 1986).

The nutritionist needs to be vigilant to avoid the real problem of "refeeding syndrome" in starved women and follow electrolytes such as phosphorous, magnesium, and potassium closely and replenish in a timely fashion. Low levels of electrolytes can result in cardiac irregularities and respiratory failure (see Chapter 20).

Hyperemesis gravidarum develops in about 2% of pregnancies (Erick, 1995) and is associated with an increase in maternal free thyroid hormone (Panesar et al., 2001) as well as several other hormones, including a variant of the HCG molecule (Goodwin, 2002). Hospitalization is usually indicated when dehydration occurs. Tube feeding may be used and should be considered before parenteral nutrition because of relatively fewer complications. Enteral nutrition does not guarantee an end to nausea, vomiting, and retching in all cases (Erick, 2006). Nasogastric feedings, percutaneous endoscopic gastrostomy (PEG) (Godil and Chen, 1998; Serrano et al., 1998), jejunostomy feedings (Erick, 1997), and PEG with a jejunal port (Irving et al., 2004) have been tried.

It is not common to give pregnant women antianxiety medications during tube insertion because of the potential of fetal risk, and it is important to respect the wishes of the client if she declines enteral nutrition. The provider needs to be sensitive to the reality that many ill women may choose pregnancy termination out of desperation as a means to eliminate nausea and vomiting (Mazzotta et al., 2001). Parenteral nutritional support may also be used in persistent cases.

One nuisance factor, which plagues 37% of women with hyperemesis, is **ptylinism** gravidarum, or excess saliva. Salivary output can be substantial and can be a source of lost electrolytes (Erick, 1998). It is not uncommon for ptylinism

to range from 500 to 1000 ml per day and needs to be considered in any hydration plan. The disability associated with hyperemesis is not insignificant. A recent study of annual U.S. health care costs estimated those from HG to be $200 million for hospitalization alone (Bailit, 2005).

Heartburn

Gastric esophageal reflux is a common occurrence during the latter part of pregnancy, and it often occurs at night. In most cases this is an effect of pressure of the enlarged uterus on the intestines and stomach, which, in combination with the relaxation of the esophageal sphincter, may result in regurgitation of stomach contents into the esophagus. Relief may occur by suggesting that the pregnant woman eat frequent small meals. Dinner plates can be changed for luncheon plates to remind a woman and her family about reduced gastric volume (see Chapter 26).

Constipation and Hemorrhoids

Pregnant women will become constipated if they fail to consume adequate water and fiber. And it is not uncommon for women in the first trimester who are being treated with Zofran (ondansetron) for nausea and vomiting to become extremely constipated. Straining during stooling—called *val salva*—increases the risk for hemorrhoids. Increased consumption of fluids, fiber-rich foods (see Appendix 41), and dried fruits (especially prunes and figs) usually controls these problems, but some women may also require a bulking type of stool softener (see Chapter 27).

Edema and Leg Cramps

Mild, physiologic edema is usually present in the extremities in the third trimester and should not be confused with the pathologic, generalized edema associated with pregnancy-induced hypertension. Normal edema in the lower extremities in pregnancy is caused by the pressure of the enlarging uterus on the vena cava, obstructing the return of blood flow to the heart. When a woman reclines on her side, the mechanical effect is removed, and extravascular fluid is mobilized and eventually eliminated by increased urine output. No dietary intervention is required.

Calcium supplementation for leg cramps during pregnancy has been used extensively, although only three studies met the criteria for analysis by the Cochrane Review, and the use of calcium for leg cramps in pregnancy is not supported (Young and Jewell, 2000). The authors suggest that the best evidence for the relief of leg cramps is use of magnesium lactate or citrate (Young and Jewell, 2000). Magnesium supplementation may relieve leg cramps because pregnancy and lactation can lead to a secondary magnesium deficiency as evidenced by low serum magnesium levels. Signs of magnesium deficiency include muscle tremor, ataxia, tetany, constipation, and cramps; thus supplemental magnesium may relieve the leg cramps associated with pregnancy or lactation (see Appendix 55).

A placebo-controlled study demonstrated that women with pregnancy-related leg cramps had low serum magnesium levels. With the administration of 122 mg of magnesium (as lactate and citrate) in the morning and 244 mg in the evening, the magnesium-treated group reported a significantly greater reduction of distress than did the control group. Interestingly, however, the low serum magnesium level initially detected in the magnesium-treated group did not return to normal levels, even though leg cramps improved.

Diabetes Mellitus

Individualized, expert care is needed for the nutritional management of the pregnant woman with diabetes. Based on a nutritional history and assessment early in pregnancy, or preferably preconception, the woman's meal plan in the form of lowered carbohydrates should be adapted for pregnancy by a skilled nutritionist as part of the health care team (see Chapter 30). The risk of PIH, macrosomia, chorioamnionitis, prematurity, intrauterine fetal demise (IUFD), and fetal morbidity is significantly greater in the pregnant women with diabetes than in the pregnant women without diabetes. Recent evidence suggests that women who do not meet the criteria to be classified as diabetic but have elevated blood glucose during pregnancy also carry significant risk for pregnancy complications, including macrosomia, prematurity, and chorioamnionitis (Scholl et al., 2001). These adverse outcomes can be avoided with specialized care, including ongoing involvement with the nutritionist, and the risk of complications can be reduced to the same level as seen in pregnant women who do not have diabetes.

Pregnancies without vascular disease can result in fetal macrosomia which is caused by *in utero* hyperglycemia from maternal blood. The fetus responds to maternal hyperglycemia by increasing its own insulin production, leading to excessive growth and adiposity. Infants born to women with long-standing type 1 diabetes who also have vascular disease may not be larger than those born to women without diabetes. Following delivery, the infant's pancreas continues to secrete elevated amounts of insulin. Since the maternal supply of glucose is no longer available, many infants of mothers with diabetes rapidly develop hypoglycemia requiring a glucose infusion.

Successful pregnancy requires adequate dietary intake to meet the growth needs of the fetus, prevent ketosis, and prevent depletion of maternal nutritional stores. Maintenance of optimal blood glucose levels with avoidance of ketosis is an important goal of therapy. Frequent glucose monitoring and appropriate insulin adjustments are crucial. Insulin requirements decrease in the first half of pregnancy because of fetal use of glucose, and the mother may need only two thirds of her usual amount. In the second half of pregnancy hormone changes induce an increase in insulin requirements of 70% to 100% over prepregnancy requirements. This increase occurs rather abruptly during the fifth month and may last through term. During this time the demands of pregnancy may impose a need for insulin in a pregnant woman with diabetes whose condition was adequately controlled by diet alone in the nonpregnant state. Frequent changes in diet and insulin dosage may be necessary. The number of snacks may need to be increased, and

for the insulin-dependent woman who is lactating, it is advised that she consume three small meals and four snacks to avoid drops in her blood glucose levels that can occur with a large milk output.

Gestational diabetes is usually diagnosed after 24 weeks' gestation and may affect as many as 5% to 10% of all pregnant women. Although symptoms are similar to those of diabetes mellitus, including glycosuria and elevated blood glucose, there is also a greater likelihood of developing preeclampsia. Infants whose mothers have gestational diabetes are at increased risk for perinatal mortality, as well as for prematurity with its attendant complications. If the mother's blood glucose is not well controlled, the infant is at risk for macrosomia, or infant birth weight greater than the 90th percentile or 4000 g. Stillborn babies at term are tragic but not uncommon. In addition, women who have experienced gestational diabetes are at future risk for type 2 diabetes mellitus within 15 years of the index pregnancy.

Currently most obstetric health care providers perform a routine 50-g oral glucose challenge at 24 to 28 weeks' gestation to screen for gestational diabetes. A value of 135 mg/dl is considered by some centers as the cutoff, whereas other centers use 140 mg/dl. The cost/benefit of a five-point difference has been debated in terms of numbers of false positives, staff resources, and treatment issues. A high suspicion to repeat and/or treat may follow if the woman is morbidly obese. Often a glucose-lactate tolerance value over 180 mg/dl in an obese woman will be the confirmatory data used to diagnosis the client with glucose intolerance of pregnancy, or gestational diabetes mellitus (GDM). If values are outside of normal range, an oral glucose tolerance test (GTT) is scheduled to confirm the diagnosis.

Gestational diabetes is treated largely through dietary changes (some calorie restriction may be necessary) and moderate exercise to maintain appropriate weight gain. Insulin is used if glucose levels do not respond to dietary manipulations. Dietary manipulation includes limiting carbohydrates at breakfast 10 to 30 grams with the addition of 2 to 3 ounces of protein mid morning to decrease hunger and increase compliance. The daily caloric needs of the client need to be configured in the dietary plan. Just counting carbohydrates is only one third of the dietary prescription; contributions from protein and fat need consideration (see Chapter 30). Blood glucose levels are often monitored four to six times a day with a goal of less than 90 g/dl for fasting and less than 120 mg/dl after meals. The oral hypoglycemic agents such as metformin are being used in some centers.

Pregnancy-Induced Hypertension

Pregnancy-induced hypertension (PIH) includes gestational hypertension and preeclampsia/eclampsia. **Gestational hypertension** is a maternal blood pressure equal to or greater than 140/90 with no proteinuria that develops after midpregnancy. These women may develop **preeclampsia,** which is defined by a systolic blood pressure of 140 or more or a diastolic blood pressure of 90 mm Hg or more and urinary protein of 300 mg or more in a 24-hr urine sample. Severe preeclampsia is defined as a systolic blood pressure of

160 or more or a diastolic blood pressure of 110 mm Hg or more and 5 g of protein in a 24-hr urine sample. Preeclampsia is associated with decreased uterine blood flow, owing to vasospasm, leading to reduced placental size, compromised fetal nourishment, and an IUGR fetus.

Measurement of umbilical blood flow is also helpful. "Absent end diastolic flow" signifies adversity to the fetus as blood flow through the umbilical cord is encountering significant resistance from the placenta. "Reversed end diastolic flow" is a more ominous finding, meaning that blood flow to the fetus is meeting such vascular resistance that it is moving in the opposite direction. In addition, preeclampsia may result in maternal end-organ damage such as liver impairment, renal impairment, cerebrovascular events, and retinal damage.

Vasospasm, intravascular volume depletion, and subsequent hemoconcentration are also present with severe PIH. The condition usually develops in the third trimester, affecting about 5% to 8% of the obstetric population, particularly women who are nulliparous, older than 40 years, obese, and black and who have a family history of PIH. Other risk factors include chronic hypertension, chronic renal disease, diabetes mellitus, a twin gestation, and homozygosity or heterozygosity for angiotensinogen gene T235. Insulin resistance syndrome has also been suggested as a cause for PIH (Solomon and Sealy, 2001).

A new theory involves low vitamin D status because vitamin D may have a role in the production of cytokines, which are also implicated in the etiology of PIH and PET. The incidence of preeclampsia is known to be increased in women with some autoimmune diseases such as type 1 diabetes and rheumatoid arthritis. There is a reduction in the levels of circulating 1,25 (OH)2D3 in preeclamptic patients compared with normotensive or chronically hypertensive controls, which may be caused by a disturbance in 1α-hydroxylation within the placenta/deciduas. Preeclampsia is more common in dark-skinned women living in northern latitudes who typically have a higher prevalence of hypovitaminosis D than is found in comparable white women. In Nordic countries the incidence of preeclampsia peaks during winter and is the lowest in summer and early autumn. As early as 1937, studies were conducted evaluating the role of vitamin D in preeclampsia management (Hypponen, 2005). Serum 25-hydroxy vitamin D should be measured in women with preeclampsia and appropriate diet changes made or supplementation added in those with low levels.

The etiology of preeclampsia is unknown, but vascular injury to the placental blood vessels has been implicated. Very young women with first pregnancy and older pregnant women are more likely to encounter the problem. Chappell et al. (2002) showed a reduction in incidence in a subsequent pregnancy with vitamin C supplementation of 1000 mg/day and vitamin E supplementation of 400 international units (IU)/day from weeks 16 to 22 of pregnancy in a study of 283 women from the United Kingdom. In the placebo group 17% of women had a recurrence of preeclampsia, whereas only 8% in the vitamin-treated group had the disease. In contrast, (Rumbold et al., 2006) a study of 1877 women in Australia failed to show any reduction in disease in women having their first pregnancy who were treated with the same dosage of both vitamins but from week 14 to 22. Another study from the United Kingdom found more low-birth-weight infants from women who took 1000 mg of vitamin C and 400 IU of vitamin E from the second trimester to term, but the incidence of preeclampsia was similar between both groups at 15% to 16% (Poston et al, 2006.) A study from India (Sharma et al., 2006) showed lower vitamin C and lycopene levels in women with severe preeclampsia. What benefits these nutrients have in reducing the incidence of or preventing preeclampsia is difficult to ascertain. These two nutrients will be studied further in a project of the Maternal-Fetal Medicine Units Network of the National Institute of Child Health and Human Development, which will enroll 10,000 low-risk U.S. women.

Eclampsia is PIH resulting in grand mal seizures. Symptoms of PIH that increase the concern for seizure are dizziness, headache, visual disturbances, facial edema, anorexia, nausea, and vomiting. Fetal death often results in women who develop eclampsia. A small percent of cases of eclampsia present in the postpartum period. Eclampsia can be fatal to the mother if not treated promptly.

Magnesium Supplementation. Magnesium supplementation has also been recommended to prevent and treat preeclampsia and eclampsia with some effectiveness.

Previous attempts to treat preeclampsia have included severe sodium restriction and diuretics. Sodium restriction and diuretics do not reduce blood pressure, limit weight gain, or reduce the amount of proteinuria in this condition; and they have no place in the treatment or prevention of preeclampsia. The use of diuretics in women with PIH would lead to fluid loss and a decrease in intravascular volume; thus further compromising the fetus. Restricted energy intake also has no role in the prevention of PIH.

Vaginal infections. Infections play a major role in premature contractions and subsequent early deliveries. Bacterial vaginosis (BV) is one such infection, affecting many pregnant women. The use of probiotics in pregnant women with BV is compelling since certain lactobacilli strains can safely colonize the vagina and displace and kill such pathogens as *Gardnerella vaginalis* and *Escherichia coli* (Reid and Bocking, 2003).

LACTATION

Exclusive breast-feeding is unequivocally the preferred method of infant feeding for the first 4 to 6 months of life. Both the American Dietetic Association and the American Academy of Pediatrics have issued position statements in support of breast-feeding (AAP, 2005; ADA reaffirmed, 2002). Research provides strong evidence that there are specific health advantages for both mother and infant (Box 5-5).

Breast-feeding is contraindicated for infants with galactosemia and mothers who have active untreated tuberculosis or are positive for human T-cell lymphotropic virus type 1 or 2, mothers who use drugs of abuse, are human immuno-deficiency virus (HIV) positive (in the United States), and who take certain medications (i.e., antimetabolites and chemotherapeutic agents). Radioactive isotopes require temporary cessation (Lawrence and Lawrence, 2005).

Although the rates of breast-feeding in the United States reached an all time low in 1970 to 25%, breast-feeding rates rose gradually to 52% in the mid 1980s. In 2001 the breast-feeding rate was at a high of 69.5% (Riordan, 2005). A number of health promotion strategies in the United States support breast-feeding including Healthy People 2010, The WIC program, and the U.S. Breastfeeding Committee (Riordan, 2005). An excellent way to promote breast-feeding is to discuss its role in decreasing the incidence or severity of a wide range of infectious diseases, including bacterial meningitis, diarrhea, and otitis media. Two studies suggest that breast-feeding can reduce the incidence of both types 1 and 2 diabetes (Malcova et al., 2006; Stuebe et al., 2005).

In 1991 the World Health Organization (WHO) and UNICEF adopted the Baby-Friendly Hospital Initiative (BFHI), a global effort to increase the incidence and duration of breast-feeding. To become "baby friendly," a hospital must show to an outside review board that it implements the "Ten Steps to Successful Breast-feeding," a guideline for mother/baby management in the hospital (Riordan, 2005). In the United States there are 55 Baby-Friendly Hospitals and Birth Centers as of July 2006 (see *Clinical Insight:* The Baby-Friendly Hospital Initiative).

Physiology of Lactation

Mammary gland growth during menarche and pregnancy prepares for lactation. The human mammary gland is illustrated in Figure 5-7. Hormonal changes markedly increase breast, areola, and nipple size. In pregnancy hormones that significantly increase ducts and alveoli influence mammary growth. Late in pregnancy the lobules of the alveolar system are maximally developed, and small amounts of **colostrum,** the thin, yellow, milky fluid rich in antibodies may be released for several weeks before term and for a few days after delivery. After birth there is a rapid drop in circulating levels of estrogen and progesterone accompanied by a rapid

---

BOX 5-5

Benefits of Breast-Feeding

Infant

Decreases incidence and/or severity of infectious diseases
   Bacterial meningitis
   Bacteremia
   Diarrhea
   Respiratory tract infection
   Necrotizing enterocolitis
   Otitis media
   Urinary tract infection
   Late-onset sepsis in preterm infants
Decreases rates of:
   Sudden infant death syndrome
   Types 1 and 2 diabetes
   Lymphoma
   Leukemia
   Hodgkin's disease
   Overweight and obesity
   Hypercholesterolemia
   Food allergies
   Asthma
Neurodevelopment
   Enhances performance on cognitive development tests
   Provides analgesia during painful procedures (heel stick for newborns)
   Promotes mother-child bonding

Mother

Decreases postpartum bleeding
More rapid uterine involution
Decreases menstrual blood loss
Increased child spacing
Earlier return to prepregnant weight
Decreases risk of breast and ovarian cancer
Possible decreased risk of postmenopausal hip fracture and osteoporosis

Adapted from American Academy of Pediatrics: Breastfeeding and the use of human milk, *Pediatrics,* 115:496, 2005.

✳ CLINICAL INSIGHT

The Baby-Friendly Hospital Initiative

Ten Steps to Successful Breast-Feeding

1. Have a written breast-feeding policy that is routinely communicated to all health care staff.
2. Train all health care staff in the skills necessary to implement this policy.
3. Inform all pregnant women about the benefits and management of breast-feeding.
4. Help the mother initiate breast-feeding within a half hour of birth.
5. Show mothers how to breast-feed and how to maintain lactation, even if they are separated from their infants.
6. Give newborn infants no food or drink other than breast milk unless medically indicated.
7. Practice rooming-in; allow mothers and infants to remain together 24 hours a day.
8. Encourage breast-feeding on demand.
9. Give no artificial teats or pacifiers (also called dummies or soothers) to breast-feeding infants.
10. Foster the establishment of breast-feeding support groups and refer mothers to them on discharge from the hospital or clinic.

From Ebrahim GJ: The baby friendly hospital initiative, *J Trop Pediatr* 39:2, 1993 by permission of Oxford University Press.

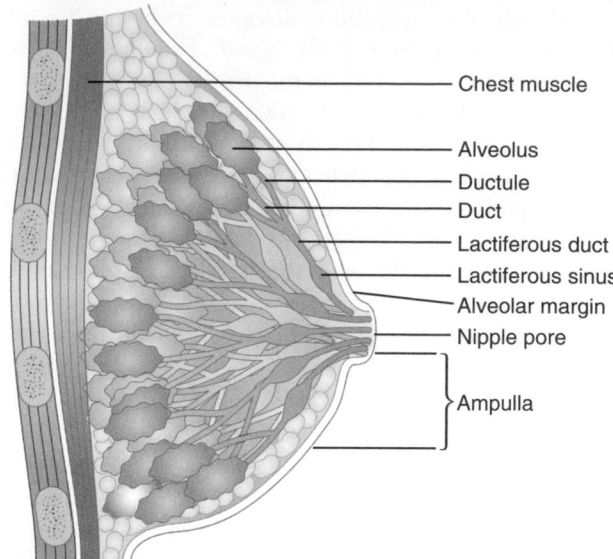

FIGURE 5-7 Structural features of the human mammary gland. The terminal glandular (alveolar) tissue of each lobule leads into the duct system, which enlarges eventually into the lactiferous duct and lactiferous sinus. The lactiferous sinuses rest beneath the areola and converge at the nipple pore.

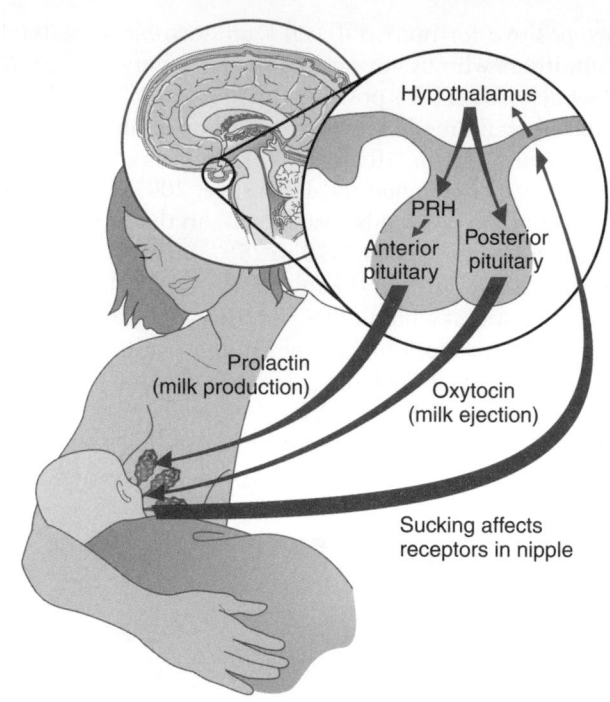

FIGURE 5-8 Physiology of milk production and the let-down reflex. *PRH,* Pituitary-releasing hormone.

increase in prolactin secretion, setting the stage for a copious milk supply.

The usual stimulus for milk production and secretion is suckling. Subcutaneous nerves of the areola send a message via the spinal cord to the hypothalamus, which in turn transmits a message to the pituitary gland, where both the anterior and posterior areas are stimulated. **Prolactin** from the anterior pituitary stimulates alveolar cell milk production, as shown in Figure 5-8. **Oxytocin** from the posterior pituitary stimulates the myoepithelial cells of the mammary gland to contract, causing movement of milk through the ducts and lactiferous sinuses, a process referred to as **let-down.**

"Let-down" is highly sensitive. Oxytocin, the milk-releasing hormone, can be released by visual, tactile, olfactory, and auditory stimuli; and even by thinking about the infant. Oxytocin secretion can also be inhibited by pain, emotional and physical stress, fatigue, and anxiety. Adrenaline release is believed to negate the effects of oxytocin on the myoepithelial cells (Lauwers and Shinskie, 2000). Women who have diabetes, are stressed during delivery, and have retained placental fragments are at risk for delayed milk production, occurring when signs of lactogenesis are absent 72 hours after birth (Lawrence and Lawrence, 2005).

Nutritional Requirements of Lactation

Lactation is nutritionally demanding, especially for the woman who nurses her infant exclusively for a number of months. Increased intake of most nutrients is advised, as Table 5-5 indicates.

Milk production is most affected by the frequency of suckling and maternal hydration. However, milk composition varies according to the mother's diet. For example, the

fatty acid composition of a mother's milk reflects her dietary intake. In addition, milk concentrations of selenium, iodine, and some of the water-soluble B vitamins are reflective of maternal diet. Breast milk of malnourished mothers has been shown to have lower levels of various nutrients, reflecting the foods available to eat. In a study from Indonesia, marginal vitamin A status was found in 54% of the breast-fed infants and in 18% of the mothers (Dijkhuizen et al., 2001). Keratomalacia has been reported in a neonate secondary to a maternal vitamin A deficiency, but this is considered rare (Gupta et al., 2005).

As gastric bypass surgery becomes more common for maternal weight management, vitamin A status before and during pregnancy, as well as during lactation, will need to be monitored. Retinal changes due to vitamin A deficiency have been reported years after gastric bypass surgery; chronic dry eyes and corneal scarring may be present (Lee et al., 2005). Since the nutritional status of the mother will affect the nutrient composition of her breast milk, it is conceivable that an exclusively breast-fed infant could suffer from suboptimal nutrition. Suboptimal nutrition is often not considered in affluent arenas; however, it does exist.

Energy

Milk production is 80% efficient: production of 100 ml of milk (about 75 kcal) requires an 85-kcal expenditure (Lawrence and Lawrence, 2005). During the first 6 months of lactation, average milk production is 750 ml/day, with a range of 550 to more than 1200ml/day (IOM, 1990). Since production is a function of the frequency, duration, and intensity of infant suckling, infants who feed well are likely to stimulate the production of larger volumes of milk.

The DRI for energy during lactation is 330 kcal greater during the first 6 months of lactation and 400 kcal greater during the second 6 months of lactation over that for a nonpregnant woman. It is the same as the RDA during the second trimester of pregnancy (IOM, 2002). The obese and overweight woman may not require the full 330 to 400 extra kcal/day. Maternal fat stores accumulated during pregnancy provide about 100 to 150 kcal to support the early months of lactation. When the reserve fat stores have been depleted, dietary energy support for lactation must be increased if the mother intends to provide all or most of her infant's nutrition through breast milk alone. During the second 6 months of lactation, production generally drops to an average of 600 ml/day or about 20 oz/day. Most infants are also consuming solid foods; thus the frequency of breast-feeding usually declines, and energy requirements for the nursing mother decline as well.

Milk production decreases in mothers who undertake rigorous calorie-restricted diets (under 1500 kcal) (Lawrence and Lawrence, 2005). However, at-risk mothers (those who are impoverished and have little money for food) can reduce their energy intake modestly to increase fat use without an adverse impact on milk production once lactation is well established. Appropriate fluid intake (i.e., drinking to thirst) and adequate rest are also needed.

Healthy breast-feeding women usually can lose as much as 1 lb/wk and still supply adequate milk to maintain their infants' growth. Breast-feeding women should be reminded of the energy expenditure required to produce milk and that exclusive breast-feeding with no reduction in calorie intake supports the loss of body fat. Women who are already lean may be at risk for reduced milk production if they restrict their energy intake. It is generally advisable for lactating women to maintain an energy intake of at least 1800 kcal/day.

Protein

The DRI suggests an additional 25 g of protein a day for lactation, or 71 g of protein a day. Clinical judgment is necessary with protein recommendations because 71 g/day may be too low in an overweight woman and too high for the woman with a lower BMI. Women with surgical delivery and women who enter pregnancy in poor nutritional shape may need additional protein. The average protein requirement for lactation is estimated from milk composition data and the mean daily volume of 750 ml, assuming an efficiency of 70% in the conversion of dietary protein to milk protein.

Carbohydrates

The EAR for carbohydrates in lactation is 160 g/day and the AI is 210 g/day (IOM, 2002). This 160 to 210 g/day is the recommended amount to provide enough calories in the diet for adequate volumes of milk and to prevent ketonemia and maintain appropriate blood glucose during lactation. The woman who has not gained the recommended amount of weight needs an individually calculated diet and may require more carbohydrates.

Lipid

The amount and type of fat in breast milk directly reflects the maternal diet. Adjustments in the maternal diet can increase or decrease specific fatty acids. Severe restriction of energy intake results in mobilization of body fat, and the milk produced has a fatty acid composition resembling that of the mother's depot fat. There is no DRI for total lipids during lactation since it depends on the amount of energy required by the mother to maintain milk production. However, present DRIs state a recommended amount of specific fatty acid for the first time because the presence of the long-chain polyunsaturated fatty acids in human milk and thus their presence in the maternal diet are crucial for the fetal and infant brain development. The AI for *n*-6 polyunsaturated fatty acids is 13 g/day, and the AI for *n*-3 polyunsaturated fatty acids is 1.3 g/day (IOM, 2002) (see *Focus On: Omega-3 Fats and Pregnancy and Lactation*).

Human milk contains 10 to 20 mg/dl of cholesterol, resulting in an approximate consumption of 100 mg/day by the infant. The amount of cholesterol in milk does not reflect the mother's diet; however, the cholesterol content of the milk decreases over time as lactation progresses.

Vitamins and Minerals

The vitamin D content of milk is related to maternal vitamin D intake and the degree of sun exposure. Numerous case reports document marginal or significant vitamin D deficiency in pregnant women and in infants of lactating women who are veiled, dark skinned or living in Northern latitudes with decreased sun exposure. Women with lactose intolerance who do not drink vitamin D–fortified milk or take a vitamin supplement may be at higher risk for vitamin D deficiency. The AI for vitamin D during lactation is 5 mcg/day (IOM, 1997). Because of reports of clinical rickets, the AAP recommends that all breast-fed infants receive an additional 200 units (5 mcg) of vitamin D daily beginning at 2 months of age (Lawrence and Lawrence, 2005). A study from Iowa evaluated breast-fed babies 280 days after birth and found that 10% of the infants had a 25-hydroxyvitamin D less than 11 ng/ml, considered deficient (Ziegler, 2006).

The *calcium* content of breast milk is not related to maternal intake, and there is no convincing evidence that maternal change in bone mineral density is influenced by calcium intake across a broad range of intakes up to 1600 mg/day. Maternal bone loss during lactation is approximately 3% to 7%, which is rapidly regained after weaning (Kalkwarf and Specker, 2002). The AI for calcium during pregnancy and lactation and in females who are not pregnant or lactating is 1300 mg/day for women less than 19 years old, 1000 mg day for 19- to 50-year-old women. The UL is the same: 2500 mg/day (IOM, 1997).

The amount of *iodine* in breast milk reflects maternal intake (see "Iodine" earlier in the chapter). The iodine levels in the Pakistani general diet have been deemed to be low (Akhter et al., 2004). The planned diets of university students in East Germany tend to contain only 50% of the daily recommended iodine intake (Brauer, 2005). Seafood has been

Omega-3 Fats and Pregnancy and Lactation

Our ancestors consumed a diet with equal amounts of omega-3 and omega-6 fatty acids. American diets are currently estimated to contain a ratio of omega-3 to omega-6 fatty acids of 1:10. This dramatic decrease in the consumption of omega-3 fatty acids over many centuries is thought to affect overall disease prevalence, as well as pregnancy outcome. The consumer is advised to follow "safe-fish" guidelines by monitoring information that is found on www.seaturtles.org/gotmercury.htm.

Fatty acids are found in all cell membranes. They compose 60% of the dry weight of fetal brain, half of which is as omega-6 and the other half as omega-3 (arachidonic acid [ARA]) and docosahexaenoic acid [DHA], respectively). Because DHA is important for the growth and development of the fetal central nervous system, including the retina, it has been suggested that the prenatal diet should include adequate amounts of preformed DHA. In fact, the new dietary reference intakes specify an amount of 1.4 g/day during pregnancy and 1.3 g/day during lactation (IOM, 2002).

The main food source of DHA is fatty, cold-water fish; and two to three fish meals per week of low-mercury fish during pregnancy appear to provide adequate amounts of DHA. However, given the recent advice that childbearing-age, pregnant, and lactating women should limit certain fish because of mercury and polychlorinated biphenyl (PCB) exposure, dietary strategies must be highly specific. Fish with elevated concentrations of DHA that are not on the Food and Drug Administration advisory are sardines. Other options to increase the DHA content in the diet of pregnant and lactating women include the consumption of omega-3–enriched eggs and the use of DHA supplements (Smuts et al., 2003). Vegetable sources of omega-3 fats include flax seeds and nuts, especially walnuts and walnut oil, although they are a less efficient way to obtain DHA. The woman allergic to fish should seek an algae source of supplemental DHA. The prenatal nutritionist needs to be alert that women may buy cod-liver oil capsules when choosing an omega-3 supplement. Cod-liver oil contains significant amounts of vitamin A, and this may be of a concern.

The breast-fed infant obtains DHA through maternal milk when the mother eats sufficient quantities of foods containing DHA. Most infant formulas now sold in the United States have ARA and DHA added. Japan has included these fatty acids in their infant formulas for years.

---

found to be one of the highest sources of iodine, but many countries may have limited access to these products. In the United States the presence of an industrial pollutant, perchlorate, has been shown to inhibit iodine uptake. Perchlorate has been found in mothers' milk as well as in the water supply (Kirk et al., 2005). This may be a reason that iodine levels in some individuals are low, despite what appears to be an adequate amount of iodine in the diet. Finally, lactating mothers who follow strict vegetarian diets devoid of adequate iodine, have been reported to have infants with transient neonatal hypothyroidism (Shaikh et al., 2003).

The requirements for *zinc* during lactation are greater than those during pregnancy. In the process of normal lactation the zinc content of breast milk drops dramatically during the first few months from 2 to 3 of mg zinc/day to 1 mg/day by the third month after birth. In zinc deficient–lactating women, normal zinc concentrations are maintained in breast milk for at least the first 2 months of lactation. The DRIs for zinc during lactation are 12 to 14 mg/day (IOM, 2001). The UL is 34 to 40 mg/day, depending on the age of the lactating woman.

Breast-Feeding an Infant

Preparation

The advantages of breast-feeding should be presented throughout the childbearing years. The process of **lactation** (milk secretion) and the benefits of breast-feeding should be a part of school health curricula. Women should be encouraged to express and discuss their opinions and feelings so that any misinformation can be corrected. During the last months of pregnancy, counseling on the process of lactation should be made available to women who have decided to breast-feed. Fathers should be encouraged to participate in counseling sessions because the emotional support they provide contributes to the success of lactation. Resources for breast-feeding support after hospital discharge should be made available at that time.

The Technique

The baby should be put to breast after birth and remain in direct skin-to-skin contact until the first feed is accomplished (AAP Policy statement, 2005). **Colostrum,** the first milk available after birth, is higher in protein and lower in fat and carbohydrate than mature milk. Colostrum provides approximately 20 kcal/oz and is a rich source of antibodies for the baby (Lawrence and Lawrence, 2005). Within 48 to 96 hours after birth the breasts become fuller and firmer as the milk volumes increase.

Breast-feeding is a learned skill for both mother and her infant. Practice, patience, and perseverance are necessary as mother and baby learn about each other. Allow the mother to choose a comfortable position so that her baby is well supported with her hand holding the lower portion of the baby's head, neck, and shoulders. With the baby close to her body, the mother aligns the nipple opposite the nose. When the mouth opens wide, the mother brings the baby's body to the breast, aiming the nipple to the back of the baby's mouth. The chin should indent the breast, and the nose may touch the breast (Figure 5-9). The baby should be allowed to nurse on the first breast until satiated and then be offered the second. Length of time at the breast should not be limited since this can prevent the establishment of successful lactation.

Lactating women may experience a tingling sensation in the breast signaling the let-down reflex. This is often accompanied by milk dripping from the other breast and occasionally, in the early days after birth, by uterine cramps, thirst, and drowsiness. It may take some time for the let-down reflex to become fully functional and conditioned. Some women never feel let-down, but swallowing by the baby is a definite sign that it has occurred. Rest or a hot shower before nursing may facilitate the let-down reflex. If the mother has too much milk, the baby may only need to nurse on one side at a feeding. Allow the baby to feed on the other breast at the next feed. If the mother experiences discomfort from a too-full breast, she can manually express or pump for comfort only. This is also an ideal opportunity for the mother to store milk for a future feeding.

To remove the baby from the breast, a finger is placed in the corner of the baby's mouth until the suction is broken. This allows the mother to prevent nipple trauma if she needs to end a feed. The need for burping is highly individualized.

Because breast milk is more easily digested, breast-feeding infants may wish to feed more often, and 8 to 12 feeds per day are common. Breast-feeding whenever the baby shows sign of feeding readiness (lip smacking, rooting, sucking movements) helps contribute to a mother's confidence in the care of her baby. During growth spurts babies often feed more often for a few days to increase the mother's supply.

Feeding time is perfectly suited for establishing and maintaining close mother-child interactions (see Figure 5-9). When she needs to be away at the usual time of a feeding, a bottle of breast milk that has been expressed earlier can be given. It is best to avoid supplemental bottles until the milk supply is established, usually around 3 to 4 weeks' after birth.

Infants who are introduced to artificial nipples in the first few weeks of life may experience "nipple preference." The sucking action required to empty a bottle is different from that needed to nurse at the breast, and the flow of milk is faster and easier to obtain. Some infants may then refuse the breast, leading to lactation difficulties. In the early weeks it is important to minimize mother-baby separation. There is no need to offer breast-fed babies additional water since 87% of breast milk is water. However, cases of hypernatremic dehydration due to suboptimal breast-feeding do occur. Most cases involve young and first-time mothers who may feel intimidated and overwhelmed at delivery, lack breast-feeding education, and are unaware of the consequences of dehydration. Extreme climactic conditions may also contribute to this problem. The consequence of hypernatremic dehydration can be permanent brain damage or death (Yldzdas et al., 2005; Rosenbloom, 2004). Therefore it is vital to evaluate the breast-feeding dyad in the hospital

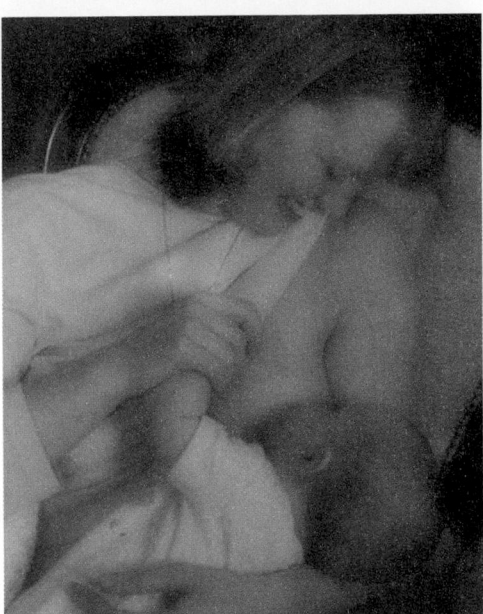

FIGURE 5-9 A nursing mother and her infant enjoy the close physical and psychologic contact that accompanies breast-feeding. *(Courtesy Kelly Carlson Atlec, Fairbanks, Alaska.)*

before discharge. Problems identified can then be addressed, and a plan of care can be implemented. All breast-fed newborns should be seen within 3 to 5 days of birth by an experienced health care professional (AAP, 2005).

Duration of Breast-Feeding

The length of time a woman breast-feeds her infant depends on her personal feelings and situation. Exclusive breast-feeding is recommended for the first 6 months but may continue for the first year or as long as it is mutually desired by mother and child (AAP, 2005). Some mothers prefer to breast-feed until the baby is weaned to a cup. This can be accomplished when the baby is 9 to 10 months of age. Some mothers choose to breast-feed much longer, letting the baby decide when to wean.

When a mother decides to wean her baby, the process should be done gradually over a period of weeks. Initially one feeding can be omitted for 3 to 4 days; then an additional feeding can be skipped. This process continues until the baby is at one feed a day (usually the night or early morning feeding). Eventually this last feeding can be discontinued. Weaning in this gradual manner is easier on the mother, avoiding engorgement of her breasts as well as easing the baby's transition to a new routine.

Exercise and Breast-Feeding

The breast-feeding mother should be encouraged to get back to exercise a few weeks' after delivery, after lactation is well established. Aerobic exercise at 60% to 70% of maximum heart rate has no adverse effect on lactation; infants gain weight at the same rate, and the mother's cardiovascular fitness improves. Exercise also improves plasma lipids and insulin response in lactating women without negating maternal or infant immune status (Lovelady, 2004).

TABLE 5-6

Drugs for Which the Effect on Nursing Infants Is Unknown but May Be of Concern*

Drug	Reported or Possible Effect
Antianxiety	
Alprazolam	None
Diazepam	None
Lorazepam	None
Midazolam	‡
Perphenazine	None
Prazepam†	None
Quazepam	None
Temazepam	‡
Antidepressant	
Amitriptyline	None
Amoxapine	None
Bupropion	None
Clomipramine	None
Desipramine	None
Dothiepin	None
Doxepin	None
Fluoxetine	Colic, irritability, feeding and sleep disorders, slow weight gain
Fluvoxamine	‡
Imipramine	None
Nortriptyline	None
Paroxetine	None
Sertraline†	None
Trazodone	None
Antipsychotic	
Chlorpromazine	Galactorrhea in mother, drowsiness and lethargy in infant, decline in developmental scores
Chlorprothixene	None
Clozapine†	None
Haloperidol	Decline in developmental scores
Mesoridazine	None
Trifluoperazine	None
Other	
Amiodarone	Possible hypothyroidism
Chloramphenicol	Possible idiosyncratic bone marrow suppression
Clofazimine	Possible transfer of high percentage of maternal dose, possible increase in skin pigmentation
Lamotrigine	Potential therapeutic serum concentrations in infant
Metoclopramide†	None described, dopaminergic blocking agent
Metronidazole	In vitro mutagen, may discontinue breast-feeding for 12-24 hr to allow excretion of dose when single-dose therapy is given to mother
Tinidazole	See *metronidazole*

Modified from American Academy of Pediatrics, Committee on Drugs: The transfer of drugs and other chemicals into human milk, *Pediatrics* 108(3): 776, 2001.

*Psychotropic drugs—the compounds listed as *anti-anxiety*, *antidepressant*, and *antipsychotic*—are of special concern when given to nursing mothers for long periods. Although very few case reports of adverse effects in breast-feeding infants are known, these drugs do appear in human milk and thus could conceivably alter short-term and long-term central nervous system function.

†Drug is concentrated in human milk relative to simultaneous maternal plasma concentrations.

‡Data not sufficient to confidently assess risk.

TABLE 5-7

Drugs That Have Been Associated With Significant Effects on Some Nursing Infants and Should Be Given to Nursing Mothers With Caution

Drug	Reported Effect*
Acebutolol	Hypotension, bradycardia, tachypnea
5-Aminosalicylic acid	Diarrhea (one case)
Aspirin (salicylates)	Metabolic acidosis (one case)
Atenolol	Cyanosis, bradycardia
Bromocriptine	Suppresses lactation; may be hazardous to the mother
Clemastine	Drowsiness, irritability, refusal to feed, high-pitched crying, neck stiffness (one case)
Ergotamine	Vomiting, diarrhea, convulsions (in doses used in migraine medications)
Lithium	One third to one half therapeutic blood concentration in infants
Phenindione	Anticoagulant: increased prothrombin and partial thromboplastin time in one infant; not used in United States
Phenobarbital	Sedation, infantile spasms after weaning from milk containing phenobarbital, methemoglobinemia (one case)
Primidone	Sedation, feeding problems
Sulfasalazine (salicylazosulfapyridine)	Bloody diarrhea (one case)

Modified from American Academy of Pediatrics, Committee on Drugs: The transfer of drugs and other chemicals into human milk, Pediatrics 108(3):776, 2001.

*Blood concentration in infant may be of clinical importance.

Former opinions that strenuous exercise resulting in lactic acid production, which "flavors" breast milk, thus making it unacceptable to the baby, have not been proven (Wright et al., 2002).

Transfer of Drugs into Human Milk

Almost all drugs taken by the mother will appear in her milk to some degree. The amount that usually transfers is quite small. Many factors influence how medications transfer into human milk: milk/plasma ratio, molecular weight of the drug, and the protein binding and lipid solubility of the drug. It is also important to consider the oral bioavailability of the drug to the infant or how much enters the infant's bloodstream (Hale, 2006).

The American Academy of Pediatrics issued a statement on the transfer of drugs and other chemicals into human milk (AAP, 2005). Many drugs (i.e., cytotoxic drugs) are known to have detrimental affects, and some drugs have unknown effects but may be of concern (i.e., antidepressants, antianxiety and neuroleptic drugs) (Table 5-6). Maternal medications usually compatible with lactation are presented in Table 5-7. Food and environmental agents that can affect breast-feeding are presented in Table 5-8.

Failure to Thrive in the Breast-Fed Infant

Insufficient milk supply is rarely a problem for the well-fed, well-rested, and unstressed mother. Sucking stimulates the flow of milk; thus feeding on demand should supply ample amounts of milk to the infant. If the baby continues to gain weight and length steadily, has at least six to eight wet diapers daily, and has frequent stools, the milk supply is probably adequate.

Occasionally, however, an infant fails to thrive while seeming to nurse properly. A variety of circumstances can be explored as likely reasons for the failure. The diagram in Figure 5-10 illustrates potential problems in the mother or the infant that should be investigated during the course of evaluation.

If the cause of the problem cannot be identified or the defined problem cannot be corrected, it may be necessary to encourage the mother to use commercial infant formula for at least partial nutritional support of the infant. A thorough assessment of the maternal diet and health habits is always necessary. Women who consume diets low in vitamin B_{12}, vitamin D, or iodine will produce milk with low levels; the result is failure to thrive in the breast-fed infant.

Sometimes the infant may become intolerant or allergic to something the mother has ingested. Cow's milk protein, notably casein, has been implicated along with peanuts. When suspicious foods are removed from the mother's diet, it is important to assess the nutritional quality of her diet and supplement her appropriately (see Chapter 29).

Other Problems of Breast-Feeding

Overweight lactating women can restrict their energy intake by 500 kcal per day by decreasing consumption of foods high in fat and simple sugars, but they must increase their intake of foods high in calcium and vitamin D, especially from fruits and vegetables (Lovelady et al., 2006).

TABLE 5-8

Food and Environmental Agents: Effects on Breast-Feeding

Agent	Reported Sign or Symptom in Infant or Effect on Lactation
Aflatoxin	None
Aspartame	Caution if mother or infant has phenylketonuria
Bromide (photographic laboratory)	Potential absorption and bromide transfer into milk
Cadmium	None reported
Chlordane	None reported
Chocolate (theobromine)	Irritability or increased bowel activity if excess amounts ($\geq$16 oz/day) consumed by mother
Dichloro-diphenyl-trichloroethane (DDT), benzene hexachlorides, dieldrin, aldrin, hepatachlorepoxide	None
Fava beans	Hemolysis in patient with glucose-y-phosphate dehydrogenase (G6PD) deficiency
Fluorides	None
Hexachlorobenzene	Skin rash, diarrhea, vomiting, dark urine, neurotoxicity, death
Hexachlorophene	None, possible contamination of milk from nipple washing
Lead	Possible neurotoxicity
Mercury, methyl mercury	Possible neurodevelopmental effects
Methylmethacrylate	None
Monosodium glutamate	None
Polychlorinated biphenyls and polybrominated biphenyls	Lack of endurance, hypotonia, sullen, expressionless facies
Silicon	Esophageal dysmotility
Tetrachlormethylene cleaning fluid (perchloroethylene)	Obstructive jaundice, dark urine
Vegetarian diet	Signs of B_{12} deficiency

Modified from American Academy of Pediatrics, Committee on Drugs: The transfer of drugs and other chemicals into human milk, *Pediatrics* 108(3):776, 2001.

Breast augmentation, a procedure in which an implant is inserted into the breast to enlarge the breast, is a common elective breast procedure. Periareolar and transareolar incisions can cause lactation insufficiency. Better lactation results occur when incisions are made under the breast or in the axilla (Riordan, 2005). These mothers should be encouraged to breast-feed, and their infants monitored for appropriate weight gain.

Reduction mammoplasty is often recommended for women with extremely large breasts who suffer from back, shoulder, or neck pain or poor body image. There are wide variations in milk production, from a little to full production, depending on the amount of tissue removed and the type of surgical incision. These mothers should also be encouraged to breast-feed and be given anticipatory guidance and support; their infants should be monitored closely for appropriate weight gain.

Low- or very low–birth-weight infants may spend time in a neonatal intensive care unit, making it a challenge to the mother who wishes to breast-feed. It is important to counsel mothers of these infants about the incidence of lactation initiation and breast milk feeding without increasing maternal stress and anxiety (Sisk et al., 2006).

There can be a number of other hurdles to overcome to breast-feed successfully. These problems and their solutions are discussed in Table 5-9.

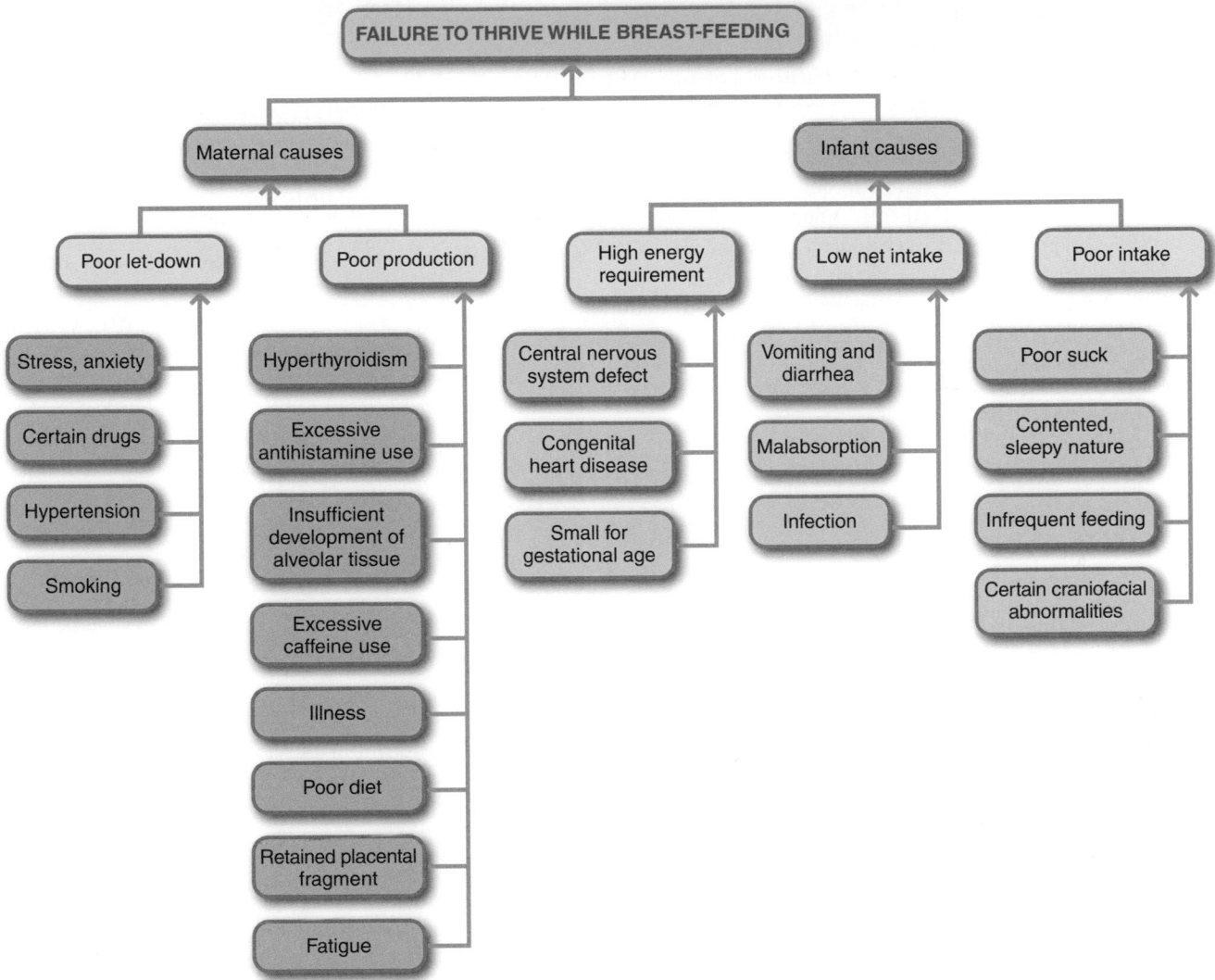

FIGURE 5-10 Diagnostic flow chart for failure to thrive in the breast-feeding infant.

TABLE 5-9

Management of Breast-Feeding Problems

Problem	Approaches to Management
Retracted nipple(s)	Before feeding the infant, roll the nipple gently between the fingers until erect.
Baby's mouth not open wide enough	Before feeding, depress the infant's lower jaw with one finger as the nipple is guided into the mouth.
Baby sucks poorly	Stimulate sucking motions by pressing upward under the baby's chin. Expression of colostrums often occurs, and the taste may stimulate sucking.
Baby demonstrates rooting but does not grasp the nipple; eventually cries in frustration	Interrupt the feeding, comfort the infant; the mother should take time to relax before trying again.
Baby falls asleep while nursing	If the infant falls asleep early in the feeding, the mother should awaken the infant by holding him or her upright, rubbing his or her back, talking to him or her, or providing similar quiet stimuli; another effort at feeding can then be made. If the baby falls asleep again, the feeding should be postponed.

✴ CLINICAL SCENARIO 1

Ana is a 45-year-old Latino woman who comes to the physician's office at 24 weeks with a diagnosis of gestational diabetes on a Friday afternoon at 3:30 pm. She is 5'2" with a prepregant weight of 150 lb and is now 160 lb with puffy ankles and in need of a dietary guidance. Although there is some language barrier, she speaks cautiously and slowly and wants to do her best to have a healthy child. She is G5P031 and had three babies born over 9 pounds in her native country. She is afraid that she will need insulin. She is eating mini-meals to try to keep her weight controlled.

✴**Nutrition Diagnosis:** Food and nutrition-related knowledge deficit related to consumption of small meals to control weight as evidenced by fear of needing insulin to control gestational diabetes.

1. Would you get an interpreter to assist you or provide her with the standard diabetes material you have in the cabinet?
2. How will you address her weight gain in the setting of her reported intake?
3. She says she is taking two of her children's chewable complete vitamin/mineral supplement because she ran out of money and she can't afford to buy anything else. How do you advise her?

✴ CLINICAL SCENARIO 2

Lucy is a 34-year-old, G2P001, woman who comes to you 12 weeks' pregnant with spontaneous twins and a 10-pound weight loss since week 6. She is 5'6" with a pregravid weight of 190 lb. History is notable for a seafood allergy. One year before pregnancy she lost 50 lb as a result of a gastric bypass operation, and 6 months ago she had a spontaneous abortion. She has had frequent bouts of nausea and vomiting.

✴**Nutrition Diagnosis:** Involuntary weight loss related to frequent bouts of nausea and vomiting as evidenced by 10-lb weight loss.

1. How would you classify her with malnutrition, and if so, which category?
2. What nutrients concern you most?
3. What are your recommendations for weight gain, and how would you create a nutritional plan to meet these goals?

✴ CLINICAL SCENARIO 3

Claire is a 23-year-old woman who has a 2-year-old child and a 10-day-old infant. She has come to the WIC clinic for certification as a breast-feeding mother. She is breast-feeding her infant every 3 hours but is concerned that he may not be getting enough milk. While with the nutritionist in the clinic, she begins to cry and talk about her sore nipples, profound fatigue, and worry. A 24-hour recall of foods eaten the day before reveals that Claire skipped breakfast and ate some microwave meals for lunch and dinner.

The nutritionist asks permission to watch Claire nurse her infant. Because she is not supporting the infant's back and buttocks firmly, the infant tugs at the nipple and causes the soreness. The nutritionist then weighs the infant and finds that he has already regained his birth weight.

✴**Nutrition Diagnosis:** Difficulty breast-feeding related to poor infant positioning as evidenced by mom's reports of fatigue and sore nipples.

1. What would you say to Claire regarding her concern that her son may not be getting enough milk?
2. What would you recommend to improve the infant's position during nursing? How would this improve the nursing experience?
3. What advice would you give Claire about her fatigue?
4. How would you design an eating plan that Claire could follow?

FOCAL POINTS

- The Dietary Guidelines for Americans provide an appropriate base for counseling women of reproductive age, but there is also need for individualized counseling.
- Whether defined problems are attributable to lack of resources, lack of knowledge, self-imposed food manipulations, genetic individuality, or a combination of these factors, solutions to problems during pregnancy and lactation can usually be found.
- A woman of reproductive age needs to know she gets but one chance to create the best baby she can; optimizing nutrition and her environment are critical ingredients.
- Nutrition status during pregnancy affects not only the gestation of the fetus, but the subsequent health of the mother and the eventual health of child
- Breast-feeding remains the best source of nutrition for newborns, and new mothers need support to breastfeed as long as possible up to 12 months.

Useful Websites

Agency for Toxic Substances and Disease Registry, Polychlorinated Biphenyls
http://www.atsdr.cdc.gov/tfacts17.html

Breastfeeding After Breast Reduction
www.BFAR.org

Centers for Disease Control, Listeriosis
http://www.cdc.gov/ncidod/dbmd/diseaseinfo/listeriosis

Center for Food Safety and Applied Nutrition, Food and Drug Administration. Consumer Advisory
http://www.cfsan.fda.gov/~dms/admehg3.html

Health Canada Advisory: Mercury levels in fish
http://www.hcsc/ca/english/archives/warnings/2001/2001

Mercury
www.seaturtles.org/gotmercury.htm or www.gotmercury.org

Virtual Embryo
www.visembryo.com

References

Akhter P et al: Assessment of iodine levels in the Pakistani diet, *Nutrition* 20:783, 2004.
American Academy of Pediatrics: Breastfeeding and the use of human milk, *Pediatrics* 115:496, 2005.
American Academy of Pediatrics, Committee on Drugs:. The transfer of drugs and other chemicals into human milk, *Pediatrics* 108:776, 2001.
American College of Obstetrics and Gynecology (ACOG): Exercise during pregnancy and the postpartum period, ACOG Committee Opinion 267:171, 2002.
American College of Obstetrics and Gynecology (ACOG): Obesity in pregnancy, Committee Opinion #315, *Obstet Gynecol* 106: 671, 2005.
American Dietetic Association: Position of the American Dietetic Association. Nutrition and lifestyle for a healthy pregnancy outcome, *J Am Diet Assoc* 102: 1479, 2002.
Armas LA et al: Vitamin D_2 is much less effective than vitamin D_3 in humans, *J Clin Endocrinolog Metab* 89:5387, 2004.
Bailey LB, Berry RJ: Folic acid supplementation and the occurrence of congenital heart defects, orofacial clefts, multiple births, and miscarriage, *Am J Clin Nutr* 81:1213S, 2005.
Bailit JL: Hyperemesis gravidarum: epidemiologic findings from a large cohort, *Obstet Gynecol* 193: 811, 2005.
Bay K et al: Testicular dysgenesis syndrome: possible role of endocrine disrupters, *Best Pract Res Clin Endocrinol Metab* 20:77, 2006.
Bech BH et al: Coffee and fetal death: a cohort study with prospective data, *Am J Epidemol* 162:983, 2005.
Bennett M: Vitamin B_{12} deficiency, infertility and recurrent fetal loss, *J Reprod Med* 46:209, 2001.
Bernstein IM et al: Morbidity and mortality among very-low-birth-weight neonates with intrauterine growth restriction, *Am J Obstet Gynecol* 182:198, 2000.
Brauer VF et al: Iodine nutrition, nodular thyroid disease, and urinary iodine excretion in a German university study population, *Thyroid* 15:364, 2005.
Carlin AM et al: Prevalence of vitamin D depletion among morbidly obese patients seeking gastric bypass surgery, *Surg Obes Relat Dis* 2(2):98, 2006.
CFSAN (Center for Safety and Applied Nutrition). www.cfsan.fda.gov/. Accessed December 1, 2006.
Chan-Cua S et al: Urinary iodine levels in term newborns and their mothers: a pilot study, *Southeast Asia J Med Pub Health* 34S:158, 2003.
Chappell LC et al:. Vitamin C and E supplementation in women at risk of preeclampsia is associated with changes in indices of oxidative stress and placental functio, *Am J Obstet Gynecol* 187:777, 2002.
Cho E et al: Dietary choline and betaine assessed by food-frequency questionnaire in relation to plasma total homocysteine concentration in the Framingham Offspring Study, *Am J Clin Nutr* 83:905, 2006.
Czeizel AE et al: Pregnancy outcomes in a randomized controlled trial of periconceptional multivitamin supplementation, Arch Gynecol Obstet 255:131, 1993.
Davis AJ et al: A severe case of ovarian hyperstimulation syndrome with liver dysfunction and malnutrition, *Eur J Gastroenterol Hepatol* 14:779, 2002.
Den Hond E and Schoeters G: Endocrine disrupters and human puberty, Int J Androl 29:264, 2006.
Dijkhuizen MA et al: Concurrent micronutrient deficiencies in lactating mothers and their infants in Indonesia, *Am J Clin Nutr* 73:786, 2001.
Eichholzer M et al: Folic acid: a public-health challenge, *Lancet* 367:1352, 2006.

Entin PL, Coffin L: Physiological basis for recommendations regarding exercise during pregnancy at high attitudes, *High Alt Med Biol* 5:321, 2004.

Erick M: Nutritional management of gestational diabetes mellitus, *Dietitians Gen Clin Pract Newsletter* IX(2):2, 1991.

Erick M: Hyperolfaction and hyperemesis gravidarum: What is the relationship? *Nutr Rev* 53:289, 1995.

Erick M: Nutrition via jejunostomy in refractory hyperemesis gravidarum: a case report, *J Am Diet Assoc* 97:1154, 1997.

Erick M: Ptylinism gravidarum: an unpleasant reality, *J Am Diet Assoc* 98:129, 1998.

Erick M: Morning sickness impact study, *Midwifery Today Int Midwife*, 59:30, Autumn 2001.

Erick M: *Managing morning sickness: a survival guide for pregnant women*, Boulder, Colo, 2004, Bull Publishing..

Erick M: Epigenetics: cutting edge science in maternal and fetal nutrition. Update of vitamin D, calcium, iron, iodine and omega 3 fatty acids. Presented at the Food, Nutrition, Conference and Exhibition of the American Dietetic Association, St Louis, Mo, October 25, 2005.

Erick, M. *Enteral nutrition and hyperemesis gravidarum: another perspective*, Women's Health and Reproductive Nutrition Practice Group newsletter, Chicago, Fall 2006, American Dietetic Association.

ESHRE Capri Workshop Group: Nutrition and reproduction in women, *Hum Reprod Update* 12:193, 2006.

Fait G et al: Effect of 1 week of oral hydration on the amniotic fluid index, *J Reprod Med* 48 (3):187, 2003.

Feron F et al: Developmental vitamin D_3 deficiency alters the adult brain, *Brain Res Bull* 65:14, 2005.

Flegal KM et al: Excess death associated with underweight, overweight and obesity, *JAMA* 293:1861, 2005.

Gharib SD et al, editors: Infertility: a guide to evaluation, treatment and counseling, Boston, 2003, Brigham and Women's Hospital.

Ghezzi F et al: Elevation in amniotic CRP is a marker for preterm deliver, *Am J Obstet Gynecol* 186:268, 2002.

Godil A, Chen YK: Percutaneous endoscopic gastrostomy for nutrition support in pregnancy associated with hyperemesis gravidarum and anorexia nervous, *J Parenter Enter Nutr* 22:238, 1998.

Goldberg BB et al: Prevalence of periconceptual folic acid use and perceived barriers to postgestational continuance of supplemental folic acid: survey from a Teratogen Information Service, *Birth Defects Res A Clin Mol Teratol* 76:193, 2006.

Goodwin TM: Nausea and vomiting of pregnancy: an obstetric syndrome, *Am J Obstet Gynecol* 185(Suppl 5):S184, 2002.

Gordon MV et al: Life-threatening milk-alkali syndrome resulting from antacid ingestion during pregnancy, *Med J Aust* 182: 350, 2005.

Greco E et al: ICSI in cases of sperm DNA damage: beneficial effect of oral antioxidant treatment, *Hum Reprod* 20:2590, 2005.

Groenen PM et al: Low maternal dietary intakes of iron, magnesium, and niacin are associated with spina bifida in the offspring, *J Nutr* 134:1516, 2004.

Grosso LM et al: Caffeine metabolites in umbilical cord blood, cytochrome P-450 1A2 activity, and intrauterine growth restriction, *Am J Epidemiol* 163:1035, 2006.

Gultepe M et al: Assessment of iodine intake in mildly iodine-deficit pregnant women by a new automated kinetic urinary iodine determination method, *Clin Chem Lab Med* 43:280, 2005.

Gupta M et al: Keratomalacia in a neonate secondary to maternal Vitamin A deficiency, *Indian J Pediatr* 72: 881, 2005.

Hale T: *Medications and mothers' milk*, Amarillo, Tx, 2006, Hale Publishing.

Hendler I et al: The preterm predication study: association between maternal body mass index and spontaneous and indicated preterm birth, *Am J Obstet Gynecol* 192: 882, 2005.

Henry RJW, Vadas RA: Spontaneous rupture of the esophagus following severe vomiting in early pregnancy: a case report, *Br J Obstet Gynecol* 93:392, 1986.

Hernandez L, Green PH. Extraintestinal manifestations of celiac disease, *Curr Gastroenterol Rep* 8 (5):383, 2006.

Hill JB et al: Acute renal failure in association with hyperemesis gravidarum, *Obstet Gynecol* 100:1119, 2002.

Houet T et al: Comparsion of women's alcohol consumption before and during pregnancy from a prospective series of 150 women, *J Gynecol Obstet Biol Reprod* 34:687, 2005.

Huerta S et al: Vitamin A deficiency in a newborn resulting from maternal hypovitaminosis A after biliopancreatic diversion for the treatment of morbid obesity, *Am J Clin Nutr* 76:426, 2002.

Hughes WL, Robinson AC: Treatment of hyperemesis gravidarum with intramuscular injections of husband's blood, *Am J Obstet Gynecol* 44:103, 1942.

Hypponen E: Vitamin D for the prevention of preeclampsia? A hypothesis, *Nutr Rev* 63:225, 2005.

Institute of Medicine, Food and Nutrition Board: *Nutrition during pregnancy*, Parts I and II, Washington, DC, 1990, National Academies Press.

Institute of Medicine, Food and Nutrition Board: *Dietary reference intakes for calcium, phosphorus, magnesium, vitamin D, and fluoride*, Washington, DC, 1997, National Academies Press.

Institute of Medicine, Food and Nutrition Board: *Dietary reference intakes for thiamin*, riboflavin, niacin, vitamin B_6, folate, vitamin B_{12}, pantothenic acid, biotin and choline, Washington, DC, 1998, National Academies Press.

Institute of Medicine, Food and Nutrition Board: *Dietary reference intakes for dietary antioxidants and related compounds*, Washington, DC, 2000, National Academies Press.

Institute of Medicine, Food and Nutrition Board: *Dietary reference intakes for vitamin A, vitamin K, arsenic, boron, chromium, copper, iodine, iron, molybdenum, nickel, silicon, vanadium and zinc*, Washington, DC, 2001, National Academies Press.

Institute of Medicine, Food and Nutrition Board: *Dietary reference intakes for energy and the macronutrients, carbohydrate, fiber, fat, and fatty acids*, Washington, DC, 2002, National Academies Press.

Irving PM et al: Percutaneous endoscopic gastrotomy with a jejunal port for severe hyperemesis gravidarum, *Eur J Gastroenterol Hepatol* 16:937, 2004.

Jednak MA et al: Protein meals reduce nausea and gastric wave dysrhythmic activity in first trimester pregnancy, *Am J Physiol* 277 (4 pt 1):G855, 1999.

Jewell D, Young G: Interventions for nausea and vomiting in early pregnancy, *Cochrane Database Syst Rev* (1):CD000145, 2002.

Kakarla N et al: Pregnancy after gastric bypass surgery and internal hernia formation, *Obstet Gynecol* 105:1195, 2005.

Kalkwarf HJ, Specker BL: Bone mineral changes during pregnancy and lactation, *Endocrine* 1:49, 2002.

Kirk AB et al: Perchlorate and iodide in dairy and breast milk, *Environ Sci Technol* 39:2001, 2005.

Lauwers J, Shinskie D: *Counseling the nursing mother,* Boston, Mass, 2000, Jones and Bartlett.

Lawrence RA, Lawrence RM: *Breastfeeding: a guide for the medical profession,* Philadelphia, 2005, Mosby.

Lee WB et al: Ocular complications of hypovitaminosis A after bariatric surgery, *Ophthalmology* 112:1031, 2005.

Lopez LB et al: Pica during pregnancy: a frequently underestimated problem, *Arch Latinoam Nutr* 54:17, 2004.

Lordo RA et al: Semi-volatile organic compounds in adipose tissue: estimated average for the US population and selected subpopulations, *Am J Pub Health* 86:1253, 1996.

Lovelady CA: The impact of energy restriction and exercise in lactating women, *Adv Exp Med Biol* 554:115, 2004.

Lovelady CA et al: The effects of dieting on food and nutrient intake of lactating women, *J Am Diet Assoc* 106:908, 2006.

Luke B: Nutrition in multiple gestations, *Clin Perinatol* 32:403, 2005.

Malcova H et al: Absence of breast-feeding is associated with the risk of type I diabetes: a case-control study in a population with rapidly increasing incidence, *Eur J Pediatr* 165:114, 2006.

Margann EF et al: Effect of maternal hydration on amniotic fluid volume, *Obstet Gynecol* 101:1261, 2003.

Marinella MA: Refeeding syndrome and hypophosphatemia, *J Intern Care Med* 20:155, 2005.

Martin JA et al: Births: preliminary data for 2001, *Natl Vital Stat Rep* 6:50(10):1, 2002.

Mason ME et al: Metabolic complicatins of bariatric surgery: diagnosis and management issues, *Gastroenterol Clin North Am* 34:25, 2005.

Mazzotta P et al: Factors associated with elective termination of pregnancy among Canadian and American women with nausea and vomiting of pregnancy, *J Psychosom Obstet Gynaecol* 22:7, 2001.

Medical Research Council (MRC) Vitamin Study Research Group: Prevention of neural tube defects: results of the Medical Research Council vitamin study, *Lancet* 338: 131, 1991.

Menacker F et al: Births to 10-14 year-old mothers, 1990-2002: trends and health outcomes, *Natl Vital Stat Rep* 53:1, 2004.

Mennes T et al: Impact of ambient air pollution on birth weight in Syndey, Australia, *Occup Environ Med* 62: 524, 2005.

Miles HL et al: Fetal origins of adult diseases: a paediatric perspective, *Rev Endocrinol Metabol Dis* 6: 261, 2005.

Munch S: Chicken or the egg? The biological-psychological controversy surrounding hyperemesis gravidarum, *Soc Sci Med* 55:1267, 2002.

National Institute for Child Health and Human Development (NICHD), National Institutes of Health: *Moderate doses of vitamin A do not pose risk of birth defects.* Available at http://www.nichd.nih.gov//new/releases/vitama.cfm, 2001, accessed December 1, 2006.

Nelen WL, et al: Hyperhomocysteinemia and recurrent early pregnancy loss: a meta-analysis, *Fertil Steril* 74:1196, 2000.

Nohr EA et al: Prepregnancy obesity and fetal death: a study within the Danish National Birth Cohort, *Obstet Gynecol* 106: 250, 2005.

Ohara N et al: The role of thyroid hormone in trophoblast function, early pregnancy maintenance, and fetal neurodevelopment, *J Obstet Gynaecol Can.* 26:982, 2004.

Oken E et al: Decline in fish consumption among pregnancy women after national mercury advisory, *Obstet Gynecol* 102:346, 2003.

Owen AL, Owen GM: Twenty years of WIC: a review of some effects of the program, *J Am Diet Assoc* 97:777, 1997.

Panesar NS et al: Are thyroid hormones or hCG responsible for hyperemesis gravidarum? A matched paired study in pregnant Chinese women, *Acta Obstet Gynecol Scand* 80:519, 2001.

Pearce EN et al: Dietary iodine in pregnant women from the Boston, Massachusetts area, *Thyroid* 14:327, 2004.

Perchlorate Environmental Contamination: *toxicological review and risk characterization (2002 External Review Draft).* US Environmental Protection Agency, Office of Research and Development, National Center for Environmental Assessment, Washington Office, Washington, DC, NCEA-1-0503, 2002.

Poston L et al: Vitamin C and vitamin E in pregnant women at risk for preeclampsia (VIP trial): randomized placebo-controlled trial, *Lancet* 367:1145, 2006.

Redmond G: Thyroid dysfunction and women's reproductive health, *Thyroid* 14:5S, 2004.

Rees S, Inder T: Fetal and neonatal origins of altered brain development, *Early Hum Dev* 81:753, 2005.

Reid G, Bocking A: The potential for probiotics to prevent bacterial vaginosis and preterm labor, *Am J Obstet Gynecol* 189:1202, 2003.

Riordan J: *Breastfeeding and human lactation,* Boston, 2005, Jones and Bartlett.

Roberts A et al: Sucralose metabolism and pharmacokinetics in man, *Food Chem Toxicol* 30:31S, 2000.

Robinson NJ et al: Coagulopathy secondary to vitamin K deficiency in hyperemesis gravidarum, *Obstet Gynecol* 92:673, 1998.

Rosenbloom AL: Permanent brain from hypernatremic dehydration in breastfed infants: patient reports, *Clin Pediatr* 43:855, 2004.

Rumbold AR et al: Vitamins C and E and risks of preeclampsia and perinatal complications, *N Engl J Med* 354:1796, 2006.

Rwebembera AA et al: Relationship between infant birth weight <2000 g and maternal zinc levels at Muhimbili National Hospital, Dar Es Salamm, Tanzania, *J Trop Pediatr* 52:118, 2005.

Scheplyagina LA: Impact of the mother's zinc deficiency on the woman's and newborn's health status, *J Trace Elem Med Biol* 19:29, 2005.

Schieve LA et al: Pre-pregnancy body mass index and pregnancy weight gain: associations with preterm delivery, The NMIHS Collaborative Study Group, *Obstet Gynecol* 96:194, 2000.

Scholl TO et al: Maternal glucose concentration influences fetal growth, gestation, and pregnancy complications, *Am J Epidemiol* 154:514, 2001.

Scialli AR, Public Affairs Committee of the Teratology Society: Teratology public affairs committee position paper: maternal obesity and pregnancy, *Birth Defects Res A Clin Mol Teratol* 76:73, 2006.

Scotland N et al: Body Mass Index, provider advice and target gestational weight gain, *Obstet Gynecol* 105:633, 2005.

Shaikh MG et al: Transient neonatal hypothyroidism due to a maternal vegan diet, *J Pediatr Endocrinol Metab* 16:111, 2003.

Sharma JB et al: Oxidative stress markers and antioxidant levels in normal pregnancy and preeclampsia, *Int J Gynaecol Obstet* 94:23, 2006.

Sheiner E et al: Pregnancy after bariatric surgery is not associated with adverse perinatal outcome, *Am J Obstet Gynecol* 190:1135, 2004.

Signorello L, McLaughlin JK: Maternal caffeine consumption and spontaneous abortion: a review of the epidemiologic evidence, *Epidemiology* 15:229, 2004.

Sisk PM et al: Lactation counseling for mothers of very low birth weight infants: effect on maternal anxiety and infant intake of human milk, *Pediatrics* 117(1):e67, 2006.

Skeaff SA et al: Are breast-fed infants and toddlers in New Zealand at risk of iodine deficiency? *Nutrition* 2:325, 2005.

Smuts CM et al: A randomized trial of docosahexanenoic acid supplementation during the third trimester of pregnancy, *Obstet Gynecol* 101:469, 2003.

Solomon CG, Seely EW: Brief review: hypertension in pregnancy: a manifestation of the insulin resistance syndrome? *Hypertension* 37: 232, 2001.

Stan C et al: Hydration for treatment of preterm labour, *Cochraine Database Syst Rev* (2), CD003096, 2002.

Stazi AV, Mantovani A: A risk factor for female fertility and pregnancy: celiac disease, *Gynecol Endocrinol* 14:454, 2000.

Stephansson O et al: Maternal weight, pregnancy weight gain, and the risk of antepartum stillbirth, *Am J Obstet Gynecol* 184:463, 2001.

Stevens-Simon C: Puberty: In Frederickson H, Wilkins L, editors: *Obstetric and gynecologic secrets*, ed 2, Philadelphia, 1997, Hanley & Belfus, pp 86-92.

Story M, Stang J, editors: *Nutrition and the pregnant adolescent: a practice reference guide*, 2000, Center for Leadership, Education, and Training in Maternal and Child Nutrition: Public Health Nutrition: Division of Epidemiology: School of Public Health, University of Minnesota. Minneapolis, 2000.

Stuebe A et al: Duration of lactation and incidence of type 2 diabetes, *JAMA* 294:2601, 2005.

Thompson T: Thiamin, riboflavin, and niacin contents of the gluten-free diet: is there cause for concern? *J Am Diet Assoc* 7:858, 1999.

van der Meer IM et al: High prevalence of vitamin D deficiency in pregnant non-Western women in The Hague, Netherlands, *Am J Clin Nutr* 84:350, 2006.

Watkins ML et al: Maternity obesity and risk for birth defects, *Pediatrics* 111:1152, 2003.

Williams CL: Epigenetics: cutting edge science in maternal and fetal nutrition: prenatal choline and folate requirements for brain and cognitive development. Presented at FNCE (Food, Nutrition Conference and Exhibition) St. Louis, Mo, October 25, 2005.

Wong WY et al: Effects of folic acid and zinc sulfate on male factor subfertility: double-blind, randomized placebo-controlled trial, *Fertil Steril* 77:491, 2002.

Woods JR: Reactive oxygen species and premature rupture of membranes: a review, Placenta Trophoblast Res 15(suppl A): S38, 2001.

Wright KS et al: Infant acceptance of breast milk after maternal exercise, *Pediatrics* 109:585, 2002.

Yao XH et al: Adult rats prenatally exposed to ethanol have increased gluconeogenesis and impaired insulin response of hepatic gluconeogenic genes, *J Appl Physiol* 100:642, 2005.

Yldzdas HY et al: May the best friend be an enemy if not recognized early: hypernatremic dehydration due to breastfeeding, *Pediatr Emerg Care* 21:445, 2005.

Young GL, Jewell D: Interventions for leg cramps in pregnancy, *Cochrane Database Syst Rev* CD000121, 2000.

Zeisel SH, Niculescu MD: Perinatal choline influences brain structure and function, *Nutr Rev* 64:197, 2006.

Zervos IA, et al: Effects of dietary vitamin A on acrosin and plasminogen activator activity of ram spermatozoa, *Reproduction* 129:707, 2005.

Ziegler EE et al: Vitamin D deficiency in breastfed infants in Iowa, *Pediatrics* 118(2):603, 2006.

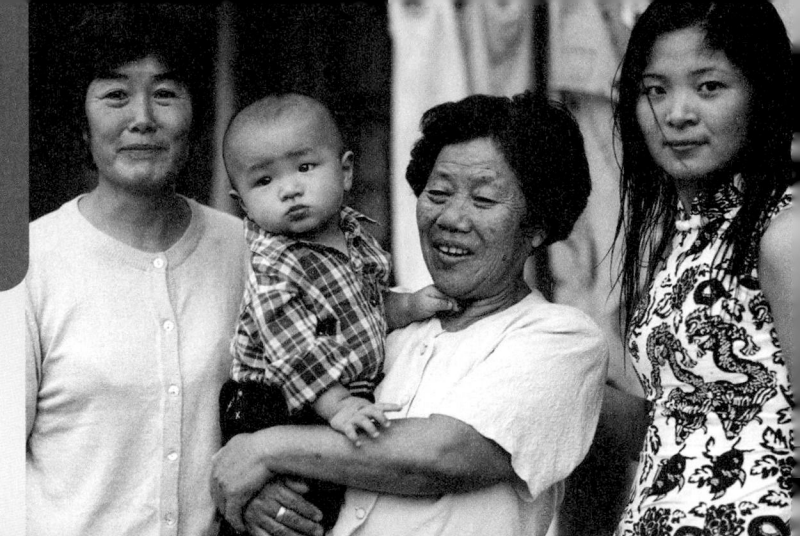

CHAPTER 6

Cristine M. Trahms, MS, RD, CD, FADA
Kelly N. McKean, MS, RD, CD

Nutrition During Infancy

KEY TERMS

arachidonic acid (ARA) a very long–chain fatty acid (C20:4n-6), known to be a derivative of linoleic acid, that is found in human milk

casein the principal protein in cow's milk

casein hydrolysate casein that has been split into smaller components by acid, alkali, or enzymes

catch-up the growth phenomenon in the first year of life that occurs when the rate of growth increases to the genetic potential

colic severe abdominal pain in infants

docosahexaenoic acid (DHA) a very long–chain fatty acid (C22:6n-3), known to be a derivative of linolenic acid, that is found in human milk

growth channel a curve of weight and length or height gain throughout the period of growth; stated as a percentile based on a growth chart

electrolytically reduced iron iron that has been fractionated into small particles for improved absorption; used in the fortification of foods

hemorrhagic disease of the newborn a self-limiting hemorrhagic disorder that develops during the first few days of life and is caused by a vitamin K deficiency; develops more frequently in breast-fed infants than in formula-fed infants

lactalbumin an easy-to-digest protein found in human milk

lactoferrin the iron-binding protein in human milk

lag-down the growth phenomenon in the first year of life that occurs when the rate of growth decreases to the genetic potential

palmar grasp an immature way of holding an object with the palm

pincer grasp a more refined and mature way (than the palmar grasp) of holding an object with the fingers

renal solute load the amount of nitrogenous waste and minerals that must be excreted by the kidney

suckle to take nourishment at the breast

whey proteins the proteins remaining in the watery fraction of milk after the curd and cream have been removed; contains lactalbumin

During the first 2 years of life, which are characterized by rapid physical and social growth and development, many changes occur that affect feeding and nutrient intake. The adequacy of infants' nutrient intakes affects their interaction with their environment. Healthy, well-nourished infants have the energy to respond to and learn from the stimuli in their environment and to interact with their parents and caregivers in a manner that encourages bonding and attachment (Trahms and Pipes, 1997).

PHYSIOLOGIC DEVELOPMENT

The length of gestation, the mother's prepregnancy weight, and the mother's weight gain during gestation determine an infant's birth weight. After birth, the growth of an infant is influenced by genetics and nourishment (Figure 6-1). Most infants who are genetically determined to be larger reach their **growth channel,** a curve of weight and length or height gain throughout the period of growth, between 3 and 6 months of age. However, many infants born at or below the tenth percentile for length may not reach their genetically appropriate growth channel until 1 year of age; this is called **catch-up** growth. Larger infants at birth who are genetically determined to be smaller grow at their fetal rate for several months and often do not reach their growth channel until 13 months of age (Smith et al., 1976). This phenomenon during the first year of life is called **lag-down** growth.

Infants lose about 6% of their body weight during the first few days of life, but their birth weight is usually regained by the seventh to tenth day. Growth thereafter proceeds at a rapid but decelerating rate. Infants usually double their birth weight by 4 to 6 months of age and triple it by the age of 1 year. The amount of weight gained by the infant during the second year approximates the birth weight. Infants increase their length by 50% during the first year of life and double it by 4 years. Total body fat increases rapidly during the first 9 months, after which the rate of fat gain tapers off throughout the rest of childhood. Total body water decreases throughout infancy from 70% at birth to 60% at 1 year. The decrease is almost all in extracellular water, which declines from 42% at birth to 32% at 1 year of age (see Figure 4-1).

The stomach capacity of infants increases from a range of 10 to 20 ml at birth to 200 ml by 1 year, enabling infants to consume more food at a given time and at less frequent intervals as they grow older. During the first weeks of life, gastric acidity decreases and for the first few months remains lower than that of older infants and adults. The rate of emptying is relatively slow, depending on the size and composition of the meal.

Although gastric secretion of pepsin remains low during the first 3 months of life, it is not a limiting factor for protein digestion. Trypsin activity in duodenal fluids is lower in infants than in older children, as is the activity of enterokinase (the enzyme responsible for the activation of trypsin) (see Chapter 1). However, the enzymatic activity is sufficient to digest the milk protein that infants normally consume.

Fat absorption varies in the neonate. Human milk fat is well absorbed, but butterfat is poorly absorbed, with fecal excretions of 20% to 48%. The fat combinations in commercially prepared infant formula are well absorbed. Human milk contains two lipases; one of them, found in the lipid fraction of milk, is essential for the milk lipid formation in the mammary gland but is of no known nutritional importance to the infant. The other lipase—bile salt–stimulated lipase—hydrolyzes triglycerides into free fatty acids and glycerol. The infant's lingual and gastric lipases hydrolyze short- and medium-chain fatty acids in the stomach. Gastric lipase also hydrolyzes long-chain fatty acids and is important in initiating the digestion of triglycerides in the stomach.

Most long-chain triglycerides pass unhydrolyzed into the small intestine, where they are broken down by pancreatic lipase. The bile salt–stimulated lipase in human milk is stimulated by the infant's bile salts and hydrolyzes the triglycerides in the small intestine. Bile salts, which are effective emulsifiers when combined with monoglycerides, fatty acids, and lecithin, aid in the intestinal digestion of fat.

The activities of the enzymes responsible for the digestion of disaccharides—maltase, isomaltase, and sucrase—reach adult levels by 28 to 32 weeks' gestation. Lactase activity (responsible for digesting the disaccharide in milk) increases near birth and reaches adult levels by birth. Pancreatic amylase, which digests starch, continues to remain low during the first 6 months after birth. If the infant consumes starch before this time, increased activity of salivary amylase and digestion in the colon usually compensate.

The neonate has functional but physiologically immature kidneys that increase in size and concentrating capacity in the early weeks of life. The kidneys double in weight by 6 months and triple in weight by 1 year of age. The last renal tubule is estimated to form between the eighth fetal month and the end of the first postnatal month. The glomerular tuft is covered by a much thicker layer of cells throughout neonatal life than at any later time, which may explain why the glomerular filtration rate is lower during the first 9 months of life than it is in later childhood and adulthood. In the neonatal period the ability to form acid, urine, and concentrate solutes is often limited. The renal concentrating capacity at birth may be limited to as little as 700 mOsm/L in some infants. Others have the concentrating capacity of adults (1200 to 1400 mOsm/L). By 6 weeks, most infants can concentrate urine at adult levels. Renal function in a normal newborn infant is rarely a concern; however, difficulties may arise in infants with diarrhea or those who are fed formula that is too concentrated (Butte et al., 2004).

NUTRIENT REQUIREMENTS

Nutrient needs of infants reflect rates of growth, energy expended in activity, basal metabolic needs, and the interaction of the nutrients consumed. Balance studies have

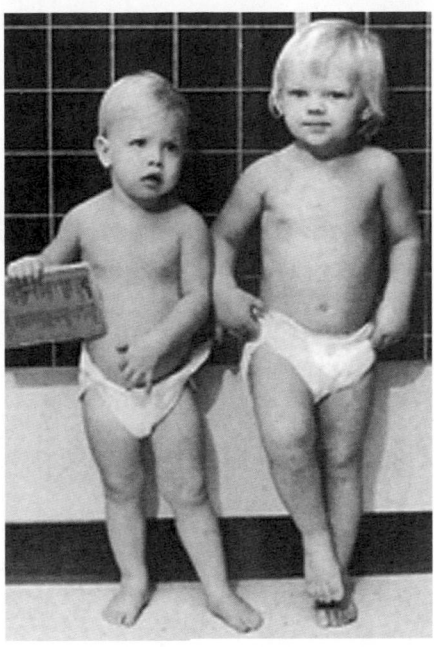

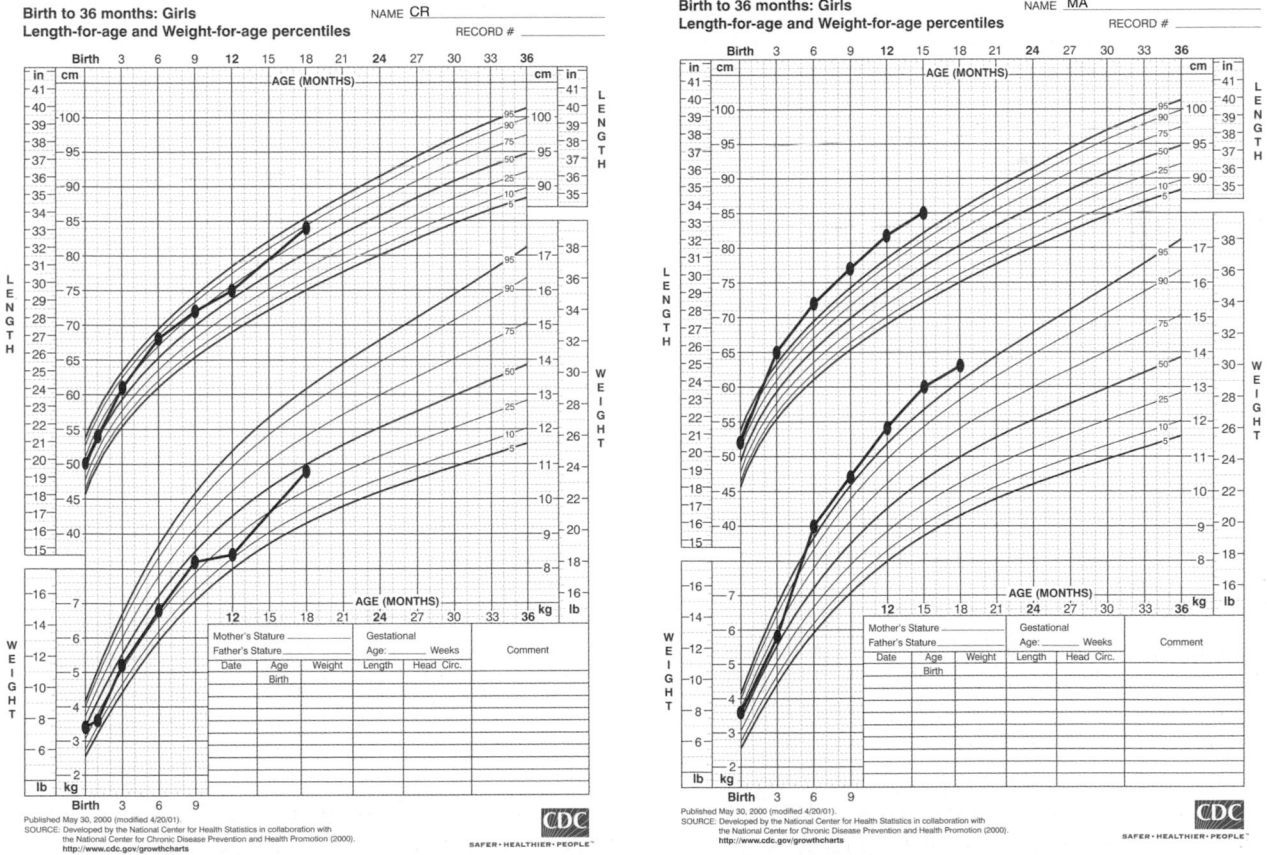

FIGURE 6-1 Two girls born just 1 month apart with only a 1-lb difference in birth weight; note the marked difference in growth. (The girls are approximately 20 months of age.) In the growth chart, note M.A.'s early catch-up growth to above the 95th percentile for height and weight by 6 months of age. In addition, note the effect of an illness on C.R.'s weight gain and linear growth at the age of 12 months, as well as the subsequent catch-up growth. *(Data from The National Center for Health Statistics, in collaboration with the National Center for Chronic Disease Prevention and Health Promotion, 2000, http://www. cdc.gov/growthcharts.)*

defined minimum acceptable levels of intakes for a few nutrients, but for most nutrients the suggested intakes have been extrapolated from the intakes of normal, thriving infants consuming human milk. The dietary reference intakes (DRIs) for infants are shown in Table 6-1.

Energy

Full-term infants who are breast-fed to satiety and infants who are fed a standard 20-kcal/oz formula generally adjust their intake to meet their energy needs when caregivers are sensitive to the infants' hunger and satiety cues. An effective

TABLE 6-1

Dietary Reference Intakes: Adequate Intakes and Recommended Dietary Allowances for Infants and Children from Birth to 3 Years

Nutrient (amount/day)	Age		
	Birth-6 mo	6 mo-1 yr	1-3 yr
Protein (g)	9.1	11	13
Energy (kcal)	M:570 F:520	M:743 F:676	M:1046 F:992
Carbohydrate (g)	60	95	130*
Fiber (g)	ND	ND	19
Water (L/day)	0.7	0.8	1.3
Total fat (g)	31	30	ND
n-6 Polyunsaturated fatty acids [omega-6, linoleic] (g)	4.4	4.6	7
n-3 Polyunsaturated fatty acids [omega-3, linolenic] (g)	0.5	0.5	0.7
Vitamin A (mcg)[†]	400	500	300*
Vitamin D (mcg)[‡]	5	5	5
Vitamin E (mg)	4	5	6*
Vitamin K (mcg)	2	2.5	30
Vitamin C (mg)	40	50	15*
Thiamin (mg)	0.2	0.3	0.5*
Riboflavin (mg)	0.3	0.4	0.5*
Niacin (mg)[§]	2	4	6*
Vitamin B_6 (mg)	0.1	0.3	0.5*
Folate (mcg)[‖]	65	80	150*
Vitamin B_{12} (mcg)	0.4	0.5	0.9*
Pantothenic acid (mg)	1.7	1.8	2
Biotin (mcg)	5	6	8
Choline (mg)	125	150	200
Calcium (mg)	210	270	500*
Phosphorus (mg)	100	275	460*
Magnesium (mg)	30	75	80*
Iron (mg)	0.27	11*	7*
Zinc (mg)	2	3*	3*
Iodine (mcg)	110	130	90*
Selenium (mcg)	15	20	20*
Fluoride (mg)	0.01	0.5	0.7
Manganese (mg)	0.003	0.6	1.2
Molybdenum (mcg)	2	3	17*
Chromium (mcg)	0.2	5.5	11
Copper (mcg)	200	220	340*

Data from Institute of Medicine, Food and Nutrition Board: *Dietary reference intakes*, Washington DC, November 2005, http://www.iom.edu/project.asp?id=4574

*RDAs and AIs may both be used as goals for individual intakes. RDAs are set to meet the needs of almost all (98%) individuals in a group. For healthy breast-fed infants, the AI is the mean intake. An AI is set instead of an RDA if there is insufficient data to set an RDA.

†Retinol activity equivalents (REA): 1 REA = 1 mcg retinol = 12 mcg β-carotene = 24 mcg α-carotene.

‡1 mcg cholecalciferol = 40 IU vitamin D.

§Niacin equivalents (NE): 1 mg niacin = 60 mg Tryptophan; for 0-6 months value is preformed niacin (not NE).

‖Dietary folate equivalents (DFE): 1 DFE = 1 mcg food folate = 0.6 mcg folate from fortified food.

method for determining the adequacy of an infant's energy intake is to carefully monitor gains in weight, length, and weight-for-length for age and plot these data on the growth charts shown in Appendix Tables 9, 10, 13, and 14. It is important to recognize that, during the first year, a catch-up or lag-down period in growth may occur.

If infants begin to experience a decrease in their rate of weight gain, do not gain weight, or lose weight, their energy and nutrient intake should be monitored carefully. If the rate of growth in length decreases or ceases, potential malnutrition, an undetected disease, or both should be investigated thoroughly. If the weight gain proceeds at a much more rapid rate than growth in length, the energy concentration of the formula, the quantity of formula consumed, and the amount and type of semisolid and table foods offered should be evaluated. The activity level of the infant should also be assessed (Campbell, 2003). Infants who are at the highest end of the growth charts for weight or body mass index, or who grow rapidly in infancy, tend to be at greater risk for obesity later in life (Baird et al., 2005).

Formula-fed infants consume more kilocalories of energy per unit of body size than breast-fed infants during the first year. Gains in weight are greater in formula-fed infants, as are increases in body mass per gram of protein intake. However, no functional advantage has been ascribed to the more rapid growth rate (Dewey et al., 1993; Heinig et al., 1993). The recently developed World Health Organization (WHO) Growth Standards use the breast-fed infant as the normative model for "prescriptive" assessment of infant growth. It is expected that these growth charts will enable clinicians to identify infants "in the process" of becoming overnourished or undernourished and lead to timely intervention (Garza, 2006).

Protein

Protein is needed for tissue replacement, deposition of lean body mass, and growth (Rodriguez, 2005). Protein requirements during the rapid growth of infancy are higher per kilogram of weight than those for adults or older children. Recommendations for protein intake are based on the composition of human milk, and it is assumed that the efficiency of human milk use is 100%.

Infants require a larger percentage of total amino acids as essential amino acids than do adults. Histidine seems to be an essential amino acid for infants, but not for adults. Tyrosine, cystine, and taurine may be essential for premature infants.

Human milk or infant formula provides the major portion of protein during the first year of life. The amount of protein in human milk is adequate for the first 6 months of the infant's life even though the amount of protein in human milk is considerably less than in infant formula. In the last 6 months of the first year, diets of infants should be supplemented with additional sources of high-quality protein such as yogurt, strained meats, or cereal mixed with formula or human milk.

Infants may receive inadequate amounts of protein if their formula is excessively diluted, a prolonged regimen

designed to treat diarrhea after an enteric illness is used, or they have multiple food allergies restricting intake (see Chapter 29).

Lipids

The current recommendation for infants younger than 1 year of age is to consume a minimum of 30 g of fat per day. This quantity is present in human milk and all infant formulas. Significantly lower fat intakes (e.g., with skim-milk feedings) may result in an inadequate total energy intake. An infant may try to correct the energy deficit by increasing the volume of milk ingested but usually cannot make up the entire deficit this way.

Human milk contains a generous amount of the essential fatty acids linoleic acid and linolenic acid, as well as the longer-chain derivatives **arachidonic acid (ARA)** (C20:4n-6) and **docosahexaenoic acid (DHA)** (C22:6n-3). Infant formulas are supplemented with linoleic acid and linolenic acid, from which ARA and DHA are derived. Increasingly, many formulas are also supplemented with ARA and DHA. Table 6-2 indicates the linoleic acid, ARA, and DHA contents of infant formulas.

Linoleic acid, which is essential for growth and dermal integrity, should provide 3% of the infant's total kilocalories, or 4.4 g/day for infants younger than 6 months of age and 4.6 g/day for infants 7 months to 1 year of age. Five percent of the kilocalories in human milk and 10% in most

TABLE 6-2

Fatty Acid Content of Selected Infant Formulas

FORMULA	(mg per 100 kcal energy)		
	Linoleic Acid	ARA	DHA
Alimentum Advance (Ross)	1900	21	8
Pregestimil (Mead Johnson)	1040	0	0
Isomil Advance (Ross)	1000	21	8
Similac Advance (Ross)	1000	21	8
Good Start Supreme Soy DHA & ARA (Nestlé)	920	32	16
Good Start Supreme DHA & ARA (Nestlé)	900	32	16
Enfamil LIPIL (Mead Johnson)	860	34	17
LactoFree LIPIL (Mead Johnson)	860	34	17
Nutramigen LIPIL (Mead Johnson)	860	34	17
Prosobee LIPIL (Mead Johnson)	860	34	17
Elecare (Ross)	800	0	0
Neocate (SHS)	677	0	0

Often there are two versions of each infant formula: one that contains DHA and ARA, and one that does not. The DHA/ARA–containing formulas, if available, were included. The linoleic acid content is the same for each comparable formula that does not contain DHA/ARA.

infant formulas are derived from linoleic acid. Smaller amounts of α-linolenic acid, a precursor of the *n*-3 fatty acids DHA and eicosapentaenoic acid (EPA), should be included. The current recommendation is 0.5 g/day during the first year of life. Because DHA can be formed by desaturation of α-linolenic acid, the importance of dietary DHA intake is uncertain. The concentration of DHA in human milk varies, depending on the amount of DHA in the mother's diet.

Recently the importance of long-chain polyunsaturated fatty acids (LCPUFAs) in infant visual and neurologic development has been studied. DHA and ARA are the major *n*-3 and *n*-6 LCPUFAs, respectively, of neural tissues; and DHA is the major fatty acid of the photoreceptor membranes of the retina. Although findings suggest that DHA and ARA positively affect visual acuity and mental and psychomotor development in premature infants (Clandinin et al., 2005; SanGiovanni et al., 2000), studies with full-term infants are less clear. For example, randomized trials reveal that DHA and ARA supplementation increases visual acuity in infants who are fed formula (Birch et al., 2005; Morale et al., 2005; Hoffman et al., 2003), but other studies have not found any effects (Auestad et al., 2003; Makrides et al., 2000). One study, in which DHA concentration was related to visual acuity at 2 and 12 months of age, seems to suggest that factors other than breast-milk sources of DHA may be important (Innis et al., 2001). The concentration of supplemented LCPUFAs may also play a significant role in the effectiveness (Uauy et al., 2003).

Carbohydrates

Carbohydrates should supply 30% to 60% of the energy intake during infancy. Approximately 40% of the energy in human milk and 40% to 50% of the energy in infant formulas is derived from lactose or other carbohydrates. Although rare, some infants cannot tolerate lactose and require a modified formula in their diet (see Chapters 27 and 44).

Botulism in infancy is caused by the ingestion of *Clostridium botulinum* spores, which germinate and produce toxin in the bowel lumen. Honey and corn syrup, occasionally used in home-prepared foods, have been identified as the only food sources of these spores in infants' diets. The spores are extremely resistant to heat treatment and are not destroyed by current methods of processing. Thus honey and corn syrup should not be fed to infants younger than 1 year of age because they have not yet developed the immunity required to resist botulism spore development.

Water

The water requirement for infants is determined by the amount lost from the skin and lungs and in the feces and urine, in addition to a small amount needed for growth. The recommended total water intake for infants, based on the DRIs, is 0.7 L/day for infants up to 6 months and 0.8 L/day for infants 7 to 12 months of age. Note that total water includes all water contained in food, beverages, and drinking water. Water requirements per kilogram of body weight are shown in Table 6-3.

TABLE 6-3	
Water Requirements of Infants and Children	
Age	**Water Requirement (ml/kg/day)**
10 days	125-150
3 mo	140-160
6 mo	130-155
1 yr	120-135
2 yr	115-125
6 yr	90-100
10 yr	70-85
14 yr	50-60

From Barness LA: Nutrition and nutritional disorders. In Behrman RE, Kliegman RM: *Nelson textbook of pediatrics*, ed 17, Philadelphia, 2003, Saunders.

Because the renal concentrating capacity of young infants may be less than that of older children and adults, they may be vulnerable to developing a water imbalance. Under ordinary conditions, human milk and formula that is properly prepared supply adequate amounts of water. However, when formula is boiled, the water evaporates and the solutes become concentrated; therefore, boiled milk or formula is inappropriate for infants. In very hot, humid environments, infants may require additional water. When other than renal losses of water are high (e.g., vomiting and diarrhea), infants should be monitored carefully for fluid and electrolyte imbalances.

Water deficits result in hypernatremic dehydration and its associated neurologic consequences (e.g., seizures, vascular damage). Hypernatremic dehydration has been reported in breast-fed infants who had a weight loss of greater than 10% of their birth weight in the first few days of life (Manganaro et al., 2001; Oddie et al., 2001). Because of the potential for hypernatremic dehydration, careful monitoring of volume of intake, weight gain, and hydration status (e.g., number of wet diapers) in all newborns is warranted.

Water intoxication results in hyponatremia, restlessness, nausea, vomiting, diarrhea, and polyuria or oliguria; seizures can also result. This condition may occur when water is provided as a replacement for milk, the formula is excessively diluted, or bottled water instead of an electrolyte solution is provided as treatment for diarrhea.

Minerals

Calcium

The previous RDA of 400 to 800 mg/day of calcium was set to meet the needs of infants fed cow's milk–based formula who retain approximately 25% to 30% of the intake. This is not applicable to breast-fed infants, who retain approximately two thirds of their calcium intake. The recommended adequate intake (AI) (the mean intake of healthy breast-fed infants) for infants 0 to 6 months of age is 210 mg/day; for infants 7 to 12 months of age the AI is 270 mg/day.

Iron

Full-term infants are considered to have adequate stores of iron for growth up to a doubling of their birth weight. This occurs at approximately 4 months of age in full-term infants and much earlier in prematurely born infants. Recommended intakes of iron increase, depending on age, growth rate, and iron stores. At 4 to 6 months of age, infants who are fed only human milk are at risk for developing a negative iron balance and may deplete their reserves by 6 to 9 months (Kim et al., 1996). Iron in human milk is highly bioavailable; however, breast-fed and formula-fed infants should receive an additional source of iron by 4 to 6 months of age. Iron-fortified cereals and infant formula are common food sources. Cow's milk is a poor source of iron and should not be given before 12 months of age.

Iron deficiency and iron deficiency anemia are common health concerns for the older infant. The prevalence of iron deficiency in children 9 months to 3 years of age who are living in the United States and the United Kingdom and are primarily among low socioeconomic and minority groups has been estimated at 30%, and the prevalence of iron deficiency anemia has been estimated at 10% or more (Eden, 2005).

Monitoring iron status is important because of the long-term cognitive effects of iron deficiency in infancy (Eden, 2005). Low hemoglobin concentrations at 8 months of age correlated with impaired motor development at 18 months of age (Sherriff et al., 2001). In addition, children with chronic iron deficiency in infancy demonstrated long-term developmental deficits and behavioral issues in early adolescence (Lozoff et al., 2000).

Zinc

Newborn infants are immediately dependent on a dietary source of zinc. Zinc is better absorbed from human milk than from infant formula. Human milk and infant formulas provide adequate zinc (0.3 to 0.5 mg per 100 kcal) for the first year of life. Other foods (e.g., meats, cereals) should provide most of the zinc required during the second year.

Fluoride

The importance of fluoride in preventing dental caries has been well documented. However, fluoride can also cause dental fluorosis, ranging from fine white lines to entirely chalky teeth (see Chapter 25). To prevent fluorosis, the tolerable upper intake level (UL) for fluoride has been set at 0.7 mg/day for infants up to 6 months and 0.9 mg/day for infants 7 to 12 months of age.

Human milk has a very low fluoride content. Commercially prepared infant cereals, wet pack cereals, and fruit juice produced with fluoridated water are significant sources of fluoride in infancy. Currently fluoride supplementation is not recommended for infants younger than 6 months of age. After tooth eruption it is recommended that fluoridated water be offered several times per day to breast-fed infants, those who receive cow's milk, and those fed formulas made with water that contains less than 0.3 mg of fluoride/L (American Academy of Pediatrics, 2004).

Vitamins

Vitamin D

Human milk derived from an adequately fed, lactating mother supplies all the vitamins the term infant needs except for vitamin D; human milk contains approximately only 20 international units (IU)/L (0.5 mcg cholecalciferol) of vitamin D. For the prevention of rickets (see Figure 3-17) and vitamin D deficiency, the American Academy of Pediatrics (AAP) recommends a vitamin D supplement of 200 IU per day for all breast-fed infants and for formula-fed infants who consume less than 500 ml/day of vitamin D–fortified formula (AAP, 2003). For infants with fair skin, regular exposure to sunlight for 30 minutes per week with the infant wearing only a diaper, or 2 hours per week if fully clothed without a hat, has been reported to be sufficient to meet vitamin D needs (Specker et al., 1985). There appears to be a higher risk of rickets among young, breast-fed infants and children with dark skin (Weisberg et al., 2004). Since a variety of environmental and family lifestyle factors can affect both sunlight exposure and absorption of vitamin D, the AAP recommendations are appropriate for all infants (see *Clinical Insight:* Sunshine, Vitamin D, and Fortification in Chapter 3).

Vitamin B$_{12}$

Milk from lactating mothers who follow a strict vegan diet may be vitamin B$_{12}$ deficient, especially if the mother followed the regimen for a long time before and during the pregnancy. Vitamin B$_{12}$ deficiency has also been diagnosed in infants breast-fed by mothers with pernicious anemia (Weiss et al., 2004) (see Chapter 31).

Vitamin K

The vitamin K requirements of the neonate need special attention. Deficiency may result in bleeding or **hemorrhagic disease of the newborn.** This condition is more common in breast-fed infants than in other infants because human milk contains only 2.5 mcg/L of vitamin K, whereas cow's milk–based formulas contain approximately twenty times this amount. All infant formulas contain a minimum of 4 mcg of vitamin K per 100 kcal of formula. The AI for infants is 2 mcg/day during the first 6 months and 2.5 mcg/day during the second 6 months of life. This can be supplied by mature breast milk, although perhaps not during the first week of life. For breast-fed infants vitamin K supplementation is necessary during that time to considerably decrease the risk for hemorrhagic disease (Greer, 2004; Greer, 2001). Many states require that infants receive an injection of vitamin K as a prophylactic measure while they are in the nursery. Previous reports that vitamin K injections may increase the risk of leukemia or cause cancer have not been supported by studies (Ross and Davies, 2000).

Supplementation

Vitamin and mineral supplements should be prescribed only after careful evaluation of the infant's intake. Commercially prepared infant formulas are fortified with all necessary vitamins; therefore formula-fed infants rarely need supplements.

◎ **FOCUS ON**

Vitamin and Mineral Supplementation Recommendations for Full-Term Infants

Iron

Breast-Fed Infants

About 1 mg/kg/day by 4 to 6 months of age, preferably from supplemental foods, and only iron-fortified formulas for weaning or supplementing breast milk

Formula-Fed Infants

Only iron-fortified formula during the first year of life

Vitamin D

Supplementation of 200 IU/day recommended for all breast-fed infants and infants consuming less than 500 ml of vitamin-D fortified formula each day, or adequate sun exposure for infants with fair skin (i.e., regular exposure to sunlight for 30 minutes per week with the infant wearing only a diaper or 2 hours per week if fully clothed without a hat) has been reported to be sufficient to meet vitamin D needs. Since a variety of environmental and family lifestyle factors can affect both sunlight exposure and absorption of vitamin D, the American Academy of Pediatrics recommendations are appropriate for all infants.

Vitamin K

Supplementation soon after birth to prevent hemorrhagic disease of the newborn

Fluoride

Intake of 0.25 mg/day after 6 months of age if water contains less than 0.3 ppm

Modified from American Academy of Pediatrics, Committee on Nutrition: *Pediatric nutrition handbook*, ed 5, Elk Grove Village, Ill, 2004.

Breast-fed infants need additional vitamin D supplementation by 2 months of age and iron by 4 to 6 months of age (see *Focus On:* Vitamin and Mineral Supplementation Recommendations for Full-Term Infants). Older infants who are fed homogenized milk need a food source or supplement of vitamin C. (Chapter 43 discusses the feeding of premature or high-risk infants and their special needs.)

MILK

Human Milk

Human milk is unquestionably the food of choice for the infant. Its composition is designed to provide the necessary energy and nutrients in appropriate amounts. It contains specific and nonspecific immune factors that support and strengthen the immature immune system of the newborn and thus protect the body against infections (Oddy, 2001). Human milk also helps prevent diarrhea and otitis media (AAP, 2005). Allergic reactions to human milk protein are rare. Moreover, the closeness of the mother and infant during breast-feeding facilitates attachment and bonding (see Figure 5-9); and breast milk provides nutritional benefits (i.e., optimal nourishment in an easily digestible and bioavailable form), decreases infant morbidity, provides maternal health benefits (e.g., lactation amenorrhea, maternal weight loss, some cancer protection), and has economic and environmental benefits (American Dietetic Association, 2005).

Population-based and meta-analysis studies indicate that breast-feeding benefits cognitive development (Angelsen et al., 2001), helps prevent childhood asthma (Dell and To, 2001; Gdalevich et al., 2001), and may help prevent children from becoming overweight as a dose-dependent effect (Hediger et al., 2001) or because it mediates maternal control over feeding (Fisher et al., 2000). For these reasons the Healthy Children 2010 objectives propose to support breast-feeding among mothers of newborn infants (see *Focus On:* Healthy Children 2010 Objectives: Nourishment of Infants).

The American Dietetic Association (ADA) and the AAP support exclusive breast-feeding for the first 6 months of life and breast-feeding supplemented by weaning foods for at least 12 months (AAP, 2005; ADA, 2005). It is important to note the ages of the infants in these recommendations; adding other foods at too young of an age decreases breast milk intake and increases early weaning (Hill et al., 1997). In addition, early introduction of foods may be a risk factor for developing type 1 diabetes mellitus–associated autoimmunity (Ziegler et al., 2003).

Breast-feeding may not be appropriate for mothers with certain infections or those who are taking medications that may have untoward effects on the infant. For example, a mother who is infected with human immunodeficiency virus (HIV) can transmit the infection to the infant (Humphrey and Iliff, 2001), and a mother using psychotropic drugs or other pharmacologic drugs may pass the medication to the infant through her breast milk (AAP, Committee on Drugs, 2001).

Composition of Human and Cow's Milk

The composition of human milk is different from that of cow's milk; for this reason, unmodified cow's milk is not recommended for infants until at least 1 year of age. Both provide 20 kcal/oz; however, the nutrient sources of the energy are different. For example, protein provides 6% to 7% of the energy in human milk and 20% of the energy in cow's milk. Human milk is 60% **whey proteins** (mainly lactalbumins) and 40% casein; by contrast, cow's milk is 20% whey and 80% casein. **Casein** forms a tough, hard-to-digest curd in the infant's stomach, whereas **lactalbumin** in human milk forms soft, flocculent, easy-to-digest curds. The amino acids taurine and cystine are present in higher concentrations in human milk than in cow's milk. These amino acids

Healthy Children 2010 Objectives: Nourishment of Infants

Healthy People 2010 is a comprehensive set of health objectives for the United States to achieve during the first decade of 2000. Healthy People 2010 identifies a wide range of public health priorities and specific, measurable objectives. The objectives have 28 focus areas, one of which is Maternal, Infant, and Child Health. The objectives related to nourishment of infants are as follows:

GOAL: Improve the health and well-being of women, infants, and families

Objective 16-19. Increase the proportion of mothers who breast-feed their infants to 75% in the early postpartum period, to 50% until their infants are 6 months old, and to 25% until their infants are 12 months old

GOAL: Promote health and reduce chronic disease associated with diet and weight

Objective 19-4. Reduce growth retardation among low-income children ages 5 years and younger to less than 5%

Objective 19-12. Reduce iron deficiency among children ages 1 to 2 years to less than 5%

GOAL: Prevent and control oral and craniofacial diseases, conditions, and injuries and improve access to related services

Objective 21-1a. Reduce the proportion of young children with dental caries in their primary teeth

The complete text of the Healthy People 2010 Objectives can be found at www.healthypeople.gov/document/.

may be essential for premature infants. Lactose provides 42% of the energy in human milk and only 30% of the energy in cow's milk.

Lipids provide 50% of the energy in human and whole cow's milk. Monounsaturated oleic acid is the predominant fatty acid in both milks. Linoleic acid, an essential fatty acid, provides 4% of the energy in human milk and only 1% in cow's milk. The cholesterol content of human milk is 10 to 20 mg/dl compared with 10 to 15 mg/dl in whole cow's milk. Less fat is absorbed from cow's milk than from human milk; a lipase in the nonfat fraction of human milk is stimulated by bile salts and contributes significantly to the hydrolysis of milk triglycerides.

All of the water-soluble vitamins in human milk reflect maternal intake. Cow's milk contains adequate quantities of the B-complex vitamins, but little vitamin C. Breast milk and supplemented cow's milk provide sufficient vitamin A. Human milk is a richer source of vitamin E than cow's milk. Human milk contains five metabolites of vitamin D, providing 20 IU/L (0.5 mcg cholecalciferol) of vitamin D activity; however, the need for additional vitamin D becomes important by 2 months of age. Cow's milk is usually fortified with 400 IU/L (10 mcg of cholecalciferol) of vitamin D.

The quantity of iron in human and cow's milk is small (0.3 mg/L). Approximately 50% of the iron in human milk but less than 1% of the iron in cow's milk is absorbed. The bioavailability of zinc in human milk is higher than in cow's milk. Cow's milk contains three times as much calcium and six times as much phosphorus as human milk, and its fluoride concentration is twice that of human milk.

The much higher protein and ash content of cow's milk results in a higher **renal solute load,** or amount of nitrogenous waste and minerals that must be excreted by the kidney. The sodium and potassium concentrations in human milk are about one third those in cow's milk, contributing to the decreased renal solute load of human milk. The osmolality of human milk averages 286 mOsm/kg, whereas that of cow's milk is 400 mOsm/kg.

Antiinfective Factors

Human milk and colostrum contain antibodies and antiinfective factors that are not present in infant formulas. Secretory immunoglobulin A (sIgA) is the predominant immunoglobulin in human milk, and it plays a role in protecting the infant's immature gut from infection. However, research indicates that breast-feeding must be maintained until the infant is at least 3 months of age to obtain this benefit (Heinig, 2001).

The iron-binding protein **lactoferrin** in human milk deprives bacteria of iron and thus slows their growth. Lysozymes, which are bacteriolytic enzymes found in human milk, destroy the cell membranes of bacteria after the peroxides and ascorbic acid that are also present in human milk have inactivated them. Breast milk enhances the growth of the bacterium *Lactobacillus bifidus*, which produces an acidic gastrointestinal environment that interferes with the growth of certain pathogenic organisms. Because of these antiinfective factors, the incidence of infections is lower in breast-fed infants than in formula-fed infants.

Formulas

Infants whose mothers are unwilling or unable to breast-feed are usually fed a formula based on cow's milk or a soy product. Many mothers may also choose to offer a combination of breast milk and formula feedings. Those infants who have special requirements receive specially designed products.

Commercial formulas made from heat-treated nonfat milk or a soy product and supplemented with vegetables fats, vitamins, and minerals are formulated to approximate, as closely as possible, the composition of human milk. They provide the necessary nutrients in an easily absorbed form. The manufacture of infant formulas is regulated by the Food and Drug Administration (FDA) through the Infant Formula Act (Nutrient Requirements for Infant Formulas, 1985). By law, infant formulas are required to have a nutrient level that is consistent with these guidelines (Table 6-4).

Formulas are also available for older infants and toddlers. However, most pediatricians believe that "older infant" formulas are unnecessary unless toddlers are not receiving adequate amounts of infant or table foods.

TABLE 6-4

Nutrient Levels in Infant Formulas As Specified by the Infant Formula Act

Specified Nutrient Component	Minimum Level Required (per 100 kcal of energy)
Protein (g)	1.8
Fat (g)	3.3
Percentage of calories	30.0
Linoleic acid (mg)	300.0
Percentage of calories	2.7
Vitamin A (international units)	250.0
Vitamin E (international units)	0.7
Vitamin D (international units)	40.0
Vitamin K (mcg)	4.0
Thiamin (mcg)	40.0
Riboflavin (mcg)	60.0
Niacin (mcg)	250.0
Ascorbic acid (mg)	8.0
Pyridoxine (mcg)	35.0
Vitamin B_{12} (mcg)	0.15
Folic acid (mcg)	4.0
Biotin (mcg) (nonmilk-based formulas only)	1.5
Pantothenic acid (mcg)	300.0
Choline (mg) (nonmilk-based formulas only)	7.0
Inositol (mg) (nonmilk-based formulas only)	4.0
Calcium (mg)	60.0
Phosphorus (mg)	30.0
Iron (mg)	0.15
Zinc (mg)	0.5
Magnesium (mg)	6.0
Manganese (mcg)	5.0
Sodium (mg)	20.0
Potassium (mg)	80.0
Iodine (mcg)	5.0
Chloride (mg)	55.0
Copper (mcg)	60.0

From Nutrient requirements for infant formulas, Final Rule (21 CFR 107), *Fed Reg* 50:45106, 1985.

The declining prevalence of anemia in infants is credited to the use of iron-fortified formula; for this reason, the AAP recommends iron-fortified formulas for all formula-fed infants. The widespread theory that iron-fortified formula may cause constipation, loose stools, **colic** (severe abdominal pain), and spitting up has not been confirmed by clinical studies (AAP, 1999). Formulas are available with and without additional iron. Table 6-5 shows the composition of various formulas, human milk, and cow's milk.

Soy-based formulas are under regular scrutiny. Infants ingesting soy formulas grow and absorb minerals as well as infants fed cow's milk–based formulas, but they are exposed to several thousand times higher levels of phytoestrogens and isoflavones than infants fed human milk or cow's milk–based formulas. The amount of soy protein isolate used in the manufacture of soy-based infant formulas determines the isoflavone content. The biologic impact of these elevated isoflavone levels on long-term infant development is not yet clear; but no evidence of altered growth, development, or reproduction has been identified (Merritt and Jenks, 2004).

Efforts are ongoing to manufacture infant formulas that closely approximate human milk. ARA and DHA are found in human milk but not in cow's milk. No current documentation shows that the growth or development of formula-fed infants is compromised when they consume formulas without ARA or DHA supplementation. Many infant formulas now have these very long–chain fatty acids added (Innis et al., 2001). The DRIs for infants recommend 0.5 g/day of omega-3 fatty acids.

Various products are available for infants who cannot tolerate the protein in cow's milk–based formulas. Soy products designed to meet all nutrient needs are recommended for (1) children in vegetarian families, (2) children with galactosemia or primary lactase deficiency and those recovering from secondary lactose intolerance, and (3) infants who may be allergic to cow's milk protein but who have not shown clinical manifestations of the allergy. These soy formulas are not recommended for children known to have protein allergies because many infants who are allergic to cow's milk protein also develop allergies to soy milk protein (AAP, 1998a) (see Chapter 29).

Infants who cannot tolerate cow's milk–based or soy products can be fed formulas made from a **casein hydrolysate,** which is casein that has been split into smaller components by treatment with acid, alkali, or enzymes. These formulas are Nutramigen, Pregestimil, and Alimentum. In addition, these formulas do not contain lactose. For infants who have food protein intolerances and cannot tolerate hydrolysate formulas, free amino acid–based formulas are available (Neocate and Elecare) (AAP, 2000). Other formulas are available for children with problems such as malabsorption or metabolic disorders (e.g., phenylketonuria) (see Chapters 7 and 44).

Whole Cow's Milk

Some parents may choose to transition their infant from formula to fresh cow's milk before 1 year of age. However, the AAP Committee on Nutrition has concluded that infants should not be fed whole cow's milk during the first year of life (AAP, 1998b). Infants who are fed whole cow's milk have been found to have lower intakes of iron, linoleic acid, and vitamin E and excessive intakes of sodium, potassium, and protein. Cow's milk may cause a small amount of gastrointestinal blood loss.

Low-fat (1% to 2%) and nonfat milk are also inappropriate for infants during the first 12 months of life. The infants may ingest excessive amounts of protein in large volumes of milk in an effort to meet their energy needs, and the decreased amount of essential fatty acids may be insufficient in

Text continued on p. 213.

TABLE 6-5

Composition of Milk and Selected Infant Formulas per Liter

Milk or Formula	Energy (kcal)	Protein (g)	Fat (g)	Carbohydrate (g)	Calcium (mg)	Phosphorus (mg)	Sodium (mEq)	Sodium (mg)	Potassium (mEq)	Potassium (mg)	Iron (mg)	Protein Source	Fat Source	Carbohydrate Source	Comments
Human milk†	700	10.3	44	69	320	140	7.4	170	13	510	0.3	Lactalbumin, casein	Human breast milk	Lactose	Protein readily digested; adequate in all nutrients except vitamin D and fluoride
Cow's Milk–Based Infant Formulas															
Similac (Ross)	676	14.0	36.5	73.0	528	284	7.1	162	18.2	710	12.2/ 4.7*	Nonfat milk, whey	High oleic safflower, soy, coconut oils	Lactose	Vitamins and minerals added
Enfamil (Mead Johnson)	670	14	35.3	72.7	520	287	7.8	180	18.4	720	12.1/ 4.7*	Nonfat milk, whey	Palm olein, soy, coconut, high oleic sunflower oils	Lactose	Vitamins and minerals added
LactoFree (Mead Johnson)	670	14.0	35.3	72.7	546	369	8.6	200	18.6	733	12.0	Milk protein isolate	Palm olein, soy, coconut, high oleic sunflower oils	Corn syrup solids	Vitamins and minerals added
Good Start Supreme (Nestlé)	670	14.7	34.2	75	429	241	7.9	181	18.5	724	10.1	Enzymatically hydrolyzed reduced-mineral whey	Palm olein, soy, coconut, high oleic safflower oils	Lactose, corn maltodextrin	Vitamins and minerals added
Cow's Milk															
Skim	357	35.0	2.0	50.0	1256	1028	23.0	524	43.0	1689	Trace	Casein	None	Lactose	Inappropriate for infants

Data from Mead Johnson Nutritionals Product Information, November 2005, http://www.meadjohnson.com/professional/prodinfo.html; Ross Product Handbook, November 2005, http://www.ross.com/productHandbook/pedNut.asp; Nestlé Infant Formulas, November 2005, http://www.verybestbaby.com/content/article.asp?section=bf&id=2001928151781575717469; and SHS North America Product Information, November 2005, http://www.shsna.com/pages/products.htm

* Without added iron.

†Based on data from USDA National Nutrient Database for Standard Reference, November 2005, http://www.nal.usda.gov/fnic/foodcomp/search/

MCT, Medium-chain triglycerides.

Continued

TABLE 6-5

Composition of Milk and Selected Infant Formulas per Liter—cont'd

Milk or Formula	Energy (kcal)	Protein (g)	Fat (g)	Carbohydrate (g)	Calcium (mg)	Phosphorus (mg)	Sodium (mEq)	Sodium (mg)	Potassium (mEq)	Potassium (mg)	Iron (mg)	Protein Source	Fat Source	Carbohydrate Source	Comments
Cow's Milk—cont'd															
2%	503	34.0	20.0	49.0	1236	965	508	22.0	1568	40.0	Trace	Casein	Butterfat	Lactose	Inappropriate for infants
Whole	624	33.0	34.0	47.0	1211	948	499	22.0	1539	39.0	Trace	Casein	Butterfat	Lactose	Inappropriate for infants younger than 12 months of age
Soy-Based Infant Formulas															
Prosobee (Mead Johnson)	670	16.6	35.3	70.7	700	553	240	10.4	800	20.5	12	Soy protein isolate with L-methionine	Palm olein, soy, coconut, high oleic sunflower oils	Corn syrup solids	Vitamins and minerals added
Isomil (Ross)	676	16.6	36.9	69.7	710	507	298	12.9	730	18.7	12.2	Soy protein isolate with L-methionine	High oleic safflower, coconut, soy oils	Corn syrup, sucrose	Vitamins and minerals added
Good Start Supreme Soy (Nestlé)	670	16.8	34.2	75	700	420	268	11.6	777	19.9	12.0	Soy protein isolate with L-methionine	Palm olein, soy, coconut, high oleic safflower oils	Corn maltodextrin, sucrose	Vitamins and minerals added
Casein Hydrolysate Formulas															
Nutramigen (Mead Johnson)	670	18.6	35.3	69	627	420	313	13.5	733	18.6	12.0	Casein hydrolysate with added amino acids	Palm olein, soy, coconut, high oleic sunflower oils	Corn syrup solids, modified corn-starch	Vitamins and minerals added

Continued

Formula											Protein source	Fat source	Carbohydrate source	Other
Pregestimil (Mead Johnson)	670	18.6	37.3	68	767	500	313	13.5	733	18.6	12.0	Casein hydrolysate with added amino acids	MCT (55%), corn, soy, high oleic safflower oils	Corn syrup solids, dextrose, modified corn-starch	Vitamins and minerals added
Alimentum (Ross)	676	18.6	37.5	69.0	710	507	298	12.9	798	20.4	12.2	Casein hydrolysate with added amino acids	Safflower, MCT (33%), soy oils	Sucrose, modified tapioca starch	Vitamins and minerals added

Amino Acid–Based Formulas

Formula											Protein source	Fat source	Carbohydrate source	Other
Elecare (Ross)	676	20.4	32.2	72.4	730	548	304	13.2	1014	25.9	12	Free L-amino acids	High oleic safflower MCT (33%), soy oils	Corn syrup solids	Vitamins and minerals added
Neonate Infant (SHS)	670	20.7	30	78	827	621	249	10.8	1035	26.5	12.3	Free L-amino acids	High oleic safflower, coconut, soy, MCT (5%) oils	Corn syrup solids	Vitamins and minerals added

Formulas for Feeding Beyond 9 Months of Age

Formula											Protein source	Fat source	Carbohydrate source	Other
Good Start 2 Supreme (Nestlé)	670	14.7	34.2	75	804	449	181	7.8	724	18.5	10.1	Enzymatically hydrolyzed reduced minerals whey	Palm olein, soy, coconut, high oleic safflower oils	Lactose, corn maltodextrin	Vitamins and minerals added

TABLE 6-5

Composition of Milk and Selected Infant Formulas per Liter—cont'd

Formulas for Feeding Beyond 9 Months of Age—cont'd

Milk or Formula	Energy (kcal)	Protein (g)	Fat (g)	Carbohydrate (g)	Calcium (mg)	Phosphorus (mg)	Sodium (mEq)	Sodium (mg)	Potassium (mEq)	Potassium (mg)	Iron (mg)	Protein Source	Fat Source	Carbohydrate Source	Comments
Good Start 2 Supreme Soy (Nestlé)	670	18.8	33.5	73	1273	710	11.6	268	19.9	777	13	Soy protein isolate with L-methionine	Palm olein, soy, coconut, high oleic safflower oils	Corn maltodextrin, sucrose	Vitamins and minerals added
Next Step (Mead Johnson)	670	17.3	35.4	70	1300	867	10.4	240	22.2	867	13.3	Nonfat milk	Palm olein, soy, coconut, high oleic sunflower oils	Corn syrup solids, lactose	Vitamins and minerals added
Next Step Prosobee (Mead Johnson)	670	22	29.3	78.7	1300	867	10.4	240	20.5	800	13.3	Soy protein isolate with L-methionine	Palm olein, soy, coconut, high oleic sunflower oils	Corn syrup solids, sucrose	Vitamins and minerals added
Similac 2 (Ross)	676	14	37.1	71.7	798	433	7.1	162	18.2	710	12.2	Nonfat milk, whey	High oleic safflower, coconut, soy oils	Lactose	Vitamins and minerals added
Isomil 2 (Ross)	676	16.6	36.9	69.7	913	609	12.9	298	18.7	730	12.2	Soy protein isolate with L-methionine	High oleic, safflower, coconut, soy oils	Corn syrup solids, sucrose	Vitamins and minerals added

preventing deficiency (AAP, 2004). In addition, substitute or imitation milks such as rice, oat, or nut milks are inappropriate and should not be fed to infants unless they are properly supplemented.

Formula Preparation

Commercial infant formulas are available in ready-to-feed forms that require no preparation, as concentrates prepared by mixing with equal parts of water, and in powder form that is designed to be mixed with 2 oz of water per level tablespoon or scoop of powder.

Infant formulas should be prepared in a clean environment. All equipment, including bottles, nipples, mixers, and the top of the can of formula, should be washed thoroughly. Formula may be prepared for up to a 24-hour period and refrigerated. Formula for each feeding should be warmed in a hot water bath, not in a microwave. Any formula warmed and not consumed at that feeding should be discarded. Any opened cans of formula should be covered, refrigerated, and used within 24 hours.

FOOD

Various commercially prepared foods and organically grown products are available for infants. These products vary widely in their nutrient value. Foods for infants should be thoughtfully selected to meet their nutritional and developmental needs.

Ready-to-serve dry infant cereals are fortified with **electrolytically reduced iron,** which is iron that has been fractionated into small particles for improved absorption. Three level tablespoons of cereal provide about 5 mg of iron or from one half to one third the amount the infant requires. Therefore cereal is usually the first food added to the infant's diet. Jarred cereal and fruit mixtures are fortified with ferrous sulfate and provide 7 to 9 mg of iron per 4.5-oz jar.

Strained and "junior" vegetables and fruits provide carbohydrates and various amounts of vitamins A and C. Vitamin C is added to numerous jarred fruits and all fruit juices. In addition, tapioca is added to several of the jarred fruits. Milk is added to the creamed vegetables, and wheat is incorporated into the mixed vegetables.

Most strained and junior meats are prepared with water. Strained meats, which have the highest energy density of any of the commercial baby foods, are an excellent source of high-quality protein and heme iron.

Numerous dessert items are also available such as puddings and fruit desserts. The nutrient composition of these products varies, but all contain excess energy in the form of sugar and modified cornstarch or tapioca starch. Most infants do not need this excess energy.

Mothers who would like to make their own infant food can easily do so by following the directions in Box 6-1. Home-prepared foods are generally more concentrated in nutrients than commercially prepared foods because less water is used. Salt and sugar should not be added to foods prepared for infants.

FEEDING

Early Feeding Patterns

Because milk from a mother with an adequate diet is uniquely designed to meet the needs of the human infant, breast-feeding for the first 6 months of life is strongly recommended. Most chronic medical conditions do not contraindicate breast-feeding.

A mother should be encouraged to nurse her infant immediately after birth. Those who care for and counsel parents during the first postpartum days should acquaint themselves with ways in which they can be supportive. Ideally, counseling and preparation for breast-feeding start in the last few months or weeks of pregnancy (see Chapter 5).

During the first few days of life, a breast-feeding infant receives colostrum, a yellow, transparent fluid that meets the infant's needs during the first week. It contains less fat and carbohydrate but more protein and greater concentrations of sodium, potassium, and chloride than mature milk. It is also an excellent source of immunologic substances.

Infants who are formula fed are likely to receive ready-to-feed formula in the hospital. At home, products that have been refrigerated such as concentrated formulas should be mixed with warm water or heated to body temperature in a water bath. Refrigerated, ready-to-feed formula also needs

---

BOX 6-1

Directions for Home Preparation of Infant Foods

1. Select fresh, high-quality fruits, vegetables, or meats.
2. Be sure that all utensils, including cutting boards, grinder, knives, and other items, are thoroughly cleaned.
3. Wash hands before preparing the food.
4. Clean, wash, and trim the food in as little water as possible.
5. Cook the foods until tender in as little water as possible. Avoid overcooking, which may destroy heat-sensitive nutrients.
6. Do not add salt or sugar. Do not add honey to food intended for infants younger than 1 year of age.*
7. Add enough water for the food to be easily puréed.
8. Strain or purée the food using an electric blender, a food mill, a baby food grinder, or a kitchen strainer.
9. Pour purée into an ice cube tray and freeze.
10. When the food is frozen hard, remove the cubes and store in freezer bags.
11. When ready to serve, defrost and heat in a serving container the amount of food that will be consumed at a single feeding.

Clostridium botulinum spores, which cause botulism, have been reported in honey; young infants do not have the immune capacity to resist this infection.

TABLE 6-6

Satiety Behaviors in Infants

Age (weeks)	Behavior
4-12	Draws head away from the nipple
	Falls asleep
	When nipple is reinserted, closes lips tightly
	Bites nipple, purses lips, or smiles and lets go
16-24	Releases nipple and withdraws head
	Fusses or cries
	Obstructs mouth with hands
	Pays more attention to surroundings
	Bites nipple
28-36	Changes posture
	Keeps mouth tightly closed
	Shakes head as if to say "no"
	Plays with utensils
	Uses hands more actively
	Throws utensils
40-52	See behaviors listed for previous age range
	Sputters with tongue and lips
	Hands bottle or cup to mother

From Pipes PL: Health care professionals. In Garwood G, Fewell R, editors: *Educating handicapped infants*, Rockville, Md, 1982, Aspen Systems.

to be warmed. Microwave heating is not recommended because of the risk of burns from formula that is too hot or unevenly heated.

Regardless of whether infants are breast-fed or formula fed, they should be held and cuddled during feedings. Once a feeding rhythm has been established, infants become fussy or cry to indicate they are hungry, whereas they often smile and fall asleep when they are satisfied (Table 6-6). Infants, not adults, should establish the feeding schedules. Initially most infants feed every 2 to 3 hours; by 4 weeks of age most feed every 4 hours. By 2 to 4 months of age infants have usually matured enough to allow the mother to omit night feedings.

Development of Feeding Skills

At birth, infants coordinate sucking, breathing, and swallowing and are prepared to **suckle** liquids from the breast or bottle, but not able to handle foods with texture. During the first year, typical infants develop head control, the ability to move into and sustain a sitting posture, and the ability to grasp, first with a **palmar grasp** and then with a refined **pincer grasp** (Figure 6-2). They develop mature sucking and rotary chewing abilities and progress from being fed to feeding themselves using their fingers. In the second year, they learn to feed themselves independently with a spoon (Figure 6-3).

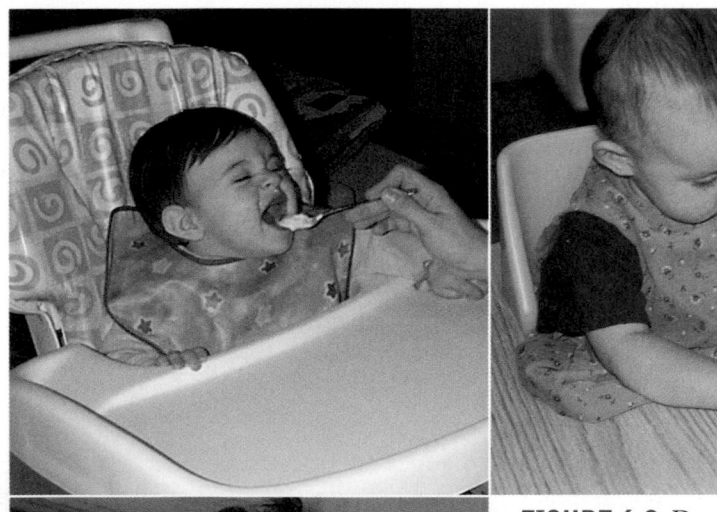
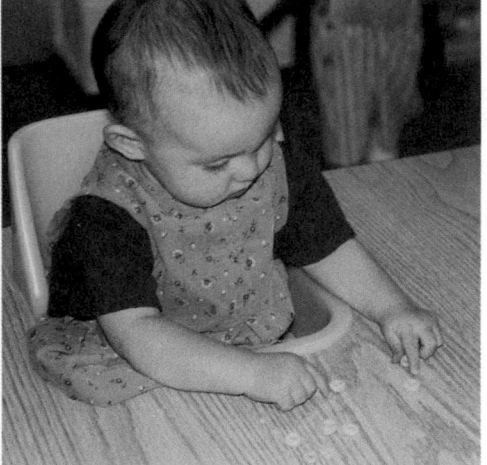
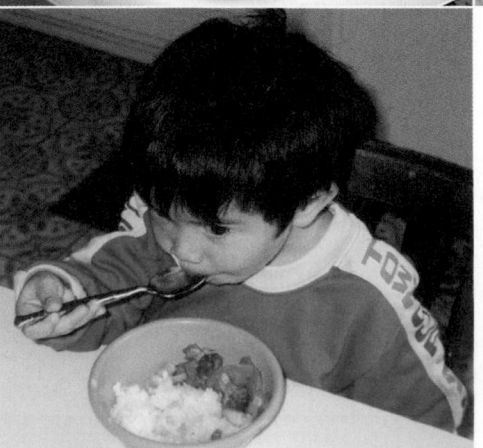

FIGURE 6-2 Development of feeding skills in infants and toddlers. **A,** This 7-month-old child shows the beginnings of involvement with feeding by anticipating the spoon. **B,** This 9-month-old girl is using a refined pincer grasp to pick up her food. **C,** This 19-month-old boy is beginning to use his spoon independently, although he is not yet able to rotate his wrist to keep food on it.

Addition of Semisolid Foods

Developmental readiness and nutrient needs are the criteria that determine appropriate times for the addition of various foods. During the first 4 months of life, the infant attains head and neck control, and oral motor patterns progress from a suck to a suckling to the beginnings of a mature sucking pattern. Puréed foods introduced during this phase are consumed in the same manner as are liquids, with each suckle being followed by a tongue-thrust swallow. Table 6-7 lists developmental landmarks and their indications for semisolid and table food introduction.

Between 4 and 6 months of age, when the mature sucking movement is refined and munching movements (up-and-down chopping motions) begin, the introduction of strained foods is appropriate. Infant cereal is usually introduced first. To support developmental progress, cereal is offered to the infant from a spoon, not combined with formula in a bottle; thereafter various commercially or home-prepared foods may be offered. The sequence in which these foods are introduced is not important; however, it is important that one single ingredient food (e.g., peaches, not peach cobbler, which has many ingredients) be introduced at a time. Introducing a single new food at a time at 2- to 7-day intervals enables parents to identify any allergic responses or food intolerances (Butte et al., 2004). Introducing vegetables before fruits may increase vegetable acceptance.

Infants demonstrate their acceptance of new foods by slowly increasing the variety and quantity of solids they accept. Breast-fed infants seem to accept greater quantities than do formula-fed infants (Sullivan and Birch, 1994). Parents who thoughtfully offer a variety of nourishing foods are more likely to provide a well-balanced diet and help their children learn to accept more flavors.

As oral-motor maturation proceeds, an infant's rotary chewing ability develops, indicating a readiness for more textured foods such as well-cooked mashed vegetables, casseroles, and pasta from the family menu. Learning to grasp—with the palmar grasp, then with an inferior pincer grasp, and finally with the refined pincer grasp—indicates a readiness for finger foods such as oven-dried toast, arrowroot biscuits, or cheese sticks (see Figure 6-2). Table 6-8 presents recommendations for adding foods to an infant's diet. Foods with skins or rinds and foods that stick to the roof of the mouth (e.g., hot dogs, grapes, bread with peanut butter) may cause choking and should not be offered to young infants.

During the last quarter of the first year, infants can approximate their lips to the rim of the cup and can drink if the cup is held for them. During the second year they gain the ability to rotate their wrists and elevate their elbows, thus allowing them to hold the cup themselves and manage a spoon. They are very messy eaters at first, but by 2 years of age most typical children skillfully feed themselves (see Figure 6-3).

Weaning from Breast or Bottle to Cup

The introduction of solids into an infant's diet begins the weaning process in which the infant transitions from a diet of only breast milk or formula to a more varied one. Weaning should proceed gradually and be based on the infant's rate of growth and developmental skills. Weaning foods should be carefully chosen to complement the nutrient needs of the infant, promote appropriate nutrient intake, and maintain growth.

Many infants begin the process of weaning with the introduction of the cup at about 6 to 9 months of age and complete the process when they are able to ingest an adequate amount of milk from a cup at 18 to 24 months of age. Parents of infants who are breast-fed may choose to transition the infant directly to a cup or have an intermittent transition to a bottle before the cup is introduced.

Early Childhood Caries

Early childhood caries (ECC), or baby bottle tooth decay, is the most common chronic disease of childhood (Douglass et al., 2004, Mouradian et al., 2000). ECC is a pattern of tooth decay that involves the upper anterior and sometimes lower posterior teeth. ECC is common among infants and children who are allowed to bathe their teeth in sugar (sucrose or lactose) throughout the day and night (see Figure 25-4). If infants are given sugar-sweetened beverages or fruit juice in a bottle during the day or at bedtime after teeth have erupted, the risk of dental caries increases (see Chapter 25). To promote dental health, infants should be fed and burped and then put to bed without milk, juice, or food. Juice should be limited to 4 to 6 oz/day for infants and young children and offered to children only from a cup (AAP, 2001).

Feeding Older Infants

As maturation proceeds and the rate of growth slows down, infants' interest in and approach to food change. Between 9 and 18 months of age most reduce their breast-milk or formula intake. They can become finicky about what and how much they eat (see *Clinical Insight:* Self-Selected Diets of Infants and Young Children).

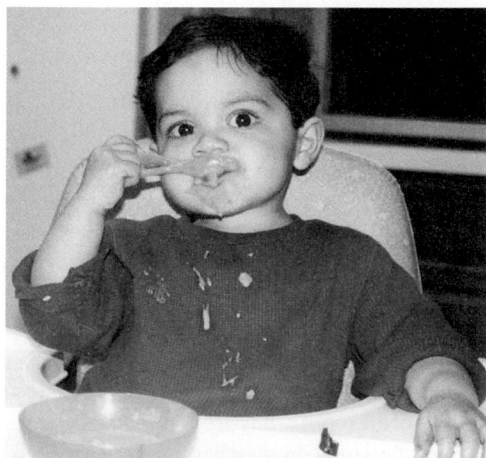

FIGURE 6-3 This 2-year-old is skilled at self-feeding because he has the ability to rotate his wrist and elevate his elbow to keep food on the spoon.

TABLE 6-7

Feeding Behaviors: Developmental Landmarks During the First 2 Years of Life

Developmental Landmarks	Change Indicated	Examples of Appropriate Foods
Tongue laterally transfers food in the mouth Shows voluntary and independent movements of the tongue and lips Sitting posture that can be sustained Shows beginning of chewing movements (up and down movements of the jaw)	Introduction of soft, mashed table food	Tuna fish; mashed potatoes; well-cooked, mashed vegetables; ground meats in gravy and sauces; soft, diced fruit such as bananas, peaches, and pears; flavored yogurt
Reaches for and grasps objects with palmar grasp Brings hand to mouth	Finger feeding (large pieces of food)	Oven-dried toast, teething biscuits; cheese sticks (Should be soluble in the mouth to prevent choking)
Voluntarily releases food (refined digital [pincer] grasp)	Finger feeding (small pieces of food)	Bits of cottage cheese, dry cereal, peas and other bite-size vegetables; small pieces of meat
Shows rotary chewing pattern	Introduction of food of varied textures from family menu	Well-cooked, chopped meats and casseroles; cooked vegetables and canned fruit (not mashed); toast; potatoes; macaroni, spaghetti; peeled ripe fruit
Approximates lips to rim of the cup	Introduction of cup for sipping liquids	
Understands relationship of container and its contents	Beginning of self-feeding (though messiness should be expected)	Food that when scooped adheres to the spoon, such as applesauce, cooked cereal, mashed potatoes, cottage cheese, yogurt
Shows increased movements of the jaw Shows development of ulnar deviation of the wrist	More skilled at cup and spoon feeding	Chopped fibrous meats, such as roast and steak Raw vegetables and fruit (introduced gradually)
Walks alone	May seek food and obtain food independently	Foods of high nutritional value
Names food, expresses preferences; prefers unmixed foods Goes on food jags Appetite appears to decrease		Balanced food choices, with child permitted to develop food preferences (Parents should not be concerned that these preferences will last forever.)

Modified from Trahms CM, Pipes P: *Nutrition in infancy and childhood*, ed 6, New York, 1997, McGraw-Hill.

In the weaning stage infants have to learn many manipulative skills, including the ability to chew and swallow solid food and use utensils. They learn to tolerate various textures and flavors of food, eat with their fingers, and then feed themselves with a utensil. Very young children should be encouraged to feed themselves (see *Clinical Insight:* A New Look at the Food Practices of Infants and Toddlers).

At the beginning of a meal, children are hungry and should be allowed to feed themselves; when they become tired, they can be helped quietly. Emphasis on table manners and the fine points of eating should be delayed until they have the necessary maturity and developmental readiness for such training.

The food should be in a form that is easy to handle and eat. Meat should be cut into bite-size pieces. Potatoes and vegetables should be mashed so that they can be eaten easily with a spoon. Raw fruits and vegetables should be in sizes that can be picked up easily. In addition, the utensils should be small and manageable. Cups should be easy to hold, and dishes should be designed so that they do not tip over easily.

Type of Food

In general, children prefer simple, uncomplicated foods. Food from the family meal can be adapted for the child and served in child-size portions. Children younger than 6 years of age usually prefer mild-flavored foods. Because a young child's stomach is small, a snack may be required between meals. Fruit, cheese, crackers, dry cereal, fruit juices, and milk contribute nutrients and energy. Children ages 2 to 6 years often prefer raw instead of cooked vegetables and fruits.

TABLE 6-8

Suggested Ages for the Introduction of Juice, Semisolid Foods, and Table Foods

| Food | Age (mo) | | |
	4-6	6-8	9-12
Iron-fortified cereals for infants	Add.		
Vegetables		Add strained.	Gradually eliminate strained foods and introduce table foods.
Fruits		Add strained.	Gradually eliminate strained foods; introduce chopped, well-cooked, or canned foods.
Meats		Add strained or finely chopped table meats.	Decrease the use of strained meats; increase the varieties of table meats offered.
Finger foods, such as arrowroot biscuits, oven-dried toast		Add foods that can be secured with a palmar grasp.	Increase the use of small finger foods as the pincer grasp develops.
Well-cooked mashed or chopped table foods prepared without added salt or sugar			Add and introduce use of spoon to infant.
Juice or formula by cup			Add.

Modified from Trahms CM, Pipes P: *Nutrition in infancy and childhood*, ed 6, New York, 1997, McGraw-Hill.

✳ CLINICAL INSIGHT

Self-Selected Diets of Infants and Young Children

If left to their own devices with a wide variety of wholesome foods at their disposal, young children instinctively choose an adequate diet. This was documented by research conducted in the late 1920s by Davis, who was attempting to demonstrate that the prevailing practice of withholding solid foods until 1 year of age was not in the best interest of the child (Davis, 1928). At the onset of the study, Davis studied three children, ages 7 to 9 months, for 6 months to 1 year. Later she studied 12 additional children for 6 months to 4½ years, during which time their diets were entirely self-selected. They were offered various fresh, unprocessed, and unseasoned foods and were allowed to eat as little or as much as they pleased of any or all items (Davis, 1939). A modern evaluation of their intakes indicates that the nutrients in the foods consumed equaled or exceeded the recommendations for all nutrients except iron.

Although some of the foods offered are unfamiliar to today's families, it seems difficult for a child with a typical appetite to fail to obtain an adequate diet when his or her choices are limited to the following: beef, lamb, chicken, liver, kidney, brains, sweetbreads, haddock, whole-wheat bread, oatmeal, barley, cornmeal, Ry-Krisp, bone marrow, bone jelly, eggs, raw milk, apples, oranges, bananas, peaches, pineapples, lettuce, cabbage, spinach, cauliflower, peas, beets, carrots, turnips, potatoes, tomatoes, and sea salt.

No desserts or snacks commonly eaten during those times were included, and certainly none of the highly refined, energy-rich, and nutrient-dilute foods available today were offered.

A preference for sweetness that is present at birth and persists throughout childhood suggests that infants who are offered dietary selections that include desserts and sweetened snack foods are unable to make the choices appropriate for a nutritious diet (Story and Brown, 1987).

However, a similar study of children ages 1½ to 4 years who were presented with wholesome foods that are common today also demonstrated the ability to select foods to meet their energy requirements. Unfortunately the nutrient adequacy of their selected diets was not determined (Birch et al., 1991).

Infants should be offered foods that vary in texture and flavor. Infants who are accustomed to many kinds of foods are less likely to limit their variety of food choices later. To add variety to an infant's diet, vegetables and fruits can be added to cereal feedings (Butte et al., 2004). It is important to offer various foods and not allow the infant to continue consuming a diet consisting of one or two favorite foods. Older infants generally reject unfamiliar foods the first time they are offered. When parents continue to offer small portions of these foods without comment, infants

✳ CLINICAL INSIGHT

A New Look at the Food Practices of Infants and Toddlers

The Feeding Infants and Toddlers Study (FITS) was a national random sample of over 2500 infants and toddlers from 4 to 24 months of age and their mothers. Applications from the FITS study update and reinforce the earlier work of Davis, Story, and Birch.

- Assuming that a variety of nutritious foods are offered to infants and toddlers, parents and caregivers should encourage self-feeding without concern for compromising energy intake and nutrient adequacy (Carruth et al., 2004b).

- Parents and caregivers should offer a variety of fruits and vegetables daily; sweets, desserts, sweetened beverages, and salty snacks should be offered only occasionally. Because family food choices influence the foods offered to infants, family-based approaches to healthy eating habits should be encouraged (Fox et al., 2004).

- By 24 months of age, 50% of toddlers were described as picky eaters. When offering a new food, caregivers need to be willing to provide 8 to 15 repeated exposures to enhance acceptance of that food (Carruth et al., 2004a).

- Infants and toddlers have an innate ability to regulate energy intake. Parents and caregivers should understand the cues of hunger and satiety and recognize that coercive admonitions about eating more or less food can interfere with the infant's or toddler's innate ability to regulate energy intake (Fox et al., 2006).

- On average, infants and toddlers were fed seven times per day, and the percentage of children reported to be eating snacks increased with age. Snack choices for infants and toddlers could be improved by delaying the introduction of and limiting foods that have a low nutrient content and are energy dense (Skinner et al., 2004).

become familiar with them and often accept them (Butte et al., 2004). It is important that fruit juice does not replace more nutrient-dense foods. If excessive amounts of juice are consumed, children may fail to thrive (Dennison, 1996) (see Chapter 7). Finally, overall energy management according to body mass index is important. Attention to diets early in life is essential to prevent cardiovascular disease later (Gidding et al., 2006).

Serving Size

The size of a serving of food offered to a child is very important. At 1 year infants eat one third to one half the amount an adult normally consumes. This proportion increases to one half an adult portion by the time the child reaches 3 years of age and increases to about two thirds by 6 years of age. Young children should not be served a large plateful of food; the size of the plate and the amount should be in proportion to their age. A tablespoon (not a heaping tablespoon) of each food for each year of age is a good guide to follow. Serving less food than parents think or hope will be eaten helps children eat successfully and happily. They will ask for more food if their appetite is not satisfied.

Forced Feeding

Children should not be forced to eat; instead, the cause for the unwillingness to eat should be determined. A typical, healthy child eats without coaxing. Children may refuse food because they are too inactive to be hungry or too active and overtired.

To avoid both overfeeding and underfeeding, parents should be responsive to the cues for hunger and satiety offered by the infant. A child who is fed snacks or given a bottle too close to mealtime (within 90 minutes) is not hungry for the meal and may refuse it (Butte et al., 2004).

Parents who support the development of self-feeding skills respond to the infant's need for assistance and offer encouragement for self-feeding; they also allow the infant to initiate and guide feeding interactions without excessive pressure on the infant for neatness in self-feeding or amount of food consumed. If a child refuses to eat, the family meal should be completed without comment, and the plate should be removed. This procedure is usually harder on the parent than on the child. At the next mealtime, the child will be hungry enough to enjoy the food presented.

Eating Environment

Young children should eat their meals at the family table; it gives them an opportunity to learn table manners while enjoying meals with a family group. Sharing the family fare strengthens ties and makes mealtime pleasant. However, if the family meal is delayed, the children should receive their meal at the usual time. When children eat with the family, everyone must be careful not to make unfavorable comments about any food. Children are great imitators of the people they admire; thus, if the father or older siblings make disparaging remarks about squash, for example, young children are likely to do the same.

- Infant growth, development and nourishment are integrally related.
- Human milk is the food of choice for infants; commercially prepared infant formulas, manufactured to approximate human milk, also promote typical growth and development.
- Nutrient needs of infants reflect rates of growth, energy expended in activity, basal metabolic needs, and the interaction of nutrients consumed.
- Infants grow rapidly in the first year of life; thus the types of infant feedings (human milk or formula), the composition of feedings, and the addition of solids to infants' diets have immediate and long-term impact.

- The use of solid foods of appropriate type and portion size support nourishment and developmental progress and sets the stage for lifelong food habits.
- The use of solid foods (with thought given to the types of foods and portion sizes served) to support nourishment and developmental progress sets the stage for lifelong food habits that promote appropriate growth and healthy food choices.

✳ CLINICAL SCENARIO 1

Lela is a 12-week-old female infant who was born by cesarean section at 42 weeks' gestation to an 18-year-old unmarried mother. Her mother gained 70 lb during the pregnancy. Lela's weight-for-length is plotted at the 95th percentile, and her length and weight continue in the same channels as at birth.

Lela's mother chose to feed Lela infant formula rather than breast-feed. Lela is offered Similac with iron that is prepared with 1 scoop of powder mixed in 2 oz of water. Lela consumes about six 8-oz bottles per day and is fed on demand. She usually sleeps during the night, but if she is fussy, her mother gives her small amounts of commercially prepared infant cereal, vegetables, and fruit.

✳**Nutrition Diagnosis:** Excessive oral food/beverage intake related to using foods to soothe baby as evidenced by weight for height above 95th percentile for age.

1. What additional information is needed to get an accurate assessment of this infant's intake?
2. When you assess Lela's growth, what are your expectations for her growth rate? Do you have concerns about her rate of growth?
3. What is Lela's estimated energy intake? Is this appropriate?
4. The American Academy of Pediatrics recommendations suggest that the addition of complimentary foods be delayed until after 4 months of age. How would you assess Lela's readiness for semisolid foods? Which infant skills would you assess in a feeding evaluation?

✳ CLINICAL SCENARIO 2

Shana is 12 months old and has been growing at the 50th percentile for weight and the 25th percentile for length since early infancy. She consumes formula from a bottle (24 oz per day of Enfamil with iron), table and finger foods (e.g.,

crackers, toast fingers, cooked carrot sticks, cooked green beans, cheese cubes, mashed potatoes, applesauce, and canned pears), and 12 to 14 oz of apple juice each day. Shana's mother wonders if Shana is drinking enough formula each day.

Continued

CLINICAL SCENARIO 2—cont'd

*Nutrition Diagnosis: Food and nutrition-related knowledge deficit related to questions concerning adequacy of formula intake as evidenced by current intake of 24 oz infant formula each day.

1. Do you need additional information to accurately assess Shana's nutrient intake?
2. Do you think Shana is drinking enough formula each day? What, if any, changes would you suggest to her mother?
3. How would you evaluate the foods offered to Shana in terms of her motor development? Her oral health? Her growth? The adequacy of her nutrient intake?
4. What suggestions might you make to Shana's mother so that she can use food to support Shana's developmental progress?

USEFUL WEBSITES

American Academy of Pediatrics
www.aap.org/

National Center for Education in Maternal and Child Health

Bright Futures: Nutrition in Practice
www.brightfutures.org/nutrition/

National Center for Health Statistics

Healthy People 2010: Objectives
   for Improving Health
www.healthypeople.gov/

University of Washington Assuring Pediatric Nutrition in the Community
http://depts.washington.edu/nutrpeds/

World Health Organization Child Growth Standards
http://www.who.int/childgrowth/standards/en/

References

American Academy of Pediatrics, Clinical Report: Prevention of rickets and vitamin D deficiency: new guidelines for vitamin D intake, *Pediatrics* 111:908, 2003.

American Academy of Pediatrics, Committee on Drugs: Transfer of drugs and other chemicals into human milk, *Pediatrics* 108:776, 2001.

American Academy of Pediatrics, Committee on Nutrition: Soy protein-based formulas: recommendations for use in infant feeding, *Pediatrics* 101:148, 1998a.

American Academy of Pediatrics, Committee on Nutrition: The use of whole cow's milk in infancy, *Pediatrics* 91:515, 1992 (reaffirmed April 1998b).

American Academy of Pediatrics, Committee on Nutrition: Iron fortification of infant formulas, *Pediatrics* 104:119, 1999.

American Academy of Pediatrics, Committee on Nutrition: Hypoallergenic infant formulas, *Pediatrics* 106:346, 2000.

American Academy of Pediatrics, Committee on Nutrition: The use and misuse of fruit juice in pediatrics, *Pediatrics* 107:1210, 2001.

American Academy of Pediatrics, Committee on Nutrition: *Pediatric nutrition handbook*, ed 5, Elk Grove Village, Ill, 2004, The Academy.

American Academy of Pediatrics, Section on Breastfeeding: Breastfeeding and the use of human milk, *Pediatrics* 115:496, 2005.

American Dietetic Association, Position of the American Dietetic Association: promoting and supporting breastfeeding, *J Am Diet Assoc* 105:810, 2005.

Angelsen NK et al: Breastfeeding and cognitive development at age 1 and 5 years, *Arch Dis Child* 85:183, 2001.

Auestad N et al: Visual, cognitive, and language assessments at 39 months: a follow-up study of children fed formulas containing long-chain polyunsaturated fatty acids at 1 year of age, *Pediatrics* 112:e177, 2003.

Baird J et al: Being big or growing fast: systematic review of size and growth in infancy and later obesity, *Br Med J* 331:929, 2005.

Birch EE et al: Visual maturation of term infants fed long-chain polyunsaturated fatty acid–supplemented or control formula for 12 mo, *Am J Clin Nutr* 81:871, 2005.

Birch L et al: The variability of young children's energy intake, *N Engl J Med* 324:232, 1991.

Butte N et al: The Start Healthy feeding guidelines for infants and toddlers, *J Am Diet Assoc* 104:442, 2004.

Campbell CM: Preventing obesity: prevention starts in infancy, *Br Med J* 326(7380):102, 2003.

Carruth BR et al: Prevalence of picky eaters among infants and toddlers and their caregivers' decisions about offering a new food, *J Am Diet Assoc* 104:S57, 2004a.

Carruth BR et al: Developmental milestones and self-feeding behaviors in infants and toddlers, *J Am Diet Assoc* 104:S51, 2004b.

Clandinin MT et al: Growth and development of preterm infants fed infant formulas containing docosahexaenoic acid and arachidonic acid, *J Pediatr* 146:461, 2005.

Davis CM: Self-selection of diet by newly weaned infants: an experimental study, *Am J Dis Child* 36:651, 1928.

Davis CM: Results of the self-selection of diets by young children, *Can Med Assoc J* 41:257, 1939.

Dell S, To T: Breastfeeding and asthma in young children: findings from a population-based study, *Arch Pediatr Adolesc Med* 155:1261, 2001.

Dennison BA: Fruit juice consumption by infants and children: a review, *J Am Coll Nutr* 15:4S, 1996.

Dewey KG et al: Breast-fed infants are leaner than formula-fed infants at 1 year of age: the DARLING study, *Am J Clin Nutr* 57:140, 1993.

Douglass JM et al: A practical guide to infant oral health, *Am Fam Physician* 70:2113, 2004.

Eden AN: Iron deficiency and impaired cognition in toddlers: an underestimated and undertreated problem, *Pediatr Drugs* 7:347, 2005.

Fisher JO et al: Breast-feeding through the first year predicts maternal control in feeding and subsequent toddler energy intakes, *J Am Diet Assoc* 100:641, 2000.

Fox MK et al: Feeding infants and toddlers study: what foods are infants and toddlers eating? *J Am Diet Assoc* 104:S22, 2004.

Fox MK et al: Relationship between portion size and energy intake among infants and toddlers: evidence of self-regulation, *J Am Diet Assoc* 106:S77, 2006.

Garza C: New growth standards for the 21st century: a prescriptive approach, *Nutr Rev* 64:S55, 2006.

Gdalevich M et al: Breast-feeding and the risk of bronchial asthma in childhood: a systematic review with meta-analysis of prospective studies, *J Pediatr* 139:261, 2001.

Gidding SS et al: Dietary recommendations for children and adolescents: a guide for practitioners, *Pediatrics* 117:544, 2006.

Greer FR: Are breast-fed infants vitamin K deficient? *Adv Exp Med Biol* 501:391, 2001.

Greer FR: Vitamin K in human milk—still not enough, *Acta Paediatr* 93:449, 2004.

Hediger ML et al: Association between infant breastfeeding and overweight in young children, *JAMA* 285:2453, 2001.

Heinig MJ: Host defense benefits of breastfeeding for the infant—effect of breastfeeding on duration and exclusivity, *Pediatr Clin North Am* 48:105, 2001.

Heinig MJ et al: Energy and protein intakes of breast-fed and formula-fed infants during the first year of life and their association with growth velocity: the DARLING Study, *Am J Clin Nutr* 58:152, 1993.

Hill PD et al: Does early supplementation affect long-term breastfeeding? *Clin Pediatr* 56:345, 1997.

Hoffman DR et al: Visual function in breast-fed term infants weaned to formula with or without long-chain polyunsaturates at 4 to 6 months: a randomized control trial, *J Pediatr* 142:669, 2003.

Humphrey J, Iliff P: Is breast not best? Feeding babies born to HIV-positive mothers: bringing balance to a complex issue, *Nutr Rev* 59:119, 2001.

Innis SM et al: Are human milk long-chain polyunsaturated fatty acids related to visual and neural development in breast-fed term infants? *J Pediatr* 139:532, 2001.

Kim SK et al: Red blood cell indices and iron status according to feeding practices in infants and young children, *Acta Paediatr* 85:139, 1996.

Lozoff B et al: Poorer behavioral and developmental outcome more than 10 years after treatment for iron deficiency anemia in infancy, *Pediatrics* 105:e51, 2000.

Makrides M et al: A critical appraisal of the role of dietary long-chain polyunsaturated fatty acids on neural indices of term infants: a randomized controlled trial, *Pediatrics* 105:32, 2000.

Manganaro R et al: Incidence of dehydration and hypernatremia in exclusively breast-fed infants, *J Pediatr* 139:673, 2001.

Merritt RJ, Jenks BH: Safety of soy-based infant formulas containing isoflavones: the clinical evidence, *J Nutr* 134:1220S, 2004.

Morale SE et al: Duration of long-chain polyunsaturated fatty acids availability in the diet and visual acuity, *Early Hum Dev* 81:197, 2005.

Mouradian W et al: Disparities in children's oral health and access to dental care, *JAMA* 284:2625, 2000.

Nutrient Requirements for Infant Formulas, Final Rule (21 CFR 107), *Fed Reg* 50:45106, 1985.

Oddie S et al: Hypernatremic dehydration and breastfeeding: a population study, *Arch Dis Child* 85:318, 2001.

Oddy WH: Breastfeeding protects against illness and infection in infants and children: a review of the evidence, *Breastfeed Rev* 9:11, 2001.

Rodriguez NR: Optimal quantity and composition of protein for growing children, *J Am Coll Nutr* 24:150S, 2005.

Ross JA, Davies SM: Vitamin K prophylaxis and childhood cancer, *Med Pediatr Oncol* 34:434, 2000.

SanGiovanni JP et al: Meta-analysis of dietary essential fatty acids and long-chain polyunsaturated fatty acids as they relate to visual resolution acuity in healthy preterm infants, *Pediatrics* 105:1292, 2000.

Sherriff A et al: Should infants be screened for anemia? A prospective study investigating the ratio between hemoglobin at 8, 12, and 18 months and development at 18 months, *Arch Dis Child* 84:480, 2001.

Skinner JD et al: Meal and snack patterns of infants and toddlers, *J Am Diet Assoc* 104:S65, 2004.

Smith D et al: Shifting linear growth during infancy: illustration of genetic factors in growth from fetal life through infancy, *J Pediatr* 89:225, 1976.

Specker B et al: Sunshine exposure and serum-25-hydroxyvitamin D concentrations in exclusively breast-fed infants, *J Pediatr* 107:372, 1985.

Story M, Brown JE: Do young children instinctively know what to eat? *N Engl J Med* 316:103, 1987.

Sullivan SA, Birch LL: Infant dietary experience and acceptance of solid foods, *Pediatrics* 93:271, 1994.

Trahms C, Pipes P: *Nutrition in infancy and childhood*, ed 6, New York, 1997, McGraw-Hill.

Uauy R et al: Term infant studies of DHA and ARA supplementation on neurodevelopment: results of randomized controlled trials, *J Pediatr* 143:S17, 2003.

Weisberg P et al: Nutritional rickets among children in the United States: review of cases reported between 1986 and 2003, *Am J Clin Nutr* 80:1697S, 2004.

Weiss R et al: Severe vitamin B_{12} deficiency in an infant associated with a maternal deficiency and a strict vegetarian diet, *J Pediatr Hematol Oncol* 26:270, 2004.

Ziegler A et al: Early infant feeding and risk of developing type 1 diabetes–associated autoantibodies, *JAMA* 290:1721, 2003.

CHAPTER 7

Betty L. Lucas, MPH, RD, CD
Sharon A. Feucht, MA, RD, CD

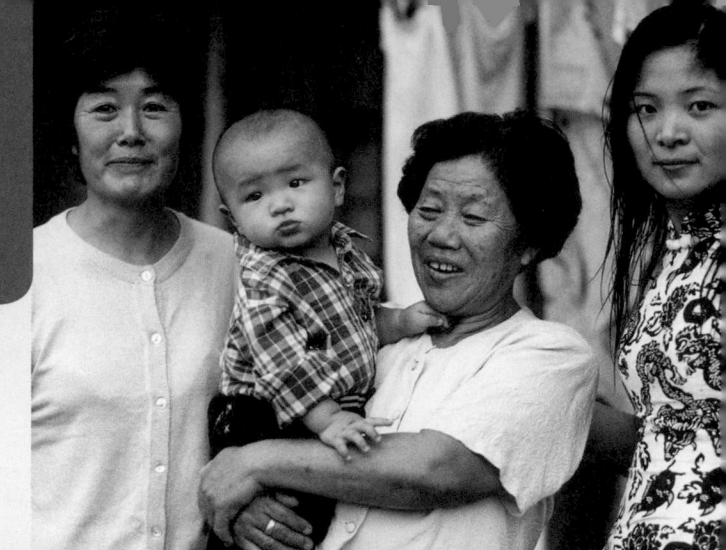

Nutrition in Childhood

adiposity rebound a phenomenon of normal growth, occurring at approximately 6 years of age, which is when a child's body fat increases

catch-up growth a higher-than-normal growth rate after a period of growth suppression as a result of extended illness or deprivation

failure to thrive (FTT) weight loss, lack of weight gain, or significant decreased velocity of weight gain in a child because of an acute or a chronic illness, a restricted diet, poor appetite, lack of food, lack of social interaction, or a harsh or disruptive environment; also called pediatric undernutrition or growth deficiency

food insecurity having limited or uncertain availability of nutritionally adequate and safe foods or a limited ability to acquire appropriate foods in socially acceptable ways

food jags periods during which foods that were previously liked are refused or a particular food is requested at every meal; common in children ages 2 to 6 years

growth channels curves of weight and height gain throughout the period of growth; stated as a percentile based on a standard growth chart

The period that begins after infancy and lasts until puberty is often referred to as the latent or quiescent period of growth—a contrast to the dramatic changes that occur during infancy and adolescence. Although physical growth may be less remarkable and proceed at a steadier pace than it did during the first year, these preschool and middle-school years are a time of significant growth in the social, cognitive, and emotional areas.

GROWTH AND DEVELOPMENT

Growth Patterns

The rate of growth slows considerably after the first year of life. In contrast to the usual tripling of birth weight that occurs in the first 12 months, another year passes before the birth weight quadruples. Likewise, birth length increases by 50% in the first year but does not double until approximately the age of 4 years. Increments of change are small compared with those of infancy and adolescence; weight typically increases an average of 2 to 3 kg (4½ to 6½ lb) per year until the child is 9 or 10 years old. Then the rate increases, signaling the approach of puberty. Height increase increments average 6 to 8 cm (2½ to 3½ inches) per year from 2 years of age until puberty.

Growth is generally steady and slow during the preschool and school-age years, but it can be erratic in individual children, with periods of no growth followed by growth spurts. These patterns usually parallel similar changes in appetite and food intake. For parents, periods of slow growth and poor appetite can cause anxiety, leading to mealtime struggles.

Body proportions of young children change significantly after the first year. Head growth is minimal, trunk growth slows substantially, and limbs lengthen considerably, all of which create more mature body proportions. Because of walking and increased physical activity, the legs straighten, and the abdominal and back muscles strengthen to support the now erect child. These changes are gradual and subtle, occurring over years.

The body composition of preschool and school-age children remains relatively constant. Fat gradually decreases during the early childhood years, reaching a minimum between 4 and 6 years of age. Children then experience the **adiposity rebound,** or increase in body weight in preparation for the pubertal growth spurt. Earlier adiposity rebound has been associated with increased adult body mass index (BMI) (Whitaker et al., 1998). Sex differences in body composition become increasingly apparent—boys have more lean body mass per centimeter of height than girls. Females have a higher percentage of weight as fat than males, even in the preschool years, but these differences in lean body mass and fat do not become significant until adolescence.

Catch-Up Growth

A child who is recovering from an illness or undernutrition and whose growth has slowed or ceased experiences a greater-than-expected rate of recovery. This recovery is referred to as **catch-up growth,** a period during which the body strives to return to the child's normal growth channel. The degree of growth suppression is influenced by the timing, severity, and duration of the precipitating cause; that is, a severe illness or prolonged nutritional deprivation during a period of rapid growth has the most dramatic impact (Berhane and Dietz, 1999).

Initial studies supported the thesis that malnourished infants who did not experience immediate catch-up growth would have permanent growth retardation. However, studies of malnourished children from developing countries who subsequently received adequate nourishment, as well as reports of children who were malnourished because of chronic disease such as celiac disease (see Chapter 27) or cystic fibrosis (see Chapter 35), have reported that these children caught up to their normal growth channels after the first year or two of life.

The nutritional requirements for catch-up growth depend on whether the child has stunted growth and is chronically malnourished or primarily wasted (i.e., has a weight deficit that exceeds the height deficit). A chronically malnourished child may not be expected to gain weight as rapidly as a child who is primarily wasted (Cunningham and McLaughlin, 1999).

Nutrient requirements, especially for energy and protein, depend on the rate and stage of catch-up growth. For instance, more protein and energy are needed during the very rapid weight gain period and for those in whom lean tissue is the major component of the weight gain. In addition to energy, other nutrients are important, including vitamin A, iron, and zinc (Villamor et al., 2002; Rivera et al., 2003). Supplementation is a low-cost, effective intervention to decrease growth retardation in those with infectious diseases.

Current growth parameters are used to determine the child's weight age (the age corresponding to the child's weight at the 50th percentile), ideal (median) weight for age, and ideal (median) weight for actual stature. Formulas are then used to calculate the minimum and maximum energy needed for catch-up growth (Cunningham and McLaughlin, 1999). After a child who is wasted catches up in weight, dietary management changes to slow the weight gain velocity to avoid excessive gain. The catch-up in linear growth reaches its peak about 1 to 3 months after treatment starts, whereas weight gain begins immediately (Cunningham and McLaughlin, 1999).

Assessing Growth

Because children are constantly growing and changing, periodic assessments allow any problems to be detected and treated early. Unfortunately, many children are seen by health care professionals only when they are ill; thus growth and development may not be the focus of care.

A complete assessment of nutritional status includes the collection of anthropometric data. This includes length or standing height, weight, and weight for length or BMI, all of which are plotted as percentiles on the Centers for Disease Control and Prevention (CDC) growth charts (see Appendixes 9 through 16). Other measurements that are less commonly used but that provide estimates of body composition include upper arm circumference and triceps or subscapular fat folds. Care should be taken to use standardized equipment and techniques for obtaining and plotting growth measurements. Charts designed for birth to 36 months of age are based on length measurements and nude weights, whereas charts used for 2- to 20-year-olds are based on standing height and weight with light clothing and without shoes (see Chapter 14).

The proportion of weight to length or height is a critical element of growth assessment. This parameter is determined by plotting the weight-for-length measurement on the CDC birth- to 36-month growth charts or calculating BMI and plotting it on the 2- to 20-year-old CDC growth charts (see Appendixes 9 through 16). Growth measurements obtained at regular intervals provide a growth pattern. One-time height and weight measurements do not allow for an interpretation of growth status. Children generally maintain their heights and weights in the same **growth channels** during the preschool and childhood years, although the channels are not well established until after 2 years of age. Individual children sometimes grow at faster or slower rates; nonetheless, they should follow along the same channels.

Regular monitoring of growth enables problematic trends to be identified early and intervention or education initiated so that long-term growth is not compromised (Story et al., 2000). Weight that increases rapidly and crosses growth channels suggests the development of obesity. Lack of weight gain or loss of weight over a period of months may be a result of undernutrition, an acute illness, an undiagnosed chronic disease, or significant emotional or family problems. Figure 7-1 demonstrates these changes in growth parameters.

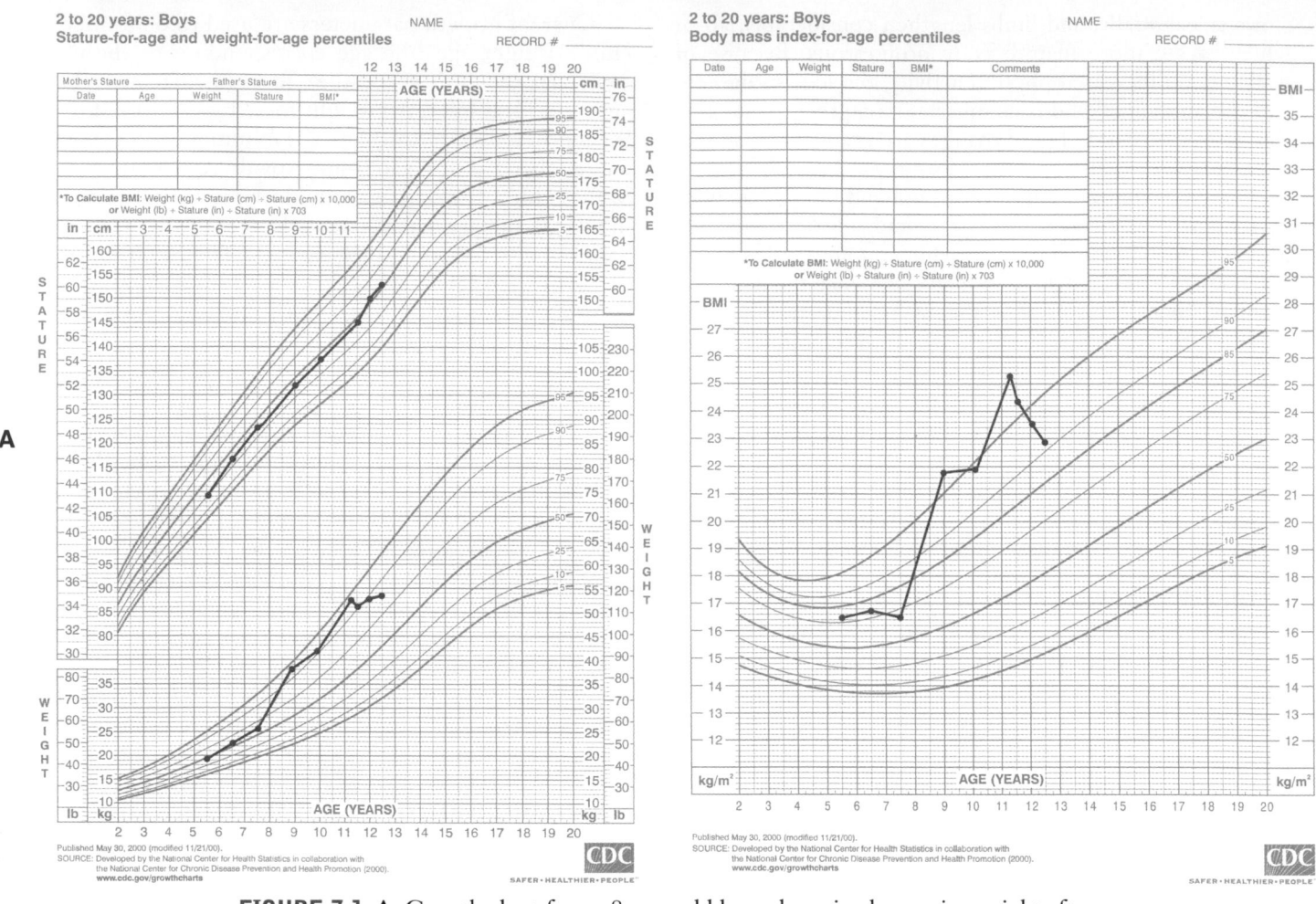

FIGURE 7-1 A, Growth chart for an 8-year-old boy who gained excessive weight after having leg surgery and being immobilized in a body cast for 2 months. The surgery and immobilization were followed by a long period of stress from family problems. At the age of 11 years, he became involved in a weight management program. *(Source of growth charts only: The National Center for Health Statistics in collaboration with the National Center for Chronic Disease Prevention and Health Promotion, 2000.)*

NUTRIENT REQUIREMENTS

Because children are growing and developing bones, teeth, muscles, and blood, they need more nutritious food in proportion to their size than do adults. They may be at risk for malnutrition when they have a poor appetite for a long period, eat a limited number of foods, or dilute their diets significantly with nutrient-poor foods.

The dietary reference intakes (DRIs) are based on current knowledge of nutrient intakes needed for optimal health (Institute of Medicine [IOM], 1997, 1998, 2000, 2001, 2002, 2004a). They include estimated average requirements (EARs), recommended dietary allowances (RDAs), adequate intakes (AIs), and tolerable upper intake levels (ULs). Most data for preschool and school-age children are values interpolated from data on infants and adults (see Table 6-1 and DRI tables inside front cover). These reference intakes are meant to improve the long-term health of the population by reducing the risk of chronic disease and preventing nutritional deficiencies. Thus, when intakes are less than the recommended level, it cannot be assumed that a particular child is inadequately nourished.

Energy

The energy needs of healthy children are determined on the basis of basal metabolism, rate of growth, and energy expenditure. Dietary energy must be sufficient to ensure growth and spare protein from being used for energy but not allow excess weight gain. Suggested intake proportions of energy are 45% to 65% as carbohydrates, 30% to 40% as fat, and 5% to 20% as protein for 1 to 3 year olds, with carbohydrates the same for 4 to 18 year olds, 25% to 35% as fat, and 10% to 30% as protein (IOM, 2002).

The new DRIs for estimated energy expenditure (EER) equations are based on studies using doubly labeled water. These equations estimate average energy requirements based on life-stage groupings for healthy individuals of

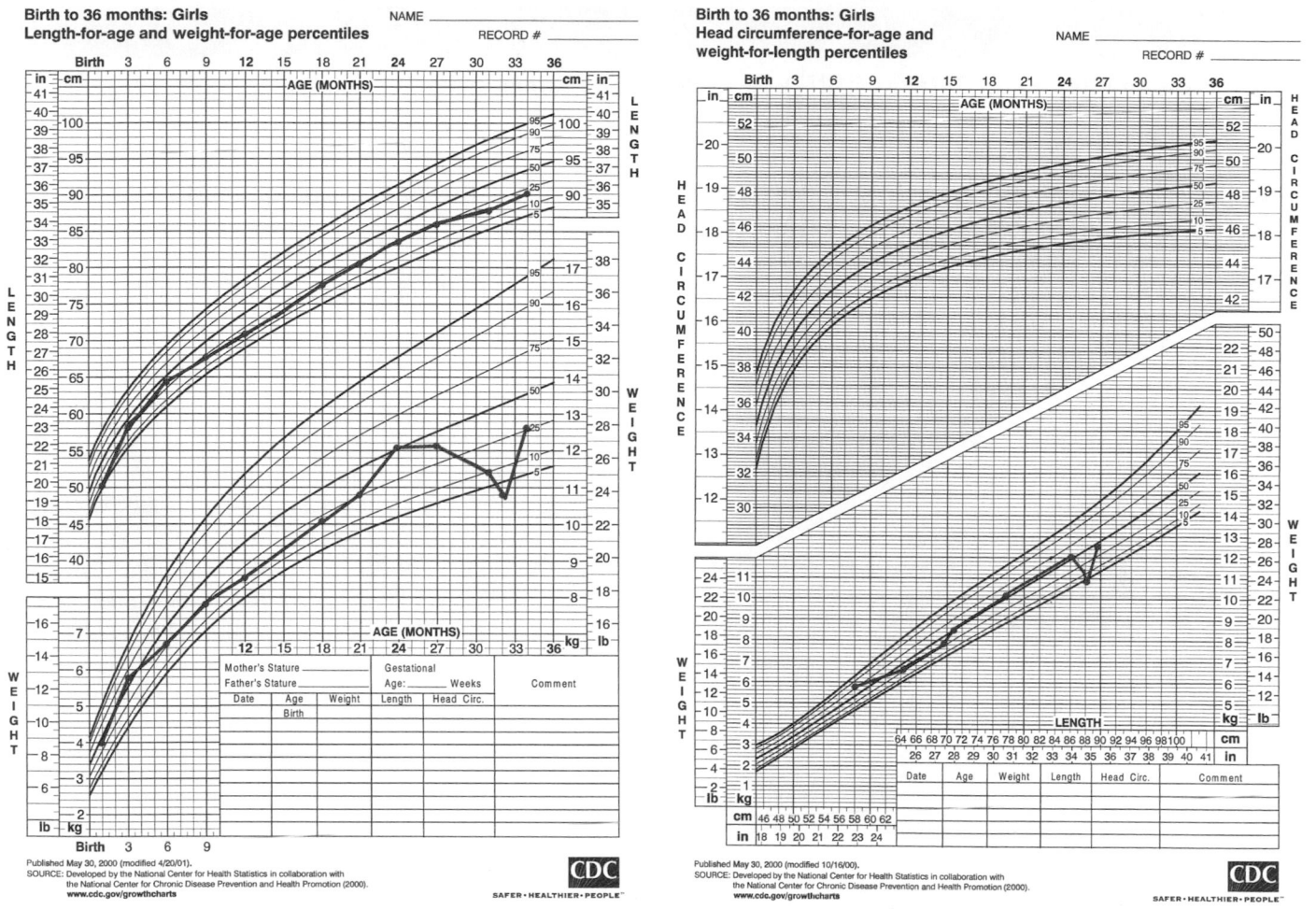

FIGURE 7-1, cont'd B, Growth chart for a 2-year-old girl who experienced significant weight loss during a prolonged period of diarrhea and feeding problems. After being diagnosed with celiac disease, she began following a gluten-free diet and entered a period of catch-up growth. (*Source of growth charts only: The National Center for Health Statistics in collaboration with the National Center for Chronic Disease Prevention and Health Promotion, 2000.*)

normal weight. Toddlers 13 through 35 months are grouped together; for older children the EERs are divided by sex and age (3 through 8 years and 9 through 18 years) (Table 7-1). The EER includes the total energy expenditure (TEE) plus energy needed for growth (see Chapter 2). The DRIs are applied to child nutrition programs and other guidelines (IOM, 2002). See Box 7-1 for examples of determining EER for two children.

On an individual basis, it can be useful to determine energy requirements using energy per kilogram of weight or per centimeter of height. Results of energy intake from a longitudinal study were 13 to 15 kcal/cm for children ages 2 to 5 years and 13 to 14 kcal/cm for girls and 16 to 17 kcal/cm for boys ages 6 to 11 years (Beal, 1970).

Protein

The need for protein per kilogram of body weight decreases from approximately 1.1 g in early childhood to 0.95 g in late childhood (Table 7-2). Protein intake can range from 5% to 30% of the energy DRI based on age. Protein deficiency is

uncommon in American children, partly because of the cultural emphasis on protein foods. National surveys show that less than 3% of children fail to meet the EAR (Moshfegh et al., 2005). Children who are most at risk for inadequate protein intake are those on strict vegan diets, with multiple food allergies, or who have limited food selections because of fad diets, behavioral problems, or inadequate access to food.

Minerals and Vitamins

Minerals and vitamins are necessary for normal growth and development. Insufficient intake can cause impaired growth and result in deficiency diseases (see Chapter 3) (the DRIs for different age-groups are listed in Table 6-1 and the inside front cover).

Iron

Children between 1 and 3 years of age are at high risk for iron deficiency anemia. The rapid growth period of infancy is marked by an increase in hemoglobin and total iron mass. Children with prolonged bottle feeding and those of Mexican-

TABLE 7-1

Energy Dietary Reference Intakes (DRIs) for Children and Adolescents

Energy Requirements	Sex/Age	Calculation (EER or TEE)	Physical Activity (PA) Coefficient (Note PAL is physical activity level)	
Estimated energy requirements (EER)	Boys and Girls, 13-35 mo	$(89 \times wt[kg] - 100) + 20^*$	Not applicable	
	Boys, 3 through 8 yr	$EER = 88.5 - 61.9 \times age [y] + PA \times (26.7 \times wt[kg] + 903 \times ht[m]) + 20^*$	PA= 1.00 if PAL is estimated to be $\geq 1.0 < 1.4$ (sedentary)	PA= 1.26 if PAL is estimated to be $\geq 1.6 < 1.9$ (active)
	Boys, 9 through 18 yr	$EER = 88.5 - 61.9 \times age [y] + PA \times (26.7 \times wt[kg] + 903 \times ht[m]) + 25^*$	PA= 1.13 if PAL is estimated to be $\geq 1.4 < 1.6$ (low active)	PA=1.42 if PAL is estimated to be $\geq 1.9 < 2.5$ (very active)
	Girls, 3 through 8 yr	$EER = 135.3 - 30.8 \times age [y] + PA \times (10.0 \times wt[kg] + 934 \times ht[m]) + 20^*$	PA= 1.00 if PAL is estimated to be $\geq 1.0 < 1.4$ (sedentary)	PA= 1.31 if PAL is estimated to be $\geq 1.6 < 1.9$ (active)
	Girls, 9 through 18 yr	$EER = 135.3 - 30.8 \times age [y] + PA \times (10.0 \times wt[kg] + 934 \times ht[m]) + 25^*$	PA= 1.16 if PAL is estimated to be $\geq 1.4 < 1.6$ (low active)	PA= 1.56 if PAL is estimated to be $\geq 1.9 < 2.5$ (very active)
For Overweight and Obese Boys and Girls 3-18 yr	Boys, 3 through 18 yr	$TEE = 114 - 50.9 \times age[y] + PA (19.5 \times wt[kg] + 1161.4 \times ht[m])$	PA= 1.00 if PAL is estimated to be $\geq 1.0 < 1.4$ (sedentary) PA=1.12 if PAL is estimated to be $\geq 1.4 < 1.6$ (low active) to be $\geq 1.9 < 4.5$ (very active)	PA= 1.24 if PAL is estimated to be $\geq 1.6 < 1.9$ (active) PA= 1.45 if PAL is estimated
Total energy expenditure (TEE) for weight maintenance	Girls, 3 through 18 yr	$TEE = 389 - 41.2 \times age[y] + PA (15.0 \times wt[kg] + 701 \times ht[m])$	PA= 1.00 if PAL is estimated to be $\geq 1.0 < 1.4$ (sedentary) PA= 1.18 if PAL is estimated to be $\geq 1.4 < 1.6$ (low active)	PA= 1.35 if PAL is estimated to be $\geq 1.6 < 1.9$ (active) PA= 1.60 if PAL is estimated to be $\geq 1.9 < 2.5$ (very active)

Adapted from Feucht S: Dietary reference intakes (DRI) review: case studies illustrating energy and protein for children and adolescent with special needs, *Nutr Focus Newsletter* 20:1, 2005.

*Energy deposition in kcal.

American descent are at highest risk for iron deficiency (Brotanek et al., 2005). In addition, the diet may not be rich in iron-containing foods. Recommended intakes must factor in the absorption rate and quantity of iron in foods, especially those of plant origin (see Chapters 3 and 31).

Calcium

Calcium is needed for adequate mineralization and maintenance of growing bone in children. The DRI for calcium for children 1 to 3 years old is 500 mg/day; for children ages 4 to 8 years it is 800 mg/day; and for those ages 9 to 18 years it is 1300 mg per day (IOM, 1997). Actual need depends on individual absorption rates and dietary factors such as quantities of protein, vitamin D, and phosphorus. Because calcium intake has very little influence on the degree of urinary calcium excretion during periods of rapid growth, children need two to four times more calcium per kilogram than adults. Since milk and other dairy products are primary sources of calcium, children who consume limited amounts of these foods are at risk for poor bone mineralization (Figure 7-2). Other calcium-fortified foods such as soy and rice milks and fruit juices are now available.

BOX 7-1

Using the Estimated Energy Requirement (EER) to Determine Energy

(Examples using Table 7-1)

1. For 13- to 35-month-old children:

$$EER \ (kcal) = (89 \times wt \ [kg] - 100) + 20$$

An 18-month-old boy has a length of 84 cm and weighs 12.5 kg

$$EER \ (kcal) = (89 \times 12.5 - 100) + 20$$

$$EER \ (kcal) = (1113 - 100) + 20$$

$$EER \ (kcal) = 1033$$

2. For females 3 through 8 years:

$$EER \ (kcal) = 135.3 - 30.8 \times age \ [y] + PA \times (10.0 \times wt \ [kg] + 934 \times ht \ [m]) + 20$$

A 6½-year-old girl is 112 cm tall, weighs 20.8 kg, and has moderate activity (physical activity [PA] coefficient of 1.31)

$$EER \ (kcal) = 135.3 - 30.8 \times 6.5 + 1.31 \times (10.0 \times 20.8 + 934 \times 1.12) + 20$$

$$EER \ (kcal) = 135.3 - 200.2 + 1.31 \times (208 + 1046.1) + 20$$

$$EER \ (kcal) = 135.3 - 200.2 + 1642.9 + 20$$

$$EER \ (kcal) = 1598$$

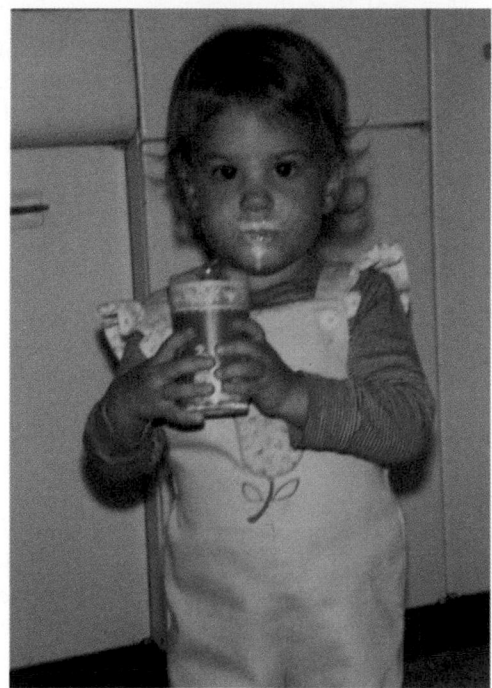

FIGURE 7-2 Milk and other dairy products supply preschool children with the calcium and vitamin D needed for growing bones.

TABLE 7-2

Protein Dietary Reference Intakes for Children through Age 13 Years

Age	Protein Grams/Day (g/day)*	Grams/Kilogram/Day
1-3 yr	13 g/day	1.10 g/kg/day
4-8 yr	19 g/day	0.95 g/kg/day
9-13 yr	34 g/day	0.95 g/kg/day

*RDA for reference individual (g/day).

Adapted from Feucht S: Dietary reference intakes (DRI) review: case studies illustrating energy and protein for children and adolescent with special needs, *Nutr Focus Newsletter* 20:1, 2005.

Zinc

Zinc is essential for growth; a deficiency results in growth failure, poor appetite, decreased taste acuity, and poor wound healing (see Figure 3-37). Because the best sources of zinc are meats and seafood, some children may regularly have a low intake (see Appendix 58). Marginal zinc deficiency has been reported in preschool and school-age children from middle- and low-income families (Roberts and Heyman, 2000). Diagnosis may be difficult because laboratory parameters, including plasma, serum, erythrocyte, hair, and urine levels are of limited value in determining zinc deficiency. Meta-analyses of randomized controlled zinc supplementation studies have demonstrated a positive impact of zinc supplementation on growth and serum zinc concentrations in prepubertal children (Brown et al., 2002). Improving zinc nutrition status by food and supplementation programs has demonstrated positive results in populations with high rates of childhood stunting and underweight (Rivera et al., 2003) (see Chapter 3).

Vitamin D

Vitamin D is needed for calcium absorption and deposition of calcium in the bones. Rickets is the bone disease resulting from too little vitamin D (see Figure 3-17). Because this nutrient is also formed from sunlight exposure on the skin, the amount required from dietary sources depends on non-dietary factors such as geographic location and time spent outside. Children living in tropical areas may need no dietary vitamin D or only 2.5 mcg (100 international units) or less for optimal calcium deposition (see Chapter 3, *Focus On: Sunshine, Vitamin D, and Fortification*). In the temperate zones some dietary source is needed. Vitamin D–fortified milk is the primary source of this nutrient; however, dairy products such as cheese and yogurt are not usually made from fortified milk. Regardless, many breakfast cereals and nondairy milks are fortified with vitamin D.

Vitamin-Mineral Supplements

Almost 50% of preschool children are given supplements (commonly a multivitamin-mineral with iron), but use usually decreases in older children (Balluz et al., 2000). Families with more education, health insurance coverage, and higher incomes generally have higher rates of supplement use, although these may not be the families who are at greatest risk for having inadequate diets. Supplements do not necessarily fulfill specific nutrient needs. For instance, although many children consume less than the recommended amount of calcium, children's vitamin-mineral supplements typically do not contain significant amounts of calcium. Careful evaluation of each pediatric supplement is suggested because many types are available and are not complete.

Evidence shows that fluoride can help prevent dental caries. If a community's water supply is not fluoridated (i.e., has <0.6 ppm), fluoride supplements are recommended from 6 months until 16 years of age (see Chapter 25). However, individual family practices should be assessed, including the child's primary source of fluids (i.e., drinking water, juices, or other beverages) and fluoride sources from day care, school, and toothpaste and mouthwash.

The American Academy of Pediatrics (AAP) does not support giving healthy children routine supplements of any vitamins or minerals other than fluoride. However, children at risk for inadequate nutrition who may benefit from supplementation include those (1) from deprived families or those who experience parental neglect or abuse; (2) with anorexia, or inadequate and capricious appetites or who consume fad diets; (3) with chronic diseases such as cystic fibrosis, inflammatory bowel disease, or renal or liver dis-

ease; and (4) who participate in dietary regimens to manage obesity (AAP, 2004).

Children who routinely take a multiple vitamin or a vitamin-mineral supplement usually do not experience negative effects if the supplement contains nutrients in amounts that do not exceed the DRIs, especially the tolerable UL values. However, children should not take megadoses, particularly of the fat-soluble vitamins, because large amounts can result in toxicity (see Chapter 3). Parents should be educated to keep vitamin-mineral supplements out of reach of children (since many look and taste like candy) to avoid excessive intake of nutrients such as iron.

Complementary nutrition therapies and herbal products are becoming more common for children, especially those with special needs such as children with Down syndrome, autism spectrum disorder, or cystic fibrosis (Harris, 2005). Practitioners should inquire as to the use of these products and therapies in nutrition assessments, be knowledgeable about their efficacy and safety, and help families determine whether they are beneficial and how to use them (see Chapter 18).

PROVIDING AN ADEQUATE DIET

Food and eating are more than the simple provision of nutrients for body growth and maintenance. The development of feeding skills, food habits, and nutrition knowledge parallels the cognitive development that takes place in a series of stages, each laying the groundwork for the next. Table 7-3 outlines the development of feeding skills in terms of Piaget's theory of child psychology and development.

TABLE 7-3

Feeding, Nutrition, and Piaget's Theory of Cognitive Development

Developmental Period	Cognitive Characteristics	Relationships to Feeding and Nutrition
Sensorimotor (birth-2 yr)	Neonate progresses from automatic reflexes to a child with intentional interaction with the environment and the beginning use of symbols.	Progression involves advancing from sucking and rooting reflexes to the acquisition of self-feeding skills. Food is used primarily to satisfy hunger, as a medium to explore the environment, and as an opportunity to practice fine motor skills.
Preoperational (2-7 yr)	Thought processes become internalized; they are unsystematic and intuitive. Use of symbols increases.	Eating becomes less the center of attention and is secondary to social, language, and cognitive growth. Food is described by color, shape, and quantity, but the child has only a limited ability to classify food into "groups."
	Reasoning is based on appearances and happenstance. The child's approach to classification is functional and unsystematic. The child's world is viewed egocentrically.	Foods tend to be categorized into "like" and "don't like." Foods can be identified as "good for you," but reasons why they are healthy are unknown or mistaken.

TABLE 7-3		
Feeding, Nutrition, and Piaget's Theory of Cognitive Development—cont'd		
Developmental Period	**Cognitive Characteristics**	**Relationships to Feeding and Nutrition**
Concrete operations (7-11 yr)	The child can focus on several aspects of a situation simultaneously.	The child begins to realize that nutritious food has a positive effect on growth and health but has a limited understanding of how or why.
	Cause-and-effect reasoning becomes more rational and systematic.	
	The ability to classify, reclassify, and generalize emerges.	
	A decrease in egocentrism permits the child to take another's view.	Mealtimes take on a social significance. The expanding environment increases the opportunities for the influences on food selection; for example, peer influence increases.
Formal operations (11 yr and beyond)	Hypothetical and abstract thought expand.	The concept of nutrients from food functioning at physiologic and biochemical levels can be understood.
	The child's understanding of scientific and theoretical processes deepens.	Conflicts in making food choices may be realized (i.e., knowledge of the nutritious value of foods may conflict with preferences and non-nutritive influences).

Intake Patterns

Children are most likely to consume inadequate amounts of calcium, iron, zinc, folate, vitamin B_6, vitamin E, magnesium and vitamin A (Roberts and Heyman, 2000; Suitor and Gleason, 2002; Moshfegh et al., 2005). However, clinical signs of malnutrition in American children are rare.

Children's food patterns have changed over the years. They drink less milk, but more of it is low-fat and nonfat milk. The total fat as a percent of energy intake has decreased but remains above recommendations with an average of 33.5%. One in four youths meets the recommended intakes for fat and saturated fat, whereas 75% meet the intake recommendations for cholesterol (Troiano et al., 2000). More energy comes from snacks, and more food is consumed in environments other than the home (French et al., 2001; ADA, 2004). Sugar consumption, including noncitrus fruit juices, carbonated beverages, and candy has increased, particularly in young children (Kranz et al., 2005a; Sebastian et al., 2005). Data from national food intake studies of children and adolescents indicate that most of their diets do not meet the national recommendations for food groups (ADA, 2004). The most recent Healthy Eating Index (HEI) reported that children ages 2 to 3 years have the highest HEI scores among all age and gender groups; as children grow older, their HEI scores decline through adolescence (Basiotis et al., 2002). Some children receive almost 50% of their energy from additional fat and sugar (Brady et al., 2000).

Population studies of nutritional status have reported an increased frequency of low nutrient intake and higher cholesterol in children from low-income families (Casey et al., 2001). In addition, inner-city, low-income children and homeless children are at more risk for poor dietary intake and lead exposure and toxicity (see *Focus On:* Childhood Lead Exposure and Toxicity: the Role of Nutrition).

Like physical growth patterns, food intake patterns are not smooth and consistent. Although subjective, appetites usually follow the rate of growth and nutrient needs. By a child's first birthday, milk consumption begins to decline. In the next year vegetable intake decreases, whereas intakes of cereals, grain products, and sweets increase. Young children often prefer softer protein sources instead of meats that are harder to chew.

Changes in food consumption are reflected in nutrient intakes. Compared with nutrient intake in infancy, that in the early preschool years shows a decrease in calcium, phosphorus, riboflavin, iron, and vitamin A. Intakes of most other key nutrients remain relatively stable. During the early school years, a pattern of consistent and steady increased intakes of most nutrients is seen until adolescence. For healthy children a wide variability of nutrient intake is seen in any age- and sex-group.

Factors Influencing Food Intake

Numerous influences, some obvious and others subtle, determine the food intake and habits of children. Habits, likes, and dislikes are established in the early years and carried through to adulthood. The major influences on food intake in the developing years include family environment, societal trends, the media, peer pressure, and illness or diseases.

◎ **FOCUS ON**

Childhood Lead Exposure and Toxicity: The Role of Nutrition

Elevated blood lead levels in toddlers and children can result in developmental regression, irritability, anorexia, gastrointestinal symptoms (e.g., abdominal pain, constipation, vomiting), and ataxia. High levels can cause growth impairment and mental retardation. Children living in poverty and non-Hispanic black children are at greatest risk, partly because they are more likely to be exposed to lead-based paint and contaminated soil, dust, and air emissions in industrial areas. Lead exposure can also result from consuming contaminated drinking water (from lead pipes or solder) and contaminated food (from lead glazing or lead crystal). Toddlers who typically put everything in their mouths and children with mental retardation who exhibit pica are exposed to lead from many environmental sources.

When correlations were found between middle-class toddler blood lead levels and the toddlers' subsequent IQ scores at ages 5 and 10, the Centers for Disease Control and Prevention (CDC) lowered the blood lead threshold to 10 mcg/dl and established screening guidelines (CDC, 1997a). There has been a decrease in the prevalence of elevated blood lead levels over the past decade, although not all at-risk children are screened (CDC, 2005).

Although the effect of lead exposure varies with its intensity and timing (with younger children being the most susceptible to its effects), blood lead levels of 10 to 25 mcg/dl can have a negative impact a child's attention, adaptive behaviors, and emotional reactivity, all of which affect learning, school achievement, and life functioning. Blood lead levels less than 10 mcg/dl can also negatively affect young children, and there is consideration of lowering the threshold to 5 mcg/dl (Bernard and McGeehin, 2003).

Because more lead is absorbed from an empty stomach, nutrition guidelines include regular meals and snacks. Increased calcium and iron intakes are also recommended to minimize the lead absorption in children with mineral deficiencies. However, the associations that have been found between high blood lead levels and calcium and iron deficiencies could also be a result of poverty and other environmental factors.

A recent study of Mexican school children found a negative association between blood lead levels and cognitive test performance, but this association was not explained by iron deficiency or anemia (Kordas et al., 2004). Because of these inconsistent results, practitioners can promote a mineral-rich diet but should not assume that it can ameliorate the negative effects of lead ingestion (Ballew and Bowman, 2001). In addition to ensuring that children at risk for lead exposure follow a nutrient-rich diet, regular screening and education should be provided, and public health policies should be developed to decrease environmental lead levels.

Family Environment

For toddlers and preschool children the family is the primary influence in the development of food habits. In young children's immediate environment, parents and older siblings are significant models. Food attitudes of parents can be strong predictors of food likes and dislikes and diet complexity in children of primary-school age. Similarities between children's and their parents' food preferences are likely to reflect genetic and environmental influences (ADA, 2004).

Contrary to common belief, young children do not have the innate ability to choose a balanced, nutritious diet; they can choose one only when presented with nutritious foods (see Chapter 6, *Clinical Insight:* Self-Selected Diets of Infants and Young Children). A positive feeding relationship includes a division of responsibility between parents and children. The parents and other adults provide safe, nutritious, developmentally appropriate food as regular meals and snacks; and the children decide how much, if any, they eat (Satter, 2000).

National trends indicate that eating together at family meals is becoming less common, partly because of family schedules, more time eating in front of the television, and the decreasing amount of time devoted to planning and preparing family meals. In a recent report school-age children and adolescents who ate more dinners with their families consumed more fruits and vegetables, less soda, and fewer fried foods than those who rarely ate dinner with their families (Gillman et al., 2000).

The atmosphere around food and mealtime also influences attitudes toward food and eating. Unrealistic expectations for a child's mealtime manners, arguments, and other emotional stress can have a negative effect. Meals that are rushed create a hectic atmosphere and reinforce the tendency to eat too fast. A positive environment is one in which sufficient time is set aside to eat, occasional spills are tolerated, and conversation that includes all family members is encouraged (Figure 7-3).

Societal Trends

Because almost three fourths of women with school-age children are employed outside the home, children eat one or more meals at child-care homes, day-care centers, or schools. In these settings all children should have access to nutritious meals served in a safe and sanitary environment that promotes healthy growth and development (ADA, 2003a; ADA, 2005). Due to time constraints, family meals may include more convenience or fast foods. However, having a mother who is employed outside the home does not seem to affect children's dietary intakes negatively.

Approximately one in five American children lives in families with incomes below the poverty line; these chil-

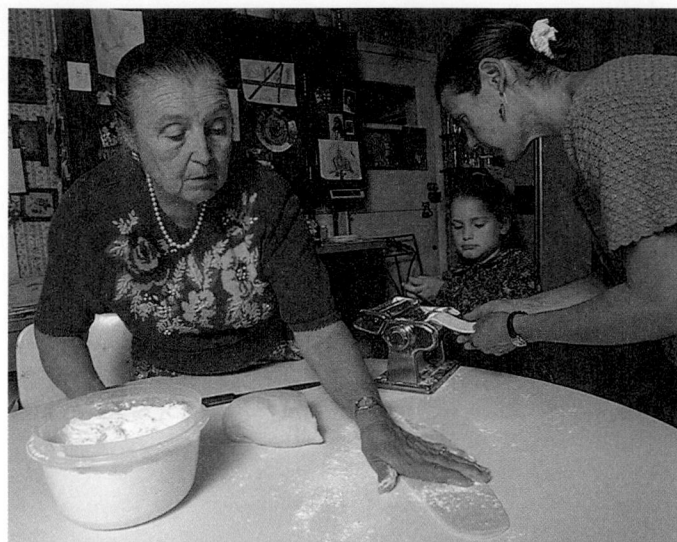

FIGURE 7-3 Three generations of Italian Americans make a pasta dinner. The custom of eating authentically prepared foods gives meals a place of prominence in this home—meals that will not be replaced with fast foods eaten on the run. *(From Leahy J, Kisilay P:* Foundations of nursing practice: a nursing process approach, *Philadelphia, 1998, Saunders.)*

dren constitute 35% of all the poor in the United States (DeNavas-Walt et al., 2005). Overall, households with children report food insecurity at almost double the rate for those without children (Nord et al., 2005). The increasing numbers of single-parent households predominantly headed by women have lower incomes and less money for all expenses, including food, than households headed by men. This phenomenon makes these families increasingly vulnerable to multiple stressors such as marginal health and nutritional status partly because of lack of jobs, child care, adequate housing, and health insurance.

Of the 11.9% of households reporting food insecurity in the United States, just over one half participated in one or more of these programs: National School Lunch, Food Stamp Program, and Special Supplemental Nutrition Program for Women, Infants and Children (WIC) (Nord et al., 2005). Of note is that the food stamp allotment for families, based on the USDA Thrifty Food Plan, does not provide adequate funds to purchase food based on the government's nutrition guidelines (Neault et al., 2005). Food insecurity also increases the risk for children less than 3 years of age to be iron deficient with anemia (Skalicky et al., 2005). Studies suggest that intermittent hunger in American children is associated with poor psychosocial function (Kleinman et al., 1998) (see *Focus On:* Childhood Hunger and Its Effect on Behavior and Emotions).

Media Messages

Food is marketed to children using a variety of techniques, including television advertising, in-school marketing, sponsorship, product placement, Internet marketing, and sales promotion. Of these, television is perhaps the most popular means worldwide with marketing to students in school be-

ing second. Both of these marketing methods have regulations to some degree. Internet marketing however, is a new market for children, and regulations are still developing (Hawkes, 2004).

By the time average American children have graduated from high school, they have watched 15,000 hours of television and spent 11,000 hours in the classroom. School-age children watch an average of 23 hours or more per week, whereas preschool children average about 27 hours per week. Forty-four percent of television advertising to children is composed of candy, sweets, and soft drinks, whereas 34% is composed of convenience and fast foods (Harrison and Marske, 2005). Compared to all other foods, there were far fewer ads for breads and cereals, fruits and vegetables, and milk products; meats, fish, and poultry had very little exposure. Snack time eating is portrayed more often than consuming food at breakfast, lunch, and dinner combined (Harrison and Marske, 2005).

Preschool children are generally unable to distinguish commercial messages from regular programs. In fact, they often pay more attention to the commercials; thus they remember and request the advertised items (Borzekowski and Robinson, 2001). As children get older, they gain knowledge about the purpose of commercial advertising and become more critical of its validity but are still susceptible to the commercial message. Media literacy education programs teach children and adolescents about the intent of advertising and media messages and how to evaluate and interpret their obvious and subtle influences.

Television can also be detrimental to growth and development because it encourages inactivity and passive use of leisure time. Indeed, television viewing and its multiple media cues to eat have been suggested as a factor contributing to excessive weight gain in school-age children and adolescents (Dietz and Gortmaker, 2001). In addition, the types of food eaten during television viewing can contribute to increased dental caries due to the continued exposure of the teeth to dense carbohydrate and sugar-laden foods (Palmer, 2005).

Peer Influence

As children grow, their world expands and their social contacts become more important. Peer influence increases with age and affects food attitudes and choices. This may result in a sudden refusal of a food or a request for a currently popular food. Decisions about whether to participate in school meals may be made more on the basis of friends' choices than on the menu. Such behaviors are developmentally typical. Positive behaviors such as a willingness to try new foods can be reinforced. Parents need to set limits on undesirable influences but also need to be realistic; struggles over food are self-defeating.

Illness or Disease

Children who are ill usually have a decreased appetite and limited food intake. Acute viral or bacterial illnesses are often short-lived but may require an increase in fluids, protein, or other nutrients. Chronic conditions such as asthma,

Childhood Hunger and Its Effect on Behavior and Emotions

It is well accepted that malnourished children are less responsive, less inquisitive, and participate in less exploratory behavior than well-nourished infants. Specific nutrient deficiencies such as iron deficiency anemia can also result in a decreased ability to pay attention and poorer problem-solving skills. Less clear is the impact of periodic hunger or **food insecurity** on a child's behavior and functioning. With recent federal welfare reform legislation and economic downturns, an increasing number of children from low-income families are at risk for limited food resources.

In the 1990s the Community Childhood Hunger Identification Project (CCHIP) conducted surveys using standardized questions and large, rigorously selected samples to categorize families as "hungry," "at risk for hunger," or "not hungry" (Kleinman et al., 1998). Results estimated that each year 8% of the children younger than 12 years of age living in the United States experience prolonged periods in which they have insufficient food. The CCHIP survey questions were incorporated into the annual Current Population Survey conducted by the U.S. Census Bureau. Data from 2004 indicated that 1.4 million households with children were food insecure, representing almost 50% of all food-insecure households (Food Research and Action Center, 2005). This survey and others suggest that the number of children in food-insecure households continues to increase.

In one study a group of 328 parents from a larger CCHIP study were asked to complete the Pediatric Symptom Checklist, which was related to their child's emotional and behavioral symptoms. "Hungry" children were three times more likely than "at risk for hunger" children and seven times more likely than "not hungry" children to have scores indicative of characteristics such as aggression, irritability, oppositional behavior, and anxiety (Kleinman et al., 1998).

Weinreb and colleagues conducted a study of hunger in homeless and low-income preschool and school-age children, using standardized tools to determine the impact on health, behavior and mental health (Weinreb et al., 2002). Severe hunger was associated with greater homelessness, more chronic illness and traumatic life events, higher levels of internalizing behavior problems, and elevated reports of anxiety and depression in school-age children. Mothers of the children reporting severe hunger were more likely to have a diagnosis of posttraumatic stress disorder (Weinreb et al., 2002). A recent longitudinal study following about 21,000 children from kindergarten through third grade found that persistent food insecurity was predictive of impaired academic outcomes, poorer social skills, and a tendency to increased BMI (Jyoti et al., 2005).

Although these studies have limitations because of other factors (e.g., stress, family dysfunction, or substance abuse) that may affect a child's functioning, a correlation exists between children's lack of sufficient food and their behavioral and academic functioning. As future studies provide more evidence of this relationship, it will be clear that social policies need to ensure the provision of children's basic needs for optimal growth and development.

---

cystic fibrosis (see Chapter 35), or chronic renal disease (see Chapter 36), may make it difficult to obtain sufficient nutrients for optimal growth. Children with these types of conditions are more likely to have behavior problems relating to food. Children requiring special diets (e.g., those who have diabetes or phenylketonuria) not only have to adjust to the limits of foods allowed, but also have to deal with issues of independence and peer acceptance as they grow older. Some rebellion against the prescribed diet is typical, especially as children approach puberty.

Feeding Preschool Children

From 1 to 6 years of age children experience vast developmental progress and acquisition of skills. One-year-old children primarily use fingers to eat and may need assistance with a cup. By 2 years of age, they can hold a cup in one hand and use a spoon well (see Figure 6-3) but may prefer to use their hands at times. Six-year-old children have refined skills and are beginning to use a knife for cutting and spreading.

As the growth rate slows after the first year of life, appetite decreases, which often concerns parents. Children have less interest in food and an increased interest in the world around them. They can develop **food jags** or periods when foods that were previously liked are refused, or they can request a particular food at every meal. This behavior may be attributable to boredom with the usual foods or may be a means of asserting newly discovered independence.

Parents may have concerns about the adequacy of their child's diet and be frustrated with their child's seemingly irrational food behavior. Struggles over control of the eating situation are fruitless; no child can be forced to eat. This period is developmental and temporary. Parents still retain control over what foods are offered, and they have the opportunity to set limits on inappropriate behaviors. Neither rigid control nor a laissez-faire approach is likely to succeed. Parents and other caregivers should continue to offer a variety of foods, including the child's favorite ones, and not make substitutions a routine. Preschool children tend to vary considerably in their meal intakes during the day, but their total daily energy intake remains fairly constant.

With smaller stomach capacity and variable appetites, preschool children eat best with small servings of food offered four to six times a day. Snacks are as important as meals in contributing to the total daily nutrient intake.

TABLE 7-4

Feeding Guide for Preschool Children*

Food	2- to 3-Year-Olds		4- to 6-Year-Olds		Comments
	Portion Size	Number of Servings	Portion Size	Number of Servings	
Milk and Dairy Products	½ cup (4 oz)	4-5	½-¾ cup (4-6 oz)	3-4	The following may be substituted for ½ cup of liquid milk: ½-¾ oz cheese, ½ cup yogurt, 2½ tbsp nonfat dry milk powder.
Meat, Fish, Poultry, or Equivalent	1-2 oz	2	1-2 oz	2	The following may be substituted for 1 oz of meat, fish, or poultry: 1 egg, 2 tbsp peanut butter, 4-5 tbsp cooked legumes.
Fruits and Vegetables		4-5		4-5	Include one green leafy or yellow vegetable for vitamin A, such as spinach, carrots, broccoli, or winter squash.
Vegetables					
Cooked	2-3 tbsp		3-4 tbsp		
Raw†	Few pieces		Few pieces		
Fruit					Include one vitamin C-rich fruit, vegetable, or juice, such as citrus juices, an orange, grapefruit sections, strawberries, melon in season, a tomato, or broccoli.
Raw	½-1 small		½-1 small		
Canned	2-4 tbsp		4-6 tbsp		
Juice	3-4 oz		4 oz		
Bread and Grain Products		3		3	The following may be substituted for 1 slice of bread: ½ cup spaghetti, macaroni, noodles, or rice; 5 saltines; 1 tortilla; or ½ bagel.
Whole-grain or enriched bread	½-1 slice		1 slice		
Cooked cereal	¼-½ cup		½ cup		
Dry cereal	½-1 cup		1 cup		

Modified from Lowenberg ME: Development of food patterns in young children. In Trahms CM, Pipes P: *Nutrition in infancy and childhood*, ed 6, St Louis, 1997, WCB/McGraw-Hill.

*This is a guide to a basic diet. Fats, oils, sauces, desserts, and snack foods provide additional kilocalories to meet the needs of a growing child. Foods can be selected from this pattern for meals and snacks.

†Do not give to children until they can chew well.

Carefully chosen snacks are dense in nutrients and least likely to promote dental caries (see Chapter 25). Wholesome snacks enjoyed by many young children include fresh fruit, cheese, raw vegetable sticks, milk, fruit juices, whole-grain crackers, dry cereal, and peanut butter sandwiches. A general rule of thumb is to offer 1 tablespoon of each food for every year of age and to serve more food according to the child's appetite. Table 7-4 is a guide for food and portion sizes and is designed to provide an adequate diet for preschoolers.

Senses other than taste play an important part in food acceptance by young children. They tend to avoid food with extreme temperatures, and some foods are rejected because of odor rather than taste. A sense of order in the food presentation is often required; many children will not accept foods that touch each other on the plate, and mixed dishes or casseroles with unidentifiable foods are not popular. Broken crackers may go uneaten or a sandwich may be refused because it is "cut the wrong way."

The physical setting of children's meals is as important as the emotional atmosphere. Their feet should be supported with no dangling, and chair height should allow a comfort-able reach to the table at chest height. Sturdy, child-size tables and chairs are ideal, or a high chair or booster seat should be used. Bowls, plates, and cups should be unbreakable and heavy enough to resist tipping. For very young children, a shallow bowl is often better than a plate for scooping. Thick, short-handled spoons and forks allow for an easier, less tiring grasp.

Young children do not eat well if they are tired; thus this should be considered when meal and play times are scheduled. A quiet activity or rest immediately before eating is conducive to a relaxed, enjoyable meal. However, children need active, large-motor activities and time in the fresh air to stimulate a good appetite.

Fruit juices, especially apple juice and juice drinks, are an increasingly common beverage for young children, at home and in group settings; they frequently replace water and milk in children's diets. In addition to altering the diet's nutrient content, excessive intake of fruit juice can result in carbohydrate malabsorption and chronic, nonspecific diarrhea (AAP, 2001). This suggests that juices, especially apple and pear, should be avoided when using clear liquids to treat acute diarrhea. For children with chronic diarrhea, a trial of restricting fruit juices may be warranted before more costly diagnostic tests are done.

Excessive fruit juice consumption (12 to 30 oz/day) has been identified as a contributing factor in some cases of failure to thrive in toddlers. A reduction in juice intake, in addition to nutritional education designed to increase total energy intake, resulted in improved growth (AAP, 2001). Excess juice intake by young preschool children may replace the consumption of higher-energy foods and decrease a child's appetite, resulting in decreased food intake and poor growth. It is also possible that large volumes of juice, combined with other dietary and activity factors, may contribute to or sustain an overweight condition in a child. The AAP recommends that fruit juice be limited to 4 to 6 oz per day for infants older than 6 months of age and toddlers and to 6 to 12 oz per day for older children and adolescents (AAP, 2001).

Many children spend part or most of their days in day-care homes or centers, preschools, or Head Start programs. Depending on the amount of time the children are in these settings, they may consume only a snack, or they may eat as many as two meals and two snacks per day. Therefore many children consume more than half of their nutrients outside the home.

Food service in group settings such as day-care centers, Head Start programs, and preschool programs in elementary schools is regulated by federal or state guidelines. Many facilities and some day-care homes may participate in the USDA Child and Adult Care Food Program. However, the quality of meals and snacks can vary greatly; parents should investigate food service when considering child-care options. In addition to providing children with optimal nutrients, a program should offer food that is appealing, safely prepared, and appropriate, incorporating cultural and developmental patterns (ADA, 2005) (see Chapters 11 and 12).

Because of peer influence, children usually eat well in group settings, which are also ideal environments for nutrition education programs during mealtimes and as the focus for various learning activities (Figure 7-4). Experiencing new foods, participating in simple food preparation, and planting a garden are activities that develop and enhance positive food habits and attitudes.

Feeding School-Age Children

Growth from ages 6 to 12 years is slow but steady, paralleled by a constant increase in food intake. Children are in school a greater part of the day; and they begin to participate in clubs, organized sports, and recreational programs. The influence of peers and significant adults such as teachers, coaches, or sports idols increases. Except for severe issues, most behavioral problems connected with food have been resolved by this age, and children enjoy eating to alleviate hunger and obtain social satisfaction.

School-age children may participate in the school lunch program or bring a lunch from home. The National School Lunch Program, established in 1946 and administered by the USDA, provides approximately one third of the DRI for students. Children from low-income families are eligible for free or reduced-price meals. In addition, the School Breakfast Program that began in 1966 is offered in about 72% of the schools that participate in the lunch program. The USDA also offers the Summer Food Service Program, which offers meals and snacks to children in programs during school vacations (see Chapter 11).

Over the years efforts have been made to decrease food waste by altering menus to accommodate student preferences, allowing students to decline one or two menu items and offering salad bars. Ongoing concerns over excessive amounts of fat, salt, and sugar in school meals resulted in changes to school meals that incorporated the Dietary Guidelines for Americans. Specific changes in the school and child nutrition programs included reducing the fat content of recipes and offering a greater variety of fresh fruits and vegetables, whole-grain products, and fewer baked items (see Chapter 11). By 1999 significantly more elementary and secondary schools were meeting the lower fat and sodium standards for school lunches (USDA, 2001). Efforts to increase participation in school lunch to more than 60% of students will require consistent messages that support healthful eating (Gross and Cinelli, 2004). School wellness policies are required by the school year 2006-2007 in those institutions that participate in school lunch and school breakfast programs. A recent survey indicated that many parents, while supporting restriction of snack foods and wanting more physical education, are unaware of the required school wellness policies (Action for Healthy Kids, 2005). The school, including the administration, teachers, students, and food service personnel together with families and the community, are encouraged to work together to support nutrition integrity in the educational setting (ADA, 2000).

Consumption of school meals is also affected by the daily school schedule and the amount of time allotted for children to eat. Children often spend considerable time waiting in line to participate in the school lunch program before consuming their meal (Bergman et al., 2000). Those children who bring lunch from home are able to devote more time to eating the food without increasing their rate of consumption (Buergel et al., 2002). A study of elementary school

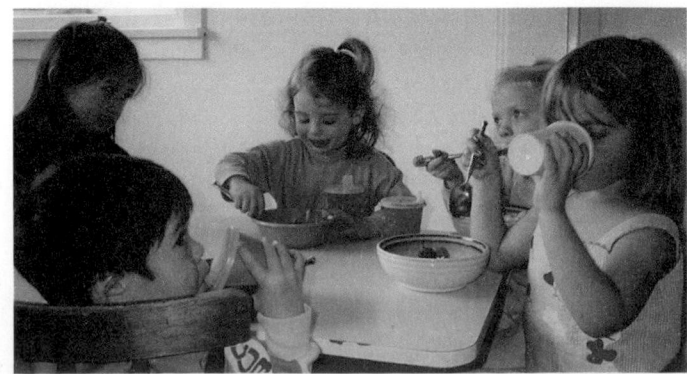

FIGURE 7-4 Children who eat with each other in an appropriate environment often eat more nutritiously and try a wider variety of foods than they do when alone.

students found that food waste significantly decreased when recess was scheduled before, rather than after, the lunch period (Getlinger et al., 1996).

Children who require a special diet because of certain medical conditions such as diabetes, hyperlipidemia, or documented food allergy are eligible for modified school meals. Children with developmental disabilities are eligible to attend public school from ages 3 to 21 years, and some of them need modified school meals (e.g., meals that are texture modified, high in calories, or low in calories). To receive modified meals, families must submit written documentation by a medical professional of the diagnosis, meal modification, and rationale. For children receiving special education services, the documentation for meals and feeding (e.g., modified meals, snacks and supplement needs, feeding therapy programs) can be incorporated as objectives in the child's individual education plan (IEP), the school education plan developed collaboratively between school personnel and the family (Horsley, 2004) (see Chapter 45).

Studies of lunches packed at home indicate that they usually provide fewer nutrients but less fat than school lunch meals. Favorite foods tend to be packed, so children have less variety. Food choices are limited to those that travel well and require no heating or refrigeration. A typical well-balanced lunch brought from home could include a sandwich with whole-grain bread and a protein-rich filling (lean meat, egg, cheese, peanut butter); fresh fruit, vegetables, or both; low-fat milk; and possibly a cookie, a graham cracker, or another simple dessert. Food safety measures (e.g., keeping perishable foods well chilled) must be observed when packing lunches for school.

Today many school-age children are responsible for preparing their own breakfasts. It is not uncommon for children to skip this meal altogether, even children in the primary grades. Children who skip breakfast tend to consume less energy and fewer nutrients than those who eat breakfast. Reviews of the effects of breakfast on cognition and school performance suggest that children who go to school without breakfast are more likely to experience performance deficits than those who eat breakfast (Rampersaud et al., 2005) (see *Focus On:* Breakfast: Does It Affect Learning?).

Snacks are commonly eaten by school-age children, primarily after school and in the evening. As children grow older and have money to spend, they tend to consume more snacks from vending machines, fast-food restaurants, and neighborhood groceries. Families should continue to offer wholesome snacks at home and support nutrition education efforts in the school. In most cases, good eating habits established in the first few years help children through this period of decision making and responsibility.

Nutrition Education

As children grow, they acquire knowledge and assimilate concepts by leaps and bounds. The early years are ideal for providing nutrition information and promoting positive attitudes about all foods. This education can be informal and natural and take place in the home with parents as models and a diet with a wide variety of foods. Food can be used in daily experiences for the toddler and preschooler and to promote the development of language, cognition, and self-help behaviors (i.e., labeling; describing size, shape, and color; sorting; assisting in preparation; and tasting).

More formal nutrition education is provided in preschools, Head Start programs, and public schools. Some programs such as Head Start have federal guidance and standards that incorporate healthy eating and nutrition education for the families involved. Nutrition education in

⊚ FOCUS ON

Breakfast: Does It Affect Learning?

The educational benefits of school meal programs and especially the role of breakfast in better school performance have been debated and discussed for decades. Experimental studies of healthy 9- to 11-year-old children have shown that those who skipped breakfast and were then given a variety of tests made more errors, had slower stimulus discrimination, and had slower memory recall (Pollitt et al., 1998). Similar studies in other countries with children who were at nutritional risk (i.e., had wasted and stunted growth) and skipped breakfast demonstrated even poorer performance on the learning tasks (Pollitt et al., 1998; Rampersaud et al., 2005). Recent school-based breakfast experiments in 9- to 11- and 6- to 8-year-old children found similar positive results with breakfast consumption (i.e., enhanced short term memory, better spatial memory, and improved processing of complex visual stimuli) (Mahoney et al., 2005), but other reports are

less supportive (Rampersaud et al., 2005). These studies suggest that brain functioning is sensitive to short-term variations in nutrient availability. A short fast may impose greater stress on young children than on adults, resulting in metabolic alterations as various homeostatic mechanisms work to maintain circulating glucose concentrations.

Both controlled trials and observational studies in the United States and developing countries have also shown that school breakfast programs result in better academic performance, achievement test scores, and attendance (Powell et al., 1998; Rampersaud et al., 2005). In addition, breakfast contributes significantly to the child's overall nutrient intake.

These studies underscore the potential benefits—not only for low-income and at-risk children but also for all school children—of a breakfast at home or school meal programs that include breakfast.

schools is less standard and frequently has minimum or no requirements for inclusion in the curriculum or the training of teachers. Recent recommendations include policies in schools promoting coordination between nutrition education; access to and promotion of child nutrition programs; and cooperation with families, the community, and health services (ADA, 2003b).

Teachers attempting to teach children nutrition concepts and information should take into account the children's developmental level. The play approach, based on Piaget's theory of learning, is one method for teaching nutrition and fitness to school-age children (Rickard et al., 1995). Many written and electronic resources on nutrition education for children exist, such as at the National Center for Education in Maternal and Child Health.

The concept of nutrition is abstract and as such may not be understood by preschoolers and most primary school children. Some nutrition curricula are too sophisticated for the children's conceptual abilities, and modifications may be necessary to make the educational experiences meaningful. Activities and information that focus on children's real-world relationships with food are most likely to yield positive results. Meals, snacks, and food-preparation activities provide children an opportunity to practice and reinforce their nutrition knowledge and demonstrate their cognitive understanding. Parental involvement in nutrition education projects can produce positive outcomes that are also beneficial in the home.

NUTRITIONAL CONCERNS

Overweight/Obesity

The increasing prevalence of overweight children is a significant and alarming public health problem. The most recent National Health and Nutrition Examination Survey (NHANES) reported an overweight (BMI higher than the 95th percentile) prevalence of 17.1% in children ages 2 to 19 years, and at risk for overweight (BMI higher than the 85th percentile but lower than the 95th percentile) prevalence of 33.6% (Ogden et al., 2006). For children 2 to 5 years of age, the prevalence is 13.9% for overweight and 26.2% for at risk for overweight (Ogden et al., 2006). This prevalence continues to increase in this decade. The national data document higher percentages of overweight and at risk for overweight for black and Mexican-American children (Ogden et al., 2006).

The terms "overweight" and "obesity" are often used interchangeably but are different. Overweight is when the weight is higher than standard for a child's stature; obese is the condition of excess fatness. Many individuals with a BMI significantly over the 95th percentile are likely obese, but BMI alone is primarily a screening tool.

Although more people are recognizing the role of inheritability in obesity development because of studies of molecular genetics and animal obesity phenotypes, the increases in the prevalence of overweight children cannot be explained by genetics alone. Factors contributing to excess energy intake for the pediatric population include ready access to eating and food establishments, eating tied to leisure activities (many of which are sedentary), children making more food and eating decisions, larger portion sizes, and inactivity (French et al., 2001).

Inactivity plays a major role in obesity development, whether it results from television and computer use, limited opportunities for physical activity, or safety concerns that prevent children from enjoying free play outdoors. Although increased television viewing has been associated with childhood overweight, a recent review suggests that the greater risk of overweight is related to television viewing plus a low activity level (Ritchie et al., 2005). Using automobiles for short trips limits children's opportunities to walk to local destinations, a phenomenon particularly relevant to children in the suburbs.

Obesity in childhood is not a benign condition, despite the popular belief that overweight children will outgrow their condition. The longer a child has been overweight, the more likely the child is to be overweight or obese during adolescence and adulthood (Goran, 2001). Consequences of overweight in childhood include psychosocial difficulties such as discrimination from others, a negative self-image, depression, and decreased socialization. In the past the health consequences of childhood overweight were thought to be manifested in adulthood, but current evidence shows that many overweight children have one or more cardiovascular risk factors such as hyperlipidemia, hypertension, or hyperinsulinemia (Freedman et al., 2001). An even more dramatic health consequence of overweight is the rapid increase in the incidence of type 2 diabetes in children and adolescents, which has a serious impact on adult health, development of other chronic diseases, and health care costs (Narayan et al., 2003) (see Chapters 21 and 30).

Determining whether growing children are obese is difficult. Some excess weight may be gained at either end of the childhood spectrum; the 1-year-old toddler and the prepubescent child may weigh more for developmental and physiologic reasons, but this extra weight is often not permanent. BMI, a useful clinical tool for screening for overweight, has limitations in determining obesity because of variability related to sex, race, body composition and maturation stage (Daniels et al., 1997). However, the CDC Growth Charts allow tracking of BMI from age 2 into adulthood; thus children can be monitored periodically, and prevention or intervention provided when the rate of BMI change is excessive. The BMI charts show the adiposity rebound, which normally occurs in children between 4 and 6 years of age. Children whose normal growth adiposity rebound occurs before 5½ years of age are more likely to weigh more as adults than those whose adiposity rebound occurs after 7 years of age. The timing of the adiposity rebound and excess fatness in adolescence are two critical factors in the development of obesity in childhood, with the latter being the most predictive of adult obesity and related morbidity (Whitaker et al., 1998).

The AAP has developed guidelines for overweight screening and assessment for children from age 2 through adolescence (Barlow and Dietz, 1998). In addition to growth parameters, other important information includes dietary intake and patterns, previous growth patterns, family history, physical activity, and family interactions.

Interventions for obesity in children have had limited impact on the childhood obesity problem, especially for black, Hispanic, and Native American populations. Success is most likely to result from programs that include comprehensive behavioral components such as family involvement, dietary modifications, nutrition information, physical activity, and behavioral strategies (Kirk et al., 2005). Incorporating behavioral intervention in obesity treatment improves outcomes and is most effective with a team approach (Epstein et al., 2001). Depending on the child, goals for weight change may include a decrease in the rate of weight gain, maintenance of weight, or, in severe cases, gradual weight loss (see Chapter 21). An individualized approach should be tailored to each child, with minimum use of highly restrictive diets or medication, except if there are significant other diseases (Barlow et al., 2002).

Intervention strategies require family involvement and support. Incorporating motivational interviewing and stages of change theory into the comprehensive program will likely be more successful (Kirk et al., 2005) (see Chapter 19). Changes to address overweight should include the child's input and choices and plans that modify the family's food and activity environment, not just the child's. Adequate energy and nutrients are needed to ensure maintenance of height velocity and nutrient stores. The hazards of treating overweight children too aggressively include alternate periods of undereating and overeating, feelings of failure in meeting external expectations, ignoring internal cues for appetite and satiation, feelings of deprivation and isolation, an increased risk for eating disorders, and a poor or an increasingly poor self-image.

Some children with special health care needs, such as those with Down syndrome, Prader-Willi syndrome, short stature, and limited mobility, are at increased risk for being overweight. Their size, level of activity, and developmental status need to be considered when estimating energy intake and providing dietary guidance to their families. Prader-Willi syndrome is a genetic disorder characterized by hypotonia in early life, short stature, cognitive delays, low energy needs, and a preoccupation with food. To avoid gaining excessive weight, children with this syndrome usually need a lower energy intake than typical for children their height; their food access must also be controlled in all situations (see Chapter 45).

Prevention of childhood obesity has become an important public health priority in the United States. The IOM has published recommendations that target families, health care professionals, industry, schools, and communities (IOM, 2004b; Kirk et al., 2005). The recommendations include schools (improved nutritional quality of food sold and served; increased physical activity, wellness education); industry (improved nutrition information for consumers, clear media messages); health care professionals (tracking BMI, providing counseling for children and families); and communities and government (better access to healthy foods, improved physical activity opportunities). Schools are a natural environment for obesity prevention, which can include nutrition and health curricula, opportunities for physical education and activity, and appropriate school meals. Recent efforts have resulted in school nutrition policies that limit the kinds of products sold in vending machines and food/beverages sold for fundraising. More research is also needed to develop effective prevention strategies that incorporate cultural competency issues for high-risk populations.

Families are key for modeling food choices, healthy eating, and leisure activities for their children. Parents influence children's environment by choosing nutrient-rich foods, having family meals (including breakfast), offering regular snacks, and spending time together in physical activity, all of which can be critical in overweight prevention. Reducing sedentary behaviors can increase energy expenditure and reduce prompts to eat; the AAP recommends limiting television and video time to no more than 2 hours per day (AAP, 2003). Parents exerting too much control over their child's food intake or promoting a restrictive diet may cause children to be less able to self-regulate and more likely to overeat when the opportunity is available (Ritchie et al., 2005). Health professionals should support positive parenting within the child's developmental level (Satter, 2005).

Underweight and Failure to Thrive

Weight loss, lack of weight gain, or **failure to thrive (FTT)** can be caused by an acute or chronic illness, a restricted diet, a poor appetite, feeding problems, a poor appetite because of constipation or medication, neglect, or a simple lack of food. Some experts prefer the terms pediatric undernutrition or growth deficiency to FTT. Infants and toddlers are most at risk for FTT and poor growth, often as a result of prematurity, medical conditions, developmental delays, inadequate parenting, or all of these. Dietary practices can also contribute to poor growth, including food restrictions in preschool children stemming from parents' concerns about obesity, atherosclerosis, or other potential health problems, and excess fruit juice intake (AAP, 2001).

A careful assessment of FTT is critical and must include the social and emotional environment of the child and any physical findings. If neglect is documented to be a contributing factor to FTT, health professionals are obligated to report the case to the local child protective services (Block and Krebs, 2005). Because of the complexity of FTT, an interdisciplinary team is ideal for assessments and interventions.

The provision of adequate energy and nutrients and nutrition education should be among the goals of the management plan. Nutrition is often one part of an overall interdisciplinary plan to assist children and their families. Attempts should be made to increase children's appetites and modify the environment to ensure optimal intake (Cunningham and McLaughlin, 1999). Frequent, small meals and snacks should be offered at regular times, using developmentally appropriate, nutrient-dense foods. This optimizes the smaller stomach capacity of the young child and provides structure and predictability for the eating environment.

Families should receive support for positive parent-child interactions, with respect for the division of responsibility in feeding and avoidance of any pressure or coercion on the child's eating.

Lack of fiber in the diet or poor bowel habits that lead to chronic constipation can result in poor appetite, diminished intake, and FTT. Adding legumes and fruits (especially dried fruits), vegetables, high-fiber breakfast cereals, bran muffins, or all of these to the diet can help relieve constipation, improve appetite, and eventually promote weight gain. Because the fiber intake of children is often low, especially in children who are picky eaters, fiber intake should always be addressed in the evaluation (see Chapter 27). If the child is also of short stature, the possibility of a zinc deficiency should be investigated (see Chapter 3).

Iron Deficiency

Iron deficiency is one of the most common nutrient disorders of childhood, affecting approximately 9% of toddlers (Looker et al., 1997). The highest prevalence of anemia in children who participate in various federally funded programs occurs in those younger than 2 years of age (Polhamus et al., 2004). Iron deficiency is less of a problem among older preschool and school-age children. Certain low-income populations and other groups such as Native Alaskans have an increased incidence of iron deficiency, even in older children (Looker et al., 1997). Possible factors associated with iron deficiency, with or without anemia, include parents' educational level and access to medical care, as well as dietary intake.

Infants with iron deficiency, with or without anemia, tend to score lower on standardized tests of mental development and pay less attention to relevant information needed for problem solving. Lozoff reevaluated 11- to 14-year-old children who had been treated for iron deficiency anemia in infancy. In addition to poor performance on developmental tests when they were 5 years old, the children continued to score lower on measures of mental and motor functioning when they were older (Lozoff et al., 2000). Another report assessed the academic performance of children 6 to 16 years of age who had iron deficiency (some with and some without anemia), and the children had lower scores on standardized academic tests (Halterman et al., 2001). These data should be considered during assessments of the nutrient quality of individual diets and in policy-making decisions intended to address the nutritional needs of low-income, high-risk children.

In addition to growth and the increased physiologic need for iron, dietary factors also play a role. For example, a 1-year-old child who continues to consume a large quantity of milk and excludes other foods may develop milk anemia. Many young preschool children do not like meat, so most of their iron is consumed in the nonheme form from fortified cereals, which is absorbed less efficiently. To enhance absorbability of nonheme iron sources, parents should be taught to increase the amount of ascorbic acid and meat, fish, and poultry in their children's diets. (See Chapter 31 for a more detailed discussion of anemia.)

Dental Caries

Nutrition and eating habits are important factors affecting dental health. An optimal nutrient intake is needed to produce strong teeth and healthy gums. The composition of the diet and an individual's eating habits (e.g., dietary carbohydrate intake, retentiveness of foods, eating frequency) are significant factors in the development of dental caries. Infants and young children who drink sweetened liquids from a bottle at bedtime or frequently throughout the day are susceptible to early childhood caries (ECC) (see Chapter 25). Dietary guidelines, including intake of two or more servings of milk products daily and limiting intake of 100% juice to four to six ounces daily with limited use of other sugared beverages to occasional use, will support lowered incidence of caries in young children (Marshall et al., 2003).

Because children tend to consume snacks regularly, those that are least cariogenic (i.e., least likely to cause caries) should be emphasized. When protein foods such as cheese, nuts, and meats are eaten with more fermentable, sticky foods, they prevent the decrease in the plaque pH that usually accompanies ingestion of these foods and may help protect the teeth against caries. For older school-age children, chewing sugarless gum after cariogenic snacks may be beneficial because it raises the salivary pH. Desserts and sweet foods should be consumed infrequently and incorporated into meals to reduce their cariogenicity. Parents are strong role models for their children and should have positive food habits and practice good dental hygiene. A toothbrush should be introduced to toddlers, and a daily oral hygiene routine developed. Because fluoride is highly effective in caries prevention, it should be supplied to children via a fluoridated water supply or a fluoride supplement (see Chapters 3 and 25).

Allergies

Food allergies usually develop during infancy and childhood and are more likely when a child has a family history of allergies. Allergic responses most often are respiratory or gastrointestinal symptoms or involve the skin, but others may include fatigue, lethargy, and behavior changes. Controversy exists over the definition of food allergy, food intolerance, and food sensitivity, and some tests for food allergies are unspecific and unequivocal (see Chapter 29).

Attention Deficit Hyperactivity Disorder

Attention deficit hyperactivity disorder (ADHD) is a clinical diagnosis based on specific criteria—excessive motor activity, impulsiveness, a short attention span, a low tolerance for frustration, and an onset before 7 years of age. Various dietary factors have been suggested as a cause of this disorder, including artificial flavors and colors, sugar, altered fatty acid metabolism, and allergies. Over the years, dietary treatments have been promoted such as the Feingold diet, the omission of sugar, allergy elimination diets, and supplements of vitamins and essential fatty acids. Little evidence exists to support these dietary interventions (see Chapter 45).

Autism Spectrum Disorders

Autism spectrum disorders (ASDs) affect 1 in 166 children and are diagnosed by impairments in three behavioral categories: social interactions, verbal and nonverbal communication, and restricted or repetitive behaviors. These impairments affect the children's nutrient intake and eating behaviors by acceptance of only specific foods, refusal of new or unfamiliar foods, increased hypersensitivities (e.g., to texture, temperature, color, and smell), and difficulty in making transitions. Children with an ASD usually refuse fruits and vegetables and may only eat a few foods from the other food groups. Although most children have normal growth parameters, their restricted diets make them at risk for marginal or inadequate nutrient intake. They are often very resistant to taking a vitamin-mineral supplement, even though they could benefit from one.

Popular nutrition interventions for ASDs include elimination diets (e.g., gluten-free/casein-free, allergy), essential fatty acid supplements, large doses of vitamins, and other alternative therapies. Despite anecdotal reports of benefits, few well-designed controlled studies have been done to test the effectiveness of these interventions, and currently there is no strong evidence of benefits (Nye and Brice, 2005; Milward et al., 2004). Behavioral nutrition interventions may increase the types of food accepted at home and school (Lucas et al., 2002). If families want to try alternative dietary therapies, nutrition professionals can help them make sure the child's diet is adequate and any supplements are safe (see Chapter 45 for further discussion of ASD, Chapter 27 for a gluten-free diet, and Chapter 29 for a casein-free diet).

PREVENTING CHRONIC DISEASE

The roots of chronic adult diseases such as heart disease, cancer, diabetes, and obesity are often based in childhood—a phenomenon that is particularly relevant to the increasing rate of obesity-related diseases such as type II diabetes, resulting from pediatric and adult obesity. To help decrease the prevalence of chronic conditions in Americans, governmental and nonprofit agencies have been promoting healthy eating habits. Their recommendations include the Dietary Guidelines for Americans, the USDA MyPyramid, the National Cholesterol Education Program (NCEP), and the National Cancer Institute Dietary Guidelines (see Chapter 12).

Dietary Fat and Cardiovascular Health

Compared with their counterparts in many other countries, American children and adolescents have higher blood cholesterol levels and higher intakes of saturated fatty acids and cholesterol. Autopsy studies demonstrate that early coronary atherosclerosis begins in childhood and adolescence and is related to high serum total cholesterol levels, low-density lipoprotein (LDL) cholesterol and very low–density lipoprotein (VLDL) cholesterol levels, and low high-density lipoprotein (HDL) levels (AAP, 2004).

The NCEP recommendations for prevention of cardiovascular disease in children older than 2 years of age are the same as those for adults: (1) no more than 30% of calories from fat (10% or less from saturated fat, up to 10% from unsaturated fat, and 10% to 15% from monounsaturated fat); and (2) no more than 300 mg of cholesterol per day. Cholesterol screening is also recommended for children with family risk factors—parents or grandparents who have had a cardiac event (heart attack, angina, or cardiac surgery) before the age of 55 years or at least one parent with a cholesterol level of 250 mg/dl or more (AAP, 2004) (see Chapter 32).

The AAP advises that children older than 2 years of age gradually adopt a lower-fat diet so that by age 5 their diet contains no more than 30% of calories from fat. Dietary trends have demonstrated a decrease in total fat, saturated fat, and percentage of calories from fat in children's diets; but at the same time overweight has increased with increased risk of cardiovascular disease (Gidding et al., 2005). A consensus statement from the American Heart Association and endorsed by the AAP provides recommendations including (1) a diet low in saturated fat and *trans*-fatty acids; increased fish intake, whole grains, vegetables and fruits; limited juice and sweetened beverages; (2) 60 minutes of moderate-to-vigorous activity daily, and (3) no more than 35% of calories from fat (Gidding, 2005). Reports have shown that from the age of 4 years to adolescence, children can consume diets that comply with the NCEP guidelines without compromising energy or nutrient intake (Gidding, 2005; Obarzanek et al., 2001). A long-term dietary intervention study demonstrated improved lipid levels and improved eating habits in children with elevated LDL cholesterol levels (Obarzanek et al., 2001; Van Horn et al., 2005). Some critics warn of the risks from broad implementation of low-fat diets for children (Olson, 2000). Although no apparent risks to growth or nutrient intake are associated with a diet meeting the guidelines, health practitioners should assess each child individually regarding total fat intake and excessive consumption of low-fat and nonfat foods (especially by preschool children) (see Chapter 32).

Calcium and Bone Health and Obesity

Osteoporosis prevention begins early by maximizing calcium retention and bone density during childhood and adolescence, when bones are growing rapidly and are most sensitive to environmental influences such as diet and physical activity (Leonard and Zemel, 2002) (see Chapter 24). Regardless, many pediatricians are not sharing information about the prevention of osteoporosis with their patients (Fleming and Patrick, 2002).

Studies suggest that to reach the maximum calcium balance during puberty children may need to consume more than the recommended amount (Abrams et al., 2004). However, mean dietary intakes of calcium are lower than the AI, with 20% to 30% of pubertal girls having intakes less than 500 mg per day (Ervin et al., 2004) (see Figure 3-28). Although calcium supplementation coupled with an average calcium dietary intake in pubertal

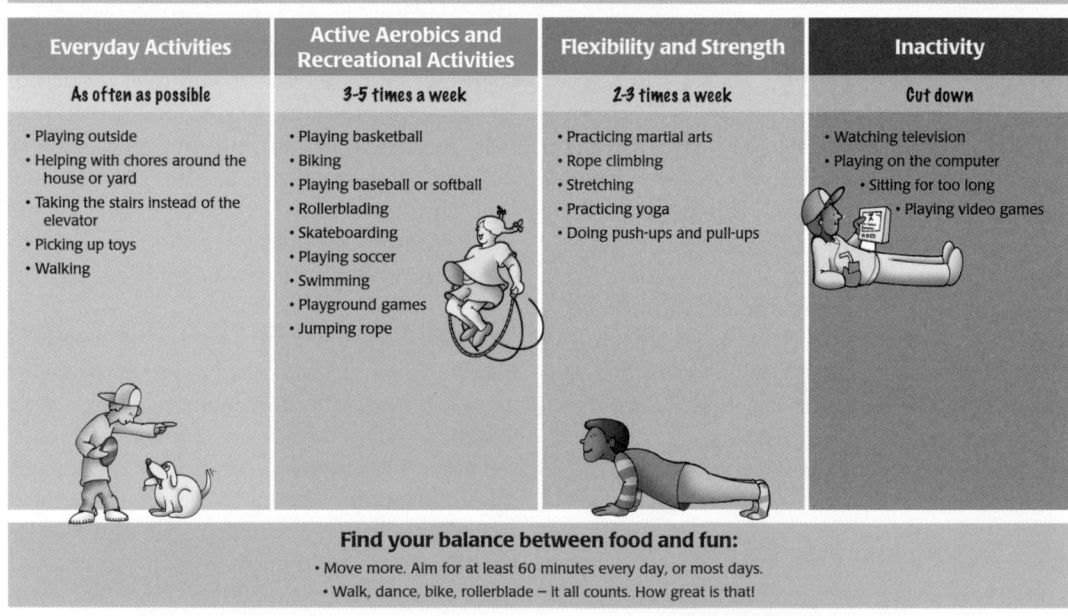

FIGURE 7-5 MyActivity Pyramid. *(This publication is adapted from USDA's MyPyramid and was funded in part by USDA's Food Stamp Program. Issued in furtherance of Cooperative Extension Work Acts of May 8 and June 30, 1914, in cooperation with the United States Department of Agriculture. L. Jo Turner, Interim Director, Cooperative Extension, University of Missouri, Columbia, Mo, July, 2006.)*

children has been shown to increase bone mineral density significantly, it is less certain whether this benefit is long term (Matkovic et al., 2005; Ervin et al., 2005). One longitudinal study of white children from infancy to 8 years of age found that bone mineral content was positively correlated with intake of protein and several minerals, suggesting that many nutrients are related to bone health in children (Bounds et al., 2005) (see Chapter 24).

Data from trials in which calcium intake was the independent variable reveal the consistent effects of higher calcium intakes on lower body fat, body weight, or both, and less weight gain during midlife (Heaney et al., 2002). Each 300-mg increase in regular calcium intake has been associated with approximately 1 kg less body fat in children and 2.5 to 3 kg lower body weight in adults. Increasing calcium intake by the equivalent of two dairy servings per day could reduce the risk of overweight substantially, perhaps by as much as 70% (Heaney et al., 2002).

Because food consumption surveys show that children are drinking more soft drinks and noncitrus juices and less milk, education is needed to encourage young people to consume an appropriate amount of calcium from food sources. Different types of reinforcement for better calcium intake are needed according to cultural and gender differences (Lytle et al., 2002).

Fiber

Education about dietary fiber and disease prevention has mainly been focused on adults, and only limited information is available on the dietary fiber intake of children. Dietary fiber is needed for health and normal laxation in children. National survey data indicate that preschool children consume a mean of 10.7 g of dietary fiber per day; school-age children consume approximately 13 g/day (USDA, 1997). This is lower than the DRI for children, which is based on the same 14 g/1000 kcal as adults (because of lack of scientific evidence for the pediatric population) (IOM, 2002). Generally, higher fiber intakes are associated with more nutrient-dense diets in young children (Kranz et al., 2005b). Education is needed to help increase fiber intake by children.

Physical Activity

A decreased level of physical activity in children has been noted for several decades, and it is thought to be a substantial contributor to obesity in children. Participation in school physical education programs has declined over time and generally decreases with increasing age (ADA, 2004). Regular physical activity not only helps control excess weight gain but also improves strength and endurance, enhances self-esteem, and reduces anxiety and stress. Activity, combined with an optimal calcium intake, is associated with increased bone mineral density in children and adolescents. Several national groups, including the IOM, have recommended that children be active for at least a total of 60 minutes a day, with activity including moderate to vigorous activities (IOM, 2002; IOM, 2004b). The CDC has developed guidelines for school and community programs to promote lifelong physical activity among young people (CDC, 1997b).

In an effort to promote dietary habits that can reduce the incidence of chronic diseases later in life, the Dietary Guidelines for Americans and the MyPyramid have been applied to children and their parents. There are also physical activity pyramids based on the new pyramid framework (ages 6 to 11). The Kid's MyActivity Pyramid promotes substituting sedentary activities for more physically active choices (Figure 7-5).

⬡ FOCAL POINTS

- Children's diets should provide enough energy to support optimal growth and development without causing excessive weight gain.
- For children's diets emphasis should be placed on fruits and vegetables, whole-grain products, low-fat dairy products, legumes, and lean meat, fish, and poultry.
- Fermentable carbohydrate intake should be controlled for good dental health.
- Adherence to general food guidelines is beneficial for children because their total fat intake decreases and their food fiber and micronutrient intake increases, resulting in a more nutrient-dense diet.

- Physical changes in the years between infancy and adolescence happen at a slower and steadier pace, and the cognitive, physical, and socio-emotional growth is significant.
- Nutrition education and resources for families and children can help establish healthy, positive eating and activity patterns that carry through during adolescence and adulthood.

✦ CLINICAL SCENARIO 1

Brian is a 7-year, 4-month-old boy who gained 15 lb during the past school year. His height is 50½, inches and his weight is 70 pounds. An evaluation revealed that Brian moved to a new home and began a new school a year ago after his parents' divorce. After-school care has been provided by an older neighbor, who loves to bake for Brian. Because he has no friends in the neighborhood, his main leisure activities have been watching television and playing video games. His mother reports that they have been relying more on take-out and fast-food meals because of the time constraints of her full-time job, and she has gained weight herself. However, she has recently started an aerobics class with a friend and is interested in developing healthier eating habits.

After joint sessions with Brian and his mother, the following goals were identified by the family: (1) explore after-school care at the local community center, which has sports activities; (2) alter shopping and food preparation to emphasize the MyPyramid and low-fat choices; (3) begin weekend swimming or bicycling for the family; and (4) limit television and video games to no more than 2 hours daily.

It is 4 months later, and most of the changes have been made, except for participating in the weekend family activity and watching less television on the weekends. However, Brian is now playing soccer, has lost 4 pounds, and has grown taller. He is 51 inches tall and weighs 66 pounds.

✳Nutrition Diagnosis 1: Physical inactivity related to lack of knowledge of after-school activities as evidenced by decreased activity after school.

✳Nutrition Diagnosis 2: Undesirable food choices related to lack of time to cook as evidenced by fast-food and take out meals several times a week

1. What recommendations should be made to prevent Brian and his mother from resuming their old habits?
2. Calculate and plot Brian's BMI over time. Discuss the changes.
3. What other activities can Brian try to help him avoid or reduce the tendency to overeat?
4. What would you suggest to promote a positive feeding relationship between Brian and his mother, considering his age and level of development?
5. How can Brian's mother alter some of his favorite recipes to lower the fat content? For example, his favorite meal is fried chicken with gravy, mashed potatoes, and ice cream.

USEFUL WEBSITES

Bright Futures in Practice: Nutrition
www.brightfutures.org/nutrition/

Eat Well, Play Hard
http://counties.cce.cornell.edu/erie/ewph.html

Growth Charts
www.cdc.gov/growthcharts/

Guidelines for Physical Activity
www.cdc.gov/nccdphp/dash/guidelines/physact.htm

MyPyramid Food Guidance System
www.MyPyramid.gov

National Center for Education in Maternal and Child Health
www.ncemch.org
http://www.mchlibrary.info/KnowledgePaths/kp_childnutr.html

Nutrition and Physical Activity
www.cdc.gov/nccdphp/dnpa/

Pediatric Nutrition Practice Group
www.pediatricnutrition.org/

References

Abrams SA et al: Calcium absorption is related to growth during puberty, *Pediatr Res* 55:181A, 2004.

Action for Health Kids: Parents' Views on School Wellness Practices, September 2005, www.actionforhealthykids.org, accessed November 20, 2005.

American Academy of Pediatrics, Committee on Nutrition: The use and misuse of fruit juice in pediatrics, *Pediatrics* 107:1210, 2001.

American Academy of Pediatrics, Committee on Nutrition: Prevention of pediatric overweight and obesity, *Pediatrics* 112:424, 2003.

American Academy of Pediatrics: *Pediatric nutrition handbook*, ed 5, Elk Grove Village, Ill, 2004, AAP.

American Dietetic Association: Position of the American Dietetic Association: Local support for nutrition integrity in schools, *J Am Diet Assoc* 100:108, 2000.

American Dietetic Association: Position of the American Dietetic Association: Child and adolescent food and nutrition programs, *J Am Diet Assoc* 103:887, 2003a.

American Dietetic Association: Position of the American Dietetic Association, Society for Nutrition Education, and American School Food Service Association-Nutrition Services: an essential component of comprehensive school health programs, *J Am Diet Assoc* 103:505, 2003b.

American Dietetic Association: Position of the American Dietetic Association: Dietary guidance for healthy children aged 2 to 11 years, *J Am Diet Assoc* 104:660, 2004.

American Dietetic Association: Position of the American Dietetic Association: Benchmarks for nutrition programs in child care settings, *J Am Diet Assoc* 105:979, 2005.

Ballew C, Bowman B: Recommending calcium to reduce lead toxicity in children: a critical review, *Nutr Rev* 59:71, 2001.

Balluz LS et al: Vitamin and mineral supplement use in the United States, Results from the Third National and Nutrition and Examination Survey, *Arch Fam Med* 9:258, 2000.

Barlow SE, Dietz WH: Obesity evaluation and treatment: expert committee recommendations, *Pediatrics* 102(3):e29, 1998.

Barlow SE et al: Treatment of child and adolescent obesity: reports from pediatricians, pediatric nurse practitioners, and registered dietitians, *Pediatrics* 110:229 (1, part 2), 2002.

Basiotis PP et al: *The Healthy Eating Index: 1999-2000*, 2002, U.S. Department of Agriculture, Center for Nutrition Policy and Promotion. CNPP-12.

Beal VA: Nutritional intake. In McCammon RW, editor: *Human growth and development*, Springfield, Ill, 1970, Charles C Thomas.

Bergman E et al: Time spent by school children to eat lunch, *J Am Diet Assoc* 100:696, 2000.

Berhane R, Dietz WH: Clinical assessment of growth. In Kessler DB, Dawson P, editors: *Failure to thrive and pediatric undernutrition*, Baltimore, 1999, Brookes Publishing.

Bernard SM, McGeehin MA: Prevalence of blood lead levels > or = 5 micro g/dl among U.S. children 1 to 5 years of age and socioeconomic and demographic factors associated with blood of lead levels 5 to 10 micro g/dl, Third National Health and Nutrition Examination Survey, 1988-1994, *Pediatrics* 112:1308, 2003.

Block RW, Krebs NF, American Academy of Pediatrics, Committee on Child Abuse and Neglect, Committee on Nutrition: Failure to thrive as a manifestation of child neglect, *Pediatrics* 116:1234, 2005.

Borzekowski DLG, Robinson TN: The 30-second effect: an experiment revealing the impact of television commercials on food preferences of preschoolers, *J Am Diet Assoc* 101:42, 2001.

Bounds W et al: The relationship of dietary and lifestyle factors to bone mineral indexes in children, *J Am Diet Assoc* 105:735, 2005.

Brady LM et al: Comparison of children's dietary intake patterns with U.S. dietary guideline, *Br J Nutr* 84:361, 2000.

Brotanek JM et al: Iron deficiency, prolonged bottle-feeding, and racial/ethnic disparities in young children, *Arch Pediatr Adolesc* 159:1038, 2005.

Buergel NS et al: Students consuming sack lunches devote more time to eating than those consuming school lunches, *J Am Diet Assoc* 102:1283, 2002.

Casey PH et al: Children in food-insufficient, low-income families: prevalence, health, and nutrition status, *Arch Pediatr Adolesc* 155:508, 2001.

Centers for Disease Control and Prevention: *Screening young children for lead poisoning: guidance for state and local public health officials*, 1997a, U.S. Department of Health and Human Services, Public Health Service.

Centers for Disease Control and Prevention, National Center for Chronic Disease Prevention and Health Promotion: *Guidelines for school and community programs to promote lifelong physical activity among young people*, 1997b, http://www.cdc.gov/nccdphp/dash/guidelines/physact.htm, accessed December 1, 2006.

Centers for Disease Control and Prevention: Blood lead levels—United States, 1999-2002, *MMWR Morb Mortal Wkly Rep* 54:513, 2005.

Cunningham KF, McLaughlin M: Nutrition. In Kessler DB, Dawson P, editors: *Failure to thrive and pediatric undernutrition*, Baltimore, 1999, Brookes Publishing.

Daniels SR et al: The utility of body mass index as a measure of body fatness in children and adolescents: differences by race and gender, *Pediatrics* 99:804, 1997.

DeNavas-Walt C et al: *U.S. Census Bureau, Current Population Reports, P60-229, Income, Poverty, and Health Insurance Coverage in the United States: 2004*, U.S. Government Printing Office, Washington, DC, 2005, http:www.census.gov/, accessed October 4, 2005.

Dietz WH, Gortmaker SL: Preventing obesity in children and adolescents, *Annu Rev Public Health* 22:337, 2001.

Epstein LH et al: Behavioral therapy in the treatment of pediatric obesity, *Pediatr Clin North Am* 48:981, 2001.

Ervin RB et al: Dietary intake of selected minerals for the United States population: 1999-2000, *Adv Data* 27:1, 2004.

Fleming R, Patrick K: Osteoporosis prevention: pediatricians' knowledge, attitudes, and counseling practices, *Prev Med* 34:411, 2002.

Food Research and Action Center: *Hunger and food insecurity in the United States*, http://www.frac.org/html/hunger_in_the_us/hunger_index.html, accessed December 12, 2005.

Freedman DS et al: Relationship of childhood obesity to coronary heart disease risk factors in adulthood: the Bogalusa Heart Study, *Pediatrics* 108:712, 2001.

French SA et al: Environmental influences on eating and physical activity, *Annu Rev Public Health* 22:309, 2001.

Getlinger MJ et al: Food waste is reduced when elementary-school children have recess before lunch, *J Am Diet Assoc* 96:906, 1996.

Gidding SS et al: Dietary recommendations for children and adolescents: a guide for practitioners: consensus statement from the American Heart Association, *Circulation* 112:2061, 2005.

Gillman MW et al: Family dinner and diet quality among older children and adolescents, *Arch Fam Med* 9:235, 2000.

Goran MI: Metabolic precursors and effects of obesity in children: a decade of progress, 1990-1999, *Am J Clin Nutr* 73:158, 2001.

Gross SM and Cinelli B: Coordinated school health program and dietetics professionals: partners in promoting healthful eating, *J Am Diet Assoc* 104:793, 2004.

Halterman JS et al: Iron deficiency and cognitive achievement among school-aged children and adolescents in the United States, *Pediatrics* 107:1381, 2001.

Harris AB: Evidence of increasing dietary supplement use in children with special health care needs: strategies for improving parent and professional communication, *J Am Diet Assoc* 105:34, 2005.

Harrison K, Marske A: Nutritional content of foods advertised during the television programs children watch most, *Am J Public Health* 95:1568, 2005.

Hawkes C: *Marketing food to children: the global regulatory environment*, Geneva, Switzerland, 2004, World Health Organization.

Heaney RP et al: Calcium and weight: clinical studies, *J Am Coll Nutr* 21(2):152S, 2002.

Horsley JW: Community Services and Programs. In: Lucas B, Feucht S, Grieger L, editors: *Children with special health care needs: nutrition care handbook*, Chicago, Ill, 2004, American Dietetic Association.

Institute of Medicine, Food and Nutrition Board: Committee on Prevention of Obesity in Children and Youth, Koplan JP, Liverman CT, Kraak VA, editors: *Preventing childhood obesity: health in the balance*, Washington, DC, 2004b, National Academies Press.

Institute of Medicine, Food and Nutrition Board: *Dietary reference intakes for calcium, phosphorus, magnesium, vitamin D, and fluoride*, Washington, DC, 1997, National Academies Press.

Institute of Medicine, Food and Nutrition Board: *Dietary reference intakes for thiamin, riboflavin, niacin, vitamin B6, folate, vitamin B12, pantothenic acid, biotin, and choline*, Washington, DC, 1998, National Academies Press.

Institute of Medicine, Food and Nutrition Board: *Dietary reference intakes for dietary antioxidants and related compounds*, Washington, DC, 2000, National Academies Press.

Institute of Medicine, Food and Nutrition Board: *Dietary reference intakes for vitamin A, vitamin K, arsenic, boron, chromium, copper, iodine, iron, manganese, molybdenum, nickel, silicon, vanadium, and zinc. dietary antioxidants and related compounds*, Washington, DC, 2001, National Academies Press.

Institute of Medicine, Food and Nutrition Board: *Dietary reference intakes for energy, carbohydrates, fiber, fat, fatty acids, cholesterol, protein, and amino acids, (macronutrients)*, Washington, DC, 2002, National Academies Press.

Institute of Medicine, Food and Nutrition Board: *Dietary reference intakes for water, potassium, sodium, chloride, and sulfate*, Washington, DC, 2004a, National Academies Press.

Jyoti DF et al: Food insecurity affects school children's academic performance, weight gain, and social skills, *J Nutr* 135:2831, 2005.

Kirk S et al: Pediatric obesity epidemic: treatment options, *J Am Diet Assoc* 105:S44, 2005.

Kleinman RE et al: Hunger in children in the United States: potential behavioral and emotional correlates, *Pediatrics* 101(1): e3, 1998.

Kordas K et al: Blood level, anemia, and short stature are independently associated with cognitive performance in Mexican school children, *J Nutr* 134:363, 2004.

Kranz S et al: Adverse effect of high added sugar consumption on dietary intake in American preschoolers, *J Pediatr* 146:105, 2005a.

Kranz S et al: Dietary fiber intake by American preschoolers is associated with more nutrient-dense diets, *J Am Diet Assoc* 105:221, 2005b.

Leonard MB, Zemel BS: Current concepts in pediatric bone disease, *Pediatr Clin North Am* 49:143, 2002.

Looker AC et al: Prevalence of iron deficiency in the United States, *JAMA* 277:973, 1997.

Lozoff B et al: Poorer behavioral and developmental outcome more than 10 years after treatment for iron deficiency in infancy, *Pediatrics* 105(4):e51, 2000.

Lucas B et al: Nutrition concerns of children with autism spectrum disorders, *Nutr Focus* 17(1):1, 2002.

Lytle LA et al: Nutrient intake over time in a multi-ethnic sample of youth, *Public Health Nutr* 5:319, 2002.

Mahoney CR et al: Effect of breakfast composition on cognitive processes in elementary school children, *Physiol Behav* 85:635, 2005.

Marshall TA et al: Dental caries and beverage consumption in young children, *Pediatrics* 112:184, 2003.

Matkovic V et al: Calcium supplementation and bone mineral density in females from childhood to young adulthood: a randomized controlled trial, *Am J Clin Nutr* 81:175, 2005.

Milward C et al: Gluten- and casein-free diets for autism spectrum disorder. *Cochrane Database Syst Rev* 2004, Issue 2, Art. No.: CD003498. DOI: 10.1002/14651858.CD003498. pub2.

Moshfegh A et al: *What we eat in America, NHANES 2001-2002: usual nutrient intakes from food compared to dietary reference intakes*, Washington, DC, 2005, U.S. Department of Agriculture, Agricultural Research Service, http://www.ars. usda.gov/SP2UserFiles/Place/12355000/pdf/ usualintaketables2001-02.pdf, accessed December 7, 2005.

Narayan KM et al: Lifetime risk for diabetes mellitus in the United States, *JAMA* 290:1884, 2003.

Neault N et al: *The real cost of a healthy diet; healthful foods are out of reach for low-income families in Boston, Massachusetts*, Boston, Ma, 2005, Boston Medical Center Department of Pediatrics, http://dcc2.bumc.bu.edu/scnappublic/HealthyDiet_Aug2005. pdf, accessed November 12, 2005.

Nord M et al: *Household food security in the United States*, USDA Economic Research Report No. ERR11, October 2005, http:// www.ers.usda.gov/publications/err11/, accessed November 21, 2005.

Nye C, Brice A: Combined vitamin B6-magnesium treatment in autism spectrum disorder. *Cochrane Database Syst Rev* 2005, Issue 4. Art. No.: CD003497, DOI: 10.1002/14651858. CD003497.pub2.

Obarzanek E et al: Long-term safety and efficacy of a cholesterol-lowering diet in children with elevated low-density lipoprotein cholesterol: seven-year results of the Dietary Intervention Study in Children (DISC), *Pediatrics* 107:256, 2001.

Ogden CL, et al: Prevalence of overweight and obesity in the United States, 1999-2004, *JAMA* 295:1549, 2006.

Olson RE: Is it wise to restrict fat in the diets of children? *J Am Diet Assoc* 100:28, 2000.

Palmer CA: Dental caries and obesity in children: different problems, related causes, *Quintessence Int* 36:457, 2005.

Polhamus B et al: *Pediatric nutrition surveillance 2003 report*, Atlanta, Ga, 2004, U.S. Health and Human Services, Centers for Disease Control and Prevention.

Pollitt E et al: Fasting and cognition in well- and undernourished school children: a review of three experimental studies, *Am J Clin Nutr* 67(suppl):779, 1998.

Powell CA et al: Nutrition and education: a randomized trial of the effects of breakfast in rural primary school children, *Am J Clin Nutr* 68:873, 1998.

Rampersaud GC et al: Breakfast habits, nutritional status, body weight, and academic performance in children and adolescents, *J Am Diet Assoc* 105:743, 2005.

Rickard KA et al: The play approach to learning in the context of families and schools: an alternative paradigm for nutrition and fitness education in the 21st century, *J Am Diet Assoc* 95:1121, 1995.

Ritchie LD et al: Family environment and pediatric overweight: What is a parent to do? *J Am Diet Assoc* 105:S70, 2005.

Rivera JA et al: The effect of micronutrient deficiencies on child growth: a review of results from community-based supplementation trials, *J Nutr* 133:4010S, 2003.

Roberts SB, Heyman, MB: Micronutrient shortfalls in young children's diets common and owing to inadequate intakes both at home and at child care centers, *Nutr Rev* 58:27, 2000.

Satter E: *Child of Mine—Feeding with love and good sense*, revised, Palo Alto, Calif, 2000, Bull Publishing Co.

Satter E: *Your child's weight: helping without harming*, Madison, Wisc, 2005, Kelcy Press.

Sebastian R et al: Changes over 25 years in the dietary intakes of children 6-19 years (abstract), *Fed Am Soc Exp Biol Jl* 19(4):A87, 2005.

Skalicky A et al: Child food security and iron deficiency anemia in low-income infants and toddlers in the United States, *Matern Child Health* J Nov 19:1-9 [Epub ahead of print], 2005.

Story M et al, editors: *Bright futures in practice: nutrition*, Arlington, Va, 2000, National Center for Education in Maternal and Child Health.

Suitor CW, Gleason PM: Using dietary reference intake–based methods to estimate the prevalence of inadequate nutrient intake among school-aged children, *J Am Diet Assoc*102:530, 2002.

Troiano RP et al: Energy and fat intakes of children and adolescents in the United States: data from the national health and nutrition examination surveys, *Am J Clin Nutr* 72:1343S, 2000.

U.S. Department of Agriculture, Agricultural Research Service Food Surveys Research Group: 1997 data tables: results from USDA's 1994-96 Continuing Survey of Food Intakes by Individuals and 1994-96 Diet and Health Knowledge Survey, http://www.barc.usda.gov/bhnrc/foodsurvey/home.html, accessed December 1, 2006.

U.S. Department of Agriculture: School Nutrition Dietary Assessment Study—II: Summary of findings, Washington, DC, 2001, USDA.

Van Horn L et al: Children's adaptations to a fat-reduced diet: the intervention study in children (DISC), *Pediatrics* 115:1723, 2005.

Villamor E et al: Vitamin A supplements ameliorate the adverse effect of HIV-1, malaria, and diarrhea/infections on child growth, *Pediatrics* 109:E6, 2002.

Weinreb L et al: Hunger: its impact on children's health and mental health, *Pediatrics* 110:E41, 2002.

Whitaker RC et al: Early adiposity rebound and the risk of adult obesity, *Pediatrics* 101(3):e5, 1998.

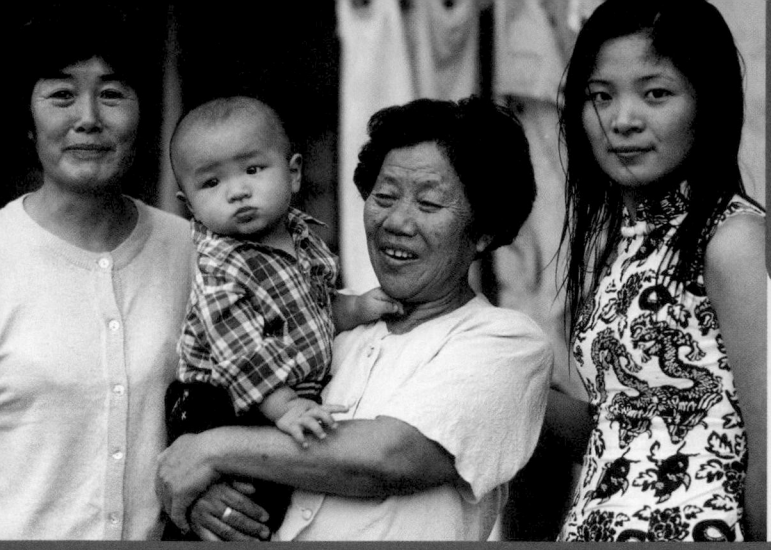

CHAPTER 8

Jamie Stang, PhD, MPH, RD

Nutrition in Adolescence

KEY TERMS

adolescence the period of life beginning with the appearance of secondary sex characteristics and ending with the cessation of somatic growth, often considered to occur between the ages of 12 and 18 or 12 and 21 years old

body image mental self-concept related to growth rate, changes in body proportions, and perception of personal body size in comparison to peers or popular media images

disordered eating abnormal behaviors related to food and eating; may include starving, bingeing, vomiting, laxative abuse, or excessive exercise accompanied by unrealistic ideas about food, a distorted body image, and psychological and developmental abnormalities

growth spurt the 18- to 24-month period of adolescence when the growth rate is the fastest

gynecologic age the number of years between the onset of menses and the current chronologic age

menarche onset of menses

peak height gain velocity the fastest rate of growth during the growth spurt

physiologic anemia of growth a low serum hematocrit or hemoglobin level that is not accompanied by decreased iron stores and is caused by rapid growth and a significant increase in lean body mass; often develops in adolescents

puberty the period during which the secondary sex characteristics begin to develop and a person becomes capable of sexual reproduction

sexual maturity rating (SMR) used to assess a person's stage of sexual development; usually expressed as sexual maturation stage or Tanner stage

Adolescence is one of the most exciting yet challenging periods in human development. Generally thought of as the period of life that occurs between 12 and 21 years of age, adolescence is a period of tremendous physiologic, psychological and cognitive transformation during which a child becomes a young adult. The gradual growth pattern that characterizes early childhood changes to one of rapid growth and development, affecting both physical and psychosocial aspects of health. Changes in cognitive and emotional functioning allow teens to become more independent as they mature. Peer influence and acceptance may become more important than family values, creating periods of conflict between teens and parents. Because all of these changes have a direct impact on the nutrient needs and dietary behaviors of adolescents, it is important that health care providers develop a full understanding of how these developmental changes of adolescence can affect nutritional status.

GROWTH AND DEVELOPMENT

Physiologic Changes

Puberty is the period of rapid growth and development during which a child physically develops into an adult and becomes capable of sexual reproduction. It is initiated by the increased production of reproductive hormones such as estrogen, progesterone, and testosterone and is characterized by the outward appearance of secondary sexual characteris-

---

Sections of this chapter were written by Bonnie A. Spear, PhD, RD, for the previous edition of this text.

TABLE 8-1

Ratings of Sexual Maturation*

	Pubic Hair	Genitalia	Corresponding Changes
Boys			
Stage 1	None	Prepubertal	
Stage 2	Small amount at outer edges of pubis, slight darkening	Beginning penile enlargement Testes enlarged to 5-ml volume Scrotum reddened and changed in texture	Increased sweat gland activity
Stage 3	Covers pubis	Penis longer Testes enlarged to 8-10 ml Scrotum enlarged	Voice changes Faint mustache/facial hair Axillary hair Beginning of peak height gain velocity (growth spurt of 6-8 inches)
Stage 4	Adult type, does not extend to thighs	Penis wider and longer Testes enlarged to 12 ml Scrotal skin darker	End of peak height gain velocity Voice deeper Possibly severe acne More facial hair Darker hair on legs
Stage 5	Adult type, spreads to thighs	Adult penis Testes enlarged to 15 ml	Significantly increased muscle mass
Girls			
Stage 1	None	No change from childhood	
Stage 2	Small amount, downy, on medial labia	Breast buds	Increased sweat gland activity Beginning of peak height gain velocity (growth spurt of 3-5 inches)
Stage 3	Increased, darker, curly	Larger, but no separation of the nipple and the areola	End of peak height gain velocity Beginning of acne Axillary hair
Stage 4	More abundant, coarse texture	Larger Areola and nipple form secondary mound	Possibly severe acne Menarche begins
Stage 5	Adult, spreads to medial thighs	Adult distribution of breast tissue, continuous outline	Increased fat and muscle mass

Modified from Tanner JM: *Growth at adolescence*, ed 2, Oxford, 1962, Blackwell Scientific Publications.

*See Appendixes 17 and 18.

tics such as breast development in females and the appearance of facial hair in males (Table 8-1).

Sexual maturity rating (SMR), also known as Tanner stage, is used to clinically assess the degree of sexual maturation during puberty. Among males SMR is based on genital and pubic hair development (Appendix 18). Among females SMR is assessed by breast and pubic hair development (Appendix 17). SMR is measured through a series of five stages, with stage 1 marking prepubertal development and stage 5 marking the completion of physical growth and development. The five stages of SMR correlate highly with other markers of growth and development during puberty such as alterations in height, weight, body composition, and endocrine functioning. A thorough understanding of the rela-

tionship between physical growth and development and SMR enables health care professionals to assess an adolescent's potential for future growth (Figure 8-1).

In general, females enter puberty earlier than males. **Menarche,** which is the onset of menses or menstruation, is often considered the hallmark of puberty among females, yet it occurs relatively late in puberty. Menarche occurs at 12.4 years in the average female; however, the onset of menses can occur anywhere between the ages of 9 and 17 years (Herman-Giddens et al., 1997; Tanner, 1962). Research suggests that there may be differences in the initiation and duration of puberty among females of different racial backgrounds. In a study of black and white females, 48% of black girls had entered SMR stage 2 by age 8 years,

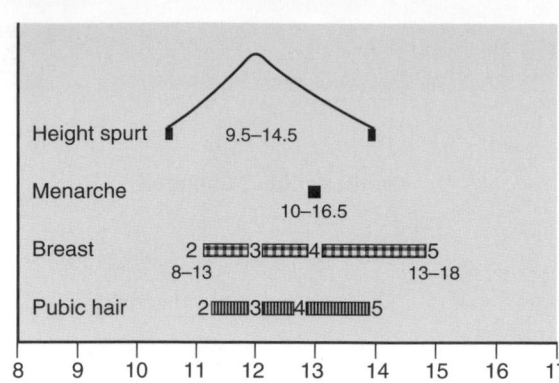

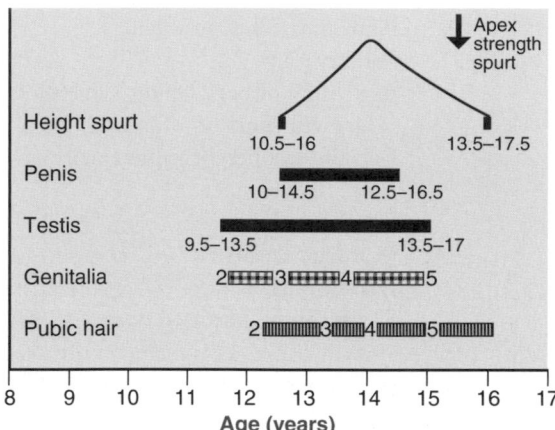

FIGURE 8-1 Sequence of events during puberty in girls (upper chart) and boys (lower chart). Breast, genitalia, and pubic hair development are numbered 2 to 5 based on the Tanner developmental stages. *(From Marshall WA, Tanner JM: Variations in the pattern of pubertal changes in boys, Arch Dis Child 45:13, 1970.)*

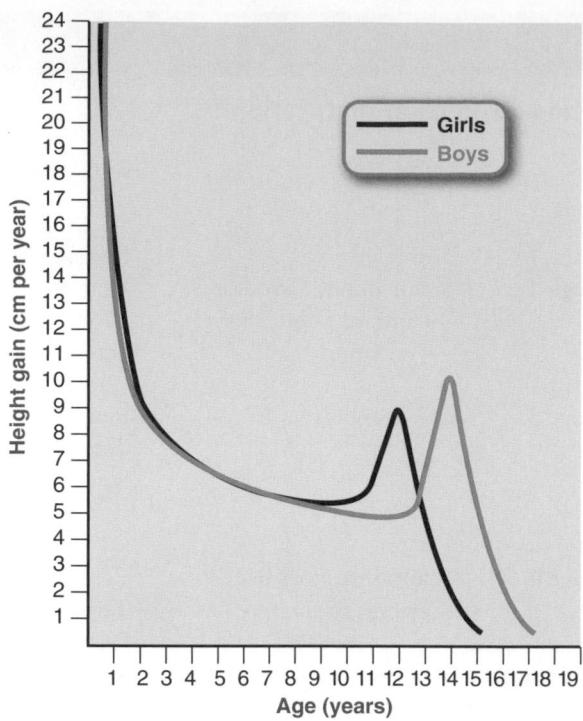

FIGURE 8-2 Typical individual velocity curves for supine length or height in boys and girls. Curves represent the growth velocity of the typical boy and girl at any given age.

whereas only 15% of their white peers had entered SMR stage 2 (Herman-Giddens et al., 1997). Initial breast development was apparent among black females by 8.8 years of age and among white females by 9.9 years. Pubic hair development had begun among black girls at age 8.7 years but did not begin in white girls for another 2 years. The age of menarche was similar among both groups of females (12.2 years for black and 12.8 years for white girls), suggesting that puberty began earlier for black girls but lasted longer.

The velocity of physical growth during adolescence is much higher than that of early childhood (Figure 8-2). On average, adolescents gain about 20% of their adult height during puberty. There is a great deal of variability in the timing and duration of growth among adolescents, as illustrated in Figure 8-3 by a group of 13-year-old males.

Linear growth occurs throughout the 4 to 7 years of pubertal development in most teens; however, the largest percentage of height is gained during an 18- to 24-month period commonly referred to as the **growth spurt.** The fastest rate of growth during the growth spurt is labeled the **peak height gain velocity.** Although growth slows after the achievement of sexual maturity, linear growth and weight acquisition continue into the late teens for females

and early 20s for males. Most girls gain no more than 2 to 3 inches after menarche, although girls who have early menarche tend to grow more after its onset than do those having later menarche.

Increases in height are accompanied by increases in weight during puberty. Teens gain 40% to 50% of adult body weight during adolescence. The majority of weight gain coincides with increases in linear height. However, it should be noted that teens may gain more than 15 pounds after linear growth has ceased. Changes in body composition accompany changes in weight and height. Males gain twice as much lean tissue as females, resulting in differentiation in percent body fat and lean body mass. Body fat levels increase from prepuberty averages of 15% for males and 19% for females to 15% to 18% in males and 22% to 26% in females. Differences in lean body mass and body fat mass affect energy and nutrient needs throughout adolescence and differentiate needs of females from those of males.

Psychological Changes

Adolescence is often depicted as a time of irrational behavior. The physical growth of puberty transforms the teen body into an adultlike form, leading adults to believe that adolescent development is complete. However, the social and emotional development of adolescence lags behind. The mismatch between how teens look and how they act may lead adults to deduce that the adolescent is "not acting his or her age." The rebellion that is associated with the

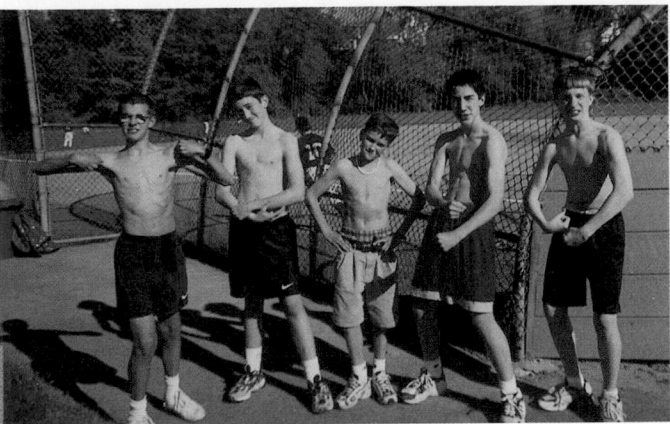

FIGURE 8-3 These boys are all 13 years old, but their energy needs vary according to their individual growth rates.

teen years is actually the manifestation of their search for independence and a sense of autonomy. Food can be, and often is, used as a means of exerting autonomy. Adolescents may choose to become vegetarian as a way to differentiate themselves from their meat-eating parents or to express their moral and ethical concerns over animal welfare or the environment. Eating fast food becomes a strong social factor for adolescents that differentiate them from their parents and older generations. In their minds, asking teens to stop eating fast food is equivalent to asking them to stop being adolescents.

Cognitive and emotional development is best understood when it is divided into three periods: early, middle, and late adolescence (Ingersoll, 1992). Each period has unique features in terms of the ability to synthesize information and apply health concepts, and this has a direct bearing on methods used when providing nutritional counseling and designing educational programs.

Early adolescence, occurring between the ages of 13 and 15, is characterized by the following:

- Preoccupation with body size, shape, and **body image** (the mental self-concept and perception of personal body size) as a result of the rapid growth and development that has occurred
- Continuation of trust and respect for adults as authority figures, however this diminishes during this phase of psychosocial development
- Strong influence of peers, especially around areas of body image and appearance, with peer pressure peaking at about 14 years of age
- Desire for autonomy but still obtaining parental approval for major decisions and still seeking parental security when experiencing stress
- Expanded cognitive ability, including abstract reasoning
- Increased spending money results in more independent purchasing power, including for snacks and meals

Middle adolescence, occurring between the ages of 15 and 17, is characterized by the following:

- Persistence of peer group influence; however, teens are influenced by fewer individuals with whom they closely bond
- Trust in adult authority and wisdom decreases
- Body image issues become less pronounced as the adolescent becomes more comfortable in his or her adultlike body shape and size
- Social, emotional, and financial independence becomes more pronounced, leading to increased independent decision making related to food and beverage intake
- Significant cognitive development occurs as abstract reasoning is nearly complete and egocentrism decreases

Late adolescence, occurring between the ages of 18 and 21, is characterized by the following:

- Abstract reasoning is fully developed; however, teens may still revert to less complex thinking patterns when they are stressed
- Future orientation, which is required to understand the link between current behavior and chronic health risks, has developed
- Social, emotional, financial, and physical independence from family occurs as teens leave home to attend college or seek full-time employment
- Development of a core set of values and beliefs that guides moral, ethical, and health-related decisions

The psychosocial development of adolescents has a direct bearing on the foods and beverages they choose. Teens in early to mid-adolescence are at risk for restricting calories as a means of dieting because of body image concerns. Because abstract reasoning ability is not yet fully developed, teens of this age are generally unable to see the relationship between their current behaviors and their future health risk. Nutrition education and counseling methods that focus on how adolescents look, such as improving skin appearance or promoting hair growth, are most likely to be effective with young teens.

NUTRIENT REQUIREMENTS

The dietary reference intakes (DRIs), which include the recommended dietary allowances (RDAs), adequate intakes (AIs), estimated average requirements (EARs), and tolerable upper intake levels (ULs) are used to determine the nutrient needs of all individuals. DRIs for adolescents are listed by chronologic age and gender. Although the DRIs provide an estimate of the energy and nutrient needs for an individual adolescent, actual need varies greatly between teens as a result of differences in body composition, degree of physical maturation, and level of physical activity. Therefore health professionals should use the DRIs as a guideline during nutritional assessment, but should rely on clinical judgment and indicators of growth and

TABLE 8-2

Estimated Energy Requirements for Male Adolescents

Age	Reference Weight (kg[lb])	Reference Height (m[in])	Estimated Energy Requirements (kcal/day)			
			Sedentary PAL*	Low Active PAL*	Active PAL*	Very Active PAL*
10	31.9 (70.3)	1.39 (54.7)	1601	1875	2149	2486
11	35.9 (79.1)	1.44 (56.7)	1691	1985	2279	2640
12	40.5 (89.2)	1.49 (58.7)	1798	2113	2428	2817
13	45.6 (100.4)	1.56 (61.4)	1935	2276	2618	3038
14	51.0 (112.3)	1.64 (64.6)	2090	2459	2829	3283
15	56.3 (124)	1.70 (66.9)	2223	2618	3013	3499
16	60.9 (134.1)	1.74 (68.5)	2320	2736	3152	3663
17	64.6 (142.3)	1.75 (68.9)	2366	2796	3226	3754
18	67.2 (148)	1.76 (69.3)	2383	2823	3263	3804

Data from Institute of Medicine, Food and Nutrition Board: *Dietary reference intakes for energy, carbohydrate, fiber, fat, fatty acids, cholesterol, protein, and amino acids,* Washington, DC, 2002, National Academies Press.

*PAL, Physical activity level. PAL categories, which are based on walking per day at 2-4 mph, are as follows: *sedentary,* no additional activity; *low active,* 1.5-2.9 miles/day; *active,* 3-5.8 miles/day; and *very active,* 7.5-14 miles/day (see Table 2-3).

physical maturation to make a final determination of an individual's nutrient and energy requirements.

Energy

Estimated energy requirements (EERs) vary greatly among males and females because of variations in growth rate, body composition, and physical activity level. EERs are calculated using an adolescent's gender, age, height, weight, and physical activity level (PAL), with an additional 25 kcal/day added for energy deposition or growth (IOM, 2002). To determine adequate energy intake (in kilocalories), physical activity assessment is required. The energy requirements allow for four levels of activity (sedentary, low active, active, and very active), which reflect the energy expended in activities other than the activities of daily living. Tables 8-2 and 8-3 show the EER (kcal/day) for each activity level based on PALs.

Adequacy of energy intake is best assessed by monitoring weight and body mass index (BMI) among adolescents. Excessive weight gain indicates that energy intake is exceeding energy needs, whereas weight loss or a drop in BMI below an established percentile curve suggests that energy intake is inadequate to support the body's needs. Groups of adolescents who are at elevated risk for inadequate energy intake include teens who "diet" or frequently restrict caloric intake to reduce body weight; individuals living in food-insecure households, temporary housing, or on the street; adolescents who frequently use alcohol or illicit drugs, which may reduce appetite or replace food intake; and teens with chronic health conditions such as cystic fibrosis, Crohn's disease, or muscular dystrophy.

Recent concerns about excessive energy intake among youths have centered on the intakes of added fats and sugars in their diets. Sweetened soft drinks are the largest contributor of added sugars in the diets of teens, contributing 37% of all added sugars for females and 41% for males (Guthrie and Morton, 2000). It is estimated that 9% of the total caloric intake of male adolescents and 8% of total caloric intake of female adolescents can be attributed to soft drink consumption (Golden, 2000; Jacobson, 1998). Counseling related to excessive energy intakes among adolescents should focus on intake of discretionary calories, especially those from added sweeteners.

Protein

During adolescence protein requirements vary with degree of physical maturation. The DRIs for protein intake are estimated to allow for adequate pubertal growth and positive nitrogen balance (IOM, 2002). Table 8-4 illustrates the protein requirements for adolescents. Actual protein needs are best determined based on a per kilogram of body weight method during puberty to account for differences in rates of growth and development among teens.

Insufficient protein intake is uncommon in the U.S. adolescent population. However, as with energy intake, food security issues, chronic illness, frequent dieting, and substance use may compromise protein intakes among adolescents. Teens who follow vegan or macrobiotic diets are another group that is at elevated risk for inadequate protein intake.

When protein intake is inadequate, alterations in growth and development are seen. In the still-growing adolescent, insufficient protein intake will result in delayed or stunted increases in height and weight. In the physically mature teen, inadequate protein intake can result in weight loss, loss of lean body mass, and alterations in body composition. Impaired immune response and susceptibility to infection may also be seen.

Carbohydrates and Fiber

Carbohydrate requirements of adolescents are estimated to be 130 g/day (IOM, 2002). The requirements for carbohydrates, as for most nutrients, are extrapolated from adult

TABLE 8-3

Estimated Energy Requirements for Female Adolescents

Age	Reference Weight (kg[lb])	Reference Height (m[in])	Estimated Energy Requirements (kcal/day)			
			Sedentary PAL*	Low Active PAL*	Active PAL*	Very Active PAL*
10	32.9 (72.5)	1.38 (54.3)	1470	1729	1972	2376
11	37.2 (81.9)	1.44 (56.7)	1538	1813	2071	2500
12	40.5 (89.2)	1.49 (58.7)	1798	2113	2428	2817
13	44.6 (91.6)	1.51 (59.4)	1617	1909	2183	3640
14	49.4 (108.8)	1.60 (63)	1718	2036	2334	3831
15	52.0 (114.5)	1.62 (63.8)	1731	2057	2362	2870
16	53.9 (118.7)	1.63 (64.2)	1729	2059	2368	2883
17	55.1 (121.4)	1.63 (64.2)	1710	2042	2353	2871
18	56.2 (123.8)	1.63 (64.2)	1690	2024	2336	2858

Data from Institute of Medicine, Food and Nutrition Board: *Dietary reference intakes for energy, carbohydrate, fiber, fat, fatty acids, cholesterol, protein, and amino acids*, Washington, DC, 2002, National Academies Press.

*PAL, Physical activity level. PAL categories, which are based on walking per day at 2-4 mph are as follows: *sedentary*, no additional activity; *low active*, 1.5-2.9 miles/day; *active*, 3-5.8 miles/day; and *very active*, 7.5-14 miles/day (see Table 2-3).

needs and should be used as a starting point for the determination of an individual adolescent's actual need. Teens who are very active or are actively growing will need additional carbohydrates to maintain adequate energy intake, whereas teenagers who are inactive or have a chronic condition that limits mobility may require fewer carbohydrates. Whole grains are the preferred source of carbohydrates because these foods provide vitamins, minerals, and fiber. Intake of carbohydrates is adequate in most teens, with less than 3% of adolescents in the United States reporting intakes less than the RDA value (Moshfegh et al., 2005).

Fiber intakes of youths are low, however, because of poor intake of whole grains, fruits, and vegetables. The AI values for fiber intake among adolescents are 31 g/day for males 9- to 13-years old, 38 g/day for males 14- to 18-years old, and 26 g/day for 9- to 18-year-old females (IOM, 2002). These values are derived from calculations that suggest that an intake of 14 g/1000 calories provides optimal protection against cardiovascular disease and cancer (IOM, 2002). Adolescents who require less energy intake due to activity restrictions may have needs that are lower than the AI values.

Data from the 2001-2002 What We Eat in America survey, which is a component of the National Health and Nutrition Examination Survey (NHANES), suggest that median intakes of fiber are 14 to 14.6 g/day for teenage males and 11.2 to 11.8 g/day for females (Moshfegh et al., 2005). The disparities noted between fiber recommendations and actual intakes suggest that more emphasis needs to be placed on educating adolescents about optimal sources of carbohydrates, including whole grains, fruits, vegetables, and legumes.

Fat

DRI values for absolute fat intake have not been established for adolescents. Instead it is recommended that fat intakes not exceed 30% to 35% of total caloric intake,

TABLE 8-4

Protein: Estimated Average Requirements and Recommended Dietary Allowances for Adolescents

Age (yr)	EAR (g/kg/day)	RDA (g/kg/day)
9-13	0.76	0.95 or 34 g/day*
14-18		
Boys	0.73	0.85 or 52 g/day*
Girls	0.71	0.85 or 46 g/day*

Data from Institute of Medicine, Food and Nutrition Board: *Dietary reference intakes for energy, carbohydrate, fiber, fat, fatty acids, cholesterol, protein, and amino acids*, Washington, DC, 2002, National Academies Press.

*Based on average weight for age.

EAR, Estimated average requirement; RDA, recommended dietary allowance.

with no more than 10% of calories coming from saturated fatty acids. However, specific recommendations for intakes of *n*-6 and *n*-3 fatty acids have been set in an attempt to ensure that teens consume adequate essential fatty acids to support growth and development, as well as to reduce chronic disease risk later in life. The AI for *n*-6 polyunsaturated fatty acids (linoleic acid) are 12 g/day for 9- to 13-year-old males, 10 g/day for 9- to 13-year-old females, 16 g/day for 14- to 18-year-old males and 11 g/day for 14- to 18-year-old females (IOM, 2002). Estimated requirements for *n*-3 polyunsaturated fatty acids (α-linolenic acid) among teens are 1.2 g/day for 9- to 13-year-old males, 1 g/day for 9- to 13-year-old females, 1.6 g/day for 14- to 18-year-old males and 1.1 g/day for 14- to 18-year-old females (IOM, 2002).

Minerals and Vitamins

Micronutrient needs of youth are elevated during adolescence to support physical growth and development. However, micronutrients involved in the synthesis of lean body mass, bone, and red blood cells are especially important during adolescence. Vitamins and minerals involved in protein, ribonucleic acid (RNA), and deoxyribonucleic acid (DNA) synthesis are needed in greatest amounts during the growth spurt; needs decline after physical maturation is complete. However, the requirements for vitamins and minerals involved in bone formation are elevated throughout adolescence and into adulthood since bone density acquisition is not completed by the end of puberty.

In general, male adolescents will require greater amounts of most micronutrients during puberty, with the exception of iron. Micronutrient intakes during adolescence are inadequate among some subgroups of teens, especially among females. Tables 8-5 and 8-6, based on the 2001-2002 What We Eat in America survey, illustrate the adequacy of micronutrient intakes among U.S. adolescents compared to DRI recommendations. These data suggest that in all age and gender categories the intakes of vitamin E, calcium and fiber are too low with teenage females between the ages of 14 and 18 years old being the ones most likely to consume inadequate intakes of the most vitamins and minerals, and will benefit the most from nutrition intervention.

Calcium

Because of accelerated muscular, skeletal, and endocrine development, calcium needs are greater during puberty and adolescence than during childhood or adult years. Bone mass is acquired at much higher rates during puberty than any other time of life; rates of bone accretion during adolescence may be four times as high as rates during early childhood or adulthood (Bonjour et al., 1991; Slemenda et al., 1994). In fact, females accrue approximately 92% of their bone mass by the age of 18 years, making adolescence a crucial time for osteoporosis prevention (IOM, 1997; Golden, 2000).

The AI for calcium is 1300 mg for all adolescents; however, there is some controversy over whether the AI may be too low for some teens. The National Institutes of Health (NIH) Consensus Development Conference Statement on Optimal Calcium Intake (1994) recommended 1200 to 1500 mg of calcium per day for adolescents 11 to 24 years of age. In their statement the committee acknowledged that a certain threshold level of dietary calcium is necessary to allow growing adolescents to achieve their genetically predetermined peak bone mass. The UL for calcium is 2000 mg/day, indicating that intakes of calcium in the range suggested by the NIH Consensus Panel would be safe for adolescents to consume.

Calcium intake declines with age during adolescence, especially among females (Harnack et al., 1999; Alaimo et al., 1994; Johnson et al., 1998). Data from the 2001-2002

TABLE 8-5

Mean Intakes of Selected Nutrients Compared to DRIs: Adolescent Males

	9- to 13-Year-Old Males		14- to 18-Year-Old Males	
	Mean Intake	**RDA/AI**	**Mean Intake**	**RDA/AI**
Vitamin A	670	600	638	700
Vitamin E	6	11	7.3	15
Thiamin	1.78	0.9	1.96	1.2
Riboflavin	2.51	0.9	2.57	1.3
Niacin	22.5	12	27	16
Vitamin B$_6$	1.87	1	2.17	1.3
Folate	644	300	683	400
Vitamin B$_{12}$	6	1.8	6.69	2.4
Vitamin C	80.2	45	100	75
Phosphorus	1431	1250	1575	1250
Magnesium	250	240	284	410
Iron	17	8	19.1	11
Zinc	13	8	15.1	11
Calcium	1139	1300	1142	1300
Sodium	3549	1500	2806	1500
Fiber	14.2	31	15.3	38

Data sources: Moshfegh AJ et al: *What we eat in America, NHANES 2001-2002: usual nutrient intakes from food compared to dietary reference intakes*, retrieved December 6, 2005, from http://www.ars.usda.gov/Services/docs.htm?docid=9098; Institute of Medicine (U.S.), Food and Nutrition Board: *Dietary reference intakes for calcium, phosphorus, magnesium, vitamin D, and fluoride*, Washington, DC, 1997 National Academies Press; Institute of Medicine (U.S.), Standing Committee on the Scientific Evaluation of Dietary Reference Intakes: *Dietary reference intakes for thiamin, riboflavin, niacin, vitamin B$_6$, folate, vitamin B$_{12}$, pantothenic acid, biotin, and choline; a report*, Washington, DC, 1998, National Academies Press; Institute of Medicine (U.S.), Food and Nutrition Board: *Dietary reference intakes for energy, and the macronutrients, carbohydrate, fiber, fat, fatty acids, cholesterol, protein and amino acids*, Washington, DC, 2002, National Academies Press.

AI, Adequate intake; *RDA*, recommended dietary allowance; *DRI*, dietary reference intake; *NA*, not available.

What We Eat in America survey determined that the median calcium intake among adolescent females fell from 865 mg/day in early adolescence to 804 mg/day by late adolescence. Among boys, median intakes were fairly steady at approximately 1140 mg/day (Moshfegh et al., 2005).

Research suggests that high soft drink consumption in the adolescent population contributes to low calcium intake by displacing milk consumption. Several studies have documented that increasing intakes of sweetened soft drinks are found to be related to decreasing numbers of servings of dairy foods and a decrease in the adequacy of calcium intake (%AI) among children and adolescents (Harnack et al., 1999; Frary et al., 2004). Interventions to promote calcium consumption among youth should focus not only on increasing dairy product intake, but also on decreasing intakes of soft drinks and increasing intakes of calcium-fortified foods such as orange juice, bread, dark-green vegetables, nuts, and ready-to-eat cereals.

Iron

Iron requirements are increased during adolescence for the deposition of lean body mass, increase in red blood cell volume, and to support iron lost during menses among females. Iron needs are highest during periods of active growth among all teens and are especially elevated after the onset of menses in adolescent females. The DRI for iron intake among females increases from 8 mg/day before age 13 (or before the onset of menses) to 15 mg/day after the onset of menses. Among adolescent males recommended intakes increase from 8 to 11 mg/day, with higher levels required during the growth spurt. Iron needs remain elevated for females after age 18, but fall back to prepubescent levels in males once growth and development is completed.

Median intakes of iron among adolescent males range from 17 mg/day in early adolescence to 19.1 mg/day in mid to late adolescence. Among females median intakes drop during adolescence from a high of 13.7 mg/day to 13.3 mg/day by mid to late adolescence. Increased needs for iron, combined with low intakes of dietary iron, place adolescent females at risk for iron deficiency and anemia. It is estimated that 9% of adolescent females 12 to 15 years old and 11% to 16% of females 16 to 19 years old are iron deficient, with 2% to 3% classified as having iron deficiency anemia (CDC, 1998).

Rapid growth may temporarily decrease circulating iron levels, resulting in **physiologic anemia of growth.** Other risk factors for iron deficiency anemia are listed in Box 8-1. During adolescence, iron deficiency anemia may impair the immune response and decrease resistance to infection. Iron deficiency anemia can also affect cognitive functioning and short-term memory (Halterman et al., 2001).

Zinc

Zinc is known to be essential for growth and sexual maturation. Although plasma zinc levels decline during pubertal development, retention of zinc increases significantly during the growth spurt. DRIs for males are 8 mg/day for 9- to

TABLE 8-6

Mean Intakes of Selected Nutrients Compared to DRIs: Adolescent Females

	9- to 13-Year-Old Females		14 to 18- Year-Old Females	
	Mean Intake	RDA/AI	Mean Intake	RDA/AI
Vitamin A	536	600	513	700
Vitamin E	5.6	11	5.6	15
Thiamin	1.44	0.9	1.4	1
Riboflavin	1.94	0.9	1.80	1
Niacin	18.5	12	18.6	14
Vitamin B$_6$	1.52	1	1.48	1.2
Folate	512	300	500	400
Vitamin B$_{12}$	4.4	1.8	4.16	2.4
Vitamin C	81.0	45	75.6	65
Phosphorous	1141	1250	1099	1250
Magnesium	215	240	206	360
Iron	13.7	8	13.3	15
Zinc	9.8	8	9.5	9
Calcium	865	1300	804	1300
Sodium	2806	1500	2799	1500
Fiber	12.3	26	11.7	26

Data sources: Moshfegh AJ et al: *What we eat in America, NHANES 2001-2002: usual nutrient intakes from food compared to dietary reference intakes,* retrieved December 6, 2005, from http://www.ars.usda.gov/Services/docs.htm?docid=9098; Institute of Medicine (U.S.), Food and Nutrition Board: *Dietary reference intakes for calcium, phosphorus, magnesium, vitamin D, and fluoride,* Washington, DC, 1997 National Academies Press; Institute of Medicine (U.S.), Standing Committee on the Scientific Evaluation of Dietary Reference Intakes: *Dietary reference intakes for thiamin, riboflavin, niacin, vitamin B$_6$, folate, vitamin B$_{12}$, pantothenic acid, biotin, and choline; a report,* Washington, DC, 1998, National Academies Press; Institute of Medicine (U.S.), Food and Nutrition Board: *Dietary reference intakes for energy, and the macronutrients, carbohydrate, fiber, fat, fatty acids, cholesterol, protein and amino acids,* Washington, DC, 2002, National Academies Press.

AI, Adequate intake; *RDA,* recommended dietary allowance; *DRI,* dietary reference intake; *NA,* not available.

BOX 8-1

Risk Factors for Iron Deficiency

Inadequate Iron Intake/Absorption/Stores

Vegetarian eating styles, especially vegan diets

Macrobiotic diet

Low intakes of meat, fish, poultry, or iron-fortified foods

Low intake of foods rich in ascorbic acid

Frequent dieting or restricted eating

Chronic or significant weight loss

Meal skipping

Substance abuse

History of iron deficiency anemia

Recent immigration from developing country

Special health care needs

Increased Iron Requirements/Losses

Heavy/lengthy menstrual periods

Rapid growth

Pregnancy (recent or current)

Inflammatory bowel disease

Chronic use of aspirin, nonsteroidal antiinflammatory drugs (e.g., ibuprofen), or corticosteroids

Participation in endurance sports (e.g., long-distance running, swimming, cycling)

Intensive physical training

Frequent blood donations

Parasitic infection

Reprinted with permission from Stang J, Story M, editors: *Guidelines for adolescent nutrition services*, Minneapolis, 2005, Center for Leadership Education and Training in Maternal and Child Nutrition, Division of Epidemiology and Community Health, School of Public Health, University of Minnesota.

13-year-olds and 11 mg/day for 14- to 18-year-olds, whereas median intakes are estimated to be 13 to 15.1 mg/day among teenage males, suggesting intakes are adequate. Among adolescent females, DRIs are set at 8 and 9 for 9- to 13-year-olds and 14- to 18-year-olds, respectively. Median intakes reported by teenage females range from 9 to 9.8 mg/day. Groups of teens who may be at risk for low intakes of zinc include those who have a low intake of animal products, including vegans, as well as teens who restrict calories or frequently diet.

Folic Acid

The DRI for folate intake among teens is 300 mcg/day for 9- to 13-year-old males and females, increasing to 400 mcg/day for 14- to 18-year-olds (IOM, 1998). The need for folate increases during later adolescence to support accretion of lean body mass and to provide AI among females of reproductive age as a preventive measure against neural tube defects. Food sources of folate should include both naturally occurring folate, found in dark green leafy vegetables and citrus fruit, as well as folic acid found in fortified grain products.

Median intakes of folate reported in the 2001-2002 What We Eat in America Survey suggest that young male adolescents consume an average of 644 mcg of folate daily, whereas older male teens consume 683 mcg/day. Female adolescents appear to be at greater risk for inadequate intake of folate, even though the median intake of folate among 9- to 13-year-old females is estimated at 512 mcg/day, and that of 14- to 18-year-old females is at 500 mcg/day, because 19% of females had intakes way below the DRI, even below the minimum requirements.

Supplement Use by Adolescents

The position statement of the American Dietetic Association (ADA) on vitamin and mineral supplementation states that consuming a wide variety of foods is preferred to nutrient supplementation as a method for obtaining adequate vitamins and minerals (ADA, 2001a). Despite this recommendation, studies show that adolescents do not consume nutrient-dense foods and usually have inadequate intakes of many vitamins and minerals.

National surveys show that 16% to 49% of adolescents report using vitamin or mineral supplements (Stang et al., 2000; O'Dea, 2003). Adolescents surveyed in these studies who used micronutrient supplements had higher mean dietary intakes of most micronutrients and carbohydrates and lower intakes of total and saturated fat than those who did not take supplements. More than one third of all adolescents had dietary intakes of vitamins A and E, calcium, and zinc that were less than 75% of the RDA. In addition, 35% of the females who did not use supplements consumed inadequate amounts of every micronutrient in the study (Stang et al., 2000).

The use of herbal and botanical supplements, as well as other forms of dietary supplements, is not well documented. One study of 78 adolescents suggests that herbal supplements were used by 18%, creatine and guarana were used by 5%, and coenzyme Q by 1% of teens (O'Dea, 2003). The use of herbs and supplements by youths is highly controversial.

FOOD HABITS AND EATING BEHAVIORS

Food habits that are seen more frequently among teens than other age-groups include irregular consumption of meals, excessive snacking, eating away from home (especially fast-food venues), dieting, and meal skipping. Many factors contribute to these behaviors, including decreasing influence of family and increasing influence of peers on food and health choices, increasing exposure to media, increasing prevalence of employment outside the home, greater discretionary spending capacity, and increasing responsibilities, leaving less time for teens to eat meals with their families. Most adolescents are aware of the importance of nutrition and the components of a healthy diet; however, there are many barriers to choosing healthy foods and beverages (Story et al., 2002b).

Teens cite taste, time, and convenience as the key factors that affect their food and beverage choices (Neumark-Sztainer et al., 1999). Lack of time to locate or prepare healthy foods is frequently mentioned as the most significant barrier to eating properly. Other factors identified as important influences on food and beverage choices by teens are the availability of food, the perceived benefits of food (e.g., energy, appearance), and the context or situation in which eating takes place.

Developmentally, many teens lack the ability to associate current eating habits with future disease risk and show little concern for their future health. Teens are often more focused on "fitting in" with their peers and will adopt health behaviors that demonstrate their quest for autonomy and make them feel more like adults such as drinking alcohol, smoking, and engaging in sexual activity. Nutrition education and counseling should focus on short-term benefits, such as improving school performance, looking good, and having more energy. Messages should be positive, developmentally appropriate, and concrete, emphasizing skills to help teens make healthy choices. Specific skills such as looking for foods with no more than 5 g of fat per serving, ordering broiled rather than fried meats, and choosing baked rather than fried snack chips are key concepts to include in nutrition education and counseling for adolescents.

Irregular Meals and Snacking

Meal skipping is a common behavior among adolescents. Meal skipping increases throughout adolescence as teens try to sleep longer in response to early school start times, try to lose weight through calorie restriction, and as their lives become busier in general. Breakfast is the most commonly skipped meal, especially among adolescent females (Story et al., 2002b). National data suggest that 24% of females and 20% of males skip breakfast on a given day (Lin et al., 1996). Breakfast is skipped by 15% of 9- to 13-year-olds; however, it is skipped by 34% of female and 28% of 14- to 18-year-old males (Gleason et al., 2001). Breakfast skipping has been associated with poor health outcomes including higher BMI, poorer concentration and school performance, and increased risk of inadequate nutrient intake, especially of calcium and fiber (Affenito et al., 2005).

Teens who skip meals often snack in response to hunger instead of eating a meal. Adolescents consume approximately two snacks per day, accounting for 25% of daily calorie intake and averaging 612 kcal/day (Jahns et al., 2001). Snack foods consumed by teens are often high in added fats, sweeteners, and sodium. Soft drinks are the most commonly consumed snacks, accounting for 6% of daily caloric intake among teens (Subar et al., 1998). Because snacking is prevalent among adolescents and snacks are often consumed in place of meals, teens should be encouraged to make healthy choices when choosing snack foods and beverages rather than to avoid snacking. Box 8-2 provides ideas for healthy snacks or meal alternatives for teens.

BOX 8-2

Teen-Friendly Healthy Snacks

Pudding made with skim milk

A glass of skim milk sweetened with a teaspoon of chocolate or strawberry syrup

Soft pretzels warmed in the microwave and topped with mustard or salsa

Sliced apples dipped in peanut butter or fat-free caramel dip

English muffin mini-pizzas (topped with tomato/pizza sauce and mozzarella cheese)

Air-popped popcorn

Peeled and sectioned oranges

Humus and pita bread

Mozzarella or string cheese

Baked tortilla chips with bean dip or salsa

Baked potato (microwaved) topped with salsa, yogurt, or fat-free sour cream

Graham crackers, animal crackers containing no *trans* fat

Frozen yogurt or juice bars

Fruit drink spritzer (half cranberry juice and half seltzer water)

Trail mix (dried fruit with nuts and seeds)

Baby carrots and low-fat ranch dressing

Low fat granola bars

Mini-rice cakes or popcorn cakes

Sandwich wraps with slices of turkey, cheese, and tomato

Adapted with permission from Stang J, Story M, editors: *Guidelines for adolescent nutrition services*, Minneapolis, 2005, Center for Leadership Education and Training in Maternal and Child Nutrition, Division of Epidemiology and Community Health, School of Public Health, University of Minnesota.

Fast Foods and Convenience Foods

Fast foods include foods from vending machines, convenience groceries, canteens, or school stores and franchised food restaurants. In a 30-day period the most common two types of stores teenagers visit are food stores, with more than 200 million visits to convenience stores and supermarkets (Figure 8-4). Fast-food restaurants and convenience stores are among the top employers of teenagers. These venues have become socially acceptable places for teens to work and spend time with their friends. The highest number of visits to fast-food restaurants occur immediately after school (Figure 8-5), and the next highest number occur during weekday dinnertime hours (see *Focus On: Where to Eat on the Way Home from School?*).

Fast foods and convenience foods tend to be low in vitamins, minerals, and fiber but high in added fat, sweeteners, and sodium. Few teens are willing to stop purchasing foods from fast-food restaurants, vending machines, or convenience stores because the low price, convenient access, and taste of fast foods appeal to adolescents (Figure 8-6). Health

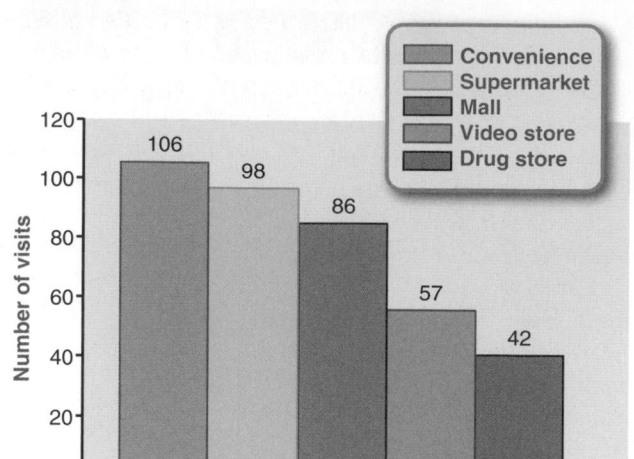

FIGURE 8-4 Store visits by teenagers in a 30-day period. *(Data from Channel One Network, New York, 2000.)*

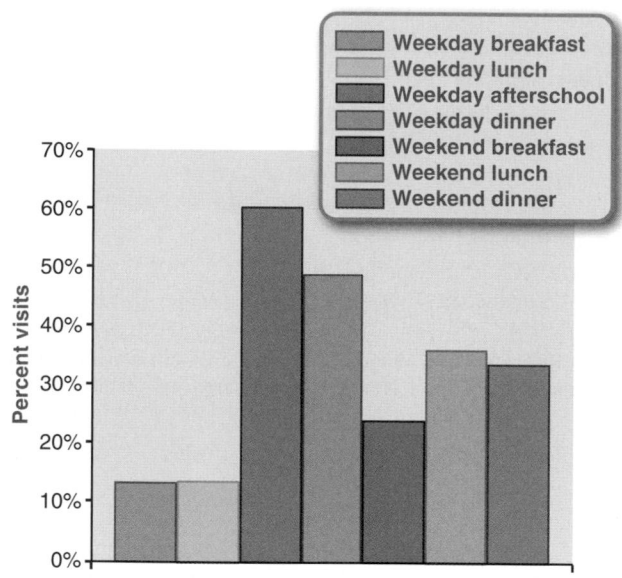

FIGURE 8-5 Fast-food restaurant visits by teenagers in a 2-week period. *(Data from Channel One Network, New York, 2000.)*

professionals should refrain from asking teenagers to not eat these foods and should instead counsel them on how to make wise and healthy choices when eating these foods. Concrete guidelines, such as choosing snacks or vending and fast-food options with fewer than 5 g of fat per serving, are easy for adolescents to remember. Teens can also be encouraged to check labels to determine if foods are made from whole grains or are high in added sweeteners or sodium.

Family Meals

The frequency with which adolescents eat meals with their families decreases with age (Gillman et al., 2000; Neumark-Sztainer et al., 2000). Teens in the seventh grade eat an average of 5.7 meals per week with their family, whereas teens in the tenth grade eat 3.5 meals with their family each week. Between 22% and 35% of adoles-

Where to Eat on the Way Home From School?

Why do so many teens eat fast food after school? One study suggests that it may be because fast-food restaurants are strategically placed close to schools. Geographic information system models were developed to examine the proximity of schools to fast-food restaurants in Chicago, Ill. The results showed that fast-food restaurants were three to four times more likely to be located close to a school than would be expected based on general locations of fast-food restaurants (Austin et al., 2005). Eighty percent of schools had a fast-food restaurant within 800 meters of the school building (approximately a 10-min walk), and 35% of the schools had fast-food restaurants within 400 meters. The clustering of fast-food restaurants was highest in higher-income areas and in areas outside of downtown. Easy access to fast-food restaurants while walking or driving home may cause teens to eat fast food more often. Health professionals need to address the neighborhood food environment of the school when developing programs to improve the eating habits of teens.

cents report that they rarely or never eat meals with their families, and about one third eat meals with their families every day. Adolescents who eat meals with their families have been found to have better academic performance and to be less likely to engage in health-risky behaviors such as drinking alcohol, smoking, and engaging in sexual activity compared to peers who do not frequently engage in family meals (U.S. Council of Economic Advisors, 2000).

Family meals not only allow for more communication between teens and their parents, but they also provide an ideal environment during which parents can model healthy food and beverage choices and attitudes toward eating. Teens who eat at home more frequently have been found to consume more fruits and vegetables and to eat fewer fried foods (Gillman et al., 2000).

Media and Advertising

Marketing to teenagers has become a multibillion-dollar business. It is estimated that the nation's approximately 23 million teenagers spend nearly $100 billion annually (Channel One Network, 2000). About one third of their annual spending is for clothing, another 22% is for entertainment, and another $15 billion is for fast foods and snacks.

According to findings from *Generation M: Media in the Lives of 8-18 year-olds*, American youths spend 6.5 hours per day, or 44.5 hours per week, with media. Almost 4 hours per day are spent watching television, DVDs and other visual media such as that from the internet, 1.75 hours per day listening to radio or recorded music, and 45 minutes per day reading magazines or books (not for school) (Kaiser Family Foundation, 2005). The majority of youths (68%) have a

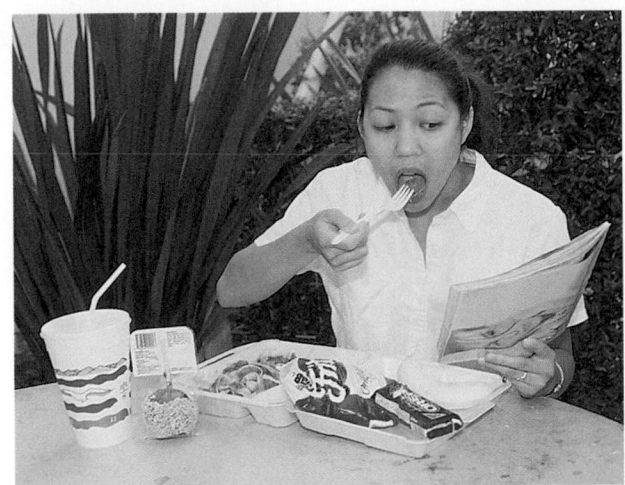

FIGURE 8-6 For teenagers who eat meals or snacks in addition to traditional meals, the choice of food is more important than the time it is eaten or place in which it is eaten. (*From Bowden VR et al:* Children and their families: the continuum of care, *Philadelphia, 1998, WB Saunders.*).

television, and 54% also have a DVD/VCR player in their bedroom. As the number of television channels that specifically target youths has increased, so has the ability for advertisers to influence their eating behaviors. It is estimated that youths view 20,000 to 40,000 television advertisements per year, so that, by the time children reach the teenage years, they have viewed 100,000 food commercials (Brown and Witherspoon, 1998; Story et al., 2002a). More than 65% of food advertisements promote beverages, candy, and fast foods. Media literacy education can and should be taught to teens to assist them in determining the accuracy and validity of media and advertising messages.

Dieting and Body Image

Body image concerns are common during adolescence. Many teens describe themselves as being overweight despite being of normal weight, signifying a disturbance in their body image. Data from the 2003 Youth Risk Behavior Survey (YRBS) found that 30% of high school students identified themselves as being overweight, despite the fact that only 13.5% were actually found to be overweight (Grunbaum et al., 2004). Body image disturbance is more common among white and Hispanic females than among males or other racial/ethnic groups (Grunbaum et al., 2004).

Poor body image can lead to weight control issues and dieting. YRBS data show that 44% of U.S. adolescents were attempting to lose weight. White and Hispanic females had the highest prevalence of dieting at 62%, followed by black females (47%), Hispanic males (37%), white males (28%), and black males (23%) (Grunbaum et al., 2004). The prevalence of dieting increased with age among females but decreased with age among males.

Forty-two percent of U.S. teens reported eating fewer calories or less fat in the previous month to either lose weight or prevent weight gain (Grunbaum et al., 2004). Two thirds of females had exercised in the previous month to lose weight or prevent weight gain compared to 49% of males. These behaviors can be viewed as healthy weight loss behaviors when used in moderation and can be a starting point for nutrition education and counseling on improving eating behaviors.

Not all dieting behaviors have the potential to improve health, however. High-risk dieting practices are used by many teens and carry with them the risk of poor nutritional status and increased risk for **disordered eating** (see Chapter 22). Fasting, or refraining from eating for more than 24 hours, was practiced by 18% of U.S. teenage females and 8.5% of teenage males in the past month as a means of dieting (Grunbaum et al., 2004). Eleven percent of females and 7% of males had used diet pills to lose weight, increasing with age among both males and females. The use of purging methods, including vomiting and laxative or diuretic use, was reported by 8% of female and 4% of male teens. The prevalence of purging behaviors was highest among Hispanic females (10%).

NUTRITION SCREENING, ASSESSMENT, AND COUNSELING

The Guidelines for Adolescent Preventive Services (GAPS) recommend that adolescents have an annual health screening to determine risk factors for acute and chronic disease. It should include screening for nutrition risk (American Medical Association, 2006). Nutrition screening should include the assessment of height, weight, and BMI to determine weight status; detection of potentially high-risk dietary habits such as vegetarianism, food allergies, and calorie restriction; and the evaluation of the presence of iron deficiency anemia (females only).

Weight, height, and BMI should be plotted using the CDC National Center for Health Statistics (NCHS) BMI tables to determine appropriateness of weight for height. Although BMI is not a direct measure of body fatness and thus cannot be used to clinically assess obesity, it is highly correlated with body fatness and is the recommended screening method for weight status among youth (Himes and Dietz, 1994; Barlow and Dietz, 1998). A BMI below the fifth percentile may signal the presence of chronic or metabolic disease, growth failure, or an eating disorder. A BMI at or above the 85th percentile, but below the 95th percentile, indicates that an adolescent is at risk for overweight, whereas a BMI at or above the 95th percentile indicates the presence of overweight. All BMI values that indicate the presence of overweight risk should be corroborated with a direct measure of body fat to determine that excessive fat, or obesity, is truly indicated.

When nutrition screening indicates the presence of nutritional risk, a full assessment should be conducted. Components of a full nutrition assessment are listed in Table 8-7. Nutrition assessment should include a complete evaluation of food intake through a 24-hour recall, dietary records, or brief food frequency questionnaire (FFQ) (see Chapter 14).

TABLE 8-7

Elements of a Nutritional Screening and Assessment for Adolescents

	Medical and Psychosocial History	Growth and Development	Diet and Physical Activity	Routine Screenings and Laboratory Tests
Components of an initial nutrition screening	Medical history Psychosocial history Socioeconomic status and history	Body mass index (BMI) Sexual maturation rating (SMR)	Meal and snacking patterns Nutrient and nonnutrient supplement use Food security Food allergies/ intolerances Special dietary practices Alcohol consumption Physical activity and competitive sports	Hemoglobin (females) Serum cholesterol or blood lipids Blood pressure
Indications for an in-depth nutritional assessment	Chronic disease Substance use Poverty and/or homelessness Depression or dysthymia Disordered eating Eating disorders Body image disorders Pregnancy or lactation	Underweight Overweight At risk for overweight Delayed sexual maturation Short stature or stunting	Food insecurity Meal skipping Inadequate micronutrient intake Excessive intake of total or saturated fat Food allergy or intolerance Vegetarian diet Use of nonnutritional or herbal supplements Competition in competitive sports Chronic dieting Fasting Alcohol consumption	Hypertension Hyperlipidemia Iron deficiency anemia Hyperglycemia

Reprinted with permission from Stang J, Story M, editors: *Guidelines for adolescent nutrition services*, Minneapolis, 2005, Center for Leadership Education and Training in Maternal and Child Nutrition, Division of Epidemiology and Community Health, School of Public Health, University of Minnesota.

The Youth Assessment Questionnaire (YAQ) is a food frequency questionnaire that was developed for and has been validated in populations of children and adolescents (Rockett et al., 1997). The adequacy of energy, fiber, macronutrients, and micronutrients should be determined as well as excessive intake of any dietary components such as sodium or sweeteners. Nutritional assessments also should include an evaluation of the nutritional environment, including parental, peer, school, cultural, and personal lifestyle factors. The attitude of the adolescent toward food and nutrition is also a primary component of a comprehensive evaluation (Stang, 2002). A prime component of nutritional counseling for adolescents is helping them overcome their perceived barriers to eating well.

Teens who live in food-insecure households, temporary housing, or shelters or who have run away from home are at especially high nutritional risk, as are adolescents who use alcohol and street drugs. It is important that health professionals working with high-risk teens develop part-

nerships with community-based food assistance programs to ensure that youths have access to a steady, nutritious food supply. Homeless teens, as well as those living in temporary shelters, will benefit from nutrition counseling focusing on lightweight, low-cost, prepackaged foods that do not require refrigeration or cooking facilities. Dried fruit, nuts, granola bars, cereal bars, tuna in pouches, and meat jerky are foods that should be available for runaway or homeless teens.

Nutrition education and counseling should be tailored to meet the specific dietary issues identified during the nutrition assessment. A teen who has been found to be overweight with type 2 diabetes will require a different type and intensity of counseling than a teen who has been diagnosed with iron deficiency anemia. Knowledge, attitude, and behavior must be addressed when guiding adolescents toward acquiring healthful food habits. For a plan to succeed, the adolescent must be willing to change; therefore an assessment of a teenager's desire to change is essential. Encourag-

TABLE 8-8

MyPyramid Recommended Number of Servings for Adolescents Ages 13 and 16 Years Based on Activity Level

	Grains (ounce)	Vegetables (cup)	Fruit (cup)	Milk (cup)	Meat/Beans (ounce)	Whole Grains (ounce)*
Males						
13 Years of Age						
≤30 min physical activity/day	6	2.5	2	3	5.5	3
30-60 min physical activity/day	7	3	2	3	6	3.5
≥60 min physical activity/day	9	3.5	2	3	6.5	4.5
16 Years of Age						
≤30 min physical activity/day	8	3	2	3	6.5	4
30-60 min physical activity/day	10	3.5	2.5	3	7	5
≥60 min physical activity/day	10	4	2.5	3	7	4
Females						
13 Years of Age						
≤30 min physical activity/day	5	2	1.5	3	5	3
30-60 min physical activity/day	6	2.5	2	3	5.5	3
≥60 min physical activity/day	7	3	2	3	6	3.5
16 Years of Age						
≤30 min physical activity/day	6	2.5	1.5	3	5	3
30-60 min physical activity/day	6	2.5	2	3	5.5	3
≥60 min physical activity/day	8	3	2	3	6.5	4

*No. of servings of whole grains are not in addition to, but included in the number of servings of grains (see www.MyPyramid.gov).

ing the desire to change usually requires most of the nutrition counselor's attention (see Chapter 19).

Information can be provided in various settings ranging from the classroom to the hospital. The clinician must understand the change process and how to meaningfully communicate this process. Parents may be included in the process and encouraged to be supportive but not intrusive (Sigman-Grant, 2002). Recommended eating plans based on recommended energy intakes for adolescents as recommended by MyPyramid, are shown in Table 8-8.

SPECIAL SITUATIONS

Vegetarian Dietary Patterns

As adolescents mature they begin to develop autonomous social, moral, and ethical values. These values may lead to vegetarian eating practices because of concerns about animal welfare, the environment, or personal health. Concerns about body weight also motivate some adolescents to adopt a vegetarian diet because it is a socially acceptable way to reduce dietary fat. Well-planned vegetarian diets that include a variety of legumes, nuts, and whole grains can provide adequate nutrients for teens who have completed the majority of their growth and development.

Vegetarian diets that become increasingly more restrictive should be viewed with caution, however, since this may signal the development of disordered eating, with the veg-

etarian diet used as a means to hide a restriction of food intake (Story et al., 2002b; Neumark-Sztainer et al., 1999). Both male and female teens who adopt vegetarian dietary patterns have been found to use more high-risk weight control behaviors, especially vomiting, to lose weight (Perry et al., 2001). Interestingly, the effects of vegetarian dietary patterns on increased risk for disordered eating behaviors appear to be stronger for males than for females.

Research has shown that vegetarian adolescents have higher intakes of iron, vitamin A, and fiber and lower intakes of dietary cholesterol than their omnivorous peers (Perry et al., 2002). Vegetarian diets that include eggs or dairy products are consistent with the Dietary Guidelines for Americans and can meet the DRIs for all nutrients. A sample eating plan to assist vegetarian teens in achieving adequate energy and nutrient intakes is listed in Table 8-9.

Vegan diets, which do not include animal products of any kind, will not provide natural sources of vitamin B_{12} and may be deficient in calcium, vitamin D, zinc, and iron. Therefore it is imperative that vegan adolescents choose foods that are fortified with these nutrients or take a daily multivitamin-mineral supplement to be sure they receive adequate micronutrients.

When adolescents become vegetarians, parents are often concerned about the diet's nutritional adequacy and especially about their children meeting their protein requirements. Parents need reassurance that a vegetarian diet can meet their children's nutritional needs, and they should receive information on the principles of healthy vegetarian eating for adolescents. In addition, parents and adolescents should be informed that overly restricted or inappropriately selected vegetarian diets can result in significant malnutrition. Iron deficiency anemia, vitamin B_{12} deficiency, and altered physical growth and development have developed in vegetarian adolescents who did not consume a wide variety of foods and beverages or did not choose adequately fortified foods (Story et al., 2002a; Sanders, 1995).

Eating Disorders

Eating disorders are the third most common chronic illness in adolescent females, with an incidence of from 1.5% to 5% (see Chapter 22). The prevalence of eating disorders has increased over the past three decades (Kreipe and Birndorf, 2000; American Dietetic Association, 2001b). Eating disorders are more commonly diagnosed in females compared to males but do occur in both genders. Athletes who compete in sports such as wrestling, dancing, track, rowing, and sports that require low body fat such as body building or gymnastics are at higher-than-average risk for developing eating disorders (Herbold and Frates, 2000).

The criteria for anorexia nervosa and bulimia nervosa are listed in Chapter 22. In general, anorexia nervosa is characterized by a dangerously low body weight, preoccupation with thinness, and restrictive dietary behaviors. Bulimia nervosa is characterized by a body weight that is close to normal, episodes of uncontrollable eating (bingeing), and efforts to eliminate calories or food from the body (purging). Numerous adolescents who have eating disorders do not meet the strict Diagnostic and Statistical Manual-IV (DSM-IV) criteria for either anorexia nervosa or bulimia nervosa but can be classified as having eating disorders not otherwise specified (EDNOS) (see Chapter 22).

Diagnostic criteria for eating disorders such as those provided by the DSM-IV may not be entirely applicable to adolescents. The wide variability in the rate, timing, and magnitude of height and weight gain during normal puberty; the absence of menstrual periods in early puberty combined with the unpredictability of menses soon after menarche; and the cognitive lack of abstract concepts limit the application of the diagnostic criteria to adolescents (Kreipe and Birndorf, 2000; American Dietetic Association, 2001b). Just as adolescents are at increased risk for developing eating disorders, they are also more vulnerable to the complications of these disorders. The impact of malnutrition on linear growth, brain development, and bone acquisition can be long-standing and irreversible. Yet with early and aggressive treatment, adolescents have the potential for a better outcome than adults who have had the disease longer (Golden, 2000).

Early identification of adolescents with disordered eating habits has been linked to a better long-term outcome, but identification can be difficult. Adolescent females who engage in weight control behaviors such as the use of laxatives and diuretics, diet pills, excessive exercise and fasting are considered to be exhibiting disordered eating behaviors. The occurrence of these behaviors should be considered a risk factor for the development of an eating disorder. Other symptoms that may signal the presence of disordered eating behaviors include recurring gastrointestinal complaints, amenorrhea, or unexplained weight loss. Overweight females have been found to be twice as likely to engage in disordered eating behaviors such as vomiting, fasting, and using diuretics or laxatives to lose weight. A screening for disordered eating can easily be done and should include questions about fear of becoming fat, amount of dieting, use of laxatives, fasting or frequently skipping meals to lose weight, fear of certain foods (e.g., foods containing fat or sugar), vomiting, bingeing, and excessive exercise (see Chapter 22).

Obesity

The incidence of obesity in teenagers is increasing with about one third of U.S. children and teens being overweight or on the brink of becoming overweight. Adolescent weight status is evaluated based on BMI (weight/height^2 [kg/m^2]) as shown in Appendixes 12 and 16. Among 12- to 19-year-olds in the United States, the prevalence of at-risk of overweight, characterized by a BMI higher than the 85th percentile but lower than the 95th percentile, is 15.5%. The prevalence of overweight (BMI ≥95th percentile) is 15%. Obesity is a complex, multifactorial health issue that is influenced by genetics, metabolic efficiency, physical activity level, dietary intake and environmental and psychosocial factors (Greger and Edwin, 2001; Christoffel and Ariza, 1998).

Adolescent obesity has both short- and long-term health consequences. Adolescents who are overweight are at higher risk for hyperlipidemia, hypertension, insulin resistance, and type 2 diabetes compared to normal weight peers (Freedman et al., 1999). Adolescents who are found

---

TABLE 8-9

Suggested Daily Food Intake Guide for Vegetarian Adolescents

Food Group	Servings/Day*
Bread, grains, cereal	9-11
Legumes	2-3
Vegetables	4-5
Fruits	4
Nuts, seeds	1
Milk, yogurt, cheese	3
Eggs (limit three/week)	½
Fats, oils (added)	4-6
Sugar (added teaspoons)	6-9

Modified from Story M, Holt K, Sofka D, editors: *Bright futures in practice: nutrition*, ed 2, Arlington, Va, 2002, National Center for Education in Maternal and Child Health.

*Age ≥11 years; 2200-2800 kcal.

to be at risk of overweight should be referred for second-level screening, which includes data on family history, blood pressure, total cholesterol level, any major change in BMI, and concerns about weight (Story et al., 2002a; Dietz and Robinson, 1998). Overweight teens should be referred for additional in-depth medical assessments to determine the presence of additional comorbidities such as sleep apnea, orthopedic disorders, metabolic syndrome, and polycystic ovarian syndrome (see Chapter 21).

Adolescent obesity has been shown to be related to long-term health outcomes as well. A 55-year follow-up of the Harvard Growth Study found an increased risk of morbidity from coronary heart disease and arteriosclerosis in men and women who were overweight as teenagers. In men who were overweight teenagers, the risk of colorectal cancer and gout increased; whereas in women who were overweight teenagers, the risk of arthritis was higher than that of their leaner counterparts (Must et al., 1992). Looking at just women, the Nurses' Health Study showed that teens who were overweight or obese at age 18 were at greater risk of dying during middle age than their healthy-weight counterparts, and the most common cause of their middle-age death was cancer followed by heart disease (van Dam et al., 2006).

Early identification of the overweight adolescent is important because treatment is most successful when the potential for growth is still available (Williams et al., 1997). To be successful, weight management programs should be family centered and behavior based and include individualized nutrition and physical activity plans, as well as behavioral counseling. Weight management programs should stress goals of healthier eating and physical activity patterns instead of weight goals to prevent excessive focus on weight, which might lead to disordered eating behaviors (Barlow and Dietz, 1998). Family members should participate in weight management programs along with adolescents (Williams et al, 1997; Greger and Edwin, 2001). Family-based programs should teach behavior modification skills, provide guidance with food choices and meal planning, and assist families in locating affordable and enjoyable physical activity options. Family therapy is an important factor in preventing progression from obesity in childhood to severe obesity in adolescence.

Concern has been expressed over the use of bariatric surgery in adolescents. Recommendations for bariatric surgery suggest that it is only appropriate in severely overweight teens (BMI >40) who have severe comorbid medical conditions and have completed most of their physical growth and development (Inge et al., 2004a). A study of adolescents who underwent bariatric surgery reported that 70% of patients experienced complications (Inge et al., 2004b). Difficulty in complying with dietary restrictions following surgery led to complications such as dumping syndrome following high carbohydrate intake, voluntary excessive food intake, meat impacted in a gastrojejunal anastamosis, and B vitamin deficiency due to poor compliance with vitamin-mineral supplementation.

Hyperlipidemia and Hypertension

The onset of cardiovascular diseases (CVDs)—coronary artery disease and essential hypertension—occurs during youth. CVD risk factors have been shown to "track" with age and predict adult risk levels (Berenson et al., 1997). CVD risk factors also tend to cluster, resulting in metabolic syndrome in some individuals. Many of the risk factors are comorbid conditions, such as obesity and high blood pressure or obesity and hyperlipidemia (see Chapter 32).

Table 8-10 lists the classification criteria for the diagnosis of hyperlipidemia among youth. When hyperlipidemia is found in teens, it is important to rule out secondary causes of hyperlipidemia when determining dietary treatment options (Table 8-11). Dietary treatment recommendations from the American Academy of Pediatrics and the National Cholesterol Education Program are listed in Table 8-12. Both recommendations encourage reduction of total and saturated fat and dietary cholesterol intakes. Table 8-13 provides a guideline for meal planning for teens who require intensive dietary therapy to lower blood lipid levels. Promoting healthy lifestyle behaviors to reduce CVD risk should include a discussion of the benefits of regular physical activity in addition to dietary recommendations.

National screening criteria for blood pressure levels among adolescents are listed in Tables 8-14 and 8-15. Teenagers 17 years of age and younger are determined to have prehypertension if their average blood pressure readings fall between the 90th and 94th percentiles. Hypertension is diagnosed when the average of three blood pressure measurements exceed the 95th percentile for age, gender, and height.

Dietary counseling and weight management are integral components of hypertension treatment. The dietary approaches to stop hypertension (DASH) eating pattern has been shown to be effective in reducing blood pressure in many individuals (Sacks et al., 2001) (see Chapter 33). In addition to the DASH diet, teens with elevated blood pressure should be counseled to reduce sodium intake to less

TABLE 8-10

Classification of LDL and Total Cholesterol Levels in Adolescents*

	Acceptable	Borderline	High
Total cholesterol (mg/dl)	<170 mg/dl	170–199 mg/dl	≥200 mg/dl
LDL cholesterol (mg/dl)	<110 mg/dl	110–129 mg/dl	(≥130 mg/dl

Source: National Cholesterol Education Program (U.S.): *Report of the expert panel on blood cholesterol levels in children and adolescents*, NIH publication no. 91-2732, Bethesda, Md, 1991, National Institutes of Health, National Heart, Lung, and Blood Institute; National Cholesterol Education Program: Cholesterol in childhood (RE9805) policy statement, *Am Acad Pediatr* 101(1):141-147, 1998, http://www.aap.org/policy/re9805.html, accessed November 10, 2006.

*Based on the average of two measurements.

LDL, Low-density lipoprotein.

TABLE 8-11

Secondary Causes of Hyperlipidemia

	Lipid Abnormality		
Anabolic steroid use	↑ LDL	↓ HDL	
Anorexia nervosa	↑ LDL		
Cigarette smoking		↓ HDL	
Diabetes	↑ LDL	↑ TG	↓ HDL
Hypothyroidism		↑ TG	
Liver disease, obstructive	↑ LDL		
Medications: corticosteroids, bile acid-binding resins, anticonvulsants, certain oral contraceptives, Accutane (isotretinoin), Depo-provera®	Varies		
Overweight or obesity	↑ LDL	↑ TG	↓ HDL
Renal disease	Varies		
Therapeutic diet: ketogenic; high carbohydrate	↑ LDL	↑ TG	
Transplant (bone marrow, heart, kidney, or liver)		↑ TG	↓ HDL

Reprinted with permission from Stang J, Story M, editors: *Guidelines for adolescent nutrition services*, Minneapolis, 2005, Center for Leadership Education and Training in Maternal and Child Nutrition, Division of Epidemiology and Community Health, School of Public Health, University of Minnesota.

than 2000 mg/day and to achieve and maintain a healthy body weight. An overview of the DASH diet is presented in Chapter 33 and discussed in detail in Appendix 33.

Physical Activity and Sports Nutrition

Physical Activity

Physical activity, along with a healthy diet, can reduce excessive body weight, enhance body composition, improve blood lipid profiles, and reduce blood pressure in adolescents. Weight-bearing physical activity plays an important role in the development of bone mass during adolescence and can help maintain the structure and functional strength of bone throughout life (Patrick et al., 2001). National recommendations for physical activity suggest that all youth should participate in moderate activity on most if not all days of the week and should engage in strenuous exercise (defined as exercise that makes a person breathe hard and sweat) at least 3 days each week (U.S. Public Health Service, 1996; Patrick et al., 2001). However, many youths do not meet these recommendations. More than one third of high school students do not meet recommendations for strenuous exercise, and more than two thirds do not meet moderate exercise recommendations (Kann et al., 2000). Physical activity has been found to decrease 26% during high school, with a 64% decline among white females and an even

greater decline among black females (Aaron et al., 2002; Kimm et al., 2002).

Teenage athletes have unique nutrient needs. Adequate fluid intake to prevent dehydration is especially critical for young athletes. In fact, heat illness is second only to head injury as a cause of reported noncardiac causes of death in secondary school athletes (Patrick et al., 2001). Young adolescents are at higher risk for dehydration because they produce more heat production during exercise but have less ability to transfer heat from the muscles to the skin (Steen, 1996). They also sweat less, which decreases their capacity to dissipate heat through the evaporation of the sweat (see Chapter 23). Adolescents with medical conditions are at increased risk for developing heat-related illness. Children or adolescents with bulimia, diarrhea, congenital heart disease, diabetes mellitus, gastroenteritis, fever, or obesity may experience excessive fluid loss. In addition, those with anorexia nervosa, cystic fibrosis, developmental disabilities, or kidney disease may be less likely to consume sufficient fluid intake (Patrick et al., 2001).

Athletes who participate in sports that use competitive weight categories or emphasize body weight are at elevated risk for the development of disordered eating behaviors. A concern among female athletes is the female athlete triad relationship, a constellation of low body weight and inadequate body fat levels, amenorrhea, and osteoporosis (see Chapter 23). Female athlete triad may lead to premature bone loss, decreased bone density, increased risk of stress fractures, and eventual infertility (Patrick et al., 2001). Sports nutrition education for teens should focus on the benefits of healthy eating, such as having extra energy and improving physical performance.

Pregnancy

Adolescent females who become pregnant are at particularly high risk for nutritional deficiencies because of elevated nutrient needs. Pregnant adolescents with a **gynecologic age** (the number of years between the onset of menses and current age) of less than 4 and those who are undernourished at the time of conception have the greatest nutritional needs. As with adult women, pregnant teens require additional folic acid, iron, zinc, calcium and other micronutrients to support fetal growth (see Chapter 5).

Recommended weight gain during pregnancy is controversial among teens. Current recommendations from the IOM recommend that teens gain at the upper end of the weight gain ranges, with a weight gain of 28 to 40 pounds for a female with a BMI less than 19.8, 25 to 35 pounds for females with a BMI 19.8 to 26, 15 to 25 pounds for females with a BMI 26.1 to 29, and 15 lb for females with a BMI greater than 29 (IOM, 1990). These recommended weight gain ranges are based largely on adult data. BMI cutoff points for underweight, at risk for overweight, and overweight among teen females are generally lower than those of adult women and those used by the IOM weight gain recommendations.

The use of the IOM BMI ranges could result in a significant number of pregnant teens being misclassified, resulting in erroneous weight gain recommendations. Therefore it is prudent for health professionals to determine the

TABLE 8-12

Dietary Recommendations for Hyperlipidemia

	Total Fat (% kcal)	Sat Fat (% kcal)	Poly Fat (% kcal)	Cholesterol (mg/day)	Mono Fat (% kcal)	Other
NCEP 1991 Children and adolescents						CHO 55% PROT 15%-20% Appropriate calories for growth and maintain desirable BW
Step-One	<30%	<10%	≤10%	<300	~10-13%	
Step-Two	<30%	<7%	≤10%	<200		
AAP 1998 Children >2 y	No more than 30%, no less than 20%	<10%		<300		If LDL still high→ <7% saturated fat <200 mg cholesterol

Adapted with permission from Stang J, Story M, editors: *Guidelines for adolescent nutrition services*, Minneapolis, 2005, Center for Leadership Education and Training in Maternal and Child Nutrition, Division of Epidemiology and Community Health, School of Public Health, University of Minnesota.

NCEP, National Cholesterol Education Program of the National Heart, Lung Blood and Lung Institute, NIH; *AAP*, American Academy of Pediatrics; *CHO*, carbohydrate; *PROT*; protein.

TABLE 8-13

NCEP Step-One Dietary Guidelines

	Ages 11-14		Ages 15-18	
Food Group	Females	Males	Females	Males
	Daily Number of Servings			
Meat, poultry, fish (oz)	6	6	6	6
Eggs per week	3	3	3	3
Dairy products (sv)	4	4	4	4
Fruits (sv)	3	3	5	3
Vegetables (sv)	4	3	4	3
Bread, cereals (sv)	9	8	12	8
Fats, oils (sv)	7	5	10	5
Sweets, modified fat desserts	4	3	4	3

Serving Size

Dairy: 1 c milk or yogurt, 1 oz cheese, ½ c dairy dessert

Fruits: 1 med piece, ½ c juice

Vegetables: ½ c raw or cooked, 1 c salad

Breads, cereals: 1 slice bread, 1 tortilla, ½ c rice or pasta, 1 muffin, 4-inch pancake

Fats, oils: 1 tsp oil or margarine, 1 Tb salad dressing

Sweets: 6 oz sugared drink, ¾ oz hard candy, 2 cookies, 1 slice cake, 1½ Tb jelly

Reprinted with permission from: Stang J, Story M, editors: *Guidelines for Adolescent Nutrition Services*. Minneapolis, 2005, Center for Leadership Education and Training in Maternal and Child Nutrition, Division of Epidemiology and Community Health, School of Public Health, University of Minnesota.

NCEP, National Cholesterol Education Program of the National Heart, Lung, and Blood Institute; *sv*, serving.

adolescent's prepregnancy BMI category using the CDC reference data and then choose the appropriate corresponding weight gain range from the IOM recommendations. The current high weight category in the IOM guidelines (BMI higher than 26) would be equivalent to the CDC at risk for overweight category (BMI at the 85th percentile or higher but less than the 95th percentile), whereas the IOM obese category (BMI >29) would be equivalent to the CDC overweight category for adolescents (95th percentile or higher). The IOM underweight status would correspond to a BMI lower than the fifth percentile among teens based on the CDC BMI percentile cutoff points.

TABLE 8-14

90th and 95th Percentiles for Blood Pressure for Adolescent Males by Height Percentiles

Age	Height %tiles* BP†	Diastolic BP (mm Hg)							Systolic BP (mm Hg)						
		5%	10%	25%	50%	75%	90%	95%	5%	10%	25%	50%	75%	90%	95%
10	90th	111	112	114	115	117	119	119	73	73	74	75	76	77	78
	95th	115	116	117	119	121	122	123	77	78	79	80	81	81	82
11	90th	113	114	115	117	119	120	121	74	74	75	76	77	78	78
	95th	117	118	119	121	123	124	125	78	78	79	80	81	82	82
12	90th	115	116	118	120	121	123	123	74	75	75	76	77	78	79
	95th	119	120	122	123	125	127	127	78	79	80	81	82	82	83
13	90th	117	118	120	122	124	125	126	75	75	76	77	78	79	79
	95th	121	122	124	126	128	129	130	79	79	80	81	82	83	83
14	90th	120	121	123	125	126	128	128	75	76	77	78	79	79	80
	95th	124	125	127	128	130	132	132	80	80	81	82	83	84	84
15	90th	122	124	125	127	129	130	131	76	77	78	79	80	80	81
	95th	126	127	129	131	133	134	135	81	81	82	83	84	85	85
16	90th	125	126	128	130	131	133	134	78	78	79	80	81	82	82
	95th	129	130	132	134	135	137	137	82	83	83	84	85	86	87
17	90th	127	128	130	132	134	135	136	80	80	81	82	83	84	84
	95th	131	132	134	136	138	139	140	84	85	86	87	87	88	89

From National High Blood Pressure Education Program Working Group on High Blood Pressure in Children and Adolescents. Fourth report on the diagnosis, evaluation, and treatment of high blood pressure in children and adolescents. *Pediatrics* 114(2):555-576, 2004.This supplement is a work of the U.S. government, published in the public domain by the American Academy of Pediatrics. Available at http://www.pediatrics.org/cgi/content/full/114/2/S2/555.

*Height percentile determined by standard growth curves.

†Blood pressure percentile determined by a single measurement.

TABLE 8-15

90th and 95th Percentiles for Blood Pressure for Adolescent Females by Height Percentiles

Age	Height %tiles* BP†	Diastolic BP (mm Hg)							Systolic BP (mm Hg)						
		5%	10%	25%	50%	75%	90%	95%	5%	10%	25%	50%	75%	90%	95%
10	90th	112	112	114	115	116	118	118	73	73	73	74	75	76	76
	95th	116	116	117	119	120	121	122	77	77	77	78	79	80	80
11	90th	114	114	116	117	118	119	120	74	74	74	75	76	77	77
	95th	118	118	119	121	122	123	124	78	78	78	79	80	81	81
12	90th	116	116	117	119	120	121	122	75	75	75	76	77	78	78
	95th	119	120	121	123	124	125	126	79	79	79	80	81	82	82
13	90th	117	118	119	121	122	123	124	76	76	76	77	78	79	79
	95th	121	122	123	124	126	127	128	80	80	80	81	82	83	83
14	90th	119	120	121	122	124	125	125	77	77	77	78	79	80	81
	95th	123	124	125	126	127	129	129	81	81	81	82	83	84	84
15	90th	120	121	122	123	125	126	127	78	78	78	79	80	81	81
	95th	124	125	126	127	129	130	131	82	82	82	83	84	85	86
16	90th	121	122	123	124	126	127	128	78	78	79	80	81	81	82
	95th	125	126	127	128	130	131	132	82	82	83	84	85	85	86
17	90th	122	122	123	125	126	127	128	78	79	79	80	81	81	82
	95th	125	126	127	129	130	131	132	82	83	83	84	85	85	86

From National High Blood Pressure Education Program Working Group on High Blood Pressure in Children and Adolescents. Fourth report on the diagnosis, evaluation, and treatment of high blood pressure in children and adolescents, *Pediatrics* 114(2):555-576, 2004. This supplement is a work of the U.S. government, published in the public domain by the American Academy of Pediatrics. Available at http://www.pediatrics.org/cgi/content/full/114/2/S2/555.

*Height percentile determined by standard growth curves.

†Blood pressure percentile determined by a single measurement.

Data from the Camden study (Scholl et al., 1997) have shown that, in general, young pregnant adolescents gain more weight than fully grown women, yet their infants weigh less. For this reason, weight gain at the upper end of recommended IOM categories is recommended for teens with a gynecologic age of less than 4. Adolescents who begin having children at a young age (i.e., while still growing themselves) may be at particular risk for developing overweight and obesity, so their weight gain should be followed closely. The Camden Study (Hediger et al., 1997) documented excessive accrual of subcutaneous fat stores at central body sites among young pregnant females, which increases the risk of CVD and other chronic diseases later in life.

Pregnant teens should have a full nutrition assessment done early in pregnancy to determine any nutrient deficiencies and to promote adequate weight gain. Referral to appropriate food assistance programs such as the Special Supplemental Food Program for Women, Infants and Children (WIC) is an important part of prenatal nutrition education.

FOCAL POINTS

- Adolescence is a period of tremendous physical and cognitive changes.
- Teens are nutritionally vulnerable because of increased need for all nutrients at a time when changes in lifestyle and food habits greatly affect nutrient intake.
- Adolescents with special needs, such as those who participate in sports, have a chronic illness, are pregnant, diet excessively, or use alcohol and drugs, are at high risk for nutritional inadequacies and have the greatest need for nutrition education and counseling.

- Educating adolescents about the optimal energy and fat intake and level of physical activity helps them to develop a healthy body and lifestyle and avoid overweight, obesity, and its comorbidities of hypertension and hyperlipidemia.

CLINICAL SCENARIO 1

Shawna is a 17-year-old female who is being seen at the pediatric clinic today for a preemployment physical. The physician has recommended that she talk with you, the nutritionist, about her eating habits because her hemoglobin level was low. When you question Shawna about her eating habits, she reveals that she skips breakfast each day because she doesn't have time to eat in the morning, but she does have a cup of coffee on her way to school at 7:15 AM. Shawna's first food intake is usually a snack from the vending machine at 10:30 AM, which consists of a candy bar or a bag of chips and a soft drink. Occasionally she purchases ala carte lunches of tacos or a burger, but generally she skips lunch. Shawna gets out of school at 2 PM and goes to work at the mall. She has a half-hour break in late afternoon, so she goes to the food court for dinner. The evening meal usually consists of one to two slices of pizza, two tacos, or one to two pieces of chicken with a soft drink. About half of the time she also orders fries or chips. When Shawna gets home from work at 9 PM, she usually has a snack of ice cream, tortilla chips, spicy cheese puffs, or microwave popcorn. She usually has a large glass of juice or lemonade with her snack.

When you suggest to Shawna that she might benefit from eating meals rather than snacks, she says she doesn't have time to cook meals, especially in the morning. She also tells you that there are no other food choices besides fast foods at the mall where she works.

⁎Nutrition Diagnosis 1: Undesirable food choices related to perceived limitations of work and school as evidenced by daily intake of high-fat, high-sugar foods

⁎Nutrition Diagnosis 2: Inadequate iron intake related to low intake of iron-containing foods as evidenced by diet history reflecting 70% of DRI for iron

1. What types of foods might you suggest to Shawna to have for breakfast? Why would you choose these foods?
2. What is the recommended iron intake for a female of Shawna's age? Does it appear that she is getting adequate iron intake from her diet? What food choices would you recommend for Shawn to increase her hemoglobin level?
3. How much calcium does a 17-year-old teen female need? What suggestions could you make to increase Shawna's calcium intake based on the foods she likes and the places she eats?
4. What types of foods might you suggest that Shawna choose at the mall fast food court to improve her nutrient intake and to help treat her anemia?

Nate is a 14-year-old male who is being seen by you today on the advice of his pediatrician. Nate's parents are divorced, and he splits his time between the two households. His mother has become increasingly concerned that he is spending too much time exercising and not enough time with his friends. His father thinks his mother is overreacting.

When you talk with Nate about his eating habits, you find out that he is a vegan. On questioning, you discover that he became a lacto ovo-vegetarian at the age of 11 because he was concerned about animal welfare. Nate's diet became increasingly restrictive over the next 2 years as he attempted to reduce the fat intake in his diet. He has been vegan for the past 14 months. His mother has been a vegetarian for as long as he can remember, but his father eats poultry and fish.

When questioned about exercise, Nate reports that he runs 1-to 2 hours a day 5 to 6 days a week. When he is not able to run due to the weather, he walks the stairs at his school or uses his father's exercise machines. Nate reports that he runs because it makes him feel good and because it helps to keep him fit. He mentions that he has begun lifting weights to try to "bulk up," but that hasn't been effective so far.

Nate's medical chart shows that his BMI percentile has dropped from the 45th percentile down to less than the 25th percentile in the past 8 to 9 months. His hemoglobin and hematocrit are at the low end of normal, and his blood pressure is low.

✳**Nutrition Diagnosis 1:** Excessive exercise related to mom's concerns that exercise is impacting social development as evidenced by running 1 to 2 hours daily and weight loss

1. What concerns do you have regarding Nate's decision to follow a vegan diet, given his age and lifestyle? On the basis of these concerns, what advice would you give him?
2. What are the energy and protein needs for a male of Nate's age? What types of foods would you recommend that he consume if he continues to follow a vegan diet?
3. What referrals would you make based on Nate's information?

USEFUL WEBSITES

Amateur Athletic Union
www.aausports.org

American Academy of Pediatrics Media Matters Program
www.aap.org/advocacy/mmcamp.htm

American Alliance for Health, Physical Education, Recreation and Dance
www.aahperd.org

American College of Sports Medicine
www.acsm.org

American School Health Association
www.ashaweb.org

Bright Futures
www.brightfutures.org

Centers for Disease Control and Prevention
www.cdc.gov

Empowered Parents
www.empoweredparents.com

International Association of Eating Disorder Professionals
www.iaedp.org

National Collegiate Athletics Association
www.ncaa.org

National Eating Disorder Association
www.nationaleatingdisorders.org

National Recreation and Parks Association
www.activeparks.org

New Mexico Media Literacy Project
www.nmmlp.org

School Nutrition Association
www.schoolnutrition.org

Vegetarian Resource Group
www.vrg.org

References

Aaron D J et al: Longitudinal study of the number and choice of leisure time physical activities from mid to late adolescence: implications for school curricula and community recreation programs, *Arch Pediatr Adolesc Med* 156(11):1075, 2002.

Affenito SG et al: Breakfast consumption by African-American and white adolescent girls correlates positively with calcium and fiber intake and negatively with body mass index, *J Am Diet Assoc* 105(6):938, 2005.

Alaimo K et al: Dietary intake of vitamins, minerals, and fiber of persons ages 2 months and over in the United States: Third National Health and Nutrition Examination Survey, Phase 1, 1988-91, *Adv Data* 258:1, 1994.

American Dietetic Association: Position of the American Dietetic Association: food fortification and dietary supplements, *J Am Diet Assoc* 101(1):115, 2001a.

American Dietetic Association: Position of the American Dietetic Association: nutrition intervention in the treatment of anorexia nervosa, bulimia nervosa, and eating disorders not otherwise specified (EDNOS), *J Am Diet Assoc* 101(7):810, 2001b.

American Medical Association: Guidelines for adolescent preventive services recommendations monograph, available at www.ama-assn.org/ama/upload/mm/39/gapsmono.pdf, accessed December 12, 2006.

Austin SB et al: Clustering of fast food restaurants around schools: A novel application of spatial statistics to the study of school environments, *Am J Publ Hlth* 95:1575, 2005.

Barlow SE, Dietz WH: Obesity evaluation and treatment: Expert Committee Recommendations. Maternal and Child Health Bureau, Health Resources and Services Administration, Department of Health and Human Services, *Pediatrics* 102(3):E29, 1998.

Bonjour J et al: Critical years and stages of puberty for spinal and femoral bone mass accumulation during adolescence, *J Clin Endocrinol Metab* 73: 555, 1991.

Brown JD, Witherspoon EM: *The mass media and American adolescents' health*, paper presented at Health Futures of Youth! Pathways to Adolescent Health, Annapolis, Md, 1998.

Centers for Disease Control and Prevention: Recommendations to prevent and control iron deficiency in the United States, *MMWR Morb Mortal Wkly Rep* 47(RR-3):1, 1998.

Channel One Network: *Teen fact book*, New York, 2000, Channel One Network.

Christoffel KK, Ariza A: The epidemiology of overweight in children: relevance for clinical care, *Pediatrics* 101(1 Pt 1):103, 1998.

Dietz WH, Robinson TN: Use of the body mass index (BMI) as a measure of overweight in children and adolescents, *J Pediatr* 132(2):191, 1998.

Frary CD et al: Children and adolescents' choices of foods and beverages high in added sugars are associated with intakes of key nutrients and food groups, *J Adolesc Health* 34(1):56, 2004.

Freedman DS et al: The relation of overweight to cardiovascular risk factors among children and adolescents: the Bogalusa Heart Study, *Pediatrics* 103(6 Pt 1):1175, 1999.

Gillman M et al: Family dinner and diet quality among older children and adolescents, *Arch Fam Med* 9:235, 2000.

Gleason P et al: *Children's diets in the mid-1990s: dietary intake and its relationship with school meal participation*, Alexandria, Va, 2001, U.S. Dept of Agriculture, Food and Nutrition Service.

Golden NH: Osteoporosis prevention: a pediatric challenge, *Arch Pediatr Adolesc Med* 154(6):542, 2000.

Greger N, Edwin CM: Obesity: a pediatric epidemic, *Pediatr Ann* 30(11):694, 2001.

Grunbaum JA et al: Youth risk behavior surveillance—United States, 2003, *MMWR Surveill Summ* 53(2):1, 2004.

Guthrie JF, Morton JF: Food sources of added sweeteners in the diets of Americans, *J Am Diet Assoc* 100(1):43, 2000.

Halterman JS et al: Iron deficiency and cognitive achievement among school-aged children and adolescents in the United States, *Pediatrics* 107(6):1381, 2001.

Harnack L et al: Soft drink consumption among U.S. children and adolescents: nutritional consequences, *J Am Diet Assoc* 99(4):436, 1999.

Hediger ML et al: Implications of the Camden Study of adolescent pregnancy: interactions among maternal growth, nutritional status, and body composition, *Ann NY Acad Sci* 817:281, 1997.

Herbold NH, Frates SE: Update of nutrition guidelines for the teen: trends and concerns, *Curr Opin Pediatr* 12(4):303, 2000.

Herman-Giddens ME et al: Secondary sexual characteristics and menses in young girls seen in office practice: a study from the pediatric research in office settings network, *Pediatrics* 99(4): 505, 1997.

Himes J, Dietz W: Guidelines for overweight in adolescent preventive services: Recommendations from an expert committee, *Am J Clin Nutr* 59(2):307, 1994.

Inge TH et al: A multidisciplinary approach to the adolescent bariatric surgical patient, *J Pediatr Surg* 39(3):442, 2004a.

Inge TH et al: Bariatric surgery for severely overweight adolescents: concerns and recommendations, *Pediatrics* 114(1):217, 2004b.

Ingersoll GM: 1992 Psychological and social development. In McAnarney ER, Kreipe RE, editors: *Textbook of adolescent medicine*, Philadelphia, 1992, Saunders.

Institute of Medicine: *Nutrition during pregnancy. Part I: Weight gain. Part 2: Nutrient Supplements*, IOM Committee on Nutritional Status During Pregnancy and Lactation, Washington, DC, 1990, National Academies Press, p 480.

Institute of Medicine: *Dietary reference intakes for calcium, phosphorus, magnesium, vitamin D, and fluoride*, Washington, DC, 1997, National Academies Press.

Institute of Medicine: *Dietary reference intakes for thiamin, riboflavin, niacin, vitamin B_6, folate, vitamin B_{12}, pantothenic acid, biotin, and choline; a report*, Washington, DC, 1998, National Academies Press.

Institute of Medicine: *Dietary reference intakes for energy, and the macronutrients, carbohydrate, fiber, fat, fatty acids, cholesterol, protein and amino acids*, Washington, DC, 2002, National Academy Press.

Jacobson MF: *Liquid candy: How soft drinks are harming Americans' health*, Washington, DC, 1998, Center for Science in the Public Interest.

Jahns L et al: The increasing prevalence of snacking among U.S. children from 1977 to 1996, *J Pediatr* 138(4):493, 2001.

Johnson R et al: The association between noon beverage consumption and the diet quality of school-age children, *J Child Nutr Manage* 22(2):95, 1998.

Kaiser Family Foundation: *Generation M: media in the lives of 8-18 year-olds*, http://www.kff.org, Kaiser Family Foundation, 2005.

Kimm SY et al: Decline in physical activity in black girls and white girls during adolescence, *N Engl J Med* 347(10):709, 2002.

Kreipe RE, Birndorf SA: Eating disorders in adolescents and young adults, *Med Clin North Am* 84(4):1027, viii-ix, 2000.

Lin BH et al: *The diets of America's children: influences of dining out, household characteristics, and nutrition knowledge,* 1996, U.S. Department of Agriculture Economic Report Number 746 (AER-746).

Moshfegh A et al: What we eat in America, NHANES 2001-2002: usual nutrient intakes from food compared to dietary reference intakes, http://www.ars.usda.gov/Services/docs.htm?docid=9098, accessed December 6, 2005.

Must A et al: Long-term morbidity and mortality of overweight adolescents: a follow-up of the Harvard Growth Study of 1922 to 1935, *N Engl J Med* 327(19): 1350, 1992.

Neumark-Sztainer D et al: Factors influencing food choices of adolescents: findings from focus-group discussions with adolescents, *J Am Diet Assoc* 99(8):929, 1999.

Neumark-Sztainer D et al: Family meals among adolescents: findings from a pilot study, *J Nutr Educ* 32: 335, 2000.

NIH: NIH Consensus conference: optimal calcium intake: NIH consensus development panel on optimal calcium intake, *JAMA* 272(24):1942, 1994.

O'Dea JA: Consumption of nutritional supplements among adolescents: usage and perceived benefits, *Health Educ Res* 18(1):98, 2003.

Patrick K et al: *Bright futures in practice: physical activity,* Arlington, Va, 2001 National Center for Education in Maternal and Child Health.

Perry CL et al: Characteristics of vegetarian adolescents in a multiethnic urban population, *J Adolesc Health* 29(6):406, 2001.

Perry CL et al: Adolescent vegetarians: how well do their dietary patterns meet the *Healthy People 2010* objectives? *Arch Pediatr Adolesc Med* 156(5): 431, 2002.

Rockett H et al: Validation of a youth/adolescent food frequency questionnaire, *Prevent Med* 26:808, 1997.

Sacks FM et al: Effects on blood pressure of reduced dietary sodium and the dietary approaches to stop hypertension (DASH) diet. DASH-Sodium Collaborative Research Group, *N Engl J Med* 344(1):3, 2001.

Sanders TA: Vegetarian diets and children, *Pediatr Clin North Am* 42(4):955, 1995.

Scholl TO et al: Maternal growth and fetal growth: pregnancy course and outcome in the Camden Study, *Ann NY Acad Sci* 817:292, 1997.

Sigman-Grant M: Strategies for counseling adolescents, *J Am Diet Assoc* 102(3 suppl):S32, 2002.

Slemenda CW et al: Influence on skeletal mineralization in children and adolescents: evidence for varying effects of sexual maturation and physical activity, *J Pediatr* 125:201, 1994.

Stang J: Assessment of nutritional status and motivation to make behavior changes among adolescents, *J Am Diet Assoc* 102 (3 suppl):S13, 2002.

Stang J et al: Relationships between vitamin and mineral supplement use, dietary intake, and dietary adequacy among adolescents, *J Am Diet Assoc* 100(8):905, 2000.

Steen SN: Timely statement of The American Dietetic Association: nutrition guidance for adolescent athletes in organized sports, *J Am Diet Assoc* 96(6):611, 1996.

Story M et al, editors: *Bright futures in practice: nutrition,* Arlington, Va, National Center for Education in Maternal and Child Health, 2002a.

Story M et al: Individual and environmental influences on adolescent eating behaviors, *J Am Diet Assoc* 102(3 Suppl): S40, 2002b.

Subar AF et al: Dietary sources of nutrients among U.S. children, 1989-1991, *Pediatrics* 102(4 Pt 1):913, 1998.

Tanner J: *Growth at adolescence,* Oxford, 1962, Blackwell Scientific Publications.

U.S. Council of Economic Advisors: *Teens and their parents in the 21st century: an examination of trends in teen behavior and the role of parental involvement,* Council of Economic Advisors White Paper, May 2000, http://clinton3.nara.gov/WH/EOP/CEA/html/Teens_Paper_Final.pdf, accessed December 17, 2001.

U.S. Public Health Service: *Physical activity and health: a report of the Surgeon General.* Washington, DC, 1996, U.S. Dept. of Health and Human Services, Centers for Disease Control and Prevention, National Center for Chronic Disease Prevention and Health Promotion; President's Council on Physical Fitness and Sports, pp xvii, 278.

van Dam RM et al: The relationship between overweight in adolescence and premature death in women, *Ann Intern Med* 145:91, 2006.

Williams CL et al: Management of childhood obesity in pediatric practice, *Ann N Y Acad Sci* 817:225, 1997.

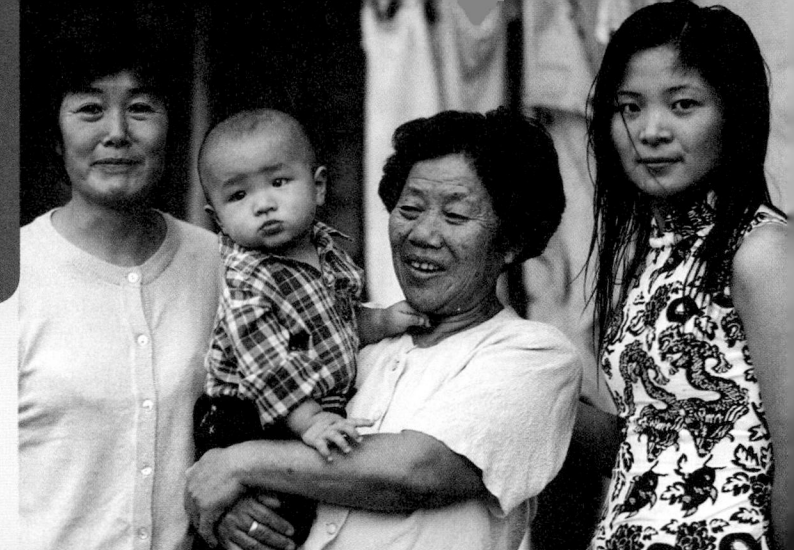

CHAPTER 9

Judith L. Dodd, MS, RD, FADA

Nutrition in the Adult Years

KEY TERMS

carotenoids a subclass of phytochemicals found in fruits and vegetables

flavonoids pigments that act as free radical scavengers in plants, may contribute to maintenance of heart health; boost antioxidant defenses

food security access by individuals to a readily available supply of nutritionally adequate and safe foods and an ensured ability to acquire acceptable foods

functional foods foods with demonstrated health benefits beyond that of basic nutrition

health-related quality of life (HRQOL) a person or group's perceived physical and mental health over time; a concept used to measure the effects on patients or clients of chronic illness or short- or long-term disabilities or illness

insulin resistance cellular resistance to insulin that results in hyperinsulinemia, or excess insulin secretion by the body in an attempt to regulate blood sugar

isoflavones phytoestrogens that may contribute to bone health; boost the immune system

lycopene one of the carotenoid phytochemicals; appears to act as a free radical scavenger

metabolic syndrome a cluster of metabolic disorders, including type 2 diabetes mellitus, hypertension, and dyslipidemia, that is characterized by insulin resistance

phytochemicals (plant chemicals) or **phytonutrients** biologically active, naturally existing substances in plants that act as natural defense systems in plants and show potential in humans for reducing risk for cardiovascular disease, cancer, and other disease states

phytoestrogens phytochemicals that are nonsteroidal estrogens; present in foods such as soy products

prebiotics nondigestible food products that stimulate the growth of bacteria already present in the colon; may improve gastrointestinal health

probiotics microbial foods or supplements that can be used to change or reestablish the intestinal flora

wellness the process of being aware of and actively working toward better health

Wellness Councils of America (WELCOA) a national non-profit organization that promotes healthier lifestyles with emphasis on adults in worksites

Sections of this chapter were written by Kimberly Mathai, MS, RD, CN, for the previous edition of this text.

SETTING THE STAGE: NUTRITION IN THE ADULT YEARS

This chapter emphasizes the background and tools for encouraging adults to set nutrition-related lifestyle goals that promote positive health and reduce risk factors. Other chapters of this text provide in-depth information about the major chronic diseases and conditions that affect the food and nutrition choices in the adult years, including cardiovascular disease (CVD), diabetes, cancer, weight control, and osteoporosis. The focus in the adult years is on assisting adults in achieving and maintaining a state of positive health or "wellness" and in making lifestyle choices to achieve the goals outlined in *Healthy People 2010* (USDHHS, 2000; CDC, 2006a).

Targeted here are nutrition- and food-related behaviors for the years following adolescence but before one is eligible to be deemed an older adult, often defined as age 65. Admittedly this is a large age span, and, like all population groups, it is heterogeneous. There are some guides and markers that the nutrition and health professional can use to meet this population's needs. The dietary reference intakes (DRIs) on the inside cover of this text provide an overview of the nutrient levels and age-groups under the DRI umbrella (see Chapter 12). Nutrient needs are similar but, as in all life stages, are affected by gender, state of health, medications, and lifestyle choices such as eating behaviors, smoking, and activity. These are markers that can be determined through assessment. Other markers are less evident and include the adult's perceptions of quality of life and motivation in the areas of nutrition and health.

A first step for dietetic and health professionals is to recognize that large segments of adults are prime targets for nutrition and health information that offers positive guidance. As with any group, adults need to be approached with information and interventions that fit their health and education needs. The American Dietetic Association (ADA) Trends survey offers some insights. This study surveyed a representative sampling of adult Americans on food, nutrition, and activity messages and their reactions to these messages. Because this survey was conducted every 2 years for 12 years, it provides a picture of the attitudes about the importance of nutrition and activity. In 2002 38% of Americans believed they had made significant adjustments in achieving a healthful and nutritious diet, an increase of 10% from the 2000 survey. Thirty percent of respondents fell into a group ADA Trends labeled as "I Know I Should, but . . . ," a drop from 40% in 2000. The remaining 32% of the respondents were in the group labeled as "Don't Bother Me." At one point in the life of the survey this group had been at a high of 40% (ADA, 2002a).

Surveys such as ADA Trends support the idea that an increasing number of adults, more females than males, are seeking nutrition information and using it to make positive lifestyle changes, and more recent information continues to support the message that adults are on a positive path. In a recent survey almost 70% of 30,000 U.S. adults said that they are trying to eat healthier foods. Almost half are looking for nutrition value and have an ongoing concern about controlling calories (Dornblaster, 2006).

A casual review of the health and nutrition information in magazines and on television reinforces the idea that nutrition and health information is "in," but consumers are selective about their personal concerns. The International Food Information Council (IFIC) Foundation Food & Health Survey (IFIC Foundation, 2006) noted that three quarters of consumers describe their overall health status in positive terms, but only 54% stated that they are satisfied with their overall health. When asked to rate the influence of diet, weight, and physical activity on their health, 92% identified physical activity and weight as independent factors affecting their perceptions of health. Eighty-nine percent included diet (food, beverages, and supplements) as another factor. Fifty-four percent described their diets as healthful but identified some areas of concern. Nearly two thirds noted that they are somewhat or very concerned about the amount and type of fat they eat, but nearly half indicated they are not trying to increase or decrease the amount. On the issue of carbohydrates, about 75% noted that they are trying to consume more fiber and whole grains (IFIC, 2006).

A 2006 Harris Poll further identified that messages regarding the potential benefits and risks of certain foods and nutrients are being heard by consumers. Messages such as the negative impact of saturated fat, *trans*-fatty acids, and sodium are acknowledged by consumers. In addition, two in five adults say they will eat more whole grains this year and will increase the fiber in their diets because of the messages they are hearing. Seventy-nine percent noted that they believe there is a link between mental acuity and their diets (Harris Interactive Poll, 2006). When it comes to eating for nutrition, more than half of the most successful new consumer products offered "better-for-you" benefits in 2006. There is a demand for foods marketed as healthful, and also there is a demand for creating and marketing foods that fit this image (Sloan, 2006).

Where consumers get their information is another factor to consider. Both the source and the message affect the scientific value, but to the adult consumer the promise of specific benefits is likely to be more important than the standard "it's good for you" message. The ADA Trends identified that television and magazines are major sources of food and nutrition information for adults. Although the Internet was noted less frequently, indications are that it is increasing in popularity, especially in the adult population ages 25 to 34 and among college graduates (ADA, 2002a). Ninety-three percent of consumers are using the labels on foods and beverages, including both the Nutrition Facts panel and other label information, to get health information. Nearly nine in ten consumers have some knowledge of the USDA-promoted MyPyramid. However, of those who know about this tool, only two in ten report customizing their diet using the MyPyramid website. There are opportunities for change by helping consumers use these tools (IFIC, 2006).

Frequently mainstream adults are ignored as a unique segment of the population needing a positive message. Preventive strategies are likely to be targeted to address the formative years of prenatal, infancy, childhood, adolescence, and young adulthood. The older adult group is likely to be targeted with health intervention strategies and quality of life messages. But the population group in the middle of the continuum, the adult age 25 to about 65, is likely to be segmented in reference to a disease state, a life event, or a lifestyle choice. For example, adults are targeted as having or being at risk for diabetes or heart disease, in need of a medication, or being pregnant or an athlete.

The adult who is not pregnant or an athlete or "sick" and who is seeking guidance on normal nutrition or prevention may be directed toward diets for chronic disease or weight loss. Such information may be a good fit when the information is based on science. Fortunately the guidance provided by such groups as the American Heart Association (AHA), the ADA, the American Diabetes Association, and the American Cancer Society (ACS) mirror what is promoted in the Nutrition and Health: Dietary Guidelines for Americans (DGA), with the AHA releasing new guidelines in 2006 (Lichtenstein et al., 2006). Adults are prime targets for information on chronic disease prevention and weight management; however, the messages may appear to be conflicting and less sensational than advice promising quick solutions. In spite of this, Health 2006, a report on U.S. health status, suggests that health education and public health programs, along with improved research and care, have contributed to changes in morbidity and mortality of the adult population (Health, 2006). It appears that U.S. adults are on a path to positive change that needs to be continued (i.e., moving from knowledge to action) (National Center for Health Statistics NCHS, 2004).

Adults in the awareness and action stages are likely to be looking for answers, often short-term fixes or reversals of a health problem. Which is best—low carb or high carb? What's the message on fat and are there "good fats?" What is a "healthy" or "unhealthy" food or diet? Guidance based on science generally addresses total diet and lifestyle rather than single nutrients or foods. The concepts of *healthful eating*, *nutrient density*, and *nutritious food* are being defined and debated by food and nutrition professionals (Drewnowski, 2005). Unfortunately these debates are fodder for media coverage, adding to the confusion and perception of mixed messages.

But adults are a population group with both the interest and the ability to seek out their own resources and answers. A search for information on choosing foods for health can result in evidence-based information such as the DGA, as well as questionable guidance based on single studies or product promotion. The combination of marketing and electronic media makes it easier to mix science with speculation and outright untruths. Adults with an interest in improving the nutritional quality of their diet may end up with incredible advice pointing to supplements or quick-fix solutions or products.

Consider the adult years as a time for health promotion, health maintenance, and disease prevention, along with the interventions that accompany the progression of chronic disease that can come with aging. It is a time for adults to take responsibility and control. The Food and Health Survey (IFIC, 2006) is the first in what is intended to be a series of benchmark studies that will provide a snapshot of consumer attitudes on food and health and provide the dietetic and health professional the information on "hot buttons" or issues of importance to consumers (IFIC, 2006). Examining this and other surveys targeting adults is critical to presenting relevant information and also initiating and reinforcing positive nutrition and health behaviors.

In 2005 the U.S. Surgeon General, Vice Admiral Richard H. Carmona, recommended:

> As a society, we can no longer afford to make poor health choices such as being physically inactive and eating an unhealthy diet; these choices have led to a tremendous obesity epidemic. As policy makers and health professionals, we must embrace small steps toward coordinated policy and environmental changes that will help Americans live longer, better, healthier lives.

THE WELLNESS YEARS

The adult years are a broad span chronologically and, like all life cycle phases, are complicated by physiologic, developmental, and social factors. Along with their genetic and social history, adults have accumulated the results of behaviors and risks from environmental factors. These factors shape the heterogeneity of the adult years. Nonetheless, the adult years are an ideal time for conveying a positive health promotion and disease prevention message. The DGA provide the framework for nutrition and health guidance, including guidance on physical activity (USDHHS, USDA, 2005a). The MyPyramid food guidance system adds more information that supports a positive and balanced message (USDA, 2005) (see Chapter 12).

These years are frequently a time of an epiphany, a sudden realization regarding one's own health. In the transitions from adolescence to early and then middle adulthood, health and wellness can take on a new importance. This may be the result of a life event or education, and the result is a triggering of an awareness that being well and staying well are important. Examples are: learning the results of a screening for blood pressure, cholesterol, or diabetes; facing the reality of death; the self-reflecting that comes when personal health or that of a peer or family member is in crisis; or realizing that clothes don't fit as well as they should. Regardless of the reason, the concept of wellness takes on a new meaning, and in the health educator's mind these events are teachable moments in which to place an accent on wellness.

Wellness, or being well, can be defined as an absence of disease, a classic but limiting definition. A more encompassing explanation is that of the **Wellness Councils of America (WELCOA),** in which wellness is described as a process that involves being aware of better health and actively working toward that goal (WELCOA, 2003). With this mindset, a state of wellness can exist at any age and can start at any point in a person's health status.

In this context wellness is more than physical health and well-being. A state of well-being includes mental and spiritual health and encompasses the ability of a person to move through Maslow's Hierarchy of Needs (Maslow, 1970). The ability to address nutrition needs within this hierarchy and engage in prevention includes having **food security** (i.e., access to a safe, acceptable and adequate source of food).

It is estimated that approximately 23 million adults and 13 million children in America live in households where there is food insecurity (Alaimo, 2005); the highest levels of food insecurity are in black and Hispanic households (CDC, 2006b). Household food insecurity in Canada is also considered to be a serious public health concern (Tarasuk, 2005). *Healthy People 2010* addresses this issue (Objective 19-18: Increase food security among U.S. households) as a part of the strategies to improve overall nutrition (CDC, 2006a, 2006b).

Participation in the Food Stamp Program is a marker of food insecurity, and one study notes that slightly over half of all Americans between the ages of 20 and 65 will at some point receive food stamps, a suggestion of the risk for food insecurity in the adult years (Rank and Hirschl, 2005). The issue of food insecurity has a special concern for women because of the role women typically have as food managers of the family. In 2003 as many as 14 million women were food insecure. Adults are known to make trades-offs between their own and their children's health, thus raising the risk that the adult woman in a food-insecure family is likely to compromise her own nutrition to meet the needs of her children (Olson, 2005). On a more global basis, a 2005 report by the Food and Agriculture Organization of the United Nations (FAO) summarizes the concerns for hunger and food security (FAO, 2005). In working with adults, food security must be appraised and addressed before attempting to set nutrition goals.

Taking the concept of wellness forward, it is important to consider that one's perceptions of personal health (both mental and physical) relate to views on wellness and perceptions of quality of life. **Health-related quality of life (HRQOL)** is a concept that can be used to measure the effects of current health conditions on a person's day-to-day life. To capture this and create a tool for professionals, the Centers for Disease Control and Prevention (CDC) measures population health-related quality of life perceptions, including the perception of "feeling healthy."

The CDC Behavioral Risk Factor Surveillance System from 1993 to 2003 revealed that adults overall reported that they felt unhealthy (physically or mentally) about 6 days a month and felt healthy and "full of energy" about 19 days a month. Those with chronic diseases and disabilities reported higher numbers of unhealthy days. Adults in lower socioeconomic levels or with less education reported more unhealthy days. Persons with existing CVD reported an average of 10 unhealthy days in the prior month compared to 5 unhealthy days in those without CVD. Adults with diabetes reported similar differences (CDC, 2000). Since one of the goals of the nutrition and health professional is to encourage a person to make a change or take action, recognizing these perceptions of the quality of life can help remove barriers and plan for interventions.

The adult years offer unique opportunities to evaluate health status, build on the positive, and change or reposition the negative factors that will affect the quality of life. A positive wellness focus can affect the health of not only the adult but also those whom they influence. Since adults are teachers, coaches, parents, caregivers, and worksite leaders, targeting the wellness-related attitudes and behaviors of adults has the potential of a multiplier effect.

NUTRITION-RELATED RISK FACTORS

Even when the emphasis is on wellness, there is a strong link to risk factors that influence morbidity and mortality. In the United States the leading causes of death and debilitation among adults include (1) heart disease, (2) cancer, (3) cerebrovascular disease, (4) chronic lung disease, and (5) diabetes (CDC, 2005a). Chronic diseases, including heart disease, stroke, cancer, and diabetes, are among the most costly and preventable of all health problems and account for one third of the years of potential life lost before age 65 and for 75% of the nation's medical care costs (CDC, 2004). Four of these chronic diseases have links to diet and lifestyle, including CVD, diabetes, certain cancers, and osteoporosis (see Chapters 32, 30, 37, and 24, respectively). Three precursors to these diseases (i.e., hypertension, hyperlipidemia, and elevated blood glucose) are often seen together with or without obesity and referred to as the metabolic syndrome (see *Clinical Insight: The Metabolic Syndrome*).

An overarching concern in all of the major chronic disease states is the relationship each has to unhealthy weight. Overweight in adults (body mass index (BMI) of 25 to 29) and obesity (BMI of 30 and above) is a major risk factor in both the prevention and the control of heart disease, stroke, diabetes, and more recently breast cancer. It is estimated that 65% of adults over age 20 are overweight or obese. This number has increased by more than 75% since 1991 (AHA and ASA, 2005) (see Chapter 21).

The achievement of a healthy weight has other implications. On the other end of the spectrum from obesity and overweight is chronic underweight, frequently accompanied by undernutrition. Anorexia nervosa is the extreme condition, a form of self-starvation that is more likely to affect young women but a condition found in both genders across the age span. An unhealthy weight or unhealthy concern about body weight not only affects overall health but in women can also affect fertility and the ability to conceive and is important to assess in the adult years (see Chapter 22).

The Metabolic Syndrome

The **metabolic syndrome** is a cluster of metabolic disorders most likely to be recognized in midlife and includes high fasting blood glucose levels, hypertension, dyslipidemia, and abdominal obesity. However, metabolic syndrome may also develop without the presence of a high body mass index. It is estimated that approximately 47 million people in the United States have metabolic syndrome (Ford et al., 2002).

A major factor in metabolic syndrome is a defect in glucose metabolism; **insulin resistance,** cellular resistance to insulin that results in hyperinsulinemia; or excess insulin secretion by the body in an attempt to regulate blood sugar (Figure 9-1).

Originally defined by Gerald Reaven, MD, it was initially known as syndrome X. Several groups, including the World Health Organization and the American Heart Association have defined metabolic syndrome as a risk factor, but not all experts agree on the definitions.

Intervention is a combination of increasing exercise; reducing body fat if necessary; and making dietary choices that are low in fat, meet goals for fiber, meet the dietary reference intakes (IOM, 1998–2004) for all minerals and vitamins, and include complex carbohydrates with limited added sugar.

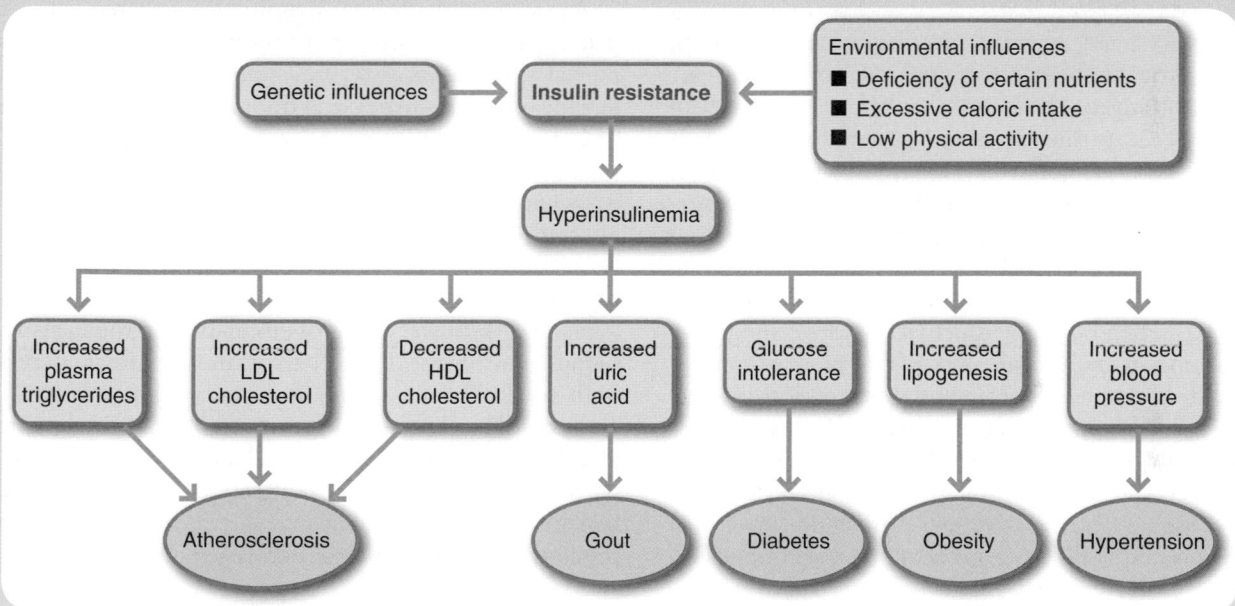

FIGURE 9-1 Pathophysiologic etiology of insulin resistance and the metabolic syndrome.

Another area targeted in *Healthy People 2010*, the DGA 2005, and MyPyramid is physical activity. Over the last 20 years there has been an increase in obesity and overweight, an issue with a direct link to calorie imbalance. It is estimated that only 44% of U.S. adults participate in regular physical activity, with 26% reporting no activity. Many of the health risks in the adult years, including coronary artery disease, certain types of cancer, hypertension, type 2 diabetes, and osteoporosis have a relationship to lack of participation in regular physical activity and poor eating behaviors. Physical activity also plays a role in managing mild-to-moderate depression and anxiety. One cannot achieve positive health without a combination of physical activity and food choices that fit personal needs for energy balance and nutrition.

Nutrition-related lifestyle choices, including activity, lay the framework for health and wellness. The health of people

living in the United States has continued to improve over the past 50 years in part because of education that has led to lifestyle changes. Life expectancy has continued to increase (projected at 77.4 years), and the morbidity and mortality rate from heart disease, cancer, and stroke has dropped (NCHS, 2004).

Implementation of *Healthy People 2010* goals is based in part on eliminating disparities that increase the health risks for affected populations. Such disparities are related to access to health care, race and ethnicity, gender, education, income level, and geographic location. Access to care is a disparity that has a major effect on a person's ability to attain wellness. Males of working age are nearly twice as likely as females to have no usual source of health care (NCHS, 2004). Chronic diseases and obesity have been shown to be more of a burden to racial minorities and women (CDC, 2004).

There is a higher incidence of heart disease, diabetes, and obesity or overweight in low-income, black, and Hispanic populations (AHA and ASA, 2005). These same population groups have limited access to preventive care, nutrition education, and guidance (USDHHS, 2000). Food insecurity and limited access to healthful foods are also disparities; usually it is more expensive to eat healthy foods than less healthy, high-calorie foods (Drewnowski, 2004; AHA and ASA, 2005). Limited skills in the areas of wise food purchasing and food preparation coupled with limited resources (both food and equipment) further complicate a person's ability to follow advice for a healthy lifestyle. This puts emphasis on adult consumer education in basic food skills. Although this chapter mainly addresses adults in the United States, the problems associated with chronic diseases are similar in other developed countries (WHO, 2003).

Emphasis: Women's Health

Combined with Canada, women comprise over 150 million, and 33% to 40% of them are in their reproductive years (ADA, 2001). Many of the issues that affect the health of women are related to the monthly hormonal shifts associated with menses. Osteoporosis, heart disease, and some cancers are disease states that are affected by specific hormones. Pregnancy and breast-feeding also have an effect on a woman's health (see Chapter 5). New research is linking the potential benefits of weight stability, lowered risk for diabetes, and better bone health, that breast-feeding may have for a woman (Stuebe et al., 2005). Therefore encouraging women to breast-feed is a potential prevention strategy for the future health of both the mother and her infant (see Figure 5-9).

Shifts of the hormones estrogen and progesterone that trigger the female reproductive cycle affect the health of women. Associated with menses is a complex set of physical and psychological symptoms known as *premenstrual syndrome (PMS)*. Reported symptoms vary but are described as general discomfort, anxiety, depression, fatigue, breast pain, and cramping. Such symptoms are reported to occur approximately a week to 10 days before the onset of menses and increase in severity into menses. Currently there is no single cause or intervention identified for PMS. Hormone imbalance, neurotransmitter synthesis defects, and low levels of certain nutrients (i.e., vitamin B_6 and calcium) have been implicated. Studies show that women supplemented with either of these nutrients reported better management of PMS than those receiving a placebo; but the size of the studies, along with other variables, limits the ability to make definitive recommendations (Wyatt et al., 1999; Thys-Jacobs et al., 1998; NIH and ODS, 2005). A diet high in sodium and refined rather than complex carbohydrates has also been reported to be associated with symptoms of PMS, but again the evidence is not complete enough to make recommendations (NIH and ODS, 2005). However, analysis of their diets and counseling of women to obtain adequate dietary levels of all nutrients, along with greater emphasis on a plant-based diet of whole grains, fruits, vegetables, lean or low fat protein sources, and low fat dairy or soy beverages, are reasonable interventions. Exercise and activity, including relaxation techniques, have also been reported as lessening the symptoms.

When menses end, either because of age or surgical removal of reproductive organs, women have special health and nutrition concerns. Peri-menopause and menopause generally begin in the late forties, although genetics, general health, and the age that menses began alter the timing of this marker. These are the signals of the end of the reproductive years and subsequent changes in hormonal balance. Typically estrogen production decreases around age 50. Endogenous estrogen circulation decreases approximately 60%, and the effects are a cessation of menses and the loss of the healthful benefits of estrogen. Even after the ovaries cease production, some estrogen, a weaker form, continues to be produced by the adrenal glands, and some is stored in adipose tissue (Barrett-Connor et al., 2002).

As estrogen decreases, symptoms associated with menopause may occur. Both the onset of menopause and the reported side effects vary. For some women it is a gradual decline in the frequency and duration of menses, whereas in others it is an abrupt cessation. The symptoms most often reported include low energy levels and vasomotor symptoms known as hot flashes. Bone, heart, and brain health are affected. The decrease in circulating estrogen limits the body's ability to remodel bones, the natural process of bone turnover. This can result in a decrease of bone mass (see Chapter 24). Lower levels of circulating estrogen also affect blood lipid levels. The result is the potential increase of both total cholesterol and low-density lipoprotein (LDL) cholesterol levels and a decrease in high-density lipoprotein (HDL) cholesterol levels (see Chapter 32). Brain function, particularly memory, is also affected; the negative changes may be postponed or alleviated, depending on the timing of the hormonal therapy (MacLennan et al., 2006).

Managing menopause using dietary means points to emphasis on plant-based foods for the potential benefits of phytoestrogens, soluble fiber, and other components, which may help to add to the regulation of blood cholesterol (see Chapter 32). Having sufficient calcium, vitamin D, vitamin K, and magnesium, using the DRI as the guideline, is important to protecting bone health (see Chapter 24). The benefits of plant estrogens such as those found in soy (isoflavones) continue to be suggested by the popular press as a way to control hot flashes (Table 9-1). At the current time research is still exploring the validity of these suggestions. Since additional weight gain is reported by some women, balance of food intake and activity and choices of nutrient-dense foods low in fat are general guidelines. Physical activity, including aerobic endeavors and both resistance and weight-bearing exercise, becomes preventive for bone health, cardiovascular health, and emotional health as well as being a way to balance calories and manage weight.

Emphasis: Men's Health

The leading causes of death among American men include heart disease, prostate cancer, and lung cancer. For the adult male a diet that supports reducing the risk for heart disease

TABLE 9-1

Functional Components in Foods

Carotenoids	
β-carotene	May neutralize free radicals that damage cells, boost antioxidant defenses
Lutein	Much discovered about its role in protecting the eyes from oxidation; also being investigated for potentially reducing the risk of colon, breast, lung, and skin cancer (www.luteininfo.com)
Lycopene	Protects prostrate health by reducing risk of prostate cancer; may also aid in preserving bone health
Diallyl sulfides	Along with promoting heart health, boosts production of enzymes that benefit the immune system
Ellagic acid	May block body's production of enzymes needed for tumor growth; causes cancer cell death in the test tube; functions as antioxidant; possible antiviral and antibacterial activities

Flavonoids	
Anthocyanins	Most studied; may neutralize free radicals, bolster antioxidant defenses, especially at the DNA level; contributes to heart health and vision and brain function by reducing oxidation of LDL cholesterol
Lignans	Acting as phytoestrogens, may boost immune function and contribute to maintaining heart health; may also help block some hormone related cancers
Limonene	Boosts levels of naturally occurring liver enzymes involved in detoxification of carcinogens
Phytic acid	May suppress oxidation reactions in the colon that produce free radicals; reduces rate of starch digestion and thus blood glycemic response; converted to related compounds in body involved in cellular communication; may be effective in slowing tumor growth
Proanthrocyandins (also called condensed tannins or procyanidins)	The active component of cranberries that contributes to urinary tract health but may also have a role in heart health
Omega-3 fatty acids	Along with being beneficial to heart health by decreasing blood clotting and preventing arrhythmias, these may contribute to mental and physical functioning
Phenols	May boost antioxidant defense while maintaining healthy vision
Phytoestrogens	Genistein and diadzein; may contribute to healthy bones, brain function, and immune function; relationship of phytoestrogens and cancers is still being debated
Plant stanols/sterols	May help bolster the benefits of a hear-healthy diet with exercise, thus reducing the risk of heart disease
Prebiotics	Nondigestible food ingredients such as dietary fibers that provide food for gut bacteria to grow on; may improve gastrointestinal health and immune function; inulin and oligofructose are the most commonly studied prebiotics
Probiotics	Beneficial bacteria that improve gastrointestinal health and may improve calcium absorption
Sulphoraphane	An isothiocynate that stimulates body to produce protective phase II enzymes; neutralizes free radicals; potential anticancer substance
Organosulfuric compounds	Believed to fight cancer cell growth; may be useful in treating arthritic joints

is especially important because males develop heart disease at a younger age than women (see Chapter 32). Regular exercise and activity are important. Along with contributing to cardiovascular health, weight-bearing exercise has a positive effect on bone health.

Of special interest is research on the benefits of certain phytochemicals, especially **lycopene,** a carotenoid that acts as a free radical scavenger, and its potential to reduce risk for heart disease and prostrate cancer (Rao and Agarwal, 2000) (see Chapter 37). In one study men with the lowest serum lycopene levels had a three times' higher risk of hav-

ing an acute coronary event or a stroke (Rissanen et al., 2001). Gianetti concluded that lycopene helped prevent atherosclerosis (Gianetti et al., 2002) (see Chapter 32). In a study of almost 48,000 health care professionals, researchers found that the subjects who reported the highest level of dietary lycopene had a 16% reduction in prostate cancer (Giovannucci et al., 2002). Recommendations are to include tomato products, a source of lycopene in the diet, and that the tomato products should be cooked and eaten with fat so that the lycopene will be more bioavailable (Millen and Quatromoni, 2001). Along with tomatoes,

TABLE 9-2

Dietary Sources of Functional Components

Functional Components	Food Sources
Carotenoids	
β-carotene	Carrots, dark orange fruits, butternut squash, cantaloupe
Lutein	Deep green vegetables, kale, spinach, collards, corn, eggs, citrus
Lycopene	Processed tomato products, guava, pink grapefruit, watermelon
Diallyl sulfides	Onions, garlic, scallions, leeks, chives
Ellagic acids	Strawberries, raspberries, pomegranates, cranberries, walnuts
Fatty acids: omega-3	Foods qualifying for a label claim of "high" source of omega-3
α-linolenic acid	Flax seeds, flax oil, walnuts, canola oil, soybean oil, Atlantic salmon, sardines in oil
Eicosapentaenoic acid	Herring, Coho salmon and wild Atlantic salmon, blue fin tuna, sardines in oil, striped bass, and sea bass
Docosahexaenoic acid	Atlantic salmon, blue fin tuna, herring, Coho salmon, striped bass, mackerel, sea bass, omega-3–enriched eggs
Flavonoids	Berries, (especially dark-colored), cherries, red grapes, tea (especially green tea), cocoa, coffee, onions, apples
Isothiocyanates	Cabbage, cauliflower, broccoli, Brussels sprouts, horseradish
Lignans	Flax seed, rye, some vegetables
Limonene	Essential oils of citrus fruits and other plants
Organosulfuric compounds	Garlic, onions, chives, citrus fruits, broccoli, cabbage, cauliflower, Brussels sprouts
Phenols	Apples, pears, citrus fruits, parsley, carrots, broccoli, cabbage, cucumbers, squash, yams, tomatoes
Phytic acid (inositol)	Wheat bran, flax seed, sesame seeds, beans and other high fiber foods
Phytoestrogens	
Isoflavones Daidzein, Genistein	Soybeans, soybean products
Plant stanols/sterols	Corn, soy, wheat, fortified foods, beverages, fortified table spreads, fortified chocolate, peanut oil
Prebiotics	Whole grains (especially oatmeal), flax and barley; greens; berries, bananas, and other fruits; legumes; onions, garlic, honey, leeks
Proanthocyandins	Cranberries, cocoa, cinnamon, peanuts, wine, grapes, strawberries, peanut skins
Probiotics	Yogurt (with active, live culture), kefir, buttermilk and other fermented dairy products; fermented vegetables such as kim chi and sauerkraut; and fermented soy products such as miso and tempeh
Soy potein	Soybeans, soy products
Synbiotics	Innovative food products containing both a prebiotic and a probiotic

pink grapefruit, watermelon, and guava are sources of lycopene (Table 9-2).

Another issue in adult men is iron intake. Unless adult men are diagnosed with iron deficiency anemia and require additional iron, they should not get additional iron from multivitamin-mineral supplements and enriched sports or energy bars or drinks. Excessive iron intake is problematic because excessive iron in the body functions as an oxidant in the body, and men and postmenopausal women do not have menstruation, pregnancy, or lactation to get rid of excess iron. A certain percentage of the population (much more prevalent in men than women) carries the genetic variant for hemochromatosis and iron overload, and in this situation iron is particularly dangerous (see Chapter 31).

IMPLEMENTATION: NUTRITION AND PREVENTION

Adults are in the ideal life cycle phase for health promotion and disease prevention nutrition advice because of the combination of life experience and influence. This group has the potential to shape personal lifestyle choices and influence those of others. The tools are in place, including the DGA, MyPyramid, and the Nutrition Facts panel on food labels (IFIC, 2004). Alternative patterns exist to support those who choose to be vegetarian or vegan (ADA and Dietitians of Canada, 2003).

Implementation of positive choices and moving people along the continuum of a healthy life style is another issue.

Studies support that most consumers are aware of the concerns associated with lifestyle and diet (IFIC, 2006). They are also aware of the implied promises for good health that come with many of the messages in circulation by the media, friends, and health professionals. However, they are unlikely to move from awareness to action without motivation stronger than another promise (IFIC, 2005). ADA Trends indicated a similar message from consumers who had yet to commit to a healthier lifestyle. When asked why they hadn't made the decision, concerns centered on not wanting to give up the foods they liked and on the fear that food that was healthy didn't taste good (ADA, 2002a). Focusing on a total diet approach of making gradual changes of food and lifestyle choices may help to reduce these obstacles (ADA, 2002b). The Small Step Program available through the U.S. Department of Health and Human Services is an example of such an approach in a simple Internet-based program (USDHHS, 2006). America on the Move is another program that puts emphasis on achievable goals while maintaining calorie balance through small changes.

However, the steps to prevention and health promotion, even when small, are personal responsibilities that cannot be legislated. Americans have many choices: what and where they eat, where they receive their information, and what they include in or remove from their lifestyle. Adults in our culture value choice: it is a right, even if it leads to poor health, chronic disease, or death.

Some issues associated with implementation of healthy choices are related to reaching adults where they live and work. The United States and other developed countries are mobile societies, and for the working adult populations much of the day is tied to a work site. There are increasing efforts in both the private and public sectors to promote positive nutrition-related behaviors for adults.

The U.S. Department of Health and Human Services report, *Prevention Makes Common "Cents,"* summarizes some of the major health issues that affect working adults, including overweight and obesity, diabetes, CVD, and asthma, noting that expenditures for U.S. health care continue to rise and much of the cost includes care of the ill worker and loss of work and productivity. Much less is spent on preventing than on diagnosis and treatment, even as there is accumulating evidence that much of the morbidity and mortality associated with these chronic diseases may be preventable through behavior and lifestyle choices (USDHHS, 2003).

FOOD TRENDS AND PATTERNS

Where one eats, who prepares it, and how much is consumed are all patterns of behavior and choice. There is no stereotypic "adult" when it comes to lifestyles. Adults may be single or partnered, with or without children, working outside the home or at home. The sit-down family meals at home have given way to eating on the run, take out, and drive through. Too little time for planning or preparation and limited cooking skills can lead to reliance on processed foods, speed-scratch cooking (combining processed with fresh ingredients), or more food prepared out of the home. Meal planning, shopping, and preparation traditionally fall to the female in the household, but more men are getting involved in these tasks (ADA, 2002b). For the health professional working with adults, this means that both males and females need to be part of the education.

It is estimated that Americans spend up to 46% of their food dollars away from home, which is up from 27% in 1962 (Variyam, 2005) and is 58% greater than away-from-home expenditures in 1992 (Stewart et al., 2004). These changing food patterns and the use of more processed and purchased foods result in an increase of foods higher in sodium, added fat and sweeteners, and a decrease in use of basic foods such as fruits, vegetables and whole grains. Portion sizes (either the amount presented or the amount chosen to eat) replace serving sizes (what is recommended as a serving by the DGA or other source), as others determine what is considered a meal or snack. Portions have become unreasonably large, as evidenced from using the tool "Portion Distortion" available at http://hin.nhlbi.nih.gov/portion/keep.htm.

Dietary changes have affected nutrition and are already reflected in the current concerns for weight and nutrient imbalances. The DGA 2005 and MyPyramid can be viewed as attempts to put more emphasis on basic, nutrient-dense rather than calorie-dense foods and total amounts of foods per day rather than numbers of servings.

So what are Americans eating? Historically the U.S. Department of Agriculture (USDA) Economic Research Service (ERS) collected and disseminated information on food consumption patterns (USDA, 2004b). This information is now being blended with information from MyPyramid (Food and Drug Association [FDA]) Health and Diet Survey and other studies to provide nutrition professionals with a snapshot of what American adults are eating. Although more food is prepared away from home than in the past, in a typical week most meals are still consumed at home. When asked how many meals were eaten away from home (including food prepared away-from home), 14% of the respondents reported none; 45%, one to three; and 26%, 4 to 7 per week (FDA, 2005).

Imbalance in the diet becomes apparent from examining USDA reports. Based on food consumption studies from 1985 to 2000, the average American dietary style is described as an hour glass rather than a pyramid (Putnam et al., 2002). Large portions of pasta and grains (mostly refined) on the bottom and generous amounts of fat and sugar at the top squeeze out the foods in the middle, especially fruits, vegetables, and low-fat dairy foods. Between 1985 and 2000 there was a jump in average daily calorie intake of 12%, an additional 300 kcal/day, and this was without the benefit of added activity or exercise (Putnam et al., 2002). By applying the estimate that each 3500 calories over basic needs can add 1 pound of body weight, one realizes that 300 added kcal a day, regardless of the food source, contributes to the Americans' propensity for weight gain.

Of the added 300 kcal a day, grain servings (mainly refined) accounted for 46%, in part due to overly generous portions. Added fats accounted for 24%, and added sugar accounted for 23% Fruits and vegetables accounted for about 8% of the additional calories, but there was a 1% decline in the calories from dairy and meat choices (Putnam et al., 2002).

Comparing trend data to the guidelines of the original Food Guide Pyramid (using a 2200-calorie diet pattern) shows that the U.S. diet has become high in refined grains and added fat and sugar and low in whole grains. The overall picture on fruits and vegetables indicates that Food Guide Pyramid number of servings recommendations are not being met and variety is limited. Five vegetables—iceberg lettuce, frozen potatoes, fresh potatoes, potato chips, and canned tomatoes—accounted for almost half of the vegetable servings. Another 19% came from dehydrated potatoes, garlic, carrots, fresh tomatoes, and fresh onions. No other vegetable accounted for more than 3% of the total number of vegetable servings. Fruit servings were also limited. Six fruits (i.e., orange juice, bananas, apple juice, fresh apples, fresh grapes, and watermelon) out of a potential 60 fruit products accounted for over 50% of the reported servings. In the meat group red meat, poultry, fish, and shellfish accounted for most of the intake. Vegetarian sources of protein such as lentils and beans, tofu, eggs, and nuts were limited. Fluid dairy food (milk) intake showed a decline while intake of cheese and yogurt increased. In 2000 two dairy group foods (cheese and whole milk) contributed half the dairy servings and 22% of the saturated fat (Putnam et al., 2002). When reviewing consumption of total fat in the diet, 56% was from added fat rather than from that found naturally in food. Shortening and margarine, major sources of *trans*-fatty acids, accounted for more than one third of the added fats (Putnam et al., 2002).

The issue of fat in the diet has many links, including amount (calories), bad types (saturated, *trans*-fat), and good types (omega-3 fats, monounsaturated) with regard to heart disease and dietary guidance. The FDA survey indicates that there is a level of recognition of the types of fat and their relationship to heart disease. Of the respondents to the Diet and Health Survey, 67% reported they had heard of *trans*-fatty acids, whereas 95% had heard of saturated fat. Sixty-one percent recognized omega-3 fatty acids as a term, and 51% of those knew that its consumption would lower the risk of heart disease. Of those who had heard of *trans*-fat, 48% were able to state that using it would raise the risk for heart disease. Seventy-eight percent of those recognizing saturated fat noted that it would raise the risk for heart disease (FDA, 2004).

As measured by consumption data, current adult diets are likely to be higher in total fat than the 30% of total calories recommended and have most carbohydrates as added sugar and refined grains; fruit and vegetable guidelines are not being met. Chicken and fish servings have increased, and animal sources outweigh plant-based protein sources. Cheese and fluid milk are the leaders in the dairy group, although the consumption of yogurt improved, whereas

milk consumption as a whole declined below the recommendations. Added fat at 65 g (equivalent to about 13 t of margarine or butter) and added caloric sweeteners with a reported intake of 31 t/day in a 2200-kcal diet were in abundance. The MyPyramid recommendation is to limit added fat to 41 g/day and added caloric sweeteners to less than 12 t/day (Putnam et al., 2002). Key nutrients that are likely to be in short supply for adults are the minerals calcium, magnesium, and potassium and vitamins A, C, and E (which play antioxidant roles in the body) (USDHHS, 2005b).

NUTRITIONAL SUPPLEMENTATION

It is the position of the ADA that the best nutritional strategy for promoting optimal health and reducing the risk of chronic disease is to wisely choose a wide variety of foods. Additional nutrients from fortified foods and/or supplements can help some people meet their nutritional needs as specified by science-based nutrition standards such as the DRI (ADA, 2005).

In making the above statement, the ADA puts food first but leaves the door open for those with nutrient needs, identified through assessment by a dietetic or health professional, to be nutritionally supplemented (ADA, 2005). Traditionally one thinks of vitamins and minerals, fiber, and protein as nutrient supplements, generally in a pill, capsule, or liquid form. The DRIs are the standards used with most adults as explained in Chapters 3 and 12 and presented on the inside cover.

However, food fortification is another form of nutrient supplementation. The level of fortified foods (such as "energy bars" or "sports drinks") in the marketplace puts another layer of potential nutrient sources in the mix with traditional supplements. Less traditional supplements such as herbals and other natural dietary "enhancers" are also added to the mix of supplementation in the marketplace and available to consumers (see Chapter 18).

Americans frequently do not meet the dietary recommendations for promoting optimal health. Several segments of the adult population fall into high-risk groups who are unlikely to meet their vitamin, mineral, or protein needs because of life stage needs (e.g., pregnancy), alcohol or drug dependency, food insecurity, chronic illness, recovery from illness, or choosing a vegan (vegetarians who eat no animal products) or nutritionally restrictive lifestyle (ADA, 2005). Other examples of persons with special needs include those with food allergies or intolerances that eliminate major food groups, persons using prescription drugs or therapies that change the way the body uses nutrients, those with disabilities that limit their ability to enjoy a varied diet, and those who are just unable or unwilling because of time or energy to prepare or consume a nutritionally adequate diet. All of these adults potentially need a nutritional supplement.

The American Medical Association (AMA) stated that all adult Americans "should consider use of a multivitamin supplement daily for chronic disease prevention" based on the fact that many Americans are not meeting the DRI for vitamins, especially the vitamins related to antioxidant function (Fletcher and Fairfield, 2002) (see Chapter 18).

From a national survey it is apparent that Americans are using supplements (ADA, 2005). Several questions come to mind when considering supplementation for adults:

1. What are their DRIs based on their health profile?
2. What is their current intake of food, including fortified foods and food-based supplements?
3. Which nutrients are likely to be compromised because of intake, lifestyle, health, or oversupplementation because of age (based on the tolerable upper limits of the DRI or decreased requirements such as iron in adult men or postmenopausal women)?
4. How can their nutritional needs be met (traditional food, fortified foods, supplements) most efficiently?

DIETARY GUIDANCE

Nutrition and Your Health: Dietary Guidelines for Americans 2005 (DGA) is the first evidence-based edition of U.S. Dietary Guidelines. Included in these guidelines is the Dietary Approaches to Stop Hypertension (DASH) Eating Plan, a healthful eating plan that incorporates much of the general guidance (see Table 33-4). A follow-up to the DGA and a companion tool is MyPyramid (see Figure 12-1); because of the excellent resources with this tool, it is more than a graphic. For adults who are Internet-savvy, there are tools that can take the basic information provided in the DGA and MyPyramid to a personal level, something that is a missing link in much general dietary guidance. For the nutrition professional, these can be accessible starting points for dietary guidance.

But nutrition professionals need to give advice beyond that found in the DGA and MyPyramid. Adherence to the DGA, measured using the USDA Healthy Eating Index (HEI), a scoring system for diet quality was associated with only a small reduction in the risks for major chronic diseases, and it was concluded that dietary guidance needs to provide more specific and comprehensive advice (McCullough et al., 2002). When more specific advice, including the health benefits of unsaturated oils and the advantages of highly colored vegetables and fruits and high-fiber whole grains, was included (the newer Alternate Healthy Eating Index AHEI), the prediction of major chronic disease risk was twice as strong as with the HEI (McCullough and Willett, 2006). This new index has been translated into the Healthy Eating Pyramid, designed by nutrition experts at Harvard School of Public Health (Willett, 2001) and is shown in Figure 9-2.

The DGA and the recommendations reflected in MyPyramid are summarized in Box 9-1 as they apply to healthy adults. See www.healthierus.gov/dietaryguidelines/ for the complete details of the DGA and MyPyramid and Chapter 12 for other guidelines for dietary planning such as the Mediterranean Pyramid (see Figure 12-4). Other chapters in this text provide disease-specific guidance for persons with chronic diseases. Ideas for counseling an adult on personalized food patterns and choices are discussed in Chapter 19.

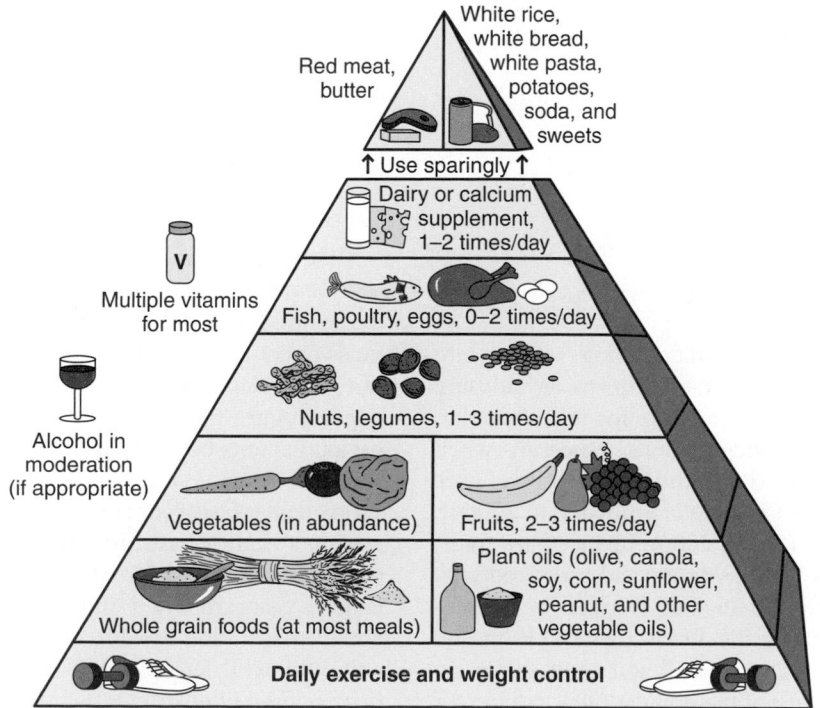

FIGURE 9-2 Healthy Eating Food Pyramid. (*From* EAT, DRINK, AND BE HEALTHY *by Walter C. Willett, M.D. Copyright © 2001, 2005 by the President and Fellows of Harvard College. Reprinted by permission of Free Press/Simon & Schuster, Inc.*)

BOX 9-1

Dietary Guidelines for Americans, 2005

Recommendations for carbohydrates

- Aim for a range of 45% to 65% of total calories, with the majority coming from complex carbohydrates such as whole grains, fruits, and vegetables to provide 14 g of fiber per 1000 calories.

Recommendations for fruits and vegetables

- Choose a variety of fruits and vegetables each day. In particular select from all vegetable subgroups (dark green, orange, legumes, starchy vegetables, and other vegetables) each week.

Recommendations for fat

- Aim for a range of 25% to 35% of total calories.
- Consume less than 10 % of calories from saturated fatty acids. Keep trans-fatty acid consumption as low as possible.
- Aim for less than 300 mg of cholesterol per day.

Recommendations for protein

- Aim for 10% to 35% of total calories.
- Choose lean protein sources, lean meat, white meat of poultry without the skin, fish, and seafood.
- Include plant sources of protein, including nuts, seeds, legumes, soy and tofu.
- Include milk and milk products. The recommendation is 3 cups per day of fat-free or low-fat milk or the equivalent (yogurt, low fat cheeses).
- If unable to use dairy products, choose calcium-fortified soy beverage or other calcium and vitamin D–fortified foods.

Limit consumption of sodium to less than 2300 milligrams a day.

Limit total discretionary calories to the amount that fits the calorie need.

- Discretionary calories are extra calories from added sugars, additional fats and oils, alcohol, and foods that are eaten in greater quantities than recommended by MyPyramid. At 2000 calories, the MyPyramid goal for discretionary calories is no more than 265 calories.
- Control portions and choose serving sizes that fit the daily calorie needs.
- The calorie recommendations for adults are presented for those age 30 years with adjustments for more calories when one is younger than age 30 and for fewer calories as one moves past age 30.

If alcohol is desired and fits the health needs, limit intake to up to one drink a day for women and up to two drinks a day for men.

Engage in regular physical activity.

- To reduce the risk of chronic disease in adulthood, 30 minutes a day of moderate-intensity activity above the usual activity is recommended most days.
- To help manage weight and prevent gradual weight gain, engage in approximately 60 minutes of moderate-vigorous intensity activity on most days of the week in concert with a balance of calorie intake.
- To sustain weight loss, participate in at least 60 to 90 minutes of daily moderate intensity–physical activity in concert with a balanced caloric intake.

Follow food safety guidelines.

Data from U.S. Department of Health and Human Services, U.S. Department of Agriculture: *Nutrition and your health: Dietary guidelines for Americans*, Washington, DC, 2005, U.S. Government Printing Office.

DIETARY ENHANCEMENTS: FUNCTIONAL FOODS

Adults interested in attaining and maintaining wellness are frequently interested in altering dietary patterns or choosing foods for added health benefits. The desire for fewer calories, multiple benefits, and risk-reducing foods, especially when children are in the home, is driving the growth in the U.S. functional foods market. That market is estimated in 2006 to be 36 billion dollars in sales (Sloan, 2006). Included are traditional foods such as whole grains, yogurt, and fruits and vegetables along with lower-fat foods and fortified or supplemented products. Sorting out the foods that fit easily and safely into one's diet requires some skill and is a role for dietetic professionals. A segment of the population is looking for ways to enhance their health; providing this information not only gains the adult's attention but also takes nutrition guidance to a higher level.

Research continues to provide information on dietary patterns and components of foods that may have added benefits for health. Many of these factors are categorized as functional foods or components (IFIC, 2004). **Functional foods** are fruits and vegetables, flax seeds, the oils of fish, whole grains, certain spices, yogurt, nuts, soy, and legumes that are associated with having benefits beyond their usual nutrient value. Helping to lower blood cholesterol or control blood sugar, serving as an antioxidant or scavenger against harmful components, promoting a healthy gastrointestinal tract, or stimulating activity of detoxification enzyme systems in the liver are examples of benefits being reported and researched for validity (see *Focus On:* Detoxification Systems).

Adults who have no major health problems that would restrict food choices can benefit from guidance on meeting the recommendations of MyPyramid and the DGA as a first step. This guidance is based on increasing the intake of fruits, vegetables (including legumes), grains (with emphasis

Detoxification Systems

Current thinking on defensive eating or a diet for optimal health is based on a system of choosing foods to protect the body. Although integrative nutrition philosophies fall into this thinking, the concept of choosing foods to optimize nutrition has a basis in all levels of nutrition guidance. The body is protected from xenobiotics (compounds foreign to the body) by natural barriers, including the GI system, the lungs, and the skin. When compounds that are potentially harmful or unknown cross these barriers, the body's detoxification systems go into play, with the result of decreasing the negative impact of the xenobiotics, drugs, or toxins. The major detoxification pathways with a food and nutrition link are the immune tissue in the gut and the enzyme systems in the liver.

The potential power of these systems to protect the body is demonstrated by a closer look at the major barrier, the gut. More than half the body's lymphoid tissue surrounds the digestive tract. Gut-associated lymphoid tissue (GALT) generates almost 70% of the body's antibodies and contains the greatest number of lymphocytes in the body (Mayer, 2000). It is the GALT immunoglobulins that prevent absorption of bacteria and viruses. Secretory immunoglobin A is a part of the major immune system of the gut and has been reported to directly deactivate enzymes and toxins from bacteria such as *Escherichia coli* (Lei and Walker, 2001). The mechanisms for the food and nutrient link are being explored, but it is suggested that phytochemicals are involved, along with more traditional nutrients that build and support the enzyme systems. Isothiocyanates found in cruciferous vegetables; organosulfuric compounds in garlic, onions, and other members of the allium family; and the components present in prebiotics (nondigestible food products that stimulate the growth of bacteria already present in the colon), and the bacteria of probiotics are examples of food choices that can affect detoxification in both prevention and healing. Eating defensively is supported by the guidance in the Dietary Guidelines of America 2005 and can be done within the parameters of a "healthful" diet (see Tables 9-1 and 9-2).

Adapted from Mathai K: Nutrition in the adult years. In Mahan K, Escott-Stump: *Krause's food, nutrition, and diet therapy*, ed 11, Philadelphia, 2004, Elsevier.

---

on whole grains), and seeds and nuts—some of the same foods believed to have components that go beyond the benefits associated with major nutrients. Most of these components that are considered dietary enhancers are associated with plant foods. **Phytochemicals or phytonutrients** (from the Greek word *phyto* for plant) are biologically active and naturally occurring chemical components in plant foods. In plants phytochemicals act as natural defense systems for their host and offer protection against microbial invasions or infections. They also provide color, aroma, and flavor, with over 2000 plant pigments identified. These include **flavonoids**, anthocyanins, and **carotenoids** (Craig, 1997; King and Young, 1999) (see Table 9-1). Soy is an example of a food of current interest for its value beyond that of being a source of quality protein. The health benefits of soy products or components of soy include reducing the risk for heart disease and certain types of cancer and reducing vasomotor symptoms (hot flashes) in menopausal females. Note that soy itself, as a plant, has no cholesterol and is a source of **isoflavones,** a **phytoestrogen** or plant estrogen. In 1999 the FDA approved a food label claim for soy, addressing its potential role in reducing the risk of heart disease. To qualify, the food needs to have 6.25 g of soy protein in one serving; be low in fat (less than 3 g); be low in saturated fat (1 g) and cholesterol (less than 20 mg); and have no more than 480 mg of sodium for an individual food, 720 mg if an entrée, and 960 mg if a meal (Henkel, 2000).

In January 2006 the AHA released the results of a review by its Nutrition Committee of 22 randomized trials on the effect of soy protein with isoflavones on serum cholesterol (Sacks et al., 2006). The committee found that soy protein and isoflavones have not been shown to lessen vasomotor symptoms of menopause and show no significant effects on HDL cholesterol or triglycerides. This report and others have also refuted the role of soy in providing a protective effect against breast cancer and question the potential of soy consumption by women at high risk for breast cancer (Maskarinec, 2005). In October 2005 a petition to the FDA for a soy protein and cancer prevention claim was withdrawn by a leader in soy products, noting that the science was being reviewed (FDA, 2005).

The current thinking on soy is an example of the questions that accompany the use of food or food components at levels beyond what would be consumed in a traditional diet (Maskarinec, 2005). The concern appears to be related to isolated components such as the isoflavones rather than on the use of soy as a quality protein with a heart-healthy profile. As a food, soy is a source of fiber with a positive heart-healthy fat profile (low in saturated fat, high in polyunsaturated fat) and other nutrients. The AHA statement notes that such foods can be part of heart-healthy guidance (Sacks et al., 2006). In addition, foods that fit the FDA label claim for soy protein have a positive nutrition profile by virtue of the label requirements, and moderate amounts of soy foods can be part of a balanced diet even for cancer survivors (Maskarinec, 2005). In 2006 the AHA revised its diet and lifestyle guidelines, recommending that soy can be used to displace animal protein and help lower intake of saturated

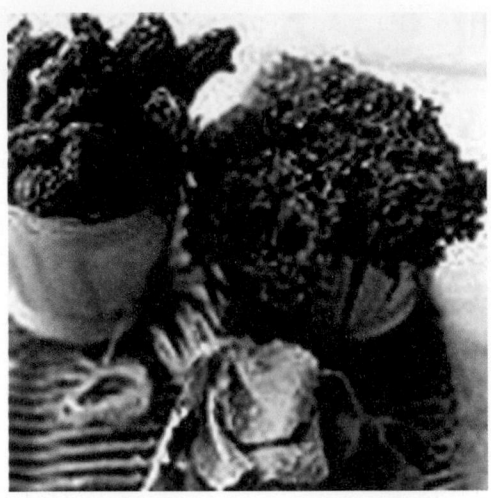

FIGURE 9-3 Functional foods and ingredients are important.

fat but that soy is not recommended as a therapy to reduce HDL cholesterol or other cardiovascular risk factors (Lichtenstein et al., 2006).

However, one cannot address dietary guidance without considering the issues of both functional components and functional foods (ADA, 2004). Rather than isolating and promoting food components, current thinking supports the emphasis of food as a package and a first source for its nutrients and potential enhancers (Figure 9-3). In the big picture it is the health status of the person, lifestyle choices, and genetics that form potential for wellness, but dietary enhancement is a tool that gains attention and helps the person move forward on the wellness continuum.

Alcohol

The idea of functional foods or components in foods that might have a protective effect on health goes beyond traditional foods to the ingestion of alcohol. For some adults the idea of the potential health benefits from alcohol is viewed as a reason to drink. Looking at the evidence, there are some benefits to moderate intake of alcohol for specific population groups, but the extent to which these benefits are related to lifestyle are still unclear.

Case-controlled and perspective studies as cited in the Report of the 2005 DGA have supported the idea that light-to-moderate intake of alcohol is associated with a lower risk for cardiovascular disease, and these benefits appear to be independent of other CVD risk factors, including age, sex, smoking habits, and body mass intake. The DGA noted that women age 55 and older and men age 45 and older at risk for heart disease were in the groups most likely to benefit (USDHHS, 2005b), whereas in younger adults it is speculated that the benefits can be offset by the increases in the risk for alcohol abuse–related accidents.

The actual cardiovascular "protective" effect of alcohol is still unclear. It may be the polyphenols in red wine (especially Pinot Noir), yet other forms of alcohol and colors of wine have also been shown to have protective effects (Markamal et al., 2003). Other factors are still being studied, including the role of nonalcoholic sources of the polyphenols such as grape juice. In addition, the question of energy intake by those who enjoy wine is a factor, and lifestyles are being explored. For example, in a Danish study of 3.5 million supermarket purchases, those who bought wine were also more likely to buy fruits, vegetables, olives, and low-fat cheeses than those who bought beer (Johansen et al., 2006). Adding to the confusion are the "French paradox" and the relationship of the health benefits of the Mediterranean Diet (see Chapter 12).

Based on the literature and the risks of potential abuse of alcohol, the best advice may be to proceed cautiously. As with any food-related advice, there is the opportunity for abuse; in the case of alcohol, this can lead to problems beyond the risks of CVD. The 2005 DGA for alcohol (i.e., "if" alcohol is consumed, it should be in moderation) is guidance that can be shared with adults who make this choice. This should accompany other guidance that one should be the legal age to use alcohol; drink responsibly; enjoy it with a healthful meal; and be medically able to use alcohol based on health, life stage (no alcohol while pregnant or breast-feeding), and medications. Moderation is defined as one drink a day for women and up to two drinks per day for males. A drink is defined as 12 oz of regular beer, 5 oz of wine, or 1.5 oz of 80-proof distilled liquor.

FOCAL POINTS

- The adult years are a prime time for nutrition and health professionals to reach adults with positive messages and interventions that encourage them to take personal responsibility for their health.
- Since this group includes the parents, teachers, coaches of youth, and the gatekeepers in both the family and the worksite, the potential effect for a wellness initiative is powerful.
- Interventions for adults will require the knowledge and skills necessary with all population groups: assessing their unique needs, involving them in planning and

setting of goals, and integrating information that meets their needs and lifestyle choices.
- Regular nutrition assessment and intervention for adults may help delay the onset or severity of chronic diseases with their costs of reduced life expectancy, increased health care utilization, and decreased quality of life.
- Today's adults have access to multiple resources besides health professionals; the possibility of misinformation must be considered along with the opportunity of gaining deeper insights and readiness for behavioral change.

✴ CLINICAL SCENARIO

Lee is a 35-year-old woman who lives in an urban neighborhood with her husband and 12-year-old daughter. She is 5 ft, 10 in tall and currently weighs 165 pounds. In the past 2 years she has gained 10 pounds. At a recent neighborhood health fair Lee's blood glucose and blood pressure screening results were higher than they had been a year ago but were still in a good range. She has a family history of heart disease and diabetes and recognizes that her weight gain is an issue. Her grandmother recently died with colon cancer. Both she and her husband work full time, and blending their schedules with that of their daughter is hectic. Lee does all the cooking and shopping, although they eat out (fast food or take out) for most lunches and at least two dinners a week. They have no regular activity or exercise. They have minimum health insurance that requires a large co-pay; thus they don't have an ongoing health care routine.

Lee made an appointment with her health care source. She asked for some dietary counseling and was asked to bring a 1-day food recall for the registered dietitian. Breakfast: egg and sausage on a bagel, coffee; mid-morning: low-fat snack bar from vending machine with coffee; lunch: double burger with cheese on a bun and large fries, diet soda; dinner: chicken and rice casserole, corn, lettuce salad with diet ranch dressing; evening: dish of ice cream.

✴**Nutrition Diagnosis 1:** Physical inactivity related to lifestyle issues as evidenced by no regular physical activity and a 10-lb weight gain

✴**Nutrition Diagnosis 2:** Undesirable food choices related to high-fat and low-fruit/vegetable intake as evidenced by diet history revealing high fat foods at every meal and average 1 fruit/vegetable each day.

1. What lifestyle factors and nutrition triggers are likely to be identified by the dietitian?
2. What foods should Lee consider, including in her diet to build a prevention-related meal plan?
3. Plan a meal pattern and two sample meals that illustrate your recommendations, including at least one at-home and away-from-home breakfast, lunch, and dinner.

USEFUL WEBSITES

America on the Move
http://aom.americaonthemove.org/site/

American Dietetic Association
http://www.eatright.org

Centers for Disease Control and Prevention Health 2004
http://www.cdc.gov/nchs/data/hus/hus04trend.pdf#pref

Dietary Guidelines for Americans
http://www.health.gov/dietaryguidelines/

FAO
http://www.fao.org/documents/show_cdr.asp?url_file=/docrep/008/a0200e/a0200e00.htm

Healthy People
www.health.gov/healthypeople/document/

Institute of Medicine (DRI)
http://www.iom.edu

Flax Council of Canada, 2006, New Flax Facts: Omega-3 Fats in Flax and Fish
www.flaxcouncil.ca

National Center for Chronic Disease Prevention and Health Promotion, Centers for Disease Control and Prevention
http://www.cdc.gov/hrqol/

U.S. Department of Agriculture: Agricultural Research Service (ARS)
http://www.ars.usda.gov/

U.S. Department of Agriculture: MyPyramid
http://www.mypyramid.gov/

U.S. Department of Health and Human Services: Small Steps
http://www.smallstep.gov

U.S. Food and Drug Administration: Health claims for soy protein
www.cfsan.fda.gov/~dms/fdsoypr.html

WELCOA Wellness Councils of America
http://www.welcoa.org/

References

Alaimo K: Food insecurity in the United States: an overview, *Topics Clinical Nutr* 20; 4:281, 2005.

American Dietetic Association (ADA) and Dietitians of Canada: Position: nutrition and women's health, available at www. Eatright.org, (Reaffirmed September, 2001; in effect until 2008).

American Dietetic Association (ADA): *Nutrition and you: Trends,* Chicago, 2002a, American Dietetic Association.

American Dietetic Association (ADA): Position of the ADA: total diet approach to communicating food and nutrition information, *J Am Diet Assoc* 102:100, 2002b.

American Dietetic Association and Dietitians of Canada: Position Paper: Vegetarian Diets, *J Am Diet Assoc* 103(6):748, 2003.

American Dietetic Association (ADA): Position of the ADA: fortification and nutritional supplements, *J Am Diet Assoc* 105(8):1300, 2005.

American Heart Association, American Stroke Association: *A nation at risk: obesity in the United States,* a statistical sourcebook funded by the Robert Wood Johnson Foundation, Stanford, CA, 2005, The Association.

Barrett-Connor E et al: *Best clinical practices. Chapter 13 from the International Position Paper on Women's health and menopause: a comprehensive approach,* National Heart, Lung, and Blood Institute, NIH Office of Research on Women's Health and the Giovanni Lorenzini Medical Science Foundation 2002, www. nhlbi.nih.gov/health/prof/heart/other/wm_menop.htm, accessed January 20, 2007.

Centers for Disease Control and Prevention (CDC), National Center for Chronic Disease: *Prevention and health promotion: measuring healthy days,* 2000, http://www.cdc.gov/hrqol, accessed January 20, 2007.

Centers for Disease Control and Prevention (CDC): *Chronic disease overview,* http://www.cdc.gov/nccdphp/overview.htm, October 2004, accessed January 20, 2007.

Centers for Disease Control and Prevention (CDC), National Center for Chronic Disease Prevention and Health Promotion: *1993-2003 Trend data on adult health-related quality of life (hrqol) by states and subgroups,* 2005a, http://www.cdc.gov/hrqol, accessed March 15, 2006.

Centers for Disease Control and Prevention (CDC): *Physical activity and good nutrition: essential elements to prevent chronic diseases and obesity,* 2005b, http://www.cdc.gov/nccdphp/aag/ aag_dnpa.htm, accessed January 20, 2007.

Centers for Disease Control and Prevention (CDC): *ABOUT DATA 2010, Healthy People 2010 Database 2006,* http://wonder. cdc.gov/data2010/. An Internet-based, current review of information on programs and progress on 2010 Objectives. This site is state, year, and focus area specific (Ongoing update, cited April, 2006a).

Centers for Disease Control and Prevention (CDC): *National vital statistic reports. June 28, 2005,* Tables A, B and 3 updated. February 15, 2006. *Table 1. Provisional number of live births and deaths,* 2006b, http://www.cdc.gov/nchs/data/nvsr/nvsr53/ nvsr53_21.pdf, accessed January 20, 2007.

Craig W: Phytochemicals: guardians of our health, *J Am Diet Assoc* 97(suppl 2):199, 1997.

Dornblaser L: Trends in the food industry, Reported at Food Marketing Institute (FMI) Trade Show, Chicago, May, 2006.

Drewnowski A: Concept of a nutritious food: toward a nutrient density score, *Am J Clin Nutr* 82:721, 2005.

Fletcher RH, Fairfield KM: Vitamins for chronic disease prevention in adults: clinical applications, *JAMA,* 287:3127, 2002.

Food and Agriculture Organization of the United Nations (FAO): *The state of food insecurity in the world,* 2005, http://www.fao. org/, accessed March 15, 2006.

Food and Drug Administration (FDA), Center for food Safety and Applied Nutrition (CFSAN): *Health and Diet Survey, 2004 Supplement,* http://www.cfsan.fda.gov/comm/~crnutri3.html, accessed November, 2005.

Food and Drug Administration (FDA): *Qualified health claims: withdrawn soy protein and cancer,* http://www.cfsan.fda.gov/~dms/ lab-qhc.html, accessed October 7, 2005.

Ford ES et al: Prevalence of the metabolic syndrome among U.S. adults: findings from the third National Health and Nutrition Examination Survey, *JAMA* 287:356, 2002.

Gianetti J et al: Inverse association between carotid intima-media thickness and the antioxidant lycopene in atherosclerosis, *Am Heart* J 143:467, 2002.

Giovannucci E et al: A prospective study of tomato products, lycopene and prostate cancer risk, *J Natl Cancer Inst* 94:391, 2002.

Harris Interactive Poll reported in Gullo K, editor: Healthcare News: Healthy eating messages appear to be resonating with consumers, according to new Harris interactive survey, Harris Interative Inc., Rochester, NY, April 5, 2006, http://www. harrisinteractive.com/news/allnewsbydate.asp?NewsID51039, accessed May 15, 2007.

Health, United States, 2006. www.cdc.gov/nchs/data/hus/hus06. pdf, accessed January 20, 2007.

Henkel J: Soy: health claims for soy protein: questions about other components, U.S. Food and Drug Administration, FDA Consumer, May-June 2000, http://www.cfsan.fda.gov/~dms/ fdsoypr.html, accessed March 15, 2007.

Institute of Medicine (IOM), National Academy of Sciences (NAS): *Dietary reference intake (DRI) series,* Washington DC, National Academies Press, 1998-2004.

International Food Information Council (IFIC): *Background on adult nutrition, health & physical activity,* April, 2005, http:// www.ific.org/nutrition, accessed March 15, 2006.

International Food Information Council (IFIC): *Background on functional foods,* IFIC Foundations, February, 2004, http://www. ific.org/nutrition, accessed May 15, 2006.

International Food Information Council (IFIC): *Food & health survey: consumer attitudes toward food, nutrition & health: a benchmark survey 2006,* Washington, DC, 2006, IFIC, http:// www.ific.org/nutrition, accessed May 15, 2006.

Johansen D et al. Food buying habits of people who buy wine or beer: cross sectional study, *Br Med J* 332(7540):519, 2006.

King A, Young G: Characteristics and occurrence of phenolic phytochemicals, *J Am Diet Assoc* 99:213, 1999.

Lei L, Walker WA: Pathologic and physiological interactions of bacteria with the gastrointestinal epithelium, *Am J Clin Nutr* 73:11245, 2001.

Lichenstein AH et al: Diet and lifestyle recommendations revision 2006: a scientific statement from the American Heart Association Nutrition Committee, *Circulation* June 19, 2006.

MacLennan AH et al: Hormone therapy, timing of initiation, and cognition in women older than 60 years: the REMEMBER pilot study, *Menopause* 13:28, 2006.

Markamal KJ et al: Roles of drinking pattern and type of alcohol consumed in coronary heart disease in men, *N Engl J Med* 348:109, 2003.

Maskarinec G: Commentary: Soy foods for breast cancer survivors and women at high risk for breast cancer, *J Am Diet Assoc* 105:10, 1524, 2005.

Maslow A: *Motivation and personality*, 2nd ed, New York, Harper, 1970.

Mayer L: Mucosal immunity and gastrointestinal antigen processing, *J Pediatr Gastroenterol Nutr* 30(suppl):4, 2000.

Millen BE, Quatromoni PA: Nutritional research within the Framingham Heart Study, *J Nutr Health Aging* 5(3):139, 2001.

McCullough ML et al: Diet quality and major chronic disease risk in men and women: moving toward improved dietary guidance, *Am J Clin Nutr* 76:1261, 2002.

McCullough ML, Willett WC: Evaluating adherence to recommended diets in adults: the Alternate Healthy Eating Index, *Publ Health Nutr* 9(1A):152, 2006.

National Center for Health Statistics (NCHS): Health, United States, 2004 with chart book on trends in the health of Americans, Hyattsville, Md, 2004, NCHS.

National Institutes of Health (NIH), Office of Dietary Supplements (ODS): Dietary supplement fact sheet: B6, Posted 12/9/2002, updated March 25, 2005, http://dietarysupplements.info.nih/gov, accessed March 30, 2005.

Olson CM: Food insecurity in women, *Topics in Clin Nutr* 20:(4):321, 2005.

Putnam J et al: U.S. per capita food supply trends: more calories, refined carbohydrates and fats, *Food Review* 25(3):2, 2002.

Rank HR, Hirschl TA: Likelihood of using food stamps during the adulthood years, *J Nutr Educ Behav* 37(3):137, 2005.

Rao AV, Agarwal S: Role of antioxidant lycopene in cancer and heart disease, *J Am Coll Nutr* 19:563, 2000.

Rissanen TH et al: Low serum lycopenc concentration is associated with an excess incidence of acute coronary events and stroke: the Kuopio ischemic heart disease risk factor study, *Br J Nutr* 85:749 2001.

Sacks F et al: Soy protein, isoflavones, and cardiovascular health: an American Heart Association Science Advisory for Professionals from the Nutrition Committee, *Circulation* 113:1034, 2006, http://www.circulationaha.org, accessed May 15, 2006.

Sloan AE: Top 10 functional food trends, *Food Technol* 60(4): 22, 2006, www.ift.org, accessed May 15, 2006.

Stewart H et al: The demand for food away from home: full-service or fast food, Agricultural Economic Report Number 829, April, 2004.

Stuebe AM et al: Duration of lactation and incidence of type 2 Diabetes, *JAMA* 294:2601, 2005.

Tarasuk V: Household food insecurity in Canada, *Topics Clin Nutr* 20(4):299, 2005.

Thys-Jacobs S et al: Calcium carbonate and the premenstrual syndrome: effects on premenstrual and menstrual symptoms. Premenstrual Syndrome Study Group, *Am J Obstet Gynecol* 179: 444, 1998.

U.S. Department of Agriculture (USDA), Economic Research Service (ERS): *Food consumption: food supply and use*, 2004b, http://www.ers.usda.gov/briefing/consumption/Supply.htm, accessed May 15, 2004.

U.S. Department of Agriculture (USDA): *MyPyramid food guidance system*, 2005, www.MyPyramid.gov, accessed May 15, 2007.

U.S. Department of Health and Human Services (USDHHS): Health finder: lifestyle changes could save millions, National Health Information Services quoting News Release, *Lancet*, October, 2005b, www.healthfinder.gov/newsletters/diabetes011606.asp #485207, accessed October 1, 2005.

U.S. Department of Health and Human Services (USDHHS): *Healthy People 2010*, ed 2, vol I, *Understanding and improving health*; vol 2, *Objectives for the nation*, Washington, DC, 2000, U.S. Government Printing Office.

U.S. Department of Health and Human Services (USDHHS): *Prevention makes common "cents,"* Washington, DC, September, 2003, http://aspe.hhs.gov/health/prevention, accessed May 1, 2003.

U.S. Department of Health and Human Services (USDHHS): *Small steps: a web-based wellness program*, http://www.smallstep.gov (ongoing update, cited April, 2006), accessed April 1, 2006.

U.S. Department of Health and Human Services, United States Department of Agriculture: *Nutrition and your health: dietary guidelines for Americans*, Washington, DC, 2005a, U.S. Government Printing Office.

Variyam JN: Economic Research Report No. (ERR4), *Nutrition labeling in the food-away from home sector: an economic assessment*, April, 2005, U.S. Department of Agriculture, Economic Research Service, http://www.ers.usda.gov/publications/ERR4, accessed May 15, 2005.

Wellness Councils of America: *The 5 smartest things you could ever do*, Omaha, Nebr, 2003, WELCOA.

Willet WC: *Eat, drink and be healthy*, New York, 2001, Simon and Schuster, www.hsph.harvard.edu/nutritionsource/pyramids.html, accessed January 20, 2007.

World Health Organization (WHO): *The world health report 2003 and fact sheet*, Copenhagen, December 2003, WHO.

Wyatt KM et al: Efficacy of vitamin B6 in the treatment of premenstrual syndrome: systematic review, *Br Med J* 318(7195):1375, 1999.

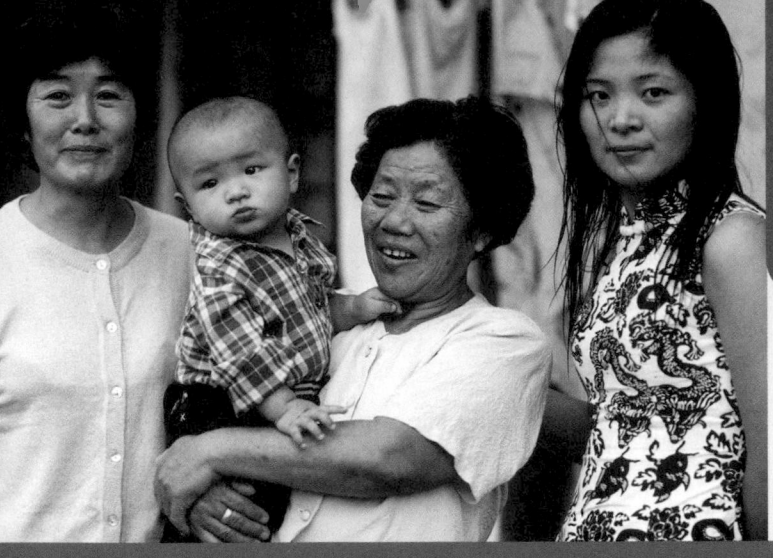

CHAPTER 10

Nancy S. Wellman, PhD, RD, FADA
Barbara J. Kamp, MS, RD

Nutrition in Aging

KEY TERMS

achlorhydria insufficient production of stomach acid

activities of daily living (ADLs) individual self-performance skills needed in everyday life; ambulation/locomotion, eating, toileting, grooming, personal hygiene, bathing

age-related macular degeneration (AMD) occurs when the macula, the center part of the retina, degrades

ageism any prejudice or discrimination against or in favor of an age-group

agerasia Greek; appearance of youth with advanced age

assisted living facilities combination of housing, personalized supportive services, and health care for those who need help with activities of daily living

atrophic gastritis chronic gastritis with atrophy of mucous membrane and destruction of peptic glands

baby boomer or boomer member of the baby-boom generation born between 1946 and 1964

cataract a clouding of the lens of the eye

diabetic retinopathy a complication of diabetes; occurs when blood vessels of the retina leak and produce spotty hemorrhages

dysgeusia loss of taste

dysphagia swallowing problems due to weakened tongue or cheek muscles

functionality ability to perform self-care, self-maintenance, and physical activities

geriatrics study of chronic diseases frequently associated with aging

gerontology scientific study of biologic, psychological, and sociologic phenomena associated with normal aging

glaucoma damage to optic nerve due to high pressure in the eye

hyposmia decreased sense of smell

one percent rule 1% decline in organ function each year starting at age 30

polypharmacy taking five or more prescriptions and/or over-the-counter drugs regularly

pressure ulcers sores that develop from continuous pressure that impedes capillary blood flow to skin and underlying tissue

presbycusis lessening of hearing acuteness due to degenerative changes in the ear

quality of life general sense of happiness and satisfaction with one's life and environment

sarcopenia age-related loss of muscle mass, strength, and function

sarcopenic obesity less visible loss of lean muscle mass in obese older persons

sedentary death syndrome (SeDs) a term describing the life-threatening health problems caused by a sedentary lifestyle, a level of inactivity below the threshold of the beneficial health effects of regular physical activity or, more simply, burning under 200 calories per day in moderate physical activity

senescence organic process of growing older and displaying the effects of increased age

skilled nursing facility defines nursing home licensed to provide the highest level of care; meets Medicare certification per 1819(a) of the federal Social Security Act

somatic mutation theory genetic mutations accumulate with age, causing cells to deteriorate and malfunction

xerostomia dryness of mouth resulting from diminished or arrested salivary secretion

Xers member of the generation born between 1965 and 1980

Sections of this chapter were written by Nancy G. Harris, MS, RN, LDN, FADA, for the previous edition of this text.

THE OLDER POPULATION

Older adults in the United States are living longer, healthier, and more functionally fit lives than ever before. Life expectancy increased by 30 years in the twentieth century. Those born today can expect to live an average of 77.6 years. Women who reach age 65 can expect to live an additional 19.8 years, and men, 16.8 years. By the year 2030 the population over age 65 will double in number from 36 to 72 million, increasing from 12.5% to 20% of the population. The fastest-growing segment of this cohort are those age 85+, currently 4.6 million and increasing to 9.6 million in 2030.

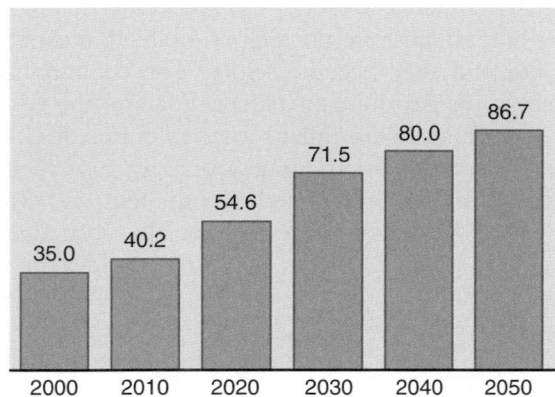

Note: The reference population for these data is the resident population (in millions).

FIGURE 10-1 Population ages 65 and over: 2000 to 2050. *(Data from U.S. Census Bureau, Current Population Reports, P23-209, 65+ in the United States: 2005, Washington, DC, 2005, U.S. Government Printing Office).*

Members of minority groups will also increase from 17% to 26% of the older population (He et al., 2005; U.S. Administration on Aging AOA, 2005) (see Figures 10-1 and 10-2 for population-related data on aging).

By 2030 the number of older adults will exceed the number of school-age children in 10 states—FL, PA, VT, WY, ND, DE, NM, MT, MA, WV. A few years ago no state had more people 65+ than those under 18. Twenty-six states will double their 65+ population by 2030, when the oldest **baby boomers** enter their 80s. Growth in the 65+ population will equal 3.5 times the U.S. growth as a whole. This demographic shift has enormous social, economic, and political implications (He et al., 2005).

Classification

Everyone knows people older than themselves, but those considered old depends a lot on one's own age. Youngsters consider their 20- or 30-something parents old. Almost everyone used to think anyone with gray hair or wrinkles or anyone who retired was old. Today hair color, wrinkles, or age 65 no longer defines old. In fact, many boomers and **Xers** have a goal to retire in their 40s or 50s—as soon as they can stockpile enough for a comfortable lifestyle.

Qualifying as an "older adult" is based on the minimum eligibility age of 65 in federal retirement programs, including Social Security. The U.S. Census Bureau uses a stratified system to define this generation-spanning age-group; those ages 65 to 74 are the young old; 75 to 84, old; and 85+, oldest old. Some consider today's new old to be those in their 90s. The 50,000 centenarians today are no longer considered unique since many of them still live independently.

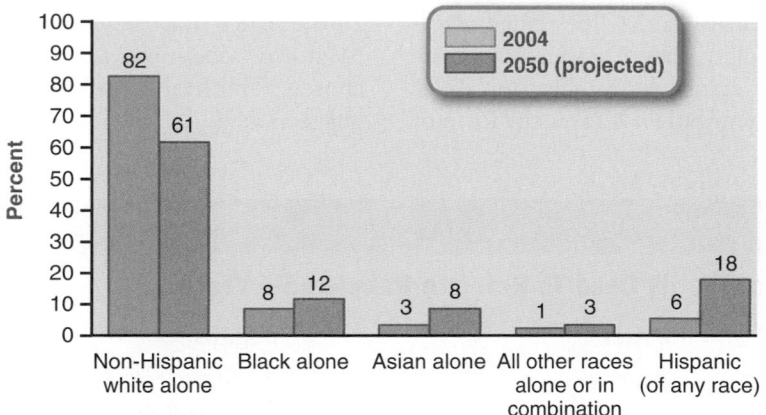

FIGURE 10-2 Percent of people ages 65 and over in poverty by sex, race, and Hispanic origin. Note: The term "non-Hispanic white alone" is used to refer to people who reported being white and no other race and who are not Hispanic. The term "black alone" is used to refer to people who reported being black or African American and no other race, and the term "Asian alone" is used to refer to people who reported only Asian as their race. The use of single-race populations in this report does not imply that this is the preferred method of presenting or analyzing data. The U.S. Census Bureau uses a variety of approaches. The race group "All other races alone or in combination" includes American Indian and Alaska Native, alone; Native Hawaiian and Other Pacific Islander, alone; and all people who reported two or more races. Reference population: These data refer to the resident population. *(U.S. Census Bureau, Population Estimates and Projections, 2004).*

Women live longer than men. They make up more than half of the young old and 69% of the oldest old. Over 75% of older men are married, whereas only 50% of older women are married. Women are three times as likely as men to be widowed, even at higher ages, where 78% of older women as compared to 35% of older men are widowed. Half of older women live alone. Hence the oft-quoted truism is that "Men die married and women die alone."

AGEISM

Ageism, a term coined in the 1960s, continues to paint a grim picture of aging. It perpetuates negative stereotypes that are exceptionally difficult to shed in age-denying, youth-worshipping America. Ageism is defined as any prejudice or discrimination against or in favor of an age-group. It has profound personal and professional consequences. Even as Americans are living longer and healthier than ever, ageism abounds due to the unrelenting quest for youth and death denial that characterizes American culture.

Ageism is tough to change, say two of the most well-known anti-ageist champions, Robert Butler and Erdman Palmore. Butler, a powerful dynamic speaker now in his 80s, founded the National Institute on Aging at the National Institutes of Health and currently heads the International Longevity Center in New York City. Palmore combats ageism by living what he preaches. He skydives and white-water rafts; he bicycles his age in miles each birthday. Now in his mid-70s, he finds it particularly annoying that our language and culture equate aging with deterioration and impairment.

Research shows that a positive attitude toward aging can actually increase life by 7½ years. A positive attitude has a greater impact on longevity than gender, socioeconomic status, loneliness, and functional health. The remedy is to delegitimize ageism in our society. Americans have internalized the negative image of aging thoroughly; for older Americans ageism is primarily negative. It takes the form of cruel imagery, jokes, language, and attitudes directed at older people. Many people take part without realizing it. Older persons are rarely if ever depicted positively in cartoons or on TV. This form of prejudice is the only one that *all* people will suffer in their lifetimes; many who believe they are not ageist probably hold some ageist attitudes based on myths, stereotypes, and misinformation.

One of the biggest fallacies regarding the older population is that they are a homogenous group. This cohort spans several generations and differs considerably based on culture, race, ethnicity, religion, language, gender, sexual orientation, income, education, employment, life experiences, marital status, living arrangement, cognitive capacity, health, and functional status. Most (95%) older adults do not live in nursing homes; most are not sick or disabled; most are not senile nor will they become senile. The commonly held misconceptions surrounding older adults are the basis for the overwhelming ageism that thrives in our country.

The stereotypes about aging people are many ranging from they are sick or disabled or impotent and without sexual desire or activity to they are socially isolated, lonely and senile. In popular American culture, consider the ageist phrase "You aren't getting older. You're getting better," in comparison to "You're getting older and better." The latter does not deny aging. Demeaning language and images in advertisements and TV programs are negative if older adults are included. To sharpen sensitivity to ageism, consider the classification of words that refer to people 65+ years (Table 10-1).

The age biases, such as *gerontophobia* and the *poor dear* syndrome, are present in the many guises of ageism in gender, workplace, cosmetic surgery, cosmetics, overweight, disabilities, minorities, health care, long-term care, education, the legal system, politics, and technology (Hendricks, 2005). *AARP Magazine* used to be called *Modern Maturity*. "Maturity" does not work anymore; thus a neutral title was chosen. The health professions need to update their language as well.

TABLE 10-1

Typical Categorization of Words Used To Refer to People 65+ Years

Positive	Neutral	Negative
Active	Adaptable	Antiquated, archaic
Experienced	Aged, aging	Cantankerous, crotchety
Independent	Dementia, demented	Difficult, rigid
Mature, powerful	Eccentric	Dying, terminal
Old master	Mature, advanced in years	Geezer, old fogey, old timer, old goat, old maid
Quick-witted	Older adult, older person	Feeble, slow, impaired
Useful	Retired	Grouchy, grumpy, peevish
Veteran	Self-sufficient	Old, childlike
Vigorous	Seasoned	Senile, senescent
Wise, venerable	Warm	Withered, wizened
Youthful	Vulnerable	Helpless, frail

From Palmore EB: *Ageism: negative and positive*, ed 2, New York, 1998, Springer Publishing.

The American Psychological Association says *elderly* is not acceptable as a noun and is considered pejorative by some as an adjective. Likewise, the American Medical Association (AMA) Manual of Style says the term should generally be avoided. Although Native Americans use "elder" as a term of respect, in our language it tends to stereotype older adults as having a common set of negative characteristics. *Senior* is considered passé, especially by today's 78 million baby boomers. The best choices are older adult, older person, older American, and older individual. YMCA organizations refer to *AOAs*, active older adults.

NUTRITION AND ITS MULTIPLE ROLES IN PREVENTION

Nutrition is comprised of three types of prevention as described in the following paragraphs. In aging it is important not to assume that nutrition care is only medical nutrition therapy. It is never too late to emphasize nutrition for health promotion and disease prevention. Older Americans, more than any other age-group, want health and nutrition information and are willing to make changes to maintain their independence and quality of life. They often need a bit more help in improving self-care behaviors. They want to know how to eat healthier, exercise safely, and stay motivated to do both.

Nutrition As Primary Prevention

The timing is right to emphasize nutrition in health promotion and disease prevention, the first steps in improving the health of older Americans. It is also an ideal time to pair healthy eating with physical activity.

Nutrition As Secondary Prevention

Nutrition as secondary prevention is risk reduction and slowing the progression of chronic nutrition-related diseases to maintain functionality and quality of life. Function-ality is a more positive way to discuss levels of disability and dependence. In aging, terms are used such as functional fitness, physical fitness, just plain fitness, and physical activity. Yet, *exercise* is a term that doesn't appeal to older adults. Many community dining centers with the Older Americans Act (OAA) Nutrition Programs are finding that fitness programs are the first thing they have offered that has attracted more people than Bingo.

Most dietitians realize that common diseases of aging—heart disease, diabetes, osteoporosis, and cancer—compromise functional fitness. But it is difficult for social service colleagues to see connections among diseases and diets and functionality. They relate heart disease and diabetes to some foods but often do not make connections to functionality, even with diabetes, in which amputation is a consequence of poor management. Similarly, age-related macular degeneration and age-related hearing loss both strongly affect function, and diet is involved in preservation of function. Cognition and mental health are affected by nutrition and hydration, as is recovery from infection or wound healing. Fractures and falls also have a food connection. We need to help older people understand that functionality is a food issue and functionality is preserved simply by eating a wide variety of healthy foods.

Nutrition As Tertiary Prevention

Medical nutrition therapy is the most common way nutrition has been related to health. Nutrition treatments for chronic diseases are covered in other chapters in this book. Newer roles for registered dietitians (RDs) in tertiary prevention include case management and discharge planning. Although case managers are strongly influenced by nutrition issues such as chewing and appetite problems, modified diets, and functional limitations, in discharge planning they infrequently consult dietitians. Dietitians who provide case management say they are comfortable handling all cases just as nurses and social workers do and, in fact, have an advantage because so many clients have nutrition-related chronic diseases (see *New Directions:* Preparing Today's Students for Tomorrow's Jobs).

⇄ **NEW DIRECTIONS**

Preparing Today's Students for Tomorrow's Jobs

Registered dietitians (RDs) are identified by the Institute of Medicine (2000) as "the single group with the standardized education and clinical training necessary to be directly reimbursed through Medicare as providers of nutrition therapy." The projected growth for dietitians is 15% overall and 70% in home and residential care. RDs have more opportunities because of the major expansion of medical nutrition therapy (MNT) under the Medicare Reform/Prescription Drug Law. The Centers for Medicare and Medicaid Services (CMS) is contracting with chronic care improvement programs for individuals with threshold nutrition-related conditions, including heart failure, diabetes, and chronic obstructive pulmonary disease.

There is a need to better prepare tomorrow's RDs for these new opportunities. A survey of 299 students in 10 large universities in California, Florida, New York, Texas, and Pennsylvania (i.e., states with the greatest number of older adults) found scant knowledge of aging (Kaempfer et al., 2002). More than half had negative views: "Older adults are set in their ways; do not adjust to new conditions easily; expect to depend on others as they grow older." Students ranked working with older adults as their least preferred choice.

Continued

⇄ **NEW DIRECTIONS**

Preparing Today's Students for Tomorrow's Jobs—cont'd

An online review of about 300 undergraduate and graduate nutrition programs (Rhee et al., 2004) found few courses on aging but more on maternal and child health. All commonly used nutrition textbooks had few pages on aging and greater focus on geriatrics (illness) and malnutrition (Wellman et al., 2004; O'Neill et al., 2005). Positive aspects of aging such as nutrition and quality of life received little emphasis. Only 10% of ageism words were positive; 36% were negative. Overall, nutrition textbooks failed to present aging comprehensively or positively.

The few courses and often ageist textbook language negatively affects attitudes and stereotypes. Other disciplines offer numerous courses and aging certificates, but only a few nutrition and aging certificate programs are available; some are online. The Commission on Dietetic Registration credentialing agency for ADA developed the Gerontologic Nutrition specialty certification examination for dietitians in 2007.

Nutrition students are encouraged to want to work with older adults because jobs are growing rapidly and financial incentives are strong. Wages are highest for direct-care RDs in long-term care. In Florida registered dietetic technicians (DTRs) in nursing homes earn more than RDs in hospitals.

Full-time RDs have been shown to improve the quality of nursing home care because their expertise is essential to prevent unintended weight loss, dehydration, and pressure ulcers. Assisted living facilities (ALFs) and continuous-care communities present job opportunities as they expand and serve more at-risk persons.

Improving knowledge and attitudes about aging takes exposure to positive RD role models and older adults in a wide variety of settings. There are opportunities in service projects, practica, internship placements, and summer externships to lead nutrition and physical activity programs at, for example, Senior Olympics; community dining centers; and retirement, assisted living, and continuous-care facilities. Volunteering at food banks on days when older adults are scheduled to pick up groceries; teaming up with volunteers who deliver meals to the frail homebound; and participating in mealtime assistance for nursing home residents who cannot eat independently are good opportunities. Student dietetic associations can sponsor activities that foster interactions across the spectrum of aging from the well active to the frail needy. Such experiences are sure to reduce ageist stereotypes, increase interest, and develop skills needed to ride America's age wave.

GERONTOLOGY + GERIATRICS = THE SPECTRUM OF AGING

Aging terminology in health care is somewhat misunderstood. Nutrition fits into the two aging domains of gerontology and geriatrics, although the traditional emphasis has focused on nutrition-related chronic diseases. **Gerontology,** the study of normal aging, derives from science, including biology, psychology, and sociology. Gerontologic nutrition focuses on health promotion, risk reduction, and disease prevention in older adults. Health-promotion programs are most often offered to older populations in communities.

Geriatrics is the study of the chronic diseases frequently associated with aging, including their diagnosis and treatment. Medical nutrition therapy for older adults is often called geriatric nutrition. Although medical nutrition therapy has commonly been practiced in hospitals, the distinction is blurring as nutrition therapy services move out of hospitals and into homes and communities.

A broader focus on nutrition in all aspects of aging is evolving, as is the focus on healthy lifestyles and disease prevention. Without increasing the emphasis on better diets and more physical activity at all ages, health care expenditures will increase even more exorbitantly as the U.S. population ages.

THEORIES ON AGING

Gerontologists (i.e., those who study aging) have a host of diverse theories about why the body ages. It is generally agreed that a loss of efficiency comes about as some cells wear out or die—and are not replaced. This is sometimes referred to as the **one percent rule** since most organ systems lose about 1% of their functioning each year starting at age 30.

No single theory can fully explain the complex processes of aging. A good theory should integrate knowledge and tell how and why phenomena are related. Broadly, theories can be grouped into two categories: predetermined and accumulated damage. Gerontologists often do not agree on a common list of aging theories. With over a dozen theories of aging, most likely more than one theory explains the heterogeneity in older populations. The more common theories are described in Table 10-2.

PHYSIOLOGIC CHANGES

Aging is a normal biologic process. However, it involves some decline in physiologic function. Organs change with age. The rates of change differ among individuals and within organ systems. It is important to distinguish between

TABLE 10-2

Aging Theories

Category	Theory	Description
Predetermination: A built-in mechanism determines when aging begins and time of death	Pacemaker theory	"Biologic clock" is set at birth that runs for a specified period of time, winds down with aging, and ends at death.
	Genetic theory	Life span is determined by heredity.
	Rate of living theory	Each living creature has a finite amount of a "vital substance," and, when it is exhausted, the result is aging and death.
	Oxygen metabolism theory	Animals with the highest metabolisms are likely to have the shortest life spans.
	Immune system theory	Cells undergo a finite number of cell divisions that will eventually cause deregulation of immune function, excessive inflammation, aging, and death.
Accumulated damage: Systemic breakdown over time	Cross-link theory	With time—proteins, DNA and other structural molecules in the body make inappropriate attachments or cross-links to each other, leading to decreased mobility, elasticity, and cell permeability.
	Wear and tear theory	Years of damage to cells, tissues, and organs eventually take their toll, wearing them out and ultimately causing death.
	Free radical theory	Accumulated, random damage caused by oxygen radicals slowly cause cells, tissues, and organs to stop functioning.
	Somatic mutation theory	Genetic mutations caused by oxidizing radiations and other factors accumulate with age, causing cells to deteriorate and malfunction.

normal changes of aging versus changes due to diseases such as atherosclerosis, with onset seen in some teenagers.

The human growth period draws to a close around age 30, when senescence begins. **Senescence** is the organic process of growing older and displaying the effects of increased age. Disease and impaired function are not inevitable parts of aging. Nevertheless, there are certain systemic changes that occur as part of growing older. These changes result in varying degrees of efficiency and functional decline. Factors such as genetics, illnesses, socioeconomics, and lifestyle all determine how aging progresses in each person. In fact, one's outward expression of age may or may not reflect one's chronologic age. The Greeks called the appearance of youth with advanced age **agerasia.** Today it may not be as rare because of surgical enhancements and cosmetic treatments, including facelifts, Botox, hair dyes, sunscreen, and a plethora of yet-to-be "age-defying cures."

Body Composition Changes

Body composition changes with aging. Fat mass and visceral fat increase, whereas lean muscle mass decreases. **Sarcopenia,** the age-related loss of muscle mass, strength, and function, can significantly impact an older adult's quality of life by decreasing mobility, increasing risk for falls, and altering metabolic rates. Sarcopenia accelerates with a decrease in physical activity, but weight-bearing exercise can slow its pace (Raguso et al., 2006). Although inactive persons have faster and greater losses of muscle

mass, sarcopenia is found in active older individuals, albeit to a lesser degree.

Currently no specified degree of lean body mass loss determines a diagnosis of sarcopenia. All losses are important because of the close connection between muscle mass and strength. By the fourth decade of life evidence of sarcopenia is detectable, and the process accelerates after about age 75 (Waters et al., 2000). **Sarcopenic obesity** is the loss of lean muscle mass in older persons with excess adipose tissue. Together the excess weight and decreased muscle mass exponentially compound to further decrease physical activity, which in turn accelerates sarcopenia. An extremely sedentary lifestyle in obese persons is a major detractor from quality of life.

Sedentary Lifestyle

Sedentary lifestyle choices can lead to a condition known as **sedentary death syndrome (SeDs).** The President's Council on Physical Fitness coined the phrase. It describes the life-threatening health problems caused by a sedentary lifestyle. *Sedentary lifestyle* can be defined as a level of inactivity below the threshold of the beneficial health effects of regular physical activity or, more simply, burning under 200 calories per day.

Healthy People 2010 includes physical activity among the leading health indicators addressed. The Surgeon General's Call to Action to Prevent and Decrease Overweight and Obesity outlines the health consequences of inactivity as greater risk for cardiovascular disease (CVD), hypertension, diabetes, dyslipidemia, obesity, overweight, and ultimately increased rates of death (USDHHS, 2001).

By age 75 one in three men and one in two women engage in *no* regular physical activity (USDHHS, 1996). Few older adults achieve the minimum recommended 30 or more minutes of moderate physical activity on 5 or more days per week. According to the Centers for Disease Control and Prevention (CDC), 28% to 34% of adults ages 65 to 74 and 35% to 44% over age 75 are inactive. This includes engaging in no leisure-time physical activity. Inactivity is more common in older people than younger people; women were more likely than men to report no leisure-time activity. The American College of Sports Medicine (ACSM) promotes that the benefit of regular physical activity in the frail and very old outweighs any associated risks (ACSM, 1998). This reassuring position asserts that exercise for older persons is neither futile nor unsafe (see *Focus On: Nutrition and Physical Activity: You Can!*)

Sensory Losses

Sensory losses affect people to varying degrees and at different ages. Genetics, environment, and lifestyle are all parts of the decline in sensory competence. Age-related alterations to the sense of taste, smell, and touch can lead to poor appetite, inappropriate food choices, and lower nutrient intake. Although some degrees of **dysgeusia**, loss of taste, and **hyposmia** (i.e., decreased sense of smell) are attributable to aging, many changes are due to medications. Other causes include conditions such as Bell's palsy; head injury; diabetes; liver and kidney diseases; hypertension; neurologic conditions, including Alzheimer's and Parkinson's; and zinc or niacin deficiency. Untreated mouth sores, tooth decay, poor dental or nasal hygiene,

and cigarette smoking also can decrease these senses. In older adults taste and smell are not completely gone, but sensation thresholds are higher. A risk when these senses are impaired is the temptation to overseason foods, especially to add more salt. Since taste and smell stimulate metabolic changes such as salivary, gastric acid, and pancreatic secretions and increases in plasma levels of insulin; decreased sensory stimulation may impair these metabolic processes (Finkelstein and Schiffman, 1999).

Oral Health

Diet and nutrition can be compromised by poor oral health (Sahyoun et al., 2003). Tooth loss, use of dentures, and **xerostomia** (i.e., dry mouth) can lead to difficulties chewing and swallowing. Oral diseases and conditions are common among Americans who grew up without the benefit of community water fluoridation and other fluoride products. Although 30% of today's adults 65 years and older no longer have any natural teeth, tooth loss is not part of normal aging. Missing, loose, or rotten teeth or poor-fitting painful dentures make it difficult to eat some foods. People with these mouth problems often prefer soft, easily chewed foods and avoid some nutritionally dense options such as whole grains, fresh fruits and vegetables, and meats.

Most older Americans take prescription and over-the-counter drugs. **Polypharmacy**, commonly taking five or more prescriptions or over-the-counter drugs, is widespread. Nutrition-related consequences are significant. For example, over 400 commonly used medications can cause dry mouth (see Chapter 16 and Appendix 31). Preparing foods that are moisture rich such as hearty soups and stews, adding sauces, and pureeing and chopping foods can all make meals easier to eat. In addition, those with poor oral health may benefit from fortified foods with increased nutrient density.

◎ FOCUS ON

Nutrition and Physical Activity: *You Can!*

Despite overwhelming evidence of benefits, few older adults engage in the recommended 30 minutes or more of moderate physical activity on most days of the week. In an effort to start older adults on the path to increased physical activity, *You Can! Steps to Healthier Aging*, part of the USDHHS *Steps to a Healthier U.S.*, was created. This initiative encourages Americans of every age to live longer, better lives by being physically active, eating health-promoting diets, getting periodic preventive screenings, and making healthy choices such as not smoking. On the premise that every step counts, The National Resource Center on Nutrition, Physical Activity, & Aging developed *Eat Better & Move More: a Guidebook for Community Programs*. This *ready-to-use* program has plans for 12 weekly sessions that encourage healthier food choices, and step counters motivate participants to walk more.

The program fits the interests and needs of older adults who need encouragement to maintain their quality of life and independence. This simple-to-implement integrated community program improves diets and activity in older adults. It is successful because small changes in diet and physical activity can make a difference at any age (see Figure 10-5).

For more information go to http://www.aoa.gov/youcan/.

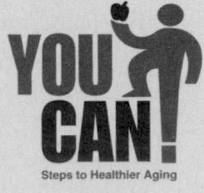

Gastrointestinal

Some gastrointestinal (GI) disorders may be age-related. Rather than ascribing any of these disorders to aging, the true clinical etiology should be determined. GI changes can negatively impact a person's nutrient intake starting in the mouth.

Decreases in taste sensation and saliva production make eating less pleasurable and more difficult. **Dysphagia** due to weakened tongue or cheek muscles can make chewing and swallowing both difficult and dangerous. Dysphagia increases the risk for aspiration pneumonia, an infection caused by food or fluids entering the lungs. Thickened liquids and texture-modified foods can help people with dysphagia eat safely. The National Dysphagia Diet is in Appendix 35 and appropriate levels of texture modification are also defined (see *Focus On: Food Texture Modification Levels*).

Gastric changes can also affect a person's ability to eat. Decreased gastric mucosa leads to an inability to resist damage such as cancer, ulcers, and infections. Gastritis causes inflammation and pain; delayed gastric emptying, discomfort. These all affect the bioavailability of nutrients and increase the risk of developing a chronic deficiency disease such as osteoporosis.

Achlorhydria is the insufficient production of stomach acid. The decline in acid can be due to age as well as **atrophic gastritis.** About 30% of those over age 50 have achlorhydria. Sufficient stomach acid and intrinsic factor are required for the absorption of vitamin B_{12}. Although substantial amounts are stored in the liver, B_{12} deficiency does occur. Symptoms, often misdiagnosed since they mimic Alzheimer's or other chronic conditions, include extreme fatigue, dementia, confusion, and tingling and weakness in the arms and legs (see Chapters 3 and 31).

The incidence of diverticulosis increases with age. Half of the population over age 60 will develop it, but only 20% of them will have clinical manifestations. The most common problems with diverticular disease are lower abdominal pain and diarrhea (see Chapter 28).

Constipation is not a disease; it is a symptom. Constipation is defined as having fewer bowel movements than usual, having difficulty or excessive straining at stool, painful bowel movements, hard stool, or incomplete emptying of the bowel. Older adults are more likely than younger adults to become constipated. Primary causes include insufficient fluids, lack of physical activity, and low intake of dietary fiber. Constipation is also caused by delayed transit time in the gut and medications. Constipation can usually be alleviated by increasing fluids, activity, and fiber (see Chapter 28).

Cardiovascular

CVD includes heart disease and stroke. Although the effects of CVD are often measured by deaths in later life, it is not a disease of aging. This nutrition-related disease has its roots in unhealthy food choices made throughout one's lifetime.

CVD is America's No. 1 cause of deaths in both genders and all racial and ethnic groups (USDHHS, 2006). CVD age-related changes are extremely variable and are highly impacted by environmental influences such as smoking, exercise, and diet. Changes include decreased arterial wall compliance, decreased maximum heart rate; decreased responsiveness to β-adrenergic stimuli, increased left ventricle muscle mass, and slowed ventricular relaxation. Studies show that lowering blood cholesterol and blood pressure reduces the risk of dying of heart disease, having a nonfatal heart attack, and needing heart bypass surgery or angioplasty (see Chapter 32).

Renal Disease

Age-related changes in renal function vary tremendously. Some older adults experience little change, whereas others can have devastating life-threatening change. On average, glomerular filtration rate, measured in creatinine clearance rates, declines by about 8 to 10 ml/min/$1.73m^2$/decade after ages 30 to 35. The resulting increase in serum creatinine concentrations should be considered when determining medication dosages. The progressive decline in renal function can lead to an inability to excrete concentrated or dilute urine, a delayed response to sodium deprivation or a sodium load, and delayed response to an acid load. Renal function is also impacted by dehydration, diuretic use, and medications, especially antibiotics.

Neurologic Function

There can be significant age-related declines in neurologic processes. Functions including cognition, steadiness, reactions, coordination, gait, sensations, and daily living tasks can decline as much as 90% or as little as 10%. On average, the brain loses 5% to 10% of its weight between the ages of 20 and 90. This loss was believed to be from a decrease in neurons, but research now indicates that unless a specific pathology is present, most if not all neurons are functional until death.

Other changes in brain physiology include widening of surface grooves, decrease in surface area, increase in number of plaques, and neurofibrillary tangles (i.e., the microscopic filaments that run through the neuron body and extend into the axon and dendrites). All these changes can

---

⊙ FOCUS ON

Food Texture Modification Levels

Level 1: Pureed: pureed, homogenous, cohesive, puddinglike

Level 2: Mechanically altered: cohesive, moist, semisolid; requires some chewing ability; ground or minced meats with fork-mashable fruits & vegetables; excludes most bread products, crackers, and other dry foods

Level 3: Advanced: Soft-solid; requires more chewing ability; easy to-cut meats, fruits, vegetables; excludes hard, crunchy fruits & vegetables, sticky foods, very dry foods

Level 4: Any solid textures

Adapted from National Dysphagia Diet: Standardization for Optimal Care

impair brain function. Again it is important to make the distinction between normal, age-related decline and impairment from conditions such as dementia. Dementia is a disease process. Memory difficulties do not necessarily indicate dementia, Alzheimer's disease, Parkinson's disease, or any mental disorder. Many changes in memory can be attributed to environmental factors, including stress, chemical exposure, and poor diet rather than to physiologic processes.

Depression

Depression can cause mental impairment that is both transient and treatable, but it is not an inevitable consequence of aging. Causes of depression vary widely form person to person. Among older persons it is often caused by other conditions such as heart disease, stroke, diabetes, cancer, and grief and stress. Depression in older people is frequently undiagnosed or misdiagnosed because symptoms are confused with other medical illnesses. Untreated depression can have serious side effects for older adults. It diminishes the pleasures of living, including eating; it can exacerbate other medical conditions; it can compromise immune function. It is associated with decreased appetite, weight loss, and fatigue. Nutritional care plays an important role in addressing this condition by providing nutrient- and calorie-dense foods, additional beverages, texture-modified foods, and favorite foods at optimal times when people are most likely to eat the greatest quantity.

Pressure Ulcers

Pressure ulcers, formerly called bedsores or decubitus ulcers, develop from continuous pressure that impedes capillary blood flow to skin and underlying tissue. Several factors contribute to the formation of pressure ulcers, but impaired mobility is key. Older adults with neurologic problems, those heavily sedated, and those with dementia are often unable to shift positions to alleviate pressure. Paralysis, sensory losses, and rigidity can all contribute to the problem. Notably malnutrition (inadequate protein) and undernutrition (inadequate energy intake) set the stage for its development and can delay wound healing. The escalating chronic nature of pressure ulcers requires vigilant attention to nutrition.

Several classification systems exist to describe pressure ulcers. The four stages of pressure ulcers, based on the depth of the sore and level of tissue involvement, are described in (Box 10-1).

Frailty and Failure to Thrive

The four syndromes known to be predictive of adverse outcomes in older adults that are prevalent in patients with frailty or "failure to thrive" include impaired physical functioning, malnutrition, depression, and cognitive impairment (Robertson and Montagnini, 2004). Symptoms of this condition include weight loss, decreased appetite, poor nutrition, dehydration, inactivity, and impaired immune function. Interventions should be directed at easily remediable contributors in the hope of improving overall functional

status. Again nutrition interventions are essential (Sarkisian and Lachs, 1996).

Hearing and Eyesight

In the United States 30% to 35% of adults ages 65 to 75 and 50% of those over age 75 have some degree of hearing loss (National Institute on Deafness, 2006). Approximately one in four older adults who need a hearing aid actually use one. The most common type of hearing loss is **presbycusis.** This loss is usually greater in the high-pitched tonal range (e.g., telephone ring). The cumulative effect of exposure to daily noises such as traffic, construction, loud music, noisy office, and machines causes a change to the inner ear complex. The change occurs slowly over time, and sufferers may not be aware of the loss.

Some vitamins may play a part in hearing loss. Vitamin B_{12}, a nutrient often found to be deficient in the diets of older adults, has been associated with increased chronic tinnitus (ringing in the ears), presbycusis, and reduced auditory brainstem response (Johnson et al., 2004). Vitamin D may have an impact on hearing loss because of the role it plays in calcium metabolism, fluid and nerve transmission, and bone structure.

Vision loss is not a part of normal aging. However, everyone's vision changes with age. For most the changes are small and correctable with glasses, improved lighting, or large print. Reading glasses often become necessary in the fourth decade of life.

Age-related macular degeneration (AMD) is the leading cause of blindness in people over age 65 in the United States; it may also be linked to an increased risk for stroke (Wong et al., 2006). AMD occurs when the macula, the center part of the retina, degrades. The result is central vision loss. The macular pigment is composed of two chemicals, lutein and zeaxanthin. A diet rich in fruits and vegetables may help delay or prevent the development of AMD. Zinc has also been shown to decrease the risk of developing AMD. Finally, correcting obesity and smoking are modifiable factors that can reduce progression of AMD (Clemons et al., 2006).

Glaucoma is damage to the optic nerve due to high pressure in the eye. It is the second most common cause of vision loss in the United States and affects approximately 3 million Americans. Hypertension, diabetes, and CVD all increase the risk of glaucoma developing.

A **cataract** is a clouding of the lens of the eye. About half of Americans 65 and older have some degree of clouding of the lens. Most common treatment is surgery; the clouded lens is removed and replaced with a permanent clear plastic lens. A diet high in antioxidants such as β-carotene, selenium, resveratrol, and vitamins C and E, may delay cataract development. Studies show that a high sodium intake may increase risk of development of cataract.

Diabetic retinopathy is a complication of diabetes. It occurs when blood vessels of the retina leak and produce spotty hemorrhages. Not all persons with diabetes develop retinopathy; blood glucose control can help protect the retina from damage.

BOX 10-1

Pressure Ulcer Stages

Suspected Deep Tissue Injury

Purple or maroon localized area of discolored intact skin or blood-filled blister due to damage of underlying soft tissue from pressure and/or shear. The area may be preceded by tissue that is painful, firm, mushy, boggy, warmer, or cooler as compared to adjacent tissue.

Deep tissue injury may be difficult to detect in individuals with dark skin tones. Evolution may include a thin blister over a dark wound bed. The wound may further evolve and become covered by thin eschar. Evolution may be rapid, exposing additional layers of tissue even with optimal treatment.

Stage I

Intact skin with non-blanchable redness of a localized area, usually over a bony prominence. Darkly pigmented skin may not have visible blanching; its color may differ from the surrounding area.

The area may be painful, firm, soft, warmer, or cooler as compared to adjacent tissue. Stage I may be difficult to detect in individuals with dark skin tones. May indicate "at risk" persons (a heralding sign of risk).

Stage II

Partial thickness loss of dermis presenting as a shallow open ulcer with a red pink wound bed without slough. May also present as an intact or open/ruptured serum-filled blister.

Presents as a shiny or dry shallow ulcer without slough or bruising. This stage should not be used to describe skin tears, tape burns, perineal dermatitis, maceration, or excoriation. Bruising indicates suspected deep tissue injury.

Stage III

Full thickness tissue loss. Subcutaneous fat may be visible but bone, tendon, or muscle are not exposed. Slough may be present but does not obscure the depth of tissue loss. May include undermining and tunneling.

Stage III, cont'd

The depth of a stage III pressure ulcer varies by anatomic location. The bridge of the nose, ear, occiput, and malleolus do not have subcutaneous tissue, and stage III ulcers can be shallow. In contrast, areas of significant adiposity can develop extremely deep stage III pressure ulcers. Bone/tendon is not visible or directly palpable.

Stage IV

Full thickness tissue loss with exposed bone, tendon, or muscle. Slough or eschar may be present on some parts of the wound bed. Often include undermining and tunneling.

The depth of a stage IV pressure ulcer varies by anatomic location. The bridge of the nose, ear, occiput, and malleolus do not have subcutaneous tissue, and these ulcers can be shallow. Stage IV ulcers can extend into muscle and/or supporting structures (e.g., fascia, tendon, or joint capsule) making osteomyelitis possible. Exposed bone/tendon is visible or directly palpable.

Unstageable

Full thickness tissue loss in which the base of the ulcer is covered by slough (yellow, tan, gray, green, or brown) and/or eschar (tan, brown, or black) in the wound bed.

Until enough slough and/or eschar is removed to expose the base of the wound, the true depth, and therefore stage, cannot be determined. Stable (dry, adherent, intact without erythema or fluctuance) eschar on the heels serves as "the body's natural (biologic) cover" and should not be removed.

From the National Pressure Ulcer Advisory Panel, 2007. Reprinted with permission. Reproduction of the National Pressure Ulcer Advisory Panel (NPUAP) materials in this document does not imply endorsement by the NPUAP of any products, organizations, companies, or any statements made by any organization or company.

All forms of vision loss can negatively affect nutritional status. Those with moderate-to-severe vision loss may have difficulty shopping for, identifying, and preparing foods and self-feeding.

Immunocompetence

As immunocompetence declines with age, immune response is slower and less efficient. Changes occur at all levels of the immune system, from chemical alterations within the cells to differences in the kinds of proteins found on the cell surface and even to mutations to entire organs. The progressive decline in T-lymphocyte function and cell-mediated immunity is a major contributor to the increased infection and cancer rates seen in aging populations (Barve et al., 2004). The mechanisms of age-related changes in immune function are not fully understood but are likely dependent on environmental factors and lifestyle choices that affect overall immune function from the molecular level to that of the entire organism (Burns, 2004). Maintaining good nutritional status promotes good immune function.

QUALITY OF LIFE

There is little agreement regarding how quality of life is defined and measured. *Healthy People 2010* defines it as a general sense of happiness and satisfaction with one's life and environment. Health-related **quality of life** is the personal sense of physical and mental health and the ability to react to factors in the physical and social environments (USDHHS, 2006). To assess health-related quality of life, common measures and scales, either general or disease-specific, can be used (Amarantos et al., 2001). The SF-36

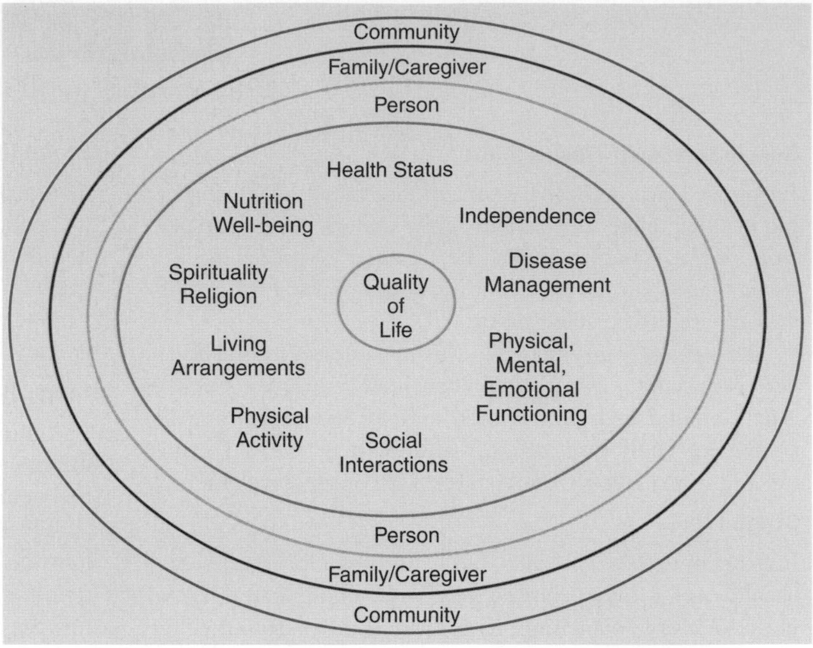

FIGURE 10-3 Factors that influence quality of life of adults 60 years and older.

is a widely used quality of life measurement and can be self-administered (Ware and Sherbourne, 1992). Because older age is often associated with health problems and decrease in functionality, quality of life issues become more relevant in the care of older adults (Amarantos et al., 2001; Ware and Sherbourne, 1992; Drewnowski and Evans, 2001).

Food and nutrition contribute to one's physiologic, psychological, and social quality of life. A measure of nutrition-related quality of life has been proposed to document quality-of-life outcomes for individuals receiving medical nutrition therapy (Barr and Schumacher, 2003). The multiple factors impacting the quality of life of adults 60 years and older are shown in Figure 10-3 (Kuczmarski and Weddle, 2005). In assessing quality of life for older individuals, dietitians should consider these variables at the personal level and also within the family and community.

Functionality

Functionality and *functional status* are terms used to describe physical abilities and limitations in, for example, ambulation (National Center for Chronic Disease Prevention and Health Promotion, 2006; Agency for Healthcare Research and Quality and Centers for Disease Control, 2006).

Functionality, the ability to perform self-care, self-maintenance, and physical activities, correlates with independence and quality of life. Disability rates among older adults are declining, but the actual number considered disabled is increasing as the size of the aging population grows. Limitations in **activities of daily living (ADLs),** or individual self-performance skills needed in everyday life, and instrumental activities of daily living (IADLs) and other measures are used to monitor physical function (see *Focus On:* Activities of Daily Living).

Many nutrition-related diseases affect functional status, especially in older individuals (Amarantos et al., 2001)

(e.g., amputations in persons with diabetes that have chronically uncontrolled dietary compliance). Inadequate nutrient intake, both excess and insufficiency, may induce or hasten decline as a result of loss of muscle mass and strength, which can have a negative effect on performing ADLs (Sharkey, 2004). Among the 87% of older adults who have one or more nutrition-related chronic diseases, consequences include impaired physical function that may cause greater disability, increased morbidity, nursing home admissions, and death (Nelson et al., 2004).

Weight Maintenance

Obesity

The prevalence of obesity in all ages has increased during the past 25 years in the United States; older adults are no exception. Obesity rates are greater among those ages 65 to 74 than among those age 75 and over. Obesity is associated with increased mortality and contributes to many chronic diseases: type 2 diabetes, heart disease, hypertension, arthritis, dyslipidemia, and cancer. Obesity causes a progressive decline in physical function, which may lead to increased frailty. Overweight and obesity can lead to a decline in IADLs.

Current data demonstrate that weight-loss therapy improves physical function, quality of life, and reduces the medical complications associated with obesity in older persons (Villareal et al., 2005). Accordingly weight loss therapies that maintain muscle and bone mass are recommended for obese older adults. Lifestyle changes that include diet, physical activity, and behavior modification techniques are the most effective. The goals of weight loss and management for adults are the same for the general population. They should include prevention of further weight gain, or reduction of body weight, and maintenance of long-term weight loss.

Weight loss of 10% of total body weight over 6 months should be the initial goal. After that, strategies for mainte-

◎ **FOCUS ON**

Activities of Daily Living

Activities of Daily Living

- Feeding
- Bed/chair transfer
- Indoor/outdoor mobility
- Dressing
- Bathing
- Toileting
- Continence

Instrumental Activities of Daily Living

- Telephone use
- Traveling
- Shopping
- Preparing meals
- Doing light housework
- Taking medication
- Money management

---

nance should be implemented. Dietary changes include an energy deficit of 500 to 1000 kcal/day. Usual caloric goals range from 1200 to 1800 kcal/day but should not be less than 800 kcal/day. It is critical for the older adult on a calorie-restricted diet to meet nutrient requirements. This may necessitate the use of a multivitamin/mineral supplement as well as nutrition education.

Underweight and Malnutrition

The prevalence of underweight among older adults is quite low. From 1999 to 2002, 2% of older men and women were underweight; older women over age 65 were three times as likely as their male counterparts to be underweight (Federal Interagency Forum, 2006). However, many older adults are at risk for undernutrition and malnutrition.

Among those hospitalized, 40% to 60% are malnourished or at risk for malnutrition, 40% to 85% of nursing home residents have malnutrition, and 20% to 60% of home care patients are malnourished (see Chapter 14). Many community-residing older persons consume fewer than 1000 kcal/day, an amount not adequate to maintain good nutrition. Some causes of undernutrition include medications, depression, decreased sense of taste or smell, poor oral health, chronic diseases, dysphagia, and other physical problems that make eating difficult. Social causes may include living alone, inadequate income, lack of transportation, and limitations in shopping for and preparing food.

Health care professionals frequently overlook protein-energy undernutrition (PEU). The physiologic changes of aging, as well as changes in living conditions and income, all contribute to the problem. Symptoms of PEU are often attributed to other conditions, leading to misdiagnosis. Some common symptoms are confusion, fatigue, and weakness. Older adults with low incomes, who have difficulty chewing and swallowing meat, who smoke, or engage in little or no physical activity are at increased risk of developing PEU. Most contributing factors are modifiable through diet and physical activity.

Older malnourished adults are at risk of refeeding syndrome, especially those who receive nutrition support (Mallet, 2002). Strategies to decrease PEU include increased caloric and protein intake. In a clinical setting nutritional oral supplements and enteral feedings may be used. Frailty is often related to micronutrient deficiencies, especially in women (Michelon et al., 2006).

In a community setting older adults should be encouraged to eat energy-dense and high-protein foods. Diet restrictions should be liberalized to offer more choices. Adding gravies and creams can increase calories and soften foods for easier chewing (Ritchie and Joshipura, 2004). Federal food and nutrition services are also available for older adults. See section on Supportive Services.

NUTRITION SCREENING

There are tools to evaluate nutrition status in older adults. The Mini Nutritional Assessment (MNA) is an efficient, innovative, noninvasive method to detect risk for malnutrition using questions and anthropometric measures to determine a malnutrition indicator score (Vellas et al., 1999).

The Nutrition Screening Initiative (NSI), a broad multidisciplinary effort led by the American Academy of Family Physicians and ADA along with a coalition of more than 25 national health, aging, and medical organizations, was founded in 1989. NSI promotes the integration of nutrition screening and earlier interventions for older adults. The initiative developed the *Determine Your Nutritional Health Checklist* as a public awareness tool to highlight the warning signs of malnutrition (Figure 10-4).

The Level I screen (see Figure 14-7) identifies those who may need preventive nutrition intervention. It can be used in many health care and social service systems. The screen calculates body mass index (BMI) and obtains information on dietary habits, living environment, and functional status. If one or more statements are checked, a referral for a complete nutrition assessment should be made.

The Level II screen (see Figure 14-8) contains specific screening measures including anthropometrics, laboratory data, drug use, clinical features, and cognitive status. This screen is used when level I identifies potential nutrition problems (Lipschitz et al., 1992).

The *Physician's Guide to Nutrition and Chronic Disease Management of Older Adults*, a popular NSI publication, emphasizes the importance of making referrals to dietitians for complex nutrition problems that Medicare reimburses. NSI promotes nutrition standards of care for The Joint Commission (TJC) and the National Committee on Quality Assurance (NCQA) and for the Agency for Healthcare Research and Quality (AHRQ).

The Warning Signs of poor nutritional health are often overlooked. Use this checklist to find out if you or someone you know is at nutritional risk.

Read the statements below. Circle the number in the yes column for those that apply to you or someone you know. For each yes answer, score the number in the box. Total your nutrition score.

DETERMINE YOUR NUTRITIONAL HEALTH

	YES
I have an illness or condition that made me change the kind and/or amount of food I eat.	2
I eat fewer than two meals per day.	3
I eat few fruits or vegetables or milk products.	2
I have three or more drinks of beer, liquor, or wine almost every day.	2
I have tooth or mouth problems that make it hard for me to eat.	2
I don't always have enough money to buy the food I need.	4
I eat alone most of the time.	1
I take three or more different prescribed or over-the-counter drugs a day.	1
Without wanting to, I have lost or gained 10 pounds in the last 6 months.	2
I am not physically able to shop, cook, and/or feed myself.	2
TOTAL	

Total Your Nutritional Score. If it's —

0–2   Good! Recheck your nutritional score in 6 months.

3–5   **You are at moderate nutritional risk.** See what can be done to improve your eating habits and lifestyle. Your office on aging, senior nutrition program, senior citizens center, or health department can help. Recheck your nutritional score in 3 months.

6 or more   **You are at high nutritional risk.** Bring this checklist the next time you see your doctor, dietitian, or other qualified health or social service professional. Talk with them about any problems you may have. Ask for help to improve your nutritional health.

Remember that warning signs suggest risk but do not represent diagnosis of any condition.

The Nutrition Checklist is based on the Warning Signs described below. Use the word DETERMINE to remind you of the Warning signs.

Disease   Any disease, illness or chronic condition which causes you to change the way you eat, or makes it hard for you to eat, puts your nutritional health at risk. Four out of five adults have chronic diseases that are affected by diet. Confusion or memory loss that keeps getting worse is estimated to affect one out of five or more of older adults. This can make it hard to remember what, when or if you've eaten. Feeling sad or depressed, which happens to about one in eight older adults, can cause big changes in appetite, digestion, energy level, weight and well-being.

Eating Poorly   Eating too little and eating too much both lead to poor health. Eating the same foods day after day or not eating fruit, vegetables, and milk products daily will also cause poor nutritional health. One in five adults skip meals daily. Only 13% of adults eat the minimum amount of fruit and vegetables needed. One in four older adults drink too much alcohol. Many health problems become worse if you drink more than one or two alcoholic beverages per day.

Tooth Loss/Mouth Pain   A healthy mouth, teeth, and gums are needed to eat. Missing, loose, or rotten teeth, or dentures which don't fit well or cause mouth sores, make it hard to eat.

Economic Hardship   As many as 40% of older Americans have incomes of less than $6,000 per year. Having less—or choosing to spend less— than $25–30 per week for food makes it very hard to get the foods you need to stay healthy.

Reduced Social Contact   One-third of all older people live alone. Being with people daily has a positive effect on morale, well-being and eating.

Multiple Medicines   Many older Americans must take medicines for health problems. Almost half of older Americans take multiple medicines daily. Growing old may change the way we respond to drugs. The more medicines you take, the greater the chance for side effects, such as increased or decreased appetite, change in taste, constipation, weakness, drowsiness, diarrhea, nausea, and others. Vitamins or minerals, when taken in large doses, act like drugs and can cause harm. Alert your doctor to everything you take.

Involuntary Weight Loss/Gain   Losing or gaining a lot of weight when you are not trying to do so is an important warning sign that must not be ignored. Being overweight or underweight also increases your chance of poor health.

Needs Assistance in Self-Care   Although most older people are able to eat, one out of every five has trouble walking, shopping, or buying and cooking food, especially as they get older.

Elder Years Above Age 80   Most older people lead full and productive lives. But as age increases, the risk of frailty and health problems increases. Checking your nutritional health regularly makes good sense.

FIGURE 10-4 Determine Your Nutritional Health Checklist. *(Courtesy Nutrition Screening Initiative, a project of the American Academy of Family Physicians, the American Dietetic Association, and the National Council of the Aging and funded in part by a grant from Ross Products Division, Abbott Laboratories, 1991.)*

The ADA and members of the NSI helped secure Medicare reimbursement for medical nutrition therapy (MNT) so that nutrition is in the Medicare Prescription Drug and Modernization Act of 2003.

NUTRITION ASSESSMENT

Some commonly used assessment measures are not necessarily accurate or feasible to use with older adults. Physical and metabolic changes of aging can yield inaccurate results. An illustration of this is anthropometric measurements (height, weight, skin-fold thickness). With aging, fat mass increases and height decreases as a result of vertebral compression (Villareal et al., 2005). An accurate height measure may be difficult in those unable to stand up straight, the bed bound, those with spinal deformations such as a Dowager's hump, and those with osteoporosis. Measuring arm span or knee height may give more accurate measurements. BMIs based on questionable heights are inaccurate. Clinical judgment is needed for accuracy.

Body composition measures may also be ineffective. Skin-fold thickness and mid-arm circumference used to detect changes in body fat are limited in their inability to distinguish between changes in fat and muscle mass, due to decreased elasticity and increased incompressibility of older skin. Mid-arm muscle circumference measures may be more accurate and sensitive to weight change than overall body composition (Wilson and Morley, 2004).

NUTRITION NEEDS

Many older adults have special nutrient requirements because aging affects absorption, use, and excretion (Kuczmarski and Weddle, 2005). The DRIs now separate the over–age 50 cohort into two groups, ages 50 to 70 and 71+. Previously published recommendations combined both in a 50+-age category. Older adults' scores were lowest for the components of the Healthy Eating Index (HEI) (see Chapter 9) measuring daily servings of fruit and milk products. Their scores were highest for HEI components measuring cholesterol intake and dietary variety (Federal Interagency Forum, 2006).

Studies suggest that older persons have low intakes of calories; total fat; fiber; calcium; magnesium; zinc; copper; folate; and vitamins B_{12}, C, E, and D (USDA, 2004; USDHHS NHANES III, 2006; USDHHS, 2004). See the inside cover for the DRI tables related to older adults.

Energy

Basal metabolic rates decrease linearly with age; this change is the result of the body composition changes discussed earlier. Energy needs decrease approximately 3% per decade. Low-kilocalorie diets are often deficient in most essential nutrients. The *Dietary Guidelines for Americans 2005* (DGA) (USDHHS/USDA, 2005) strongly encourage older adults to select nutrient-dense foods that provide substantial amounts of micronutrients for the calories supplied (Box 10-2; see Box 9-1).

Protein

Protein needs do not usually change with age, although the research is not conclusive (Lucas and Heiss, 2005). Protein intake in excess of the recommended dietary allowance (RDA) for older adults is associated with increased bone-mineral density when calcium intake is adequate, and does not appear to compromise renal health in older individuals with normal renal function. Protein requirements can vary because of chronic disease. Balancing needs and restrictions is a challenge, particularly in health care facilities. Protein absorption may decrease with aging as the body may make less protein. However, this does not mean that protein intake should be routinely increased. Because of the general decline in kidney function, excess protein could unnecessarily stress kidneys.

Carbohydrates

Current dietary guidelines recommend that approximately 45% to 65% of the total daily calories should come from carbohydrates. Emphasis is on increasing intake of complex carbohydrate sources such as legumes, vegetables, whole grains, and fruits to provide fiber and essential vita-

---

BOX 10-2

Dietary Guidelines for Americans, 2005: Key Recommendations for Older Adults

- Consume vitamin B_{12} in its crystalline form (i.e., fortified foods or supplements).
- Consume extra vitamin D from vitamin D–fortified foods and/or supplements.
- Consult a health care provider about weight loss strategies before starting a weight-reduction program to ensure appropriate management of other health conditions.
- Participate in regular physical activity to reduce functional declines associated with aging and to achieve the other benefits of physical activity identified for all adults.
- Aim to consume no more than 1500 mg of sodium per day and meet the potassium recommendation (4700 mg/day) with food.
- Do not eat or drink raw (unpasteurized) milk or any products made from unpasteurized milk, raw or partially cooked eggs or foods containing raw eggs, raw or undercooked meat and poultry, raw or undercooked fish or shellfish, unpasteurized juices, and raw sprouts.
- Only eat certain deli meats and frankfurters that have been reheated to steaming hot.

Data from U.S. Department of Agriculture and U.S. Department of Health and Human Services: *Nutrition and your health: dietary guidelines for Americans*, ed 5, Garden Bulletin No. 232, 2000.

mins and minerals. Constipation is a serious concern for many older adults. The DGA stress the importance of increasing dietary fiber for improving laxation, especially in older adults.

Lipids

The DGA recommend keeping fat intake between 20% to 35% of total calories, with most from polyunsaturated and monounsaturated sources. The *Guidelines* also advise consuming less than 10% of calories from saturated fats, less than 300 mg/day of cholesterol, and eating *trans*-fats as little as possible. Lower intakes of fat, less than 7% saturated fat and less than 200 mg/day cholesterol may be recommended for older adults with elevated low-density lipoprotein cholesterol. However, it should be noted that severe restriction of fats alter the taste, texture, and enjoyment of food and can negatively impact the overall diet, weight, and quality of life.

Vitamins and Minerals

Although much remains to be known, understanding the vitamin and mineral requirements, absorption, use, and excretion in aging has increased greatly in the past decades. The challenge for older adults is to increase vitamin and mineral intake in relation to total caloric intake. Oxidative processes affect aging, reinforcing the central role antioxidants play in maintaining health throughout life. Most chronic diseases begin earlier in life. Therefore it is essential to encourage younger people to improve their diets so they enter later life in better health.

Vitamin B_{12}

Older adults are at risk for deficiency because of low intakes of vitamin B_{12}–rich sources and the decline in gastric acid, which aids in releasing vitamin B_{12} from protein. The DGA recommend that those over age 50 eat foods fortified with the crystalline form of vitamin B_{12} such as in fortified cereals or supplements.

Vitamin D

People over age 50 may be at increased risk of vitamin D deficiency (Holick, 2002). The skin does not synthesize vitamin D as efficiently and the kidneys are less able to convert vitamin D to its active hormone form. As many as 30% to 40% of older adults who have had a hip fracture are vitamin D insufficient (Office of Dietary Supplements, 2006). The DGA recommend that those at high risk, including older adults and dark-skinned individuals, should consume substantially higher levels of vitamin D to maintain serum 25-hydroxy-vitamin D levels at 80 nmol/L. To attain these levels, supplementation may be necessary.

Vitamin E

Most Americans, especially older adults, should increase their intake of vitamin E–rich foods. Preliminary studies show that the antioxidant properties may help prevent or delay cataract growth (Pham and Plakogiannis, 2005).

Folate

Folate may be important in lowering homocysteine levels, a possible risk marker for atherothrombosis, Alzheimer's disease and Parkinson's disease (Irizarry et al., 2005). Folate fortification of grain products has greatly improved folate status. Of course, when supplementing with folate, it is important to monitor B_{12} levels.

Calcium

The older adult's dietary calcium requirement may be increased due to decreased absorption that occurs with aging. Only 4% of women and 10% of men over age 60 reach the daily calcium recommendation. DGAs recommend that older adults pay more attention to this nutrient.

Potassium

According to the DGA, a potassium-rich diet can blunt the effect of sodium on blood pressure. Older adults are encouraged to meet the potassium recommendation of 4700 mg/day with food, especially fruits and vegetables.

Sodium

Older adults are at risk of both hypernatremia and hyponatremia. Hypernatremia can be a consequence of dietary excess and dehydration. Hyponatremia can result from fluid retention. The DGA recommend that older adults aim to consume no more than 1500 mg/day of sodium.

Zinc

There is no universally accepted method for assessing zinc status. Although most older adults have intakes below the current RDA, they do not display overt zinc deficiency. Low zinc intake is associated with impaired immune function, anorexia, loss of sense of taste, delayed wound healing, and pressure ulcer development.

Water

Maintenance of fluid balance is essential for normal physiologic functions at all ages. Hydration status of older adults is often tenuous. As discussed earlier, the lean body mass decrease with age impacts the percentage of water in the body. It can diminish from 60% to 50% total body weight. Dehydration in older adults can be caused by decreased fluid intake, decreased kidney function, or increased losses due to increased urine output from medications, including laxatives or diuretics. Fluid intake of at least 1500 ml/day ensures proper hydration.

Symptoms of dehydration are electrolyte imbalance, altered drug effects, headache, constipation, blood pressure change, dizziness, confusion, and dry mouth and nose. Older adults are at increased risk of dehydration because of their impaired sense of thirst, fear of incontinence, and dependence on others to get beverages. Dehydration in older adults is often unrecognized because it can present as falls, confusion, change in level of consciousness, weakness or change in functional status, or fatigue.

MEDICARE BENEFITS

Prescription Benefits: Part D

Beginning in 2006 everyone eligible for Medicare, regardless of income, health status, or prescription drug usage, has access to prescription drug coverage. Part D subsidizes prescription drugs for the disabled and those over age 65. To meet the diverse needs of individual beneficiaries, the beneficiary must choose from among several coverage options. Part D is administered through different plans by private companies, unions, etc., whose plans must be approved by the Centers for Medicare and Medicaid Services (CMS). Plans differ by drugs covered, price, and delivery method. Number and types of plans differ from state to state. The monthly premium averages about $32 for the standard Medicare plan, but the exact amount depends on the plan chosen. Drug plans must offer at least two prescription drugs in each of 112 different illness/injury/affliction categories. Not every drug is covered by every drug plan.

In 2007, approximately 8 million of the 23 million eligible have enrolled. The plan has the greatest benefit for the poorest old, who have often been forced to choose among food, rent, heat, and medications. It is anticipated that the wider availability of drug coverage will improve disease management, but without vigilance an increase in unfavorable drug-nutrient and drug-drug interactions may also occur. Dietitians can play a vital role in the monitoring of older adult medication usage (see Figure 16-1).

Medical Nutrition Therapy Benefits

MNT became a Medicare benefit in January 2002. Medicare covers nutrition services by a registered dietitian for those with diabetes or preend-stage renal disease. In December 2003 two new provisions were added that expanded the MNT provided through Medicare to include preventive services and chronic care improvement.

Preventive services took effect for new Medicare beneficiaries in 2005. Each new beneficiary has 6 months after joining Medicare to get an initial preventive physical examination. The examination includes a physical measuring of height, weight, and blood pressure and an electrocardiogram. It also includes education, counseling, and a referral with respect to screening and other preventive services. One of the specified preventive services required under the law is MNT offered by a qualified registered dietitian.

In an effort to maintain health and reduce hospitalizations, *chronic care improvement* (CCI) was initiated early in 2006. The CMS contracts with CCI programs to provide the benefit. The benefit is administered by CCI programs and not directly by CMS. Individuals with certain conditions, including heart failure, diabetes, chronic obstructive pulmonary disease, or other diseases or conditions as selected by CMS, will be eligible for participation (ADA, 2006). Figure 10-5 shows an active senior citizen who manages her chronic disease with exercise and diet.

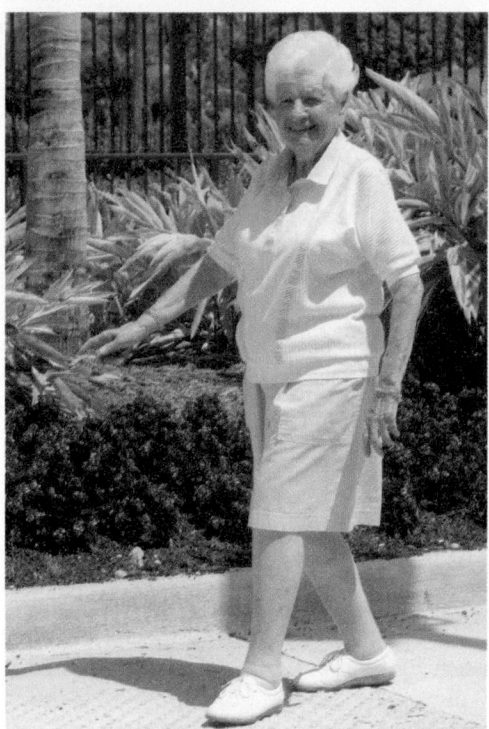

FIGURE 10-5 An active, healthy older American managing her diabetes with nutrition and exercise.

SUPPORTIVE SERVICES

Older Americans Act Nutrition Program

The OAA nutrition program is the largest, most visible, federally funded community-based nutrition program for older persons. Primarily a state-run program, it has few federal regulations and considerable variation in state-to-state policies and procedures. This nutrition program provides congregate and home-delivered meals, nutrition screening, education, and counseling, as well as an array of other supportive and health services. Although frequently called *Meals-on-Wheels*, that term accurately refers *only* to the home-delivered meals.

The OAA nutrition program, available to persons age 60 and over, is targeted to those in greatest economic and social need, with particular attention to low-income minorities and rural individuals. To receive home-delivered meals, an individual must be assessed to be homebound or otherwise isolated. These services can be a primary source of support for many older adults who would not receive services under other income-based programs. It is the chief gap-filling service system for individuals who may be slightly over the poverty line.

In the USDHHS, the AoA administers the OAA programs through an Aging Network that includes 57 State Units on Aging, 655 Area Agencies on Aging, thousands of local providers under Title III, 233 Tribes and Tribal Organizations representing American Indian and Alaskan Natives, and two organizations serving Native Hawaiians under Title VI. All other nutrition assistance programs are housed in the U.S. Department of Agriculture (USDA).

Over half of the OAA annual budget supports the nutrition program that provides about 250 million congregate and home-delivered meals to approximately 3 million older adults annually. Home-delivered meals have grown to about 54% of all meals served, and at least 41% of the programs have waiting lists (Mathematica Policy Research, Inc, 1996b). The OAA funds about 44% of the cost of congregate and 30% of the cost of home-delivered meals. These federal funds are highly leveraged by state and local monies and services. Participants themselves contribute 20% toward the cost of congregate and home-delivered meals. The average cost of a Titles III and VI meal, including donated labor and supplies, ranges from $5 to $7 (Mathematica Policy Research, Inc, 1996a).

Today the nutrition program is closely linked to home- and community-based care (HCBC) systems through cross-referrals and the coordination of service delivery by the Aging Network. Since older adults are being discharged earlier from hospitals and nursing homes, many require a care plan that includes home-delivered meals and other nutrition services (e.g., nutrition screening, assessment, education, counseling, and care planning). Many states are enrolling Medicaid beneficiaries in HMOs, using Medicaid HCBC waivers, and creating state-funded programs to provide necessary HCBC medical, social, and supportive services, including home-delivered meals and nutrition education and counseling services (Kuczmarski and Weddle, 2005; Mallet, 2002).

At congregate sites the Nutrition Program is a foundation service that provides access and linkages to other community-based services. It is the primary source of food and nutrients for many program participants. It presents opportunities for active social engagement and meaningful volunteer roles. Home-delivered meals are among the most critical and necessary in-home services provided to vulnerable older adults, who are usually older, poorer, more likely to be women, and significantly functionally impaired and who usually have several chronic illnesses or disabling conditions that may be managed by nutrition interventions.

Inadequate nutrient intake affects approximately 37% to 40% of community-dwelling individuals 65 years of age and older (Federal Interagency Forum, 2006). The OAA Nutrition Program is important in reaching the *Healthy People 2010* goals, which are to improve the quality and years of healthy life and to reduce health disparities that exist because of differences in gender, race, or ethnicity, income or education, disability, or living location. Substantial disparities in cause of death exist among racial and ethnic groups and between genders (www.cdc.gov/nchs/nhanes.htm). The OAA Nutrition Program successfully targets individuals at nutrition risk, including those who are of advanced age, of poor income status, and live alone, as well as racial/ethnic minorities. About 25% of participants are minorities—almost twice the national percentage.

The OAA nutrition program has not received the research and evaluation attention that a program its size deserves, but the most recent national evaluation showed the positive impact. Participants had higher daily intakes of key nutrients than similar nonparticipants. The meals are nutritionally dense per calorie and each meal supplies more than 33% of the RDAs (an OAA requirement) and provides 40% to 50% of daily intakes of most nutrients (Ponza et al, 1996).

USDA Food Assistance Programs

Several USDA food and nutrition assistance programs (www.fns.usda.gov/fns/default.htm) are available to older adults. All USDA programs are means tested (i.e. recipients must meet income criteria). As MNT moves out of hospitals and nursing homes into home and community systems these food assistance programs become more important.

Food Stamp Program

The mandate of the Food Stamp Program (FSP), the largest USDA food assistance program, is to end hunger and improve nutrition and health of low-income Americans. Beneficiaries use electronic debit cards to purchase certain foods at authorized retail food stores. The FSP is operated by state and local welfare offices under USDA guidance.

Currently FSP serves 21 million individuals. However, only one in three eligible adults over age 65 participates. Approximately 20% of food stamp households include an older adult. Among the many reasons for low FSP participation rates by older adults is the myth that they only qualify for $10 monthly benefit. In reality, the average benefit is $44 for older adults living alone and $116 for households with an older adult.

Food Stamp Nutrition Education Program

The goal of FSP nutrition education is to improve the likelihood that FSP participants will make healthy choices within a limited budget and choose active lifestyles consistent with the current DGA and MyPyramid. State Cooperative Extension, nutrition education networks, public health departments, welfare agencies, and university centers generally provide FSP nutrition education. Unfortunately little outreach specific to older adults is offered.

Commodity Supplemental Food Program

Commodity Supplemental Food Program (CSFP) strives to improve the health of low-income Americans by supplementing their diets with nutritious USDA commodity foods. It provides food and administrative funds to states to supplement diets. Currently 33 states and two tribal organizations participate. In states CSFP administration may be located in public health; nutrition services; health services; education; family and children; housing; community service; environmental nutrition; Women, Infants and Children (WIC) services; or agriculture departments. Eligible populations include adults over age 60 with incomes less than 130% of the poverty level. Local CSFP agencies determine applicant eligibility, distribute the foods, and provide nutrition education. The food packages do not provide a complete diet but may be good sources of nutrients frequently lacking in low-income diets. In 2005 the 460,000 older adults served equal 90% of those served by CSFP (www.fns.usda.gov/pd/fdpart.htm).

Seniors' Farmers Market Nutrition Program

Seniors' Farmers Market Nutrition Program (SFMNP) is administered by state departments of agriculture, aging and disability services, health and human service, markets, public health, state unit on aging, or state food and nutrition services. SFMNP provides coupons to low-income older individuals to purchase fresh, unprepared foods at farmers' markets, roadside stands, and community-supported agriculture programs. It provides eligible older adults with local seasonal access to fresh fruits, vegetables, and herbs. It is also increases domestic consumption of agricultural commodities and specifically helps support and create more farmers' markets, roadside stands, and community-supported agriculture programs. Annual benefits to the 802,000 older participants average $25 annually and are available during local harvest seasons.

Child and Adult Care Food Program

The Child and Adult Care Food Program (CACFP) serves nutritious meals and snacks to eligible children and older adults in participating child-care centers, day-care homes, and adult day centers. Centers can serve breakfast, lunch, supper and snack. Meals are composed of 1 cup milk, 1 to 2 pieces of fruits or vegetables, grain, and meat or meat alternative. Portion sizes vary by age-group. Breakfast must include three components; lunch, all four components; supper, three components; and snack, two of the four components. Meals served must meet these minimum requirements to be reimbursable.

Emergency Food Assistance Program

The Emergency Food Assistance Program (TEFAP) is a commodity food distribution program. The USDA buys food, including processing and packaging, and ships it to the states' distributing agencies. The program was designed to help reduce federal food inventories and storage costs while assisting the needy. Each state's allotment depends on the number of its low-income and unemployed population. States provide food to local agencies, usually food banks, which in turn distribute the food to soup kitchens and food pantries that directly serve those needing food assistance. These organizations distribute the commodities for household consumption or use the foods to prepare and serve meals in a congregate setting. Since TEFAP tracks amounts of food distributed nationally, there are no data regarding the number of recipients.

Food Distribution Program on Indian Reservations

Food Distribution Program on Indian Reservations (FDPIR) is a commodity food distribution program that at times, such as in the winter when travel is impossible, is used instead of food stamps. USDA purchases and ships commodity foods to Indian tribal organizations and state

agencies based on orders from a list of available foods. Administering agencies store and distribute the food, determine applicant eligibility, and provide nutrition education to recipients. USDA provides the administering agencies with funds for program administrative costs. In 2003 FDPIR served 107,000 people, 15% of whom were age 60+.

Medicaid and Nutrition Services

The Social Security Act suggests seven core HCBS waiver program services: case management, homemaker services, home health aide services, personal care services, adult day health, habilitation, and respite care. Note that nutrition service is not a core Medicaid service. Older persons who are eligible for nursing home placement are not usually able to shop for food, store food safely, or plan and prepare nutritionally appropriate meals. Thus a strong argument can be made to fund all or some meals and nutrition services based on health and nutrition risk criteria. Yet, only 38 states include meals and/or nutrition services among the specified benefits available through Medicaid waivers. Approved nutrition services include home-delivered meals, nutrition risk reduction counseling, and nutritional supplements as appropriate.

LONG-TERM LIVING: SUBSIDIZED HOUSING, ASSISTED LIVING, AND SKILLED CARE FACILITIES

About 5% or 1.75 million older adults live in self-described senior housing of various types, many of which have supportive services available to their residents. Some but not all have OAA nutrition programs on site, although older adults in subsidized high-rise apartments often have greater unmet needs than those who reside in traditional community housing (Moore, 1991).

Assisted living facilities (ALFs) generally serve the fastest growing population segment—those ages 85 and older. The estimated 33,000 licensed ALFs are home to about a million persons. They combine housing and personalized supportive and health care for those who need help with ADLs. Often residents move to ALFs when they can no longer safely live alone, have some cognitive impairment, and require supervision and "cueing" about their daily routine. ALFs usually involve the resident's family, neighbors, and friends. Care is provided in ways that promote maximum independence and dignity. Assisted living residences cost less than nursing home care. Residents are encouraged to maintain active social lives with planned activities, exercise classes, religious and social functions, and field trips directed by the facilities.

Recent studies have found that comprehensive state regulations for food and nutrition services in ALFs are rare. Most are virtually unregulated (Chao and Dwyer, 2004). Emphasizing that food and nutrition matter at every age, it is essential that support for nutrition and quality of life extend beyond food availability and safety. Dietitian expertise is needed for nutrition assessment and care planning to meet special dietary needs such as type and amounts of macronutrients and micronutrients, texture modifications, and quality of life aspects related to food and nutrition.

Surprisingly only 4.5% or 1.6 million live in the approximately 18,000 **skilled nursing facilities,** commonly called nursing homes. The percentage of the population that lives in skilled nursing facilities increases dramatically with age: 1.1% of those 65 to 74 years; 4.7%, 75 to 84 years; and 18.2%, 85+ (US AoA, 2005). These percentages have declined since 1990, likely due to improved health, substitution of caretaking in ALFs, growth of in-home health care due to Medicaid reform, and availability of hospice (He et al., 2006). Facilities must undergo certification by CMS.

The average size of nursing homes is increasing, and more residents are there for short-stay, postacute care (Decker, 2005). Thus more comprehensive medical nutrition therapy is needed. Nutritional care within long-term living facilities must be directed toward identifying and responding to changing physiologic and psychological needs over time that protect against avoidable decline. Attractive and palatable food served in an atmosphere that encourages eating independence, or assistance with eating provided when necessary, helps to promote nutritional well-being. For older adults overall health goals may not warrant implementation of strict therapeutic diets that are often unpalatable and lessen quality of life (Neidert, 2005). In instances such as terminal care for hospice patients, interventions may be limited to providing comfort foods and emotional support for family and friends.

In 1987 Congress approved the initial nursing home reform legislation as a part of the Omnibus Reconciliation Act (OBRA) to improve care quality for nursing home residents by strengthening standards that must be met for Medicaid reimbursement. Nursing homes are required to conduct periodic assessments to determine the residents' needs; to provide services that ensure residents maintain the highest practical physical, mental and psychological well-being; and to ensure that no harm is inflicted.

Surveyors from regulatory agencies use CMS criteria to evaluate nursing homes' care. They have the authority to immediately close down a facility if many violations or substandard care, neglect, or abuse are noted. For consultant dietitians it may be difficult to provide all the necessary services if on-site time is limited. Facilities are now often encouraged to hire full-time RDs to provide more comprehensive medical nutrition therapy.

Primary to Tertiary Nutrition Prevention in Nursing Homes

Involuntary weight loss, pressure ulcers, and dehydration are avoidable in nursing homes if one emphasizes primary nutrition prevention, not just tertiary treatment after the fact. Secondary prevention could be an emphasis on walking to reduce sarcopenia and risk of falling. A focus on adequate hydration could decrease mental confusion. Tertiary prevention is commonplace since today's nursing homes are yesterday's hospitals and today's hospitals are really intensive care units. Minimum nutrition consultant hours allowing only time to chart but not to see residents enable some nursing homes to keep their insurance, but this should not be the case.

An RD Council for Quality Nursing Home Care shares best practice information and works to improve long-term care practice through advocacy and research. It is involved with 250,000 beds nationwide. Staffing for a facility or particular building is based on resident acuity and number of admissions per month. One study of weight loss as a quality measure showed that the difference between high and low weight loss in nursing homes is in the attention to dining programs and provision of feeding assistance (Simmons et al., 2003). However, the adequacy and quality of feeding assistance care needed improvement in all the nursing homes studied.

Since there is generally better continuity of care when provided by regular employees of a facility or company, whether full- or part-time, one can deduce that more attention to nutrition-related services is likely if RDs are regular employees rather than consultants in many instances. Medicaid reform is focusing on avoiding its long-standing institutional bias. Today only the frailest, sickest older adults are being admitted to nursing homes. Thus it is apparent that RD services should be more universally available in home- and community-based systems that serve older adults who previously would have been in institutions.

- One in five Americans will be age 65+ by 2030.
- Growing older is not synonymous with decrepitude, and believing so is "ageist." Health professionals need to distinguish the consequences of normal aging from those of chronic diseases.
- Functionality, independence and quality of life of older adults are dramatically affected by malnutrition, and many of its causes are avoidable or remediable.
- Nutritional care for health promotion, risk reduction and disease prevention can benefit all older adults; the positive role of nutrition in daily food choices is an important concept
- More than any other age group, older adults want nutrition and health information and are willing to make changes to maintain their independence and quality of life; they want to know how to eat healthier, exercise safely, and stay motivated to do both.
- Almost nine in ten older adults can benefit from MNT for chronic diseases. Therefore, individualized MNT provided by an RD should be central to the care management of persons with diabetes, hypertension, dyslipidemia, or a combination of these conditions, as well as under- and overweight, osteoporosis, COPD, some types of cancers, and dementia.
- Nutrition screening, assessment, intervention, and monitoring are key elements of the total health package that should be available to all older persons.

✹ CLINICAL SCENARIO 1

NG is a 76-year old widow who lives alone. She qualifies for and receives a hot lunch 5 days per week from the Older Americans Act Nutrition Program (commonly called *Meals-on-Wheels*). Her daughter and neighbor help with grocery shopping and preparation of other meals.

NG dislikes salty foods and complains about the taste of soups her neighbor prepares. She enjoys cooked vegetables, finding them easy to chew, and drinks a glass of milk every evening for her bones. However, recently she has exhibited signs of dehydration and some confusion.

During a severe storm her electricity went out. Her usual home-delivered meal cannot be delivered because of flooding. The Nutrition Program had provided an emergency meal in case of a disaster, but she ate the meal 2 weeks ago as a substitute for her neighbor's soup.

NG's daughter is out of town. Her neighbor visits after the storm. NG seems tired and confused. Her neighbor wants to help but is unsure what food to prepare or if the food and water in the refrigerator are safe. At present she is unable to cook anything because of the power outage. The neighbor has volunteered to go to the store and pick up a few shelf-stable items.

✳**Nutrition Diagnosis:** Limited access to adequate safe food related to contamination of available foods as evidenced by neighbor's report of power failure and no shelf-stable foods

1. Considering nutritional factors, why might NG sound tired and confused?
2. What shelf-stable items would be appropriate for NG, given her dislike for salty foods?
3. What could be appropriate substitutes for NG's usual glass of milk?
4. How long can food be kept in the refrigerator and freezer when the power is out?
5. What agencies could NG and her neighbor contact for help?

✹ CLINICAL SCENARIO 2

The following case illustrates the benefits that an older person might receive from various assistance programs. NOTE: the annual benefit from each program varies greatly; expenditures can easily exceed income when health care, prescription drugs, housing, and other costs are higher than average.

SD, a 79-year-old overweight widow in good health with hypertension, worked part-time after raising children. Her husband, a moderate wage earner, died of a heart attack at age 66. Most of their modest savings went to pay his medical bills and prescriptions. SD receives a monthly Social Security benefit of $875 per month. She also receives $3500 annually ($291 monthly) from her husband's pension. She does not own her home and pays $460 per month rent (≈41% of her income). Monthly SD spends $155 on food; $115 on utilities; and $65 on transportation, clothing, home maintenance, and toiletries. Annual health care expenses total $3568 and include monthly out-of-pocket expenses of $157 for insurance, $80 for prescription drugs, $50 on medical services, and $14 on medical supplies. Estimates for out-of-pocket health costs are likely low and will increase over the next few years as health care costs increase. Medicare premiums also rise as health care costs rise. After expenses are paid, SD has only $70. The table illustrates her situation:

⁎**Nutrition Diagnosis:** Limited access to food related to limited income as evidenced by only $70 disposable income available after all expenses are paid

1. What federal agencies are available to help? Consider Older Americans Nutrition Programs, food stamps, Senior Farmer's Market Nutrition Program.
2. Design a menu for 7 days of meals and snacks that are easy to prepare and reasonable in cost.

Description	Monthly Income ($)	Monthly Expense ($)
Social Security	875	
Widow's pension	291	
Rent		460
Food		155
Utilities		115
Misc., transportation, clothing, etc.		65
Health insurance		157
Drugs/medication		80
Medical services		50
Medical supplies		14
BALANCE	70	

Federal Nutrition Assistance

Older Americans Nutrition Program: Value of meals	100	
Food Stamps	50	
CSFP	17	
Actual retail value generally higher		
Senior Farmer's Market Food Program	2	
Note: $25 average annual benefit ÷ 12		
TOTAL VALUE	169	

USEFUL WEBSITES

Administration on Aging
http://www.aoa.gov

Agency for Healthcare Research and Quality
http://www.ahrq.gov/

American Association of Retired Persons (AARP)
http://www.aarp.org

American Association of Homes and Services for the Aging
http://www.aahs.org

American Geriatrics Society
http://www.americangeriatrics.org

Centers for Medicare and Medicaid Services (CMS)
http://www.cms.hhs.gov/

Dietary Reference Intakes: The Essential Guide
http://www.nap.edu/catalog/11537.html

International Longevity Center
http://www.ilcusa.org/

Meals on Wheels Association of America, Inc. (MOWAA)
http://www.mowaa.org/

Mini Nutritional Assessment
http://www.nestle-nutrition.com/tools/mna.aspx

National Association of Area Agencies
on Aging (n4a)
http://www.n4a.org/

National Association of Nutrition
and Aging Services Programs (NANASP)
http://www.nanasp.org

National Citizen's Coalition for Nursing
Home Reform
http://www.nccnhr.org/static_pages/Citizens_groups_list.cfm

National Institute on Aging (NIA)
http://www.nih.gov/nia

National Resource Center on Nutrition,
Physical Activity & Aging
http://nutritionandaging.fiu.edu/

Nutrition Screening Initiative
http://www.aafp.org/online/en/home/clinical/nsi.html

Nutrition Management and Restorative Dining
for Older Adults, U.S. Health Care Financing
Administration
http://www.hcfa.gov/medicaid/siq/siqnhpg.htm

OAA Nutrition Program
www.aoa.gov/prof/aoaprog/nutrition/nutrition.asp

Seniors and Food Safety–Preventing Foodborne
Illness, Food and Nutrition Service,
U.S. Department of Agriculture
http://www.cfsan.fda.gov/~dms/seniors.html

White House Conference on Aging, 2005
http://www.whcoa.gov/

References

Agency for Healthcare Research and Quality and the Centers for Disease Control: Physical activity and older Americans: benefits and strategies, June 2002, http://www.ahrq.gov/ppip/activity.htm, accessed June 1, 2006.

Amarantos E et al: Nutrition and quality of life in older adults, *J Gerontol A Biol Sci Med Sci* 56:5, 2001.

American College of Sports Medicine: Position stand: exercise and physical activity for older adults, *Med Sci Sports Exerc* 30:992, 1998.

American Dietetic Association: Medicare reform act provisions impacting MNT, 2006, http://www.eatright.org/cps/rde/xchg/ada/hs.xsl/advocacy_5534_ENU_HTML.htm?dologin=1, accessed June 1, 2006.

Barr J, Schumacher G: Using focus groups to determine what constitutes quality of life in clients receiving medical nutrition therapy: first steps in the development of a nutrition quality-of-life survey, *J Am Diet Assoc*;103:844 2003.

Barve S et al: Aging and immunity. In: Bales CW, Ritchie CS, editors: *Handbook of clinical nutrition and aging*, Totowa, NJ, 2004, Humana Press.

Burns EA: Effects of aging on immune function, *J Nutr Health Aging*; 8(1):9 2004.

Chao S, Dwyer J: Food and nutrition services in assisted living facilities: boon or big disappointment for elder nutrition? *Generations J Am Soc Aging* 28(3):72, 2004.

Clemons TE et al: Cognitive impairment in the age-related eye disease study: AREDS report no. 16, *Arch Ophthalmol* 124(4):537, 2006.

Decker FH: *Nursing homes, 1977-1999: what has changed, what has not?* Hyattsville, Md, 2005, USDHHS National Center for Health Statistics.

Drewnowski A, Evans WJ: Nutrition, physical activity, and quality of life in older adults: summary, *J Gerontol Series A: Biol Sci Med Sci* 56:89, 2001.

Federal Interagency Forum on Aging-Related Statistics: *Older Americans 2006: key indicators of well-being*, Federal Interagency Forum on Aging-Related Statistics, Washington, DC, May 2006, U.S. Government Printing Office, http://www.agingstats.gov/, accessed June 1, 2006.

Finkelstein JA, Schiffman SS: Workshop on taste and smell in the elderly: an overview, *Physiology Behav* 66:173, 1999.

He W et al: U.S. Census Bureau, Current Population Reports, P23-209, 65+ in the United States: 2005, U.S. Government Printing Office, Washington, DC, http://www.census.gov/prod/2006pubs/p23-209.pdf, accessed December 1, 2005.

Hendricks J: Ageism in the new millennium, *Generations, J Am Soc Aging* Fall:28, 2005.

Holick MF: Vitamin D: the underappreciated D-lightful hormone that is important for skeletal and cellular health, *Curr Opin Endocrinol Diabetes* 9:87, 2002.

Institute of Medicine, Committee on Nutrition Services for Medicare Beneficiaries: *The role of nutrition in maintaining health in the nation's elderly: evaluating coverage of nutrition services for the Medicare population*, 2000, Washington, DC, National Academies Press.

Institute of Medicine, Food and Nutrition Board: DRI table for older adults, as compiled by the National Resource Center on Nutrition, Physical Activity & Aging, http://nutritionandaging.fiu.edu, accessed January 10, 2007.

Irizarry MC et al: Association of homocysteine with plasma amyloid beta protein in aging and neurodegenerative disease, *Neurol* 65: 1402, 2005.

Johnson MA et al: Hearing loss and nutrition in older adults. In Bales CW, Ritchie CS: *Handbook of clinical nutrition and aging*, Totowa, NJ, 2004, Humana Press.

Kaempfer D et al: Dietetics students' low knowledge, attitudes, and work preferences toward older adults indicate need for improved education about aging, *J Am Diet Assoc* 102:197, 2002.

Kuczmarski MF, Weddle DO: American Dietetic Association Position Statement: nutrition across the spectrum of aging, *J Am Diet Assoc* 105:616, 2005.

Lipschitz DA, et al: An approach to nutrition screening for older American—Nutrition Screening Initiative, Part 3, American Family Physician, 1992, http://www.findarticles.com/p/articles/mi_m3225/is_n2_v45/ai_12019311, accessed June 1, 2006.

Lucas M, Heiss CJ: Protein needs of older adults engaged in resistance training: a review, *J Aging Phys Act* 13:223, 2005.

Mallet M: Refeeding syndrome, *Age Aging* 31:65, 2002.

Mathematica Policy Research, Inc: *Serving elders at risk, the older Americans act nutrition programs: national evaluation of the elderly nutrition program 1993-1995, vol I: Title III evaluation findings,* Washington, DC, 1996a, U.S. Department of Health and Human Services.

Mathematica Policy Research, Inc: *Serving elders at risk, the older Americans act nutrition programs: national evaluation of the elderly nutrition program 1993-1995, volume ii: title vi evaluation finding,* Washington, DC, 1996b, U.S. Department of Health and Human Services.

Michelon E et al: Vitamin and carotenoid status in older women: associations with the frailty syndrome, *J Gerontol A: Biol Sci Med Sci* 61:600, 2006.

Moore ST: Integrating housing and long-term care services for the elderly: a social marketing approach, *Health Mark Q* 9 (1-2):129, 1991.

National Center for Chronic Disease Prevention and Health Promotion: Physical Activity and Health, A Report of the Surgeon General, 2006, www.cdc.gov/nccdphp/sgr/sgr.htm, accessed June 1, 2006.

National Institute on Deafness and Other Communicative Disorders, National Institutes of Health: 2006, http://www.nidcd.nih.gov/health/hearing/presbycusis.htm#what), accessed June 1, 2006.

Neidert KC: American Dietetic Association Position Statement: Liberalization of the diet prescription improves quality of life for older adults in long-term care, *J Am Diet Assoc* 105:1955, 2005.

Nelson ME et al: The effects of multidimensional home-based exercise on functional performance in elderly people, *J Gerontol* 59A:154, 2004.

Office of Dietary Supplements, NIH Clinical Center, National Institutes of Health: Dietary supplement fact sheet: vitamin D, http://ods.od.nih.gov/factsheets/vitamind.asp#h5, accessed June 1, 2006.

O'Neill PS et al: Aging in community nutrition, diet therapy, and nutrition and aging textbooks. *Gerontol Geriatr Educ* 25:65, 2005.

Pham DQ, Plakogiannis R: Vitamin E supplementation in Alzheimer's disease, Parkinson's disease, tardive dyskinesia, and cataract, Part 2. *Ann Pharmacother* 39:2065, 2005.

Ponza M et al: Serving Elders at Risk: The Older Americans Act Nutrition Programs - National Evaluation of the Elderly Nutrition Program, 1993-1995, executive summary, U.S. Department of Health and Human Services, 1996.

Raguso CA et al: A 3-year longitudinal study on body composition changes in the elderly: role of physical exercise. *Clin Nutr* 25:573, 2006.

Rhee LQ et al: Continued need for increased emphasis on aging in dietetics education, *J Am Diet Assoc* 104:645, 2004.

Ritchie CS, Joshipura K: Oral health in nutrition. In Bales CW, Ritchie CS, editors: *Handbook of clinical nutrition and aging,* Totowa, NJ, 2004, Humana Press.

Robertson RG, Montagnini M: Geriatric failure to thrive, *Am Fam Physician* 70:343, 2004.

Sahyoun NR et al: Nutritional status of the older adult is associated with dentition status, *J Am Diet Assoc* 103:61, 2003.

Sarkisian CA, Lachs MS: "Failure to Thrive" in older adults, *Ann Intern Med* 124:1072, 1996, http://www.annals.org/cgi/content/full/124/12/1072, accessed June 1, 2006.

Sharkey JR: The influence of nutritional health on physical function: a critical relationship for homebound older adults, *Generations, J Am Soc Aging* 28(3):34, 2004.

Shea JD: Pressure sores: classification and management, *Clin Orthop Relat Res* 112:89, 1975.

Simmons SF et al: The minimum data set weight-loss quality indicator: does it reflect differences in care processes related to weight loss? *J Am Geriatr Soc* 51:1410, 2003.

U.S. Administration on Aging: Profile of older Americans 2005, http://www.aoa.gov/prof/Statistics/statistics.asp, accessed December 1, 2005.

U.S. Department of Agriculture, Center for Nutrition Policy and Promotion: Quality of diets of older Americans, Nutrition Insight 29, June 2004, www.cnpp.usda.gov/insights.html, accessed June 1, 2006.

U.S. Department of Health and Human Services: NHANES III, www.cdc.gov/nchs/nhanes.htm, accessed June 1, 2006.

U.S. Department of Health and Human Services: *Physical activity and health: a report of the Surgeon General,* Atlanta, Ga, 1996, Centers for Disease Control and Prevention (CDC), National Center for Chronic Disease Prevention and Health Promotion, www.cdc.gov/nccdphp/sgr/sgr.htm, accessed June 1, 2006.

U.S. Department of Health and Human Services: *The Surgeon General's call to action to prevent and decrease overweight and obesity,* Rockville, Md, 2001, USDHHS Public Health Service; U.S. Government Printing Office.

U.S. Department of Health and Human Services: *The 2004 Surgeon General's report on bone health and osteoporosis,* www.surgeongeneral.gov/library/bonehealth/docs/Osteo10sep04.pdf, accessed June 1, 2006.

U.S. Department of Health and Human Services and U.S. Department of Agriculture: *Dietary Guidelines for Americans, 2005,* ed 6, Washington, DC, 2005, U.S. Government Printing Office, available at http://www.healthierus.gov/dietaryguidelines/, accessed December 1, 2005.

Vellas B et al: Mini nutritional assessment (MNA): Research and practice in the elderly, *Nestle Nutrition Workshop Series—* Clinical and Performance Programme, vol. 1, 1999, Basel, Switzerland, TS Karger.

Villareal DT et al: Obesity in older adults: technical review and position statement of the American Society for Nutrition and The Obesity Society, *Am J Clin Nutr* 82:923, 2005.

Ware JE, Sherbourne CD: The MOS 36-item short-form health survey (SF-36), I: conceptual framework and item selection, *Med Care* 30:473, 1992.

Waters DL et al: Sarcopenia: current perspectives, *J Nutr Health Aging* 4:133, 2000.

Wellman NS et al: Aging in introductory and life cycle nutrition textbooks, *Gerontol Geriatr Educ* 24:67, 2004.

Wilson MG, Morley JE: Nutritional assessment and support in chronic disease management. In Bales CW, Ritchie CS: *Handbook of clinical nutrition and aging,* Totowa, NJ, 2004, Humana Press, pp 77-101.

Wong TY et al: Age-related macular degeneration and risk for stroke, *Ann Intern Med* 145:98, 2006.

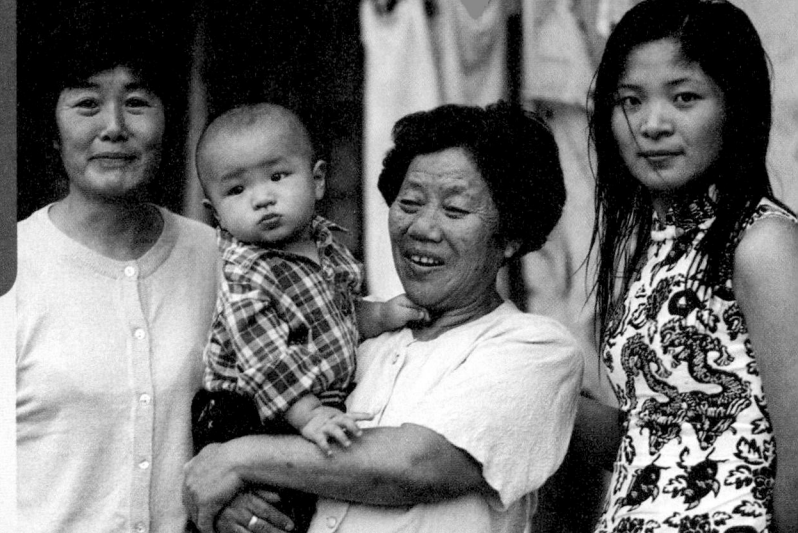

Judith L. Dodd, MS, RD, FADA*
Cynthia Taft Bayerl, MS, RD, LDN*

Nutrition in the Community

KEY TERMS

avian influenza (bird flu) a disease caused by influenza viruses that occur naturally among wild migratory birds with the potential of infecting domestic poultry; there is no evidence that this is transmitted by cooked poultry that has reached 165° internal temperature

biosecurity precautions taken to minimize the risk of introducing an infectious agent into a population

bioterrorism the deliberate use of microorganisms or toxins from living organisms to induce death or disease

community assessment one of the three public health core functions that involves all of the activities related to the concept of community diagnosis (surveillance, identifying needs, analyzing the causes of problems, collecting and interpreting data, case finding, monitoring and forecasting trends, research, and evaluation of outcomes)

DHS The Department of Homeland Security, a federal agency established in 2002 with a commitment to the safety of our country; works closely with other agencies on the safety of food and water and through FEMA to protect the public health in the event of a natural or man-made disaster

FEMA The Federal Emergency Management Agency, a unit of the DHS with links to health; safe housing; and water, food, and worker safety in the event of a natural or man-made disaster

foodborne illnes an illness acquired as the result of consumption of contaminated foods; commonly and incorrectly referred to as "food poisoning"; bacteria, toxic products of bacteria, viruses, parasites, chemicals, or poisons naturally occurring in some animals and plants that may cause illness

food security access by individuals to a readily available supply of nutritionally adequate and safe foods and an ensured ability to acquire acceptable foods

Hazard Analysis Critical Control Points (HACCP) a systematic approach to the identification, evaluation, and control of food safety hazards; involves identifying any biologic, chemical, or physical agent that is reasonably likely to cause illness or injury in the absence of its control as it pertains to food production

National Food and Nutrition Survey (NFNS) the January 2002 merge of the NHANES and the CSFII; known as What We Eat in America

National Health and Nutrition Examination Survey (NHANES) a population-based survey that collects information from medical history, physical measurements, biochemical evaluation, physical examination, and dietary intake of a representative sample of U.S. population groups; a responsibility of the National Center for Health Statistics of DHHS; initiated in the early 1960s, NHANES studies are now continuous

National Nutrient Data Bank the primary U.S. resource of information on the nutrient content of foods

National Nutrition Monitoring and Related Research (NNMRR) Act a law passed in 1993 to provide organization, consistency, and unification to the survey methods that monitor the food habits and nutrition of the U.S. population

pandemic a worldwide outbreak of any disease in numbers clearly in excess of normal; a rapid outbreak for which there is no natural immunity or immediately available treatment or prevention; one concern is avian or bird flu

policy development one of the three public health core functions; the process by which society makes decisions about problems, chooses goals and prepares the means to reach them, handles conflicting views about what should be done, and allocates resources

*With assistance from Rachel Kossover, MPH.

309

primary prevention a disease prevention strategy that targets generally healthy individuals to decrease the probability that they will develop a disease or disability

public health assurance one of the three core public health functions; addresses the implementation of legislative mandates, maintenance of statutory responsibilities, support of crucial services, regulation of services and products provided in both the public and private sector, and maintenance of accountability

secondary prevention a disease prevention strategy that focuses on detection, diagnosis, and intervention early in the disease process to minimize detrimental and disabling effects

tertiary prevention rehabilitation of an individual to optimal function by correcting or ameliorating the health defect or disability from a disease; may involve medical treatment

USDHHS The U.S. Department of Health and Human Services, a federal agency formerly the U.S. Department of Health, Education, and Welfare; houses The Food and Drug Administration (FDA) and Centers for Disease Control and Prevention (CDC)

What We Eat in America the name for the National Food and Nutrition Survey which includes the NHANES and CFSII

Community nutrition is an evolving area of practice with the broad focus of serving the population at large. Although this practice area encompasses the goals of public health, in the United States the current model has been shaped and expanded by prevention and wellness initiatives that evolved in the 1960s. Since the thrust of community nutrition is to be both proactive and responsive to the needs of the community, disaster planning, promoting safety of the food and water supply, and addressing risk factors related to obesity have shaped emphasis areas.

Historically public health was defined as "the science and art of preventing disease, prolonging life, and promoting health and efficiency through organized community effort, so organizing these benefits as to enable every citizen to realize his birthright of health and longevity" (Winslow, 1920). The public health approach, also known as a population-based or epidemiologic approach, differs from the clinical or patient care model generally seen in hospitals and other clinical settings. In the public health model the client is the community, a geopolitical entity. The focus of the traditional public health approach is **primary prevention** (health promotion) as opposed to **secondary prevention** (risk reduction) or **tertiary prevention** (treatment and rehabilitation) (Egan, 1994). Changes in the health care system, technology, and attitudes of the nutrition consumer have been influencers in expanding the responsibilities of community nutrition.

A 1988 groundbreaking report of the Institute of Medicine (IOM) reinforced the concept that the scope of community nutrition is a work in progress (IOM, 1988). This report defined a mission and delineated roles and responsibilities for practicing community nutrition that are still the basis for this area of practice. The scope of community-based nutrition encompasses efforts to prevent disease and promote positive health and nutritional status for individuals and groups in settings where they live and work. The focus is on well-being and building potential for the best possible quality of life. "Well-being" goes beyond the usual constraints of physical and mental health and includes other factors that affect the quality of life within a community. Community members need a safe environment and adequate housing, food, income, employment, and education. This philosophy echoes the IOM intent that the mission of community nutrition is to fulfill society's interest in ensuring conditions in which people can be healthy.

The potential audience for programming and services is any segment of the population, and the program or service should reflect the diversity of the designated community. Politics, geography, culture, ethnicity, ages, genders, socioeconomic issues, and overall health status help to define a community. Along with primary prevention, community nutrition provides links to programs and services with goals of disease risk reduction and rehabilitation. Heart-healthy cooking classes and demonstrations are an example of multifaceted programming and services offered under the community nutrition umbrella. Depending on the audience, the program is primary prevention (the general public), secondary prevention (sessions for people at high risk for heart disease) or tertiary prevention (support groups for those with cardiovascular disease).

In the traditional model, funding sources for public health efforts were monies allocated from official sources (government) at the local, state, or federal level. Part of the changing "turf" in the community is the sharing of the responsibility for meeting the mission. Currently nutrition programs and services are funded alone or in partnership between a broad range of sources, including public (government), private, and voluntary health sectors. As public source funding has declined, the need for private funding has become more crucial. In the example, heart-healthy cooking classes might receive funding from the American Heart Association (a voluntary, nonprofit agency), a health care insurer (nonprofit or for-profit agency), a supermarket or business (for-profit entity), or a demonstration grant from a government source. The potential size and diversity of a designated "community" makes collaboration critical. A single agency may be unable to fund or deliver the full range of services. In addition, it is likely that the funding will be services or product (in-kind) rather than cash. Creative funding and management skills are crucial for a community practitioner.

NUTRITION PRACTICE IN THE COMMUNITY

Nutrition professionals recognize that successful delivery of food and nutrition services involves actively engaging people in their own community. The pool of nutrition professionals delivering medical nutrition therapy and nutrition education in community-based or public health facilities continues to expand. Although the settings may vary, there are three core functions in community nutrition practice. In addition, the objectives of *Healthy People 2010* offer a common framework of measurable public health outcomes that can be used to assess the overall health of a community (*Healthy People 2010*, 2000).

The three "core" functions of public health are: community assessment, policy development, and public health assurance (IOM, 1988). These areas are also the components of community nutrition practice, especially community assessment, also known as *needs assessment*, as it relates to nutrition. The findings of needs assessments shape policy development and the components of ensuring that the nutritional health of the public is protected.

Although there is shared responsibility for completion of the core functions of public health, the IOM report designates that personnel of the official state health agencies have primary responsibility for this task. Under this model state public health agencies, in conjunction with community organizations and leaders, have responsibility for assessing the

capacity of their state to perform the essential functions of public health nutrition and for supporting both attainment and monitoring of the goals and objectives of *Healthy People 2010*.

Local health agencies are charged with protecting the health of their population groups by ensuring that effective service delivery systems are in place. The role of the federal government is to support the development and dissemination of public health knowledge and to provide funds to strengthen the capacity to carry out the core functions. Box 11-1 lists the federal agencies that are relevant to food and nutrition concerns of the community.

The expansion of community-based practice beyond the scope of traditional public health has opened new employment opportunities for nutrition professionals. Such professionals are found in agencies or organizations that provide primary care, promote health, and prevent chronic disease in the community. Nutrition professionals also serve as consultants or maintain community-based private practices. Some settings for community nutrition in practice are public health agencies (state and local); the WIC

BOX 11-1

Government Agencies Related to Food and Nutrition

Central Website for Access to All U.S. Government Information on Nutrition
http://www.nutrition.gov

Centers for Disease Control and Prevention
1600 Clifton Road, NE
Atlanta, GA 30333
Phone: (404) 639-3311
http://www.cdc.gov

Environmental Protection Agency
Ariel Rios Building
1200 Pennsylvania Avenue, NW
Washington, DC 20460
Phone: (202) 260-2090
http://www.epa.gov

Federal Trade Commission
Public Reference Branch
600 Pennsylvania Avenue, NW
Room 130
Washington, DC 20580
Phone: (202) 326-2222
http://www.ftc.gov

Food and Agriculture Organization of the United Nations
Viale delle Terme di Caracalla
00100 Rome, Italy
http://www.fao.org

Food and Drug Administration
Office of Public Affairs
5600 Fishers Lane
Rockville, MD 20857-0001
Phone: (888) 463-6332
http://www.fda.gov

Food and Drug Administration Advisory Committees
Phone: (800) 741-8138
Food Advisory Committee, ext. 10564
National Center for Toxicological Research Science Advisory Committee, ext. 12559
http://www.fda.gov/nctr/

Food and Drug Administration Center for Food Safety and Applied Nutrition
Phone: (800) FDA-4010
http://www.vm.cfsan.fda.gov

National Cancer Institute
NCI Public Inquiries Office
6116 Executive Boulevard, MSC8322
Suite 3036A
Bethesda, MD 20892-8322
Phone: (301) 496-6641
http://www.nci.nih.gov

National Health Information Center
PO Box 1133
Washington, DC 20013-1133
Phone: (800) 336-4797
http://www.health.gov/nhic

Continued

BOX 11-1

Government Agencies Related to Food and Nutrition—cont'd

National Institutes of Health
Office of Communications and Public Liaison
1 Center Drive, MSC0188
Building 1, Room 344
Bethesda, MD 20892
Phone: (301) 496-4461
http://www.nih.gov

National Institutes of Health
Office of Dietary Supplements
31 Center Drive, MSC2086
Building 31, Room 1B29
Bethesda, MD 20892-2086
Phone: (301) 435-2920
E-mail: ods@nih.gov
http://dietary-supplements.info.nih.gov

National Marine Fisheries Service
National Oceanic Atmospheric Administration Office
  of Public and Constituent Affairs
1305 East-West Highway, #1W514
Silver Spring, MD 20910
Phone: (301) 713-1208
http://www.nmfs.noaa.gov

USDA Center for Nutrition Policy and Promotion
3101 Park Center Drive
Room 1034
Alexandria, VA 22302-1594
Phone: (703) 305-7600
http://www.usda.gov/cnpp

USDA Food and Nutrition Service
Public Information Staff
3101 Park Center Drive
Room 819
Alexandria, VA 22302-1594
Phone: (703) 305-2286
http://www.fns.usda.gov/fns

USDA Food Safety and Inspection Service
1400 Independence Avenue, SW
Room 2932—South
Washington, DC 20250-3700
Meat and Poultry Hotline: (800) 535-4555
http://www.fsis.usda.gov

Gateway to Government Food Safety Information
http://www.foodsafety.gov

USDA National Agriculture Library
Food and Nutrition Information Center
10301 Baltimore Avenue
Beltsville, MD 20705-2351
Phone: (301) 504-5719
http://www.nal.usda.gov/fnic

World Health Organization
Headquarters Office in Geneva (HQ)
Avenue Appia 20
1211 Geneva 27
Switzerland
Telephone: (+ 00 41 22) 791 21 11
Fax: (+00 41 22) 791 31 11
Telex: 415 416
Telegraph: UNISANTE GENEVA
http://www.who.org

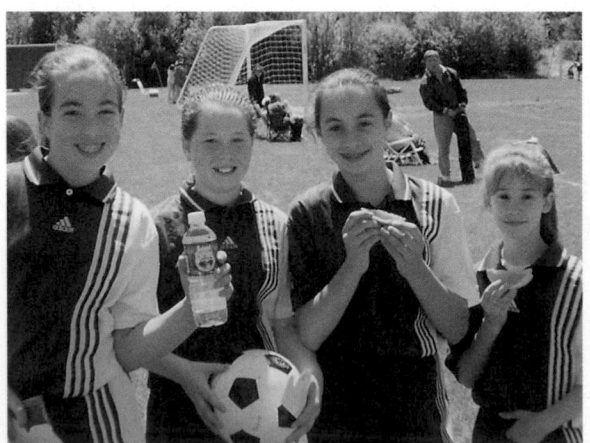

FIGURE 11-1 Working with girls on a soccer team, community nutritionists can encourage them to make better food choices and improve their nutrition.

program; services for senior adults; community health centers; early intervention programs, Head Start; health maintenance organizations and health insurers; food pantries and shelters; physicians' offices; and schools (Bayerl and Ries, 1995) (Figure 11-1).

Effective practice in the community requires a nutrition professional who understands the impact of economic, social, and political issues on health. Since many community-based efforts are funded or guided by legislation and the resulting regulations and public policies, community practice also requires an understanding of the legislative process and an ability to translate policies into action (see *Focus On:* Legislation and Advocacy). In addition, community practice requires a working knowledge of funding sources and resources at the federal, state, regional, and local level.

◎ FOCUS ON

Legislation and Advocacy

Nutrition and health professionals can be valuable advocates for legislation (local, state, or federal) that supports the nutritional well-being of the population, especially those who are underserved or underrepresented. This can be accomplished by:

- Visiting, writing, or calling legislators and their aides to provide important information and establish communication links
- Encouraging community members to provide testimony on their successes or the consequences when medical nutrition therapy or nutrition services are not available or are limited by funding; this is especially important when legislation is pending
- Inviting legislators to visit local agencies, schools, or hospital sites to showcase the benefits of nutrition services provided by qualified professionals
- Serving on campaign committees, donating time and money, or running for office

For more information, contact the American Dietetic Association at http://www.eatright.org/gov.

NEEDS ASSESSMENT FOR COMMUNITY-BASED NUTRITION SERVICES

Nutrition services should be organized to meet the needs of a "community." Once a community has been defined, a **community assessment** or needs assessment can be used to shape the planning, implementation, and evaluation of nutrition services. An assessment is a current snapshot of the community and is useful in identifying the health risks or areas of greatest concern to community well-being. To be effective, a needs assessment must be a dynamic document that is responsive to changes in the community. Since a plan is only as good as the research used to shape the decisions, a mechanism for ongoing review and revision should be built into the planning.

A needs assessment is based on objective data, including demographic information and health statistics. When possible, information should represent the community's diversity and be segmented by such factors as age, gender, socioeconomic status, disability, and ethnicity. Examples of information to be gathered include current morbidity and mortality statistics; number of low-birth-weight infants, deaths attributed to chronic diseases with a link to nutrition, and health risk indicators such as incidence of smoking or obesity. *Healthy People 2010* outlines leading health indicators, several of which can impact nutritional status. Health indicators are then used to create target objectives. The *Healthy People 2010* leading health indicators are listed in

---

BOX 11-2

Healthy People 2010:
Leading Health Indicators

Physical activity
Overweight and obesity
Tobacco use
Substance abuse
Responsible sexual behavior
Mental health
Injury and violence
Environmental quality
Immunization
Access to health care

From *Healthy People 2010: national health promotion and disease prevention objectives,* Washington, DC, 2000, U.S. Department of Health and Human Services.

Box 11-2 (*Healthy People 2010*, 2000). Subjective information such as input from community members and leaders and health and nutrition professionals can be useful in supporting the objective data or in emphasizing questions or concerns. The process mirrors what the business world knows as market research.

In addition to studying the health indicators of the community and conducting interviews with community leaders, accessible community resources and services should be catalogued. In nutrition planning the goal is to determine who and what are available to community members when they need food- or nutrition-related products or services. What services are available in the areas of medical nutrition therapy (screening, assessment, monitoring), nutrition and food education, and child care or homemaker skills training? Are there safe areas for exercise or recreation? Is there access to transportation? Is there compliance with disability legislation? In the area of **food security,** or access by individuals to a readily available supply of nutritionally adequate and safe foods, are programs such as food stamps, food pantries, congregate and home-delivered meals, child nutrition programs, and supermarkets and other food sources available and being used? Are mechanisms in place for emergencies that might affect access to adequate and safe food and water?

At first glance some of the data gathered in this process may not appear to relate directly to nutrition, but an experienced community nutritionist or a community-based advisory group with public health professionals can help connect this information to nutrition- and diet-related issues. Often the nutritional problems identified in a review of nutrition indicators are associated with dietary inadequacies, excesses, or imbalances that can be triggers for disease risk. Examples of trigger areas are: presence of risk factors for cardiovascular disease; diabetes and stroke, including elevated blood cholesterol and lipids, inactivity, smoking, elevated blood glucose, high body mass index (BMI), and elevated blood pressure; risk factors for osteoporosis; evidence of eating disorders; high levels of teenage pregnancy; and evidence of hunger and food insecurity. Careful attention should be paid to the special needs of adults and children with disabilities or other lifestyle-limiting conditions. Access to safe and adequate amounts of food and water can be interrupted by something as simple as a power outage or as complex as a disaster. Once evaluated, the information is used to propose needed services, including medical nutrition therapy (MNT) as discussed in other chapters, as part of the strategy for improving the overall health of the community.

Sources for Needs Assessment Information

Census information is a starting point for beginning a needs assessment. Morbidity and mortality and other health data collected by state and local public health agencies, the Centers for Disease Control and Prevention (CDC), and the National Center for Health Statistics (NCHS) are useful. Federal agencies and their state program administration counterparts are data sources; these agencies include the U.S. Department of Agriculture (USDA), **U.S. Department of Health and Human Services (USDHHS),** and the Administration on Aging (AoA). Local providers such as community hospitals; Women, Infants and Children (WIC) and child care agencies; and health centers, as well as universities with a public health or nutrition department are additional sources of information. Volunteer organizations such as the March of Dimes, the American Heart Association (AHA), the American Diabetes Association, and the American Cancer Society (ACS) maintain population statistics. Health insurers are a source for current information related to health care consumers and geographic area. Inclusion of community leaders and other professionals in the needs assessment process aids in gaining access to these resources and information.

The face of the community and its resources are constantly in flux. Technology has made it simpler to access current data, and much of the information is available at Internet websites. It is critical that community practitioners know how to locate relevant resources and evaluate the information for validity and reliability. Knowing the background and intent of any data source and identifying the limitations and the dates when the information was collected are critical points to consider when selecting and using such sources.

NATIONAL NUTRITION SURVEYS

Nutrition and health surveys at the federal and state level are basic data sources. Such surveys are useful in providing information on the dietary status of a population, the nutritional adequacy of the food supply, the economics of food consumption, and the effects of food assistance and regulatory programs. Public guidelines for food selection such as The Dietary Guidelines for Americans (DGA) (see Box 9-1) are based on surveys. The data are also used in policy setting; program development; and funding at the national, state, and local levels. Until the late 1960s, the USDA was the primary source of food and nutrient consumption data. Although much of the data collection is still at the federal level, other agencies and states are now generating information that provides comprehensive information on the health and nutrition of the public.

National Health and Nutrition Examination Survey (NHANES)

The **National Health and Nutrition Examination Survey (NHANES)** provides a framework for describing the health status of the nation. Sampling the noninstitutionalized population, the initial study began in the early 1960s, with subsequent studies on a periodic basis from 1971 to 1994. Beginning with the eighth study in 1999, NHANES is collected on a continuous basis. The process includes interviewing approximately 6000 individuals each year in their homes and following up with about 5000 individuals with a complete health examination. Dietary information is collected and released as What We Eat in America.

Since its inception, each successive NHANES has included changes or additions that make the survey more responsive as a measurement of the health status of the population. NHANES I to III include (1) medical history, (2) physical measurements, (3) biochemical evaluation, (4) physical signs and symptoms, and (5) diet information using food frequency questionnaires and a 24-hour recall. Some past design changes added special population studies to increase information on underrepresented groups such as the 1982-1984 Hispanic HANES (Woteki et al., 1988; Kuczmarski et al., 1994). NHANES III (1988–1994) included a large proportion of persons age 65 years and older. This information enhanced understanding of the growing and changing population of senior adults.

Currently reports are released in 2-year cycles (NCHS, 2005a). In 2009 and 2010 oversampling will include persons with a low income, those over the age of 60, blacks, and Hispanic Americans (NCHS, Proposal Guidelines, 2005b).

Information on past and current NHANES is available through the National Center for Health Statistics (NCHS) of the CDC (see Box 11-1).

Nationwide Food Consumption Survey

The Nationwide Food Consumption Survey (NFCS) of USDA monitored the nutrient intake of a representative sampling of the U.S. public. The NFCS compiled information on food consumption of households and individuals using a food use and food cost questionnaire about food eaten at home and away from home over a 3-day period. The first survey was conducted in 1935, and the data were updated approximately every 10 years until 1988. The information collected is still quoted (Nutrition Monitoring, 1989).

Continuing Survey of Food Intake of Individuals: Diet and Health Knowledge Survey

The Continuing Survey of Food Intake of Individuals (CSFII) was a nationwide dietary survey instituted in 1985 by the USDA. In 1990 CSFII became part of the USDA National Nutrition Monitoring System. The Diet and

Health Knowledge Survey (DHKS), a telephone follow-up to CFSII, began in 1989. Information from previous surveys is available from 1985 to 1986, 1989 to 1991, and 1994 to 1996 (USDA, CSFII, 1998).

The DHKS was designed as a personal interview questionnaire that allowed individual attitudes and knowledge about healthy eating to be linked with reported food choices and nutrient intakes. Early studies focused on dietary history and a 24-hour recall of adult men and women ages 19 to 50. The 1989 and 1994 surveys questioned men, women, and children of all ages and included a 24-hour recall (personal interview) and a 2-day food diary. Household data for these studies were determined by calculating the nutrient content of foods reported to be used in the home during the survey. These results were compared with nutrition recommendations for persons matching in age and gender. The information derived from the CSFII and DHKS is still useful for decision makers and researchers in monitoring the nutritional adequacy of American diets, measuring the impact of food fortification on nutrient intakes, tracking trends, and developing dietary guidance and related programs. By January 2002 both surveys had merged with NHANES to become the **National Food and Nutrition Survey (NFNS)** or **What We Eat in America**.

What We Eat in America

The integrated survey, What We Eat in America, is collected as part of NHANES. Food intake data are linked to health status from other NHANES components, allowing for exploration of relationships between dietary indicators and health status. The DHHS is responsible for sample design and data, whereas the USDA is responsible for the survey's dietary data collection methodology, maintenance of the database used to code and process the data, and data review and processing.

National Nutrition Monitoring and Related Research Act

In 1990 Congress passed Public Law 101-445, the **National Nutrition Monitoring and Related Research (NNMRR) Act**. This law is seen as an umbrella to provide organization, consistency, and unification to the survey methods that monitor the food habits and nutrition of the U.S. population (Sims, 1993). The intent is to coordinate efforts of the 22 federal agencies that implement or review nutrition services or surveys. Areas of nutrition monitoring include food supply determinations, household and individual dietary surveys, nutritional and health assessments, and other related research (Wotecki, 2003).

Data obtained through NNMRR are used to direct research activities, develop programs and services, and make policy decisions regarding regulation and evaluation of nutrition-related programs (Wotecki, 2003). Food labeling, food and nutrition assistance programs, food safety, and education activities are areas shaped by the information gathered under the NNMRR. Reports of the various activities are issued approximately every 5 years. The reports summarize dietary, nutritional, and related health markers

of Americans and the nutritional quality of the food they consume. The activities under NNMRR provide information on trends in nutrition and health, knowledge, attitude and behavior, food composition, and food supply determinants (FASEB, 1995; Kuczmarski, 1994). Nutrition monitoring reports can be obtained through the National Agricultural Library database.

Nutrition Screening Initiative

The Nutrition Screening Initiative (NSI) was created in 1990 by a partnership of the American Dietetic Association (ADA), the American Academy of Family Physicians (ACFP) and the National Council on the Aging (NCA). The goal was to promote improved nutrition and nutrition care for the older population. NSI was a response to studies indicating that early detection and interventions addressing nutrition-related problems could improve the quality of life and reduce hospitalizations. Products resulting from NSI include a series of validated screening tools that can be used to assess senior adults living independently. The initial screen is a self-assessment for the older adult or a nonprofessional (see Figure 10-4). The Level 1 screen is designed to be used by nonprofessionals with some guidance from professionals and can help identify warning signs of nutritional risk, such as altered body weight, eating habits, living environment, and functional status (see Figure 14-7).

Levels 2 and 3 screens provide more comprehensive nutritional assessment to be used by nutrition and health care professionals (see Figure 14-8). By the year 2000 the screening tools had been used with more than 300,000 individuals nationwide. The information collected using these screens built a valuable database on senior adults and guidance for community-based caregivers (NSI, 1997). The NSI is no longer funded as a separate initiative, but the validated tools and data collected using these tools continue to be a valuable resource. Chapters 10 and 14 describe the NSI in greater detail.

National Nutrient Data Bank

The **National Nutrient Data Bank**, maintained by the USDA, is the United States' primary resource of information on the nutrient content of foods. The source of the information is from private industry, academic institutions, and government laboratories. Historically the information was published as the series *Agriculture Handbook 8*. Currently the databases are available to the public on tapes and on the Internet. The bank is updated frequently and includes supplemental sources, the databases from other countries, and links to other sites. This data bank is a standard and updated source of nutrient information for commercial references and data systems. When using sources other than the USDA site, it is important to check the sources and the dates of the updates for evidence that these sources are reliable and current.

Centers for Disease Control and Prevention

The CDC is a component of the DHHS. It monitors the nation's health, detects and investigates health problems, and conducts research to enhance prevention. The CDC is also a source of information on health for travelers outside of the United States. Housed at CDC is the *National Center for Health Statistics*, which is the lead agency for NHANES, as well as for information on mortality, morbidity, BMI, and other health-related measures. Hard copies of reports and publications are available to professionals through a publications list or the website (see Box 11-1).

NATIONAL NUTRITION GUIDELINES AND GOALS

Policy development, the process by which society makes decisions about problems, chooses goals and prepares the means to reach them, frequently includes health priorities, and often dietary guidance. Table 11-1 lists some landmark reports that have influenced the development of dietary guidance or affected the content and scope of health priorities. This section provides a brief overview of some of these reports that have shaped dietary guidance.

Healthy People and the Surgeon General's Report on Nutrition and Health

Healthy People, a 1979 report of the Surgeon General, Promoting Health/Preventing Disease: Objectives for the Nation, outlined the prevention agenda for the nation with a series of health objectives to be accomplished by 1990 (*Healthy People*, 1979; Promoting Health, 1980). In 1988 *The Surgeon General's Report on Nutrition and Health* further stimulated the health promotion and disease prevention movement. This detailed report included information on dietary practices and health status. Along with specific health recommendations, there was documentation of the scientific basis for each. Since the focus included implications for the individual as well as for future public health policy decisions, this report has remained a useful reference and tool.

Healthy People 2000: National Health Promotion and Disease Prevention Objectives and *Healthy People 2010* are the next generations of these landmark public health efforts. Both reports outline the progress made on previous objectives and set new objectives for the next decade (Healthy People 2000, and Healthy People, 2010) (Box 11-3).

TABLE 11-1

History of Dietary Recommendations for the U.S. Public

Publication	Year	Organization or Agency	Recommendation
Food for Young Children	1916	USDA	First U.S. government dietary guidance pamphlet
Food Guide	1917	USDA	Five food groups: flesh, starches, fats, watery fruits and vegetables, sweets
Food Guide	1933	USDA	Twelve food groups
Recommended Dietary Allowances	1941	FNB/NAS	Recommended intakes for known nutrients
Food Guide	1946	USDA	"Basic 7" food groups
Food for Fitness (daily food guide)	1958	USDA	"Basic 4" food groups based on RDA*
Dietary Goals for the United States, ed 1	1977	Senate Select Committee on Nutrition and Human Needs	First government publication to address macronutrient intake and excess
Dietary Goals for the United States, ed 2	1978	Senate Select Committee on Nutrition and Human Needs	Refined recommendations of first edition
Nutrition and Your Health: Dietary Guidelines for Americans	1980	USDA/DHHS	Generic recommendations similar in content to the *Dietary Goals* without specified amounts
Toward Healthful Diets	1980	FNB/NAS	Similar to *Dietary Guidelines* and goals except for fat recommendations
Various guidelines on nutrition	1980	AMA, AHA, NCI, American Society for Clinical Nutrition, NAS	Several organizations published similar recommendations

During the evaluation phase for setting the 2010 objectives, it was determined that the United States has made progress in reducing the number of deaths from cardiovascular disease, stroke, and certain cancers. Dietary evaluation indicated a slight decrease in total dietary fat intake. However, during the last decade there has been an increase in the number of persons who are overweight or obese, a risk factor for cardiovascular disease, stroke, and other leading chronic diseases and causes of death. The midcourse review of accomplishing the 2010 objectives is being assembled to provide an update on progress, including information by regions and states.

Reducing the incidence of overweight and obesity and increasing physical activity are targeted priorities in 2010

TABLE 11-1

History of Dietary Recommendations for the U.S. Public—cont'd

Publication	Year	Organization or Agency	Recommendation
Diet, Nutrition, and Cancer	1982	Committee on Diet, Nutrition, and Cancer; NRC; NAS	Dietary guidelines to reduce risk of cancer
Nutrition and Your Health: Dietary Guidelines for Americans, ed 2	1985	USDA/DHHS	
National Cholesterol Education Program (NCEP): Adult Treatment Panel I	1987	DHHS/NHLBI	Guidelines for the clinical treatment of patients with hyperlipoproteinemia
NCI Dietary Guidelines: Rationale	1988	DHHS/NCI	Recommendations to reduce risk of cancer
Nutrition and Your Health: Dietary Guidelines for Americans, ed 3	1990	USDA/DHHS	
Food Guide Pyramid	1992	USDA/HNIS	New eating guide based on RDA that also considers salt, fat, and sugar
NCEP: Adult Treatment Panel II	1994	DHHS/NHLBI	Established categories of risk; more aggressive clinical measures for patients at a higher risk for coronary heart disease
Dietary Guidelines for Americans, ed 4	1995	USDA/DHHS	
Dietary Reference Intakes	1996	FNB/NAS	Reference values for nutrient intake; contain three components: estimated average requirement (EAR), recommended dietary allowance (RDA), and tolerable upper intake level (UL)
Dietary Guidelines for Americans, ed 5	2000	USDA/DHHS	Guidelines grouped into three categories: (1) aim for fitness, (2) build a healthy base, and (3) choose sensibly (the ABC approach)
Americans Heart Association Eating Plan for Healthy Americans	2000	AHA	Dietary guidelines to reduce the risk of hypertension, hyperlipoproteinemia, and overweight and obesity
NCEP: Adult Treatment Panel III	2001	DHHS/NHLBI	Adds recommendations for primary prevention of hyperlipoproteinemia in people with multiple risk factors
Dietary Guidelines for Americans, ed 6	2005	USDA/DHHS	Simplifies recommendations and clarifies role of physical activity in addition to diet.

*Recommended dietary allowances (RDAs) revised approximately every 5 years since 1943.

AHA, American Heart Association; *AMA*, American Medical Association; *DHHS*, Department of Health and Human Services; *FNB*, Food and Nutrition Board; *HNIS*, Human Nutrition and Information Services; *NAS*, National Academy of Sciences; *NCI*, National Cancer Institute; *NHLBI*, National Heart, Lung, and Blood Institute.

for all segments of the population (Table 11-2). Other areas continuing to be targeted are improving the health of minorities, increasing breast-feeding, and reducing the incidence of iron deficiency anemia (Healthy People, 2010) (Figure 11-2). The evaluations of past objectives and current updates of the 2010 can be found at the website.

Dietary Guidelines for Americans

Senator George McGovern and The Senate Select Committee on Nutrition and Human Needs presented the first Dietary Goals for the United States in 1977 (Senate Select Committee, 1977). In 1980 the goals were modified and issued jointly by the DHHS and the USDA as the DGA. Updated every 5 years, the current revision is the sixth edition, *Dietary Guidelines for Americans 2005* (see Box 9-1). The original guidelines were a response to an increasing national concern for the rise in overweight, obesity, and chronic diseases with a nutrition cause (diabetes, coronary artery disease, hypertension, and certain cancers). The approach continues to be one of health promotion and disease prevention, with special attention paid to

specific population groups. Activity and exercise, as well as food safety, are a part of the guidance (Dietary Guidelines for Americans, 2005).

The 2005 DGA are evidence-based science rather than statements based on "advice." The report of the expert committee recommending revisions to the DGA provides scientific documentation useful to health practitioners. The DGA have become a central theme in community nutrition assessment, program planning, and evaluation, and they are incorporated into programs such as School Lunch and Congregate Meals. More information on the DGA is included in Chapters 9 and 12.

Other Dietary Guidance

Until the release of the DGA, dietary guidance was likely to have a specific disease approach (see Table 11-1). The AHA guidelines were updated in 2000 and provide guidance for persons at risk for hypertension and coronary artery disease. The National Heart, Lung, and Blood Institute (NHLBI) provided landmark guidelines for identifying and treating hyperlipoproteinemia in 1987, updated in 2001 (ADA, 2002). Chapters 32 and 33 provide clinical insights on implementing these guidelines for individuals.

The National Cancer Institute (NCI) landmark report *Diet, Nutrition and Cancer* led to Dietary Guidelines for Cancer Prevention (NRC, 1982). These were updated and broadened, combining recommendations on energy balance, nutrition, and physical activity (NCI, 2004). The ACS and the American Institute for Cancer Research (AICR) are continuing sources for recommendations and information (see Chapter 37), along with the NCI.

With the release of the DGA 2005 and its evidence-based approach, recommendations concerning dietary guidance are providing a more synchronized message to the community. The common theme is that a diet lower in fat, especially saturated fat, with emphasis on foods that are sources of fiber, complex carbohydrates, and lean or plant-based proteins is desirable. The message is based on food choices for optimal health, with emphasis on whole grains, fruits and vegetables, leaner dairy and animal protein sources, and use of more plant-based protein sources. Essential to this message is emphasis on appropriate portion sizes and calorie choices related to a person's physiologic needs. Exercise and activity guidance has become an accepted part of dietary guidance.

A consumer-friendly single health guideline was released in 1991 as a part of "5-A-Day for Better Health." The sponsors were the NCI, the National Institutes of Health (NIH), and the Produce for Better Health Foundation. The guidance is built around fruits and vegetables being naturally low in fat and good sources of fiber, several vitamins and minerals, and phytochemicals. In keeping with the evidence-based DGA 2005, the message has been expanded to "Eat five to nine servings of fruits and vegetables a day to promote good health" (USDHHS, 2005a). The latest promotion "Fruits and Veggies: More Matters," is an attempt to increase intake above five to nine servings per day.

TABLE 11-2

Healthy People 2010 Focus Area 19: Nutrition and Overweight

Weight Status and Growth

19-1	Increase the proportion of adults who are at a healthy weight.
19-2	Reduce the proportion of adults who are obese.
19-3	Reduce the proportion of children and adolescents who are overweight or obese.
19-4	Reduce growth retardation among low-income children under age 5 years.

Food and Nutrient Consumption

19-5	Increase the proportion of persons ages 2 years and older who consume at least two daily servings of fruit.
19-6	Increase the proportion of persons ages 2 years and older who consume at least three daily servings of vegetables, with at least one third being dark green or orange vegetables.
19-7	Increase the proportion of persons ages 2 years and older who consume at least six daily servings of grain products, with at least three being whole grains.
19-8	Increase the proportion of persons ages 2 years and older who consume less than 10% of calories from saturated fat.
19-9	Increase the proportion of persons ages 2 years and older who consume no more than 30% of calories from total fat.
19-10	Increase the proportion of persons ages 2 years and older who consume 2400 mg or less of sodium daily.
19-11	Increase the proportion of persons ages 2 years and older who meet dietary recommendations for calcium.

Iron Deficiency and Anemia

19-12	Reduce iron deficiency among young children and females of childbearing age.
19-13	Reduce anemia among low-income pregnant females in their third trimester.
19-14	Reduce iron deficiency among pregnant females.

Schools, Worksites, and Nutrition Counseling

19-15	Increase the proportion of children and adolescents ages 6 to 19 years whose intake of meals and snacks at school contributes to good overall dietary quality.
19-16	Increase the proportion of worksites that offer nutrition or weight management classes or counseling.
19-17	Increase the proportion of physician office visits made by patients with a diagnosis of cardiovascular disease, diabetes, or hyperlipidemia that includes counseling or education related to diet and nutrition.

Food Security

19-18	Increase food security among U.S. households and in so doing reduce hunger.

From *Healthy People 2010: national health promotion and disease prevention objectives,* Washington, DC, 2000, U.S. Department of Health and Human Services.

Other Focus Areas with objectives pertaining to nutrition include: 1-Access to Quality Health Services; 2-Arthritis, Osteoporosis and Chronic Back Conditions; 3-Cancer; 4-Chronic Kidney Disease; 5-Diabetes; 7-Educational and Community-Based Programs; 10-Food Safety; 11-Health Communication; 12-Heart Disease and Stroke; 16-Maternal, Infant and Child Health; 18-Mental Health and Mental Disorders; 22-Physical Activity and Fitness; and 26-Substance Abuse.

The Recommended Dietary Allowances and Dietary Reference Intakes

The recommended dietary allowances (RDAs) were developed in 1943 by the Food and Nutrition Board of the National Research Council of the National Academy of Sciences. Until 1989 the RDAs were revised approximately every 10 years. The first tables were developed at a time when the U.S. population was recovering from a major economic depression and World War II; nutrient deficiencies were a concern (Food and Nutrition Board, 1989). The philosophy was to develop guidelines that would promote optimal health, with a goal of nutrient intakes set at a level to lower the risk of nutrient deficiencies. As the food supply and the nutrition needs of the

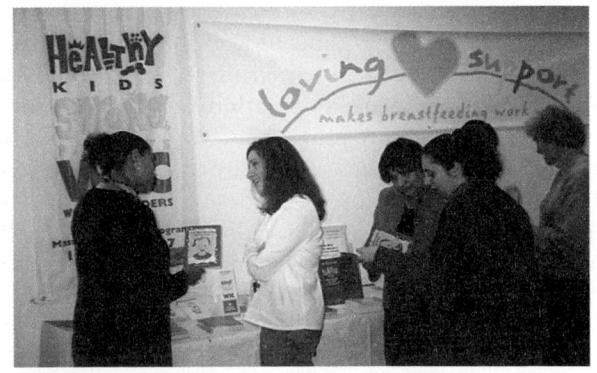

FIGURE 11-2 Strategies for reaching 2010 objectives: breast-feeding works. Using a health fair to encourage women to breast-feed.

population changed, the intent of the RDAs was adapted to preventing nutrition-related disease.

The RDAs have always reflected gender, age, and life-phase differences. There have been additions of nutrients and revisions of the age-groups. However, the recent revisions are a major departure from the single list some professionals still view as the RDAs. Beginning in 1998 a new umbrella of nutrient guidelines known as the dietary reference intakes (DRIs) was introduced. Included in the DRIs are RDAs, as well as new designations, including guidance on safe upper limits of certain nutrients. The research supporting these values provides a framework for assessment and planning (IOM, 2000). As a group the DRIs are being evaluated, expanded, and revised at intervals, thus making these tools more reflective of current research and population base needs (IOM, 2006). See Chapter 12 for complete discussion of the DRIs.

Food Guides

In 1916 the USDA initiated the idea of food grouping in the pamphlet, *Food for Young Children*. Food grouping systems have changed in shape (wheels, boxes, and pyramids) and numbers of groupings (four, five, and seven groups), but the intent has remained (i.e., to present an easy guide for healthful eating). The current guide, released in 2005, is an Internet-based tool called *MyPyramid.gov: Steps to a Healthier You* (USDA, MyPyramid) (see Figure 12-1). In September 2005 a companion *MyPyramid for Kids* was released with a target audience of children. Like other current public health tools, this food guidance system has a focus on health promotion and disease prevention (USDA, 2006; Davis et al., 2001).

FOOD ASSISTANCE
AND NUTRITION PROGRAMS

Public health assurance addresses the implementation of legislative mandates, maintenance of statutory responsibilities, support of crucial services, regulation of services and products provided in both the public and private sector, and maintenance of accountability. This includes providing for food security, which translates into having access to an adequate amount of healthful and safe foods. Although there is a documented increase in obesity and overweight in the U.S. population, a segment of the population is at risk for hunger and undernutrition. The ADA addressed the issues related to U.S. food and nutrition security in a position paper describing the impact of hunger and undernutrition on vulnerable groups such as infants, children, pregnant women, and older Americans (ADA, 2006). Access requires that food be readily available and that there are resources to obtain the food. Historically public health nutritionists have advocated for food and nutrition programs that link consumers to adequate and safe food. These programs are described in Table 11-3.

FOODBORNE ILLNESS

The 2000 edition of the DGA was the first to include food safety. This is an important step in linking the safety of the food and water supply with health promotion and disease prevention and acknowledges the potential for **foodborne illness** to cause both acute illness and long-term chronic complications (Wotecki, 2001). Since 2000 all revisions of the DGA have made food safety a priority.

Each year there are an estimated 76 million cases of foodborne illness in the United States. The majority of foodborne illness outbreaks reported to the CDC result from bacteria, followed by viral outbreaks, chemical etiology, and parasitic etiology (ADA, 2003b). Segments of the population are particularly susceptible to foodborne illnesses, with vulnerable individuals more likely to become ill and experience serious complications as a result of illness. Some of the nutritional complications associated with foodborne illness include reduced appetite and reduced nutrient absorption from the gut.

Persons at increased risk for foodborne illnesses include young children; pregnant women; older adults; persons who are immunocompromised because of AIDS/HIV, steroid use, chemotherapy, diabetes mellitus, or cancer; alcoholics; persons with liver disease, decreased stomach acidity, autoimmune disorders, or malnutrition; persons who take antibiotics; and persons living in institutionalized settings. Costs associated with foodborne illness include those related to investigation of foodborne outbreaks and treatment of victims, employer costs due to lost productivity, and food industry losses due to lower sales and lower stock prices (ADA, 2003b). Table 11-4 describes common foodborne illnesses and their signs and symptoms, timing of onset, duration, causes, and prevention.

All food groups have foods associated with food safety issues. There are public health concerns about microbial contamination of fruits and vegetables that are either farmed organically or imported from another country, as is common in the United States' increasingly global food supply. Other factors that may contribute to increased foodborne illness incidence include new methods of food production and distribution and increased reliance on commercial food sources (ADA, 2003b). Improperly cooked meats can harbor organisms that can trigger a foodborne illness. Even properly cooked meats have the potential to cause foodborne illness if the food handler allows raw meat juices to contaminate other foods during preparation (Wotecki, 2001). Sources of a foodborne illness outbreak vary, depending on such factors as the type of organism involved, the point of contamination, the duration of food-holding periods, and the temperature during holding.

One approach to combating foodborne illness is targeted food safety public education campaigns. However, the model for food safety has expanded beyond the individual consumer and now includes government, the food industry, and the general public. Several government agencies provide information through websites with links to the CDC, USDA's Food Safety and Inspection Service (FSIS),

Text continued on p. 330

TABLE 11-3

U.S. Food Assistance and Nutrition Programs

Program Name	Goal/Purpose	Services Provided	Target Audience	Eligibility	Funding	Level of Prevention*
After-School Snack Program	Provides reimbursement for snacks served to students after school	Provides cash reimbursement to schools for snacks served to students after the school day snacks must contain two of four components: fluid milk, meat/meat alternate, vegetable or fruit or full-strength juice, whole grain or enriched bread	Children under 18 whose school sponsors a structured, supervised after-school enrichment program and provides lunch through the NSLP	School programs located within the boundaries of eligible low-income areas may be reimbursed for snacks served at no charge to students	U.S. Department of Agriculture (USDA)	Primary, secondary
Child and Adult Care Food Program	Provides nutritious meals and snacks to infants, young children, and adults receiving day care services as well as infants and children living in emergency shelters	Provides commodities or cash to help centers serve nutritious meals that meet federal guidelines	Infants, children, and adults receiving day care at child-care centers, family day care homes, and homeless shelters		USDA FNS	Primary, secondary
Commodity Supplemental Food Program	Provides no-cost monthly supplemental food packages composed of commodity foods to populations perceived to be at nutritional risk	Provides food packages; nutrition education services are available often through Extension Service Programs; program referrals provided	Generally children ages 5-6, postpartum nonbreast-feeding mothers from 6-12 months' postpartum, seniors 60+	Between 130% and 185% of the poverty guideline	USDA FNS	Primary, secondary
Disaster Feeding Program	Makes commodities available for distribution to disaster relief agencies	Commodities are provided to disaster victims through congregate dining settings and direct distribution to households	Those experiencing a natural disaster	Those experiencing a natural disaster	USDA FNS	Primary

*Level of prevention rationale: Programs that provide food only are regarded as primary; programs that provide food, nutrients at a mandated level of recommended dietary allowances or an educational component are regarded as secondary; and programs that used health screening measures on enrollment were regarded as tertiary.

Continued

TABLE 11-3

U.S. Food Assistance and Nutrition Programs—cont'd

Program Name	Goal/Purpose	Services Provided	Target Audience	Eligibility	Funding	Level of Prevention*
The Emergency Food Assistance Program (TEFAP)	Commodities are made available to local emergency food providers for preparing meals for the needy or for distribution of food packages	Surplus commodity foods are provided for distribution	Low-income households	Low-income households at 150% of the Federal Poverty Income Guideline	USDA FNS	Primary
Emergency Food and Shelter Program (EFSP)	Funds are used to purchase food/shelter to supplement and extend local services	EFSP provides funding for: the purchase of food products, operation costs associated with mass feeding and shelter, limited rent or mortgage assistance, providing assistance for first month's rent, limited off-site emergency lodging, and limited utility assistance	Those in need of emergency services	Primary	Federal Emergency Management Agency (FEMA)	Primary
Head Start	Provides agencies and schools with support and guidance for half- and full-day child development programs for low-income children	Programs receive reimbursement for nutritious meals and snacks and USDA-donated commodities, support for curriculum, social services and health screenings	Low-income children ages 3–5; parents are encouraged to volunteer and be involved	Same as NSLP	USDA (food) DHHS (health)	Primary Secondary
National School Breakfast Program	Provides nutritionally balanced, low-cost or free breakfasts to children enrolled in participating schools	Participating schools receiving cash subsidies and USDA-donated commodities in return for offering breakfasts that meet same criteria as school lunch and offering free and reduced-price meals to eligible children	Children preschool age through grades 12 in schools; children and teens 20 years of age in residential child-care and juvenile correctional institutions	Same as NSLP	USDA FNS	Primary, secondary

Program	Description	Target audience	Eligibility	Agency	Level of prevention
National School Lunch Program (NSLP)	Provides nutritionally balanced, low-cost or free lunches to children enrolled in participating schools	Participating schools receive cash subsidies and USDA-donated commodities in return for offering lunches that meet dietary guidelines and ⅓ of RDA for protein, iron, calcium, vitamins A and C, and calories and for offering free and reduced-price meals to eligible children	Children preschool age through grade 12 in schools; children and teenagers 20 years of age and younger in residential childcare and juvenile correctional institutions	185% of Federal Poverty Income Guideline for reduced-price lunches; 130% for free lunches	USDA FNS	Primary, secondary
Nutrition Program for the Elderly/ Area Agencies on Aging	Provides commodity and cash assistance to programs providing meal services to older adults	Provides nutritious meals for older adults through congregate dining or home-delivered meals	Older adults	No income standard applied	DHHS administers through state and local agencies; USDA cash and commodity assistance	Primary
Seniors' Farmers Market Nutrition Program	Providing fresh, nutritious, unprepared, locally grown fruits, vegetables, and herbs from farmers' markets, roadside stands, and community-supported agriculture programs to low-income seniors	Coupons for use at authorized farmers' markets, roadside stands, and community supported agriculture programs (foods that are not eligible for purchase with coupons by seniors are: dried fruits or vegetables, potted plants and herbs, wild rice, nuts, honey, maple syrup, cider and molasses)	Low-income adults over the age of 60	Low-income seniors with household incomes not exceeding 195% of the Federal Poverty Income Guideline	USDA FNS	Primary
Special Milk Program	Provides milk to children in participating schools who do not have access to other meal programs	Provides cash reimbursement for milk with vitamins A and D at RDA levels served at low or no cost to children; milk programs must be run on nonprofit basis	Same target audience as School Lunch and School Breakfast Programs	Eligible children do NOT have access to other supplemental foods programs	USDA FNS	Primary, secondary

*Level of prevention rationale: Programs that provide food only are regarded as primary; programs that provide food, nutrients at a mandated level of recommended dietary allowances or an educational component are regarded as secondary; and programs that used health screening measures on enrollment were regarded as tertiary.

Continued

TABLE 11-3

U.S. Food Assistance and Nutrition Programs—cont'd

Program Name	Goal/Purpose	Services Provided	Target Audience	Eligibility	Funding	Level of Prevention*
Summer Food Service Program	Provides healthy meals (per federal guidelines) and snacks to eligible children when school is out, using agriculture commodity foods	Reimburses for up to two or three meals and/or snacks served daily free to eligible children when school is not in session; cash based on income level of local geographic area or of enrolled children	Infants and children 18 years of age and younger served at variety of feeding sites		USDA FNS	Primary, secondary
Women, Infants and Children (WIC) Special Supplemental Nutrition Program for Women, Infants and Children	Providing supplemental foods to improve health status of participants	Nutrition education, free nutritious foods (protein, iron, calcium, vitamins A and C), referrals, breast-feeding promotion	Pregnant, breast-feeding and postpartum women up to 1 year Infants, children up to 5 yrs	185% of Federal Poverty Income Guideline nutritional risk	UDSA FNS, home state support	Primary, secondary, tertiary
WC Farmers Market Nutrition Program (FMNP)	Providing fresh, unprepared, locally grown fruits and vegetables to WIC recipients, and to expand the awareness, use of and sales at farmers' markets	FMNP food coupons for use at participating farmers' markets stands; nutrition education through arrangements with state agency	Same as WIC recipients	Same as WIC recipients	USDA FNS	Primary

*Level of prevention rationale: Programs that provide food only are regarded as primary; programs that provide food, nutrients at a mandated level of recommended dietary allowances or an educational component are regarded as secondary; and programs that used health screening measures on enrollment were regarded as tertiary.

TABLE 11-4

Common Foodborne Illnesses

Illness	Signs and Symptoms	Onset and Duration	Causes and Prevention	Comments
Bacillus cereus	Watery diarrhea, abdominal cramping, vomiting	6-15 hours after consumption of contaminated food; duration 24 hours in most instances	Meats, milk, vegetables, and fish have been associated with the diarrheal type; vomiting-type outbreaks have generally been associated with rice products; potato, pasta and cheese products; food mixtures such as sauces, puddings, soups, casseroles, pastries, and salads may also be a source	*B. cereus* is a gram-positive, aerobic spore former
Campylobacter jejuni	Diarrhea (often bloody), fever, and abdominal cramping are key symptoms	2-5 days after exposure; duration 2-10 days	Drinking raw milk or eating raw or undercooked meat, shellfish, or poultry; to prevent exposure, avoid raw milk and cook all meats and poultry thoroughly; it is safest to drink only pasteurized milk; the bacteria may also be found in tofu or raw vegetables. Hand-washing is important for prevention; wash hands with soap before handling raw foods of animal origin, after handling raw foods of animal origin, and before touching anything else; prevent cross-contamination in the kitchen; proper refrigeration and sanitation are also essential	Top source of foodborne illness; some people develop antibodies to it, but others do not. In persons with compromised immune systems, it may spread to the bloodstream and cause sepsis; may lead to arthritis or to Guillian-Barré syndrome (GBS); 40% of GBS in the United States is caused by campylobacteriosis and affects the nerves of the body, beginning several weeks after the diarrheal illness; can lead to paralysis that lasts several weeks and usually requires intensive care

Continued

Adapted with permission from Escott-Stump S: *Nutrition and diagnosis-related care*, ed 6, Baltimore: Lippincott Williams & Wilkens, 2008. Other sources: http://www.cdc.gov/health/diseases; http://www.cfsan.fda.gov/~mow/intro.html, accessed July 1, 2006.

TABLE 11-4

Common Foodborne Illnesses—cont'd

Illness	Signs and Symptoms	Onset and Duration	Causes and Prevention	Comments
Clostridium botulinum	Muscle paralysis caused by the bacterial toxin: double or blurred vision, drooping eyelids, slurred speech, difficulty swallowing, dry mouth, and muscle weakness; infants with botulism appear lethargic, feed poorly, are constipated, and have a weak cry and poor muscle tone	In foodborne botulism symptoms generally begin 18-36 hours after eating contaminated food; can occur as early as 6 hours or as late as 10 days; duration days or months	Home-canned foods with low acid content such as asparagus, green beans, beets, and corn; outbreaks have occurred from more unusual sources such as chopped garlic in oil, hot peppers, tomatoes, improperly handled baked potatoes wrapped in aluminum foil, and home-canned or fermented fish Persons who home-can should follow strict hygienic procedures to reduce contamination of foods; oils infused with garlic or herbs should be refrigerated; potatoes that have been baked while wrapped in aluminum foil should be kept hot until served or refrigerated; because high temperatures destroy the botulism toxin, persons who eat home-canned foods should boil the food for 10 minutes before eating	If untreated, these symptoms may progress to cause paralysis of the arms, legs, trunk, and respiratory muscles; long-term ventilator support may be needed Throw out bulging, leaking, or dented cans and jars that are leaking; safe home-canning instructions can be obtained from county extension services or from the U.S. Department of Agriculture; honey can contain spores of *C. botulinum* and has been a source of infection for infants; children younger than 12 months old should not be fed honey
Clostridium perfringens	Nausea with vomiting, diarrhea, and signs of acute gastroenteritis lasting 1 day	Within 6-24 hours from the ingestion	Ingestion of canned meats or contaminated dried mixes, gravy, stews, refried beans, meat products, and unwashed vegetables Cook foods thoroughly; leftovers must be reheated properly or discarded	
Cryptosporidium parvum	Watery stools, diarrhea, nausea, vomiting, slight fever, and stomach cramps	2-10 days after being infected	Contaminated food from poor handling Hand washing is important	Protozoa causes diarrhea among immune-compromised patients
Enterotoxigenic Escherichia coli (ETEC)	Watery diarrhea, abdominal cramps, low-grade fever, nausea and malaise	With high infective dose, diarrhea can be induced within 24 hours	Contamination of water with human sewage may lead to contamination of foods; infected food handlers may also contaminate foods; dairy products such as semi-soft cheeses may cause problems, but this is rare	More common with travel to other countries; in infants or debilitated elderly persons, electrolyte replacement therapy may be necessary

Organism	Symptoms	Onset/Duration	Food Sources/Prevention	Comments
Escherichia coli: O157:H7 *Enterohemorrhagic E. coli (EHEC)*	Hemorrhagic colitis (painful, bloody diarrhea)	Onset is slow, usually approximately 3–8 days after ingestion. Duration 5–10 days	Undercooked ground beef and meats, from unprocessed apple cider, or from unwashed fruits and vegetables; sometimes water sources; alfalfa sprouts, unpasteurized fruit juices, dry-cured salami, lettuce, spinach, game meat, and cheese curds. Cook meats thoroughly, use only pasteurized milk, and wash all produce well	Antibiotics are not used because they spread the toxin further; the condition may progress to hemolytic anemia, thrombocytopenia, and acute renal failure, requiring dialysis and transfusions; hemolytic uremic syndrome (HUS) can be fatal, especially in young children; there are several outbreaks each year, particularly from catering operations, church events, and family picnics; *E. coli* O157:H7 can survive in refrigerated acid foods for weeks (Mayerhauser, 2001)
Listeria monocytogenes (LM)	Mild fever, headache, vomiting, and severe illness in pregnancy; sepsis in the immuno-compromised patient; meningoencephalitis in infants; and febrile gastroenteritis in adults	Onset 2–30 days. Duration variable	Processed, ready-to-eat products such as undercooked hot dogs, deli or lunchmeats, and unpasteurized dairy products; postpasteurization contamination of soft cheeses such as feta or Brie, milk, and commercial coleslaw; cross-contamination between food surfaces has also been a problem. Use pasteurized milk and cheeses; wash produce before use; reheat foods to proper temperatures; wash hands with hot, soapy water after handling these ready-to-eat foods; discard foods by their expiration dates	May be fatal. Caution must be used by pregnant women, who may pass the infection on to their unborn child (Wotecki, 2001)
Norovirus	Gastroenteritis with nausea, vomiting, and/or diarrhea accompanied by abdominal cramps; headache, fever/chills, and muscle aches may also be present	24 to 48 hours after ingestion of the virus, but can appear as early as 12 hours after exposure	Foods can be contaminated either by direct contact with contaminated hands or work surfaces that are contaminated with stool or vomit or by tiny droplets from nearby vomit that can travel through air to land on food; although the virus cannot multiply outside of human bodies, once on food or in water, it can cause illness; most cases occur on cruise ships	Symptoms are usually brief and last only 1 or 2 days; however, during that brief period, people can feel very ill and vomit, often violently and without warning, many times a day; drink liquids to prevent dehydration

Continued

TABLE 11-4

Common Foodborne Illnesses—cont'd

Illness	Signs and Symptoms	Onset and Duration	Causes and Prevention	Comments
Salmonella	Diarrhea, fever, and abdominal cramps	12-72 hours after infection Duration usually 4-7 days	Ingestion of raw or undercooked meat, poultry, fish, eggs, unpasteurized dairy products; unwashed fruits and raw vegetables (melons and sprouts) Prevent by thorough cooking, proper sanitation, and hygiene	There are many different kinds of *Salmonella* bacteria; *Salmonella typhimurium* and *Salmonella enteritidis* are the most common in the United States. Most people recover without treatment, but some have diarrhea that is so severe that the patient needs to be hospitalized; this patient must be treated promptly with antibiotics; the elderly, infants, and those with impaired immune systems are more likely to have a severe illness
Shigellosis	Bloody diarrhea, fever, and stomach cramps	24-48 hours after exposure Duration 4-7 days	Milk and dairy products; cold mixed salads such as egg, tuna, chicken, potato, and meat salads Proper cooking, reheating, and maintenance of holding temperatures should aid in prevention; careful hand washing is essential	This is caused by a group of bacteria called *Shigella*; may be severe in young children and the elderly; severe infection with high fever may be associated with seizures in children younger than 2 years old
Staphylococcus aureus	Nausea, vomiting, retching, abdominal cramping, and prostration	Within 1-6 hours; rarely fatal Duration 1-2 days	Meat, pork, eggs, poultry, tuna salad, prepared salads, gravy, stuffing, cream-filled pastries Cooking does not destroy the toxin; proper handling and hygiene are crucial for prevention	Refrigerate foods promptly during preparation and after meal service

	Symptoms	Onset/Duration	Foods	Comments
Streptococcus pyogenes	Sore and red throat, pain on swallowing; tonsillitis, high fever, headache, nausea, vomiting, malaise, rhinorrhea; occasionally a rash occurs	Onset 1–3 days	Milk, ice cream, eggs, steamed lobster, ground ham, potato salad, egg salad, custard, rice pudding, and shrimp salad; in almost all cases, the foodstuffs were allowed to stand at room temperature for several hours between preparation and consumption	Entrance into the food is the result of poor hygiene, ill food handlers, or the use of unpasteurized milk. Complications are rare; treated with antibiotics
Vibrio vulnificus	Vomiting, diarrhea, or both; illness is mild	Gastroenteritis occurs about 16 hours after eating contaminated food. Duration about 48 hours	Seafood, especially raw clams and oysters, that has been contaminated with human pathogens; although oysters can only be harvested legally from waters free from fecal contamination, even these can be contaminated with *V. vulnificus* because the bacterium is naturally present	This is a bacterium in the same family as those that cause cholera; it yields a *Norovirus*; it may be fatal in immuno-compromised individuals
Yersinia enterocolitica	Common symptoms in children are fever, abdominal pain, and diarrhea, which is often bloody; in older children and adults, right-sided abdominal pain and fever may be predominant symptom and may be confused with appendicitis	1–2 days after exposure. Duration 1–3 weeks or longer	Contaminated food, especially raw or undercooked pork products; postpasteurization contamination of chocolate milk, reconstituted dry milk, pasteurized milk, and tofu are also high-risk foods; cold storage does not kill the bacteria. Cook meats thoroughly; use only pasteurized milk; proper hand washing is also important	Infectious disease caused by the bacterium *Yersinia*; in the United States most human illness is caused by *Y. enterocolitica*; it is most often in young children. In a small proportion of cases, complications such as skin rash, joint pains, or spread of bacteria to the bloodstream can occur

the Environmental Protection Agency (EPA), the National Institute of Allergy and Infectious Diseases (NIAID) of the National Institutes of Health, and the Food and Drug Administration (FDA) (see Useful Websites).

An integral strategy to reduce foodborne illness is risk assessment and risk management. Risk assessment entails hazard identification, characterization and exposure; risk management covers risk evaluation, option assessment and implementation, and monitoring and review of progress. One formal program, organized in 1996, is the **Hazard Analysis Critical Control Points (HACCP)**, a systematic approach to the identification, evaluation, and control of food safety hazards. HACCP involves identifying any biologic, chemical, or physical agent that is reasonably likely to cause illness or injury in the absence of its control as it pertains to food production. It also involves identifying points at which control can be applied, thus preventing or eliminating the food safety hazard or reducing it to an acceptable level. Restaurants and health care facilities are obligated to use HACCP procedures in their food handling practices.

There is an increased communication of potential risks to health care professionals with direct patient contact, as well as those involved in community education. Those who serve populations at the greatest risk for foodborne illness have a special need to be involved in the network of food safety education and to communicate this information to their clients.

FOOD AND WATER SAFETY

Although individual educational efforts are effective in raising awareness of food safety issues, food and water safety must be examined on a national, systems-based level. *Healthy People 2010* includes objectives relating to food and water safety: reducing disease related to foodborne pathogens and pesticide and allergen exposure, promoting food-handling practices that support food safety, reducing disease incidence associated with water, and reducing food- and water-related exposure to environmental pollutants (*Healthy People 2000*). These continue to be monitored and updated as strategies are implemented to reach the objectives (*Healthy People 2010*, 2004a). The ADA Position Paper, *Food and Water Safety*, provides further evidence of these linkages and notes the role of dietetics professionals (ADA, 2003b).

Contamination

Adoption of the HAACP regulations, food quality assurance programs, handling of fresh produce guidelines, technologic advances designed to reduce contamination, increased food supply regulations, and a greater emphasis on food safety education has contributed to a substantial decline in foodborne illness. A current concern illustrates the importance of food safety (i.e., a **pandemic** [population wide] influenza outbreak related to **avian influenza [bird flu]**). Although the risks and the controls are still being determined, there is one precaution related to controlling risk: the issue of meeting food safety standards. People cannot become infected with avian

flu by eating properly handled and cooked eggs or poultry (McNally, 2006). Using appropriate hand-washing techniques, properly handling poultry and eggs, washing utensils and surfaces to lessen the risk of cross-contamination, and using food thermometers to make sure that a cooked food reaches an internal temperature of 165° F are steps that should be encouraged by nutrition and health professionals.

Controls and precautions in the area of limiting potential contaminants in the water supply are of continuing importance. Water contamination with arsenic, lead, pesticides, mercury, chlorine, herbicides and *Escherichia coli* has been repeatedly highlighted by the media. It has been estimated that many public water systems, built using early twentieth-century technology, will need to invest over $138 billion over the next 20 years to ensure continued safe drinking water (ADA, 2003b). The effect on the potential safety of foods that have contact with these contaminants is an ongoing issue being monitored by advocacy and professional groups and governmental agencies.

Of interest to many is the issue of the potential hazards of ingestion of seafood that has been in contact with methyl mercury present naturally in the environment and released into the air from industrial pollution. Mercury has accumulated in bodies of water (i.e., streams, rivers, lakes, and oceans) and in the flesh of seafood in these waters (USFDA/EPA, 2004). The body of knowledge on issues such as this is constantly being updated, and there are now recommendations to restrict the consumption of certain fish such as shark, mackerel, tilefish, tuna, and swordfish by pregnant women (CFSAN, 2007) (see Chapter 5 for further discussion). Other contaminants in fish, polychlorinated biphenyls (PCBS) and dioxin are also of concern (Mozaffarian and Rimm, 2006).

The issues surrounding use of pesticides and contaminants in the water supply affecting produce are further concerns (see *Focus On:* Is it Really Organic, and Is It Healthier?). Both the EPA and the Center for Food Safety and Applied Nutrition (CFSAN) websites are sources for ongoing monitoring and guidance. In addition, food and water safety and foodborne illness issues are monitored by state and local health departments. There are precautions in place at the federal, state, and local levels that need to be addressed by dietetics professionals whose role includes advocacy, as well as communication and education, to help the public and the local officials understand the risks and the importance of carrying out programs for food and water safety and protection.

Bioterrorism

The threat of **bioterrorism,** the deliberate use of microorganisms or toxins from living organisms to induce death or disease, and the nation's food and water supplies have made food **biosecurity,** or precautions to minimize risk, an issue of concern when addressing preparedness planning (Bruemmer, 2003). The CDC has identified seven foodborne pathogens as having the potential to be used by bioterrorists to attack the food supply: tularemia, brucellosis, *Clostridium botulinum* toxin, epsilon toxin of *Clostridium perfringens*, *Salmonella*, *E. coli*, and *Shigella*. These pathogens, along with potential

Is It Really Organic and Is It Healthier?

The popularity of organic and natural foods continues to increase with the growth of ethical consumerism. Environmental, social, and political issues are as important as nutrition in organic farming and whether a consumer decides to "go organic." The organic food industry represents just over 2% of food sales in the United States and is growing at the rate of 20% per year.

There is a legal definition for the word *organic*. As of October 2002, a food designated as Aorganic@ has met production and handling standards identified and regulated by the USDA; in the marketplace the food is labeled with the word Aorganic@ or a sticker with the USDA Organic seal.

For a food to earn the designation Aorganic@, 95% or more of the ingredients must be organic and must have been produced in fields that use renewable resources and conserve soil and water to enhance environmental quality. The other 5% of ingredients must be nonagricultural substances on an approved list that are not available in an organic form.

Aorganic@ meat, poultry, eggs, and dairy come from animals grown without antibiotics or growth hormones and fed 100% organic feed. Organic milk is one of the most popular organic foods chosen by consumers. Fruits and vegetable are grown without conventional pesticides, petroleum-based fertilizers, or sewage sludge–based fertilizers. The land on which organic crops are grown is required to be pesticide and herbicide free for 3 years before a crop is harvested. In addition, bioengineering or genetic modification or ionizing radiation cannot be used in the production of the food. For a product or farm to use the designation Aorganic@, a government-approved certifier must inspect the farm or processor; obtaining this designation is voluntary (USDA, 2002).

Products labeled "made with organic ingredients" must contain at least 70% organic ingredients, but they may not use the USDA seal. Processed products that contain less than 70% organic ingredients can list those ingredients as organic, but they cannot be labeled as organic.

Is organic food healthier? In terms of promoting organic agriculture as environmentally sustainable agriculture, it is. But there is no conclusive evidence that organically grown foods are more nutritious or concentrated in nutrients than conventionally grown foods, except perhaps for vitamin C, which may be higher in organically grown leafy vegetables and potatoes (Magkos et al., 2003). One study comparing organically grown vs. conventionally grown marion berries, strawberries, and corn showed statistically greater amounts of phenolic compounds (phytonutrients with antioxidant capabilities) in the organically grown produce compared to that conventionally grown (Asami et al., 2003).

One study of children eating either conventional or organic foods found that, after eating organic foods for just 5 days, the levels of organophosphorous pesticide metabolites in their urine fell to undetectable levels. As the authors state, eating organic certainly changed the children's exposure to, if not their risk for, cancers that may be linked to pesticide exposure (Lu et al., 2006).

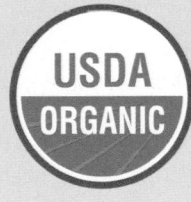

water contaminants such as mycobacteria, *Legionella*, *Giardia*, viruses, arsenic, lead, copper, methyl butyl ether, uranium and radon, are the targets of federal systems put in place to monitor the safety of the food and water supply. Current surveillance systems are designed to detect foodborne illness outbreaks resulting from food spoilage, poor food handling practices, or other unintentional sources, but they were not designed to identify an intentional attack.

Consequences of a compromised food and water supply would be physical, psychological, political, and economic. Compromise could occur with food being the primary agent such as a vector to deliver a biologic or chemical weapon or with food being a secondary target, leaving an inadequate food supply to feed a region or the nation. Intentional use of a foodborne pathogen as the primary agent might be mistaken as a routine outbreak of foodborne illness. Distinguishing normal illness fluctuation from an intentional attack depends on having in place a system for preparedness planning, rapid communication, and central analysis.

With the food supply as a secondary target, there may be limited access to food and water, social disruption, and self-imposed quarantine. These situations require a response different from the traditional approach to disaster relief, during which it is assumed that hungry people will seek assistance and have confidence in the safety of the food that is offered (Bruemmer, 2003). Experience with the series of hurricanes in 2005 emphasizes the need to provide access to a safe food and water supply in emergencies and disasters. In the event of a disaster, dietetics professionals can play a key role by being aware of their environment, knowing available community and state food and nutrition resources, and participating in coordination and delivery of relief to victims of the disaster.

Because of their training, registered dietitians can also take a global approach to identifying measures for ensuring a safe food supply and be effective members of preparedness planning groups when planning for the possibility of an attack or an outbreak. They can assist in the identification of population subgroups with unique nutritional risks and in communication and dissemination of information to identified groups. Their knowledge of correct food-handling practices to avoid foodborne illness would be critical during the time of an attack (Bruemmer, 2003).

Dietetics and health professionals working in food service will be expected to assist in planning for distribution of food in an emergency situation, choosing food distribution sites, establishing temporary kitchens, preparing foods with limited resources, and keeping prepared food safe to eat through HAACP procedures (Puckett and Norton, 2003). FoodNet to track foodborne illness incidence and trends and PulseNet for early detection of foodborne illness outbreaks are useful resources in this situation (Peregrin, 2002) (see Table 11-5 for these resources and others).

DISASTER PLANNING

Several agencies within the federal government share the responsibility of ensuring food and water safety. Planning, surveillance, detection, response, and recovery are the key components of public health preparedness. The key agencies are the USDA, the Department of Homeland Security **(DHS)** and the Federal Emergency Management Agency (FEMA), the CDC and the Food and Drug Administration (FDA).

In conjunction with DHS, USDA operates Protection of the Food Supply and Agricultural Production (PFSAP), and Ready.gov. PFSAP takes on issues dealing with food production, processing, storage, and distribution. It addresses threats against the agricultural sector and border surveil-

TABLE 11-5

Food and Water Safety Resources

American Egg Board	http://www.aeb.org
American Dietetic Association	http://www.eatright.org/ada/files/avian_flu.pdf
American Meat Institute	http://www.meatami.com
Center For Food Safety And Applied Nutrition (CFSAN) Food and Drug Administration	http://www.cfsan.fda.gov
CFSCAN—Food and Water Safety—Disasters	http://www.cfsan.fda.gov/~dms/fsdisas.html
Centers for Disease Control and Prevention	http://www.cdc.gov
CDC Disaster	http://www.bt.cdc.gov/disasters/
Federal Emergency Management Agency (FEMA)	http://www.fema.gov
Food Chemical News	http://www.foodchemicalnews.com
Food Marketing Institute	http://www.fmi.org
Food Marketing Institute—Bird Flu	http://www.fmi.org/foodsafety/avian_flubrochure.htm
FoodNet	http://www.cdc.gov/foodnet/
Food Preservation and Safety, Iowa State University	http://www.foodpres.com
Foundation for Food Irradiation Education	http://www.food-irradiation.com
Government Food Safety Information Gateway	http://www.foodsafety.gov
Grocery Manufacturers of America	http://www.gmabrands.org
International Food Information Council	http://ific.org/food
National Broiler Council	http://www.eatchicken.com
National Cattleman's Beef Association	http://www.ncanet.org
National Institutes of Health	http://www.nih.gov
National Food Safety Database	http://www.agen.ufl.edu/foodsaf/foodsaf.html
National Restaurant Association Educational Foundation	http://www.edfound.org
The Partnership for Food Safety Education	http://www.fightbac.org.main.cfm
Produce Marketing Association	http://www.pma.com
PulseNet	http://www.cdc.gov/pulsenet/whatis.html
U.S. Department of Agriculture	http://www.usda.gov
U.S. Department of Agriculture Food Safety and Inspection Service	http://www.fsis.usda.gov
U.S. Department of Education	http://www.ed.gov
U.S. Department of Health and Human Services	http://os.dhhs.gov
U.S. Environmental Protection Agency (EPA) Office of Ground and Drinking Water	http://www.epa.gov/safewater
U.S. Environmental Protection Agency (EPA) Seafood Safety	http://www.epa.gov/ost/fish
U.S. Food and Drug Administration	http://www.fda.gov
U.S. Poultry and Egg Association	http://www.poultryegg.org

NOTE: Specific websites often change because of updating. Go to the home website and use a search to find the document.

lance. PFSAP conducts food safety activities concerning meat, poultry, and egg inspection and provides laboratory support, research, and education on outbreaks of foodborne illness. Ready.gov (www.ready.gov) is an education tool informing the public on how to prepare for a national emergency, including possible terrorist attacks. In addition, the USDA Food Safety and Inspection Service (FSIS) operates the PrepNet (Food Threat Preparedness Network) and the Food Biosecurity Action Team (F-Bat). PrepNet ensures effective coordination of food security efforts, focusing on preventive activities to protect the food supply. F-Bat assesses potential vulnerabilities along the farm-to-table continuum, provides guidelines to industry on food security and increased plant security, strengthens FSIS's coordination and cooperation with law enforcement agencies, and enhances security features of FSIS laboratories (Bruemmer, 2003).

CDC has three operations relating to food security and disaster planning: PulseNet, FoodNet, and the Centers for Public Health Preparedness. PulseNet is a national network of public health laboratories that performs DNA fingerprinting on foodborne bacteria, assists in detecting foodborne illness outbreaks and tracing them back to their source, and provides linkages among sporadic cases. FoodNet is the Foodborne Diseases Active Surveillance Network, which functions as the principle foodborne disease component of the CDC's Emerging Infections Program, providing active laboratory-based surveillance. The Centers for Public Health Preparedness funds academic centers linking schools of public health with state, local, and regional bioterrorism preparedness and public health infrastructure needs (Bruemmer, 2003).

CFSAN in the Food and Drug Administration is concerned with regulatory issues such as seafood HAACP, safety of food and color additives, safety of foods developed through biotechnology, food labeling, dietary supplements, food industry compliance, and regulatory programs to address health risks associated with foodborne chemical and biologic contaminants. CFSAN also runs cooperative programs with state and local governments.

FEMA, under the DHS, provides emergency support functions after a disaster or emergency. FEMA identifies food and water needs, arranges delivery, and provides assistance with temporary housing and other emergency services. Agencies that assist FEMA include USDA, Department of Defense, USDHHS, EPA, and General Services Administration. Major players include voluntary agencies such as the American Red Cross, the Salvation Army, and community-based agencies and organizations.

Disaster management is evolving as it is tested by both man-made and natural disasters. The efforts following the hurricanes in the late summer and early fall of 2005 are examples of both of the systems that are in place and the gaps. This is an area that has great need of the organizational and professional skills and the knowledge of food and nutrition professionals (ADA, 2005).

◉ FOCAL POINTS

- The three activities of public health, community assessment, policy development and public health assurance apply to the nutritional health of a community.
- Promoting a positive health profile in the community crosses the life cycle and includes all aspects of food and nutrition.
- The broad issues in today's community continue to be the same as in the past, but the scope of practice has expanded with the needs of a rapidly changing community that communicates in new and faster ways.
- The complexity of today's environment and the interfacing of health promotion, disease prevention, and community safety all impact the nutritional health of a community.
- Nutrition services provided by qualified and enthusiastic nutrition professionals with the goal of optimization of the nutritional health of the community can have a powerful effect on the total well-being of that community.
- Registered dietitians and other health professionals are essential translators of food, nutrition, and health information into food choices and patterns; they can work together to develop eating patterns and habits that promote health.

⬡ CLINICAL SCENARIO 1

You are employed as a health professional in a community center. MB has been referred to you to discuss the results of her pregnancy test, which reveals that she is 6 weeks' pregnant. She wants to be enrolled into prenatal care because she has many concerns regarding the health of her baby and herself. During the intake interview you learn more about MB's family. MB is 17 years old. She lives with her mother (a single parent) and her sister, age 4. MB was born in the United States; but her mother speaks limited English, works in a minimum-wage job, and has recently been diagnosed with type 2 diabetes. You refer MB to case management services to discuss enrollment of the family into primary care services at your facility and for possible referral into other community-based services.

Continued

✳ CLINICAL SCENARIO 1—cont'd

✳Nutrition Diagnosis: Nutrition-related knowledge deficit related to no previous nutrition education regarding type 2 diabetes as evidenced by elevated postprandial blood glucose levels

1. What community health and nutrition programs would benefit MB?
2. What referrals might be possible for her 4-year-old sister and her mother?

3. What health and nutrition programs are available in your community to promote optimal health and education of infants and children? What are the eligibility guidelines?
4. In addition to nutrition programs, what other health and safety programs and resources are available in your community for this family? (Consider issues related to food and water safety, budgeting assistance, and food assistance.)

✳ CLINICAL SCENARIO 2

LJ is a single mom who is in her second trimester of pregnancy. LJ has a 2-year-old with food allergies and a 4-year-old. The family has Medicaid benefits.

✳Nutrition Diagnosis: Knowledge deficit related to WIC eligibility as evidenced by lack of awareness of potential program for assistance during pregnancy.

1. Contact *either* the WIC or Food Stamp Program in your area. Introduce yourself as a nutrition student. Tell them that as part of your studies you need to find our more about the application process and would like to complete an application for your case study family. This may entail you visiting the program talking with the staff and/or communicating with staff by phone or email.

2. Complete the following information and be prepared to discuss with your fellow classmates:
   - What WIC benefits are available to this family?
   - What type of nutrition education is available to LJ for herself?
   - What nutrition benefits are available for her children?
3. Be prepared to discuss what other programs and resources are available in your community which would support LJ and her children to improve their nutritional status (e.g. food pantry, food stamps, primary care educational program for children)

✳ CLINICAL SCENARIO 3

Dietitians and nutritionists play an important role in emergency preparedness. The role of qualified nutrition professionals will vary with the type of emergency of disaster (e.g., hurricane, flood, foodborne illness outbreak, ice storm). As an emerging nutrition professional you can play a role within your own family and community by helping them to prepare safe and adequate food for an emergency.

Your family is composed of seven members: two parents, one infant on infant formula, one school-age child, one teenager, and two grandparents. The grandparents are on moderate food restrictions that reduce sugar and sodium. Review information on emergency preparedness information from the American Red Cross (www.redcross.org) and the Department of Home Land Security (www.dhs.gov.org) and propose an emergency food package for your family that includes food and water and supplies, including menus for 7 days.

✳Nutrition Diagnosis: Lack of access to safe foods and water related to no planning as evidenced by insufficient preparation and food and water supplies for emergencies.

1. What steps can you take to design a plan?
2. How many days of food and water should be available?
3. How concerned are you about expiration dates?

Additional Resources: Along with the references cited in this chapter, see American Dietetic Association Media Release September 12, 2005: *Disasters and Emergencies: Are You Prepared?* ADA Position Paper Food and Water Safety (http://www.eatright.org).

USEFUL WEBSITES

American Heart Association
http://www.americanheart.org/

CDC website
http://www.cdc.gov/

Dietary Guidelines for Americans
http://www.health.gov/dietaryguidelines/dga2005/report/

Dietary Reference Intakes
http://www.iom.edu/

Environmental Protection Agency's fish website
www.epa.gov/ost/fish

FEMA
http://www.dhs.gov/dhspublic

Food Safety
http://www.foodsafety.gov/~fsg/fsgdisas.htm
http://www.bt.cdc.gov/disasters/foodwater.asp

FDA Center for Food Safety and Applied Nutrition (CFSAN)
http://cfsan.fda.gov/~dms/fsterrqa.html

Head Start
http://www.acf.dhhs.gov/programs/hsb/

Healthy People 2010
http://web.health.gov/healthypeople

MyPyramid
http://mypyramid.gov

National Center for Health Statistics
http://www.cdc.gov/nchs

National Academy Press website
http://www.nap.edu/catalog (IOM, 2006)

USDA Nutrient Database
http://www.ars.usda.gov/nutrientdata

What We Eat in America
http://www.barc.usda.gov/bhnrc/foodsurvey/home.htm

References

American Dietetic Association Media Release: Disasters and emergencies: are you prepared? American Dietetic Association offers advice on stocking supplies for safety, September 12, 2005, http://www.eatright.org.

American Dietetic Association (ADA): Position of the American Dietetic Association: the role of registered dietitians and dietetic technicians, registered in health promotion and disease prevention programs, *J Am Diet Assoc* 106:1875, 2006.

American Dietetic Association (ADA): Position of the American Dietetic Association: addressing world hunger, malnutrition, and food insecurity, *J Am Diet Assoc* 103:1046, 2003a.

American Dietetic Association (ADA): Position of the American Dietetic Association: Food and water safety, *J Am Diet Assoc* 103:1203, 2003b (Reaffirmed in 2005, and in effect until 2007).

American Dietetic Association (ADA): Position of the American Dietetic Association: food insecurity and hunger in the United States, *J Am Diet Assoc* 106:446, 2006.

Asami DK et al: Comparison of the total phenolic and ascorbic acid content of freeze-dried and air-dried marionberry, strawberry, and corn grown using conventional, organic, and sustainable agricultural practices, *J Agric Food Chem* 51:1237, 2003.

Bayerl C, Ries J: EARLY START: *Nutrition services in early intervention*, Boston, 1995, Department of Public Health.

Bruemmer B: Food biosecurity, *J Am Diet Assoc* 103:687, 2003.

Center for Food Safety and Applied Nutrition (CFSAN), USDHHS, Food and Drug Administration, http://cfsan.fda.gov/~dms/admehg3.html, accessed January 15, 2007.

Davis CA et al: Past, present, and future of the food guide pyramid, *J Am Diet Assoc* 101:881, 2001.

Dietary Guidelines for Americans 2005: www.health.gov/DietaryGuidelines/dga2005/document, accessed January 15, 2007.

Egan M: Public health nutrition: a historical perspective, *J Am Diet Assoc* 94:298, 1994.

Federation of American Societies for Experimental Biology (FASEB), Interagency Board for Nutrition Monitoring and Related Research: *Third report on nutrition monitoring in the United States: executive summary*, Washington, DC, 1995, U.S. Government Printing Office.

Food and Nutrition Board, National Research Council, NAS: *Recommended dietary allowances*, ed 10, Washington, DC, 1989, National Academies Press.

(FNS) Food and Nutrition Service on-line: *Nutrition assistance programs*, Washington, DC, 2004, USDA, http://www.fns.usda.gov/fns, accessed December 1, 2005.

Healthy People: *The Surgeon General's Report on health promotion and disease prevention*, Washington, DC, 1979, U.S. Department of Health and Human Services.

Healthy People 2000: National health promotion and disease prevention objectives, Washington, DC, 1990, U.S. Department of Health and Human Services.

Healthy People 2010: National health promotion and disease prevention objectives, Washington, DC, 2000, U.S. Department of Health and Human Services.

Healthy People 2010: National health promotion and disease prevention progress reviews on focus areas, Washington, DC, 2004a, U.S. Department of Health and Human Services, http://www.cdc.gov/nchs/hphome.htm. Also see CDC update for data at http://wonder.cdc.gov/data2010/, accessed July 1, 2006.

Healthy People 2010: National health promotion and disease prevention progress review— focus area 10 food safety, Washington, DC, 2004b: U.S. Department of Health and Human Services.

Institute of Medicine (IOM), Committee for the Study of Public Health: *The future of public health: a vision of public health in America: an attainable level*, Washington, DC, 1988, National Academies Press.

Institute of Medicine (IOM), National Academy of Sciences (NAS): *Dietary reference intakes: applications in dietary assessment*, Washington, DC, 2000, National Academies Press.

Institute of Medicine (IOM), National Academy of Sciences (NAS): *Dietary reference intakes: the essential guide to nutrient requirements*, Washington DC, 2006: National Academies Press, http://www.nap.edu, accessed July 1, 2006.

Kuczmarski M et al: Update on nutrition monitoring activities in the United States, *J Am Diet Assoc* 94:753, 1994.

Lu C et al: Organic diets significantly lower children's dietary exposure to organophosphorus pesticides, *Environ Health Perspect* 114:260, 2006.

Magkos F et al: Organic food: nutritious food or food for thought? A review of the evidence, *Int J Food Sci Nutr* 54:357, 2003.

Mayerhauser CM: Survival of enterohemorrhagic *Escherichia coli* O157:H7 in retail mustard, *J Food Protect* 64:783, 2001.

Mozaffarian D and Rimm EB: Fish intake, contaminants, and human health: evaluating the risks and the benefits, *JAMA* 296:1885, 2006.

McNally L: American Dietetic Association Hot Topics: Avian bird flu and our food, May, 2006, http://www.eatright.org, accessed July 1, 2006.

National Cancer Institute, U.S. National Institutes of Health: Energy Balance: The complex interaction of diet, physical activity and genetics in cancer prevention and control, January 20, 2004, http://www.cancer.gov; and optimizing energy balance to reduce the cancer burden, http://plan2005.cancer.gov/energy.html, accessed December 1, 2005.

National Center for Health Statistics (NCHS): National Health and Nutrition Examination Survey (NHANES) background history, 2005a, http://www.cdc.gov/nchs/about/major/nhanes/bhistory.htm, accessed December 1, 2005.

National Center for Health Statistics (NCHS): National Health and Nutrition Examination Survey (NHANES) research proposal guidelines, 2005b, http://www.cdc.gov/nchs/nhanes.htm, accessed December 1, 2005..

National Research Council (NRC), Committee on Diet, Nutrition and Cancer: *Diet, nutrition and cancer*, Washington, DC, 1982, National Academies Press.

Nutrition Monitoring Division, Human Nutrition Information Service: USDA nationwide food consumption survey: Continuing survey of food intakes by individuals—1986, *Nutr Today* 24(5):35, 1989.

Nutrition Screening Initiative (NSI): *The role of nutrition in chronic disease care*, Washington DC, 1997, Greer, Margolis, Mitchell, Burns and Associates.

Peregrin T: Bioterrorism and food safety: what nutrition professionals need to know to educate the American public, *J Am Diet Assoc* 102:14, 2002.

Puckett R, Norton C: *Disaster and emergency preparedness in food service operations*, Chicago 2003, American Dietetic Association, available at http://www.eatright.org.

Senate Select Committee on Nutrition and Human Needs: *Dietary goals for the United States*, Publ No.052-070-03913-2, Washington, DC, 1977, U.S. Government Printing Office.

Sims L: *Research aspects of public policy in nutrition generating research questions to determine the impact of nutritional, agricultural and health care policy and regulation on the health and nutrition status of the public: the research agenda for dietetics conference proceedings*, Chicago, 1993, The American Dietetic Association.

U.S. Department of Agriculture (USDA): *Continuing survey of food intakes by individuals (CSFI) 1994–96*, Beltsville, Md, 1998, USDA.

U.S. Department of Agriculture (USDA): Organic food standards and labels, the facts, Washington DC, 2002, http://www.ams.usda.gov/nop/Consumers/brochure.html, accessed December 1, 2005.

U.S. Department of Health and Human Services (USDHHA) Institutes of Health: 5 a day, 2005a, http://www.5aday.gov, accessed December 1, 2005.

U.S. Department of Health and Human Services, U.S. Department of Agriculture: *Dietary guidelines for Americans, 2005*, ed 6, Washington, DC, 2005b, U.S. Government Printing Office.

U.S. Department of Agriculture (USDA), Agricultural Research Service (ARS): *Nutrient data laboratory*, Beltsville, Md, 2006 and ongoing, USDA, http://www.ars.usda.gov/nutrientdata, accessed July 1, 2006.

U.S. Food and Drug Administration (FDA) and U.S. Environmental Protection Agency (EPA): What you need to know about mercury in fish and shellfish, 2006, available in several languages at http://www.epa.gov/ost/fish, accessed July 1, 2006.

Winslow CEA: The untilled field of public health, *Mod Med* 2:183, 1920.

Wotecki CE et al: National Health and Nutrition Examination Survey—NHANES: plans for NHANES III, *Nutr Today* 23(1):25, 1988.

Wotecki CE et al: Keep food safe to eat: healthful food must be safe as well as nutritious, *J Nutr* 131:502S-509S, 2001.

Wotecki CE: Integrated NHANES: uses in national policy, *J Nutr* 133:582S, 2003.

CHAPTER 12

Sylvia Escott-Stump, MA, RD, LDN
Robert Earl, DrPH, RD

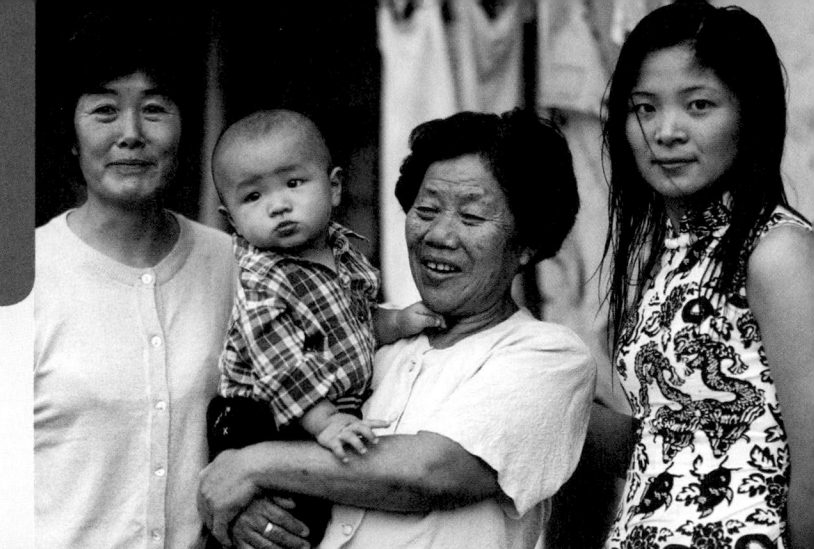

Guidelines for Dietary Planning

KEY TERMS

adequate intake (AI) the recommended daily intake level based on observed or experimentally determined approximations of nutrient intake by a group (or groups) of healthy people; used when a recommended dietary allowance cannot be determined

daily reference values (DRVs) a set of food labeling reference values for which no nutrient recommendation previously existed; established for fat, saturated fatty acids, cholesterol, total carbohydrate, protein, dietary fiber, sodium, and potassium

daily value (DV) reference term on food labels to aid consumers in selecting a healthy diet; consists of two sets of references—the reference daily intakes (RDIs) and daily reference values (DRVs)—expressed as percentages

Dietary Guidelines for Americans (DGA) dietary recommendations that promote health and reduce risk of chronic disease for people ages 2 years and older

dietary reference intake (DRI) an overall term designed to encompass the four specific types of nutrient recommendations (adequate intake [AI], estimated average requirement [EAR], recommended dietary allowance [RDA], and tolerable upper intake level [UL]); used for nutrient recommendations for the United States and Canada

estimated average requirement (EAR) nutrient intake value that is estimated to meet the requirements of half the healthy individuals in a group

estimated safe and adequate daily dietary intake (ESADDI) recommended intake ranges of nutrients for which not enough information is available to establish a recommended dietary allowance

health claim any claim on a food package label or other label (such as an advertisement) of a food, including fish and game meat, that characterizes the relationship of any nutrient or other substance in the food to a disease or health-related condition

Healthy Eating Index (HEI) summary measure of overall diet quality; designed to assess and monitor the dietary status of Americans

MyPyramid Food Guidance System translates the Dietary Guidelines for Americans and nutrient recommendations into a visual form of the types and amounts of food to eat each day; new system incorporates physical activity into daily patterns

nutrition facts label nutrient content information on food products designed to help consumers (4 years of age and older) select foods to incorporate into a healthy diet using the MyPyramid Food Guidance System and Dietary Guidelines for Americans

recommended dietary allowance (RDA) the amount of a nutrient needed to meet the requirements of almost all (97% to 98%) of the healthy population

reference daily intakes (RDIs) set of dietary references for vitamins and minerals on food labels based on the 1968 recommended dietary allowances; replaces the U.S. recommended daily allowances that were previously used with nutrition labeling on food products

tolerable upper intake level (UL) the highest daily intake amount of a nutrient that is likely to pose no risk of adverse health effects for almost all individuals in the general population

Sections of this chapter were written by Susan T. Borra, RD, and Paul R. Thomas, EdD, RD, for previous editions of this text.

An appropriate diet is adequate and balanced and considers the individual's characteristics such as age and stage of development, taste preferences, and food habits. It also reflects the availability of foods, socioeconomic conditions, storage and preparation facilities, and cooking skills. An adequate and balanced diet meets all the nutritional needs of an individual for maintenance, repair, living processes, growth, and development. It includes energy and all nutrients in proper amounts and in proportion to each other. The presence or absence of one essential nutrient may affect the availability, absorption, metabolism, or dietary need for others. The recognition of nutrient interrelationships provides further support for the principle of maintaining variety in foods to provide the most complete diet.

With increasing knowledge of diet and disease links that lead to premature disability and mortality among Americans, an appropriate diet is now considered one that helps reduce the risk of developing chronic degenerative diseases and conditions. In this era of vastly expanding scientific knowledge and information about food components, the way the public thinks about food intake for health promotion and disease prevention is changing rapidly. In addition to traditional nutrient requirements, the public often hears references to functional foods, which are foods or food components that provide more benefits than basic nutritional benefits. Dietitians and other health professionals are essential translators of food, nutrition, and health information into dietary choices and patterns for groups and individuals. See Conceptual Framework on the inside back cover.

According to the Food and Nutrition Board, choosing various foods to meet dietary recommendations should provide adequate amounts of the nutrients that do not have well-defined recommended levels. A varied diet also ensures that a person is consuming sufficient amounts of food constituents that, although not defined as nutrients, have biologic effects and may influence health and susceptibility to disease. Examples include dietary fiber and carotenoids, as well as lesser known phytochemicals (substances found in plant products) such as isothiocyanates in broccoli or other cruciferous vegetables and lycopene in tomato products (see Tables 9-1 and 9-2). Diets rich in phytochemicals may help reduce the risk of developing certain types of cancer, but their exact mechanisms are not totally understood.

DETERMINING NUTRIENT NEEDS

Worldwide Guidelines

Numerous standards serve as guides for planning and evaluating diets and food supplies for individuals and population groups. Many countries have issued guidelines appropriate for the circumstances and needs of their populations. The Food and Agriculture Organization (FAO) and the World Health Organization (WHO) of the United Nations have established international standards in many areas of food quality and safety, as well as dietary and nutrient recommendations. In the United States the Food and Nutrition Board (FNB) of the Institute of Medicine (IOM) has led the development of nutrient recommendations since the 1940s. Since the mid-1990s, nutrient recommendations developed by the FNB have been used by the United States and Canada. The U.S. Department of Agriculture (USDA) and Department Health and Human Services (DHHS) have a shared responsibility for issuing dietary recommendations, collecting and analyzing food composition data, and formulating regulations for nutrition information on food products. In Canada, Health Canada is the agency responsible for Canadian dietary recommendations and food labeling regulations.

Dietary Reference Intakes

American standards for nutrient requirements have been the recommended dietary allowances (RDAs) established by the FNB of the IOM. They were first published in 1941 and most recently revised between 1997 and 2002. Each revision incorporates the most recent research findings. In 1993 the FNB developed a framework for the development of nutrient recommendations, called **dietary reference intakes (DRI)**. DRIs encompass four types of nutrient recommendations for healthy individuals: adequate intake (AI), estimated average intake (EAR), RDA, and tolerable upper intake level (UL).

DRI reports for nutrients are now complete. Nutrition and health professionals should also use the most updated food composition databases and tables and inquire whether data used in computerized nutrient analysis programs have been revised to include the most up-to-date information.

Components

The DRI model expands the previous RDA, which focused only on levels of nutrients for healthy populations to prevent deficiency diseases. To respond to scientific advances in diet and health throughout the life cycle, the DRI model now includes four reference points.

The **adequate intake (AI)** is a nutrient recommendation based on observed or experimentally determined approximation of nutrient intake by a group (or groups) of healthy people when sufficient scientific evidence is not available to calculate an RDA or an EAR. The **estimated average requirement (EAR)** is the average requirement of a nutrient for healthy individuals; a functional or clinical assessment has been conducted, and measures of adequacy have been made at a specified level of dietary intake. An EAR is the amount of a nutrient with which approximately one half of individuals would have their needs met and one half would not. The EAR should be used for assessing the nutrient adequacy of populations, not individuals.

The **recommended dietary allowance (RDA)** presents the amount of a nutrient needed to meet the requirements of almost all (97% to 98%) of the healthy population of individuals for whom it was developed. An RDA for a nutrient should serve as a goal for intake for individuals, not as a benchmark of adequacy of diets of populations. Finally the **tolerable upper intake level (UL)** has been established for many nutrients to reduce the risk of adverse or toxic effects from increased consumption of nutrients in concentrated forms—either alone or combined with others (not in food)—or from enrichment and fortification. A UL is the highest level of daily nutrient intake

TABLE 12-1

Acceptable Macronutrient Distribution Ranges

Nutrient	AMDR (Percentage of Energy as kcal/day)			AMDR Sample Diet Adult, 2000-kcal/day Diet	
	1-3 Years	4-18 Years	>19 Years	% Reference*	g/Day
Protein†	5-20	10-30	10-30	10	50
Carbohydrate	45-65	45-65	45-65	60	300
Fat	30-40	25-35	25-35	30	67
α-Linolenic acid (*n-3)‡	0.6-1.2	0.6-1.2	0.6-1.2	0.8	1.8
Linoleic acid (n-6)	5-10	5-10	5-10	7	16
Added sugars§	≤25% of total calories			500	125

Modified from Food and Nutrition Board, Institute of Medicine: Dietary reference intakes for energy, carbohydrate, fiber, fat, fatty acids, cholesterol, protein, and amino acids, Washington, DC, 2002, National Academies Press.

*Suggested maximum.

†Higher number in protein AMDR is set to complement AMDRs for carbohydrate and fat, not because it is a recommended upper limit in the range of calories from protein.

‡Up to 10% of the AMDR for a-linoenic acid can be consumed as EPA, DHA, or both (0.06%-0.12% of calories).

§Reference percentages chosen based on average dietary reference intake (DRI) for protein for adult men and women, then calculated back to percentage of calories. Carbohydrate and fat percentages chosen based on difference from protein and balanced with other federal dietary recommendations.

that is unlikely to have any adverse health effects on almost all individuals in the general population. The DRIs for the macronutrients, vitamins and minerals, including the Uls are presented on the inside front cover and opening page of this text. The acceptable macronutrient distribution ranges based on energy intake are shown in Table 12-1.

Target Population

Each of the nutrient recommendation categories in the DRI system is used for specific purposes among individuals or populations. The EAR is used for evaluating the nutrient intake of populations. The new RDA can be used for individuals. Nutrient intakes between the RDA and the UL may further define intakes that may promote health or prevent disease in the individual.

Age- and Sex-Groups

Because nutrient needs are highly individualized depending on age, sexual development, and the reproductive status of females, the DRI framework has 10 age-groupings, including age-group categories for children, men and women 51 to 70 years of age, and those over 70 years of age. It separates three age-group categories each for pregnancy and lactation—less than 18 years, 19 to 30 years, and 31 to 50 years of age.

Reference Men and Women

The requirement for many nutrients is based on body weight. The RDAs are listed according to reference men and women of designated height and weight. These values for age-sex groups of individuals older than 19 years of age are based on actual medians obtained for the American population by the third National Health and Nutrition Examination Survey (NHANES) III, 1988 to 1994. Although this does not necessarily imply that these weight-for-height

values are ideal, at least they make it possible to define recommended allowances appropriate for the largest number of people. The reference heights and weights for children and adults in the U.S. are shown in Table 12-2.

Estimated Safe and Adequate Daily Dietary Intakes

Numerous nutrients are known to be essential for life and health, but data for some are insufficient to establish a recommended intake. Intakes for these nutrients are **estimated safe and adequate daily dietary intakes (ESADDI)**. Most intakes are shown as ranges to indicate that not only are specific recommendations not known, but also at least the upper and lower limits of safety should be observed.

NUTRITIONAL STATUS OF AMERICANS

Food and Nutrient Intake Data

Twenty-two federal agencies collect information about the dietary and nutritional status of Americans and the relationship between diet and health. This effort is coordinated by the USDA and DHHS through the National Nutrition Monitoring and Related Research Program (NNMRRP) (FASEB, 1995). The NHANES and the Continuing Survey of Food Intakes by Individuals (CSFII) are the cornerstone surveys of the NNMRRP (see Chapter 11).

Overall the nutritional quality of the American diet shows that the population is slowly changing eating patterns and adopting more healthy diets, although gaps exist between consumption and government recommendations among population subgroups. Intake of total fat, saturated fatty acids, and cholesterol has decreased among some

TABLE 12-2

Reference Heights and Weights for Children and Adults in the United States

Sex	Age	Previous Median Body Mass Index* (BMI) (kg/m²)	New Median BMI† (kg/m²)	New Median Reference Height† cm (in)	New Reference Weight‡ kg (lb)
Male, female	2-6 mo	—	—	62 (24)	6 (13)
	7-12 mo	—	—	71 (28)	9 (20)
	1-3 yr	—	—	86 (34)	12 (27)
	4-8 yr	15.8	15.3	115 (15)	20 (11)
Male	9-13 yr	18.5	17.2	144 (57)	36 (79)
	14-18 yr	21.3	20.5	174 (68)	61 (134)
	19-30 yr	24.4	22.5	177 (70)	70 (154)
Female	9-13 yr	18.3	17.4	144 (57)	37 (81)
	14-18 yr	21.3	20.4	163 (64)	54 (119)
	19-30 yr	22.8	21.5	163 (61)	57 (126)

From Dietary Reference Intakes: *Applications in dietary planning*, Washington DC, 2003, The National Academies Press, http://www.iom.edu/CMS/3788/4003/4733.aspx.

*Taken from male and female median BMI and height-for-age data from the Third National Health and Nutrition Examination Survey (NHANES III), 1988-1994; used in earlier DRI reports.

†Taken from new data on male and female median BMI and height-for-age data from the Centers for Disease Control and Prevention/National Center for Health Statistics Growth Charts.

‡Calculated from CDC/NCIIS Growth Charts, median BMI and median height for ages 4 through 19 years.

portions of the population. The average consumption of servings of fruits and vegetables has risen to four per day, approaching the recommendation of five servings per day. However, many Americans experience food insecurity, or hunger from not getting enough to eat (see Chapter 11).

Nutrition-related health measurements indicate that overweight and obesity are increasing from lack of physical activity. The number of people with acceptable serum cholesterol levels is increasing, although some individuals still have high levels, a major risk factor for coronary heart disease. Hypertension remains a major public health problem in middle-age and older adults; among non-Hispanic blacks it increases the risk of stroke and coronary heart disease. Osteoporosis develops more often among non-Hispanic whites than non-Hispanic blacks or Mexican Americans.

Healthy Eating Index

The Center for Nutrition Policy and Promotion of the USDA releases the **Healthy Eating Index (HEI)** to measure how well people's diets conform to recommended healthy eating patterns. The index provides a picture of foods people are eating, the amount of variety in their diets, and compliance with specific recommendations in the Dietary Guidelines for Americans (DGA). The HEI is designed to assess and monitor the dietary status of Americans by using data from the CSFII and evaluating 10 components, each representing different aspects of a healthy diet. The dietary components used in the evaluation include grains, vegetables, fruits, milk, meat, total fat, saturated fat, cholesterol sodium, and variety. Data from the HEI over time show that Ameri-

cans are reducing total fat and saturated fat in their diets and eating a wider variety of foods but still need to eat more fruit, drink more milk or calcium and vitamin D concentrated beverages, and reduce their sodium intake. Women generally have scores higher than men, and children ages 2 to 3 have the highest HEI scores. The overall healthy eating index (HEI) score ranges from 0 to 100. In 1989 the overall HEI score was 61.5, in 1996 it was 63.8, and it remained the same in 2000. Of the U.S. population, 10% had a good diet with a rating of 80 or higher, 74% had diets that needed improvement, and 16% had poor diets with scores less than 51 (Basiotis et al., 2002). The Healthy Eating Index 2005 can be used to assess the diet of an individual also (Table 12-3).

Nutrition Monitoring Report

At the request of the DHHS and USDA, the Expert Panel on Nutrition Monitoring was established by the Life Sciences Research Office of the Federation of American Societies for Experimental Biology (FASEB) to review the dietary and nutritional status of the American population. The report of the committee summarized the results of data from NHANES II, Hispanic HANES, and the Nationwide Food Consumption Survey (NFCS) and CSFII surveys. In general, the committee concluded that the food supply in the United States is abundant, although some people may not receive enough nutrients for various reasons. Nutrient intakes are most likely to be low in persons living below the poverty level. Intakes of nutrients reported to be low in the general population are even lower in the poverty group. Key food components that are identified as current or potential public health issues are listed in Table 12-4.

TABLE 12-3

Healthy Eating Index 2005 Components and Standards for Scoring*

Component	Maximum Points	Standard for Maximum Score	Standard for Minimum Score of Zero
Total fruit (includes 100% juice)	5	≥0.8 cup equiv per 1000 kcal	No fruit
Whole fruit (not juice)	5	≥0.4 cup equiv per 1000 kcal	No whole fruit
Total vegetables	5	≥1.1 cup equiv per 1000 kcal	No vegetables
Dark green and orange vegetables and legumes†	5	≥0.4 cup equiv per 1000 kcal	No dark green or orange vegetables or legumes
Total grains	5	≥3.0 oz equiv per 1000 kcal	No grains
Whole grains	5	≥1.5 oz equiv per 1000 kcal	No whole grains
Milk‡	10	≥1.3 cup equiv per 1000 kcal	No milk
Meat and beans	10	≥2.5 oz equiv per 1000 kcal	No meat or beans
Oils§	10	≥12 g per 1000 kcal	No oil
Saturated fat	10	≤7% of energy‖	≥15% of energy
Sodium	10	≤0.7 g per 1000 kcal‖	≥2 g per 1000 kcal
Calories from solid fat, alcohol and added sugar (SoFAAS)	20	≤20% of energy	≥50% of energy

From U.S. Department of Agriculture, Center for Nutrition Policy and Promotion: *Healthy eating index 2005*, available at www.cnpp.usda.gov, accessed April 16, 2007.

*Intakes between the minimum and maximum levels are scored proportionately, except for saturated fat and sodium (see ‖).

†Legumes counted as vegetables only after meat and beans standard is met.

‡Includes all milk products, such as fluid milk, yogurt, and cheese.

§Includes nonhydrogenated vegetable oils and oils in fish, nuts, and seeds.

‖Saturated fat and sodium get a score of 8 for the intake levels that reflect the 2005 Dietary Guidelines: <10% of calories from saturated fat and 1.1 g of sodium per 1000 kcal, respectively.

TABLE 12-4

Food Components and Public Health Concerns

Food Component	Relevance to Public Health
Energy	Median reported energy intakes in the 1988 to 1991 CSFII were below recommended levels, yet many adolescents and adults are overweight. The high prevalence of overweight indicates that an energy imbalance exists among Americans because of physical inactivity and underreporting of energy intake or food consumption in national surveys.
Total fat, saturated fat, and cholesterol	Intakes of fat, saturated fatty acids, and cholesterol among all age-groups older than 2 years of age were higher than recommended levels (<30% of calories for total fat and 8% to 10% of calories for saturated fatty acids). Cholesterol intakes were generally within the recommended range of 300 mg/dl or less.
Alcohol	Intake of alcohol is a public health concern because it displaces food sources of nutrients and has potential health consequences.
Iron and calcium	Low intakes of iron and calcium continue to be a public health concern, particularly among infants and females of childbearing age. Prevalence of iron deficiency anemia was higher among these groups than among other age- and sex-groups. Low calcium intake is a particular concern among adolescent girls and adult women in most racial and ethnic groups.
Sodium	Sodium intake continues to exceed government recommendations of 2400 mg/day in most age- and sex-groups.
Other nutrients at potential risk	Some population or age-groups may consume insufficient amounts of total carbohydrate and carbohydrate constituents such as dietary fiber; protein; vitamin A; antioxidant vitamins (vitamins C and E) carotenoids; folate, vitamins B_6 and B_{12}; magnesium, potassium, zinc, copper, selenium, phosphorus, and fluoride. Intakes of polyunsaturated and monounsaturated fatty acids, *trans*-fatty acids, and fat substitutes may be unbalanced.

NATIONAL GUIDELINES FOR DIET PLANNING

Within the past 30 years, attention has been focused increasingly on the relationship of nutrition to chronic diseases and conditions. Although this interest derives somewhat from the rapid increase in number of older adults and their longevity, it is also prompted by the desire to prevent premature deaths from diseases such as coronary heart disease, diabetes mellitus, and cancer. Approximately two thirds of deaths in the United States are caused by chronic disease.

Current Dietary Guidance in the United States and Canada

Eating can be one of life's greatest pleasures. People eat for enjoyment and to obtain energy and nutrients. Although many genetic, environmental, behavioral, and cultural factors affect health, diet is equally important for promoting health and preventing disease.

In 1969, then President Nixon convened the White House Conference on Nutrition and Health (White House, 1970). Increased attention was being given to prevention of hunger and disease. The development of dietary guidelines in the United States began with the 1977 report of the U.S. Senate Select Committee on Nutrition and Human Needs called *Dietary Goals for the United States* (U.S. Senate Select Committee on Nutrition and Human Needs, 1977).

In addition to these dietary guidelines, several other important government or expert reports have addressed dietary recommendations for healthy Americans. Previous Surgeon General's Reports on Nutrition and Health and the National Academy of Sciences (NAS) have provided similar qualitative or quantitative dietary recommendations. In Canada, dietary recommendations are prepared by Health Canada (see *Clinical Insight:* Nutrition Recommendations for Canadians).

Guidelines directed toward prevention of a particular disease, such as those from the National Cancer Institute, the American Diabetes Association, The American Heart Association, and the National Heart, Lung, and Blood Institute's cholesterol education guidelines, contain recommendations unique to particular conditions. The American Dietetic Association (ADA) (2002) published a position statement stating that all foods can fit into a healthful diet when the total diet, or overall pattern of food eaten, is consumed in moderation with appropriate portion sizes and combined with regular physical activity. The various guidelines, summarized in Box 12-1 can be used by health counselors throughout most of the developed world.

Implementing the Guidelines

The task of planning nutritious meals centers on including the essential nutrients in sufficient amounts as outlined in the newest DRIs, in addition to appropriate amounts of energy, protein, carbohydrate (including fiber and sugars), fat (especially saturated and *trans*-fats), cholesterol, and salt. Suggestions are included to help people meet the specifics of the recommendations. When specific numeric recommendations differ, they are presented as ranges.

The **MyPyramid Food Guidance System,** shown in Figure 12-1, offers a method for determining appropriate patterns for daily food choices based on servings from the five major food groups. The MyPyramid system replaces the Food

---

✷ CLINICAL INSIGHT

Nutrition Recommendations for Canadians

The revision to Canada's Food Guide to Healthy Eating was released in 2007 and developed age- and gender-specific food intake patterns. These age- and gender-specific suggestions include 4 to 7 servings of vegetables and fruits, 3 to 7 servings of grain products, 2 to 3 servings of milk or milk alternatives, and 1 to 3 servings of meat or meat alternatives. Unlike MyPyramid in the United States, Canada's Eating Well with Canada's Food Guide contains four food groupings presented in a rainbow shape (Health Canada, 2007) (see Figure 12-2). Tips include:

- Consume no more than 400-450 mg of caffeine per day.
- Eat at least one dark green and one orange vegetable each day.
- Make at least half of grain products comsumed each day whole grain.
- Compare the Nutrition Facts table on food labels to choose products that contain less fat, saturated fat, *trans* fat, sugar, and sodium.

- Drink skim, 1% or 2% milk, or fortified soy beverages each day. Check the food label to see if the soy beverage is fortified with calcium and vitamin D.
- Include a small amount (30-45 ml [2-3 Tbsp]) of unsaturated fat each day to get the fat needed.
- Limit the intake of soft drinks, sports drinks, energy drinks, fruit drinks, punches, sweetened hot and cold beverages, and alcohol.
- Eat at least two Food Guide Servings of fish each week.
- Build 30-60 minutes of moderate physical activity into daily life for adults and at least 90 minutes a day for children and youth.

Data from Health Canada: Eating well with Canada's food guide, ©Her Majesty the Queen in Right of Canada, represented by the Minister of Healthy Canada, 2007, available at www.hc-sc.gc.ca/fn-an/food-guide-aliment, accessed February 8, 2007.

BOX 12-1

Universal Prescription for Health and Nutritional Fitness

- Adjust energy intake and exercise level to achieve and maintain appropriate body weight.
- Eat a wide variety of foods to ensure nutrient adequacy.
- Increase total carbohydrate intake; increase complex carbohydrate intake.
- Eat less total fat and less saturated fat.
- Eat more fiber-rich foods.
- Eat more fruits and vegetables.
- Eat fewer high cholesterol foods.
- Eat fewer high-sodium foods.
- Reduce intake of concentrated sugars.

- Drink alcohol in moderation or not at all.
- Meet the recommended dietary allowance (RDA) for calcium, a recommendation especially important for adolescents and women.
- Meet the RDA for iron, a recommendation especially for children, adolescents, and women of childbearing age.
- Limit protein to no more than twice the RDA.
- If using a daily multivitamin, choose dietary supplements that do not exceed the dietary reference intake.
- Drink fluoridated water.

Anatomy of MyPyramid

One size doesn't fit all

USDA's new MyPyramid symbolizes a personalized approach to healthy eating and physical activity. The symbol has been designed to be simple. It has been developed to remind consumers to make healthy food choices and to be active every day. The different parts of the symbol are described below.

Activity
Activity is represented by the steps and the person climbing them, as a reminder of the importance of daily physical activity.

Moderation
Moderation is represented by the narrowing of each food group from bottom to top. The wider base stands for foods with little or no solid fats or added sugars. These should be selected more often. The narrower top area stands for foods containing more added sugars and solid fats. The more active you are, the more of these foods can fit into your diet.

Personalization
Personalization is shown by the person on the steps, the slogan, and the URL. Find the kinds and amounts of food to eat each day at MyPyramid.gov.

Proportionality
Proportionality is shown by the different widths of the food group bands. The widths suggest how much food a person should choose from each group. The widths are just a general guide, not exact proportions. Check the Web site for how much is right for you.

Variety
Variety is symbolized by the 6 color bands representing the 5 food groups of the Pyramid and oils. This illustrates that foods from all groups are needed each day for good health.

Gradual Improvement
Gradual improvement is encouraged by the slogan. It suggests that individuals can benefit from taking small steps to improve their diet and lifestyle each day

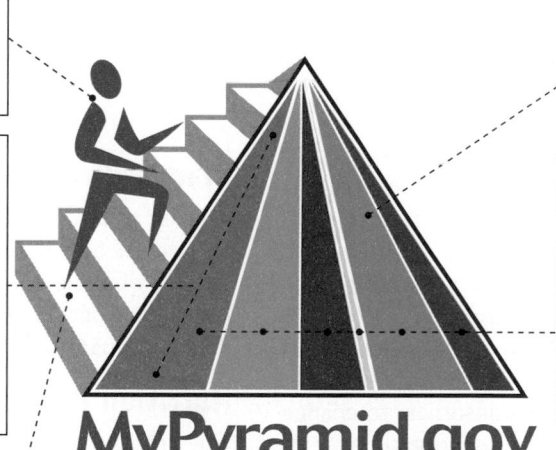

MyPyramid.gov
STEPS TO A HEALTHIER YOU

For a 2,000-calorie diet, you need the amounts below from each food group. To find the amounts that are right for you, go to MyPyramid.gov.

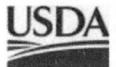

U.S. Department of Agriculture
Center for Nutrition Policy and Promotion
April 2005 CNPP-16

GRAINS	VEGETABLES	FRUITS	OILS	MILK	MEAT & BEANS
Eat 6 oz. every day	Eat 2½ cups every day	Eat 2 cups every day		Get 3 cups every day; for kids aged 2 to 8, it's 2	Eat 5½ oz. every day

FIGURE 12-1 MyPyramid Food Guidance System adds physical activity for public awareness. *(U.S. Department of Agriculture and U.S. Department of Health and Human Services, available at http://www.mypyramid.gov/, accessed August 2, 2006).*

Guide Pyramid, which was highly visible but not clearly understood by the public.

For comparison, Eating Well with Canada's Food Guide is shown in Figure 12-2. To help people select an eating pattern that achieves specific health promotion or disease prevention objectives, nutritionists should assist individuals in making food choices (e.g., to reduce fat, to increase fiber).

Dietary recommendations have evolved during the past 30 years. Although numerous federal agencies are involved in the issuance of dietary guidance, USDA and DHHS lead the effort. Following the Senate's Dietary Goals report, the **Dietary Guidelines for Americans (DGA)** was first published in 1980. The guidelines were revised in 1985 (second edition), 1990 (third edition), 1995 (fourth edition), 2000 (fifth edition) and the most recent guidelines were released in 2005. With the passage of the Nutrition Monitoring Act in 1990, the dietary guidelines are now required to be reviewed every 5 years.

The DGA are designed to motivate consumers to change their eating and activity patterns by providing them with positive, simple messages. Using consumer research, the DGA develop messages that expand the influence of the dietary guidelines to encourage consumers to adopt them and ultimately change their behaviors. The messages reach out to consumers' motivations, individual needs, and life goals and can be used in education, counseling, and communications initiatives. Box 12-2 lists the nine focus areas, Box 9-1 in Chapter 9 gives a summary of them, and the website provides full details and background information (see *Useful Websites*).

FOOD LABELING

To help consumers make choices between similar types of food products that can be incorporated into a healthy diet, the Food and Drug Administration (FDA) established a voluntary system of providing selected nutrient information on food labels. The regulatory framework for nutrition information on food labels was revised and updated by the USDA (which regulates meat and poultry products and eggs) and the FDA (which regulates all other foods) with enactment of the Nutrition Labeling and Education Act (NLEA) in 1990. The labels became mandatory in 1994.

Mandatory Nutrition Labeling

As a result of the NLEA, nutrition labels must appear on most foods except products that provide few nutrients (such as coffee and spices), restaurant foods, and ready-to-eat foods prepared on site, such as supermarket bakery and deli items (FDA, 1993). Providing nutrition information on many raw foods is voluntary. However, the FDA and USDA have called for a voluntary point-of-purchase program in which nutrition information is available in most supermarkets. Nutrition information is provided through brochures or point-of-purchase posters for the 20 most popular fruits, vegetables, and fresh fish and the 45 major cuts of fresh meat and poultry.

Nutrition information for foods purchased in restaurants is widely available at the point of purchase or from Internet sites or toll-free numbers. Ready-to-eat unpackaged foods in delicatessens or supermarkets may provide nutrition information voluntarily. However, if nutrition claims are made, nutrition labeling is required at the point of purchase.

If a food makes the claim of being organic, it also must meet certain criteria and labeling requirements. In 2002 the government regulations were established for organic food labeling (see *Focus On:* Is it Really Organic and Is it Healthier? in Chapter 11).

Standardized Serving Sizes

Serving sizes of products are set by the government based on reference amounts commonly consumed. For example, a serving of milk is 8 oz, and a serving of salad dressing is 2 tbsp. Standardized serving sizes make it easier for consumers to compare the nutrient contents of similar products.

Nutrition Facts Label

The **nutrition facts label** on a food product provides information on its per-serving calories and calories from fat. The label then lists the amount (in grams) of total fat, saturated fat, cholesterol, sodium, total carbohydrate, dietary fiber, sugar, and protein. For most of these nutrients the label also shows the percentage of the **daily value (DV)** supplied by a serving. A product's content of vitamins A and C, calcium, and iron is listed in terms of DV percentage only. DVs show how a product fits into an overall diet by comparing its nutrient content with recommended intakes of those nutrients.

It is important to remember that DVs are not recommended intakes for individuals; no one nutrient standard applies to everyone. They are simply reference points to provide some perspective on daily nutrient needs. DVs are based on a 2000-kcal diet; however, the bottom of the nutrition label also provides the DVs for a 2500-kcal diet. For example, individuals who consume diets supplying more or fewer calories can still use the DVs as a rough guide to ensure that they are getting adequate amounts of vitamin C but not too much saturated fat.

Recommended Number of Food Guide Servings per Day

	Children			Teens		Adults			
Age in Years	2-3	4-8	9-13	14-18		19-50		51+	
Sex	Girls and Boys			Females	Males	Females	Males	Females	Males
Vegetables and Fruit	4	5	6	7	8	7-8	8-10	7	7
Grain Products	3	4	6	6	7	6-7	8	6	7
Milk and Alternatives	2	2	3-4	3-4	3-4	2	2	3	3
Meat and Alternatives	1	1	1-2	2	3	2	3	2	3

The chart above shows how many Food Guide Servings you need from each of the four food groups every day.

Having the amount and type of food recommended and following the tips in *Canada's Food Guide* will help:

- **Meet your needs for vitamins, minerals and other nutrients.**
- **Reduce your risk of obesity, type 2 diabetes, heart disease, certain types of cancer and osteoporosis.**
- **Contribute to your overall health and vitality.**

What is One Food Guide Serving?
Look at the examples below.

Oils and Fats

- Include a small amount – 30 to 45 mL (2 to 3 Tbsp) – of unsaturated fat each day. This includes oil used for cooking, salad dressings, margarine and mayonnaise.
- Use vegetable oils such as canola, olive and soybean.
- Choose soft margarines that are low in saturated and trans fats.
- Limit butter, hard margarine, lard and shortening.

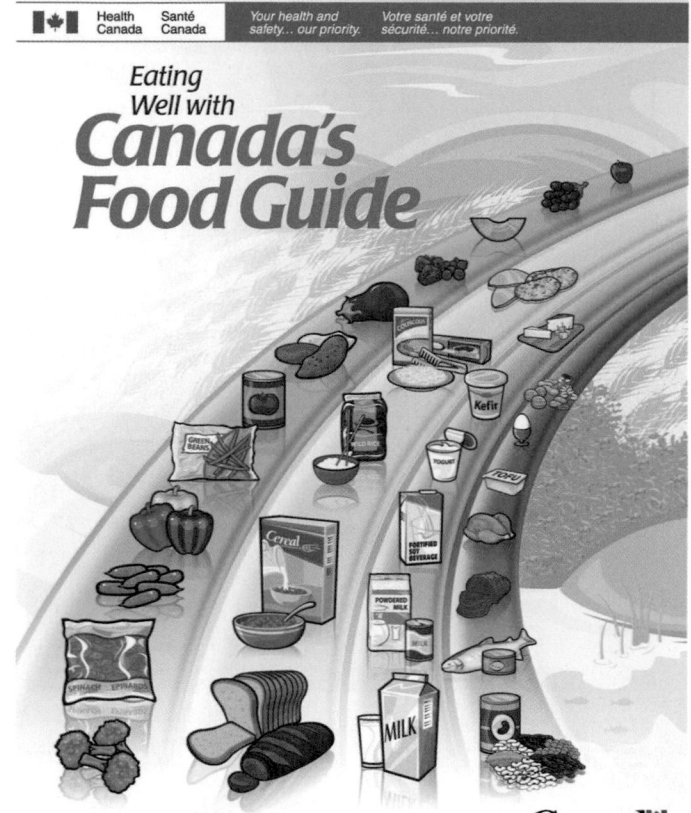

FIGURE 12-2 Eating Well with Canada's Food Guide. *(Reprinted with permission from Health Canada. Data from Health Canada: Eating well with Canada's food guide, ©Her Majesty the Queen in Right of Canada, represented by the Minister of Healthy Canada, 2007, available at www.hc-sc.gc.ca/fn-an/food-guide-aliment, accessed February 8, 2007.* *Continued*

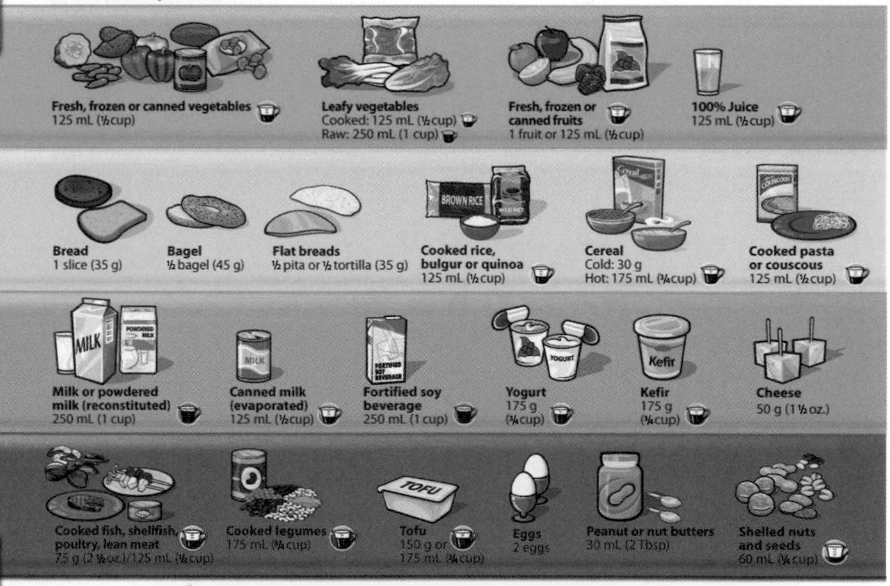

Make each Food Guide Serving count...
wherever you are – at home, at school, at work or when eating out!

▸ **Eat at least one dark green and one orange vegetable each day.**
  - Go for dark green vegetables such as broccoli, romaine lettuce and spinach.
  - Go for orange vegetables such as carrots, sweet potatoes and winter squash.

▸ **Choose vegetables and fruit prepared with little or no added fat, sugar or salt.**
  - Enjoy vegetables steamed, baked or stir-fried instead of deep-fried.

▸ **Have vegetables and fruit more often than juice.**

▸ **Make at least half of your grain products whole grain each day.**
  - Eat a variety of whole grains such as barley, brown rice, oats, quinoa and wild rice.
  - Enjoy whole grain breads, oatmeal or whole wheat pasta.

▸ **Choose grain products that are lower in fat, sugar or salt.**
  - Compare the Nutrition Facts table on labels to make wise choices.
  - Enjoy the true taste of grain products. When adding sauces or spreads, use small amounts.

▸ **Drink skim, 1%, or 2% milk each day.**
  - Have 500 mL (2 cups) of milk every day for adequate vitamin D.
  - Drink fortified soy beverages if you do not drink milk.

▸ **Select lower fat milk alternatives.**
  - Compare the Nutrition Facts table on yogurts or cheeses to make wise choices.

▸ **Have meat alternatives such as beans, lentils and tofu often.**

▸ **Eat at least two Food Guide Servings of fish each week.***
  - Choose fish such as char, herring, mackerel, salmon, sardines and trout.

▸ **Select lean meat and alternatives prepared with little or no added fat or salt.**
  - Trim the visible fat from meats. Remove the skin on poultry.
  - Use cooking methods such as roasting, baking or poaching that require little or no added fat.
  - If you eat luncheon meats, sausages or prepackaged meats, choose those lower in salt (sodium) and fat.

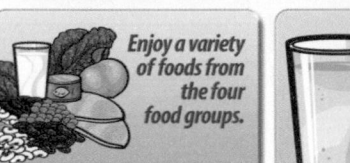

Enjoy a variety of foods from the four food groups.

Satisfy your thirst with water!
Drink water regularly. It's a calorie-free way to quench your thirst. Drink more water in hot weather or when you are very active.

* Health Canada provides advice for limiting exposure to mercury from certain types of fish. Refer to www.healthcanada.gc.ca for the latest information.

Advice for different ages and stages...

Children

Following *Canada's Food Guide* helps children grow and thrive.

Young children have small appetites and need calories for growth and development.

- Serve small nutritious meals and snacks each day.
- Do not restrict nutritious foods because of their fat content. Offer a variety of foods from the four food groups.
- Most of all... be a good role model.

Women of childbearing age

All women who could become pregnant and those who are pregnant or breastfeeding need a multivitamin containing **folic acid** every day. Pregnant women need to ensure that their multivitamin also contains **iron**. A health care professional can help you find the multivitamin that's right for you.

Pregnant and breastfeeding women need more calories. Include an extra 2 to 3 Food Guide Servings each day.

Here are two examples:
- Have fruit and yogurt for a snack, or
- Have an extra slice of toast at breakfast and an extra glass of milk at supper.

Men and women over 50

The need for **vitamin D** increases after the age of 50.

In addition to following *Canada's Food Guide*, everyone over the age of 50 should take a daily vitamin D supplement of 10 µg (400 IU).

Eat well and be active today and every day!

The benefits of eating well and being active include:
- Better overall health.
- Lower risk of disease.
- A healthy body weight.
- Feeling and looking better.
- More energy.
- Stronger muscles and bones.

Be active

To be active every day is a step towards better health and a healthy body weight.

Canada's Physical Activity Guide recommends building 30 to 60 minutes of moderate physical activity into daily life for adults and at least 90 minutes a day for children and youth. You don't have to do it all at once. Add it up in periods of at least 10 minutes at a time for adults and five minutes at a time for children and youth.

Start slowly and build up.

Eat well

Another important step towards better health and a healthy body weight is to follow *Canada's Food Guide* by:
- Eating the recommended amount and type of food each day.
- Limiting foods and beverages high in calories, fat, sugar or salt (sodium) such as cakes and pastries, chocolate and candies, cookies and granola bars, doughnuts and muffins, ice cream and frozen desserts, french fries, potato chips, nachos and other salty snacks, alcohol, fruit flavoured drinks, soft drinks, sports and energy drinks, and sweetened hot or cold drinks.

Read the label
- Compare the Nutrition Facts table on food labels to choose products that contain less fat, saturated fat, trans fat, sugar and sodium.
- Keep in mind that the calories and nutrients listed are for the amount of food found at the top of the Nutrition Facts table.

Limit trans fat

When a Nutrition Facts table is not available, ask for nutrition information to choose foods lower in trans and saturated fats.

Take a step today...

✓ Have breakfast every day. It may help control your hunger later in the day.
✓ Walk wherever you can – get off the bus early, use the stairs.
✓ Benefit from eating vegetables and fruit at all meals and as snacks.
✓ Spend less time being inactive such as watching TV or playing computer games.
✓ Request nutrition information about menu items when eating out to help you make healthier choices.
✓ Enjoy eating with family and friends!
✓ Take time to eat and savour every bite!

For more information, interactive tools, or additional copies visit *Canada's Food Guide* on-line at:
www.healthcanada.gc.ca/foodguide

or contact:

Publications
Health Canada
Ottawa, Ontario K1A 0K9
E-Mail: publications@hc-sc.gc.ca
Tel.: 1-866-225-0709
Fax: (613) 941-5366
TTY: 1-800-267-1245

Également disponible en français sous le titre :
Bien manger avec le Guide alimentaire canadien

This publication can be made available on request on diskette, large print, audio-cassette and braille.

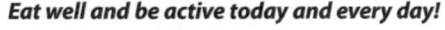

Nutrition Facts
Per 0 mL (0 g)

Amount	% Daily Value
Calories 0	
Fat 0 g	0 %
Saturates 0 g	0 %
+ Trans 0 g	
Cholesterol 0 mg	
Sodium 0 mg	0 %
Carbohydrate 0 g	0 %
Fibre 0 g	0 %
Sugars 0 g	
Protein 0 g	

Vitamin A	0 %	Vitamin C	0 %
Calcium	0 %	Iron	0 %

How do I count Food Guide Servings in a meal?

Here is an example:

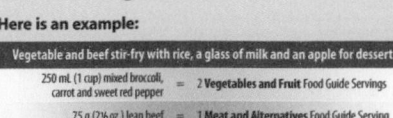

Vegetable and beef stir-fry with rice, a glass of milk and an apple for dessert		
250 mL (1 cup) mixed broccoli, carrot and sweet red pepper	=	2 **Vegetables and Fruit** Food Guide Servings
75 g (2½ oz.) lean beef	=	1 **Meat and Alternatives** Food Guide Serving
250 mL (1 cup) brown rice	=	2 **Grain Products** Food Guide Servings
5 mL (1 tsp) canola oil	=	part of your **Oils and Fats** intake for the day
250 mL (1 cup) 1% milk	=	1 **Milk and Alternatives** Food Guide Serving
1 apple	=	1 **Vegetables and Fruit** Food Guide Serving

FIGURE 12-2, cont'd Eating Well with Canada's Food Guide.

TABLE 12-5

Reference Daily Intakes

Nutrient	Amount
Vitamin A	5000 IU
Vitamin C	60 mg
Thiamin	1.5 mg
Roboflavin	1.7 mg
Niacin	20 mg
Calcium	1 g
Iron	18 mg
Vitamin D	400 IU
Vitamin E	30 IU
Vitamin B_6	2 mg
Folic acid	0.4
Vitamin B_{12}	6 mcg
Phosphorus	1 g
Iodine	150 mcg
Magnesium	400 mg
Zinc	15 mg
Copper	2 mg
Biotin	0.3 mg
Pantothenic acid	10 mg
Selenium	70 mcg

From Center for Food Safety & Applied Nutrition: *A food labeling guide*, College Park, Md, 1994, U.S. Department of Agriculture, revised 1999.

TABLE 12-6

Daily Reference Values (DRVs)

Food Component	DRV	Calculation
Fat	65 g	30% of kcal
Saturated fat	20 g	10% of kcals
Cholesterol	300 mg	Same regardless of kcal
Carbohydrates (total)	300 g	60% of calories
Fiber	25 g	11.5 g per 1000 kcal
Protein	50 g	10% of kcal
Sodium	2400 mg	Same regardless of kcal
Potassium	3500 mg	Same regardless of kcal

NOTE: The DRVs were established for adults and children over 4 years old. The values for energy yielding nutrients below are based on 2,000 calories per day.

From Center for Food Safety & Applied Nutrition: *A food labeling guide*, College Park, Md, 1994, U.S. Department of Agriculture, revised 1999.

The DVs exist for nutrients for which RDAs already exist (in which case they are known as **reference daily intakes [RDIs]**) (Table 12-5) and for which no RDAs exist (in which case they are known as **daily reference values [DRVs]** [Table 12-6]). However, food labels use only the term "daily value." RDIs provide a large margin of safety; in general, the RDI for a nutrient is greater than the RDA for a specific age-group. The term *RDI* replaces the term *U.S. RDAs* used on previous food labels.

The previously mentioned nutrients must be listed on the food label. Nutrients that a manufacturer or processor may voluntarily disclose include those for which a DV has been established such as monounsaturated and saturated fat, potassium, vitamins such as thiamin and riboflavin, and minerals such as iodine and magnesium. As new DRIs are developed in various categories, labeling laws are updated. Figure 12-3 shows a sample nutrition facts label.

Nutrient Content Claims

Nutrient content terms such as reduced sodium, fat free, low calorie, and healthy must now meet government definitions that apply to all foods (Box 12-3). For example, *lean* refers to a serving of meat, poultry, seafood, or game meat with less than 10 g of fat, less than 4 g of saturated fat, and less than 95 mg of cholesterol per serving or per 100 g. Extra lean meat or poultry contains less than 5 g of fat, less than 2 g of saturated fat, and the same cholesterol content as lean, per serving, or per 100 g of product.

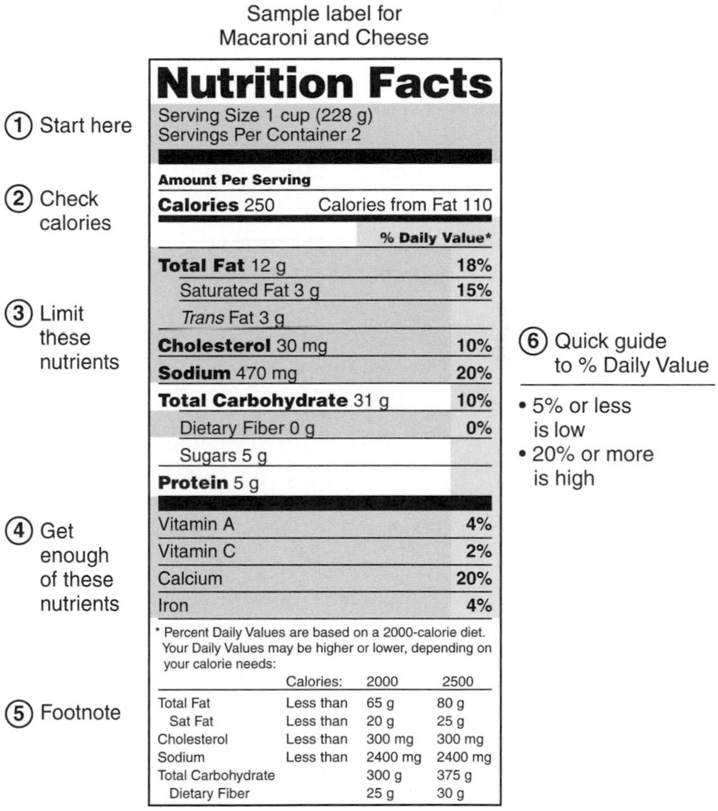

FIGURE 12-3 Nutrition facts label information. (*Source: U.S. Food and Drug Administration, available at http://www.cfsan.fda. gov/~dms/foodlab.html#twoparts, accessed August 2, 2006.*)

Health Claims

A **health claim** is allowed only on appropriate food products that meet specified standards. The government requires that health claims be worded in ways that are not misleading (e.g., the claim cannot imply that the food product itself helps prevent disease). Health claims cannot appear on foods that supply more than 20% of the DV for fat, saturated fat, cholesterol, and sodium. The following is an example of a health

BOX 12-3

Nutrient Content Claims

Free: This term means that a product contains no amount of, or only trivial or "physiologically inconsequential" amounts of, one or more of these components: fat, saturated fat, cholesterol, sodium, sugar, and calories. For example, "calorie-free" means fewer than 5 calories per serving, and "sugar-free" and "fat-free" both mean less than 0.5 g per serving. Synonyms for "free" include "without," "no" and "zero." A synonym for fat-free milk is "skim."

Low: This term can be used on foods that can be eaten frequently without exceeding dietary guidelines for one or more of these components: fat, saturated fat, cholesterol, sodium, and calories.

- **Low fat**: 3 g or less per serving
- **Low saturated fat**: 1 g or less per serving
- **Low sodium**: 140 mg or less per serving
- **Very low sodium**: 35 mg or less per serving
- **Low cholesterol**: 20 mg or less and 2 g or less of saturated fat per serving
- **Low calorie**: 40 calories or less per serving

Synonyms for low include "little," "few," "low source of," and "contains a small amount of."

- **Lean and extra lean:** These terms can be used to describe the fat content of meat, poultry, seafood, and game meats.

  Lean: less than 10 g fat, 4.5 g or less saturated fat, and less than 95 mg cholesterol per serving and per 100 g.

  Extra lean: less than 5 g fat, less than 2 g saturated fat, and less than 95 mg cholesterol per serving and per 100 g.

High: This term can be used if the food contains 20% or more of the daily value for a particular nutrient in a serving.

Good source: This term means that one serving of a food contains 10% to 19% of the daily value for a particular nutrient.

Reduced: This term means that a nutritionally altered product contains at least 25% less of a nutrient or of calories than the regular, or reference, product. However, a reduced claim can't be made on a product if its reference food already meets the requirement for a "low" claim.

Less: This term means that a food, whether altered or not, contains 25% less of a nutrient or of calories than the reference food. For example, pretzels that have 25% less fat than potato chips could carry a "less" claim. "Fewer" is an acceptable synonym.

Light: This descriptor can mean two things:

- First, that a nutritionally altered product contains one-third fewer calories or half the fat of the reference food. If the food derives 50% or more of its calories from fat, the reduction must be 50% of the fat.
- Second, that the sodium content of a low-calorie, low-fat food has been reduced by 50%. In addition, "light in sodium" may be used on food in which the sodium content has been reduced by at least 50%.
- The term "light" still can be used to describe such properties as texture and color, as long as the label explains the intent (e.g., "light brown sugar" and "light and fluffy."

More: This term means that a serving of food, whether altered or not, contains a nutrient that is at least 10% of the daily value more than the reference food. The 10% of daily value also applies to "fortified," "enriched" and "added" "extra and plus" claims, but in these cases the food must be altered.

Data from Food and Drug Administration, available at http://www.fda.gov/opacom/backgrounders/foodlabel/newlabel.html#nutri, accessed August 2, 2006.

BOX 12-4

Health Claims for Diet-Disease Relationships

- Calcium and a reduced risk of osteoporosis
- Dietary fat and an increased risk of cancer
- Dietary saturated fat and cholesterol and an increased risk of coronary heart disease
- Fiber-containing grain products, fruits, and vegetables and a reduced risk of cancer
- Fruits, vegetables, and grain products that contain fiber and a reduced risk of coronary heart disease
- Sodium and an increased risk of hypertension
- Potassium and a decreased risk of hypertension
- Fruits and vegetables and a reduced risk of cancer

- Folic acid during pregnancy and a reduced risk of neural tube defects
- Sugar alcohols and a reduced risk of dental caries
- Soluble fiber from certain foods, such as whole oats and psyllium seed husk, and heart disease
- Stanol and sterol esters (in vegetable oil spreads and salad dressings) and a reduced risk of coronary heart disease

Data from Food and Drug Administration, available at http://www.fda.gov/opacom/backgrounders/foodlabel/newlabel.html#nutri, accessed August 2, 2006.

claim for dietary fiber and cancer: "Low-fat diets rich in fiber-containing grain products, fruits, and vegetables may reduce the risk of some types of cancer, a disease associated with many factors." Box 12-4 lists health claims that manufacturers can use to describe food-disease relationships.

CULTURAL ASPECTS OF DIETARY PLANNING

To plan diets for individuals or groups that are appropriate from a health and nutrition perspective, it is important that nutritionists and health professionals develop cultural awareness (cultural competency) and use resources that are targeted to the specific client or group. Numerous popula-tion subgroups in the United States and throughout the world have specific cultural, ethnic, or religious beliefs and practices to consider. These groups have their own set of dietary practices or beliefs, which are important when considering dietary planning.

The Mediterranean Diet

Cultural, ethnic, or religious rules can have an effect on access to food, food choices, preparation, and storage methods. For example, the Mediterranean Diet Pyramid has been developed to represent the eating pattern of the Mediterranean culture and to demonstrate a reasonable diet for reducing chronic disease (Figure 12-4) (see *Focus On:* The Mediterranean Diet: Is It Good for All of Us?). Cultural aspects of dietary planning may also include vegetarianism, ethnic heritage practices, and religious customs or rules.

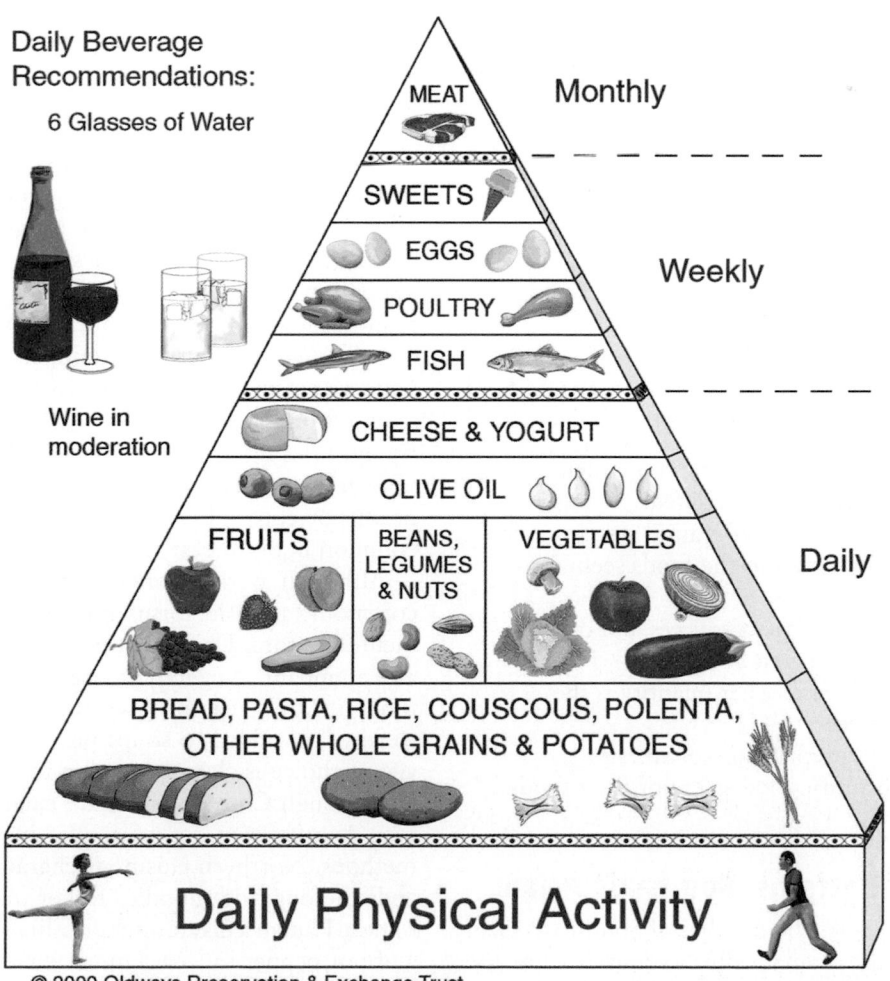

FIGURE 12-4 The Traditional Healthy Mediterranean Diet Pyramid. (*Courtesy Oldways Preservation and Exchange Trust. Adapted from: http://www.oldwayspt.org/, accessed March 13, 2007.*)

The Mediterranean Diet: Is It Good for All of Us?

The Mediterranean Diet has received attention because of its potential for protecting the body against cardiovascular disease and cancers. The diet is rich in fruits, vegetables, whole grains, and sources of monounsaturated and polyunsaturated fatty acids (such as omega-3 fatty acids).

A trial involving this diet was conducted as part of the Lyon Diet Heart Study; 605 patients with coronary heart disease who had already had a heart attack were randomly selected to follow either a Mediterranean-type diet or a control diet (Hakim, 1998). Those following the Mediterranean pattern ate less delicatessen food, beef, pork, butter, and cream and more vegetable oils, vegetable oil margarine-type spreads, and olive oil. The control diet was similar to the Step 1 American Heart Association (AHA) Prudent Diet (30% energy from fat). Compared with the control diet, the Mediterranean diet provided more fiber, vitamin C, and omega-3 fatty acids both from fish and as α-linolenic acid from walnuts, seeds, and herbs and less cholesterol and saturated fatty acids. Participants were monitored for 4 years, and at the end there was a 50% to 75% reduction in risk for another heart attack. The risk ratios were also lower for cancers, and overall mortality rates. More use of these strategies in dietary planning may be beneficial in U.S. populations when combined with adequate daily physical activity.

CULTURAL DIETARY PATTERNS

Table 12-7 lists common cultural dietary patterns. The following questions may help nutritionists accommodate food habits while meeting dietary recommendations:

- Which individual foods are the major components of the food or mixed dish to be classified?
- To which food groups in the MyPyramid system or the Mediterranean Diet Pyramid do the foods seem most related?
- What are the important nutrient sources and their contribution to overall nutrient adequacy?
- How is the food used, and in what quantity is the food typically consumed?
- Do any food handling, preparation, or storage considerations compromise food safety or limit food choices?

Common Dietary Patterns: Southeast Asian

During the past few decades the number of Southeast Asian refugees has increased dramatically worldwide. In the United States immigrants from Southeast Asia have become the third largest ethnic group after blacks and Hispanics.

Among these immigrants are numerous groups, each with a distinct language, culture, and food habits. From Laos, Cambodia, and Vietnam come the native ethnic groups, as well as Muslims and ethnic Chinese. From Laos, Thailand, and Southern China come the nomadic hill people, the Hmong (Tripp, 1982). Urban and rural immigrants may have lifestyles that differ considerably even when the people come from the same country.

The traditional Hmong (Southeast Asian) diet is high in complex carbohydrates and low in refined carbohydrates, predominantly from rice that is eaten at every meal. The Southeast Asian Hmong diet includes large amounts of fruits, vegetables, and soy products (mostly tofu), and smaller amounts of meat, poultry, and fish. Common spices include lemon grass, coriander, chili peppers, green onion, basil, cilantro, ginger, and garlic. Lemon and lime juice often are used in place of salad dressings and salt; soy and fish sauces and monosodium glutamate (MSG) are common seasonings (American Dietetic Association [ADA] and American Diabetes Association, 1999).

Although lactose intolerance has been reported to be a problem in many Southeast Asians, many adults are able to drink it in small amounts without any discomfort. If the immigrants are refugees, they may be at nutritional risk because of low access to food supplies and parasitic anemias. General malnutrition, hypertension, dental caries, and iron deficiency anemia have been identified as problems among incoming refugees.

Common Dietary Patterns: Chinese

In Chinese culture food plays a vital role in preventing and treating diseases and addressing certain health conditions. The traditional Chinese diet is much richer in carbohydrates (i.e., rice) and includes various meats, poultry, and seafood in small quantities. The Chinese diet obtains more than 80% of its calories from grains, legumes, and vegetables; 20% from animal protein, fruits, and fats. Northern Chinese cuisine may include more noodles, dumplings, and steamed buns made from wheat flour. Stir-frying, deep-fat frying, braising, roasting, smoking, and steaming are common food preparation techniques. When foods are fried, peanut or corn oil is used rather than lard, which is more common in Southeast Asian cuisine.

Although pork is often a mainstay, soybeans are also commonly used in forms including sprouts, dried, or fermented as tofu. Dairy products are rarely consumed. Fruits are abundant. Vegetables are also frequent in the diet, though rarely eaten raw; they are generally stir-fried, steamed, or added to soups just before serving. The beverage of choice is clear, hot green tea.

Although Chinese meals are eaten communally, each region has its own set of foods, ingredients, and cooking methods. Northern cuisine is characterized by garlic, leeks, and scallions, with noodles rather than rice. In the Western region Hunan cuisine includes liberal use of chili peppers and hot pepper sauces. Hunan dishes are spicier and oilier than dishes in other regions. Southern Chinese cuisine, or Cantonese, includes primarily steamed and stir-fried dishes

Text continued on p. 358

TABLE 12-7

Cultural Dietary Patterns

Culture	Bread, Cereal, Rice, and Pasta Group	Vegetable Group	Fruit Group	Milk, Yogurt, Cheese Group	Meat, Poultry, Fish, Dry Beans, Eggs, and Nuts Groups	Fats, Oils, and Sweets
Native American	Blue corn flour (ground dried blue corn kernels) used to make cornbread, mush dumplings; fruit dumplings (walakshi); fry bread (biscuit dough deep fried); ground sweet acorn; hominy; tortillas; wheat and rye products; wild rice	Artichokes, cacti, chili, mushrooms, nettles, onions, potatoes, pumpkin, squash, sweet potatoes, tomatoes, wild greens, turnips, and yucca	Dried wild berries, cherries, and grapes; berries, elderberries, persimmons, plums, and rhubarb	None in traditional diet	Bear, buffalo, deer, elk, moose, rabbit, and squirrel; duck, goose, quail, and wild turkey; a variety of fish, legumes, nuts, and seeds	Tallow and lard Maple sugar and pine sugar
Northern European	Barley, hops, oat, rice, rye, and wheat products	Artichokes, asparagus, beets, Brussels sprouts, cabbage, carrots, cauliflower, celery, cucumbers, eggplant, fennel, green peppers, kale, leeks, mushrooms, olives, onions, peas, potatoes, radishes, spinach, turnips, and watercress	Apples, apricots, cherries, currants, gooseberries, grapes, lemons, melons, oranges, peaches, pears, plums, prunes, raspberries, rhubarb, and strawberries	Cheese (made from cow, sheep, and goat milk), cream, milk, sour cream, and yogurt	Beef, lamb, oxtail, pork, rabbit, veal, and venison; chicken, duck, goose, pheasant, pigeon, quail, and turkey; a wide variety of fish, legumes, and nuts	Butter, lard, margarine, olive oil, vegetable oil, and salt pork; honey and sugar

Continued

Used with permission as modified from Kittler PG, Sucher KP: *Food and culture*, ed 4, Belmont Calif, 2004, Thomson and Wadsworth; and Grodner M et al: *Foundations and clinical applications of nutrition: a nursing approach*, ed 4, St Louis, 2006, Mosby.
Common food choices associated within these cultural groups are noted, and individuals may also consume other foods.

TABLE 12-7

Cultural Dietary Patterns—cont'd

Culture	Bread, Cereal, Rice, and Pasta Group	Vegetable Group	Fruit Group	Milk, Yogurt, Cheese Group	Meat, Poultry, Fish, Dry Beans, Eggs, and Nuts Groups	Fats, Oils, and Sweets
Cuban and Puerto Rican	Rice; starchy green bananas, usually fried (plantain)	Beets, breadfruit, chayote, chili peppers, eggplant, onion, tubers (yucca), white yams (boniato)	Coconuts, guava, mango, oranges (sweet and sour), prune and mango paste	Flan, hard cheese (queso de mano)	Chicken, fish, (all kinds and preparations, including smoked, salted, canned, and fresh), shellfish, legumes (all kinds, especially black beans), pork (fried), sausage (chorizo), calf brain, beef tongue	Olive and peanut oil, lard, coconut
South American	Amaranth (corn, rice, quinoa) and wheat products	Ahipa, arracacha, calabaza, cassava, green peppers, hearts of palm, kale, okra, oca, onions, rosella, squash, sweet potatoes, yacon, and yams	Avocadoes, abiu, acerola, apples, banana, caimito, casimiroa, cherimoya, feijoa, guava, grapes, jackfruit, jabitocaba, lemons, limes, lulo, mammea, mango, melon, olives, oranges, palm fruits, papaya, passion fruit, peaches, pineapple, pitanga, quince, sapote, and strawberries	Cheese and milk	Beef, frog, goat, guinea pig, llama, mutton, pork, and rabbit; chicken, duck, turkey and a variety of fish, shellfish, and nuts	Palm oil, olive oil, and butter; sugar cane, brown sugar, and honey
Chinese	Rice and related products (flour, cakes, and noodles); noodles made from barley, corn, and millet; wheat and related products (breads, noodles, spaghetti, stuffed noodles [won ton] and filled buns [bow])	Bamboo shoots, cabbage (nappa), celery, Chinese turnips (lo bok), dried daylil ies, dry fungus (Black Juda's ear); leafy green vegetables including kale, cress, mustard greens (gai choy), chard (bok choy), amaranth greens (yin choy), wolfberry leaves (gou gay), and Chinese beans	Apples, bananas, custard apples, coconuts, dates, longan, figs, grapes, kumquats, lime, litchi, mango, muskmelon, oranges, papaya, passion fruit, peaches, persimmons, pineapples, plums, pomegranates, pomelos, tangerines, and watermelon	Milk (cows, buffalo, and soymilk)	Beef, lamb, and pork; chicken, duck, quail, squab, a large variety of fish and shellfish, in addition to legumes and nuts	Lard; peanut, soy, sesame and rice oil; honey, rice or barley malt, palm sugar, sorghum sugar, and dehydrated cane juice

	Breads and Cereals	Vegetables	Fruits	Milk Products	Meats and Meat Substitutes	Fats
		broccoli (gai lan); eggplant, lotus tubers, okra, snow peas, stir-fried vegetables (chow yuk), taro roots, white radish (daikon), and yams				
Japanese	Rice and rice products, rice flour (mochiko), noodles (comen/soba), buckwheat and millet	Artichoke, asparagus, bamboo shoots (takenoko), burdock (gobo), cabbage (nappa), eggplant, horseradish (wasabi), mizuna, mushrooms (shiitake, matsutake, nameko), Japanese parsley (seri), lotus root (renkon), pickled cabbage (kimchee), pickled vegetables, seaweed (laver, nori, wakame, kombu), snow peas, spinach, sweet potato, vegetable soup (mizutaki), watercress, white radish (daikon)	Pearlike apple (nasi), apricots, bananas, cherries, figs, grapefruit (yuzu), kumquats, lemons, limes, persimmons, plums, pineapples, strawberry, and tangerine (mikan)	Milk, butter, and ice cream	Beef, deer, lamb, port, rabbit, veal; fish and shellfish, including dried fish with bones, raw fish (sashimi), and fish cake (kamaboko); a variety of poultry (chicken, duck, goose, turkey) and legumes (black beans, red beans, soybeans—as tofu, fermented soybean and sprouts)	Lard; soy, sesame, rapeseed and rice oil; honey and sugar
Korean	Barley, buckwheat, millet, rice and wheat products	Bamboo shoots, bean sprouts, beets, cabbage, chives, chrysanthemum leaves, cucumber, eggplant, fern, green onion, green pepper, leeks, lotus root, mushrooms, onion, perilla, seaweed, spinach, sweet potato, turnips, water chestnut, watercress, and white radish	Apples, Asian pears, cherries, dates, grapes, melons, oranges, pears, persimmons, plums, and tangerines	Very little, if any, consumption	Beef, oxtail, pork, chicken, pheasant, and a variety of fish, shellfish, legumes, and nuts	Sesame oil and vegetable oil; honey and sugar

Continued

TABLE 12-7
Cultural Dietary Patterns—cont'd

Culture	Bread, Cereal, Rice, and Pasta Group	Vegetable Group	Fruit Group	Milk, Yogurt, Cheese Group	Meat, Poultry, Fish, Dry Beans, Eggs, and Nuts Groups	Fats, Oils, and Sweets
Filipino	Noodles, rice, rice flour (mochiko), stuffed noodles (won ton), white bread (pan de sal)	Amaranth, bamboo shoots, beets, burdock root, cassava, Chinese celery, dark green leafy vegetables (malunggay and salvyot), eggplant, garlic, green peppers, hearts of palm, hyacinth bean, kamis, leek, mushrooms, okra, onion, sweet potatoes (camotes), turnips, and root crop (gabi)	Apples, avocadoes, banana, bitter melon (ampalaya), breadfruit, coconut, guavas, jackfruit, limes, mangoes, papaya, pod fruit (tamarind), pomelos, rambutan, rhubarb, star fruit, tamarind, tangelo (naranghita), and watermelon	White cheese, evaporated cow or goat milk, and soy milk	Beef, carabao, goat, pork, monkey, organ meats, and rabbit; fish, dried fish (dilis); egg roll (lumpia), fish sauce (alamang and bagoong); legumes such as mung beans, bean sprouts, chickpeas; and soybean curd (tofu)	Coconut oil, lard, and vegetable oil; brown and white sugar, coconut, and honey
Pacific Islanders	Rice and wheat products	Arrowroot, bitter melon, burdock root, cabbage, carrot, cassava, daikon, eggplant, ferms, green pepper, horseradish, jute, kohlrabi, leeks lotus root, mustard greens, green onions, seaweed, spinach, squashes, sweet potato, taro, water chestnuts, and yams	Acerola cherries, apples, apricot, avocado, banana, breadfruit, coconut, guava, jackfruit, kumquat, litchis, loquat, mango, melons, papaya, passion fruit, peach, pear, pineapple, plum, prune, strawberries, and tamarind	Very little, if any, consumption	Beef, pork, chicken, duck, squab, turkey; a variety of fish, shellfish, and legumes	Butter, coconut oil, lard, sesame oil, and vegetable oil; sugar
South Asian	Rice, wheat, buckwheat, corn, millet, and sorghum products	Agathi flowers, amaranth, artichokes, bamboo shoots, beets, bitter melon, Brussels sprouts, cabbage, collard greens, cucumbers, drumstick plant, eggplant, lotus root, manioc, mushrooms, okra, pandanus, plantain flowers, sago palm, spinach, turnips, yams, water chestnuts, water convulus, and water lilies	Apples, apricots, avocadoes, bananas, coconut, dates, figs, grapes, guava, jackfruit, limes, litchis, loquats, mangoes, melon, nongus, oranges, papaya, peaches, pears, persimmons, pineapple, plums, pomegranate, pomelos, star fruit, sugar cane, tangerines, and watermelon	Milk (evaporated and fermented products), cheese, and milk-based desserts	Beef, goat, mutton, pork, chicken, duck, and a variety of fish, seafood, legumes, and nuts	Coconut oil, ghee, mustard oil, peanut oil, sesame seed oil, and sunflower oil; sugar cane, jaggery, and molasses

| Jewish (both cultural and religious customs) | Bagel, buckwheat groats (kasha), dumplings made with matzoh meal (matzoh balls or knaidelach), egg bread (challah), noodle or potato pudding (kugel), crepe filled with farmer cheese and/or fruit (blintz), unleavened bread or large cracker made with wheat flour and water (matzoh) | Potato pancakes (latkes); vegetable stew made with sweet potatoes, carrots, prunes, and sometimes brisket (tzimmes); beet soup (borscht) | A mixture of fish formed into balls and poached (gefilte fish); smoked salmon (lox) | Chicken fat |

with a lot of fish and shellfish. As Chinese adopt traditional American foods, their diet begins to include more sweets such as cookies, chocolate, soft drinks, and snacks.

Common Dietary Patterns: Hispanic Cultures

Hispanics are the most rapidly growing ethnic group in the United States, and Mexican-Americans are the largest subgroup of Hispanics. Hispanic cuisine is based on the concept of foods having "hot" and "cold" properties and on beliefs about the contribution of food to health and well-being (ADA and ADA 1998). "Cold" foods include most vegetables, tropical fruits, dairy products, and inexpensive cuts of meat. "Hot" foods include chili peppers, garlic, onions, most grains, expensive cuts of meat, oils, and alcohol. For example, pregnancy is considered a "hot" condition; thus "hot" foods upset the stomach. Therefore some Hispanics may not eat chili peppers while pregnant for cultural reasons rather than because of safety issues for the mother or developing fetus. Depending on the part of the world, the main dishes of Hispanic diets may include meat (pork, veal, sausage), poultry, or fish. Rice and tortillas are mainstays of the diet, as are fruits and vegetables. Milk and cheese are consumed when available. Fried foods are often eaten and may need to be limited for medical reasons. Chili peppers are commonly used and are a rich source of vitamin C. Chili peppers can range from mild to very hot and from small to very large.

Common Dietary Patterns: Native Americans

Native Americans (American Indians and Alaska Natives) often live on federal Indian reservations and in small rural communities. In this culture food has great religious and social significance for celebrations and ceremonies. Food is more of a social or religious obligation than simple nourishment. Common foods may be prepared and used in different ways in various regions and tribal organizations. Fry bread (fried dough) is a central part of American Indian cuisine and is eaten with foods such as stews, soups, and bean dishes. Fried foods are generally prepared with lard.

Corn is the carbohydrate staple of the American Indian diet, in addition to protein-rich dried beans. Fruits and vegetables were traditionally gathered from the wild but are also cultivated on small farms. Lamb (mutton), goat, game, and poultry are more common than pork or beef. Diabetes is a big problem in natives consuming the modern American diet (see *Focus On*: Diabetes Does Discriminate, in Chapter 30).

Common Dietary Patterns: Alaska Natives

The Alaska Native diet consists of a mixture of traditional foods and American prepared and processed foods. The diet is high in protein and fat since it is based on meat, fish, sea mammals, and game as staple foods. Seaweed, willow leaves, and sour dock are some of the few edible plants consumed. Since obesity and diabetes mellitus are common, it is important to merge cultural sensitivity with diet and health issues.

Dietary Patterns of Specific Religious Groups

Another major consideration is religious beliefs that affect dietary patterns (Table 12-8).

Jewish Food Customs, Dietary Laws, and Holidays

The Jewish dietary laws are biblical ordinances that include rules regarding food, chiefly about the selection, slaughter, and preparation of meat. Animals allowed to be eaten (clean) are quadrupeds that have cloven hooves and chew cud, specifically cattle, sheep, goats, and deer. Permissible fowl are chicken, turkey, goose, pheasant, and duck. All animals and fowl must be inspected for disease and killed by a ritual slaughterer according to specific rules. Only the forequarter of the quadruped may be used, except when the hip sinew of the thigh vein can be removed, in which case the hindquarter is also allowed.

Blood is forbidden as food because blood is synonymous with life. The traditional process of koshering meat and poultry removes all blood before cooking. Koshering involves soaking meat in water, salting it thoroughly, allowing it to drain, and then washing it three times to remove the salt. Foods that have been prepared in this way can carry a kosher designation.

Meat and milk cannot be combined in the same meal. Milk or milk-related foods can be eaten immediately before a meal but not with a meal. After eating meat, a person must wait 6 hours before consuming milk products. Because of the rules related to separating meat and milk products, those in traditional orthodox Jewish homes must keep two completely separate sets of dishes, silver, and cooking equipment—one for meat meals and one for dairy meals. Only fish with fins and scales can be eaten; thus no shellfish or eel is permissible. Fish can be eaten with dairy or meats. Eggs can also be combined with meat or milk. However, an egg yolk containing a drop of blood cannot be eaten because the blood is considered a chick embryo, or a sign of a new life.

Fruits, vegetables, cereal products, and all of the other foods that generally comprise a diet can be consumed with no restrictions. Bakery products and prepared food mixtures must be produced under acceptable kosher standards.

The most important of the Jewish holy days is the Sabbath, or day of rest, which is observed from sundown on Friday until sundown on Saturdays. The Friday night meal is the most special of the week and usually includes fish and chicken. No food is allowed to be cooked or heated on Saturday; thus all food eaten on the Sabbath is cooked on Friday and either kept warm in the oven or eaten cold. Festival holidays include Rosh Hashanah (the New Year) in September; Succoth, the fall harvest holiday; Chanukah (the Feast of Lights) in midwinter; and Purim, a joyous holiday in spring. Each holiday has certain associated food delicacies. Yom Kippur, the Day of Atonement, occurs 10 days after Rosh Hashanah and is a day of fasting from all food and drink from sundown on the eve of the holiday to sundown on the holiday. Pregnant females and those who are ill do not fast.

TABLE 12-8

Religious Dietary Practices

	Buddhist	Hindu	Jewish	Moslem	Christian Roman Catholic	Christian Eastern Orthodox	Christian Mormon	Christian Seventh Day Adventist
Beef	A	X						A
Pork	A	A	X	X				X
Meats, all	A	A	R	R	R	R		A
Eggs/dairy	O	O	R			R		O
Fish	A	R	R			R		A
Shellfish	A	R	X			O		X
Alcohol		A		X			X	X
Coffee/tea				A			X	X
Meat and dairy at same meal			X					
Leavened foods			R					
Ritual slaughter of meats			+	+				
Moderation	+			+				+
Fasting*	+	+	+	+	+	+	+	

Modified from Kittler PG, Sucher KP: *Food and culture*, ed 4, Belmont, Ca, 2004, Thomson and Wadsworth; and Escott-Stump S: *Nutrition and diagnosis-related care*, Baltimore, Md, 2008, Lippincott Williams & Wilkins.

*Fasting varies from partial (abstention from certain foods or meals) to complete (no food or drink).

X, Prohibited or strongly discouraged; A, avoided by the most devout; R, some restrictions regarding types of foods or when a food may be eaten; O, permitted, but may be avoided at some observances; +, practiced.

Passover, a spring commemorative festival lasting 8 days, includes special dietary requirements. During the Passover holiday leavened bread or cake is prohibited. Matzo, (i.e., unleavened bread) is eaten, and all cake and baked products are made of flour from ground-up matzo or potato starch and leavened only with beaten egg whites. No salt is allowed in traditional Passover matzo. Variations of fried matzo or matzo-meal pancakes are prepared with generous amounts of fat.

Muslim Food Customs, Dietary Laws, and Holidays

Islam promotes the concept of "eating to live." Muslims are advised to stop eating while they are still hungry and always to share food. Although many foods are allowed, certain codes must be observed, and some dietary restrictions exist. The flesh of animals slaughtered in a humane way as outlined by Islamic law is considered *halal* (according to Islamic law). All meat to be consumed as food must be slaughtered with a ritual letting of blood while speaking the name of God. The slaughter can be done by anyone—no special person is designated for this function. Muslims eat kosher meat products because they know that they have been slaughtered properly. If an animal is slaughtered improperly, the meat becomes *haram*, or forbidden. Pork and pork products such as gelatin are prohibited, as are alcoholic beverages and alcohol products (e.g., vanilla extract or other alcohol-based food or flavoring extracts).

Although all foods not specifically prohibited are allowed to be eaten, certain foods are recommended such as milk, dates, meat, seafood, sweets, honey, and olive oil. Prayers are offered before any food is eaten. Muslims fast every year during the month of Ramadan, which occurs during the ninth month of the Islamic lunar calendar. Muslims fast completely from dawn to sunset and eat only twice a day—before dawn and after sunset. The end of Ramadan is marked by the Feast of Breaking the Fast (Eid-ul-Fitr). Muslims are also encouraged to fast 3 days of every month. Menstruating, pregnant, or lactating females are not required to fast but must make up the fasting days at some other time.

Vegetarianism

Vegetarian diets are increasing in popularity. Those who choose them may be motivated by philosophic, religious, or ecologic concerns or a desire to have a healthier lifestyle. Considerable evidence attests to the health benefits of a vegetarian diet. Studies of Seventh-Day Adventists indicate that the diet results in lower rates of type 2 diabetes, breast and colon cancer, and cardiovascular and gallbladder disease.

Of the millions of Americans who profess to be vegetarians, many eliminate "red" meats but eat fish, poultry, and dairy products. A lacto-vegetarian does not eat meat, fish, poultry, or eggs but does consume milk, cheese, and other dairy products. A lacto-ovo-vegetarian also consumes eggs. A true vegetarian, or vegan, does not eat any food of animal origin. The vegan diet is the only vegetarian diet that has any real risk of obtaining inadequate nutrition, but this risk can be avoided by careful planning.

Vegetarian diets tend to be lower in iron than omnivorous diets, although the nonheme iron in fruits, vegetables, and unrefined cereals is usually accompanied either in the food or in the meal by large amounts of ascorbic acid that aids in iron assimilation. Vegetarians do not have a greater risk of iron deficiency than those who are not vegetarians (ADA, 1997). Vegetarians who consume no dairy products may have low calcium intakes, and vitamin D intakes may be inadequate among those in northern latitudes where there is less exposure to sunshine (see *Focus On:* Sunshine, Vitamin D, and Fortification in Chapter 3). The calcium in some vegetables is inactivated by the presence of oxalates. Although phytates in unrefined cereals also can inactivate calcium, this is not a problem for Western vegetarians, whose diets tend to be based more on fruits and vegetables than on the unrefined cereals of Middle Eastern cultures. Long-term vegans may develop megaloblastic anemia because of a deficiency of vitamin B_{12}, found only in foods of animal origin. The high levels of folate in vegan diets may mask the neurologic damage of a vitamin B_{12} deficiency. Vegans should have a reliable source of vitamin B_{12} such as fortified breakfast cereals, soy beverages, or a supplement.

Although most vegetarians meet or exceed the requirements for protein, their diets tend to be lower in protein than those of omnivores. This lower intake may help vegetarians retain more calcium from their diets. Furthermore, lower protein intake usually results in lower dietary fat because many high-protein animal products are also rich in fat (ADA, 1997).

Well-planned vegetarian diets are safe for infants, children, and adolescents and can meet all of their nutritional requirements for growth. They are also adequate for pregnant and lactating females. The key is that the diets be well planned. Vegetarians should pay special attention to ensure that they get adequate calcium, iron, zinc, and vitamins B_{12} and D. Calculated combinations of complementary protein sources is not necessary, especially if protein sources are reasonably varied.

FOCAL POINTS

- The latest science behind nutrient needs and requirement along with educational level, lifestyle patterns and socioeconomic status go into development of dietary guidelines, food guides, nutrition labeling and other educational material to provide information and direction on food and activity choices for individuals and groups.
- The cultural, ethnic and religious backgrounds of individuals and groups are highly influential in food choices and meal planning, and must be considered when translating eating guidelines into the lifestyle choices.
- With a knowledge of dietary planning, nutrient needs, and food and nutrient information, as well as developed skills in counseling, dietetic counselors and health professionals are essential translators of food, nutrition, and health information into food choices and patterns for groups or individuals.

CLINICAL SCENARIO 1

Marty is a 45-year-old Jewish man who emigrated from Israel to the United States 3 years ago. He follows a strict kosher diet. In addition, he does not drink milk but does consume other dairy products. He has a body mass index (BMI) of 32 and a family history of heart disease. He has come to you for advice on increasing his calcium intake.

*Nutrition Diagnosis: Knowledge deficit related to calcium as evidenced by request for nutrient and dietary information

1. What type of dietary guidance would you offer Marty?
2. What type of dietary plan following strict kosher protocols would meet his daily dietary needs and promote weight loss?
3. What suggestions would you offer him about dietary choices for a healthy heart?
4. Which special steps should Marty take to meet calcium requirements without using supplements?
5. How can food labeling information be used to help Marty meet his weight loss and nutrient goals and incorporate his religious dietary concerns?

CLINICAL SCENARIO 2

Nan is a 20-year-old college student who has decided to become a vegetarian for nonreligious reasons. She does not eat red meat, chicken, fish, or dairy products. She is 5 ft, 2 in and weighs 95 lb. Her health is stable, but she does have low serum levels of iron, zinc, and vitamin B₁₂. Her blood pressure is 90/75 mm Hg. She has been referred to the nutrition clinic for counseling about changing some of her dietary habits.

Nutrition Diagnosis: Inadequate intake of iron, zinc, and vitamin B_{12} related to omission of animal foods as evidenced by low serum levels

1. What type of dietary guidance would you offer Nan?
2. Nan is at risk for developing deficiencies of which nutrients?
3. Plan a 3-day menu for Nan that excludes the foods she does not eat but provides adequate amounts of the key nutrients she needs.
4. What other dietary health-related advice would you give Nan?

USEFUL WEBSITES

American Dietetic Association
www.eatright.org

Center for Nutrition Policy and Promotion, USDA
www.usda.gov/cnpp/

Centers for Disease Control, NHANES Survey
www.cdc.gov/nchs/nhanes.htm

Dietary Guidelines for Americans
www.health.gov/DietaryGuidelines

Eat Smart, Play Hard
http://www.fns.usda.gov/eatsmartplayhardkids/

Ethnic and Cultural Food Guides
www.nal.usda.gov/fnic/etext/000023.html#xtocid2381818

Food and Drug Administration, Center for Food Safety and Applied Nutrition
www.cfsan.fda.gov

Food and Nutrition Information Center, National Agricultural Library, USDA
www.nal.usda.gov/fnic/

Health Canada
http://www.hc-sc.gc.ca/fn-an/index_e.html

Healthy Eating Index
http://www.cnpp.usda.gov/

Institute of Medicine, National Academy of Sciences
http://www.iom.edu/

International Food Information Council
http://ific.org

MyPyramid Food Guidance System
http://www.mypyramid.gov/

National Center for Health Statistics
www.cdc.gov/nchs/nhanes.htm

Nutrition.gov (U.S. government nutrition site)
www.nutrition.gov

U.S. Department of Agriculture
www.usda.gov

References

American Dietetic Association: Position of the American Dietetic Association: vegetarian diets, *J Am Diet Assoc* 97:1317, 1997.

American Dietetic Association: Position of the American Dietetic Association: total diet approach to communicating food and nutrition information, *J Am Diet Assoc* 102:100, 2002.

American Dietetic Association and American Diabetes Association: *Mexican American food practices, customs, and holidays, Ethnic and Regional Food Practices Series*, Chicago, 1998b, American Dietetic Association.

American Dietetic Association and the American Diabetes Association: *Hmong American food practices, customs, and holidays, Ethnic and Regional Food Practices Series*, Chicago, 1999, American Dietetic Association.

Federation of American Societies for Experimental Biology, Life Sciences Research Office: Third report on nutrition monitoring in the United States, Prepared for the Interagency Board for Nutrition Monitoring and Related Research, Washington, DC, 1995, U.S. Government Printing Office.

Food and Drug Administration: Focus on food labeling, Special Issue of FDA Consumer Magazine, Department of Health and Human Services Pub No (FDA) 93-2262, Washington, DC, May 1993, U.S. Government Printing Office.

Hakim I: Mediterranean diets and cancer prevention, *Arch Intern Med* 158(11):1169, 1998.

Health Canada: Eating well with Canada's food guide, ©Her Majesty the Queen in Right of Canada, represented by the Minister of Healthy Canada, 2007, available at www.hc-sc.gc. ca/fn-an/food-guide-aliment, accessed February 8, 2007.

Tripp RR: World refugee survey, 1982, New York, 1982, U.S. Committee for Refugees.

U.S. Department of Agriculture, Center for Nutrition Policy and Promotion: *Healthy eating index 2005*, available at www.cnpp. usda.gov, accessed April 16, 2007.

U.S. Senate Select Committee on Nutrition and Human Needs: *Dietary goals for the United States*, ed 2, Washington, DC, U.S. Senate, 95th Congress, first session, December 1977.

White House: *White House conference on food, nutrition, and health*, Final report, Washington, DC, 1970, U.S. Government Printing Office.

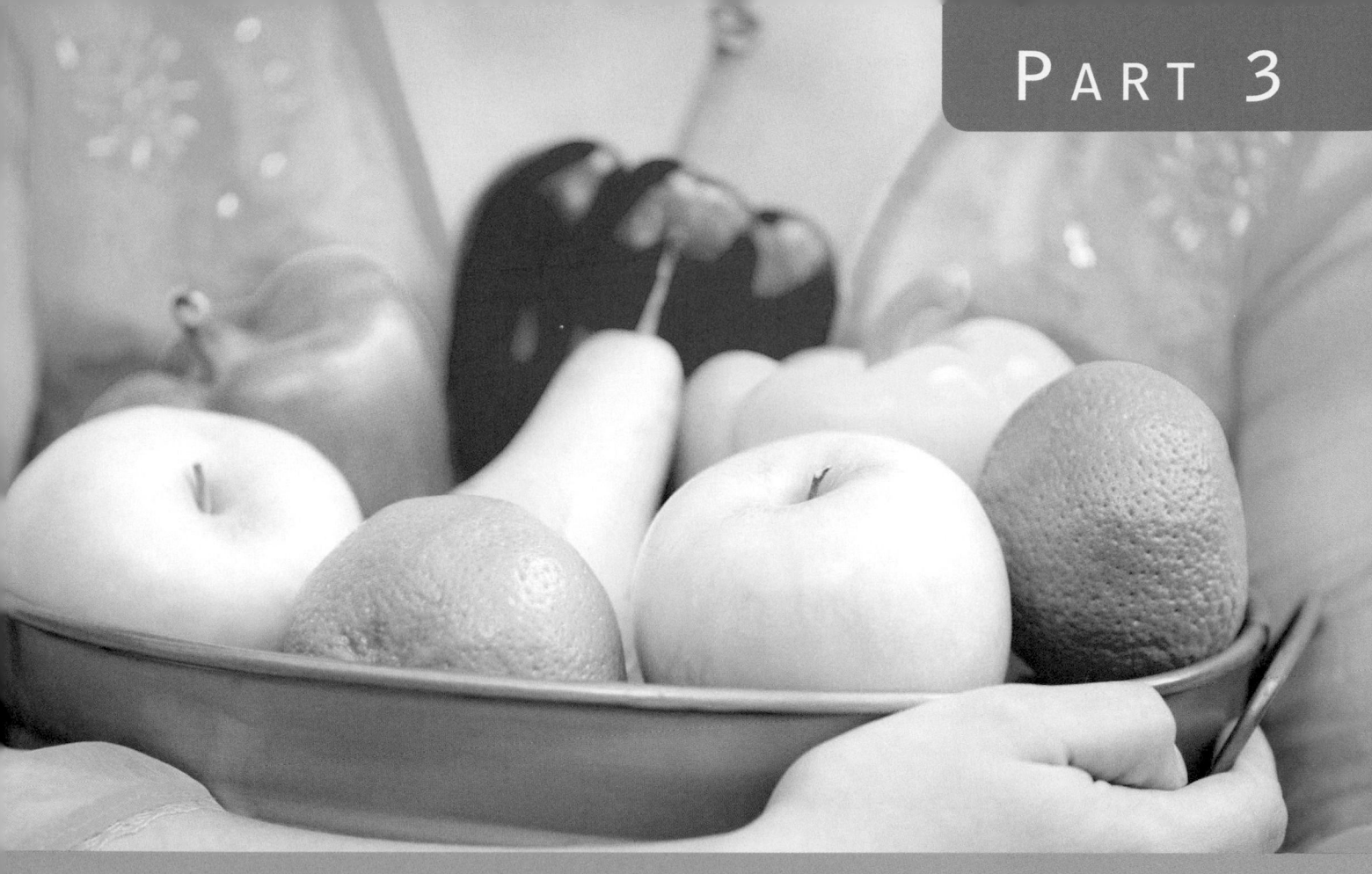

PART 3

Nutrition Care Process

THE type of nutrition care provided for an individual depends on the presence of disease or risk of potential disease, the environment, the stage of growth and development, and socioeconomic issues. It will include an assessment of the factors affecting the adequacy of nutritional intake and the current nutritional status, and the identification of nutrition diagnoses. Manipulation of the diet, provision of enteral or parenteral support, or intervention in the form of counseling or education and coordination of care are the possible interventions that may be selected according to the etiology of the problem. In most cases institutions will have established standards of care or practice guidelines that describe recommended actions in the nutrition care process. These standards often serve as a basis for assessing the quality of care provided to the patient.

The chapters in this section begin discussions of the formal nutrition care process, including an overview of nutritional genomics, followed by chapters related to assessment of nutrition status; selection of nutrition diagnoses; and interventions to solve problems or improve nutritional status. The final steps of the nutrition care process pertain to monitoring and evaluation, which are specific to the individual patient or client and relate to the signs and symptoms identified in the assessment.

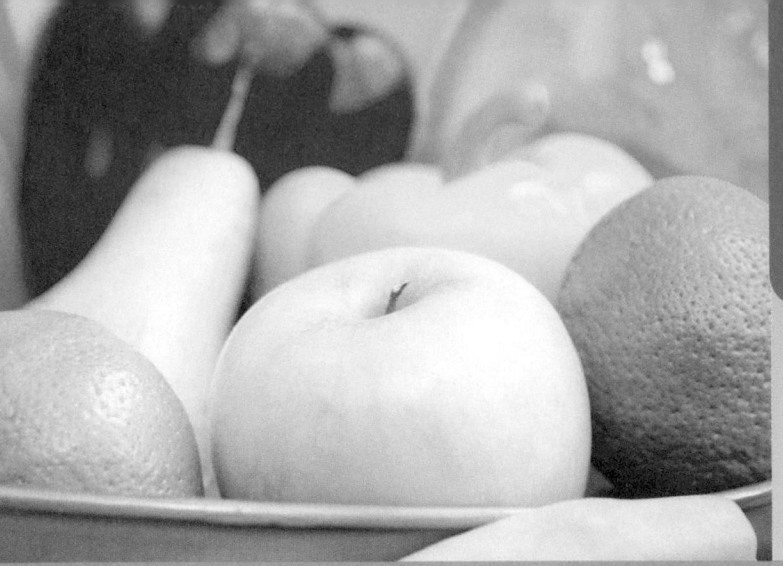

Assessment: Nutritional Genomics

KEY TERMS

alleles variants of a gene; refers to the different variations in DNA sequence that a gene may have within a population

autosomal-dominant refers to inheritance resulting when an allele on an autosome gives rise to a phenotype that is essentially the same whether a single copy of the allele is present (heterozygous, "carrier") or two copies are present (homozygous)

autosomal-recessive refers to inheritance resulting when a mutant allele carried on an autosome gives rise to a phenotype only when two copies of that allele are present; when only a single copy is present, the phenotype of the dominant normal allele masks that of the recessive mutant allele

autosome one of the 22 pairs of nonsex (X or Y) chromosomes

bioactive food components nutrients and other food components that convey information to the genetic material and effect a change in gene expression, such as by serving as ligands for signal transduction or for transcription control of gene expression

chromosomes subunits of DNA that are composed of DNA and protein; a means of packaging the large amount of DNA into the nucleus of a cell; humans have 23 pairs of chromosomes, and each gene has an address at a discrete location on a specific chromosome

codon a set of three nucleotides in deoxyribonucleic acid (DNA) arranged side-by-side; specifies an amino acid in the gene's protein product or a signal to start or stop transcription

conditionally essential referring to a nutrient that is required to be present in the diet of individuals who, because of their genetic makeup, need it in higher amounts for optimal body function rather than other individuals who, because of genetic makeup, are able to internally produce enough of the nutrient

deletion loss of genetic material; may be loss of a portion of a chromosome or a single nucleotide

deoxyribonucleic acid (DNA) the genetic material for humans and most organisms; consists of two strands of nucleotide building blocks arranged side by side on each strand; a linear arrangement of nucleotides that encodes the information needed to create and operate a living organism

dominant description of genes with characteristics that are expressed when only a single copy of allele is present

epigenetics heritable changes to the genome that do not alter the DNA sequence itself

ELSI ethical, legal, and social implications/issues of genetic research; initiative of the Human Genome Project to ensure that genetic information is used positively and fairly

exons the sequence of DNA nucleotides within a gene that codes for the amino acid sequence of the gene's protein product

genes a segment of DNA that encodes the instructions for synthesizing a protein

genetic code the combination of codons that specify the amino acids used to synthesize proteins

genetic engineering the alteration of genetic material, typically by recombinant DNA technology

genetics the science of how traits are inherited

gene variants changes in the typical sequence of nucleotides at a particular locus; although technically a mutation, terminology is evolving such that "mutation" connotes a harmful consequence, whereas "gene variant" connotes a change that in itself is not harmful but has a consequence to the functioning of the organism; changes in genes influenced by nutrition and other lifestyle choices are typically referred to as "gene variants" rather than "mutations"

genome the total of an organism's genetic information

genomic imprinting process by which the phenotype is influenced by whether an allele is inherited from the mother or the father; technically: epigenetic modification of a parental allele (or the chromosome on which it resides) in the gamete or zygote, resulting in differential expression of the two alleles in the somatic cells of the offspring

genomics a broader concept of genetics that includes not only genes, their proteins, and associations with diseases, but also the interaction among susceptibility factors and environmental factors and the potential for multiple genes, proteins, and environmental factors to influence health and well-being

genotype an individual's unique genetic makeup

heterozygous two different alleles at a single genetic locus; such an individual is called a heterozygote ("carrier"); in classical genetics a heterozygote has one normal/common allele and one variant/mutant allele; in nutrigenomics terminology, a heterozygous individual may have the more common allele and a variant allele or two different variant alleles

homozygous two identical alleles at a single genetic locus; such an individual is called a homozygote; in classical genetics a homozygote has either two normal alleles or two mutant alleles; in nutrigenomics terminology, a homozygous individual may have two normal/common alleles or two copies of the same variant allele

Human Genome Project a multinational collaborative effort to completely identify the sequence of nucleotides in the DNA of human beings and numerous other organisms, associate this sequence with genes and their protein products, and identify the function of these proteins

intervening sequences DNA sequences between two genes; most of DNA in humans, and function unknown

introns DNA sequences between two exons; these sequences are transcribed into mRNA and then removed before the translation of mRNA into its encoded protein

karyotype a visual display of chromosomes arranged in pairs according to size, from largest to smallest, followed by the X and Y chromosomes at the end

ligands molecules or cofactors that bind to another chemical entity to form a larger complex, such as small molecules binding to a receptor, a transcription factor, or the catalytic site of an enzyme; results in a change of activity, either activation or inhibition

maternal inheritance a trait is passed from mother to child; see mitochondrial inheritance

Mendelian inheritance the predictable inheritance pattern of a single gene trait; named after Gregor Mendel, who first described the rules of inheritance for single gene traits

messenger RNA (mRNA) a class of ribonucleic acid (RNA) in which the information in double-stranded DNA is converted into a single-stranded RNA molecule composed of nucleotides containing the sugar ribose, the mineral phosphorus, and one of four nitrogen-containing bases (adenine, cytosine, guanine or uracil); serves as an intermediary between DNA and the protein it encodes and directs the amino acid sequence of the protein being synthesized

metabolomics the study of how metabolites formed from cellular metabolism can be used as biomarkers for diagnostic and therapeutic purposes; useful in nutritional genomics as a means of monitoring efficacy of therapeutic interventions

mitochondrial inheritance the inheritance pattern of a trait carried on mitochondrial DNA, which is typically passed from mother to child

mutations changes in the DNA sequence that may change the protein whose synthesis is directed by the information in the DNA sequence; if the change alters the function of the protein significantly, a disease can result

nucleotide the building block of DNA and RNA; consists of the sugar ribose, the mineral phosphorus, and a nitrogen-containing purine or pyrimidine base; in DNA the base is adenine, cytosine, guanine, or thymine; in RNA it is adenine, cytosine, guanine, or uracil

nutrigenetics the study of the impact of an individual's genetic variants on their metabolic and physiologic function (i.e., on such parameters as level of nutrients required, ability to digest and absorb food, susceptibility to various diseases)

nutrigenomics abbreviation for nutritional genomics

nutritional genomics the study of the consequences of the influence of nutrients and other bioactive food components on the expression of the genetic material; also called nutrigenomics

pedigree a visual method of tracing the inheritance of traits through multiple generations of a family

penetrance the proportion of a population that has a disease-causing genotype and expresses the associated phenotype; when that proportion is less than 100%, the gene is said to have reduced penetrance

peroxisome proliferator-activated receptors (PPARS) antioxidants that protect against oxidative stress and inflammation; may be useful in reducing atherosclerosis

pharmacogenomics the study of the way genetic variations in key drug-metabolizing enzymes affect drug efficacy and safety; the genetic uniqueness of each individual confers different drug-metabolizing abilities; thus the same dosage of a drug may be toxic for one person, effective for another, and ineffective for another

phenotype the measurable expression of a gene, such as a physical trait or the level of a protein in a blood sample

polymorphism refers to one of multiple variations of a gene's sequence

post-transcriptional processing involves preparing the mRNA molecule for translation into protein, which involves removal of introns, capping of the 5-prime end, and the addition of a poly-adenosine "tail" to the 3-prime end of the mRNA

post-translational processing some proteins are synthesized in their precursor (or "pro" form) and must have chemical moieties added (e.g., carbohydrates) or removed (e.g., one or more amino acids) before becoming an active molecule

promoter a specific DNA sequence within a gene, just before the coding region, to which RNA polymerase can bind and transcribe the DNA into mRNA; an important region of a gene in terms of regulating gene expression

Continued

proteins molecules composed of amino acids; carry out the work of the living cell by serving as enzymes, receptors, transporters, hormones, antibodies, or communicators

proteomics the study of the structure and function of proteins in living organisms

recessive description of genes that are not expressed when only a single copy of an allele is present and that only express their phenotype when two copies are present

recombinant DNA hybrid DNA made from two different sources by cutting out a segment of DNA from one organism and inserting it into the DNA of another; recombinant DNA technology is also called genetic engineering

response element a DNA sequence in the 5-prime (5′) end of a gene (the regulatory region) to which transcription and other regulatory proteins can bind and control the expression of that gene

restriction endonucleases (restriction enzymes) bacterial enzymes that recognize a specific DNA sequence and cut the DNA at that location; bacteria contain thousands of these enzymes, and each has a particular DNA recognition site; useful as "molecular scissors" for precisely excising a sequence of DNA that can then be transferred into the DNA of another organism; some single nucleotide polymorphisms used for diagnostic purposes involve changes within restriction sites

sex chromosomes in humans, the X and Y chromosomes

sex-linked traits carried in the X or Y chromosome in humans, ranging from a change in a single nucleotide to the gain or loss of an entire chromosome

single nucleotide polymorphism (SNP) a type of structural variant of DNA that results from a change to the base component of a single nucleotide; when such a variant occurs in greater than 1% of a population, it is called a single nucleotide polymorphism

transcription the process of transferring information encoded in DNA to RNA; mRNA serves as an intermediary between DNA and the amino acid sequence of the protein to be synthesized

transcription factors proteins that bind to response elements within the 5-prime end of a gene to increase or decrease transcription of DNA into mRNA; bioactive components in food can bind to transcription factors and thereby influence gene expression

translation the process of transferring information encoded in mRNA into the amino acid sequence of a protein

xenobiotics chemicals that are foreign to the body

X-linked dominant an inheritance pattern in which an allele carried on the X chromosome gives rise to the variant phenotype in women when only one copy of the allele is present (this terminology is not relevant to males since they have only a single copy of the X chromosome)

X-linked recessive an inheritance pattern in which an allele carried on the X chromosome gives rise to the variant phenotype in women only when two copies of the allele are present; in males only a single copy of the allele is needed to give rise to the phenotype since male human beings have only a single copy of the X chromosome and will typically express the phenotype if their X chromosome carries the variant allele

Y-linked inheritance refers to an inheritance pattern resulting from an allele carried on the Y chromosome; expressed only in males

Nutrition professionals have long been intrigued and more than a little puzzled by the fact that one person can be lean and have an identical twin who is overweight, that the Pima Indians living in northern Mexico are lean even though their genetic counterparts in the American southwest are obese and have a high incidence of type 2 diabetes, and that a low-fat diet can reduce blood lipid levels in many people but not in everyone. What has become obvious is that, although people's genetic makeup sets the stage for one's susceptibilities to various illnesses, environmental factors such as nutrition and other lifestyle choices determine who among the susceptible actually develops a disease. The role of nutrients and other biologically active food components on gene expression is the focus of an exciting field of nutrition called nutritional genomics, often shortened to "nutrigenomics."

Genetic research is rapidly clarifying the association between genes and physiologic function. Mistakes in the genes are being correlated with dysfunction and disease. This evolving appreciation for the central role of genetics in health and disease is having a significant impact on the way health is viewed. As the details of the connections among genes, their protein products, and disease unfold, the focus of the health care system is shifting. During the past 50 years the focus has been on treating manifest disease, and physicians have had increasingly sophisticated drugs and technologies available with which to meet this challenge. However, with the understanding that disease is genetically based but environmentally influenced, the focus is on targeted intervention and prevention based on an understanding of the genes and environmental factors involved and the metabolic and physiologic consequences of their interactions.

The first practical applications of this changed focus in health care involved the medical and pharmaceutical aspects of acute care, but nutrition therapy is expected to figure prominently as a cornerstone of preventive care. Genetic research is helping to clarify the pathogenesis of disease, which includes the influence of bioactive components in food. From these advances will come diagnostic tests and susceptibility profiles that, coupled with genetic testing and family history analysis, will allow health care professionals to predict those at risk for particular disorders. Nutrition can mitigate the harmful effects of many genetic errors that result in disease, from supplying missing metabolites to altering gene expression. Thus nutrition therapy will become an increasingly important therapeutic tool for maximizing health and minimizing the risk of disease in susceptible individuals.

Perhaps more important, nutritional genomics will allow detection and intervention to promote health and prevent disease. The expectation is that, by analyzing individuals' genotypes at birth or prenatally, disease susceptibilities will be known from an early age and can be factored into the nutrition and lifestyle choices available to individuals throughout their lives. Beyond minimizing or preventing disease is the potential for maximizing human potential. Armed with extensive knowledge of one's potential and the associated lifestyle choices, humans will have the option to live to their full genetic potential throughout a long, healthy life.

The role of the nutrition professional in this new era of health promotion and disease prevention is pivotal. Nutrition professionals will play a prominent role in recommending preventive therapy using nutrition and lifestyle approaches. Increasingly nutrition recommendations will be customized to the genetic uniqueness of individuals and their particular disease susceptibilities and functional abilities. Nutrition professionals need to have a firm foundation in genetics, the associations among genes, disease, and environmental influences, and the role of nutrients and other food components in the modulation of gene expression.

THE HUMAN GENOME PROJECT

The **Human Genome Project** has been the impetus for this fundamental shift to integrating genetic principles into health care (see Useful Websites). This project began in 1990 as a multinational cooperative effort, with the goal of identifying each of the nucleotides in the deoxyribonucleic acid (DNA) that makes up the genetic material of human beings (the human **genome**). This aspect of the project was completed in 2003, in time to mark the 50-year anniversary of the identification of DNA as the genetic material. Currently the focus in laboratories throughout the world is on (1) cataloging the number of genes represented by the 3 billion nucleotides that make up human DNA; (2) identifying the protein products of each of these genes (functional units within the genome that contain information for making proteins) and understanding their function (the science of **proteomics**); (3) associating variations in genes with specific diseases; (4) understanding the way genes, proteins, and environmental factors interact to cause the physiologic dysfunction that results in disease; and (5) identifying metabolites that are useful in monitoring disease progression (the science of **metabolomics,** see German, 2005; German et al., 2003), and for nutritional applications. The expectation is that this type of detailed knowledge will lead to an understanding of ways to prevent disease and help people stay healthy.

Additional goals include sequencing the genomes of other organisms that are used as model systems in the laboratory to explore the molecular basis of disease and addressing the ethical, legal, and social implications **(ELSI)** of genetic research. This latter focus has been a strong commitment of the project from the beginning (see *Focus On:* ELSI: Ethical, Legal, and Social Implications of Genetics Research). The project has resulted in rapid progress in developing new technologic tools that are needed for the successful practical application of genetic technology within health care; improving their accuracy and speed; and lowering their cost. Sophisticated computer technology that can handle the vast amount of data generated by genetic technology has been developed and is the backbone of the new field called *bioinformatics*. In addition, project goals include the challenges of educating genetic scientists and clinicians and integrating the results of genetic research into clinical practice.

Clinical Applications

Much of the knowledge and many of the technologic advances gained from the Human Genome Project have clinical applications. Knowing the gene associated with a particular disease and its DNA sequence, its protein product, and the function of its protein product in promoting health or illness provides the basis for diagnostic assays. For example, tumors that appear identical physically can be distinguished by their genetic profiles. This distinction is important for effective therapy because different types of tumors respond to different therapeutic approaches. Not only can such assays be used to definitively reach a diagnosis, they also can be used for detection in those without symptoms, which allows interventions to be initiated before the symptoms of a disease become apparent.

Similarly, the information gained from the Human Genome Project has been pivotal in developing diagnostic assays to determine gene variations among people in terms of their drug-metabolizing enzymes (i.e., the science of **pharmacogenomics**). Each human being has the same basic set of drug-metabolizing enzymes, but the genes responsible for these enzymes can have numerous variations, which means that the resulting enzyme function varies also. One drug may have the intended effects on one person, be ineffective for another person, and actually be harmful to a third person. The ability to assess an individual's genetic makeup as it relates to the major drug-metabolizing genes helps the physician select the drug and dosage that will have the desired effect on that individual. Like drugs, food requires numerous enzymatic processes in order to be digested, absorbed, and used by the body's cells. The ability to tailor food to the genetic makeup of individuals is expected to be an important application of genetic research, similar to the applications of pharmacogenomics.

Another aspect of genetic research relevant to nutrition professionals is the applicability of the research to food production and safety. The field of food biotechnology is based on targeted manipulation of the genetic material of food crops and animals and on diagnostics for detecting contaminating organisms. Although modern biotechnology began long before the Human Genome Project, many of the

◎ FOCUS ON

ELSI: Ethical, Legal, and Social Implications of Genetics Research

Genetic technology gives humans the power to read the information in each of their genes and tell them who is likely to remain healthy or become ill—and with which type of illness. Genetic technology also gives humans the power to change their genetic information through gene therapy. Not surprisingly such power raises many concerns. From its inception, the Human Genome Project has addressed such implications of genetic research. Professionals from diverse disciplines are working together to identify and address the ethical, legal, and social implications (ELSI) that are emerging.

Among the issues being addressed are: (1) ways to ensure that genetic information about an individual will be used fairly and that the individual's privacy will be protected; (2) the best ways to implement genetic technologies into the practice of health care to ensure more targeted therapy with increased benefits and decreased side effects; (3) ways to handle the many developing ethical issues; and (4) the best ways to educate health care professionals so that they can meet the growing demand for genetics-savvy practitioners.

Protecting the privacy of the individual is of paramount concern. People are extremely concerned that genetic information can be misused (e.g., they might be discriminated against based on their genotypic profile). Federal legislation helps to ensure that such discrimination does not occur, but

it is likely to take some time before people are comfortable with the way genetic information is used. Ready and open access to such information is critical if the benefits of pre-symptomatic testing are to be realized. Ideally a person's genotypic profile should be just another important piece of information in analyzing health risk—like height, weight, and blood pressure. Reaching this point will take a concerted effort on many fronts.

In considering how best to implement genetic technologies into the practice of health care, the issue becomes "who should be tested?" Ethical issues abound. For example, should individuals be tested for a disease for which there is no cure? Do parents have the right to have their children, if they are minors, tested for a genetic disease without the children's consent? Do they have the right to withhold the results from the children? Should gene therapy be allowed on reproductive cells so that any corrected genes can be inherited by subsequent generations? Should human cloning be allowed? The basis of health care is becoming more intertwined with genetics and genetic technology, so what is the best way to educate those who are already in practice as health care professionals? What changes are needed so that future health care practitioners can be properly educated?

---

same basic genetic techniques are used, and the progress in streamlining genetic technology has had a beneficial effect on food biotechnology development.

GENOTYPE AND NUTRITION ASSESSMENT

The application expected to have the most dramatic impact on the way nutrition professionals approach their work is the ability to associate a **genotype,** an individual's unique genetic makeup, with that person's susceptibility to a particular disease. Genetic science and nutritional science are identifying the influence of specific food components and other environmental factors on gene expression. As this knowledge unfolds, protocols will be developed to guide the nutrition professional in the most efficacious therapy for ameliorating or, ideally, preventing the development of various nutrition-related diseases. Clients will arrive for nutrition counseling sessions with their genetic profiles in hand.

Nutrition professionals will need to be able to read the genotypes and know which diseases clients are susceptible to and which therapeutic approaches will be most effective in reducing their susceptibility. If nutrition professionals are going to be prepared for the era of genomic medicine, they must

build a foundation in genetics, biochemistry, metabolism, and other aspects of nutrition science. A number of overviews of genomics and its applications to nutrition are available (Afman and Müller, 2006; Corella and Ordovas, 2005; DeBusk, 2003; DeBusk et al., 2005; DeBusk and Joffe, 2006; German et al., 2005; Gillies, 2003; Kaput and Rodriquez, 2004; Kauwell 2005; Müller and Kersten, 2003; Olson, 2003; Ordovas and Mooser, 2004; Ordovas, 2006; Stover, 2003; Stover, 2004; Trujillo et al., 2006; van Ommen, 2004).

GENETIC FUNDAMENTALS

It is assumed that the reader has a basic understanding of DNA as the genetic material for humans and of chromosomal and molecular genetics (see *Focus On: DNA Transcription and RNA Translation* in Chapter 3). Among the key concepts at the chromosomal level are the packaging of DNA into chromosomes within the nucleus, the processes of meiosis and mitosis, autosomal and sex-linked inheritance, linkage and the mapping of genes, and chromosomal mutation and its consequences. At the molecular level, key basic concepts include: (1) the fact that information is encoded in DNA and must be decoded and converted into proteins that do the work of the cells through the processes of transcription, post-transcriptional processing, transla-

DNA, The Molecule of Life

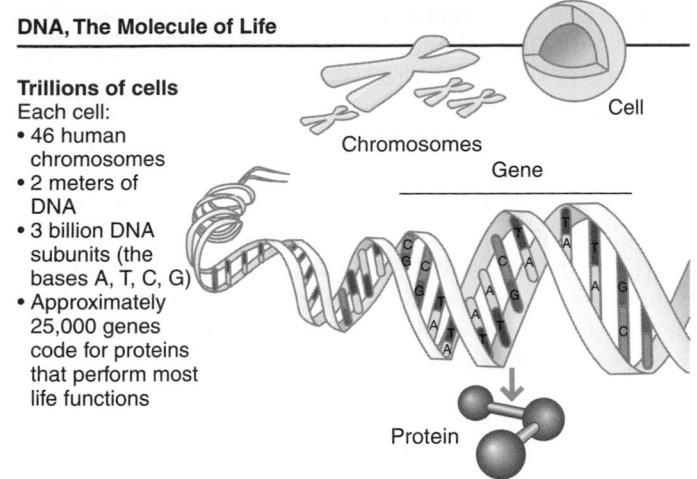

Trillions of cells
Each cell:
- 46 human chromosomes
- 2 meters of DNA
- 3 billion DNA subunits (the bases A, T, C, G)
- Approximately 25,000 genes code for proteins that perform most life functions

Cell

Chromosomes

Gene

Protein

FIGURE 13-1 Cells are the fundamental working units of every living system. All the instructions needed to direct their activities are contained within the chemical deoxyribonucleic acid (DNA). *(From U.S. Department of Energy; Human Genome Program: www.ornl.gov/hgmis.)*

tion, and post-translational processing; (2) the nature of a gene as the regulatory region (and its controlling elements, transcription factors, promoter sequence) and coding region (and its exons and introns); and (3) the concept of changes in the DNA nucleotide sequence and the impact on phenotype, including susceptibility to disease. Figures 13-1 through 13-5 review these fundamental genetic principles.

Figure 13-1 depicts DNA as the source of encoded information critical for operating the myriad of cells in the body and shows how the major components involved in decoding this information are interrelated. Figure 13-2 highlights the complex process of DNA replication required to faithfully duplicate each DNA base pair when synthesizing new strands of DNA for each new cell. Figure 13-3 focuses on the process of decoding the information in a gene by showing the important connection between the base sequence in the gene's DNA and the amino acid sequence of the protein that the gene encodes. In Figure 13-4 the impact of a change in the DNA base sequence on the protein's structure and function is illustrated. Sequence variations may cause major disruption to function and result in a disease state or in the minor differences that lead to physical and functional variability between individuals (Figure 13-5). Some of these minor differences do not affect health and others increase the risk of developing a disease.

Genetics and Genomics; Nutrigenetics and Nutrigenomics

Genetics is the science of inheritance. Historically genetics has focused on identifying the mechanisms by which traits are passed from parent to child, focusing on eye color and other readily observable characteristics. Certain rare diseases were found to be inherited from generation to generation; thus genetic disease came to be thought of as a separate disease category. Today scientists realize that, di-

DNA Replication Prior to Cell Division

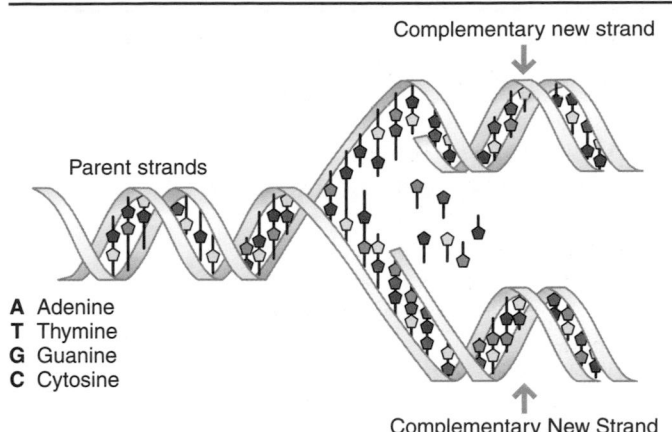

Complementary new strand

Parent strands

A Adenine
T Thymine
G Guanine
C Cytosine

Complementary New Strand

FIGURE 13-2 Each time a cell divides into two daughter cells, its full genome is duplicated; for humans and other complex organisms, this duplication occurs in the nucleus. During cell division the deoxyribonucleic acid (DNA) molecule unwinds, and the weak bonds between the base pairs break, allowing the strands to separate. Each strand directs the synthesis of a complementary new strand, with free nucleotides matching up with their complementary bases on each of the separated strands. Strict base-pairing rules are adhered to (i.e., adenine will pair only with thymine [an A-T pair] and cytosine with guanine [a C-G pair]). Each daughter cell receives one old and one new DNA strand. The cells' adherence to these base-pairing rules ensures that the new strand is an exact copy of the old one. This minimizes the incidence of errors (mutations) that may greatly affect the resulting organism or its offspring. *(From U.S. Department of Energy; Human Genome Program: www.ornl.gov/hgmis.)*

DNA Genetic Code Dictates Amino Acid Identity and Order

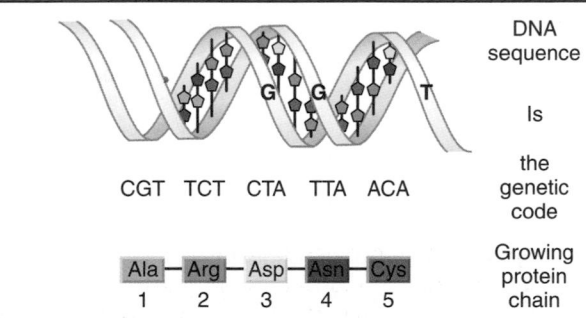

DNA sequence

Is

the genetic code

CGT TCT CTA TTA ACA

Ala — Arg — Asp — Asn — Cys
1   2   3   4   5

Growing protein chain

FIGURE 13-3 All living organisms are composed largely of proteins. Proteins are large, complex molecules made up of long chains of subunits called *amino acids.* Twenty different kinds of amino acids are usually found in proteins. Within the gene, each specific sequence of three deoxyribonucleic acid (DNA) bases (codons) directs the cells protein-synthesizing machinery to add specific amino acids. For example, the base sequence ATG codes for the amino acid methionine. Since 3 bases code for 1 amino acid, the protein coded by an average-sized gene (3000 bp) will contain 1000 amino acids. The genetic code is thus a series of codons that specify which amino acids are required to make up specific proteins. *ATG: A*, adenine; *T*, thymine; *G*, guanine; *bp*, base pairs. *(From U.S. Department of Energy; Human Genome Program: www.ornl.gov/hgmis.)*

DNA Sequence Variation in a Gene Can Change the Protein Produced by the Genetic Code

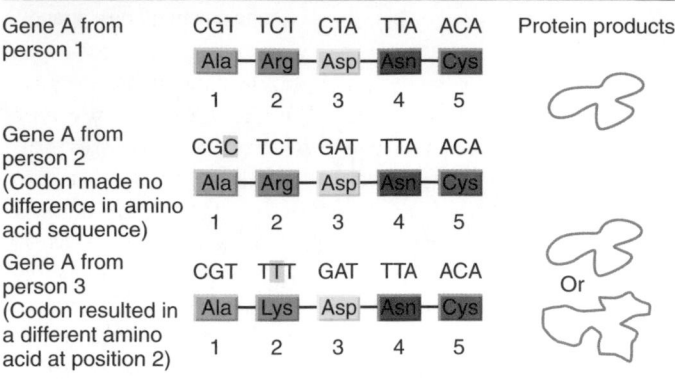

FIGURE 13-4 Some variations in a person's genetic code will have no effect on the protein that is produced; others can lead to disease or an increased susceptibility to a disease. *(From U.S. Department of Energy; Human Genome Program: www.ornl. gov/hgmis.)*

Health or Disease?

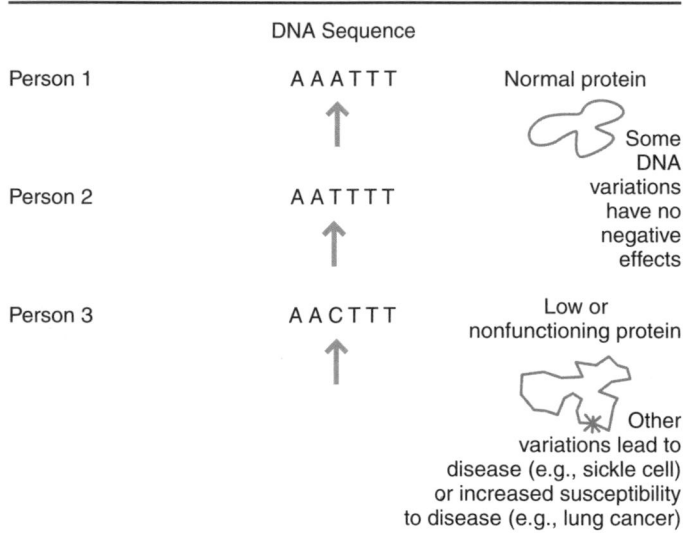

FIGURE 13-5 It is estimated that human beings differ from each other in only 0.1% of the total sequence of nucleotides that comprise deoxyribonucleic acid (DNA). These variations in genetic information are thought to be the basis for the physical and functional differences between individuals. *(From U.S. Department of Energy; Human Genome Program: www.ornl.gov/hgmis.)*

rectly or indirectly, all disease is connected to the information in the genes.

As a result, the science of genetics has significantly expanded in scope and includes the whole set of genetic information in an organism—its genome—and the interactions of the various genes and their protein products with each other and the environment. **Genomics** more accurately describes this complex, interactive situation. Whereas genetics was initially concerned with diseases that arose from a mistake in a single gene, genomics is more concerned with today's chronic diseases that result from the influence of multiple genes and multiple factors. Increasing emphasis is

being placed on determining the way various environmental factors influence whether individuals develop diseases to which they are susceptible.

Nutrigenetics concerns the study of how an individual's particular genetic variants affect function. For example, an individual with a particular variant in the 5,10-methylenetetrahydrofolate reductase (MTHFR) gene is likely to require more folate for optimal health than an individual with the more common version of this gene. Diet and other lifestyle choices will be geared towards the particular variants an individual has. On the other hand, **nutritional genomics** (often shortened to **"nutrigenomics"**) is the study of the impact of the environment on genes and their protein products, of how bioactive food components trigger changes in gene expression in response to the environment in which the organism lives.

Genetic Basics

Deoxyribonucleic acid (DNA) is the genetic material of all living organisms. The molecule is a double helix consisting of two strands of **nucleotide** subunits held together by hydrogen bonds. Each subunit contains the sugar deoxyribose, the mineral phosphorus, and one of four nitrogenous bases: adenine (A), thymine (T), guanine (G), or cytosine (C). The nucleotides are arranged side by side, and it is this linear arrangement that determines the particular information encoded in a stretch of DNA. In humans approximately 3 billion nucleotides make up the genome, which is housed in the nucleus of cells. A **gene** is a sequence of nucleotides that encodes the information for synthesizing a **protein**. An average gene is 3,000 nucleotides, and the human genome contains approximately 20,000 to 25,000 genes (www.ornl. gov/hgmis/project/info.html; Venter et al, 2001). Long stretches of nucleotides are often found between one gene and the next along the chromosome. Such sequences are called **intervening sequences** and comprise the majority of the DNA in humans. These sequences do not code for proteins, and their function is currently unknown.

To be useful to the cells, information in the DNA must first be decoded and translated into **proteins,** which perform the work of the organism at the cellular level. Information decoding occurs in two steps: (1) the process of **transcription,** during which the enzyme ribonucleic acid polymerase (RNA polymerase) converts DNA into an intermediate molecule **(messenger RNA [mRNA]),** and (2) a subsequent **translation** step in which the information encoded within the mRNA directs the assembly of amino acids into the protein molecule according to a universal **genetic code.** Genes have a common structure, with a **promoter** region where the binding of the RNA polymerase is controlled, which in turn controls transcription; and a coding (informational) region where the RNA polymerase transcribes the DNA into mRNA. Within the gene are sequences of nucleotides **(exons)** that correspond to the order of the amino acids in the gene's protein product. Each set of three nucleotides in the exon make up a **codon,** and each codon specifies an amino acid in the protein. A gene also contains **introns,** which are sequences interspersed between exons that do not code for amino acids. RNA polymerase transcribes the exons and introns into mRNA, which then must be processed **(post-transcriptional processing)** so that the introns are removed before the protein is synthesized. Some proteins need further **post-translational processing** before they are active, such as occurs with glycoproteins and with proenzymes and prohormones that must be cleaved before becoming active.

Upstream from the 5-prime end of the promoter region is the regulatory region, where control of the transcriptional process takes place. Within this region are sequences called **response elements** that serve as binding sites for regulatory proteins such as **transcription factors** and their bound **ligands.** The binding of transcription factors triggers the recruitment of additional proteins to form a protein complex that in turn changes the expression of that gene by changing the conformation of the promoter region and increases or decreases the ability of RNA polymerase to attach and begin transcription. The array of response elements within the promoter region can be quite complex, allowing for the binding of multiple transcription factors that in turn fine-tune the control of gene expression. It is through the binding of transcription factors to response elements that environmental factors such as the bioactive components in food convey to a gene that more or less of its protein product is needed.

The proteins coded for by the genes provide the metabolic machinery for the cells. They have various roles, such as enzymes, receptors, transporters, antibodies, hormones, and communicators. Changes within a gene can alter the amino acid sequence of the protein. Such changes in the DNA are technically called **mutations,** which historically have been associated with the concept of severely impairing the function of that protein and creating dysfunction within the cells. It only takes one change in a single nucleotide to cause a devastating disease. For example, in those with sickle cell disease a single nucleotide change causes a single amino acid change in the hemoglobin molecule, resulting in severe anemia and considerable pain, which is believed to result from a combination of the defective hemoglobin molecules being unable to carry adequate oxygen to the cells and the sickled, pointed shape of the defective hemoglobin as it moves through the blood vessels (see Chapter 31).

Changes in the DNA are the basis for evolution; thus clearly not all mutations are harmful; some actually improve function, and many, referred to as *silent mutations*, have no effect. Further, in the genomics era, researchers have found that many genes occur in slight variations on the "normal" (most common) version. The resulting proteins typically function slightly differently from the more common version but aren't enough in themselves to cause a debilitating disease. Such changes are also mutations but have come to be called **"gene variants"** to distinguish them from single gene changes that typically have a more detrimental effect. It's a matter of magnitude: "mutation" connotes significant difference that is typically deleterious, whereas "gene variant" connotes simply a difference, which has an impact but is not in itself sufficient to cause serious harm to the organism.

Thus genes exist in slightly different forms called **alleles.** As a result, genes have protein products with differing amino acid sequences (isoforms) and often different functions. When a particular allele exists in greater than 1% of the population, it is called a genetic **polymorphism,** and the gene is said to be polymorphic. Polymorphism is an important concept because it explains why human beings, although 99.9% alike genetically, are distinctively different. The 0.1% difference is sufficient to explain the obvious physical variations among humans. It is also the basis for more subtle differences that may not be readily observable, such as in the functional ability of a key metabolic enzyme. Such variations are thought to underlie many of the inconsistencies in therapeutic outcomes and nutritional intervention research, despite the relationships suggested by large epidemiologic studies.

The **single nucleotide polymorphism (SNP)** is the structural variant best studied to date. However, ongoing analysis of the human genome suggests that other structural variations may also play an important role in the genotypic and phenotypic variation among humans (Feuk et al., 2006). Loss or gain of nucleotides, duplication of sequences of nucleotides, and copy number variants also appear to have important functional consequences.

This finding of genetic variation within a population is changing the focus in health care from diagnostics to therapeutics. Each person is susceptible to a different set of diseases, handles environmental toxins differently, metabolizes molecules differently, and has slightly different nutritional requirements. These exciting discoveries are revolutionizing the way people think about health and disease and the clinical aspects of medicine, pharmacology, and nutrition. They have laid the foundation for personalized therapy in many aspects of health care.

Modes of Inheritance and Penetrance

Mendelian Inheritance

Each cell nucleus contains a complete set of genetic material (genome), divided among 22 pairs of **chromosomes,** called **autosomes,** and 2 **sex chromosomes,** for a total of 46 chromosomes. During mitosis (cell division) all 46 are duplicated and distributed to each new cell. During meiosis one member of each of the autosome and sex chromosome pairs is distributed to each haploid egg or sperm; the full set of 46 chromosomes is reconstituted on fertilization.

Because genes are carried on chromosomes, the rules governing the distribution of chromosomes during mitosis and meiosis also govern the distribution of genes. These rules describe the **Mendelian inheritance** of a gene, named after Gregor Mendel, who first deduced that the inheritance of traits was governed by a predictable set of rules. It is possible to track a gene through multiple generations by knowing these rules of inheritance. This transmission can be depicted as a **pedigree,** which shows the journey of a gene through multiple generations of a family and can be used to predict the probability of a gene being inherited by a particular family member. When the gene of interest is associated with a disease, pedigrees are helpful in predicting the probability that an individual will inherit the disease. The Family History Initiative implemented by the U.S. Surgeon General focuses on helping people construct their family pedigrees (see http://www.hhs.gov/familyhistory).

The Mendelian modes of inheritance are logical and predictable as a result of the distribution of chromosomes during meiosis. Autosomal refers to traits carried on one of the 22 pairs of autosomes; **sex-linked** refers to traits carried on either the X or Y chromosome. There are five classic modes of inheritance (Table 13-1). An individual's **genotype** obeys the laws of inheritance, but the **phenotype** (the measurable expression of the genotype) may not because of the following. Each gene in an individual is present in two copies (alleles), one on each chromosome. When the alleles are the same (either both normal/common or both mutant/variant), the individual is said to be **homozygous** for that gene. If the alleles are different (one normal, one mutant or two different mutant alleles), the individual is **heterozygous.**

Dominance and recessiveness refer to whether or not a trait is expressed in an individual that has one common (normal) allele and one variant (mutant) allele. Genes with characteristics that are expressed when only a single copy of an allele is present are called **dominant** (i.e., the phenotype of the variant allele is the predominant one). Alleles that do not dominate the genotype when only a single copy is present are called **recessive.** The changed allele is present in the genome but it is not expressed unless two copies are present.

Further confounding the nomenclature is the concept of penetrance. Even when a pedigree suggests that a gene should cause a particular individual to display a certain phenotype, the disease may not be evident. Such a gene is said to have reduced **penetrance,** meaning that not everyone who has the gene expresses it in a measurable form. Penetrance is a fascinating concept and of particular interest to nutrition professionals because it is likely the result of environmental factors modulating the expression of the gene,

which suggests that modifying such factors can potentially improve outcomes for those with some disorders.

Mitochondrial Inheritance

In addition to the genetic material in the nucleus, the mitochondria in each cell also contain DNA that gives rise to a limited number of proteins. The majority of these genes are involved in housekeeping needs related to maintenance of the mitochondrion and its energy-producing activities. As with nuclear DNA, changes in mitochondrial genes can lead to disease. For example, Wolfram syndrome, a form of diabetes with associated deafness, was one of the earliest disorders to be traced to mitochondrial DNA. Presently over 60 diseases that result from changes in mitochondrial DNA have been identified. For details of mitochondrially inherited disorders, search the Online Mendelian Inheritance in Man database at www.ncbi.nlm.nih.gov/omim.

Traits resulting from mitochondrial genes have a characteristic inheritance pattern, but it is non-Mendelian because mitochondria and their genetic material typically pass from mother to child, a mode of inheritance called **mitochondrial inheritance** or **maternal inheritance.** This biologic principle has become the basis for anthropologic studies that trace lineage and population migration patterns through the centuries. It also has provided a way to trace familial diseases caused by gene defects in mitochondrial DNA. However, as with other biologic processes, occasional mistakes occur; reports exist of mitochondrial DNA being passed from father to child. This phenomenon was first noted in mice and has subsequently been reported in humans (Gyllensten et al., 1991; Schwartz and Vissing, 2002).

Disease at the Chromosomal Level

In addition to changes in the DNA that occur within a single gene, disease can be caused by changes in the number of chromosomes or the arrangement of the DNA within a chromosome. Such disorders are detected by means of a **karyotype,** a visualization of all the chromosomes in picture form. Because chromosomes contain thousands of genes, such changes are typically harmful to the individual and often fatal. Examples of nonfatal chromosomal abnormalities include trisomy 21 (Down syndrome), trisomy 18 (cri du chat syndrome), and Klinefelter's syndrome, in which an extra chromosome 21, 18, or X is present, respectively. In addition, females with Turner's syndrome have only a single X chromosome. These disorders result from the gain or loss of all or a significant portion of a chromosome. Nutrition professionals play an important role in the therapy of such individuals because they typically have oral-motor problems that affect their nutritional status and cause growth problems in early life. Later in development, obesity is common in those with trisomy 21, Klinefelter's syndrome, and Turner's syndrome; and nutrition therapy is helpful in controlling weight and preventing the diabetes and cardiovascular complications that typically accompany obesity.

In contrast to syndromes caused by extra chromosomes, some syndromes are caused by the loss of a portion of a chromosome (a partial **deletion**); examples include

TABLE 13-1	
Classic Modes of Inheritance	
Mode of Inheritance	**Related Disorders**
Autosomal-dominant	Albright hereditary osteodystrophy, Marfan syndrome, familial hypercholesterolemia
Autosomal-recessive	Inborn errors of metabolism such as phenylketonuria, tyrosinemia, maple syrup urine disease
X-linked dominant	Fragile X syndrome
X-linked recessive	Nephrogenic diabetes insipidus, adrenoleukodystrophy, Duchenne muscular dystrophy disorder
Y-linked	Retinitis pigmentosa

Williams syndrome (chromosome 7 deletion), Beckwith-Wiedemann syndrome (chromosome 11 deletion), and some types of Prader-Willi and Angelman syndromes (chromosome 15 deletions). Those with these syndromes often have feeding difficulties and require the assistance of a knowledgeable nutrition professional. Williams syndrome is characterized by cardiac defects that have nutritional implications. Beckwith-Wiedemann syndrome is characterized by organ overgrowth, including an oversized tongue, which leads to feeding difficulties and for many infants hypoglycemia. Prader-Willi and Angelman's syndromes typically have abnormal feeding behaviors. Many more chromosomal disorders that have nutritional consequences are known. In people with such abnormalities, therapy is often complicated by mental retardation, ranging from mild to severe. The expertise of a knowledgeable nutrition professional is invaluable in mitigating the detrimental effects of these disorders on nutritional status (see Chapter 45).

Epigenetics and Genomic Imprinting

Prader-Willi and Angelman's syndromes can be used to illustrate an additional genetic phenomenon, known as **epigenetics,** specifically genomic imprinting. Epigenetics is characterized by alterations to the DNA molecule that affect gene expression but do not change the nucleotide sequence (Egger et al., 2004; Holliday, 2005; Santos et al., 2005). There are at least three known mechanisms involved: (1) DNA methylation, (2) histone modification, and (3) genomic imprinting. The covalent attachment of methyl groups to CpG dinucleotides within the regulatory region of genes results in silencing of transcription of that gene. This mechanism appears to be useful for silencing DNA that is not needed in a particular cell type or that, when activated, may result in abnormal growth that can lead to cancer. On a larger scale, histone proteins are important in silencing large regions of chromosomes and thereby multiple genes. Covalent modification of histone proteins by processes such as acetylation, methylation, phosphorylation, or ubiquitination are critical to whether chromosomal DNA can decondense and become available for transcription.

Genomic imprinting is an epigenetic phenomenon that results when the genetic change is the same but different phenotypes result, depending on whether an allele (or chromosome region) was inherited from the mother or the father. In some forms of Prader-Willi and Angelman's syndromes, when both abnormal alleles are inherited from the mother, the child develops Prader-Willi. When both abnormal alleles are inherited from the father, the result is Angelman's. Both syndromes are characterized by intellectual disabilities, but Prader-Willi individuals also experience a lack of perception of satiety, which leads to overeating and lifelong challenges with morbid obesity.

Epigenetics, including gene silencing and genomic imprinting, is under active investigation presently and is explored more thoroughly in reviews by Egger et al., 2006; Feinberg et al., 2006; Mathers, 2005; Santos et al., 2005; and Waterland and Jirtle, 2004. In addition to their association with the disorders described here, these epigenetic phenomena have implications for the development of cancer.

Disease at the Molecular Level

Insight into disease at the molecular level has been among the major advances of genetic research and its applications to health care, and form the majority of situations related to nutritional genomics. Changes in the DNA at the molecular level usually involve a single nucleotide change or several nucleotides within a single gene. Typically one nucleotide is substituted for another, or a nucleotide is added to or deleted from the DNA sequence, but larger-scale changes involving the deletion or addition of multiple nucleotides can also occur. These changes can occur within the regulatory region or the protein coding region of the gene. Alterations in the regulatory region may increase or decrease the quantity of protein produced or alter the ability of the gene to respond to environmental signals. Alterations in the coding region may affect the amino acid sequence of the protein, which in turn can affect the conformation and function of the protein.

The vast majority of human genes reside on nuclear chromosomes and are transmitted by Mendelian inheritance. The **autosomal-dominant** single gene disorders that have nutritional implications include several that result in oral-motor problems, growth problems, increased weight gain, and occasionally difficulties with constipation. Examples include Albright hereditary osteodystrophy, which commonly results in dental problems, obesity, hypocalcemia, and hyperphosphatemia; chondrodysplasias, which often result in oral-motor problems and obesity; and Marfan syndrome, which promotes cardiac disease susceptibility and excessive growth and its concomitant nutritional needs. Familial hypercholesterolemia results in a defective low-density lipoprotein (LDL) receptor and elevated levels of cholesterol, which leads to atherosclerosis.

Genetic Metabolic Disorders

Autosomal-recessive disorders are by far the most common of the Mendelian inherited disorders and include numerous metabolic disorders of amino acid, carbohydrate, and lipid metabolism—disorders called *inborn errors of metabolism* (see Chapter 44 for an in depth treatment of these disorders). Dietary modification is a primary treatment modality for these disorders. Phenylketonuria (PKU) is a classic example of this type of disorder. The gene coding for the enzyme phenylalanine hydroxylase is defective, leading to an inability to convert the amino acid phenylalanine to tyrosine. Lifelong dietary restriction of phenylalanine enables individuals with PKU to live into adulthood and enjoy a quality life. Tyrosinemia is a similar disorder of amino acid metabolism caused by a mutation in the gene for the enzyme fumarylacetoacetate hydrolase. Dietary restriction of tyrosine and phenylalanine is essential to prevent the accumulation of these amino acids. In maple syrup urine disease, the metabolic defect is branched-chain α-keto acid decarboxylase, a multimeric enzyme complex encoded by six genes.

A mutation in any one of these genes can result in accumulation of α-keto acids in the urine, which produces an odor similar to maple syrup. Failure to limit branched-chain amino acid intake leads to mental retardation, seizures, and death (see Chapter 44).

Another inborn error of amino acid metabolism, classic homocystinuria, is of particular interest because it led to the realization that an elevated blood level of homocysteine is an independent risk factor for cardiovascular disease, an idea originally proposed by McCully in 1969. A defect in the vitamin B$_6$–requiring enzyme cystathionine β-synthase prevents the conversion of homocysteine to cystathionine. Homocysteine accumulates and can promote atherosclerosis and form homocystine, which leads to abnormal collagen cross-linking and osteoporosis. Nutrition therapy is multipronged, depending on the specific genetic defect. Some individuals have an enzyme defect that requires a high concentration of the vitamin B$_6$ cofactor for activity. Others are not responsive to B$_6$ and need a combination of folate, vitamin B$_{12}$, choline, and betaine to convert homocysteine to methionine; and others must limit their methionine intake. At least three forms of homocystinuria exist, each requiring a different nutritional approach. The ability to use genetic analysis to distinguish these similar disorders has been a technologic advance (see Chapters 15 and 31).

Autosomal-recessive inborn errors of carbohydrate metabolism include galactosemia and hereditary fructose intolerance. A mutation in the gene encoding galactose-1-phosphate uridyl transferase prevents the sugar galactose from being converted to glucose. Dietary restriction of galactose prevents its accumulation and the accompanying failure to thrive, developmental delay, and hepatic insufficiency. In hereditary fructose intolerance, fructose cannot be converted to glucose because of a defect in the gene encoding fructose 1,6-biphosphate aldolase. Breast-fed infants are typically asymptomatic until fruit is added to the diet. Nutrition therapy involves the elimination of fructose and the fructose-containing disaccharide sucrose (see Chapter 44).

Autosomal-recessive disorders of lipid metabolism also exist. The most common is a deficiency of medium-chain acyl-coenzyme A (acyl-CoA) dehydrogenase. Nutrition therapy centers around preventing the accumulation of toxic fatty acid intermediates that, when not controlled, can lead to death (see Chapter 44 and Isaacs and Zand, 2006).

Sex-Linked Disorders

Examples of X-linked disorders with nutritional implications include the **X-linked dominant** fragile X syndrome and the **X-linked recessive** nephrogenic diabetes insipidus, adrenoleukodystrophy, and Duchenne muscular dystrophy disorders. Fragile X syndrome is characterized by developmental delays and mental retardation. The name *fragile X* comes from the discovery that cells grown in a culture medium deficient in the B vitamin folic acid break near the tip of the long arm of the X chromosome. Whether folate nutriture influences the in vivo expression of this syndrome is unclear. Individuals with X-linked recessive nephrogenic diabetes insipidus are unable to concentrate urine and exhibit polyuria and polydipsia. This disorder is usually detected in infancy and can manifest as dehydration, poor feeding, vomiting, and failure to thrive. X-linked recessive adrenoleukodystrophy results from a defect in the enzyme that breaks down very long–chain fatty acids. These fats accumulate and lead to brain and adrenal dysfunction and ultimately motor dysfunction. X-linked recessive Duchenne muscular dystrophy is characterized by fatty infiltration of muscles and extreme muscle wasting. Children are typically confined to a wheelchair by age 11 and need assistance with feeding.

Y-linked inheritance disorders involve male sex determination and physiologic "housekeeping functions." To date no nutrition-related disorders have been conclusively assigned to the Y chromosome.

Progressing beyond knowing the chromosomal position of a disease trait to associating the disease with a particular gene and understanding its functional consequences has required the development of sophisticated genetic technologies for analyzing the molecular basis of changes in DNA. One of the key technologic advances has been **recombinant DNA,** which has allowed major progress in terms of studying genes, their functions, and the regulation of their expression. Using bacteria-derived **restriction endonucleases (restriction enzymes),** researchers can cut the DNA in precise places along the nucleotide chain, isolate the DNA fragments from one organism, and insert them into the genetic material of another.

This basic approach has been the cornerstone of many molecular techniques that are now routinely used. It is the foundation for **genetic engineering** and the production of human therapeutic proteins such as insulin and growth hormone. It paved the way for DNA sequencing, which is used to identify the sequence of nucleotides within a gene and pinpoint the exact location of any change. Recombinant DNA is also the basis for diagnostic tests that can detect variation in DNA sequences that predict disease susceptibilities. Still another important application is its role in gene therapy, by which a corrected gene sequence can be introduced into the cells of an individual with a disease-causing mutation.

Additional genetic technologies that have been critical in the development of molecular medicine and the ability to associate genes with diseases include transgenic technology and single nucleotide polymorphisms (SNPs, pronounced "snips") technology. The transgenic mouse is an example of a model system, which is an experimental approach used in research laboratories to explore questions that cannot be readily addressed in a human being, such as the need to control mating partners and timing or to control nutrient intake. Because the mouse and human share many of the same genes, the ability to manipulate the genetic material of the mouse and examine the impact on metabolism and physiologic function has been invaluable for understanding health and disease in the human.

Several approaches are used with transgenic mice. In the "knockout" mouse, a gene is altered ("knocked out") so that the normal protein is no longer made. Alternatively a gene can be altered so that it expresses too much or too little of its product. Regulatory sequences can be altered so that a gene no longer responds appropriately to environmental signals. In these ways the normal function of a gene can be determined, the effects of over expressing or under expressing a gene can be studied, and the details of the communication process between signals outside the organism and the genetic material inside the organism can be determined. Transgenic mice are particularly valuable for studying gene-diet interactions.

SNPs are a common type of gene variant found in greater than 1% of the population. It is the cumulative effect of these subtle variations and other types of gene variations that is thought to distinguish one member of a species from another. A growing number of SNPs are being identified that are linked to an increased susceptibility to disease. Once such an association has been confirmed, diagnostic screening tests can be developed, which allow for early detection of disease susceptibility. When coupled with appropriate therapeutic interventions, the potential exists for minimizing the impact of the disease as well as potentially preventing its manifestation. It is these types of changes in the DNA that are increasingly of interest to nutrition professionals.

Food and dietary supplement choices, exercise habits, alcohol and tobacco use, and approaches to handling chronic stressors are all important lifestyle choices that individuals need to consider when attempting to minimize their risk of developing disease and maximizing their genetic potential. A genetics-savvy nutrition professional is invaluable in helping people understand their disease susceptibilities and their options for enjoying lifelong health.

Disease at the Mitochondrial Level

Human mitochondrial DNA codes for 13 proteins and the 2 ribosomal RNAs and 22 transfer RNAs needed to synthesize these proteins (Report of the Committee of the Human Mitochondrial Genome, 2002). A major function of mitochondria is to produce cellular energy through the respiratory system. Not surprisingly, alterations in mitochondrial DNA are typically degenerative, affect tissues with a high demand for oxidative phosphorylation, and have considerably varied clinical manifestations, including neurologic disease, cardiomyopathy, and skeletal myopathy (MITOMAP, 2005; Shoffner and Wallace, 1992). Maternally inherited diabetes and deafness have also been traced to changes in mitochondrial DNA (MITOMAP, 2005).

GENETICS AND NUTRITION THERAPY

Each of the above examples concerning the impact of chromosomal and single-gene mutations on nutrition status illustrates the importance of nutrition therapy to individuals with these disorders. Nutrition professionals have long played valuable roles in caring for individuals with these

disorders and will continue to do so as states steadily expand their newborn screening programs to initiate appropriate nutrition therapies as early as possible in the life of the infant. In addition to this role in classical genetic applications to nutrition, the rapid development of nutritional genomics is expanding the role of the nutrition professional beyond these rare disorders and into the more prevalent chronic diseases such as cardiovascular disease, cancer, diabetes, inflammatory disorders, osteoporosis, and many others.

Progress in identifying gene variants associated with particular chronic disorders and understanding the interaction of **bioactive food components** with these variants has led to the need for nutrition professionals that can interpret genetic screening information and link the findings to appropriate nutrition interventions. Nutrition professionals will be needed as nutrigenomics practitioners and as coaches to assist individuals in making informed lifestyle choices and integrating them into their daily lives. Overviews of this emerging science and its relevance to nutrition professionals are provided by several authors (Kauwell, 2005; Mutch et al., 2005; DeBusk and Joffe, 2006).

As with any evolving science, early research often generates a bewildering array of seemingly unrelated facts. It's helpful to construct an organized "big-picture" framework on which to "hang" facts as they emerge and to continue to fill in the framework over time as the picture becomes clearer. One approach that works well is to organize nutritional genomics in terms of the ways in which bioactive food components affect genetic outcomes: (1) by influencing *metabolic processes*, either by supplying components that are in inadequate supply due to genetic limitations or by eliminating components that trigger harmful reactions, again as the result of genetic limitations, and (2) by influencing *gene expression*, either directly by interacting with transcription factors or indirectly by serving as transducers for signal transduction cascades that ultimately influence transcription. In the following section examples of each of these roles of bioactive components in food will be explored.

Nutritional Genomic Influences on Metabolic Processes

The interplay between nutrition and genetics varies from being straightforward to being intriguingly complex. The most straightforward is the direct correlation between a faulty gene, a defective protein, a deficient level of a metabolite, and a resultant disease state that is passed on through Mendelian inheritance and is responsive to nutrition therapy. Nutrition professionals are quite familiar with this type of interaction in that the inborn errors of metabolism discussed earlier are good examples of such interactions (see Chapter 44). The use of diet to supply essential nutrients is another such example. Certain amino acids, fatty acids, vitamins, and minerals cannot be synthesized by the body and must be provided through the diet to prevent dysfunction and disease. For example, human beings lack the enzyme gulonolactone oxidase and cannot synthesize vitamin C. If dietary vitamin C intake is below needed levels, individuals are at risk for developing scurvy. Similarly, human beings are unable to synthesize the essential amino and fatty acids and must obtain these essential nutrients from the diet.

Although nutrition professionals have long known of the need for supplying essential nutrients through the diet (or risk disease consequences), what's new is an understanding of the genetic basis for these nutrient requirements and the realization that nutrition therapy can circumvent genetic limitations by supplying the missing nutrients. This realization provides a hint of what is to come in nutritional genomics (i.e., nutrition therapy as a tool for compensating for changes in the DNA that lead to disease susceptibility).

At the molecular level a change in the DNA may affect the conformation of a protein and prevent it from binding with its substrate, resulting in the disease states discussed previously. Conformational changes may also alter the affinity of a protein for its nutrient cofactor. Approximately 50 metabolic reactions that involve enzymes with decreased affinities for their cofactors and that require high levels of a nutrient to restore function have been identified (Ames et al., 2002). Most of the supplementation levels are well in excess of the normally recommended levels, which highlights the importance of remembering that each individual is genetically unique and has distinct metabolic needs. Although generalized guidelines for recommended nutrient levels are helpful, individuals may have genetic variants that require them to consume significantly more or less of certain nutrients than the general recommendation. It is becoming possible to look at nutrients as being **conditionally essential** in some individuals. This refers to a nutrient that is required to be present in the diet of individuals who, because of their genetic makeup need it in higher amounts for optimal body function than other individuals who because of genetic makeup are able to internally produce enough of the nutrient. This approach to establishing global dietary recommended intakes based on genetic makeup is another area of nutritional genomics that is under active investigation (Stover, 2006).

A well-established example of the need to tailor nutrition recommendations to genotype is illustrated with the enzyme MTHFR, which produces the biologically active form of folate (5-methyltetrahydrofolate). Folate is essential for the conversion of the metabolic intermediate homocysteine to *S*-adenosylmethionine, a critical methyl donor to numerous metabolic reactions, including those involved in synthesizing nucleic acids (see Chapter 31). A common variation in the MTHFR gene is the 677C>T gene variant, which involves substitution of thymine for cytosine at position 677. The resultant enzyme is thermolabile and has reduced activity, causing homocysteine to accumulate (Kang et al., 1988). An elevated blood level of homocysteine is an independent risk factor for vascular disease (see Chapter 32). It also increases the risk of neural tube defects in developing fetuses, which led to required fortification of cereal grains with folate in the United States to ensure adequate levels in women of childbearing age (see Chapter 5).

This gene variant has implications for people of all ages, however. The extent to which homocysteine accumulates and responds to supplementation with one or more of the B vitamins folate, B_2, B_6, and B_{12}, as well as the forms of folate that are most effective, is related to the genotype of the individual (Bailey et al., 2002; Fohr et al., 2002; Kauwell et al., 2000a, 2000b). A recent study by this group extended the complexity of homocysteine metabolism by demonstrating that B_{12} genotype was also important (von Castel-Dunwoody et al., 2005). Such findings suggest that nutrient recommendations tailored to genotype would be beneficial.

In addition to mutations in enzymes involved in metabolic pathways, disease-causing changes can occur in genes coding for other types of proteins such as transport proteins, membrane receptors, hormones, and transcription factors. Mutations that increase the transport of iron (hereditary hemochromatosis) or copper (Wilson's disease) to higher than normal levels have nutritional implications (see Chapter 31). Mutations in vitamin D receptors are associated with deleterious effects on bone health but also more globally throughout the body since vitamin D is a hormone involved in several different metabolic and regulatory processes. Errors in the gene coding for insulin can result in structural changes in the insulin hormone and lead to dysglycemia, as can mutations in the insulin receptor. Many proteins such as kinases, cytokines, and transcription factors that are involved in critical signaling cascades are subject to mutational changes and altered activities.

Nutritional Genomic Influences on Gene Expression

In addition to compensating for metabolic limitations, nutrients and other bioactive food components can influence gene expression. This ability has long been known from studies with lower organisms, such as the *lac* and *tryp* operons in bacteria. In these situations the organism "senses" the presence of a nutrient in its external environment and alters its gene expression accordingly. In the case of lactose, the proteins required to use lactose as an energy source are induced by transcriptional regulation of the genes that code for the lactose transport system and the enzyme that degrades lactose into glucose and galactose. The opposite occurs when tryptophan is present in the environment: the organism inhibits the endogenous biosynthesis of tryptophan by inhibiting transcription of the genes that encode tryptophan biosynthetic proteins. In this way even the most primitive organisms monitor and respond to their environment to deploy their resources most efficiently.

Not surprisingly, higher organisms have similar mechanisms by which they monitor the environment that bathes their cells and alter cellular activity as needed. An example is the response of cells to the presence of glucose. Insulin is secreted and binds to its receptor on the surface of skeletal muscle cells and initiates a stepwise biochemical signaling cascade that causes the translocation of GLUT 4, the receptor that admits glucose into muscle cells. Similarly, a drop in blood sugar levels triggers the release of epinephrine and glucagon that, in turn, bind to cell surface receptors in the liver and skeletal muscle and, through signal transduction, stimulate glycogen breakdown to glucose to restore blood sugar levels.

Nutrients and other bioactive food components can also serve as **ligands**, molecules that bind to specific sequences (response elements) within a gene's regulatory region. Binding results in a change in gene expression through the regulation of the transcription process. Transcription may be turned on or off, or it may be modulated in terms of increasing or decreasing the rate. Examples of such food components are the polyunsaturated omega-3 fatty acids. These fats are important in decreasing inflammation. In addition to serving as precursors for the synthesis of antiinflammatory eicosanoids, they also serve to decrease the expression of key genes that lead to inflammatory cytokine production such as tumor necrosis factor–α and the interleukin-1 family of genes. The role of omega-3 and other polyunsaturated fatty acids in regulating the expression of genes involved in lipid metabolism has become increasingly clear (Jump, 2004; Sampath and Ntambi, 2004; Sampath and Ntambi, 2005).

The omega-3 and omega-6 fatty acids have also been found to serve as ligands for the **peroxisome proliferator-activated receptor (PPAR)** transcription factors. The PPARs function as lipid sensors and regulate lipid and lipoprotein metabolism; glucose homeostasis; and cell proliferation and differentiation, especially of adipocytes; and the formation of foam cells from monocytes. They are known to be important in insulin resistance and obesity caused by a high-fat diet (Hihi et al., 2002; Kadowaki et al., 2002).

The PPARgamma isoform is the best studied to date and plays a critical role in adipocyte differentiation and gene expression. To influence the expression of the genes under its control, this transcription factor must first complex with a second transcription factor, the retinoic X receptor (RXR). Once each has bound its ligand, omega-3 or omega-6 fat and retinoic acid (vitamin A derivative), respectively, the PPAR-RXR complex can then bind to a specific DNA sequence (response element) within the regulatory region of the gene. Binding results in a conformational change in the structure of the DNA molecule that results in RNA polymerase being able to bind and transcribe the PPARgamma-regulated genes, leading to a host of lipogenic and proinflammatory activities. The thiazolidenedione (TZD) class of drugs act as PPARgamma agonists and mimic this effect, thereby serving as useful drugs for insulin resistance and type 2 diabetes.

PPARgamma and RXR are just two members of the 48-member nuclear family of receptors, including the RXRs, PPARs, the liver X receptors (LXRs), the farnesoid X receptor, the constitutive androstane receptor (CAR), the sterol regulatory element binding proteins (SREBPs), and the nuclear vitamin D receptor (VDRnuc). These nuclear receptors serve as transcription factors, and their ligands are either provided by the diet or made endogenously, such as cholesterol, steroid hormones, bile acids, **xenobiotics** (foreign chemicals such as mercury or lead), and the active form of vitamin D (Chawla et al., 2001; Jacobs and Lewis, 2002).

Identifying the genetic and biochemical mechanisms underlying health and disease provides the basis for developing individualized intervention and prevention strategies. In the case of the omega-3 fatty acids, researchers are actively seeking conditions under which dietary omega-3s can be used to decrease inflammation and increase insulin sensitivity.

Complex Genetic-Nutrition Connections

In contrast to most single gene disorders in which the change in the DNA is known, the abnormal protein can be identified and analyzed, and the resulting phenotype is clearly defined, chronic disorders (e.g., cardiovascular disease, cancer, diabetes, osteoporosis, inflammatory disorders) are far more complex. First, they involve multiple genes, each of which comes in more than one variation, that likely contribute in small ways to the overall condition rather than have the dramatic impact that is more typical with single-gene disorders. Second, the genes are more likely to be influenced by environmental factors, which makes the resulting phenotype murkier than with single-gene disorders. An individual might have gene variants that predispose to a particular chronic disorder but, depending on that individual's nutritional and other lifestyle choices, the disorder may or may not develop.

Genetic Variability

Certainly it's far more challenging to pin down the details of such disorders when multiple genes and environmental factors are involved. Nutrition professionals are similarly challenged in working with clients with these nutrition-related disorders in terms of the heterogeneity of responses to the same therapeutic approach. Given the genetic variability among individuals in a population, the high degree of variability in client response to nutrition therapy should not be surprising. Despite these challenges, the upsides of such disorders are that the gene variants involved affect the magnitude of response rather than create a life-threatening situation and many of the variants are responsive to diet and other lifestyle parameters. These genes and their variants are of most interest to nutrition professionals in the era of nutritional genomics because they confer susceptibility to disease but that susceptibility can be minimized through informed lifestyle choices.

The major focus of nutritional genomics research is on identifying (1) gene-disease associations, (2) the dietary components that influence these associations, (3) the mechanisms by which dietary components exert their effects, and (4) the genotypes that benefit most from particular dietary choices. The practical applications of this research include a new set of tools that nutrition professionals can use to identify disease susceptibilities and a growing body of knowledge that will form the basis for developing strategies for disease prevention and intervention that are specifically targeted to the underlying genetic mechanisms.

The following section takes a brief look at some of the key diet-related genes and their known variants and how these variants affect the person's response to diet. Keep in mind that chronic diseases involve complex interactions among genes and bioactive food components, and unraveling the details will require population and intervention studies large enough to have the statistical power needed to draw meaningful conclusions. Although what is known today is but the tip of the iceberg compared to what will come in the years ahead, it is clear that integrating knowledge of gene variants into dietary recommendations for populations and individuals will increasingly play a role in nutrition counseling and policy making.

Cardiovascular Disease

Nutrition professionals who work with clients with dyslipidemia know firsthand the high degree of individual variability of responses to the widely recommended dietary interventions. These therapies are used primarily to lower elevated blood levels of LDL cholesterol (LDL-C), raise high-density lipoprotein cholesterol (HDL-C), and lower triglycerides (TGs). The standard dietary approach is a diet low in saturated fat and cholesterol, with increased content of polyunsaturated fats. Response across a population has been quite varied, ranging from reduced LDL-C levels and TGs in some, to decreased HDL-C levels to elevated TGs. Further, some have had their LDL-C levels respond dramatically to dietary oat bran and other soluble fibers, whereas others have had more modest responses. In some a low-fat diet has caused a shift to a lipid pattern that is more atherogenic than the original one (first reported by Dreon et al. in 1994). With the advent of nutritional genomics, it's becoming clear that an individual's genetic makeup (genotype) is an important factor in this response and that dietary interventions must be matched to genotypes to effect the intended lipid-lowering responses. The underlying basis for the seemingly inconsistent results is the genetic heterogeneity of the population being studied.

A number of such genes have already been identified and include those involved with postprandial lipoprotein and triglyceride response, homocysteine metabolism, hypertension, blood-clotting, and inflammation. Among the genes that have been the most extensively studied in terms of their gene-diet interactions are those that code for apolipoprotein E (APOE), apolipoprotein A-1 (APOA-1), cholesterol esteryl transport protein (CETP), hepatic lipase (LIPC), lipoxygenase-5 (ALOX5), perilipin (PLIN), MTHFR, angiotensinogen (AGT), the interleukin-1 family (IL1), interleukin-6 (IL6), and tumor necrosis factor-α (TNF-α).

Data from the Framingham Study provide an example of how knowing the client's genetic variants can be helpful in developing effective nutritional interventions (Marín et al., 2002; Ordovas et al., 2002a). The APOA-1 gene codes for apolipoprotein A-1, the primary protein in HDL (see Chapters 15 and 32 for a discussion of this laboratory assessment). One of the variants that has been identified to be diet-related is −75G>A, in which the typical guanine has been replaced with an adenine at position 75 within the regulatory region of the APOA-1 gene (the "−" sign denotes a position before the first nucleotide—position "0"—of the gene's coding region). In women with the more common G allele, increasing dietary polyunsaturated fat (PUFA)

levels from less than 4% of total energy to 4% to 8% to greater than 8% resulted in a corresponding decline in HDL levels as PUFA levels increase. However, in women with the A allele, increasing PUFA concentrations increased HDL levels. The effect was most dramatic in those with two copies of the A allele and intermediate in those with one copy. The practical application is that manipulating the PUFA levels will have different effects on HDL levels, depending on which variant an individual has.

A sampling of other diet-responsive gene variants that have implications for nutrition therapy related to preventing and treating cardiovascular disease include APOE gene variants and the responses to dietary fat, soluble fiber, and alcohol (Corella et al., 2001; Corella and Ordovas, 2005; Nicklas et al., 2002; Masson et al., 2003; Djoussé, 2004); APOE variants and the response of LDL and HDL to exercise training (Taimela et al., 1996, Hagberg et al., 2000); CETP variants and effects on HDL levels, lipid-modifying response to statin drugs, and response of lipid parameters to physical activity (Corella et al., 2001; Brousseau et al., 2002; Masson et al., 2003; Winkelmann et al., 2003; Ayyobi et al., 2005); APOE, CETP, and APOA-IV gene variants and low HDL levels (Miltiadous et al., 2005); effect of LIPC gene variants on HDL levels and modification by saturated fat (Ordovas et al., 2002b; Zhang et al., 2005); ALOX5 variants and response to omega-3 and omega-6 fats on atherogenesis (Dwyer et al., 2004); and variants of the PLIN gene as they relate to susceptibility to obesity and response to dietary fats (Qi et al., 2004a, 2004b). In addition, cardiovascular disease is an inflammatory disorder (Ridker, 2004; Libby and Theroux, 2005). Not surprisingly, variants of genes such as TNF-α and IL1 and IL6 impact cardiovascular disease susceptibility (Padovani et al., 2000; Humphries et al., 2001). See Kornman et al. (2004) for an overview of genetic variation and inflammation in reference to nutrigenomics.

In addition, progress is being made in understanding the role of genetic variants in hypertension, including intriguing results that suggest that some genotypes respond better to the Dietary Approaches to Stop Hypertension (DASH) diet than others and that some genotypes result in blood pressure that is not responsive to dietary sodium restriction (Hunt et al., 1998; Svetkey et al., 2001; Gu et al., 2005). Knowing the genotype of clients provides additional important information as to how they are likely to respond to particular dietary interventions. (For excellent reviews of nutritional genomics applications to cardiovascular disease, see Corella and Ordovas, 2005; Ordovas and Mooser, 2004.)

Immune Health and Cancer

Much ongoing research, including that conducted at the National Cancer Institute, relates to gene-diet interactions and carcinogenesis (Go et al., 2003; Davis and Hord, 2005; Davis and Milner, 2004; Junien and Gallou, 2004; Kim and Milner, 2003; Ulrich, 2005; Trujillo et al., 2006; Wargovich and Cunningham, 2003). One of the key mechanisms by which the body protects against cancer is detoxification, the process of neutralizing potentially harmful molecules (see *Focus On*: Detoxification Systems in Chapter 9). Among the better-characterized genes involved in various aspects of detoxification are the cytochrome P450 isozymes (CYPs), glutathione *S*-transferases (GSTs), and superoxide dismutases (SOD1, SOD2, SOD3). The CYP and GST genes are part of the liver's phase I and phase II detoxification system; the SOD genes code for proteins that dismantle the reactive oxygen species superoxide. Each of these genes has nutritional implications, and variants have been identified that result in decreased detoxification. Nutritional genomics provides the basis for analyzing the genotypes of individuals and directing nutrition therapy in such a way that it protects against cancer by augmenting endogenous detoxification activity.

Other Chronic Diseases

Although nutritional genomics applications have made more progress to date in reference to cardiovascular disease and cancer, research is underway for many other chronic disorders as well. Candidate genes, gene variants, and diet-gene interactions are being investigated for type 2 diabetes, osteoporosis, and obesity. Populations differ in the types and frequencies of the gene variants that are present and therefore differ in the dietary approaches most appropriate for intervention and prevention. As gene variants and their health implications are being identified, attention is also being paid to examining the frequency of particular variants among populations. These findings will be helpful in developing effective dietary approaches.

⊙ FOCAL POINTS

- The genetic revolution has ushered in an exciting era, one in which many new opportunities are expected for nutrition professionals with expertise in nutritional genomics.
- The molecular basis of disease provides the means for personalizing therapy, with the expectation of increased therapeutic efficacy as the outcome.
- As genetics is integrated into health care, medical, pharmacologic and nutritional therapies will become more oriented toward the genotype of each person. Nutrition assessment and intervention will be the keys to preventing or mitigating the expression of diseases for which an individual is susceptible.
- Medical nutrition therapy is the key to improving the quality of life for those individuals who have already developed a disease because specific nutrients will be used to alter biochemical outcomes.
- Nutrition professionals will gain a deeper understanding of the underlying genetic and biochemical basis for disorders and will be able to apply new tools that will focus on preventing disease through early detection and intervention.

✴ CLINICAL SCENARIO 1

Jared and Matthew are identical twins who grew up together but have lived apart since college. Jared stayed in the Northeast and majored in accounting. He is now a certified public accountant in a high-profile accounting firm, working long hours in a stressful environment. Matthew went to school on the West Coast, where he studied nutrition and exercise physiology and now manages the wellness program at a large fitness center. At age 30 the two brothers are noticeably different in weight and body shape. Jared has a BMI of 36. Jared has developed central obesity, hypertension, and problems with blood sugar regulation, all signs of a tendency toward developing type 2 diabetes. Matthew is lean and has a normal blood pressure and normal blood sugar regulation.

✴**Nutrition Diagnosis:** Overweight/obesity in Jared related to possible genetic susceptibility, overeating with snacks and consumption of large meals as evidenced by central obesity and body mass index of 36

1. Because they are identical twins, would you have expected the two brothers to have similar health profiles?
2. How would you expect their diets to be different?
3. What is going on? Does Matthew not have the same genetic susceptibilities that Jared has? If not, why not? If so, why doesn't Matthew exhibit the same phenotype as Jared?
4. What would you advise Jared to do to decrease his genetic susceptibility to diabetes?

✹ CLINICAL SCENARIO 2

Maria is in her early thirties and planning to have a child before too long. Recently the ethnic community in which she lives has begun an awareness campaign to alert the population that it is now well established that this particular ethnic group has an increased frequency of the MTHFR 677C>T gene variant and to educate residents about their options for minimizing any negative effects of having this variant.

✶Nutrition Diagnosis: Nutrition-related knowledge deficit related to nutrigenetic counseling for pregnancy as evidenced by client questions about nutrition and high-risk pregnancy

1. Would nutrigenetic testing be of help to Maria? If not, why not? If so, in what ways might testing be beneficial?
2. If she has the gene variant MTHFR 677C>T, what are the implications for Maria?
3. As a nutrition professional, what would be your advice to her?

Useful websites

Basic Genetics and Genomics
www.genome.gov
www.ncbi.nlm.nih.gov/omim
www.ornl.gov
www.ornl.gov/sci/techresources/Human_Genome/
  publicat/primer2001/
www.ornl.gov/hgmis/publicat/primer2001

Core Competencies in Genetics Essential for All Health Care Professionals
www.nchpeg.org/core/core.asp

Ethical, Legal, and Social Issues
www.ornl.gov/hgmis/elsi/elsi.html
www.genome.gov/ELSI
www.utoronto.ca/jcb/home/main.htm

Family History Initiative
www.hhs.gov/familyhistory

Genetic Counseling
www.nsgc.org/
www.gradschools.com/biomed_health.html

Genetics Glossaries
www.genome.gov/
www.ornl.gov/TechResources/Human_Genome/glossary

Human Genome Project
www.genome.gov
www.ornl.gov/hgmis/project/info.html
www.ornl.gov/sci/techresources/Human_Genome/hg5yp/
  index.shtml

National Center for Biotechnology Information
www.ncbi.nlm.nih.gov/omim

Nutritional Genomics
http://cancergenome.nih.gov
www.nugo.org
www.nutrigenomics.nl
www.nutrigenomics.org.nz
www.nutrigenomics.psu.edu
www.nutrigenomics.ucdavis.edu

Public Health and Genetics
www.cdc.gov/genomics

References

Afman L, Müller M: Nutrigenomics: from molecular nutrition to the prevention of disease, *J Am Diet Assoc,*106:569, 2006.

Ames BN et al: High-dose vitamin therapy stimulates variant enzymes with decreased coenzyme binding affinity (increased Km): relevance to genetic disease and polymorphisms, *Am J Clin Nutr* 75:616, 2002.

Ayyobi AF et al: Cholesterol ester transfer protein (CETP) Taq1B polymorphism influences the effect of a standardized cardiac rehabilitation program on lipid risk markers, *Atherosclerosis* 181:363, 2005.

Bailey LB et al: Vitamin B_{12} status is inversely associated with plasma homocysteine in young women with C677T and/or A1298C methylenetetrahydrofolate reductase polymorphisms, *J Nutr* 132:1872, 2002.

Brousseau ME et al: Cholesteryl ester transfer protein TaqI B2B2 genotype is associated with higher HDL cholesterol levels and lower risk of coronary heart disease end points in men with HDL deficiency: Veterans Affairs HDL, Cholesterol Intervention Trial, *Arterioscler Thromb Vasc Biol* 22:1148, 2002.

Chawla A et al: Nuclear receptors and lipid physiology: opening the X-files, *Science* 294:1866, 2001.

Corella D et al: Alcohol drinking determines the effect of the APOE locus on LDL-cholesterol concentrations in men: the Framingham Offspring Study, *Am J Clin Nutr* 73:736, 2001.

Corella D, Ordovas JM: Single nucleotide polymorphisms that influence lipid metabolism: interaction with dietary factors, *Annu Rev Nutr* 25:341, 2005.

Davis CD, Hord NG: Nutritional "omics" technologies for elucidating the role(s) of bioactive food components in colon cancer prevention, *J Nutr* 135:2694, 2005.

Davis CD, Milner J: Frontiers in nutrigenomics, proteomics, metabolomics and cancer prevention, *Mutat Res* 551:51, 2004.

DeBusk RM: *Genetics: the nutrition connection*, Chicago, 2003, American Dietetic Association.

DeBusk R, Joffe Y: *It's Not Just Your Genes!* San Diego, 2006, BKDR.

DeBusk RM et al: Nutritional genomics in practice: where do we begin? *J Am Diet Assoc* 105:589, 2005.

Djoussé L, et al: Apolipoprotein E polymorphism modifies the alcohol-HDL association observed in the National Heart, Lung, and Blood Institute Family Heart Study, *Am J Clin Nutr* 80:1639, 2004.

Dreon DM et al: Low-density lipoprotein subclass patterns and lipoprotein response to a reduced-fat diet in men, *FASEB J* 8:121, 1994.

Dwyer JH et al: Arachidonate5-lipoxygenase promoter genotype, dietary arachidonic acid, and atherosclerosis, *N Engl J Med* 350:29, 2004.

Egger G et al: Epigenetics in human disease and prospects for epigenetic therapy, *Nature* 429:457, 2004.

Feinberg AP et al: The epigenetic progenitor origin of human cancer, *Nat Rev Genet* 7: 21, 2006.

Feuk L et al: Structural variation in the human genome, *Nat Rev Genet* 7:85, 2006.

Fohr IP et al: 5,10-Methylenetetrahydrofolate reductase genotype determines the plasma homocysteine-lowering effect of supplementation with 5-methyltetrahydrofolate or folic acid in healthy young women, *Am J Clin Nutr* 75:275, 2002.

German JB: Genetic dietetics: nutrigenomics and the future of dietetics practice, *J Am Diet Assoc* 105:530, 2005.

German JB et al: Metabolomics in practice: emerging knowledge to guide future dietetic advice toward individualized health, *J Am Diet Assoc* 105:1425, 2005.

German JB et al: Personal metabolomics as a next generation nutritional assessment, *J Nutr* 133:4260, 2003.

Gillies PJ: Nutrigenomics: the Rubicon of molecular nutrition, *J Am Diet Assoc* 103:S50, 2003.

Go VL et al: Diet, nutrition, and cancer prevention: the postgenomic era, *J Nutr* 133:3830S, 2003.

Gu CC et al: Haplotype association analysis of AGT variants with hypertension-related traits: the HyperGEN Study, *Hum Hered* 60:164, 2005.

Gyllensten U et al: Paternal inheritance of mitochondrial DNA in mice, *Nature* 352:255, 1991.

Hagberg JM et al: APO E gene and gene-environment effects on plasma lipoprotein-lipid levels, *Physiol Genomics* 4:101, 2000.

Hihi AK et al: PPARs: transcriptional effectors of fatty acids and their derivatives, *Cell Mol Life Sci* 59:790, 2002.

Holliday R. DNA methylation and epigenotypes, *Biochemistry (Moscow)* 70:612, 2005.

Humphries SE et al: The interleukin-6 -174 G/C promoter polymorphism is associated with risk of coronary heart disease and systolic blood pressure in healthy men, *Eur Heart J* 22:2243, 2001.

Hunt SC et al: Angiotensinogen genotype, sodium reduction, weight loss, and prevention of hypertension: trials of hypertension prevention, phase II, *Hypertension* 32:393, 1998.

Isaacs JS, Zand DJ: Single-gene autosomal recessive disorders and Prader-Willi syndrome: an update for food and nutrition professionals, *J Am Diet Assoc* 107:466, 2007.

Jacobs MN, Lewis DF: Steroid hormone receptors and dietary ligands: a selected review, *Proc Nutr Soc* 61:105, 2002.

Jump DB: Dietary polyunsaturated fatty acids and regulation of gene transcription, *Curr Opin Lipidol* 13:155, 2002.

Junien C, Gallou C: Cancer nutrigenomics, *World Rev Nutr Diet* 93:210, 2004.

Kadowaki T et al: The role of PPARgamma in high-fat diet–induced obesity and insulin resistance, *J Diabetes Complications* 16:41, 2002.

Kang et al: Intermediate homocysteinemia: a thermolabile variant of methylenetetrahydrofolate reductase, *Am J Hum Genet* 43:414, 1988.

Kaput J, Rodriguez RL: Nutritional genomics: the next frontier in the postgenomic era, *Physiol Genomics* 16:166, 2004.

Kauwell GPA: Emerging concepts in nutrigenomics: a preview of what is to come, *Nutr Clin Pract* 20:75, 2005.

Kauwell GP et al: Methylenetetrahydrofolate reductase mutation (677C→T) negatively influences plasma homocysteine response to marginal folate intake in elderly women, *Metabolism* 49:1440, 2000a.

Kauwell GP et al: Folate status of elderly women following moderate folate depletion responds only to a higher folate intake, *J Nutr* 130:1584, 2000b.

Kim YS, Milner JA: Nutritional genomics and proteomics in cancer prevention. Proceedings of a conference, September 5-6, 2002, Bethesda, Md, *J Nutr* 133:2399S, 2003.

Kornman KS et al: Genetic variations and inflammation: a practical nutrigenomics opportunity, *Nutrition* 20:44, 2004.

Libby P, Theroux P: Pathophysiology of coronary artery disease, *Circulation* 111:3481, 2005.

Marín C et al: Effects of the human apolipoprotein A-I promoter G-A mutation on postprandial lipoprotein metabolism, *Am J Clin Nutr* 76:319, 2002.

Masson LF et al: Genetic variation and the lipid response to dietary intervention: a systematic review, *Am J Clin Nutr* 77:1098, 2003.

Mathers JC: Nutrition and epigenetics: how the genome learns from experience, *Br Nutr Foundation Nutr Bull* 30:6-12, 2005.

McCully KS: Vascular pathology of homocysteinemia: implications for the pathogenesis of arteriosclerosis, *Am J Pathol* 56:111, 1969.

Miltiadous G et al: Gene polymorphisms affecting HDL-cholesterol levels in the normolipidemic population, *Nutr Metab Cardiovas Dis* 15:219, 2005.

MITOMAP, map of the mitochondrial genome, available at http://www.mitomap.org/, accessed 2005.

Müller M, Kersten S: Nutrigenomics: goals and strategies, *Nature Rev* 4:315-322, 2003.

Mutch DM et al: Nutrigenomics and nutrigenetics: the emerging faces of nutrition, *FASEB J* 19:1602, 2005.

Nicklas BJ et al: Effects of apoliprotein E genotype on dietary-induced changes in high-density lipoprotein cholesterol in obese postmenopausal women, *Metabolism* 51:853, 2002.

Olson RE: Nutrition and genetics: an expanding frontier, *Am J Clin Nutr* 78: 201, 2003.

Ordovas JM: Nutrigenetics, plasma lipids and cardiovascular risk, *J Am Diet Assoc* 106:1074, 2006.

Ordovas JM, Mooser V: Nutrigenomics and nutrigenetics, *Curr Opin Lipidol* 15:101, 2004.

Ordovas J et al: Dietary fat intake determines the effect of a common polymorphism in the hepatic lipase gene promoter on high-density lipoprotein metabolism, *Circulation* 106:2315, 2002a.

Ordovas JM et al: Polyunsaturated fatty acids modulate the effects of the APOA1 G-A polymorphism on HDL-cholesterol concentrations in a sex-specific manner: the Framingham Study, *Am J Clin Nutr* 75:38, 2002b.

Padovani JC et al: Gene polymorphisms in the TNF locus and the risk of myocardial infarction, *Thromb Res* 100:263, 2000.

Qi L et al: Genetic variation at the perilipin (PLIN) locus is associated with obesity-related phenotypes in white women, *Clin Genet* 66:299, 2004a.

Qi L et al: Gender-specific association of a perilipin gene haplotype with obesity risk in a white population, *Obes Res* 12:1758, 2004b.

Report of the Committee of the Human Mitochondrial Genome, 2002, www.mitomap.org/mitomap/report.html, accessed May 1, 2006.

Ridker PM: High-sensitivity C-reactive protein, inflammation, and cardiovascular risk: from concept to clinical practice to clinical benefit, *Am Heart J* 148:S19, 2004.

Sampath H, Ntambi JM: Polyunaturated fatty acid regulation of gene expression, *Nutr Rev* 62:333, 2004.

Sampath H, Ntambi JM: Polyunsaturated fatty acid regulation of genes of lipid metabolism, *Annu Rev Nutr* 25:317, 2005.

Santos KF et al: The prima donna of epigenetics: the regulation of gene expression by DNA methylation, *Braz J Med Biol Res* 38:1531, 2005.

Schwartz M, Vissing J: Paternal inheritance of mitochondrial DNA, *N Engl J Med* 347:576, 2002.

Shoffner JM, Wallace DC: Mitochondrial genetics: principles and practice, *Am J Hum Genet* 51:1179, 1992.

Stover PJ: New paradigms for nutrient control of genome translation, *Nutr Rev* 61:427, 2003.

Stover P: Nutritional genomics, *Physiol Genomics* 16:161, 2004.

Stover PJ: Influence of human genetic variation on nutritional requirements, *Am J Clin Nutr* 83:436S, 2006.

Svetkey LP et al: Angiotensinogen genotype and blood pressure response in the Dietary Approaches to Stop Hypertension (DASH) study, *J Hypertens* 19:1949, 2001.

Taimela S et al: The effect of physical activity on serum total and low-density lipoprotein holesterol concentrations varies with apolipoprotein E phenotype in male children and young adults: the Cardiovascular Risk in Young Finns Study, *Metabolism* 45:797, 1996.

Trujillo E et al: Nutrigenomics, proteomics, and the dietetics professional, *J Am Diet Assoc* 106:403, 2006.

Ulrich CM: Nutrigenetics in cancer research—folate metabolism and colorectal cancer, *J Nutr* 135:2698, 2005.

van Ommen B: Nutrigenomics: exploiting systems biology in the nutrition and health arenas, *Nutrition* 20:4, 2004.

Venter JC et al: The sequence of the human genome, *Science* 291:1304, 2001.

von Castel-Dunwoody KM et al: Transcobalamin 776C->G polymorphism negatively affects vitamin B_{12} metabolism, *Am J Clin Nutr* 81:1436, 2005.

Wargovich MJ, Cunningham JE: Diet, individual responsiveness and cancer prevention, *J Nutr* 133:2400S, 2003.

Waterland RA, Jirtle RL: Early nutrition, epigenetic changes at transposons and imprinted genes, and enhanced susceptibility to adult chronic disease, *Nutrition* 20:63, 2004.

Winkelmann BR et al: Haplotypes of the cholesteryl ester transfer protein gene predict lipid-modifying response to statin therapy, *Pharmacogenomics J* 3:284, 2003.

Zhang C et al: Interactions between the −514C→T polymorphism of the hepatic lipase gene and lifestyle factors in relation to HDL concentrations among U.S. diabetic men, *Am J Clin Nutr* 81:1429, 2005.

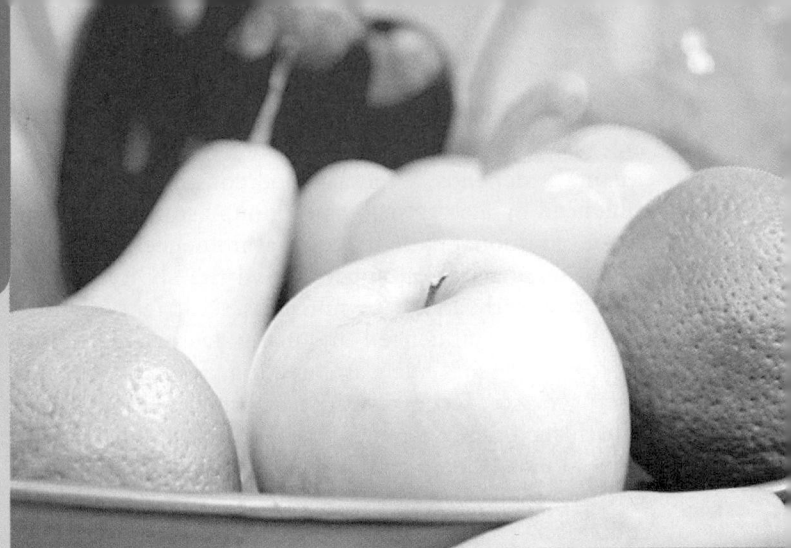

CHAPTER **14**

Kathy Hammond, MS, RN, RD, LD, CNSD

Assessment: Dietary and Clinical Data

KEY TERMS

24-hour recall a method of dietary assessment in which an individual is asked to remember everything eaten during the previous 24 hours

ageusia loss of sense of taste

anosmia loss of sense of smell

anthropometry the science of measuring the size, weight, and proportions of the human body

bioelectrical impedance analysis (BIA) a precise body composition analysis technique that uses a small electrical current to estimate total body water, fat-free mass, fat mass, and body cell mass

body mass index (BMI) weight (kg)/height (m)^2; a definition of the degree of adiposity

dietary history a detailed dietary record; may include a 24-hour recall, food frequency questionnaire, food diary, and other information such as weight history, previous diet changes, use of supplements, and food intolerances

dietary intake data data about food consumption, including information on appetite, eating patterns, and estimations of typical nutrient intake

dysgeusia diminished or distorted sense of taste

food diary a written record of the amounts of all foods and liquids consumed during a set time, usually 3 to 7 days; often includes information on eating time, place, and situation

food frequency questionnaire a method of dietary assessment in which the data collected relate to how often and in what amount foods are consumed (e.g., servings per week, month, or year)

height-for-age curve assessment of stature and change in stature for a child at a specific age and over time, compared with a norm

nutrient intake analysis (NIA) a process by which food, beverage, and supplement intake is evaluated for nutrient content over a specified period of time

nutrition assessment the science of determining nutrition status by analyzing an individual's medical, dietary, and social history; anthropometric data; biochemical data; clinical data; and drug-nutrient interactions

nutrition screening a process used to identify nutritional problems and risk factors

nutrition status a measurement of the extent to which an individual's physiologic need for nutrients is being met

waist circumference the distance around the smallest girth below the rib cage and above the umbilicus (belly button); provides a risk prediction for obesity-related disease; used in patients with a body mass index of up to 35

weight-for-age curve assessment of weight and change in weight for a child at a specific age and over time, compared with a norm

weight-for-length curve a standard for evaluating the growth of children that gives the percentile rankings for weight according to specific lengths or heights but disregarding age

An individual's **nutrition status** reflects the degree to which physiologic needs for nutrients are being met. Nutrient intake depends on actual food consumption, which is influenced by factors such as economic situation, eating behavior, emotional climate, cultural influences, effects of various disease states on appetite, and the ability to consume and absorb adequate nutrients. Nutrient requirements are also influenced by many factors, including physiologic stressors such as infection, acute or chronic disease processes, fever, or trauma; normal anabolic states of growth such as pregnancy or rehabilitation; body maintenance and well-being; and psychological stress. The balance between nutrient intake and nutrient requirements is the nutrition status.

When adequate nutrients are consumed to support the body's daily needs and any increased metabolic demands, the person moves into optimal nutrition status as shown in Figure 14-1. This status promotes growth and development, maintains general health, supports activities of daily living, and helps protect the body from disease and illness. Appropriate assessment techniques can detect a nutritional deficiency in the early stages of development, allowing dietary intake to be improved through nutrition support and counseling before a more severe condition develops.

A nutrition status assessment should be performed routinely for any individual. However, the type of assessment for those who are basically healthy differs from assessments for those who are critically ill. Persons at nutritional risk can be identified on the basis of screening information that is routinely obtained at the time of admission to a hospital or nursing home or after returning to home-based care. Information obtained in the nutrition assessment is used to design an individual nutrition care plan (see Chapter 17). A thorough nutrition assessment increases the effectiveness of nutrition intervention, education, and counseling (see Chapter 19).

NUTRITION IMBALANCE

Nutrition is an important factor in the etiology and management of several major causes of death and disability in contemporary society. Table 14-1 shows the top ten causes of death in 2002 identified for race.

Several of the leading causes of death, including cardiovascular disease (atherosclerotic heart disease and hypertension), cerebrovascular disease (stroke), diabetes, and some types of cancer, have a strong link with the type and amount of food consumed (USDHHS, 2000). Nutrition is also significant in major diseases such as obesity, anemia, and osteoporosis. In addition, cirrhosis of the liver and some accidents may be associated with excessive alcohol intake. Modifications in dietary intake may assist in the prevention of some diseases and events or their precursors, particularly overweight and obesity.

States of nutritional deficiency or excess occur when the nutrient intake is not balanced with specific requirements for optimal health. Within the safe range of intake, homeostatic mechanisms allow the body to use nutrients equally effectively, with no detectable advantage being gained by a

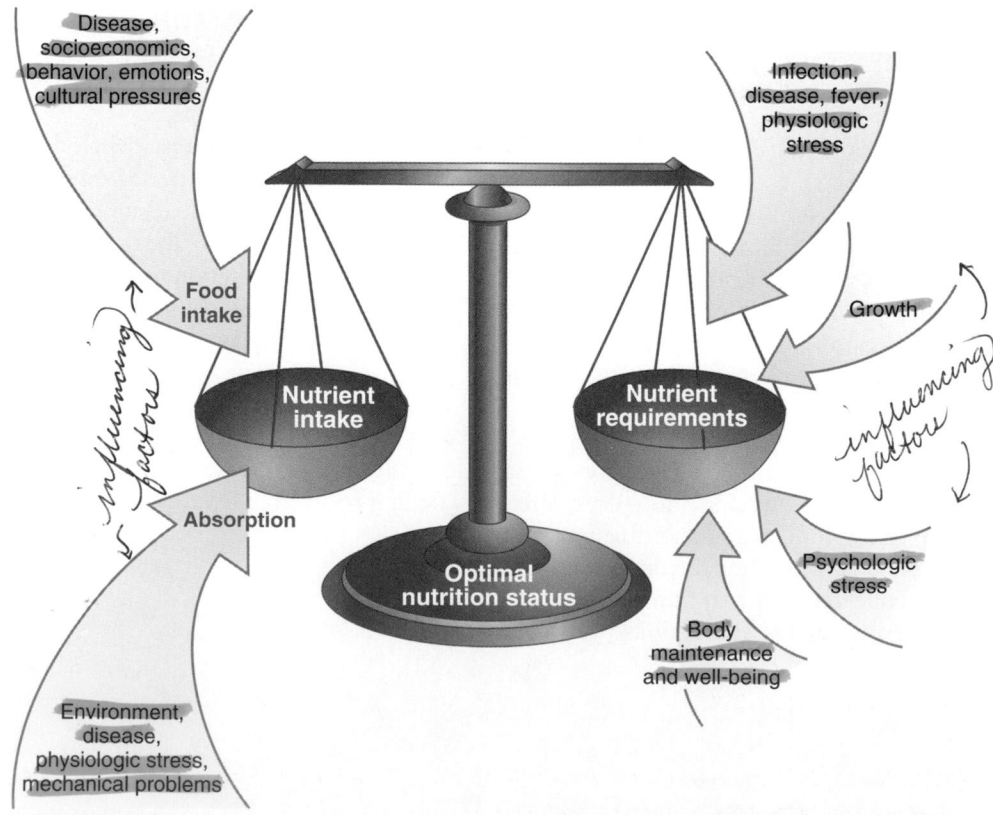

FIGURE 14-1 Optimal nutrition status: a balance between nutrient intake and nutrient requirements.

given level of intake. As nutritional deficiencies or excesses develop, adaptations are made to achieve a new steady state without any significant loss in physiologic function (see Figure 14-1). As the intake departs further from the accepted range, the organism accommodates to the changing supply of nutrients by reducing its function or changing the size or status of the affected body compartments. The nutrition status of an individual is determined by identifying the presence or absence of these adaptations (see Chapter 17 and Appendix 29). For example, before iron deficiency anemia develops (and is diagnosed by measures of hematocrit, hemoglobin, and appropriate clinical signs), a gradual diminution in iron stores can be diagnosed on the basis of increased iron absorption, decreased serum ferritin levels, or bone marrow evaluation (see Chapter 31).

When nutritional reserves are depleted or nutrient intake is inadequate to meet the body's daily metabolic needs, a state of undernutrition develops. Nutrient deficiency may stem from inadequate ingestion, impaired digestion or absorption, dysfunctional metabolic processing, or increased excretion of essential nutrients. Infants, children, pregnant females, individuals with low incomes, hospitalized persons, and older adults are at the greatest risk for becoming undernourished. Undernourishment may result in impaired growth and development, lowered resistance to infection, poor wound healing, and poor clinical outcome from disease or trauma with increased morbidity and mortality.

It is estimated that in academic hospitals in the United States, 25% of patients show some type of malnutrition, generalized wasting, or protein depletion. Other studies show that approximately 50% of hospitalized patients exhibit signs of moderate malnutrition (Pfau and Rombeau, 2000). Pichard and colleagues (2004) found low fat-free mass in 37% of those hospitalized for 1 to 2 days and in 56% of those hospitalized for more than 12 days, and concluded that severe nutritional depletion was evident in those with a length of stay greater than 12 days.

Overnutrition also presents major nutritional problems manifesting as obesity and related disease states such as diabetes, atherosclerotic heart disease, hypertension, and the metabolic syndrome. These conditions may also result in poor clinical outcomes with increased morbidity and mortality. Overweight and obesity have reached epidemic proportions in the United States with one third of all adults classified as obese; among children and teens ages 6 to 19, 16% are overweight (NCHS, 2004). Today almost twice as many children and approximately three times as many adolescents are overweight than were overweight in 1980. These staggering statistics are associated with approximately 300,000 deaths per year related to overweight and obesity (USDHHS, 2001).

Assessing the obese injured patient presents a challenge. Current assessment screening tools identify one at risk only if undernourished and, using this concept, would place the

TABLE 14-1

Ranking of the Leading Causes of Death in the United States, 2002

All Causes	Rank for All Races, Both Sexes, All Ages	Rank for White Race, Both Sexes, All Ages	Rank for Hispanic, Both Sexes, All Ages	Rank for Black, Both Sexes, All Ages	Rank for Native American, Both Sexes, All Ages
Heart diseases	1	1	1	1	1
Malignant neoplasms	2	2	2	2	2
Cerebrovascular diseases	3	3	4	3	5
Chronic lower respiratory	4	4	8	8	7
Accidents, unintentional injuries	5	5	3	5	3
Diabetes mellitus	6	6	5	4	4
Influenza and pneumonia	7	7	9	—	9
Alzheimer's disease	8	8	—	—	—
Nephritis, nephritic syndrome, nephrosis	9	9	—	9	—
Septicemia	10	—	—	10	—
Suicide	—	10	—	—	8
Chronic liver disease or cirrhosis	—	—	6	—	6
Assault or homicide	—	—	7	6	10
Conditions originating in prenatal period	—	—	10	—	
AIDS or HIV disease	—	—	—	7	

From Kochanek KD et al: *Final data for 2002: national vital statistics reports* (vol 53, no. 5), Hyattsville, Md, 2004, National Center for Health Statistics.

Key: — indicates that a ranking was not in the top ten causes for the category.

AIDS, Acquired immune deficiency syndrome; *HIV*, human immunodeficiency virus.

DEVELOPMENT OF DEFICIENCY

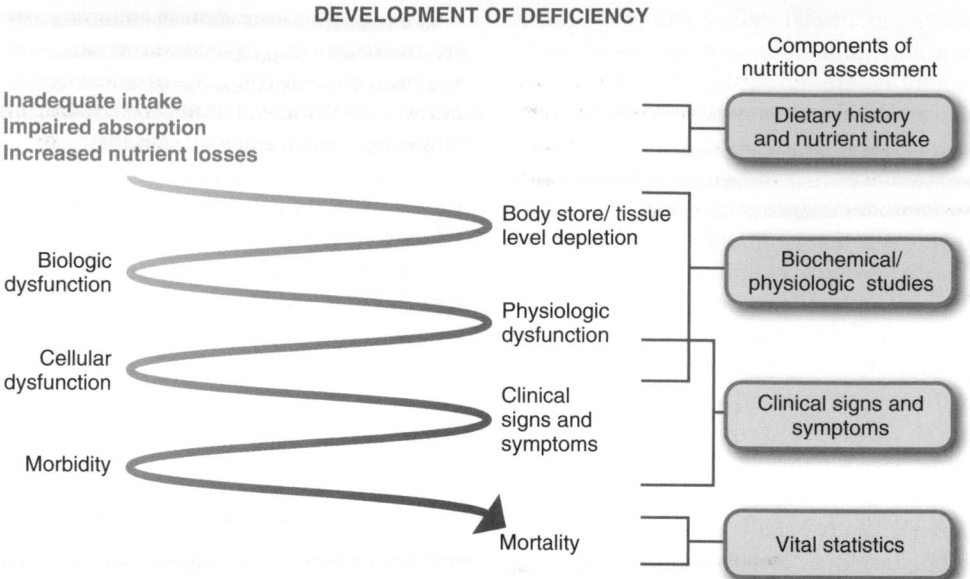

FIGURE 14-2 Development of clinical nutritional deficiency with corresponding dietary, biochemical, and clinical evaluations.

TABLE 14-2

Nutritional Risk Factors

Category	Factors
Food and nutrient intake patterns	• Calorie and protein intake greater or less than that required for age and activity level • Vitamin and mineral intake greater or less than that required for age • Swallowing difficulties • Gastrointestinal disturbances • Unusual food habits (e.g., pica) • Impaired cognitive function or depression • Nothing by mouth for more than 3 days • Inability or unwillingness to consume food • Increase or decrease in activities of daily living • Misuse of supplements • Inadequate transitional feeding, tube feeding or parenteral nutrition, or both • Bowel irregularity (e.g., constipation, diarrhea) • Restricted diet • Feeding limitations
Psychological and social factors	• Low literacy • Language barriers • Cultural or religious factors • Emotional disturbances associated with feeding difficulties (e.g., depression) • Limited resources for food preparation or obtaining food and supplies • Alcohol or drug addiction • Limited or low income • Lack of or inability to communicate needs • Limited use or understanding of community resources
Physical conditions	• Extreme age: adults older than 80 years, premature infants, very young children • Pregnancy: adolescent, closely spaced, or three or more pregnancies

obese patient with injuries at minimum or no risk and less likely to be rescreened over time. This results in the potential for increases in morbidity. Obesity is associated with low-grade inflammation and the presence of inflammatory markers such as C-reactive protein and proinflammatory cytokines. This inflammatory state results in comorbidities such as coronary heart disease (Davidson and Smith, 2004; Haffner and Taegtmeyer, 2003). More appropriate tools of assessment are needed to accurately assess this population (see Chapter 21).

The concepts of nutritional well-being and the continuum of nutritional health are essential. Evaluation for specific nutrient deficiencies consists of a review of dietary and medical histories, weight, physical examination, laboratory evaluation (see Chapter 15), and review of the use of medications and herbal products (see Chapters 16 and 17). Figure 14-2 illustrates the general sequence of steps leading to nutritional decline and the development of a nutritional deficiency, as well as areas in which an assessment can iden-tify problems and clinical intervention can prevent poor nutrition before it develops.

Many different factors help measure whether a person is at nutritional risk. Factors to consider include food and nutrient intake patterns, psychosocial factors, physical conditions associated with particular disease states and disorders, biochemical abnormalities, and medication regimens (ADA, 2006) (Table 14-2).

Nutrition screening and assessment are integral parts of the nutrition care process (NCP) which has four phases: (1) assessment of nutrition status; (2) identification of nutritional diagnoses; (3) medical nutrition therapy (MNT) interventions such as dietary change, nutritional supplements, education, counseling, or referrals, and (4) monitoring and evaluation of the effectiveness of the interventions (American Dietetic Association, 2006). To provide cost-effective MNT in today's health care environment, it is important to first identify patients who are at nutritional risk. Nutrition screening is the first step in this process.

TABLE 14-2

Nutritional Risk Factors—cont'd

Category	Factors
Physical conditions—cont'd	• Alterations in anthropometric measurements: marked overweight or underweight for height, age, or both; head circumference less than normal; depressed somatic fat and muscle stores; amputation • Fat or muscle wasting • Obesity or overweight • Chronic renal or cardiac disease and related complications • Diabetes and related complications • Pressure ulcers or altered skin integrity • Cancer and related treatments • Acquired immune deficiency syndrome • Gastrointestinal complications (e.g., malabsorption, diarrhea, digestive or bowel changes) • Catabolic or hypermetabolic stress (e.g., trauma, sepsis, burns, stress) • Immobility • Osteoporosis, osteomalacia • Neurologic impairments, including impairment in sensory function • Visual impairments
Abnormal laboratory values	• Visceral proteins (e.g., albumin, transferrin, prealbumin) • Lipid profile (cholesterol, high-density lipoproteins, low-density lipoproteins, triglycerides) • Hemoglobin, hematocrit, and other hematologic tests • Blood urea nitrogen, creatinine, and electrolyte levels • Fasting serum blood glucose level • Other laboratory indexes as indicated
Medications	• Chronic use • Multiple and concurrent administration (polypharmacy) • Drug-nutrient interactions and side effects

Data from Council on Practice, Quality Management Committee: ADA's definitions for nutrition screening and nutrition assessment, *J Am Diet Assoc* 94:838, 1994.

NUTRITION SCREENING

Ideally everyone should undergo periodic nutrition status screening throughout the life span, not just during illness. The components of nutrition screening may vary slightly from one setting to another. A more thorough assessment follows screening when nutritional risks are identified.

Nutrition screening precedes the nutrition care process (see Chapter 17). The purpose of a nutrition screen is to quickly identify individuals who are malnourished or at nutritional risk and determine whether a more detailed assessment is warranted (Charney, 2005; ASPEN, 2002). The nutrition screen can usually be completed by a dietetic technician, nurse, physician, or other qualified health care professional. In most settings the nutrition screen is completed by a health professional other than the dietitian. Once completed, patients who are at nutritional risk are usually referred to a registered dietitian.

A nutrition screening tool should be simple, easy to complete; inclusive of routine data readily available; cost-effective; and effective in identifying nutrition problems that require further assessment. In a survey of clinical nutrition managers, the most common criteria used for screening included patient history of weight loss, current nutrition support, skin breakdown, poor intake, and chronic use of modified diets (Chima, 2006). Further information collected during a nutrition screen depends on (1) the setting in which the information is obtained (e.g., home, clinic, hospital), (2) the life cycle or disease type, (3) available data, (4) a definition of risk priorities, and (5) the goals of the screening process. Finally the tools must be reliable (consistent between measures of the same factor, such as weight) and valid; validity verifies that the measure tests what it is supposed to test.

Regardless of the information gathered, the goal of screening is to identify individuals who are at nutritional risk, those likely to become at nutritional risk, and those

---

NUTRITION SERVICES SCREENING ASSESSMENT FORM

Admission Date: _____   ADDRESSOGRAPH

Medical Record Review

Diagnosis _____ Age _____

Ht. _____ Wt. _____ IBW _____ % IBW _____ UBW _____ % UBW _____

Albumin _____ Other Labs _____

Appetite: >50%   ≤50%   Poor

Medication _____

Other _____

Diet Order_____Date_____ Diet Order_____ Date_____ Diet Order_____ Date_____

Evaluation Criteria (Check all that apply)

☐ Loss of appetite >48 hr.

☐ Difficulty chewing/swallowing

☐ Significant food allergies/intolerances

☐ Malnourished appearance

☐ Length of stay ≥7 days

☐ >65 years of age with a surgery this admission

☐ <50% meals consumed

☐ Modified diet _____

Pt. identified to be at nutritional risk based on meeting >2 criteria above.

Plan

Pt. not at high nutritional risk at this time. Basic nutritional care services and follow-up will be provided per policy.

☐ Pt. seen for snacks/food preferences.

☐ Pt. to receive comfort measures only. No intervention planned unless requested/ordered by staff or pt.

☐ Pt./care provider familiar with dietary modifications. No education planned.

☐ Other _____

X _____

   Signature   Date

Nutrition Services Screening Assessment Form

3/97
Piedmont Graphics

Original - Chart
Yellow - Department

FIGURE 14-3 Nutrition screening form. *IBW,* Ideal body weight; *UBW,* usual body weight. *(Courtesy Northside Hospital, Atlanta, Ga.)*

who need further assessment. Several screening tools exist. Figure 14-3 is an example of a nutrition screen used in an acute-care hospital or residential setting, whereas the questionnaire in Figure 14-4 is used in a perinatal service, and Figure 14-5 is an example of a screen that could be used in a pediatric practice.

One of the most recent screening tools available is the Malnutrition Universal Screening Tool (MUST) developed

---

Perinatal Nutrition Screening/Assessment Form

ADDRESSOGRAPH

SCREENING CRITERIA FOR POTENTIAL NUTRITIONAL RISK *(full assessment if one checked)*

SCREENING CRITERIA FOR POTENTIAL NUTRITIONAL RISK

ANTEPARTUM

☐ Obstetrical Condition (Multiple Gestation, PIH, IUGR, Diabetes, Hyperemesis, Anemia)
☐ Chronic/Systemic Condition Affecting Nutritional Status or Intake
☐ Adolescence (≤17 years)   ☐ Inappropriate Weight Change
☐ Albumin ≤2.5 mg/dl   ☐ Therapeutic or Limited Diet
☐ Lack of Knowledge re Pregnancy Diet   ☐ Length of Stay ≥5 days

POSTPARTUM

☐ Gestational Diabetes this Pregnancy   ☐ Albumin ≤2.5 mg/dl   ☐ Hg <8.0 g/dl

Breastfeeding mother meeting the following criteria:
     ☐ ≤17 Years Old
     ☐ Therapeutic or Limited Diet
     ☐ Lack of Knowledge re Lactation Diet
     ☐ Multiple Birth with Infants in Special Care Nursery

COMPREHENSIVE ASSESSMENT

Weight Gain/Expected Weight Gain _____

Cultural/Social Concerns _____

Activity Level _____

Plans to Breastfeed? ☐ Yes ☐ No

Other _____

Diagnosis _____ Parity _____ EGA/EDC _____

Medical/Obstetrical History _____

Age _____ Ht _____ Pregravid Wt _____ BMI _____ Current Wt _____

Medications _____ Vitamin/Mineral Supplements _____

Physical Exam _____ GI Function _____

Food Allergies/Intolerance _____ Diet Order _____

Labs _____

Estimated Energy Needs _____ Protein _____ Other _____

Adequacy of Intake/Evaluation of Nutritional Status _____

_____

_____

_____

FIGURE 14-4 Perinatal nutrition screening and assessment form. *BMI,* Body mass index; *EGA,* estimated gestational age; *EDC,* estimated date of confinement; *PIH,* pregnancy-induced hypertension; *IUGR,* intrauterine growth retardation. *(Courtesy Northside Hospital, Atlanta, Ga.)*

Shriners Burns Hospital
Rehabilitation Nutrition Screening Form

Date: _____   Level _____

Name: _____   Unit# _____

Age _____   ___ M ___ F

Birthdate _____

Reason for admission _____

Weight _____   _____ %NCHS
Height _____   _____ %NCHS

Recent weight loss/gain   ____Y   ____N
If yes, intended   ____Y   ____N
   How much _____
   Time frame _____

Recent: ____ Nausea   ____ Vomiting   TX: ____
          ____ Diarrhea   ____ Constipation
          ____ HX of anemia   ____ Change in appetite
          ____ Dentition concerns ____ Difficulty swallowing

Food allergies   ____N ____Y   _____

Diet restrictions   ____N ____Y   _____

Cooking facilities   ____ Stove   ____ Refrigerator

Drinks   ____ Bottle   ____ Straw   ____ Sippee cup   ____ Cup

Vitamin supplementation   ____N   ____Y Type ____
                                         Reason ____

Medications   ____N   ____Y Type(s) ____
                             Reason ____

Caretaker/relationship _____

Nutritional concerns stated by patient/caretaker:

Nutritional intervention proposed:

FIGURE 14-5 Pediatric screening and assessment form. (*Courtesy Shriners Burn Hospital, Cincinnati, Ohio.*)

by Stratton and colleagues (2004) to assess malnutrition in hospital inpatients and outpatients rapidly and easily, yet accurately and completely. MUST is designed to be used by multiple disciplines rather than by a specific group of professionals. Three independent criteria are used: current weight using body mass index (BMI), unintentional weight loss using specific cutoff points, and acute disease effect on nutrition intake for greater than 5 days. These three components work better together to predict outcome rather than the individual components. Once the scores are added, the overall risk of malnutrition can be determined using three categories: 0 = low risk; 1= medium risk; and 2 and above = high risk. Management guidelines can then be followed (Stratton et al., 2004) (Figure 14-6).

The Nutrition Screening Initiative (NSI) developed assessment tools to bring focus to the nutritional care given to older adults (AAFP, 2006). These tools are simple, brief, and generic; are designed to be flexible, and have been validated in outpatient (primary care) settings (Charney, 2005). Three tools are available that focus attention on nutrition in older adults: The DETERMINE Your Nutritional Health checklist is an awareness tool designed to highlight the warning signs of poor nutrition status (see Figure 10-4); the level I screen (Figure 14-7) highlights individuals who should be referred for a more comprehensive nutritional or medical follow-up; and the level II screen (Figure 14-8) highlights more serious nutrition or medical problems.

NUTRITION ASSESSMENT

Nutrition assessment is a comprehensive evaluation carried out by a registered dietitian for defining nutrition status using medical, social, nutritional, and medication histories; physical examination; anthropometric measurements; and laboratory data (see Chapter 15). Nutrition assessment involves interpretation of data from the nutrition screen and incorporates additional information. The purpose of assessment is to gather adequate information in which to make a professional judgment about nutrition status (Lacey and Pritchett, 2003; ASPEN, 2002). The nutrition assessment is the first step in the Nutrition Care Process (Lacey, 2003) (Table 14-3; see Appendix 5 and Chapter 17).

Information gathered depends on the particular setting, present health status of the individual or group, how data is related to particular outcomes, whether it is an initial or follow-up assessment, and recommended practices (ADA, 2005). Once the nutrition assessment process is complete and a nutrition diagnosis made, the nutrition plan of care can be developed. Once interventions are chosen, they can be implemented as tailored for the appropriate setting (e.g., hospital, clinic, home).

The goals of nutrition assessment are to (1) identify individuals who require aggressive nutrition support, (2) restore or maintain an individual's nutrition status, (3) identify appropriate MNT, and (4) monitor the efficacy of these interventions.

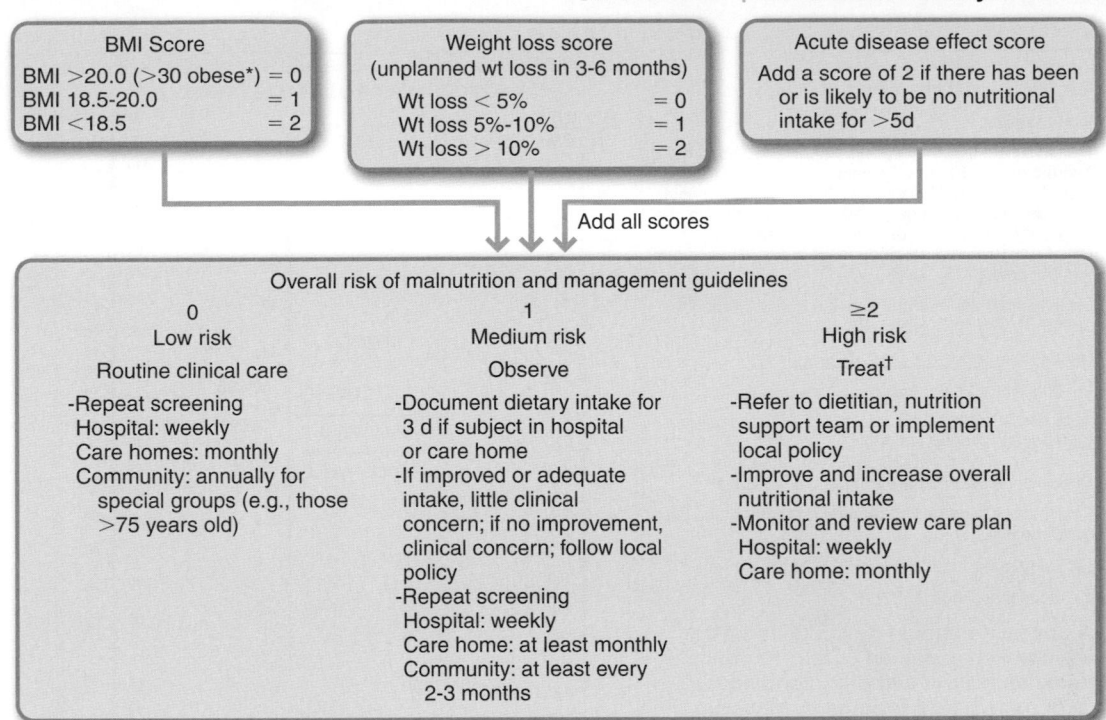

FIGURE 14-6 The Malnutrition Universal Screening Tool ('MUST') for adults **MAG**. Record malnutrition risk category, presence of obesity and/or need for special diets and follow local policy: for those identified at risk. (*Courtesy Professor Marinos Elia, Editor; BAPEN, 2003 ISBN 1 899467 70X. Copies of the full report are available from the BAPEN Office, Secure Hold Business Centre, Studley Road, Redditch, Worcs BN98 7LG Tel: 01527 457850.*)

If unable to obtain height and weight, alternative measurements and subjective criteria are provided (Elia, 2003).

*In the obese, underlying acute conditions are generally controlled before treatment of obesity.

†Unless detrimental or no benefit is expected from nutritional support (e.g., imminent death).

Patients with acute or chronic illnesses have the potential for malnutrition and should be evaluated further. Malnutrition is not uncommon in those who are obese, cachexic, older, or have undergone trauma and in whom nutritional intervention is neglected. Furthermore, the nutrition status of patients who are hospitalized for longer than 2 weeks deteriorates (see *Focus On: Malnutrition in Hospitals*).

Histories

The information collected about individuals or populations is used as part of the nutrition status assessment. Frequently the information is in the form of histories—medical, social, medication, and dietary.

Medical History

The medical history usually includes the following information: chief complaint, present and past illness, current health, allergies, past or recent surgeries, family history of disease, psychosocial data, and a review of problems—by body system—from the patient's perspective (Hammond, 1998). These histories usually provide much insight into nutrition-related problems. Alcohol and drug use, increased metabolic needs, increased nutritional losses, chronic disease, recent major surgery or illness, disease or surgery of the gastrointestinal (GI) tract, and recent significant weight loss all may contribute to malnutrition. In older patients an additional review is recommended to detect mental deterioration,

Text continued on p. 395

◎ FOCUS ON

Malnutrition in Hospitals

In a landmark article Butterworth (1974) showed that malnutrition could indeed be found in the United States—in hospitals, where it was frequently not recognized. Over the course of the next few years, malnutrition was noted in many hospitalized patients, and attempts were made to evaluate its severity and reverse its course. Between 35% to 65% of patients admitted to hospitals today may be malnourished.

The past 30 years have seen periods of heightened awareness and periods of minimum awareness. Much of the heightened awareness centered around the development of aggressive and effective techniques for nutrition support such as improved enteral tube feeding and parenteral nutrition. With only minimum training in nutrition (e.g., nutrition courses spread throughout the curriculum or having very few hours in nutrition studies) offered in many medical schools, physicians graduate with little practical knowledge about nutrition and therefore little awareness of malnutrition. To maintain a high level of awareness, physician education programs in nutrition should be conducted regularly and dietetics practitioners in those settings must continually bring the patient's nutrition status and care to the forefront in team discussions of the patient's overall care planning and implementation.

LEVEL I SCREEN

Body Weight

Measure height to the nearest inch, and weigh to the nearest pound. Record the values below and mark them on the Body Mass Index (BMI) scale to the right. Then use a straightedge (ruler) to connect the two points and circle the spot where this straight line crosses the center line (body mass index). Record the number below.

Healthy older adults should have a BMI between 24 and 27.

Height (in): _____

Weight (lb): _____

Body Mass Index: _____
(number from center column)

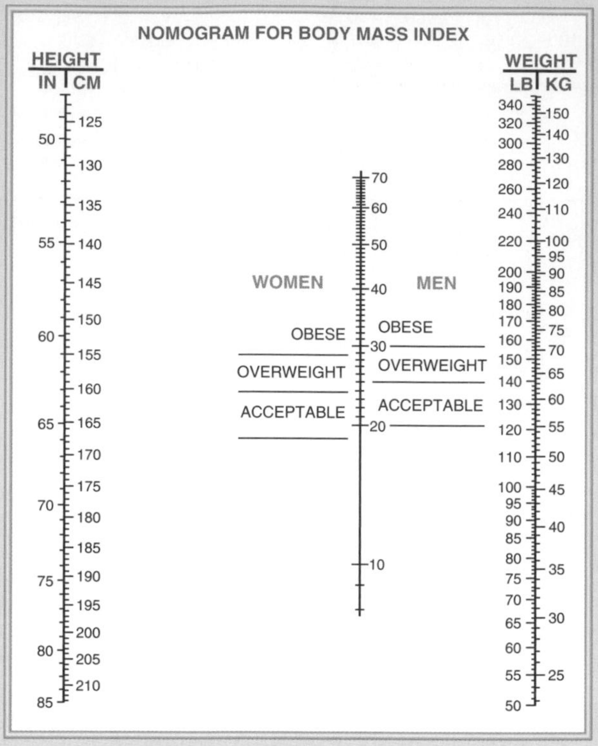

Check any boxes that are true for the individual:

☐ Has lost or gained 10 pounds (or more) in the past 6 months.

☐ Body mass index <24

☐ Body mass index >27

A physician should be contacted if the individual has gained or lost 10 pounds unexpectedly or without intending to during the past 6 months. A physician should also be notified if the individual's body mass index is above 27 or below 20.

For the remaining sections, please ask the individual which of the statements (if any) is true for him or her and place a check by each that applies.

Eating Habits

☐ Does not have enough to eat each day

☐ Usually eats alone

☐ Does not eat anything on one or more days each month

☐ Has a poor appetite

☐ Is on a special diet

☐ Eats vegetables two or fewer times daily

☐ Eats milk or milk products once or not at all daily

☐ Eats fruit or drinks fruit juice once or not at all daily

☐ Eats breads, cereals, pasta, rice, or other grains five or fewer times daily

☐ Has difficulty chewing or swallowing

☐ Has more than one alcoholic drink per day (if woman); more than two drinks per day (if man)

☐ Has pain in mouth, teeth, or gums

Living Environment

☐ Lives on an income of less than $6000 per year (per individual in the household)

☐ Lives alone

☐ Is housebound

☐ Is concerned about home security

☐ Lives in a home with inadequate heating or cooling

☐ Does not have a stove and/or refrigerator

☐ Is unable or prefers not to spend money on food (<$25–$35 per person spent on food each week)

NOMOGRAM FOR BODY MASS INDEX

Functional Status

Usually or always needs assistance with (check all that apply):

☐ Bathing

☐ Dressing

☐ Grooming

☐ Toileting

☐ Eating

☐ Walking or moving about

☐ Traveling (outside the home)

☐ Preparing food

☐ Shopping for food or other necessities

If you have checked one or more statements on this screen, the individual you have interviewed may be at risk for poor nutritional status. Please refer this individual to the appropriate health care or social service professional in your area. For example, a dietitian should be contacted for problems with selecting, preparing, or eating a healthy diet, or a dentist if the individual experiences pain or difficulty when chewing or swallowing. Those individuals whose income, life-style, or functional status may endanger their nutritional and overall health should be referred to available community services: home-delivered meals, congregate meal programs, transportation systems, counseling services, day-care programs, etc.

Please repeat this screen at least once each year — sooner if the individual has a major change in his or her health, income, immediate family (e.g., spouse dies), or functional status.

FIGURE 14-7 Level I screen. *(Courtesy NSI, Washington, DC and Ross Products Division, Abbott Laboratories, Columbus, Ohio.)*

LEVEL II SCREEN

Complete the following screen by interviewing the patient directly and/or by referring to the patient chart. If you do not routinely perform all of the described tests or ask all of the listed questions, please consider including them, but do not be concerned if the entire screen is not completed. Try to conduct a minimal screen on as many older patients as possible; and try to collect serial measurements, which are extremely valuable in monitoring nutritional status. Please refer to the manual for additional information.

Anthropometrics

Measure height to the nearest inch and weigh to the nearest pound. Record the values below and mark them on the Body Mass Index (BMI) scale to the right. Then use a straightedge (paper, ruler) to connect the two points and circle the spot where this straight line crosses the center line (body mass index). Record the number below. Healthy older adults should have a BMI between 24 and 27; check the appropriate box to flag an abnormally high or low value.

Height (in): _____

Weight (lb): _____

Body Mass Index: _____
(number from center column)

Please place a check by any statement regarding BMI and recent weight loss that is true for the patient:

☐ Body mass index <20

☐ Body mass index >27

☐ Has lost or gained 10 pounds (or more) in the past 6 months.

Record the measurement of mid-arm circumference to the nearest 0.1 centimeter and of triceps skinfold to the nearest millimeter (mm).

Mid-arm circumference (cm): _____

Triceps skinfold (mm): _____

Mid-arm muscle circumference (cm): _____

Refer to the table and check any abnormal values:

☐ Mid-arm muscle circumference <10th percentile

☐ Triceps skinfold <10th percentile

☐ Triceps skinfold >95th percentile

Note: mid-arm circumference (cm) − {0.314 × triceps skinfold (mm)} = mid-arm *muscle* circumference (cm)

Percentile	Men		Women	
	55–65 y	65–75 y	55–65 y	65–75 y
Arm circumference (cm)				
10th	27.3	26.3	25.7	25.2
50th	31.7	30.7	30.3	29.9
95th	36.9	35.5	38.5	37.3
Arm muscle circumference (cm)				
10th	24.5	23.5	19.6	19.5
50th	27.8	26.8	22.5	22.5
95th	32.0	30.6	28.0	27.9
Triceps skinfold (mm)				
10th	6	6	16	14
50th	11	11	25	24
95th	22	22	22	36

For the remaining sections, please place a check by any statements that are true for the patient.

Laboratory Data

☐ Serum albumin below 3.5 g/dl

☐ Serum cholesterol below 160 mg/dl

☐ Serum cholesterol above 240 mg/dl

Drug Use

☐ Three or more prescription drugs, OTC medications, and/or vitamin/mineral supplements daily

Clinical Features
Presence of (check all that apply)

☐ Problems with mouth, teeth, or gums

☐ Difficulty chewing

☐ Angular stomatitis

☐ Glossitis

☐ History of bone pain

☐ History of bone fractures

☐ Skin changes (dry, loose, nonspecific lesions, edema)

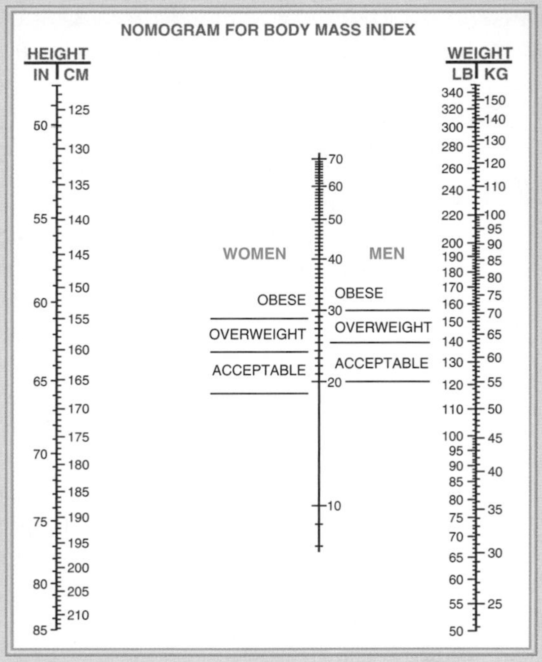

NOMOGRAM FOR BODY MASS INDEX

HEIGHT IN/CM — WEIGHT LB/KG

WOMEN   MEN

OBESE   OBESE

OVERWEIGHT   OVERWEIGHT

ACCEPTABLE   ACCEPTABLE

LEVEL II SCREEN   Name: Date:

Eating Habits

☐ Does not have enough to eat each day

☐ Usually eats alone

☐ Does not eat anything on one or more days each month

☐ Has poor appetite

☐ Is on a special diet

☐ Eats vegetables two or fewer times daily

☐ Eats milk or milk products once or not at all daily

☐ Eats fruit or drinks fruit juice once or not at all daily

☐ Eats breads, cereals, pasta, rice, or other grains five or fewer times daily

☐ Has more than one alcoholic drink per day (if woman); more than two drinks per day (if man)

Living Environment

☐ Lives on an income of less than $6000 per year (per individual in the household)

☐ Lives alone

☐ Is housebound

☐ Is concerned about home security

☐ Lives in a home with inadequate heating or cooling

☐ Does not have a stove and/or refrigerator

☐ Is unable or prefers not to spend money on food (<$25–$35 per person spent on food each week)

Functional Status
Usually or always needs assistance with (check all that apply)

☐ Bathing   ☐ Walking or moving about

☐ Dressing   ☐ Traveling (outside the home)

☐ Grooming   ☐ Preparing food

☐ Toileting   ☐ Shopping for food or other necessities

☐ Eating

Mental/Cognitive Status

☐ Clinical evidence of impairment (e.g., Folstein <26)

☐ Clinical evidence of depressive illness (e.g., Beck Depression Inventory >15, Geriatric Depression Scale >5)

FIGURE 14-8 Level II screen. (*Courtesy NSI, Washington, DC and Ross Products Division, Abbott Laboratories, Columbus, Ohio.*)

TABLE 14-3

Nutrition Care Process: Step 1: Nutrition Assessment

Basic definition and purpose	Nutrition Assessment is the first step of the Nutrition Care Process. Its purpose is to obtain adequate information to identify nutrition-related problems. It is initiated by referral and/or screening of individuals or groups for nutritional risk factors. Nutrition assessment is a systematic process of verifying and interpreting data to make decisions about the nature and cause of nutrition-related problems. The specific types of data gathered in the assessment vary, depending on (a) practice settings, (b) individual's/group's present health status, (c) how data are related to outcomes to be measured, (d) recommended practices such as ADA's Evidenced-Based Guides for Practice, and (e) whether it is an initial assessment or a reassessment. Nutrition assessment requires making comparisons between the information obtained and reliable standards (ideal goals). Nutrition assessment is an ongoing, dynamic process that involves not only initial data collection but also continual reassessment and analysis of patient/client/group needs. Assessment provides the foundation for the nutrition diagnosis at the next step of the Nutrition Care Process.
Data sources/ tools for assessment	Referral information and/or interdisciplinary records Patient/client interview (across the life span) Community-based surveys and focus groups Statistical reports; administrative data Epidemiologic studies
Types of data collected	Nutritional adequacy (dietary history/detailed nutrient intake) Health status (anthropometric and biochemical measurements, physical and clinical conditions, physiologic and disease status) Functional and behavioral status (social and cognitive function, psychological and emotional factors, quality-of-life measures, change readiness)
Nutrition assessment components	Review dietary intake for factors that affect health conditions and nutrition risk Evaluate health and disease condition for nutrition-related consequences Evaluate psychological, functional, and behavioral factors related to food access, selection, preparation, physical activity, and understanding of health condition Evaluate patient's/client's/group's knowledge, readiness to learn, and potential for changing behaviors Identify standards by which data will be compared Identify possible problem areas for making nutrition diagnoses
Critical thinking	The following types of critical thinking skills are especially needed in the assessment steps: Observing for nonverbal and verbal cues that can guide and prompt effective interviewing methods Determining appropriate data to collect Selecting assessment tools and procedures (matching the assessment methods to the situation) Applying assessment tools in valid and reliable ways Distinguishing relevant from irrelevant data Distinguishing important from unimportant data Validating the data Organizing and categorizing the data in a meaningful framework that relates to nutrition problems Determining when a problem requires consultation with or referral to another provider
Documentation of assessment	Documentation is an ongoing process that supports all of the steps in the Nutrition Care Process Quality documentation of the assessment step should be relevant, accurate, and timely; inclusion of the following information would further describe quality assessment documentation: Date and time of assessment Pertinent data collected and comparison with standards Patient's/client's/group's perceptions, values, and motivation related to presenting problems Changes in patient's/client's/group's level of understanding, food-related behaviors, and other clinical outcomes for appropriate follow-up Reason for discharge/discontinuation if appropriate
Determination for continuation of care	If on completion of an initial or reassessment it is determined that the problem cannot be modified by further nutrition care, discharge or discontinuation from this episode of nutrition care may be appropriate

From Lacey K, Pritchett E: Nutrition care process and model: ADA adopts road map to quality care and outcomes management, *J Am Diet Assoc* 103(8):1064, 2003.

constipation or incontinence, poor eyesight or hearing, slowed reactions, major organ diseases, effects of prescription and over-the-counter drugs, and physical disabilities (see Table 14-2).

Social History

Social aspects of the medical history may also relate to nutrition status (e.g., information pertaining to socioeconomic status, the individual's ability to purchase food independently, whether the person is living or eating alone, physical or mental handicaps, smoking, or drug or alcohol addiction. In older adults, confusion caused by environmental changes, unsuitable housing conditions, lack of socialization at meals, psychological problems, or poverty may add to the risks.

Knowledge of various cultures is important during the interviewing process to meet the needs of diverse groups of clients (Curry, 2000). Components or factors that affect a person's cultural values include religious beliefs; rituals; symbols; language; dietary practices; education; communication style; views on health, wellness, and illness; and racial identity. Establishing a bond with clients of different cultures is important for positive outcomes (Heineken and McCoy, 2000) (see *Clinical Insight:* Cultural Awareness, and Chapter 12).

Medication History

Food and drugs interact in many ways that affect nutrition status and drug therapy effectiveness; thus a medication history is an important part of any nutrition assessment. Those who are older, are chronically ill, have a history of marginal or inadequate nutritional intake, or are receiving multiple drugs for a period are susceptible to drug-induced nutritional deficiencies. The effects of drug therapy can be altered by specific foods and the timing of food and meal consumption (see Chapter 16 and Appendix 31). Use of herbal products may also alter the effects of medications (see Chapter 18).

Nutrition or Diet History

Anorexia, **ageusia** (loss of the sense of taste), **dysgeusia** (diminished or distorted taste), **anosmia** (loss of smell), excessive alcohol intake, poor-fitting dentures, fad dieting, chewing or swallowing problems, frequent meals away from home, adverse food and drug interactions, cultural or religious restrictions of diet, an inability to eat for more than 7 to 10 days, intravenous fluid therapy for more than 5 days, or feeding dependence can lead to inadequate nutrient intake and nutritional inadequacy. For many older adults the inability to eat independently, denture problems, changes in taste and smell, long-established poor food habits, food fads, and inadequate knowledge of nutrition are common problems. Alternative nutrition therapies, including use of megadoses of vitamins and minerals, various herbs, macrobiotic diets, probiotics, and amino acid supplements, must be addressed because they have an effect on the person's nutritional and overall health care. Box 14-1 lists some questions in a nutrition questionnaire.

⬡ **CLINICAL INSIGHT**

Cultural Awareness

A cross-cultural assessment tool that includes the following questions can be used in the acute-care setting, home, or other care sites and may be useful in addressing sensitive issues during the initial assessment. If the patient is an immigrant, you may want to ask the following:

- How is this kind of illness treated in your country?
- How would you describe this problem you have? Or, is there someone else I should talk to?
- What does this sickness do to you?
- How long have you had the problem? Why has the problem happened to you?
- Why do you think the problem began when it did?
- What do you think is wrong, out of balance, or causing the problem?
- What has been done so far?
- What do you think will help your problem clear up? What should be done?
- What does your family think should be done?
- Apart from me, who else do you think can help get you better?
- How serious do you think this situation or problem is?

Data from Heineken J, McCoy N: Establishing a bond with clients of different cultures, *Home Healthcare Nurs* 18(1):45, 2000.

A **dietary history** is perhaps the best means of obtaining dietary intake information, and refers to a review of an individual's usual patterns of food intake and the food selection variables that dictate the food intake. See Box 14-2 for the kind of information collected from a dietary history.

Dietary Intake Data. **Dietary intake data** are assessed either by collecting retrospective intake data as with a 24-hour recall or food frequency questionnaire or summarizing prospective intake data, as with a food record kept for a number of days by an individual or the caretaker. Each method has specific purposes, strengths, and weaknesses. The choice depends on the purpose and setting in which the assessment is completed. The goal is to determine the nutrient content of the food and the appropriateness of the intake for a particular individual. The prospective method involves recording data at the time the food is consumed or shortly thereafter.

Daily Food Record or Diary. A daily food record, or **food diary,** involves documenting dietary intake as it occurs and is often used in outpatient clinic settings. Usually a food diary is completed by the individual client (Figure 14-9). A food record is usually most accurate if the food and amounts eaten are recorded at the time of consumption. The individual's nutrient intake is then calculated and averaged at the end of the desired period (usually 3 to 7 days) and compared

BOX 14-1

Nutrition Questionnaire

1. Height: _____ Usual weight: _____ Actual weight: _____
2. Have you had a recent weight loss of greater than 10 lb within 30 days?
3. Have you followed a weight reduction diet? _____ yes _____ no
   If yes, how long ago?_____
4. Have you had a recent change in appetite? _____ yes _____ no
5. Do you have any problems with: swallowing? _____ yes _____ no
   chewing? _____ yes _____ no
   nausea? _____ yes _____ no
   diarrhea? _____ yes _____ no
   vomiting? _____ yes _____ no
   constipation? _____ yes _____ no
6. Do you follow any special diet? _____ yes _____ no
   If yes, what type of diet?_____
7. What, if any foods are you allergic to? _____
8. Do you take any vitamin/mineral supplements? _____ yes _____ no
   If yes, please list:_____
9. Do you take any medications? _____ yes _____ no
   If yes, please list:
   Prescription   *Over-the-counter*

Food Diary: DAY _____				
MEAL Foods (list)	AMOUNT EATEN	HOW PREPARED	WHERE EATEN (home, work, etc.)
Breakfast:			
Snack:			
Lunch:			
Dinner:			
Snack:			

Food Supplements   Cans/Day: _____ Name: _____
Vitamins/Mineral Supplement:_____

FIGURE 14-9 Food diary.

BOX 14-2

Dietary History Information

Economics

Income: frequency and steadiness of employment
Amount of money for food each week or month
Individual's perception of financial adequacy for meeting
    food needs
Eligibility for food stamps and cost of stamps
Public aid assistance status

Physical Activity

Occupation: type, hours/week, shift, energy expenditure
Exercise: type, amount, frequency (seasonal?)
Sleep: hours/day (uninterrupted?)
Handicaps

Ethnic or Cultural Background

Influence on eating habits
Religion
Education

Home Life and Meal Patterns

Number in household (eat together?)
Person who does shopping
Person who does cooking
Food storage and cooking facilities (e.g., stove, refrigerator)
Type of housing (e.g., home, apartment, room)
Ability to shop and prepare foods

Appetite

Good, poor, any changes
Factors that affect appetite
Taste and smell perception (any changes?)

Attitude toward Food and Eating

Disinterest in food
Irrational ideas about food, eating, or body weight
Parental interest in child's eating

Allergies, Intolerances, or Food Avoidances

Foods avoided and reason for avoidance
Length of time of avoidance
Description of problems caused by foods

Dental and Oral Health

Problems with chewing
Foods that cannot be eaten
Problems with swallowing, salivation, food sticking

Gastrointestinal Factors

Problems with heartburn, bloating, gas
Problems with diarrhea, vomiting, constipation, distention
Frequency of problems
Home remedies
Antacid, laxative, or other drug use

Chronic Disease

Treatment
Length of treatment time
Dietary modification: self-imposed or physician prescribed,
    date of modification, education, compliance with diet

Medication and Supplements and Herbal Remedies

Vitamin and/or mineral supplements: frequency of
    administration, type, amount
Medications: type, amount, frequency of administration,
    length of time on medication
Herbal remedies: type, amount, purpose

Recent Weight Change

Loss or gain: how many pounds and over what length
    of time?
Intentional or nonvolitional

Dietary or Nutritional Problems (as Perceived by Patient)

---

with dietary reference intakes (DRIs) (see Chapter 12 or inside front cover) or guidelines in the MyPyramid Guide (see Figure 12-1).

Food Frequency Questionnaire. The **food frequency questionnaire** is a retrospective review of intake frequency (i.e., food consumed per day, per week, or per month). For ease of evaluation the food frequency chart organizes foods into groups that have common nutrients. Because the focus of the food frequency questionnaire is the frequency of consumption of food groups rather than of specific nutrients, the information obtained is general, not specific, for certain nutrients. During illness food consumption patterns can change, depending on the stage of illness. Therefore it is helpful to complete food frequency questionnaires for the period immediately before hospitalization and before illness to obtain a complete and accurate history. Box 14-3 shows a

food frequency questionnaire. Another example of a more specific quantified questionnaire is online at http://www.fhcrc.org/science/shared_resources/nutrition/ffq/gsel.pdf.

24-Hour Recall. The **24-hour recall** method of data collection requires individuals to remember the specific foods and amounts of foods they consumed in the past 24 hours. The information is then analyzed by the person or professional gathering the information. Problems commonly associated with this method of data collection include (1) an inability to recall accurately the kinds and amounts of food eaten, (2) difficulty in determining whether the day being recalled represents an individual's typical intake, and (3) the tendency for persons to exaggerate low intakes and underreport high intakes of foods. Concurrent use of food frequency and 24-hour recall questionnaires (i.e., doing a cross-check) improves the accuracy of intake estimates.

BOX 14-3
General Food Frequency*

1. Do you drink milk? If so, how much?   What kind?   Whole   Skim   Low-fat
2. Do you use fat? If so, what kind?   How much?
3. How often do you eat meat?   Eggs?   Cheese?   Beans?
4. Do you eat snack foods? If so, which ones?   How often?   How much?
5. Which vegetables (in each group) do you eat?   How often?
   - a. Broccoli   Green peppers   Cooked greens   Carrots   Sweet potatoes
   - b. Tomatoes   Raw cabbage
   - c. Asparagus   Beets   Cauliflower   Corn   Cooked cabbage   Celery   Peas   Lettuce
6. Which fruits do you eat? How often?
   - a. Apples or applesauce   Apricots   Bananas   Berries   Cherries   Grapes or grape juice
     Peaches   Pears   Pineapple   Plums   Prunes   Raisins
   - b. Oranges, orange juice   Grapefruit   Grapefruit juice
7. Bread and cereal products
   - a. How much bread do you usually eat with each meal? How much between meals?
   - b. Do you eat cereal? (daily? weekly?) What type?   Cooked   Dry
   - c. How often do you eat foods such as macaroni, spaghetti, and noodles?
   - d. Do you eat whole-grain breads and cereals? How often?
8. Do you use salt? Do you salt your food before tasting it? Do you cook with salt? Do you crave salt or salty foods?
9. How many teaspoons of sugar do you use daily? Include sugar on cereal, fruit, toast, and in beverages such as coffee and tea.
10. Do you eat desserts? How often?
11. Do you drink sugar-containing beverages such as soda pop or sweetened juice drinks? How often? How much?
12. How often do you eat candy or cookies?
13. Do you drink water? How often during the day? How much each time? How much water do you drink each day?
14. Do you use sugar substitutes in packet form or in drinks? What type do you use? How often?
15. Do you drink alcohol? Which type: beer, wine, liquor? How often? How much?
16. Do you drink caffeinated beverages? How often? How much per day?

*To determine the frequency of food consumption, the following pattern of questions may be useful. However, questions may need to be modified based on information from the 24-hour recall. For instance, if a woman states that she drank a glass of milk the day before, do not ask, "Do you drink milk?" rather, "How much milk do you drink?" Record answers with the appropriate time frame designated (e.g., 1/day, 1/wk, 3/mo) or as accurately as possible. The frequency may need to be recorded as "occasionally" or "rarely" if the patient cannot be more specific.

Reliability and validity of dietary recall methods are important issues to address (Kant, 2002). When attention is directed toward the diet, people may consciously or unconsciously alter their intake either to simplify recording or impress the interviewer, thus decreasing the information's validity. The validity of dietary recall information from obese individuals is often questionable because they tend to underreport their intake. The same can be true for children, patients with eating disorders, those who are critically ill, those who abuse drugs or alcohol, individuals who are confused, and those whose intake may be unpredictable. Table 14-4 describes the advantages and disadvantages of the various methods used to obtain accurate dietary intake data.

Nutrient Intake Analysis

A **nutrient intake analysis (NIA)** is also referred to as a nutrient intake record or calorie count, depending on the information collected and the analysis done. The NIA is a tool used in various in-patient settings to identify nutritional inadequacies by monitoring intakes before deficiencies develop. Information about actual intake is collected through direct observation or an inventory of foods eaten based on observation of what remains on the individual's tray or plate after a meal. Tube feeding, either parenteral or enteral is also recorded.

NIAs should be recorded for at least 72 hours to reflect variations in intake that may occur from day to day. Complete records for this period usually accurately reflect an average intake for most individuals. If the record is incomplete, it may be necessary to extend the duration of the intake until a full 72-hour record can be completed. It should be kept in mind that eating habits or meals consumed during the weekend and during the week may differ. The record of total intake can then be analyzed for its nutrient content, using one of several available computerized methods.

Anthropometry

Anthropometry involves obtaining physical measurements of an individual and relating them to standards that reflect the growth and development of the individual. These physical measurements are another component of the nutrition assessment and are useful for evaluating overnutrition or

TABLE 14-4

Methods of Obtaining Dietary Intake Data

Method	Advantages	Disadvantages
Nutrient intake analysis	Allows actual observation of food	May yield inconsistent and subjective estimates consumption Possible variation in portion size
Daily food record or diary	Provides daily record of food consumption Can provide information on quantity of food, how food is prepared, and timing of meals and snacks	Variable literacy skills of participants Requires ability to measure or judge portion size Actual food intake possibly influenced by the recording process Questionable reliability of records
Food frequency	Easily standardized Can be beneficial when considered in combination with usual intake Provides overall picture of intake	Requires literacy skills Does not provide meal pattern data Requires knowledge of portion sizes
24-hour recall	Quick Easy	Relies on memory Requires knowledge of portion sizes May not represent usual intake Requires interviewing skills

Data from *Diet manual and nutrition practice guidelines: a manual of the Georgia Dietetic Association*, Section 5.5-5.3, 2004.

undernutrition. They can be used to monitor the effects of nutrition intervention.

Individuals conducting these measurements should be trained in the proper technique; if more than one professional is conducting these measurements, measures of accuracy between them should be established. Measurements of accuracy can be established by several clinicians taking the same measurement and comparing results. It may take more than 20 practice sessions to become proficient (Lee and Nieman, 2003).

Anthropometric data are most valuable when they reflect accurate measurements and are recorded over a period of time. Valuable measurements are height, weight, skin-fold thicknesses, and girth measurements. Head circumference and length are commonly used in pediatric populations. Birth weight and ethnic, familial, and environmental factors affect these parameters and should be taken into consideration when anthropometric measures are evaluated.

Interpretation of Height and Weight

Reference standards in current use are based on a statistical sample of the U.S. population. Therefore an individual measurement shows how a person's measurement compares with that of the total population, not with an established standard.

Height and weight measurements of children are evaluated against various norms. They are recorded as percentiles, which reflect the percentage of the total population of children of the same sex who are at or below the same height or weight at a certain age. Children's growth at every age can be monitored by mapping data on growth curves, known as **height-for-age,** length-for-age, **weight-for-age,** and **weight-**

BOX 14-4

Using Height and Weight To Assess a Hospitalized Patient's Nutritional Status

- Measure, do not just ask a person's height
- Measure weight (at admission, current, and usual).
- Determine percentage of weight change over time (weight pattern).
- Determine percentage above or below usual or ideal body weight.

for-length curves. Appendixes 9 through 16 describe percentiles and growth charts for infants, children, and adolescents up to the age of 20 years. Height and weight are useful in determining nutrition status in adults. Both should be measured because the tendency is to overestimate height and underestimate weight, resulting in an underestimation of the relative weight or BMI. In addition many adults are shrinking as a result of osteoporosis, joint deterioration, and poor posture, and this should be noted (Box 14-4).

Length and Height

Height measurements are valuable when used in conjunction with other anthropometric and clinical assessment measurements. Various methods may be used to measure length and height. Measurements of height can be obtained using a direct or an indirect approach. The direct method involves a measuring rod, or statiometer, and the person must be able to stand or recline flat. Indirect methods, including arm span (see

Figure 45-2), recumbent length (using a tape measure), and knee height measurements (see Figure 45-1), may be options for those who cannot stand or stand straight such as individuals with scoliosis, kyphosis (curvature of the spine), cerebral palsy, muscular dystrophy, contractures, or paralysis or those who are bedridden (see Appendix 20). Recumbent height measurements made with a tape measure while the person is in bed may be appropriate for individuals in institutions who are comatose, critically ill, or unable to be moved. However, this method can only be used with patients who do not have musculoskeletal deformities or contractures.

Sitting heights (see Figure 45-1) are used for children who cannot stand, and recumbent length measurements are used for infants and children younger than 2 or 3 years of age. Ideally these young children should be measured using a length board as demonstrated in Figure 14-10. Recumbent lengths in children age 3 and under should be recorded on the Birth to 36 month growth grids, while standing heights of children age 2 to 3 years should be recorded on the 2 to 20 years growth grids (see Appendixes 9 to 16). Recording on the proper growth grids provides a record of a child's gain in height over time and compares the child's height with that of other children of the same age. The rate of length or height gain reflects long-term nutritional adequacy.

Weight

Weight is another measure that is easy to obtain but is very telling. In children it is a more sensitive measure of nutritional adequacy than height, and it reflects recent nutritional intake. Weight also provides a crude evaluation of overall fat and muscle stores (Hopkins, 1993). Body weight is obtained and interpreted using various methods, including BMI, usual weight, and actual weight.

Ideal weight for height from reference standards such as the Metropolitan Life Insurance Tables from 1959 and 1983 and the National Health and Nutrition Examination Survey (NHANES) percentiles is no longer used. Usual body weight (UBW) is a more useful parameter than ideal body weight for those who are ill. Comparing the present weight to the UBW allows weight status changes to be assessed. One problem with using a UBW measurement is that it is dependent on the patient's memory.

Actual body weight is the weight measurement obtained at the time of examination. This measurement may be influenced by changes in the individual's fluid status. Weight loss (in pounds or kilograms) can reflect dehydration but can also reflect an immediate inability to meet nutrition requirements and thus may indicate nutritional risk. The percentage of weight loss is highly indicative of the extent and severity of an individual's illness. The following formula (Blackburn, 1977) is useful in determining the percentage of recent weight loss:

Significant weight loss: 5% loss in 1 month, 7.5% loss in 3 months, 10% loss in 6 months

Severe weight loss: >5% weight loss in 1 month, >7.5% weight loss in 3 months, >10% weight loss in 6 months

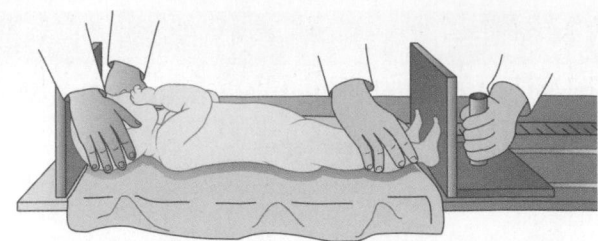

FIGURE 14-10 Measurement of the length of an infant. Crown-to-heel length of children 3 years and younger should be measured as follows: (1) Lay the child on a ruled board that has an attached piece of wood at one end and a movable piece at the other. (2) Stretch the child out on the board for the most accurate measurement. (3) Place the movable end flat against the bottom of the child's foot and read the length from the side of the board.

Another method for determining the percentage of weight loss is to determine an individual's current weight as a percentage of the usual weight. Minimum weight for survival is 48% to 55% of UBW (Buchman, 1997). The percentage of UBW or ideal body weight can be used to assess the degree of malnutrition as follows:

- Patients with weight within 85% to 90% of UBW: mild malnutrition
- Patients with weight within 75% to 84% of UBW: moderate malnutrition
- Patients with weight less than 74% of UBW: severe malnutrition

To determine whether an adult's weight is appropriate for height, the practitioner should look at the BMI of the individual.

Body Mass Index

The Quetelet's index (W/H^2), the most widely used height-weight index (Lee and Nieman, 2003), is commonly referred to as the **body mass index (BMI)** and is a validated measure of nutrition status. The BMI calculation requires weight and height measurements and, based on the result, it can indicate overnutrition or undernutrition. BMI accounts for differences in body composition by defining the level of adiposity and relating it to height, thus eliminating dependence on frame size (Stensland and Margolis, 1990). BMI can be calculated using any of the following formulas:

- Metric formula: BMI = Weight (kg) ÷ Height (m)²

- English formula: BMI = Weight (lb) ÷ (Height [in] × Height [in]) × 703

Nomograms: Also available to calculate BMI are various charts (see Appendix 23.) Further, Appendixes 11 and 15 allow for the plotting of the BMI on a growth grid used with children ages 2 to 20 years) (see *Clinical Insight:* Calculating BMI and Determining Appropriate Body Weight).

The BMI has the least correlation with body height and the highest correlation with independent measures of body fat for adults, including older adults. The BMI does not

CLINICAL INSIGHT

Calculating BMI and Determining Appropriate Body Weight

Example: Woman who is 5' 8" (1.72 m) tall and weighs 185 pounds (lb) (84 kg)

Step 1: Calculate current BMI:

Formula: Weight (kg) 84 kg ÷ Height (1.72 m) ×
(Metric)   (1.72 m) = 84 ÷ 84/2.96 m² =
                                       28.4 = overweight

Step 2: Appropriate weight range to have a BMI that falls between 18.5 and 24.9

18.5   (18.5) × (2.96) = 54.8 kg = 121 pounds
24.9   (24.9) × (2.96) = 73.8 kg = 162 pounds

Appropriate weight range = 121 – 162 lb or 54.8 – 73.8 kg

Formula (English) Weight (lb) ÷ (Height [in] × (Height [in] × 703

Body Composition

Differences in skeletal size and the proportion of lean body mass can contribute to body weight variations among individuals of similar height. For example, muscular athletes may be classified as overweight because their excess muscle mass, not their adipose mass, increases their weight. Older adults tend to have lower bone density and therefore may weigh less than younger adults of the same height. Indirect methods for measuring body composition include triceps skin-fold (TSF), midarm muscle circumference (MAMC), and midarm circumference (MAC) (Shopbell et al., 2001).

The health professional must know that these measures are useful in the assessment of individuals over time but not in critical- and acute-care settings because changes in body fluid and composition may influence the results. When conducting body composition measurements, strict adherence to established protocols must be followed to yield accurate results. For example, most North American investigators use the right side of the body to take skin-fold measurements, and the standards are based on this. The methods used to gather meaningful data should be considered carefully (Lee and Nieman, 2003).

Subcutaneous Fat (Skin-Fold Thickness)

The fat-fold or skin-fold thickness measurement is a means of assessing the amount of body fat in an individual. It is practical in clinical settings, although its validity depends on the accuracy of the measuring technique (Box 14-5) and repetition of measurements over time. If changes are going to occur, they take 3 to 4 weeks. This measurement bases total body fat estimates on the assumption that 50% of body fat is subcutaneous (Figure 14-11). Accuracy decreases with increasing obesity.

The skin-fold sites identified as most reflective of body fatness are over the triceps and the biceps, below the scapula, above the iliac crest (suprailiac), and on the upper thigh. The triceps skin-fold and subscapular measurements are the most useful because the most complete standards and methods of evaluation are available for these sites (Figures 14-12 and 14-13) (see Appendixes 24-26) and the EVOLVE website for various tables related to arm and skin-fold measurements). Figure 14-14 shows the measurement of the suprailiac crest skin-fold.

Circumference Measurements

If more complete information on actual body composition is needed, additional anthropometric data can be obtained. These data include additional skin-fold and circumference measurements. Depending on the setting of patient care, some measurements may be more appropriate than others. For example, in the acute-care setting where the patient has more acute pathophysiologic changes going on such as daily fluid shifts, measures of arm circumference and triceps skin-fold measurements are not usually performed. But in the long-term setting or home setting, these measurements can be tracked over time (e.g., monthly or quarterly) and provide valuable information on long-term nutrition status.

measure body fat directly but correlates with the direct body fat measures such as underwater weighing and dual x-ray absorptiometry (DEXA) (Keys et al., 1972) (Mei et al., 2002). BMI ranges are based on the relationships between body weight, disease processes, and mortality (CDC, 2002).

Standards classify a BMI for an adult at less than 18.5 as underweight, a BMI between 25 and 29 as overweight, and a BMI greater than 30 as obese. A healthy BMI for adults is considered between 18.5 and 24.9 (Centers for Disease Control and Prevention, 2002) (see Table 21-2). Although a strong correlation exists between total body fat and BMI, individual variations need to be recognized before the final assessment (Shopbell et al., 2001). Differences in race, sex, and age must be considered when evaluating the BMI (Sanchez et al., 2000; Tam et al., 1999).

BMI values tend to increase with age (Vaccarino and Krumholz, 2001). Recent studies report an association between BMI and mortality for nonhospitalized patients 65 years of age and older, but the data do not support the BMI range of 25 to 27 as a risk factor for all-cause and cardiovascular mortality. The conclusion is that federal guideline standards for ideal weight (BMI of 18.5 to less than 25) may be too restrictive for older adults. Careful interpretation of risk factors must be part of the total assessment (see Chapter 10).

Appendixes 12 and 16 present the grids for recording BMI measurements and changes for children and adolescents over time. The method of calculation of BMI in children and teens is the same as that for adults, but the interpretation is different as is shown on these tables. For example, a BMI of only 17 is very appropriate for a 10-year-old girl (see Appendix 19).

BOX 14-5

Skin-Fold Measurement Techniques

1. Take measurement on the right side of the body.
2. Mark the site to be measured and use a flexible, nonstretchable tape.
3. The tape measure can be used to locate the midpoints on the body.
4. Firmly grasp the skin fold with the thumb and index finger of the left hand about 1 cm or ½ inch proximal to the skin-fold site, pulling it away from the body.
5. Hold the caliper in the right hand, perpendicular to the long axis of the skin fold and with the caliper's dial face up. Place the caliper tip on the site and about 1 cm or ½ inch distal to the fingers holding the skin fold. (Pressure from the fingers does not affect the measurement.)
6. Do not place the caliper too deeply into the skin fold or too close to the tip of the skin fold.
7. Read the caliper approximately 4 seconds after pressure from the measurer's hand has been released from the lever. Exerting force longer than 4 seconds results in smaller readings because fluids are forced from the compressed tissue. Measurements should be recorded to the nearest 1 mm.
8. Take a minimum of two measurements at each site to verify results. Wait 15 seconds between measurements to allow the skin-fold site to return to normal. Maintain pressure with thumb and index finger during measurements.
9. Do not take measurements immediately after the person has exercised or if the person is overheated because the shift in body fluid makes the result larger.
10. When measuring obese clients, it may be necessary to use both hands to pull the skin away while a second person makes the measurement. If the calipers do not fit, another technique may be required.

Data from Lee RD, Nieman DC: *Nutritional assessment*, ed 3, New York, 2003, McGraw-Hill.

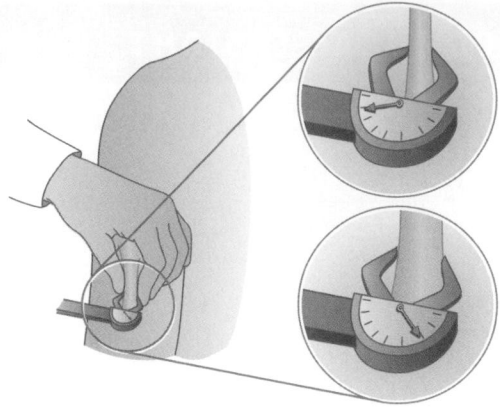

FIGURE 14-11 Skin-fold calipers measuring the thickness of subcutaneous fat (in millimeters), giving a rough measurement of adiposity. Measurements are read counterclockwise. (*Courtesy Dorice Czajka-Narins, PhD.*)

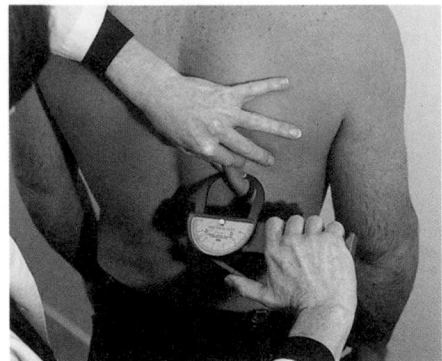

FIGURE 14-12 Measurement of the subscapular skin-fold thickness.

Because of the recognition that fat distribution is an indicator of risk, circumferential or girth measurements are used more frequently today. The presence of excess body fat around the abdomen out of proportion to total body fat is considered a risk factor for ailments associated with obesity and the metabolic syndrome. Waist circumference measurements are often used.

The older method, waist-to-hip circumference ratio (WHR) is used to detect possible signs of excess fat deposition (lipodystrophy) in those infected with the human immunodeficiency virus (HIV); it is used less often today, but a ratio of 0.8 or above indicates risk in a woman, and 1 and above indicates risk in a man.

Waist Circumference. **Waist circumference** is obtained by measuring the distance around the smallest area below the rib cage and above the umbilicus with the use of a nonstretchable tape measure. Waist circumference measurements assess abdominal fat content. A measurement of greater than 40 inches (102 cm) for men and greater than 35 inches (88 cm) for women is an independent risk factor for disease (Centers for Disease Control and Prevention, 2002). These measurements may not be as useful for those less than 60 inches tall or with a BMI of 35 or above (Centers for Disease Control and Prevention, 2002). Figure 14-15 shows the proper location to measure waist (abdominal) circumference.

Midarm Circumference. MAC is measured in centimeters halfway between the acromion process of the scapula and the olecranon process at the tip of the elbow as shown in Figure 14-13, *A.* Combining MAC with TSF measurements allows indirect determination of the arm muscle area (AMA) and arm fat area (AFA) (see Appendixes 25 and 26). Bonefree AMA is calculated by using the formula shown in Figure 14-16; for men, a factor of 10 is subtracted from the AMA, whereas for women a factor of 6.5 is subtracted (Frisancho, 1984).

The AMA, or bone-free muscle area, is a good indication of lean body mass and thus an individual's skeletal protein reserves. The AMA is important in growing children and is

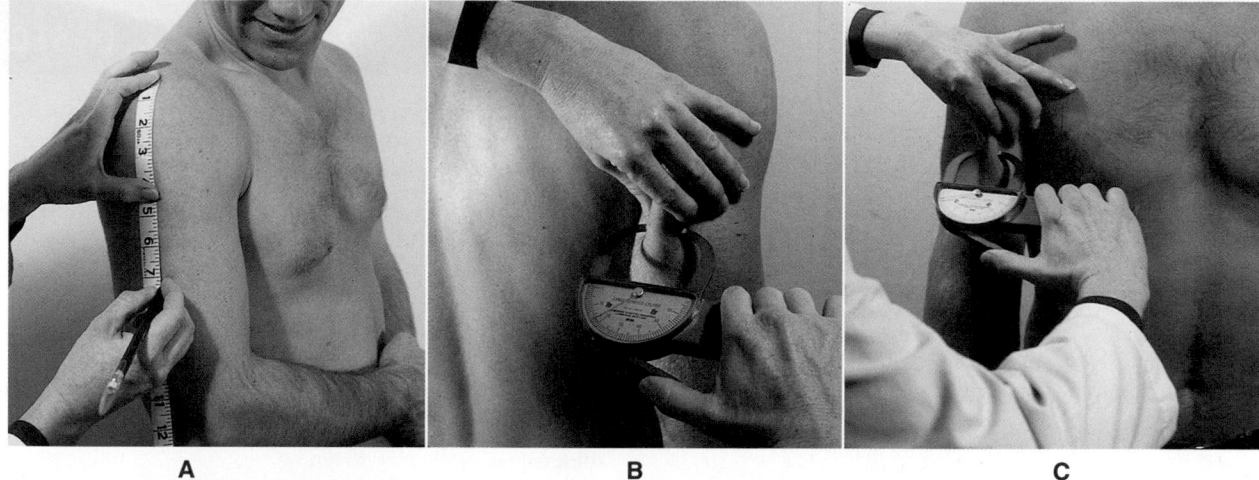

FIGURE 14-13 A, Measurement and marking of the midpoint between the acromion process at the shoulder and the olecranon process at the elbow. **B,** Measurement of the triceps skin-fold (in mm) at the marked midpoint, and **C,** measurement of the biceps skin-fold (in mm) at the marked midpoint.

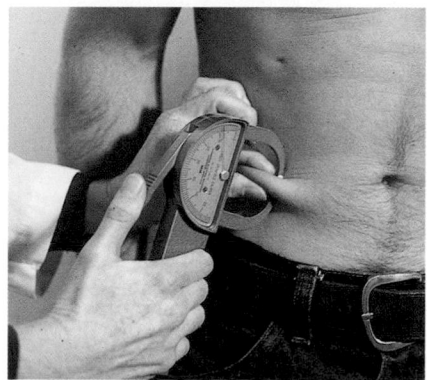

FIGURE 14-14 Measurement of the supraliac crest skin-fold (in mm) above the bony prominence of the iliac crest and across from the navel.

especially valuable in evaluating possible protein-energy malnutrition as a result of chronic illness, stress, an eating disorder, multiple surgeries, or an inadequate diet (see EVOLVE website).

Head Circumference. Head circumference measurements are useful in children younger than 3 years of age, primarily as an indicator of nonnutritional abnormalities. Undernutrition must be very severe to affect head circumference (see *Clinical Insight:* Head Circumference).

Calf Circumference. Measurements of calf circumference, combined with other anthropometric measures, can be used to estimate body weight in older adults (Lohman et al., 1988).

Other Methods of Measuring Body Composition

Underwater Weighing. A more direct measure of determining whole-body density is densitometry, which includes underwater (hydrostatic) weighing. Underwater weighing is based on Archimedes' principle: the volume of an object

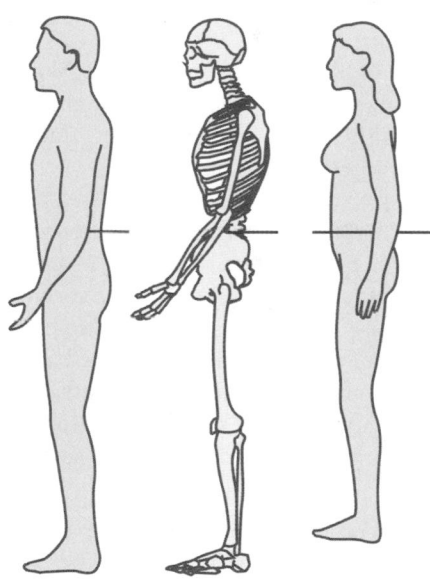

FIGURE 14-15 Measuring tape position for waist (abdominal) circumference measurement. *(From www.nhlbi. nih.gov/guidelines/obesity/e_txtbk/txgd/4142.htm.)*

submerged in water equals the volume of water the object displaces. Once the volume and mass are known, the density can be calculated. Although this method is considered the gold standard (Indorato, 2001), it is not always practical, involves significant training to perform, and requires considerable cooperation on the part of those being measured because they must be submerged under water and remain motionless long enough for the measurements to be made (Lee and Nieman, 2003).

Total Body Potassium. Total body potassium can be used to study body composition because more than 90% of the body's potassium is found in fat-free tissues. Measurements are made with a special counter that is fitted with multiple gamma-ray detectors interfaced with a computer that is

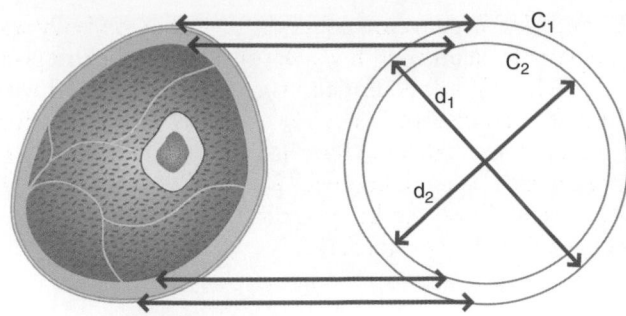

$$AA \ (mm^2) = \pi/4 \times d_1^2 \text{ where } d_1 = C_1/\pi$$
$$AMA \ (mm^2) = (C_1 - \pi T)^2/4\pi = (C_1 = \pi T)^2/12.56$$
$$AFA \ (mm^2) = AA - AMA$$
$$\text{Bone-free } AMA - AMA - 10 \text{ for males}$$
$$\text{Bone-free } AMA - AMA - 6.5 \text{ for females}$$

FIGURE 14-16 Upper arm area *(AA)*, upper arm muscle area *(AMA)*, and upper arm fat area *(AFA)* are derived from measurements of upper arm circumference in centimeters *(C1)* and triceps skin-fold *(T)* in millimeters.

expensive and not always readily available. Not all researchers agree on the exact concentration of potassium in fat-free tissue and the differences between sexes, during the aging process, and in obese individuals.

Neutron Activation Analysis. The neutron activation analysis allows measurements of the body's calcium, iodine, hydrogen, sodium, chloride, phosphorus, carbon, and nitrogen contents (Lee and Nieman, 2003). Neutron activation measures lean body mass. The analysis is based on the assumption that fat-free tissue conducts electricity better than fat (Shopbell et al., 2001). This type of measurement is expensive and impractical in a daily clinical setting.

Bioelectrical Impedance Analysis. **Bioelectrical impedance analysis (BIA)** is a body composition analysis technique based on the principle that relative to water, lean tissue has a higher electrical conductivity and lower impedance than fatty tissue because of its electrolyte content. BIA has been found to be a reliable measurement of body composition (fat-free mass and fat mass) when compared with BMI or skin-fold measurements or even height and weight measurements (Kyle et al., 2001). BIA involves attaching electrodes to the right hand, wrist, ankle, and foot of a patient and passing a small electrical current through the body.

The BIA method is popular as a means of assessment because it is safe, noninvasive, portable, and rapid. For accurate results the patient should be well hydrated; have not exercised in the previous 4 to 6 hours; and have not consumed alcohol, caffeine, or diuretics in the previous 24 hours. If the person is dehydrated, a higher percentage of body fat than really exists is measured. Fever, electrolyte imbalance, and extreme obesity also affect the reliability of measurements (Shronts et al., 1998). Depending on the type of system used, additional recommendations for the person being measured include drinking two to four glasses of wa-

⬥ **CLINICAL INSIGHT**

Head Circumference

Indications

Head circumference is a standard measurement for serial assessment of growth in children from birth to 36 months and in any child whose head size is in question.

Equipment

Paper or metal tape measure (cloth can stretch) marked in tenths of a centimeter since growth charts are listed in 0.5 cm increments.

Technique

1. The head is measured at its greatest circumference.
2. The greatest circumference is usually above the eyebrows and pinna of the ears and around the occipital prominence at the back of the skull.
3. More than one measurement may be necessary since the shape of the head can affect the location of the maximum circumference.
4. Compare the measurement with the National Center for Health Statistics (NCHS) standard curves for head circumference (see Appendixes 10 and 14).

Data from Hockenberry MJ, Wilson D: *Wong's nursing care of infants and children*, ed 8, St. Louis, 2007, Mosby.

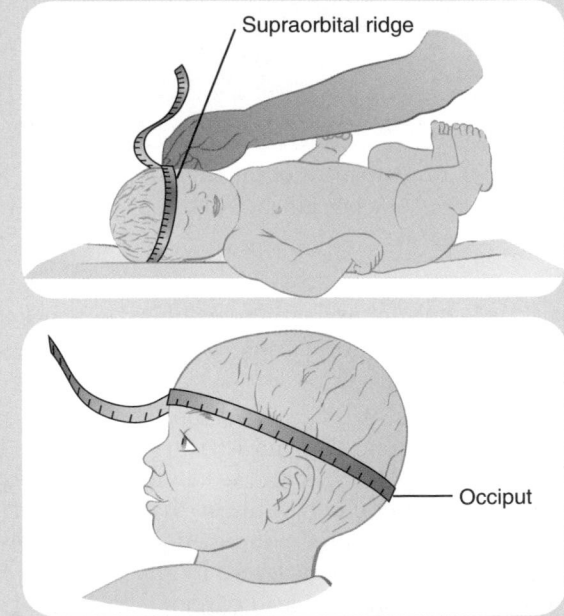

ter approximately 2 hours before the test and emptying the bladder just before the test is given (Indorato, 2001).

Several companies manufacture BIA systems, and the different systems have different advantages. For example, the Bodystat require sensors to be attached at the wrist and ankle (Figure 14-17), whereas other systems such as the Tanita use a "stand-on" sensor and another uses a hand-held sensor. Professional systems range in price from $1200 to $5000, and software packages add an additional cost. Personal

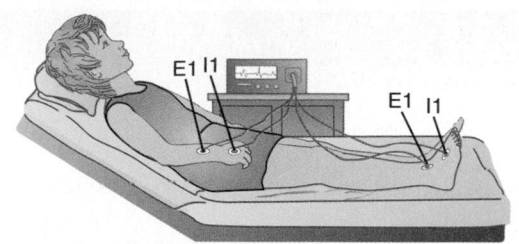

FIGURE 14-17 Bioelectrical impedance analysis (BIA).

models for home use range from $49 to $250. Professionals who would like to use BIA equipment need to speak with the various manufacturers to decide which system is best for their particular practice; factors to consider include details such as cost; ages and types of clients seen; ease of transport; and convenience (Indorato, 2001).

Computed Tomography. Computed tomography, or CT scan, has been useful for studying nutrition status. It has been particularly helpful for assessing the deposition of subcutaneous and intraabdominal fat, which aids in determining nutritional risk associated with morbidity and mortality. It does involve the use of ionizing radiation.

Ultrasound and Magnetic Resonance Imaging. Magnetic resonance imaging (MRI) can be used to measure the size of visceral organs, the size of the skeleton, and the amount and distribution of intraabdominal fat. MRI has several advantages, two of which are that it is noninvasive and involves no ionizing radiation, which makes it safe for children, females of childbearing age, and multiple studies on the same individual. The disadvantages of MRI include expense and limited availability (Lee and Nieman, 2003; Shopbell et al., 2001).

Dual-Energy X-Ray Absorptiometry. DEXA is a means of assessing bone mineral density and can be used for measuring fat and boneless lean tissue. The energy source in DEXA is an x-ray tube that contains an energy beam (Lee and Nieman, 2003). The amount of energy loss depends on the type of tissue through which the beam passes; the result can be used to measure mineral, fat, and lean tissue compartments (Shopbell et al., 2001). DEXA is easy to use, emits low levels of radiation, is relatively available in the hospital setting, and requires little cooperation from the patient, thus making it a useful tool. Differences in hydration status and the presence of bone or calcified soft tissue can result in inaccurate measurements (Lee and Nieman, 2003).

Air Displacement Plethysmogram. Air displacement plethysmogram (ADP) relies on measurements of body density to estimate body fat and fat-free masses. ADP with the BOD-POD (see Figure 2-3) is a new densitometry technique found to be an accurate method to measure body composition (Aleman-Mateo et al., 2004). ADP appears to be a reliable instrument in body composition assessment; it is of particular interest in the pediatric and obese individual, areas which require further study (Fields et al., 2005). In addition, ADP is convenient and does not rely on body water content to determine body density and body composition, which makes it potentially useful in those adults with end-stage renal disease (Flakoll et al., 2004). However, further research is needed in understanding possible sources of measurement error (Fields et al., 2005). The use of a BOD-POD is usually based on budget, the patient population, and the experience of the clinician.

NUTRITION-FOCUSED PHYSICAL EXAMINATION

A nutrition-focused physical examination is an important component of overall nutrition assessment because some nutritional deficiencies may not be identified by other assessment approaches. Some signs of nutritional deficiency are not specific and must be distinguished from those with a nonnutritional etiology.

Physical Signs

A systems approach is used when performing the examination, which should be conducted in an organized, logical way that progresses from head to toe to ensure efficiency and thoroughness. The examination moves from a global to a more defined or focused examination based on the results of the medical and nutrition histories. The nutrition-focused physical examination is tailored for each patient. In other words, every body system may not have to be assessed in all people; clinical judgment guides this decision (Hammond, 1998).

Equipment

The extent of the nutrition-focused physical examination dictates the necessary equipment. Any or all of the following may be used: a stethoscope, a penlight or flashlight, a tongue depressor, scales, a reflex hammer, calipers, a tape measure, a blood pressure cuff, and an ophthalmoscope.

Examination Techniques

Four basic physical examination techniques are used during the nutrition-focused physical examination. These techniques include inspection, palpation, percussion, and auscultation (Table 14-5).

Findings

Some significant nutritional findings from the physical examination that should alert the clinician to the need for further assessment and intervention may include temporal wasting, proximal muscle weakness, depleted muscle bulk, dehydration, overhydration, poor wound healing, and chewing or swallowing difficulties. The appearance of the skin should be evaluated for any pallor, scaly dermatitis, wounds, quality of wound healing, bruising, and hydration status. Membranes (conjunctiva or pharynx) should be examined for integrity, hydration, pallor, and bleeding (see *Clinical Insight:* Hydration Status).

TABLE 14-5

Physical Examination Techniques

Technique	Description
Inspection	General observation that progresses to a more focused observation using the senses of sight, smell, and hearing; most frequently used technique
Palpation	Tactile examination to feel pulsations and vibrations; assessment of body structures, including texture, size, temperature, tenderness, and mobility
Percussion	Assessment of sounds to determine body organ borders, shape, and position; not always used in a nutrition-focused physical examination
Auscultation	Use of the naked ear or a stethoscope to listen to body sounds (e.g., heart and lung sounds, bowel sounds, blood vessels)

From Hammond K: Nutrition focused physical assessment, *Support Line* 18(4):4, 1996.

Special attention should be given to the areas where signs of nutritional deficiencies appear (e.g., skin, hair, teeth, gums, lips, tongue, eyes, and genitalia [in men]). The hair, skin, and mouth are susceptible because of the rapid cell turnover of epithelial tissue. Mucosal changes in the GI tract are indicated by problems such as diarrhea and anorexia. Symptoms of nutrient deficiencies may or may not be apparent during the physical examination. Many signs result from a lack of several nutrients, as well as from non-nutritional causes. Appendix 29 discusses the physical examination and findings in more detail. Potential nutrition diagnosis codes for classifying nutritional problems can be found on EVOLVE.

Immune Function

Skin testing, or delayed hypersensitivity reactivity (DHR), and total lymphocyte count (TLC) are two measures of immune function that can be used as screening and assessment parameters. DHR measures cell-mediated immunity and involves the intradermal injection of small amounts of antigen, most commonly tuberculin, *Candida* organisms, mumps, or trichophytin, just under the skin to determine the person's reaction. A healthy person reacts with induration, indicating that exposure has probably taken place and immunocompetence is intact; no reaction may be associated with malnutrition. DHR is not useful for individuals with an electrolyte imbalance, an infection, cancer, liver disease, renal failure, trauma, or immunosuppression (Shopbell et al., 2001). DHR is not always a useful component of the nutrition assessment for hospitalized patients (Shronts et al., 1998). TLC is also an indicator of immune function reflective of B and T cells (see Chapter 15).

Handgrip Dynamometry

Handgrip dynamometry can provide a baseline nutritional assessment of muscle function by measuring grip strength and endurance and is useful in serial measurements. Measurements are expressed as a percentage of a standard for men and women (Guenter et al., 1989):

Men: 48.8 ± 7.0 kg; Women 34.4 ± 4.7 kg

Biochemical Analysis

Biochemical tests are the most objective and sensitive measures of nutrition status, but not all are appropriate. Caution must be used when interpreting results because they can be affected by disease state and therapy. Chapter 15 and Appendix 30 provide a complete discussion of the role of laboratory data in nutritional assessment.

CLASSIFYING MALNUTRITION

Once a nutrition assessment is completed, the extent of nutritional adequacy, deficiency, or excess is apparent. Malnutrition can then be classified based on several indexes, including body weight, body fat, somatic and visceral protein stores, and laboratory values.

Once the nutrition assessment is completed and the nutrition status determined, a nutrition diagnosis can be established, followed with appropriate interventions and determination of outcomes (see Chapter 17). Implementing a nutritional care plan involves defining the nutrition problem to be addressed (based on assessment), identifying the appropriate nutrition diagnoses, establishing therapeutic goals or desired outcomes, determining appropriate interventions to be implemented as they relate to the nutrition therapy goals, identifying the educational needs of the patient, and formulating a plan for monitoring and evaluation.

In many cases the plan of care is included on the nutrition assessment form (see Figure 14-18 for a sample assessment form).

Date:	Time:	Age:	Sex:

NUTRITION ASSESSMENT
Adm. Medical Diagnosis:_____
PMHx:_____

Current Relevant Labs:

Significant Meds:

Anthropometrics:
Ht:_____ Est. Dry Wt:_____ BMI:_____
Admit Wt:_____ IBW:_____ % IBW:_____
Current Wt:_____ Usual BW:_____ % Usual BW:_____
　　　　　　　　　　　　 Wt Hx:_____

Patient/Family Interview:
_____
_____

Intake/Digestive Problems		**Physical & Mental Status**	**Metabolic Stressors**	**Access** ☐ PO
☐ Anorexia	☐ Diarrhea	☐ Hearing impaired	☐ Post-op/surgery	☐ NGT ☐ NJT
☐ Chewing problem:	☐ Food allergy/Intol		☐ Fever/infection	☐ OGT ☐ GT
_____		☐ Limited vision	☐ Wounds	☐ JT ☐ GJT
☐ Swallowing problem			☐ Trauma/fracture	☐ PEG ☐ HICKMAN
_____		☐ Dementia	☐ Sepsis	☐ PORTACATH
☐ Poor dentition	☐ Assist w/ Meals	☐ Language barrier	☐	☐ PICC
☐ Nausea	☐ ETOH/Drugs	☐ Mental status changes	Other_____	
☐ Vomiting	☐ NPO____days	☐ N/A		
☐ Constipation	☐ Aspiration precautions			

Diet Prior to Admission:　　　　　　　　　　　**Current Diet Rx:**

☐ Adequately nourished　　☐ Obese　　☐ At risk for malnutrition　　☐ Malnourished
☐ Physical appearance _____

Est. needs based on:　　　　kcals: _____ Pro.:_____ Fluid:_____ ml
NUTRITION DIAGNOSTIC STATEMENTS: (PES: Problem, Etiology, Signs/Symptoms)　　Nutrition risk level _____ (low-moderate-high)
Problem _____
Related to _____
As evidenced by _____

Problem _____
Related to _____
As evidenced by _____

NUTRITION INTERVENTION:
Short-term goal _____
Long-term goal _____
Food-Nutrition Therapy: _____

Education: _____

Counseling: _____

Coordination of Care: _____

Expected outcome:　☐ Patient will increase PO intake to 50%-75% of meals/supplements consistently within____days.
　　　　　　　　　☐ Patient will tolerate tube feeding/PN goal of _____within ____days.
　　　　　　　　　☐ Patient will meet at least 75% of estimated needs from all sources of nutrient intake within____days.
　　　　　　　　　☐ Other: _____
☐ Patient/family aware of interventions
MONITORING/EVALUATION:
☐ I&0 sheet　　☐ Labs_____
☐ Patient rounds　　☐ Patient care team rounds　　☐ Other_____

SIGNATURE: Registered/Licensed Dietitian _____ Pager #_____

FIGURE 14-18 Sample nutrition assessment form.

✳ CLINICAL INSIGHT

Hydration Status

It is important to recognize the fluid volume status of an individual during the nutrition-focused physical examination. Fluid disturbances can be associated with other imbalances such as electrolyte imbalance.

Fluid Volume Deficit

From the history: Note any excessive loss of water and electrolytes from vomiting, diarrhea, excessive laxative abuse, fistulas, GI suction, polyuria, fever, excessive sweating, and edema (third-space fluid shifts). Fluid volume deficit can also be caused by decreased intake, which may be prominent in those with anorexia, nausea, depression, and inability to gain access to fluids.

Associated characteristics: Characteristics of a fluid volume deficit include weight loss that occurs over a short period, decreased skin and tongue turgor, dry mucous membranes, postural hypotension, a weak and rapid pulse, slow-filling peripheral veins, a decrease in body temperature (95° to 98° F), decreased urine output, cold extremities, disorientation, changes in laboratory test results (e.g., a blood urea nitrogen [BUN] level elevated out of proportion to serum creatinine, elevated hematocrit) (see Chapter 4).

Fluid Volume Excess

From the history: Note any history of renal failure, congestive heart failure, cirrhosis of the liver, or Cushing's syndrome; excess use of sodium-containing intravenous fluids; and excessive intake of sodium-containing food or medication products.

Associated characteristics: Characteristics of fluid volume excess include weight gain that occurs over a short period, peripheral edema, distended neck veins, slow emptying of peripheral veins, rales in lungs, polyuria, ascites, pleural effusion, a bounding and full pulse, changes in laboratory test results (e.g., decreased BUN, decreased hematocrit), and in severe cases pulmonary edema.

Data from Methany N: *Fluid and electrolyte balance: nursing considerations,* Philadelphia, 1992, Lippincott.

◉ FOCAL POINTS

- Nutrition screening is needed to identify those individuals who would benefit from more in-depth nutrition assessment, intervention and follow-up.
- Careful and meticulous nutrition assessment is an important tool in patient management.

- Adaptations of the exact content of the screening and assessment will vary according to the patient's medical diagnosis and clinical setting.
- A skilled registered dietitian uses the screening and assessment process to make the best possible decisions about the specific nutritional diagnoses, interventions, desired outcomes and evaluation.

✳ CLINICAL SCENARIO 1

Carl is a 32-year-old man who is 5 ft, 9 in tall. He was diagnosed as having acquired immune deficiency syndrome (AIDS) 1 year ago. In the past year his weight has gradually decreased from a usual weight of 175 lb to the current low of 130 lb. His visceral proteins are depleted, and a triceps skinfold measurement reveals a body fat value that is 55% of standard. Carl's oral intake ability has gradually decreased; he can only take sips of an enteral supplement and occasional bites of food.

✱**Nutrition Diagnosis:** Inadequate oral food/beverage intake related to poor appetite and inability to eat as evidenced by loss of 45 lb in 12 months and intake much less than requirements

1. Is Carl exhibiting a degree of undernutrition? If so, classify the extent of malnutrition he has.
2. Carl's current weight is what percentage of his usual body weight?
3. What is Carl's body mass index?
4. Develop a nutrition assessment questionnaire for Carl.

⬡ CLINICAL SCENARIO 2

Laverne, a 66-year-old black woman, has contacted you to set up an outpatient nutrition screening appointment. She has a 20-year history of diabetes mellitus, a 10-year history of colon cancer, and hypertension. She is 5 ft, 8 in tall and weighs 203 lb. Her current medications are gluconase and a diuretic. (She does not know its name.)

＊Nutrition Diagnosis: Overweight/obesity related to poor food choices as evidenced by a BMI of 31

1. What would you include in a nutrition assessment for Laverne?
2. How would you identify her medications?
3. What anthropometry measurement would you take and how would you interpret it?
4. If you need more details, what questions would you ask her physician?
5. What other information do you need to develop a nutrition care plan?

USEFUL WEBSITES

Bioelectrical impedance
www.odp.od.nih.gov/consensus/ta/015/015_statement.htm

Centers for Disease Control and Prevention
www.cdc.gov/nchs/about/major/nhanes/growthcharts/charts.htm
www.cdc.gov/nchs/nhanes.htm
www.cdc.gov/nccdphp/dnpa/obesity/basics.htm

Maternal and Child Health Bureau (MCHB) Training Modules
www.depts.washington.edu/growth/

National Heart, Lung, and Blood Institute
www.nhlbi.nih.gov/index.htm

National Institutes of Health
www.cc.nih.gov/nutr.care.htm

U.S. Department of Agriculture
www.nal.usda.gov/fnic/etext/000108.html

References

Aleman-Mateo H et al: Determination of body composition using air displacement plethysmography, anthropometry and bio-electrical impedance in rural elderly Mexican men and women, *J Nutr Health Aging* 8(5):344, 2004.

American Academy of Family Physicians: Nutrition Screening Intitiative, http://www.aafp.org/online/en/home/clinical/nsi.html, accessed August 7, 2006.

American Dietetic Association: Nutrition assessment. In *ADA Nutrition Care Manual On-line*, Chicago, 2005, American Dietetic Association.

American Dietetic Association: Medical nutrition therapy, http://www.eatright.org/ada/files/chartofmntvsnuted12905pm.pdf, accessed August 7, 2006.

ASPEN Board of Directors: Guidelines for the use of parenteral and enteral nutrition in adults and pediatric patients, *JPEN J Parenter Enteral Nutr*, 26(supl 1):ISA, 2002.

Blackburn GL: Nutritional and metabolic assessment of the hospitalized patient, *JPEN J Parenter Enteral Nutr* 1:11, 1977.

Buchman AL: *Handbook of nutritional support*, Baltimore, 1997, Williams & Wilkins.

Butterworth CE: The skeleton in the hospital closet, *Nutr Today* March/April, p 4, 1974.

Centers for Disease Control and Prevention: Basics about overweight and obesity, 2002, www.cdc.gov/nccdphp/dnpa/obesity/basics.htm.

Charney P: Nutrition screening and assessment in older adults, *Today's Dietitian* 7(5):10, 2005.

Chima C: *Nutrition screening practices in health care organizations: a pilot survey*, Clinical Nutrition Management electronic newsletter, Chicago, 2006, American Dietetic Association, http://www.cnmdpg.org/index_875.cfm, accessed August 7, 2006.

Curry KR: Multicultural competence in dietetics and nutrition, *J Am Diet Assoc* 100:1142, 2000.

Davidson I, Smith S: Nutritional screening: pitfalls of nutrition screening in the injured obese patient, *Proc Nutr Soc* 63:421, 2004.

Elia M: *Screening for malnutrition: a multidisciplinary responsibility. development and use of the 'malnutrition universal screening tool' ('MUST') for adults*, Worcester, England, 2003, Redditch.

Fields DA et al: Air-displacment plethysmography: here to stay, *Curr Opin Clin Nutr Metabol Care* 8(6):624, 2005.

Flakoll PJ et al: Bioelectrical impedance vs air displacement plethysmography and dual-energy X-ray absorptiometry to determine body composition in patients with end-stage renal disease, *JPEN J Parenter Enteral Nutr* 28(1):13, 2004.

Frisancho AR: New standards of weight and body composition by frame size and height for assessment of nutritional status of adults and the elderly, *Am J Clin Nutr* 40:808, 1984.

Guenter PA et al: Anthropometric measurements. In Rombeau JL et al, editors: *Atlas of nutritional support techniques*, Boston, 1989, Little, Brown.

Haffner S, Taegtmeyer H: Epidemic obesity and the metabolic syndrome, *Circulation* 108:1541, 2003.

Hammond KA: The history and physical exam. In Matarese LE, Gottschlich M, editors: *Contemporary nutrition support practice*, Philadelphia, 1998, Saunders.

Heineken J, McCoy N: Establishing a bond with clients of different cultures, *Home Healthcare Nurs* 18(1):45, 2000.

Hopkins B: Assessment of nutritional status. In Gottschlich MM, Matarese LE, Shronts EP, editors: *Nutrition support dietetics*, ed 2, Silver Spring, Md, 1993, American Society for Parenteral and Enteral Nutrition.

Indorato D: Body composition analysis, *Today's Dietitian* 3:9, 2001.

Kant AK: Nature of dietary reporting by adults in the third National Health and Nutrition Examination Survey, 1988-1994, *J Am Coll Nutr* 21:315, 2002.

Keys A et al: Indices of relative weight and obesity, *J Chronic Dis* 25:329, 1972.

Kyle UG et al: Fat-free mass percentiles in 5225 healthy subjects aged 15 to 98 years, *Nutrition* 17(7):8, 2001.

Lacey K, Pritchett E: Nutrition care process and model: ADA adopts road map to quality care and outcomes management, *J Am Dietetic Assoc* 103(8):1061, 2003.

Lee RD, Nieman DC: *Nutritional assessment*, ed 3, New York, 2003, McGraw-Hill.

Lohmann TG et al, editors: *Anthropometric standardization reference manual*, Champaign, Ill, 1988, Human Kinetics Publishers.

Mei Z et al: Validity of body mass index compared with other body-composition screening indexes for the assessment of body fatness in children and adolescents, *Am J Clin Nutr* 75:978, 2002.

National Center for Health Statistics: *Leading causes of death, National Vital Statistics*, available at http://www.cdc.gov/nchs/data/dvs/LCWK2_2002.pdf, accessed July 18, 2004.

Pfau PR, Rombeau JL: Nutrition, *Med Clin N Am* 84:1209, 2000.

Pichard C et al: Nutritional assessment: Lean body mass depletion at hospital admission is associated with an increased length of stay, *Am J Clin Nutr* 79(4):613, 2004.

Sanchez AM et al: Reduced mortality associated with body mass index (BMI) in African-Americans relative to Caucasians, *Ethn Dis* 10(1):24, 2000.

Shopbell et al: Nutrition screening and assessment. In Gottschlich M et al, editors: *The science and practice of nutrition support: American Society for Parenteral and Enteral Nutrition*, Dubuque, Iowa, 2001, Kendall/Hunt.

Shronts EP et al: Nutrition assessment. In Merritt RS et al, editors: *The A.S.P.E.N. nutrition support practice manual*, Silver Spring, Md, 1998, American Society for Parenteral and Enteral Nutrition.

Stensland SH, Margolis S: Simplifying the calculation of body mass index for quick reference, *J Am Diet Assoc* 90:856, 1990.

Stratton RJ et al: Malnutrition in hospital outpatients and inpatients: prevalence, concurrent validity and ease of use of the 'malnutrition universal screening tool' ('MUST') for adults, *Br J Nutr* 92(5):799, 2004.

Tam SY et al: Body mass index is different in normal Chinese and Caucasian infants, *J Pediatr Endocrinol Metab* 12:507, 1999.

U.S. Department of Health and Human Services: *Healthy People 2010*, Washington, DC, 2000.

U.S. Department of Health and Human Services: *The Surgeon General's call to action to prevent and decrease overweight and obesity*, Rockville, Md, 2001, Office of the Surgeon General.

Vaccarino HA, Krumholz HM: An evidence-based assessment of federal guidelines for overweight and obesity as they apply to elderly persons, *Arch Intern Med* 161:1194, 2001.

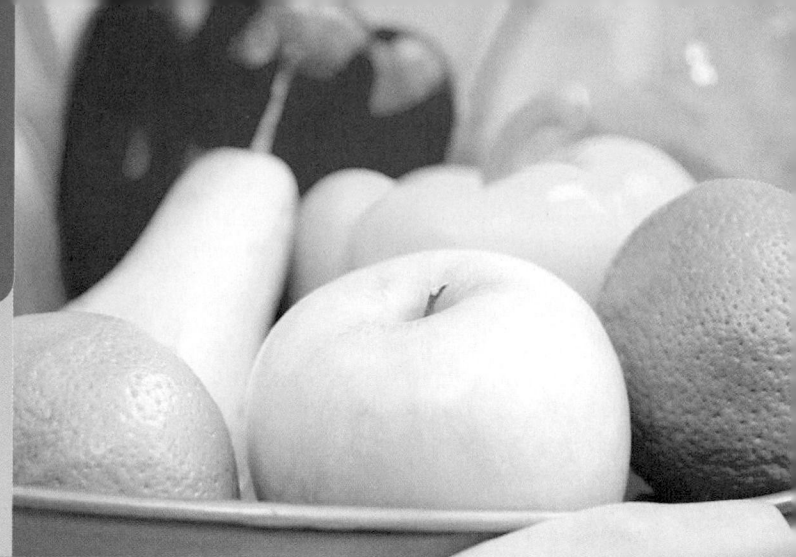

CHAPTER **15**

Mary Demarest Litchford, PhD, RD, LDN

Assessment: Laboratory Data

KEY TERMS

albumin the most abundant (55% to 65% of total) plasma protein; a negative acute-phase respondent with a long half-life ($t_{1/2}$ = 21 days); maintains plasma oncotic pressure and acts as a transport protein

anemia of chronic and inflammatory diseases (ACD) a condition of impaired iron use in which functional iron (i.e., hemoglobin) is low, but tissue iron (i.e., ferritin) is normal or high; due to raised cytokine levels, shortened erythrocyte survival, and impaired bone marrow response

basic metabolic panel (BMP) eight blood tests used for screening

complete blood count (CBC) analysis and description of the red blood cells

comprehensive metabolic panel (CMP) 14 blood tests, including all the tests in the basic metabolic panel used for screening

C-reactive protein (CRP) acute-phase protein that increases in infectious diseases, inflammatory disorders, malignancy, and tissue trauma

creatinine a chemical breakdown product of creatine phosphate; used as a marker of renal function and muscle mass

differential count part of white blood cell count that enumerates each of the specific classes of leukocytes

ferritin a protein that sequesters iron in a form readily activated for transport; found primarily in the liver and other iron storage sites; plasma ferritin is proportional to intracellular ferritin and useful in assessing iron status

functional assay the appraisal of nutrient pool size by measurement of the activity of a biochemical or physiologic activity dependent on a specific nutrient

hematocrit the measure of the percentage of red blood cells in total blood volume

hemoglobin measure of the total amount of hemoglobin, the oxygen-carrying pigment of red blood cells, in the peripheral blood

high-density lipoprotein (HDL) subtypes five types of HDL (HDL2a, HDL2b, HDL2c, HDL3a, and HDL3b) that provide different levels of protection against cardiovascular disease

high-sensitivity C-reactive protein (hs-CRP) a special CRP test to detect slight elevations of CRP, which are associated with increased risk for occlusive cardiovascular diseases, peripheral vascular disease, and end-stage kidney disease

homocysteine an amino acid that is an intermediate in the synthesis of methionine and the methyl group donor, *S*-adenosylmethionine; because the *S*-adenosylmethionine cycle requires vitamin B_{12} and folate, deficiencies in these vitamins are associated with hyperhomocysteinemia, an independent risk factor for occlusive cardiovascular disease

lp(a) 'lipoprotein little a' a highly atherogenic low-density lipoprotein fraction

macrocytic anemia a condition marked by a mean red cell volume of greater than 100 femtoliters (fl); most often caused by vitamin B_{12} or folate deficiencies

microcytic anemia a condition marked by a mean red cell volume of less than 80 femtoliters (fl); commonly associated with iron deficiency

negative acute-phase respondents a group of plasma proteins, including albumin and prealbumin (transthyretin), the concentrations of which decrease during inflammatory conditions (the acute-phase reaction)

Sections of this chapter were written by Timothy H. Carlson, PhD, RD, NRCC, for the previous edition of this text.

nutrition-specific laboratory data tests on body fluids (e.g., plasma, serum, saliva), tissues (e.g., whole blood, cells, hair, nails), and waste (e.g., urine, feces, sweat) that are performed by controlled physical, chemical, biochemical, molecular, diagnostic, or microscopic examination primarily to provide information about nutrient pool status

oxidative stress the balance between the formation of toxic, free radical oxidation products and the reactions that convert these compounds to benign end products

pattern A LDL low-density lipoprotein subclass that is buoyant and less dense (per mg cholesterol) and is the least atherogenic of the LDL subclasses

pattern B LDL low-density lipoprotein subclass that is small and dense (per milligram of cholesterol) and is the most atherogenic of the LDL subclasses

positive acute-phase respondents a group of plasma proteins, including C-reactive protein and alpha 1-acid glycoprotein (orosomucoid), the concentrations of which increase during inflammatory states (the acute-phase reaction)

prealbumin (PAB) a negative acute-phase respondent plasma protein that is also called transthyretin (TTHY); binds thyroxine and retinol-binding protein and is commonly used to monitor protein-energy status; because of its short half-life ($t_{1/2}$ = 2 days), it rapidly responds to improving protein-energy status

reactive oxidation species (ROS) free radical species, including hydrogen peroxide (H_2O_2), superoxide radicals (O^{2-}), and hydroxyl radicals (OH) that are formed during metabolic processes or metabolism of xenobiotic compounds

retinol-binding protein (RBP) a negative acute-phase respondent plasma protein with a half-life ($t_{1/2}$ = 12 hours) the concentration of which correlates with protein-energy status; binds and transports retinol

static assay appraisal of nutrient pool size by direct measurement of the nutrient in a biologic fluid, tissue, or waste

total iron-binding capacity (TIBC) a measurement of the potential for plasma to bind ferric ion (Fe[III])+)

transferrin the plasma protein that transports iron from one organ to another; a negative acute-phase respondent that has a medium half-life ($t_{1/2}$ = 8 days) and is responsive to protein-energy status

urinalysis physical and/or chemical examination of the urine to screen for infections and diseases that result in the appearance of abnormal metabolites in the urine

Laboratory tests are ordered to diagnose diseases, evaluate treatment plans, monitor medication effectiveness, and evaluate medical nutrition therapy (MNT). Acute illness or injury can trigger dramatic changes in laboratory test results, including rapidly deteriorating nutrition status. However, chronic diseases that develop slowly over time also influence these results, but it is unclear how much lifestyle choices and genetics or combinations of additional factors contribute to the current condition.

DEFINITIONS AND USEFULNESS OF NUTRITION LABORATORY DATA

Laboratory assessment is a stringently controlled process. It involves analyzing control samples, with predetermined analyte concentrations, with every batch of patient specimens. The results obtained from the control samples analyzed with a particular batch of patient samples must compare favorably with the predetermined acceptable values before the patient data are considered valid. Laboratory data are the only objective data used in nutritional assessment that are "controlled"—that is, the validity of the method of its measurement is checked each time a specimen is assayed by also assaying a sample with a known value (Figure 15-1).

Laboratory-based nutritional testing, used to estimate nutrient availability in biologic fluids and tissues, is critical for assessment of both clinical and subclinical nutrient deficiencies. As shown in Figure 15-2, the size of a nutrient pool can vary continuously from frankly deficient, to adequate, to toxic. Most of these states can be assessed in the laboratory so that nutritional intervention can occur before frank deficiency occurs (Litchford, 2005). Furthermore, the patient's response to nutritional intervention by laboratory measurement of the body's nutrient pool or function can be assessed sooner, before clinical or anthropometric changes take place (see Appendix 30).

The nutrition professional can use laboratory data to support subjective judgment and clinical assessment findings. Furthermore, because numeric values do not themselves connote personal judgment, this kind of data can often be passed on to a patient or client without implicit or perceived blame. Laboratory test results provide objective data to use in the nutrition care process to assess nutrition status, identify nutrition diagnoses, and monitor and evaluate nutrition care outcomes.

Single test results must be evaluated in light of the patient's current medical condition, medications, lifestyle choices, age of the patient, hydration status, fasting status at the time of

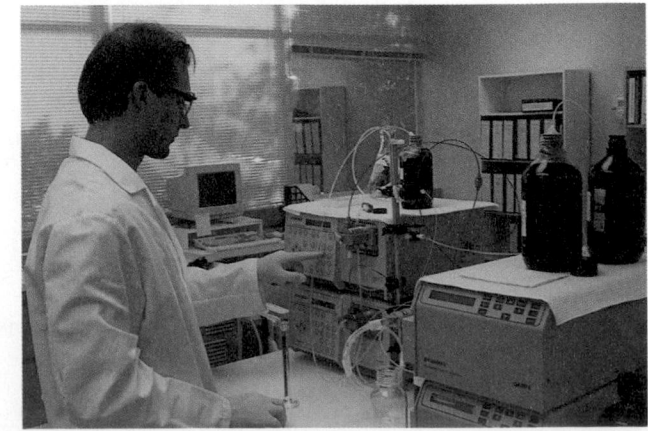

FIGURE 15-1 A technician sets up a high-performance liquid chromatography (HPLC) assay to measure various vitamins and carotenoids.

the specimen collection, and reference standards used by the clinical laboratory. Single test results are useful for screening or to confirm an assessment based on changing clinical, anthropometric, and dietary status. Comparison of current test results to historic baseline test results from the same laboratory is preferred, if available. Changes in laboratory test results that occur over time are an objective measure of the impact of MNT or pharmacologic interventions.

Specimen Types

Ideally the specimen to be tested reflects the total body content of the nutrient to be assessed. However, the best specimen may not be readily available.

The most common specimens for analysis for nutrients and nutrient-related substances are the following:

- Whole blood: collected with an anticoagulant if entire content of the blood is to be evaluated; none of the elements are removed; contains red blood cells, white blood cells, and platelets suspended in plasma
- Serum: the fluid obtained from blood after the blood has been clotted and then centrifuged to remove the clot and blood cells
- Plasma: the transparent (slightly straw colored) liquid component of blood, composed of water, blood proteins, inorganic electrolytes, and clotting factors
- Blood cells: separated from anticoagulated whole blood for measurement of cellular analyte content
- Erythrocytes (red blood cells)
- Leukocytes (white blood cells) and leukocyte fractions
- Blood spots: dried whole blood from finger or heel prick that is placed on paper and can be used for selected hormone tests and other tests such as infant phenylketonuria screening
- Other tissues (obtained from scrapings or biopsy samples)
- Urine (from random samples or timed collections): contains a concentrate of excreted metabolites
- Feces (from random samples or timed collections): important in nutritional analyses when nutrients are not absorbed and therefore are present in fecal material

Less commonly used specimens include the following:

- Saliva: noninvasive medium that has a fast turnover and currently is used to evaluate functional adrenal stress and hormone levels
- Nails: easy-to-collect tissue that may be of value in determining exposure to toxic metals; usually a poor indicator of actual body levels of nutrients
- Hair: an easy-to-collect tissue that is usually a poor indicator of actual body levels of nutrients; may have value in determining exposure to toxic metals
- Sweat: classically used for presence of cystic fibrosis

The latter specimens have significant drawbacks, including potential contamination from contact with the environment and lack of standardized procedures for processing, assay, and quality control. Nutrient levels or indices may be less than the amounts that can be measured accurately and precisely (see *Clinical Insight:* Hair Analysis). However, because these specimens can be collected at the point of care, considerable research is being done to improve their usefulness.

Assay Types

The two fundamental types of laboratory assays are static assays and functional assays. **Static assays** measure the actual level of nutrient in the specimen. Examples of this kind of assay include serum iron, white blood cell ascorbic acid, and hair zinc. Although this kind of assay has the advantage of being absolutely specific for the nutrient of interest, specimen nutrient concentrations do not reflect the amount of that substance stored in body pools that are not sampled. The other major limitation of static assays is that recent dietary intake can influence the amount of a nutrient found in serum, plasma, or any other fluid or tissue. This problem can be overcome, at least partially, by collecting the specimen when the person is fasting. An overnight (8- to 12-hour) fast is usually adequate.

Functional assays quantitatively measure a biochemical or physiologic activity that depends on the nutrient of interest. This type of assay can be very sensitive for a nutrient at its functional site. A good example of a functional assay is serum ferritin. The concentration of ferritin released into the blood is a function of the iron present in the cellular

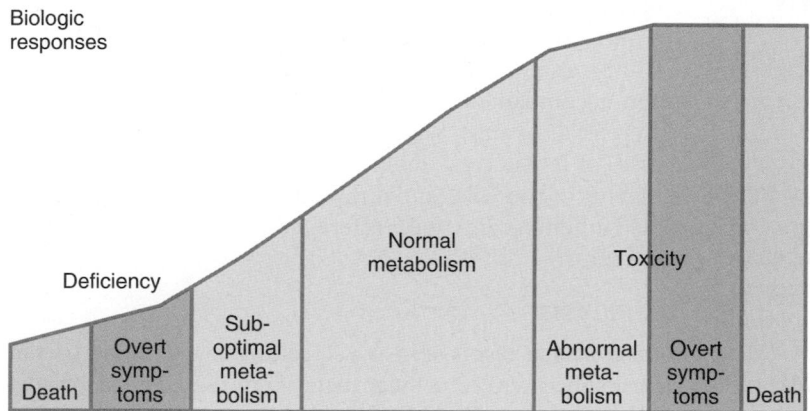

FIGURE 15-2   The size of a nutrient pool can vary continuously from frankly deficient, to adequate, to toxic.

✸ CLINICAL INSIGHT

Hair Analysis

Hair analysis is not particularly useful for assessing levels of minerals such as sodium, magnesium, phosphorus, potassium, calcium, iron, and iodine because good tests already exist for evaluating body functions related to these minerals. However, hair analysis may be helpful in assessing levels of trace elements such as zinc, copper, chromium, and manganese—for which measurements of functional status are not well developed—and levels of cadmium and lead, which have negative biologic effects. Hair can be used for DNA testing and may be useful in the future as a noninvasive methodology to predict genetic predisposition to disease and effectiveness of MNT (see Chapter 13).

However, to be clinically useful, hair analysis procedures must be refined and standardized, and "normal" values for hair mineral content defined and accepted. Currently hair analysis is more useful in experimental efforts than in clinical medicine. The technique is most useful when used to analyze levels of a single element rather than several elements at one time because the probability of an abnormal test result increases as the specificity of the test decreases.

Even if hair analysis results are judged to be "abnormal," it is not known whether these results reflect abnormal exposure to an element and thus a cause of the disease, or whether the abnormal result is an effect of the disease. Use of hair dyes and other chemical processes may also affect results. No evidence shows that nutritional therapy based on hair analysis is of any benefit.

DNA, Deoxyribonucleic acid.

BOX 15-1

Two Common Groups of Laboratory Tests

Basic Metabolic Panel (BMP) Includes:

Glucose
Calcium
Sodium
Potassium
CO_2 (carbon dioxide, bicarbonate)
Chloride
Blood urea nitrogen (BUN)
Creatinine

Comprehensive Metabolic Panel (CMP) Includes:

Glucose
Calcium
Sodium
Potassium
CO_2 (carbon dioxide, bicarbonate)
Chloride
Blood urea nitrogen (BUN)
Creatinine
Albumin
Total protein
Alkaline phosphate (ALP)
Alanine aminotransferase (ALT)
Aspartate aminotransferase (AST)
Bilirubin

storage pool. Unfortunately functional assays are not always specific for the nutrient of interest because many physiologic and biochemical functions depend on various biologic factors in addition to the specific nutrient.

NUTRITION INTERPRETATION OF ROUTINE MEDICAL LABORATORY TESTS

Clinical Chemistry Panels

Laboratory tests are ordered as panels or groupings of tests or as individual tests. The most commonly ordered groups of tests are the **basic metabolic panel (BMP)** and the **comprehensive metabolic panel (CMP)** that include groups of laboratory tests defined by the Centers for Medicare and Medicaid Services for reimbursement purposes. The BMP includes eight tests used for screening, and the CMP includes all the tests in the basic metabolic panel and six additional tests (Box 15-1). Table 15-1 briefly explains these

tests, but the information is not exhaustive, and reference norms may vary; see the various textbooks on the topic and Appendix 30 to obtain more detailed information.

Clinical chemistry panels used in conjunction with health history, physical examination findings, anthropometric data, and dietary intake data can be helpful in screening for nutrition-related health conditions and monitoring MNT. Used in this way, these panels can provide **nutrition-specific laboratory data** that allows dietitians to complete nutrition assessments.

The Complete Blood Count

Another panel of tests that is commonly available for review by nutritionists is the **complete blood count (CBC)**. The CBC or analysis and description of the red blood cells is often accompanied by a **differential count** (often called a differential, or diff), which enumerates each of the specific classes of leukocytes. Table 15-2 provides a list of the basic elements of the CBC and differential (which are collectively called a hemogram), with reference ranges and explanatory comments.

Urinalysis

The **urinalysis** test is used as a screening or diagnostic tool to detect substances or cellular material in the urine associated with different metabolic and kidney disorders. Urinalysis data are qualitative or semiquantitative, and much of the data re-

TABLE 15-1

Constituents of the Common Serum Chemistry Panels

Analytes	Reference Range*	Significance
Serum electrolytes		
Na⁺	135-145 mEq/L†	Of general interest in monitoring various patients, such as those receiving total parenteral nutrition or who have renal conditions, chronic obstructive pulmonary disease, uncontrolled diabetes mellitus (DM), various endocrine disorders, ascitic and edematous symptoms, or acidotic or alkalotic conditions; decreased K⁺ associated with diarrhea, vomiting or nasogastric aspiration, some drugs, licorice ingestion, and diuretics; increased K⁺ associated with renal diseases, crush injuries, infection, and hemolyzed blood specimens
K⁺	3.6-5 mEq/L†	
Cl⁻	101-111 mEq/L†	
HCO₃⁻ (or total CO₂)	21-31 mEq/L†	
Glucose	70-99 mg/dl (fasting)	Fasting glucose >125 mg/dl indicates DM (oral glucose tolerance tests are not needed for diagnosis); fasting glucose >100 mg/dl is indicator of insulin resistance
		Monitor levels along with triglycerides in those receiving total parenteral nutrition for glucose intolerance
Creatinine	0.6-1.2 mg/dl; 53-106 µmol/L (males) 0.5-1.1 mg/dl; 44-97 µmol/L (females)	Increased in those with renal disease and decreased in those with PEM (i.e., blood urea nitrogen/creatinine ratio >15:1)
Blood urea nitrogen (BUN) or urea	5-20 mg urea nitrogen/dl 1.8-7 mmol/L	Increased in those with renal disease and excessive protein catabolism; decreased in those with liver failure and negative nitrogen balance and in females who are pregnant
Albumin	3.5-5 mg/dl	Decreased in those with liver disease or acute inflammatory disease
Serum enzymes		
Alanine aminotransferase (ALT)	4-36 units/L at 37° C; 4-36 units/L	Increased in those with any of a variety of malignant, muscle, bone, intestinal, and liver diseases or injuries
Gamma glutamyltransferase	4-25 units (females) 12-38 units (males	
Alkaline phosphatase (ALP)	30-120 units/L; 0.5-2.0 µKat/L	AST and ALT useful in monitoring liver function in those receiving total parenteral nutrition
Aspartate aminotransferase (AST)	0-35 international units/L; 0-.58 µKat/L	
Bilirubin	Total bilirubin 0.3-1.0 mg/dL; 5.1-17.0 µmol/L Indirect bilirubin 0.2-0.8 mg/dL; 3.4-12.0 µmol/L Direct bilirubin 0.1-0.3 mg/ dL; 1.7-5.1 µmol/L	Increased in association with drugs, gallstones, and other biliary duct diseases; intravascular hemolysis and hepatic immaturity; decreased with some anemias
Total calcium	8.5-10.5 mg/dl	Hypercalcemia associated with endocrine disorders, malignancy, and hypervitaminosis D
		Hypocalcemia associated with vitamin D deficiency and inadequate hepatic or renal activation of vitamin D, hypoparathyroidism, magnesium deficiency, renal failure, and nephrotic syndrome
Phosphorous (phosphate)	3-4.5 mg/dl	Hypophosphatemia associated with hypoparathyroidism and decreased intake; hyperphosphatemia associated with hyperparathyroidism, chronic antacid ingestion, and renal failure

*Reference ranges may vary slightly among laboratories.

† mEq/L = 1 mmol/L.

PEM, Protein-energy malnutrition.

Continued

TABLE 15-1

Constituents of the Common Serum Chemistry Panels—cont'd

Analytes	Reference Range*	Significance
Total cholesterol	<200	Decreased in those with protein-calorie malnutrition, liver diseases, and hyperthyroidism
Triglycerides	40-160 mg/dl (age and sex dependent)	Increased in those with glucose intolerance (e.g., in those receiving total parenteral nutrition who have combined hyperlipidemia) or in those who are not fasting

* Reference ranges may vary slightly among laboratories.

† mEq/L = 1 mmol/L.

TABLE 15-2

Constituents of the Hemogram: Complete Blood Count and Differential

Analytes	Reference Range*	Significance
Red blood cells	$4.3\text{-}5.9 \times 10^6/\text{mm}^3$ (men) $3.5\text{-}5.9 \times 10^6/\text{mm}^3$ (women)	In addition to nutritional deficits, may be decreased in those with hemorrhage, hemolysis, genetic aberrations, marrow failure, or renal disease or who are taking certain drugs; not sensitive for iron, vitamin B_{12} or folate deficiencies
Hemoglobin concentration	14-17 g/dl (men) 12-15 g/dl (women) <11 g/dl (pregnant females) 14-24 g/dl (newborns)	In addition to nutritional deficits, may be decreased in those with hemorrhage, hemolysis, genetic aberrations, marrow failure, or renal disease or who are taking certain drugs; not sensitive for iron, vitamin B_{12} or folate deficiencies
Hematocrit	42%-52% (men) 35%-47% (women) <33% (pregnant females) 44%-64% (newborns)	In addition to nutritional deficits, may be decreased in those with hemorrhage, hemolysis, genetic aberrations, marrow failure, or renal disease or who are taking certain drugs; not sensitive for iron, vitamin B_{12} or folate deficiencies
Mean cell volume (MCV)	80-99 fl 96-108 fl (newborns)	Decreased (microcytic) in presence of iron deficiency, thalassemia trait and chronic renal failure, anemia of chronic disease; increased (macrocytic) in presence of vitamin B_{12} or folate deficiency and genetic defects in DNA synthesis; neither microcytosis nor macrocytosis sensitive to marginal nutrient deficiencies
Mean cell hemoglobin (MCH)	27-31 pg/cell 23-34 pg (newborns)	Causes of abnormal values similar to those for MCV
Mean cell hemoglobin concentration (MCHC)	32-36 g/dl 32-33 g/dl (newborns)	Decreased in those with iron deficiency and thalassemia trait; not sensitive to marginal nutrient deficiencies
White blood cell count (WBC)	$5\text{-}10 \times 10^3/\text{mm}^3$ (>2 yr) $6\text{-}17 \times 10^3/\text{mm}^3$ (<2 yr) $9\text{-}30 \times 10^3/\text{mm}^3$ (newborns)	Increased (leukocytosis) in those with infection, neoplasia, and stress decreased (leucopenia) in those with PEM, autoimmune diseases, or overwhelming infections or who are receiving chemotherapy or radiation therapy
Differential	55%-70% neutrophils 20-40% lymphocytes 2-8% monocytes 1%-4% eosinophils 0.5%-1% basophils	*Neutrophilia:* Ketoacidosis, trauma, stress, pus-forming infections, leukemia *Neutropenia:* PEM, aplastic anemia, chemotherapy, overwhelming infection *Lymphocytosis:* Infection, leukemia, myeloma, mononucleosis *Lymphocytopenia:* Leukemia, chemotherapy, sepsis, AIDS *Eosinophilia:* Parasitic infestation, allergy, eczema, leukemia, autoimmune disease *Eosinopenia:* Increased steroid production *Basophilia:* Leukemia *Basopenia:* Allergy

*Reference ranges may vary slightly among laboratories.

PEM, Protein-energy malnutrition.

TABLE 15-3

Chemical Tests in a Urinalysis

Analyte	Expected Value	Significance
Specific gravity	1.010-1.025 mg/ml	Can be used to test and monitor the concentrating and diluting abilities of the kidney; low in those with diabetes insipidus, glomerulonephritis, or pyelonephritis; high in those with vomiting, diarrhea, sweating, fever, adrenal insufficiency, hepatic diseases, or heart failure
pH	6-8 (normal diet)	Acidic in those with a high-protein diet or acidosis (e.g., uncontrolled diabetes mellitus [DM] or starvation), during administration of some drugs, and in association with uric acid, cystine, and calcium oxalate kidney stones; alkaline in individuals consuming diets rich in vegetables or dairy products and in those with a urinary tract infection, immediately after meals, with some drugs, and in those with phosphate and calcium carbonate kidney stones
Protein	2-8 mg/dl	Marked proteinuria in those with nephrotic syndrome, severe glomerulonephritis, or congestive heart failure; moderate in those with most renal diseases, preeclampsia, or urinary tract inflammation; minimal in those with certain renal diseases or lower urinary tract disorders
Glucose	Not detected (2-10 g/dl in DM)	Positive in those with DM; rarely in benign conditions
Ketones	Negative	Positive in those with uncontrolled DM (usually type 1); also positive in those with a fever, anorexia, certain GI disturbances, persistent vomiting, or cachexia or who are fasting or starving
Blood	Negative	Indicates urinary tract infection, neoplasm, or trauma; also positive in those with traumatic muscle injuries or hemolytic anemia
Bilirubin	Not detected	Index of unconjugated bilirubin; increase in those with certain liver diseases (e.g., gallstones)
Urobilinogen	0.1-1 units/dl	Index of conjugated bilirubin; increased in those with hemolytic conditions; used to distinguish among hepatic diseases
Nitrite	Negative	Index of bacteriuria
Leukocyte esterase	Negative	Indirect test of bacteriuria; detects leukocytes

flects the urinary tract status. However, some urinalysis data have broader medical and nutritional significance. For example, glycosuria suggests abnormal carbohydrate use and possibly diabetes. The full urinalysis includes a record of (1) the appearance of the urine, (2) the results of basic tests done with chemically impregnated reagent strips (often called dipsticks) that can be read visually or by an automated reader, and (3) the microscopic examination of urine sediment. Table 15-3 provides a list of the chemical tests performed in a urinalysis and their significance.

ment. Overhydration is caused by an increase in capillary hydrostatic pressure or capillary permeability, a decrease in colloid osmotic pressure, or physical inactivity. Laboratory measures of hydration status include serum sodium, blood urea nitrogen, serum osmolality, and urine specific gravity. Although the laboratory is important, decisions regarding hydration should only be made in conjunction with other information from physical examination and the clinical condition of the patient (see Chapter 14, especially *Clinical Insight: Hydration Status*).

ASSESSMENT OF HYDRATION STATUS

Disorders of fluid balance include dehydration and overhydration. Dehydration is a state of negative fluid balance caused by decreased intake, increased losses, and fluid shifts. Overhydration, or edema, occurs when there is an increase in the extracellular fluid volume. The fluid shifts from the extracellular compartment to the interstitial fluid compart-

ASSESSMENT FOR PROTEIN-CALORIE MALNUTRITION

Hormonal and Cell-Mediated Response to Stress

Acute illness or trauma causes inflammatory stress, leading to the need to rapidly determine requirements for nutrition intervention (see Chapter 39). These conditions trigger the release of cytokines such as interleukin-1, interleukin-6, and tumor necrosis factor (TNF). The cytokines reorient hepatic synthesis of plasma proteins and increase the breakdown of muscle protein to meet the demand for protein and energy during the inflammatory response. The acute-phase proteins regulate inflammatory mediator levels during inflammation in response to demand and opsonize bacteria, foreign organisms, particles, or other cells, making them more susceptible to the action of phagocytes. Acute-phase proteins are proteins, the levels of which fluctuate in response to tissue injury such as trauma, myocardial infarction, acute infections, malignancy, burns, and chronic inflammation (e.g., Crohn's disease or rheumatoid arthritis).

Proteins that are designated **negative acute-phase respondents**, such as albumin, transferrin, prealbumin (transthyretin), and retinol-binding protein, decrease during the acute-phase response. Others, designated **positive acute-phase respondents** such as C-reactive protein, α-1 antichymotrypsin, α_1-antitrypsin, haptoglobins, ceruloplasmin, serum amyloid A, fibrinogen, ferritin, complement components C3 and C4, and orosomucoid, increase to varying degrees. The change in the levels of these proteins is generally proportional to the severity of the tissue injury associated with the trauma, infection, or other physiologic insult (Fuhrman et al., 2004). The decrease in the plasma levels of albumin and in the levels of the other negative acute-phase proteins that occurs during the acute phase is caused by (1) down-regulation of gene expression and translation, (2) increases in catabolism, (3) transport to extravascular pools, and (4) a probable reduction in synthesis caused by decreased levels of dietary essential amino acids. The shift of albumin (and similarly sized negative acute-phase proteins) to the extravascular space during the acute inflammatory response is different from the process that occurs during uncomplicated starvation (marasmus) without inflammatory stress. In the latter, even though albumin synthesis decreases somewhat, plasma albumin is maintained by a shift of albumin from the extravascular space into the plasma.

More than 300 proteins have been identified in human plasma. Box 15-2 shows how acute-phase respondent proteins and proteins that have been studied as indicators of protein nutrition status fit into a functional classification of plasma proteins.

Nitrogen Balance

Nitrogen balance studies can only reflect the balance between exogenous nitrogen intake (orally, enterally, or parenterally) and renal removal of nitrogen-containing compounds (urinary, fecal, wound), and other nitrogen sources. Nitrogen balance studies are not a measure of protein anabolism and catabolism because true protein turnover studies require consumption of labeled (stable isotope) protein to track protein use. Even if useful, nitrogen balance studies are difficult because valid 24-hour urine collections are tedious unless the patient has a catheter. In addition, changes in renal function are common in patients with inflammatory metabolism, making standard nitrogen balance

---

BOX 15-2

Classification of Certain Plasma Proteins by Function*

Immunoglobulins

IgG, IgA, IgM, IgD, IgE

Complement Components

C1q, C1r, C1s, C2, **C3**, **C4**, C5, C6, C7, C8, and C9; properdin; factors D, H, I, and P; C4bp; S-protein; C8bp

Coagulation and Fibrinolytic Factors

Fibrinogen; prothrombin; factors V, VII, VIII, IX, XI, XII, and XIII; protein C and protein S; prekallikrein; HMW-kininogen; von Willebrand's factor; plasminogen

Enzyme Inhibitors

α1-antitrypsin, α2-macroglobulin, inter-α-trypsin inhibitor antithrombin III, C1-inhibitor, **α1-chymotrypsin,** α2-antiplasmin, heparin cofactor II, cystatin C, pregnancy-associated α2-glycoprotein, tissue factor pathway inhibitor (lipoprotein-associated coagulation inhibitor [LACI])

Lipid Transport–Associated Proteins

Apoproteins A-I, A-II, B, C-I, C-II, C-III, D, and E; β2-glycoprotein I; **serum amyloid A**

Transport Proteins

Albumin, prealbumin transthyretin, transferrin, retinol-binding protein, thyroxin-binding protein, vitamin D–binding protein, sex hormone–binding protein, transcobalamin I, transcobalamin II, corticosteroid-binding globulin, transcortin, **hemopexin, haptoglobin, ceruloplasmin**

Proteins of Uncertain or Other Functions

α₁-Acid glycoprotein (orosomucoid), α₁B-glycoprotein, serum amyloid P component, α₁-microglobulin, Zn-α₂-glycoprotein, fibronectin, α-HS-glycoprotein, histidine-rich glycoprotein, **CRP**

*Positive acute-phase proteins are shown in **bold** type; negative acute-phase proteins are in *italics*; proteins that are used in protein-energy assessment are underlined. Note that the positive acute-phase proteins are distributed among almost all functional classes, whereas the main negative acute-phase proteins are transport proteins.

---

calculations inaccurate without calculation of nitrogen retention (Gottschlich et al., 2001).

It is clear that the acutely ill patient is losing protein rapidly due to the inflammatory process. However, it is unclear if increasing exogenous protein intake will attenuate the loss of endogenous protein. One study concluded that nutrition support combined with physical therapy may reduce loss of muscle mass in acutely ill hospitalized patients (Vanek, 1998). Clinicians using nitrogen balance to estimate protein flux in critically ill patients must remember the limitations of these studies and that positive nitrogen balance may not mean that protein catabolism has decreased, particularly in

Nitrogen Balance Calculations

Nitrogen balance = nitrogen intake − nitrogen losses

Nitrogen intake = protein intake/6.25 (or appropriate conversion factor)

Nitrogen losses = urinary urea nitrogen (UUN) + Nonurea urinary nitrogen (1-2 g) + fecal nitrogen (1-2 g) + miscellaneous losses from skin, sweat, etc. ($\approx$1 g or 0.1-0.5 g/m^2)

Nitrogen balance (in grams) = (protein intake in grams) − (UUN excretion in grams + 3-5 g) × 6.25 g of nitrogen per gram of protein (or appropriate conversion factor)

Measurement of nitrogen balance is most accurate in patients who receive a defined nutrient intake (e.g., enteral or parenteral nutrition). The conversion factor commonly used for dietary protein is 6.25 g nitrogen per gram of protein. Refer to product literature or website link for specific conversion factors for enteral or parenteral products.

inflammatory (disease and trauma) conditions. Adequate nutrition cannot circumvent the inflammatory metabolism. See Box 15-3 for calculation of nitrogen balance.

Hepatic Transport Proteins

Unlike nitrogen balance measurements that assess only short-term changes in whole body protein status, plasma protein levels integrate protein synthesis and degradation over longer periods. Albumin, prealbumin (or transthyretin), retinol-binding protein, and other transport proteins are synthesized in the liver and represent approximately 3% of total body protein. Serum levels of albumin and prealbumin have traditionally been used as part of nutrition assessment; however, levels should always be evaluated carefully in view of the patient's clinical condition. During stress and illness, albumin and prealbumin may decrease as part of the inflammatory response as mentioned previously and not represent nutrition status.

Levels of both albumin and prealbumin may remain normal or near normal during uncomplicated starvation as redistribution from the interstitium to the plasma occurs. For these reasons, a well-nourished but stressed patient may have low levels of the hepatic transport proteins, whereas a patient who has had significant weight loss and undernutrition may have normal or close to normal levels.

Albumin

Albumin is synthesized by the liver at a rate of 8 to 14 g/day and accounts for approximately 60% of total serum proteins. The major purpose of albumin is to maintain colloidal osmotic pressure; providing approximately 80% of colloidal osmotic pressure of the plasma. When serum albumin levels decrease, the water in plasma moves to the interstitial compartment, leading to edema. The loss of plasma fluid results in hypovolemia, which in turn triggers renal retention of water and sodium. In addition to its role in maintaining oncotic pressure, albumin transports major blood constituents, hormones, enzymes, medications, minerals, ions, fatty acids, amino acids, and metabolites.

Transferrin

Transferrin is a negative acute-phase respondent, but it has a shorter half-life ($t_{1/2}$ = 8 days) than albumin (Table 15-4). Levels diminish with acute inflammatory reactions, malignancies, collagen vascular diseases, and liver diseases.

In addition to being responsive to dietary protein, the plasma transferrin level is controlled by the size of the iron storage pool. When iron stores are depleted, transferrin synthesis increases. Transferrin levels reflect both protein and iron status.

Although the half-life of transferrin is shorter than that of albumin, it still does not respond rapidly enough to changes in nutrient intake to be useful in acute-care settings. This, in addition to its nonspecificity, makes transferrin only slightly more useful than albumin as a marker of protein status.

Prealbumin

Prealbumin (PAB) is a negative acute-phase reactant protein with a short half-life ($t_{1/2}$ = 2 days). PAB is a transport protein synthesized by the liver and transported in the serum as a complex of retinol-binding protein and vitamin A. PAB is also called transthyretin (TTHY) and thyroxine-binding prealbumin. It is secondary to thyroxine-binding globulin in the transportation of the thyroid hormones triiodothyronine (T_3) and thyroxine (T_4).

Clinicians often believe that PAB is a sensitive indicator of protein deficiency and of improvement in protein status with refeeding. However, PAB levels are often maintained in "uncomplicated" malnutrition and decreased in well-nourished individuals who have undergone recent stress or trauma. When malnutrition is significant, the serum PAB may not decrease. Serum PAB is not greatly affected by iron deficiency, mild renal or liver disease, or fluid compartment shifts, and it is not influenced by the administration of exogenous albumin. However, as renal and liver disease compromise organ function, the PAB levels may not reflect overall protein status. Serum levels decrease with inflammation, malignancy, and protein-wasting diseases of the intestines or kidneys. Serum levels also decrease in the presence of a zinc deficiency because zinc is required for hepatic synthesis and secretion of PAB. Zinc status, based on dietary intake and medical history, in addition to inflammation, should be taken into account when interpreting low plasma PAB levels.

In some cases of nephrotic syndrome, PAB levels are increased. Proteinuria is common in nephrotic syndrome, causing hypoproteinemia (see Chapter 36). Since PAB is rapidly synthesized, a disproportionate percentage of PAB can exist in the blood when other proteins take longer to produce (Litchford, 2006). During pregnancy the changed

TABLE 15-4

Properties of Proteins Commonly Used in Protein-Energy Assessments

Protein	Approximate Half-Life	Reference Range
Albumin	3 wk	3.5-5.0 g/dl; 35-50 g/L
Transferrin	8-10 days	
Female		250-380 mg/dl; 2.50-3.8 g/L
Male		215-365 mg/dl; 2.15-3.65 g/L
Prealbumin	2 days	15-36 mg/dl; 150-360 mg/L
Retinol-binding protein	12 hr	2.6-7.6 mg/dl; 1.43-2.86 μmol/L

estrogen levels stimulate PAB synthesis, and its level may increase (see Chapter 5).

Retinol-Binding Protein

Another protein with a short half-life ($t_{1/2}$ = 12 hr) that has been used to assess nutrition status is **retinol-binding protein (RBP),** a small plasma protein that does not pass through the renal glomerulus because it circulates in a complex with PAB. As implied by its name, RBP binds retinol, and transport of this vitamin A metabolite seems to be its exclusive function (see Figure 3-13). RBP is synthesized in the liver and released with retinol. After RBP releases retinol in peripheral tissue, its affinity for PAB decreases, leading to dissociation of the PAB-RBP complex and filtration of apo-RBP by the glomerulus. The protein is then catabolized in the renal tubule.

The plasma RBP concentration has been shown to decrease in uncomplicated protein calorie malnutrition. However, confounding the interpretation of RBP levels is its actions in those with acute inflammatory stress. RBP is a negative acute-phase protein, meaning that RBP may not reflect protein status in acutely stressed patients; however, it is not as affected by inflammatory stress as albumin, transferrin, or PAB.

The simultaneous secretion of RBP and retinol from the liver means that retinol status also complicates the interpretation of reduced RBP values. RBP cannot reliably be used to assess protein status when the vitamin A status is compromised.

The use of RBP in assessing protein-energy malnutrition (PEM) is complicated by the normal catabolism of apo-RBP by the kidney. Patients with renal failure are likely to have elevated RBP levels, regardless of their protein-energy status, because the RBP is not being catabolized by the renal tubule (see Chapter 36).

RBP4 is an adipocyte-derived peptide of RBP that influences glucose homeostasis. Animal models demonstrate increased levels in obesity and insulin resistance, suggesting a possible relationship between these conditions. RBP4 may be an emerging biomarker for obesity and insulin-resistant diabetes (Yang et al., 2005; Graham, 2006).

C-Reactive Protein

Evaluation of nutrition status of acutely ill patients exhibiting inflammatory stress is difficult because commonly used measures of assessment are negative acute-phase reactant proteins. Use of inflammatory biomarkers such as **C-reactive protein (CRP)** is helpful to predict when the hypermetabolic period of the inflammatory response wanes. CRP is a nonspecific marker and reflects any type of inflammation. As long as inflammatory markers are elevated, the albumin and PAB are useless as measures of nutrition status.

Although the exact function of CRP is unclear, it increases in the initial stages of acute stress—usually within 4 to 6 hours of surgery or other trauma. Furthermore, its level can increase as much as 1000-fold, depending on the intensity of the stress response. When the CRP level begins to decrease, the patient has entered the anabolic period of the inflammatory response, and more intensive nutrition therapy may be beneficial. Ongoing assessment and follow-up is required to address changes in nutrition status.

Recent interest in CRP has been generated by the observation that slightly increased levels of the protein are associated with increased risk for the development of disease associated with atherosclerosis (Blake and Ridker, 2001), and evidence shows that nutrition affects this response (Liu et al., 2002). This chronic subclinical inflammation of atherosclerosis is marked by a moderate increase in serum CRP. A different test, **high-sensitivity C-reactive protein (hs-CRP),** is used to measure these slightly elevated CRP levels (see "Inflammation" later in the chapter).

Creatinine

Creatinine is formed from creatine, a compound found almost exclusively in muscle tissue, and has been used to assess somatic (muscle) protein status. Creatine is synthesized from the amino acids glycine and arginine with addition of a methyl group from the folate- and cobalamin-dependent methionine-S-adenosylmethionine-homocysteine cycle. As creatine phosphate (CP) it is a high-energy phosphate buffer and provides for a constant supply of adenosine triphosphate (ATP) for muscle contraction. When creatine is dephosphorylated, some of it is spontaneously converted to creatinine by an irreversible, nonenzymatic reaction. Creatinine has no specific biologic function; it is continuously released from the muscle cells and excreted by the kidneys with little reabsorption. When a patient follows a meat-restricted diet, the size of the somatic (muscle) protein pool is directly proportional to the amount of creatinine excreted. This means that men generally excrete larger amounts of creatinine than women, and that individuals with greater muscular development excrete larger amounts than those who are less muscular. Total body weight is not proportional to creatinine excretion, but muscle mass is.

Creatinine excretion rate is related to muscle mass, as shown by the following equation:

$$\text{Muscle mass} = k + k' \times \text{Urinary creatinine}$$
$$\text{where } k \text{ and } k' = \text{Empirical constants}$$

Using computed tomography as the gold standard, the following equation is used:

$$\text{Skeletal muscle mass (kg)} = 4.1 + 18.9 \times$$
$$\text{24-hr creatinine excretion (g/day)}$$

This equation works well for most individuals but not for body builders, and it has not been tested with sick or injured patients.

The use of creatinine to assess somatic protein status is confounded by omnivorous diets. As already mentioned, creatine is stored in muscle; so muscle meats, which are rich in creatine, and the creatinine that is formed from dietary creatine cannot be distinguished from endogenously produced creatinine. Another factor confounding interpretation of urinary creatinine data is that daily creatinine excretion varies significantly within individuals, probably because of sweat losses. In addition, the test is based on 24-hour urine collections, which are difficult to obtain. Because of these limitations, urinary creatinine concentration as a marker of muscle mass is typically used only in research.

Immunocompetence

PEM is associated with impaired immunocompetence, including depressed cell-mediated immunity, phagocyte dysfunction, decreased levels of complement components, reduced mucosal secretory antibody responses, and lower antibody affinity. Assessing immunocompetence in critically ill patients may be useful in determining the extent of the inadequate nutrition and disease. Assessing immunocompetence is also useful in the patient who is being treated for allergies, as is discussed in Chapter 29.

There is no single marker for immunocompetence except for the clinical outcome of infection or allergic response. Laboratory markers with a high degree of sensitivity include vaccine-specific serum antibody production, delayed-type hypersensitivity response (DHR), vaccine-specific or total secretory IgA in saliva, and the response to attenuated pathogens. Less sensitive markers include natural killer cell cytotoxicity, oxidative burst of phagocytes, lymphocyte proliferation, and the cytokine pattern produced by activated immune cells. Using a combination of markers is currently the best approach to measure immunocompetence (Albers et al., 2005).

LABORATORY DATA FOR NUTRITIONAL ANEMIAS

Anemia is a condition characterized by a reduction in the number of erythrocytes per unit of blood volume or a decrease in the hemoglobin of the blood to below the level of usual physiologic need. By convention, anemia is defined as a hemoglobin concentration below the 95th percentile for healthy reference populations of men, women, or age-grouped children. Anemia is not a disease but a symptom of various conditions, including extensive blood loss, excessive blood cell destruction, or decreased blood cell formation. It is observed in many hospitalized patients and is often a symptom of a disease process; its etiology should be investigated.

Clinical nutritionists are primarily concerned with distinguishing between nutritional anemia caused by nutritional inadequacies and anemia caused by other factors (see Chapter 31). Hydration management problems can mask nutritional anemias or result in falsely low blood values.

Classification of Anemia

Nutritional deficits are a major cause of decreased hemoglobin and erythrocyte production. The initial descriptive classification of anemia is derived from the hematocrit value or complete blood count (CBC) as explained in Table 15-2 and associated calculations. Anemias associated with a mean red blood cell volume of less than 80 fl (femtoliters) are called microcytic, whereas those with values of 80 to 99 fl are termed normocytic, and those associated with values of 100 fl or more are macrocytic (see Chapter 31).

Data from the CBC are helpful in differentiating nutritional causes of anemia. **Microcytic anemia** is most often associated with iron deficiency, whereas **macrocytic anemia** is generally caused by either folate- or vitamin B_{12}–deficient erythropoiesis. However, because of the low specificity of these indexes, additional data are needed to distinguish between the various nutritional causes of microcytic and macrocytic anemias and their nonnutritional causes such as thalassemia trait and chronic renal insufficiency. Normocytic anemia is associated with inadequate iron use, most commonly in the **anemia of chronic and inflammatory diseases (ACD)**. This type of anemia is associated with rheumatic diseases, chronic infection, cancer, severe tissue injury, multiple fractures, and Hodgkin's disease. ACD does not respond to iron supplementation.

Other information from the CBC that helps to differentiate the nonnutritional causes of anemia includes leukocyte, reticulocyte, and platelet counts. When these are low, marrow failure is indicated; high counts are associated with anemia caused by leukemia or infection. Erythrocyte sedimentation rate (ESR) is ordered when symptoms are nonspecific and inflammatory autoimmune diseases are suspected. Reticulocytes are large, nucleated, immature red blood cells that are released in small numbers with mature cells. When red blood cell production rates increase, reticulocyte counts also increase. Any time anemia is accompanied by a high reticulocyte count, elevated erythropoietic activity in response to bleeding should be considered. In such cases, stool specimens can be tested for occult blood to rule out chronic gastrointestinal (GI) blood loss. Other causes of a high reticulocyte count include intravascular hemolysis syndromes and an erythropoietic response to therapy for iron, vitamin B_{12}, or folic acid deficiencies.

Normocytic or microcytic anemia may be caused by chronic or acute blood loss. Refer to the recent medical history for corroborating evidence such as recent surgery, injury, or positive occult stool tests. However, in those with hemolytic anemias and early iron deficiency anemia, the red blood cell size may still be normal (see Table 31-1).

Macrocytic anemias include megaloblastic anemia or folate deficiency and pernicious anemia or vitamin B_{12} deficiency. The presence of macrocytic red blood cells requires evaluation of both folate and vitamin B_{12} status. Both nutrients arrest deoxyribonucleic acid (DNA) synthesis by preventing the formation of thymidine monophosphate at different steps of the synthetic pathway. The effects of either nutrient deficiency are impairment of red blood cell synthesis and maturation of red blood cells, causing large, nucleated cells to be released into the circulation. Although pernicious anemia is categorized as a macrocytic normochromic anemia, approximately 40% of the cases are normocytic.

Iron Deficiency Anemias

Hematocrit or Packed Cell Volume and Hemoglobin

Hematocrit (Hct) and hemoglobin (Hgb) are part of a routine CBC and are used together to evaluate iron status. **Hematocrit** is the measure of the percentage of red blood cells in total blood volume. Usually the Hct percentage is three times the Hgb concentration in grams per deciliter. The Hct value is affected by an extremely high white blood cell count and hydration status. Individuals living in high altitudes often have increased values. It is common for individuals over the age of 50 to have slightly lower levels than younger adults.

The **hemoglobin** concentration is a measure of the total amount of Hgb in the peripheral blood. It is a more direct measure of iron deficiency than Hct because it quantifies total Hgb in red blood cells rather than a percentage of total blood volume. Hgb and Hct are below normal in the four types of nutritional anemias and should always be evaluated in light of other laboratory values and recent medical history (see Table 31-1).

Serum Iron

Serum iron measures the amount of circulating iron that is bound to transferrin. However, it is a relatively poor index of iron status because of large day-to-day changes, even in healthy individuals. Diurnal variations also occur, with the highest concentrations occurring midmorning (from 6 AM to 10 AM), and a nadir, averaging 30% less than the morning level, occurring midafternoon. Serum iron should be evaluated in light of other laboratory values and recent medical history to definitively assess iron status.

Total Iron-Binding Capacity and Transferrin Saturation

Total iron-binding capacity (TIBC) is a direct measure of all proteins available to bind mobile iron and is dependent on the number of free binding sites on the plasma iron-transport protein transferrin. Each transferrin molecule binds ferric ions (Fe[III]) at each of two binding sites and two bicarbonate

ions at separate sites. Intracellular iron availability regulates the synthesis and secretion of transferrin. Therefore the plasma transferrin concentration increases in those with iron deficiency. In addition, when the amount of stored iron available for release to transferrin decreases and dietary iron intake is low, saturation of transferrin decreases.

In people with sufficient iron levels, the normal plasma transferrin concentration is 215 to 380 mg/dl (2.15 to 3.80 g/L). Since transferrin has two iron-binding sites and iron has an atomic weight of 56 daltons, the expected TIBC is 2800 to 5600 mg/L (280 to 560 mg/dl). However, the range of normal TIBC values is 250 to 460 mg/dl (45 to 82 µmol/L), indicating that full occupation of all transferrin binding sites does not occur. Because bicarbonate binding by transferrin is required to activate iron binding fully, loss of this ion from the serum when it sits in a collection tube or when there is intrinsically inadequate amounts of it could explain the incomplete saturation of transferrin, even in the presence of excess iron. Because of this discrepancy, direct correlation of TIBC with transferrin level is not a 1:1 relationship.

There are exceptions to the general rule that transferrin saturation decreases and TIBC increases in patients with iron deficiency. For example, TIBC increases in those with hepatitis. It also increases in people with hypoxia, women who are pregnant, or those taking oral contraceptives or receiving estrogen replacement therapy. On the other hand, TIBC decreases in those with malignant disease, nephritis, and hemolytic anemias. Furthermore, the plasma level of transferrin may be decreased in those with PEM, fluid overload, and liver disease. Thus, although TIBC and transferrin saturation are more specific than Hct or Hgb values, they are not perfect indicators of iron status.

An additional concern about the use of serum iron, TIBC, and transferrin saturation values is that normal values persist until frank deficiency actually develops. Thus these tests cannot detect decreasing iron stores and preanemic iron deficiencies.

Ferritin

Ferritin is the storage protein that sequesters the iron normally gathered in the liver (reticuloendothelial system), spleen, and marrow. As the iron supply increases, the intracellular level of ferritin increases to accommodate iron storage. A small amount of this ferritin leaks into the circulation. This ferritin can be measured by assays that are available in most clinical laboratories. In individuals with normal iron storage, 1 ng/ml of serum ferritin is approximately 8 mg of stored iron. Therefore measurement of ferritin that has leaked into the serum is an excellent indicator of the size of the body's iron storage pool.

Effect of Inflammation on Ferritin

Ferritin can act as a positive acute-phase reactant protein and may be elevated in conditions that do not reflect iron stores such as acute inflammation, infections, metastatic cancer and lymphoma. Cytokines and other inflammatory mediators can increase ferritin synthesis, ferritin leakage from cells, or both. Elevations in ferritin occur 1 to 2 days after the onset of the acute illness and peak at 3 to 5 days. If iron deficiency also exists, it may not be diagnosed because the level of ferritin would be falsely elevated.

ACD is the primary condition in which ferritin fails to correlate with iron stores (Haurani, 2002; Ozatli et al., 2000). ACD, a common form of anemia in hospitalized patients, occurs in those with inflammatory, infectious, and neoplastic disorders (Bron et al., 2001). It occurs during inflammation because red cell production decreases as the result of inadequate mobilization of iron from its storage sites. This is apparently caused by the release of cytokines such as interleukin-1 and TNF, which also inhibit division of erythroid progenitors and may inhibit erythropoietin production. In those with arthritis, depletion of stored iron develops partly because of reduced absorption of iron from the gut. Also the regular use of nonsteroidal antiinflammatory drugs can cause occult GI blood loss. This form of anemia is usually mild and normocytic.

However, in 30% to 50% of patients, hypochromic (i.e., having inadequate amounts of Hgb), microcytic red cells are made, serum iron levels and TIBC are low, and iron stores are normal or elevated. Because iron stores do not decrease, normal amounts of ferritin should be present in the plasma. However, in some cases iron stores may be depleted, but inflammatory mediators may cause ferritin levels to remain normal. Patients with chronic inflammatory diseases such as rheumatoid arthritis may have reduced or deficient stores. ACD has many forms and must be distinguished from iron deficiency anemia so that inappropriate iron supplementation is not initiated.

Serum Transferrin Receptor Test

Serum transferrin receptor (sTfR) test is a measure of iron status that is not affected by inflammatory status. The transferrin receptor protein binds holotransferrin (transferrin-Fe[III]) during cellular iron uptake. When cellular iron levels decrease, synthesis of sTfR increases. sTfR reflects the amount of this protein on the surface of cells, and an increase in serum levels correlates with iron deficiency. This test is useful to detect and determine the etiology of iron deficiency in inflammatory states, to evaluate erythropoiesis in individuals receiving erythropoietin treatment, and to evaluate iron status during pregnancy. It is not helpful in assessing iron status in patients with coexisting enhanced erythropoiesis conditions such as megaloblastic anemia or thalassemia. It is also not as sensitive or specific as serum ferritin for differentiating iron deficiency anemia from anemia of chronic and inflammatory diseases in elderly patients with anemias.

Macrocytic Anemias Associated with B Vitamin Deficiencies

Macrocytic anemias include megaloblastic anemia or folate deficiency and pernicious anemia or vitamin B_{12} deficiency. The nutritional causes of macrocytic anemia are related to the availability of folate and vitamin B_{12} (cobalamin) in the bone marrow and require evaluation of both folate and vitamin B_{12} status. Both nutrients arrest DNA synthesis by preventing the formation of thymidine monophosphate. Folate and vitamin B_{12} are used at different steps of the synthetic pathway. The effect of either nutrient deficiency is impairment of red blood cell synthesis and maturation of red blood cells, causing large, nucleated cells to be released into the circulation (see Chapter 31).

Static Tests for Folate and Vitamin B_{12} Status

Evaluation for macrocytic anemia includes static measurement of folate and vitamin B_{12} deficiency in blood. They can be assayed using tests of the ability of the patient's blood specimen to support the growth of microbes that require either folate or vitamin B_{12}, radiobinding assays, or immunoassays.

Folate is most often simultaneously measured in whole blood (i.e., combined plasma and blood cells) and in the serum alone. The difference between whole blood folate and serum folate levels is then used to calculate the red blood cell folate concentration. Red blood cell folate concentration is a better indicator of folate status than serum folate, although the latter is the variable generally measured (Chernecky and Berger, 2004). However, considerable evidence shows that a serum sample obtained after scrupulous fasting is as good for assessing folate status as red blood cell folate levels. The advantage of the serum measurement is that it is considerably less laborious and less expensive.

Vitamin B_{12} is measured in the serum, and all indications are that the serum level gives as much information about vitamin B_{12} status as does the red blood cell level. Methylmalonic acid levels in serum or urine are also useful to assess B_{12} status.

Homocysteine. Folate and vitamin B_{12} are required for the synthesis of *S*-adenosylmethionine, the biochemical precursor involved in the transfer of one-carbon (methyl) groups during many biochemical syntheses. *S*-adenosylmethionine is synthesized from the amino acid methionine by a reaction that includes the addition of a methyl group and the purine base adenine (from ATP). For example, when *S*-adenosylmethionine donates a methyl group for the synthesis of thymine, choline, creatine, epinephrine, and protein and DNA methylation, it is converted to *S*-adenosyl homocysteine. After losing the adenosyl group, the remaining **homocysteine** can either be converted to cysteine by the vitamin B_6–dependent transsulfuration pathway or converted back to methionine in a reaction that depends on folate and vitamin B_{12} (see Figure 31-5).

When either folate or vitamin B_{12} is lacking, the homocysteine-to-methionine reaction is virtually blocked, causing homocysteine to build up in the affected tissue and spill into the circulation. The vitamin B_6–dependent transsulfuration pathway can metabolize excess homocysteine. Therefore an elevated homocysteine level is expected to indicate either genetic defects involved in the enzymes that catalyze these reactions or a deficiency in folate, vitamin B_{12}, or vitamin B_6. Homocysteine has been shown to be very sensitive to folate and vitamin B_{12} deficiency (Savage et al., 2000).

Methylmalonic Acid (MMA). Once a genetic cause is ruled out, the most straightforward biochemical method for differentiating folate and vitamin B_{12} deficiencies is to monitor the hyperhomocysteinemia by measuring the serum or urinary methylmalonic acid (MMA) level. The latter metabolite is formed during the degradation of the amino acid valine and odd-chain fatty acids. MMA is the side product in this metabolic pathway that increases when the conversion of methylmalonic CoA to succinyl CoA is blocked by lack of vitamin B_{12}, a coenzyme for this reaction. Therefore deficiency leads to an increase in the MMA pool, which is reflected by the serum or urinary MMA level.

The urinary MMA test is more sensitive than the serum B_{12} test because it indicates true tissue B_{12} deficiency. The serum MMA test may give falsely high values in renal insufficiency and intravascular volume depletion. The urinary MMA test is the only B_{12} deficiency assay that has been validated as a screening tool (Morris et al., 2005).

The advantage that homocysteine and MMA testing has over assaying serum vitamin B_{12} levels or serum and red cell folate levels is that homocysteine and MMA tend to detect impending vitamin deficiencies better than the static assays. This is especially important when assessing the status of certain patients such as vegans or older adults, who could have vitamin B_{12} deficiency associated with central nervous system impairment.

Vitamin B_{12} and the Schilling Test

If vitamin B_{12} status is compromised, the Schilling test may be used to detect defects in vitamin B_{12} absorption. The patient is given an oral dose of radiolabeled cobalamin and an injection of unlabeled vitamin. The vitamin saturates vitamin B_{12} storage sites so that all of the radiolabeled vitamin absorbed is excreted in the urine within approximately 24 hours. If less than the expected amount of radioactivity appears in the urine, vitamin B_{12} malabsorption is confirmed. The test can then be repeated with administration of a combination of radiolabeled cobalamin and intrinsic factor. If urinary radioactivity reaches the expected levels, intrinsic factor deficiency is the cause of the malabsorption.

Folate malabsorption may also develop. Folate is absorbed in the jejunum, and its malabsorption has several causes; but a specific test for folate absorption has not been developed (see Chapter 3). However, the presence and extent of deficiency should be assessed in patients with celiac disease or those with a history of long-term use of certain medications, including anticonvulsants and sulfasalazine (see Chapter 16 and Appendix 31). Alcohol consumption interferes with folate use. See Chapter 13 for discussion of genetic markers affecting folate absorption.

MARKERS OF MALABSORPTION

Malabsorption syndrome is a condition in which several nutrients are abnormally absorbed (see Chapter 27). In almost all such disorders, fat is not absorbed normally. The etiology of malabsorption may be from diverse causes, including pancreatic exocrine insufficiency, cystic fibrosis, celiac disease, gastric surgery, reduced bile salt secretion, a wide variety of conditions associated with abnormal intestinal mucosa such as some food allergies, short-gut syndrome, infection, lymphatic obstruction, some cardiovascular diseases, certain drugs, and unexplained causes associated with diseases not commonly considered to affect the GI tract.

Fecal Fat

Laboratory tests for confirming fat malabsorption begin with the Sudan stain for fecal fat. Over 95% of patients with steatorrhea have a positive test. Proof of malabsorption by quantitative fecal fat determination involves chemical analysis of a 24-hour stool specimen. However, simpler tests to screen for steatorrhea include blood carotene level and urinary *d*-xylose determinations. Carotone comes in two primary forms: α and β-carotene. Carotene can be stored in the liver and converted to vitamin A as needed. Lower-than-normal levels may indicate a diet inadequate in β-carotene or a problem with intestinal absorption of fat-soluble substances, including β-carotene. This often indicates steatorrhea.

d-xylose is absorbed primarily by a passive mechanism and is slowly metabolized in the body so that urinary excretion should reflect the ability of the mucosa to absorb it. Drawbacks of urinary *d*-xylose testing include intolerance of the test and variations in urinary excretion due to delayed gastric emptying or impaired renal function. *d*-xylose may be metabolized by bacteria if there is proximal bacterial overgrowth in stasis syndrome. A very low blood carotene, or a low urinary *d*-xylose excretion after an oral dose of xylose, suggests significant loss of jejunal mucosal function. The accuracy of both of these tests in confirming malabsorption is only 75%. These tests tend to miss mild malabsorption and are impacted by other coexisting diseases (Saunders et al., 2006).

Fat-Soluble Vitamins

Fat malabsorption may also result in impaired absorption of vitamins A, E, D, and K. Factors including low luminal pH, bile salts below the critical micellar concentration, and inadequate triglyceride hydrolysis can interfere with normal bile salt micelle formation, causing impaired absorption of fat-soluble vitamins. See Appendix 30 for further discussion of tests for assessing specific vitamin adequacy.

Vitamin D

Individual vitamin D status can be estimated by measuring plasma 25-hydroxyvitamin D (25-OH-D_3) levels. This test defines vitamin D sufficiency as the lowest threshold value for plasma 25-(OH)D_3 (around 80 nmol/L or 30 ng/ml) that prevents secondary hyperparathyroidism, increased bone turnover, bone mineral loss, or seasonal variations in plasma parathyroid hormone. Vitamin D deficiency is defined as values below this level. Serum levels even higher at 90-100 nmol/L (36-40 ng/ml) are recommended by some (Bischoff-Ferrari et al., 2006). A deficiency may be caused by inadequate dietary intake, inadequate exposure to sunlight (see *Focus On*: Sunshine, Vitamin D and Fortification in Chapter 3), or malabsorption of vitamin D that can also lead to secondary malabsorption of calcium. Any type of steatorrhea may lead to calcium malabsorption because calcium forms insoluble, unabsorbable salts with long-chain fatty acids. Calcium malabsorption occurs in chronic renal failure because renal hydroxylation is required to activate vitamin D, which promotes synthesis of a calcium-binding protein in intestinal absorptive cells (Mosekilde, 2005).

CHRONIC DISEASE RISK ASSESSMENT

Lipid Indices of Cardiovascular Risk

Serum lipoprotein and cholesterol levels are directly implicated in the development of atherosclerosis and are affected by modifiable factors, including diet. The National Cholesterol Education Program (NCEP) Adult Treatment Panel (ATP III) has established guidelines for serum levels of total cholesterol, low-density lipoprotein (LDL) cholesterol, and high-density lipoprotein (HDL) cholesterol that are associated with risk of coronary heart disease (CHD) or cardiovascular disease (CVD) (Grundy et al., 2004) (see Chapter 32). Patients undergoing lipid assessments should be fasting (for a recommended 12 hours) at the time of blood sampling. Fasting is necessary primarily because triglyceride levels rise and fall dramatically in the postprandial state, and LDL cholesterol values are calculated from measured total serum cholesterol and HDL cholesterol concentrations. This calculation, based on the Friedewald equation, is most accurate when triglyceride concentrations are less than 400 mg/dl. The Friedewald equation gives an estimate of fasting LDL cholesterol levels that is generally within 4 mg/dl of the true value when triglyceride concentrations are less than 400 mg/dl.

Direct methods of measuring serum LDL cholesterol levels such as density-gradient ultracentrifugation, vertical ultracentrifugation (VAP) and sequential gradient ultracentrifugation are available and quickly replacing the Friedewald equation for LDL cholesterol measurement. Ultracentrifugation tests, which also require a fasting blood sample, provide all the information found in a traditional lipid panel (total cholesterol, direct measured LDL-C, HDL-C, and triglycerides) along with LDL density (i.e., Pattern A versus Pattern B), intermediate density lipoprotein (IDL), HDL subtypes, very low–density lipoprotein (VLDL) density, and Lp(a). Based on the prevalence of expanded lipid abnormalities in cardiac patients, the additional information provided by these tests can improve the ability to predict the risk of patients developing cardiovascular disease (see Box 15-4). For example, **Pattern A LDL** is large, buoyant and less dense (per milligram of cholesterol) and is the least atherogenic of the LDL subclasses. **Pattern B LDL** is small and dense (per milligram of cholesterol) and is the most atherogenic of the LDL subclasses. **Lp(a) 'lipoprotein little a'** is another highly atherogenic LDL fraction similar in chemical structure to plasminogen, the precursor of the proteolytic enzyme plas-

---

BOX 15-4

Lipid and Lipoprotein Cardiovascular Disease Risk Factors

Patterns of LDL Fractions

Pattern A: Least atherogenic of the LDL subclasses
Pattern B: Most atherogenic of the LDL subclasses

Patterns of HDL Subtypes

HDL_2: Most protective subtype
HDL_3: Least protective subtype and possibly atherogenic
IDL: Elevated levels are atherogenic
VLDL density: Remnants are atherogenic
Triglyceride concentrations: Elevated levels are atherogenic
Lp(a): Elevated levels are atherogenic
apoprotein B: Increased concentration is atherogenic
apoprotein A-I: Decreased concentration is atherogenic
hs-CRP: Elevated levels, without acute or chronic inflammatory condition, are atherogenic
Serum homocysteine: Increased; greater risk
RBP4: Elevated levels may identify early insulin resistance and associated cardiovascular risk factors

HDL, High-density lipoprotein; *hs-CRP,* high sensitivity C-reactive protein; *IDL,* intermediate-density lipoprotein; *LDL,* low-density lipoprotein; *RBP4,* retinol-binding protein 4; *VLDL,* very low–density lipoprotein.

---

min. Individuals with elevated Lp(a) appear to have a much higher risk for CHD. In circulation there are five distinct **high-density lipoprotein (HDL) subtypes:** HDL_{2a}, HDL_{2b}, HDL_{2c}, HDL_{3a}, and HDL_{3b}. The cardioprotection from HDL is attributable mainly to the HDL_{2b} subfraction, and in fact elevated HDL_{3b} may actually be associated with an increased risk of CHD. A high total HDL secondary to HDL_{3b} elevation is not cardioprotective and may likewise warrant more aggressive LDL lowering. Pharmacologic interventions and MNT interventions have been successful in modifying the lipid subfraction profiles (see Chapter 32).

Inflammation

Markers of inflammation, hs-CRP and homocysteine levels have been identified as risk factors for CVD independent of lipid status. Although there is about a 40% individual variation in CRP levels, values >0.5 mg/dl should be repeated to avoid inappropriate interpretation. In addition, it is prudent to wait at least 2 weeks after an acute or chronic inflammatory event or tissue trauma to measure hs-CRP. Interpretation of hs-CRP is more meaningful when individual hs-CRP levels are compared to quartiles (25% segments) or quintiles (20% segments) of the population than when they are related to relative risk. Several studies have shown that, in apparently healthy adults, an hs-CRP value that places an individual in the highest quintile of the otherwise "healthy" population is associated with a two to four times higher risk of atherosclerosis, stroke, myocardial infarction, or peripheral vascular disease (Table 15-5).

Many individuals who die of atherosclerotic disease do not have abnormal lipoprotein cholesterol and triglyceride concentrations. One possible explanation for this is that many factors may be involved in the development of atherosclerosis. Recent research strongly supports the hypothesis that an elevated plasma concentration of the sulfur-containing amino acid homocysteine is an independent risk factor for developing CVD (see Chapter 32). Homocysteine is elevated in folate deficiency, vitamin B_{12} deficiency and is associated with an increased risk for end-stage renal disease, ischemic heart disease, cerebrovascular disease, peripheral arterial disease, and venous thrombosis that is independent of lipid levels.

Although homocysteine plays an important role in the synthesis of methionine, the bulk of the current research suggests that when cellular homocysteine leaks into the circulation, even in slightly elevated amounts, the risk of CHD, stroke, peripheral vascular disease, and venous thrombosis and pulmonary embolism increases significantly (Bønaa et al., 2006). Just as the mechanism for the effect of plasma lipoproteins on the development of atherosclerosis was initially unclear, the mechanism of the effects of homocysteine on atherogenesis is not completely clear.

Currently homocysteine testing is not standardized, and normal ranges vary. However, levels less than 12 (mol/L are optimal, levels 12-15 µmol/L are borderline, and levels higher than 15 µmol/L are considered high risk for vascular disease. Men tend to have higher homocysteine levels than women, possibly due to higher creatinine values and greater muscle mass. Even individuals with a plasma homocysteine concentration within the population reference (normal) range may be at increased risk for developing CVD. In addition, almost all individuals can reduce their homocysteine levels by adding vitamin B supplements to their diet, and evidence now suggests that replacing fat intake with fruits and vegetables can also produce a significant decrease in serum homocysteine levels. However, numerous studies have not demonstrated that lowering homocysteine levels using vitamin B supplements has reduced the risk for CVD.

Indices of Oxidative Stress

Many diseases, including CVD, Alzheimer's disease, Parkinson's disease, inflammatory bowel disease, cancer, as well as aging, are initiated by **oxidative stress** as evidenced by free radical oxidation of lipids, nucleic acids, or proteins (Figure 15-3). Oxidative stress is imposed on cells as a result of three factors: (1) an increase in oxidant generation, (2) a decrease in antioxidant protection, or (3) a failure to repair oxidative damage. Cell damage is caused by **reactive oxygen species (ROS).** ROS are either free radicals, reactive anions containing oxygen atoms, or molecules containing oxygen atoms that can either produce free radicals or are chemically activated by them (Blanck et al., 2003). These products include the superoxide radical (O_2^-), hydroxyl radical (OH), and hydrogen peroxide (H_2O_2). The formation of ROS is sometimes, but not always, mediated by certain essential trace elements (e.g., iron, copper, chromium, and nickel).

In the case of CVD, the ROS react with unsaturated fatty acids in LDL, creating lipid peroxides, another free radical species. Like all free radicals, lipid peroxides initiate the oxidation of other compounds, including apolipoprotein, the protein present in lipoproteins. This oxidation leads to the formation of free radical products throughout the large, heterogeneous lipoprotein particle. Cells associated with the arterial wall ingest the resulting oxidized lipoproteins. Once present in these cells, additional metabolism of this modified complex does not seem to occur. Over time, other pathophysiologic responses stabilize the deposited oxidized lipoprotein as atherosclerotic plaque (Hulthe and Fagerberg, 2002) (see Chapter 32).

Antioxidant Status

An indirect way of assessing the level of oxidative stress is to measure the levels of antioxidant compounds present in

TABLE 15-5

Cardiovascular Disease Risk and hs-CRP

Quintile	hs-CRP mg/dl	Relative Risk of CVD*
1	<0.07	1.0
2	0.07-0.11	1.2
3	0.12-0.19	1.4
4	0.20-0.38	1.7
5	0.39-1.50	2.2

CVD, Cardiovascular disease; *hs-CRP*, high sensitivity C-reactive protein.

* Risk associated with hs-CRP alone.

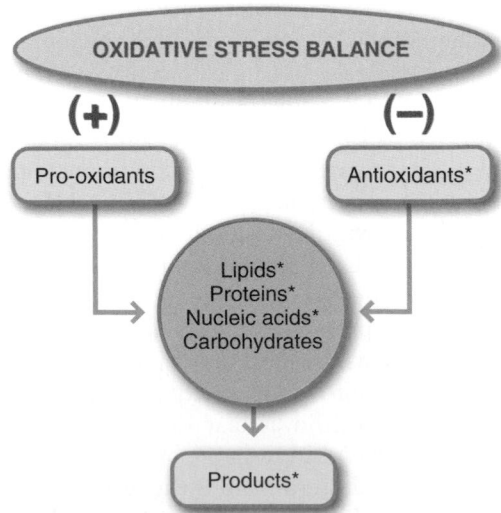

FIGURE 15-3 Steps in maintaining the balance between pro-oxidants (reactive oxygen species) and antioxidants. The compounds marked with an asterisk (*) have been used as markers of oxidative stress balance.

body fluids. Oxidative stress is related to levels of the following:

- Antioxidant vitamins (tocopherols and ascorbic acid)
- Minerals with antioxidant roles (e.g., selenium)
- Dietary phytochemicals with antioxidant properties (e.g., carotenoids)
- Endogenous antioxidant compounds and enzymes (e.g., superoxide dismutase, glutathione)

More precisely, the concentration of these compounds correlates with the balance between their intake and production and their use during the inhibition of free radical compounds.

Markers of Oxidative Stress

Biomarkers of oxidative stress status and inflammation have been associated with many chronic conditions and risk factors. Measurement of intracellular antioxidant thiols such as glutathione can be estimated using the free oxygen radical test (FORT) via spectrophotometric techniques on specimens obtained from finger sticks. However, further standardization of protocols for assays and methods of combining and integrating multiple panels of biomarkers of oxidative stress and inflammation are needed to facilitate evaluation of biomarkers for risk factor prediction. Although some intervention studies examining the effects of diet and exercise on biomarkers of oxidative stress and inflammation have been done, the data have been inconclusive, and more studies are needed to understand the underlying biology to help direct future development of therapies (Harrison and Nieto, 2004).

The most commonly used chemical markers of oxidative stress are presented in Table 15-6. Some tests measure the presence of one class of free radical products, and others measure the global antioxidant capacity of plasma or a plasma fraction. These tests have been promoted on the assumption that knowledge of the total antioxidant capacity of the plasma or plasma fraction might be more useful than knowledge of the individual concentrations of free radical markers or antioxidants. This total antioxidant activity is determined by a test that assesses the combined antioxidant capacities of the constituents. Unfortunately, the results of these tests include the antioxidant capacities of compounds such as uric acid and albumin, which are not compounds of interest. In other words, no one type of assay is likely to provide a global picture of the oxidative stress to which an individual is exposed. A new method being considered, which may become useful in the future, is a method which uses Raman spectroscopy in the Biophotonic Antioxidant Laser scanner (see *New Directions:* Raman Spectroscopy Used to Measure Antioxidant Capacity).

Despite this lack of correlation or specificity of assays of oxidative stress, two assays seem promising. One is the immunoassay of oxidatively modified LDL particles (see Table 15-6). Because it measures a product that may directly participate in atherogenesis, this assay may allow a specific correlation of CVD risk with dietary and supplemental antioxidant consumption. The second assay is the measurement of the compounds F_2 isoprostanes either in plasma or urine (Harrison and Nieto, 2004). This test measures the presence of a continuously formed free radical compound that is produced by free radical oxidation of specific polyunsaturated fatty acids. Isoprostanes are prostaglandin-like compounds that are produced by free radical mediated peroxidation of lipoproteins. Elevated isoprostane levels are associated with oxidative stress, and clinical situations of oxidative stress such as hepatorenal syndrome, rheumatoid arthritis, atherosclerosis, and carcinogenesis (Roberts and Fessel, 2004).

TABLE 15-6		
Markers of Oxidative Stress		
Class	**Functions**	**Comment**
Class I: Antioxidant Markers		
Vitamin C (plasma or leukocyte)	Specific inhibitor of water-soluble radicals	Measured by chromatography, capillary electrophoresis, or an automated enzymatic assay
α-Tocopherol	Inhibitor of lipid peroxidation	Measured by chromatography or capillary electrophoresis
γ-Tocopherol	An inhibitor of the nitrous oxide radical	Measured by chromatography or capillary electrophoresis
Carotenoids	Primarily inhibitors of lipid peroxidation	Measured by chromatography; includes α- and β-carotenes, lycopene, cryptoxanthin, zeaxanthin, and lutein
Class II: Endogenous Systems		
Glutathione assay	Detoxifies the ROS hydrogen peroxide (H_2O_2)	Measured by plasma or erythrocyte glutathione or ratio of reduced to oxidized glutathione

LDL, Low-density lipoprotein; *NA*, not applicable; *ROS*, reactive oxidation species.

Continued

TABLE 15-6

Markers of Oxidative Stress—cont'd

Class	Functions	Comment
Class III: Global Tests of Antioxidant Capacity		
LDL oxidative susceptibility	Reflects the concentration of antioxidants in LDLs	In vitro determination of the rate of formation of LDL oxidation products called *conjugated dienes*
Oxygen radical absorbance capacity (ORAC)	NA	Measures decrease in fluorescence over time; reflects the total antioxidant capacity of the specimen
Total peroxyl radical trapping parameter (TRAP)	NA	Measures total antioxidant capacity; reflects the levels of uric acid and albumin
2,2′-Azino-bis (3-ethyl benzytiazoline-sulfonic acid) (ABTS)	NA	ABTS assay in commercial by available kit; also called *total antioxidant status (TAS)*
Class IV: Products of Free Radical Reactions		
Modified LDL	NA	Immunoassay of oxidized LDL proteins; may directly reflect risk of atherosclerosis; may become commercially available, allowing assay to be performed by clinical laboratories
Isoprostane	No known function	Primary form, isoprostane $F_{2\alpha}$, measured by chromatography or an immunoassay that is available commercially and can be rapidly performed
Thiobarbituric acid reactive substances (TBARS)	NA	A colorimetric assay that is easy to perform but not specific for oxidation products; measures products of lipid peroxidation called *aldehydes* (e.g., malondialdehyde)

LDL, Low-density lipoprotein; *NA,* not applicable, *ROS,* reactive oxidation species.

⇄ NEW DIRECTIONS

Raman Spectroscopy Used to Measure Antioxidant Capacity

Noninvasive measurements of clinical parameters are always preferable to those requiring blood, urine, or tissue. Raman spectroscopy is just such a measurement technique and may become widely used in the future. Using a laser light that is pointed toward the fat pad of the palm, as the laser light penetrates the skin, the amount of carotenoids (all-trans-beta-carotene, lycopene, alpha-carotene, gamma-carotene, phytoene, phytofluene, sepapreno-betacarotene, 7,7′-dihydro-beta-carotene, astaxanthin, canthaxanthin, zeaxanthin, lutein, beta-apo8′carotenal, violaxanthins, and rhodoxanthin) is measured at the cellular level. Because all carotenoids have a carbon backbone with alternating carbon double and single bonds, the vibration of these bonds can be detected with Raman spectroscopy. Raman spectroscopy has been used to assess carotenoids in precancerous skin lesions as well as in the retina to assess early stages of macular degeneration (Ermakov et al., 2005). Carotenoids are powerful antioxidants, and because they are part of the "antioxidant network," a measure of their presence can give a good assessment of the antioxidant capacity of the cell. The Raman spectroscopy score also correlates inversely with urinary isoprostanes, a measure of oxidative stress (Carlson et al., 2006).

Serum carotenoids significantly correlate with skin carotenoids, as measured using Raman spectroscopy and the Biophotonic Laser scanner (Smidt et al., 2004; Zidichouski et al., 2004). Serum carotenoids are a good measure of the absorptive capacity of the individual (see Chapter 3). Thus an individual with a diet high in fruits and vegetables and therefore large amounts of dietary carotenoids usually has a high carotenoid antioxidant score. The antioxidant score, or the numeric result from this scan, can be used to determine how well a person is processing carotenoid antioxidants and whether the antioxidants are reaching the cell where they exert their protective functions. The number, which seems to be in the range of 25,000 and higher in those with optimal health, increases with greater consumption of carotenoid-containing fruits and vegetables, consumption of carotenoid-containing nutritional supplements, smoking cessation, and loss of excess body fat (Carlson et al., 2006). The measurement is quick, easy, and inexpensive, making it a likely assessment tool for nutrition professionals in the future.

FOCAL POINTS

- Laboratory data, essential components of the nutrition assessment, and diagnosis and are used to screen, assess for specific nutrient deficiencies, and formulate risk assessment.
- Practitioners must use the wealth of routinely available laboratory data to support nutrition diagnoses and to monitor and evaluate nutrition intervention.

- Because laboratory data are increasing the knowledge of the mechanisms involved in the development of chronic disease, new tests are constantly being developed to identify risk earlier and their clinical usefulness becomes proven.
- Timing of initiation of laboratory tests is based on the patient's clinical condition due to age, history, illness, or injury.

CLINICAL SCENARIO 1

Chandra is seen at County Hospital emergency room. She has a long history of eating disorders and substance abuse. In the last 3 years she has had bleeding gastric ulcers and Crohn's disease. She works at an upscale restaurant as a dishwasher. One of the benefits of her job is one free meal the days she works. Chandra keeps very little food in her apartment and eats most meals at fast-food restaurants when she is not at work. Chandra has called in sick to work for the past 3 days. She has a poor work history, and her employer questions her motives for missing work. Her employer told her if she is really too sick to come to work, she must see her doctor for a medical release to return to work.

The ER doctor orders laboratory tests and Chandra is admitted to the hospital. Her medical profile today is:

Age	**42 years old**
Height	5'1"
Weight	85 lb
Frame	Small
PAB	9 mg/dl; 90 mg/L
Alb	2.8 g/dl; 28 gm/L
Hgb	6 g/dl; 3.73 mmol
Serum Fe	52 μg/dl; 9.31 μmol/kg
MCV	71 μm^3; 71 fL
Ferritin	180 ng/ml; 180 μg/L
AST	23 units/L; 0.38 μKat/L
ALT	28 units/L
FBG	92 mg/dl; 5.11 mmol/L
BUN	40 mg/dl; 14.28 mmol/L
Creatinine	0.6 mg/dl; 53.04 μmol/L
Na	149 mEq/L; 149 mmol/L
Osmolality	287 mOsm/kg/H$_2$O; 287 mmol/kg/H$_2$O

Chandra is referred for medical nutrition therapy. Assess her nutrition status using the data provided.

✳Nutrition Diagnosis: Altered laboratory values related to substance abuse and disordered eating pattern as evidenced by low proteins and signs of anemia.

1. Estimated Chandra's energy and protein needs based on her anthropometric data.
2. Considering Chandra's medical history, what does her laboratory report for hemoglobin, MCV, ferritin, and serum Fe suggest?
3. What does her laboratory report for AST and ALT values suggest?
4. What does her laboratory report for sodium, BUN, creatinine, and osmolality suggest about her hydration status?
5. What does her laboratory report for BUN and creatinine suggest about her renal status?

Chandra is scheduled for a series of tests. She is given intravenous fluids, two pints of blood and is NPO. The preliminary findings indicate several tumors obstructing the small intestine. Exploratory surgery is scheduled tomorrow.

6. How would you expect Chandra's laboratory tests to change 24 hours after major surgery?
7. What additional laboratory tests would be helpful for a comprehensive nutrition assessment?

✴ CLINICAL SCENARIO 2

Uriel is seen at the Southeastern Medical Clinic today complaining of fatigue, chest pains, and shortness of breath after he plays basketball. He works as a landscaping contractor. Uriel has a history of high blood pressure and takes medication daily. He is concerned about his risk for heart disease. He has gained 18 pounds this year after quitting smoking and divorcing his wife. He eats breakfast and lunch at fast-food restaurants. His favorite foods are biscuits, fried meat sandwiches, and French fries. His father prepares the evening meal. Uriel reports drinking three to five beers nightly while watching television. He sees his five children on weekends and holidays. He has moved in with his father until he can afford a new place to live. His medical profile is a follows: 49-year-old Hispanic male; Height: 5' 5"; Weight: 195 lbs, large frame.

Laboratory Report

Glucose	155 mg/dl; 8.6 mmol/L
Calcium	10 mg/L; 2.5 mmol/L
Sodium	140 mEq/L; 140 mmol/L
Potassium	3.5 mEq/L; 35 mmol/L
CO_2	25 mEq/L; 25 mmol/L
Chloride	101 mEq/L; 101 mmol/L
BUN	44 mg/dl; 15.7 mmol/L
Creatinine	2.6 mg/dl; 230 μmol/L
Albumin	2.8 g/dl; 28 g/L
Total protein	4.8 g/dl; 48 g/L
ALP	88 international units/L; 1.47 μKat/L
AST	22 international units/L; 0.37 μKat/L
ALT	24 international units/L; 24 units/L
Bilirubin	0.7 mg/dl; 12 μmol/L
Total serum cholesterol	205 mg/dl; 5.3 mmol/L
HDL cholesterol	70 mg/dl; 1.8 mmol/L
LDL cholesterol	110 mg/dl; 2.85 mmol/L
Triglycerides	350 mg/dl
Homocysteine	18 μmol/L
Blood pressure	166/99 mm Hg

Uriel is referred for medical nutrition therapy. Assess his nutrition status based on the data provided.

✴**Nutrition Diagnosis:** Altered laboratory values related to recent weight gain and smoking cessation as evidenced by elevated blood pressure, symptoms of metabolic syndrome, and dietary recall.

1. Based on the health history, social history, fasting laboratory report and medical profile, what risk factors does he have for chronic diseases?
2. Considering Uriel's medical profile, what does his laboratory report for glucose, BUN, sodium, potassium, and creatinine suggest?
3. What does his laboratory report for ALP, AST and ALT suggest?
4. What does his lipid profile and homocysteine suggest?
5. Uriel's physician orders a vertical ultracentrifugation test. What additional information will this test provide his physician?

USEFUL WEBSITES

National Center for Health Statistics, National Health and Nutrition Examination Survey–NHANES
www.cdc.gov/nchs/nhanes

National Cholesterol Education Program–NCEP, ATPIII Guidelines
www.nhlbi.nih.gov/guidelines/cholesterol/index.htm

The Merck Manual of Diagnosis and Therapy Section I–Nutritional Disorders
www.merck.com/pubs/mmanual/section1/sec1.htm

References

Albers R et al; Markers to measure immunomodulation in human nutrition intervention studies. *Br J Nutr* 94(3):452, 2005.

Bischoff-Ferrari HA et al: Estimation of optimal serum concentrations of 25-hydroxyvitamin D for multiple health outcomes, *Am J Clin Nutr*, 84:18, 2006.

Blake GJ, Ridker PM: Novel clinical markers of vascular wall inflammation, *Circ Res* 89:763, 2001.

Blanck HM et al: Laboratory issues: use of nutritional biomarkers, *J Nutr* 133(suppl 3):888S, 2003.

Bønaa KH et al: Homocysteine lowering and cardiovascular events after acute myocardial infarction, *N Engl J Med* 354:1578, 2006.

Bron D et al: Biological basis of anemia, *Semin Oncol* 28(2suppl 8):1S, 2001.

Carlson JJ et al: Associations of antioxidant status, oxidative stress with skin carotenoids assessed by Raman spectroscopy (RS), *FASEB J* 20:1318, 2006.

Chernecky CC, Berger BJ: *Laboratory tests and diagnostic procedures*, ed 4, Philadelphia, 2004, Saunders.

El-Sohemy A et al: Individual carotenoid concentrations in adipose tissue and plasma as biomarkers of dietary intake, *Am J Clin Nutr* 76:172, 2002.

Ermakov IV et al: Resonance Raman detection of carotenoids antioxidants in living human tissue, *J Biom Opt* 10(6):064028, 2005.

Fuhrman MP et al: Hepatic proteins and nutrition assessment, *J Am Diet Assoc* 104:1258, 2004.

Gottschlich MM et al (editors): *The science and practice of nutrition support: a case-based core curriculum*, Dubuque, Ia, 2001, Kendall/Hunt Publishing.

Graham TE et al: Retinol-binding protein 4 and insulin resistance in lean, obese, and diabetic subjects, *N Engl J Med* 354:2552, 2006.

Grundy S et al: Implications of recent clinical trials for the National Cholesterol Education Program Adult Treatment Panel III Guidelines, *Circulation* 110:227-239, 2004.

Harrison DG, Nieto FJ: NHLBI Workshop on Oxidative Stress/Inflammation meeting proceedings, Bethesda, Md, November 29, 2004, http://www.nhlbi.nih.gov/meetings/workshops/oxidative-stress.htm, accessed October 1, 2006.

Haurani FI: Interpretation of serum ferritin in anemia of chronic disease, *Am J Hematol* 69:296, 2002.

Hulthe J, Fagerberg B: Circulating oxidized LDL is associated with subclinical atherosclerosis development and inflammatory cytokines (AIR Study), *Arterioscler Thromb Vasc Biol* 122(7):1162, 2002.

Litchford, MD: *Common denominators of declining nutritional status*, Greensboro, NC, 2005, CASE Software & Books, 2005.

Litchford MD: *Practical applications in laboratory assessment of nutritional status*, Greensboro, NC, 2006, CASE Software & Books.

Liu S et al: Relation between a diet with a high glycemic load and plasma concentrations of high-sensitivity C-reactive protein in middle-aged women, *Am J Clin Nutr* 75:492, 2002.

Morris MC et al: Dietary folate and B_{12} intake and cognitive decline among community-dwelling older persons, *Arch Neurol* 62:641, 2005.

Mosekilde L: Vitamin D and the elderly, *Clin Endocrinol* 62(3):265, 2005.

Ozatli D et al: Erythrocytes: anemias in chronic liver diseases, *Hematology* 5:69, 2000.

Roberts LJ, Fessel JP: The biochemistry of the isoprostane, neuroprostane, and isofuran pathways of lipid peroxidation, *Chem Phys Lipids* 128:173, 2004.

Saunders DR et al: Univ of Washington, Division of Gastroenterology: the gut course: small bowel, 2006, http://www.uwgi.org/gut/smallbowel_02.asp, accessed October 1, 2006.

Savage DG et al: Etiology and diagnostic evaluation of macrocytosis, *Am J Med Sci* 319:343, 2000.

Smidt CR et al: Non-invasive Raman spectroscopy measurement of human carotenoid status, *FASEB J* 18:A480 (Abstract), 2004.

Vanek VW: The use of serum albumin as a prognostic or nutritional marker and the pros and cons of IV albumin therapy, *Nutr Clin Pract* 13:110, 1998.

Yang Q et al: Serum retinol binding protein 4 contributes to insulin resistance in obesity and type 2 diabetes, *Nature* 436:356, 2005.

Zidichouski et al: Clinical validation of a novel Raman spectroscopic technology to non-invasively assess carotenoid status in humans, *Am Coll Nutr* 23:468, 2004.

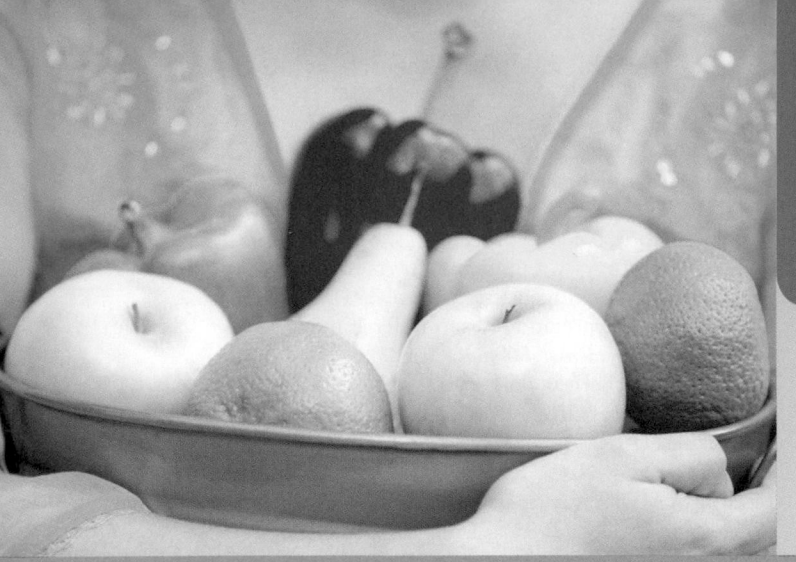

CHAPTER 16

Zaneta M. Pronsky, MS, RD, LDN, FADA,
Sr. Jeanne P. Crowe, PharmD, RPH

Assessment: Food-Drug Interactions

KEY TERMS

absorption the process of movement of a drug from the site of administration into the systemic circulation

acetylation a conjugation reaction involving the hepatic enzyme acetyl transferase, which metabolizes and inactivates amines, hydrazines, and sulfonamides

adsorption the adhesion of drug molecules to the surface of another substance by physical or chemical attraction

bioavailability the degree to which a drug or other substance reaches the general circulation and becomes available to the target organ or tissue

biotransformation the metabolism of drugs by reactions such as oxidation, reduction, hydrolysis, or conjugation

black box warning the most serious warning required by the Food and Drug Administration on drug labels; such warnings appear in a box surrounded by a black border at the beginning of the label information

cytochrome P-450 enzyme system a multienzyme system in the smooth endoplasmic reticulum of numerous tissues that is involved in phase I of liver detoxification and is the major catalyst of drug biotransformation reactions

drug-nutrient interaction the result of the action between a drug and a nutrient that would not happen with the nutrient or the drug alone

excipient substance added to a drug, such as a buffer, binder, filler, diluent, disintegrant, glidant, flavoring, dye, preservative, suspending agent, or coating; also called inactive ingredient

food-drug interaction a broad term that includes drug-nutrient interactions and the effect of a medication on nutritional status

half-life the amount of time it takes for the blood concentration of a drug to decrease by one-half its steady-state level

pharmacodynamics the study of the physiologic and biochemical effects of a drug or combination of drugs

pharmacogenomics the study of genetically determined variations that are revealed solely by the effects of drugs in the body

pharmacokinetics the movement of a drug through the body by absorption, distribution, metabolism, and excretion

physical incompatibility a food-drug interaction involving granulation, gel formation, or separation of the enteral nutritional product when food and drug are combined

polypharmacy the use of multiple drugs to treat one or more health conditions

pressor agents organic compounds, including tyramine, dopamine, phenylethylamine, and histamine, that cause vasoconstriction and an increase in blood pressure

side effect adverse effect, reaction, or any undesirable outcome of a drug

unbound fraction the amount of a drug that is not bound to serum proteins, is able to leave the vasculature, and produces a pharmacologic effect at a target organ

The management of many diseases requires drug therapy, frequently involving the use of multiple drugs. Food-drug interactions can change the effects of drugs, and the therapeutic effects or side effects of medications can affect the nutrition status of an individual. Alternatively, the diet and use of supplements, genetic makeup, or the nutritional status of the patient can decrease the efficacy of a drug or increase its toxicity.

The terms *drug-nutrient interaction* and *food-drug interaction* are often used interchangeably. In actuality, drug-nutrient interactions are some of the many possible food-drug interactions. **Drug-nutrient interactions** include specific changes to the pharmacokinetics of a drug caused by a nutrient(s) or changes to the kinetics of a nutrient(s) caused by a drug. **Food-drug interactions** is a broader term that also includes the effects of a medication on nutritional status. Nutritional status may be impacted by the side effects of a medication, which could include an effect on appetite or the ability to eat.

For clinical, economic, and legal reasons, it is important to recognize food-drug interactions. Food-drug interactions that reduce the efficacy of a drug can result in longer or repeated stays in health care facilities, the use of multiple drugs, and deterioration of the patient because of the effects of the disease. Additional health problems can occur because of long-term drug-nutrient interactions. An example of this type of interaction would be the long-term effects of corticosteroids on calcium metabolism and resulting osteoporosis. Medical team members should be aware that therapeutically important food-drug interactions can do the following:

- Alter the intended response to the medication
- Cause drug toxicity
- Alter normal nutritional status

Awareness of these interactions enables the health care professional and patient to work together to avoid or minimize problems (Box 16-1).

BOX 16-1

Benefits of Minimizing Drug Interactions

Medications achieve their intended effects.
Patients do not discontinue their drug.
The need for additional medication is minimized.
Fewer caloric or nutrient supplements are required.
Adverse side effects are avoided.
Optimal nutritional status is preserved.
Accidents and injuries are avoided.
Disease complications are minimized.
The cost of health care services is reduced.
There is less professional liability.
Licensing agency requirements are met.

From *Food-medication interactions*, ed 14, Birchrunville, Pa, 2006, Food-Medication Interactions.

The Joint Commission (TJC) requires education about "the safe and effective use of medications." In the publication *2005 Comprehensive Accreditation Manual for Hospitals* education section is Standard PC.6.10: "The patient is educated about the safe and effective use of medication . . . (and) . . . nutrition interactions, modified diets, or oral health . . . " Education about safe and effective use of medications must include food-drug interactions as applicable.

PHARMACOLOGIC ASPECTS OF FOOD-DRUG INTERACTIONS

Medication is administered to produce a pharmacologic effect in the body or, more specifically, in a target organ or tissue. To achieve this goal, the drug must move from the site of administration to the bloodstream and eventually to the site of drug action. In due course the drug may be changed to active or inactive metabolites and ultimately eliminated from the body. An interaction between the drug and food, a food component, or a nutrient can alter this process at any point. Food-drug interactions may be divided into two broad types: (1) pharmacodynamic interactions, which affect the pharmacologic action of the drug; and (2) pharmacokinetic interactions, which affect the movement of the drug into, around, or out of the body.

Pharmacodynamics

Pharmacodynamics is the study of the biochemical and physiologic effects of a drug. The mechanism of action of a drug might include the binding of the drug molecule to a receptor, enzyme, or ion channel, resulting in the observable physiologic response. Ultimately this response may be enhanced or attenuated by the addition of other substances with similar or opposing actions.

Pharmacokinetics is the study of the time course of a drug in the body involving the absorption, distribution, metabolism (biotransformation), and excretion of the drug. **Absorption** is the process of the movement of the drug from the site of administration to the bloodstream. This process depends on: (1) the route of administration, (2) the chemistry of the drug and its ability to cross biologic membranes, (3) the rate of gastric emptying (for orally administered drugs) and gastrointestinal movement, and (4) the quality of the product formulation. Food, food components, and nutrition supplements can interfere with the absorption process, especially when the drug is administered orally.

Distribution occurs when the drug leaves the systemic circulation and travels to various regions of the body. Body areas of distribution vary with different drugs, depending on the drug's chemistry and ability to cross biologic membranes. The rate and extent of blood flow to an organ or tissue strongly affect the amount of drug that reaches the area. Many drugs are highly bound to plasma proteins such as albumin. The bound fraction of drug does not leave the vasculature and therefore does not produce a pharmacologic effect. Only the **unbound fraction** is able to produce an effect at a target organ.

A drug is eliminated from the body as either an unchanged drug or a metabolite of the original compound. The major organ of metabolism, or **biotransformation,** in the body is the liver, although other sites contribute to a lesser degree. One of the more important enzyme systems that facilitate drug metabolism is the **cytochrome P-450 enzyme system.** This is a multienzyme system in the smooth endoplasmic reticulum of numerous tissues that is involved in phase I of liver detoxification (see *Focus On*: Detoxification Systems in Chapter 9). Substances such as food or dietary supplements, which either increase or inhibit the activity of this enzyme system, can significantly change the rate or extent of drug metabolism. The general tendency of the process of metabolism is to transform a drug from a lipid-soluble to a more water-soluble compound that can be handled more easily by the kidneys and excreted in the urine.

Renal excretion is the major route of elimination for drugs and drug metabolites either by glomerular filtration or tubular secretion. To a lesser extent drugs may be eliminated in bile and other body fluids. Under certain circumstances, such as a change in urinary pH, drugs that have reached the renal tubule may pass back into the bloodstream. This process is known as tubular resorption. The recommended dose of a drug generally assumes normal liver and kidney function. The dose and/or dosing interval of an excreted drug or active metabolite must be adjusted to meet the degree of renal dysfunction in patients with kidney disease (see Chapter 36).

RISK FACTORS FOR FOOD-DRUG INTERACTIONS

Patients must be assessed individually for the effect of food on drug action and the effect of drugs on nutrition status. Interactions can be caused or complicated by **polypharmacy,** nutrition status, genetics, underlying illness, special diets, nutrition supplements, tube feeding, herbal or phytonutrient products, alcohol intake, drugs of abuse, non-nutrients in food, excipients in drugs or food, allergies, or intolerances. Poor patient compliance and physicians' prescribing patterns further complicate the risk. Drug-induced malnutrition occurs most commonly during long-term treatment for chronic disease, and older patients are at a particularly high risk for many reasons (see *Focus On*: Food-Drug Interactions in Older Adults).

Existing malnutrition also places patients at greater risk for drug-nutrient interactions. Protein alterations—specifically low albumin levels—and changes in body composition secondary to malnutrition can affect drug disposition by altering protein binding and drug distribution. Patients with active neoplastic disease or active acquired immune deficiency syndrome (AIDS) with significant anorexia and wasting are at special risk because of the high prevalence of malnutrition in these groups. The presence of the tumor and resulting illness may lead to reduced intake. Treatment modalities such as chemotherapy and radiation may exacerbate nutritional disturbances. Cisplatin (Platinol-AQ) and other cytotoxic agents commonly cause nausea, vomiting, diarrhea, anorexia, and reduced food intake.

Drug disposition can be affected by alterations in the gastrointestinal tract, such as vomiting, diarrhea, hypochlorhydria, mucosal atrophy, and motility changes. Malabsorption caused by intestinal damage from disease such as cancer, celiac disease, or inflammatory bowel disease creates greater potential for food-drug interactions.

Body composition is an important consideration in determining drug response. In obese or older patients, the proportion of adipose tissue to lean body mass is increased. In theory, accumulation of fat-soluble drugs such as the long-acting benzodiazepines (e.g., diazepam [Valium]) is more likely to occur. Accumulation of a drug and its metabolites in adipose tissue may result in prolonged clearance and increased toxicity. In older patients this interaction may be complicated by decreased hepatic clearance of the drug (Ritschel and Kearns, 1999).

The developing fetus, infant, and pregnant woman are also at high risk for drug-nutrient interactions (see Tables 5-6 and 5-7). Many drugs have not been tested on these populations, making it difficult to assess the risks of negative drug effects, including food-drug interactions.

Pharmacogenomics

Genetic variations in an enzyme or enzyme system affect individual response to specific drug(s). **Pharmacogenomics** involves genetically determined variations that are revealed solely by the effects of drugs and can be a driver for nutrigenomics as discussed in Chapter 13 (Ghosh et al., 2007). Examples that have food-drug interaction ramifications are G6PD (glucose-6-phosphate dehydrogenase) enzyme deficiency, warfarin (Coumadin) resistance, and slow inactivation of isoniazid (INH) or phenelzine (Nardil). Warfarin resistance can affect individual requirements for and response to warfarin.

Slow inactivation of INH or phenelzine are examples of the effect of slow acetylation. **Acetylation** is a conjugation reaction that metabolizes and inactivates amines, hydrazines, and sulfonamides. "Slow acetylators" are persons who metabolize these drugs more slowly than average because of inherited lower levels of the hepatic enzyme acetyl transferase. Therefore unacetylated drug levels remain higher for longer periods in these persons than in those who are "rapid acetylators." For example, the **half-life** of INH for fast acetylators is about 70 minutes, whereas the half-life is more than 3 hours for slow acetylators (Roth, 1995). A dose of drug prescribed normally for fast acetylators can be toxic for slow acetylators. Elevated blood levels of affected drugs in slow acetylators increase the potential for food-drug interactions. Slow inactivation of INH increases the risk of pyridoxine deficiency and pe-

Food-Drug Interactions in Older Adults

Older patients are more likely to be taking multiple drugs, both prescription and over-the-counter, than are younger patients. They have a higher risk of food-drug interactions because of physical changes related to aging, such as the increase in the ratio of fat tissue to lean body mass, a decrease in liver mass and blood flow, and impairment of kidney function. Illness, cognitive or endocrine dysfunction, and ingestion of restricted diets also increase this risk. Malnutrition and dehydration affect drug kinetics. The use of herbal or phytonutrient products has increased significantly in all developed countries, including use by older adults. Drugs of abuse or excessive alcohol intake are often missed in the older patient.

Central nervous system side effects of drugs can interfere with the ability or desire to eat. Drugs that cause drowsiness, dizziness, ataxia, confusion, headache, weakness, tremor, or peripheral neuropathy can lead to nutritional compromise, particularly in older patients. Recognition of these problems as a drug side effect rather than a consequence of disease or aging is often overlooked.

Care must be taken to evaluate intake of interacting nutrients (in the oral diet, supplements, or tube feedings) when specific drugs are used. Examples are vitamin K with warfarin (Coumadin); calcium and vitamin D with alendronate (Fosamax); and potassium, sodium, and magnesium with loop diuretics such as furosemide (Lasix). Parkinson's patients may be concerned with the amount and timing of protein intake because of interaction with levodopa (Sinemet, Dopar) (Duarte et al., 1993). The interdisciplinary team, which includes the physician, pharmacist, nurse, and dietitian, must work together to plan and coordinate the medication regimen and diet and nutritional supplements to preserve optimal nutrition status and minimize food-drug interactions (Figure 16-1).

ripheral neuropathy. Slow inactivation of phenelzine, a monoamine oxidase (MAO) inhibitor, increases the risk for hypertensive crisis if foods high in tyramine are consumed (Box 16-2). Dapsone (DDS) and hydralazine (Apresoline) are also metabolized by acetylation and affected by inherited differences in acetylase enzymes.

Deficiency of G6PD is an X-chromosome–linked deficiency of G6PD enzyme in red blood cells. It can lead to neonatal jaundice, hemolytic anemia, or acute hemolysis. Most common in African, Middle Eastern, and Southeast Asian populations, it is also called favism. Fava (Vicia faba) beans or pollen can cause acute hemolysis in some G6PD-deficient persons, particularly those of Mediterranean origin. Some drugs such as aspirin, sulfonamides, and antimalarial drugs can cause hemolysis and acute anemia. There have been several reports of acute hemolysis induced in G6PD deficiency because of high-dose vitamin K or ascorbic acid (Rees et al., 1993). Therefore the potential exists for food-drug interactions in G6PD deficiency resulting from the ingestion of fava beans (also called broad beans), vitamin C, or vitamin K.

Another factor that affects drug metabolism is genetically different activity of CYP enzymes. "Slow metabolizers" may have less of a specific enzyme or their enzyme(s) may be less active. Such individuals have a higher risk of adverse drug effects. Slow CYP2D6 metabolizers make up approximately 5% to10% of whites, whereas approximately 20% of Asians are CYP2C19 poor metabolizers. Tests are now available to analyze deoxyribonucleic acid (DNA) to determine variations in the activity of these two enzymes. CYP2D6 and CYP2C19 metabolize about 25% of all drugs, including many antipsychotics, antidepressants, and narcotics. Slow metabolizers achieve a higher blood level with usual doses

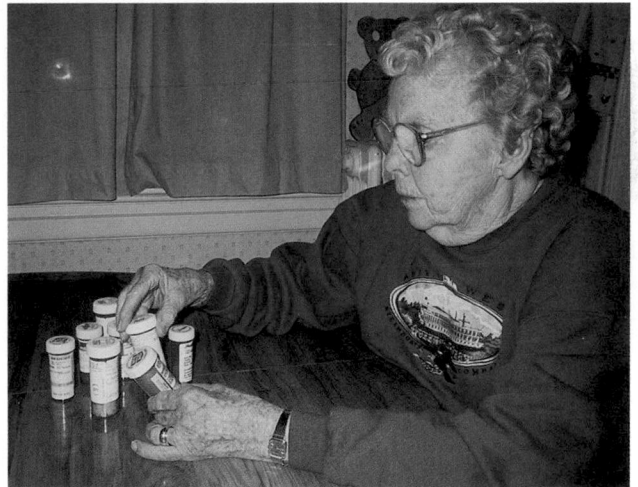

FIGURE 16-1 As a result of the increased potential for illness with aging, older adults often take multiple drugs, both prescription and over-the-counter preparations. This places them at increased risk for drug-drug and food-drug interactions.

of such drugs, whereas fast metabolizers may have an unpredictable response as a result of rapid metabolism of the drug (Med Lett, 2005).

Drug response genotyping will help determine which drugs will be most effective, depending on an individual's genetic makeup (DeBusk, 2003) (see Chapter 13). The ability to predict response to specific drugs will help to determine effective treatment for cancer, mental illness, and even pain management. Genotyping will help reduce adverse drug reactions, including food medication interactions.

BOX 16-2

Pressor Agents in Foods and Beverages
(Tyramine, Dopamine, Histamine, Phenylethylamine)

Avoid with monoamine oxidase inhibitor (MAOI) medications - Phenelzine [Nardil], Tranyl cypromine [Parnate], Isocarboxazid [Marplan], Selegiline [Eldepryl in doses > 10 mg/day], and the antibiotic Linezolid [Zyvox].

Foods That Must Be Avoided

Aged cheeses (e.g., cheddar, blue, Gorgonzola, Stilton)

Aged meats (e.g., dry sausage such as salami, mortadella, Chinese dried duck)

Soy sauce

Fermented soya beans, soya bean paste, teriyaki sauce

Tofu/fermented bean curd, tempeh

Miso

Fava (broad) beans or pods, snow pea pods (contain dopamine)

Sauerkraut, kim chee

Tap beer, Korean beer

Concentrated yeast extracts (Marmite)

Banana peel

All casseroles made with aged cheese

Meats, fish or poultry stored longer than 3-4 days in the refrigerator

Foods That May Be Used with Caution

Red or white wine 2-4 oz per day

Coffee, cola*

Pizza (homemade or gourmet pizzas may have higher content)

Bottled beer, two 12-oz bottles, maximum

Alcohol-free beer, two 12-oz bottles, maximum

Liquers or distilled spirits (two 1½ oz servings per day)

Foods Not Limited (based on current analyses)

Unfermented cheeses (cream, cottage, ricotta, mozzarella, processed American if refrigerated less than 2–3 weeks)

Smoked white fish, salmon, carp, or anchovies

Pickled herring

Fresh meat poultry or fish

Canned figs, raisins

Fresh pineapple

Beetroot, cucumber

Sweet corn, mushrooms

Salad dressings, tomato sauce

Worcestershire sauce

Baked raised products, English cookies

Boiled egg, yogurt, junket, ice cream

Avocado, figs, banana, raspberries

Brewer's yeast (vitamin supplements)

Curry powder

Peanuts, chocolate

Packaged or processed meats (e.g., hot dogs, bologna, liverwurst), although they should be stored in refrigerator immediately and eaten as soon as possible; histamine content is highest in improperly stored or spoiled fish, tuna

From Pronsky ZM: *Food medication-interactions*, ed 13, Birchrunville, Pa, 2004, Food-Medication Interactions.

*Contains caffeine, a weak pressor agent, in quantities >500 mg/day may exacerbate reactions.

EFFECTS OF FOOD ON DRUG THERAPY

Drug Absorption

The presence of food and nutrients in the stomach or lumen of the intestinal tract has the potential to reduce the absorption of a drug. Examples of a critically significant reduction in drug absorption are the antiosteoporosis drugs alendronate (Fosamax), risedronate (Actonel), or ibrandronate (Boniva). Absorption is negligible if these drugs are given with food and reduced by 60% if taken with coffee or orange juice. The manufacturer's instructions for alendronate or risedronate are to take the drug on an empty stomach with plain water at least 30 minutes before any other food, drink, or medication. Ibrandronate must be taken at least 60 minutes before any other food, drink, or medication. However, in one study **bioavailability** was reduced by 40% when 10 mg of alendronate was taken 30 to 60 minutes instead of

2 hours before breakfast (Fosamax, 2001). Alendronate and risedronate are now available in daily and weekly formulations, whereas ibrandronate is available in daily or a once monthly formulation.

The absorption of the iron from supplements may be decreased by 50% when taken with food. Iron is best absorbed when taken with 8 oz of water on an empty stomach. If iron must be taken with food to avoid gastrointestinal distress, it should not be taken with bran, eggs, high-phytate foods, fiber supplements, tea, coffee, dairy products, or calcium supplements, because each of these can decrease iron absorption (see Chapter 3).

Various mechanisms may contribute to the reduction in the rate or extent of drug absorption in the presence of food or nutrients. The presence and type of meal or food ingested influence the rate of gastric emptying. Gastric emptying may be delayed by the consumption of high-fiber meals and meals with high fat content. In general, a delay in drug absorption is not clinically significant as long as the extent of absorption is not affected. However, delayed absorption of antibiotics or analgesics may be clinically significant. Chelation reactions occur between certain medications and divalent or trivalent cations, such as iron, calcium, magnesium, zinc, or aluminum, and the absorption of drugs may be reduced by chelation with one of these metal ions.

The antibiotics ciprofloxacin (Cipro) and tetracycline (Achromycin-V or Sumycin) form insoluble complexes with calcium in dairy products or calcium-fortified foods and beverages; calcium, magnesium, zinc, or iron supplements; or aluminum in antacids, thus preventing or reducing the absorption of both drug and nutrient (Neuhofel et al., 2002). The optimal approach to avoid this interaction is to stop noncritical supplements for the duration of the antibiotic prescription. If this is not possible, particularly with magnesium or with long-term antibiotic use, it is advisable to give the drug at least 2 hours before or 6 hours after the mineral.

Adsorption, or the adhesion to food or a food component, is another mechanism by which drug absorption is slowed or reduced. A high-fiber diet may decrease the absorption of tricyclic antidepressants such as amitriptyline (Elavil), leading to loss of therapeutic effect of the antidepressant because of the adsorption of the drug to the fiber. Likewise, the cardiovascular drug digoxin (Lanoxin) should not be taken with high-phytate foods such as wheat bran or oatmeal.

Gastrointestinal pH is an important factor for the absorption of some drugs. Any situations resulting in changes in gastric acid pH, such as achlorhydria or hypochlorhydria, may reduce drug absorption. An example of such an interaction is the failure of ketoconazole (Nizoral) to clear a *Candida* infection in patients with human immune deficiency virus (AIDS) or in persons taking potent acid-reducing agents for gastroesophageal reflux disease (GERD). Ketoconazole achieves optimal absorption in an acid medium. Because of the high prevalence of achlorhydria in patients infected with AIDS, dissolution of ketoconazole tablets in the stomach is reduced, leading to impaired drug absorption (Welage et al., 1995). This is also a concern with hypochlorhydria in persons receiving chronic acid suppression therapy, such as antacids, histamine 2 (H_2) receptor antagonists (e.g., famotidine [Pepcid]), or proton-pump inhibitors (e.g., omeprazole [Prilosec]). Ingestion of ketoconazole with an acidic liquid such as cola or a dilute HCl solution may improve bioavailability in these patients. The absorption of delavirdine (Rescriptor), an antiretroviral agent, is also reduced in patients with achlorhydria. Such patients should take it with orange or cranberry juice to decrease gastric pH.

The presence of food in the stomach enhances the absorption of some medications, such as the antibiotic cefuroxime axetil (Ceftin) or the antiretroviral drug saquinavir (Fortovase or Invirase). These drugs are prescribed to be taken after a meal to reduce the dose that must be taken to reach an effective level. The bioavailability of cefuroxime axetil is substantially greater (52% versus 37%) when taken with food, compared with taking it in the fasting state.

Maximum blood levels of saquinavir increased twofold in one study after the consumption of a heavy breakfast (940 to 1000 calories and 54 to 57 g of fat).

Medication and Enteral Nutrition Interactions

Continuous enteral feeding is an effective method of providing nutrients to patients who are unable to swallow or eat adequately (see Chapter 20). Use of the feeding tube to administer medication can cause problems, however. When liquid medications are mixed with enteral feeding formulas, incompatibilities may occur. Types of **physical incompatibility** include granulation, gel formation, and separation of the enteral product, frequently resulting in clogged feeding tubes and interruption of the delivery of nutrition to the patient. Examples of drugs that can cause granulation and gel formation are thioridazine (Mellaril) solution, chlorpromazine (Thorazine) concentrate, ferrous sulfate elixir, guaifenesin (Robitussin expectorant), and pseudoephedrine (Sudafed) cough syrup. Emulsion breakage also commonly occurs when acidic pharmaceutical syrups are added to enteral formulas. This reaction is more common in enteral formulas with intact protein and less common with hydrolyzed protein or free amino acids (Burns et al., 1988; Thomson and Rollins, 1991).

Most compatibility studies of medication and enteral products have focused on the effect of the drug on the integrity of the enteral product. More important is the effect of the enteral product on the bioavailability of the drug. This area requires much more research as the placement of feeding tubes becomes a more common practice. Bioavailability problems are common with phenytoin (Dilantin) and tube feeding. Because blood levels of phenytoin are routinely performed to monitor the drug, much information exists about the reduction of phenytoin bioavailability when given with enteral feedings, and individual variability is significant. Recommendations to separate phenytoin suspension from tube-feeding formulas are common. Stopping the tube feeding before and after the phenytoin dose is generally suggested, but recommendations vary from 1- to 4-hour intervals. The most common is a 2-hour feeding-free interval before and after the dose of phenytoin is administered (Au Yeung and Ensom, 2000).

Information may not be readily available concerning a drug and enteral product interactions even though the manufacturer may have unpublished information about their drug's interaction with enteral products. Checking with the manufacturer's medical information department may yield more information for the clinician.

Drug Distribution

Albumin is the most important drug-binding protein in the blood. Low serum albumin levels, often the result of inadequate protein intake and poor nutrition, provide fewer binding sites for highly protein-bound drugs. Fewer binding sites mean that a larger free fraction of drug will be present in the serum. Only the free fraction (unbound fraction) of a drug is able to leave the vasculature and exert a

5-phosphate. Particularly in patients with low pyridoxine intake, this interaction may cause pyridoxine deficiency and peripheral neuropathy. Pyridoxine supplementation (25 to 50 mg/day) is generally recommended with the prescription of INH because it is prescribed for at least 6 months at a time. Some other drugs that function as pyridoxine antagonists are hydralazine (Apresoline), penicillamine, levodopa (Dopar), and cycloserine (Seromycin).

Methotrexate (MTX or Rheumatrex) is a folic acid antagonist used to treat cancer and rheumatoid arthritis. Without folic acid, DNA synthesis is inhibited, cell replication stops, and the cell dies. Pyrimethamine (Daraprim), used to treat malaria and ocular toxoplasmosis, is also a folic acid antagonist. These drugs bind to and inhibit the enzyme dihydrofolate reductase, preventing conversion of folate to its active form (see Chapter 3), which eventually can lead to megaloblastic anemia as a result of folate deficiency (see Chapter 31). Leucovorin (folinic acid, the reduced form of folic acid) is used with folic acid antagonists to prevent anemia and gastrointestinal damage, especially with chemotherapy such as high-dose methotrexate. Leucovorin does not require reduction by dihydrofolate reductase; thus, unlike folic acid, it is not affected by folic acid antagonists. Therefore leucovorin may "rescue" normal cells from MTX damage by competing for the same transport mechanisms into the cells. However, for patients with rheumatoid arthritis who are receiving low-dose MTX therapy, studies show that administration of daily folic acid supplements or folinic acid can lower toxicity without affecting efficacy of the drug (Ortiz et al., 1998).

Nutrient Excretion

Some drugs can either increase or decrease the urinary excretion of nutrients. Drugs can increase the excretion of a nutrient by interfering with nutrient resorption by the kidneys. For instance, most clinicians know that loop diuretics such as furosemide (Lasix) or bumetanide (Bumex) increase the excretion of potassium; but these diuretics also increase the excretion of magnesium, sodium, chloride, and calcium. Potassium supplements are routinely prescribed with loop diuretics. In addition, clinicians need to consider supplements of magnesium and calcium, especially with long-term drug use, high doses of the diuretics, or poor dietary intake. Electrolyte and magnesium blood levels should be monitored. Prolonged use of high-dose diuretics, particularly by older patients on low-sodium diets, can cause sodium depletion. Hyponatremia may be overlooked in older patients because the mental confusion that is symptomatic of sodium depletion may be misdiagnosed as organic brain syndrome or dementia. Thiazide diuretics such as hydrochlorothiazide (HCTZ) increase the excretion of potassium and magnesium but reduce the excretion of calcium by enhancing renal resorption of calcium. High-dose HCTZ plus calcium supplementation may result in hypercalcemia.

Potassium-sparing diuretics such as spironolactone (Aldactone) or triamterene (Dyrenium) increase excretion of sodium, chloride, and calcium. Blood levels of potassium can rise to dangerous levels if patients also take potassium supplements or suffer from renal insufficiency. Antihypertensive angiotensin-converting enzyme (ACE) inhibitors such as enalapril (Vasotec) or fosinopril (Monopril) decrease potassium excretion, leading to increased serum potassium levels. The combination of a potassium-sparing diuretic and an ACE inhibitor increases the danger of hyperkalemia.

Corticosteroids such as prednisone decrease sodium excretion, resulting in sodium and water retention. Conversely, enhanced excretion of potassium and calcium is caused by these drugs; so a low-sodium, high-potassium diet is recommended. Calcium and vitamin D supplements are generally recommended with long-term corticosteroid use to prevent osteoporosis, such as might be the case for a person with asthma, lupus, or rheumatoid arthritis. With corticosteroid use this risk is important because it appears that not only is calcium lost in the urine, but corticosteroids may impair intestinal calcium absorption and the bone-building activity of osteoblasts (Lems et al., 1998).

Phenothiazine-class antipsychotic drugs such as chlorpromazine (Thorazine) increase excretion of riboflavin and can lead to riboflavin deficiency in those with poor dietary intake (Pinto and Rivlin, 1987).

A well-recognized complication associated with the use of cisplatin is the development of acute hypomagnesemia resulting from nephrotoxicity and renal magnesium wasting. As many as 90% of patients are affected (Lajer and Daugaard, 1999). Hypocalcemia, hypokalemia, and hypophosphatemia are also common. Both intravenous magnesium supplementation via rectal treatment or post-treatment hydration and oral magnesium supplements taken between chemotherapeutic courses have been used to prevent magnesium depletion. Results of the efficacy of each approach vary (Sartori et al., 1993). Hypomagnesemia can result from cisplatin use even with high-dose magnesium replacement therapy. Hypomagnesemia can persist for months or even years after the final course. When any drugs known to cause hypomagnesemia are administered, preventive treatment is warranted (Atsmon and Dolev, 2005).

MODIFICATION OF DRUG ACTION BY FOOD AND NUTRIENTS

Food or nutrients can alter the intended pharmacologic action of a medication by enhancing the medication effects or by opposing it. The classic example of an enhanced drug effect is the interaction between monoamine oxidase inhibitors (MAOIs) such as phenelzine sulfate (Nardil) or tranylcypromine (Parnate) and **pressor agents** such as dopamine, histamine, and especially tyramine. These biologically active amines are normally present in many foods (see Box 16-2), but they rarely constitute a hazard because they are deaminated rapidly by MAO and diamine oxidases. Inhibition of MAO by medication prevents the breakdown of tyramine and other pressor agents. Tyramine is a vasoconstrictor that raises blood pressure. Significant ingestion of high-tyramine foods such as aged cheeses and cured meats while being treated with an MAOI antidepressant can cause a hypertensive crisis (increased heart rate, flushing, headache, stroke, and even death) (Gardner et al., 1996). This reaction may be avoided with use of a transdermal system that bypasses the gastrointestinal tract (Blob et al., 2007).

Caffeine in foods or beverages (see Appendix 39) increases the adverse effects of stimulant drugs such as amphetamines, methylphenidate (Ritalin, Concerta), or theophylline, causing nervousness, tremor, and insomnia. Conversely, the central nervous system (CNS) stimulatory properties of caffeine can oppose or counteract the antianxiety effect of tranquilizers such as lorazepam (Ativan).

Warfarin (Coumadin) is an oral anticoagulant that reduces the hepatic production of four vitamin K–dependent clotting factors by inhibiting the conversion of vitamin K to a usable form. Because this is a competitive interaction, the ingestion of vitamin K in the usable form will oppose the action of warfarin and allow the production of more clotting factors. To achieve an optimal level of anticoagulation, a balance must be maintained between the dose of the drug and the ingestion of vitamin K. Counseling of a person taking oral anticoagulation therapy should include medical nutrition therapy (MNT) to maintain a consistent dietary vitamin K intake rather than prohibiting all high–vitamin K foods, such as dark green leafy vegetables (Johnson, 2005) (see Appendix 50). Coenzyme Q10, St. John's wort or avocado also counteract the effect of warfarin. Ingestion of other substances may enhance the anticoagulant effect of warfarin. These substances include onions, garlic, quinine, papaya, mango, or vitamin E supplements in doses greater than 400 IU. Certain herbal products such as dong quai, which contain coumarin-like substances, or ginseng, which is a platelet inhibitor, also enhance the effect of the warfarin. Enhancement of the anticoagulation effects of warfarin may lead to serious bleeding events (Greenblatt and von Moltke, 2005).

Alcohol

Ethanol combined with certain medications will produce additive toxicity, affecting various body organs and systems. Ethanol combined with CNS-depressant medications such as a benzodiazepine (e.g., diazepam [Valium]) or a barbiturate (e.g., phenobarbital) may produce excessive drowsiness, incoordination, and other signs of CNS depression.

In the gastrointestinal tract ethanol acts as a stomach mucosal irritant. Combining ethanol with drugs that cause the same effect such as aspirin or other NSAIDs (ibuprofen [Advil or Motrin]) may increase the risk of gastrointestinal ulceration and bleeding. Because of the hepatotoxic potential of ethanol, it should not be combined with medications that also exhibit a risk of hepatotoxicity such as acetaminophen (Tylenol), amiodarone (Cordarone), or methotrexate (Rheumatrex) (Lieber, 1994).

Ethanol can inhibit gluconeogenesis, particularly when consumed in a fasting state. Inhibition of gluconeogenesis will prolong a hypoglycemic episode caused by insulin or an oral hypoglycemic agent such as glyburide (Diabeta, Micronase) (Van de Wiel, 2004).

The combination of disulfiram (Antabuse) and ethanol produces a potentially life-threatening reaction characterized by flushing, rapid heartbeat, palpitations, and elevation of blood pressure. Disulfiram inhibits aldehyde dehydrogenase, an enzyme necessary for the normal catabolism of ethanol by the liver. As a result of this enzyme inhibition, high levels of acetaldehyde accumulate in the blood. Symptoms such as flushing, headache, and nausea appear within 15 minutes of alcohol ingestion. Because these symptoms are unpleasant, the drug is sometimes used as an aid to prevent alcoholics from returning to drinking. However, because these symptoms may also be life threatening, candidates for this drug must be chosen carefully. Other medications, when ingested concurrently with ethanol, may produce disulfiram-like reactions. Some of these medications are the antibiotics metronidazole (Flagyl) and cefoperazone (Cefobid), the oral hypoglycemic agent chlorpropamide (Diabinese), and the antineoplastic agent procarbazine (Matulane).

Ethanol can also affect the physical characteristics of a medication. The Food and Drug Administration (FDA) recently required a change in the labeling of the extended-release capsules of morphine sulfate, brand names Avinza or Kadian. The label now includes a **black box warning** that patients must not consume alcoholic beverages or take Avinza or Kadian with medications containing alcohol. If taken with alcohol, the extended-release beads of morphine can dissolve rapidly, delivering a potentially fatal dose of morphine.

EFFECTS OF DRUGS ON NUTRITION STATUS

The desired effects of medications often are accompanied by effects that are considered undesirable or **side effects.** Side effects are often an extension of the desired effects, such as bacterial overgrowth, as a result of use of an antibiotic. Overgrowth of *Clostridium difficile* causes pseudomembranous colitis. Suppression of natural oral bacteria may lead to oral yeast overgrowth, or candidiasis (see Chapter 27).

Oral, Taste, and Smell

Many drugs affect the ability to taste or smell foods (Box 16-3). Drugs can cause an alteration in taste sensation (dysgeusia), reduced acuity of taste sensation (hypogeusia), or an unpleasant aftertaste, any of which may affect food intake. The mechanisms by which drugs alter the chemical senses are not well understood. They may alter the turnover of taste cells or interfere with transduction mechanisms inside taste cells. They may also alter neurotransmitters in the CNS that process chemosensory information (Schiffman, 1994). Common drugs that cause dysgeusia include the antihypertensive drug captopril (Capoten), the antiretroviral amprenavir (Agenerase), the antineoplastic cisplatin (Platinol-AQ), and the anticonvulsant phenytoin. When exploring taste changes related to medication use it is always important to consider

BOX 16-3

Examples of Drugs That Cause Altered Taste, or Dysgeusia

Antiasthmatics

Beclomethasone (Beconase, Vancenase)
Terbutaline (Brethine, Bricanyl)

Antineoplastics

Carboplatin (Paraplatin)
Cisplatin (Platinol-AQ)
Dactinomycin (Actinomycin-D)
Fluorouracil (5-FU) (Adrucil)
Interferon alfa 2a (Roferon-A)
Methotrexate (Methotrexate, Rheumatrex)
Oxaliplatin (Eloxatin)

Antiinfectives

Amprenavir (Agenerase)
Cefuroxime (Ceftin, Zinacef)
Clarithromycin (Biaxin)
Clotrimazole (Mycelex)
Didanosine (Videx)
Ethionamide (Trecator-SC)
Metronidazole (Flagyl)
Pyrimethamine (Daraprim)
Pentamidine isethionate (NebuPent, Pentam 300)
Rifabutin (Mycobutin)

Cardiac Drugs

Acetazolamide (Diamox)
Captopril (Capoten)
Gemfibrozil (Lopid)
Quinidine (Quinaglute Dura, Quinidex Extentabs, Quinora)

Central Nervous System Drugs

Clomipramine (Anafranil)
Eszopiclone (Lunesta)
Levodopa (Dopar, Larodopa)
Phenytoin (Dilantin)
Phentermine (Adipex-P, Fastin, Ionamin)
Sumatriptan succinate (Imitrex)

Miscellaneous

Disulfiram (Antabuse)
Docusate sodium (Colace)
Etidronate disodium (Didronel)
Selenium (Se)

From Pronsky, ZM: *Food-medication interactions*, ed 14, Birchrunville, Pa, 2006, Food-Medication Interactions.

changes in zinc absorption related to the medication. An underlying zinc deficiency may affect the sense of taste (Heckmann and Lang, 2006).

Captopril (Capoten) may cause a metallic or salty taste and the loss of taste perception. The antibiotic clarithromycin (Biaxin) enters the saliva. The drug itself has a bitter taste that stays in the mouth as long as the drug is present in the body. An unpleasant or metallic taste has been reported by up to 34% of patients taking the sleep aide eszopiclone (Lunesta).

Antineoplastic drugs, used in chemotherapy for cancer, affect cells that reproduce rapidly, including the mucous membranes. Inflammation of the mucous membranes, or mucositis, occurs and is manifest as stomatitis (mouth inflammation), glossitis (tongue inflammation), or cheilitis (lip inflammation and cracking). Mucositis can be extremely painful to the point that patients are not able to eat or even drink (see Figure 37-4). Aldesleukin, also called interleukin-2 (Proleukin), paclitaxel (Taxol), and carboplatin (Paraplatin), are examples of antineoplastic agents that commonly cause severe mucositis.

Anticholinergic drugs (Box 16-4) compete with the neurotransmitter acetylcholine for its receptor sites, thereby inhibiting transmission of parasympathetic nerve impulses. This results in decreased secretions, including salivary secretions, causing dry mouth (xerostomia). Tricyclic antidepressants such as amitriptyline (Elavil), antihistamines such as diphenhydramine (Benadryl), and antispasmodic bladder

control agents such as oxybutynin (Ditropan) are particularly problematic. Dry mouth immediately causes loss of taste sensation. Long-term dry mouth can cause dental caries and loss of teeth, gum disease, stomatitis, and glossitis, as well as nutritional imbalance and undesired weight loss (Friedlander et al., 2003) (see Chapter 25).

Gastrointestinal Effects

Gastrointestinal irritation and ulceration are serious problems with many drugs. The antiosteoporosis drug alendronate (Fosamax) is contraindicated in patients who are unable to sit upright for at least 30 minutes after taking it because of the danger of esophagitis. NSAIDs such as ibuprofen (Advil, Motrin) or aspirin can cause stomach irritation, dyspepsia, gastritis, ulceration, and sudden serious gastric bleeding, sometimes leading to fatalities. Fluoxetine (Prozac) and other selective serotonin reuptake inhibitors (SSRIs) can also cause serious gastric irritation, leading to hemorrhage, especially when aspirin or NSAIDs are also used (Yuan et al., 2006) (Box 16-5).

Antineoplastic drugs, used to treat cancer, often cause severe nausea and vomiting. Severe, prolonged nausea and vomiting, lasting as long as a week, have been reported with cisplatin (Platinol-AQ). Dehydration and electrolyte imbalances are of immediate concern. Weight loss and malnutrition are common long-term effects of these drugs, although it is often difficult to distinguish these effects from the com-

BOX 16-4

Examples of Drugs With Anticholinergic Effects

Antiemetics, Antivertigo Agents

Dimenhydrinate (Dramamine)
Meclizine (Bonine, Antivert)
Scopolamine (Transderm Scop)

Antihistamines

Clemastine (Tavist)
Cyproheptadine (Periactin)
Diphenhydramine (Benadryl)
Hydroxyzine HCl (Atarax)
Hydroxyzine pamoate (Vistaril)
Promethazine (Phenergan)

Antiparkinson Agents

Benztropine (Cogentin)
Trihexyphenidyl (Artane)

Bladder Anticholinergics

Flavoxate (Uripas)
Oxybutynin (Ditropan)
Tolterodine (Detrol)
Trospium (Sanctura)

Gastrointestinal Antispasmodics

Atropine
Dicyclomine (Bentyl)
Glycopyrrolate (Robinul)
L-Hyoscyamine (Levsin)
Propantheline (Pro-Banthine)

Inhalation Solution

Ipratropium (Atrovent)

Psychotropics

Antipsychotics, Phenothiazines
Chlorpromazine (Thorazine)
Mesoridazine (Serentil)
Thioridazine HCl (Mellaril)

Antipsychotics, Atypical
Clozapine (Clozaril)
Olanzapine (Zyprexa)

Antipsychotics, Typical
Haloperidol (Haldol)
Perphenazine (Trilafon)
Thiothixene (Navane)

Antidepressants, Tricyclic
Amitriptyline (Elavil)
Clomipramine (Anafranil)
Doxepin (Sinequan)
Imipramine (Tofranil)

Antidepressants, Monoamine Oxidase Inhibitors
Isocarboxazide (Marplan)
Phenelzine (Nardil)
Tranylcypromine (Parnate)

From Pronsky ZM: *Food medication interactions*, ed 14, Birchrunville, Pa, 2006, Food Medication Interactions.

plications of the disease itself (see Chapter 37). Serontonin antagonists such as ondansetron (Zofran) help to reduce these GI side effects.

Drugs can cause changes in bowel function that can lead to constipation or diarrhea. Narcotic agents such as codeine and morphine (MS Contin, MSIR, Avinza) cause a nonproductive increase in smooth muscle tone of the intestinal muscle wall, thereby decreasing peristalsis and causing constipation. Drugs with anticholinergic effects decrease intestinal secretions, slow peristalsis, and cause constipation (see Box 16-4). The atypical antipsychotic clozapine (Clozaril), tricyclic antidepressant amitriptyline (Elavil), and antihistamine diphenhydramine (Benadryl) cause constipation and possibly impaction. Patients should be closely monitored and kept adequately hydrated.

Destruction of intestinal bacteria leads to diarrhea (Box 16-6), possibly because of the overgrowth of *C. difficile*, causing pseudomembranous colitis. Some drugs are used to inhibit intestinal enzymes, such as the diabetic drugs acarbose (Precose) and miglitol (Glyset), which are α-glucosidase inhibitors. Such action leads to a delayed and reduced rise in postprandial blood glucose levels and plasma insulin responses. The major adverse effect is gastrointestinal intolerance, specifically diarrhea, flatulence, and cramping secondary to both the osmotic effect and bacterial fermentation of undigested carbohydrates in the distal bowel.

Orlistat (Xenical), now available over the counter (OTC), a lipase inhibitor for weight loss, reduces the absorption of fat by binding to lipase in the intestine, thereby inhibiting its action. Consequently, fecal fat excretion is increased, a factor that contributes to the gastrointestinal complaints associated with the drug, specifically oily spotting, increased fecal urgency, and possible fecal incontinence. A low-fat diet of no more than 30% of calories from fat is essential. Fat intake should be distributed among all three meals. Orlistat is not an appetite suppressant, and some persons may find it difficult to maintain a low-fat diet. Sufficient counseling and support is needed for success with this medication. Attention should also be given to potential malabsorption of fat soluble vitamins A, D, E and K and carotenoids requiring the presence of fat for optimal absorption.

Obviously any of these problems, from dry mouth, to gastrointestinal irritation, to constipation or diarrhea, can negatively affect food intake and nutrient absorption and nutrition status (see Chapter 14).

BOX 16-5

Examples of Drugs That Cause Gastrointestinal Bleeding and Ulceration

Antiinfectives

Amphotericin B (Abelcet, AmBisome, Amphotec, Fungizone)

Ganciclovir sodium (Cytovene)

Antineoplastics

Aldesleukin interleukin-2 (Proleukin)

Fluorouracil (5-FU) (Adrucil)

Leuprolide acetate (Lupron)

Imatinib mesylate (Gleevec)

Leuprolide (Lupron)

Mitoxantrone (Novantrone)

Methotrexate (Methotrexate, Rheumatrex)

Vinblastine sulfate (Velban)

Bisphosphonates

Alendronate (Fosamax)

Ibandronate (Boniva)

Pamidronate (Aredia)

Risedronate (Actonel)

Immunosuppressants

Corticosteroids (Prednisone)

Myophenolate mofetil (CellCept)

Miscellaneous

Bromocriptine (Parlodel)

Donepezil (Aricept)

Fluoxetine (Prozac)

Fluvoxamine (Luvox)

Levodopa (Dopar)

Paroxetine (Paxil)

Sertraline (Zoloft)

Trazodone HCl (Desyrel)

NSAIDs, Analgesics, Antiarthritics

Aspirin/acetylsalicylic acid (Bufferin, Ecotrin)

Celecoxib (Celebrex)

Diclofenac sodium (Cataflam, Voltaren)

Etodolac (Lodine)

Ibuprofen (Advil, Motrin)

Indomethacin (Indocin)

Ketoprofen (Orudis)

Meloxicam (Mobic)

Nabumetone (Relafen)

Naproxen (Naprosyn, Anaprox, Aleve)

Sulindac (Clinoril)

From Pronsky ZM: *Food-medication interactions*, ed 14, Birchrunville, Pa, 2006, Food-Medication Interactions.

Appetite Changes

Drugs can suppress appetite (Box 16-7), leading to undesired weight changes, nutritional imbalance, and growth retardation in children. In the past the stimulant drug dextroamphetamine (Dexedrine) was used as an appetite suppressant. Because of the potential for abuse, the use of amphetamines for appetite suppression is no longer legal. Dextroamphetamine is now only indicated for treatment of attention-deficit hyperactivity disorder (ADHD) or narcolepsy.

In general, most CNS stimulants, including the amphetamine mixture (Adderall) and methylphenidate (Ritalin, Concerta), suppress appetite or cause frank anorexia. These drugs are used extensively to treat ADHD in children and may cause weight loss and inhibit growth (see Chapter 7).

Sibutramine (Meridia) and phentermine (Adipex-P, Ionamin), structurally related to amphetamines, are used as appetite suppressants. These drugs are indicated for short-term use, along with a reduced-calorie diet and exercise, in obese patients (i.e., patients with a body mass index [BMI] greater than 30) or in overweight patients (BMI greater than 27) if additional risk factors such as hypertension, diabetes, or hyperlipidemia are present.

A major side effect of stimulant drugs is hypertension. Thus they are often contraindicated for hypertensive patients or those who have seizures or cardiac disease. Because hypertension is common among obese persons, these con-

traindications may limit the use of stimulants in obese or overweight hypertensive patients.

CNS side effects can interfere with the ability or desire to eat. Drugs that cause drowsiness, dizziness, ataxia, confusion, headache, weakness, tremor, or peripheral neuropathy can lead to nutritional compromise, particularly in older or chronically ill patients. Recognition of these problems as a drug side effect rather than a consequence of disease or aging is often overlooked.

Many medications stimulate appetite and lead to weight gain (Box 16-8). Antipsychotic drugs such as clozapine (Clozaril), olanzapine (Zyprexa), tricyclic antidepressant drugs such as amitriptyline (Elavil), and the anticonvulsant divalproex (Depakote) often lead to weight gain. Patients complain of a ravenous appetite and the inability to "feel full." Weight gains of 40 to 60 lb in a few months are not uncommon. Corticosteroid use is associated with dose-dependent body weight gain in many patients. Sodium and water retention, as well as appetite stimulation, causes weight increases with corticosteroids. MNT is essential, as is routine exercise.

Appetite stimulation is desirable for patients suffering from wasting (cachexia) resulting from disease states such as cancer or HIV/AIDS (Tisdale, 2006). Drugs indicated as appetite stimulants or antiwasting agents are the hormone megestrol acetate (Megace, Megace ES), human growth hormone somatropin (Serostim), the anabolic steroid oxandro-

BOX 16-6

Examples of Drugs That Cause Diarrhea

Antibiotics

Amoxicillin (Amoxil)
Amphotericin B (Abelcet, AmBisome, Amphotec, Fungizone)
Ampicillin
Atovaquone (Mepron)
Azithromycin (Zithromax)
Cefdinir (Omnicef)
Cefixime (Suprax)
Cefuroxime (Ceftin Zinacef)
Cephalexin (Keflex)
Clofazimine (Lamprene)
Clindamycin (Cleocin)
Levofloxacin (Levaquin)
Linezolid (Zyvox)
Meropenem (Merrem IV)
Metronidazole (Flagyl)
Quinine sulfate (Quinine)
Rifampin (Rifadin)
Penicillin
Pyrimethamine (Daraprim)
Tetracycline HCl (Achromycin-V, Sumycin)

Antigout Agents

Colchicine (Colchicine)

Antineoplastics

Aldesleukin/interleukin-2 (Proleukin)
Capecitabine (Xeloda)
Carboplatin (Paraplatin)
Fluorouracil (5-FU) (Adrucil)
Imatinib mesylate (Gleevec)
Irinotecan (Camptosar)
Methotrexate (Methotrexate, Rheumatrex)
Mitoxantrone (Novantrone)
Paclitaxel (Taxol)

Antiviral Agents

Amprenavir (Agenerase)
Didanosine (Videx)
Lopinavir (Kaletra)
Nelfinavir (Viracept)
Ritonavir (Norvir)
Stavudine (Zerit)
Foscarnet (Foscavir)

Gastrointestinal Agents

Lactulose (Chronulac)
Magnesium magonate (Milk of Magnesia)
Metoclopramide HCl (Reglan)
Misoprostol (Cytotec)
Casanthranol and docusate sodium (Peri-Colace)
Sorbitol
Orlitstat (Xenical)

Oral Hypoglycemic Agents

Acarbose (Precose)
Metformin (Glucophage)
Miglitol (Glyset)

From Pronsky ZM: *Food-medication interactions*, ed 14, Birchrunville, Pa, 2006, Food-Medication Interactions.

lone (Oxandrin), and the marijuana derivative dronabinol (Marinol). Drugs also used as appetite stimulants, although not FDA-indicated as such, are the anabolic steroids oxymetholone (Anadrol-50) and nandrolone (Deca-Durabolin), the antihistamine cyproheptadine (Periactin), and the hormone testosterone (Androderm, Virilon). The omega-3 fatty acid, eicosapentaenoic acid (EPA) has been suggested as an appetite stimulant. While some studies have not shown improvement in appetite or weight gain (Jatoi et al., 2004 and Fearon et al., 2006), one has shown improvement in cachexia (Stehr and Heller, 2006). Obviously this is an area of further study. With the successful advent of highly active antiretroviral therapy (HAART), lipodystrophy is often a problem for HIV/AIDS patients. Debate about an accurate definition of lipodystrophy is ongoing. Redistribution of body fat, fat wasting, glucose intolerance, hypertension, and hyperlipidemia are common aspects of this syndrome. Antidiabetic drugs such as metformin (Glucophage) and rosiglitazone (Avandia) are used to normalize glucose and insulin levels. Antihyperlipidemic drugs such as atorvastatin (Lipitor), pravastatin (Pravachol) or fenofibrate (Tricor) are used to control elevated triglycerides and/or cholesterol.

Organ System Toxicity

Drugs can cause specific organ system toxicity such as hepatotoxicity, nephrotoxicity, pulmonary toxicity, neurotoxicity, ototoxicity, ocular toxicity, pancreatitis, or cardiotoxicity. MNT may be indicated as part of the treatment of these toxicities. Although all toxicities are of concern, hepatotoxicity and nephrotoxicity are addressed here because drugs

BOX 16-7

Examples of Drugs That Cause Anorexia

Antiinfectives

Amphotericin B (Abelcet, AmBisome, Amphotec, Fungizone)
Atovaquone (Mepron)
Cidofovir (Vistide)
Didanosine (ddI) (Videx)
Ethionamide (Trecator-SC)
Fomivirsen (Vitravene)
Foscarnet sodium (Foscavir)
Hydroxychloroquine sulfate (Plaquenil)
Metronidazole (Flagyl)
Pentamidine isethionate (NebuPent, Pentam 300)
Pyrimethamine (Daraprim)
Sulfadiazine
Zalcitabine (HIVID)

Antineoplastics

Aldesleukin/interleukin-2 (Proleukin)
Bleomycin sulfate (Blenoxane)
Capecitabine (Xeloda)
Carboplatin (Paraplatin)
Cytarabine (ara-C) (Cytosar-U)
Dacarbazine (DTIC-Dome)
Fluorouracil (Adrucil) (5-FU)
Hydroxyurea (Hydrea)
Imatinib mesylate (Gleevec)
Irinotecan HCl (Camptosar)
Methotrexate (MTX)
Vinblastine sulfate (Velban)
Vinorelbine tartrate (Navelbine)

Bronchodilators

Albuterol sulfate (Proventil, Ventolin)
Theophylline (Elixophyllin, Slo-Phyllin, Theo-24, Theobid, Theolair, Uniphyl)

Cardiovascular Drugs

Amiodarone HCl (Cordarone)
Acetazolamide (Diamox)
Hydralazine HCl (Apresoline)
Quinidine (Quinaglute Dura, Quinidex Extentabs, Quinora)

Stimulants

Amphetamines (Adderall, Dexedrine)
Methylphenidate HCl (Ritalin, Concerta)
Phentermine (Adipex-P, Fastin, Ionamin)

Miscellaneous

Fluoxetine (Prozac, Sarafem)
Galantamine (Reminyl)
Naltrexone HCl (ReVia)
Oxycodone (Oxycontin)
Rivastigmine (Exelon)
Sibutramine HCl (Meridia)
Sulfasalazine (Azulfidine)
Topiramate (Topamax)

From Pronsky ZM : *Food-medication interactions*, ed 14, Birchrunville, Pa, 2006, Food-Medication Interactions.

are eliminated from the body predominately through the liver and kidney.

Examples of drugs that cause hepatotoxicity (liver damage) leading to hepatitis, jaundice, hepatomegaly, or even liver failure are amiodarone (Cordarone), amitriptyline (Elavil), lovastatin (Mevacor) and other "statin" antihyperlipidemic drugs, divalproex (Depakote), carbamazepine (Tegretol), methotrexate, kava, niacin, and sulfasalazine (Azulfidine). Monitoring of hepatic function through routine blood work for liver enzyme levels is generally prescribed with use of these drugs (see Table 15-1).

Nephrotoxicity (kidney damage) may change the excretion of specific nutrients (see cisplatin) or cause acute or chronic renal insufficiency, which may not resolve with cessation of drug use. Examples of drugs that often cause nephrotoxicity are antiinfectives amphotericin B (especially with intravenous desoxycholate form [Fungizone]) and cidofovir (Vistide), as well as antineoplastics cisplatin (Plaquenil-AQ), gentamicin (Garamycin), ifosfamide (Ifex), methotrexate, and pentamidine (Pentam 300). Adequate or extra prehydration, often administered intravenously, is prescribed to reduce renal tox-

icity. For example, with cidofovir, 1 L of intravenous normal saline (0.9% NaCl) is infused 1 to 2 hours before infusion of the drug. If tolerated, up to an additional liter may be infused after the drug infusion. Oral probenecid (Benemid) is also prescribed with cidofovir to reduce nephrotoxicity.

Glucose Levels

Many drugs affect glucose metabolism, causing hypoglycemia or hyperglycemia and in some cases frank diabetes (Box 16-9) (Pandit et al., 1993). The mechanisms of these effects vary from drug to drug and from individual to individual. Drugs may stimulate glucose production or impair glucose uptake. They may inhibit insulin secretion, decrease insulin sensitivity, or increase insulin clearance. Glucose levels may be affected by changes in other parameters, such as hypokalemia induced by thiazide diuretics or weight gain induced by antipsychotic medications (Izzedine et al., 2005). Corticosteroids, particularly prednisone, prednisolone, and hydrocortisone, are diabetogenic because of increased gluconeogenesis, but they also cause insulin resistance and therefore inhibit glucose uptake.

BOX 16-8

Examples of Drugs That Increase Appetite

Psychotropics

Alprazolam (Xanax)
Benzodiazepine antianxiety agents
Chlordiazepoxide (Librium)

Antipsychotics, Typical

Haloperidol (Haldol)
Perphenazine (Trilafon)
Thiothixene (Navane)
Thioridazine HCl (Mellaril)

Antipsychotics, Atypical

Clozapine (Clozaril)
Olanzapine (Zyprexa)
Quetiapine Fumarate (Seroquel)
Risperidone (Risperdal)

Antidepressants, Tricyclic

Amitriptyline HCl (Elavil)
Clomipramine HCl (Anafranil)
Doxepin HCl (Sinequan)
Imipramine HCl (Tofranil)
Selegiline (Eldepryl) only in doses >10 mg/day

Antidepressants, MAOI

Isocarboxazide (Marplan)
Phenelzine sulfate (Nardil)
Tranylcypromine sulfate (Parnate)

Antidepressants, Other

Mirtazapine (Remeron)
Paroxetine (Paxil)

Anticonvulsants

Divalproex/valproic acid (Depakote/Depakene)
Gabapentin (Neurontin)

Hormones

Corticosteroids (cortisone, methylprednisolone, prednisone)
Human growth hormone/somatropin (Serostim)
Medroxyprogesterone acetate (Provera, Depo-Provera)
Megestrol acetate (Megace)
Oxandrolone (Oxandrin)
Oxymetholone (Anadrol-50)
Testosterone (Androderm, Testoderm)

Miscellaneous

Cyproheptadine (Periactin)
Dronabinol (Marinol)

From Pronsky ZM: *Food-medication interactions*, ed 14, Birchrunville, Pa, 2006, Food-Medication Interactions.

BOX 16-9

Examples of Drugs That Affect Glucose Levels

Antidiabetes (Lower or Normalize Glucose Levels)

Acarbose (Precose)
Exenatide (Byetta)
Glimepiride (Amaryl)
Glipizide (Glucotrol)
Glyburide (DiaBeta)
Insulin (Humulin)
Metformin (Glucophage)
Miglitol (Glyset)
Neteglinide (Starlix)
Pioglitazone HCl (Actos)
Pramlinitide (Symlin)
Repaglinide (Prandin)
Rosiglitazone maleate (Avandia)

Drugs That Can Cause Hypoglycemia

Disopyramide (Norpace) antiarrhythmic
Pentamidine isethionate (Pentam 300) antiprotozoal
Quinine antimalarial
Ethanol

Drugs That Can Increase Glucose Levels

Antiretroviral agents, protease inhibitors
Amprenavir (Agenerase)
Nelfinavir mesylate (Viracept)
Ritonavir (Norvir)
Saquinavir (Invirase, Fortovase)

Diuretics, Antihypertensives

Furosemide (Lasix)
Hydrochlorothiazide (HCTZ, HydroDIURIL, Microzide)
Indapamide (Lozol)

From Pronsky ZM: *Food-medication interactions*, ed 14, Birchrunville, Pa, 2006, Food-Medication Interactions.

Continued

BOX 16-9

Examples of Drugs That Affect Glucose Levels—cont'd

Hormones

Corticosteroid (cortisone, prednisone)
Danazol (Danocrine)

Estrogen or Estrogen/Progesterone (Hormone Replacement Therapy)

Medroxyprogesterone (Cycrin, Provera, Depo-Provera)
Megestrol acetate (Megace)
Nandrolone decanoate (Deca-Durabolin)
Octreotide acetate (Sandostatin)

Oral Contraceptives

Oxandrolone (Oxandrin)
Oxymetholone (Anadrol-50)

Miscellaneous

Niacin (nicotinic acid) antihyperlipidemic
Baclofen (Lioresal) skeletal muscle relaxant
Caffeine (No-Doz) stimulant
Clofazimine (Lamprene) antibiotic
Clozapine (Clozaril) antipsychotic
Olanzapine (Zyprexa) antipsychotic
Cyclosporine (Neoral, Sandimmune) immunosuppressant
Interferon alfa-2a (Roferon-A) antineoplastic

From Pronsky ZM: *Food-medication interactions*, ed 14, Birchrunville, Pa, 2006, Food-Medication Interactions.

Second-generation antipsychotics, particularly clozapine (Clozaril) or olanzapine (Zyprexa), have been reported to cause treatment-emergent hyperglycemia. Recently the FDA added a labeling requirement for a warning of "Hyperglycemia and Diabetes" for all second-generation antipsychotics.

EXCIPIENTS AND FOOD-DRUG INTERACTIONS

An **excipient** is added to drug formulations for its action as a buffer, binder, filler, diluent, disintegrant, glidant, flavoring, dye, preservative, suspending agent, or coating. Excipients are also called inactive ingredients (Box 16-10). Hundreds of excipients are approved by the FDA for use in pharmaceuticals. Several common excipients have potential for interactions in persons with an allergy or enzyme deficiency. Often just one brand of a drug or one formulation or strength of a particular brand may contain the excipient of concern. For example, tartrazine, listed as yellow dye No. 5, is used in Cleocin (brand of clindamycin) capsules in the 75- and 150-mg strengths but not in the 300-mg strength. Reglan (brand of metoclopramide) 5-mg tablets contain lactose, but the 10-mg tablets do not. Prometrium (micronized progesterone) capsules contain peanut oil and lecithin, whereas other progesterone forms do not. Prometrium labeling includes a warning that anyone allergic to peanuts should not use the drug (see Chapter 29).

Lactose is commonly used as a filler in many pills and capsules. The amount of lactose may be significant enough to cause gastrointestinal problems for lactase-deficient patients, particularly those on multiple drugs throughout the day (see Chapter 27).

Patients with celiac disease have gluten sensitivity and must practice lifelong abstinence from wheat, barley, rye, and oats (which may be contaminated with gluten). They are particularly concerned with the composition and source of excipients such as wheat starch or flour, which might contain gluten. Only a few pharmaceutical companies guarantee their products to be gluten-free. Excipients such as dextrin and sodium starch glycolate are usually made from corn and potato, respectively, but can be made from wheat or barley. For example, the excipient dextrimaltose, a mixture of maltose and dextrin, is produced by the enzymatic action of barley malt on corn flour (Crowe and Falini, 2001; Kibbe, 2000). The source of each drug ingredient, if not specified, should be checked with the manufacturer.

Finally some drug brands may contain enough excipient to be nutritionally significant (Table 16-1), such as vitamin E in Agenerase (amprenavir), magnesium in Accupril (quniapril), calcium in Fibercon or Fiber-Lax (calcium polycarbophil), and soybean oil lipid emulsion in propofol (Diprivan). Proprofol is commonly used long term for sedation of patients in the intensive care unit. Its formulation includes 10% emulsion, which contributes 1.1 kcal/ml. When infused at doses up to 9 mg/kg/hr in a patient weighing 70 kg, for instance, it may contribute an additional 1663 kcal/day from the emulsion. For a patient receiving total parenteral nutrition, limiting the use of long-chain fatty acids and using medium chain triglycerides (MCT) oil may be recommended while he or she is taking propofol (Dubey and Kumar, 2005). Specific brands or formulation(s) of a specific brand provide significant amounts of sodium and therefore may be contraindicated for patients who need to limit sodium.

BOX 16-10

Examples of Potential Interactive Drug Excipients

Albumin (egg or human): May cause allergic reaction. Human albumin is a blood product.

Alcohol (ethanol): Central nervous system (CNS) depressant used as a solvent. All alcohol and alcohol-containing products and drugs must be avoided with medications such as disulfiram (Antabuse) or limited with other drugs to prevent additive CNS or hepatic toxicity. Most elixirs contain 4% to 20% alcohol. Some solution, syrup, liquid, or parenteral forms contain alcohol.

Aspartame: A nonnutritive sweetener composed of the amino acids aspartic acid and phenylalanine. Phenylketonuria (PKU) patients lack the enzyme phenylalanine hydroxylase. If aspartame is ingested in significant quantities by PKU patients, accumulation of phenylalanine causes toxicity to brain tissue (see Chapter 44).

Lactose: Lactose is used as a filler. The natural sweetener in milk, lactose is hydrolyzed in the small intestine by the enzyme lactase to glucose and galactose. Lactose intolerance (due to lactase deficiency) results in gastrointestinal distress when lactose is ingested (see Chapter 27). Lactose in medications may cause this reaction.

Mannitol: The alcohol form of the sugar mannose, used as a filler. Mannitol is absorbed more slowly, yielding half as many calories per gram as glucose. Because of slow absorption, mannitol can cause soft stools and diarrhea.

Saccharin: Nonnutritive sweetener. Extensive human research has found no evidence of carcinogenicity.

Sorbitol: The alcohol form of sucrose. Absorbed more slowly than sucrose, sorbitol inhibits the rise in blood glucose. Because of slow absorption, sorbitol can cause soft stools or diarrhea.

Starch: Starch from wheat, corn, or potato is added to medication as a filler, binder, or diluent. Celiac disease patients have a permanent intolerance to gluten, a protein in wheat, barley, rye, and a contaminant of oat. In celiac disease, gluten causes damage to the lining of the small intestine (see Chapter 27).

Sucrose: Sweetener. Significant source of simple carbohydrate and calories.

Sulfites: Sulfiting agents are used as antioxidants. Sulfites may cause severe hypersensitivity reactions in some people, particularly asthmatics (see Chapter 29). They include sulfur dioxide, sodium sulfite, and sodium and potassium metabisulfite. The Food and Drug Administration (FDA) requires the listing of sulfites when present in foods or drugs.

Tartrazine: Tartrazine is yellow dye No. 5 color additive, which causes severe allergic reactions in some people (1 in 10,000) (see Chapter 29). The FDA requires the listing of tartrazine when it is present in foods or drugs.

Vegetable oil: Soy, sesame, cottonseed, corn, or peanut oil is used in some parenteral drugs as a nonaqueous vehicle. Hydrogenated vegetable oil is a tablet/capsule lubricant. May cause allergic reactions in sensitive people (see Chapter 29).

Modified from Pronsky ZM: Potential interactive ingredients. In Pronsky ZM: *Food-medication interactions*, ed 14, Birchrunville, Pa, 2006, Food-Medication Interactions.

TABLE 16-1

Examples of Drugs That Contain Nutritionally Significant Ingredients

Trade Name	Generic Name	Ingredient	Nutritional Significance
Accupril	Quinapril	Magnesium carbonate Magnesium stearate	Provides 50-200 mg magnesium daily
Accutane	Isotretinoin	Drug is related to vitamin A; contains soybean oil	Avoid vitamin A or β-carotene May cause allergic reaction
Agenerase	Amprenavir	Vitamin E	1744 international units in adult daily dose
Atrovent (inhaler)	Ipratropium Bromide	Soya lecithin	May cause allergic reaction
Fibercon/ Fiber-Lax	Calcium olycarbophil	Calcium polycarbophil	100-mg Ca/tablet up to 6 tablets/ day = 600 mg calcium total

Data from Pronsky ZM: *Food-medication interactions*, ed 13, Birchrunville, Pa, 2004, Food-Medication Interactions.

Continued

TABLE 16-1

Examples of Drugs That Contain Nutritionally Significant Ingredients—cont'd

Trade Name	Generic Name	Ingredient	Nutritional Significance
Marinol	Dronabinol	Sesame oil	May cause allergic reaction
Phazyme	Simethicone	Soybean oil in capsule	May cause allergic reaction
Prometrium	Micronized progesterone	Peanut oil	May cause allergic reaction
Diprivan	Propofol	10% soybean oil emulsion	Oil is significant caloric source
		Egg yolk phospholipids	May cause allergic reaction
Videx	Didanosine	Sodium buffer in powder	≥2760 mg Na/adult daily dose
Zantac	Ranitidine	Sodium in *prescription* granules and tablets; Zantac 75 (nonprescription) is sodium free	350-730 mg Na/adult daily dose

MEDICAL NUTRITION THERAPY

MNT can be divided into prospective and retrospective. Prospective includes all MNT offered when the patient first starts a drug. Retrospective concerns evaluation of symptoms to determine whether medical problems might be the result of food-drug interactions.

A diet history must be obtained, including information about the use of OTC (nonprescription) drugs, alcohol, vitamin and mineral supplements, and herbal or phytonutrient supplements (see Figure 18-6). The patient should be evaluated for genetic characteristics, weight and appetite changes, altered taste, and gastrointestinal problems (see Chapter 14).

Prospective drug information and MNT include basic information about the drug: the name, purpose, and duration of prescription of the drug plus when and how to take the drug. This information includes whether to take the drug with or without food. Specific foods and beverages to avoid while taking the drug and potential interactions between drug and vitamin or mineral supplements need to be emphasized. For instance, the patient taking tetracycline (Achromycin-V or Sumycin) or ciprofloxacin (Cipro) should be warned not to combine the drug with milk, yogurt, or supplements containing divalent cations, calcium, iron, magnesium, zinc, or vitamin-minerals containing any of these cations.

Potential significant side effects must be delineated, and possible dietary suggestions to relieve the side effects should be described. For instance, information about a high-fiber diet with adequate fluids should be part of MNT about an anticholinergic drug such as oxybutynin (Ditropan), which often causes constipation.

Conversely, diarrhea can be controlled by the use of psyllium (Metamucil) or probiotics, such as *Lactobacillus acidophilus* (Lactinex), particularly for antibiotic-associated diarrhea even in children (Szajewska et al., 2006).

Patients should be warned about potential nutritional problems, particularly when dietary intake is inadequate, such as hypokalemia with a potassium-depleting diuretic. Dietary changes that may alter drug action should be included, such as the effect of an increase in foods high in vitamin K on warfarin action. Special diet information, such as a low-cholesterol, low-fat, limited-sugar diet with atorvastatin (Lipitor) or other antihyperlipidemic drugs, is essential information. Written information should list medication ingredients such as nonnutrient excipients in the medication (see Box 16-10). Examples include lactose, starch, tartrazine, aspartame, and alcohol. Patients with lactose intolerance, celiac disease, allergies, phenylketonuria, or alcoholism need to avoid or limit one or more of these ingredients.

Prospective MNT should cover potential concerns with OTC drugs and herbal/natural products (Herr, 2005). It is important to emphasize that the pharmacokinetic and pharmacodynamic interactions explained in this chapter occur with all medications, whether obtained by prescription, OTC, or as natural/herbal products.

Retrospective MNT addresses the possibility of food-drug interactions. To determine whether a patient's symptoms are the result of a food-drug interaction, a complete medical and nutrition history is essential, including prescription and nonprescription drugs, vitamin-mineral supplements, and herbal or phytonutrient products. The date of beginning to take the drug(s) versus the date of symptom onset is significant information. It is important to identify the use of nutrition supplements such as enteral products or significant dietary changes such as fad diets during the course of drug prescription (see Figure 18-6).

Finally it is important to investigate the reported incidence of side effects (by percentage as compared with a placebo). For example, vomiting occurs in 1.5% of those taking omeprazole (Prilosec) compared with 4.7% of those taking a placebo. Therefore in a patient treated with omeprazole, it would be appropriate to consider other causes for vomiting. A rare drug effect is less likely to be the reason for a negative symptom than an effect that is common.

FOCAL POINTS

- Because of the importance of food-drug interactions in the effectiveness of medication and the overall health care provided, various strategies have been undertaken at health care facilities to meet the TJC requirements for food-drug interaction counseling.
- A sample policy statement would read: "Patients discharged on modified diets receive written instructions and individualized counseling before discharge, including food-drug interaction counseling when indicated" and educational materials should be available.

- Materials for use with patients should be approved by the medical team, including registered dietitians and pharmacists.
- The dietitian should consider food-drug interactions in the patient on several medications and in whom nutritional status cannot be maintained or is deteriorating.
- Documentation in the medical record is required when instruction has been given, including assessment of the patient's comprehension, ability, and willingness to follow instructions.

CLINICAL SCENARIO 1

Henry is a 31-year-old man who began to suffer seizures after a head trauma injury from a motorcycle accident at the age of 18. For the first 2 years after the accident, he was prescribed various anticonvulsant regimens. The combination of phenytoin (Dilantin), 300 mg daily, and phenobarbital, 120 mg daily, has proven to be the most effective therapy to control his seizures. Henry has been stabilized on this regimen for the last 11 years.

Henry is a senior computer programmer for a large corporation. He is 6 feet 2 inches tall and weighs 182 lb. Henry admits to having an aversion for exercise and athletics. In his free time, he enjoys reading, playing computer games, and watching television. During the past year, Henry has broken his left femur and tibia on two separate occasions. He broke his femur when he missed the bottom step on the stairway in his office building. Several months later he broke his tibia when he tripped over a broken branch in his yard. Henry recently complained to his orthopedic surgeon about hip and pelvic pain of several weeks' duration. An orthopedic examination with x-rays, bone scan, and Dexa scan revealed that Henry is suffering from osteomalacia. A review of Henry's typical diet reveals a nutritionally marginal diet that commonly includes fast foods and frozen dinners. His diet is generally deficient in fresh fruits, vegetables, and dairy products.

***Nutrition Diagnosis:** Food-medication interaction related to inadequate calcium and vitamin D intake while taking anticonvulsant medications as evidenced by osteomalacia

1. Is osteomalacia common in young men?
2. How does Henry's lifestyle contribute to the development of osteomalacia?
3. What vitamin or mineral deficiency may have contributed to the current state of Henry's bones?
4. Describe the food-drug interaction that has contributed to Henry's osteomalacia.
5. What medical nutritional therapy would you recommend for Henry?

⬡ CLINICAL SCENARIO 2

Emma is a 79-year-old woman who suffered an embolic stroke from previously undetected atrial fibrillation. In the hospital she was noted to have left-sided weakness, slurred speech, and minimum difficulty with word finding. Because Emma was still in atrial fibrillation on admission to the hospital, the decision was made to begin anticoagulation therapy with warfarin (Coumadin). The plan for Emma was to transfer her to the local rehabilitation hospital for physical, occupational, and speech therapy as soon as she was physically stable. Her prognosis was considered good for full recovery.

A psychosocial consult in the rehabilitation facility revealed a 5-feet 1-inch, 119-lb woman who was anxious to regain her independence and return to her home, where she lives alone. A son and daughter live within a 10-mile radius and are willing to participate in their mother's care once she returns home.

While Emma was hospitalized, her warfarin dose remained stable at 2.5 mg daily. Her international normalized ratio (INR) was measured consistently between 2 and 3 during the 3-week period in the hospital and the rehabilitation facility. Once Emma returned to her own home, she began having her blood drawn to monitor her INR a minimum of twice a week. At this point, however, her INR is constantly changing. Each change in INR necessitates a change in her dose of warfarin. At times the INR is higher than 3, and Emma is instructed to hold the warfarin until the next blood draw. At other times the INR is below 2, and the dose of warfarin is increased.

✳ Nutrition Diagnosis: Food-medication interaction related to fluctuating vitamin K intake while on warfarin as evidenced by varying INR

1. How do you account for the difference in the stability of Emma's state of anticoagulation before and after her discharge? What questions would you ask Emma to discover the reasons for the fluctuation in her anticoagulation state?
2. What instruction about warfarin and diet should Emma have received before her discharge?
3. List dietary factors that can affect the pharmacologic action of warfarin.
4. What vitamins or supplements can interact with warfarin?
5. Emma would like to take ginseng to try to improve her memory since her stroke. Is this a safe idea? What would you advise Emma to do?

USEFUL WEBSITES

Access to MedLine
www.ncbi.nlm.nih.gov/entrez/query.fcgi
www.pubmed.com

DRUGFACTS.com
www.factsandcomparisons.com/

FDA Center for Drug Evaluation and Research
www.fda.gov/cder/

Food and Nutrition Information Center
www.nal.usda.gov/fnic/

Food Medication Interactions
www.foodmedinteractions.com

Grapefruit-Drug Interactions
www.powernetdesign.com/grapefruit/

Newly Approved Medications
http://www.centerwatch.com/patient/drugs/druglist.html

NIH Patient Handouts
www.cc.nih.gov/ccc/patient_education/

Project Inform's Drug Interactions (HIV/AIDS)
www.projinf.org/fs/drugin.html

References

Atsmon J, Dolev E: Drug-induced hypomagnesemia: Scope and management, *Drug Saf* 28:763, 2005.

Au Yeung SCS, Ensom MHH: Phenytoin and enteral feedings: does evidence support an interaction? *Ann Pharmacother* 34:896, 2000.

Blob LF et al: Effects of a tyramine-enriched meal on blood pressure response in healthy male volunteers treated with selegiline transdermal system 6 mg/24 hr, *CNS Spectr* 12:25, 2007.

Burns P et al: Physical compatibility of enteral formulas with various common medications, *J Am Diet Assoc* 88:1094, 1988.

Clark JH, et al: Serum beta-carotene, retinol, and alpha-tocopherol levels during mineral oil therapy for constipation, *Am J Dis Child* 141:1210, 1987.

Crawford P: Best practice guidelines for the management of women with epilepsy, *Epilepsia* 46:117, 2005.

Crowe JP, Falini NP: Gluten in pharmaceutical products, *Am J Health Syst Pharmacol* 58(5):396, 2001.

DeBusk R: *Genetics: the nutrition connection*, Chicago, 2003 American Dietetic Association.

Duarte J et al: Efficiency of the protein redistribution diet in the anti-parkinsonian effect of l-dopa, *Neurologia* 8:248, 1993.

Dubey PK, Kumar A: Pain on injection of lipid-free propofol and propofol emulsion containing medium-chain triglyceride: a comparative study, *Anesth Analg* 101:1060, 2005.

Egashira K et al: Pomelo-induced increase in the blood level of tacrolimus in a renal transplant patient, *Transplantation* 75:1057, 2003.

Faucheron JL, Parc R: Non-steroidal anti-inflammatory drug induced colitis, *Int J Colorectal Dis* 11:99, 1996.

Fearon KC et al: Double-blind, placebo-controlled, randomized study of eicosapentaenoic acid diester in patients with cancer cachexia, *J Clin Oncol* 24:3401, 2006.

Force RW, Nahata MC: Effect of histamine H-2 receptor antagonists on vitamin B₁₂ absorption, *Ann Pharmacother* 26:1283, 1992.

Fosamax package insert: West Point, Pa, September 2001, Merck.

Friedlander AH et al: Late-life depression: it's oral health significance, *Int Dent J* 53:41, 2003.

Gardner DM et al: The making of a user friendly MAOI diet, *J Clin Psychol* 57(3):99, 1996.

Ghosh D et al: Pharmacogenomics and nutrigenomics: Synergies and differences, *Eur J Clin Nutr* Jan 10, 2007.

Greenblatt DJ, von Moltke LL: Interaction of warfarin with drugs, natural substances and foods, *J Clin Pharmacol* 45:127, 2005.

Heckmann JG, Lang CJ: Neurological causes of taste disorders *Adv Otorhinolaryngol* 63:255, 2006.

Herr SM: Herb-drug interaction handbook, ed 3, Nassau, NY, 2005, Church Street Books.

Hori H et al: Grapefruit juice-fluvoxamine interaction: Is it risky or not? *J Clin Psychopharmacol* 23:422, 2003.

Izzedine H et al: Drug-induced diabetes mellitus, *Expert Opin Srug Saf* 4:1097, 2005.

Jatoi A et al: An eicosapentaenoic acid supplement versus megestrol acetate versus both for patients with cancer-associated wasting, *J Clin Oncol* 22:2469, 2004.

Johnson MA: Influence of vitamin K on anticoagulant therapy depends on vitamin K status and the source and forms of vitamin K, *Nutr* Rev 63:91, 2005.

Kibbe AH, editor: *Handbook of pharmaceutical excipients*, ed 3, Washington, DC, 2000, American Pharmaceutical Association.

Lajer H, Daugaard G: Cisplatin and hypomagnesemia, *Cancer Treat Rev* 35(1):47, 1999.

Lems WK et al: Pharmacological prevention of osteoporosis in patients on corticosteroid medication, *Ned Tijdschr Geneeskd* 142 (34):1904, 1998.

Lieber CS: Mechanisms of ethanol-drug nutrition interactions, *J Toxicol Clin Toxicol* 32(6):631, 1994.

Lilja JJ et al: Duration of effect of grapefruit juice on the pharmacokinetics of the CYP3A4 substrate simvastatin, *Clin Pharmacol Ther* 68:384, 2000.

Malhotra S et al: Seville orange juice-felodipine interactions: comparison with dilute grapefruitjuice and involvement of furocoumarins, *Clin Pharmacol Ther* 89(1):14, 2001.

Med Lett: AmpliChip CYP450 tes, *Med Lett Drugs Ther* 47 (1215-1216):71, 2005.

Neuhofel AL et al: Lack of bioequivalence of ciprofloxacin when administered with calcium-fortified orange juice: a new twist on an old interaction, *J Clin Pharmacol* 42:461, 2002.

Nicolaidou P et al: Effects of anticonvulsant therapy on vitamin D status in children: prospective monitoring study, *J Child Neurol* 21:2005, 2006.

Ortiz Z et al: The efficacy of folic acid and folinic acid in reducing methotrexate gastrointestinal toxicity in rheumatoid arthritis: a metaanalysis of randomized clinical trials, *J Rheumatol* 25 (1):36, 1998.

Pandit MK et al: Drug-induced disorders of glucose tolerance, *Ann Intern Med* 118:529, 1993.

Pelton R et al: *Drug-induced nutrient depletion handbook*, ed 2, Hudson, Ohio, 2001, Lexi-Comp.

Pinto JT, Rivlin RS: Drugs that promote renal excretion of riboflavin, *Drug Nutr Inter* 5:143, 1987.

Pronsky ZM: *Food medication interactions*, ed 14, Birchrunville, Pa, 2006, Food Medication Interactions.

Rees DC et al: Acute haemolysis induced by high dose ascorbic acid in glucose-6-phosphate dehydrogenase deficiency, *Br Med J* 306(6881):841, 1993.

Ritschel WA, Kearns GL: *Handbook of basic pharmacokinetics*, ed 5, Washington DC, 1999, American Pharmaceutical Association.

Roth JA: Drug metabolism. In Smith CM, Reynard AM, editors: *Essentials of pharmacology*, Philadelphia, 1995, Saunders.

Sartori S et al: Changes in intracellular magnesium concentrations during cisplatin chemotherapy, *Oncology* 50:230, 1993.

Schiffman S: Changes in taste and smell: drug interactions and food preferences, *Nutr Rev* 52(suppl 8):S11, 1994.

Sica DA: Interaction of grapefruit juice and calcium channel blockers, *Am J Hyperts* 19:768, 2006.

Stehr SN, Heller AR: Omega-3 fatty acid effects on biochemical indices following cancer surgery, *Clin Chim Acta* 373:1, 2006.

Szajewska H et al: Probiotics in the prevention of antibiotic associated diarrhea in children: a meta-analysis of randomized controlled trials, *J Pediatr* 149:367, 2006.

Thomson C, Rollins C: Enteral feedings and medication incompatibilities, *Support Line* 113(3):9, 1991.

Tisdale MJ: Clinical anticachexia treatments, *Nutr Clin Pract* 21:168, 2006.

Valley M et al: Emerging peptide therapeutics for inflammatory diseases, *Curr Pharm Biotechnol* 7:241, 2006.

Van de Wiel A: Diabetes mellitus and alcohol, *Diabetes Metab Res Rev* 20:263, 2004.

Walter-Sack I, Klotz U: Influence of diet and nutritional status on drug metabolism, *Clin Pharmacokinet* 31(1):47, 1996.

Welage LS et al: Alterations in gastric acidity in patients infected with HIV, *Clin Infect Dis* 21:1431, 1995.

Yuan Y et al: Selective serotonin reuptake inhibitors and risk of upper GI bleeding: confusion or confounding? *Am J Med* 119:719, 2006.

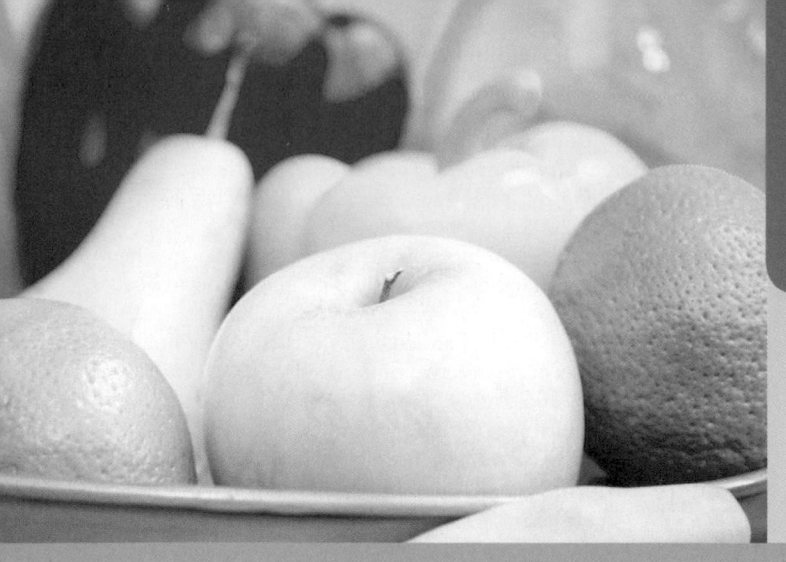

CHAPTER 17

Pamela Charney, PhD, RD, CNSD
Sylvia Escott-Stump, MA, RD, LDN
L. Kathleen Mahan, MS, RD, CDE

Nutrition Diagnosis and Intervention

KEY TERMS

A-D-I-M-E an acronym for the steps of the nutrition care process—assessment, nutrition diagnosis, intervention, monitoring and evaluation

advance directives guidelines established by a patient allowing a designated person(s) to make medical decisions if the patient loses decision-making capabilities; may include items such as use of mechanical ventilation or feeding tubes

case management process to ensure timely, efficient, cost-effective achievement of patient goals

diet or nutrition prescription designates the type, amount, texture, and frequency of feeding, meals or supplements; may limit or increase amounts of carbohydrate, protein, fat, alcohol, fluid, vitamins, minerals, or phytonutrients

discharge planning team planning for education, counseling, and resources needed by the patient following hospitalization as part of the continuum of nutrition care

disease management a disease-specific standardized approach to patient care, primarily used in an outpatient setting

evidence-based guides for practice protocols that include a stringent review of research summarized in evidence tables and conclusion statements that reflect the strength of the science

Health Insurance Portability and Accountability Act (HIPAA) federal law in which Title 1 protects workers when they change jobs and Title 2 improves efficiency and privacy related to electronic data exchange in health care; protects patient confidentiality

managed-care organizations (MCOs) mechanism for financing and organizing health care delivery in which providers and payers have predetermined payments for care provided

nutrition assessment the process by which the nutritional status of an individual is determined; usually includes diet history and intake data, laboratory data, physical examination and health history, anthropometric data, psychosocial data, and intake of nutrient and herbal supplements

nutrition care process (NCP) a systematic problem-solving method used to critically think and make decisions to address nutrition-related problems and provide safe and effective quality nutrition care

nutrition diagnoses nutrition problems specifically resolved by registered dietitians; not to be confused with medical diagnoses

palliative care comfort measures for terminally ill patients

patient-centered objective a statement of what the patient will achieve or be able to do when the objective is met

patient-focused care (PFC) care that is organized around the patient as the central focus of the team, the "customer" of health services

preferred provider organization (PPO) an organization that has negotiated a contract that specifies a favored status in providing health care services for a specific population group

problem, etiology, and signs/symptoms (PES) designated for each nutrition diagnosis

standards of care practice guidelines that are established by a facility to ensure that, at a minimum, reasonable care is rendered; often used in litigation to compare practices in facilities of similar size, staffing, and region

The Joint Commission (TJC) a peer review organization that evaluates health care institutions and ensures their compliance with established minimum standards

utilization management cost-efficient patient care management with a focus on reducing excessive use of diagnostic or therapeutic tests, procedures, and services

Sections of this chapter were written by Cynthia M. Brylinsky, MS, RD, LDN, for the previous edition of this text.

Nutrition care is an organized group of activities allowing identification of nutritional needs and provision of care to meet these needs. The **nutrition care process (NCP)** was established by the American Dietetic Association (ADA) as a standardized process for provision of nutrition care and includes four steps: assessment of nutritional status, identification of the nutrition diagnosis (problems), implementation of relevant interventions, and monitoring and evaluation of the nutrition care outcomes (Lacey and Pritchett, 2003). It is referred to as **A-D-I-M-E**.

THE NUTRITION CARE PROCESS AND MEDICAL NUTRITION THERAPY

Comprehensive nutrition care involves many different health care practitioners—the physician, registered dietitian (RD), nurse, pharmacist, physical or occupational therapist, social worker, speech therapist, and case manager—and all may be integral in achieving desired outcomes, depending on the care setting. The patient is also an integral part of the NCP. A collaborative approach helps to ensure that care is coordinated and that all team members and the patient are aware of goals and priorities. Coordinating the activities of health care professionals requires documentation of the process, as well as regular discussions to allow for the communication and interaction necessary for complete nutritional care. Patients benefit from interdisciplinary decision making regarding nutritional and medical concerns. Team conferences, formal or informal, are useful in all settings, whether the patient or client is receiving care in the home, the community, a long-term care facility, a clinic, or a hospital.

Nutrition Screening and Assessment

Nutrition screening precedes the NCP and provides a mechanism to identify patients who would benefit from nutrition assessment. **The Joint Commission (TJC),** a peer review organization that evaluates health care institutions and ensures their compliance with established minimum standards, requires that nutrition risk be identified in hospitalized patients within 24 hours of admission but does not mandate a method to accomplish screening.

Many health care facilities have developed some sort of multidisciplinary admission assessment form. One efficient mechanism for completing the nutrition screen is to incorporate the screen into this admission assessment since it is not necessary that an RD complete the nutrition screen. The nutrition risk screen should be designed to be quick, easy to administer, and cost-effective while maintaining accuracy needed to identify those patients needing nutrition intervention. Patients identified "at risk" during the admission screen should be referred to the RD for nutrition assessment. Table 17-1 lists information that is frequently included in a nutrition screen; nutrition screening forms should be accurate, sensitive, and concise.

Rescreening should occur at regular intervals during hospitalization because there may be a relationship between length of stay and worsening nutrition status. Policies for repeating the nutrition screen should take into account the average length of time a patient will stay at the facility.

Nutrition assessment involves the gathering and evaluation of medical, family and genetic history, social information, nutritional, herbal and medication histories, physical examination and laboratory data (see Chapters 13 through 16). Selection of the correct nutrition diagnosis is guided from a thorough assessment of these factors. Patients with nutrition deficits may have higher risk for morbidity, increased length of hospital stay, and infectious complications. Nutrition-related complications can lead to a significant increase in costs associated with hospitalization, lending support to the early identification of nutrition problems followed by prompt intervention (see Figure 14-18).

Nutrition Diagnosis

After assessment of nutrition status using all of the available data, **nutrition diagnoses** (problems or needs) are identified, prioritized, and documented in the medical record. Many facilities use standardized formats to facilitate communication of information gathered in the nutrition assessment and nutrition diagnosis. A nutrition diagnosis includes identification of the **problem, etiology, and signs/symptoms (PES)** in a simple, clear statement. Box 17-1 presents the nutrition care process applied to a patient, JW.

Nutrition Intervention

The nutrition intervention relates to the etiology and translates assessment data into activities that will enable the patient or client to meet established objectives. Intervention can begin once the nutrition diagnosis is identified and objectives are determined. Interventions may include food and nutrition therapies (changing the diet prescription, providing food or nutrition supplements, initiating a tube feeding for a patient who cannot eat), nutrition education, counseling, or coordination of care such as providing referral for financial or food resources. The care process is a continuous one; the initial plan may change as the condition of the patient changes, as new needs are identified, or if the patient does not respond to interventions implemented.

Interventions should be specific; they are the "what, where, when, and how" of the care plan (ADA, 2007). For example, in the patient with "evident protein-energy malnutrition," an objective might be to increase calorie intake. This could be implemented through provision of high-calorie, high-protein foods via small, frequent meals and snacks; or by providing a supplement or milk shake between meals. Plans should be communicated to the health care team and the patient to ensure understanding of the plan and its rationale. Thorough communication by the RD increases the likelihood of adherence to the plan. Box 17-2 describes the interventions for patient JW.

TABLE 17-1

Standard of Care for Nutrition Risk Screening

Action	Responsible Party	Documentation
Assess weight status	Admitting health care professional	Check yes or no on admission screen.
Has the patient lost weight without trying before admission?		
Assess gastrointestinal (GI) symptoms	Admitting health care professional	Check yes or no on admission screen.
Has the patient had GI symptoms keeping him or her from usual intake over the past 2 weeks?		
Determine need to consult RD	Admitting health care professional	If either screening criterion is "yes," consult RD for nutrition assessment.

BOX 17-1

Applying the Nutrition Care Process for Patient JW: A-D-I-M-E

JW is a 70-year-old white man admitted for cardiac bypass surgery. The nutrition risk screen reveals that he has lost weight without trying and has been eating poorly for several weeks before admission, leading to referral to the registered dietitian (RD) for nutrition assessment (Step 1 of the nutrition care process).

Assessment: Chart review and patient interview reveals the following data:

Laboratory data and medications:
    Glucose and electrolytes: within normal limits (WNL)
    Albumin: 3.8 g/dl
    Cholesterol/triglycerides: WNL
    Medications: Inderal

Anthropometric data:
    Height: 70″
    Weight: 130 lb (15 lb weight loss over 3 months)

Nutrition interview findings:
    Caloric intake: 1200 kcal/day (less than energy requirements as stated in the recommended dietary allowances)
    Meals: irregular throughout the day; drinks coffee frequently

Medical history:
    History of hypertension, thyroid dysfunction, asthma, prostate surgery

Psychosocial data:
    JW lives alone in his own home. He lost his wife 3 months ago, and for the past 6 months he rarely sits down to a cooked meal.

Diagnoses: Several nutrition problems are identified. He has been consuming fewer calories than he requires and has little interest in eating. RD determines his nutrition

diagnosis: (1) *Involuntary weight loss related to missing meals as evidenced by loss of 15 lbs over 3 months.* This nutrition diagnosis may be quite different from his medical problem list since it is specific to the patient's nutrition status and identifies a problem that the RD is responsible for treating independently. The RD might also have selected the nutrition diagnosis of (2) *Inadequate oral food and beverage intake;* however, because JW is hospitalized, his weight loss can impact wound healing from the upcoming surgery; thus weight loss would be the more important nutrition diagnosis.

Interventions: Identification of the nutrition diagnosis allows the RD to focus the nutrition intervention on treatment of the etiology of the problem (in this case the missing meals). Goal setting is the first step, and short-term and long-term plans are established.

In this case one goal would be to increase JW's caloric intake by 300 kcal/day to facilitate weight gain. To facilitate change, goals must be agreeable to the patient; so the RD involves JW in determining the calorie goal and how best to achieve it. It is often helpful to offer several choices to empower the patient to decide which choice is most suitable. When a patient is not able to be involved (e.g., the patient is being fed by nasogastric tube), the RD may need to discuss the planned nutrition intervention with the physician. If the RD establishes this goal without communicating with the physician and others on the health care team, an identified goal might be made that would not be appropriate.

In the education process the client and the RD must jointly establish achievable goals. For example, one objective in dealing with a client being counseled on weight loss would be to agree on both short-term and long-term weight goals. Objectives should be expressed in behavioral terms and stated in terms of what the patient will do or achieve when the

BOX 17-1

Applying the Nutrition Care Process for Patient JW: A-D-I-M-E—cont'd

objectives are met. Objectives should reflect the educational level and the economic and social resources available to the patient and the family. Objectives should also be stated in quantifiable terms to facilitate evaluation. For example, a **patient-centered objective** in this case would be: "After instruction JW will be able to identify three nutrient-dense foods." This is more appropriate than "I will teach JW how to identify nutrient-dense foods," which states the objective but does not make JW responsible for learning and behavioral change.

The objectives for JW's nutrition diagnoses are stated as follows:

***Nutrition Diagnosis 1:** Involuntary weight loss

Objectives:
(1) During the hospitalization JW will maintain his current weight; following discharge he will begin to slowly gain weight up to a target weight of 145 lb.
(2) JW will modify his diet to include adequate calories and protein through the use of nutrient-dense foods to prevent further weight loss and eventually promote weight gain.

***Nutrition Diagnosis 2:** Inadequate oral food and beverage intake

Objectives:
(1) While in the hospital JW will include nutrient-dense foods in his diet, especially when his appetite is limited.
(2) Following discharge JW will attend a local senior center for lunch on a daily basis to help improve his socialization and caloric intake.

From the stated objectives specific intervention activities are identified such as identifying particular foods or supplements that JW will consume while in the hospital as related to objectives for diagnosis 1, or referring to social service to help JW find transportation to the senior center for lunch on a daily basis. The interventions can also include education of JW and his family. Nutrition care plans are often based on standards in the profession, such as medical nutrition therapy protocols or **evidence-based guides for practice,** which summarize the evidence for a given medical condition (see *Focus On:* "Evidence-Based Medicine in Nutrition Practice"). Final steps include implementation of the intervention and determination of a means for monitoring and evaluating the results.

Monitoring: Choosing the means for monitoring if the interventions, and nutritional care activities have met the objectives or goals is important. For JW, monitoring could include weekly weight measurements and nutrient intake analyses while he is in the hospital and biweekly weight measurements at the senior center or clinic when he is back at home.

Evaluation: Evaluation of the monitoring criteria will provide the RD with information on outcomes, and this should occur over time. If nutrition status is not improving, which in this case would be evidenced by JW's weight records, and the goals are not being met, it is important to reassess JW and perhaps develop new goals and definitely create plans for new interventions.

Documentation is important in all aspects of the care plan; it ensures communication between all disciplines involved in the care of the patient or client.

Monitoring and Evaluation of Nutrition Care

The last step in the NCP is to monitor and then evaluate the care provided. This step makes the nutrition care plan dynamic and responsive to the patient's needs. If objectives are written in measurable behavioral terms, evaluation is relatively easy since new behavior is being measured against a behavior that has already been defined. For example, monitoring of JW in the sample case might include weekly reviews of his dietary intake with analysis for calories. If they reveal daily intakes of less than 1800 kcal, an evaluation might be: "JW was not able to increase his calorie intake to 1800 kcal due to his inability to cook." A revision in the care plan at this point might include the following: "JW will be provided a referral to local agencies (Meals on Wheels) that

can assist with provision of meals at home." This new intervention is then implemented and it is monitored and evaluated to determine whether the objective is now being met.

The goal of nutrition care is to meet the nutritional needs of the patient; thus the interventions must be monitored, and the meeting of the objectives evaluated frequently. This ensures that unmet objectives are addressed and that care is evaluated and modified as needed.

When the evaluation reveals that objectives are not being met or that new needs have arisen, the process begins again with reassessment, identification of new nutrition diagnoses, and formulation of a new nutrition care plan. For example, in JW's case during his hospitalization, high-calorie snacks were provided. However, monitoring of this intervention

◎ FOCUS ON

Evidence-Based Medicine in Nutrition Practice

Evidence-based medicine is described as use of current "best evidence" in making decisions about the care of individual patients. "Best evidence" may include research, consensus statements, and other evidence to support the practice. Medical nutrition therapy (MNT) evidence-based nutrition guides are available through the American Dietetic Association (ADA) to assist dietetic practitioners in providing nutrition care (ADA, 2007). ADA's evidence analysis library (http://www.adaevidencelibrary.com) provides the RD with the best evidence available to answer questions that arise in provision of nutrition care. These guidelines include major recommendations, background information, and a reference list.

The MNT process and the expected outcomes can be communicated to managed-care organizations, insurance companies, administrators, and other health care providers using evidence provided from the guidelines. A *Summary Page* summarizes the entire MNT process and includes the number of encounters typically needed, the expected length of time for each encounter, and the length of the intervals between encounters. *Outcomes* are defined as the result of the performance (or nonperformance) of a function or process; specifically "what" happened to the client. Outcome assessment factors include three elements: (1) clinical assessment factors (anatomic and physiologic elements such as biochemical parameters, anthropometric parameters, and clinical signs and symptoms); (2) behavioral assessment factors or therapeutic lifestyle changes (changes in the client's behavior related to food selection, preparation, and physical activity that may ultimately result in changes in clinical or functional outcomes); and (3) expected outcomes (type of change antici-

pated such as improvement in abnormal laboratory values, decreasing blood pressure, or decreasing weight). An *Ideal/Goal Value* section lists values for control or improvement of the disease or condition as defined and supported in the literature. The *Flowchart* provides a one-page visual overview of the process, including specific information to be obtained before the initial encounter, data to be assessed, self-management training expectations, and communications to the primary care provider or another appropriate health care provider. The *Encounter Process* section provides details of the MNT protocol by encounter with specific factors outlined, such as nutrient calculations, self-management training materials, and appropriate communications to other health care providers. This information is extremely valuable for staff orientation, competence verification, and training.

Nutrition Progress Notes are specific to the diagnosis and are designed to document the intervention and outcomes of MNT as outlined in the encounter process. This standardized form includes: *Expected Outcome; Intervention Provided to Meet Goal*; and *Goals Reached*. The *Compliance Potential* is recorded for each encounter and includes evaluation for comprehension, receptivity, and adherence potential. The *Conclusion Statements* summarize the evidence and reflect how strong the evidence is for that particular nutrition care recommendation.

Use of the evidence-based guides establishes more standardized, predictable practice. They may also create research questions for obtaining information needed in the profession. To gain access to the evidence analysis library and for further information on the protocols, go to the ADA website at www.eatright.org.

BOX 17-2

Applying the Nutrition Care Process—Interventions for JW

Nutrition interventions for each objective might be stated as follows:

For Unintentional Weight Loss: JW and the registered dietitian will determine the likely cause of his weight loss.
Intervention: JW will make an effort to eat 3 meals a day plus a bedtime snack.
Intervention: JW will increase his energy intake to 1800 kcal/day and complete a 3-day food record for analysis of adequacy.

For Inadequate Oral Food/Beverage Intake: JW will recognize the impact of his poor appetite on his weight and nutrition status.
Intervention: JW will include at least one nutrient-dense food with meals, especially when his appetite is minimal.

Intervention: JW will be referred to social service for assistance in identifying transportation for getting him to the senior center for lunch daily to improve his socialization and appetite.

This process of defining interventions is continued for every objective of each problem. Care must be taken to not overwhelm JW but rather to implement changes incrementally as he achieves success. Focusing on high-priority objectives and formulating short-term and long-term goals can help make the objectives list more manageable. The interventions just described would be implemented over several sessions to allow JW to focus his efforts on the items of highest priority. Once a high-priority intervention has been successfully accomplished, additional changes may be pursued.

reveals that JW's usual eating pattern does not include snacks; thus he was not consuming them. The evaluation showed this to be an ineffective intervention. JW agrees to a new intervention—the addition of one more food to his meals. Further monitoring and evaluation will be needed to ascertain if this new intervention improves his intake.

DOCUMENTATION: THE NUTRITION CARE RECORD

Medical nutrition therapy (MNT) or nutrition care provided must be documented in the health or medical record. The medical record is a legal document; if interventions are not recorded, it is assumed that they have not occurred. Documentation affords the following advantages:

- Ensures that nutrition care will be relevant, thorough, and effective by providing a record that identifies the problems and sets criteria for evaluating the care

- Allows the entire health care team to understand the rationale for nutrition care, the means by which it will be provided, and the role each team member must play to reinforce the plan and ensure its success

Notes in the medical record serve as a communication tool, verifying important information for evaluation of health care delivery, as well as for accreditation and peer review (see *Focus On:* The Joint Commission).

CHARTING AND DOCUMENTATION

The medical record serves as a tool for communication among members of the health care team and typically includes sections for physician orders, medical history and physical examinations, laboratory test results, consults, and progress reports. Although the format of the medical record varies, depending on facility policies and procedures, in most settings all professionals document care in the medical record. Medical records can also be either paper based or electronic as more

⊙ FOCUS ON

The Joint Commission

The Joint Commission (TJC) is the predominately accrediting body that sets standards for health care. It seeks to improve the quality of patient care in various health settings such as hospitals, long-term care organizations, health care networks, home care organizations, ambulatory care organizations, assisted living facilities and organizations offering mental health services. This is accomplished through a set of standards, adherence to which is measured by formal facility surveys and evaluations. Accreditation by TJC is voluntary but is highly regarded in terms of its impact on third-party payment and its effect on confidence rating by the community, physician recruitment, and fulfillment of portions of state/federal licensure/certification requirements. To earn and maintain accreditation, an organization must undergo and pass an on-site survey by a TJC survey team at least every 3 years.

Accreditation focuses on the facility's actual performance of important governance, managerial, clinical, and support functions (i.e., those functions that directly affect the delivery of quality patient care). It also focuses on the continual improvement in an organization's performance of these functions. Standards are provided in an "Accreditation Manual for Hospitals" document, which is updated and revised on a yearly basis. This document consists of three sections: (1) patient-focused functions, (2) organization-focused functions, and (3) structures with functions. Its approach is a functional one, and all departments and disciplines must be familiar with relevant issues found in applicable chapters. Most chapters contain standards that affect the care provided by a dietitian.

The section on "Care of the Patient" contains standards that apply specifically to medication use, rehabilitation, anesthesia, operative and other invasive procedures, and special treatments, as well as nutrition care standards. The focus of the nutrition care standards is provision of appropriate nutrition care in a timely and effective manner using an interdisciplinary approach (i.e., involvement of physicians, registered dietitians, nurses, pharmacists, and other disciplines as appropriate).

Appropriate care is considered to include screening of patients for nutrition needs, assessing and reassessing patient needs, developing a nutrition care plan, ordering and communicating the diet order, preparing and distributing the diet order, monitoring the process, and continually reassessing and improving the nutrition care process. A facility can define who, when, where, and how the process is accomplished; but TJC specifies that a qualified dietitian must be involved in establishing this process. A plan for the delivery of nutrition care may be as simple as providing a regular diet for a patient who is not at nutritional risk or as complex as managing tube feedings in a ventilator-dependent patient, which involves the collaboration of multiple disciplines.

The accreditation process typically involves an on-site survey that lasts for several days. During this survey adherence to standards is ascertained through interviews, review of documents (including patient medical records), and visits to patient care and other areas. Registered dietitians are actively involved in the survey process. Standards set by TJC play a large role in influencing the standards of care delivered to patients in all health care disciplines. For more information, see the TJC website: www.jointcommission.org.

and more facilities are converting to an electronic medical record. The RD must ensure that all aspects of nutrition care are summarized succinctly in the medical record.

More and more facilities are introducing electronic health records (EHRs). EHRs offer several benefits over paper charts, including accessibility, legibility, data management, and efficiency in providing care. The RD should be involved in all aspects of the transition from paper to EHR, including development of nutrition screens used for patient admission, assessment, and progress notes. It is easier to customize screens and drop-down menus at the preimplementation stage than to try to edit programs after they are in use.

The medical record and the information it contains are important for hospital care audits, professional standards reviews, patient education, and other efforts to maintain quality health care. RDs may also maintain a separate record of nutrition care provided. The record kept by the dietitian may be useful when patients are frequently readmitted or when a patient is transferred to a different unit (and thus to a different dietitian). Figure 17-1 is an example of a nutrition care record that may be used by a dietitian.

The medical record also serves as the basis for evaluating the care delivered. The RD provides information relative to nutrition status, nutrition interventions, and the goals of nutrition therapy. Information shared should be useful to other members of the health care team. The RD must be aware of facility policies regarding documentation (Klein et al., 1997) and that the record is a permanent legal, confidential document. The following are general guidelines for documentation in the hospital setting:

- All entries should be written in black pen or typewritten. Soft felt pens, multicolored pens, and pencils should not be used.

Patient ID: _____

Referring Physician: _____ Service: _____

Age: _____ Gender: _____ Height: _____ Weight: _____

ASSESSMENT

Weight history: _____ Weight goal: _____ Ideal Weight: _____

Activity Level: _____ Medications: _____

Past History: _____

Lab values: _____

Nutrient Requirements: _____ Nutrient Intake: _____

Current Diet Order: _____ Education/Counseling Needs: _____

NUTRITION DIAGNOSIS

_____

_____

NUTRITION INTERVENTION

_____

_____

_____

NUTRITION MONITORING/EVALUATION

_____

_____

RD Signature: _____ Date: _____

FIGURE 17-1 Sample nutrition care form.

- Documentation should be complete, clear, concise, objective, legible, and accurate.
- Entries should include date, time, and service. Each page should include the patient's name and hospital number (most facilities use a stamp for this purpose).
- Entries should be in chronologic order and be consecutive.
- The first word of every statement should be capitalized, with periods placed at the end of each thought. Complete sentences are not necessary, but grammar and spelling should be correct.
- All entries should be consistent and noncontradictory.
- All entries must be signed at the end and should include credentials (e.g., *J.Wilson, R.D.*). No one should ever chart or sign the medical record for another individual.
- Personal opinions and comments criticizing or casting doubt on the professionalism of others should never be included in the medical record.
- Documentation must be done at the time of the actual procedure or service. Entries should never be made in advance of a task performed.
- Late entries should be identified as such, including the actual date and time of the entry and the date and time it should have been recorded.
- Medical record entries should always be legible. When correcting an error, NEVER:
  Use White-Out, correction tape, or self-adhesive labels.
  Obliterate an entry by use of a thick marker or pen strokes.
  Add notes after the fact without accurately authenticating, dating, and referencing the original entry.
  Remove the original and replace it with a copy.
- Minor errors (e.g., in transcription, spelling, one word) can be corrected by drawing a single line through the error, entering the correction, and initialing and dating the correction.
- If information is accidentally omitted, write "see addendum" by the original entry, add the date and initial, and write the addendum in the medical record, identified as an addendum with the date and time of the original entry.

Formats for Medical Record Charting

Problem-oriented medical records (POMRs) are used in many facilities. The POMR is organized according to the patient's primary problems. Entries into the medical record can be done in many styles. One of the most common forms is the subjective, objective, assessment, and plan (SOAP) note. In many clinical facilities this is being replaced with the acronym A-D-I-M-E, to reflect the steps of the nutrition care process (assessment, diagnosis, interventions, monitoring, and evaluation). Table 17-2 lists charting content and Box 17-3 gives an example of an initial chart entry.

Other documentation styles include diagnosis, assessment, plan (DAP); problem, intervention, evaluation (PIE); problem, etiology, symptoms (PES); intervention, evaluation, and revision (IER); history, observation, assessment, plan (HOAP); screen, assess, plan (SAP); subjective, objective, analysis/assessment, plan, intervention, evaluation and revisions (SOAPIER); and focus/DAR charting (a positive instead of negative perspective on a problem with data, action, and review.)

The important factor is the content of the documentation, not necessarily the style. All entries made by the dietitian should address the issues of nutrition status and needs. Notes must be written efficiently, and they must be able to engage the physician and other health care team members to take action to achieve the desired nutrition care outcomes. *Focus On:* Coding for Malnutrition highlights key information that is helpful to include to ensure that malnutrition is adequately addressed in the patient's medical record (see also EVOLVE website).

Electronic charting has been in existence for some time, but its use is rapidly becoming more common. Computer documentation can reduce duplication and repetition of information, save time, and offer new tools for decision making, such as providing prescription renewal reminders or potential drug interaction alerts for care providers. Brevity in charting, regardless of the style used, is important. In one study of the use of abbreviated charting style, physicians were found to more readily implement brief dietitian recommendations than lengthy ones (Grace-Farfaglia and Rosow, 1995). Physicians have responded favorably to A-D-I-M-E charting.

One last consideration for charting and use of medical records is the **Health Insurance Portability and Accountability Act (HIPPA)** of 1996, which states that all health

---

TABLE 17-2

A-D-I-M-E Chart Content

Assessment Subjective	Information provided by patient, family, or significant other
	Significant nutritional history
	Pertinent socioeconomic, cultural information
	Level of physical activity
	Current dietary intake (in terms of nutrients)
	Reported height and weight
	Patient's comprehension and motivation toward behavioral change

Continued

TABLE 17-2

A-D-I-M-E Chart Content—cont'd

Assessment

Objective	Factual, reproducible observations (i.e., anthropometric and laboratory data)
	Diagnosis
	Measured height, weight
	Age
	Weight loss or weight gain patterns
	Desirable weight or realistic goal weight
	Pertinent clinical data (nausea, vomiting, diarrhea)
	Diet order
	Pertinent medications
	Calculation of nutrient needs
	Assessment of laboratory data as they apply to nutrition/hydration status
	Assessment of medications as they affect nutrition status
Nutrition Diagnosis	Interpretation of the patient's status based on subjective and objective data; evaluation of the food and nutritional history as it pertains to medical condition
	Determination of the patient's nutritional problem and its etiology, signs, and symptoms

Interventions

Goals	Short and long-term objectives, as designed with patient/client, family, and caregivers
Plan	Diagnostic studies needed; suggestions for gaining further pertinent data, work-up, data gathering
Treatment	Medical nutrition therapy: changes, additions, alterations in foods, nutrients, fluids
Education	Sharing of information to help the patient/client and family understand the condition and needed changes
Counseling	Offering individualized assistance and tips for self-care management and monitoring
Care Management	Consultations with other health care providers, referrals to other providers or agencies; recommendations for nutrition care in new settings and discharge planning
Monitoring and Evaluation	Outcome evaluation to determine level of success, improvement in signs and symptoms, resolution of nutrition diagnoses
	Evaluation of patient or client's ability to function independently without frequent or intense registered dietitian interventions
	Measurable goal evaluations selected and monitored

A-D-I-M-E, Assessment, diagnosis, interventions, monitoring, evaluation.

BOX 17-3

Clinical Nutrition

Nutrition Assessment

- Pt is 66-year-old female admitted with abdominal pain: Ht: 62 cm; Wt: 56 kg; IBW: 52-58 kg
- Labs noted: Na 134, calcium 8, total protein 5.8, albumin 3
- EEN: 1568-1680 calories (28-30 cal/kg) and 56-73 g protein (1-1.3 g/kg)
- Current diet is low residue with pt consuming 25% of meals recorded
- Consult for education received

Nutrition Diagnosis

- Food and nutrition related knowledge deficit related to lack of prior exposure to information as evidenced by client having no prior knowledge of need for low-residue diet (NB-1.1)

Nutrition Intervention

- Education: Will provide pt with written and verbal instruction on low-residue diet
- Goals: Pt will be able to develop 1-day menu using dietary restrictions

  Pt will be able to identify good sources of calcium and protein from list of foods appropriate for low-residue diet

  Pt will ask appropriate questions and verbalize understanding of dietary modifications

Nutrition Monitoring

- Before discharge, will follow up with pt regarding questions about diet.

J Wilson, RD 1/1/07 10:15 AM

Coding for Malnutrition

International Classification of Disease (ICD) codes were developed in the late 1800s as a mechanism to monitor and track mortality rates. The ICD coding system has been revised and updated several times; the version used in the United States at this time is the ICD-9-CM (clinical modification), whereas other countries use the ICD-10 codes. Medical records departments review medical records and assign codes to identify diagnoses, as well as complicating factors (commonly referred to as "comorbidities") to determine reimbursement by third-party payers. The presence of comorbid factors can increase reimbursement. Commonly pulmonary, gastrointestinal, endocrine, mental disorders, and cancer can lead to malnutrition as a comorbid factor. Codes frequently used to classify malnutrition include:*

260—kwashiorkor (severe protein deficiency; marked by changes in of skin and hair pigment)[†]

261—nutritional marasmus (severe tissue wasting or loss of subcutaneous fat)[†]

262—other severe protein-calorie malnutrition (nutritional edema without mention of dyspigmentation of skin and hair)

263—other and unspecified protein-calorie malnutrition

263.0—malnutrition of a moderate degree

263.1—malnutrition of a mild degree

263.2—arrested development following protein-calorie malnutrition (nutritional dwarfism)

263.8—other protein-calorie malnutrition

263.9—unspecified protein-calorie malnutrition

Coordinated nutrition care and coding for malnutrition are important elements in patient services. Use of MNT guides established by the American Dietetic Association may improve client outcomes. Depending on the primary medical diagnosis and other comorbidities, identification of malnutrition can lead to improved reimbursement.

*Adapted from the World Health Organization's International Classification of Diseases, ICD-10, http://www.cdc.gov/nchs/about/otheract/icd9/abticd10.htm.

† Mainly used in pediatric populations. For the nutrition care process, Code 261 is "evident protein-caloric malnutrition."

---

care providers ensure the protection of patient privacy. Although HIPAA does not prevent sharing of patient data required for an incident of care, patients must be notified if their medical information is to be shared outside of the care process or if protected information (e.g., address, email, income) is to be shared.

INFLUENCES ON NUTRITION CARE

The health care environment has undergone considerable change related to the provision of care and reimbursement in the last decade. Governmental influences, cost containment issues, changing demographics, and the changing role of the patient as a "consumer" have influenced the health care arena. These changes in the delivery of health care have resulted in new parameters that affect the provision of MNT.

Managed care organizations (MCOs) finance and deliver care through a contracted network of providers in exchange for a monthly premium. (MCOs) have changed health care reimbursement from a fee-for-service system to one in which fiscal risk is borne by health care organizations and physicians. **Preferred-provider organizations (PPOs)**, health maintenance organizations (HMOs), and MCOs have changed the face of health care in recent years. Strategies used by MCOs, PPOs, and HMOs are intended to contain health care costs while providing efficient and effective care that is of consistently high quality. To accomplish this, practice guidelines (or **standards of care**) are often used. These sets of recommendations serve as a guide for defining appropriate care for a patient with a specific diagnosis or medical problem. They help to ensure consistency and quality for both providers and clients in a health care system and, as such, are specific to an institution or health care organization.

Case management is a process that strives to promote the achievement of patient care goals in a cost-effective, efficient manner. It is an essential component in MCO and HMO efforts toward delivering care in a manner that provides a positive experience for the patient and ensures achievement of clinical outcomes while using resources wisely. Case management involves assessing, evaluating, planning, implementing, coordinating, and monitoring care, especially in patients with chronic disease or those who are at high risk; it typically occurs in an inpatient setting (Figure 17-2). Case management is most appropriate for patients who present a complex picture in terms of their health; economic status; and social, emotional, and psychological care, not necessarily in terms of the acuity or severity of their condition (Laramee, 1995).

Critical pathways are a key component in case management systems. They identify essential elements that should occur in the patient's care and define a timeframe in which each activity should occur to maximize patient outcomes. **Disease management** is a disease-specific approach to patient care that focuses on the outpatient setting (Biesemeier, 1997). The goal is to prevent disease progression or exacerbations and to reduce the frequency and severity of disease symptoms and complications. Education is an important component as are other strategies that maximize compliance

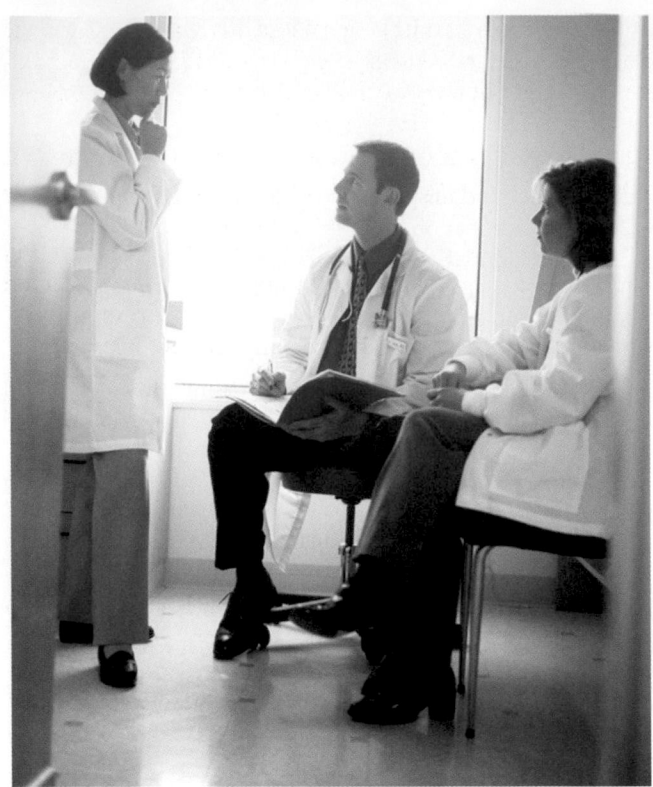

FIGURE 17-2 Dietitian working with medical team members to resolve nutritional issues.

with disease treatment. Educating a patient with type 1 diabetes regarding control of blood glucose levels would be an example of a disease management strategy; it is aimed at decreasing the complications associated with the disease (nephropathy, neuropathy, and retinopathy) and the frequency with which the client needs to access the care provider, especially on an emergent basis. Decreasing the number of emergency room visits related to hypoglycemic episodes is a sample goal.

Utilization management is a system that strives for cost efficiency by eliminating or reducing unnecessary tests, procedures, and services. A manager is usually assigned to a group of patients and is responsible for ensuring adherence to preestablished criteria.

One of the largest influences on health care delivery in the last decade has been the change in the method of payment for services provided. There are several common methods of reimbursement: cost-based reimbursement, negotiated bids, and diagnostic-related groups (DRGs). Under the DRG system, a facility receives payment for a patient's admission based on the principal diagnosis, secondary diagnosis (comorbid conditions), surgical procedure (if appropriate), and the age and gender of the patient.

Approximately 500 DRGs cover the entire spectrum of medical diagnoses and surgical treatments. DRGs allow a hospital to receive the same amount for a specific stay regardless of the number of studies, procedures, or the length of stay. It is to the advantage of the facility to manage pa-

tient care prudently in these cases. Nutrition screening can be very important in identifying patients who are malnourished or nutritionally compromised. Early identification of these factors allows for timely intervention and helps prevent the comorbidities often seen with malnutrition, which may cause the length of stay (and thus cost) to increase.

Patient-focused care (PFC) has changed how care is delivered to a patient by focusing on the patient's needs and perspective rather than the caregiver's assumptions. It drastically reduces the number of individuals with whom the patient comes in contact by decentralizing services and cross-training personnel in efforts to increase the continuity and quality of care provided. Hospitals have moved to PFC to overcome the fragmentation in care that has occurred as health care has become more specialized. How PFC is delivered varies from institution to institution, but its basic elements focus on the patient's needs, cost-effectiveness of care, reduction in work steps, and more direct patient care. Team membership varies but usually includes both skilled (licensed) and unskilled (unlicensed) personnel. Cross-training is important in making the model work. Typically only patient care services that require highly specialized expertise remain centralized.

Staffing is the last factor that affects the success of nutrition care. Clinical dietitians may be centralized (all are part of a core nutrition department) or decentralized (individual dietitians are part of a unit/service that provides care to patients), depending on the model adopted by a specific institution. Certain departments such as food service, accounting, and human resources remain centralized in most models because some of the functions for which these departments are responsible are not directly related to patient care. Dietitians should be involved in the planning and instituting of PFC to ensure that MNT is considered as part of any redesign of patient care (see Figure 17-2).

NUTRITION INTERVENTION: FOOD AND NUTRIENT DELIVERY

Therapeutic diets are based on a general, adequate diet that has been modified as necessary to provide for individual requirements, such as digestive and absorptive capacity, alleviation or arrest of a disease process, and psychosocial factors. In general, the therapeutic diet should vary as little as possible from the individual's normal diet. Personal eating patterns and food preferences should be recognized, along with socioeconomic conditions, religious practices, and any environmental factors that influence food intake, such as where the meals are eaten and who prepares them (see "Cultural Aspects of Dietary Planning" in Chapter 12).

A nutritious and adequate diet can be planned in many ways. One foundation of such a diet is the MyPyramid Food Guidance System (see Chapter 12). This is a basic plan; additional foods or more of the foods listed are included to provide additional energy and increase the intake of required nutrients for the individual. The Dietary Guidelines for Americans are also used in meal planning and to promote wellness. The Dietary Reference Intakes (DRIs) and specific nutrient Recommended Dietary Allowances (RDAs) are formulated for healthy persons, but they are also used as a basis for evaluating the adequacy of therapeutic diets. Nutrient requirements specific to a particular person's genetic makeup, disease state, or disorder must always be kept in mind during diet planning.

The Nutrition or Diet Prescription

The **diet or nutrition prescription** designates the type, amount, and frequency of feeding based on the individual's disease process and disease management goals. The prescription may specify a caloric level or other restriction to be implemented. It may also limit or increase various components of the diet, such as carbohydrate, protein, fat, alcohol, specific vitamins or minerals, phytonutrients, fiber or water.

Energy Allowance

Appetite regulates body weight with surprising accuracy in most normally active people. However, it is not always valid or reliable in disease, and energy needs may need to be calculated by a variety of methods (see Chapter 2). When necessary, actual measurement of the basal or resting metabolic rate using a metabolic cart and indirect calorimetry can be very useful (see Figure 2-5) in determining energy requirements. Other methods for calculating energy requirement include calculating the required number of kcal/day or calculating the percentage increase over basal metabolic demands (see Chapter 2 and inside front cover). The RD is responsible for determining if the patient's illness warrants an increased energy allowance based on diagnosis and illness severity. Sections of this text dealing with disease states review energy needs related to specific conditions or illnesses. The general or regular hospital diet should be planned to meet the energy needs for most healthy adults of normal weight.

Protein Allowance

The RDA for protein is 0.8 g/kg of body weight for adults (see Chapter 3 and inside front cover). This level is usually considered adequate for previously well-nourished individuals who are ambulatory or who require only brief periods of hospitalization. Protein requirements may be altered due to infection, fever, trauma, burns, and surgery. General or regular hospital diets should provide a level of protein slightly higher than requirements for normal adults since many hospitalized patients will have increased protein needs. Sections of this text dealing with disease states review protein needs related to specific conditions or illnesses.

Minerals and Vitamins

Appropriate levels of vitamins and minerals for stressed individuals are difficult to accurately determine. In times of stress, inadequacies of nutrients may be countered with mobilization of body stores, decreased losses, increased absorption, or improved use. Individual responses vary; and true deficiencies with clinical signs and symptoms may take weeks, months, or even years to develop. Biochemical measurements for identifying inadequacies at early stages are still being developed (see Figure 15-2).

To determine appropriate levels of vitamin and mineral intakes, the following should be considered: (1) requirements for healthy individuals; (2) nature of the disease or injury; (3) body stores of specific nutrients; (4) normal and abnormal losses through the skin, urine, or intestinal tract; and (5) drug-nutrient interactions. These factors are discussed further in the chapters relating to nutrition care for various disease states and in Chapter 15.

Fluids

A healthy adult at rest and not perspiring needs 1800 to 2500 ml/day (2+ quarts) of water (or approximately 1 ml/kcal consumed) to provide for urinary excretion and replace insensible fluid losses. Optimal convalescence demands adequate tissue hydration. Additional fluids must be given to replace water lost by excessive perspiration, vomiting, diarrhea, tube drainage, or other conditions marked by increased water loss (see Table 4-1). If sufficient water cannot be taken in orally, it must be supplied intravenously, usually along with electrolytes (see Chapter 4). The RD should check recorded intake and output (I&O) records to ensure that fluid needs are being met.

Modifications of the Normal Diet

Normal nutrition is the foundation on which therapeutic diet modifications are based. Regardless of the type of diet prescribed, the purpose of the diet is to supply needed nutrients to the body in a form that it can handle. Adjustment of the diet may take any of the following forms:

- Change in consistency of foods (liquid diet, pureed diet, low-fiber diet, high-fiber diet)
- Increase or decrease in energy value of diet (weight-reduction diet, high-calorie diet)
- Increase or decrease in the type of food or nutrient consumed (sodium-restricted diet, lactose-restricted diet, fiber-enhanced diet, high-potassium diet)
- Elimination of specific foods (allergy diet, gluten-free diet)
- Adjustment in the level, ratio, or balance of protein, fat, and carbohydrate (diet for diabetes, ketogenic diet, renal diet, cholesterol-lowering diet)
- Rearrangement of the number and frequency of meals (diet for diabetes, postgastrectomy diet)
- Change in route of delivery of nutrients (enteral or parenteral nutrition).

Foods as Nutrient Sources

Evaluation of general and modified diets requires knowledge of the nutrients contained in different foods. In particular, it is helpful to be aware of the nutrient-dense foods that contribute to dietary adequacy. Chapter 3 and Appendixes 46-58 provide more detailed information on specific minerals and vitamins and the foods that contain them.

Often a vitamin-mineral supplement is necessary to meet the patient's needs when the diet is limited (see Chapter 18).

NUTRITION CARE FOR THE HOSPITALIZED PATIENT

Food is an important part of nutrition care. Attempts should be made to honor patient preferences (including cultural preferences as discussed in Chapter 12, providing a pleasant atmosphere, and arranging for assistance with eating when needed). Imagination and ingenuity in menu planning are essential when planning meals acceptable to a varied patient population. Attention to color, texture, composition, and temperature of the foods, coupled with a sound knowledge of therapeutic diets, is required for menu planning. However, to the patient, good taste and attractive presentation are the most important elements. When possible, patient selection of menus results in the delivery of food that will most likely be consumed. The ability to make food selections gives the patient an option in an otherwise limiting environment.

Standard Diets Used in Hospitals or Health Care Facilities

All hospitals or health care institutions have basic, routine diets designed for uniformity and convenience of service. These standard diets are based on the foundation of an adequate diet pattern with nutrient levels as derived from the DRIs. The diets should be as realistic as possible yet ensure that nutrition needs of patients are met. The most important consideration of the type of diet offered is providing foods that the patient is willing and able to eat and that fit in with any required dietary restrictions. Shortened lengths of stay in many health care settings result in the need to optimize intake of calories and protein and this often translates into a relatively liberal approach to therapeutic diets. This is especially true when the therapeutic restrictions might compromise intake and subsequent recovery from surgery, stress, or illness.

Types of standard diets vary but can generally be classified as general or regular, modified consistency, or liquid. These diets are used routinely for patients and serve as a foundation for more diversified therapeutic diets.

Regular/General Diet

In some institutions a diet that has no restrictions is referred to as the "regular" or "house" diet. It is used when the patient's medical condition does not warrant any limitations. This diet is a basic, adequate, general diet of approximately 1600 to 2200 kcal; it usually contains 60 to 80 g of protein, 80 to 100 g of fat, and 180 to 300 g of carbohydrate. Although there are no particular food restrictions, some facilities have instituted regular diets that are low in fat, saturated fat, cholesterol, sugar, and salt to follow the dietary recommendations for the general population. In other facilities the diet focuses on providing foods the patient is willing and able to eat, with less focus on restriction of nutrients. Many institutions have a selective menu that allows the patient certain choices; the adequacy of the diet varies based on the patient's selections.

Clear Liquid Diet

Clear liquid diets are seldom used these days. They furnish fluids, some electrolytes, and small amounts of energy and consist of clear liquids such as tea, broth, carbonated beverages, clear fruit juices, and gelatin. Milk and liquids prepared with milk are omitted, as are fruit juices that contain pulp. Carbonated beverages such as ginger ale and hot beverages such as tea and broth are usually well tolerated. The average clear liquid diet contains 500 to 600 kcal, 5 to 10 g of protein, minimum fat, 120 to 130 g of carbohydrate, and small amounts of sodium and potassium. It is inadequate in calories, fiber, and all other essential nutrients and should be used only for short periods of time.

The clear liquid diet does not meet fluid needs for most patients. Fluids and electrolytes are often replaced intravenously until the diet can be advanced to a more nutritionally adequate one. Although there is little scientific evidence supporting the use of clear liquid diets as transition diets immediately after surgery (Jeffery et al., 1996), they are still often used in that way.

Consistency Modifications

Further modifications in consistency may be needed for patients who have limited chewing or swallowing ability. Chopping, mashing, pureeing, or grinding food modifies its texture. See Chapter 41 and Appendix 35 for more information on consistency modifications and for neurologic changes in particular.

Food Intake

Food served does not necessarily represent the actual intake of the patient. Prevention of iatrogenic malnutrition in the health care setting requires observation and monitoring of the adequacy of patient intake. If food intake is inadequate, measures should be taken to provide foods or supplements that may be better accepted or tolerated. Regardless of the type of diet prescribed, both the food served and the amount actually eaten must be considered to obtain an accurate determination of the patient's energy and nutrient intake. Nourishments and calorie-containing beverages consumed between meals are also considered in the overall intake. It is important that the RD maintain communication with nursing and food service personnel to determine adequacy of intake. In the past, calorie counts were often ordered; however, calorie counts are often inaccurate and incomplete. Similar information can be obtained by attending patient care rounds, talking to the patient or family, and discussing with the nursing staff.

Psychological Factors

Meals and between-meal nourishments are often highlights of the day and are anticipated with pleasure by the patient. Mealtime should be as positive an experience as possible.

Whatever setting the patient is eating in should be comfortable for the patient. Food intake is encouraged in a pleasant room with the patient in a comfortable eating position in bed or sitting in a chair located away from unpleasant sights or odors. Eating with others often promotes better intake.

Arrangement of the tray should reflect consideration of the patient's needs. Dishes and utensils should be in a convenient location. Independence should be encouraged in those who require assistance in eating. The caregiver can accomplish this by asking patients to specify the sequence of foods to be eaten and having them participate in eating, if only by holding their bread. Even visually impaired persons can eat unassisted if they are told where to find foods on the tray. Patients who require feeding assistance should be fed when the foods are still at an optimal temperature. The feeding process requires about 20 minutes as a general rule.

Poor acceptance of foods and meals may be caused by unfamiliar foods, a change in eating schedule, improper food temperatures, the patient's medical condition, or the effects of medical therapy. Food acceptance is improved when personal selection of menus is encouraged. Patients should be given the opportunity to share concerns regarding meals, which may improve acceptance and intake.

In encouraging acceptance of a therapeutic diet, the attitude of the caregiver is important. The nurse who understands that the diet contributes to the restoration of the patient's health will communicate this conviction by actions, facial expressions, and conversation. Patients who understand that the diet is important to the success of their therapy and recovery usually accept it more willingly.

When the patient must adhere to a therapeutic dietary program indefinitely, an interdisciplinary approach will help him or her achieve nutritional goals. Because they have frequent contact with patients, nurses play an important role in a patient's acceptance of nutrition care. Ensuring that the nursing staff is aware of the nutrition care plan can greatly improve the probability of success.

Intervention: Nutrition Education

Nutrition education is an important part of the MNT provided to many patients. The goal of nutrition education is to help the patient acquire the knowledge and skills needed to make changes, including modifying behavior to facilitate sustained change. Nutrition education and resultant dietary changes implemented by the patient result in many benefits. One of the most important benefits is the control of the disease or symptoms, but other benefits such as improved health status, improved quality of life, and decreased health care costs may also result when dietary changes are successful. As the average length of hospital stays has decreased, the role of the in-patient dietitian in educating inpatients has changed to providing "survival" skills. These survival skills include basic types of foods to limit, timing of meals, and portion sizes. Follow-up outpatient counseling regarding details of the diet should reinforce the basic counseling given during hospitalization. See Chapter 19 for detailed information on counseling, and Chapter 20 for managing home nutrition support.

Intervention: Coordination of Care

Nutrition care continues as a part of **discharge planning** when the patient returns home or goes to a long-term care facility or rehabilitation center. Education, counseling, and mobilization of resources to provide home care and nutrition support are included as components of discharge procedures. Completing a discharge nutritional summary for the next caregiver is imperative for optimal care. Appropriate discharge documentation includes a summary of nutrition therapies and outcomes; pertinent information such as weights, laboratory values, and dietary intake; potential drug-nutrient interactions; expected progress or prognosis; and recommendations for follow-up services. The amount and type of instruction given, the patient's comprehension of the instruction, and the expected degree of adherence to the prescribed diet must be included. An effective discharge plan increases the likelihood of a positive outcome for the patient.

A variety of resources, including home health care agencies, are available to provide services related to nutrition, including enteral or parenteral nutrition at home. Follow-up monitoring may be needed to provide continuity of care in the new setting or to ensure a smooth transition back to the original health care site, should readmission be necessary.

Regardless of the setting to which the patient is discharged, effective coordination of care begins on day 1 of a hospital or nursing home stay and continues throughout the institutionalization. The patient should be included in every step of the planning process whenever possible to ensure that decisions made by the health care team reflect the desires of the patient.

Whenever necessary, the RD refers the patient or client to other caregivers, agencies, or programs for follow-up care or services.

NUTRITION CARE OF THE TERMINALLY ILL OR HOSPICE PATIENT

Maintenance of comfort and quality of life are most typically the goals of nutrition care for the terminally ill patient. Dietary restrictions are rarely appropriate. Nutrition care should be mindful of strategies that facilitate symptom and pain control. Recognition of the various phases of dying—denial, anger, bargaining, depression, and acceptance—will help the health care practitioner understand the patient's response to food and nutrition support.

The decision as to when life support should be terminated often involves the issue of whether to continue enteral or parenteral nutrition. With **advance directives**, the patient can advise family and health care team members of his or her individual preferences with regard to end-of-life issues. Food and hydration issues may be discussed, such as whether or not tube feeding should be initiated or discontinued and under what circumstances. Nutrition support should be continued as long as the patient is competent to make this choice (or if specified in the patient's advance directives).

Palliative care encourages the alleviation of physical symptoms, anxiety, and fear while attempting to maintain the patient's ability to function independently. Hospice home care programs allow the patient to stay at home and delay or avoid hospital admission. Quality of life is the critical component. A dietitian's intervention may benefit the patient and family as they adjust to issues related to the approaching death. Families who might be accustomed to a modified diet should be reassured if they are uncomfortable about easing dietary restrictions. Ongoing communication and explanations to the family are important and helpful.

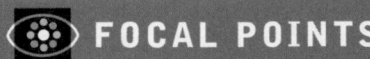 **FOCAL POINTS**

- The astute dietetics professional provides nutrition care in a predictable, step-wise manner in order to provide services that meet the needs of clients.
- Use of the Nutrition Care Process provides the dietetics professional with a framework to develop and maintain optimum nutrition care, support, and service
- Use of the model (Assessment, Nutrition Diagnosis, Intervention, Monitoring and Evaluation, or A-D-I-M-E) will help in achieving the best possible outcomes for patients and their families.
- Like other professions, the dietetics profession uses standardized language and diagnostic terms.
- Documentation of nutrition diagnoses is an area of practice that will solidify the position of nutrition care in all practice settings, whether for individuals, groups, or populations.

 CLINICAL SCENARIO

Mr. B, a 47-year-old man, 6 ft 2 in tall and weighing 200 lb, is admitted to the hospital with chest pain. Three days after admission, during the nutrition screening process, it is discovered that Mr. B has gained 30 pounds over the last 2 years. Review of the medical record reveals the following laboratory data: LDL: 240 (desirable <130), HDL 30 (desirable >65), triglyceride 350 (desirable <200). Blood pressure is 120/85. Current medications: multivitamin/mineral daily. Cardiac catheterization is scheduled for tomorrow. Diet is poor; skips meals and eats very large dinner meals.

✳**Nutrition Diagnosis:** Altered nutrition-related laboratory values related to undesirable food choices as evidenced by hyperlipidemia with elevated LDL and low HDL

1. What other information do you need to develop a nutrition care plan?
2. Was nutrition screening completed in a timely manner? Discuss the implications of timing of screening vs. implementing care.
3. Develop a chart (A-D-I-M-E) note based on the above information and the interview you conduct with the patient.
4. What nutrition care goals would you develop for this patient during his hospital stay?
5. What goals would you develop for this patient after discharge? Discuss how the type of health care insurance coverage the patient has might influence this plan.

Useful Websites

American Dietetic Association
www.eatright.org

Managed Care Information Center
http://www.themcic.com/

The Joint Commission
www.jointcommission.org

Tufts University Nutrition
www.navigator.tufts.edu

Wikipedia: Nutrition Care Process
http://en.wikipedia.org/wik:/Nutrition_Care_Process

References

American Dietetic Association: *Nutrition diagnosis and intervention: standardized language for the nutrition care process,* Chicago, Il, 2007, American Dietetic Association.

Biesemeier C: Case manager/registered dietitian partnerships: teaming up to achieve positive patient outcomes, *J Care Mgmt* 3:72, 1997.

Grace-Farfaglia P, Rosow P: Automating clinical dietetics documentation, *J Am Diet Assoc* 95:688, 1995.

Jeffery KM et al: The clear liquid diet is no longer necessary in the routine postoperative management of surgical patients, *Am J Surg* 62:167, 1996.

Klein CJ et al: Physicians prefer goal-oriented note format more than three to one over other outcome focused documentation, *J Am Diet Assoc* 97:1306, 1997.

Lacey K, Pritchett E: Nutrition care process and model: ADA adopts road map to quality care and outcomes management, *J Am Diet Assoc,* 103:1061, 2003.

Laramee S: Case management: an overview, *Clin Nutr Mgmt Newslett* 14(4):1, 1995.

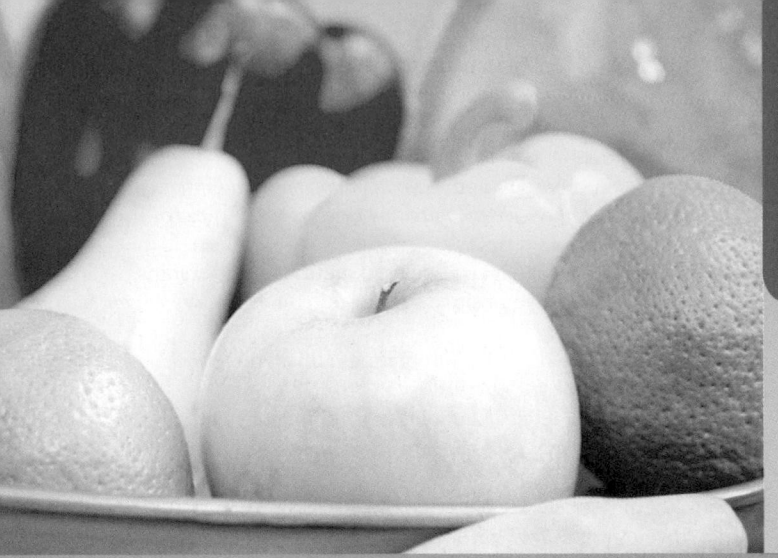

CHAPTER 18

Cynthia A. Thomson, PhD, RD

Intervention: Dietary Supplementation and Integrative Care

KEY TERMS

acupuncture use of thin needles inserted into points on the meridians to stimulate the body's vital energy

botanicals plants (including their leaves, flowers, stems, rhizomes, or roots) that are used for medicinal purposes

chi (Qi) a term in traditional Oriental medicine that means life-force energy; the center of the body's functions

chiropractic a healing system that involves manual manipulation of the musculoskeletal system to improve the normal functioning of the nervous system, which in turn is thought to promote health

Commission E Monographs therapeutic monographs on phytomedicines developed in Germany by an expert commission of scientists and health care professionals

complementary and alternative medicine (CAM) approaches to healing (health-related methods and practices) that are not generally within the scope of conventional medicine; nonstandard medicine; includes but is not limited to botanical use, mind-body approaches, musculoskeletal manipulation, energy medicine, and nutrition-diet interventions

dietary supplement a product (other than tobacco) intended to supplement the diet that bears or contains one or more of the following dietary ingredients: a vitamin; a mineral; an herb or other botanical; an amino acid; a dietary substance for use by man to supplement the diet by increasing the total daily intake; or a concentrate, metabolite, constituent, extract, or combination of these ingredients

Dietary Supplement Health and Education Act of 1994 (DSHEA) a law that defines dietary supplements with provisions related to the marketing of these products

health claim a written claim on the dietary supplement label that has two essential components: (1) a *substance* and (2) a *disease* or health-related condition; describes the relationship between these two components; a statement lacking either one of these components does not meet the regulatory definition; must meet the significant scientific agreement standard and requires prenotification of the Food and Drug Administration

holistic therapies treatments that emphasize the healing force of nature and the body's ability to self-heal

homeopathy a medical system based on the theory that substances in large doses that produce symptoms of a disease in healthy people will cure the same symptoms when administered in very dilute amounts

integrative medicine a holistic approach to health that combines complementary and alternative therapies with conventional medicine; nutrition care is considered a primary therapy within this model of medical practice

meridians a concept in traditional Chinese medicine related to channels of energy

moxibustion the application of heat along meridian acupuncture points to affect chi (Qi) and blood to balance substances and organs

naturopathy a therapeutic system that uses natural methods of healing (i.e., light, heat, air, water, and massage); modalities of naturopathy include phytomedicines, nutrition, nutritional and dietary supplements, and natural forces

pharmacognosy the science of natural substances and their physical, botanical, and biochemical properties and applications

phytotherapy the science of using plant-based medicines to prevent or treat illness

qualified health claim a label health claim based on emerging scientific evidence that, on review of the scientific evidence by the FDA, is approved for use on a food or dietary supplement label; disclaimers required to communicate level of scientific evidence to support claim

Sections of this chapter were written by Ruth M. DeBusk, PhD, RD, and Kimberly Mathai, for previous editions of this text.

structure-function claim a claim on a label that states how a substance affects a structure or function in the body or characterizes the mechanism by which a substance acts to maintain such structure or function

subluxation the dislocation of part of the body, which is thought to interfere with normal nerve function; chiropractic focuses on identifying and removing these interferences

traditional Oriental medicine a form of medicine based on the concept that energy, also termed chi (Qi) or life-force energy, is the center of body functions; wellness is a function of the balanced and harmonious flow of chi; illness or disease results from disturbances in this flow

INTEGRATIVE MEDICINE

Complementary and alternative medicine (CAM) refers to those practices that are not an integral or generally customary part of the practice of conventional medicine. This would include such treatment methodologies as acupuncture, meditation, naturopathy, and chiropractic care. **Integrative medicine** is defined slightly differently than CAM in that it is focused on the combined use of conventional and CAM approaches, and is defined as the comprehensive integration of appropriate complementary approaches along with conventional medical approaches into the care of the whole person with the goal of achieving optimal health outcomes.

Integrative medicine has been defined specifically as healing-oriented medicine that considers the whole person (body, mind, spirit) and all aspects of lifestyle. Emphasis is placed on the therapeutic relationship and all appropriate therapies, both conventional and alternative. Inherent in this approach to care is the need for a multidisciplinary approach that spans beyond conventional medicine practitioners in which patients and health care providers are partners in promoting wellness. The scope of care includes wellness and prevention, and, when illness does occur, a reliance on less invasive approaches is emphasized. Yet integrative care is evidence based, critically evaluating all medical and healing approaches.

Complementary, alternative, adjunctive, or integrative therapies are not new. In fact, their roots can be traced to early Greek and Chinese cultures. Although natural therapies are often described as being "cutting edge," they are actually much older than conventional Western medical interventions. Experts estimate that herbal remedies and ayurveda, the traditional medicine of India, are more than 5000 years old.

CAM therapies are considered holistic. **Holistic therapies,** derived from the Greek word *holos,* meaning "whole," are based on the theory that health is a vital dynamic state, reflecting a profound will and wisdom to maintain wellness rather than just the absence of disease. *Vis mediatrix*

naturae, the healing force of nature, is the underlying precept of holistic medicine. According to this precept, all living things can self-heal, and organisms have inherent self-defense mechanisms against illness. According to the National Center for Complementary and Alternative Medicine (NCCAM) classification scheme, CAM can be grouped as (1) alternative medical systems such as naturopathy, traditional Chinese Medicine, ayurveda, and homeopathy; (2) mind-body therapies such as meditation, prayer, art or music therapy and cognitive behavior therapy; (3) biologically based therapies such as the use of herbs, whole foods diets, and nutrient supplementation; (4) manipulative therapies such as massage, chiropractic medicine, osteopathy, and yoga; and (5) and whole medical systems based on energy therapies such as qi gong, magnetic therapy, reiki (Figure 18-1).

Increasingly health care practitioners, including dietetics professionals, are involved in the provision of care based on an integrative approach; and nutrition therapy and dietary supplementation are modalities practiced in the context of CAM and integrative medicine. Several diet-based therapies are listed in the descriptors of CAM modalities, including the Ornish diet, the Zone diet, the Atkins diet, the Pritikin diet, as well as macrobiotic and vegetarian diets, when the National Health Interview Survey was conducted in 2002. See Table 18-1 for descriptions of modalities identified as within the scope of CAM.

Use of Complementary and Alternative Therapies

The use of CAM therapies to enhance conventional medical practices has been increasing in the United States since the 1960s, and it is well recognized that a significant number of Americans use some form of CAM therapy even more frequently than primary care physicians. Data from the Alternative Health/Complementary and Alternative Medicine supplement to the 2002 National Health Interview Survey (NHIS) showed that among the 31,044 American adults surveyed, 74.6% report ever using CAM and 62.1% report use of CAM within the previous 12 months (Barnes et al., 2004). Megavitamin use is among the most common of CAM practices. Use was shown to be greatest among women, people with higher education, and people who were hospitalized in the previous 12 months (NCCAM, 2005).

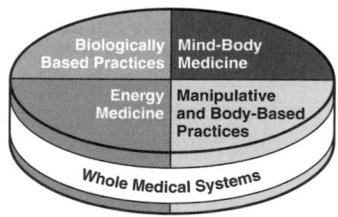

FIGURE 18-1 Classification of Complementary and Alternative Medicine Therapies. *(From Barnes P et al:* Complementary and alternative medicine use among adults, United States 2002, *CDC Advance Data Report #343, May 27, 2004.)*

The Food and Drug Administration has published tips for the dietary supplement user in making informed choices regarding which supplements to consider taking. Tips include advice regarding: (1) assessment of present diet; (2) informing health care providers of dietary supplement use; (3) potential medication–dietary supplement interactions; (4) reporting of adverse events; and (5) as-

sessment of the validity of information. See Box 18-3 for issues to consider when choosing a botanical.

Resources for Clinicians

As awareness of dietary supplement use expands within the health care community, the number of evidence-based resources available to clinicians is also growing consider-

Supplement	Type/Brand	Dose	Frequency	Length of use	Reason for use
Multi-nutrient supplements					
Multivitamin					
Multivitamin-mineral					
Antioxidant vitamin complex					
B vitamin complex					
Single Nutrients					
Vitamin C					
Vitamin E					
Folic acid					
Other:					
Mineral/Mineral combinations/Trace elements					
Calcium (including antacids)					
Calcium with vitamin D					
Calcium with vitamin D and magnesium					
Magnesium					
Iron					
Selenium					
Zinc					
Other:					
Food Constituents or herbals					
Coenzyme Q10					
Echinacea					
Evening primrose oil					
Fish oil or omega-3 fats					
Garlic					
Glucosamine/chondroitin					
Mixed carotenoids					
Mushroom extracts					
Milk thistle					
Other:					
Supplements taken for the following health conditions					
Arthritis/joint health					
Bone health					
Cancer prevention					
Fatigue/low energy					
Heart health					
Memory loss					
Menopausal symptoms					
Prostate health					
Sports conditioning					
Weight loss					
Other:					
Other:					

FIGURE 18-6 Dietary supplement intake assessment form.

ably. It is advisable that clinicians have access to at least one on-line resource that is updated at regular intervals. Resources that provide reference to the original research are also preferable. In addition, accessing available medical literature search engines is also advised, given that there are a growing number of studies being published in peer-reviewed literature. Finally identifying health care providers and researchers who are actively working in this area can be invaluable in terms of increasing awareness of safety issues, understanding mechanisms of biologic activity, and assessing the level of evidence for clinical efficacy.

BOX 18-3

Guidelines for Choosing Botanical Products

1. Be sure the choice of a botanical is appropriate to the health care goals and compatible with any prescription and over-the-counter medications or other dietary supplements. Information is available at www.consumerlab.com for validation of specific product brands on the market.
2. Investigate the quality of the manufacturer whose product is being considered. At a minimum, it is important to know that the retail suppliers carry only manufacturers that adhere to high-quality standards or that the health care professional recommending a product is knowledgeable about the quality of dietary supplements. One of the questions to ask is how herbs are grown, selected, stored, and processed to ensure absence of microbial contamination, proper identification, and potency.
3. Investigate the potential for pesticide contamination, which can be minimized by choosing organically grown herbs whenever possible.
4. Investigate the claims being made about the products and avoid products with exaggerated claims associated with them.
5. Use the dietary supplement label to obtain important information, including:
   - The complete botanical name of the product to confirm that this is the appropriate botanical.
   - The part of the plant used to prepare the product, confirming that it is the part that contains the active components.
   - The concentration of the botanical or nutrient and whether the concentration is appropriate for obtaining the reported benefits of the product (i.e., neither too weak nor too strong).
   - The daily dosage needed to obtain the desired effect.
   - A lot number, which is helpful if problems arise because it allows the product to be tracked through each stage of the manufacturing process.
   - An expiration date.
   - A recognized seal of approval that indicates Good Manufacturing Practices have been used in the production of the product and that the product has passed independent analyses confirming that the label accurately represents the product.
   - A toll-free number for contacting the manufacturer in the event of adverse reactions.
6. After determining that a manufacturer and its product meet these standards, compare prices among products of similar quality. Prices can vary widely.

Adapted from DeBusk RM: A practical guide to herbal supplements for nutrition practitioners, *Topics Clin Nutr* 16:53, 2001.

⚙ FOCAL POINTS

- Complementary and alternative medicine (CAM) therapies such as acupuncture, moxibustion, chiropractic, naturopathy, and phytotherapy are commonly practiced in the United States.
- Most CAM therapies emphasize a holistic approach to health and promote the body's ability to heal itself.
- Dietary supplementation is one of the most common of alternative or complementary therapies used in the U.S.
- Efforts to test the efficacy of dietary supplements in clinical trials are expanding and resources to stay abreast of current research in this area are now available.
- Registered dietitians are obliged to be sufficiently well informed and to advise their patients responsibly regarding CAM therapies and the safe use of dietary supplements.

✴ CLINICAL SCENARIO 1

Ellen is 66 years old and has been diagnosed as having hypertension, hypercholesterolemia, and type 2 diabetes. She has been referred by her physician for nutritional counseling, with a specific request from the referring physician that you evaluate any herbal preparations she is taking. At the initial consult, Ellen tells you she is taking the following dietary supplements: garlic pills, ginseng, ginkgo, and St. John's wort, along with the following medications: warfarin, a tricyclic antidepressant, and blood pressure–lowering medication.

✴Nutrition Diagnosis: Excessive bioactive substance intake related to daily intake of multiple supplements as evidenced by intake of supplements that conflict with medications (e.g. warfarin, garlic, and antidepressant containing St. John's wort).

1. What recommendations would you make about Ellen's diet?
2. What additional questions would you ask regarding Ellen's supplements?
3. List potential adverse interactions between the botanicals and the prescription drugs. How would you counsel Ellen?

✴ CLINICAL SCENARIO 2

Matthew is a 43-year-old highly successful sales representative for a major medical company. He enjoys the competitive nature of his job, travels a lot, and is knowledgeable about health care. Matthew "eats healthy," is at a normal weight, jogs daily, and takes a number of dietary supplements to improve his energy level, to manage his stress, to help him sleep, and to protect against heart disease (his father had a heart attack in his 50s). He takes a high-potency daily multivitamin-multimineral with extra vitamin E and B vitamins for stress, a caffeine-containing supplement to give him energy, St. John's wort and kava for anxiety, valerian at night to help him sleep, and vitamin E and omega-3 fatty acids to protect against heart disease.

✴Nutrition Diagnosis: Excessive B-vitamin and vitamin E-intake related to self-report of supplement intake as evidenced by intake exceeding DRI levels.

1. Which foods would you recommend to help Matthew achieve his health goals?
2. What questions would you ask Matthew about the supplements he's taking?
3. Which other complementary approaches might be appropriate to help Matthew accomplish his health goals?
4. How would you counsel Matthew?

USEFUL WEBSITES

Arthritis Foundation Supplement Guide
http://www.arthritis.org/conditions/supplementguide/
  herbs.asp

CAM on PubMed
http://nccam.nih.gov/camonpubmed/

Computer access to research on dietary supplements
http://dietary-supplements.info.nih.gov/Research/
  CARDS_Database.aspx

Consumer Lab
http://www.consumerlab.com/

Food and Drug Administration—Dietary supplement advice
http://www.fda.gov/fdac/features/2002/202_supp.html

International Food Information Council
http://www.IFIC.org

MedWatch
http://www.fda.gov/medwatch/

National Center for Complementary and Alternative Medicine
http://nccam.nih.gov/

Office of Dietary Supplements
http://dietary-supplements.info.nih.gov/

References

Allam MF, Lucane RA: Selenium supplementation for asthma, *Cochrane Database Syst Rev* CD003538, 2004.

Allen SJ et al: Probiotics for treating infectious diarrhea, *Cochrane Database Syst Rev*, CD003048, 2004.

Ang-Lee MK et al: Herbal medicines and perioperative care, *JAMA* 286:208, 2001.

Archer SL: Association of dietary supplement use with specific micronutrient intakes among middle-aged American men and women: the INTERMAP Study, *J Am Diet Assoc* 105:1106, 2005.

Atallah AN et al: Calcium supplementation during pregnancy for preventing hypertensive disorders and related problems, *Cochrane Database Syst Rev*, (1):CD001059, 2002.

Avenell A et al: Selenium supplementation for critically ill adults, *Cochrane Database Syst Rev*, CD003703 October 18, 2004.

Barnes P et al: *Complementary and alternative medicine use among adults, United States 2002*, CDC Advance Data Report No. 343, May 27, 2004.

Birks J et al: Ginkgo biloba for cognitive impairment and dementia, *Cochrane Database Syst Rev*, CD003120, 2002.

Bjeclakovic G et al: *Cochrane Database Syst Rev* 18(4):CD004183, 2004.

Blumenthal M, editor: *The Complete German Commission E Monographs: Therapeutic Guide to Herbal Medicines*, Elsevier, St. Louis, 2000.

Chernoff R: Micronutrient requirements in older women, *Am J Clin Nutr* 81(5):1204S, 2005.

Cohen MH et al: Policies pertaining to complementary and alternative medical therapies in a random sample of 39 academic health centers, *Alternative Ther Health Med* 11(1):36, 2005a.

Cohen MH et al: Emerging credentialing practices, malpractice liability policies, and guidelines governing complementary and alternative medical practices and dietary supplement recommendations: a descriptive study of 19 integrative health care centers in the United States, *Arch Intern Med* 165(3): 289, 2005b.

DeBusk RM: *Herbs as medicine: what you should know*, Tallahassee, Fla, 2000, PR Treadwell.

Dietary Supplement Health and Education Act of 1994, Public law 103-417, October 25, 1994.

Dwyer JT et al: Dietary supplements in weight reduction, *J Am Diet Assoc* 105:80S, 2005.

Eberhart LHJ et al: Ginger does not prevent postoperative nausea and vomiting after laparoscopic surgery, *Anesth Analg* 96:995, 2003.

Eichenberger JM et al: Longitudinal patterns of vitamin and mineral supplement use in young white children, *J Am Diet Assoc* 105:763, 2005.

Ernst E: Efficacy of ginger for nausea and vomiting: a systematic review of randomized clinical trials, *Br J Anaesth* 84:367, 2000.

Ernst E: The efficacy of herbal medicine-an overview, *Fundamental Clin Pharmacol* 19: 405, 2005.

Evans JR: Antioxidant vitamin and mineral supplements for age-related macular degeneration, *Cochrane Database Syst Rev* CD00254, 2002.

Fletcher RH, Fairfield KM: Vitamins for chronic disease prevention in adults: clinical applications, *JAMA* 287: 3127, 2002.

Foote JA: Factors associated with dietary supplement use among healthy adults of five ethnicities: the Multiethnic Cohort Study, *Am J Epidemiol* 157(10):888, 2003.

Gillespie WJ et al: Vitamin D and vitamin D analogues for preventing fractures associated with involutional and post-menopausal osteoporosis, *Cochrane Database Syst Rev* CD000227, 2001.

Graham RE et al: Use of complementary and alternative medical therapies among racial and ethnic minority adults: results from the 2002 National Health Interview Survey, *J Natl Med Assoc* 97(4):535, 2005.

Gunther S: Demographic and health-related correlates of herbal and specialty supplement use, *J Am Diet Assoc* 104:27, 2004.

Hilton M, Stuart E: Ginkgo biloba for tinnitus, *Cochrane Database Syst Rev*, CD003852, 2004.

Holmquist C: Multivitamin Supplements Are Inversely Associated with Risk of Myocardial Infarction in Men and Women-Stockholm Heart Epidemiology Program (SHEEP), *J Nutr* 133:2650-2654, 2003.

Hooper L et al: Omega 3 fatty acids for prevention and treatment of cardiovascular disease, *Cochrane Database Syst Rev*, CD003177, October 18, 2004.

Huppert FA, Van Hiekerk JK: Dehydroepiandrosterone (DHEA) supplementation for cognitive function, *Cochrane Database Syst Rev*, CD000304 2001.

Jacobs EJ et al: Multivitamin use and colorectal cancer incidence in a U.S. cohort: does timing matter? *Am J Epidemiol* 158(7):621, 2003.

Jasti S: Dietary supplement use in the context of health disparities: cultural, ethnic and demographic determinants of use, *J Nutr* 133(6):2010S, 2003.

Jepson RG et al: Cranberries for preventing urinary tract infections, *Cochrane Database Syst Rev*, CD001321, 2004.

Jepson RG et al: Garlic for peripheral arterial occlusive disease, *Cochrane Database Syst Rev*, CD000095, 2000.

Karp RJ et al: The appearance of discretionary income: influence on the prevalence of under and over nutrition, *Int J Equity Health* 28:4, 2005.

Kumar NB et al: Use of complementary/integrative nutritional therapies during cancer treatment: implications in clinical practice, *Cancer Control* 9:236, 2002.

Ledikwe JH et al: Dietary patterns of rural adults are associated with weight and nutritional status, *J Am Geriatr Soc* 52(4):589, 2004.

Linde K et al: St John's wort for depression, *Cochrane Database Syst Rev*, CD000448 April 18, 2005.

Malourf M et al: Folic acid with or without vitamin B_{12} for cognition and dementia, *Cochrane Database Syst Rev*, CD004514, 2003.

Manusirivithaya S et al: Antiemetic effect of ginger in gynecologic oncology patients receiving cisplatin, *Int J Gynecol Cancer* 14:1063, 2004

McKay DL: The effects of a multivitamin/mineral supplement on micronutrient status, antioxidant capacity and cytokine production in healthy older adults consuming a fortified diet, *J Am College Nutr* 19(5): 613, 2000.

Melchart D et al: Echinacea for preventing and treating the common cold, *Cochrane Database Syst Rev*, CD000530, 2000.

Millen AE: Use of vitamin, mineral, nonvitamin, and nonmineral supplements in the United States: the 1987, 1992, and 2000 National Health Interview Survey results, *J Am Diet Assoc* 104:942, 2004.

National Center for Complementary and Alternative Medicine (NCCAM): *NCCAM funding: appropriations history,* www.nccam.nih.gov/news/camsurvey.htm, accessed December 8, 2005.

Picciano FM: Who is using dietary supplements and what are they using? Presented at the Food, Nutrition Conference Expo, St. Louis, October 21, 2005.

Pittler MH, Ernst E: Kava extract for treating anxiety, *Cochrane Database Syst Rev,* CD003383, 2003.

Ram FS et al: Vitamin C supplementation for asthma, *Cochrane Database Syst Rev,* CD000993, 2004.

Rambaldi A et al: Milk thistle for alcoholic and/or hepatitis B or C virus liver diseases, *Cochrane Database Syst Rev,* CD003620, April 18, 2005.

Shea B et al: Calcium supplementation on bone loss in postmenopausal women, *Cochrane Database Syst Rev,* CD004526, 2004.

Simpson N, Roman K: Complementary medicine use in children: extent and reasons: a population-based study, *Br J Gen Pract* 914, 2001.

Sommerfield T, Hyatt WR: Omega-3 fatty acids for intermittent claudication, *Cochrane Database Syst Rev,* CD003833, 2004.

Thomson CA et al: Practice Paper of the American Dietetic Association: Dietary supplements, *J Am Diet Assoc* 105(3):460, 2005.

Thomson CA et al: Proposed guidelines regarding the recommendation and sale of dietary supplements, *J Am Diet Assoc* 102(8):1158, 2002.

Tindle HA et al: Trends in use of complementary and alternative medicine by U.S. adults: 1997-2002, *Altern Ther Health Med* 11(1):42, 2005.

Weingarten MA et al: Dietary calcium supplementation for preventing colorectal cancer and adenomatous polyps, *Cochrane Database Syst Rev,* CD003548, 2004.

Wilt T et al: Serenoa repens for benign prostatic hyperplasia, *Cochrane Database Syst Rev,* CD001423 2002.

Wyatt G, Post-White J: Future direction of complementary and alternative medicine (CAM) education and research, *Semin Oncol Nurs* 21(3):215, 2005.

Zeng X et al: Ginkgo biloba for acute ischaemic stroke, *Cochrane Database Syst Rev,* CD003691, October 19, 2005.

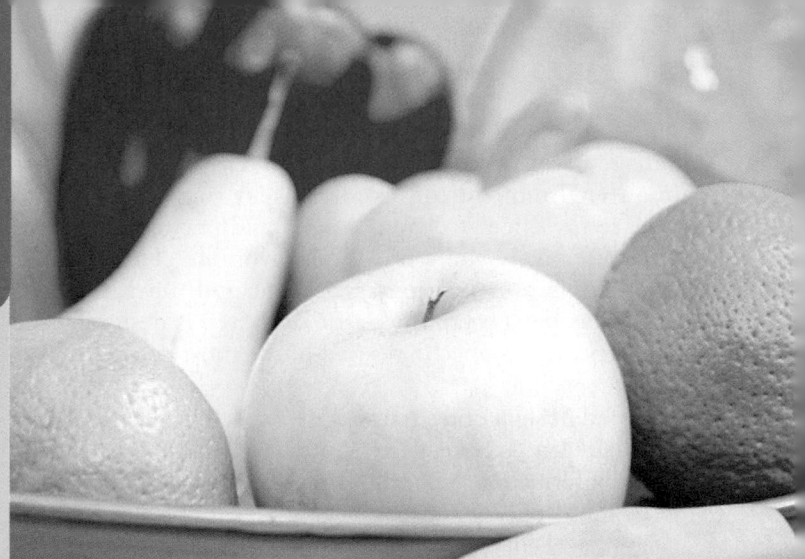

CHAPTER 19

Linda G. Snetselaar, RD, LD, PhD

Intervention: Counseling for Change

KEY TERMS

affirms supports the client's change efforts

alignment presenting a supportive statement to a client indicating that the counselor understands and is empathetic

ambivalence a client's mixed feelings about difficult change-modifying behaviors

cognitive-behavioral therapy therapy in which maladaptive thoughts (cognitions) are modified; problem-solving and coping skills are enhanced

cultural sensitivity respecting and understanding the attitudes, values, and beliefs of others; willingness to use cultural knowledge while interacting with clients

discrepancy strategy that identifies conflicting feelings when change results in both positive and negative consequences

double-sided reflection statement from the counselor describing a discrepancy between the client's current and previous words that provides ideas for open discussion to facilitate change

empathy technique by which the counselor accepts a client's feelings of turmoil about making changes

motivational interviewing (MI) counseling style designed to achieve the willingness to change within a client; responsibility is assigned to the client, but the counselor style is persuasive and supportive

negotiation strategy whereby the client and counselor interaction allows for a compromise designed to achieve a specific goal

normalization statement indicating that the client's behavior is perfectly within reason and normal; validates the client's reaction to a given situation

reflective listening guessing at what a client feels and stating that feeling; promotes understanding on the part of the counselor

reframing strategy whereby the counselor changes the client's interpretation of the same basic data that he or she has given and offers a new viewpoint

self-efficacy client's belief in his or her ability to carry out change

self-management strategy whereby the counselor facilitates the ability to change through the client's decisions

self-monitoring client's recording of behavior changes

transtheoretical model (TM) or **stages of change model** that describes behavior change as a process in which individuals progress through a series of six distinct stages: precontemplation, contemplation, preparation, action, maintenance, and relapse

The author would like to thank Victoria Poppelaars, MS, RD, LD, for her assistance in writing the multicultural section in this chapter.

People are motivated to change through their ability to manage their own behaviors. The nutrition counselor sets up an environment that is a transient support system to prepare the client to handle social and personal demands more effectively while providing favorable conditions for change. After a nutrition assessment and nutrition diagnosis have been established, the next step is designing the intervention. Counseling is one of the most complex types of intervention.

Different skills and strategies are needed to offer individualized guidance. Several steps are used: raising awareness, giving information (education), addressing client concerns, providing dietary guidelines, correcting misinformation, encouraging clients to visualize themselves in a healthier lifestyle, substituting positive behaviors for unhealthy ones, identifying barriers to success, offering encouragement, supporting a strong sense of **self-efficacy,** a client's belief in his or her

ability to carry out change, and providing social support. Equally as important as the client's sense of self-efficacy is the understanding by the counselor of his or her own psychological issues and background (see *Clinical Insight:* The Counselor Looks Within). Being aware of personal biases and approaches allows the counselor to be more effective in understanding what the client needs in order to move forward.

SOCIAL BEHAVIOR AND CULTURAL COMPETENCY

Social Behavior

Behavior does not occur in a vacuum. Consider what a person is giving up if he or she makes a change. There are

---

✳ CLINICAL INSIGHT

The Counselor Looks Within

Before entering a counseling relationship, the counselor should look inward and consider how the following factors affect his or her own thinking and how they impact the client:

Relationship Between Sense of Self and Life Choices
- Personal attributes for healthy change
- Extrinsic versus intrinsic motivation
- Defining success–personal preference

Barriers and Complexities to Life Enhancing Changes
- Distorted or irrational beliefs versus rational thinking
- The internal critic
- Ambivalence (desire versus should)
- Diffused sense of self

Origin and Influences on Thinking and Beliefs
- Gender, race, cultural scripts and expectations
- Parenting style
- Conformity versus autonomy
- Adversity and unmet needs
- Loss of own voice and individuality

Connecting Thoughts, Feelings and Beliefs
- Vicious cycle–remaining stuck versus unhealthy choices
- Why change fails
- Stages of change

Behavioral Outcome and Protecting the Fragile Self
- Procrastination
- Victimization
- Perfectionism
- Avoidance
- Escapism
- Defensiveness
- Apathy
- Excessive anger

Common Clinical Manifestations
- Depression
- Anxiety disorders
- Addictions
- Inability to self-regulate
- Unhealthy belief system

Strategies to Motivate Change
- Focus on negative outcome of choices
- Fear tactics
- Categorizing or labeling
- Giving advice
- Education alone: knowledge doesn't solve the problem
- Fostering dependency
- Reinforcing irrational beliefs
- Extrinsic rewards

Template for Change
- Challenge personal distorted beliefs
- Guidelines and questions that reinforce rationality
- Techniques for strengthening efficacy
- Acquire cognitive and behavioral skills to manage anxiety
- Negotiate behavioral plans that work

Effective Facilitator Skills
- Modeling, that is, walk the talk
- Facilitate internal motivation

"costs" and "benefits" of adopting new behaviors, and counselors must keep an open mind and consider the social milieu in which the client lives. Partners, families, colleagues, the media, and other influences all impact behavior. Ignoring the impact of one's culture (neighborhood, beliefs, background experiences) on behavior has adverse consequences for efforts at individual and social change (Shinn and Touhey, 2003).

Multicultural Counseling

Multicultural awareness is the first step toward becoming competent in nutrition counseling. Evaluation of one's own beliefs and attitudes and being comfortable with the differences (race, ethnicity, beliefs, culture, and food practices) that may exist between oneself and clients is the first and most important step (see Tables 12-7 and 12-8 in Chapter 12).

Current demographic trends have created a growing need for cultural competence in all professions. One of the most essential competencies in the delivery of health care is effective multicultural communication. In the United States the racial and ethnic composition of the population is rapidly changing. Between the years 1980 and 1990 there was an increase in all the ethnic populations except the white group (Sockalingam, 2002). By the year 2080 it is estimated that 51.1% of the total U.S. population will be composed mostly of Hispanics, followed by blacks and Asians (Tate, 2003).

Intercultural communication is a complex field that not only encompasses language but also the context in which words are interpreted, including posture, gestures, concepts of time, spatial relationships, the role of the individual within a group, status and hierarchy of persons, and the setting (Satia-Abouta, 2005). Each culture involves a series of values, ideas, assumptions, and beliefs about life and a common system of encoding and decoding verbal and nonverbal messages (Ulrey and Amason, 2001). It is easy for miscommunication to occur when individuals of different cultures interact with one another.

Generally clients do not share the terminology, norms, and assumptions of the health care profession culture. Therefore it is a challenge to communicate sensibly and effectively to promote health, relieve discomfort, and save lives (Robinson, 2002). Clients often only understand 59% of what they are told, and not surprisingly this percentage is lower for native Spanish-speaking clients (Ulrey and Amason, 2001).

Ineffective communication in health care can result in incorrect diagnoses, noncompliance with treatment, unnecessary pain and suffering, and even death (Van Wieringen et al., 2002). **Cultural sensitivity** or awareness involves respecting and understanding the attitudes, values, and beliefs of others; willingness to use cultural knowledge while interacting with clients; and considering culture during discussions and recommendations for treatment (Ulrey and Amason, 2001).

Verbal messages communicate content, whereas nonverbal messages convey information about relationships. The way in which cultures combine verbal and nonverbal messages to transmit a message determines the context of the communication (Kittler and Sucher, 2001). See Table 19-1 for differences in cultural styles.

The role of the individual within the cultural group can also greatly impact health care delivery. Clients from individual-oriented cultures enjoy confidentiality and privacy of individual health care issue; whereas clients from group-oriented cultures require greater participation of their families and relatives in decisions affecting health and illness.

Spatial relationships vary among cultures and among individuals. For example, Latinos enjoy personal closeness with friends and acquaintances. Middle Easterners prefer to be within 2 feet of whomever they are communicating with so they can observe their eyes. Blacks are likely to be offended if a person tries to increase the distance between them. Intercultural communication is most successful when preferences are understood (Kittler and Sucher, 2001).

Movements such as gestures, facial expressions, and postures are often the cause of confusion and misinterpretations in intercultural communication. Good posture is an important sign of respect in nearly all cultures. Rules regarding eye contact are usually complex and vary according to issues such as gender, distance apart, and social status.

A good way to develop rapport is by finding out how the client prefers to be addressed. Although in America it is common to call strangers and acquaintances by their given names, nearly all other cultures expect a more respectful approach. Listening sensitivity, sharing control, accepting differences, demonstrating sincere concern, respecting other cultures, seeking feedback, and being natural and honest are strategies important to achieving patient compliance and satisfaction (Kittler and Sucher, 2001; Patterson, 2004).

When working with clients who are limited in English, always use common terms, avoiding those with multiple meanings and avoiding slang. Always speak directly to the client, even when using a translator, and watch the client for nonverbal responses during the translation.

Many dietetics professionals have not developed appropriate counseling skills and may have little or no preparation in applying cultural concepts to practice. Consequently cultural factors may be neglected in dietary assessment and interventions. The universal system of counseling (Patterson, 2004) suggests that all counselors should be competent in five basic techniques (Table 19-2). Using all of these techniques will help make the counseling sessions more effective and satisfying for all parties.

THE INDIVIDUAL CLIENT AND MODELS FOR BEHAVIORAL CHANGE

Health professionals can support individuals in making sustainable lifestyle changes by using a range of behavioral techniques: assessing readiness to change; cognitive restructuring; realistic goal setting; strategies for dietary change

TABLE 19-1

Cultural Communication Styles

	Native Americans	Asians	Latinos	Middle Easterners	Whites	Blacks
	Speak slowly and softly	Speak softly	Speak softly; many perceive normal white voice as yelling	Speak softly	Speak loudly, fast; control of listener	Speak fast, with affect and rhythm
	Indirect gaze when speaking and listening	Avert eyes as sign of respect	Avert eyes as sign of respect	Direct gaze, man to man and woman to woman, but woman may avert eyes with man	Eye contact when speaking and listening; staring rude	Direct eye contact when speaking (may avert if prolonged); look away when listening
	Seldom make responses to indicate listening or offer encouragement to continue; rarely interject	Seldom make responses to indicate listening or offer encouragement to continue; rarely interject	Seldom make responses to indicate listening or offer encouragement to continue; rarely interject	Facial gestures responsive	Head nodding, murmuring	Interject often (turn taking)
	Delayed auditory (silence valued)	Mild auditory delay (silence valued)	Mild auditory delay	Mild auditory delay	Quick response	Quicker response
	Expression restrained	Polite, restrained; articulation of feelings considered immature	Men restrained, women expressive	Very expressive, emotional	Task-oriented, focused	Very expressive, demonstrative
	Prefer direct approach	Prefer indirect approach; may appear indifferent	Prefer indirect approach	Prefer indirect approach	Prefer direct approach, minimum small talk	Respectful, prefer direct approach
	Rarely ask questions; yes/no responses considered complete	Rarely ask questions	Will ask questions when encouraged	Will ask polite questions	Will ask direct questions	Assertive questioning
	Smile, handshake (not vigorous) customary greeting	Touching between strangers considered inappropriate	Shake hands, embrace, kiss cheeks, pat backs, sit and stand closer	Numerous greeting rituals, mild handshake; sit or stand very close, frequent touching (but not backslapping), use hands while speaking	Firm handshake, smile greeting; moderate touching (shoulder patting, backslapping)	Firm handshake, smile, hugging, kissing greeting; reluctance to touch may be interpreted as personal rejection

From Kittler PG, Sucher KP: *Food and culture*, ed 3, Belmont, Calif, 2001, Wadsworth, Thomson Learning, Inc, pp. 56-57. Reprinted with permission.

TABLE 19-2

Competencies for Effective Intercultural Counseling

Respect for the client	Having trust in the client and his or her capability of making choices and decisions, and solving problems
Genuineness	The counselor is a real person, not an all-knowing, objective expert
Empathic understanding	The ability to convey empathy in a culturally consistent and meaningful manner
Communication of empathy, respect, and genuineness to the client	The conditions must be felt, recognized, and perceived by the client if they are to be effective
Structuring	The counselor should define and structure his or her role to the client; there should be an indication of what, how, and why he or she intends to do the proposed interaction or program

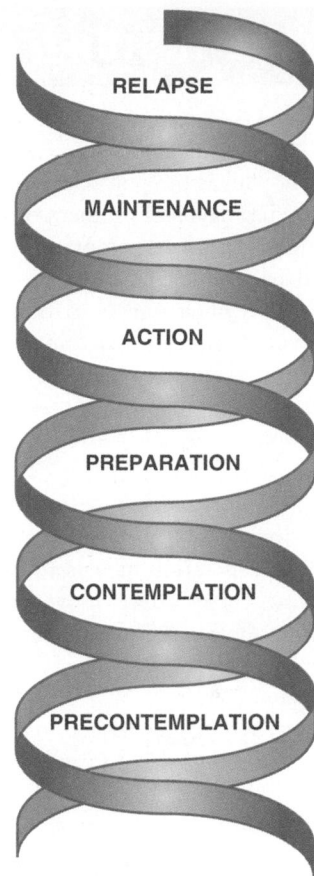

FIGURE 19-1 A spiral model of the stages of change. In changing, a person moves up this spiral to maintenance. If relapse occurs, he or she must reenter the spiral again at some point.

and increased physical activity; self-monitoring; stimulus control; relapse management; and ongoing support (Costain and Croker, 2005). Several of these techniques are described in the following paragraphs.

Transtheoretical Model of Change

The **transtheoretical model (TM),** or **stages of change model,** has been used for many years to alter addictive behaviors. The TM describes behavior change as a process in which individuals progress through a series of six distinct stages of change, as shown in Figure 19-1: (1) precontemplation, (2) contemplation, (3) preparation, (4) action, (5) maintenance, and (6) relapse (Prochaska and DiClemente, 1982, 1984, 1986; Prochaska et al., 1992, 1994; Sigman-Grant, 1996) (see *Clinical Insight:* Stages of Change).

Research data have shown that the value of the TM is in determining in which stage an individual is and then using change processes matched to that stage (Resnicow et al., 2006). Behavior change is more successful using this approach rather than the traditional model of assigning the same intervention techniques to everyone, regardless of the readiness or stage of change.

Traditional nutrition counseling focuses on the change process matched to the action and maintenance stages. This works well for persons who are actively trying to make a behavior change. However, most individuals with a problem dietary behavior are in a preaction stage that includes one of the following: precontemplation, contemplation, or preparation. These individuals are not yet ready to change (Sandoval et al., 1994; Sporny and Contento, 1995).

The traditional approach mistakenly assumes that the patient is already in the action or maintenance stage; this

may be one of the reasons for lack of success in long-term maintenance of many intervention programs (Resnicow et al., 2006; Prochaska et al., 1994). Additional behavioral trials are needed to choose the best health-related behavioral programs (Glasgow et al., 2006; Howard et al., 2006). For example, "augmented" care (dietary and exercise advice, prescriptions, and three dietary recalls every 6 months) seems to promote better long-term results than traditional care (Logue et al., 2005).

Cognitive-Behavioral Therapy

Cognitive-behavioral therapy (CBT) (Dobson, 1998) assumes that thinking affects behavior, that relevant beliefs may be identified and altered, and that desired behavior change may be achieved through changes in thinking (cognition). Cognitive restructuring has been helpful for many individuals.

CBT is an effective treatment for body-image difficulties and disorders because it promotes changes that are generalized to improved self-esteem, eating attitudes, and social anxiety. It is also useful to apply CBT in group therapy (e.g., to improve adherence to fluid restrictions among dialysis patients [Sharp et al., 2005] and to help weight-concerned smokers maintain smoking abstinence [Clark et al., 2005]).

Stages of Change

Precontemplation: This is the point at which the patient has not even contemplated having a problem or needing to make a change. A person in the precontemplative stage needs information and feedback to raise his or her awareness of the problem and possibility of change. Nutrition advice for eating changes is counterproductive at this point.

Contemplation: Once some awareness of the problem arises, the person enters a period of ambivalence: the contemplation stage. The contemplator seesaws between reasons to change and reasons to stay the same. At this stage the counselor works with the patient on advantages and disadvantages of making dietary changes.

Preparation: The preparation stage is a window of opportunity that either allows the patient to move forward or fall back into contemplation. At this point, the patient needs help in finding a change strategy or goal that is acceptable, achievable, and appropriate.

Action: The patient engages in actions that bring about change. At this point the goal is to produce a change in the problem area.

Maintenance: During this stage, the challenge is to sustain the change accomplished by previous action and to prevent relapse.

Relapse: If relapse occurs, the individual's task is to start the change process again rather than become stuck in this stage. Slips and relapses are normal, expected occurrences as a person seeks to change any long-standing pattern of behavior. The goal is to resume action efforts.

Data from Prochaska JO, Di Clemente CC: Transtheoretical therapy: toward a more integrative model of change, *Psychother Theory Res Pract* 20:161, 1982.

Motivational Interviewing

Motivational interviewing (MI) can be used to help clients recognize and begin to resolve their concerns and problems. The clients are responsible for making the changes. The goal is to increase intrinsic motivation so that clients are able to express the rationale for the changes. Persuasion and support are key elements of this style of counseling (Miller and Rollnick, 1991).

The following concepts are important to consider in facilitating dietary changes:

- People make behavioral changes only when they are ready to change.
- The nutrition intervention, including both the content and nutritionist's style, is a powerful determinant of resistance and denial, as well as motivation, in persons who want to make changes in their diet.
- People cycle through different phases of changing and maintaining their dietary modifications.

- Specific and distinctly different interventions are needed for people who are in phases of motivation that signal readiness, ambivalence, and a desire to remain in their current state.
- Ambivalence is a key deterrent to behavior change and can be resolved through intervention.
- Resistance and denial get in the way of meeting behavioral goals.

Studies point to the positive influence of MI on changes in dietary behavior. However, the literature lacks descriptions of randomized controlled trials using MI as a sole treatment modality for dietary behavior change. Although MI is useful in overcoming resistance and establishing clear motivation, once an individual is ready to make a change, other strategies such as behavioral therapy and cognitive behavioral therapy are needed (Resnicow et al., 2005a, 2005b, 2006). Larger, well-designed, randomized clinical trials using MI strategies are needed. In the meantime, use of MI has been shown to have a positive effect in many behavior change studies (Resnicow and Campbell, 2004).

ACTIVITIES THAT FACILITATE BEHAVIOR CHANGE

A variety of principles are important when determining what facilitates behavior change. The following six steps are important when working with individuals who struggle with behavior change:

1. Express empathy
2. Understand cultural factors
3. Develop discrepancy
4. Avoid arguments or defensiveness
5. Roll with resistance
6. Support self-efficacy

Each of these steps is described in further detail in the following sections.

Expressing Empathy

Empathy, counselor acceptance of what a client feels in times of turmoil, can often result in change. Acceptance facilitates change. A woman wrote a letter to her nutritionist saying that she wanted to stop working on her dietary changes. Life was too complicated, and the dietary changes were more than she could handle. The nutritionist reviewed potential scenarios to assist in solving this problem. One certainly was to take the woman's word seriously and allow her to drop out of the diet intervention process. Another was to immediately call the woman to discuss the letter, always indicating acceptance of the woman's concerns.

Beyond this acceptance is a skillful form of **reflective listening,** which allows the woman to describe her thoughts and feelings, while the nutritionist reflects back understanding. Many clients have no one with whom to discuss problems in their lives. This opportunity to have someone listen and understand the emotions behind the words is crucial to eventual dietary change. The intensity of reflective listening skills far outweighs the detail of knowledge about a nutrition topic and will result in greater levels of dietary change.

As clients review situations in their lives and lack of time for dietary changes, the counselor will hear **ambivalence.** On the one hand, clients want to make changes; on the other hand, they want to pretend that change is not important. Ambivalence is normal.

Client: I feel totally worthless. On one hand I want to follow this new eating pattern, and on the other I want to eat spontaneously, not worrying about decreasing my fat intake.

Nutrition Counselor: Your feelings are normal. You are having a difficult time merging new and old habits. This happens to many people.

Developing Discrepancy

An awareness of consequences is important. Identifying the advantages and disadvantages of modifying a behavior, or developing **discrepancy**, is a crucial process in making changes.

Client: I want to follow the new eating pattern, but so many things get in the way.

Nutrition Counselor: Let's make a list of the positives and negatives of following this new eating pattern.

Avoiding Arguments or Defensiveness

Arguments are counterproductive. A counselor's urges may lead in the direction of defending one's own ideas, but the result is frequently defensiveness on the part of the client. When a client resists, this is the signal to the counselor to change strategies.

Client: I just can't do everything right now. I just can't.

Nutrition Counselor: You are the best judge of what you can do. Perhaps we need to step back and wait for things in your life to calm down. Let's talk about what you can do and eliminate those things that are too difficult at this time. We can look at ways to meet your goals in the future. Now is the time to take care of pressing issues.

Rolling with Resistance

Invite new perspectives without imposing them. The client is a valuable resource in finding solutions to problems. Perceptions can be shifted, and the counselor's role is to help with this process. For example, a client who is wary of describing why she is not ready to change may become much more open to change if she sees openness to her resistive behaviors. When it becomes okay to discuss resistance, the rationale for its original existence may seem less important.

Client: I just feel that my level of enthusiasm for following the diet is low. It all seems like too much effort.

Nutrition Counselor: I appreciate your concerns. At this point in following a new diet, many people feel the same way. Tell me more about your concerns and feelings.

Supporting Self-Efficacy

Belief in the possibility of change is an important motivator. The client is responsible for choosing and carrying out personal change. Hope exists when there are alternative approaches to a problem.

Client: I just feel hopeless sometimes when I try to follow the diet.

Nutrition Counselor: Look at the progress you have made in 6 months. Your food records are a testimony to how much you have been able to change your eating habits. You can learn from your setbacks and do better in the future.

These concepts, along with other intervention models, shape the content of each contact described in the following motivational intervention model. This model is made up of an integration of the following theories: TM (Prochaska and DiClemente, 1982, 1986), MI (Miller and Rollnick, 1991), brief negotiation (Watson and Tharp, 1989), and behavioral self-management.

MOTIVATIONAL INTERVENTION MODEL

Interventions require careful planning by the counselor to be effective. The first step in an intervention is interviewing. Skills in knowing how to elicit information about eating habits are important as the assessment of the client's diet proceeds. The key to obtaining vital information that will later dictate treatment strategies involves initially establishing a counseling relationship.

Interviewing

The purpose of the client interview is to obtain information. A series of questions are asked in a nonthreatening manner to obtain background information that will guide the session. The session is opened with appropriate introductions of all individuals to one another. The client states why he or she is there. The counselor usually begins with broad, open-ended questions and closes the interview with closed-ended, follow-up questions.

First Session

The first session is an important time to establish the counseling relationship. The environment should be conducive to privacy, and there should be a plan for reduction of interruptions (e.g., no telephone calls, staff, or other patients knocking on the door). The counselor should be seated in a manner that reflects interest in the client, such as sitting directly across from one another in chairs without a desk as a barrier.

Communication skills and body language are also important (see *Clinical Insight:* Body Language and Communication Skills).

In an initial visit the counselor introduces the subject of the session. The following are samples:

- "The purpose of this visit is to see how you are doing in covering your dietary carbohydrate intake with insulin."
- "In looking at your monitoring tools, it seems that you have had excellent progress at some times and at other times it may have been more difficult."
- "Could we talk about your diet records to identify problems which we could solve?"

CLINICAL INSIGHT

Body Language and Communication Skills

Active listening forms the basis for effective nutrition counseling. There are two aspects to effective listening: nonverbal and verbal. Nonverbal listening skills consist of varied eye contact, attentive body language, a respectful but close space, adequate silence, and encouragers. Eye contact is direct yet varied. Lack of eye contact implies that the counselor is too busy to spend time with the client. When the counselor leans forward slightly and has a relaxed posture and avoids fidgeting and gesturing, the client will be more at ease. Showing the client respectful but close space is another important nonverbal message. Silence can give the client time to think and provide positive time for the counselor to contemplate what the client has said. Shaking one's head in agreement can be a positive encourager, leading to more conversation. Moving forward slightly toward the client is an encourager that allows for more positive interaction.

Verbal components of listening include keeping the focus on the client by demonstrating a willingness to listen. Often the nutritionist feels obligated to solve a problem or give advice. These two desires can decrease the time left for active listening. Emphasize questions that are open to detailed descriptions. Use questions that begin with "what," "how," "why," and "could."

Two types of encouragers are important in counseling: paraphrasing and summarizing. Paraphrasing is a brief repeat of the essence of what the speaker has said, using fresh and concise wording. It is not parroting or word-swapping. Paraphrasing is not easy and requires careful listening and caring. Summarizing is more lengthy than paraphrasing because it uses more information and summarizes what has been said over a period of time. In general, it is important to establish the interactive relationship before beginning the actual process of nutrition counseling.

The following approaches might be used during a follow-up contact:

- "I talked to you about a month ago to see how you were doing with your carbohydrate levels for each meal and insulin dosage."
- "I'd like to see if you have made any changes or had any further thoughts on meeting your saturated fat–intake goals."

To make the stages of change model less complicated, an alternative is to view the stages in terms of three phases:

Stage 1: Not ready to change
Stage 2: Unsure about meeting goals
Stage 3: Ready to change

To identify in which of these three stages a patient is, it is important to assess the patient's situation (Figure 19-2).

Assessment

The purpose of assessment is to identify the client's stage of change and to provide appropriate help in facilitating change. The assessment should be completed in the first visit if possible. If conversation extends beyond the designated time for the session, the assessment steps should be completed at the next session. The stage of readiness for change should be assessed and documented.

Establishing Rapport

To build rapport, one begins by asking one or two questions that are relevant to important aspects of the client's life.

- "Tell me about how _____ (e.g., hobby or interest) is going?"
- "We have about _____ minutes to meet today. I thought we might talk about how you're doing with your dietary changes. How does this sound to you?"

Assessment of Current Eating Behavior

Determining present eating habits provides ideas on how to change in the future. See Chapter 14 for details on dietary assessment. A few questions used to assess current eating behavior follow.

- "How do you limit the amount of saturated fat in your diet now?"
- "Would you say that you are eating a low–saturated fat diet now?"
- "During the past 6 months have you thought about changes that you could make to reduce the amount of saturated fat in your diet?"
- "In the next month do you plan to make any changes to reduce the amount of saturated fat in your diet?"

It is important to review client's recording of behavior changes, or **self-monitoring** tools or assess where the client sees his or her adherence level. Food diaries help identify eating habits and potential modifications.

Using a ruler that allows the client to select his or her level of adherence to the diet is one method of allowing client participation in the discussion of dietary adherence. You might say, "The ruler will help us see where you are in terms of changing your diet. On a scale of 1 to 12, to what extent would you say you are meeting your goal of changing your diet in the past month? (1 = absolutely never; 12 = absolutely always)."

Explore eating behaviors by using the following statements:

• "Tell me about your progress so far."
• "Why did you choose that number on the ruler? Why did you not choose 1? Why did you not choose 12?"

• "How do you generally feel about following this new eating pattern?"

Always provide positive confidence-building statements:

• "It is great that you _____."
• "You've worked really hard at this."

To elicit responses from the client on ideas about where changes in the diet need to occur, it is helpful to provide feedback on the client's progress toward a goal. Show the client an example of his or her progress. Indicate what the

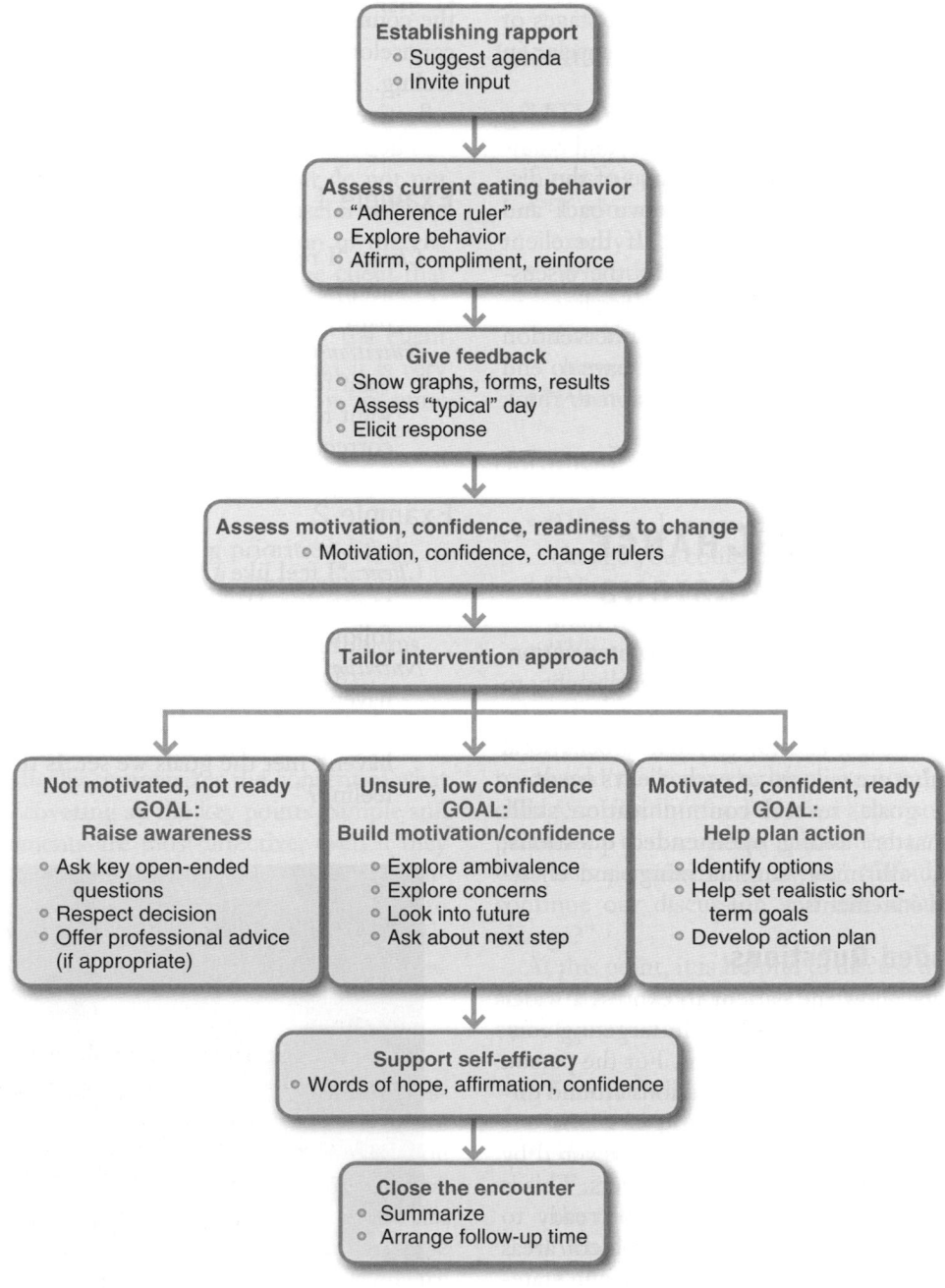

FIGURE 19-2 Algorithm of motivational intervention. *(Data from Miller WR, Rollnick S, editors: Motivational interviewing: preparing people for change, ed 2, New York, 2002, Guilford Press.)*

To show real understanding about what the client is saying, summarizing the statements about his or her progress, difficulties, possible reasons for change, and what needs to be different to move forward, is beneficial. This paraphrasing will allow the patient to rethink his or her reasoning about readiness to change. The mental processing provides new ideas that can promote actual change.

Ending the Session

Counselors often expect a decision and at least a goal-setting session when working with a client. However, it is important in this stage to realize that traditional goal setting will result in feelings of failure on both the part of the client and the nutritionist.

If the client is not ready to change, respectful acknowledgment of this decision is important. The counselor might say, "I can understand why making a change right now would be very hard for you. The fact that you are able to indicate this as a problem is very important, and I respect your decision. Our lives do change, and, if you feel differently later on, I will always be available to talk with you. I know that, when the time is right for you to make a change, you will find a way to do it."

When the session ends, the counselor will let the client know that the issues will be revisited after he or she has time to think. Expression of hope and confidence in the client's ability to make changes in the future, when the time is right, will be beneficial. Arrangements for follow-up contact can be made at this time.

With a client who is not ready to change it is easy to become defensive and authoritarian. At this point it is important to avoid pushing, persuading, confronting, coaxing, or telling the client what to do. It is reassuring to a nutritionist to know that change at this level will often occur outside the office. The client is not expected to be ready to do something during the visit (see *New Directions: The RD Counselor as Life Coach*).

UNSURE-ABOUT-CHANGE COUNSELING SESSIONS

The only goal in this stage of change is to build readiness to change. This is the point at which changes in eating behavior can escalate. This "unsure" stage is a transition from not being ready to deal with a problem eating behavior to preparing to continue the change. It involves summarizing the client's perceptions of the barriers to a healthy eating style and how they are eliminated or circumvented to achieve change.

A restatement of the client's self-motivational statements assists in setting the stage for success. The client's ambivalence is discussed, listing the positive and negative aspects of change. The counselor can restate any statements that the client has made about intentions or plans to change or to do better in the future.

The RD Counselor as Life Coach

More and more registered dietitian (RD) nutrition counselors are turning to life coaching to enhance nutrition counseling skills and increase client success. Coaching moves the focus away from the RD as the expert who tells the client what to do, to realizing that clients do know how they want to accomplish their goals. Many clients already know the information the RD provides, but the RD can be most valuable by helping them apply that information.

Life coaching involves asking questions to help clients look within to answer the questions they didn't think of. It is not therapy; it is simply asking questions without an agenda. It is taking the client from where he or she is currently to where he or she wants to be. It is helping the client accomplish more sooner.

For more information on coaching and credentialing for coaches, contact the International Coaching Federation, the lead professional organization for life coaches at http://www.coachfederation.org/eweb/.

Courtesy of Marjorie Geiser, RD, NSCA-CPT

One crucial aspect of this stage is the process of discussing thoughts and feelings about current status. Use of open-ended questions encourages the client to discuss dietary change progress and difficulties. Change is promoted through discussions focused on possible reasons for change. The counselor might ask the question: "What would need to be different to move forward?"

This stage is characterized by feelings of ambivalence. The counselor should encourage the client to explore ambivalence to change by thinking about "pros" and "cons." Some questions to ask are:

- "What are some of the things you like about your current eating habits?"
- "What concerns you about your current eating habits?"
- "What are some of the good things about making a new or additional change?"
- "What are some of the things that are not so good about making a new or additional change?"

By trying to look into the future, the counselor can help a client see new and often positive scenarios. As a change facilitator, the counselor helps to tip the balance away from being ambivalent about change toward considering change, by guiding the client to talk about what life might be like after a change, anticipating the difficulties as well as the advantages.

An example of an opening to generate discussion with the client follows: "I can see why you're unsure about making new or additional changes in your eating habits. Imagine that you decided to change. What would that be like? What would you want to do?" The counselor then summarizes the client's statements about the "pros" and "cons" of making a change and includes any statements about wanting, intending, or planning to change.

The next step is to negotiate a change. There are three parts to the **negotiation** process. The first is setting goals. Set broad goals at first and hold more specific nutritional goals until later. "How would you like things to be different from the way they are?" and "What is it that you would like to change?"

The second step is to consider options. The counselor asks about alternative strategies and options and then asks the client to choose from among them. This is effective because, if the first strategy does not work, the client has other choices. The third step is to arrive at a plan, one that has been devised by the client. The counselor touches on the key points and the problems and then asks the client to write down the plan.

To end the session the counselor asks about the next step, allowing the client to describe what might occur next in the process of change. The following questions provide some ideas for questions that might promote discussion:

- "Where do you think you will go from here?"
- "What do you plan to do between now and the next visit?"
- "Where does this leave you now?"

Arranging for the Next Contact

The counselor must take this process slowly and not assume that the client is ready to change. In a rush to help, counselors often give advice too soon. An astute counselor will avoid giving advice about change and will not feel badly if the client does not agree to change. The counselor might offer the following: "You say you're unsure about what to do. I will not push you into a decision. It is up to you. Take your time to think about it. Let me know if you want to talk about it again. You have made changes in the past, and you are the best judge of when it is the best time to consider change."

READY-TO-CHANGE COUNSELING SESSIONS

The major goal in this stage of change is to collaborate with the client to set goals for change that include a plan of action. The nutrition counselor provides the client with the tools to use in meeting nutrition goals.

This is the stage of change that is most often assumed when a counseling session begins. To erroneously assume this stage means that inappropriate counseling strategies set the stage for failure. The *assumption of this stage often results in lack of adherence on the part of the client and discouragement on the part of the nutritionist.*

Initially it is important to discuss the client's thoughts and feelings about where he or she stands relative to current dietary change status. Use of open-ended questions helps the client confirm and justify the decision to make a change. The following questions may elicit information about feelings toward change:

- "Tell me why you picked _____ on the ruler."
- "Why did you pick _____ instead of 1 or 12?"
- "Give me some ideas for why you think you are ready to change."

Helping the client to identify change options by asking if he or she would like to change and what a first step might be is an effective method. The following questions might help the client identify options:

- "What could you do to change your eating habits?"
- "Is this feasible?"
- "How do you see things turning out if you make these changes?"

This is the stage in which goal setting is extremely important. Here the counselor helps the client set a realistic and achievable short-term goal. "Let's do things gradually. What is a reasonable first step?"

Action Plan

Following goal setting, an action plan is set to assist the client in mapping out the specifics of goal achievement. Identifying a network to support dietary change is important. What can others do to help?

Early identification of barriers to adherence is important. If barriers are identified, plans can be formed to help eliminate these roadblocks to adherence.

Many clients fail to notice when their plan is working. Ask the clients to summarize their plans and identify markers of success. The counselor then documents the plans for discussion at future sessions and ensures that the clients also have their plans in writing.

The session should be closed with an encouraging statement and reflection about how the client identified this plan personally. Indicate that each person is the expert about his or her own behavior. Compliment the patient on carrying out the plan. Ways to express these ideas to clients are:

- "You are working very hard at this, and it's clear that you're the expert about what is best for you. You can do this!"
- "Keep in mind that change is gradual and takes time. If this plan doesn't work, there will be other plans to try."

Arranging for the Next Contact

The key point to remember for this stage is to avoid telling the client what to do. Clinicians often want to provide advice. However, it is critical that the client express ideas of what will work best. "There are a number of things you could do, but what do you think will work best for you?"

RESISTANCE BEHAVIORS AND POTENTIAL STRATEGIES TO MODIFY THEM

Irrespective of concerted efforts toward assessing readiness to change and affirming action and supporting change, the nutrition counselor will still be confronted with resistance behaviors. Resistance to change is the most consistent emotion or state that will be faced when dealing with clients who have difficulty with dietary adherence. Following are examples of resistance to change.

In one type of resistance the client contests the accuracy, expertise, or integrity of the nutrition counselor. In another type the client directly challenges the accuracy of what the nutrition counselor has said (i.e., the accuracy of the nutrition content). In a third type the client discounts the nutrition counselor by questioning his or her personal authority and expertise. Finally the nutrition counselor may be confronted with a hostile client. Below are examples of these types of behaviors.

Resistance may also surface as interrupting, when the client breaks in during a conversation in a defensive manner. In this case the client may speak while the nutrition counselor is still talking without waiting for an appropriate pause or silence. In another more obvious manner the client may break in with words intended to cut off the nutrition counselor's discussion.

When clients express an unwillingness to recognize problems, cooperate, accept responsibility, or take advice, they may be denying a problem. Some clients blame other people for their problems (e.g., a wife may blame her husband for her inability to follow a diet).

Clients may disagree with the nutrition counselor when a suggestion is offered, but they frequently provide no constructive alternative. This includes the familiar "Yes but . . .," which explains what is wrong with the suggestion but offers no alternative.

Clients try to excuse their behavior. They may say, "I want to do better, but my life is always in a turmoil since my husband died 3 years ago." An excuse that was once acceptable is reused even when it is no longer a factor in the woman's life.

Some clients will make pessimistic statements about themselves or others. This is done to dismiss an inability to follow an eating pattern by excusing poor compliance as just a given due to past behaviors. "My husband will never help me." "I have never been good at sticking with a goal. I'm sure I won't do well with it now."

In some cases clients are reluctant to accept options that may have worked for others in the past. They express reservations about information or advice given. "I just don't think that will work for me." Some clients will express a lack of willingness to change or an intention not to change. They make it very clear that they want to stop the dietary regimen.

Often clients show evidence of not following the nutrition counselor's advice. Clues that this is happening include using a response that does not answer the question, providing no response to a question, or changing the direction of the conversation.

These types of behavior can occur within a counseling session as clients move from one stage to another. They are not necessarily stage specific, although most are connected with either the not ready or unsure-about-change stages. A variety of strategies are available to assist the nutrition counselor in dealing with these difficult counseling situations. These strategies include: reflecting, double-sided reflection, shifting focus, agreeing with a twist, emphasizing personal choice, and reframing. Each of these options is described in the following paragraphs.

Reflecting

In reflecting the counselor identifies the client's emotion or feeling and reflects it back. This allows the client to stop and reflect on what was said. An example of this type of counseling skill is: "You seem to be very frustrated by what your husband says about your food choices."

Double-Sided Reflection

In **double-sided reflection** the counselor will use ideas that the client has expressed previously to show the discrepancy between the client's current words and the previous ones. For example:

Client: "I am doing the best I can." (Previously this client stated that she sometimes just gives up and doesn't care about following the diet.)

Nutrition Counselor: "On the one hand you say you are doing your best, but on the other hand I believe I recall that you said you just felt like giving up and didn't care about following the diet. Do you remember that? Was that point in time different than now?"

Shifting Focus

Clients may hold onto an idea that they think is getting in the way of their progress. The counselor might question the feasibility of continuing to focus on this barrier to change when other barriers may be more appropriate targets. For example:

Client: "I will never be able to follow this low–saturated fat diet as long as my grandchildren come to my house and want snacks."

Nutrition Counselor: "Are you sure that this is really the problem? Is part of the problem that you like those same snacks?"

Client: "Oh, you are right. I love them."

Nutrition Counselor: "Could you compromise? Could you ask your grandchildren which of this long list of low–saturated fat snacks they like and then buy them?"

Agreeing With a Twist

This strategy involves offering agreement, but then moving the discussion in a different direction. The counselor agrees with a piece of what the client says but then offers another perspective on his or her problems. This allows the opportunity to agree with her statement and her feeling, but then to redirect the conversation onto a key topic. For example:

Client: "I really like eating out, but I always eat too much, and my blood sugars go sky high."

Nutrition Counselor: "You are in the majority when you say that you like eating out. Now that you are retired it is easier to eat out than to cook. I can understand that. What can we do to make you feel great about eating out so that you can still follow your eating plan and keep your blood glucose values in the normal range?"

Reframing

With **reframing** the counselor changes the client's interpretation of the basic data by offering a new perspective. The counselor repeats the basic observation that the client has provided and then offers a new hypothesis for interpreting the data. For example:

Client: "I gave up trying to meet my dietary goals because I was having some difficulties when my husband died, and I have decided now that I just cannot meet those strict goals."

Nutrition Counselor: "I remember how devastated you were when he died and how just cooking meals was an effort. Do you think that this happened as a kind of immediate response to his death and that you might have just decided that all of the goals were too strict at that time?" (Pause)

Client: "Well, you are probably right."

Nutrition Counselor: "Could we look at where you are now and try to find things that will work for you now to help you in following the goals we have set?"

These strategies to help in dealing with the resistant client offer tools to ensure that nutrition counseling is not ended without appropriate attempts to turn difficult counseling situations in a positive direction.

Self-Efficacy and Self-Management

Counselors should always emphasize that any future action belongs to the client. Any advice given can be taken or disregarded. This emphasis on personal choice helps clients avoid feeling trapped and confined by the discussion. Encouraging in the client self-efficacy and **self-management,** the ability to change through his or her own decisions is and important and worthy goal of any counseling, including nutrition counseling. For more details on counseling skills for dietitians, use the latest Nutrition Care Process tools from the American Dietetic Association.

◉ FOCAL POINTS

- Counseling is a critical step in facilitating nutrition therapy self-management for clients and includes strategies for conveying expertise and theoretical knowledge so that the client can incorporate it into his or her life.
- Counseling involves studying the client's feelings, experiences, thoughts, beliefs, and attitudes and creating a strong connection, which allows guidance on the challenging journey of behavioral change.
- Any counseling relationship for the purpose of behavioral change begins with assessment of the client's readiness to change; too often this is forgotten and the client is left frustrated and the counselor feeling ineffective.
- Counseling can be rewarding, but at the same time it represents one of the greatest challenges for health care professionals.

✱ CLINICAL SCENARIO 1

Jane S. has struggled with changing her dietary fat intake and keeping her carbohydrate intake consistent over the past several months. She is concerned that she hasn't been doing well and wants to stop following the new style of eating and forget that she has type 2 diabetes.

✱**Nutrition Diagnosis:** Limited adherence to nutrition-related recommendations related to frustration with new eating plan as evidenced by food records showing no change and inconsistent carbohydrate intake

1. Reword this statement to indicate your own thoughts about the patient's statement above. What are some summarizing statements that you might make? What other open-ended questions could you ask to determine intention to change?
2. What does the patient's initial statement indicate about her stage of change? What patient conversation do these questions pertain to?
3. What are other directions you might take this interview to elicit self-motivational statements?
4. What are some problem recognition questions?
5. What questions would you ask to elicit patient concerns?
6. What questions might you ask to determine the patient's optimism relative to change?

⬡ CLINICAL SCENARIO 2

Mrs. Lee is originally from mainland China. She has been living in your area for several years and has numerous health problems, including high blood pressure and glaucoma. You have been asked to counsel her about making changes in her diet. Because her vision is poor, she will not be able to use printed materials that you have in your office that have been translated into Chinese.

∗Nutrition Diagnosis: Impaired ability to prepare food and meals related to inability to see as evidenced by patient report and history of glaucoma

1. What steps should you take to make her comfortable with this session?
2. Should you invite family members to attend the counseling session? Why or why not?
3. What tools might be useful to help Mrs. Lee understand portions or types of food that she should select?
4. Would a supermarket tour be useful? Why or why not?
5. What other types of information will be needed to help Mrs. Lee?

USEFUL WEBSITES

American Counseling Association
http://www.counseling.org/

American Dietetic Association—Nutrition Diagnosis and Intervention
http://eatright.org/

Counseling Relationships—Code of Ethics
http://www.counseling.org/resources/codeofethics.htm#ce

Cultural Competency
http://www.thinkculturalhealth.org/

Cultural Competency Resources
http://www.thinkculturalhealth.org/online_resources.asp

Cultural Competency with Adolescents
http://www.ama-assn.org/ama1/pub/upload/mm/39/culturallyeffective.pdf

Institute for Life Coach Training
http://www.lifecoachtraining.com/

International Coaching Federation
http://www.coachfederation.org/eweb/

Journal of Counseling Psychology
http://www.apa.org/journals/cou/

Office of Minority Health
http://www.omhrc.gov/

References

Clark MM et al: Body image treatment for weight concerned smokers: a pilot study, *Addict Behav* 30:1236, 2005.

Costain L, Croker H: Helping individuals to help themselves, *Proc Nutr Soc* 64(1):89, 2005.

Dobson KS: *Handbook of cognitive-behavioral therapies*, New York, 1998, Guilford Press.

Glasgow RE et al: Practical behavioral trials to advance evidence-based behavioral medicine, *Ann Behav Med* 31(1):5, 2006.

Howard BV et al: Low-fat dietary pattern and risk of cardiovascular disease: the Women's Health Initiative Randomized Controlled Dietary Modification Trial, *JAMA* 295(6):655, 2006.

Kittler PG, Sucher KP: *Food and culture*, ed 3, Belmont, Calif, 2001, Wadsworth, Thomson Learning.

Logue E et al: Transtheoretical model-chronic disease care for obesity in primary care: a randomized trial, *Obes Res* 13(5):917, 2005.

Miller W, Rollnick S: *Motivational interviewing: preparing people to change addictive behaviors*, New York, 1991, Guilford Press.

Patterson CH: Do we need multicultural counseling competencies? *J Mental Health Counseling* 26(1):67-73, 2004.

Prochaska JO, DiClemente CC: Transtheoretical therapy: toward a more integrative model of change, *Psychother Theory Res Pract* 20:161, 1982.

Prochaska JO, DiClemente CC: *The transtheoretical approach: crossing traditional boundaries of change*, Homewood, Ill, 1984, Dorsey Press.

Prochaska J, DiClemente C: Toward a comprehensive model of change. In Miller WR, Heather N, editors: *Treating addictive behaviors: processes of change*, New York, 1986, Plenum.

Prochaska JO et al: In search of how people change, *Am Psychol* 47:1102, 1992.

Prochaska JO et al: *Changing for good*, New York, 1994, William Morrow.

Resnicow K et al: Motivational interviewing for pediatric obesity: Conceptual issues and evidence review, *J Am Diet Assoc* 106:12, 2024, 2006.

Resnicow K, Campbell MK: Body and soul: a dietary intervention conducted through African-American churches, *Am J Prevent Med* 27:97, 2004.

Resnicow K et al: Results of Go Girls: a nutrition and physical activity intervention for overweight African-American adolescent females conducted through black churches, *Obes Res* 13(10):1739, 2005a.

Resnicow K et al: Results of the Healthy Body Healthy Spirit Trial, *Health Psychology* 24:339, 2005b.

Robinson M: *Communication and health in a multi-ethnic society*, Bristol, UK, 2002, Policy Press.

Sandoval WM et al: Stages of change: a model for nutrition counseling, *Topics Clin Nutr* 9:64, 1994.

Satia-Abouta J: Dietary acculturation: applications to nutrition research and dietetics, *J Am Diet Assoc* 102(8):1105, 2005.

Sharp J et al: A cognitive behavioral group approach to enhance adherence to hemodialysis fluid restrictions: a randomized controlled trial, *Am J Kidney Dis* 45:1046, 2005.

Shinn M, Toohey SM: Community contexts of human welfare, *Annu Rev Psychol* 54:427, 2003.

Sigman-Grant M: Stages of change: a framework for nutrition interventions, *Nutr Today* 31:162, 1996.

Sockalingam S: *Cultural competence in developing health promotion and intervention strategies: rhetoric or reality*, 2002, Northwest Obesity Prevention Project. http://depts.washington.edu/obesity/DocReview/Suganya/basedoc.html, accessed June 1, 2004.

Sporny LA, Contento IR: Stages of change in dietary fat reduction: social psychological correlates, *J Nutr Educ* 27:191, 1995.

Tate DM: Cultural awareness: bridging the gap between caregivers and Hispanic patients, *J Contin Educ Nurs* 35(5):213, 2003.

Ulrey KL, Amason P: Intercultural communication between patients and health care providers: an exploration of intercultural communication effectiveness, cultural sensitivity, stress and anxiety, *Health Communication* 13(4):449, 2001.

Van Wieringen JCM et al: Intercultural communication in general practice, *Eur J Public Health* 12(1):63-68, 2002.

Watson DL, Tharp RG: *Self-directed behavior: self-modification for personal adjustment*, ed 5, Pacific Grove, Calif, 1989, Brooks/Cole.

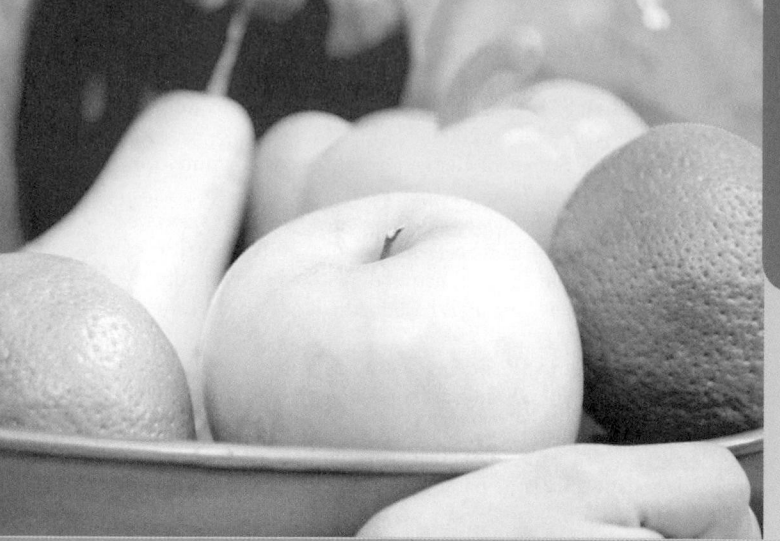

CHAPTER 20

Charles Mueller, PhD, RD, CNSD, CDN
Abby S. Bloch, PhD, RD, FADA

Intervention: Enteral and Parenteral Nutrition Support

KEY TERMS

bolus feeding infusion of up to 500 ml of enteral formula into the stomach over 5 to 20 minutes, usually with a large-bore syringe

catheter a fine tube that can be threaded into the lumen of a blood vessel for infusion of fluids or withdrawal of blood

central parenteral nutrition (CPN) vein, usually the superior vena cava

continuous drip infusion enteral formula administration into the gastrointestinal tract via pump, usually over 8 to 24 hours per day

cyclic central parenteral nutrition administration of total parenteral nutrition solution for 12 to 18 consecutive hours, usually at night, followed by a 6- to 12-hour period of no infusion

enteral nutrition provision of nutrients into the gastrointestinal tract through a tube when oral intake is inadequate

gastrointestinal decompression prevention of gaseous inflation (distention) of the gastrointestinal tract by the application of intermittent or continuous negative pressure (suction) through a nasogastric tube

hemodynamic stability the ability of a patient to maintain adequate blood pressure

intermittent drip feeding enteral formula administered at specified times throughout the day; generally in smaller volumes and at a slower rate than a bolus feeding but in larger volumes and at a faster rate than continuous feedings

lumen the interior area of a tube, catheter, or blood vessel

monomeric when referring to protein and carbohydrate, the form in which the nutrient has been hydrolyzed into its smaller parts

needle-catheter jejunostomy feeding opening used to provide small-bore needle insertion into the jejunum at time of surgery

osmolarity the number of milliosmoles of solute (particles) per liter of solution

osmolality the number of milliosmoles of solute (particles) per kilogram of solvent

parenteral nutrition provision of nutrients intravenously

percutaneous endoscopic gastrostomy (PEG) feeding tube, the insertion of which into the stomach involves using an endoscope and pulling the tube through a small incision in the abdominal wall

percutaneous endoscopic jejunostomy (PEJ) feeding tube inserted into the jejunum using an endoscopic technique

peripheral parenteral nutrition (PPN) delivery of nutrients into a smaller peripheral vein

pulmonary aspiration inadvertent inspiration into the lungs of body fluids such as vomitus from the stomach

rebound hypoglycemia low blood sugar resulting from abrupt cessation of total parenteral nutrition solutions

refeeding syndrome low serum levels of potassium, magnesium, and phosphorus with severe, potentially lethal outcome that results from the too-rapid infusion of substrates, particularly carbohydrate, into the plasma with the consequent release of insulin and shift of electrolytes into the intracellular space as glucose moves into the cells for oxidation and there is reduction in salt and water excretion

stoma artificially created opening between a body cavity and the body's surface that has healed

transitional feeding the process of progressing from one method of nutrition support to another or to oral feeding

Nutrition support is the delivery of formulated enteral or parenteral nutrients to appropriate patients for the purpose of maintaining or restoring nutritional status. **Enteral nutrition** refers to the provision of nutrients into the gastrointestinal tract through a tube or **catheter** when oral intake is inadequate. In certain instances enteral nutrition may include the use of formulas as oral supplements or meal replacements. **Parenteral nutrition** is the provision of nutrients intravenously.

RATIONALE AND CRITERIA FOR APPROPRIATE NUTRITION SUPPORT

Historically the use of enteral nutrition for acutely ill, postoperative, or posttrauma patients rested on evidence of bowel function as indicated by bowel sounds and flatus. These signs verify colonic motility. However, small bowel motility returns much sooner, within hours of surgery and trauma, and is the primary site of nutrient absorption. The feeding technique described by Abbott and Rawson (1939) required small bowel motility but not colonic and gastric motility. Using this technique requires **gastrointestinal decompression,** the prevention of gaseous inflation (distention) of the gastrointestinal tract by the application of intermittent or continuous negative pressure (suction) through a nasogastric tube. With this and concomitant small bowel feeding, enteral nutrition is now implemented in patients with small bowel function who previously were supported parenterally because their gastrointestinal function was assumed to be inadequate. Most practitioners agree that enteral nutrition presents fewer risks than parenteral nutrition and provides advantages to the patient that parenteral nutrition does not. Parenteral nutrition is reserved for patients with a nonfunctional or severely diminished (by virtue of surgery, obstruction, or infarction) small bowel.

Animal models and clinical observations in humans during enteral and parenteral nutrition support have focused on several perceived advantages of using enteral as opposed to parenteral nutrition in critical care settings: better gastrointestinal barrier function, preserved gastrointestinal immunity, and decreased rates of infection presumably unrelated to the gastrointestinal tract. The first observation led to the hypothesis that parenteral nutrition ("bowel rest") versus enteral nutrition, particularly during acute and critical illness, causes a breakdown of the gastrointestinal mucosal barrier and increases its permeability to bacteria and endotoxins, in turn contributing to sepsis syndrome and multiple organ dysfunction syndrome (Deitch, 1992) (see Chapter 39). This hypothesis has not been substantiated in humans (Lipman, 1995; Sedman, 1995).

The second observation focuses on the use of enteral as opposed to parenteral nutrition to preserve gastrointestinal immunity or gut-associated lymphoid tissue (GALT) activity, which may be compromised by bowel rest or parenteral nutrition (Jabbar et al., 2003) (see Chapter 27). GALT comprises half of total body immunity; immunoglobulin production is secreted across the gastrointestinal mucosa to defend against pathogenic substances in the gastrointestinal **lumen.** Despite considerable evidence of this phenomenon in animal models (Genton et al., 2005), it has not been substantiated in humans (Buchman et al., 1995). Nevertheless there is considerable evidence in animal and (indirectly) in human models that enteral nutrition preserves mucosal immunity in conditions of critical illness. These mechanisms maintain not only gastrointestinal (mucosal) immunity with enteral nutrition in the critically ill but also pulmonary (mucosal) immunity to both bacterial and viral infections. This may account for the observation in critically ill trauma patients that the incidence of infection, particularly pulmonary infections, is increased in parenterally as opposed to enterally fed patients (Moore et al., 1992; Kudsk et al., 1992).

There is no evidence suggesting that stable patients who are dependent on parenteral nutrition automatically translocate bacteria, become septic, or develop organ dysfunction (Jeejeebhoy, 2001). Such patients usually have less than 2 to 3 ft (60 to 100 cm) of functioning small bowel available for absorption of nutrients. For these persons, parenteral nutrition is life-sustaining therapy, and the risks of parenteral nutrition are outweighed by the benefit.

Criteria should be applied to select appropriate candidates for nutrition support (Table 20-1). Enteral nutrition should be used in patients who have at least 2 to 3 ft of functional gastrointestinal tract, who are or will become malnourished, and in whom oral intake is inadequate to restore or maintain optimal nutritional status. Parenteral nutrition should be used in patients who are or will become malnourished and who do not have sufficient gastrointestinal function to be able to restore or maintain optimal nutritional status (Matarese and Gottschlich, 2002). Figure 20-1 presents an algorithm for selecting enteral and parenteral nutrition routes.

These guidelines would seem to make the selection of the best type of nutrition support an easy decision; however, this is not always the case. For example, not all access methods reviewed here are universally available in all health care settings. Therefore, if a specific type of small bowel access is not available for enteral nutrition, parenteral nutrition may be the only realistic option. Often parenteral nutrition is used temporarily until adequate gastrointestinal function can support either enteral nutrition or oral intake. In this situation a combination of feeding methods is used (see "Transitional Feeding" later in the chapter).

Although methods of nutrition support can be standardized for the course of certain disease states or treatments, it is important to note that every patient presents an individual challenge and nutrition support must often be adapted to unanticipated developments or complications. The optimal treatment plan requires interdisciplinary collaboration that

TABLE 20-1

Conditions That Often Require Nutrition Support

Recommended Route of Feeding	Condition	Typical Disorders
Enteral nutrition	Impaired nutrient ingestion	Neurologic disorders
		HIV/AIDS
		Facial trauma
		Oral or esophageal trauma
		Congenital anomalies
		Respiratory failure
		Cystic fibrosis
		Traumatic brain injury
		Anorexia and wasting with severe eating disorder
	Inability to consume adequate nutrition orally	Hyperemesis of pregnancy
		Hypermetabolic states such as with burns
		Comatose states
		Anorexia in congestive heart failure, cancer, COPD, ED
		Congenital heart disease
		Impaired intake after orofacial surgery or injury
		Spinal cord injury
	Impaired digestion, absorption, metabolism	Severe gastroparesis
		Inborn errors of metabolism
		Crohn's disease
		Short bowel syndrome with minimum resection
	Severe wasting or depressed growth	Cystic fibrosis
		Failure to thrive
		Cancer
		Sepsis
		Cerebral palsy
		Myasthenia gravis
Parenteral nutrition	Gastrointestinal incompetency	Short bowel syndrome—major resection
		Severe acute pancreatitis
		Severe inflammatory bowel disease
		Small bowel ischemia
		Intestinal atresia
		Severe liver failure
		Major gastrointestinal surgery
	Critical illness with poor enteral tolerance or accessibility	Multiorgan system failure
		Major trauma or burns
		Bone marrow transplantation
		Acute respiratory failure with ventilator dependency and gastrointestinal malfunction
		Severe wasting in renal failure with dialysis
		Small bowel transplantation, immediate after surgery

AIDS, Acquired immune deficiency syndrome; *COPD*, chronic obstructive pulmonary disease; *ED*, eating disorder; *HIV*, human immunodeficiency virus.

is closely aligned with the overall patient care plan. In a few instances nutrition support may be warranted but physically impossible to implement within the overall patient care plan. Conversely, nutrition support may be achievable but may not be warranted because of the prognosis, unacceptable risk, or the patient's right to self-determination.

ENTERAL NUTRITION

By definition, enteral means "within or by the way of the gastrointestinal tract." For the purpose of the chapter, enteral means "tube feeding." When a patient has been determined to be a candidate for enteral nutrition, the appropriate route of access for tube placement is selected (see Figure 20-1). Enteral

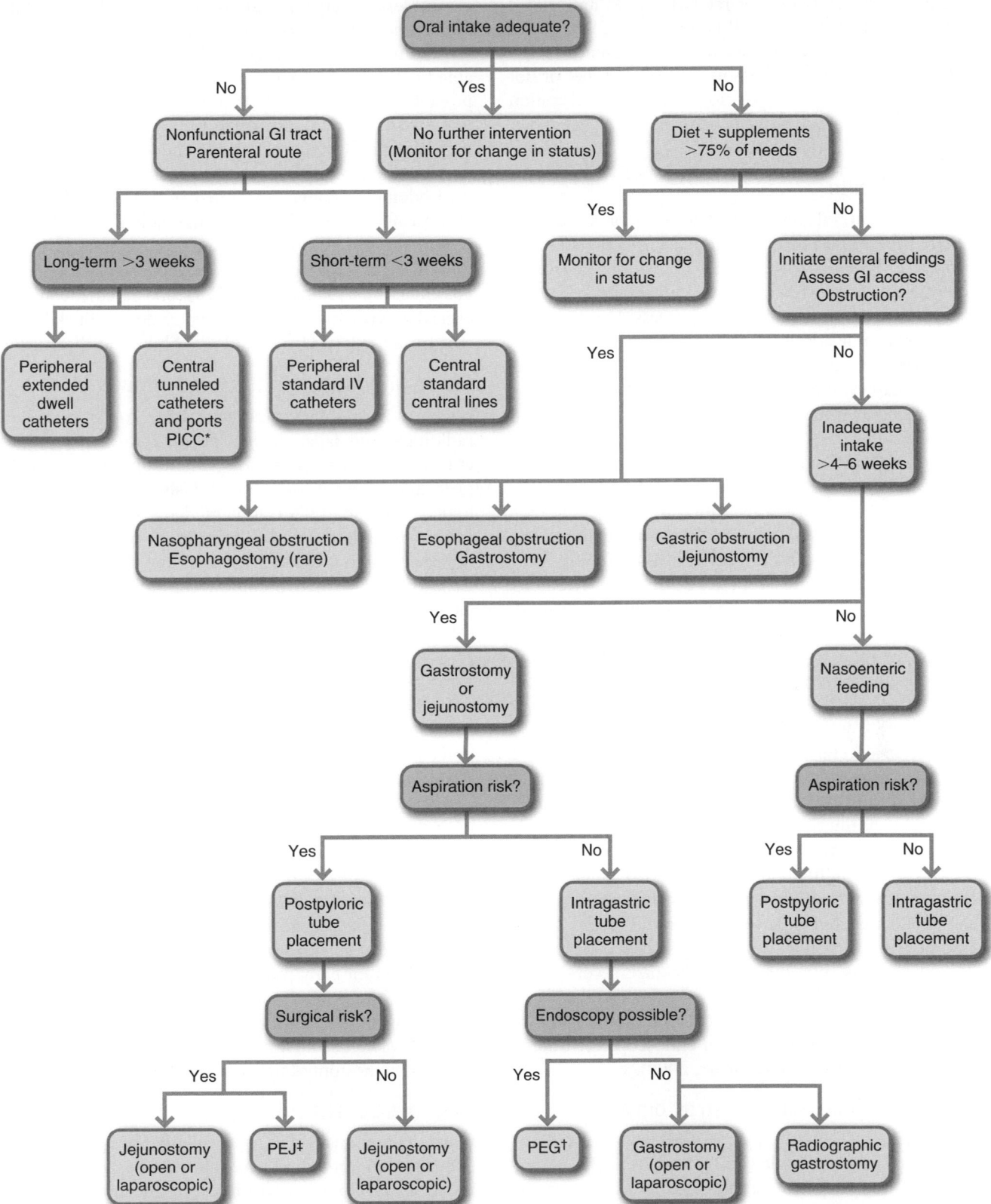

FIGURE 20-1 Algorithm for route selection for nutrition support. (*Modified from Gorman RC, Morris JB: Minimally invasive access to the gastrointestinal tract. In Rombeau JL, Rolandelli RH, editors:* Clinical nutrition: enteral and tube feeding, *Philadelphia, 1997, Saunders; and Zibrida JM, Carlson SJ: Transitional feedings. In Gottschlich MM et al:* Nutrition support dietetics core curriculum, *ed 2, Silver Spring, Md, 1993, American Society for Parenteral and Enteral Nutrition*).

access selection depends on several factors: (1) anticipated length of time enteral feeding will be required, (2) degree of risk for aspiration or tube displacement, (3) presence or absence of normal digestion and absorption, (4) whether or not there is a planned surgical intervention, and (5) administration issues such as formula viscosity and volume.

Access
Nasogastric Route

For short-term enteral nutrition of up to 3 or 4 weeks, a nasogastric tube passed through the nose into the stomach is appropriate. Patients with normal gastrointestinal function tolerate this method, which takes advantage of normal digestive, hormonal, and bactericidal processes in the stomach. Feedings can be administered by bolus injection or intermittent or continuous infusions (see "Administration" later in this chapter). Soft, flexible, and well-tolerated polyurethane or silicone tubes of various diameters, lengths, and design features may be used, depending on formula characteristics and feeding requirements. More complete descriptions of feeding tube characteristics are available elsewhere.

Tube placement is verified by aspirating gastric contents in combination with auscultation of air insufflation into the stomach or radiographic confirmation of the tube tip location. Techniques for placing a tube are described by Metheny and Meert (2004). When soft, small-bore tubes are used, aspiration of gastric contents must be performed cautiously to prevent the tube from collapsing (see *New Directions:* Dietitians Placing Enteral Feeding Tubes).

Nasoduodenal or Nasojejunal Route

For short-term enteral nutrition support of up to 3 to 4 weeks in patients with gastric motility disorders, esophageal reflux, or persistent nausea and vomiting, nasoenteric tubes placed postpylorically (into the small bowel) are appropriate. These tubes have various design features such as weighted or nonweighted tips and stylets to guide placement. The nasoenteric tube is passed through the nose and esophagus and inserted into the stomach. The tip of the tube migrates into the small bowel via peristaltic activity. In critically ill patients tube migration can take several days, causing feeding delays. Radiologic verification of tube placement is the preferred method of confirmation to ensure safety. Tubes can also be placed with endoscopic or fluoroscopic guidance (Metheny and Meert, 2004).

Percutaneous Endoscopic Gastrostomy or Jejunostomy

The **percutaneous endoscopic gastrostomy (PEG)** is a non-surgical technique for placing a tube directly into the stomach through the abdominal wall, performed using an endoscope and with the patient under local anesthesia. Tubes are endoscopically guided from the mouth into the stomach or the jejunum and then brought out through the abdominal wall (using local anesthesia) to provide the access route for enteral feedings. The PEG is the preferred access route for patients requiring tube feeding for more than 3 to 4 weeks because of its ease in providing feeding while causing the

patient less anxiety and self-consciousness. The short procedural time required for insertion, limited need for anesthesia, and minimum wound complications also make it preferable for the physician and others caring for the patient. It is possible to convert a PEG to a gastrojejunostomy by threading a small bore tube through the PEG tube into the jejunum using either fluoroscopy or endoscopy.

After the initial PEG tube has been used successfully and the abdominal **stoma** site healed, it can be replaced with a "low-profile" device that allows the patient more freedom of movement and convenience, such as ease in showering or wearing tight clothing. It is also possible to place a **percutaneous endoscopic jejunostomy (PEJ)** tube percutaneously; however, this procedure requires a higher degree of skill and carries greater risk (Kirby et al., 1998; Shike and Bloch, 1998).

Other Minimally Invasive Techniques

High-resolution video cameras have made percutaneous radiologic and laparoscopic gastrostomy and jejunostomy enteral access an option for patients in whom endoscopic procedures are contraindicated. Using fluoroscopy, a radiologic technique, tubes can be guided visually into the stomach or the jejunum and then brought out through the abdominal wall to provide the access route for enteral feedings. Laparoscopic or fluoroscopic techniques are used in some facilities and offer alternative options for enteral access (Nikolaidis, 2005; Oliveira, 2003).

Surgically Placed Enterostomies

Surgical gastrostomies and jejunostomies are placed in patients requiring enteral support who are undergoing a surgical procedure or in whom endoscopic and radiologic techniques are not possible. The simplest surgical procedures for placing a gastrostomy tube are the Stamm and Witzel techniques. A more permanent method is the Janeway procedure. Surgical gastrostomy tubes have virtually the same use as PEGs (Kirby et al., 1998; Shike and Bloch, 1998). The Witzel jejunostomy and **needle-catheter jejunostomy** (creating a feeding opening by a small-bore needle insertion into the jejunum at time of surgery) are short-term small bowel access methods. They are usually used for early postoperative enteral nutrition in combination with gastric decompression. The small lumen size of the needle-catheter jejunostomy can be problematic because it is easily dislodged and not all formulas flow readily through it. Surgical jejunostomies have the same problems.

Multiple Lumen Tubes

Gastrojejunal dual tubes are available for either endoscopic or surgical placement. These tubes are designed for patients in whom prolonged gastrointestinal decompression is anticipated. The tube has one lumen for decompression, and the other lumen is used to feed into the small bowel. These tubes are used for early postoperative feeding. For a summary of access sites, see Figure 20-2.

Formula Composition

A wide variety of enteral feeding products are commercially available. Evaluation of the suitability and efficacy of

⇄ **NEW DIRECTIONS**

Dietitians Placing Enteral Feeding Tubes

It is accepted that enteral feeding is preferred over parenteral feeding whenever it is possible. However, safely gaining timely enteral access can often be a challenge; and, if it doesn't happen, the patient can receive parenteral rather than more appropriate and physiologically beneficial enteral feeding. The nutrition support dietitian (NSD) is an ideal clinician to place bedside enteral feeding tubes because she or he is aware of the patient's specialized nutritional requirements and is typically the patient's advocate for the optimal feeding regimen and delivery method.

Placement of small bowel feeding tubes (SBFTs) is an invasive procedure (see following procedure) that requires specialized training, demonstrated competency, and delineated clinical privileges. The NSD interested in placing SBFTs should make sure that state licensure laws do not prohibit this practice by an NSD. Most states do not delineate which practices can and cannot be performed by the NSD. The NSD should also ensure that the health care facility wants the NSD to place these tubes and that it will facilitate the proper training and performance of periodic competency assessments of the NSD that are recorded in personnel files. The NSD and the facility also need to ensure proper insurance coverage for this clinical activity. Inclusion of this privilege in the NSD's job description will aid with this necessary coverage.

Although placing SBFTs can add to the burden of a daily workload of an NSD, it has many potential personal benefits in addition to the patient benefits previously mentioned. Personal benefits include increased self-esteem and job satisfaction, job flexibility and retention, increased perceived value of the NSD by the other members of the health care team, and potentially increased compensation of the NSD.

Procedure: SBFT Placement
Supplies

10-Fr feeding tube, with stylet, 43 inch, *nonweighted*
60-ml syringe with Luer Lock
Water-soluble lubricant
Silk tape
Cup with warm water
Towel and gloves
Stethoscope

Procedure

This procedure takes approximately 10-45 minutes.

1. Position patient on his or her back or in sitting position if tolerated, with the head of bed at 30 degrees or more (if tolerated). Drape towel over patient's chest.
2. Administer 10 mg IV metoclopramide into the already placed IV line.
3. Using the tube, measure the patient for gastric placement (usually 50-65 cm).
4. Insert the feeding tube into the patient's nostril or mouth, adding lubricant as needed. Advance the tube to the predetermined length. If the patient is awake and alert, encourage the patient to relax and swallow as the tube is advanced.
5. Check gastric placement by instilling 15-20 ml of air, using a syringe, and simultaneously auscultate over the epigastric area with a stethoscope. Repeat this procedure over the lungs to ensure gastric rather than pulmonary placement.
6. Once gastric placement is confirmed and if patient has a preexisting nasogastric tube (NGT), remove it.
7. Advance the feeding tube approximately 5-10 cm every 3-5 minutes, rotating the tube in a clockwise fashion. Tape the tube in place after every advancement.
8. After each advancement instill 20 ml of air and auscultate on left, mid, and right abdomen to determine location and direction of tube movement. Pull back on the syringe to obtain aspirate, if available, and note the color and consistency of the aspirate. Flush the tube with 20 ml of warm water with each advancement.
9. Advance the tube to the eventual 95- to 100-cm marking. Tape the feeding tube securely in place and obtain an abdominal radiograph to confirm small bowel placement.
10. On radiograph confirmation reinsert the NGT if desired.
11. Remove stylet wire from feeding tube and follow standard feeding administration and tube care procedures.

Courtesy Gail Cresci, MS, RD, CNSD, Assistant Professor Surgery, Co-Director Surgical Nutrition Service, Medical College of Georgia, Augusta, Ga.

---

products, whether for individual or institutional use, is increasingly complex. As more products become available, with claims for pharmacologic effects, clinical evidence for new products must be evaluated before a decision is made to use a formula.

The suitability of a feeding formula for a patient should be evaluated based on the following characteristics: (1) functional status of the patient's gastrointestinal tract, (2) physical characteristics of the formula such as osmolarity and viscosity, (3) energy and nutrient content, (4) digestion and absorption capability of the patient, (5) other clinical considerations of the patient such as fluid and electrolyte status and organ/system function, and (6) cost-effectiveness. Small bowel feeding requires careful selection of formula because of sensitivity to osmolarity and absorptive function of the small bowel (Figure 20-3). See Chapter 43 for a similar discussion on feeding infants and an algorithm for formula selection.

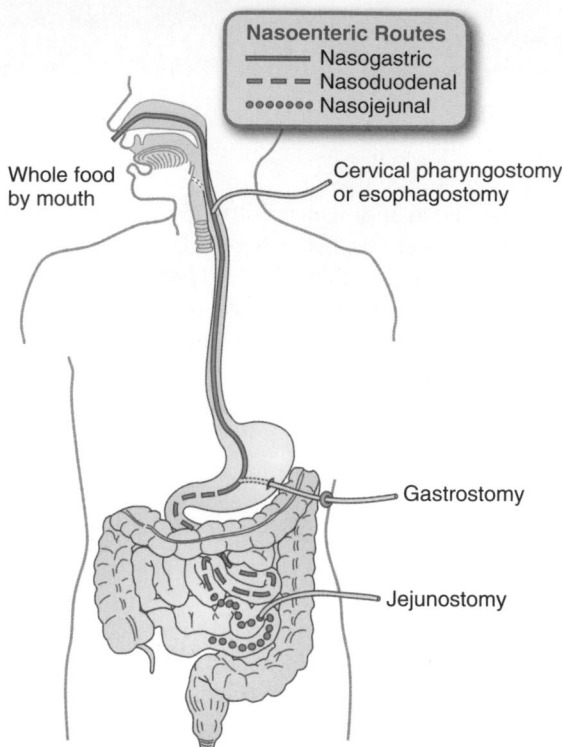

FIGURE 20-2 Diagram of enteral tube placement.

Formulas are classified in a variety of ways, usually based on protein or overall macronutrient composition (see Appendix 32). Most patients with a variety of clinical conditions tolerate standard formulas intended to meet the nutritional requirements of general patient populations. The formulas are lactose free, contain 1 kcal/ml, and are used as over-the-counter oral supplements and tube-feeding formulas. Standard formulas are often concentrated to provide 1.5 to 2 kcal/ml when fluid restriction is required for patients with cardiopulmonary, renal, and hepatic failure. Formulas intended for use as supplements to oral diets are flavored and contain simple sugars for palatability. Although rare, blenderized formulas from natural foods or commercially prepared are an alternative to standard formulas, but maintenance of aseptic technique is essential to prevent bacterial contamination.

High-nitrogen formulas are used for patients with increased protein requirements such as those with burns, fistulas, sepsis, or trauma. Chemically defined formulas are specialized **monomeric** formulas that have been hydrolyzed to contain short-chain carbohydrate or simple sugars and peptides or amino acids. They are used for patients with conditions of maldigestion or malabsorption. Chemically defined formulas are low in fat and often supplemented with medium-chain triglycerides that can be readily absorbed into the hepatoportal circulation. Exclusive extended use of these formulas can lead to an essential fatty acid deficiency. Originally these formulas were referred to as "elemental" to describe their monomeric components of protein and carbohydrate, which were amino acids and simple sugars, respectively. Subsequently these formulas contain protein fragments (dipeptides, tripeptides, or oligopeptides).

Chemically defined formulas can be viewed as disease-specific formulas when prescribed for conditions of malabsorption and maldigestion such as pancreatitis, short bowel syndromes, or HIV/AIDS related gastrointestinal pathology. Disease-specific formulas are also available for patients who have renal, hepatic, or cardiopulmonary disease, immunosuppression, glucose intolerance, or special needs such as wound healing. The efficacy of disease-specific formulas is controversial since evidence for the necessity of these products is limited by few controlled studies. They are generally much more expensive than standard formulas.

Carbohydrates, protein, fat, fiber, and micronutrient modules can be added to enteral formulas as a supplement. New enteral formulas can be compounded from modules to provide specific nutrient requirements. However, these methods require more labor and increase risk of microbial contamination that may discourage facilities from using modular compounding systems.

Protein

Standard formulas contain biologically complete, intact proteins such as caseinate, lactalbumin, beef, and soy protein isolate. Formulas containing peptide fragments and amino acids are derived from the hydrolysis of casein, whey, lactalbumin, or soy. These formulas have a higher osmolarity (number of particles per liter of solution) because of the hydrolyzed protein.

The form of protein (intact or hydrolyzed) that is most efficiently digested and absorbed by the gastrointestinal tract is controversial. High-protein formulas increase nitrogenous waste excretion by the kidneys, and this process requires adequate amounts of fluid, which is particularly important in patients who cannot communicate thirst.

Glutamine and arginine, both contained in standard enteral formula protein sources, may be conditionally essential amino acids under conditions of trauma and critical illness. Glutamine is the primary carrier of nitrogen derived from skeletal muscle and energy substrate for enterocytes and lymphocytes. It has been supplemented in enteral formulas for a potential role in preserving gastrointestinal integrity and immunity. Arginine has immune-enhancing properties and a role in collagen synthesis and wound healing. Evidence for use of these two amino acids as enhancements to immune function, gastrointestinal integrity, and wound healing remains controversial (Peng et al., 2004; Williams et al., 2002).

Carbohydrates

The percentage of total calories provided as carbohydrates in enteral formulas varies from 30% to 90%, depending on the condition for which the product was designed. Pulmonary and diabetic products are usually low in carbohydrates in contrast to chemically defined formulas, which are high in (simple) carbohydrate. Carbohydrate sources used in formulas are pureed fruits and vegetables, corn syrup solids, corn and tapioca starch hydrolysates, maltodextrins, sucrose, fructose, and glucose. Similar to protein, the carbohydrate source and degree of hydrolysis affect osmolarity.

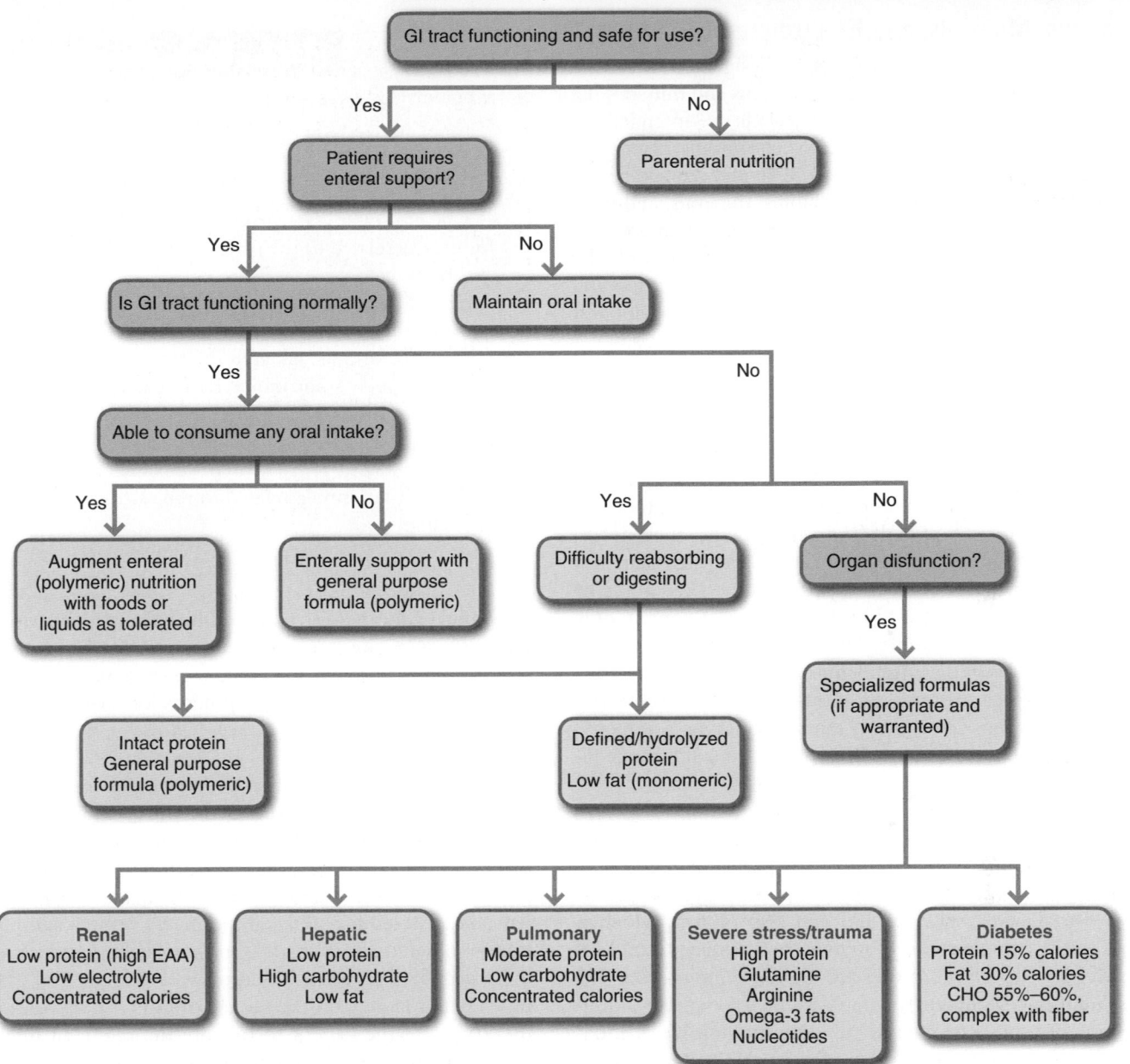

FIGURE 20-3 Algorithm for enteral formula selection. *(Modified from Zibrida JM, Carlson SJ: Transitional feedings. In Gottschlichg MM et al.:* Nutrition support dietetics core curriculum, *ed 2, Silver Spring, Md, 1993, American Society for Parenteral and Enteral Nutrition, and Rolandelli RH et al.:* Clinical nutrition: enteral and tube feeding, *ed 4, Philadelphia, 2005, Saunders.)*

Lactose is not used as a carbohydrate source in most formulas because lactase deficiency is common in acutely ill patients. Fiber or carbohydrate that cannot be digested by human enzymes, although digested by colonic microflora into short-chain fatty acids, is frequently added to enteral formulas. Fibers are classified as water soluble (pectins and gums) or water insoluble (cellulose or hemicellulose) (see Chapters 1 and 3). The effectiveness of different fibers in enteral formulas used to treat gastrointestinal symptoms in acutely ill patients is controversial (Gottschlich, 2006).

Lipid

Lipid provides 1.5% to 55% of the total kilocalories in enteral formulas, but most formulas have between 30% and 40% of their total kilocalories provided by lipids, usually from corn, soy, sunflower, safflower or canola oils. Chemically defined formulas usually have minimum amounts of lipid.

Approximately 2% to 4% of the daily calories in the form of linoleic acid is necessary to prevent essential fatty acid deficiency. Research suggests that high dosages of linoleic acid may suppress immune function. Short- and medium-chain saturated fatty acids, monounsaturated fatty acids, and omega-3 polyunsaturated fatty acids have been included in disease-specific formulas as alternatives to the high linoleic acid-containing vegetable oil in formulas. Omega-3 fatty acids have been included in disease-specific formulas because of their modulating effect on immune function.

Vitamins, Minerals, and Electrolytes

Most but not all available formulas are designed to meet the dietary reference intakes (DRIs) for vitamins and minerals if a sufficient volume is taken. However, DRIs are intended for healthy populations, not for acute or chronically ill populations. Formulas intended for use in renal and hepatic failure are intentionally low in specific vitamins, minerals, and electrolytes. In contrast, disease-specific formulas often are supplemented with antioxidant vitamins and minerals with the intention of improving immune function and accelerating wound healing. Electrolytes are provided in relatively modest amounts compared with the oral diet and may require supplementation when diarrhea or drainage losses occur.

Fluid

Fluid needs for adults can be estimated at 1 ml of water per kilocalorie, or 30 to 35 ml/kg of usual body weight (see Chapter 4). Without an additional source of fluid, tube-fed patients may not get enough free water to meet their needs, particularly when concentrated formulas are used. Standard (1 kcal/ml) formulas contain approximately 85% water by volume, but concentrated (2 kcal/ml) formulas contain only about 70% water by volume. All sources of fluid being given to a patient receiving enteral nutrition, including feeding tube flushes, medications, and intravenous fluids, should be considered when determining and calculating a patient's intake. Additional water can be provided through the feeding tube as needed.

Osmolarity

The size and number of the nutrient particles in a liter of solution define its **osmolarity.** General-purpose formulas have osmolarities between 300 and 500 mOsm, which is close to the osmolarity of blood and body fluids. Osmolarities of concentrated formulas are higher, ranging from 400 to 700 mOsm. **Osmolality** is stated as the the number of milliosmoles of solute (particles) per kilogram of solvent, and is usually not used to define the concentration of a formula. Chemically defined formulas are as high as 900 mOsm/L. Box 20-1 summarizes the factors to consider when selecting an enteral formula.

Administration

The three common methods of tube-feeding administration are bolus feeding, intermittent drip, and continuous drip. Method selection is based on the patient's clinical status and quality of life considerations. One method can serve as a transition to another method as the patient's status changes.

Bolus

The feeding modality of choice when patients are clinically stable with a functional stomach is the syringe bolus method. Syringe **bolus feedings** administered over 5 to 20 minutes are more convenient and less expensive than pump or gravity bolus feedings and should be encouraged when tolerated. A 60-ml syringe is used to infuse the formula. If bloating or abdominal discomfort develops, the patient is encouraged to wait 10 to 15 minutes before proceeding with the remainder

---

BOX 20-1

Factors to Consider When Choosing an Enteral Formula

Gastrointestinal function

The type of protein, fat, carbohydrate, and fiber in the formula as related to the patient's digestive and absorptive capacity

Caloric and protein density of the formula (i.e., kcal/ml, g protein/ml, and kcal:nitrogen ratio)

Ability of the formula, taken in the amounts tolerated, to meet the patient's nutritional requirements

Sodium, potassium, magnesium, and phosphorus content of the formula, especially for patients with cardiopulmonary, renal, or hepatic failure

Viscosity of the formula related to tube size and method of feeding

---

of formula allocated for that feeding. The patient with normal gastric function can usually tolerate 500 ml of formula at each feeding. Three or four bolus feedings per day can provide the daily nutritional requirements for most patients.

Intermittent Drip

Quality-of-life issues are often the reason for the initiation of **intermittent drip feeding** regimens, which allow mobile patients more free time and autonomy compared with continuous drip infusions. These feedings can be given by pump or gravity drip. A schedule is based on four to six feedings per day administered for 20 to 60 minutes. Formula administration is initiated at 100 to 150 ml per feeding and increased incrementally as tolerated. Success with this method of feeding depends largely on the degree of mobility, alertness, and motivation of the patient to tolerate the regimen. Intermittent feedings, as well as bolus feedings, should not be used with patients at high risk for **pulmonary aspiration.**

Continuous Drip

Continuous drip infusion of formula requires a pump. This method is appropriate for patients who do not tolerate large-volume infusions during a given feeding such as those occurring with bolus or intermittent methods. Patients with compromised gastrointestinal function because of disease, surgery, antineoplastic therapy, or other physiologic impediments are candidates for continuous drip infusion. Patients with small bowel access should also be fed by continuous drip infusion. The feeding rate goal, in milliliters per hour, is set by dividing the total daily volume by the number of hours per day of administration (usually 18 to 24 hours). Feeding is started at one quarter to one half the goal rate and advanced every 8 to 12 hours to the final volume. Formulas with osmolarities between 300 and 500 mOsm/kg can be started at full strength. Hyperosmolar formulas should be advanced conservatively to ensure tolerance. Dilution of formulas is not necessary.

Modern enteral pumps are small and easy to handle. Many pumps are battery operated for up to 8 hours in addition to being electrically powered, allowing flexibility and mobility for the patient. Most pumps have a complete delivery system available, including bags and tubing compatible with proper pump operation.

Complications and Monitoring
Complications

Abdominal leakage of gastric contents from a gastrostomy site can cause skin erosion and skin breakdown, leading to infection and peritonitis; however, fewer than 10% of patients experience serious complications. Other complications can be prevented or managed with careful patient monitoring (Farwell et al., 2002). Box 20-2 provides a comprehensive list of complications associated with enteral nutrition.

Aspiration is a concern for patients receiving enteral nutrition and is also a controversial topic since many experts believe the issue is not aspiration of formula into the airway, but aspiration of throat contents and saliva. Nevertheless, to minimize the risk of aspiration, patients should be positioned with their heads and shoulders above their chests during and immediately after feeding.

There is confusion in the literature as to the efficacy of checking gastric residuals because procedures are not standardized, and the practice of checking residuals does not protect the patient from aspiration. Stable patients, especially those who have been fed by tube for long periods of time, do not need residuals checked regularly. Also it is difficult to aspirate the stomach contents, and the residuals may contain more secretions and gastric fluids than formula. In critically ill patients the best methods for decreasing the risk of aspiration are elevating the head of the bed, continuous subglottic suctioning and oral decontamination (McClave et al., 2002; Metheny, 2002; McClave and Snider, 2002; Scolapio, 2002).

Blue dye (Food, Drug and Cosmetic [FD&C] Blue No 1) added to enteral formulas has been used to detect aspiration of formula for years. Recently this practice has become controversial. Reports indicate that some critically ill patients have discoloration of the skin, urine, serum or other body fluids after ingestion of the blue dye and that some have died within days of dye ingestion. Although a causal relationship between blue dye and adverse reaction has not been described, many hospitals have discontinued its use. In 2003 the Food and Drug Administration issued a public health bulletin concerning discoloration and death in patients receiving enteral formulas (American Dietetic Association, 2004).

Diarrhea is a common complication associated with enteral nutrition. However, the most likely causes of diarrhea among enterally fed patients are bacterial overgrowth, antibiotic therapy, and gastrointestinal motility disorders associated with acute and critical illness and not the enteral nutrition. Hyperosmolar medications such as magnesium-containing antacids, sorbitol-containing elixirs, and electrolyte supplements can also contribute to diarrhea. Adjustment of medications or administration methods can frequently correct the diarrhea. The addition of soy polysaccharide, a prebiotic, pectin, and other

---

BOX 20-2
Complications of Enteral Nutrition

Access Problems

Pressure necrosis/ulceration/stenosis
Tube displacement/migration
Tube obstruction
Leakage from ostomy/stoma site

Administration Problems

Regurgitation
Aspiration
Microbial contamination

Gastrointestinal Complications

Nausea/vomiting
Distention/bloating/cramping
Delayed gastric emptying
Constipation
High gastric residuals
Diarrhea
Osmotic
Secretory
Medications
Treatment/therapies
Hypoalbuminemia
Maldigestion/malabsorption
Formula choice/rate of administration

Metabolic Complications

Refeeding syndrome
Drug-nutrient interactions
Glucose intolerance/hyperglycemia/hypoglycemia
Hydration status—dehydration/overhydration
Hyponatremia
Hyperkalemia/hypokalemia
Hyperphosphatemia/hypophosphatemia
Micronutrient deficiencies

Data from Hamaoui E, Kodsi R: Complications of enteral feeding and their prevention. In Rombeau JL, Rolandelli RH, editors: *Clinical nutrition: enteral tube feeding*, Philadelphia, 1997, Saunders; and Ideno KT: Enteral nutrition. In Gottschlich MM et al, editors: *Nutrition support dietetics core curriculum*, Silver Spring, Md, 1993, American Society for Parenteral and Enteral Nutrition.

---

fibers, bulking agents, probiotics, and antidiarrheal medications can also be beneficial.

Among stable patients receiving enteral nutrition, constipation can be a problem. Fiber-containing formulas or stool-bulking medication may be helpful, and adequate fluid must be provided. Gastrointestinal motility should be assessed because diarrhea can coexist with constipation, usually when there is also an impaction.

Monitoring

Patients receiving enteral nutrition are monitored to prevent and correct complications. In addition, monitoring the patient's actual intake and tolerance is necessary to ensure

Monitoring the Patient Receiving Enteral Nutrition

Weight (at least 3 times/wk)
Signs and symptoms of edema (daily)
Signs and symptoms of dehydration (daily)
Fluid intake and output (daily)
Adequacy of enteral intake (at least 2 times/wk)
Abdominal distention and discomfort
Gastric residuals (every 4 hr) if appropriate
Serum electrolytes, blood urea nitrogen, creatinine, (2-3 times/wk)
Serum glucose, calcium, magnesium, phosphorus, (weekly or as ordered)
Stool output and consistency (daily)

that nutrition goals are achieved and maintained. During routine patient care actual feeding time is commonly lost from the patient's prescribed feeding schedule as a result of (1) a dislodged tube, (2) gastrointestinal intolerance, (3) medical procedures requiring discontinuation of feeding, and (4) difficulties with the feeding tube position.

Monitoring metabolic and gastrointestinal tolerance, hydration status, and nutritional status is extremely important for the tube-fed patient; Box 20-3 gives guidelines. Practice guidelines, institutional protocols, and standardized ordering procedures are helpful to ensure optimal, safe provision of enteral nutrition support. Figure 20-4 displays an enteral nutrition order form.

PARENTERAL NUTRITION

Parenteral nutrition is the provision of nutrients directly into the bloodstream intravenously. Assuming that a patient is an appropriate candidate for parenteral nutrition, it is then necessary to choose between central and peripheral access (see Figure 20-1). Central access refers to catheter tip placement in a large, high-blood-flow vein such as the superior vena cava; this is **central parenteral nutrition (CPN).**

Peripheral access refers to catheter tip placement in a small vein typically in the arm. Many clinicians do not use **peripheral parenteral nutrition (PPN)** because they argue that it is short-term therapy with minimum impact on nutritional status; they believe that central access is required for effective parenteral nutrition. Others argue that PPN can be used as a supplemental feeding or in a transitional phase to enteral or oral feeding. Newer peripheral devices have made it possible to infuse PPN with a single catheter placed for up to a month.

Peripheral veins cannot tolerate concentrated solutions; therefore diluted larger-volume infusions are often necessary to meet nutritional requirements. Volume-sensitive patients such as those with cardiopulmonary, renal, or hepatic failure are not good candidates for PPN. Additional helpful information for appropriate access selection is previous access history, edema or skin damage at the access site, medical and medication history, coagulation time, need for additional infusions, peripheral vein condition, functional status, and lifestyle (Sachs et al., 2005). See Chapter 43 for discussion related to the feeding low-birth-weight infants.

Access

Peripheral Access

Nutrient solutions not exceeding 800 to 900 mOsm/kg of solvent can be infused through a routine peripheral intravenous catheter placed in a vein in good condition. Protocols for dressing changes and rotation of the site are used to prevent the principal complication of peripheral catheters—thrombophlebitis.

A more recent development in peripheral catheter technology is the extended dwell catheter. These catheters are sometimes called midline or midclavicular catheters, depending on their position. Extended dwell catheters require a vein large enough to advance the catheter 5 to 7 inches into the vein. These catheters can remain at the original site for 3 to 6 weeks and have made PPN a more feasible option in patients with veins large enough to tolerate the catheter (Krzywda et al., 2005).

Short-Term Central Access

Catheters used for CPN ideally consist of a single lumen. If central access is needed for other reasons such as hemodynamic monitoring, drawing blood samples, or giving medications, multiple-lumen catheters are available. To reduce the risk of infection, the catheter lumen used to infuse CPN should be reserved for only that purpose. Catheters are most commonly inserted into the subclavian vein and advanced until the catheter tip is in the superior vena cava, using strict aseptic technique. Alternatively, an internal or external jugular vein catheter can be used with the same catheter tip placement. However, the motion of the neck makes this site much more difficult for maintaining the sterility of a dressing. Radiologic verification of the tip site is necessary before infusion of nutrients can begin. Strict infection control protocols should be used for catheter placement and maintenance (Krzywda et al., 2005). Figure 20-5 shows alternative venous access sites for CPN; femoral placement is also possible.

Long-Term Central Access

A commonly used long-term catheter is a "tunneled" catheter. These single- or multiple-lumen catheters are placed in the cephalic, subclavian, or internal jugular veins and fed into the superior vena cava. A subcutaneous tunnel is created so that the catheter exits the skin several inches away from its venous entry site. Another type of long-term catheter is a port device that is implanted under the skin where the catheter would normally exit at the end of the subcutaneous tunnel. A special needle must access the entrance port. Ports can be single or double; an individual port is equivalent to a lumen.

ENTERAL NUTRITION SUPPORT ORDER
Date: _____ Time: _____
DX: _____
Reason for TF: _____

ENTERAL NUTRITION SUPPORT ORDERS:
1. ROUTE: Check tube type
   ( ) NGT   ( ) PEG/G-TUBE   ( ) PEG/JTUBE

2. FORMULA: Check the desired formula

Formula	kcal/cc		Formula	kcal/cc
( ) General purpose	1.0		( ) Fiber enriched	1.0
( ) General purpose/ High Nitrogen	1.2-1.4		( ) Monomeric	1.0

3. METHOD OF FEEDING: Check the desired schedule.
   ( ) Schedule A: Bolus Feeding Via Syringe/Gravity Bag
      1. 8:00 PM 240 cc formula
          12:00 PM 240 cc formula
          4:00 PM 240 cc formula
          8:00 PM 240 cc formula
      2. Water can be added to gravity bag depending on hydration needs.
      3. As tolerated, registered dietitian to advance feeding and adjust water to meet goal rates.
      4. Formula progression to goal: _____
         _____
         _____
         _____

   ( ) Schedule B: Pump
   1. Begin full strength 30 cc/hr × 8 hr.
   2. If tolerated after 8 hr, advance to 50cc/hr × 24 hr.
   3. As tolerated, registered dietitian to advance feeding and adjust water to meet goal rates.
   4. Formula progression to goal:
      _____
      _____
      _____
      _____
      _____

   ( ) Schedule C: Tube Feeding Protocol Via Gravity Bag
      1. Schedule: 6:00 AM   2:00 PM
                          10:00 AM   6:00 PM
                                     10:00 PM
      2. Initial feeding - 240 cc water.
         At next scheduled time - 240 cc Formula + 240 cc water.
      3. As tolerated, registered dietitian to advance feeding and adjust water to meet goal rates.
      4. Formula progression to goal:

4. ( ) ALTERNATE ORDERS:
        CONSULT REGISTERED DIETITIAN TO
        DETERMINE FORMULA AND SCHEDULE:

        1. Formula: _____
        2. Schedule: _____
           _____
           _____
           _____

REGISTERED DIETITIAN:

1. NUTRITIONAL GOAL:

Formula: _____
Calories: _____
Protein: _____
Vitamins/Minerals: _____
_____
_____

2. RECOMMENDATIONS:
_____
_____
_____

Registered Dietitian: _____

ENTERAL NUTRITION SUPPORT GUIDELINES:
PHYSICIAN:
1. PLACEMENT: Confirm placement of NGT by abdominal x-ray.
2. MEDICATIONS: Identify via enternal feeding tube:
   A. Consult pharmacist to verify appropriate form of medication.
   B. 30 cc water flush before and after each medication.
   C. Administer each medication separately.
3. FLUID BALANCE: Patient fluid requirements and intake should be assessed, include IV, water flush, and water available from tube feeding (formula is approximately 80% free water).
4. LABORATORY WORK-UP:
   A. Initial: Na, K, CO_2, C1, BUN, Creat, Mg, Ca, Phos.
   B. Thereafter: As needed.

FIGURE 20-4 Enteral nutrition order form. (*Courtesy Memorial-Sloan Kettering Cancer Center, New York, NY.*)

The latest development in catheter technology is a peripherally inserted central catheter (PICC). This catheter is inserted into a vein in the antecubital area of the arm and threaded into the subclavian vein with the catheter tip placed in the superior vena cava. Nonphysician trained professionals can insert a PICC, whereas placement of a tunneled catheter is a surgical procedure (Krzywda et al., 2005).

Both tunneled catheters and PICCs can be used for extended therapy in the hospital and are frequently used for home infusion therapy. Their greatest advantage for patients is better mobility and time away from infusion, which can be cycled at intervals. They also minimize risk of infection because the tunnel creates a barrier between the entry of the catheter into the skin and into the vein. Care of long-term catheters requires specialized handling and extensive patient education.

Nutrition Solutions
Protein

Commercially available standard solutions are composed of all the essential amino acids and only some of the nonessential crystalline amino acids. Nonessential nitrogen is provided principally by the amino acids alanine and glycine, usually without aspartate, glutamate, cysteine, and taurine. Specialized solutions with adjusted amino acid content are available for pediatric patients and patients with renal or liver disease. These specialized solutions are used infrequently because of their expense and the lack of conclusive research data supporting the efficacy of their use. Individual amino acid additives such as glutamine and arginine are used for research purposes, but they have not been approved for general clinical use in parenteral solutions.

The concentration of amino acids in these solutions ranges from 3% to 20%. Thus a 10% solution of amino acids supplies 100 g of protein per liter. The percentage of a solution is usually expressed at its final concentration after dilution with other nutrient solutions. The caloric content of amino acid solutions is approximately 4 kcal/g of protein provided. About 15% to 20% of total energy intake should come from protein (Kumpf et al., 2005).

Carbohydrates

Carbohydrates are supplied as dextrose monohydrate in concentrations ranging from 5% to 70%. The dextrose monohydrate yields 3.4 calories per gram. As with amino acids, a 10% solution yields 100 g of carbohydrates per liter of solution. The use of carbohydrates (100 g daily for a 70-kg person) ensures that protein is not catabolized for energy during conditions of normal metabolism.

Maximum rates of carbohydrate administration should not exceed 5 mg/kg/min. Excessive administration can lead to hyperglycemia, hepatic abnormalities, and increased ventilatory drive (see Chapter 35). Calculation of osmolarity of a parenteral solution may be useful to ensure venous tolerance (Kumpf et al., 2005) (see *Clinical Insight:* Calculating the Osmolarity of a Parenteral Nutrition Solution).

Lipid

Lipid emulsions, available in 10% and 20% concentrations, are composed of aqueous suspensions of soybean or safflower oil, with egg yolk phospholipid as the emulsifier. The three-carbon molecule, glycerol, which is water soluble, is added to the emulsion to provide osmolarity. Glycerol is oxidized and yields 4.3 kcal/g. A 10% emulsion provides 1.1 kcal/ml; a 20% emulsion provides 2 kcal/ml. About 10% of calories per day from fat emulsions provide the 2% to 4% of calories from linoleic acid required to prevent essential fatty acid deficiency. Soybean and safflower oils are rich (about 40%) sources of linoleic acid.

Linoleic acid alters prostaglandin metabolism, thereby producing both proinflammatory and immunosuppressive effects, particularly at high doses and at faster infusion rates (Mizock and DeMichele, 2004). Therefore infusion of currently available parenteral lipid emulsions over 24-hour periods at a maximum of 1 g of lipid per kilogram per 24 hours is recommended to avoid deleterious effects.

General guidelines for daily requirements for electrolytes are given in Table 20-2, for vitamins in Table 20-3, and for trace elements in Table 20-4. Because parenterally administered vitamins and trace elements do not go through the digestive and absorptive processes, these recommendations are lower than the DRIs. Parenteral solutions also represent

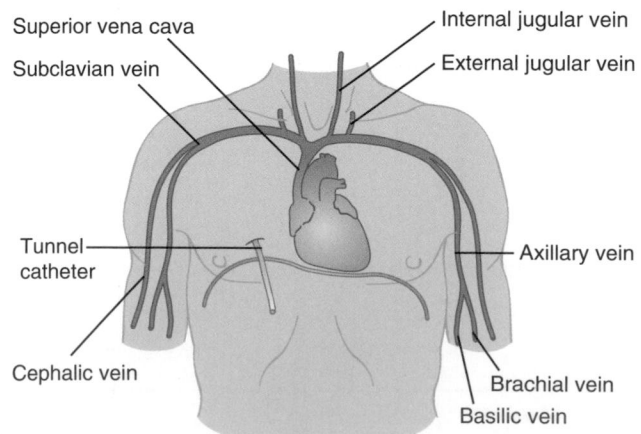

FIGURE 20-5 | Venous sites from which the superior vena cava may be accessed.

✳ CLINICAL INSIGHT

Calculating the Osmolarity of a Parenteral Nutrition Solution

1. Multiply the grams of dextrose per liter by 5.
   Example: 50 g of dextrose × 5 = 250 mOsm/L.
2. Multiply the grams of protein per liter by 10.
   Example: 30 g of protein × 10 = 300 mOsm/L
3. Fat is isotonic and does not contribute to osmolarity.
4. Electrolytes further add to osmolarity.
   Total osmolarity = 250 + + 300 = 550 mOsm/L.

a significant portion of total daily fluid and electrolyte intake. Once a solution is prescribed and initiated, minor to major adjustments for proper fluid and electrolyte balance may be necessary, depending on the stability of the patient. The choice of the salt form of electrolytes (e.g., chloride, acetate) has an impact on acid-base balance.

Iron is also not normally part of parenteral infusions because it is not compatible with lipids and may enhance certain bacterial growth. When needed, it is given separately to stable home care patients as iron dextran.

Fluid

Fluid needs for parenteral and enteral nutrition are calculated similarly. Maximum volumes of CPN rarely exceed 3 L, with typical prescriptions of 1.5 to 3 L daily. In critically ill patients volumes of prescribed CPN should be closely coordinated with their overall care plan. The administration of other medical therapies requiring fluid administration, such as intravenous medications and blood products, necessitates careful monitoring. Patients with cardiopulmonary, renal, and hepatic failure are especially sensitive to fluid administration.

Compounding Methods

Parenteral nutrition prescriptions require preparation or compounding by competent pharmacy personnel under laminar airflow hoods using aseptic techniques. Prescriptions are compounded in two general ways. One method compounds all components except the fat emulsion, which is infused separately. Solutions are usually mixed in one bag at a 1:1 dextrose-to-amino acid volume ratio. The second method combines the lipid emulsion with the dextrose and amino acid solution and is referred to as a *total nutrient admixture* or 3-in-1 solution.

Institutions frequently use standardized solutions, which are compounded in batches, thus saving labor and lowering costs; however, flexibility for individualized compounding should be available when warranted (Kumpf et al., 2005). Standard order forms are often useful (Table 20-5).

A number of medications, including antibiotics, vasopressors, narcotics, diuretics, and many other commonly administered drugs, can be compounded with parenteral nutrition solutions. In practice this occurs infrequently because it requires specialized knowledge of physical compatibility or incompatibility of the solution contents. The most

TABLE 20-2

Daily Electrolyte Requirements During Total Parenteral Nutrition—Adults

Electrolyte	Parenteral Equivalent of RDA	Standard Intake
Calcium	10 mEq	10-15 mEq
Magnesium	10 mEq	8-20 mEq
Phosphate	30 mmol	20-40 mmol
Sodium	N/A	1-2 mEq/kg + replacement
Potassium	N/A	1-2 mEq/kg
Acetate	N/A	As needed to maintain acid-base balance
Chloride	N/A	As needed to maintain acid-base balance

From National Advisory Group on Standards, and Practice Guidelines for Parenteral Nutrition, ASPEN: Safe practices for parenteral nutrition formulations, *JPEN J Parenter Enteral Nutr* 22(2):49, 1998.

N/A, Not applicable.

TABLE 20-3

Adult Parenteral Multivitamins: Comparison of Guidelines and Products

Vitamin	NAG-AMA Guidelines	FDA Requirements	MVI-12	MVI-13 (Infuvite) Baxter
A (retinol)	3300 units (1 mg)	3300 units (1 mg)	3300 units (1 mg)	3300 units (1 mg)
D (ergocalciferol cholecalciferol))	200 units (5 mcg)	200 units (5 mcg)	200 units (5 mcg)	200 units (5 mcg)
E (mcg-tocopherol)	10 units (10 mg)	10 units (10 mg)	10 units (10 mg)	10 units (10 mg)
B$_1$ (thiamin)	3 mg	6 mg	3 mg	6 mg
B$_2$ (riboflavin)	3.6 mg	3.6 mg	3.6 mg	3.6 mg
B$_3$ (niacinamide)	40 mg	40 mg	40 mg	40 mg
B$_5$ (dexpanthenol)	15 mg	15 mg	15 mg	15 mg
B$_6$ (pyrodoxine)	4 mg	6 mg	4 mg	6 mg
B$_{12}$ (cyanocobalamin)	5 mcg	5 mcg	5 mcg	5 mcg
C (ascorbic acid)	100 mg	200 mg	100 mg	200 mg
Biotin	60 mcg	60 mcg	60 mcg	60 mcg
Folic acid	400 mcg	600 mcg	400 mcg	600 mcg
Vitamin K		150 mcg	0	150 mcg

From *Fed Reg* 66(77): April 20, 2000.

NAG, National Advisory Group; *AMA*, American Medical Association; *FDA*, U.S. Food and Drug Administration; *MVI-12* and *MVI-13*, multivitamin supplements.

Centers for Disease Control and Prevention, O'Grady NP et al: *Guidelines for the prevention of intravascular catheter-related infections*, August 9, 2002, http://www.cdc.gov/mmwr/preview/mmwrhtml/rr5110a1.htm, accessed January, 2006.

Comprehensive accreditation manual for hospitals 2006: *The official handbook (CAMH)*, Oakbrook Terrace, Ill, 2006, The Joint Commission.

Deitch EA: Multiple organ failure, *Ann Surg* 216:117, 1992.

Farwell DG et al: Predictors of perioperative complications in head and neck patients, *Arch Otolaryngol Head Neck Surg* 128:505, 2002.

Genton L et al: Enteral feeding preserves gut Th-2 cytokines despite mucosal cellular adhesion molecule-1 blockade, *JPEN J Parenter Enteral Nutr* 29(1):44, 2005.

Gottschlich MM: Adult enteral nutrition: formulas and supplements. In Buchman A, editor: *Clinical nutrition in gastrointestinal disease*, Thoroughfare, NJ, 2006, Slack Inc.

Jabbar A et al: Gut immunology and the differential response to feeding and starvation, *Nutr Clin Pract* 18:461, 2003.

Jeejeebhoy KN: Enteral and parenteral nutrition: evidence-based approach, *Proc Nutr Soc* 60:399, 2001.

Kirby DF et al: Enteral access and infusion equipment. In Merritt R: *The ASPEN nutrition support practice manual*, Silver Spring, Md, 1998, American Society for Parenteral and Enteral Nutrition, 1998.

Kraft MD et al: Review of the refeeding syndrome, *Nutr Clin Pract* 20:625, 2005.

Krzywda EA et al: Parenteral nutrition access and infusion equipment. In Merritt R editor: *The ASPEN nutrition support practice manual*, ed 2, Silver Spring, Md, 2005, American Society for Parenteral and Enteral Nutrition.

Kudsk KA et al: Enteral versus parenteral feeding: effects on septic morbidity after blunt and penetrating abdominal trauma, *Ann Surg* 215:503, 1992.

Kumpf VJ et al: Parenteral nutrition formulations: preparation and ordering. In Merritt R, editor: *The ASPEN Nutrition support practice manual*, ed 2, Silver Spring, Md, 2005, American Society for Parenteral and Enteral Nutrition.

Lipman TO: Bacterial translocation and enteral nutrition in humans: an outsider looks in, *JPEN J Parenter Enteral Nutr* 19:156, 1995.

Matarese LE, Gottschlich MM: *Contemporary nutrition support practice*, ed 2, St Louis, 2002, Saunders.

McClave SA, Snider HL: Clinical use of gastric residual volumes as a monitor for patients on enteral tube feeding, *JPEN J Parenter Enteral Nutr* 26:43S, 2002.

McClave SA et al: North American Summit on Aspiration in the Critically Ill Patient: consensus statement, *JPEN J Parenter Enteral Nutr* 26:80, 2002.

Merritt R, editor: *The ASPEN nutrition support practice manual*, ed 2, Silver Spring, Md, 2005, American Society for Parenteral and Enteral Nutrition.

Metheny NA: Risk factors for aspiration, *JPEN J Parenter Enteral Nutr* 26(6):26S, 2002.

Metheny NA, Meert KL: Monitoring tube feeding placement, *Nutr Clin Pract* 19:487, 2004.

Mizock BA, DeMichele SJ: The acute respiratory distress syndrome: role of nutritional modulation of inflammation through dietary lipids, *Nutr Clin Pract* 19:563, 2004.

Moore FA et al: Early enteral feeding compared with parenteral reduces postoperative septic complications, *Ann Surg* 216:172, 1992.

Mueller C, Nestle M: Regulation of medical foods: toward a rational policy, *Nutr Clin Pract* 10:8, 1995.

Naylor CJ et al: Does a multidisciplinary total parenteral nutrition team improve patient outcomes? A systematic review, *JPEN J Parenter Enteral Nutr* 28:251, 2004.

Nikolaidis P et al: Practice patterns of nonvascular interventional radiology procedures at academic centers in the United States? *Acad Radiol* 12:1475, 2005.

Oliveira L: Laparoscopic stoma creation and closure, *Semin Laporosc Surg* 10:191, 2003.

Peng X et al: Effects of enteral supplementation with glutamine granules on intestinal mucosal barrier function in severely burned patients, *Burns* 30:135, 2004.

Sachs GS et al: Parenteral nutrition implementation and management. In Merritt R, editor: *The ASPEN nutrition support practice manual*, ed 2, Silver Spring, Md, 2005, American Society for Parenteral and Enteral Nutrition.

Sands MJ: Vascular access in the adult home infusion patient, *JPEN J Parenter Enteral Nutr* 30:S57, 2006.

Scolapio JS: Methods for decreasing risk of aspiration pneumonia in critically ill patients, *JPEN J Parenter Enteral Nutr* 26:58S, 2002.

Sedman PC et al: Preoperative total parenteral nutrition is not associated with mucosal atrophy or bacterial translocation in humans, *Br J Surg* 82:1663, 1995.

Shike M, Bloch AS: Enteral nutrition, *Gastrointest Endosc Clin North Am* 8(3):529, 1998.

Somogyi-Zalud E et al: The use of life-sustaining treatments in hospitalized persons aged 80 and older, *J Am Geriatr Soc* 50:930, 2002.

Williams JZ et al: Effect of a specialized amino acid mixture on human collagen deposition, *Ann Surg* 236:369, 2002.

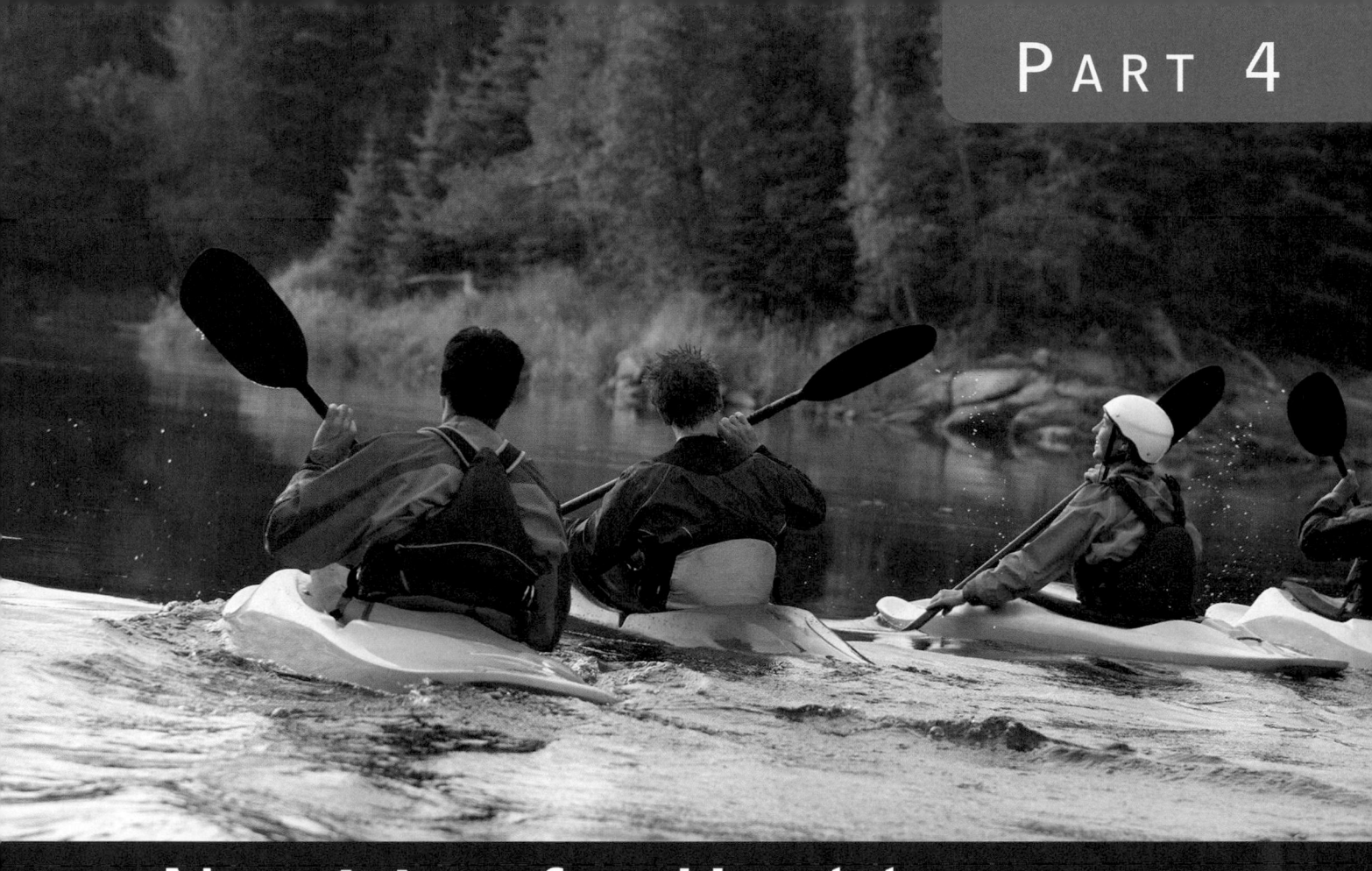

PART 4

Nutrition for Health and Fitness

T**HE** chapters in this section reflect the evolution of nutritional science, from the identification of nutrient requirements and the practical application of this knowledge to the concepts that relate nutrition to the prevention of chronic and degenerative diseases and optimization of health and performance.

The relationship between nutrition and dental disease has long been recognized. In more recent decades the possibility of reducing the incidence of osteoporosis by emphasizing appropriate nutrition has accumulated supportive evidence. The role of nutrition in reducing inflammation, now recognized as a contributor to chronic disease, is recent, but supports the awareness of diet in disease prevention. Understanding the role of nutrition in sports and in optimizing performance has led to dietary and exercise practices generally applicable to a rewarding lifestyle.

The opportunities for members of an affluent society to choose from a great variety of foods can easily lead to an overabundant intake of energy. Efforts to reduce body weight, widely pursued with varying degrees of enthusiasm and diligence, are often disheartening, making the knowledge presented here so important in nutrition practice. Frustration with dieting and stress often lead to eating disorders, which are increasing in frequency and require attention and understanding from the nutrition professional. Weight management and exercise form the basis for a great deal of nutrition in health, fitness, and disease prevention.

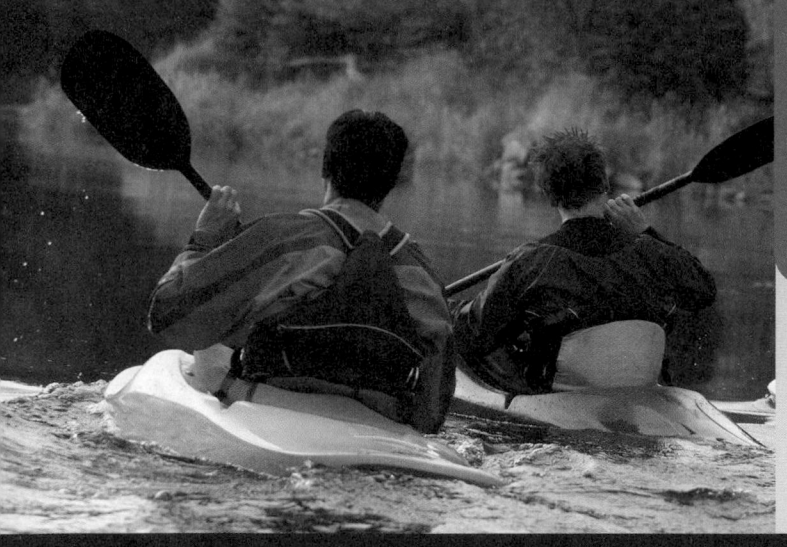

CHAPTER 21

Molly Gee, MEd, RD
L. Kathleen Mahan, MS, RD, CDE
Sylvia Escott-Stump, MA, RD, LDN

Weight Management

KEY TERMS

adipocyte a cell that synthesizes and stores triglycerides; fat cell

adipocytokines proteins released by the adipose cell into the bloodstream that act as signaling molecules and influence metabolism

android fat deposition deposition of fat around the waist and upper abdomen; "apple-shape" fat distribution

bariatric surgery gastroplasty, gastric bypass, and biliopancreatic diversion, operations for the purpose of stomach size reduction or malabsorption for the purpose of weight reduction

body mass index (BMI) a mathematical formula that correlates with body fat and is expressed as weight in kilograms divided by height in meters squared (BMI = kg/m²)

brown adipose tissue (BAT) fat located in the scapular area that is involved in heat production for cold adaptation and possibly burning off excess energy

catecholaminergic referring to the brain neurotransmitters norepinephrine, epinephrine, and dopamine

comorbidities conditions associated with obesity that usually worsen as the degree of obesity increases and often improves as the obesity is successfully treated

essential fat fat in the internal organs, bone marrow, and nerve tissues that is necessary for survival; about 3% to 12% of body weight

extreme or morbid obesity a state of adiposity in which body weight is 100% above the ideal body weight; a body mass index of 40 or greater

fat mass the fat from all body sources, including fat in the brain, skeleton, and adipose tissue

gastric bypass a surgical procedure in which the size of the stomach is reduced by a stapling procedure and the small intestine is connected to the smaller stomach pouch through a new opening

gastroplasty a surgical procedure in which the size of the stomach is reduced with a row of staples across the top half of the stomach with a small opening left into the distal stomach

gynoid fat distribution deposition of fat in the thighs and buttocks; "pear-shape" fat distribution

hormone-sensitive lipase (HSL) an enzyme in the adipose cell that is responsible for the hydrolysis of triglyceride into fatty acids and glycerol, which then leave the adipose cell and enter the circulation

hyperphagia a period of overeating

hyperplasia increase in tissue size by an increase in the number of cells

hypertrophy increase in tissue size by an increase in cell size

hypophagia a period of undereating

incretins gastrointestinal hormones that increase the amount of insulin released from the beta cells of the pancreas after eating and slow the rate of absorption by reducing gastric emptying

lean body mass (LBM) the part of the body free of adipose tissue; includes the skeletal muscles, water, bone, and a small amount of essential fat in the internal organs, bone marrow, and nerves

lifestyle modification change in the antecedents, behaviors, and consequences associated with eating habits, exercise, or thinking patterns

lipogenesis the conversion of glucose and intermediates into fat

lipoprotein lipase (LPL) an enzyme on the luminal side of the capillary that facilitates transport of lipid from the blood into the adipose cell

---

Sections of this chapter were written by Idamarie Laquatra, PhD, RD, for the previous edition of this text.

liposuction aspiration of fat deposits out of the body by means of a small incision through which a tube is fanned out into the adipose tissue

metabolic syndrome (MetS) a condition associated with glucose intolerance, insulin resistance, hyperlipidemia, and hypertension; strongly linked to abdominal obesity

obesity a state of adiposity in which body fatness is above the ideal; a body mass index of 30 to 39.9

overweight a state in which weight exceeds a standard based on height; a body mass index of 25 to 29.9 or greater

sensory-specific satiety a decline in the pleasantness of a food as it is consumed

storage fat the fat that accumulates under the skin and around internal organs

underweight a body weight 15% to 20% below the accepted weight standard; a body mass index of less than 18.5

very low–calorie diet (VLCD) a diet providing 800 kcal or less per day

visceral adipose tissue (VAT) fat accumulation in the intraabdominal (under the peritoneum) cavity

white adipose tissue (WAT) repository for triglycerides; a cushion to protect body organs and an insulator to preserve body heat

yo-yo effect the process of losing and gaining weight several times throughout a lifetime; often characterized by increased fatness with each cycle

Body weight is the sum of bone, muscle, organs, body fluids, and adipose tissue. Some or all of these components are subject to normal change as a reflection of growth, reproductive status, variation in exercise levels, and the effects of aging. Maintaining a constant body weight is orchestrated by a complex system of neural, hormonal, and chemical mechanisms that keeps the balance between energy intake and energy expenditure within fairly precise limits. Abnormalities of these mechanisms, many of which are not completely understood, result in exaggerated weight fluctuations. Of these, the most common are overweight and obesity. Although the inability to gain weight can also be a problem, underweight is usually secondary to another disease state. However, it is often accompanied by an eating disorder or psychological problem (see Chapter 22). In the elderly or in children unintentional weight loss can be especially detrimental and should be assessed and treated early to prevent malnutrition and other undesirable consequences.

BODY WEIGHT COMPONENTS

Body weight is often described in terms of its composition, and different models have been advanced to estimate body fat. Traditionally a two-compartment model has been used, dividing the body into the **fat mass,** the fat from all body sources including the brain, skeleton, and adipose tissue, and the fat-free mass (FFM). FFM can be divided into wa-

ter, protein, and mineral components (Wagner and Heyward, 2000). FFM is often used interchangeably with lean body mass (LBM), but it is not exactly the same.

Lean body mass (LBM) is the part of the body free of adipose tissue and includes the skeletal muscles, water, bone, and a small amount of essential fat in the internal organs, bone marrow, and nerve tissues. LBM is higher in men than in women, increases with exercise, and is lower in older adults. It is the major determinant of the resting metabolic rate. It follows that a decrease in lean tissue could hinder the progress of weight loss. Therefore, with respect to long-term effectiveness of weight-loss programs, the loss of fat mass while maintaining FFM and thus the resting metabolic rate (RMR) seems desirable (Stiegler and Cunliffe, 2006). Water, which makes up 60% to 65% of body weight, is the most variable component of LBM, and the state of hydration can induce fluctuations of several pounds in body weight.

Muscle and even skeletal mass adjust to some extent to support the changing burden of adipose tissue. Studies on the composition of excess weight gained showed that the LBM of the body accounts for an average of 29% of the excess weight in the obese person (Pierson et al., 1997).

Body Fat

Fat in the body is categorized as either "essential" or "storage." **Essential fat,** which is necessary for normal physiologic functioning, is stored in small amounts in the bone marrow, heart, lung, liver, spleen, kidneys, muscles, and lipid-rich tissues in the nervous system. In men, about 3% of body fat is considered essential. In women essential fat is higher, about 12%, because it also includes sex-specific body fat in the breasts, pelvic regions, and thighs.

The primary energy reserve of the body is the fat stored as triglycerides in depots made up of adipose tissue. This **storage fat** accumulates under the skin and around the internal organs to protect them from trauma. Most storage fat is considered "expendable." The totality of fat stores in adipocytes is capable of extensive variation, thus allowing for changing requirements of growth, reproduction, and aging as well as fluctuations in environmental and physiologic circumstances such as the availability of food and the demands of physical exercise. The range of total body fat (essential fat plus storage fat) expressed as a percentage of total body weight that is associated with optimum health is 8% to 24% in males and 21% to 35% in females (Gallagher et al., 2000), although professional and elite athletes have body fats much lower than those of the average person (Figure 21-1).

Adipose Tissue Structure

Adipose tissue is located primarily under the skin, in the mesenteries and omentum, and behind the peritoneum. Although it is primarily fat, adipose tissue is also composed of small amounts of protein and water. Adipose tissue exerts a profound influence on whole-body homoeostasis.

There are two types of adipose tissue in mammals: white adipose tissue and brown adipose tissue. **White adipose tissue (WAT)** stores energy as a repository for triglycerides, serves as a cushion to protect abdominal organs, and insulates the body

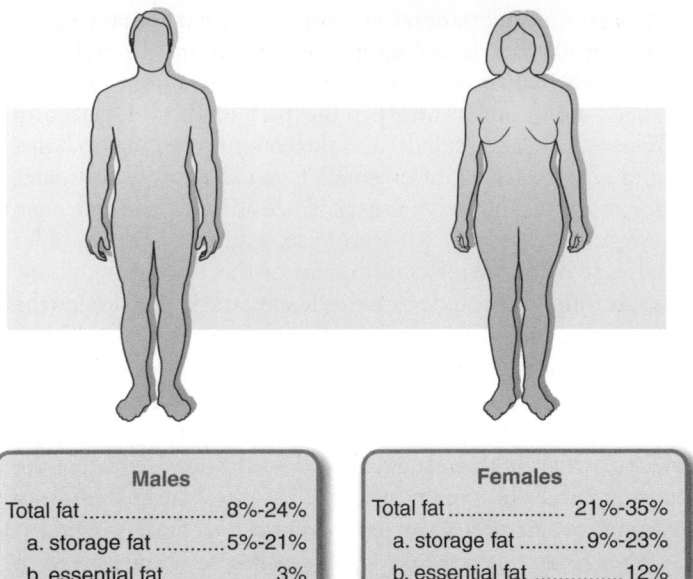

Males	
Total fat 8%-24%	
a. storage fat 5%-21%	
b. essential fat 3%	
Muscle 44.8%	
Bone 14.9%	
Remainder 16.3%-32.3%	

Females	
Total fat 21%-35%	
a. storage fat 9%-23%	
b. essential fat 12%	
Muscle 38%	
Bone 12%	
Remainder 15%-29%	

FIGURE 21-1 Behnke's theoretic body composition model for a man and a woman with healthy percentage body-fat ranges. *(Data from Gallagher D et al: Healthy percentage body-fat ranges: an approach for developing guidelines based on body mass index, Am J Clin Nutr 72:694, 2000.)*

to preserve heat. Carotene gives it a slight yellow color. **Brown adipose tissue (BAT),** seen in infants and in very small amounts in adults, occurs primarily in the scapular and subscapular areas. The brown color is due to extensive vascularization. In animals it appears to be involved in heat production as a means of adapting to cold and possibly of dissipating excess energy. Its function in humans remains poorly understood, but it is possible that BAT is a key regulator of energy expenditure (Hansen and Kristiansen, 2006).

Adipocytes, Hypertrophy, and Hyperplasia

The mature **adipocyte** consists of a large central lipid droplet surrounded by a thin rim of cytoplasm, which contains the nucleus and the mitochondria; these cells store fat in quantities equal to 80% to 95% of their volume. Adipose tissue increases either by increasing the size of cells already present when lipid is added **(hypertrophy)** or by increasing the number of cells **(hyperplasia).** Weight gain may be the result of hypertrophy, hyperplasia, or a combination of the two.

The fat depots can expand as much as 1000 times through hypertrophy alone, a process that can occur at any time as long as space is available in the adipocytes. Hyperplasia occurs primarily as a part of the growth process during infancy and adolescence, but it can also occur in adulthood when the fat content of existing cells has reached capacity. When weight is reduced as a result of trauma, illness, starvation, or changes in diet and exercise, fat cell size decreases; fat cell number does not.

Fat Cell Development

The greatest level of fatness in normal growth (about 25%) occurs at the age of 6 months. In lean children, fat cell size then decreases; however, this decrease does not occur in obese children. At the age of 6 years in lean children, increase in fatness occurs (adiposity rebound), with the increase being greater in girls than in boys. An early adiposity rebound occurring before 5.5 years is predictive of a higher level of adiposity at 16 years of age and in adulthood, a relationship that appears to occur regardless of the child's adiposity at 1 year of age. A later rebound is correlated with normal adult weight (Rolland-Cachera, 2005). Cell number increases in both lean and obese children throughout childhood into adolescence, but the number increases faster in obese children than in lean children. After adolescence, increases in body fat occur primarily by an increase in fat cell size. Contrary to old theories, the number of fat cells can increase throughout life; however, cell numbers do not increase until maximum cell size is reached. The number of cells does not decrease with weight loss. Prevention is the key, because once fat is gained and maintained over time, it is more difficult to lose.

Fat Storage

Most depot fat comes directly from dietary triglycerides, evidenced by the fact that fatty acid composition of adipose tissue mirrors the fatty acid composition of the diet. Excess dietary carbohydrate and protein are also converted to fatty acids in the liver by means of a comparatively inefficient process, **lipogenesis.**

Composition of the diet has been the focus of intense study. Under normal feeding conditions little dietary carbohydrate is used to produce adipose tissue, and it requires about three times as much energy to convert excess energy from carbohydrate to fat storage as it does to convert excess energy from dietary fat to fat storage. When high-carbohydrate diets are fed, however (in particular when the carbohydrate is in the form of simple sugars), lipogenesis does occur but does not represent a significant contribution to fat stores (McDevitt et al., 2001).

However, surplus carbohydrate energy makes individuals fatter not by lipogenesis but by suppressing fat oxidation (Hellerstein, 2001). Data from several sources indicate that Americans eat too many calories, even though they eat less fat than was consumed 30 years ago (Willett, 2002). Therefore recommendations simply to reduce dietary fat are inappropriate; total calories remain critical as the variable for weight management.

Lipoprotein Lipase

Dietary triglyceride is transported to the liver as a part of chylomicrons and is removed from the blood by the enzyme **lipoprotein lipase (LPL),** which sits on the luminal side of the capillary and facilitates removal of lipid from the blood and its entry through the capillary wall into the adipose cell. Triglycerides, synthesized in the liver from free fatty acids, travel as part of very low–density lipoprotein (VLDL) particles and are removed from the blood in the periphery by LPL. The enzyme hydrolyzes triglycerides into free fatty acids and glycerol. Glycerol proceeds to the liver, and fatty acids enter the adipocyte, where they are reesterified into triglycerides. When needed by other cells, the latter are hydrolyzed once again to fatty acids and glycerol through the action of **hormone-sensitive lipase (HSL)** within the adipose cell, and they are released and enter the circulation.

Hormones affect LPL activity in different adipose tissue regions. Estrogens appear to stimulate LPL activity in the gluteofemoral adipocytes and thus promote fat storage in this area, an effect that is seldom seen in obese men. This may be for the specific purpose of providing for childbearing and lactation. In the presence of sex steroid hormones, a normal distribution of body fat exists; with a decrease in sex steroid hormones, as occurs with aging and menopause or gonadectomy, there is a tendency to increase central obesity (Mayes and Watson, 2004). With weight loss there is a reduction in adipose tissue LPL levels and there is an improvement in lipid metabolic risk factors (Nicklas et al., 2000).

REGULATION OF BODY WEIGHT

Regulatory systems such as neurochemicals, body-fat stores, protein mass, hormones, and postingestion factors all play a role in regulating intake and weight. Some evidence suggests that regulation takes place on both a short- and a long-term basis. Short-term regulation governs consumption of food from meal to meal; long-term regulation is controlled by the availability of adipose stores and hormone responses. Total calories are more important than any single macronutrient.

Short- and Long-Term Regulation

Short-term controls are concerned primarily with factors governing hunger, appetite, and satiety. Satiety is associated with the postprandial state when excess food is being stored. Hunger is associated with the postabsorptive state when those stores are being mobilized. Physical triggers for hunger are much stronger than those for satiety, and it is easier to override the signals for satiety.

A study investigated the effects of aging on the mechanisms of body energy regulation in an attempt to determine the causes of unexplained weight loss in older persons (Roberts et al., 1994). Healthy younger and older men of normal weight consumed a typical diet and performed usual activities. When either overfeeding or underfeeding interventions were made, the younger men exhibited spontaneous **hypophagia** (undereating) or **hyperphagia** (overeating) to alter body weight accordingly. The older men did not have the same responsiveness to changes in caloric intake. Findings from this study suggest that older persons are more vulnerable to unexplained weight losses or gains because of their inability to control spontaneous short-term changes in food intake. Yet age alone should not preclude weight loss treatment in older adults; careful evaluation of risks and benefits is needed.

Long-term regulation seems to involve a feedback mechanism in which a signal from the adipose mass is released when "normal" body composition is disturbed, as when weight loss occurs. These proteins, released by the adipose cell into the bloodstream, act as signaling molecules and are referred to as **adipocytokines.** This factor may play a greater role in younger persons than in older adults.

Set-Point Theory

Fat storage in nonobese adults appears to be regulated in a manner that preserves a specific body weight. In both animals and humans deliberate efforts to starve or overfeed are followed by a rapid return to the original body weight, as though the latter constitutes a "set point" that is amenable to physiologic influences. If this is true, some forms of obesity could be the result of an abnormally established set point; however, data are not conclusive in this area of research. Body weight remains remarkably stable despite variations, possibly from internal regulatory mechanisms that are genetically determined. Some studies suggest that body weight can be displaced only temporarily and that resting metabolic rate lowers, resulting in body weight returning. Other studies do not show an adaptive metabolic response to weight loss. Instead, a transient reduction in energy expenditure is observed with energy restriction that normalizes on return to energy balance conditions (Weinsier et al., 2000). The controversy continues.

Factors Regulating Energy Intake and Body Weight

Dietary Thermogenesis and the Thermic Effect of Food

The components of energy expenditure are the resting energy expenditure (REE), often expressed as RMR; the energy expended in voluntary activity; and the thermic effect of food (TEF), also called diet-induced thermogenesis (DIT) or specific dynamic action (SDA) of food. TEF is the increment in energy expenditure above RMR due to the processing of food for use and storage (see Chapter 2 for a detailed discussion).

Meal size, meal composition, the nature of the previous meal, insulin resistance, physical activity, and aging all influence TEF. For example, a single bout of aerobic exercise enhances TEF related to a carbohydrate meal (Denzer and Young, 2003). Workers who work and eat at night may have a different metabolic efficiency.

Resting Metabolic Rate

The RMR explains 60% to 70% of total energy expenditure. RMR declines with age and with restriction of energy intake. When the body is suddenly deprived of adequate energy, such as with involuntary or deliberate starvation or semistarvation, the RMR adapts to conserve energy against an unpredictable future by dropping rapidly, by as much as 15% in 2 weeks. When adequate food intake is restored, the RMR returns to baseline levels (Ravussin and Swinburn, 1992).

WEIGHT IMBALANCE: OBESITY AND OVERWEIGHT

Obesity and overweight are a result of an imbalance between food consumed and physical activity. National data have shown an increase in the calorie consumption of adults and no change in physical activity patterns. But obesity is a complex issue related to lifestyle, environment, and genes. Many underlying factors have been linked to the increase in obesity prevalence, such as increasing portion sizes; eating out more often; increasing television or computer viewing or electronic gaming time; changing labor markets; and fear of crime, which prevents outdoor exercise. Overweight adolescents often become obese adults; obese individuals are at increased risk for **comorbidities** of type 2 diabetes, hypertension, stroke, certain cancers, infertility, and other conditions.

Prevalence

The United States has the highest prevalence of obesity among the developed nations. It is not alone in terms of trends; increases in the prevalence of overweight and obesity among children and adults have been observed throughout the world. The latest estimates of overweight and obesity among children and adults are based on measured weights and heights from the National Health and Nutrition Examination Survey (NHANES), which is conducted by the Centers for Disease Control and Prevention's (CDC's) National Center for Health Statistics (CDC, 2007).

An estimated 66% of U.S. adults are overweight, and 32% are obese. In addition, 17% of children and adolescents between ages 2 and 19 years are overweight. Prevalence is higher in black and Hispanic populations, especially in Mexican-Americans (CDC, 2007) (Figure 21-2).

Disparities also exist within genders. The prevalence of overweight and obesity is higher in women who are members of racial and ethnic minorities compared with non-Hispanic white women. Non-Hispanic black women (81.6%) have a higher prevalence of overweight and obesity compared with men (69.1%). This picture reverses in non-Hispanic white men and women, with men having a higher prevalence of overweight and obesity (70.6%) compared with women (58%). Mexican-American women (75.4%) and men (76.1%) have similar rates of overweight and obesity.

The obesity "epidemic," as many health professionals label it, is now pervasive throughout the United States. According to the CDC *Behavioral Risk Factor Surveillance System Survey Data* one can see how this epidemic has developed. As shown in Figure 21-3, in 1990 no states had obesity rates of 15% or greater, whereas just 15 years later in 2005 only four states had obesity prevalence rates less than 20%. Seventeen states had prevalence rates equal to or greater than 25%, with three of those having prevalences equal to or greater than 30% (Louisiana, Mississippi, and West Virginia).

Weight Management Throughout the Life Span

Balancing energy intake and energy expenditure is the basis of weight management throughout life. The *2005 Dietary Guidelines for Americans* (see Chapters 9 and 12) provide science-based advice for eating a healthy diet and being physically active to promote health, psychological well-being, and a healthy body weight. A key recommendation is to prevent gradual weight gain over time by making small decreases in food and beverage calories and increasing physical activity. **Lifestyle modification,** where individuals become aware of the triggers for their eating behaviors in order to manage them more effectively, is also recommended.

Although it may sound simple, this feat can be extraordinarily difficult. Researchers in the area of weight management believe that part of the reason for the failure of many persons to balance energy intake and expenditure is the lack of tools that accurately assess either one (Hill, 2000). Future technologic progress will allow people to readily access

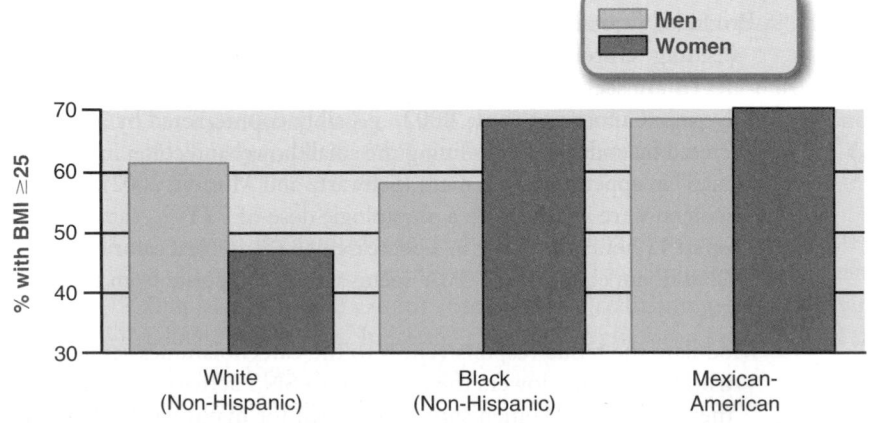

FIGURE 21-2 Age-adjusted prevalence of overweight or obesity in selected groups. *(Modified from U.S. Department of Health and Human Services:* The Surgeon General's call to action to prevent and decrease overweight and obesity, *Rockville, Md, 2001, U.S. Department of Health and Human Services, Public Health Service, Office of the Surgeon General; and Centers for Disease Control and Prevention (CDC), National Center for Health Statistics [NCHS], and National Health and Nutrition Examination Survey [NHANES].)*

tools that clearly demonstrate the impact of their behaviors on energy balance. Patterns of healthful eating and regular physical activity should begin in childhood and continue throughout adulthood. The aging process introduces special challenges to the energy balance equation. As a result of a lower RMR caused in part by a loss of FFM, energy balance must be maintained by adjusting or reducing caloric intake and increasing physical activity to prevent weight gain as individuals age.

Weight and Longevity

Prolonged calorie restriction (CR) increases life span and slows aging in rodents and other animals. The apparent generality of the longevity-increasing effects of CR has prompted speculation that similar results could be obtained in humans (see *New Directions:* Will Eating Less Make You Live Longer? in Chapter 2). Some recent findings from a short 6-month study suggest that two biomarkers of longevity (fasting insulin level and body temperature) are decreased by prolonged calorie restriction in humans and support the theory that metabolic rate is reduced beyond the level expected from reduced metabolic body mass (Heilbronn et al., 2006). However, longevity evolves as part of a life history, and the physiologic mechanisms that determine longevity are complex, and the benefits of calorie restriction

are expected to be minor (Phelan and Rose, 2006). More long-term studies are needed to determine if CR can slow down the aging process.

Assessment

Overweight is a state in which weight exceeds a standard based on height; **obesity** is a condition of excessive fatness, either generalized or localized. It is possible to be obese at a weight within normal limits according to standard tables, just as it is possible to be overweight without being obese. However, in most people, overweight and obesity parallel each other.

Overweight and obesity are assessed in a variety of ways. In the past, the tables of the Metropolitan Life Insurance Company were widely used to establish a standard of ideal body weight (IBW). Currently the most commonly used methods include (1) determination of the **body mass index (BMI)** or Quetelet Index (W/H2), in which W is weight in kilograms and H is height in meters, and (2) waist circumference. Waist-to-hip ratio (WHR) is seldom used.

Waist circumference over 40 inches in men and over 35 inches in women signifies increased risk equal to a BMI of 25 to 34.9 (NIH, 1998). When waist circumference and percentage of fat are included together, they are significant predictors of heart failure and risk associated with obesity

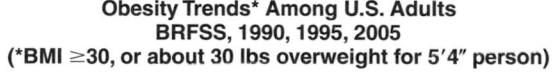

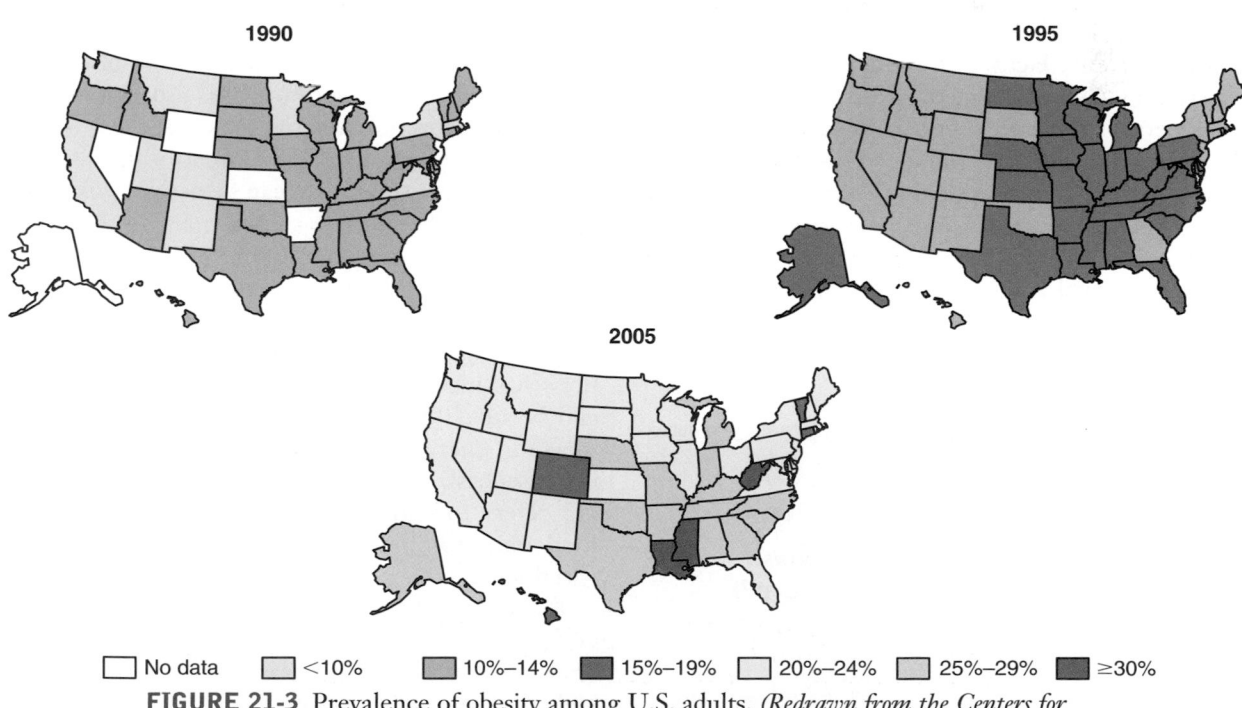

FIGURE 21-3 Prevalence of obesity among U.S. adults. *(Redrawn from the Centers for Disease Control and Prevention (CDC) Behavioral Risk Factor Surveillance System Survey, based on data from Mokdad AH et al.: The spread of the obesity epidemic in the United States, 1991-1998, JAMA 282:1519-1522, 1999; Mokdad AH et al.: The continuing epidemics of obesity and diabetes in the United States, JAMA 286:1195-1200, 2001; Mokdad AH et al.: Prevalence of obesity, diabetes, and obesity-related health risk factors, 2001, JAMA 289:76-79, 2003; Morbidity and Mortality Weekly Report: State-specific prevalence of obesity among adults, United States, 2005, MMWR Morb Mortal Wkly Rep 55:36, 2006.)*

(Nicklas et al., 2006). Waist circumference is the strongest independent correlate of insulin sensitivity index (ISI) in older adults, and waist circumference is a better predictor of adiposity. These findings support the measurement of waist circumference to assess health risk among older adults (Racette et al., 2006a) (see Figure 14-15 in Chapter 14).

The National Institutes of Health (NIH) clinical guidelines classify individuals with a BMI of 25 as overweight. Persons who have a BMI of 30 or higher are classified as obese (NIH, 1998). Overweight and obesity as defined by the NIH are shown in Table 21-2.

Optimal BMI, in terms of longevity, varies with race, gender and age, contributing to the debate over what BMI level or distribution should be considered ideal in terms of mortality risk. Simulating BMI progression over time has a substantial impact on health outcomes and should be modeled in future health economic analyses of overweight and obesity (Newby et al., 2006). These and other body fatness assessment methods are discussed in detail in Chapter 14. Tables for determining BMI are presented in Appendix 23.

Etiology

The nature and causes of obesity are the subject of intensive and continuing research. Both environmental and genetic factors are involved in a complex interaction, which also includes psychological and cultural influences, as well as physiologic regulatory mechanisms. Over the years many hypotheses have evolved to explain why some people become fat whereas others remain lean and why it is so difficult for reduced-obese persons to maintain the weight loss that was achieved. The fact that no single theory can completely explain all manifestations of obesity or apply consistently to all persons underscores the complex nature of this condition. Heredity and environment influence both the input and output of energy.

Heredity

Many of the hormonal and neural factors involved in normal weight regulation are determined genetically. These include the short- and long-term signals that determine sa-

tiety and feeding activity. Small defects in their expression or interaction could contribute significantly to weight gain. The number and size of fat cells, regional distribution of body fat, and RMR are also influenced by genes.

The first studies of the role of inheritance in obesity estimated it to be from 66% to 80% and from studies of twins it seems to confirm that genes determine 50% to 70% of the predisposition to the development of obesity (Prentice, 2005). The number of genes, markers, and chromosomal regions associated with obesity phenotypes includes genes on every chromosome except the Y chromosome (Pérusse et al., 2001). Still remaining is the task of identifying the combination of genes and mutations that contribute most to human obesity and defining the environmental promoters (Bray, 1998).

Although numerous genes are involved in obesity, several have received much attention—the ob gene, the GAD_2 gene, the FTO gene, and the β3-adrenoreceptor gene. The ob gene produces leptin, and mutations in the mouse ob gene result in obesity. The β3-adrenoreceptor gene, located primarily in the adipose tissue, is thought to regulate RMR and fat oxidation in humans. The FTO gene predisposes to diabetes by its effect on body mass (Frayling et al., 2007).

It has been suggested that typical obesity is so heterogeneous and polygenic that there will be no major genes; rather, 20 or more common gene variants may contribute a small genetic burden (Shuldiner and Sabra, 2001).

Factors Affecting Weight Gain

Although genes appear to increase vulnerability to obesity, other determinants must be present for obesity to occur. Dietary and activity patterns are also primary causes of weight problems in industrial societies; there is a mismatch between lifestyle and genetic makeup.

Excessive energy intake can be active or passive. Active overeating in Western societies is partly the result of excessive portion sizes that are accepted as the norm. The portions and calories that restaurants and fast-food outlets offer for one meal often exceed a person's energy needs for the entire day. In fact, the number of large-size portions has increased dramatically since the 1970s (Young and Nestle, 2002). Data from NHANES III suggest that intake of energy-dense, nutrient-poor foods results in an increased risk of overeating (Kant, 2000). Passive overeating refers to eating energy-dense diets; the amount of food may not be excessive, but the calorie content is (Prentice, 2001).

Research supports the fact that food and its taste elements evoke pleasure responses, and the endless variety of food available at any time at a reasonable cost can contribute to higher calorie intake because people eat more when offered a variety of choices than when a single food is available. Normally, as foods are consumed, they become less pleasant. This decline is known as **sensory-specific satiety** and is associated with a shift to other food choices during the meal (Rolls and Drewnowski, 1996). An example of overriding this principle is the all-you-can-eat buffet in which the diner reaches satiety for one food but has a plethora of choices for the "next

TABLE 21-2

Classification of Overweight and Obesity

Classification	Body Mass Index (kg/m²)
Underweight	<18.5
Normal	18.5-24.9
Overweight	25.0-29.9
Obesity, class I	30.0-34.9
Obesity, class II	35.0-39.9
Extreme obesity, class III	≥40

From National Institutes of Health, National Heart, Lung, and Blood Institute: *Clinical guidelines on the identification, evaluation, and treatment of overweight and obesity in adults—the evidence report*, NIH Publication No. 98-4083, 1998.

course." Although sensory-specific satiety can promote the intake of a more varied and nutritionally balanced diet, it can also lead to overconsumption.

The effect of eating more calories than needed is compounded by low energy expenditure. The sedentary nature of the American society is a factor in the growing problem of obesity. Fewer Americans are exercising, and more time is being spent in low-energy activities such as watching television, using the computer, and driving to activities.

Health Risks

Obesity has been directly linked with mortality and many chronic ailments, including diabetes, heart disease, hypertension, hyperlipidemia, gallbladder disease, and some cancers. Moderately high BMI in adolescence is correlated with premature death in younger and middle-age women (van Dam et al., 2006). Findings from the 24-year-old Nurse's Health Study showed that increased adiposity and reduced physical activity are strong independent risk factors for death in women. Adiposity (BMI greater than 25) predicted a higher risk of death regardless of the level of physical activity. In other words, being physically active did not protect from the risk of being overweight (Hu et al., 2004).

Estimates using mortality data from the NHANES surveys show that thousands of deaths are related to obesity. However, the health consequences of this increasing rate of obesity have not been fully clarified. Increases in diabetes are related to obesity, but increases in life expectancy and slight decreases in heart disease mortality seem to confound expectations about the effects of rising obesity rates (Flegal, 2005). However, on the basis of several large studies, the optimal BMI with the least risk for mortality is a BMI of 23 to 24.9. Above and below this there seems to be increased mortality risk (Jee et al., 2006; Adams et al., 2006). The optimal range for longevity still appears to be within the range of 20.5 to 24.9.

A subset of obese persons who are metabolically normal seems to exist. This subgroup has uncomplicated obesity and appears to have early-onset obesity, hyperplasia of normal adipocytes, and normal quantities of visceral fat (Sims, 2001). In general, however, obesity can be viewed as metabolically unhealthy. Chronic diseases such as heart disease, type 2 diabetes, hypertension, stroke, gallbladder disease, sleep apnea, certain cancers, and osteoarthritis tend to worsen as the degree of obesity increases (Shape Up America! and American Obesity Association, 2001).

An increasingly recognized condition associated with obesity is nonalcoholic fatty liver disease, which may progress to end-stage liver disease (Angulo, 2002). Obesity is also a risk factor for cancer, infertility, poor wound healing, and poor antibody response to hepatitis B vaccine. The costs of obesity are staggering. Health economists estimate costs of overweight and obesity to account for nearly 10% of total annual U.S. medical expenditures, equivalent to $92.6 billion; Medicare and Medicaid financed half of these costs (Finkelstein et al., 2004).

Healthy People 2010 objectives recognize the public health implications of overweight and obesity in our soci-

ety (see Chapter 11). The objectives include ambitious targets to increase the proportion of adults who are at a healthy weight and to reduce the proportion of adults, children, and adolescents who are obese. Underscoring the concern that overweight and obesity increase the risk for heart disease, diabetes, cancers, and other chronic health problems, the Surgeon General released in 2001 a "Call to Action," noting that gains made in other areas of public health are marginalized if overweight and obesity increases are not reversed (USDHHS, 2001).

In 2002 the Internal Revenue Service (IRS) issued a new rule qualifying obesity as a disease, allowing taxpayers to claim weight-loss expenses as a medical deduction if undertaken at a physician's direction to treat an existing disease. Although not all obese persons who have weight-loss expenses qualify for the deduction, the government now recognizes the immense impact of obesity on the health and financial well-being of the country.

Regional Distribution of Fat and Metabolic Syndrome

Regional patterns of fat deposit are controlled genetically and differ between and among men and women. Two major types of fat deposition are currently recognized: excess subcutaneous truncal-abdominal fat (android) and excess gluteofemoral fat (gynoid). Excess subcutaneous fat on the trunk, particularly in the abdominal area, is **android** or "apple-shape" obesity and is more common among men. Aging is also an important factor in visceral obesity, or excessive accumulation of **visceral adipose tissue (VAT)** under the peritoneum and in the intra-abdominal cavity. Studies indicate that this type of obesity is highly correlated with insulin resistance (NIH, 1998).

The Third Report of the National Cholesterol Education Program (NCEP) Expert Panel (ATP III) defined the **metabolic syndrome (MetS)** as having three or more of the following abnormalities: waist circumference more than 102 cm (40 in) in men and more than 88 cm (35 in) in women; serum triglycerides of at least 150 mg/dl; high-density lipoprotein (HDL) level less than 40 mg/dl in men and less than 50 mg/dl in women; blood pressure 135/85 mm Hg or higher; or serum glucose 110 mg/dl or higher (see Chapter 32). The International Diabetes Federation (IDF) has proposed a new definition of the metabolic syndrome that emphasizes central adiposity as determined by ethnic group-specific thresholds of waist circumference. Findings from a study to estimate the prevalence of this syndrome using the IDF definition demonstrated a higher prevalence estimate of the metabolic syndrome than that estimate based on the NCEP definition. The IDF definition leads to higher estimates of prevalence in all of the demographic groups, especially among Mexican-American men (Ford et al., 2002).

Regional body fat distribution has an important influence on metabolic and cardiovascular risk factors. Increased visceral fat is a risk factor for coronary artery disease (CAD), dyslipidemia, hypertension, stroke, and type 2 diabetes (Gower et al., 2006). In addition to general obesity, greater visceral adipose tissue is independently associated with the

◉ FOCUS ON

Polycystic Ovary Syndrome

Polycystic ovary syndrome (PCOS), an endocrine disorder characterized by hyperandrogenism and insulin resistance, affects 5% to 10% of women of reproductive age (McKittrick, 2000). Symptoms include erratic menstrual periods, chronic anovulation resulting in multiple ovarian cysts, infertility, acne, hirsutism (hair growth), and alopecia (hair loss). Interviews with women who have PCOS indicate that it is a deeply stigmatizing condition, making them feel abnormal and less feminine (Kitzinger and Willmott, 2002). PCOS is closely associated primarily with android obesity (Scalzo, 2000). The insulin resistance and resultant hyperinsulinemia in PCOS increase the risk of cardiovascular disease, type 2 diabetes, and the reproductive cancers (i.e., endometrial and ovarian). Treatment is symptom oriented (Legro, 2002): an individualized diet, an exercise plan to promote weight loss and normalize insulin levels, and medications to alleviate symptoms such as antihyperglycemia medications. Persons with PCOS often have disordered eating patterns.

metabolic syndrome in older men and women, particularly among those of normal body weight (Goodpaster, 2005).

Gynoid fat distribution, the "pear shape," is created by heavier deposits of fat around the thighs and buttocks. Gynoid obesity is more common in women, and the fat deposits are presumably energy reserves to support the demands of pregnancy and lactation. Women with the gynoid type of obesity do not develop the impairments of glucose metabolism seen in obese women of the same weight who carry their fat in the abdominal area.

Combinations of abdominal fat accumulation and gluteofemoral fat accumulation are also seen, particularly in women. Postmenopausal women more closely follow the male pattern of abdominal fat stores and are at increased risk for blood glucose, lipid, and pressure abnormalities. In both men and women who were obese during adolescence, rates of cardiovascular disease and diabetes are increased. Risks are increased with polycystic ovary syndrome (see *Focus On: Polycystic Ovary Syndrome*).

Discrimination

Widespread bias and discrimination based on weight have been documented in education, employment, and health care. Like other forms of prejudice, this most likely is because of a lack of understanding of the chronic disease of obesity and the medical consequences. Despite laws designed to prevent discrimination based on appearance, unfavorable attitudes and practices persist.

The impact of weight bias on overweight children and adolescents deserves special attention. There is growing evidence that overweight children experience adverse social,

educational, and psychological consequences as a result of weight bias (Latner et al., 2005). Further research on the presence and impact of weight bias against children is needed to guide interventions.

Recent studies have also documented automatic negative associations with obese people among health professionals and exercise science students and among obese individuals themselves (Brown, 2006; Carr and Friedman, 2005). A plan for continued education of the medical and nonmedical communities is essential to break down the barriers caused by ignorance and indifference. Patient support groups play an important role in the ongoing battle to correct the negative effect of these attitudes on the obese person.

MANAGEMENT OF OBESITY IN ADULTS

The management of obesity has evolved over the years as more research has increased knowledge of weight regulation. Initially clinicians focused entirely on weight loss, and little was known about weight maintenance. It was assumed that if people could just lose the weight, maintenance would easily follow. It soon became clear that focusing on weight loss without attention to weight maintenance was inappropriate, unfair, and possibly harmful to anyone trying to manage his or her weight.

Treatment has also evolved. Years ago an energy-restricted diet represented the only treatment. Eventually lifestyle modifications were added after research supported their inclusion. Finally the importance of physical activity was recognized, not just as a component for weight loss but also as an essential ingredient for weight maintenance after weight loss.

Today a chronic disease-prevention model that involves both lifestyle interventions and interdisciplinary team therapies from physicians, dietitians, exercise specialists, and behavior therapists offers the best treatment opportunity. Weight-reduction programs with the most promise of success integrate healthier food choices, exercise, and lifestyle modification. Pharmacologic treatment and surgical intervention are appropriate in some circumstances but are not a substitute for the necessary changes in eating and physical activity pattern (see *Pathophysiology and Care Management Algorithm: Management of Obesity*). The ADA Evidence Analysis provides reliable treatment guidelines (ADA, 2007).

Goals of Treatment

The goal of obesity treatment should be refocused from weight loss alone to weight management, defined as attaining the best weight possible in the context of overall health. Achieving ideal body weight or percentage of body fat is not always realistic or desirable, and under some circumstances it may not be appropriate at all. Depending on the type and severity of the existing obesity and the age and lifestyle of the individual, successfully reducing body weight varies from a being a relatively simple matter to being virtually impossible.

PATHOPHYSIOLOGY AND CARE MANAGEMENT ALGORITHM

Management of Obesity

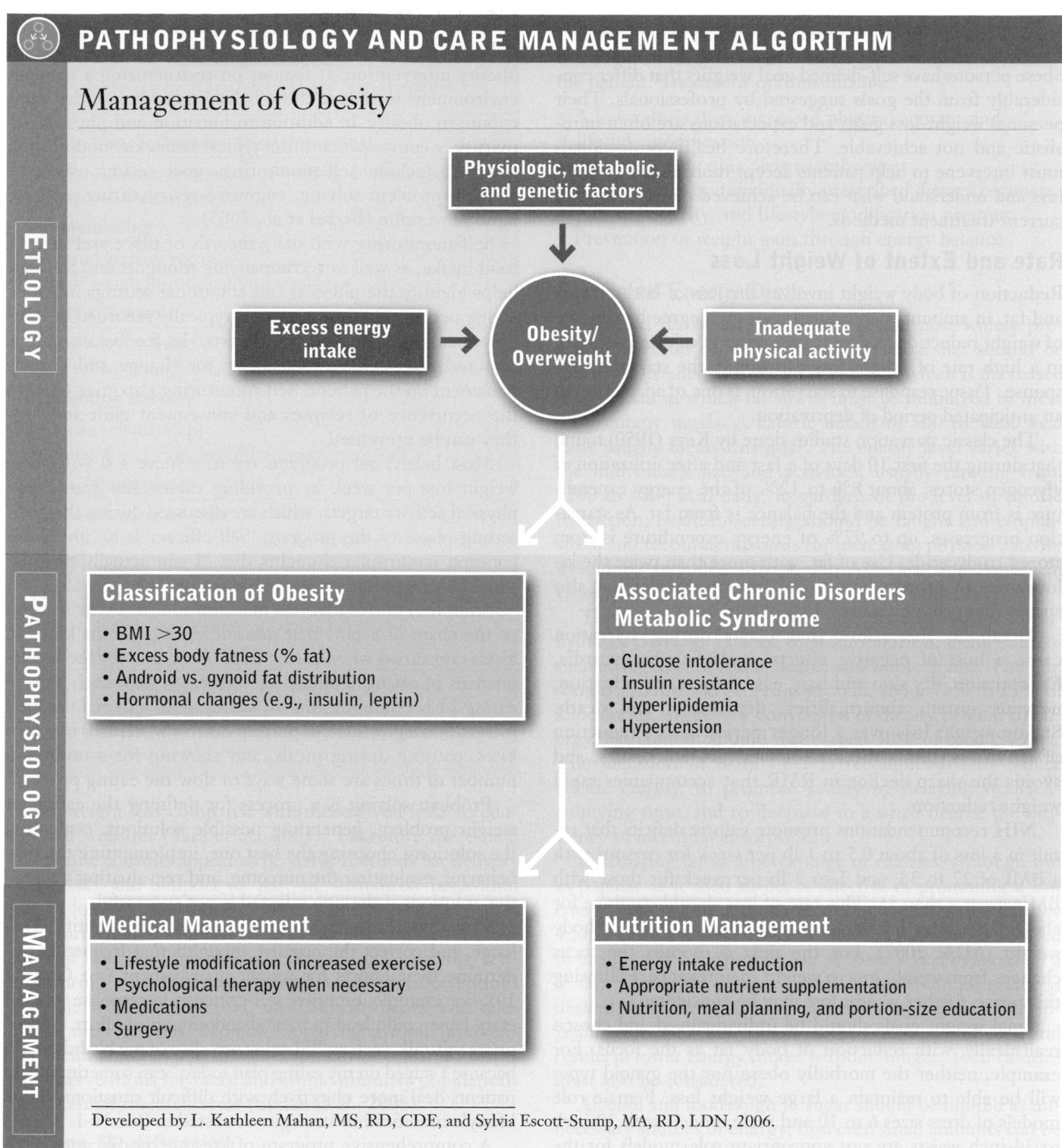

ETIOLOGY

Physiologic, metabolic, and genetic factors

Excess energy intake → Obesity/ Overweight ← Inadequate physical activity

PATHOPHYSIOLOGY

Classification of Obesity

- BMI >30
- Excess body fatness (% fat)
- Android vs. gynoid fat distribution
- Hormonal changes (e.g., insulin, leptin)

Associated Chronic Disorders Metabolic Syndrome

- Glucose intolerance
- Insulin resistance
- Hyperlipidemia
- Hypertension

MANAGEMENT

Medical Management

- Lifestyle modification (increased exercise)
- Psychological therapy when necessary
- Medications
- Surgery

Nutrition Management

- Energy intake reduction
- Appropriate nutrient supplementation
- Nutrition, meal planning, and portion-size education

Developed by L. Kathleen Mahan, MS, RD, CDE, and Sylvia Escott-Stump, MA, RD, LDN, 2006.

Maintaining present body weight or achieving a moderate loss is beneficial. Obese persons who lose even small amounts of weight (5% to 10% of initial body weight) are likely to improve their health in the short run by reducing the severity of the comorbidities associated with obesity (Anderson and Konz, 2001). A review of studies in which patients experienced a 10% or less weight reduction showed that they also had improved glycemic control, reduced blood pressure, and reduced cholesterol levels.

The critical question of whether modest weight losses, if maintained, would have a long-term impact remains unanswered. The initial effects on glycemic control were greater than the long-term effects, supporting the role of energy restriction as well as weight loss in glycemic improvement (Anderson and Konz, 2001). The maintenance of improvements at 1 year supports the prediction that long-term improvements in body weight could have a long-term effect on glycemic control.

no evidence that using artificial sweeteners reduces food intake or results in better rates of weight loss.

Vitamin and mineral supplements that meet age-related requirements are usually recommended with weight-reduction programs that provide less than 1200 kcal for women or 1800 kcal for men. It is difficult to choose foods to maintain this calorie level and meet all nutritional requirements every day.

Formula Diets and Meal Replacement Programs

Formula diets, or meal replacements, are commercially prepared, ready-to-use, portion-controlled foods or drinks. These meal replacements can be found over the counter in drug stores, supermarkets, and franchised weight loss centers or in a clinical setting as drinks, pre-packaged meals (entrees), or meal bars. They are designed to be part of a low-calorie diet. The goal of using meal replacements is to provide structure and replace other foods likely to be higher in calorie content. Per serving, most meal replacements include 0 to 5 g of fiber; 10 to 14 g of protein; various amounts of carbohydrate, depending on whether they are artificially sweetened; 0 to 10 g of fat: and 25% to 30% of RDAs for vitamins and minerals. Usually shakes are milk or soy based and may be high in calcium. They range from 150 to 250 kcal/8 oz. Some shakes are prepared using a blender at home and are made with a purchased protein powder (either soy, milk, or rice protein concentrate) that usually has added vitamins and minerals and sometimes fiber, to which fruit or fruit juice is added for the carbohydrate, and oil such as olive, canola or flaxseed, for the fat. For people who have difficulty with self-selection or portion control, meal replacements (e.g., liquid meals, meal bars, calorie-controlled packaged meals) may be used as part of the diet component of a comprehensive weight management program. Substituting one or two daily meals or snacks with meal replacements is a successful weight loss and weight maintenance strategy (ADA, 2007).

Commercial Programs

Millions of Americans turn to commercial weight-loss or self-help programs in search of permanent weight loss. The more caloric-restricted programs are usually medically supervised in a health care setting. As Table 21-3 illustrates, the programs vary considerably. Some require the use of proprietary prepackaged low-fat meals. Prepackaged diets appeal to some people because they allow them to avoid making choices about food. Some provide classes on self-introspection, behavior modification, and nutrition.

TABLE 21-3

Popular Commercial Diet Programs

Name	Foods or Products	Education	Teachers/Counselors	Maintenance
VLCD Programs				
Health Management Resources (HMR) www.yourbetterhealth.com	Special drink, multidisciplinary team	1½-hr weekly group meetings with registered dietitian (RD) and midweek phone calls	MDs, health educators, registered nurses, RDs, exercise physiologists	Weekly meetings for 18 mo
Medifast www.med.fast.net	Special drink; physician supervised	Weekly individual sessions Weekly group meetings	Supervised by MDs	Weekly meetings for 5 mo
Optifast www.optifast.com	Special drink; physician supervised	Weekly individual sessions with MD 1½-hr weekly group meetings One meeting with RD	MDs, registered nurses, RDs, and psychologists at most locations	No time limit, begins at 20th week
Diet Programs				
Diet Center www.dietcenter.com	Regular food	Daily individual sessions	Trained staff	Maintenance: weekly meetings for the first 3 mo; biweekly for months 4-6; monthly for months 6-12
Jenny Craig www.jennycraig.com	Prepackaged foods	14 1-hr video group classes; weekly individual sessions	RDs and psychologists	Monthly meetings for 6 mo or 1 yr

Use of the Internet has spawned a new generation of commercial programs. A randomized, controlled trial of overweight adults with BMI of 25 to 36 indicated that the Internet can be used successfully to deliver a weight-loss program if it includes behavioral therapy with weekly contact and individualized feedback (Tate et al., 2001). The importance of a tailored approach was the conclusion of a randomized controlled trial (RCT) comparing an Internet-based tailored weight management program with an information-only Internet weight management program based in an integrated health care setting (Rothert, 2006).

With the exception of Weight Watchers, the evidence to support the use of the major commercial and self-help weight loss programs is suboptimal. The reported results

---

TABLE 21-3

Popular Commercial Diet Programs—cont'd

Diet Programs—cont'd

Nutri/System www.nutrisystem.com	Prepackaged foods	30-min weekly group meetings; 10-min weekly individual sessions	College graduates	1-yr transition diet; program and regular foods
Weight Watchers www.weightwatchers.com	Regular food	45-min weekly group meetings	Program graduates	Weekly meetings for 6 wk; free meetings if maintain goal weight
The Solution www.shapedown.com	Regular food	Weekly 2-hr group meetings	RDs and psychologists certified by the program	Monthly meetings for 6 mo or 1 yr; continuation with weekly meetings as necessary; no time limit

Internet-Based Diets

Cyberdiet www.DietWatch.com and www.Cyberdiet.com	Regular food	Personal and professional eCounseling provide weekly meal plans and nutrition and fitness report cards Professional eCounseling provides biweekly chats with an RD in chat rooms, bulletin boards; e-newsletter also available	Registered dietitians; also uses the expertise of physiologists, fitness trainers, culinary chefs, MDs, and psychologists	Maintenance program available once personal goals are met
eDiets www.ediets.com	Regular food	Weekly meal plan and exercise routines Chat rooms, bulletin boards, e-newsletter available	RDs, registered nurses, fitness trainers, counselors, psychologists	Maintenance meal plans are available
Nutrio www.nutrio.com	Regular food	Daily and weekly meal plans; exercise and nutrition logs, community message boards and e-newsletter	RDs, exercise physiologists, and psychologists	Maintenance meal plans available

VLCD, Very low–calorie diet.

are probably a best-case scenario because many studies did not control for high attrition rates. Controlled trials are needed to assess the efficacy and cost-effectiveness of most commercial programs (Tsai and Wadden 2005).

In summary, it is important to evaluate all weight loss programs for sound nutritional practices. Consumers are savvy, and many programs have begun to collect data on the effects of treatment, including dropout rates, success rates, and maintenance data.

Extreme Energy Restriction and Fasting

Extreme energy-restricted diets provide fewer than 800 kcal per day, and starvation or fasting diets provide fewer than 200 kcal per day. Fasting is seldom prescribed as a treatment; however, it is frequently invoked as a part of religious or protest regimen or in a personal effort to lose weight. Under these circumstances it is seldom continued long enough to produce the serious neurologic, hormonal, and other side effects that accompany prolonged starvation. More than 50% of the rapid weight reduction is fluid, which often leads to serious hypotension problems. Accumulation of uric acid can precipitate episodes of gout; gallstones can also occur. Sometimes what starts as extreme energy restriction to lose weight leads to an eating disorder, often anorexia nervosa (see Chapter 22).

Very Low–Calorie Diets

Diets providing 200 to 800 kcal are classified as **very low–calorie diets (VLCDs).** Little evidence suggests that intakes of fewer than 800 calories daily are of any advantage. Most VLCDs are hypocaloric but relatively rich in protein (0.8-1.5 g/kg IBW per day); they are designed to include a full complement of vitamins, minerals, electrolytes, and essential fatty acids, but not calories; they are given in a form that completely replaces usual food intake; and they are usually given for a period of 12 to 16 weeks Their major advantage is rapid weight loss. Because of potential side effects, prescription of these diets is reserved for persons with a BMI above 30 for whom other diet programs with psychotherapy have been unsuccessful. Occasionally VLCDs may be indicated for persons with a BMI of 27 to 30 who have comorbidities or other risk factors.

The VLCD that first became popular in the early 1970s resulted in several deaths; however, improved formulation with respect to protein quality has led to their acceptability and safety for those whose obesity is potentially life-threatening. The VLCDs can lead to an increase of urinary ketones that interfere with the renal clearance of uric acid, resulting in increased serum uric acid levels, often manifested as gout. Higher serum cholesterol levels resulting from mobilization of adipose stores pose a risk of gallstones. Additional adverse reactions that are common include cold intolerance, fatigue, light-headedness, nervousness, euphoria, constipation or diarrhea, dry skin, thinning reddened hair, anemia, and menstrual irregularities. Some of these are typical of triiodothyronine (thyroid) deficiency.

In 1998 the NIH recommended against using VLCDs for weight-loss therapy because the deficits are too great and nutritional inadequacies will occur unless VLCDs are supplemented with vitamins and minerals (NIH, 1998). In addition, a recent metaanalysis of VLCDs compared to LCDs showed that, even though there were significantly greater weight losses with the VLCDs in the short term, there were no significant differences in the weight losses in the long term (Gilden and Wadden, 2006). Thus there does not seem to be reason to recommend these VLCDs over more moderate calorie restriction except in very rare instances. For those who have lost weight on a VLCD, limiting dietary fat intake and maintaining physical activity are both important factors for the prevention of weight regain based on 3-year follow-up study. To promote better weight loss outcomes, patients should limit their fat intake to less than 30% of calories, and increase high activity levels.

Popular Diets and Practices

Each year, new approaches to weight loss find their way to the consumer through the popular press and media. Some of the programs are sensible and appropriate, whereas others emphasize fast results with minimum effort. Some of the proposed diets would lead to nutritional deficiencies over an extended period; however, the potential health risks are seldom realized because the diets are usually abandoned after a few weeks. Diets that emphasize fast results with minimum effort encourage unrealistic expectations, setting the dieter up for failure, subsequent guilt, and feelings of helplessness at ever managing the weight problem.

The U.S. Department of Agriculture Research Education and Economics supported a scientific review of popular diets to assess their efficacy for weight loss and weight maintenance, as well as their effect on metabolic parameters, psychological well-being, and reduction of chronic disease (Freedman et al., 2001). Diets were divided into categories on the basis of their macronutrient content and included high-fat, low-carbohydrate; moderate-fat, balanced–nutrient reduction; and low- and very-low-fat diets. A summary is shown in Table 21-4.

The low-carbohydrate, high-fat diet restricts carbohydrates to less than 20% of calories (and often less than 10% in the beginning), and fat constitutes 55% to 65% of calories, with protein making up the balance. Protein obtained from animal sources means that fat, saturated fat, and cholesterol intakes are high. Although these diets feature high ketone production, they suppress appetite to only a minor degree. The initial rapid weight loss from diuresis is secondary to the carbohydrate restriction. Examples of carbohydrate-restricted diets include *Dr. Atkins' New Diet Revolution* and *The Carbohydrate Addict's Diet.*

The *"Zone"* and the *"South Beach Diet"* both restrict carbohydrates to no more than 40% of total calories, with fat and protein providing 30% of calories each. This particular diet composition is claimed to keep insulin in check, which is blamed for fat storage. The diet includes generous amounts of fiber and fresh fruits and vegetables. There is attention to the kind of fat, with emphasis on monounsaturated and polyunsaturated fat and limitation of saturated fat. Weight loss ensues not because insulin is kept in a narrow range, but because calories are restricted.

TABLE 21-4

Results of U.S. Department of Agriculture Scientific Review of Popular Diets

Area	Finding
Weight loss	Diets that reduce caloric intake result in weight loss; all popular diets result in short-term weight loss if followed.
Body composition	All low-calorie diets result in a loss of body fat. In the short term, high-fat, low-carbohydrate ketogenic diets cause a greater loss of body water than body fat.
Nutritional adequacy	• High-fat, low-carbohydrate diets are low in vitamins E and A, thiamin, B_6, and folate, and the minerals calcium, magnesium, iron, and potassium. They are also low in dietary fiber. • Very low–fat diets are low in vitamins E and B_{12} and the mineral zinc. • With proper food choices, a moderate-fat, balanced nutrient–reduction diet is nutritionally adequate.
Metabolic parameters	• Low-carbohydrate diets cause ketosis and may significantly increase blood uric acid concentrations. • Blood lipid levels decline as body weight decreases. • Energy restriction improves glycemic control. • As body weight declines, blood insulin and plasma leptin levels decrease. • As body weight declines, blood pressure decreases.
Hunger and compliance	No diet was optimal for reducing hunger.
Effect on weight maintenance	Controlled clinical trials of high-fat, low-carbohydrate, low-fat, and very low–fat diets are lacking; therefore no data are available on weight maintenance after weight loss or long-term health benefits or risk.

From Freedman M et al: Popular diets: a scientific review, *Obes Res* 9(suppl 1):1S, 2001.

Moderate-fat, balanced–nutrient reduction diets contain 20% to 30% of calories from fat, 15% to 20% of calories from protein, and 55% to 60% of calories from carbohydrate (Freedman et al., 2001). *Volumetrics*, a program in this category, focuses on the energy density of foods. Foods high in water content have a low energy density. These include fruits, vegetables, low-fat milk, and cooked grains, as well as lean meats, poultry, fish and beans. Low–water containing foods that are energy dense such as potato chips, crackers, and fat-free cookies are restricted. A 1-year clinical trial incorporating two servings of low–energy dense soups resulted in a 50% greater weight loss (Rolls et al., 2005).

Very low–fat diets are those containing less than 10% of calories from fat, and low-fat diets contain 10% to 19% of calories from fat (Freedman et al, 2001). *Dr. Dean Ornish's Program for Reversing Heart Disease* and *The Pritikin Program* fall into this category. These diets produce rapid weight loss and are very restrictive. A popular variation limits fat to 20% of total energy intake. Because fat provides more than two times the energy per gram as protein or carbohydrate (9 kcal versus 4 kcal), an effective diet can be one that includes extensive controls on this nutrient.

In 1998 the NIH released *Clinical Guidelines on the Identification, Evaluation, and Treatment of Overweight and Obesity in Adults—the Evidence Report*. The intent of the guidelines is to provide evidence for the effects of treatment on overweight and obesity. The guidelines are directed to physicians and associated health professionals in clinical practice, health care policy makers, and clinical investigators (NIH, 1998).

In October 2000 the National Heart, Lung, and Blood Institute (NHLBI) in cooperation with the North American Association for the Study of Obesity (NAASO) released *The Practical Guide: Identification, Evaluation, and Treatment of Overweight and Obesity in Adults* based on the *1998 Clinical Guidelines* publication. The practical guide provides tools for the clinician to manage overweight and obese adults (NIH and NAASO, 2000).

The American Dietetic Association examined the question of the effectiveness of the popular low-carbohydrate (less than 35% of calories) diets (e.g., Atkins, South Beach). A review of 14 accepted studies demonstrated that consumption of ad libitum low-carbohydrate diets (only the intake of carbohydrate is limited) and reduced-calorie diets both result in lower caloric intake. However, ad libitum low-carbohydrate diets often result in greater body weight loss and fat loss in the first 6 months, but after 1 year these differences are no longer significant.

Exercise

Excess body fatness is a result of an imbalance between energy intake and energy expenditure, and physical activity is an extremely important part of a weight-management program. By increasing LBM in proportion to fat, exercise helps to balance the loss of LBM and reduction of RMR that inevitably accompany even a well-managed weight-reduction program. Numerous other positive side effects include strengthening cardiovascular integrity, increasing sensitivity to insulin, and expending additional energy and therefore calories.

Physical activity is the most variable component of energy expenditure. Increases in energy expenditure through exercise and other forms of physical activity are important components of effective interventions to enhance weight loss and the prevention of weight regain. Adequate levels of exercise and physical activity to achieve this appear to be 60 to 90 minutes daily, which is recommended by the USDA. This is also the amount of activity reported by those in the National Weight Control Registry (NWCR) who have kept off at least 10% of their weight for at least a year.

Overweight and obese adults should be counseled to gradually increase to these levels of exercise and physical activity. There is evidence that, even if an overweight or obese adult is unable to achieve this level of activity, significant health benefits can be realized by participating in at least 30 minutes of daily activity of moderate intensity (ADA, 2007). Therefore it is important to have interventions that target these levels of physical activity to improve health-related outcomes and to facilitate long-term weight control (Jakicic, 2006).

A combination of aerobic and resistance training is recommended. Resistance training increases LBM, adding to the RMR and the ability to use more of the energy intake, and it increases bone mineral density, which is especially important for women (see Chapter 24). Aerobic exercise is important for cardiovascular health, as well as for the calorie expenditure and creation of an energy deficit and therefore fat loss. In addition to the physiologic benefits of exercise are the relief of boredom, increased sense of control, and improved sense of well-being (Figure 21-4).

The RMR is elevated by aerobic exercise. Except after fairly high levels of intensity or large amounts of exercise, RMR returns to resting levels within an hour or so following exercise. Energy expenditure during this period represents replacement of muscle glycogen, as well as the effects of hormonal changes and the increase in metabolic processing of fuel stores. In adults within the normal physical activity index range, the time spent at activities with low and moderate intensity determines the physical activity level; high-intensity activity is not required to increase overall activity energy expenditure (Westerterp and Plasqui, 2004).

Contrary to popular belief, spot reduction (i.e., reducing fat in one area of the body) is not possible with exercise; fat is burned from the largest concentrations of adipose tissue. Another misconception is that exercise is counterproductive because it increases the desire to eat. Consistency is key to realizing the health and weight-management benefits of exercise. Previous exercise recommendations for health called for 20 to 60 minutes of moderate- to high-intensity endurance exercise performed three or more times weekly. It now appears that most health benefits can be gained by physical activity of moderate intensity (enough to expend 200 kcal daily) accumu-

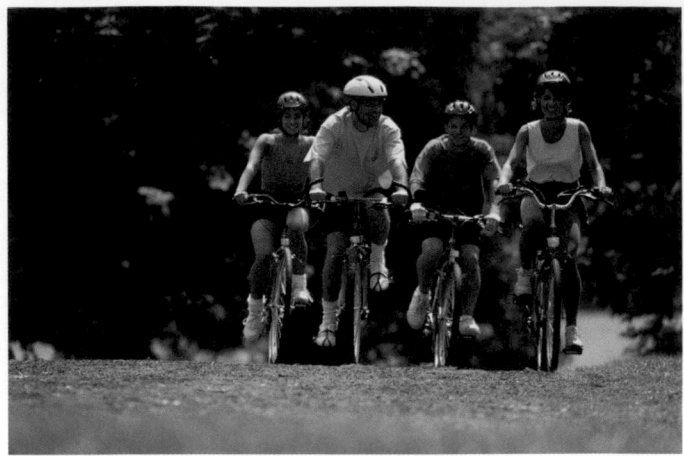

FIGURE 21-4 Cycling is an excellent aerobic activity to include in a weight-reduction program. (© *2006 Jupiter Images Corporation.*)

lated in intermittent short bouts. It is best to maintain cardiovascular health at maximum level, regardless of weight, by 20 to 30 minutes of high-intensity activity 4 to 7 days per week (Institute of Medicine, 2002).

Pharmaceutical Management

Appropriate pharmacotherapy can augment diet, physical activity, and behavior therapy as treatment for patients with a BMI of 30 or higher or patients with 27 or higher who also have significant risk factors or disease. These agents can decrease appetite, reduce absorption of fat, or increase energy expenditure. As with any drug treatment, physician monitoring for efficacy and safety is necessary.

Medications currently available can be categorized as central nervous system (CNS)-acting agents and non–CNS-acting agents. The CNS-acting agents fall into the categories of catecholaminergic agents, serotoninergic agents, and combination catecholaminergic-serotoninergic agents. Common side effects of CNS-acting agents are dry mouth, headache, insomnia, and constipation.

Currently only sibutramine (Meridia) and orlistat are approved by the Food and Drug Administration (FDA) for long-term use in the treatment of obesity. Sibutramine is a combination of catecholaminergic and serotoninergic agents, which inhibit the reuptake of serotonin and norepinephrine in the CNS to increase satiety, reduce hunger, and lessen the drop in metabolic rate that often occurs with weight loss. Because of its stimulation of the sympathetic nervous system, patients taking sibutramine may experience cardiovascular side effects, and it is not appropriate for patients with a history of CAD and related disorders.

Numerous studies demonstrate the efficacy of sibutramine as a weight-loss and weight-maintenance agent for obesity in Type 2 diabetes (Li et al., 2005). However, its safety is still uncertain (Norris et al., 2005).

Sibutramine should not be used in combination with certain antidepressant agents such as monoamine oxidase inhibitors or selective serotonin reuptake inhibitors or other central acting agents such as pseudoephedrine or ephedra. The interaction may cause elevated blood pressure.

Catecholaminergic (related to brain neurotransmitters norepinephrine, epinephrine, and dopamine) drugs act on the brain, increasing the availability of norepinephrine. Table 21-5 lists catecholaminergic agents used for short-term weight loss. Drug Enforcement Agency (DEA) Schedule II anorexic agents such as amphetamines have a high potential for abuse and are not recommended for obesity treatment. DEA Schedule III agents also pose abuse potential that should be carefully considered. Commonly used DEA Schedule IV catecholaminergic agents such as phentermine have a low potential for abuse. Because of its effects on blood pressure, phentermine is prescribed with caution in patients even with mild hypertension.

Serotoninergic agents act by increasing serotonin levels in the brain. Two drugs in this category, fenfluramine (commonly used in combination with phentermine and known as fen-phen) and dexfenfluramine were removed from the market in 1997 after concerns were raised regarding the possible side effects of cardiac valvulopathy, regurgitation, and primary pulmonary hypertension. Further studies clarified the valvular abnormalities (Khan et al., 1998). The over-the-counter medication phenylpropanolamine (PPA) was used for many years as an appetite suppressant. In 2000 scientists at Yale University released the final report of the Hemorrhagic Stroke Project (HSP) suggesting that PPA increases the risk for hemorrhagic stroke. As a result, the Food and Drug Administration (FDA) asked firms that market drugs containing PPA to discontinue them voluntarily. In 2005 the FDA issued a notice of proposed rulemaking (notice) for over-the-counter nasal decongestants and weight control products containing PPA preparations, reclassifying PPA as not safe or effective.

Orlistat, a non–CNS-acting agent, does not suppress the appetite. Orlistat inhibits gastrointestinal lipase, which reduces approximately one third the amount of fat that is absorbed from food. Depending on the fat content of a person's diet, this lowered absorption can represent 150 to 200 kcal/day. The reduction in lipid absorption with orlistat causes concern for the absorption of fat-soluble vitamins. Supplements of these vitamins are typically recommended, with care to separate the dosing of orlistat and the supplement by 2 hours or more. Research in adults has shown minimum effects of orlistat on serum concentrations of vitamins A, E, and D.

Reviews of trials in which participants were administered typical doses of orlistat along with lifestyle therapy found an incremental weight loss of 3 to 5 kg in orlistat-treated patients compared with control patients (McTigue, 2003; Arterburn, 2004; O'Meara, 2004). Side effects are gastrointestinal in nature: oily spotting, fecal urgency, and flatus with discharge. Health benefits include reduced LDL cholesterol and elevated HDL cholesterol, improved glycemic control, and reduced blood pressure.

In summary, pharmacotherapy is not a "magic pill" to cure obesity. Dietitians should collaborate with other health professionals regarding the use of FDA approved pharmacotherapy (ADA, 2007). Not all individuals respond, but for patients who do respond, clinical trials suggest that a weight loss of about 2 to 20 kg can be expected usually during the first 6 months of treatment. Medication without lifestyle modification is less effective.

Several potential new drugs targeting weight loss and obesity through the CNS pathways or peripheral adiposity signals are in early-phase clinical trials. Drug treatment is likely to change significantly because of the availability of new pharmacotherapies to regulate eating behaviors, nutrient partitioning, and energy expenditure (Ioannides-Demos, 2005). Natural weight-loss aids hold varying degrees of promise for weight loss (see *Focus On:* Natural Weight-Loss Aids).

TABLE 21-5

Available Catecholaminergic Agents

Agent	Trade Name	Daily Dosage (mg)*
Schedule II Agents		
Amphetamine	Biphetamine	10-15
Phenmetrazine HCl	Preludin	75
Schedule II Agents		
Benzphetamine HCl	Didrex	25-50 to 75-150
Phendimetrazine tartrate	Bontril	105
	Slow-Release	105
	Bontril	105
	Prelu-2	105
	Plegine	105
	X-Trozine	105
	Extended Release X-Trozine	
Schedule IV Agents		
Diethylpropion HCl (Amfepramone)	Tenuate	75
	Tenuate dospan	75
Mazindol HCl	Sanorex	1-3
	Mazanor	1-3
Phentermine HCl	Adipex-P	37.5
	Fastin	30
	Obenix	37.5
	Oby-Cap	30
	Oby-Trim	30
	Zantryl	30
Phentermine resin	Ionamin	30†

From Shape Up America! (www.shapeup.org) and American Obesity Association: *Guidance for treatment of adult obesity*, ed 3, Bethesda, Md, 2001, Shape Up America! and American Obesity Association.

*Represents recommended daily intake. Ranges represent initial dose to maximum dose. Titration may be indicated, depending on each patient's therapeutic response.

†Usual dosage. Some patients may respond to half this dosage.

⊚ FOCUS ON

Natural Weight-Loss Aids

Americans are constantly being told that "diets don't work." The lure of a quick and easy solution to the challenge of weight management is strong, and the market for natural weight-loss aids is booming. Many patients want fast results. Currently none of the 50 individual weight-loss supplements meet criteria for effective or recommended use (Sharpe et al., 2006; Saper et al., 2004). What are the product claims and what are the facts?

Chitosan: These indigestible compounds are over-the-counter weight-loss agents. Claims are that chitosan blocks fat absorption. There are no positive effects (Guerciolini et al., 2001).

Chromium: According to the claims, chromium should promote fat loss and increase lean body mass. Chromium potentiates the action of insulin in carbohydrate, lipid, and protein metabolism, although the exact mechanism is not known. Small studies suggest that there may be some benefit (Nachtigal et al., 2005).

Dehydroepiandrosterone (DHEA): Among other claims, DHEA is supposed to promote weight loss. Problems noted with DHEA include liver cancer in rats. Supplementation can lead to increased insulin resistance, the growth of unwanted hair, and a drop in high-density lipoprotein cholesterol, increasing the risk for heart disease (see Chapter 32).

Garcinia cambogia: Hydroxycitric acid is the active ingredient in garcinia cambogia, and it is promoted to reduce the body's ability to store fat. Citric acid is a component of the tricarboxylic acid (Krebs) cycle. There is no evidence that it promotes fat or weight loss.

Ma huang: Ma huang (ephedra) promoters claimed benefits such as weight loss, increased energy, performance enhancement, and increased LBM. Ma huang is a central nervous system stimulant; it increases blood pressure and heart rate and is hazardous to those with heart ailments, diabetes, hypertension, and thyroid conditions. When combined with caffeine-containing herbs (kola nut, guarana, and mat), ma huang can be especially hazardous. The Food and Drug Administration received more than 100 reports of adverse reactions ranging from heart attacks to hepatitis and several deaths, and it has been removed from the market.

Senna: Senna leaves are the dried leaflets of plants found in Egypt and India. Senna is a potent cathartic. Use of this herb, which induces diarrhea, can lead to low potassium levels. Three deaths have been associated with senna use.

Other products: Because of insufficient or conflicting evidence regarding the efficacy of conjugated linoleic acid, ginseng, glucomannan, green tea, L-carnitine, psyllium, pyruvate, and St. John's wort in weight loss, it is important to caution patients about the use of these supplements (Saper et al., 2004).

Other Nonsurgical Approaches

The nondiet paradigm maintains that the body will attain its natural weight if the individual eats healthfully, becomes attuned to hunger and satiety cues, and incorporates physical activity. This approach focuses on achieving health rather than attaining a certain weight. Advocates for the nondiet approach promote size acceptance and maintaining respect for the diversity of body shapes and sizes. Given the evidence that a 5% to 10% loss of initial weight can result in health benefits, that many persons set weight-loss goals that are unrealistic, and that fat discrimination continues to plague society, this approach may help some persons to develop a better relationship with food and a healthier perspective about their bodies.

Although hypnosis and acupuncture are popular with some, there is no definitive support for these practices. What they might do is help people relax and deal with psychological stress without eating to soothe themselves when they are not physiologically hungry.

Surgical Procedures

Bariatric surgery is an accepted form of treatment for extreme or class III obesity with a BMI of 40 or greater, or a BMI of 35 or greater with comorbidities (NIH, 2000). Each year approximately 140,000 of the 9 million Ameri-

can adults classified as extremely obese receive bariatric surgery (AHRQ, 2004).

Some surgical procedures are restrictive because they decrease the amount of food entering the gastrointestinal tract. This is known as gastroplasty and includes vertical-banded gastroplasty and gastric banding. Other surgical procedures are restrictive *and* cause malabsorption because they also prevent food from being absorbed from the gastrointestinal tract. These include Roux-en-Y gastric bypass and biliopancreatic diversion with duodenal switch.

Before any extremely obese person is considered for surgery, failure of a comprehensive program that includes calorie restriction, exercise, lifestyle modification, psychological counseling, and family involvement should be demonstrated. Failure is defined as an inability of the patient to reduce body weight by one third and body fat by one half and an inability to maintain any weight loss achieved. Such patients have intractable morbid obesity and should be considered for surgery. Before surgery the patient should be evaluated extensively with respect to physiologic and medical complications, psychological problems such as depression and poor self-esteem, and the extent of motivation. Counseling sharply improves the outcomes for both dieting and drug therapy in this population (Wadden and Sarwer, 2006).

Postoperative follow-up includes evaluation at regular intervals by the surgical team and a registered dietitian. In addition, behavioral or psychological support is necessary. Lifelong follow-up on the part of the patient and surgeon, including involvement of the patient's primary physician, is essential (NIH, 1998).

Gastroplasty and Gastric Bypass

Gastroplasty reduces the size of the stomach by applying rows of stainless-steel staples to partition the stomach and create a small gastric pouch, leaving only a small opening (0.8-1.0 cm) into the distal stomach. This opening may be banded by a piece of mesh to prevent it from enlarging during the years after surgery. Vertical-banded gastroplasty is the most popular form of gastroplasty. Another popular gastroplasty is the lap-band gastroplasty or gastric banding in which the band creating the reduced stomach pouch is able to be adjusted so that the opening to the rest of the stomach can be made smaller or enlarged, depending on the weight reduction and clinical progress of the patient. The band, filled with saline, has a tube exiting from it to the surface of the belly just under the skin; this allows for the injection of additional fluid or reducing the fluid into the lap band (Figure 21-5).

Gastric bypass involves reducing the size of the stomach with the stapling procedure but then connecting a small opening in the upper portion of the stomach to the small intestine by means of an intestinal loop. Mason and Ito developed the original operation in the late 1960s (Mason and Ito, 1969). There have been numerous improvements since the original operation, and the most successful modification is the Greenville Gastric Bypass, also known as the Roux-en-Y gastric bypass (RYGBP) (Figure 21-5).

Both gastroplasty and gastric bypass procedures have the effect of reducing the amount of food that can be eaten at one time and producing early satiety. The new stomach capacity may be as small as 20 to 30 ml, about 1 oz, or about 2 tablespoons. After surgery the patient's diet progresses from clear liquid, to full liquid, to puree, soft, and finally to a regular diet as tolerated, with emphasis on protein intake (Table 21-6).

The most frequent complications of gastric surgery are bloating of the pouch, nausea, and vomiting. A postsurgical food record noting the tolerance for specific foods in particular amounts helps in devising a program to avoid these episodes. Attention to vitamin and mineral supplementation, particularly calcium, folate, iron, and vitamin B_{12} is advised. Another problem that may arise after gastric bypass is ice-cube pica. Iron deficiency anemia is the likely cause and should be corrected (Kushner and Shanta Retelny, 2005).

Because use of the lower part of the stomach is omitted, the gastric bypass patient may also have dumping syndrome (see Chapter 26) as food empties quickly into the duodenum. The symptoms of tachycardia, sweating, and abdominal pain are so negative that they motivate the patient to make the appropriate behavioral changes and refrain from overeating. However, patients tend to choose liquids, and weight loss can be deterred by drinking too much calorically dense liquid such as milk shakes and soft drinks. Eventually the pouch expands to accommodate 4 to 5 oz at a time.

Completion of the surgery does not end the need for treatment; in fact, the procedure is considered to create malnutrition, and lifelong follow-up and regular monitoring by a multidisciplinary team of health care professionals is needed. Monitoring should include an assessment of body-fat loss, potential anemia, and deficiencies of potassium, magnesium, folate, and vitamin B_{12}, especially in patients with gastric bypass, but intake of all vitamins and minerals should be monitored (see Chapter 15). Usually multivitamin-mineral supplementation is necessary.

The results of gastric surgery are favorable, and there are fewer complications than with the intestinal bypass surgery practiced during the 1970s. On average the reduction of excess body weight after gastric restriction surgery correlates to about 30% to 40% of initial body weight. Weight-loss surgery can improve several of the obesity-related diseases or comorbidites, including hypertension, type 2 diabetes mellitus, osteoarthritis, back pain, dyslipidemia, cardiomyopathy, nonalcoholic steatohepatitis, and sleep apnea. Bariatric surgery also improves self-image and employability and depression (Sugerman, 2001; Dixon et al., 2003).

In addition to the greater absolute weight loss observed, the gastric bypass tends to have safe and sustainable results with significant resolution of serious comorbidities (Rubenstein, 2002; Sjostrom et al., 2004). RYGBP significantly improves hypertension, hyperlipidemia, and type 2 diabetes and may also improve kidney function. Patients with higher presurgical BMIs are at greater risk for postsurgical complications. A prospective study that compared weight loss, complications, and early outcome of co-morbidity resolution in patients who underwent laparoscopic gastric bypass (LGBP) versus laparoscopic adjustable silicone gastric banding (LASGB) showed similar improvements in comorbidities. Early after surgery, LGBP patients lose more weight than LASGB patients, but further follow-up is needed to determine the relative long-term efficacy of these procedures (Kim et al., 2006).

Liposuction

Liposuction (or liposculpture) involves aspiration of fat deposits by means of a 1- to 2-cm incision through which a tube is fanned out into the adipose tissue. The most successful operations are performed on younger persons with only small amounts of fat to be removed, where the elastic properties of the skin are able to allow tightening over the aspirated areas. It is not usually a weight-reduction technique but rather a cosmetic surgery because usually only about 5 lb of fat are removed at a time. Not all cases provide the anticipated outcome; and deaths, severe infections, cellulitis, and hemorrhage have been noted to occur. Recently liposuction is being used as more aggressive treatment of obesity with as much as 50 lb of fat removed using an incision and removal of the fat on the abdomen followed with a "tummy tuck" and removal of excess skin. It is proposed that

Eating disorders are debilitating psychiatric illnesses characterized by a persistent disturbance of eating habits or weight control behaviors that result in significantly impaired physical health and psychosocial functioning. American Psychiatric Association (APA) diagnostic criteria are available for anorexia nervosa (AN), bulimia nervosa (BN), eating disorder not otherwise specified (EDNOS), and binge eating disorder (BED). Night eating syndrome (NES), childhood eating disturbances, and the female athlete triad are also characterized by disordered eating and weight control behaviors (see Chapters 21 and 23).

DIAGNOSTIC CRITERIA

Anorexia Nervosa

A core clinical feature of **anorexia nervosa (AN)** is voluntary self-starvation resulting in emaciation. The reported lifetime prevalence of AN among women is 0.3 to 3.7%, depending on how strictly diagnostic criteria are defined (APA, 2006). Among males estimated prevalence is about one tenth that of females (Yager and Andersen, 2005). AN is more prevalent in Westernized, postindustrialized societies; however, transnational migration and modernization are expected to result in a more global distribution of eating disorders (Becker, 2004), including third world countries (Miller and Pumariega, 2001).

Initial presentation of AN typically occurs during adolescence or young adulthood; however, later onset (i.e., initial onset at age 25 or older) may develop in response to adverse life events. Incidence rates for AN among middle-age women (over age 50) account for less than 1% of newly diagnosed AN patients (APA, 2006). Etiology varies for this disorder, but there seems to be a genetic component, as well as environmental and psychosocial factors (Bulik et al., 2006).

Criteria for the establishment of a diagnosis of AN were first published in 1972 by Feighner and associates. The APA first published criteria for the diagnosis of AN in 1980; however, it was not until 1987 that the APA recognized AN and BN as two separate and distinct clinical entities. See Box 22-1 for the most current diagnostic criteria for AN.

The **Diagnostic and Statistical Manual of Mental Disorders, TR-IV (DSM-TR-IV)** specifies "refusal to maintain a body weight at or above a minimally normal weight for age and height (e.g., . . . body weight less than 85% of that expected)." The weight deficit may occur secondary to purposeful weight loss or manifest as failure to gain weight during periods of linear growth in children and adolescents. Growth records should be obtained to determine if the child has fallen off his or her growth curve. If stunting has occurred, the weight deficit should be calculated using the premorbid height percentile.

Determination of "minimally normal weight" is problematic. Metropolitan Life Insurance Company weight standards are often used; however, recommended weight for height differs between the 1959 and 1983 tables. Dietitians often calculate desirable body weight using the Hamwi method (see Chapter 14). This is not recommended in patients with an eating disorder (ED) because it calculates a "normal" body weight much lower than other standards. For children and adolescents ages 11 to 17 years, normal body weight should be determined from the National Center for Health Statistics weight and height tables (see Appendices 12 and 16) and the Body Mass Indices (BMI) for age in Appendix 23.

Patients with AN have **body image distortion**, causing them to feel fat despite their often cachectic state. Some individuals feel overweight all over, whereas others are overly concerned about the fatness of a specific body part such as the abdomen, buttocks, or thighs.

Amenorrhea, defined as the absence of at least three consecutive menstrual cycles in postmenarcheal women, is not an ideal criterion for AN because some patients continue to menstruate at a very low body weight (Mitchell et al., 2005). Development of AN during prepubescence may result in arrested sexual maturation and delayed menarche (primary amenorrhea). Young adolescent males with AN may have estrogen and testosterone deficiency and arrested growth and sexual development.

AN can be categorized into two diagnostic subtypes: restricting and binge eating/purging. The *restricting* type is characterized by food restriction without binge eating or **purging** (self-induced vomiting or misuse of laxatives, enemas, or diuretics). The *binge eating/purging* is characterized by regular episodes of binge eating or purging behavior. AN may initially present as the restricting subtype; however, migration to binge eating/purging subtype may occur as duration of illness progresses.

Psychological features associated with AN include perfectionism, compulsivity, harm avoidance, feelings of ineffectiveness, inflexible thinking, overly restrained emotional expression, and limited social spontaneity (APA, 2000). Several psychiatric conditions may also coexist with AN, and these include major depression, **dysthymia** (chronic mild depression), anxiety disorders, obsessive-compulsive disorder, personality disorders, and substance abuse. Lifetime comorbid depression and dysthymia have been reported in 50% to 75% of AN patients (APA, 2006).

Symptoms of depression may remit during the course of nutrition rehabilitation and weight restoration. However, the suicide rate is greater among individuals with AN than in the general population; thus ongoing psychiatric assessment is essential (APA, 2006). More than 40% of AN patients also have obsessive-compulsive disorder (OCD). Onset of OCD frequently predates AN, and many patients remain symptomatic despite weight restoration (APA, 2006).

Five percent to twenty percent of patients with anorexia nervosa die from their illness; half of those patients die of medical complications (Steinhausen, 2002). Malnutrition, dehydration, and electrolyte abnormalities may precipitate death by inducing heart failure or fatal arrhythmias (McCallum et al., 2006).

Bulimia Nervosa

Bulimia nervosa (BN) is a disorder characterized by recurrent episodes of binge eating followed by one or more inappropriate compensatory behaviors to prevent weight gain.

BOX 22-1

American Psychiatric Association Diagnostic Criteria

Anorexia Nervosa (AN)

A. Refusal to maintain body weight at or above a minimally normal weight for age and height (e.g., weight loss leading to maintenance of body weight less than 85% of that expected; or failure to make expected weight gain during period of growth, leading to body weight less than 85% of that expected)

B. Intense fear of gaining weight or becoming fat, even though underweight

C. Disturbance in the way in which one's body weight or shape is experienced, undue influence of body weight or shape on self-evaluation, or denial of the seriousness of the current low body weight

D. In postmenarcheal females, amenorrhea (i.e., the absence of at least three consecutive menstrual cycles)
   1. *Restricting type*: During the current episode of AN, the person has not regularly engaged in binge eating or purging behavior.
   2. *Binge eating/purging type*: During the current episode of AN, the person has regularly engaged in binge eating and purging behavior.

Bulimia Nervosa (BN)

A. Recurrent episodes of binge eating. An episode of binge eating is characterized by both of the following:
   1. Eating, in a discrete period of time (e.g., within any 2-hour period), an amount of food that is definitely larger than most people would eat during a similar period of time and under similar circumstances
   2. A sense of lack of control over eating during the episode (e.g., a feeling that one cannot stop eating or control what or how much one is eating)

B. Recurrent inappropriate compensatory behavior to prevent weight gain, such as self-induced vomiting; misuse of laxatives, diuretics, enemas, or other medications; fasting; or excessive exercise

C. The binge eating and inappropriate compensatory behaviors both occur, on average, at least twice a week for 3 months

D. Self-evaluation is unduly influenced by body shape and weight.

E. The disturbance does not occur exclusively during episodes of AN.
   1. *Purging type:* During the current episode of BN, the person has regularly engaged in self-induced vomiting or the misuse of laxatives, diuretics, or enemas.
   2. *Nonpurging type:* During the current episode of BN, the person has used other inappropriate compensatory behaviors such as fasting or excessive exercise but has not regularly engaged in self-induced vomiting or the misuse of laxatives, diuretics, or enemas.

Eating Disorder Not Otherwise Specified (EDNOS)

This category is for disorders of eating that do not meet criteria for any specific eating disorder.
For example:
   1. For females, all of the criteria for AN are met except that the individual has regular menses.
   2. All of the criteria for AN are met except that, despite significant weight loss, the individual's current weight is in the normal range.
   3. All of the criteria for BN are met except that the binge eating and inappropriate compensatory mechanisms occur at a frequency of less than twice a week or for a duration of less than 3 months.
   4. The regular use of inappropriate compensatory behavior by an individual of normal body weight after eating small amounts of food.
   5. Repeatedly chewing and spitting out, but not swallowing, large amounts of food.

Binge Eating Disorder (BED)

A. Recurrent episodes of binge eating in the absence of the regular use of inappropriate compensatory behaviors characteristic of BN

B. Binge episodes must occur at least 2 days per week for a period of 6 months.

From American Psychiatric Association: *Diagnostic and statistical manual of mental disorders, DSM-IV-TR*, ed 4, (text revision) Washington, DC, 2000, American Psychiatric Association.

These behaviors include self-induced vomiting, laxative misuse, diuretic misuse, compulsive exercise, or fasting. The lifetime prevalence of BN among young adult women in the United States is 1% to 3%. The rate of occurrence in males is approximately one tenth that in females (APA, 2000).

Unlike AN patients with binge and purge subtype, patients with BN are typically within the normal weight range, although some may be slightly underweight or overweight. Like their AN counterparts, these individuals place considerable importance on body shape and size, and they are often frustrated by their inability to attain an underweight state.

It is commonly thought that vomiting is the predominant feature of BN; however, it is the binge eating behavior that is central to the diagnosis. A **binge** is consumption of an unusually large amount of food in a discrete period (usually ≤2 hours). There is a sense of lack of control over the eating episode. Although the amount of food and caloric content of a binge vary, binges are often in the range of 1000 to 2000 calories (Fairburn and Harrison, 2003). Patients with BN typically binge on foods that are otherwise avoided such as snack foods and desserts; however, some binge on extremely large portions of low calorie foods such as fruit and salad.

Patients may report a binge episode when the amount of food consumed is clearly not excessive. Although these "subjective binges" may not support a diagnosis of BN, clearly these individuals have feelings about their eating behavior that merit further exploration.

BN patients engage in compensatory behaviors intended to offset food binges. The choice of compensatory behaviors further classifies BN into purging and nonpurging subtypes. Patients with *purging type BN* regularly engage in self-induced vomiting or the misuse of laxatives, enemas, or diuretics. Those with *nonpurging type BN* do not regularly engage in purging behaviors but rather fast or excessively exercise to compensate for their binge. To meet full *DSM-TR IV* criteria for BN bingeing, both binge eating and recurrent inappropriate compensatory behaviors must occur, on average, at least twice a week for 3 months. Current APA diagnostic criteria for BN are listed in Box 22-1.

Adverse emotional states such as labile mood, frustration, anxiety, and impulsivity are often found in patients with BN. Psychiatric comorbidities, including major depression, dysthymia, anxiety disorders, personality disorders, substance abuse, and self-injurious behaviors, are also common in BN. Compared to AN, BN patients are usually embarrassed and distressed by their symptoms, making it easier to engage them in treatment.

Etiologies proposed for the development of BN include addictive, family, socio-cultural, cognitive-behavioral, and psychodynamic models (APA, 2006). BN, with or without comorbid psychiatric illness, should be treated and monitored by a mental health professional. However, only a minority of individuals with BED are actually treated in mental health services (Hoek, 2006).

Eating Disorder Not Otherwise Specified

Approximately half of the individuals with eating disorders fall into the **eating disorder not otherwise specified (EDNOS)** diagnostic group. Essentially these individuals meet most, but not all, of the criteria for AN or BN (e.g., a female meeting all diagnostic criteria for AN except amenorrhea; a previously obese patient who, despite extreme weight loss, pathologic eating behavior, and amenorrhea fails to meet the AN criterion of body weight less than 85% of expected; a person who binges and purges, but with less frequency or for a shorter period of duration, than is specified for BN; or the individual who does not binge but vomits after eating a normal-size meal or snack). Clinically the EDNOS patient should receive treatment consistent with reasonable and customary care for either AN or BN. Inadequate treatment may lead to the development of full-criteria AN or BN. In addition, patients who meet criteria for BED, a diagnostic group for research purposes only, would be clinically diagnosed with EDNOS. See Box 22-1 for APA diagnostic criteria for EDNOS.

Binge Eating Disorder

Research criteria for **binge eating disorder (BED)** are listed in Box 22-1. Binge eating, similar to that seen in BN, is characteristic of BED; however, there are no inappropriate compensatory behaviors after the binge. Binge episodes must occur at least 2 days per week for a period of 6 months.

Persons with BED experience a feeling of powerlessness over their eating, similar to that felt by BN patients. Significant emotional distress characterized by feelings of disgust, guilt, and depression occurs after a binge. Onset of BED generally occurs in late adolescence or in the early twenties, with women being 1.5 times more likely to develop this disorder than men.

Most patients with this disorder are overweight, with 15% to 50% prevalence among participants in weight-control programs (APA, 2000). Patients with BED may have a higher lifetime prevalence of major depression, substance abuse, and personality disorders. In addition, some also have **night eating syndrome (NES),** consuming more than half of daily energy intake during and after dinner but before breakfast, and sleep disorders. Many of these individuals seek bariatric surgery (Allison et al., 2006).

Eating Disorders in Childhood

Onset of eating disorders most typically occurs during adolescence and young adulthood. When an eating disorder is suspected in a child or young teen, use of DSM criteria may be problematic because clinical presentation often differs from that seen in older adolescents and young adults. Complaints of nausea, abdominal pain, and difficulty in swallowing may coexist with concerns about weight, shape, and body fatness. Food avoidance, self-induced vomiting, and excessive exercise may occur, but laxative misuse is uncommon.

Any child or adolescent practicing unhealthy weight-control practices or thinking obsessively about food, body weight or shape, or exercise may be at risk for an eating disorder. Other obsessive behaviors and depression may coexist in these children as well. Early onset AN may result in delayed or stunted growth, osteopenia, and osteoporosis (APA, 2006). AN has been reported in children as young as 7 years of age. The male-to-female ratio may be higher in this younger age-group, and it appears in many different cultures and ethnic groups. BN in children is rare (APA, 2006).

The relationship between problematic childhood eating behaviors and subsequent development of eating disorders in later life is of concern. A 17-year longitudinal study of 800 children showed that eating conflicts, struggles with food, and unpleasant meals were risk factors for the development of an eating disorder in adolescence or young adulthood (Kotler et al., 2001). However, other childhood eating problems such as not eating, disinterest in food, picky eating, eating too little, and eating too slowly failed to predict subsequent development of an eating disorder.

There is a need for developmentally appropriate diagnostic criteria, screening instruments, and validated treatments for children and younger adolescents. The term *eating disturbance* versus *eating disorder* has been suggested (Bryant-Waugh, 2000). See Table 22-1 for descriptions of childhood eating disturbances, including childhood AN and BN.

TABLE 22-1

Childhood Eating Disturbances

Eating Disturbance	Characteristics
Anorexia nervosa	Determined food avoidance
	Weight loss or failure to gain weight during the period of preadolescent growth (10-14 yr) in the absence of any physical or other mental illness
	Any two or more of the following:
	Preoccupation with body weight
	Preoccupation with energy intake
	Distorted body image
	Fear of fatness
	Self-induced vomiting
	Extensive exercising
	Laxative abuse
Bulimia nervosa	Binge eating followed by purging, restricting, excessive exercise, or laxative abuse rarely seen in childhood
Food avoidance emotional disorder	A primary emotional disorder resulting in avoidance of food
	Weight loss, or failure to gain developmentally appropriate amounts of weight
	No preoccupation with weight and shape
	Absence of body image distortion
	May have comorbid medical disorders/diseases
Selective eating	Food intake limited to a very small number of foods
	May be rigid about the brand of food, or its place of purchase
	Food choices tend to be carbohydrates
	Selective eating hinders participation in social situations that include eating
	Attempts to increase variety in diet are met with extreme resistance
	Age-appropriate gains in weight and height
	No preoccupation with weight and shape
	Absence of body image distortion
	No fear of choking or gagging (see functional dysphagia)
Restrictive eating	Characteristically eats a smaller than normal amount of food
	Disinterested in eating
	No intentional food restriction
	Normal balance of carbohydrates, protein, and fats in diet
	Absence of mood disorder
	Height and weight within normal limits but at the lower end of percentiles
	May have difficulty meeting increased energy requirement during puberty
	No preoccupation with weight and shape
	Absence of body image distortion
Food refusal	Episodic, situational, or intermittent food refusal
	No preoccupation with weight and shape
	Absence of body image distortion
	Emotional issues, such as unhappiness or worry, may be the underlying cause
Functional dysphagia	Food avoidance, particularly foods of a certain type or texture
	Fear of swallowing, vomiting, choking
	An aversive event may precipitate the disorder
	No preoccupation with weight and shape
	Absence of body image distortion
Pervasive refusal syndrome	Profound and pervasive refusal to eat, drink, walk, talk, or engage in self-care
	May be underweight and dehydrated
	May be a form of posttraumatic stress disorder
	Rare but potentially life threatening
	Usually requires hospitalization

From Bryant-Waugh R: Overview of eating disorders. In Lask B, Bryant-Waugh R, editors: *Anorexia nervosa and related eating disorders in childhood and adolescence*, ed 2, East Sussex, UK, 2000, Psychology Press.

Eating Disorders in Athletes

Competitive athletes are at great risk for the development of eating disorders. Females who participate in activities that emphasize a lean body type (e.g. gymnastics, figure skating, distance running, crew, and ballet dancing) and male bodybuilders and competitive wrestlers may be particularly vulnerable.

Internal and external pressures to achieve or maintain an unrealistically low body weight underlie the development of the **female athlete triad** (see Chapter 23). The triad is a serious syndrome consisting of disordered eating, amenorrhea, and osteoporosis. Disordered eating may present in the form of chronic undereating and episodic bouts of fasting, binge eating, and purging. Parents, trainers, and coaches who are overly invested in the athlete's performance may ignore or even encourage disordered eating and dieting behaviors. Although the exact relationship between the triad and clinical eating disorders is not fully understood, athletes meeting criteria for the triad would also meet criteria for EDNOS (APA, 2006).

Eating Disorders in Individuals with Diabetes Mellitus

When an individual with type 1 or type 2 diabetes mellitus (DM) develops an eating disorder, complex medical, nutritional, and psychological management is required. Those with type 1 DM are more likely to have AN, BN, or EDNOS, whereas those with type 2 DM are more likely to have BED (APA, 2006). Binge eating, purging, and intermittent periods of food restriction make it difficult to stabilize blood glucose levels in individuals with type 1 DM, resulting in increased occurrence of medical crises and medical complications. Furthermore, insulin omission and underdosing for the purpose of weight loss may represent a specific subtype of purging behavior in insulin-dependent patients with eating disorders (APA, 2006).

TREATMENT APPROACH

Treatment of eating disorders requires a multidisciplinary approach that includes psychiatric/psychological, medical, and nutrition interventions. Treatment, provided at several levels of care depending on severity of illness, includes inpatient hospitalization, residential treatment, day hospitalization, intensive outpatient treatment, and outpatient treatment.

Inpatient treatment can be provided on a psychiatric or medical unit, and a behavioral protocol developed specifically for the management of eating-disordered patients is highly recommended. Residential eating disorder treatment facilities also provide 24-hour care; however, they are usually not equipped to manage medically or psychiatrically unstable patients. Day treatment programs provide specialized multidisciplinary care, including meals. Patients initially attend day treatment for 6 to 8 hours a day, 5 to 7 days per week.

The least intensive form of treatment is outpatient care; however, this still requires the ongoing, coordinated effort of physicians, psychotherapists, and nutritionists. Intensive outpatient treatment programs provide several hours of multidisciplinary care several times per week.

The Practice Guideline for the Treatment of Patients with Eating Disorders (APA, 2006) provides comprehensive guidelines for the formulation and implementation of treatment plans in patients with AN, BN, EDNOS, and BED. These guidelines provide specific treatment recommendations (e.g., nutritional rehabilitation, medical management, psychological interventions, medication management) and level of care guidelines for patients with eating disorders. In addition, the Society for Adolescent Medicine (SAM, 2003), the American Academy of Pediatrics (AAP, 2003), and the American Dietetic Association (ADA, 2001) have published policy statements and positions regarding guidelines for effective treatment of eating disorders.

CLINICAL CHARACTERISTICS AND MEDICAL COMPLICATIONS

Although eating disorders are classified as psychiatric illnesses, they are associated with significant medical complications, morbidity, and mortality. Numerous physiologic changes result from the weight-control habits of patients with AN and BN (Table 22-2). Some are minor changes that occur secondary to reduced energy intake; some are pathologic alterations that may have long-term consequences; and a few represent potentially life-threatening conditions.

Anorexia Nervosa

Patients with AN have a typical and distinctive appearance (Figure 22-1). Their cachectic and prepubescent body habitus often makes them look younger than their age. Common physical findings include **lanugo**, soft, downy hair growth, dry and brittle hair, **hypercarotenemia**, cold intolerance, and cyanosis of the extremities.

Protein-energy malnutrition with resultant loss of lean body mass is associated with reduced left ventricular mass and systolic dysfunction in AN. Cardiovascular complications include bradycardia (heart rate less than 60 beats/min), orthostatic hypotension, and cardiac arrhythmias (Romano et al., 2003).

Gastrointestinal complications secondary to starvation include delayed gastric emptying, decreased small bowel motility, and constipation. Complaints of abdominal bloating and a prolonged sensation of abdominal fullness complicate the refeeding process.

A serious medical complication found in both male and female patients is osteopenia (reduced bone mineral density [BMD]), the precursor of osteoporosis. A cross-sectional, community-based study of 214 adult females with AN showed that 52% had osteopenia, 34% had osteoporosis in

TABLE 22-2

Medical Complications of Eating Disorders

	AN		BN	
	Restricting	Binge-Eating Purging	Purging	Nonpurging
Fluid and Electrolyte Imbalance				
Hypokalemia		√	√	
Hyponatremia		√	√	
Hypochloremic alkalosis		√	√	
Elevated BUN	√	√	√	√
Inability to concentrate urine	√	√		
Decreased glomerular filtration rate	√	√		
Ketonuria	√	√	√	√
Cardiovascular and Electrocardiographic Abnormalities				
Bradycardia	√	√		
Orthostatic hypotension	√	√	√	√
Arrhythmias	√	√	√	√
Prolonged QT interval	√	√	√	
T wave abnormalities	√	√	√	
Conduction defects	√	√	√	
Ipecac cardiomyopathy		√	√	
Mitral valve prolapse	√	√		
Congestive cardiac failure	√	√		
Pericardial effusion	√	√		
Gastrointestinal				
Parotid hypertrophy		√	√	
Perimolysis and increased incidence of dental caries		√	√	
Constipation	√	√	√	
Bloody diarrhea		√	√	
Delayed gastric emptying	√	√	√	√
Intestinal atony	√	√	√	√
Esophagitis		√	√	
Mallory-Weiss tears		√	√	
Esophageal or gastric rupture		√	√	
Perforation/rupture of stomach		√	√	
Barrett esophagus		√	√	
Fatty infiltration and focal necrosis of liver	√	√		
Superior mesenteric artery syndrome	√	√		
Gallstones	√	√	√	√
Skeletal				
Osteopenia	√	√	?	?
Fractures	√	√	?	?
Dermatologic				
Acrocyanosis	√	√		
Yellow dry skin (hypercarotenemia)	√	√		
Brittle hair and nails	√	√		
Lanugo	√			
Russell sign (calluses over the knuckles)		√	√	
Pitting edema	√	√	√	√

From Fisher M et al.: Eating disorders in adolescents: a background paper, *J Adolesc Health* 16:420, 1995.

AN, Anorexia nervosa; *BN*, bulimia nervosa; *BUN*, blood urea nitrogen; T_3 triiodothyronine.

Continued

TABLE 22-2

Medical Complications of Eating Disorders—cont'd

	AN		BN	
	Restricting	Binge-Eating Purging	Purging	Nonpurging
Endocrine				
Growth retardation and short stature	√	√		
Delayed puberty	√	√		
Amenorrhea	√	√		
Low T₃ syndrome	√	√		
Decreased capacity to concentrate urine 2° to ↓ vasopressin secretion	√	√		
Hypercortisolism	√	√		
Hematologic				
Mild anemia	√	√		
Leukopenia	√	√		
Thrombocytopenia	√	√		
Low sedimentation rate	√	√		
Impaired cell-mediated immunity	√	√		
Neurologic				
Seizures	√	√	√	√
Myopathy	√	√	√	
Peripheral neuropathy	√	√		
Cortical atrophy	√	√		

one or more skeletal sites, and 30% had self-reported histories of fractures (Miller et al., 2005). Other studies suggest that reduced BMD occurs in more than 90% of adolescent and young women with AN (Golden, 2005). Hormone replacement therapy and biphosphonates such as alendronate have no proven efficacy in underweight females with AN (Golden et al., 2005). At present, the recommended treatment is weight gain and supplementation with calcium and vitamin D (APA, 2006).

Children and adolescents with AN develop unique medical complications that affect normal growth and development such as growth retardation, reduction in peak bone mass, and structural abnormalities in the brain (SAM, 2003).

Bulimia Nervosa

Clinical signs and symptoms of BN are more difficult to detect because patients are usually of normal weight and secretive in behavior. When vomiting occurs, there may be clinical evidence such as (1) scarring of the dorsum of the hand used to stimulate the gag reflex, known as *Russell's sign*; (2) parotid gland enlargement; and (3) erosion of dental enamel with increased dental caries resulting from the frequent presence of gastric acid in the mouth.

Chronic vomiting can result in dehydration, alkalosis, and hypokalemia. Common clinical manifestations include sore throat, esophagitis, mild hematemesis (vomiting blood), abdominal pain, and subconjunctival hemorrhage. More serious gastrointestinal complications include Mallory-Weiss esophageal tears, rare occurrence of esophageal rupture, and acute gastric dilation or rupture. Ipecac, used to induce vomiting, may cause irreversible myocardial damage and sudden death.

Laxative abuse may lead to dehydration, elevation of serum aldosterone and vasopressin levels, rectal bleeding, intestinal atony, and abdominal cramps. Diuretic abuse may lead to dehydration and hypokalemia. Cardiac arrhythmias can occur secondary to electrolyte and acid-base imbalance caused by vomiting, laxative, and diuretic abuse. Although the profound amenorrhea associated with AN is uncommon in BN, menstrual irregularities may occur (Figure 22-1).

PSYCHOLOGICAL MANAGEMENT

Eating disorders are complex psychiatric illnesses that require psychological assessment and ongoing treatment. Evaluation of the patient's cognitive and psychological stage of development, family history, family dynamics, and psychopathology is essential for the development of a comprehensive psychosocial treatment program.

The long-term goals of psychosocial interventions in AN are (1) to help patients understand and cooperate with their nutritional and physical rehabilitation; (2) to help patients

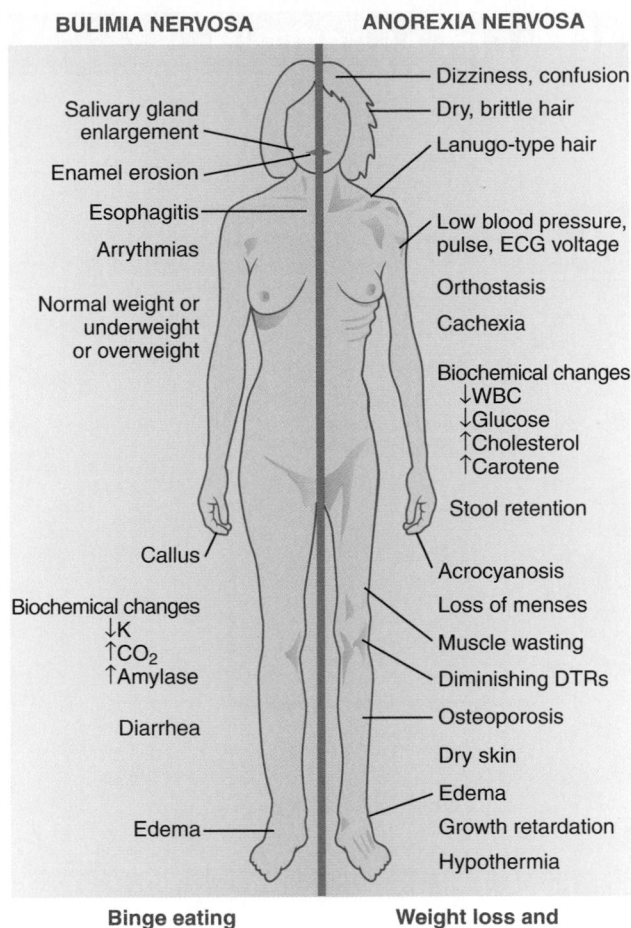

BULIMIA NERVOSA

ANOREXIA NERVOSA

Salivary gland enlargement

Enamel erosion

Esophagitis

Arrythmias

Normal weight or underweight or overweight

Callus

Biochemical changes
↓K
↑CO$_2$
↑Amylase

Diarrhea

Edema

Dizziness, confusion

Dry, brittle hair

Lanugo-type hair

Low blood pressure, pulse, ECG voltage

Orthostasis

Cachexia

Biochemical changes
↓WBC
↓Glucose
↑Cholesterol
↑Carotene

Stool retention

Acrocyanosis

Loss of menses

Muscle wasting

Diminishing DTRs

Osteoporosis

Dry skin

Edema

Growth retardation

Hypothermia

Binge eating and purging

Weight loss and malnutrition

FIGURE 22-1 Physical and clinical signs and symptoms of bulimia nervosa and anorexia nervosa. *DTRs,* Deep tendon reflexes; *ECG,* electrocardiogram; *WBC,* white blood cell.

understand and change behaviors and dysfunctional attitudes related to their eating disorders; (3) to improve interpersonal and social functioning; and (4) to address psychopathology and psychological conflicts that reinforce or maintain eating-disordered behaviors. In the acute stage of illness, malnourished AN patients are typically negativistic and obsessional, making it difficult to conduct formal psychotherapy. At this stage of treatment, psychological management is often focused on positive behavioral reinforcement of weight restoration. This includes praise for positive efforts, reassurance, coaching, and encouragement.

Inpatient treatment programs often use behavioral reinforcers that link attainment of privileges such as physical activity (versus bed rest), off-unit passes, visitation privileges, and phone privileges with attainment of targeted weight gain and improved eating behaviors. Once acute malnutrition has been corrected and weight restoration is underway, the AN patient is more likely to benefit from psychotherapy.

Psychotherapeutic treatment is frequently required for at least 1 year and in some cases for several years. Family therapy may be more beneficial than individual therapy in adolescents who have been sick for 3 years or less. Compared with AN patients, individuals with BN are generally

more distressed by their illness and are typically more accepting of psychological interventions.

Psychotherapy can help the patient understand and change core dysfunctional thoughts, attitudes, motives, conflicts, and feelings related to his or her eating disorder. Associated psychiatric conditions, including deficits in mood, impulse control, and self-esteem, as well as relapse prevention, should be addressed in the psychotherapeutic treatment plan.

Cognitive behavioral therapy (CBT) is considered the most effective single intervention in the treatment of acute symptoms of BN, but clinicians often combine elements of several psychotherapeutic approaches throughout the course of treatment (APA, 2006). Adjunctive family therapy and marital therapy may be beneficial in some cases.

Psychological measures, including validated questionnaires and interview instruments, are often used to evaluate individuals with (suspected) eating disorders. Self-reports are generally used for the purpose of screening, whereas structured interview instruments are used to determine a diagnosis. Representative instruments for assessment of eating disorders include the Eating Attitudes Test (EAT), Eating Disorder Inventory (EDI-II), Eating Disorder Examination (EDE and EDE-Q4), Eating Disorders Questionnaire (EDQ), and the Yale-Brown-Cornell Eating Disorder Scale (YBC-EDS).

NUTRITION REHABILITATION AND COUNSELING

Nutrition rehabilitation includes nutrition assessment, medical nutrition therapy (MNT), nutrition counseling, and nutrition education (see *Pathophysiology and Care Management Algorithm:* Anorexia Nervosa). Although the eating disorders are distinct illnesses, similarities exist in nutritional consequences and nutritional management.

NUTRITION ASSESSMENT

Nutrition assessment routinely includes a diet history and the assessment of biochemical, metabolic, and anthropometric indices of nutrition status (Figure 22-2).

Diet History

Guidelines should include assessment of energy intake, macronutrient and micronutrient consumption, eating attitudes, and eating behaviors (Box 22-2). Patients with AN generally consume less than 1000 kcal per day. They often "calorie count," but generally overestimate their food and energy intake. Assessment of typical energy intake will prevent overfeeding or underfeeding at the inception of nutritional rehabilitation and will open a dialogue regarding caloric requirements during the refeeding and weight maintenance phases of nutritional rehabilitation.

Energy intake in BN can be unpredictable. The caloric content of a binge, the degree of caloric absorption after a

PATHOPHYSIOLOGY AND CARE MANAGEMENT ALGORITHM

Anorexia Nervosa

ETIOLOGY

```
Distorted          ←   Coexisting        →   Preoccupation
body image             psychiatric disorder     with weight
```

```
Inadequate                              Excessive
energy intake                           physical activity
```

Body Weight Deficit
<85% of expected

PATHOPHYSIOLOGY

Diagnosis

APA diagnostic criteria

Classification

• Restricting type
• Binge eating/purging type

Clinical Findings

• Fluid and electrolyte imbalances
• Cardiovascular disorders
• Gastrointestinal disorders
• Osteopenia
• Dermatologic disorders
• Endocrine disturbance
• Hematologic disorders
• Neurologic disorders

MANAGEMENT

Medical Management

• Monitor organ function (especially cardiovascular)
• Monitor anthropometric status
• Monitor electrolytes
• Psychological counseling
• Monitor and treat fluid and electrolyte imbalances
• Antidepressant or other appropriate medication

Nutrition Management

• Nutrition assessment
• Correct malnutrition with oral feedings if possible; tube feeding if necessary
• Appropriate vitamin and mineral supplementation
• Nutrition, counseling, and education

Algorithm content developed by John J.B. Anderson, PhD, and Sanford C. Garner, PhD, 2000.

purge, and the extent of calorie restriction between binge episodes make assessment of total energy intake quite challenging. Bulimic patients assume that vomiting is an efficient mechanism for eliminating calories consumed during binge episodes; however, study of the caloric content of food ingested and purged in a feeding laboratory revealed that, as a group, 17 BN subjects consumed a mean of 2131 ($\pm$1154) kcal during a binge and vomited only 979 ($\pm$1003) kcal afterward (Kaye et al., 1993).

The notion that a binge, and thus calories consumed during the binge, can be completely purged is a common misconception among patients. As a rule of thumb, patients

EATING DISORDER ASSESSMENT

Date of birth: _____

DIAGNOSIS:

☐ Anorexia Nervosa
☐ Bulimia Nervosa
☐ Eating Disorder NOS

Hospitalizations for eating disorder:

☐ In-patient
☐ Day patient
☐ Out-patient
☐ Intensive out-patient

WEIGHT HISTORY
Wt. loss: # lb _____ From _____ To _____
Minimum weight at current height _____
Maximum weight at current height _____
IBW: _____ %IBW: _____ %Wt loss: _____ BMI%: _____

ANTHROPOMETRIC PROFILE
Skinfolds (mm): _____
Triceps: _____ Biceps: _____ Subscapular: _____
Suprailiac: _____
Sum of sites (mm): _____ % Body fat: _____ TSF%: _____
MAC (cm): _____ MAMC (cm): _____ MAMC%: _____

BODY IMAGE: _____
_____
_____

FOOD ALLERGIES: _____
_____
_____

24-HOUR RECALL: _____
_____
_____
_____
_____
_____
_____
_____
_____
_____

FLUID INTAKE: _____
_____

VITAMIN/MINERAL SUPPLEMENTS: _____
_____

OTHER SUPPLEMENTS: _____
_____

SUGAR AND FAT SUBSTITUTES: _____
_____

MISCELLANEOUS: Chewing gum: _____
Hard candy: _____
Condiments: _____
_____

BINGES: # per day _____ # per week _____
Duration per episode: _____
Binge foods: _____
_____
Approximate kcal/binge: _____

SELF-INDUCED VOMITING:
Times per day: _____ Method: _____

LAXATIVES:
Type/brand: _____ Amount: _____
Duration of use: _____ Frequency of use: _____

DIURETICS:
Type: _____ Amount: _____
Duration of use: _____ Frequency of use: _____

EXERCISE:
Type: _____
Minutes/day: _____ Times/week: _____ _____
Purpose of exercise: _____

MENSTRUAL HISTORY:
Age of menarche: _____
Last menstrual period: _____

MEDICATIONS (prescription and over-the-counter):
_____
_____
_____

BOWEL FUNCTION: _____
_____

FIGURE 22-2 Sample nutrition assessment form for eating disorders.

should be advised that approximately 50% of energy consumed during a binge is retained.

Inadequate energy intake results in decreased consumption of carbohydrate, protein, and fat. Patients with AN were historically described as carbohydrate restrictors, but at present there is a tendency to avoid fat-containing foods (Affenito et al., 2002; Hadigan et al., 2000). Observed food intake in thirty patients revealed that patients with AN consumed significantly less fat (15% to 20% of calories) than healthy controls (Hadigan et al., 2000).

Percent of calories contributed by protein may be in the average to above-average range, but the adequacy of intake will be relative to total caloric consumption. For example, the percentage of calories may remain the same, but as the calorie intake continues to drop, the actual amount of protein falls also.

Many AN patients follow vegetarian diets, and this affects both the quality and quantity of protein consumption. One study found that 47% of an AN population were vegetarians, but the specific type of vegetarianism (e.g., vegan, lacto-ovo)

Assessment of Nutrient Intake

1. Calories
   A. Compare intake with DRI (inside front cover)
   B. Estimate typical intake in AN
   C. Determine average intake and range of intake in BN
   D. Determine hidden sources (e.g., gum, hard candy)
2. Macronutrients
   A. Carbohydrate
      (1) Determine percent kcal intake
      (2) Compare intake to DRI intake
      (3) Simple
      (4) Complex
      (5) Fiber: water-soluble versus water-insoluble
   B. Protein
      (1) Determine percent kcal intake
      (2) Compare intake with DRI
      (3) Evaluate vegetarian diet for high biologic value sources
   C. Fat
      (1) Determine percent kcal intake
      (2) Source of essential fatty acid
      (3) Compare intake to DRI
3. Micronutrients
   A. Vitamins
      (1) Water-soluble
      (2) Fat-soluble
      (3) Identify supplements
   B. Minerals
      (1) Calcium
      (2) Iron
      (3) Zinc
      (4) Identify supplements
4. Fluid
   A. Determine total daily consumption
   B. Identify sources
5. Miscellaneous
   A. Alcohol
   B. Caffeine
   C. Amount and type of nonnutritive sweeteners and fat substitutes
   D. Other nutritional supplements (i.e., herbal supplements)

From Luder E, Schebendach J: Nutrition management of eating disorders, *Top Clin Nutr* 8:53, 1993.

AN, Anorexia nervosa; *BN*, bulimia nervosa; *DRI*, dietary reference intake.

was not reported (Hadigan et al., 2000). The majority of AN vegetarians adopt this practice during the course of their illness, so vegetarianism may simply be a covert method of limiting foods, particularly those containing fat. The nutritionist should determine if the adoption of vegetarian food choices predated the development of AN and whether family members also follow a vegetarian diet. Many nutritional rehabilitation programs do not allow the recovering anorexic to continue with vegetarianism during treatment, whereas others allow it, especially if the anorexic was vegetarian with family members before developing AN.

Chaotic eating, ranging from restriction to bingeing is a hallmark feature of disordered eating. Because of day-to-day variability, a 24-hour recall is not particularly useful. To assess energy intake, it is helpful to estimate daily food consumption over the course of a week. First determine the number of non-binge days (which may include restrictive and normal intake days) and approximate their caloric content; then determine the number of binge days and approximate caloric content and deduct 50% of the caloric content of binges that are purged (vomited); finally, average the caloric intake over the 7-day period. Determination of this average energy intake, as well as the range of intake, will be useful information for the counseling process.

Inadequate caloric intake, limited variety in the diet, and poor food group representation result in inadequate vitamin and mineral consumption in AN and BN patients. In general, micronutrient intake parallels macronutrient intake; thus AN patients who consistently restrict dietary fat are at greater risk for inadequate essential fatty acid intake and fat-soluble vitamin intake. Based on a 30-day diet history, Hadigan et al. (2000) found that more than 50% of thirty AN patients failed to meet DRI requirements for vitamin D, calcium, folate, vitamin B_{12}, magnesium, copper, and zinc. Nutrient intake in patients with BN varies with the cycle of binge eating and restriction. Patients with AN and BN should be queried about the use of vitamin and mineral supplements.

When obtaining a diet history, typical fluid intake should also be determined because abnormalities in fluid balance are prevalent in this population. Some patients severely restrict intake because they are intolerant of feeling full after fluid ingestion, whereas others drink excessive amounts, attempting to stave off hunger. Extremes in fluid restriction or consumption may require monitoring of urine specific gravity and serum electrolytes.

Eating Behavior

Characteristic attitudes, behaviors, and eating habits seen in AN and BN are shown in Box 22-3. Food aversions, common in this population, include red meat, baked goods, desserts, added fats, and fried foods. Patients with eating disorders often regard specific foods or groups of foods as absolutely "good" or absolutely "bad." Irrational beliefs and dichotomous thinking about food choices should be identified and challenged throughout the treatment process.

In the assessment, it is important to determine unusual or ritualistic behaviors, which may include ingestion of food in an atypical manner or with nontraditional utensils; unusual food combinations; or the excessive use of spices, vinegar, lemon juice, and artificial sweeteners. Meal spacing and length of time allocated for a meal should also be deter-

BOX 22-3

Assessment of Eating Attitudes, Behaviors, and Habits

1. Eating attitudes
   A. Food aversions
   B. Safe, risky, forbidden foods
   C. Magical thinking
   D. Binge trigger foods
   E. Ideas on appropriate amounts of food
2. Eating behaviors
   A. Ritualistic behaviors
   B. Unusual food combinations
   C. Atypical seasoning of food
   D. Excessive and atypical use of non-caloric sweeteners
   E. Atypical use of eating utensils
3. Eating habits
   A. Intake pattern
      (1) Number of meals and snacks
      (2) Time of day meals and snacks are consumed
      (3) Duration of feedings
      (4) Eating environment—where and with whom
      (5) How consumed—sitting or standing
   B. Avoidance of particular food groups
   C. Variety of foods consumed
   D. Fluid intake—restricted or excessive

From Schebendach J, Nussbaum M: Nutrition management in adolescents with eating disorders, *Adolesc Med: State of the Art Rev* 3(3):545, 1992.

mined. Many patients will save their self-allotted food ration until late in the day; others are fearful of eating past a certain time of day.

Many BN patients eat quickly, reflecting their difficulties with satiety cues. In addition, BN patients may identify foods they fear will trigger a binge episode. The patient may have an all-or-nothing approach to "trigger" foods. Although the patient may prefer avoidance, assistance with reintroduction of controlled amounts of these foods at regular times and intervals is helpful.

Many AN patients eat in an excessively slow manner, often playing with their food and cutting it into small pieces. This is sometimes regarded as a tactic to avoid food intake, but it may also be an effect of starvation (Keys et al., 1950).

Laboratory Assessment

The marked cachexia of AN may lead one to expect biochemical indices of malnutrition, but this is rarely the case. Compensatory mechanisms are remarkable, and laboratory abnormalities may not be observed until the illness is far advanced.

Significant alterations in visceral protein status are uncommon in AN. Indeed, adaptive phenomena that occur in chronic starvation are aimed at the maintenance of visceral protein metabolism at the expense of the somatic compartment. Serum albumin levels are generally within normal limits but may be masked by dehydration in early treatment (Swenne, 2004).

Despite consumption of a typically low fat, low-cholesterol diet, some AN patients initially present with elevated serum cholesterol levels (APA, 2006). Nevertheless, this does not warrant the continuation of a fat- and cholesterol-restricted diet during nutritional rehabilitation. If hyperlipidemia predated the development of AN, or if a strong family history of hyperlipidemia is identified, the patient should be reassessed after weight restoration and a period of weight stabilization. Low blood levels of essential fatty acids may contribute to the physical and mental symptoms of the disorder (Ayton, 2004).

Patients with BN may also have abnormal lipid levels. Patients with BN are prone to eating low-fat, low-energy foods during the restriction phase and high-fat, high-sugar foods during binge episodes. Premature prescription of a low-fat, low-cholesterol diet may only reinforce this dichotomous approach to eating. Care must be taken to balance extremes in the types and amounts of foods consumed. An accurate lipid profile can be obtained only after a period of dietary stabilization. Patients with BN may also have difficulty complying with the fast required for an accurate lipid profile.

Low serum glucose results from a deficit of precursors needed for gluconeogenesis and glucose production. Thyroid hormone production tends to be normal, but the peripheral deiodination of thyroxin favors formation of the less metabolically active reduced triiodothyronine (rT_3) rather than triiodothyronine (T_3) resulting in **low T_3 syndrome.** This metabolic state is characteristic of AN and typically resolves with weight restoration. Thyroid replacement is not recommended (APA, 2006).

Vitamin and Mineral Deficiencies

Hypercarotenemia is a common finding in AN, attributed to mobilization of lipid stores, catabolic changes caused by weight loss, and metabolic stress. Excessive dietary intake of carotenoids is less common. Normalization of serum carotene occurs during the course of nutrition rehabilitation.

Despite obviously deficient diets, reports of clinical and biochemical findings of true deficiency diseases are uncommon. The decreased need for micronutrients in a catabolic state, use of vitamin supplements, and selection of micronutrient-rich foods may be protective. Documented cases of riboflavin, vitamin B_6, thiamin, niacin, folate, and vitamin E deficiencies have been reported in lower-weight and more chronically ill patients with AN (Castro, 2004; Prousky, 2003).

Iron deficiency anemia is also uncommon in AN. Iron requirements are decreased secondary to amenorrhea and the overall catabolic state. The true picture may be masked by hemoconcentration resulting from dehydration in early treatment (Swenne, 2004). Once refeeding has been initiated, hemoglobin concentration may decrease from baseline values (Swenne, 2004). Zinc deficiency may also occur secondary to inadequate energy intake, avoidance of red meat, and the adoption of vegetarian food choices.

AN, past and present, is associated with a high prevalence of osteopenia and osteoporosis in both males and females. Although low estrogen and testosterone levels and weight loss are the primary causes, concurrent dietary deficiencies of calcium, magnesium, and vitamin D contribute to the overall pathogenesis. Dual x-ray absorptiometry to determine the degree of impaired bone mineralization is recommended (see Chapter 24).

Fluid and Electrolyte Balance

Vomiting and laxative and diuretic use can result in significant fluid and electrolyte imbalances in patients with eating disorders. Laxative use may result in hypokalemia, and diuretic use can also cause hypokalemia and dehydration. Vomiting may result in dehydration, hypokalemia, and alkalosis with hypochloremia. Hyponatremia is another serious complication but is seen less frequently.

Urine concentration is decreased, and urine output is increased in semistarvation. Edema may occur in response to malnutrition and refeeding. Depletion of glycogen and lean tissue is accompanied by obligatory water loss that reflects characteristic hydration ratios. For example, the obligatory water loss associated with glycogen depletion may be in the range of 600 to 800 ml. Varying degrees of fluid intake, ranging from restricted to excessive, may affect electrolyte values in AN patients.

Energy Expenditure

Resting energy expenditure (REE) is characteristically low in malnourished AN patients (de Zwaan et al., 2002). Weight loss, decreased lean body mass, energy restriction, and decreased leptin levels have been implicated in the pathogenesis of this hypometabolic state. Refeeding increases REE in malnourished AN patients. However, in some cases the increase in REE is excessive and presents as metabolic resistance to weight gain. Anxiety level, abdominal pain, hyperactivity, and cigarette smoking may also be associated with this phenomenon (Van Wymelbeke et al., 2004). An exaggerated diet-induced thermogenesis (DIT) has also been reported in AN during the course of refeeding (de Zwann et al., 2002). This further contributes to metabolic resistance to weight gain during the early course of nutritional rehabilitation in AN.

Patients with BN can have unpredictable metabolic rates. Dietary restraint between episodes of binge eating may place bulimic patients in a state of semistarvation (resulting in a hypometabolic rate). However, binge eating followed by purging can increase the metabolic rate secondary to a preabsorptive release of insulin, which activates the sympathetic nervous system (de Zwann et al., 2002).

Baseline and follow-up assessment of REE is clinically useful throughout the course of nutritional rehabilitation of AN and BN patients (Schebendach, 2003). Recent advances in handheld devices such as the MedGem and BodyGem make measurement of energy expenditure possible in a clinical setting (see Chapter 2).

Anthropometric Assessment

Patients with AN have protein-energy malnutrition characterized by significantly depleted adipose and somatic protein stores but a relatively intact visceral protein compartment. These patients meet the criteria for a diagnosis of severe protein-energy malnutrition. A goal of nutritional rehabilitation is restoration of body fat and fat-free mass. Although these compartments do regenerate, the extent and rate vary.

Percent body fat can be estimated from the sum of four skin-fold measurements (triceps, biceps, subscapular, and suprailiac crest) using the calculations of Durnin and colleagues (Durnin and Rahaman, 1967; Durnin and Womersley, 1974). This method has been validated against underwater weighing to assess percentage of body fat in adolescent girls with AN (Probst, 2001). A more accurate measurement of percentage of body fat can be obtained from underwater weighing or from a dual-energy x-ray absorptiometry (DEXA) scan equipped with body composition software; however, these methods are not generally available in an office or clinic setting (see Chapter 14).

Bioelectrical impedance analysis (BIA) is more readily available, but shifts in intracellular and extracellular fluid compartments in patients with severe eating disorders may affect the accuracy of body fat measurement. To improve the validity of BIA (see Figure 14-17) measurement in AN patients, the measurement should be done in the morning before ingestion of all food and liquid, using a reclining chair that is always reclined to the same position to prevent differential pooling of fluids (Sunday and Halmi, 2003).

For practical purposes the midarm muscle circumference, derived from midarm circumference and triceps skinfold measurements, can be easily obtained and compared with sex- and age-matched population standards (see Chapter 14). Baseline and follow-up measurements should be obtained during nutritional rehabilitation.

Body weight is assessed and routinely monitored in patients with eating disorders. In AN weight gain is necessary. In BN the short-term goal should be weight maintenance. Although weight loss may be warranted, this cannot be addressed until chaotic eating patterns are stabilized.

Rate of weight gain in AN may be affected by hydration status, glycogen stores, metabolic factors, and changes in body composition (Box 22-4). Rehydration and replenished glycogen stores contribute to weight gain during the first few days of refeeding. Thereafter weight gain results from increased lean and fat stores. It is generalized that one needs to increase or decrease caloric intake by 3500 kcal to cause a 1-lb change in body weight, but the true energy cost depends on the type of tissue gained. More energy is required to gain fat versus lean, but weight gain may be a mix of fat and lean tissue.

Although total body fat normalizes after short-term weight restoration, it may not be normally distributed (Mayer et al., 2005; Grinspoon 2001). When weight-restored AN patients were compared to body mass index (BMI)–matched normal controls, it was found that, although total adipose tissue did not differ significantly between the two groups, body fat was disproportionately deposited around the waist and abdominal cavity in the weight-restored adult female AN patients (Mayer et al., 2005). However, central accumulation of fat after weight gain was not observed after weight restoration in adolescents with AN (Misra et al., 2003).

Changes in body fat distribution after long-term maintenance of weight restoration and after weight restoration in male AN patients are not known. Variables that may affect the type of tissue gained include the stage of growth and development, degree of baseline malnutrition, duration of illness, duration of weight restoration, gender, genetics, physical activity, and possibly the type and rate of refeeding.

The anthropometric status of patients with eating disorders should be assessed and monitored regularly (see Chapter 14). The patient's goal weight can be determined by various methods, none of which is perfect. The height, weight, and BMI tables of the National Center for Health Statistics (NCHS) should be used to assess boys and girls up to 20 years of age (see Appendices 12 and 16). A bone age can be obtained in adolescents with stunted height to determine catch-up growth potential.

If a patient is hospitalized, a daily preprandial, early-morning weight should be obtained. On an outpatient basis a gowned weight should be obtained on the same scale, at approximately the same time of day, at least once a week in early treatment. Before weigh-in the patient should void, and urine specific gravity should be checked for dehydration or fluid loading. If the patient claims to be unable to provide a urine specimen, the physician should examine the patient to see whether the bladder is full. Patients may resort to deceptive tactics (water loading, hiding heavy objects on their person, and withholding urine and bowel movements) to make a mandated weight goal.

MEDICAL NUTRITION THERAPY AND COUNSELING

Treatment of AN may begin at one of four levels of care (Figure 22-3), depending on the severity of malnutrition, degree of medical and psychiatric instability, duration of illness, and growth failure. Some AN patients begin treatment with inpatient hospitalization and are stepped down to a less intensive level of treatment as weight restoration and nutritional rehabilitation progress. Other AN patients begin treatment on an outpatient basis; however, if adequate weight restoration does not occur, they are generally stepped up to a more intensive level of care.

In BN treatment typically begins and continues on an outpatient basis. On occasion a BN patient may be directly admitted to an intensive outpatient or day treatment program. However, inpatient hospitalization is relatively uncommon and generally is of short duration and for the specific purpose of fluid and electrolyte stabilization. The registered dietitian (RD) is an essential part of the treatment team at all levels of care.

Anorexia Nervosa

The goals of nutrition rehabilitation include correction of biologic and psychological sequelae of malnutrition; restoration of body weight; and normalization of eating patterns, eating behaviors, and hunger/satiety cues. Hospital-based programs or residential treatment is warranted when the AN patient is medically unstable, severely malnourished, or growth retarded (APA, 2006; SAM, 2003). Under these circumstances

---

BOX 22-4

Factors Affecting Rate of Weight Gain in Anorexia Nervosa

1. Fluid balance
   A. Polyuria seen in semistarvation
   B. Edema
      (1) Starvation
      (2) Refeeding
   C. Hydration ratios in tissues
      (1) Glycogen: 3-4:1
      (2) Protein: 3-4:1
2. Metabolic rate
   A. Resting energy expenditure
   B. Postprandial energy expenditure
3. Energy cost of tissue gained
   A. Adipose tissue
   B. Lean body mass
4. Previous obesity
5. Physical activity

From Schebendach J, Nussbaum M: Nutrition management in adolescents with eating disorders, *Adolesc Med: State of the Art Rev* 3(3):545, 1992.

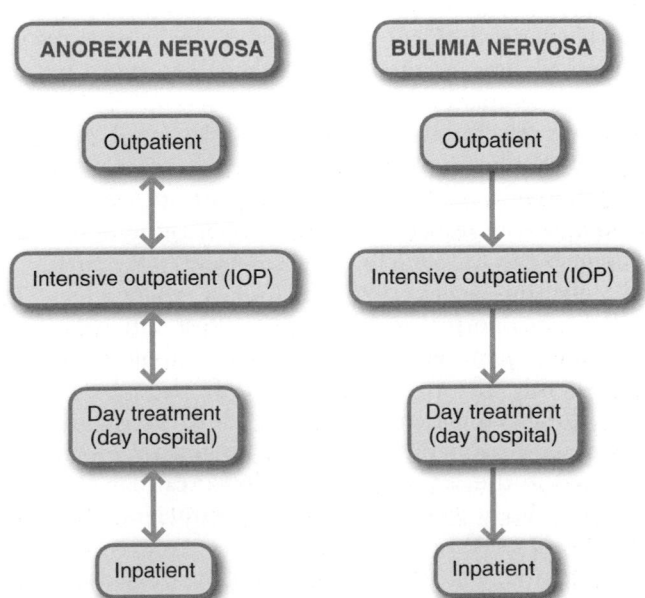

FIGURE 22-3 Nutrition counseling in the continuum of care in eating disorders.

caloric prescriptions are determined by the medical doctor or treatment team.

Institutions vary with respect to their menu-planning protocol. In some institutions the meal plan and food choices are initially fixed without patient input. As treatment progresses and weight is restored, the patient generally assumes more responsibility for menu planning. In other inpatient programs the patient participates in menu planning from the beginning of treatment. Some institutions have established guidelines that the patient must comply with to maintain the "privilege" of menu planning. Guidelines may require a certain type of milk (e.g., whole vs. low fat), and the inclusion of specific types of foods such as added fats, animal proteins, desserts, and snacks. A certain number of servings from the different food groups may be prescribed at different calorie levels. Meal-planning systems also vary among treatment programs. Some design their own, others use food group exchanges or the MyPyramid system, and some formulate an individualized meal plan for each patient.

There are no outcome studies to suggest that one method of meal planning is superior to another, and treatment programs tend to have their own philosophy about menu planning. Despite differences in protocol, AN patients consistently find it difficult to make food choices. The RD can be extremely helpful in providing a structured meal plan and guidance in the selection of nutritionally adequate meals of adequate variety and caloric density.

In an outpatient setting the treatment team obviously has less control over the AN patient's food choices, energy intake, and energy distribution. Under these circumstances the RD must use counseling skills to begin the process of developing a plan for nutritional rehabilitation. AN patients are typically precontemplative and, at best, ambivalent about making changes in eating behavior, diet, and body weight; some are defiant and hostile on initial presentation. At this point the nutrition counselor, using motivational interviewing techniques can help the AN patient resolve ambivalence toward the idea of change and move beyond the precontemplative stage (Box 22-5).

Weight restoration is critical to recovery in AN. Effective nutritional rehabilitation and counseling must ultimately result in weight gain and improved eating attitudes and behaviors. A comprehensive review of nutrition counseling techniques can be found in Chapter 18 and in Herrin (2003) and Stellefson-Meyer (1999) (see *Clinical Insight:* Does Eating Behavior Normalize After Weight Restoration?).

The treatment plan of an AN patient should include an expected rate of weight gain. Gains of 2 to 3 lb/week for the hospitalized patient and 0.5 to 1 lb/week for the outpatient are reasonable and attainable goals. Calorie prescriptions in the range of 1000 to 1600 kcal/day (30 to 40 kcal/kg of body weight per day) are sufficient to initiate weight gain (APA, 2006).

To promote controlled weight gain, the caloric prescription must be progressively increased. Increasing the energy intake by 100 to 200 calories every 2 to 3 days is generally well tolerated (APA, 2006); however, some inpatient treatment programs increase the caloric prescription in 500-calorie increments (Yager and Andersen, 2005).

Aggressive refeeding of severely malnourished AN patients (i.e., those weighing less than 70% standard body weight) may precipitate life-threatening complications of the refeeding syndrome during the first week of oral, nasogastric, or intravenous refeeding (Ornstein et al., 2003) (see Chapter 3). Manifestations of the syndrome are fluid and electrolyte imbalance; cardiac, neurologic, and hematologic complications; and sudden death. High-risk patients need to be carefully monitored with daily measurements of serum phosphorus, magnesium, potassium, and calcium for the first 5 days of refeeding and every other day for several weeks thereafter. Supplemental phosphorus, magnesium, and potassium may be given orally or intravenously.

Continued weight gain requires progressive increases in caloric intake, and consumption of 70 to 100 kcal/kg of body weight daily may be needed in some AN patients (APA, 2006). Changes in REE, DIT, and the type of tissue gained are all factors. In addition, the energy cost of physical activity must be considered because many AN patients expend significant amounts of energy in physical activity and or fidgeting behavior (de Zwann et al., 2002).

In general, caloric prescriptions in the range of 3000 to 4000 kcal/day may be needed later in the course of weight

---

BOX 22-5

Principles of Motivational Interviewing

1. Express empathy:
   Acceptance facilitates change.
   Skillful reflective listening is fundamental.
   Ambivalence on the part of the client is normal.
2. Develop discrepancy:
   Client, not the counselor, should present the arguments for change.
   Change is motivated by a perceived discrepancy between present behavior and important personal goals or value.
3. Roll with resistance:
   Avoid arguing for change.
   Resistance is not directly opposed.
   New perspectives are invited but not imposed.
   Client is a primary resource in finding answers and solutions.
   Resistance is a signal (to the counselor) to respond differently.
4. Support self-efficacy:
   A person's belief in the possibility of change is an important motivator.
   Client, not the counselor, is responsible for choosing and carrying out change.
   The counselor's own belief in the person's ability to change becomes a self-fulfilling prophecy.

From Miller WR, Rollnick S: *Motivational interviewing: preparing people for change*, ed 2, New York, The Guildford Press, 2002, pp. 33-42.

✳ CLINICAL INSIGHT

Does Eating Behavior Normalize After Weight Restoration?

Disturbances in eating behavior and weight loss are characteristic features of AN. Successful treatment of the AN patient results in weight gain, but do disturbed eating behaviors also normalize during the process of weight restoration?

Sysko and colleagues (2005) studied twelve hospitalized AN patients and compared them with normal healthy controls. All twelve AN patients were tested shortly after admission to an inpatient treatment program, and eleven were retested after weight restoration (greater than or equal to 90% of IBW). To test the eating behavior of patients and controls, subjects were given a large, sealed, 83 fl oz opaque container of strawberry yogurt shake, which provided approximately 1 calorie per gram. Subjects could not see how much shake was in the container, and they were not informed of the quantity or the caloric content. Instructions specified that participants could drink as much shake as they liked and that the shake would replace their lunch meal for that day. In AN patients mean shake consumption was 104 ± 102 g when they were at their low weight and 178 ± 203 g after weight restoration; these amounts were not significantly different. Normal control subjects consumed significantly more than did AN patients at both time points, and the average meal size was 490 ± 188 g. Despite weight restoration and significant improvement in psychological symptoms, AN patients exhibited a persistent disturbance in eating behavior. The authors concluded that nutritional rehabilitation and weight restoration may not resolve the core eating difficulties in AN. This may contribute to the high relapse rate seen in this population.

---

restoration, and male AN patients may require even more—4000 to 4500 kcal/day (APA, 2006). Patients who require extraordinarily high energy intakes should be questioned or observed for discarding of food, vomiting, exercising, and excessive physical activity, including fidgeting. After the goal weight is attained, the caloric prescription may be slowly decreased to promote weight maintenance. However, caloric prescriptions may remain at higher levels in adolescents with the potential for continued growth and development.

AN patients receiving care in less structured treatment settings such as outpatient treatment programs may be particularly resistant to formalized meal plans. A practical approach may be the addition of 200 to 300 calories per day to the patient's typical (baseline) energy intake. However, the nutritionist must carefully query and assess intake since these patients typically overestimate their food and energy consumption (Hadigan et al., 2000).

Once the caloric prescription is calculated, a reasonable distribution of macronutrients must be determined (Box 22-6). Patients may express multiple food aversions. Ex-

---

BOX 22-6

Guidelines for Medical Nutrition Therapy of Anorexia Nervosa

1. Caloric prescription:
   A. Initial weight gain
      (1) Start at 30 to 40 kcal/kg/day (approximately 1000 to 1600 kcal/day)
      (2) Assess risk for refeeding syndrome
   B. Controlled weight gain phase
      (1) Increase prescription in small, progressive increments to promote expected rate of controlled weight gain (e.g., 2-3 lb/wk for inpatients, 0.5 to 1 lb/wk for outpatients)
      (2) Late treatment: 70 to 100 kcal/kg/day
          Females: 3000 to 4000 kcal/day
          Males: 4000 to 4500 kcal/day
      (3) If patient requires a higher kcal prescription, evaluate for vomiting, discarding food, increased exercise, increased motor activity, increased REE/DIT
   C. Weight maintenance phase
      (1) Adults: 40 to 60 kcal/kg/day
      (2) Ongoing growth and development in children and adolescents: 40-60 kcal/kg/day
2. Macronutrients
   A. Protein
      (1) Minimum intake = RDA in g/kg ideal body weight
      (2) 15% to 20% kcal
      (3) High biologic value sources
   B. Carbohydrate
      (1) 50% to 55% kcal
      (2) Encourage insoluble fiber for treatment of constipation
   C. Fat
      (1) 25% to 30% kcal
      (2) Encourage small increases in fat intake until goal can be attained
      (3) Provide source of essential fatty acid
3. Micronutrients
   A. 100% RDA multivitamin with minerals supplement
   B. Note that iron-containing preparations may aggravate constipation

From Luder E, Schebendach J: Nutrition management of eating disorders, *Top Clin Nutr* 8:48, 1993.

DIT, Diet-induced thermogenesis; *RDA,* recommended dietary allowance; *REE,* resting energy expenditure.

---

treme avoidance of dietary fat is common, but continued omission will make it difficult to provide concentrated sources of energy needed for weight restoration. A dietary fat intake in the range of 25% to 30% of calories is recommended. This can be accomplished easily when AN patients are treated on inpatient units or in day hospital programs.

However, on an outpatient basis small progressive increases in dietary fat intake rather than a set optimal amount right away may be met with less resistance.

Although some patients will accept small amounts of added fat (such as salad dressing, mayo, or butter), many do better when the fat content is less obvious (as in cheese, peanut butter, granola, and snack foods). Encouraging the gradual change from fat-free products (fat-free milk) to low-fat products (1% or 2% milk) and finally to full-fat items (whole milk) is also acceptable to some patients. Focusing on good fat rather than saturated fat is another useful tip.

A protein intake in the range of 15% to 20% of total calories is recommended. To ensure adequacy the minimum protein prescription should equal the recommended dietary allowance (RDA) for age and sex in grams per kilogram of *ideal* body weight (see inside front cover). Vegetarian diets are often requested but should be discouraged during nutritional rehabilitation.

Carbohydrate intake in the range of 50% to 55% of calories is well tolerated. Sources of insoluble fiber should be included for optimal health, but also to relieve the constipation frequently seen in this population.

Although vitamin and mineral supplements are not universally prescribed, the potential for increased needs during the anabolic phase must be considered. A vitamin and mineral supplement providing 100% of the RDA is recommended, but iron-containing preparations may aggravate constipation in some patients. Care must be taken throughout the refeeding process to ensure a reasonable variety of intake. Particular attention to the inclusion of calcium-rich foods along with extra vitamin D is recommended because of the increased risk of osteopenia and osteoporosis (see Chapter 24).

Delayed gastric emptying with complaints of abdominal distention and discomfort after eating are common in AN. In early treatment intake is generally low and can be tolerated in three meals per day. However, as the caloric prescription increases, between-meal feedings become essential. The addition of an afternoon or evening snack may relieve the physical discomfort associated with larger meals, but some patients express feelings of guilt for "indulging" between meals. Commercially available, defined-formula liquid supplements containing 30 to 45 calories per fluid ounce are often prescribed once or twice daily (see Appendix 32). Patients are fearful that they will become accustomed to the large amount of food required to meet increased caloric requirements; thus use of a liquid supplement is appealing because it can easily be discontinued when the goal weight is attained.

Bulimia Nervosa

Bulimia nervosa is described as a state of dietary chaos, characterized by periods of uncontrolled, poorly structured eating, which are often followed by a periods of restrained food intake. The nutritionist's role is to help develop a reasonable plan of controlled eating while assessing the patient's tolerance for structure. Since BN patients are hospitalized infrequently, nutrition counseling will most likely begin in an outpatient treatment setting.

In BN much of the patient's eating and purging behavior is aimed at weight loss. Although weight reduction may be a reasonable long-term goal, immediate goals must be interruption of the binge-and-purge cycle, restoration of normal eating behavior, and stabilization of body weight. Attempts at dietary restraint for the purpose of weight loss typically exacerbate binge/purge behavior in BN patients.

Patients with BN have varying degrees of metabolic efficiency, which must be taken into account when prescribing the baseline diet. Assessment of REE along with clinical signs of a hypometabolic state such as a low T_3 level and cold intolerance are useful in determining the caloric prescription. If a low metabolism is suspected, a caloric prescription of 1500 to 1600 calories daily is a reasonable place to start. Another technique that is helpful in establishing an initial caloric prescription is to base it on the patient's present intake by using the following method:

1. For a typical week ask the patient to estimate the number of binge/purge days, binge/nonpurge days, moderate-intake days, and restrained-intake days.
2. Have the patient describe a typical food intake on a binge/purge day, a binge/nonpurge day, a moderate-intake day, and a restrained-intake day.
3. Estimate 50% of the caloric intake on the binge/purge days and 100% of caloric intake on the binge/nonpurge days, moderate-intake days, and restrained-intake days.
4. Calculate the total caloric intake over the 7-day period.
5. Calculate an average daily intake. The RD can then formulate an initial eating and meal plan based on this estimated average daily intake.

Body weight should be monitored with a goal of stabilization. If the patient's weight is stabilized on a lower-than-average caloric intake, small but consistent increases in the caloric intake should be prescribed every 1 to 2 weeks. This will induce incremental increases in the metabolic rate (Schebendach, 2003).

BN patients need a great deal of encouragement to follow weight-maintenance versus weight-loss diets. They must be reminded that attempts to restrict caloric intake may only increase the risk of binge eating and that their pattern of restrained intake followed by binge eating has not facilitated weight loss in the past.

A balanced macronutrient intake is essential for the provision of a regular meal pattern. This should include sufficient carbohydrates to prevent craving and adequate protein and fat to promote satiety. In general, a balanced diet providing 50% to 55% of the calories from carbohydrate, 15% to 20% from protein, and 25% to 30% from fat is reasonable. Small amounts of dietary fat should be encouraged at each meal. As is the case with AN, this may be better tolerated when provided in a less obvious manner, such as in peanut butter, cheese, or whole milk.

Adequacy of micronutrient intake relative to the caloric prescription and variety of intake should be assessed. A multivitamin–mineral preparation may be prescribed to ensure adequacy, particularly in the initial phase of treatment (Box 22-7).

Bingeing, purging, and restrained intake often impair recognition of hunger and satiety cues. The cessation of purging behavior coupled with a reasonable daily distribution of calories at three meals and prescribed snacks can be instrumental in strengthening these biologic cues. Many patients with BN are afraid to eat earlier in the day, fearful that these calories will contribute to caloric excess if they binge later. They may also digress from their meal plans after a binge, attempting to restrict intake to balance out the binge calories. Patience and support are essential in this process of making positive changes in their eating habits.

Cognitive behavioral therapy (CBT), a highly structured psychotherapeutic method used to alter attitudes and problem behaviors by identifying and replacing negative, inaccurate thoughts and changing the rewards of the behavior, is the treatment of choice in BN (APA, 2006). When applied to an eating disorder, CBT is typically a 20-week intervention that consists of three distinct and systematic phases of treatment: (1) establishing a regular eating pattern; (2) evaluating and changing beliefs about shape and weight; and (3) preventing relapse.

When the BN patient is receiving CBT, the RD can be instrumental in helping the patient to establish a regular meal pattern (phase 1). However, the RD and the psychotherapist must maintain active communication to avoid overlap in the counseling sessions. If the BN patient is engaged in a type of psychotherapy other than CBT, the RD should incorporate more CBT skills into the nutrition counseling sessions (Herrin, 2003).

Patients with BN are typically more receptive and less resistant to nutrition counseling than the AN patient and less likely to present in the precontemplation stage of change. Suggested strategies for nutrition counseling at the precontemplation, contemplation, preparation, action, and maintenance stages are given in Table 22-3.

BOX 22-7

Guidelines for Medical Nutrition Therapy of Bulimia Nervosa

1. Caloric prescription for weight maintenance
   A. Provide 1500 to 1600 kcal/day diet if patient is hypometabolic
   B. Provide DRI for energy if metabolic rate is normal
   C. Monitor body weight and adjust caloric prescription for weight maintenance
   D. Avoid weight reduction diets until eating patterns and body weight are stabilized
2. Macronutrients
   A. Protein
      (1) Minimum intake = RDA in g/kg ideal body weight
      (2) 15% to 20% kcal
      (3) High biologic value sources
   B. Carbohydrate
      (1) 50% to 55% kcal
      (2) Encourage insoluble fiber for treatment of constipation
   C. Fat
      (1) 25% to 30% kcal
      (2) Provide source of essential fatty acids
3. Micronutrients
   A. 100% RDA multivitamin with minerals supplement
   B. Note that iron-containing preparation may aggravate constipation

From Luder E, Schebendach J: Nutrition management of eating disorders, *Top Clin Nutr* 8:48, 1993.

RDA, Recommended dietary allowance; *RDI*, reference daily intake.

TABLE 22-3

Counseling Strategies Using the Stages of Change Model in Eating Disorders

Stage of Change	Counseling Strategies
Precontemplation	• Establish rapport • Assess nutrition knowledge, beliefs, attitudes • Conduct thorough review of food likes/dislikes, safe/risky foods, forbidden foods (assess reason), binge/purge foods • Assess physical, anthropometric, metabolic status • Assess level of motivation • Use motivational interviewing techniques • Decisional balance: weigh costs and benefits of maintaining current status vs. costs and benefits of change

Modified from Stellefson-Myers E: *Winning the war within: nutrition therapy for clients with anorexia or bulimia nervosa*, Dallas, Tex, 1999, Helm Publishing.

Continued

TABLE 22-3

Counseling Strategies Using the Stages of Change Model in Eating Disorders—cont'd

Stage of Change	Counseling Strategies
Contemplation	• Identify behaviors to change; prioritize • Identify barriers to change • Identify coping mechanisms • Identify support systems • Discuss self-monitoring tools: food and eating behavior records • Continue motivational interviewing technique
Preparation	• Implement: nutrition-focused cognitive behavioral therapy (CBT) • Implement self-monitoring tools: food and eating behavior records • Determine list of alternative behaviors to bingeing and purging
Action	• Develop a plan of healthy eating • Reinforce positive decision making, self-confidence, and self-efficacy • Promote positive self-rewarding behaviors • Develop strategies for handling impulsive behaviors, high-risk situations, and "slips" • Continue CBT • Continue self-monitoring
Maintenance/relapse	• Identify/strategies; management of high-risk situations • Continue positive self-rewarding behaviors • Reinforce coping skills and impulse control techniques • Reinforce relapse prevention strategies • Determine/schedule follow-up sessions needed for maintenance/reinforcement of positive changes in eating behavior and nutrition status

BOX 22-8

Patient Monitoring

1. Body weight
   A Establish goal weight
   B. Determine
      (1) Acceptable rate of weight gain in AN
      (2) Maintenance weight range in BN
   C. Monitor weight
      (1) Inpatient
         a. Daily, or every other day
         b. Gowned
         c. Preprandial
         d. Postvoid
         e. Obtain urine specific gravity
         f. Obtain additional, random, afternoon, or evening weight if fluid loading is suspected
      (2) Day treatment
         a. May vary, depending on diagnosis, age of patient, and treatment setting (i.e., daily, several times per week, once per week)
         b. Gowned
         c. Postvoid
         d. Same time of day
         e. Same scale
         f. Obtain urine specific gravity
      (3) Outpatient
         a. Once every 1-2 wk in early treatment, less frequently in mid- to late treatment
         b. Gowned
         c. Postvoid
         d. Same time of day
         e. Same scale
         f. Obtain urine specific gravity
2. Height
   A. Obtain baseline (NCHS percentile for children and adolescents)
   B. Monitor: every 1-2 mo in patients with growth potential
3. Anthropometric measurements (optional)
   A. Obtain baseline
      (1) Skinfolds; triceps, biceps, subscapula, suprailiac
      (2) Midarm circumference
      (3) Midarm muscle circumference
   B. Monitor
      (1) Inpatient: as medically indicated
      (2) Outpatient: as medically indicated

BOX 22-8

Patient Monitoring—cont'd

4. Resting and postprandial energy expenditure (optional)
   Obtain baseline
   Monitor
   (1) Inpatient: as medically indicated
   (2) Outpatient: as medically indicated
5. Outpatient diet monitoring
   A. Anorexia nervosa
      Daily food record to include:
      (1) Food
      (2) Fluid: caloric and noncaloric, alcohol
      (3) Artificial sweeteners
      (4) Eating behavior: time, place, how eaten, with whom
      (5) Exercise

B. Bulimia nervosa
   Daily food record to include:
   (1) Food
   (2) Fluid: caloric and non-caloric, alcohol
   (3) Artificial sweeteners
   (4) Eating behavior: time, place, how eaten, with whom
   (5) Emotions/feelings when eating
   (6) Foods eaten at a binge
   (7) Time and method of purge
   (8) Exercise

From: Luder E, Schebendach J: Nutrition management of eating disorders, *Top Clin Nutr* 8:48, 1993.

AN, Anorexia nervosa; *BN,* bulimia nervosa; *NCHS,* National Center for Health Statistics.

Binge-Eating Disorder

Strategies for treatment of BED include nutrition counseling and dietary management, individual and group psychotherapy, and medication. Some treatment programs focus primarily on nutrition counseling and weight loss. Although successful weight loss and decreased frequency of binge eating episodes may result, relapse occurs often. Other treatment programs focus primarily on reduction of binge episodes rather than weight loss. Self-acceptance, improved body image, increased physical activity, and better overall nutrition are also goals of treatment in BED.

Monitoring Nutritional Rehabilitation

Guidelines for monitoring the nutritional management of patients with AN are indicated in Box 22-8. The health professional, patient, and family must be realistic about treatment, which is often a long-term process. Although outcomes may be favorable, the course of treatment is rarely smooth, and clinicians must be prepared to monitor progress carefully.

NUTRITION EDUCATION

Patients with eating disorders may appear quite knowledgeable about food and nutrition. Despite this, nutrition education is an essential component of their treatment plan. Indeed, some patients spend significant amounts of time reading nutrition-related information, but their sources may be unreliable, and their interpretation potentially distorted by their illness. Malnutrition may impair the patient's ability to assimilate and process new information. Early- and mid-adolescent development is characterized by the transition from concrete to abstract operations in problem solving and directed thinking, and normal developmental issues must be considered when teaching adolescents with eating disorders (see Chapter 8).

Nutrition education materials must be thoroughly assessed to determine if language and subject matter are bias free and appropriate for AN and BN patients. For example, literature provided by many health organizations promotes a low-fat diet and low-calorie lifestyle for the prevention and treatment of chronic disease. This material would be in direct conflict with a treatment plan that encourages increased caloric and fat intake for the purpose of nutritional rehabilitation and weight restoration.

Although the interactive process of a group setting may have advantages, these topics can also be effectively incorporated into individual counseling sessions. Topics for nutrition education are suggested in Box 22-9.

PROGNOSIS

Relapse rates after weight restoration in AN are high, with as many as 50% of patients requiring rehospitalization within 1 year of inpatient treatment (Walsh et al., 2006). Follow-up studies suggest that two thirds of AN patients will have enduring morbid food and weight preoccupation (APA, 2006). In general, adolescents have better outcomes than adults, and younger adolescents have better outcomes than older adolescents.

Mortality rates in AN are among the highest in psychiatric illnesses, and women with AN are reportedly 12 times more likely to die than women of similar ages in the general population (APA, 2006). Outcomes studies in treated BN patients suggest a short-term success rate of 50% to 70%; however, relapse rates in the range of 30% to 85% have also been reported (APA, 2006).

BOX 22-9

Topics for Nutrition Education

1. Impact of malnutrition on growth and development
2. Impact of malnutrition on behavior
3. Set-point theory
4. Metabolic adaptation to dieting
5. Restrained eating and disinhibition
6. Causes of bingeing and purging
7. What does "weight gain" mean?
   - A. Glycogen storage
   - B. Fluid balance
   - C. Lean body mass
   - D. Adipose tissue
8. Impact of exercise on caloric expenditure
9. Ineffectiveness of vomiting, laxatives, and diuretics in long-term weight control
10. Portion control
11. Food exchange system
12. Social dining and holiday dining
13. MyPyramid food guidance system
14. Hunger and satiety cues
15. Interpreting food labels
16. Nutrition misinformation

From Schebendach J, Nussbaum MP: Nutrition management in adolescents with eating disorders, *Adolesc Med State Art Rev* 3(3):545, 1992.

FOCAL POINTS

- Anorexia nervosa and bulimia nervosa must be understood and appreciated as potentially chronic disorders characterized by periods of relapse.
- Refeeding in eating disorders requires the collaborative effort of medical and mental heath professionals, with the support of friends and family.
- Nutritional rehabilitation can correct some (i.e., hypometabolic state, vital sign instability) but not all (organ mass, bone mass, and growth) of the pathophysiologic consequences of malnutrition in eating disorders.
- Successful long-term treatment can take years, and the expectation of a quick cure should be dispelled.

CLINICAL SCENARIO 1

Sara is a 13-year-old girl. Her height is 61 in, and her weight is 72 lb. Sara began menstruating at age 12 but has not menstruated for the past 5 months. Laboratory data: glucose, 62 mg/dl; albumin, 4.6 g/dl; cholesterol, 240 mg/dl; phosphorus, 2.3 mg/dl; T_3-radioimmunoassay (RIA), 78 ng/dl; ESR, 2 mm/hr. Anthropometric status: Skin folds: triceps, 4 mm; biceps, 2 mm; subscapular, 5 mm; suprailiac, 4 mm; midarm circumference, 18 cm; midarm muscle circumference, 16.7 cm.

Sara's maximum weight was 103 lb 8 months ago. She was concerned that her hips and thighs were fat and started to eliminate snacks and desserts from her diet. Sara was pleased with her "willpower." She then decided to eat heart healthy and excluded all sources of dietary fat. About 5 months ago Sara eliminated red meat, poultry, and seafood, claiming that a vegetarian diet was a healthier option. As she lost weight, Sara became increasingly more concerned about her body shape and size. Her diet became more restricted in the amount and variety of intake, providing about 650 kcal per day. Sara's family expressed concern about her eating behaviors. She would ritualistically cut small portions of food into many pieces and spend up to an hour consuming one small meal. After eating Sara expressed considerable guilt about overeating and often cried.

Some days she barely ate at all, consuming only large amounts of water and diet soda. Despite her limited caloric intake, Sara's parents were amazed at her energy level. She continued to play soccer (1 to 2 hours daily, 5 days a week), did regular calisthenics (leg lifts and sit-ups, 30 minutes daily), and went running each morning (5 to 7 miles).

> **✳Nutrition Diagnosis:** Disordered eating pattern related to restricting foods as evidenced by rituals surrounding meals and foods and low weight for height
>
> 1. What are some possible medical complications that Sara may develop secondary to self-starvation?
> 2. Discuss laboratory values and what you might expect to happen to these indices during refeeding.
> 3. Determine Sara's desirable body weight, goal weight for treatment, and recommended rate of weight gain.
> 4. Calculate Sara's initial caloric prescription and discuss how you arrived at this. How might this change over time and why?
> 5. Plan a sample menu.

✳ CLINICAL SCENARIO 2

Jennifer is a 19-year-old woman. Her height is 65 in. and her weight is 138 lb. Laboratory data: glucose, 82 mg/dl; albumin, 4.2 g/dl; cholesterol, 180 mg/dl; potassium, 2.7 mmol/L; serum CO_2, 31 mmol/L. Anthropometric status: Skin folds: triceps, 20 mm; biceps, 7 mm; subscapular, 10 mm; suprailiac, 13 mm; midarm circumference, 26.7 cm; midarm muscle circumference, 20.4 cm.

Jennifer has always been unhappy with her weight. She went on every fad diet throughout high school and lost some weight but always regained it. About 1 year ago, Jennifer began binge eating. Binge episodes now occur three to four times per week. During these binges Jennifer consumes about 1500 to 2000 kcal in a 2-hour period. Binge foods include ice cream, cookies, potato chips, and other foods. Jennifer describes them as "fattening and unhealthy." After binge eating Jennifer feels extremely guilty, and vomiting is immediately self-induced. Jennifer always tries to eat as little as possible the next day, sometimes consuming only 700 or 800 kcal. Three months ago Jennifer started to overdose on laxatives about three times a week. She occasionally uses over-the-counter diet pills, but they never really help. Jennifer feels fat in her abdomen, buttocks, and thighs. Her physical activity includes 100 sit-ups and 100 leg lifts three or four times per week.

✳**Nutrition Diagnosis:** Disordered eating pattern related to binging and purging as evidenced by self-induced vomiting following binge episodes accompanied by guilt and restricted eating

1. What are some possible medical complications that Jennifer may develop secondary to binge eating and her compensatory behaviors?
2. Discuss her laboratory values and what you might expect to happen to these indices during rehabilitation.
3. Determine Jennifer's ideal body weight and goal weight for short-term and long-term treatment.
4. Calculate Jennifer's initial caloric prescription and discuss how you arrived at this.
5. Plan a sample menu.
6. Discuss how you would handle foods that Jennifer considers binge "trigger" foods.
7. What would you suggest for Jennifer to help control her episodes of vomiting, laxative use, and diet pill use?

USEFUL WEBSITES

Academy for Eating Disorders: For Professionals Working in the Area of Eating Disorders
www.aedweb.org

National Association of Anorexia Nervosa and Associated Disorders (ANAD)
http://www.anad.org

National Eating Disorders Association
http://www.nationaleatingdisorders.org

References

Affenito SG et al: Macronutrient intake in anorexia nervosa: the National Heart, Lung, and Blood Institute Growth and Health Study, *J Pediatr* 141:701, 2002.

Allison KC et al: Night eating syndrome and binge eating disorder among persons seeking bariatric surgery: prevalence and related features, *Surg Obes Relat Dis* 2(2):153, 2006.

American Academy of Pediatrics: Policy statement: identifying and treating eating disorders, *Pediatrics* 111:204, 2003.

American Dietetic Association: Nutrition intervention in the treatment of anorexia nervosa, bulimia nervosa, and other eating disorders, *J Am Diet Assoc* 106:2073, 2006.

American Psychiatric Association: *Diagnostic and statistical manual for mental disorders*, cd 4, text revision, Washington, DC, 2000, APA Press.

American Psychiatric Association: *Practice guidelines for the treatment of patients with eating disorders*, ed 3, *Am J Psychiatry* 2006, Website for members: www.Psych.org/edu/cme/pgeatingdisorders3rdedition.cfm, accessed October 1, 2006.

Ayton AK: Dietary polyunsaturated fatty acids and anorexia nervosa: is there a link? *Nutr Neurosci* 7:1, 2004.

Becker AE: New global perspectives on eating disorders, *Cult Med Psychiatry* 28:433, 2004.

Bryant-Waugh R: Overview of the eating disorders. In Lask B, Bryant-Waugh R, editors: *Anorexia nervosa and related eating disorders in childhood and adolescence*, ed 2, East Sussex, UK, 2000, Psychology Press.

Bulik CM et al: Prevalence, heritability, and prospective risk factors for anorexia nervosa, *Arch Gen Psychiatry* 63(3):305, 2006.

Castro J et al: Persistence of nutritional deficiencies after short-term weight recovery in adolescents with anorexia nervosa, *Int J Eat Disord* 35:169, 2004.

de Zwann M et al: Research on energy expenditure in individuals with eating disorders: a review, *Int J Eating Disord* 31:361, 2002.

Durnin JVGA, Rahaman MM: The assessment of the amount of body fat in the human body from measurements of skinfold thickness, *Br J Nutr* 21:681, 1967.

Durnin JVGA, Womersley J: Body fat assessed from total body density and its estimation from skinfolds thickness: measurements of 481 men and women aged from 16 to 72 years, *Br J Nutr* 32:77, 1974.

Fairburn CG, Harrison PJ: Eating disorders, *Lancet* 361:407, 2003.

Feighner JP et al: Diagnostic criteria for use in psychiatric research, *Arch Gen Psychiatry* 26:57, 1972.

Golden NH et al: Alendronate for the treatment of osteopenia in anorexia nervosa: a randomized, double-blind, placebo-controlled trial, *J Clin Endocrinol Metabol* 90:3179, 2005.

Grinspoon S et al: Changes in regional fat distribution and the effects of estrogen during spontaneous weight gain in women with anorexia nervosa, *Am J Clin Nutr* 73:865, 2001.

Hadigan CM et al: Assessment of macronutrient and micronutrient intake in women with anorexia nervosa, *Int J Eating Disord* 28(3):284, 2000.

Herrin M: *Nutrition counseling in the treatment of eating disorders*, New York, 2003, Brunner-Routledge.

Hoek HW: Incidence, prevalence and mortality of anorexia nervosa and other eating disorders, *Curr Opin Psychiatry* 19(4):389, 2006.

Kaye WH et al: Amounts of calories retained after binge eating and vomiting, *Am J Psychiatry* 150:969, 1993.

Keys A et al: *The biology of human starvation*, vols 1 and 2, Minneapolis, 1950, University of Minnesota Press.

Kotler LA et al: Longitudinal relationships between childhood, adolescent, and adult eating disorders, *J Am Acad Child Adolesc Psychiatry* 40:1434, 2001.

Mayer L et al: Body fat redistribution after weight gain in women with anorexia nervosa. *Am J Clin Nutr* 81:1286, 2005.

McCallum K et al: How should the clinician evaluate and manage the cardiovascular complications of anorexia nervosa? *Eating Disord* 14(1):73, 2006.

Miller KK et al: Medical findings in outpatients with anorexia nervosa, *Arch Intern Med* 165:561, 2005.

Miller MN, Pumariega AJ: Culture and eating disorders: a historical and cultural review, *Psychiatry* 64(2):93, 2001.

Miller WR, Rollnick S: *Motivational interviewing: preparing people for change*, ed 2, New York, 2002, Guilford Press.

Misra S et al: Regional body composition in adolescents with anorexia nervosa and changes with weight recovery, *Am J Clin Nutr* 77:1361, 2003.

Mitchell JE et al: Diagnostic criteria for anorexia nervosa: looking ahead to DSM-V, *Int J Eating Disord* 37:S95, 2005.

Ornstein RM et al: Hypophosphatemia during nutritional rehabilitation in anorexia nervosa: implications for refeeding and monitoring, *J Adoles Health* 32:83, 2003.

Probst M et al: Body composition of anorexia nervosa patients assessed by underwater weighing and skin-fold thickness measurements before and after weight gain, *Am J Clin Nutr* 73:190, 2001.

Prousky JE: Pellagra may be a rare secondary complication of anorexia nervosa: a systematic review of the literature, *Alternative Med Rev* 8:180, 2003.

Romano C et al: Reduced hemodynamic load and cardiac hypotrophy in patients with anorexia nervosa, *Am J Clin Nutr* 77:388, 2003.

Schebendach J: The use of indirect calorimetry in the clinical management of adolescents with nutritional disorders, *Adoles Med* 14:77, 2003.

Society for Adolescent Medicine: Position paper: eating disorders in adolescents, *J Adolesc Health* 33:96, 2003.

Steinhausen HC The outcome of anorexia nervosa in the 20th century, *Am J Psychiatry* 159:1284, 2002.

Stellefson-Meyer E: *Winning the war within: nutrition therapy for clients with anorexia or bulimia nervosa*, Dallas, Tex, 1999, Helm Publishing.

Sunday SR, Halmi KA: Energy intake and body composition in anorexia and bulimia nervosa, *Phys Behav* 78:11, 2003.

Swenne I: The significance of routine laboratory analyses in the assessment of teenage girls with eating disorders and weight loss, *Eating Weight Disord* 9:269, 2004.

Sysko R et al: Eating behavior among women with anorexia nervosa, *Am J Clin Nutr* 82:296, 2005.

Van Wymelbeke V et al: Factors associated with the increase in resting energy expenditure during refeeding in malnourished anorexia nervosa patients, *Am J Clin Nutr* 80:1469, 2004.

Walsh BT et al: Fluoxetine after weight restoration in anorexia nervosa: a randomized controlled trial, *JAMA* 295(22):2605-2612, 2006.

Yager J, Andersen AE: Anorexia nervosa, *N Engl J Med* 353:1481, 2005.

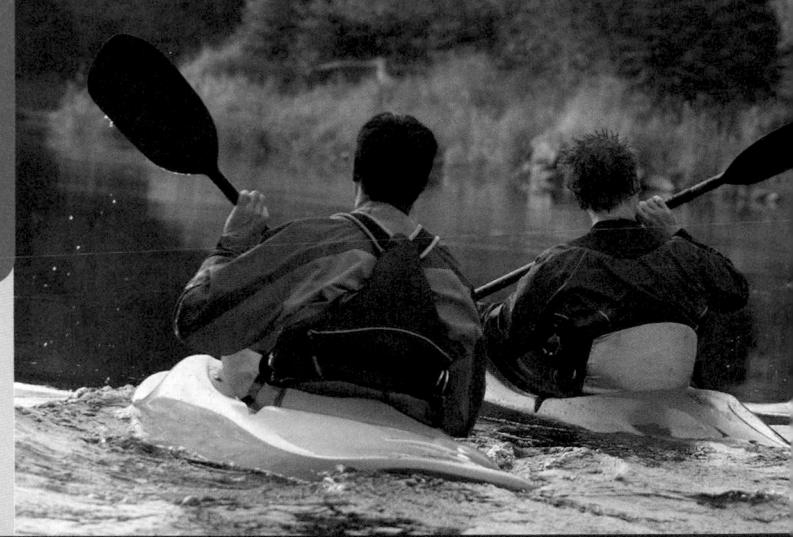

CHAPTER 23

Lisa Dorfman, MS, RD, CSSD, LMHC

Nutrition for Exercise and Sports Performance

KEY TERMS

actomyosin a complex of the proteins actin and myosin occurring in muscle

adenosine diphosphate (ADP) a nucleotide involved in energy metabolism; it is produced by the hydrolysis of ATP and converted back to ATP by the processes of oxidative phosphorylation

adenosine triphosphate (ATP) a nucleotide occurring in all cells; involved in energy transfer; energy currency of the cell

aerobic metabolism the transfer of usable energy through oxidative phosphorylation in the respiratory chain in the presence of oxygen

anabolic effects drug-induced growth or thickening of the body's nonreproductive tract tissues, including skeletal muscle, bones, the larynx, and vocal cords, and decrease in body fat

anaerobic metabolism the production of energy from glucose without the presence of oxygen

androgenic effects a drug-induced growth of the male reproductive tract and the development of secondary sexual characteristics

creatine phosphate (CP) an important temporary storage form of high-energy phosphate in muscle cells

ergogenic aid a substance or practice that increases energy or work output

female athlete triad a pattern in strenuously exercising athletes of estrogen deficiency and athletic amenorrhea, disordered eating; low body fat, and loss of bone mass

glycemic index the ratio of the area under the blood glucose curve resulting from ingestion of a given quantity of a carbohydrate and the area under the curve after the ingestion of the same quantity of carbohydrates as glucose or white bread

glycogen the form of carbohydrate storage in animals

glycogen loading (glycogen supercompensation) a combination of exercise and a high-carbohydrate diet that enables muscles to store glycogen beyond their normal capacity

glycogenolysis the hydrolysis of glycogen to yield glucose

glycolysis the breaking down of glucose with or without the presence of oxygen into simpler compounds, chiefly pyruvate or lactate

hypohydration when water loss is greater than water intake and there is a body water deficit

lactic acid a product of anaerobic glucose metabolism

mitochondria spherical components in the cytoplasm of cells that are the principal sites of the generation of energy in the form of ATP; they contain the enzymes of the Krebs and fatty acid cycles and the respiratory pathway

myoglobin a ferrous protoporphyrin protein similar to hemoglobin, but with only one iron atom per molecule instead of four; contributes to the color of muscle and acts as a store of oxygen

respiratory exchange ratio (RER) the amount of CO_2 produced by the body divided by the amount of O_2 consumed by the body in metabolizing the dietary intake

sports anemia a transient anemia seen in heavily training athletes characterized by a decrease in the red blood cell count, hemoglobin concentration, and packed cell volume, but with normal red blood cell morphology

thermoregulation the body's system for maintaining appropriate temperatures by transferring heat from the body core to the skin, where it is dissipated through convection, radiation, sweat production, and evaporation

Vo2max a measure of maximum oxygen uptake; liters of oxygen consumed per kilogram of body weight per minute

Sections of this chapter were written by Jacqueline R. Berning, PhD, RD, for the previous edition of this text.

Successful athletic performance is a combination of favorable genetics, desire, proper training, and a sensible approach to nutrition. Whether an athlete is recreational or elite, young or mature, the importance of nutrition as a contributing factor to success in training and competition has been recognized for decades.

Athletes attempting to gain a competitive edge will try almost any dietary regimen or artificial means, including nutritional supplements and oral or injectable medications, in the hope of reaching a new level of wellness or physical performance. Research suggests that athletes can benefit from nutrition education and intervention from nutrition experts—increasing knowledge, self-efficacy, and improvement in overall dietary change (Abood et al., 2006). Unfortunately there is much misinformation regarding a proper diet for physically active persons. Health professionals and the Internet are the most reported information sources for athletes. Family members, friends, physicians, or pharmacists guide supplement decision making for females; athletes, store nutritionists, fellow athletes, friends, or coaches, impact the choices of male athletes (Froiland et al., 2004; Kristiansen et al., 2005).

ENERGY PRODUCTION

The human body must be supplied continuously with energy to perform its many complex functions. As a person's energy demands increase with exercise, the body must provide additional energy, or the exercise will cease. Two metabolic systems supply energy for the body: one dependent on oxygen (**aerobic metabolism**), and the other independent of oxygen (**anaerobic metabolism**). Both systems provide energy; however, the use of one system over the other depends on the duration, intensity, and type of physical activity.

Adenosine Triphosphate

The body obtains its continuous supply of fuel through an energy-rich compound called **adenosine triphosphate (ATP)**, which is the fuel used for all the energy-requiring processes found within the cells of the body. ATP has been called the energy currency of the cell.

The energy produced from the breakdown of ATP provides the fuel that activates the processes of muscle contraction. The energy from ATP is transferred to the contractile filaments (myosin and actin) in the muscle, which form an attachment of actin to the cross-bridges on the myosin molecule, thus forming **actomyosin.** Once activated, the myofibrils slide past each other and cause the muscle to contract.

Resynthesizing Adenosine Triphosphate

Although ATP is the main currency for energy in the body, it is stored in limited amounts. In fact, only about 3 oz of ATP is stored in the body at any one time. This provides only enough energy for several seconds of exercise. ATP must continually be resynthesized to provide a constant energy source during exercise. When ATP loses a phosphate, thus releasing energy, the resulting **adenosine diphosphate (ADP)** is enzymatically combined with another high-energy phosphate from **creatine phosphate (CP)** to resynthesize ATP. The concentration of high-energy CP in the muscle is five times that of ATP.

Creatine kinase is the enzyme that catalyzes the reaction of CP with ADP and inorganic phosphate to produce creatine and regenerate ATP. It is the fastest and most immediate means of replenishing ATP, and it does so without the use of oxygen (anaerobic). Although this system has great power, it is time limited because of the concentration of CP found in the muscles (see "Creatine" later in the chapter).

The energy released from this ATP-CP system will only support an all-out exercise effort of a few seconds, such as in a power lift, tennis serve, or sprint. If the all-out effort continues for longer than 8 seconds or if moderate exercise is to proceed for longer periods, an additional source of energy must be provided for the resynthesis of ATP (Figure 23-1). The production of ATP carries on within the muscle cells through two important pathways: anaerobic or aerobic metabolism.

Anaerobic or Lactic Acid Pathway

The next energy pathway for supplying ATP for more than 8 seconds of physical activity is the process of anaerobic **glycolysis.** In this pathway the energy in glucose is released without the presence of oxygen. **Lactic acid** is the end product of anaerobic glycolysis. Without the production of lactic acid, glycolysis would shut down. A coenzyme called nicotinic acid dehydrogenase (NAD) is in limited supply in this pathway. When NAD is limited, the glycolytic pathway cannot provide constant energy. By converting pyruvic acid to lactic acid, NAD is freed to participate in further ATP synthesis. The amount of ATP furnished is relatively small (the process is only 30% efficient). This pathway contributes energy during an all-out effort lasting up to 60 to 120 seconds. Examples would be a 440-yard sprint and many sprint swimming events.

Although this process provides immediate protection from the consequences of insufficient oxygen, it cannot continue indefinitely. When exercise continues at intensities beyond the body's ability to supply oxygen and convert lactic acid to fuel, lactic acid accumulates in the blood, eventually lowering the pH to a level that interferes with enzymatic action, leading to fatigue. Research shows that lactic acid can be removed from the muscle; transported into the bloodstream; and eventually converted to energy in muscle, liver, or brain; or it is converted to glycogen. This conversion to **glycogen** occurs in the liver and to some extent in muscle, particularly among trained athletes.

The amount of ATP produced through glycolysis is small compared with that available through aerobic pathways. Substrate for this reaction is limited to glucose from blood sugar or the glycogen stored in the muscle. Liver glycogen contributes but is limited in amount.

Aerobic Pathway

Production of ATP in amounts sufficient to support continued muscle activity for longer than 90 to 120 seconds requires the input of oxygen. If sufficient oxygen is not pres-

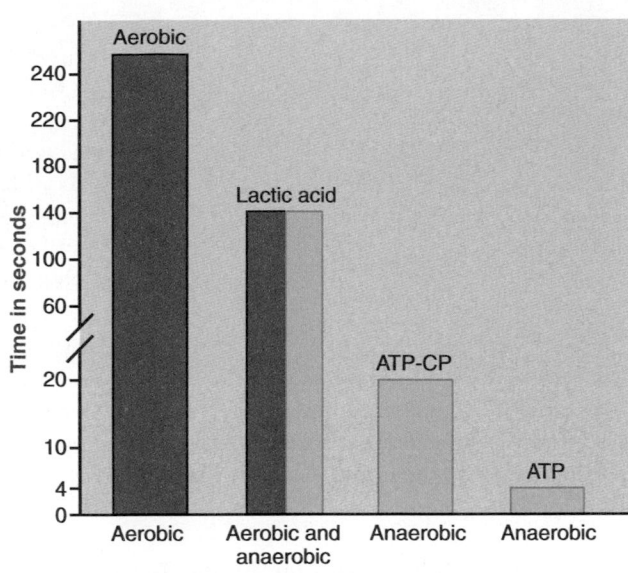

FIGURE 23-1 Classification of activities based on duration of performance and the predominant pathways of energy production. One can see that the duration of activity can continue much longer when energy is produced by aerobic metabolism.

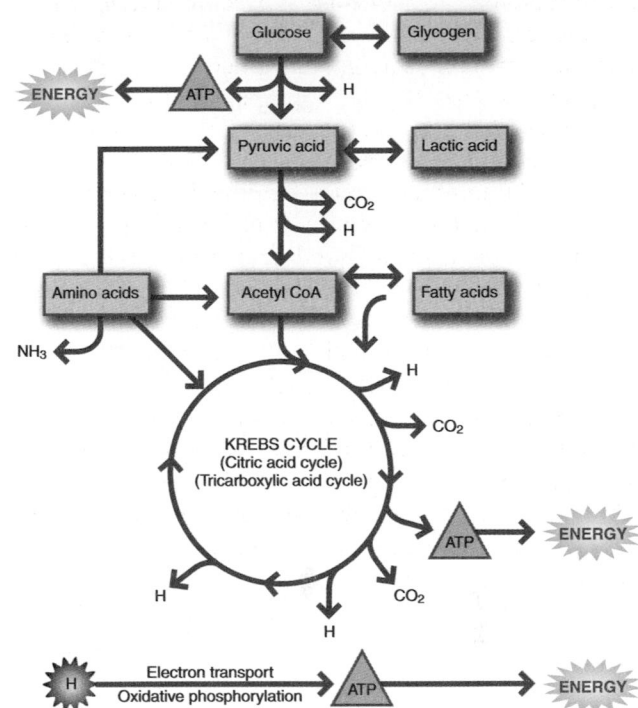

FIGURE 23-2 Pathways of energy production. *ATP*, Adenosine triphosphate; *CoA*, coenzyme A; *H*, hydrogen atoms.

ent to combine with hydrogen in the electron transport chain, no further ATP is forthcoming. Therefore the oxygen furnished through the process of respiration is of vital importance.

In the aerobic pathway glucose can be broken down far more efficiently for energy, producing 18 to 19 times more ATP. In the presence of oxygen, pyruvate is converted to acetyl coenzyme A (CoA), which enters the **mitochondria.** In the mitochondria acetyl CoA goes through the Krebs cycle, which generates 36 to 38 ATP per molecule of glucose (Figure 23-2).

The aerobic pathway can also provide ATP by metabolizing fats and proteins. β-Oxidation of fatty acids derived from lipolysis provides a large amount of acetyl CoA, which enters the Krebs cycle and provides enormous amounts of ATP. Proteins may be catabolized into acetyl CoA or Krebs cycle intermediates, or they may be directly oxidized as another source of ATP.

Aerobic metabolism is limited by the availability of substrate, a continuous and adequate supply of oxygen, and the availability of coenzymes. At the onset of exercise and with the increase in exercise intensity, the capability of the cardiovascular system to supply adequate oxygen is a limiting factor, and this is largely due to the level of conditioning.

Energy Continuum

Although each of the preceding systems produces ATP for the exercising muscle, a person who is exercising may use one or more energy pathways for the physical activity. For example, at the beginning of any physical activity, ATP is produced anaerobically. As exercise continues, the lactic acid system is producing ATP for exercise. If the person continues to exercise and does so at a moderate intensity for a prolonged period, the aerobic pathway will become the dominant pathway for fuel. On the other hand, the anaerobic pathway provides most of the energy for short-duration, high-intensity exercise such as sprinting; the 200-m swim; or high-power, high-intensity moves in basketball, football, or soccer.

The production of ATP for exercise is on a continuum that depends on the availability of oxygen. Other factors that influence oxygen capabilities, and thus energy pathways, are the capacity for intense exercise and its duration. These two factors are inversely related. For example, an athlete cannot perform high-power, high-intensity moves over a prolonged period. To do this, he or she would have to decrease the intensity of the exercise in order to increase the duration (Figure 23-3).

The aerobic pathway cannot tolerate the same level of intensity as the duration increases because of the decreased availability of oxygen and accumulation of lactic acid. As the duration of exercise increases, power output decreases. The contribution of energy-yielding nutrients must be considered also. As the duration of exercise lengthens, the contribution of fats as an energy source becomes greater. The opposite is true for high-intensity exercise. As intensity increases, the body relies increasingly on carbohydrates as its fuel source.

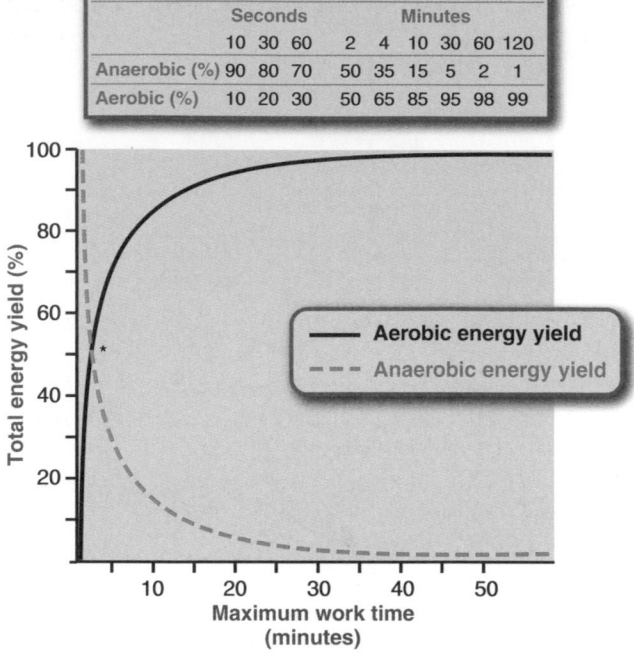

Duration of maximum exercise								
	Seconds			Minutes				
	10	30	60	2	4	10	30	60	120
Anaerobic (%)	90	80	70	50	35	15	5	2	1
Aerobic (%)	10	20	30	50	65	85	95	98	99

FIGURE 23-3 Relative contribution of aerobic and anaerobic energy during maximum physical activity of various durations. Note that 90 to 120 seconds of maximum effort requires 50% of the energy from each of the aerobic and anaerobic processes. This will also be the point when the lactic acid pathway for energy production will be at its maximum.

FUELS FOR CONTRACTING MUSCLES

Sources of Fuel

Protein, fat, and carbohydrate are all possible sources of fuel for muscle contraction. The glycolytic pathway is restricted to glucose, which can originate in dietary carbohydrates or stored glycogen, or it can be synthesized from the carbon skeletons of certain amino acids through the process of gluconeogenesis. The Krebs cycle is fueled by three-carbon fragments of glucose; two-carbon fragments of fatty acids; and carbon skeletons of specific amino acids, primarily alanine and the branched-chain amino acids. All these substrates can be used during exercise; however, the intensity and duration of the exercise determine the relative rates of substrate use (see Figure 23-2). Other factors determining which type of fuel the muscle will use during exercise are the fitness level of the individual, the gender of the individual, and the dietary intake (McArdle et al., 2004).

Intensity

The intensity of the exercise is particularly important in determining what fuel will be used by contracting muscles. High-intensity, short-duration exercise has to rely on anaerobic production of ATP. Because oxygen is not available for anaerobic pathways, only glucose and glycogen can be broken down anaerobically for fuel. When glycogen is broken down anaerobically, it is used 18 to 19 times faster than

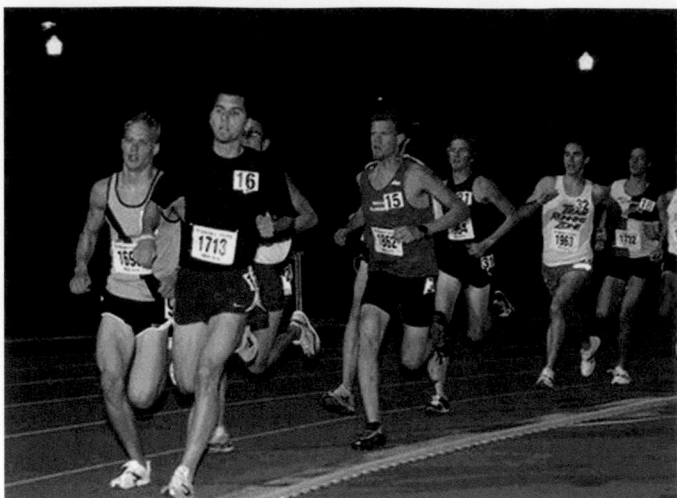

FIGURE 23-4 Running is a high-intensity exercise where both carbohydrates and fat are used as fuels, depending on the speed and length of the event. (*Courtesy Richard Andrews, Titusville, Fl.*)

when glucose is broken down aerobically. Persons who are performing in high-intensity workouts or competitive races may run the risk of running out of muscle glycogen before the event or exercise is done as a result of its high use.

Sports that use both the anaerobic and aerobic pathways also have a higher glycogen use rate and, like anaerobic athletes, athletes in these sports also run the risk of running out of fuel before the race or exercise is finished. Sports such as basketball, football, soccer, and swimming are good examples of activities in which athletes have a higher glycogen usage rate because of their intermittent bursts of high-intensity sprints and running drills. In moderate-intensity sports or exercise such as jogging, hiking, aerobic dance, gymnastics, cycling, and recreational swimming, about half of the energy for these activities comes from the aerobic breakdown of muscle glycogen, whereas the other half comes from circulating blood glucose and fatty acids.

Moderate- to low-intensity exercise such as walking is fueled entirely by the aerobic pathway; thus, a greater proportion of fat can be used to create ATP for energy. Fatty acids cannot supply ATP during high-intensity exercise because fat cannot be broken down fast enough to provide the energy. Also, fat provides less energy per liter of oxygen consumed than does glucose (4.65 kcal/L of O_2 versus 5.01 kcal/L of O_2). Therefore, when less oxygen is available in high-intensity activities, there is a definite advantage for the muscles to be able to use glycogen because less oxygen is required to produce energy from glycogen (Figure 23-4).

In general, both glucose and fatty acids provide fuel for exercise in proportions depending on the intensity and duration of the exercise and the fitness of the athlete. Exertion of extremely high intensity and short duration draws primarily on reserves of ATP and CP. High-intensity exercise that continues for more than a few seconds depends on anaerobic glycolysis. During exercise of low-to-moderate intensity (60% of maximum oxygen uptake, **Vo₂max**), energy is derived mainly from fatty acids. Carbohydrate becomes a

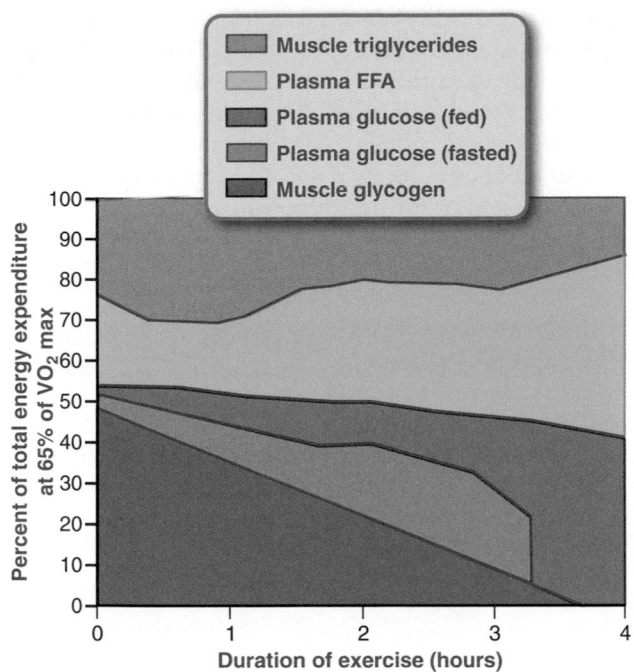

FIGURE 23-5 Sources of energy during 4 hours of exercise. *FFA*, Free fatty acid.

larger fraction of the energy source as intensity increases until, at an intensity level of 85% to 90% Vo₂max, carbohydrates from glycogen is the principal energy source, and the duration of activity is limited (Figure 23-5).

Duration

The duration of a training session determines the substrate used during the exercise bout. For example, the longer the time spent exercising, the greater the contribution of fat as the fuel. Fat can supply up to 60% to 70% of the energy needed for ultraendurance events lasting 6 to 10 hours. As the duration of exercise increases, the reliance on aerobic metabolism becomes greater, and a greater amount of ATP can be produced from fatty acids. However, fat cannot be metabolized unless a continuous stream of some carbohydrates is also available through the energy pathways. Therefore muscle glycogen and blood glucose are the limiting factors in human performance of any type of intensity or duration.

Effect of Training

The length of time an athlete can oxidize fatty acids as a fuel source is related to the athlete's conditioning, as well as the exercise intensity. In addition to improving cardiovascular systems involved in oxygen delivery, training increases the number of mitochondria and the levels of enzymes involved in the aerobic synthesis of ATP, thus increasing the capacity for fatty acid metabolism. Increases in mitochondria with aerobic training are seen mainly in the type IIA (intermediate fast-twitch) muscle fibers. These fibers quickly lose their aerobic capacity with the cessation of aerobic training, reverting to the genetic baseline.

These changes from training result in a lower **respiratory exchange ratio (RER),** the amount of CO_2 produced divided by the amount of O_2 consumed, lower blood lactate and catecholamine levels, and a lower net muscle glycogen breakdown at a specific power output. These metabolic adaptations enhance the ability of muscle to oxidize all fuels, especially fat.

NUTRITIONAL REQUIREMENTS OF EXERCISE

Energy

The most important component of successful sport training and performance is to ensure adequate calorie intake to support energy expenditure and maintain strength, endurance, muscle mass and overall health. Energy and nutrient requirements vary with weight, height, age, sex, and metabolic rate and with the type, frequency, intensity, and duration of training and performance.

Individuals who participate in an overall fitness program (i.e., 30 to 40 min/day, three times per week) can generally meet their daily nutritional needs by following a normal diet providing 25 to 35 kcal/kg/day or roughly 1800 to 2400 calories a day. However, the 50-kg athlete engaging in more intense training of 2 to 3 hours/day five to six times a week or high-volume training of 3 to 6 hours in one to two workouts per day 5 to 6 days a week may expend up to an additional 600 to 1200 calories a day, thus requiring 50 to 80 kcal/kg/day or roughly 2500 to 4000 kcal/day. For elite athletes or heavier athletes, daily calorie needs can reach 150 to 200 kcal/kg, or roughly 7,500 to 10,000 calories a day, depending on the volume and intensity of different training phases.

Meeting caloric needs for many fitness-minded and or elite, intensely training individuals can present challenges. For working individuals, balancing daily training schedules with work and family responsibilities can compromise the quantity, quality, and timing of meals, which can greatly impact energy and strength levels and overall health. In the elite athlete, consuming enough food at regular intervals without compromising performance is challenging and particularly so for the collegiate athlete, for whom school schedules, budgets, cafeteria schedules, travel requirements, and a varying appetite can further complicate the situation.

Meeting the daily energy needs and the appropriate macronutrient distribution for active individuals may necessitate the use of sports bars, drinks, and convenience foods and snacks in addition to whole foods and meals. Dietitians need to be flexible in accommodating lifestyles and eating behaviors when designing meal plans for the athlete who wants to maximize sport performance.

Convenience Supplements

This category includes all easy-to-carry, easy-to-consume, and easy-to-digest meal-replacement powders (MRPs), ready-to-drink supplements (RTDSs), energy bars, and energy gels. This group of supplements represents the largest segment—approximately 50% to 70% of the industry's sales (Kreider et al., 2003). These products are typically fortified with 33% to 100% of the recommended daily allowances (RDAs) for vitamins and minerals; provide varying amounts and types of carbohydrates, protein, and fat; and are ideal for athletes on the run literally, providing a portable, easy-to-consume food that can be used pericompetitively, while traveling, at work, in the car, or throughout the day at a multievent meet such as in track and field, swimming, diving, or gymnastics.

Many fitness-minded and athletic individuals use these products as a convenient way to enhance their current diet, (i.e., as a snack to help them to gain or lose weight). These products are generally regarded as safe; however, when they are substituted in the place of whole foods on a regular basis, they can deny the athlete of a well-balanced diet. They may also contain excesses of sugars, fats, and protein and banned substances such as caffeine, ephedra, and other botanicals; thus caution should be used for the professional or collegiate athlete and or for health reasons. Table 23-1 provides a list of some of the popular and convenient sports bars, gels, and drinks available.

TABLE 23-1

Recommendations for Use of Sport Foods

Sport Food	Characteristics	Guidelines For Consumption In Exercise		
		Before	**During**	**After**
Sports drink	CHO: 5%-7% by volume (about 14 g/8 oz) Sodium: 20-30 mEq/L (110-165 mg/8 oz) Multiple carbohydrates with high glycemic indices	0.5 L (16 oz) 1 hr before exercise	150-300 ml every 15-20 min (20-40 oz/hr)	24 oz/lb of body weight lost
High CHO energy drink	CHO: >13% by volume (more than 50 g/8 oz) Optional B vitamins: thiamin, niacin, and riboflavin at 10%-40% of RDA	0.5 L (16 oz) 2-5 hr before exercise	Typically not advised for use during the event	Immediately after and at 1-hr intervals to deliver 1 g CHO/kg of body weight
Sports bar	CHO: >70% of total kcal High glycemic index Fat: low (1-2 g/bar) or absent Vitamins and minerals not critical component	One bar 2 hr before exercise	Usually not advised except for those desiring solid foods during long-duration events	One to two bars immediately after exercise and with daily meals as desired
Sports shake	CHO: >65% of total kcal (>18 g/100 ml) High glycemic index Fat: not to exceed 25% of total kcal Protein: 15%-20% of total kcal Vitamins and minerals: optional at low levels (10%-40% of RDA)	0.5 L (16 oz) 2-5 hr before exercise	Not recommended	Immediately after to deliver 1 g CHO/kg body weight and as a supplement to daily meals
Energy gel	CHO: >50% by volume (>50 g/100 ml or 15 g/oz) Vitamins and minerals: trace or absent Avoid those with herbs	1 packet before exercise; consume adequate fluid to promote absorption	If overall fluid intake is adequate, enough to supply 30-60 g CHO/hr	Immediately after exercise and at 1-hr intervals to deliver 1 g CHO/kg body weight
Shot bloks	Organic electrolyte chew Gelatin consistency CHO: 24 g/1 oz 3 bloks =100 cal electrolytes	NA	3-6 bloks every hour with water	NA
Sports beans	14 beans =100 cal CHO: 25 g/1 oz 10% DV of vitamins B_1, B_2, B_3 20% DV of vitamins C and E	NA	Up to 14 pieces per hour for energy	NA

Modified from Gatorade Sports Science Exchange Roundtable: *Sport foods for athletes: what works?* vol 9, no 2, Chicago, 1998, Gatorade Sports Science Institute.

CHO, Carbohydrate; *DV,* daily value; *NA,* not applicable.

WEIGHT MANAGEMENT

In efforts to maximize performance, many athletes alter normal energy intake to either gain or lose weight. Although such efforts are sometimes appropriate, weight-reduction programs may involve elements of risk. For some young athletes achievement of an unrealistic light weight may jeopardize growth and development. Chronic dieting of female athletes, many of whom are dancers and gymnasts, can lead to eating disorders, delayed menarche, amenorrhea, and potential osteoporosis (see Chapters 22 and 24).

The goal weight of an athlete should be based on body fatness (see Chapters 14 and 21). Adequate time should be allowed for a slow, steady weight loss of about 1 to 2 lb each week over several weeks. Weight loss should be achieved before the competitive season begins to ensure maximum strength. In addition, the exercise should be of moderate intensity because at this level a greater proportion of energy is derived from fat than carbohydrate and the exercise can be sustained longer.

Weight gain should be achieved through a gradual increase in energy intake combined with a strength training program to maximize muscle weight gain over fat gain. A realistic goal is ½ to 1 lb weekly. Fat intake should not exceed 30% of kilocalories from fat, and protein should be 1 to 1.5 g/kg of body weight.

Appropriate programs for weight management are discussed in Chapter 21. Because pressure to have the perfect body for a sport, which for many sports (e.g., gymnastics, track, swimming, diving, rowing, beach volleyball, dancing, and figure skating) means leanness for both performance and appearance, unrealistic dieting and eating disorders are common. The pursuit of thinness leading to calorie restriction is especially evident in women involved in college athletics, where the pressure to perform, contribute to the team, and maintain scholarship eligibility is great. The professional working with an elite athlete with an eating disorder must remember the tremendous motivation from the desire to perform well in the sport (see Chapter 22).

MACRONUTRIENTS

Individuals engaging in a general fitness program can typically meet their macronutrient needs by consuming a normal diet of 45% to 55% of calories from carbohydrates (3 to 5 g/kg/day), 10% to 15% from protein (0.8 to 1 g/kg/day) and 25% to 35% from fat (0.5 to 1.5 g/kg/day). However, depending on the training regimen, athletes involved in moderate-to-high volume training need greater amounts of carbohydrates and protein to meet macronutrient needs. A minimum intake of at least 50%, but ideally 60% to 70%, of their total calories (5 to 8 g/kg/day or 250 to 1200 g/day for 50- to 150-kg athletes) should be met by carbohydrates. The remaining calories should be obtained from protein (10% to 15%) and fat (20% to 30%) (Kreider et al., 2003).

These percentages are only guidelines for estimating macronutrient requirements; however, specific recommendations with respect to carbohydrates, proteins, and fat should be used when counseling an active individual or athlete. When energy intake is high (more than 4500 calories/day), even a diet containing only 50% of the calories from carbohydrates would provide 500 g of carbohydrates, which is sufficient to maintain muscle glycogen stores. Similarly, if protein intake in this high-calorie diet were low, at 10% of calories, absolute protein intake would still exceed the recommendation for a 70-kg athlete. Thus specific recommendations based on an individual's body size, body composition, sport, and gender may be more useful than using a guideline based on a proportion. Calories and nutrients should come from a wide variety of foods on a daily basis.

CARBOHYDRATES

The first source of glucose for the exercising muscle is its own glycogen store. When this is depleted, **glycogenolysis** and then gluconeogenesis (both in the liver) maintain the glucose supply. During endurance exercise that exceeds 90 minutes such as marathon running, muscle glycogen stores become progressively lower. When they drop to critically low levels, high-intensity exercise cannot be maintained. In practical terms the athlete is exhausted and must either stop exercising or drastically reduce the pace. Athletes often refer to this as "hitting the wall."

Glycogen depletion may also be a gradual process, occurring over repeated days of heavy training, in which muscle glycogen breakdown exceeds its replacement, as well as during high-intensity exercise that is repeated several times during competition or training. For example, a distance runner who averages 10 miles per day but does not take the time to consume enough carbohydrates in his or her diet, or the swimmer who completes several interval sets at above his or her maximum oxygen consumption, can both deplete glycogen stores rapidly. A high-carbohydrate or **glycogen loading (glycogen supercompensation)** diet can help athletes maximize glycogen stores and be able to continue endurance performance.

The amount of carbohydrates required depends on the athlete's total daily energy expenditure, type of sport, gender, and environmental conditions. It is preferable to provide recommendations for daily carbohydrate intake in grams relative to body mass and allow flexibility for the athlete to meet these targets within the context of their energy needs and other dietary goals. Carbohydrate intake ranges of 5 to 7 g/kg/day for general training needs and 7 to 10 g/kg/day for the increased needs of endurance athletes are suggested (Kreider et al., 2003). For example, a 70-kg (154-lb) athlete would consume 350 to 700 g of carbohydrates daily. Table 23-1 lists several products that could be consumed during or after exercise for the maintenance of blood glucose or for glycogen resynthesis.

Types of Carbohydrates

Even though the impact of different sugars on performance, substrate use, and recovery has been studied extensively, the optimal type of carbohydrate for the athlete is still debatable. The question of which type of carbohydrate is better for athletic performance may be better understood if the carbohydrate is classified by its physiologic reaction in the body or by its glycemic index rather than by its structure. The **glycemic index** represents the ratio of the area under the blood glucose curve resulting from the ingestion of a given quantity of carbohydrates and the area under the glucose curve resulting from the ingestion of the same quantity of white bread or glucose (see Chapter 30). Appendix 43 lists the glycemic indices and glycemic loads for several foods.

Studies concerning whether the glycemic index of carbohydrates in the preexercise meal affects performance are not conclusive. Preliminary work has demonstrated that a diet based on high–glycemic index (HGI) carbohydrate foods promoted greater glycogen storage in the first 24 hours of recovery after strenuous exercise than an equal amount of carbohydrate eaten in the form of low–glycemic index (LGI) foods (Siu and Wong, 2004). Metabolic responses to high glycemic index (HGI) and low glycemic index (LGI) meals consumed during the immediate post exercise period (within 30 minutes following prolonged exercise) were not different as long as sufficient carbohydrates were consumed. However, higher insulin concentrations observed following the HGI meal later in the recovery period (after 2 hours) did facilitate further muscle glycogen resynthesis (Stevensen, 2005). While HGI food choices may facilitate recovery, the jury is still out as to whether there is a difference between the impact of HGI versus LGI on performance.

Carbohydrate Intake Before, During, and After Exercise

Preexercise Meal

The preevent or pretraining meal serves two purposes. It keeps the athlete from feeling hungry before and during the exercise bout, and it maintains optimal levels of blood glucose for the exercising muscles. A preexercise meal can improve performance compared with exercising in a fasted state. Athletes who train early in the morning before eating or drinking risk developing low liver glycogen stores, and this can impair performance, particularly if the exercise regimen involves endurance training.

Carbohydrate feedings before exercise can help to restore suboptimal liver glycogen stores, which may be called on during prolonged training and high-intensity competition. While allowing for personal preferences and psychological factors, the preevent meal should be high in carbohydrates, nongreasy, and readily digested. Fat should be limited because it delays stomach emptying time and takes longer to digest. A meal eaten 3.5 to 4 hours before competition should be limited to 25% of the kilocalories from fat. Closer to the event, the fat content should be less than 25%. Exercising with a full stomach also may cause indigestion, nausea, and vomiting.

The pregame meal should be eaten 3 to 4 hours before an event and should provide 200 to 350 g of carbohydrates

(4 g/kg). Allowing time for partial digestion and absorption provides a final addition to muscle glycogen, additional blood sugar, and also relatively complete emptying of the stomach. To avoid gastrointestinal distress, the carbohydrate content of the meal should be reduced the closer the meal is to the exercise. For example, 4 hours before the event it is suggested that the athlete consume 4 g of carbohydrate per kilogram of body weight, whereas 1 hour before the competition the athlete would consume 1 g of carbohydrate per kilogram of body weight.

Commercial liquid formulas providing an easily digested high-carbohydrate fluid are popular with athletes and more than likely do leave the stomach faster. Other appropriate pregame meals are toast or plain bagel with jelly, a baked potato, plain spaghetti, dry cereal, or a low-sugar fruit smoothie prepared with a protein powder. Foods high in fiber, fat, and lactose for some will cause gastrointestinal distress (e.g., bloating, gas, or diarrhea) and should be avoided before competition. Box 23-1 suggests preevent meals based on time of competition.

Athletes should always practice and use what works best for them by experimenting with foods and beverages during practice sessions and planning ahead to ensure that they have these foods available when they compete.

Carbohydrate Intake During Exercise

Carbohydrates consumed during endurance exercise lasting longer than 1 hour ensures the availability of sufficient amounts of energy during the later stages of exercise, improves performance, and enhances feeling of pleasure during and following exercise (Backhouse et al., 2005).

Carbohydrate feeding does not prevent fatigue; rather, it simply delays it. During the final minutes of exercise when muscle glycogen is low and athletes rely heavily on blood glucose for energy, their muscles feel heavy, and they must concentrate to maintain exercise at intensities that are ordinarily not stressful when muscle glycogen stores are full. Glucose ingestion during exercise has also been shown to spare endogenous protein and carbohydrates in fed cyclists without glycogen depletion (van-Hamont et al., 2005). Thus consuming an exogenous carbohydrate during endurance exercise helps to maintain blood glucose and improve performance.

The form of carbohydrate does not seem to matter physiologically; some athletes prefer to use a sports drink, whereas others prefer to eat a solid or gel and consume water. If a sports drink with carbohydrates is consumed during exercise, the rate of carbohydrate ingestion should be about 26 to 30 g every 30 minutes, an amount equivalent to 1 cup of a 6% to 8% carbohydrate solution taken every 15 to 20 minutes. This ensures that 1 g of carbohydrate will be delivered to the tissues per minute at the time fatigue sets in. It is unlikely that a carbohydrate concentration of less than 5% is enough to help performance, but solutions with a concentration greater than 10% are often associated with abdominal cramps, nausea, and diarrhea.

Several studies explore the possibility of combining protein and carbohydrates in a sport fluid or snack for

BOX 23-1

Examples of PreEvent Meals

For athletes who compete in events such as track or swimming meets or soccer, basketball, volleyball, and wrestling tournaments all day, nutritious, easy-to-digest food and fluid choices may be a problem. The athlete should consider the amount of time between eating and performance when choosing foods during all-day events. Suggested precompetition menus include the following:

1 hr or Less Before Competition—About 100 kcal

One of These Choices:

Fresh fruit such as a banana or orange slices
Half of a sports energy bar such as PowerBar
½ plain bagel or English muffin
Crackers such as saltines or Melba toast
Small box of cereal such as Corn Flakes, Rice Krispies or Total
8-12 oz of a sports drink such as Gatorade, PowerBar Endurance Sports Drink

2 to 3 Hours Before Competition—About 300-400 kcal

One of These Choices:

½ of turkey sandwich on white bread with baked chips
½ bagel with low sugar jelly and 1 banana
2 pancakes with lite or sugar-free syrup and berries
32 fluid oz of a sports drink such as Gatorade, PowerBar Endurance Sports Drink or 32 oz endurance drink with protein such as Endurox or Accelerade
1 low-sugar smoothie with berries, banana, and 1 scoop soy or whey protein
1 sports energy bar, 1 cup sports drink, 1 cup water

3 to 4 Hours Before Competition—About 700 kcal

One of these selections:

Scrambled egg whites with white toast/low sugar jam and banana
1 bagel with fat-free or low-fat cream cheese and low sugar jelly and 1 banana
1 6-in turkey sub on Italian bread with lettuce/tomato and mustard
1 3-oz grilled chicken breast with small baked potato, roll, and water
2 cups plain pasta with 1 plain roll
1 can of low fat sport shake with no more than 25 g protein, 1 sports bar, 1 banana, water

---

improving performance, muscle protein synthesis and net balance, and recovery. A small amount of amino acids ingested in small amounts alone or in conjunction with carbohydrates before or after exercise appears to improve net protein balance and may stimulate protein synthesis and improve net protein balance at rest during exercise and postexercise recovery (Koopman et al., 2004; Millard-Stafford et al., 2005).

Carbohydrate Intake After Exercise

On average, only 5% of the muscle glycogen used during exercise is resynthesized each hour following exercise. Accordingly, at least 20 hours will be required for complete restoration after exhaustive exercise, provided about 600 g of carbohydrates are consumed. The highest muscle glycogen synthesis rates have been reported when large amounts of carbohydrates (1 to 1.85 g/kg/hr) are consumed immediately after exercise and at 15- to 60-minute intervals thereafter for up to 5 hours after exercise. When carbohydrate ingestion is delayed by several hours, muscle glycogen synthesis may drop by as much as 50% (Jentjens and Jeukendrup, 2003). Delaying carbohydrate intake for too long after exercise will reduce muscle glycogen resynthesis.

It also appears that the consumption of carbohydrates with a high glycemic index results in higher muscle glycogen levels 24 hours after exercise compared with the same amount of carbohydrates provided as foods with a low glycemic index. Adding about 5 to 9 g of protein with every 100 g of carbohydrate eaten after exercise may further increase glycogen resynthesis rate, provide amino acids for muscle repair and promote a more anabolic hormonal profile (Millard-Stafford et al., 2005).

Many athletes find it difficult to consume food immediately after exercise. Usually when body or core temperature is elevated, appetite is depressed, and it is difficult to consume carbohydrate-rich foods. Many athletes find it easier and simpler to drink their carbohydrates rather than eat them or to consume easy-to-eat carbohydrate-rich foods such as fruit pops, bananas, oranges, melon, or apple slices.

PROTEIN

There has been considerable debate regarding the protein needs of athletes. For individuals involved in general fitness programs, the 2002 RDAs for protein of 0.66 g/kg body weight daily for 14- to 18-year olds and 0.80 to 1 g/kg body weight daily for adults, which is 12% to 15% of energy intake, will suffice (Institute of Medicine, 2002) (see Inside Front Cover). However, research over the last decade has indicated that athletes engaged in intense training need to consume about 1.5 to two times the RDA of protein in their diet (1.5 to 2g/kg/day to maintain protein balance. Inadequate protein intake can result in negative nitrogen balance, which can increase protein metabolism and lead to muscle wasting, training intolerance, and retarded recovery (Dunford, 2006).

If the need for protein during exercise is slightly elevated above that for sedentary persons, the usual protein intake of the population will more than meet these needs. Reports of food intake in athletes and nonathletes consistently indicate that protein represents from 12% to 20% of total energy intake or 1.2 to 2 g of protein per kilogram of body weight daily. The exception to the rule will be small, active women who may consume a low-energy intake in conjunction with an exercise or training program. Although these women may consume close to the RDA for protein in conjunction with the restricted energy intake, it may be inadequate to maintain lean body mass.

Consuming more protein than the body can use is not necessary and should be avoided. When athletes consume diets that are high in protein, they compromise their carbohydrate status and therefore may affect their ability to train and compete at peak levels. High-protein intakes can also result in diuresis and potential dehydration. Protein foods are often also high in fat, and consumption of excess protein can create difficulty in maintaining a low-fat diet. In addition, the hypercalciuric effect of high-protein diets is still considered by some a significant factor in calcium balance, and until the controversy is settled, a conservative approach is advised (see Chapter 24).

Protein Needs for Resistance Exercise

Sufficient data have established that the study of protein needs with resistance exercise is divided into two areas: the need for maintenance (minimum protein required to accomplish nitrogen equilibrium), and the need for increasing lean tissue (positive nitrogen balance). For bodybuilders or persons interested in increasing body mass, the mythology of increased protein needs is rampant.

Strategies to increase the concentration and availability of amino acids after resistance exercise such as timing of snacks and meals have become an area of interest and may impact overall protein synthesis (see *Clinical Insight:* How Does Type, Timing, and Amount of Protein Affect Muscle Hypertrophy?).

✺ CLINICAL INSIGHT

How Does Type, Timing, and Amount of Protein Affect Muscle Hypertrophy?

Although many factors appear to contribute to overall muscle hypertrophy, nutritional factors that control protein synthesis during exercise are not well understood, leaving experts in discord about the type, amount, and timing of meals to enhance protein synthesis and muscle hypertrophy (Kerksick and Leutholtz, 2005). Resistance training and diet consistently appear to play a role in postworkout muscle protein synthesis.

Many studies support the fact that supplementation of free-form amino acids or whole or intact forms of protein can enhance training adaptations when combined with resistance training. A 2005 study with resistance-trained participants for 14 weeks demonstrated that the administration of a protein supplement resulted in greater increases in cross-sectional muscle size of types I and II fibers and greater increase in squat height (Anderson et al., 2005). In another study a postexercise trial, including a mixture of carbohydrate and whey protein consumed 1 hour after exercise, resulted in a more immediate and overall greater protein synthesis response; whereas the addition of free essential amino acids before and after exercise also was shown to cause a rapid increase in protein synthesis and balance (Kerksick and Leutholtz, 2005). Tipton et al. (2004) compared 20 g of whey protein to 20 g of casein protein taken within 1 hour after a resistance training bout and found both to be equally effective in producing protein balance.

Hyperaminoacidemia, along with an increase in insulin when blood flow is increased, appears to offer maximum stimulation of muscle protein synthesis (Bohe et al., 2003). Although the optimal amount of amino acids to ingest for maximum protein synthesis is not known, a recent study examined the impact of a 25 g of whey and casein protein solution before and after a strength-training session (STS). The study found that, when consumed 30 minutes before an STS, there were significant increases in growth hormone, testosterone, free fatty acids, and serum insulin, and significantly increased postexercise oxygen consumption and respiratory exchange ratio during the 2 hours after exercise; hence there was a more anabolic environment for muscle growth (Hulmi et al., 2005).

Kerksick and colleagues summarized the doses in the studies they reviewed using 6 g of essential amino acids (EAAs) only, 6 g of EAAs + 6 g of nonessential amino acids, 12 g of EAAs, 17.5 g of whey protein, 20 g of casein protein, 20 g of whey protein, 40 g of mixed amino acids, and 40 g of EAAs. All had similar increases in protein synthesis and balance. Therefore, for athletes interested in muscle hypertrophy, it appears that the neither the type nor the amount of protein matters if the day's total amount is within the recommended range for resistance-training athletes of 1.2 to 2 g of protein per kilogram of body weight per day. Sports nutrition professionals can use these data to construct preworkout and postworkout formulas to enhance the resistance training sessions of their clients.

FAT

Even though maximum performance is impossible without muscle glycogen, fat also provides energy for exercise. Fat is the most concentrated source of food energy and supplies more than twice as many calories (9 kcal/g) by weight as protein (4 kcal/g) or carbohydrate (4 kcal/g) (see Chapter 3). Fat provides essential fatty acids that are necessary for cell membranes, skin, hormones, and transport of fat-soluble vitamins. The body has total glycogen stores (both muscle and liver) equaling about 2600 calories, whereas each pound of body fat supplies 3500 calories. This means that an athlete weighing 74 kg (163 lb) with 10% body fat has 16.3 lb of fat, which equals 57,000 calories.

Fat is the major, if not most important, fuel for light- to moderate-intensity exercise. Although fat is a valuable metabolic fuel for muscle activity during longer aerobic exercise and performs many important functions in the body, no attempt should be made to consume more fat over the usual amount unless the athlete is eating less than 15% of calories from fat. In addition, athletes who consume a high-fat diet typically consume fewer calories from carbohydrate.

The makeup of the exercising person's diet will also determine which substrate is used during an exercise bout. If an athlete is consuming a high-carbohydrate diet, he or she will use more glycogen as fuel for the exercise. If the diet is high in fat, more fat will be oxidized as a fuel source. Fat oxidation rates have been shown to decline after the ingestion of high-fat diets, partly because of adaptations at the muscle level and decreased glycogen stores. Fasting longer than 6 hours optimizes fat oxidation; however, the ingestion of carbohydrates in the hours before or at the beginning of an exercise session augments the rate of fat oxidation significantly when compared with fasting conditions (Achten and Jeukendrup, 2004).

Exercise intensity and duration are important determinants of fat oxidation. Fat oxidation rates decrease when exercise intensity becomes high. Maximum rates of fat oxidation are reached at exercise intensities between 59% and 64% of Vo_2max in trained athletes and at intensities of 47% to 52% Vo_2max in the general population (Achten and Jeukendrup, 2004). A high-fat diet has been shown to compromise high-intensity performance even when a high-fat diet regimen is followed by a carbohydrate loading before high-intensity performance (Havemann et al., 2005). The mode and duration of exercise can also affect fat oxidation, with running increasing fat oxidation more than cycling and endurance training (Achten and Jeukendrup, 2004).

Long-term use of a high-fat diet has been well documented as having negative health effects. Following a low-fat, high-carbohydrate diet is also important for health reasons because a high-fat diet is associated with cardiovascular disease, obesity, diabetes, and some types of cancers. Athletes should consume 20% to 30% of their calories from fat. Severe fat restriction (15% or less of energy intake) may limit performance and is not advised.

VITAMINS AND MINERALS

The need for vitamins and minerals in exercise has been reviewed by several researchers with the consensus that, unless an individual is deficient in a given nutrient, supplementation with that nutrient does not have a major effect on performance. Several nutrients are of concern in athletes, however, including folate, the other B vitamins, calcium, and zinc. A daily intake of less than one third of the RDA for several of the B vitamins (B_1, B_2 and B_6) and vitamin C, even when other vitamins are supplemented in the diet, may lead to a significant decrease in Vo_2max and the anaerobic threshold in less than 4 weeks (Williams, 2004). Because many women athletes are also vegetarians, iron and specifically vitamin B_{12} may be of additional concern in this subgroup (Dorfman, 2000). Athletes involved in heavy training may need more of several vitamins such as B_1, B_2, and B_6 because they are involved in energy production. Iron and calcium are the two minerals most likely to be low in the diet, especially in young athletes.

It has usually been assumed that, if the athlete meets requirements for increased energy, the vitamin and mineral requirements will also be satisfied. Although this may be true in most cases, many athletes may have poor intakes of vitamins and minerals. Training and work schedules, unplanned low-nutrient snacks, infrequent nutrient-dense meals, and overall low calorie intakes due to body weight and appearance concerns may cause inadequate intakes of vitamins and minerals.

When limited to 100% of the DRIs, vitamin supplementation is generally regarded as safe; however, excess amounts of several vitamins may contribute to serious health problems and tolerable upper limits have been established for many vitamins. Athletes need to understand that more is not always better. The National Academy of Sciences has established the dietary reference intakes (DRIs) for vitamins and minerals as a guide for determining nutritional needs. The DRIs are the daily amounts of nutrients recommended for practically all healthy persons to promote optimal health (see Chapter 12 and inside front cover).

B Vitamins

Increased energy metabolism creates a need for more of the B vitamins that serve as part of coenzymes involved in the energy cycles. Studies have shown that athletes can become depleted in some B vitamins, and in these athletes dietary change or supplementation improves exercise performance. For some athletes such as wrestlers, gymnasts, or rowers who consume low-calorie diets for long periods, a B-vitamin supplement to meet the RDA may be appropriate. There is no evidence that supplementing the well-nourished athlete with more B vitamins will increase performance

A deficiency of vitamin B_{12}, found only in animal foods, could develop in a vegetarian athlete after several years of a strict vegan intake (see Chapter 3); a vitamin B_{12} supplement is warranted for these individuals (Dorfman, 2000). Two studies on endurance athletes investigated the possibility of altered B_{12} metabolism based on serum homocysteine concentrations, although further investigation is recommended before supplements are advised (Herrmann et al., 2003, 2005).

The intake of folic acid is marginal for a large portion of the U.S. population and could be low in an athlete whose consumption of whole fruits and vegetables is low. If diets of athletes reflect those of the general population, they could easily not contain the recommended number of fruits and vegetables rich in folate. A folate supplement to meet the RDA is recommended for such athletes or the inclusion of wheat, grain, and fortified products to boost dietary intakes of folate.

Antioxidants

Antioxidants have been studied individually and collectively for their potential to enhance exercise performance or to prevent exercise-induced muscle tissue damage (Williams, 2004). Cells continuously produce free radicals and reactive oxidation species (ROS) as a part of metabolic processes (see Chapters 3, 9 and 15). Physical exercise may be associated with a 10- to 20-fold increase in whole body oxygen intake, whereas in active peripheral skeletal muscles during exercise, it may increase by as much as 100- to 200-fold (Sen, 2001). Oxidative stress has been shown to increase the oxidative processes in the muscle during exercise, leading to increased generation of lipid peroxides and free radicals. The magnitude of stress depends on the ability of the body's tissues to detoxify ROS.

Free radicals are neutralized by antioxidant defense systems that play an important role in protecting the cell membrane from oxidative damage. These systems include catalase; superoxide dismutase; glutathione peroxidase; nonenzymatic antioxidants such as vitamins A, E, and C; the mineral selenium; and phytonutrients such as carotenoids (see Chapters 9 and 15).

Whether exercise increases the need for additional antioxidants in the diet is unclear (Urso and Clarkson, 2003). It appears that, although supplements or a diet high in antioxidants may improve performance in deficient individuals, supplementation does not seem to enhance performance in well-nourished individuals or those with adequate amounts of antioxidants. Watson and colleagues compared antioxidant-restricted diets and high-antioxidant diets of 17 trained athletes running for 40 minutes (acute high-intensity exercise) and found an increased rate of perceived exertion, significantly higher levels of oxidative stress markers, and up to 1 hour of recovery in those with antioxidant-deficient diets (Watson et al., 2005).

Vitamins with antioxidant activity, particularly vitamin C, vitamin E, and β-carotene, neutralize free radicals. The question is whether they enhance recovery from exercise (Konig et al., 2001). In one study 90 days' supplementation with a daily antioxidant cocktail of 500 mg of vitamin E, 30 mg of β-carotene, and during the last 15 days 1 g of vitamin C, increased plasma concentrations of E, β-carotene, and C by 1.6, 10, and 1.2 times respectively; and there was a significantly higher glutathione versus glutathione disulfide ratio in neutrophils, suggesting enhancement of antioxidant activity (Tauler et al., 2002).

Antioxidant nutrients may have a role in enhancing recovery from exercise and maintaining optimal immune response, but there is no consistent evidence that they improve performance per se. The available evidence suggests that antioxidant supplementation has favorable effects on markers of lipid peroxidation after exercise. Although the physiologic implications of this effect remain to be elucidated, the prudent use of an antioxidant supplement may provide insurance against a suboptimal diet and the increased stress that physical activity puts on the immune system (Venkatraman and Pendergast, 2002). A diet rich in fruits and vegetables can ensure an adequate intake of antioxidants.

Vitamin C

Vitamin C is involved in a number of important biochemical pathways that are important to exercise metabolism and the health of athletes. Exercise generally causes a transient increase in circulating ascorbic acid levels in the hours following exercise but a decline below preexercise levels in the days after prolonged exercise (Peake, 2003). The effect of vitamin C supplementation on performance has received considerable attention, mainly because athletes consume vitamin C in large quantities, often because of the volume of food they consume. In studies in which athletes were deficient in vitamin C, supplementation improved physical performance, but a thorough analysis of these studies supports the general conclusion that vitamin C supplementation does not increase physical performance capacity in subjects with normal body levels of vitamin C (Peake, 2003). On the other hand, because exercise is a stressor to the body, some nutritionists recommend that the active individual may need more vitamin C than the DRI.

Vitamin E

Vitamin E is used widely as a supplement by athletes who hope to improve performance. Recent research is showing vitamin E to have a protective effect against exercise-induced oxidative injury and the acute immune response changes that exercise produces. Researchers found that supplementation with vitamin E enhances the immune response, preventing changes similar to those of infectious disease seen after exercise. Over the course of an exercise season with intense workouts and competition, vitamin E supplementation at the level of 200 to 450 IU daily may help to prevent oxidative injury. However, further studies are recommended (Williams, 2004).

Iron

Iron has one of the most critical implications for sport performance. As a component of hemoglobin, it is instrumental in transporting oxygen from the lungs to the tissues. It performs a similar role in **myoglobin**, which acts within the muscle as an oxygen acceptor to hold a supply of oxygen readily available for use by the mitochondria. Iron is also a vital component of the cytochrome enzymes involved in the production of ATP. Thus it follows that iron deficiency anemia limits aerobic endurance and the capacity for work;

however, partial depletion of iron stores in the liver, spleen, and bone marrow, as evidenced by low serum ferritin levels, can have a detrimental effect on exercise performance, even when anemia is not present (see Chapters 15 and 31).

Although iron deficiency anemia is not frequently seen among athletes, suboptimal iron stores as assessed by serum ferritin levels are relatively common (Sinclair and Hinton, 2005). Athletes at risk for developing low iron stores are the rapidly growing male adolescent; the female athlete with heavy menstrual losses; the athlete with an energy-restricted diet; distance runners who may have increased gastrointestinal iron loss, hematuria, hemolysis caused by foot impact, and myoglobin leakage; and those training heavily in hot climates with heavy sweating. All athletes, especially female long-distance runners and vegetarians, should be screened periodically to assess their iron status.

Heavy training can also cause a transient decrease in serum ferritin and hemoglobin that may be experienced by some athletes, especially in the conditioning phase of the sport (Spodaryk, 2002). This was once called **sports anemia**, but erythrocyte morphology remains normal, and performance does not appear to deteriorate. These decreases in serum ferritin and hemoglobin are a result of an increase in plasma volume, which causes a hemodilution and appears to have no effect on performance (see Chapter 31).

Some athletes, especially long-distance runners, experience gastrointestinal bleeding. Iron loss through gastrointestinal bleeding can be detected by fecal hemoglobin assays. The percentage of runners who experience gastrointestinal bleeding is significant and is related to the intensity and duration of the exercise, the ability of the athlete to stay hydrated, how well the athlete is trained, and whether he or she has taken nonsteroidal antiinflammatory drugs, particularly ibuprofen, before the competition (Peters et al., 2001).

The iron concentration of sweat during exercise ranges from 0.13 to 0.42 mg/L. Waller and Haymes (1996) observed that the iron concentration in sweat is lower in a hot environment (35° C) than in a thermoneutral environment (26° C). Because sweating is greater in the heat, the same amount of sweat iron was lost during 1 hour of exercise in both environments, with male athletes losing three times as much sweat iron as female athletes. They also found that, as the exercise time continued, less iron was lost in the sweat. Sweat iron concentration decreased significantly from 30 to 60 minutes, which suggests that much of the iron lost in sweat is done early in the exercise bout. Iron supplementation can be beneficial in improving iron stores of athletes who are iron depleted, but the effects on aerobic performance of nonanemic athletes are equivocal. Because large doses of iron (75 mg/day) may be toxic in persons with the genetic disorder hemochromatosis (see Chapter 31), such supplements should be used only by those diagnosed as iron depleted or anemic. At present the data do not support the value of iron supplementation for either treating or preventing sports anemia; however, testing serum ferritin may be useful in assessing iron stores in athletes. If true iron depletion is present, iron supplementation along with vitamin C to enhance its absorption is appropriate. Oral iron therapy

is effective and maintains performance in runners who are deficient in iron but not anemic (see Chapter 31).

Some athletes experience iron deficiency without anemia, a condition with normal hemoglobin levels but reduced levels of serum ferritin. Serum ferritin levels in the range of 20 to 30 ng/ml have been considered a marker of iron deficiency (see Chapter 15). Iron supplementation may restore serum ferritin to normal, but studies indicate it may not have an impact on performance (Williams, 2005).

Calcium

Osteoporosis is a major health concern, especially for women. Although the disease has been regarded as a problem of older women, young women, especially those who have had interrupted menstrual function, may be at risk for decreased bone mass.

In 1997 the American College of Sports Medicine (ACSM) identified the **female athlete triad** as a disturbing pattern emerging in women's athletics. It is characterized by estrogen deficiency, evidenced as amenorrhea, disordered eating and low body fat, and loss of bone mass (see Chapter 22). Some women who exercise strenuously stop menstruating, a condition known as athletic amenorrhea. Unfortunately the exact cause of amenorrhea has not been fully determined, but probably many factors are involved. The two most current theories are that the excessive exercise is an "energy drain" that may lead to a hypothalamic dysfunction or that excess cortisol levels (in response to stress) inhibit the release of gonadotropins (Loucks, 2001). Regardless of the cause, the lack of estrogen has a negative impact on bone, and, if the estrogen deficiency persists, bone loss may be substantial, and bone may never be regained.

Strategies to promote the resumption of menses include estrogen replacement therapy, weight gain, and reduced training. Diet modification to include more calcium, vitamin D, and magnesium is also instituted. Regardless of menstrual history, most female athletes need to increase their calcium and vitamin D3 intake (Bonjour, 2005). Low-fat and nonfat dairy products, calcium-fortified fruit juices, calcium-fortified soy milk, and tofu made with calcium sulfate are all good sources. Amenorrheic athletes who need 1500 mg of calcium daily may require supplementation with calcium and vitamin D (see Chapter 24).

FLUIDS

Maintaining fluid balance requires the constant integration of input from hypothalamic osmoreceptors and vascular baroreceptors so that fluid intake matches or modestly exceeds fluid loss (Murray, 2006). Proper fluid balance maintains blood volume, which in turn supplies blood to the skin for body temperature regulation. Because exercise produces heat, which must be eliminated from the body to maintain appropriate body temperatures, regular fluid intake is essential for maintaining a body temperature that maximizes performance. Any fluid deficit that is incurred during an exercise session can potentially compromise the subsequent exercise bout if adequate fluid replacement is not addressed (Shirreffs et al., 2004).

The body maintains appropriate temperatures by means of a system referred to as **thermoregulation.** As heat is generated in the muscles during exercise, it is transferred via the blood to the body's core. Increased core temperature results in increased blood flow to the skin, where, in cool-to-moderate ambient temperatures, heat is transferred to the environment by convection, radiation, and evaporation.

Environmental conditions have a large impact on thermoregulation. When ambient temperatures range from warm to hot, the body must dissipate the heat generated from exercise, as well as the heat absorbed from the environment. When this occurs, the body relies solely on the evaporation of sweat to maintain appropriate body temperatures. Thus maintaining hydration becomes crucial when ambient temperatures reach or exceed 36° C (96.8° F). The hotter the temperature, the more important sweating is for body heat dissipation.

Humidity affects the body's ability to dissipate heat to a greater extent than air temperatures. As humidity increases, the rate at which sweat evaporates decreases, which means more sweat drips off the body without transferring heat from the body to the environment. Combining the effects of a hot, humid environment with a large metabolic heat load produced during exercise taxes the thermoregulatory system to its maximum. Ensuring proper and adequate fluid intake is key to reducing the risk of heat stress.

Fluid Balance

Body fluid balance is regulated by mechanisms that reduce urinary water and sodium excretion, stimulate thirst, and control the intake and output of both water and electrolytes. In response to dehydration, *antidiuretic hormone* (vasopressin; ADH) and the renin-angiotensin II–aldosterone system increase water and sodium retention by the kidneys and provoke an increase in thirst. These hormones maintain the osmolality, sodium content, and volume of extracellular fluids and play a major role in the regulation of fluid balance (see Chapters 4 and 36).

Water losses throughout the course of the day include those from sweat and the respiratory tract, plus losses from the kidneys and gastrointestinal tract. When fluid is lost from the body in the form of sweat, plasma volume decreases and plasma osmolality increases. The kidneys, under hormonal control, regulate water and solute excretion in excess of the obligatory urine loss. However, when the body is subjected to hot environments, whether the heat load is imposed internally or externally, certain hormonal adjustments occur to maintain body function. Some of these adjustments include the body's conservation of water and sodium and the release of ADH by the pituitary gland to increase water absorption from the kidneys. These changes cause the urine to become more concentrated, thus conserving fluid and making the urine a dark gold color. This feedback process helps to conserve body water and blood volume.

At the same time, *aldosterone* is released from the adrenal cortex and acts on the renal tubules to increase the resorp-tion of sodium, which helps maintain the correct osmotic pressure. These reactions also activate thirst mechanisms in the body. However, in situations in which water losses are increased acutely such as in athletic workouts or competition, the thirst response can be delayed, making it difficult for athletes to trust their thirst to ingest enough fluid to offset the volume of fluid lost during training and competition. A loss of 1.5 to 2 L of fluid is necessary before the thirst mechanism kicks in, and this level of water loss already has a serious effect on temperature control. Athletes need to rehydrate on a timed basis rather than as a reaction to thirst, and it should be enough to maintain the preexercise weight.

Daily Fluid Needs

Daily fluid intake recommendations for sedentary individuals vary greatly because of the wide disparity in daily fluid needs created by body size, physical activity, and environmental conditions (Grandjean et al., 2003). The 2004 DRI for water and electrolytes identify the adequate intake for water to be 3.7 L/day in males (130 oz/ day, 16 cups of fluid/day) and 2.7 L/day for females (95 oz/day, about 12 cups/day) (Institute of Medicine, 2004). Approximately 20% of the daily water need comes from water found in foods (i.e., fruits and vegetables); the remaining 80% is provided by beverages, including water, juice, milk, coffee, tea, soup, sports drinks, and soft drinks.

When individuals work, train, and compete in warm environments, their fluid needs can increase to more than 10 L/day. The water required to excrete the urea from protein metabolism and excess electrolyte intake adds to the daily needs. However, for active individuals this volume is relatively small (130 ml/1000 kcal) and inconsequential since usually they are consuming more than 2 L each day (Murray, 2006).

Fluid Replacement

Several opinions are published by a variety of professional organizations that address fluid and electrolyte replacement before, during, and after exercise. A summary of these recommendations can be found in Box 23-2. The groups that developed these statements include The American College of Sports Medicine, National Athletic Trainers Association, American Academy of Pediatrics, American Dietetic Association and the Dietitians of Canada, International Marathon Directors Association, Inter-Association Task Force on External Heat Illnesses, and USA Track and Field. Although specific recommendations among the groups differ slightly, their main intent is to keep athletes well hydrated. When possible, fluid should be consumed at rates that closely match sweating rate, although, when that is not possible, some athletes can tolerate losses of up to 2% of body weight without significant risk to physical well-being or performance when the environment is cold (Coyle, 2004). However, when the temperature is hot, a 2% loss can impair performance.

It appears that plain water is not the best beverage to consume following exercise to replace the water lost as sweat (Murray, 2006). The replacement of electrolytes, particularly sodium, as well as water, is essential for complete

BOX 23-2

Summary of Guidelines for Proper Hydration

General Guidelines

Monitor fluid losses: Weigh in before and after practice, especially during hot weather and the conditioning phase of the season.

Do not restrict fluids before, during, or after the event.

Do not rely on thirst as an indicator of fluid losses.

Drink early and at regular intervals throughout the activity

Do not consume alcohol before, during, or after exercise since it may act as a diuretic and prevent adequate fluid replenishment.

Discourage caffeinated beverages a few hours before and after physical activity because of their diuretic effect

Before Exercise

Drink about 400 to 600 ml (14 to 22 oz) of water or sports drink (approximately 17 oz), 2 to 3 hr before the start of exercise.

During Exercise

Drink 150 to 350 ml (6 to 12 oz) of fluid every 15 to 20 min, depending on race speed, environmental conditions, and tolerance; no more than 1 C (8 to 10 oz) every 15 to 20 min), although individualized recommendations must be followed.

After Exercise

Drink 25% to 50% more than existing weight loss to ensure hydration 4-6 hours after exercise.

Drink 450 to 675 ml (16 to 24 oz) of fluid for every pound of body weight lost during exercise.

If an athlete is participating in multiple workouts in 1 day, then 80% of fluid loss must be replaced before the next workout.

Electrolyte Replacement

Sodium: 0.5 to 0.7 g/L in activity longer than 1 hour to enhance palatability and the drive to drink and to reduce the risk of hyponatremia and minimize risk of muscle cramps.

Data from Murray R: Fluid, electrolytes, and exercise. In Danford M, editor: *Sports nutrition: a practice manual for professionals,* ed 4, Washington, DC, 2006, American Dietetic Association.

rehydration. Several studies have illustrated the importance of including sodium in fluid replacement solutions, especially when compared with excessive intake of plain water (Hew, 2005; Noakes et al., 2005). For events lasting more than 2 hours, sodium should be added to the fluid to replace losses and to prevent hyponatremia.

Sodium

Several researchers have found that rehydration with water alone dilutes the blood rapidly, increases its volume, and stimulates urine output. The importance of ensuring euhy-dration before exercise and the potential benefits of temporary hyperhydration with sodium salts is an important issue (Shirreffs et al., 2004). Sodium losses can also contribute to heat cramping. Research with football players showed that sodium loss as measured by sweat rates and sweat electrolyte losses during two-a-day practices in August was twice as high (5 to 9 teaspoons of salt) in cramp prone players as in noncrampers (Stofan et al., 2005). Besides these individual variations, the intensity and duration of workouts also appear to play a role in the amount of sodium loss.

For effective restoration of fluid balance, the consumption of a volume of fluid in excess of sweat loss and replacement of electrolyte, particularly sodium, losses are essential (Shirreffs, 2004). Blood dilution lowers both sodium and the volume-dependent part of the thirst drive, thus removing much of the drive to drink and replace fluid losses.

Water-soluble electrolytes such as sodium can also move rapidly across the proximal intestines. During prolonged exercise lasting more than 4 to 5 hours, including sodium in replacement fluids increases palatability and facilitates fluid uptake in the intestines as sodium (along with carbohydrates) is actively transported from the lumen to the bloodstream. Water replacement in the absence of supplemental sodium during extended exercise can lead to hyponatremia or decreased plasma sodium concentrations. Research suggests that exercise-induced hyponatremia may result from fluid overloading during a prolonged exercise session of 4 hours (Twerenbold et al., 2004). Hyponatremia is associated with individuals who drink plain water in excess of their sweat losses or who are less physically conditioned and produce a more salty sweat. As plasma sodium levels fall below 130 mEq/L, symptoms of hyponatremia may occur, which can include lethargy, confusion, seizures, or loss of consciousness. Hyponatremia can be minimized by drinking sodium-containing fluids frequently enough to provide 680 mg of sodium per hour (Twerenbold et al., 2004).

Potassium

Another electrolyte that is involved with maintaining body fluids is potassium. Potassium is the major ion of the intracellular fluid. As the major electrolyte inside the body's cells, potassium works in close association with sodium and chloride in maintaining body fluids and in generating electrical impulses in the nerves and muscles, including the heart. Potassium balance, like sodium balance, is also regulated by aldosterone. Potassium regulation in the body is precise, and deficiencies are rare, although they may occur during fasting, episodes of diarrhea, and diuretic use. Loss of potassium from skeletal muscle has been implicated in fatigue.

Most researchers agree that there is little loss of potassium through sweat, although, compared with sodium, which is reduced considerably by the time sweat reaches the skin surface, potassium concentration is equal to or greater than that in the blood plasma. Although aldosterone acts on sweat glands to increase the resorption of sodium, potassium secretion is unaffected. The potassium loss of 32 to 48 mEq/day does not appear to be significant and can easily be replaced by diet.

Fluid Absorption

Most athletes believe that as soon as they ingest a fluid, it is rehydrating their system; however, the speed at which fluid is absorbed depends on a number of different factors, including the amount, type, temperature, and osmolality of the fluid consumed and the rate of gastric emptying.

Because glucose is actively absorbed in the intestines, it can markedly increase both sodium and water absorption. A carbohydrate-electrolyte solution was able to enhance exercise capacity by elevating blood sugar, maintaining high rates of carbohydrate oxidation, preventing central fatigue, and reducing perceived exertion (Byrne et al., 2005).

Early studies indicate that water absorption is maximized when luminal glucose concentrations range from 1% to 3% (55 to 140 mM); however, most sports drinks contain two to three times this quantity without causing adverse gastrointestinal symptoms. To determine the concentration of carbohydrate in a sports drink, the grams of carbohydrate or sugar in a serving is divided by the weight of a serving of the drink, which is usually 240 g, the approximate weight of 1 cup of water. A 6% carbohydrate drink contains 14 to 16 g of carbohydrate per 8 oz (1 cup) of drink (Figure 23-6).

Cold water is preferable to warm water because it attenuates changes in core temperature and peripheral blood flow, decreases sweat rate, and speeds up gastric emptying time. It is also absorbed more quickly.

Youth

Young children are more likely to participate in physical activities that are less than 60 minutes in duration since many youth soccer, t-ball, and basketball games last less than 60 minutes. Children, like adults, do not drink enough when offered fluids ad libitum during exercise in hot and humid climates; but children differ from adults in that, for any given level of dehydration, their core temperatures rise faster than those of adults, putting them at far greater risk for heat stress. Children who participate in sports activities must be taught to prevent dehydration by drinking above and beyond thirst and at frequent intervals (e.g., every 20 minutes) (Petrie et al., 2004; Unnithan and Goulopoulou, 2004).

A rule of thumb is that a child 10 years of age or younger should drink until he or she does not feel thirsty and then should drink an additional half a glass (⅓ to ½ cup). Older children and adolescents should follow the same guidelines; however, they should consume an additional cup of fluid (8 oz). When relevant, regulations for competition should be modified to allow children to leave the playing field periodically to drink.

One of the hurdles to getting children to consume fluids is to provide fluids they like. Providing a sports drink that will maintain the drive to drink and rehydrate them is the key to preventing active children from becoming dehydrated.

Older Athletes

Older, mature, or masters-level athletes are also at risk for dehydration and need to take precautions when exercising or staying fit. **Hypohydration** (when water loss is greater than water intake and there is a body water deficit) in older individuals can affect circulatory and thermoregulatory function to a greater extent and may be caused by the lower skin blood flow, causing core temperature to rise.

Because the thirst drive is reduced in older adults, they need to be educated about drinking adequately before exercise and drinking fluids well before they become thirsty. Female athletes need to drink more than males during interval exercise in the heat. For both genders fluid balance is maintained better when palatable carbohydrate and electrolyte solutions were offered (Baker et al., 2005).

Altitude and Hydration

Unacclimated individuals undergo a plasma volume contraction when acutely exposed to moderately high altitude. This is the result of increased renal sodium and water excretion and decreased voluntary sodium and water intake. Respiratory losses are increased by high ventilatory rates and typically dry air. The result is an increase in serum hematocrit and hemoglobin, which increases the oxygen-carrying capacity of the blood but at the cost of reduced blood volume, stroke volume, and cardiac output.

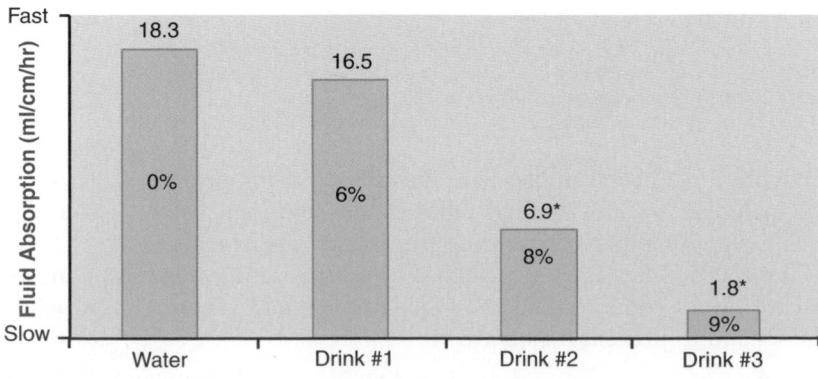

FIGURE 23-6 Intestinal absorption of sports drinks based on carbohydrate concentration. *(Modified from Ryan AJ et al: Effect of hypohydration on gastric emptying and intestinal absorption during exercise, J Appl Physiol 84:1581, 1998.)*

* $p < 0.05$ slower than water and Drink #1.
Water and Drink #1 were not statistically different from each other.

Fluid requirements increase as a result. With acclimation, red blood cell production increases and plasma and blood volume return to prealtitude levels.

OTHER CONSIDERATIONS

Alcohol

Alcohol is a central nervous system depressant. Pure alcohol supplies 7 kcal/g and is a source of energy that is metabolized more like fat. For alcohol to be used by muscle, it must first be metabolized in the liver. Alcohol consumption immediately before or during exercise has a detrimental effect on athletic performance, even though, by reducing feelings of insecurity, tension, and discomfort, it may cause the athlete to believe that he or she is performing better. Some athletes incorrectly believe that because alcohol contains carbohydrates, they can load up on beer to improve their performance. Perceptual motor performance, gross motor skills, balance, and coordination are affected by alcohol consumption.

Alcohol may cause reduced glucose secretion from the liver, which may lead to hypoglycemia and early fatigue during endurance exercise. Alcohol may also be a contributing factor to hypothermia if consumed during exercise in cold weather.

Alcohol should not be used to replace fluids immediately after exercise because of its diuretic effect and adverse effects on blood glucose and glycogen levels. Chronic alcohol use causes the loss of many nutrients important for performance and health, including thiamin, vitamin B_6, and calcium (see Chapter 28).

Caffeine

Caffeine contributes to endurance performance, apparently because of its ability to enhance mobilization of fatty acids and thus conserve glycogen stores. Caffeine may also directly affect muscle contractility, possibly by facilitating calcium transport. It could reduce fatigue as well by reducing plasma potassium accumulation, which contributes to fatigue. Probably some ergogenic effects occur at doses of 6.5 mg/kg of body weight when taken before endurance exercise; however, caffeine does not seem to offer any benefits before high-intensity exercise. Because of this potential ergogenic effect, caffeine is banned by the

International Olympic Committee (IOC), although the banned level is much higher than that needed to enhance performance. An energy-enhancing effect is seen with only 1.5 to 3 mg of caffeine per pound (3.3 to 6.6 mg/kg). For a 150-lb man this is equivalent to only one 10-oz cup of coffee. As fluid replacement beverages, tea, iced tea, coffee, cola, caffeinated water, and some of the new caffeine-containing energy drinks are poor choices because of their diuretic effect and variable carbohydrate content. The diuretic action of caffeine could have negative consequences for athletes with excessive water needs or for those participating in long-distance events who do not want to have to urinate during the event.

As a restricted drug by the IOC, caffeine is considered a doping agent if the intake results in urine caffeine concentrations above 12 mg/L.

ERGOGENIC AIDS

Ergogenic aids include any training technique, mechanical device, nutrition practice, pharmacologic method, or physiologic technique that can improve exercise performance capacity and training adaptations. The use of ergogenic aids in the form of dietary supplements is widespread in all sports. Many athletes, whether recreational, elite, or professional, use some form of dietary supplementation (e.g., substances obtainable by prescription or by illegal means or others marked as supplements, vitamins, or minerals) to improve athletic performance or to assist with weight loss (Dhar et al., 2005). Research suggests that 50% to 98.6% of university athletes use some form of supplements as ergogenic aids (Froiland et al., 2004; Kristiansen et al., 2005; Neiper, 2005).

Reasons for supplement use differ between genders. In one study female athletes reported taking supplements for their health or to overcome an inadequate diet, whereas men were more likely to take supplements to improve speed and agility or strength and power or for weight/muscle gain (Froiland et al., 2004). Health reasons (45%), immune system enhancement (40%), and performance improvement (25%) have also been cited as reasons for supplement use (Neiper, 2005). The most common supplements used by athletes are described in Tables 23-2 and 23-3.

Athletes are bombarded with advertisements and testimonials from other athletes and coaches about the effects of

Text continued on p. 606.

TABLE 23-2

Ergogenic Aids

Ergogenic Aid	Reported Action/Claim	Research on Ergogenic Effects	Side Effects	Legality
α-ketoglutarate	Intermediate in Krebs cycle	Some evidence as anticatabolic after surgery; unclear in training	None	Legal
α-lipoic acid (ALA)	Enzyme found in mitochondria involved in energy production	No studies with humans for sport; used in Europe with persons with diabetes to treat insulin resistance and neuropathy	None	Legal

Continued

TABLE 23-2

Ergogenic Aids—cont'd

Ergogenic Aid	Reported Action/Claim	Research on Ergogenic Effects	Side Effects	Legality
Amino Acids				
Arginine	Protein synthesis; precursor to creatine and potential to increase growth hormone (GH); precursor to nitric oxide (NO)	Little evidence; some rationale for athletic improvement may be to the result of role as precursor to NO; some improvement in cardiac patients on protocol of 1.5 g/10 kg of body weight for 7 days	None	Legal
Branched-chain amino acids	Decrease mental fatigue Decrease exercise-induced protein degradation and muscle enzyme release	Some evidence that decreased fatigue may occur at higher altitudes.	Mild	Legal
Essential amino acids (EAAs)		Limited; suggests 3-6 g of EAAs before exercise; stimulates protein synthesis	Same as protein	Legal
Glutamine	Boosts immunity; GH stimulates protein and glycogen synthesis	May boost immunity with branched-chain amino acids and enriched whey	None	Legal
HMB β-Hydroxy-β-methyl-butyrate	Anticatabolic; enhances recovery by stimulating protein and glycogen synthesis	Minimum gains in strength and lean body mass in untrained athletes and the elderly; possibly catabolic with prolonged exercise; mixed reports in trained subjects	None with short-term use	Legal
Chokeberry juice	Enhances endogenous antioxidant defense system	Limits exercise-induced oxidative damage to red blood cells	None reported	Legal
Chitosan	Inhibits fat and lowers cholesterol	No evidence in humans	None reported	Legal
Citrus aurantium, bitter orange, synephrine	Increase metabolism	No evidence of weight-reducing properties	None reported	Legal
Ciwujia aka Siberian ginseng Eleutherococcus senticosus (ES)	Improve cardiorespiratory fitness (CF), fat metabolism (FAM), and endurance performance	Mixed; limited research shows improvement in CF, FAM, EP, although studies flawed	None reported	Legal
Chondroitin sulfate	Builds and grows cartilage	No studies that it is effective in treating arthritis or joint damage or helps torn ligaments or cartilage	None	Legal
Ephedrine, other sympathomimetics Pseudoephedrine, Ma huang	Stimulate central nervous system; increase energy	With caffeine, increase energy, time to exhaustion; increase metabolism without exercise; without caffeine, no benefits	Restlessness, nervousness, tachycardia; arrhythmias; hypertension; death	Banned by National Football League, National Collegiate Athletic Association, International Olympic Committee

TABLE 23-2

Ergogenic Aids—cont'd

Ergogenic Aid	Reported Action/Claim	Research on Ergogenic Effects	Side Effects	Legality
Glucosamine	Serves as nonsteroidal antiinflammatory drug alternative	Readily absorbed; benefit in reducing pain and need for medication	None reported	Legal
Green tea extract	Antioxidant; increases energy expenditure	Limited; may increase energy expenditure compared with caffeine	Same as caffeine	Legal
Human growth hormone	Anabolic effect on muscle growth; increases fat metabolism	Limited ergogenic benefits	Significant and dangerous	Illegal
Methylsulfonyl methane (MSM)	Metabolite of dimethylsulfoxide, a solvent used topically for analgesic and antiinflammatory properties	Little evidence of effectiveness for pain in humans	None	Legal
Nitric oxide (NO)	Promotes a "muscle pump," signals muscle growth and speeds recovery	No evidence that NO promotes muscle growth synthesis or improves muscle strength	None	Legal
Orthinine-α-ketoglutarate	Anabolic/catabolic	Limited; may improve protein balance, gains in bench press, but no significant gains in muscle mass, GH, squat strength, or training volume	None reported	Legal
Oxygenated beverages	Increase aerobic metabolism, decrease lactic acid, improve endurance	Performance hydration and blood oxygenation unaffected by oxygenated water	None	Legal
Ribose	3-carbon carbohydrate; involved in synthesis of adenosine triphosphate	Limited; can increase exercise capacity in heart patients; no value of exercise capacity in trained or untrained subjects	None reported	Legal
Sodium bicarbonate	Buffers lactic acid production; delays fatigue	Increases body's ability to buffer lactic acid during sub max exercise for events lasting 1-7 min	Stomach distress: bloating, diarrhea; dangerous in high doses; alkalosis	Legal
Sodium phosphate	Buffer	Some; increases Vo_2max and anaerobic threshold by 5%-10%; improves endurance	Stomach distress	Legal
Tribulus terrestris	Increases endogenous steroid production (LH); promotes skeletal hypertrophy	Mixed; no effect on strength or change in body composition	Potentially dangerous at high doses	Legal
Vanadyl sulfate (Vanadium)	Trace mineral; may effect protein and glucose metabolism	No effect on strength training or muscle mass during training	None reported	Legal

TABLE 23-3

Supplements Commonly Used by Athletes

Author	Athletes	Supplement Types	Frequency
Kristiansen M et al. (2005)	University	Sports drinks, carbohydrate gels, protein powder creatine	98.6%
Froiland K et al. (2004)	University	Energy/sports drinks, calorie replacements	73%, 61.4%
		Creatine and vitamin C	37.2%, 32.4%
	Males	Ginseng, amino acids, glutamine, β-hydroxy-β-methylbutyrate, weight gainers	
	Females	Calcium and multivitamins	
Herbold NH et al. (2004)	Females	Supplement use 1 time/month	65.4%
	Varsity	Multivitamin, minerals, iron	36%
		Amino acid/protein	12%
		Herbal/botanical	17%

dietary supplements on performance. Until 1994 dietary supplements were regulated in the same manner as food, consequently monitored by the Food and Drug Administration (FDA). However, many were frustrated with the restrictions of the FDA; as a result, Congress passed the Dietary Supplement Health and Education Act (DSHEA) in 1994, which protected dietary supplements from being required to demonstrate proof of efficacy or safety (Kreider et al., 2004; Dhar et al., 2005) (see Chapter 18). Under this act the FDA no longer has regulatory control of supplements, which are defined as *any product taken by mouth that contains a dietary ingredient intended to supplement the diet.* They are now classified as foods, not as food additives or drugs, and include vitamins, minerals, amino acids, herbs or botanicals, substances such as glandulars, enzymes, organic tissues, and metabolites. Manufacturers are allowed to publish limited information about the benefits of dietary supplements in the form of statements of support, as well as so-called structure and function claims. This results in a great deal of printed material that can be confusing to athletes at the point of sale of nutritional products.

Research suggests that the Internet, family members, friends, physicians, or pharmacists guide supplement choices for female athletes; whereas the store nutritionist, fellow athletes, friends, or coachs, advise on supplement decisions for the male athlete (Froiland et al., 2004; Kristiansen et al., 2005). Many believe that ergogenic aids will improve their performance and assist in recovery. As in the past and probably in the future, many of these ergogenic aids are not supported by scientific studies. In fact, many act only as placebos.

Many of these supplements confer no performance or health benefit, and some may actually be detrimental to both performance and health when taken for prolonged periods. They may contain excessive doses of potentially toxic ingredients or contain significant amounts of ingredients not approved by the IOC, the World Anti-Doping Agency, the National Collegiate Athletic Association (NCAA), Major League Baseball, and the National Football League (NFL) (Maughan, 2005). Recent research suggests that performance-enhancing substances such as anabolic-androgenic steroids, tetrahydrogestrinone, and androstene-dione (andro); stimulants such as ephedra; and nonsteroidal agents such as recombinant human erythropoietin (rHuEPO), human growth hormone (HGH), creatine, and β-hydroxy-β-methylbutyrate (HMB) may cause serious side effects, including adverse cardiovascular changes and sudden death (Dhar et al., 2005). A list of commonly used supplements and their claims and validity can be found in Table 23-2.

Regardless of the reasons for supplement use, sports nutritionists need to know how to evaluate the scientific merit of articles and advertisements about exercise and nutrition products so they can separate marketing hype from scientifically based training and nutrition practices.

Muscle-Building Supplements

Muscle-building supplements include creatine, HMB, prohormones, branched-chain amino acids (BCAA), essential amino acids (EAA), glutamine, protein, high calorie powders and/or protein fortified beverages and bars, and other compounds listed in Table 23-1.

Amino Acids

Protein or amino acid supplementation in the form of powders or pills is not necessary and should be discouraged. Taking large amounts of protein or amino acid supplements can lead to dehydration, hypercalciuria, weight gain, and stress on the kidney and liver. Taking single amino acids or in combination, such as arginine and lysine, may interfere with the absorption of certain other essential amino acids. An additional concern is that substituting amino acid supplements for food may cause deficiencies of other nutrients found in protein-rich foods such as iron, zinc, niacin, and thiamin.

Athletes and coaches need to realize that amino acid supplements taken in large doses have not been tested in human subjects, and no margin of safety is available. It is important for the health professional to develop a strategy to approach and discuss this supplement use effectively with both athletes and coaches.

β-Hydroxy-β-Methylbutyrate (HMB)

HMB is an important compound made in the body and a metabolite of the essential amino acid leucine. Supplementing with 1.5 g to 3 g/day of calcium HMB has been reported to increase muscle mass by approximately 0.5 to 1 kg over that of controls during 3 to 6 weeks of strength training, particularly in untrained athletes initiating training and the elderly (Kreider et al., 2003). Several studies done with both animals and humans have found that subjects supplemented with HMB have less stress-induced muscle protein breakdown. In one study the volunteers supplemented with HMB had greater strength gains compared with the control group. However, it is interesting to point out that the control group started out much stronger than the HMB-supplemented group; therefore it is not surprising that the control group, who were more highly trained, had lesser strength gains from the same exercise protocol than the lesser-trained experimental HMB group. The effects of HMB supplementation in trained athletes is less clear, with most studies reporting nonsignificant gains in muscle mass, possibly as a result of a greater variability in response to HMB supplementation (Palisin and Stacy, 2005). Additional research is necessary to determine the effectiveness of this dietary supplement in athletes.

Creatine

Creatine is an amino acid normally produced in the body from arginine, glycine, and methionine. Most of the creatine in the diet comes from meat, but half of the body's supply is manufactured in the liver and kidneys. It supplies most of the energy for short-term, maximum exercise such as base running and stealing, swinging the bat, and throwing. When creatine stores in the muscles are depleted, ATP synthesis is prevented, and energy can no longer be supplied at the rate required by the working muscle (see "Resynthesizing Adenosine Triphosphate" earlier in chapter). In normal healthy persons about 40% of muscle creatine exists as free creatine; the remainder combines with phosphate to form creatine phosphate (CP), which serves as the cell's energy tank to provide rapid phosphate bond energy to resynthesize ATP as mentioned earlier. About 2% of the body's creatine is broken down to creatinine before excretion by the kidneys daily. For meat eaters, dietary intake of creatine is about 1 g daily. The body also synthesizes about 1 g of creatine per day, for a total production of approximately 2 g daily. The normal daily excretion of creatine is about 2 g for most persons. It appears that vegetarians may be at the highest risk of not having enough creatine. Vegetarian athletes with lower stores of creatine demonstrate a greater uptake of creatine after supplementation than athletes with higher stores.

Creatine supplementation elevates muscle creatine levels and facilitates the regeneration of creatine phosphate (CP), which in turn helps to regenerate ATP. Numerous studies have indicated that creatine supplementation increases body mass or muscle mass during training with few untoward effects (Kreider et al., 2003).

Creatine absorption appears to be enhanced when consumed with a high-carbohydrate sports drink or juice. One study assessed the effects of creatine supplementation in 25 NCAA Division I football athletes who were engaged in resistance training. Participants in the study who received the recommended loading dosage mixed with 500 ml of Gatorade compared with a placebo showed that supplementation concurrent with resistance and anaerobic training positively affected cell hydration status and enhanced performance variables such as strength, peak torque, knee flexion, percent torque decrement, anaerobic power, and capacity.

Once creatine is taken up by the muscles, it is trapped within the muscle tissue. It is estimated that muscle creatine stores decline slowly and will still be elevated 2 to 3 months after ingestion of 20 g for 5 days. Whereas the original loading of creatine used the regimen of 20 g for 5 days, current thought is to do away with the loading phase and simply consume creatine at a lower dose of 2 to 5 g daily. Human muscle appears to have an upper limit of creatine storage; thus creatine presumably will be of little benefit to someone with an already high concentration of muscle creatine or to one who has been ingesting high doses of creatine for many weeks.

Creatine supplementation does not enhance endurance activities, but it is associated with an increase in body weight and lean body mass of around 2 to 6 lb, which is due either to fluid retention or enhanced skeletal muscle synthesis. This weight gain might interfere with the performance of some athletes. Although there are no scientific reports of dangerous side effects, there have been anecdotal descriptions of athletes who have had muscle strains and pulls and dehydration problems while taking creatine supplements. This is a bigger problem for athletes who play in hot, humid environments and for those who do not drink enough water.

Because creatine is an amino acid, some have suggested that supplementation may cause renal stress or liver damage, although no studies have reported this consequence. There is no evidence of this when supplementation is at recommended doses of 5 g/day.

Prohormones

Androstenedione, 4 androstenediol, 19-nor-4-androstenedione, 19-nor-4-androstenediol, 7-keto dehydroepiandrosterone (DHEA) and 7-keto DHEA are naturally derived precursors to testosterone and other anabolic steroids. Androstenedione is an anabolic androgenic steroid used to increase blood testosterone levels for the purpose of increasing strength and lean body mass, although there is no research that androstenedione or its related compounds has that effect in humans.

Prohormones are popular among bodybuilders because of their belief that they are natural boosters of anabolic hormones. Although theoretically prohormones may increase testosterone levels, there is no evidence that these compounds affect training adaptations in younger men with normal hormone levels. Many studies indicate that they may even increase estrogen levels and LDL cholesterol levels and reduce HDL cholesterol.

Dehydroepiandrosterone. DHEA is a weak androgen and product of dehydroandrosterone-3-sulfate (DHEA-S) and is used to elevate testosterone levels. It is precursor to the more potent androgens testosterone and dihydrotestosterone. Although DHEA-S is the most abundant circulating

Performance Enhancement

Performance enhancement supplements are pills, drinks, bars, or gels that improve speed, strength, or performance or minimize or delay fatigue. Supplements already described to help build body mass and reduce weight or excess body fat may also enhance exercise performance.

Erythropoietin. Erythropoietin (EPO) is commonly used to keep up the body's production of red blood cells in patients with bone marrow suppression such as patients with leukemia or who are receiving chemotherapy or those with renal failure (see Chapters 36 and 37). In athletes injections are used to increase the serum hematocrit and oxygen-carrying capacity of the blood and thus enhance Vo_2max and endurance (Rush, 2004). EPO use as an ergogenic aid is difficult to detect because it is a hormone produced by the kidneys, although newer blood tests can detect its use. Typically athletes with elevated hematocrit have been banned from endurance sports for suspected EPO misuse; however, despite its ban by the IOC, it is still commonly abused. Drastically high hematocrit combined with exercise-induced dehydration can lead to thick or viscous blood, which can lead to coronary or cerebral vascular occlusions, heart attack, or stroke. EPO can also cause elevated blood pressure, flulike symptoms, and elevated potassium levels (Rush, 2004).

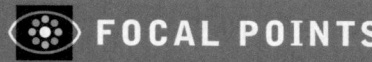

FOCAL POINTS

- Nutrition plays a role in training and conditioning, competition, and overall sports performance. It can also help to prevent injuries, enhance recovery from exercise, help maintain body weight, and improve overall health.
- Professionals in the field need to have a good working knowledge and understanding of exercise science and sports nutrition so they can help their clients perform close to their potential, whether they are competitive athletes or weekend warriors just trying to maintain health.
- Registered dietitians who desire to work with recreational or competitive athletes need to keep abreast of the latest trends in ergogenic aids, many of which are nutritional.
- A new credential called the Certified Specialist in Sports Dietetics (CSSD) has been established for dietitians who meet the educational and professional criteria to take a national examination and become certified through the Commission on Dietetic Registration (CDR).

CLINICAL SCENARIO 1

Maria is a 47-year-old wife and mother of three teenagers. She is a dedicated long-distance triathlete. Her daily 5:30 AM workout during the week includes 15 to 20 minutes of stretching, 1 hour of running approximately 8 to 9 miles in the heat and humidity of South Florida, and another 15 to 20 minutes of cool down. On weekends she adds an additional 1 to 2 hours of workout time of additional running, cycling, swimming, or a brick workout of a run-swim-run or run-bike-run. Her periodization of training is on a four-quarter cycle, with two endurance base-building periods and two speed periods each year. She races one to two times each month (e.g., from the sprint triathlon of 0.25-mile swim, 10-mile bike, 3-mile run to the Ironman [2.4-mile swim, 112-mile bike, 26.2-mile run]).

Maria works as a medical receptionist and must be in the office by 8 AM. She often skips breakfast in lieu of driving her kids to school, eats lunch from the local "healthy" fast-food restaurant, and eats dinner while carpooling kids from sports, while preparing dinner, while reading, or while watching TV with her husband.

Within the past 6 months Maria feels run down. She suspects it may be due to her schedule or the beginning of the perimenopausal period. Maria would like to have more energy during training and the remainder of the day but finds it difficult to eat more food without gaining body fat.

She needs quick, easy, and practical meal suggestions and is open to supplementation if her diet cannot meet her daily dietary needs.

✳Nutrition Diagnosis: Knowledge deficit related to preparation of easy, nutritious meals for an active lifestyle as evidenced by diet and activity records and request for information.

1. What seems to be the cause of Maria's energy problems—eating schedule? Skipped meals? Menopause?
2. What are some easy-to-consume complete meals that Maria can eat in the car on the way to work?
3. What kinds of foods and beverages can Maria take to training that can assist with the recovery process and her energy levels?
4. How much protein would Maria need for her weight of 130 lb, height of 5 ft 6 in, and activity level?
5. What types of fast, convenience foods can Maria order at the office or prepare at home to take to work that will help her enhance her glycogen stores and build her energy reserve.
6. Can Maria benefit from eating smaller meals and snacks throughout the day to keep her energy levels high?
7. What types of nutrition issues might Maria be facing over the next few years as she enters menopause? What key nutrients will she need to emphasize?

CLINICAL SCENARIO 2

Ben is a 21-year-old active college student who is interested in building muscle mass and losing body fat. His height is 5 ft 8 in, and his weight is 160 lb. He cannot understand why he is not losing body fat since he works out twice a day, includes resistance training and cardiovascular exercise, and eats the following:

Before breakfast:
> 1 protein bar with 45 g of protein and 300 calories

After workout:
> 1 protein drink with 30 g of protein

Breakfast:
> 1 protein smoothie with berries and 60 g of protein
> 1 oatmeal with 1 whey protein scoop (25 g of protein)

Snack:
> 3 oz bologna or ham

Lunch:
> 1 turkey sandwich with 6-9 oz of protein, lettuce, and tomato
>
> Before afternoon workout:
> 1 protein bar with 60 g of protein

After workout:
> Protein drink with 45 g of protein

Dinner:
> ½ chicken, string beans, and a lettuce salad with olive oil

Ben says that, although he is very disciplined, he has weekend splurges of a pizza and a six-pack of beer, as well as chips, ribs, and nuts during football, basketball, and baseball season. He does not work out on the weekends.

✳**Nutrition Diagnosis:** Excessive protein intake related to frequent intake of protein bars and supplemental beverages, as evidenced by an intake of 265 gm of protein per day from these products compared to RDA of 55 to 75 gm per day for normal growth and development.

1. How many grams of protein is Ben consuming? What is his protein per kilogram of body weight consumption? Can this be a contributing factor to his difficulty with losing body fat?
2. What level of protein intake would you recommend for him? Is this different from the RDA for normal growth and development? Are there healthier sources of protein that he can consume?
3. What is the calorie cost of his weekend splurges? Are they in excess of his calorie needs? And, if so, by how much? What type of recovery beverages and protein dosages may be more suitable for Ben to consume? What additional questions would you ask Ben about his bars and supplements?
4. What nutrients are in deficient amounts in Ben's diet? Including what foods in his diet would be beneficial?
5. What are other changes Ben can make on the weekends? What foods and exercise will help him reduce his body fat and manage his weight better?

USEFUL WEBSITES

American College of Sports Medicine
www.acsm.org

American Council on Exercise
www.acefitness.org

American Sport Education Program
www.americanrunning.org

Australian Institute of Sport
www.ausport.gov.au

ConsumerLab.com
www.consumerlab.com

Gatorade Sports Science Institute
www.gssiweb.com

International Society of Sports Nutrition
www.theissn.org

Sports and Cardiovascular and Wellness Dietitians (SCAN) of the American Dietetic Association
www.scandpg.org

Supplement Watch, Inc.
www.supplementwatch.com

Sport Science
www.sportsci.org

References

Abood DA et al: Nutrition education intervention for college female athletes, *J Nutr Educ Behav* 36:135, 2006.

Achten J, Jeukendrup AE: Optimizing fat oxidation through exercise and diet, *Nutrition* 20(7-8):716, 2004.

Anderson LL et al: Effect of resistance training and combined with timed ingestion of protein muscle fiber size and muscle strength, *Metabolism* 54:151, 2005.

Backhouse SH et al: Effect of carbohydrate and prolonged exercise on affect and perceived exertion, *Med Sci Sports Exerc* 37:1768, 2005.

Bahrke MS, Yesalis CE: Abuse of anabolic androgenic steroids and related substances in sport and exercise, *Curr Opin Pharmacol* 4:614, 2004.

Baker LB, et al: Sex differences in voluntary fluid intake by older adults during exercise, *Med Sci Sports Exerc* 37:789, 2005.

Berning J, Steen S: *Nutrition for sport & exercise*, ed 2, Gaithersburg, Md, 1998, Aspen Publishers, Inc.

Bohe J: Human muscle protein synthesis is modulated by extracellular not intramuscular availability, *J Physiol* 552:315-324, 2003.

Borer KT: Physical activity in the prevention and amelioration of osteoporosis in women: interaction of mechanical, hormonal and dietary factors, *Sports Med* 35:779, 2005.

Broeder CE: Oral andro-related prohormone supplementation: do the potential risks outweigh the benefits? *Can J Appl Physiol* 28:102, 2003.

Broeder CE et al: The andro project: the physiological and hormonal influences of androstenedione supplementation in men 35-65 years old participating in a high intensity resistance training program, *Arch Intern Med* 160(20):3093, 2000.

Byrne C et al: Water versus carbohydrate electrolyte replacement during loaded marching under heat stress, *Mil Med* 170 (8):715-721, 2005.

Clarke AS, Henderson LP: Behavioral and physiological responses to anabolic-androgenic steroids, *Neurosci Biobehav Rev* 27:413, 2003.

Coyle EF: Fluid and fuel intake during exercise, *J Sports Sci* 22:39, 2004.

Dhar R et al: Cardiovascular toxicities of performance-enhancing substances in sports, Mayo Clin Proc 80(10):1307-1315, 2005.

DiLuigi L et al: Androgenic-anabolic steroids abuse in males, *J Endocrinol Invest* 28 (Suppl 3):81S, 2005.

Dorfman L: *The vegetarian sports nutrition guide*, New York, 2000, John Wiley & Sons.

Dunford M: *Sports nutrition: a practice manual for professionals*, ed 4, Chicago, 2006, American Dietetic Association.

Evans NA: Current concepts in anabolic-androgenic steroids, *Am J Sports Med* 32:534, 2004.

Froiland K et al: Nutrition supplement use among college athletes and their sources of information, *Int J Sport Nutr Exerc Metabol* 14(1):104-120, 2004.

Grandjean AC et al: Hydration: issues for the 20th century, *Nutr Rev* 61:261-, 2003.

Hartgens F, Kuipers H: Effects of androgenic-anabolic steroids in athletes, *Sports Med* 34:513, 2004.

Havemann L et al: Fat adaptation followed by carbohydrate loading compromises high intensity sprint performance, *J Appl Physiol* 100:194, 2005.

Herbold NH et al: Traditional and nontraditional supplement use by collegiate female varsity athletes, *Int J Sport Nutr Exerc Metab* 14:586, 2004.

Herrmann M et al: Homocysteine increases during endurance exercise, *Clin Chem Lab Med* 41:1518, 2003.

Herrmann M et al: Altered vitamin B_{12} status in recreational endurance athletes, *Int J Sport Nutr Exerc Metabol* 15:433, 2005.

Hew TD: Women hydrate more during a marathon race: hyponatremia in the Houston Marathon: a report on 60 cases, *Clin J Sport Med* 15:148, 2005.

Hulmi JJ et al: Protein ingestion prior to strength exercise affects blood hormones and metabolism, *Med Sci Sports Exerc* 37: 1990, 2005.

Institute of Medicine, Food and Nutrition Board: *Dietary reference intakes (DRIs) for energy and the macronutrients, carbohydrate, fiber, fat, fatty acids, cholesterol, protein and amino acids,* Washington, DC, 2002, National Academies Press.

Institute of Medicine, Food and Nutrition Board: *Dietary reference intakes (DRIs) for water, potassium, sodium and chloride and sulfate,* Washington, DC, 2004, National Academies Press.

Jentjens R, Jeukendrup A: Determinants of post-exercise glycogen synthesis during short-term recovery, *Sports Med* 33:117, 2003.

Kerksick C, Leutholz B: Nutrient administration and resistance training, *J Int Soc Sports Nutr* 2(1):50, 2005.

Konig D et al: Exercise and oxidative stress: significance of antioxidants with reference to inflammatory, muscular, and systemic stress, *Exerc Immunol Rev* 7:108, 2001.

Koopman R et al: Combined ingestion of protein and carbohydrate improves protein balance during ultra-endurance exercise, *Am J Physiol Endocrinol Metabol* 287(4)E:712, 2004.

Kreider R et al: Long-term creatine supplementation does not significantly affect clinical markers of health in athletes, *Mol Cell Biochem* 244:95, 2003.

Kristiansen M et al: Dietary supplement use by university athletes at a Canadian university, *Int J Sports Nutr Exerc Metab* 15:195, 2005.

Leder BZ et al: Oral androstenedione administration and serum testosterone concentrations in young men, *JAMA* 283:779, 2000.

Maughan RJ: Contamination of dietary supplements and positive drug tests in sport, *J Sports Sci* 23:883, 2005.

McArdle W et al: *Exercise physiology*, ed 5, Baltimore, Md, 2004, Williams & Wilkins.

Millard-Stafford et al: Recovery from run training: efficacy of a carbohydrate-protein beverage? *Int J Sports Exerc Metabol* 15:610, 2005.

Murray R: Fluids, electrolytes, and exercise. In Danford M, editor: *Sports nutrition: a practice manual for professionals,* ed 4, Washington, DC, 2006, American Dietetic Association.

Neiper A: Nutritional supplement practices in UK junior national track and field athletes, *Br J Sports Med* 39:645, 2005.

Noakes TD et al: Three independent biological mechanisms cause exercise-associated hyponatremia: evidence from 2,135 weighed competitive performances, *Proc Natl Acad Sci* 102:18550, 2005.

Palisin T, Stacy JJ: Beta-hydroxy-methylbutyrate and its use in athletics, *Curr Sports Med Rep* 4:220, 2005.

Peake JM: Vitamin C: effects of exercise and requirements with training, *Int J Sport Nutr Exerc Metabol* 13:125, 2003.

Peters HP et al: Potential benefits and hazards of physical activity and exercise on the gastrointestinal tract, *Gut* 48:435, 2001.

Petrie HJ et al: Nutritional concerns for the child and adolescent competitor. *Nutrition,* 20:620, 2004.

Rush S: Just say no, *Am College Sport Med Health Fitness J* 8(2): 22, 2004.

Sen CK: Antioxidants in exercise nutrition, *Sports Med* 31:891, 2001.

Shirreffs SM et al: Fluid and electrolyte for preparation and recovery from training and competition, *J Sport Sci* 22(1):57, 2004.

Sinclair L, Hinton P: Prevalence of iron deficiency with and without anemia in recreationally active men and women, *J Am Diet Assoc* 105:975, 2005.

Siu PM, Wong SH: Use of the glycemic index: effects on feeding patterns and exercise performance, *J Physiol Anthropol Appl Human Sci* 23(1):1, 2004.

Spodaryk K: Iron metabolism in boys involved in intensive physical training, *Physiol Behav* 75(1-2):201, 2002.

Stevensen E, et al: The metabolic responses to high carbohydrate meals with different glycemic indices consumed during recovery from prolonged exercise, *Int J Sport Nutr Exerc Metabol* 15:291, 2005.

Stofan J et al: Sweat and sodium losses in NCAA football players: a precursor to heat cramps? *J Sport Nutr Exerc Metabol* 15:641, 2005.

Tauler P et al: Diet supplementation with vitamin E, vitamin C and beta carotene cocktail enhances basal neutrophil antioxidant enzymes in athletes, *Pflugers Arch* 443:791, 2002.

Trenton AJ, Currier GW: Behavioral manifestations of anabolic steroid use, *CNS Drugs* 19(7):571, 2005.

Twerenbold R et al: Effects of different sodium concentrations in replacement fluids during prolonged exercise in women, *Br J Sports Med* 38:790, 2004.

Unnithan VB, Goulopoulou S: Nutrition for the pediatric athlete, *Curr Sports Med Rep* 3(4):206, 2004.

Urhausen A et al: Are the cardiac effects of anabolic steroid use in strength athletes reversible? *Heart* 90:473, 2004.

vanHamont D et al: Reduction in muscle glycogen and protein utilization with glucose feeding during exercise, *Int J Sport Nutr Exerc Metabol* 15:350, 2005.

Venkatraman JT, Pendergast DR: Effect of dietary intake on immune function in athletes, *Sports Med* 32:323, 2002.

Waller MF, Haymes EM: The effects of heat and exercise on sweat iron loss, *Med Sci Sport Exerc* 28:197, 1996.

Watson TA et al: Antioxidant restriction and oxidative stress in short-duration exhaustive exercise, *Med Sci Sports Exerc* 37:63, 2005.

Williams M: Dietary supplements and sports performance: introduction and vitamins, *J Int Soc Sports Nutr* 1(2):1, 2004.

Williams M: Dietary supplements and sport performance: minerals, *J Int Soc Sports Nutr* 2(1):43, 2005.

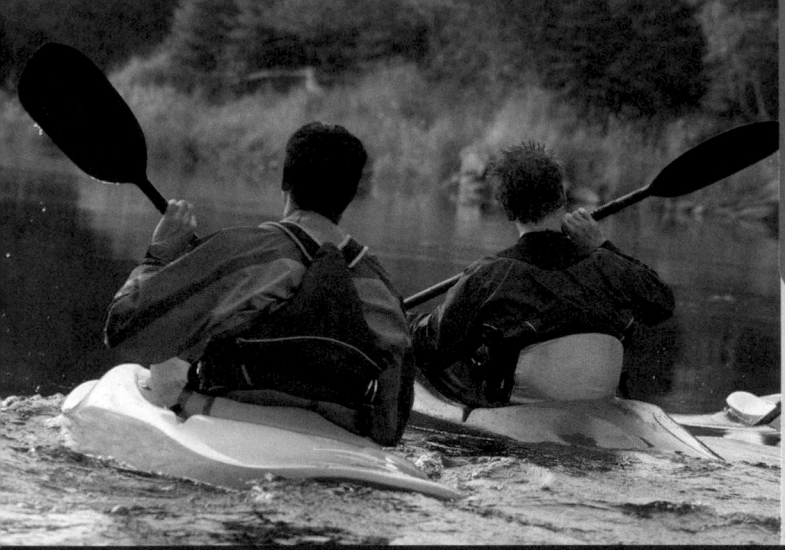

CHAPTER 24

John J. B. Anderson, PhD

Nutrition and Bone Health

KEY TERMS

age-related osteoporosis (type 2) loss of bone mineral density in both cortical and trabecular bone that occurs in elderly of both sexes after age 70; characterized by hip and vertebral fractures, the latter may lead to back pain, loss of height, and "dowager's hump"

bisphosphonates drugs that act on osteoclasts to inhibit their resorption of bone tissue; examples include etidronate, alendronate, and pamidronate

bone densitometry measurement of bone using tissue absorption of x-rays (photons) by an instrument called a dual-energy x-ray absorptiometer

bone markers molecules or portions of molecules derived from bone tissue that can be measured in blood serum or urine; matrix markers include portions of collagen molecules, whereas bone cell markers include enzymes such as alkaline phosphatase

bone mineral content (BMC) bone accumulated before end of growth cessation; BMC is expressed in grams of mineral per centimeter of bone

bone mineral density (BMD) a measurement of bone mass after developmental period is complete; bone mineral density is expressed in grams per centimeter squared of bone

bone modeling the process by which bones grow in size and change their longitudinal and cross-sectional dimensions; bone formation by osteoblasts precedes bone resorption by osteoclasts; formation and resorption are usually spatially separated

bone remodeling the process by which bone is continually dismantled and reformed to repair itself, grow, adapt to external strains, and furnish calcium for other body needs

calcium homeostasis maintenance of serum calcium concentration at a set level; bone furnishes calcium ions for other tissue needs by calcium ion transfer from bone fluid to blood and by resorption of bone tissue via osteoclasts

calcidiol 25-hydroxy vitamin D; made in the liver; the precursor to 1,25 dihydroxy vitamin D

calcitriol 1,25-dihydroxy vitamin D, (1,25 (OH)2vit D); the hormonal form of vitamin D

cortical bone the compact bone of the shaft that surrounds the medullary cavity of the long bones

estrogen receptor (ER) cellular molecule that binds to estrogens, selective estrogen receptor modulators, and phytoestrogens before delivering these molecules to nuclear DNA for initiation of events typical of estrogen stimulation of the cell

estrogen replacement therapy (ERT) administration of estrogen molecules to replace the natural hormone, which declines drastically after menopause; now used only for treating menopausal symptoms

hydroxyapatite a crystalline structure composed of calcium phosphate and calcium carbonate in an organic collagen matrix that gives strength and rigidity to bones

intermittent parathyroid hormone (PTH) therapy action of PTH (as a drug) at low concentrations on osteoblasts to increase cell proliferation and stimulate new bone formation, which results in increased bone mineral density

osteoid the organic protein structure matrix of bone that gives strength and flexibility; consists mainly of collagen

osteoblast a bone cell responsible for the formation of bone

osteocalcin a vitamin K–dependent bone-specific protein that is released into blood from the resorbed bone matrix as well as from the osteoblasts that make it

osteoclast a bone cell responsible for the resorption and removal of bone

osteocyte a bone cell derived from an osteoblast that gets buried in mineralized bone after the bone forms; it maintains communication with osteoblasts on bone surfaces by cell processes passing through canaliculi

osteomalacia a condition of impaired mineralization caused by vitamin D and calcium deficiency

osteopenia too little bone mass during any stage of life

osteoporosis a loss of bone tissue to the point that the specific skeletal site is unable to sustain ordinary strains where a fracture may develop

peak bone mass (PBM) the greatest amount of bone accumulated at any age; typically peak bone mass occurs by approximately 30 years of age, but in some individuals it may appear at an earlier or even a later age

phytoestrogens estrogen-like molecules derived from soybeans, clover, flaxseeds, and other plant sources; isoflavone and lignan molecules act on estrogen receptors more like selective estrogen receptor modulators than true estrogens

postmenopausal or **estrogen/androgen deficient (type 1) osteoporosis** a loss of bone mineral density after significant declines of sex hormones, especially estrogens in women; involves primarily the trabecular bone tissue; characterized by fractures of the distal radius and ulna and crush fractures of the lumbar vertebrae

secondary osteoporosis a loss of bone density secondary to another disease, such as liver or renal disease

selective estrogen receptor modulator (SERM) molecules, including a specific class of drugs, that act on estrogen receptors in osteoblasts to promote the maintenance of bone tissue, but without undesirable effects on reproductive tissues that lead to breast or uterine cancers; examples include tamoxifen and raloxifene

trabecular bone (cancellous bone) the spongy bone found primarily in the knobby ends of the long bones, the iliac crest, scapula, and vertebrae

Adequate nutrition is essential for the development and maintenance of the skeleton (i.e., bone health). Although diseases of the bone such as osteoporosis and **osteomalacia** (a condition of impaired mineralization caused by vitamin D and calcium deficiency) have complex etiologies, the development of these diseases can be minimized by providing adequate amounts of nutrients throughout the life cycle. Of these diseases, osteoporosis is the most common and destructive of productivity and quality of life.

The number of people over 65 years in the United States is projected to reach almost 25% of the population by 2020, greatly increasing the numbers at risk for osteoporosis and doubling or tripling the number who will experience a hip fracture (Surgeon General's Report, 2004). The average life expectancy in the United States early in the 21st century is almost 81 years for women and 74 for men. As a result of the increasing numbers of elderly, osteoporosis with resulting hip fractures has become more significant in both morbidity and mortality in the United States, as well as in cost. For example, a 50-year-old woman will have a 50% chance of having an osteoporosis-related fracture during the remainder of her life (Cummings and Melton, 2002).

Although the use of bone-building nutrients is necessary even after the onset of osteoporosis, the benefits of adequate intakes of calcium and other nutrients during adulthood and the early life period of bone growth and development are still significant.

BONE STRUCTURE AND BONE PHYSIOLOGY

Bone is a term used to mean both an organ, such as the femur, and a tissue, such as trabecular bone tissue. Each bone (organ) contains bone tissues of two major types, trabecular and cortical. These tissues undergo bone modeling during growth (height gain) and bone remodeling after growth ceases.

Composition of Bone

Bone consists of an organic matrix or **osteoid**, primarily collagen fibers, in which salts of calcium and phosphate are deposited in combination with hydroxyl ions in crystals of **hydroxyapatite**. The cablelike tensile strength of collagen and the hardness of hydroxyapatite combine to give bone its great strength. Other components of the bone matrix include osteocalcin, osteopontin, and several other matrix proteins.

Types of Bone Tissue

Approximately 80% of the skeleton consists of compact or cortical bone tissue. Shafts of the long bones contain primarily **cortical bone**, which consists of osteons or Haversian systems that undergo continuous but slow remodeling, and both contain an outer periosteal layer of compact circumferential lamellae and an inner endosteal layer of trabecular tissue. The remaining 20% of the skeleton is **trabecular** or **cancellous bone** tissue, which exists in the knobby ends of the long bones, the iliac crest of the pelvis, the wrists, scapulas, vertebrae, and the regions of bones that line the marrow. Trabecular bone tissue is less dense than cortical bone tissue as a result of an open structure of interconnecting bony spicules that resemble a sponge in appearance; thus trabecular bone is also called spongy bone or spongiosa.

The elaborate interconnecting components (columns and struts) of trabecular bone tissue add support to the cortical bone tissue shell of the long bones and provide a large surface area that is exposed to circulating fluids from the marrow and is lined by a disproportionately larger number of cells than cortical bone tissue. Therefore trabecular bone tissue is much more responsive to estrogens or the lack of estrogens than cortical bone tissue (Figure 24-1). The loss of trabecular bone tissue late in life is largely responsible for the occurrence of fractures, especially those of the spine.

Bone Cells

Osteoblasts are responsible for the formation or production of bone tissue, and **osteoclasts** govern the resorption or breakdown of bone (also see "Bone Modeling and Bone

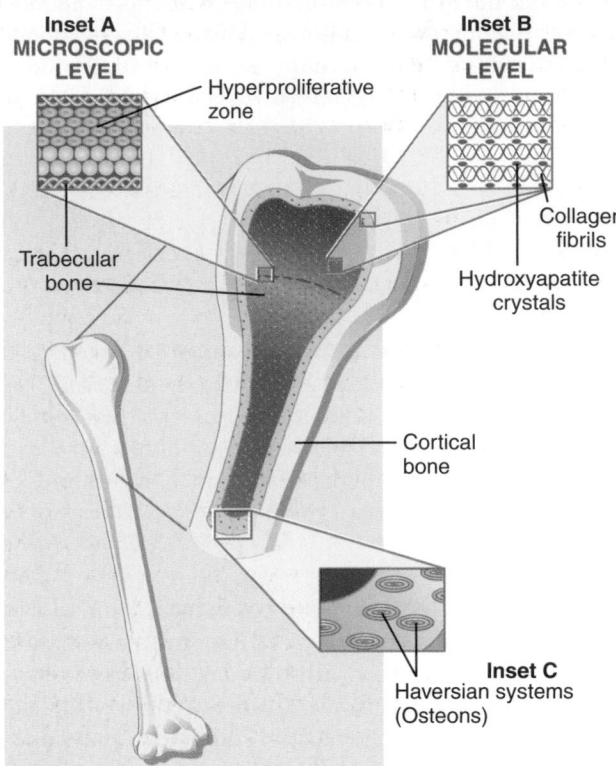

FIGURE 24-1 Schematic diagram of the structure of a long bone (hemisection of a long bone, such as the tibia). The ends of the long bones contain high percentages of trabecular (cancellous) bone tissue, whereas the shaft contains predominately cortical bone tissue. *Inset A* includes an enlarged section (approximately 100-fold) of the growth plate (epiphysis) and the subjacent hyperproliferative zone containing cartilage cells stacked like coins. Mineralization in this zone produces the primary spongiosa which is subsequently modeled by osteoblasts and osteoclasts to form the mature trabecular bone tissue. (Cartilage is replaced by bone in this region.) *Inset B* includes a section of collagen molecules (triple helices) surrounded by mineralized deposits (dark spheroids) at a magnification of approximately 1,000,000-fold. These collagen-mineral complexes exist in both trabecular and cortical bone tissues in association with other matrix proteins (not shown). *Inset C* shows the cross-section of half of the mid-shaft of a long bone (magnification approximately 10-fold). This section of cortical bone tissue contains vertical Haversian systems (osteons) that run parallel with the shaft axis (many are required to extend this system from one end of the shaft to the other). At the center of each osteon is a canal that contains an artery that supplies bone tissues with nutrients and oxygen, a vein for removing wastes, and a nerve for returning afferent relays to the brain. The lamellar structure of Haversian systems not only adds strength to the bone, but these units also undergo remodeling, which permits both repair of microfractures and adaptation to loads (strains) of the body bearing on the bone. *(Copyright John J.B. Anderson and Sanford C. Garner.)*

TABLE 24-1

Functions of Osteoblasts and Osteoclasts

Osteoblasts	Osteoclasts
Bone Formation	**Bone Resorption**

Synthesis of matrix proteins
  Collagen type 1 (90%)
  Osteocalcin and
    others (10%)
  Mineralization
Communication
  Secretion of cytokines
    that act on osteoblasts
	Degradation of bone
	  tissue via enzymes and
	  acid (H+) secretion
	Communication
	Secretion of cytokine
	    that act on osteoclasts

Remodeling" later in the chapter). The functions of these two cell types are listed in Table 24-1.

Two other important cell types also exist in bone tissue, **osteocytes** and bone-lining cells, both of which are derived from osteoblasts. The origin of the osteoblasts and osteoclasts is from primitive precursor cells found in bone marrow. These precursor or stem cells are now known to be stimulated by hormones and growth factors as part of their recruitment to bone tissue and differentiation to become mature functional bone cells.

Calcium Homeostasis

Bone tissue serves as a reservoir of calcium and other minerals that are used by other tissues of the body. **Calcium homeostasis**, or the process of maintenance of a constant serum calcium concentration, is almost totally reliant on this bone tissue source of calcium when the diet is inadequate. Bone tissue is also slowly dynamic, since it undergoes bone turnover via both modeling early in life and remodeling after skeletal growth (height gain) ceases.

Although 99% of the body calcium is found in the skeleton, the remaining 1% is critical to a great variety of indispensable life processes. The concentration of calcium in blood and other extracellular fluids is regulated by complex mechanisms that balance calcium intake and excretion with bodily needs. When calcium intake is not adequate, homeostasis is maintained by drawing on mineral from the bone to keep the serum calcium ion concentration at its set level (i.e., approximately 10 mg/dl). Depending on the amount of calcium required, homeostasis can be accomplished by drawing from two major skeletal sources: readily mobilizable calcium ions in the bone fluid or, through the process of osteoclastic resorption, from the bone tissue itself. The daily turnover of skeletal calcium ions (i.e., transfers in and out of bone) is surprisingly high, which supports the dynamic activity of bone tissue in calcium homeostasis.

Adaptation of the homeostatic mechanism regulating blood calcium concentration is achieved through two calcium-regulating hormones, parathyroid hormone (PTH) and 1,25 dihydroxy vitamin D3 (calcitriol). This calcium-regulatory system works more efficiently early in life, especially during the first few decades, but the efficiency undergoes a gradual decline in later life. For example, within a few years following menopause, urinary calcium losses from the body increase, but intestinal absorption of calcium does not increase sufficiently to offset the losses. Endogenous PTH activity, which directly contributes to bone loss, increases in both males and females during the decades of the 60s and beyond, even though PTH measurements typically remain within the normal range but at the high end. Calcium supplements typically help reduce the serum PTH concentration in elderly subjects.

The hormonal form of vitamin D, **calcitriol**, also plays an adaptational role by increasing the efficiency of intestinal calcium absorption in the upper half of the small bowel when dietary calcium is inadequate. This hormone is especially critical in the prepubertal and postpubertal growth years of girls and boys who have less than recommended intakes of calcium. However, it is much less effective in improving intestinal calcium absorption by women a decade or so after the onset of the menopause, even though serum calcitriol concentrations are elevated.

Calcitriol also has a direct effect on osteoblasts to increase the formation of several bone matrix proteins and other local factors needed for new bone formation and the suppression of bone degradation. The "bone-formation" effect of vitamin D only operates at reasonable intakes, (i.e., up to 1000 to 2000 units/day). At higher daily intakes calcitriol actually acts on osteoblasts to increase production of a molecule that stimulates osteoclastic activity. Thus, depending on total intake of vitamin D, calcitriol has a dual role in bone tissue (Table 24-2). The intake of vitamin D should be monitored closely, along with serum 25-hydroxy vitamin D, with a critical review of medication and dietary and supplemental intakes.

Bone Modeling

Bone modeling is the term applied to the growth of the skeleton until mature height is achieved. For example, during bone modeling long bones elongate and widen by undergoing great internal changes as well as external expansions in their structures. In modeling the process of formation of new bone tissue occurs first and is followed by the resorption of old tissue. In long bones growth occurs both at terminal epiphyses (growth plates that undergo hyperproliferation) and circumferentially in lamellae; at each location cells undergo division and contribute to the formation of new bone tissue (see Figure 24-1).

Bone modeling is typically completed in girls by ages 16 to 18 and in boys by ages 18 to 20. After growth (height gain) ceases, gains in bone tissue may continue by the process known as bone consolidation. The major event of the skeleton in early life is growth, whereas in later life it is the loss of bone (Figure 24-2). This concept underlines the inevitable decline of bone mass in the late stages of life: early gain and later loss.

TABLE 24-2		
Effects of Low vs. High Vitamin D Intake on Bone		
Vitamin D Intake	**Effect on Bone Cells**	**Effect on Bone Tissue**
Low (≈0.1 mg/kg)	Osteoblasts increase	Bone formation increases synthesis of osteocalcin and mineralization
High (≈1-5 mg/kg)	Osteoblasts decrease	Bone formation decreases, leading to increase in activity of osteoclasts

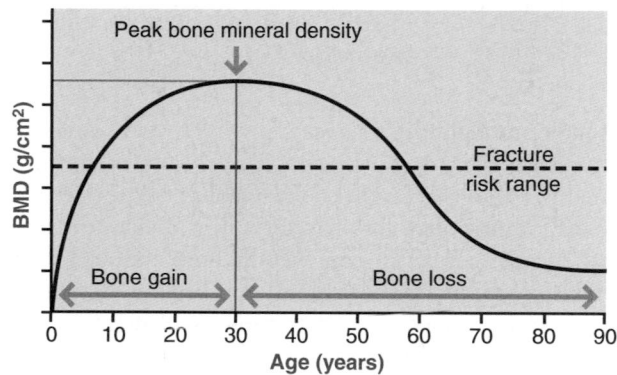

FIGURE 24-2 The early gain and later loss of bone in females. Peak bone mineral density (BMD) is typically achieved by age 30. Menopause occurs at approximately age 50 or within a few years after. Postmenopausal women typically enter the fracture risk range after age 60. Men have a more gradual decline in BMD, which starts at 50 years. *(Copyright John J.B. Anderson and Sanford C. Garner.)*

Bone Remodeling

After skeletal growth is completed, bone continuously undergoes remodeling in response to strains on the skeleton, adapts to changes in lifestyle factors and dietary intakes, maintains the set calcium concentration in extracellular fluids, and repairs microscopic fractures that occur over time. About 4% of the total bone surface is involved in remodeling at any given time as new bone is renewed continually at specific loci throughout the skeleton. Even in the mature skeleton, bone remains a dynamic tissue. Normal bone turnover is illustrated in Figure 24-3.

Both types of bone tissue are subject to the remodeling process, although the greater proportion occurs in the trabecular bone, especially at those sites located in areas subject to the greatest weight-bearing strains. Remodeling of both cortical and trabecular bone tissues occurs in response to both strains and the microscopic fractures that result from the gradual strain-related deterioration of bone tissue.

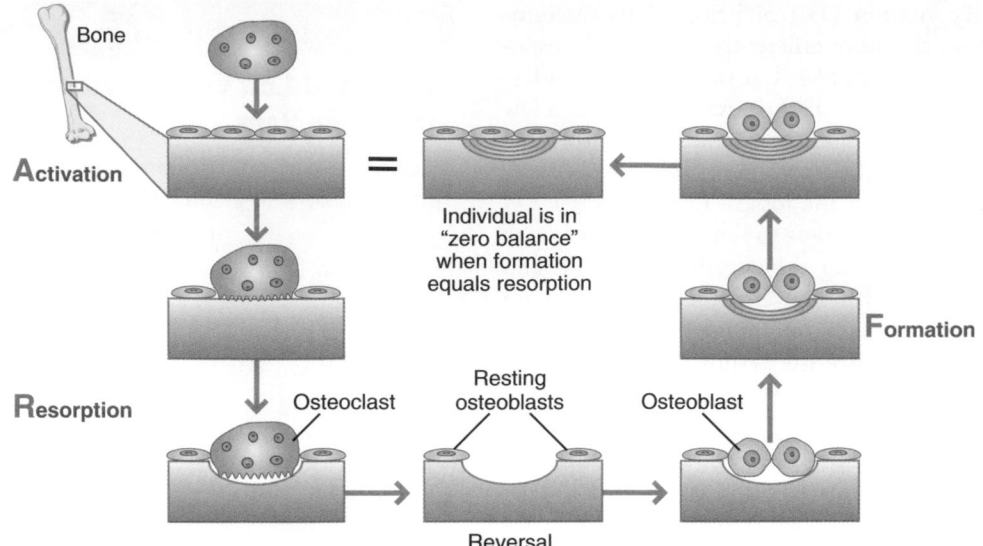

FIGURE 24-3 Normal bone turnover in healthy adults. (*Copyright John J.B. Anderson and Sanford C. Garner.*)

Bone remodeling is a process in which bone is continuously resorbed through the action of the *osteoclasts* and reformed through the action of the *osteoblasts*. After activation by specific hormones and cytokines, this dynamic turnover of bone tissue results in new healthy bone tissue. First, osteoclasts resorb both the mineral and organic components of bone by forming small cavities on bone surfaces; formation of new bone tissue follows. The resorptive process is rapid, and it is completed within a few days, whereas the refilling of these cavities by osteoblasts is slow (i.e., on the order of 3 to 6 months or even as long as a year or more in the elderly).

Trabecular bone especially declines following the menopause because of unopposed osteoclastic activity. In normal young adults the resorption and formation phases are tightly coupled, and the amount of bone mass is maintained at zero balance. In the elderly bone loss involves an uncoupling of the phases of bone remodeling with an increase of resorption over formation; bone loss occurs.

The remodeling process is initiated by the *activation* of preosteoclastic cells in the bone marrow. Interleukin (IL)-1 and other cytokines released from bone-lining cells (inactive osteoblasts) are considered to act as the triggers in the activation process of precursor stem cells in bone marrow. The preosteoclast cells from the bone marrow migrate to the surfaces of bone while differentiating into mature osteoclasts. The osteoclasts then cover a specific area of trabecular or cortical bone tissue. Acids and proteolytic enzymes released by the osteoclasts *resorb* both bone mineral and matrix on the surface of trabecular bone or cortical bone.

The *rebuilding* or *formation* stage involves secretion of collagen and other matrix proteins by the osteoblasts, also derived from precursor stem cells in bone marrow. Collagen polymerizes to form mature triple-stranded fibers, and other matrix proteins are secreted. Within a few days salts of calcium and phosphate begin to precipitate on the collagen fibers, developing into crystals of hydroxyapatite.

When the resorption and formation phases are in balance, the same amount of bone tissue exists at the completion of the formation phase as at the beginning of the resorption phase (see Figure 24-3). The benefit to the skeleton of this remodeling is the renewal of bone (i.e., new bone) without any microfractures. However, when dietary calcium is low, osteoclastic resorption becomes relatively greater than formation by osteoblasts because of a persistently elevated PTH concentration in blood (Figure 24-4). Then, large amounts of bone tissue are removed and typically not fully replaced. The net result is a decrease in both bone mineral content (BMC) and bone mineral density (BMD).

The action of PTH in promoting activity of the osteoclasts is countered by estrogen, which reduces the response of osteoblasts to PTH. PTH acts directly on osteoblasts which increase the production of IL-6 and other cytokines that in turn stimulate osteoclasts to resorb bone. Estrogen helps to block the production of PTH-stimulated cytokines. These steps of bone remodeling are illustrated in Figure 24-5.

Calcitonin, a vestigial hormone, may directly inhibit osteoclast activity (i.e., resorption), but the significance of its physiologic role in human subjects is not clear (see Chapter 3). However, calcitonin does have an important role as a drug for reducing bone resorption. Transient times between the onset of resorption and the completion of formation after a strong stimulation of activation typically takes 3 to 6 months in adolescents and young adults but 12 months or longer in later adulthood.

Bone Markers

Bone markers exist for both bone formation and bone resorption. Plasma bone-specific alkaline phosphatase is a marker of bone formation, although total plasma alkaline phosphatase may also be used. Markers of bone resorption include plasma cross-linked collagen telopeptides, urinary

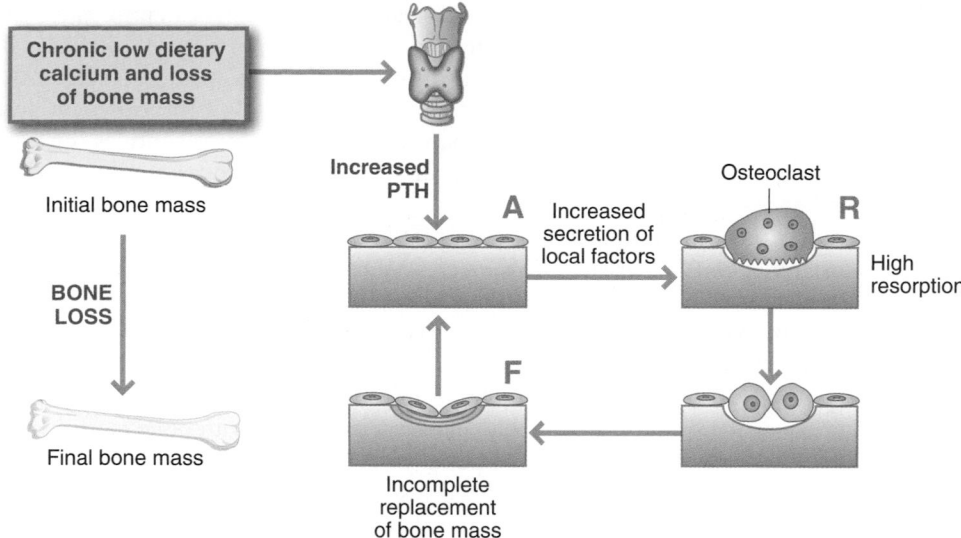

FIGURE 24-4 Effects of persistently elevated serum concentration of parathyroid hormone (PTH) on bone mass. *(Copyright John J.B. Anderson and Sanford C. Garner.)*

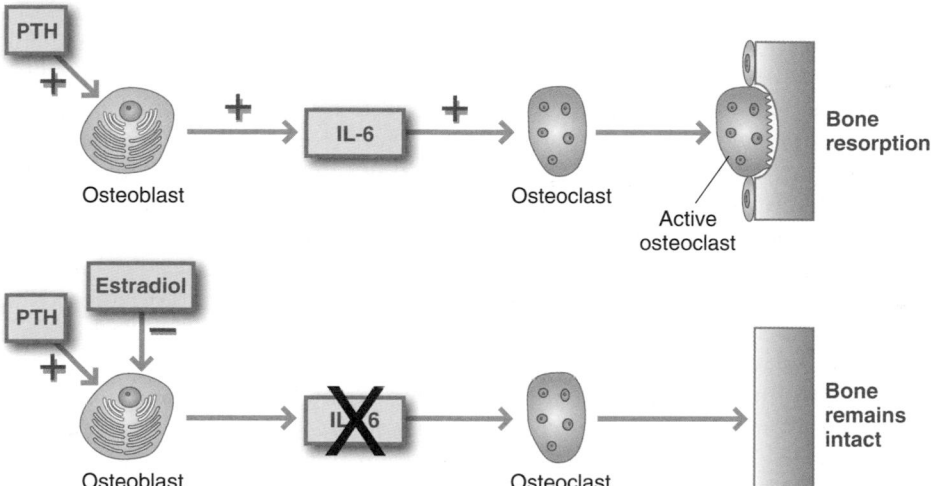

FIGURE 24-5 Interaction between osteoblasts and osteoclasts in bone remodeling. The role of parathyroid hormone (PTH) in stimulating osteoclasts to resorb bone *(upper)* is contrasted with the inhibitory action of estrogens on osteoblasts that negate the action of PTH *(lower)* *(Copyright John J.B. Anderson and Sanford C. Garner.)*

N-telopeptides (NTXs), and plasma tartrate-resistant acid phosphatase (TRAP). Osteocalcin, considered a bone formation marker, is also released following the resorption of bone matrix; therefore interpretation of its blood values is complicated by both formation and resorption, which typically occur simultaneously at several different skeletal sites.

BONE MASS

Bone mass is a generic term that refers to bone mineral content but not to bone mineral density. **Bone mineral content (BMC)** is more appropriately used in assessing the amount of bone accumulated before the cessation of growth (height gain), whereas **bone mineral density (BMD)** is better used to describe bone after the developmental period is completed. These measurements are often used interchangeably, but BMD is more useful for monitoring bone changes in adults. However, neither BMC nor BMD provides information on the microarchitectural (three-

dimensional) structural quality of bone tissue (i.e., index of risk of fracture).

Measurement of Bone Mineral Content and Bone Mineral Density

Bone densitometry measures bone mass on the basis of tissue absorption of photons produced by one or two monoenergetic x-ray tubes. Dual-energy x-ray absorptiometry (DEXA) is available in most hospitals and many clinics for the measurement of the total body and regional skeletal sites such as the lumbar vertebrae and the proximal femur (hip). Results of BMC measurements are expressed as grams of mineral per centimeter and BMD in grams per centimeter squared is calculated from the BMC divided by the width of the bone at the measurement site.

Computerized tomography (CT) may also be used to measure BMD (a true volumetric density) of the spine, but this technique has not yet been developed to measure the limbs. In the near future, more penetrating instruments are expected that will be able to assess both bone density and the 3-D quality of the bone tissue at different skeletal sites.

Ultrasound Measurements of Bone

Quantitative ultrasound measurements of the heel bone (calcaneus) and the kneecap are now possible. Measurements by ultrasound machines provide information on two properties, elasticity and strength of bone, which cannot be assessed by DEXA. The ultrasound values are not equivalent to the BMD measurements because ultrasound assesses the properties of collagen in the organic matrix rather than the mineral phase of bone tissue. Ultrasound instruments actually measure the velocity of sound waves transmitted through bone and broadband ultrasound attenuation (BUA). Measurements at the calcaneus correlate well with BMD measurements at this same skeletal site, meaning that low values by DEXA are typically mirrored by low values of BUA. Therefore ultrasound is about as good as DEXA in predicting the risk of fracture.

Accumulation of Bone Mass

During the growth periods of childhood and puberty and into early adulthood, formation exceeds the resorption of bone. **Peak bone mass (PBM)** is reached by 30 years of age or so (see Figure 24-2). The long bones stop growing in length by approximately age 18 in females and age 20 in males, but bone mass continues to accumulate for a few more years by a process known as consolidation (i.e., filling-in of osteons in the shafts of long bones). The age when BMD acquisition ceases varies, depending not only on diet but also on physical activity and strain loading on the skeleton (Wosje et al., 2000). The consumption of both calcium supplements and calcium-enriched foods contributes to increased bone accumulation in the young. In young adult women who have children, the loading related to lifting and carrying of children may also improve skeletal mass and density.

Peak Bone Mass

PBM is greater in men than in women because of their larger frame size. BMC, but not necessarily BMD, is typically lower in women. Both the lean and fat components of body composition contribute to these differences in bone mass. BMD is also greater in blacks and Hispanics than in whites and Asians, a factor that may be related to larger muscle mass. Hereditary factors also contribute to the extent of accumulation of PBM.

PBM is also related to both dietary calcium intakes and weight-bearing physical activity (Wosje et al., 2000). Calcium intake appears to be a critical factor in the early postmenarcheal growth of girls, especially under conditions of vitamin D insufficiency (Abrams et al., 2005; Tylavsky et al., 2005). The contribution of weight-bearing exercise to PBM during the growth and development period may be greater than that of calcium alone. Whether an interaction exists between these two variables is not yet clear, but a positive interaction between them appears to favorably affect measurements of BMD (Wosje et al., 2000).

Physical activity seems to be the most robust individual determinant of bone mass and BMD when it starts around the time of puberty and continues through adolescence.

When combined with adequate dietary calcium, physical activity appears to play a large supporting role in the development (i.e., early gains in bone mass) and subsequently in the maintenance of bone later in life in both men and women. Also, women who use oral contraceptives for several years may benefit after the menopause by having greater bone mass.

Finally, *body weight* (or body mass index) is a good indicator of greater BMC and BMD. Studies that adjusted for other factors reported that body weight was the most consistent factor related to bone mass, both in young adult and elderly women. The component of body composition more closely associated with bone mass is the lean body mass (skeletal muscle especially), which is correlated with bone mass during adulthood and especially during the later years of life. Sarcopenia, or age-related loss of skeletal muscle, and osteopenia are typically seen together in the elderly (Walsh et al., 2005).

Loss of Bone Mass

Age is an important determinant of BMD. If the age of a woman is known, her vertebral bone mass may be predicted with an accuracy of $\pm10\%$ (see *Clinical Insight:* Postmenopausal Women at High Risk for Hip Fracture).

At approximately age 40 BMD begins to diminish gradually in both sexes, but bone loss increases greatly in women after age 50 or the time of the menopause. A continuous loss thereafter in postmenopausal women occurs at rate of 1% to 2% per year over the next decade. Men continue to have bone loss, but at a much lower rate than women of the same age until age 70, when the loss rates are about the same for both genders. Loss of bone mass is the result of changes in the hormone-directed mechanisms that govern bone remodeling.

Cortical bone tissue and trabecular bone tissue undergo different patterns of aging. Loss of cortical bone eventually plateaus and may even cease late in life. Trabecular bone loss begins in both sexes as early as 40 years of age. Premenopausal loss of trabecular bone in women is much greater than that of cortical bone. Loss of both kinds of bone accelerates in women after the menopause, although trabecular bone is also lost at a much higher rate than cortical bone. Differences between normal and osteoporotic bone—both trabecular and cortical tissues—are shown in Figure 24-6.

The accelerated bone loss rate of 2% to 3% per year continues for between 5 and 10 years after menopause, and then the rate declines gradually to 0.5% to 1% per year thereafter. Some postmenopausal women lose bone at an even faster rate (Figure 24-7).

The typical bone loss in elderly females amounts to approximately 300 mg of calcium per day that is lost in both the urine and feces. If calcium balance is to be maintained, this amount must be replaced by absorbed calcium from the diet each day. Older women without estrogen lose more calcium in their urine than premenopausal women—as much as 100 mg more per day.

Calcium absorption is governed to a large extent by need and access to vitamin D; the body of an elderly person theoretically can adapt to reduced intakes of calcium to maintain

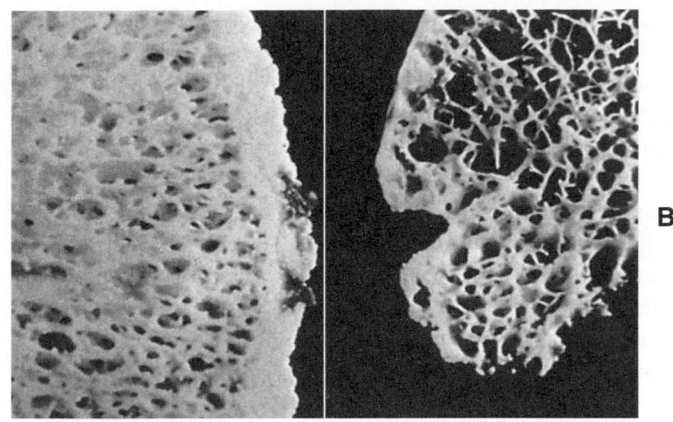

A   **B**

FIGURE 24-6 Difference between normal bone **(A)** and osteoporotic bone **(B)**. *(From Maher AB, Salmond SW, Pellino TA:* Orthopaedic nursing, *Philadelphia, 1994, Saunders, p. 469.)*

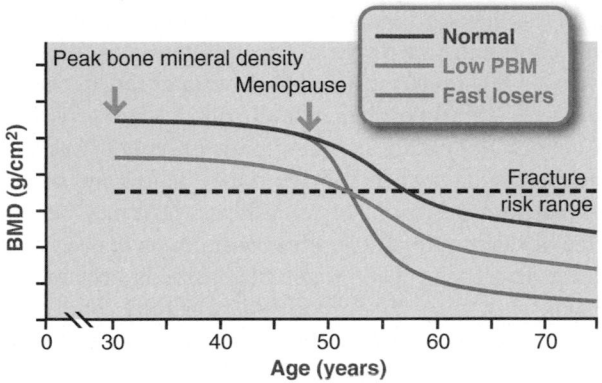

FIGURE 24-7 Variable patterns of bone loss of females following the onset of menopause at approximately 50 years of age. The rapid loss of bone mineral density (BMD) in some women referred to as *fast losers* is contrasted to the loss of *slow losers.* Women who develop low peak BMD have less bone mass than women with normal BMD, but they also can lose BMD either as slow or fast losers. *(Copyright John J.B. Anderson and Sanford C. Garner.)*

⬟ **CLINICAL INSIGHT**

Postmenopausal Women at High Risk for Hip Fracture

It is important to identify women who are at risk of developing osteoporosis as early as possible so that measures can be taken to monitor bone status and to prevent further bone loss. Since low bone mineral density (BMD) is a major risk factor for osteoporosis, its assessment is clinically useful. Assessment of bone status based on the existence of one or more risk factors such as age, height, weight, smoking status, alcohol consumption, drug use, calcium intake, exercise, frame size, and selected bone markers is not sufficiently accurate. BMD as measured by bone densitometry is more clinically useful. Typically total body BMD and the regional sites such as the proximal femur and lumbar vertebrae are measured by dual-energy x-ray absorptiometry. The machines that make these measurements are now readily available. Fees for the measurements are reasonable, and the procedures are safe and entail very low radiation exposure. In addition, the measurements are both precise and accurate. Low BMD itself is a risk factor for osteoporotic fractures.

A BMD measurement of an at-risk woman entering menopause (before becoming estrogen deficient) serves as a baseline for subsequent measurements as the individual becomes increasingly estrogen deficient and loses bone mass. This information helps physicians and patients make decisions about the need for and use of drug therapy such as bisphosphonates, parathyroid hormone drugs, and selective estrogen receptor modulators. For males or females on long-term glucocorticosteroid therapy, a BMD measurement may indicate the need for treatment with a bone-preserving medication or calcitonin.

---

calcium homeostasis, but at the expense of a loss of bone tissue. However, the vitamin D–adaptive mechanism involving calcitriol typically becomes less efficient with older age. In elderly women not on bone-conserving drug therapy, the achievement of calcium balance seldom occurs, even though calcium homeostasis can maintain a normal serum calcium concentration. This slightly negative calcium balance results because the action of hormones and other factors responsible for maintaining calcium balance—as well as the absorption of calcium—becomes less efficient with age. The decreased intestinal calcium absorption in females after 65 years of age and presumably in males of similar ages invariably leads to negative calcium balance.

The normal bone loss that occurs with aging in both sexes is related to the decline of osteoblastic function such as the reduced production of collagen, osteocalcin, osteopontin, and other matrix proteins. As a result of the uncoupling of the remodeling process, osteoclastic resorption ex-

ceeds formation with an increasing differential. Bone loss in men accelerates in later years, typically in ages 60 through 79, as other body functions begin to decline as well. The reason for bone loss in men is presumed to result from a decline in gonadal androgen production (i.e., testosterone).

Changes leading to age-related (type II) osteoporosis in both men and women are not well understood. Impaired calcitriol activity in the small intestine of older women is one important factor.

NUTRITION AND BONE

Not only are calcium, phosphate, and vitamin D essential for normal bone structure and function, but several other micronutrients also have essential roles in the development and maintenance of bone (Ilich and Kerstetter, 2000; Nieves, 2005). Nonnutrient plant molecules such as phytoestrogens

TABLE 24-3		
Recommended Intakes of Bone-Related Nutrients for Adults		
	Per Day	
Calcium	1500 mg/day for postmenopausal women, 1000-1200 for younger women	
Vitamin D	600-1000 units	
Magnesium	400-600 mg	
Manganese	2-5 mg	
Zinc	15 mg	
Boron	3 mg	
Copper	2-3 mg	
Vitamin K	500 mcg	

have been hypothesized to improve bone mass and density in postmenopausal women and older men, but most investigations of these dietary components have not supported the hypothesis.

Recommendations for the intakes of calcium and several bone-related nutrients by adults are shown in Table 24-3.

Calcium Intake

Calcium from Foods

Calcium intake in the primary prevention of osteoporosis has received much attention. The Institute of Medicine recommendations for calcium, vitamin D, and a few other nutrients are given as adequate intakes (AIs), because only the mean requirements for calcium and vitamin D during the stages of the life cycle could be quantified. The AI for calcium from preadolescence (age 11 years) through adolescence (up to 19 years) was increased to 1300 mg/day in the latest report. AIs for calcium are the same for each gender across the life cycle (see the dietary recommended intakes on inside front cover).

Calcium intakes typically do not meet the recommended AI for all ages beyond 11 years, especially females. According to NHANES data (NHANES, 2007), teen and adult women consume considerably less than the current AIs. Men are more likely to consume somewhat greater amounts than females, but they also do not meet the recommended levels after 50 years of age. These deficits translate, on average, into the need for roughly an additional 500 mg/day for teenage females and adult women.

Food sources are recommended first for supplying calcium needs because of the coingestion of other essential nutrients. Reaching AI levels of calcium from foods should be the first goal, but if insufficient amounts of calcium from foods are consumed, supplements of calcium should then be ingested to reach the age-specific AI.

Calcium from Supplements

Numerous studies of calcium supplementation in all age-groups and especially in females have typically shown sig-

nificant increases in spinal and total body BMD. A few studies have followed up the subjects who gained BMD on earlier supplementation, but without further supplements of calcium the mean BMD values of the treated groups reverted back to the mean values of the control groups. These reports suggest that the higher intakes need to be consumed consistently to maintain any gains in BMD from calcium supplements alone. Thus the question still remains of whether a brief 1-year gain in BMD resulting from a calcium supplement during early life (i.e., teenage years) may translate into later protection against osteoporosis. But it seems more likely that keeping the gains in BMD accrued before age 20 may best be met by a combination of regular physical activity *and* a reasonable consistent daily calcium intake that approaches the current AI.

Calcium Bioavailability

Calcium bioavailability from foods is generally similar to that of supplements. Calcium bioavailability from supplements containing various anion combinations is very good; however, a few preparations that contain citrate as the anion may have a slightly higher bioavailability.

Calcium bioavailability from foods is generally good, but from a few foods such as spinach it may be low and adversely affect calcium nutrition status. Wheat bread may be a good source of calcium for those who consume several servings of bread a day; green leafy vegetables such as broccoli, kale, and bok choy also have good bioavailability; and calcium from soybeans is very well absorbed. However, spinach and a few other high oxalate–containing vegetables have low calcium bioavailability. The consumption of dairy products, especially high-calcium milks, cheeses, and yogurts, appears to be the best way for most individuals to meet their daily calcium requirements. However, it is not the only way; nondairy sources of calcium such as almonds, tofu, calcium-fortified nondairy milks and juices, and dark-green leafy vegetables are excellent options.

Additional benefits of meeting calcium requirements from foods alone are that the foods containing calcium are also rich in several other nutrients needed for health in general, and for bone health in particular, and that the consumption of a calcium-rich diet from foods is also a marker of a balanced intake with respect to practically all micronutrients. The amount of calcium in major food sources is listed in Table 24-4.

Calcium Bioavailability from Calcium Supplements

Calcium bioavailability from calcium supplements depends on the anion used, but practically all calcium-containing supplements currently on the market have good bioavailability. Calcium citrate malate supplements appear to be absorbed slightly more efficiently than calcium carbonate and other calcium supplements, but the difference is typically only a couple of percentage points. Calcium carbonate can have a constipating effect that may be minimized by dividing the dose and taking more fluids and fiber. High-dose calcium supplements may reduce the absorption of

TABLE 24-4

Calcium in Selected Foods

Food/Portion	Calcium (mg)
Tofu, regular, ½ cup	434
Yogurt, part skim, 1 c	415
Sardines, in oil, drained, 3 oz	372
Collard greens, cooked, 1 c	357
Ricotta cheese, ½ c	337
Nonfat milk, 1 c	302
Pudding, vanilla 1 c	298
Whole milk, 1 c	291
Custard, 1 c	297
Buttermilk, 1 c	286
Ice milk, soft serve, 1 c	274
Swiss cheese, 1 oz	272
Turnip greens, cooked 1 c	249
Rhubarb, cooked, 1 c	212
Cheddar cheese, 1 oz	204
Spinach, cooked, 1 c	200
Pumpkin pie, ⅛ of 9-inch pie	150
Refried beans, canned, 1 c	141

Data from USDA Nutrient Database for Standard Reference, Release 18: *Nutrient Lists*, 2005, available at www.ars.usda.gov/Services/docs. htm?decid=9673, accessed September 1, 2006.

BOX 24-1

Potential Risks Associated With Excessive Calcium Supplementation

Contamination of bone meal or dolomite supplements with cadmium, mercury, arsenic, or lead
Urinary tract or renal stones in susceptible individuals
Hypercalcemia or milk alkali syndrome from extremely high intakes (>4000 mg/day)
Deficiency of iron and other mineral divalent cations resulting from decreased absorption
Constipation

---

nonheme iron and possibly zinc, magnesium, and other divalent cations, but additional evidence is needed to substantiate these potentially adverse interactions. Box 24-1 lists potential risks of calcium supplementation.

Calcium Fortification of Foods

This is another way to increase the consumption of calcium by females. Calcium is currently being added to some brands of orange juice and many brands of non-dairy milks at about 300 mg (30% DV)/1 cup of juice and to breads and other foods. Foods are considered to be a more preferable way to provide calcium than supplements because of the other nutrients contained in foods; therefore fortified foods should become more carefully factored into the diet toward achieving the total recommended calcium intake.

Vitamin D Intake

Adequate vitamin D intake is important, but there is still question about the exact amount to recommend. Excess needs to be avoided (see Chapter 3). Excessive vitamin D supplementation can induce hypercalcemia and raise the risk of soft-tissue calcifications, especially in the kidneys. However, excessive vitamin D intake is unusual; the far more common situation in the United States is inadequate vitamin D intake. The AIs for vitamin D across the life cycle are given in the DRIs inside front cover (see Appendix 51 for a table of food sources of vitamin D).

Sunlight exposure for skin biosynthesis of vitamin D may be a critical but typically insufficient source for el-derly people who commonly obtain little vitamin D from their foods and who live far from the equator. The skin of older individuals is less efficient in producing vitamin D following exposure to ultraviolet (UV) light because the skin is thinner in the elderly and it contains fewer cells that can synthesize vitamin D. In addition, elderly subjects living in nursing homes and similar institutions typically have little exposure to sunlight. Those who live at northern latitudes in the United States and Canada are at increased risk of osteoporosis because of limited UV light during winter months, leading to reduced serum vitamin D, increased serum PTH, and increased bone resorption (Pasco et al., 2004).

Vitamin D deficiency is associated with secondary hyperparathyroidism and increased bone turnover. Because low calcium intakes contribute to an elevation of serum PTH, bone resorption is also increased to keep the serum calcium ion concentration in the normal range (see Chapter 3).

Low levels of 25-hydroxy vitamin D have been found in free-living elderly women, as well as those living in nursing homes. Results from several studies suggest that supplementation of elderly subjects with vitamin D, even without a supplement of calcium, contributes to increased BMD or reductions in fractures. When the serum 25-hydroxy vitamin D status is normal, a calcium intake of 800 units/day may be adequate for the maintenance of bone and overall calcium metabolism, even in Iceland (Steingrimdottir et al., 2005). In studies of high calcium–consuming populations in Scandinavia, the Netherlands, and northern England, vitamin D supplements of elderly subjects have had little or no effect on BMD because serum 25-hydroxy vitamin D levels were generally adequate or higher (Tfelt-Hansen and Torring, 2004; Porthouse et al., 2005).

The winter-summer cycle of vitamin D formation by the skin in individuals in the higher latitudes of the northern hemisphere is thought to play a major role in the development of low bone mass during the postmenopausal period in women and at a later age in men. Vitamin D insufficiency even exists in 9- to 11-year-old girls in Maine whose serum **calcidiol** (formed in the liver and a precursor to calcitriol) concentration decreased 28% and serum PTH increased 15% between September and March (Sullivan et al., 2005).

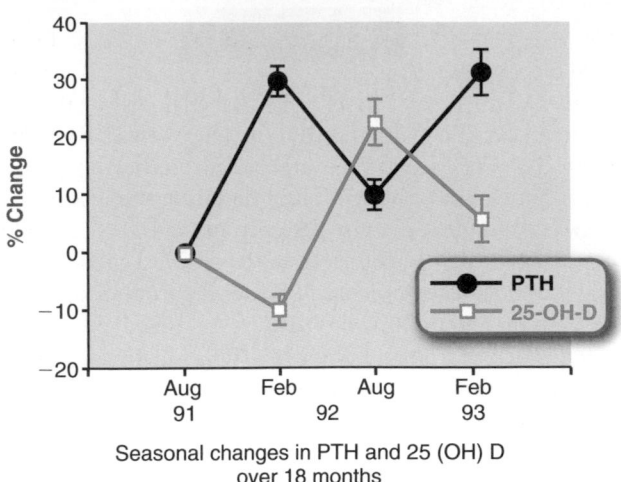

Seasonal changes in PTH and 25 (OH) D
over 18 months

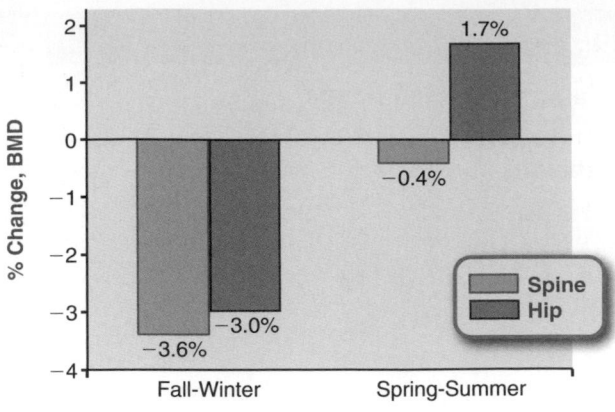

Percent change in bone mineral density of spine
and femoral neck in 15 older rural Maine
women, from fall-winter to spring-summer

FIGURE 24-8 Seasonal changes in parathyroid hormone (PTH), calcidiol (25-hydroxy vitamin D [25[OH]D]), and bone mineral density (BMD). *(Adapted with permission of the American Society for Bone and Mineral Research from Rosen et al., Bone Miner 25:83, 1994.)*

Similar results have been reported for other populations of children and adults living in northerly latitudes. Figure 24-8 illustrates the seasonal changes in serum 25-hydroxy vitamin D and PTH plus the BMD changes of vertebrae (spinal) and the hip.

Calcium and vitamin D supplements are often given together to elderly people to reduce the circulating concentration of PTH when it is at the upper end of the normal range (or possibly beyond this limit in a small percentage of elderly hyperparathyroid subjects). The combination of a daily supplement of calcium (1000 mg) and vitamin D (400 units) slightly improves BMD, but fractures are not statistically different between treated postmenopausal women and those receiving placebo (Jackson et al., 2006). Perhaps more vitamin D is necessary.

The combination of adverse seasonal effects on vitamin D production in the skin and low dietary intakes of vitamin D is now considered to be a major determinant of low BMD and increased risk of hip fractures among the elderly. Low calcium intakes generally accompany low vitamin D status in the United States because so few consume fish rich in vitamin D or D-fortified foods, especially milk.

Vitamin D supplementation reduces falls in ambulatory elderly women (Bischoff-Ferrari et al., 2004). The long-held concept that vitamin D improves skeletal muscle strength may be a component of the decline in falls, but further research is needed to establish this D-muscle relationship. Vitamin D supplementation of 1000 units/day is considered to be very safe (Vieth et al., 2007), and this amount is considerably below the UL of 2000 units for vitamin D. In fact, the UL for vitamin D is now considered to be well below the amount of vitamin D that can be safely taken as a daily supplement, which may be as much as 10,000 IU per day (Hathcock et al., 2007).

Because of this increasing prevalence of inadequate intake, a consensus of vitamin D investigators in the United States now recommends 700 to 800 units/day of vitamin D for adults to keep circulating 25-hydroxy vitamin D (calcidiol) within the normal range (i.e., ≈30 ng/ml [74.8 nmol/L] or higher) (Holick, 2005; Bischoff-Ferrari et al., 2005). A serum 25-hydroxy vitamin D greater than 200 ng/ml indicates a vitamin D toxic state. In the populations of the United States and Canada where calcium intakes may not be adequate, both calcium and vitamin D supplements seem reasonable, especially in the winter months.

Phosphate Intake

Phosphate salts are available in practically all foods, whereas calcium is not so available in the food supply. The simple act of eating provides a rather constant amount of phosphate (i.e., roughly 1000 to 1200 mg/day for adult females and 1200 to 1400 for males). The actual phosphorus intake in the United States may be even higher because of the "hidden" phosphates in foods that are provided by various salts used in processing by food manufacturers (Anderson et al., 2006). Proportionate amounts of calcium are not consumed unless a conscious effort is made to select enough servings of the few calcium-rich foods. Both calcium and phosphate ions in the ratio of about 1:1 are needed for the mineralization of bone.

Excessive phosphorus intake as phosphates can greatly alter the calcium-to-phosphate ratio, especially if calcium intakes are low. Too much phosphate compared to calcium lowers the serum calcium ion concentration, which then stimulates PTH; if this pattern of intake becomes chronic, bone loss is thought to follow over long periods of time (see Figure 24-4). The possible adaptation to a diet low in calcium but adequate in phosphorus has not been established, and most research supports the concept that an elevation of serum PTH, induced by a high phosphorus or a low vitamin D intake, results in bone loss.

Protein Intake

Protein is generally considered to have an anabolic effect on bone. A high dietary protein intake over a 2-week period has little or no effect on calcium metabolism or bone turnover in healthy adult women (Kerstetter et al., 2005). On the other hand, a chronic low protein intake contributes to low levels of serum albumin, which lowers both serum IGF-1 and serum calcium, a situation in which fracture patients may be especially vulnerable.

These two aspects of protein intake—high versus low—on bone health can be explained by two distinct metabolic actions of proteins and their absorbed amino acids: an anabolic effect on bone and a catabolic effect on bone resulting from the generation of an acid load. In most diets the two effects generally offset each other; but at extremes of intake, either very high or very low, one metabolic action will dominate and affect BMC and BMD (Sebastian, 2005).

A normal adult protein intake of approximately 1 g/kg of body weight maintains the serum PTH concentration within a healthy range (Kerstetter et al., 2000) if calcium intake is also at or near the recommended intake. Children and adolescents may need a similar protein intake to support optimal skeletal growth (Alexy et al., 2005). IGF-1 production drives the anabolic effect without excessive generation of net acid resulting from the catabolism of the amino acids; the difference between the anabolic effect and the catabolic action results in bone gain or bone loss (Sebastian, 2005). On the other hand, a low protein intake, such as in undernutrition, generates a decreased serum concentration of IGF-1 (Ammann et al., 2000).

Animal protein increases urinary losses of calcium following each meal containing large amounts of animal protein and over lengthy periods of high animal protein consumption, whereas a plant-based diet (e.g., one rich in soy protein) has little effect on urinary calcium losses because of the production of a neutral or basic urine (Wengreen et al., 2004) (see *Clinical Insight:* Acid Ash and Alkaline Ash Diets in Chapter 36). However, urinary calcium losses have been suggested to be similar for both plant and animal proteins following relatively long-term consumption (Bonjour, 2005). Therefore the relationship between protein and calcium remains unsettled.

Magnesium Intake

More than 50% of the magnesium in the body is found in bone tissue, but the role of this mineral in bone functions is poorly understood. The largest percentage of the magnesium ions in bone exists in the bone fluids, but a smaller fraction of these ions is bound in the bone crystals, probably at the surfaces only. A small percentage of the magnesium ions are located within bone cells, where they serve as enzyme cofactors, as in all other cells. Magnesium dietary deficits seem to have little effect on bone tissue, but one report suggests that adequate intakes of magnesium improve BMD (Ryder et al., 2005).

Vitamin K Intake

Vitamin K is an essential micronutrient for bone health. Its role in posttranslational modification of several matrix proteins, including osteocalcin, is now well established. **Osteocalcin,** a bone-specific protein made by osteoblasts, requires vitamin K for its posttranslational carboxylation (i.e., maturation). This molecule is secreted into the bone matrix, where the roles of osteocalcin are not well characterized, except that it appears to be involved in the mineralization process—perhaps acting to stop the formation of crystals to prevent overmineralization. Some osteocalcin is also secreted by osteoblasts directly into the circulating blood.

A second way that osteocalcin enters blood is following bone resorption and the release of these molecules; in this way, osteocalcin serves as a serum bone marker for predicting the risk of a fracture. Many elderly individuals, perhaps as high as 50%, have inadequate intakes of vitamin K, primarily because their consumption of dark-green leafy vegetables is so low. In one study vitamin K supplementation of postmenopausal women was shown to retard bone loss (Braam et al., 2003). Therefore an optimal intake of this fat-soluble vitamin, especially later in life, may be important for bone health, the reduction of fractures, and calcium homeostasis (Vermeer et al., 2004). It is important to consider the vitamin K intake in older persons who may also be taking blood-thinning medications. Therapeutic INR ranges are achieved with vitamin K in low dose supplementation, and fluctuations are few (Ford et al., 2007) (see Chapter 16).

Vitamin A (Retinol) Intake

Vitamin A consumption is generally considered to be beneficial to bone growth and maintenance. However, results of recent epidemiologic studies suggest that excessive retinal consumption, but not from carotenoids per se, may contribute to hip fractures (Feskanich et al., 2002; Promislow et al., 2002; Michaelsson et al., 2003; Wengreen et al., 2004). Two reports did not find an association between vitamin A and increased risk of fractures (Rejnmark et al., 2004; Barker et al., 2005). Nevertheless, concern remains that the combined intakes of supplemental vitamin A and vitamin A from fortified foods may be too high in the United States, especially in health-conscious postmenopausal white females. The window of safe consumption of vitamin A is fairly narrow, but it may be even narrower for the elderly (Anderson, 2002).

Trace Mineral Intakes

Relatively few studies are available about the effects of trace elements on bone. Iron, zinc, copper, manganese, and boron may function in bone cells, but their specific roles in preventing bone loss are not well established. In one study the supplementation of several trace elements (copper, fluoride, manganese, and zinc) along with calcium for 1 year resulted in a reduced loss of lumbar BMD compared to the greater loss in a control group receiving only calcium (Nieves, 2005). The skeletal roles of several trace elements are briefly noted.

Boron

Boron appears to be used by osteoblasts for bone formation, but little information exists on whether boron is absolutely required (Palacios, 2006).

Copper

Copper is needed for an enzyme that increases the cross-linking of collagen and elastin molecules, and it may have roles in other enzymes of bone cells. Because of the changes induced in the two matrix proteins by low copper intakes, bone mineralization may also be reduced, especially in the elderly.

Fluoride

Fluoride ions enter the hydroxyapatite crystals of bone as substitutes for hydroxyl ions. Within narrow limits of safety (less than 2 ppm), fluoride ions have little impact on increasing the hardness of bone mineral. At intakes of 2 ppm or greater, fluoride is considered to produce bone that is subject to increased microfractures because of the change in the properties of the hydroxyapatite crystals. Water containing 1 ppm of fluoride does not help bone like it does tooth surfaces; to get an increase in BMD from more fluoride than in the usual diet requires several ppm, which increases the risk of fluorosis and poorly mineralized bone (Palmer and Anderson, 2000).

Iron

Iron serves as a catalytic cofactor for the vitamin C–dependent hydroxylations of proline and lysine in collagen maturation. Iron also has other roles in osteoblasts and osteoclasts in mitochondrial oxidative-phosphorylation, as well as in other heme- and nonheme-containing enzymes, similar to the needs of other cells in the body.

Manganese

Manganese is required for the biosynthesis of mucopolysaccharides in bone matrix formation, and it also acts as a cofactor in energy-generating reactions.

Zinc

Zinc is essential for several critical enzymes in osteoblasts that are essential for collagen synthesis and other products. In addition, an important enzyme in osteoblasts, alkaline phosphatase, requires zinc for its activity.

Intakes of Other Dietary Components

Several other dietary factors associated with bone loss have been identified. It is not yet clear how quantitatively important any of these factors are in the typical U.S. diet (Ilich and Kerstetter, 2000).

Dietary Fiber

Excessive *dietary fiber intake* may interfere with calcium absorption, but any interference is considered extremely small in the typical low-fiber U.S. diet. Vegans who may consume as much as 50 g of fiber a day would be the most likely individuals to have a significant depression in intestinal calcium absorption (see Chapter 3).

Sodium

High sodium intakes, particularly in association with a low calcium intake, can contribute to osteoporosis because they result in increased calcium excretion (Massey, 2005).

Potassium Bicarbonate

In postmenopausal women an oral dose of potassium bicarbonate sufficient to neutralize endogenous acid improves calcium balance and bone. Decreased bone resorption and an increased rate of bone formation result. The skeleton serves as a buffer to help regulate acid-base balance, and a high-acid diet may contribute to the progressive decline in bone mass and osteoporosis (Tucker et al., 2001; Sebastian, 2005) (see *Clinical Insight:* Acid Ash and Alkaline Ash Diets in Chapter 36).

Vegetarian Diets

Vegetarian diets may be more beneficial for bone than animal diets for proteins, but they may provide less calcium than animal diets. Vegetarian diets may also contribute to a lower lifetime exposure to estrogens, which could increase the risk of osteoporotic fractures. Polyphenols and other plant antioxidants, abundant in plant foods, may benefit the optimal functioning and health of bone cells. In general, fruits and vegetables provide many bone-healthy nutrients; potassium is considered an especially powerful protector of bone because of its role in generating an alkaline ash (New et al., 2000; Tucker et al., 2001) (see *Clinical Insight:* Acid Ash and Alkaline Ash Diets in Chapter 36).

Isoflavones

The isoflavones in soybeans, which function both as estrogen agonists and antioxidants in bone cells, have been shown to be able to inhibit bone resorption in female animal models without ovaries, but they have been without effect in young adult females with normal estrogen status (Anderson et al., 2002). Perimenopausal and postmenopausal women have been reported in a few studies to have modest skeletal benefits from isoflavones because of low serum estrogen concentrations (Alekel et al., 2000; Arjmandi et al., 2003), but other investigators have not been able to show skeletal benefits with isoflavone supplementation.

Caffeine and Carbonated Beverages

The relationship of moderate consumption of caffeine to osteoporosis has not been clearly established. *Excessive* caffeine intake may have a deleterious effect on BMD (Ruffing et al., 2006). Intake of colas but not other carbonated beverages is also associated with lower BMD (Tucker et al., 2006).

Alcohol

Alcohol (ethanol) intake at high doses (more than two drinks a day) has adverse effects on the skeleton (Kanis et al., 2005). However, heavy alcohol consumption may be accompanied by poor dietary intake and cigarette smoking, which may be contributing factors.

OSTEOPENIA AND OSTEOPOROSIS

Osteoporosis may have its origin in early life during the period of skeletal growth and PBM accumulation. Statistics indicate that women are about four times more likely than men to develop osteoporosis, although with aging both genders gradually lose bone mass and become more vulnerable, especially to hip fractures, as they age. Women have almost twice the hip fracture rate as men, but the men's rate will catch up as the average life span of males continues to increase. Practically everyone over 80 years of age can be said to be osteoporotic and at risk for a hip fracture. The World Health Organization (WHO) defines osteoporosis in terms of decline in BMD (Table 24-5).

Definitions of Osteopenia and Osteoporosis

When BMD falls sufficiently below healthy values (1 standard deviation [SD] according to WHO standards) **osteopenia** exists. **Osteoporosis** occurs when the BMD becomes so low (greater than 2.5 SDs below healthy values) that the skeleton is unable to sustain ordinary strains. A study of 200,000 women 50 years or older who have had BMD measurements (or related measurements) at routine office visits showed that roughly 40% were classified as osteopenic and 7% as osteoporotic, according to WHO values (Siris et al., 2001). This alarming finding suggests that many perimenopausal women are at risk of fractures because of low BMD, which remains the single most predictive risk factor for fractures.

Prevalence of Osteoporotic Fractures

Although it is difficult to estimate rates of osteoporosis, approximately 25 million women and 12 million men are classified as osteoporotic. More than 1.5 million osteoporotic fractures occur annually, which represents a cost of billions of dollars in health care and rehabilitation services. Half of these osteoporosis-related fractures involve the vertebrae; 250,000 are fractures of the hip, which typically result in incapacitation, long-term nursing care, and a 20% death rate within a year of the fracture.

Types of Osteoporosis

The two types of primary or involutional osteoporosis are distinguished in general by sex, the age at which fractures occur, and the kinds of bone involved. However, osteoporosis should be considered to be a disease with a broad spectrum of variants forms of the disorder. Only for simple distinction is the classification of the two types used here (Table 24-6).

Postmenopausal or **estrogen/androgen deficient (type 1) osteoporosis** occurs in women within a few years of menopause, and it primarily involves loss of trabecular bone tissue because of a cessation of ovarian production of estrogens. Men may also develop type 1 osteoporosis during adulthood if they have a significant decline in androgen production, but in practice such cases are rare. This osteoporosis is characterized by fractures of the distal radius (Colles' fractures) and "crush" fractures of the lumbar vertebrae that are often painful and deforming.

Acceleration of the process that occurs in women after menopause is directly related to the lack of estrogen. BMC and BMD measurements of the lumbar spine of women with postmenopausal osteoporosis may be as much as 25% to 40% lower than in age-matched nonosteoporotic control women of the same age range. Other bone sites with a preponderance of trabecular bone such as the pelvis, ribs, and proximal femur also display low BMD.

Age-related osteoporosis (type 2) occurs around age 70 and beyond, and it affects both sexes; older men are increasingly at risk for hip fractures. Both types of bone tissue, cortical and trabecular, undergo remodeling, but the greater degree of remodeling occurs in trabecular tissue. In the elderly period the processes of bone resorption and bone formation become uncoupled. Fractures of the hips characterize this osteoporosis, but vertebral fractures continue to increase with age. A dramatic increase in hip fractures occurs late in life, and almost all women beyond 80 years of age are at risk of hip fracture. Wedge fractures of vertebrae typically lead to back pain, loss of height, spinal deformity, and kyphosis or "dowager's hump" (Figure 24-9).

Many women lose several inches in height between 50 and 80 years of age. Fractures may occur during ordinary activities, such as lifting a sack of groceries or stepping over a shower opening, but a large percentage of the hip fractures result from a fall. Although age-associated osteoporosis affects both sexes, women are more severely affected because they have a smaller skeletal mass than men and they live longer. Hip fractures affect nearly 20% of postmenopausal women up to age 80 and almost 50% of those beyond that age, and the hip fracture numbers are steadily increasing in men.

Secondary osteoporosis results when an identifiable drug (see Box 24-2 and Chapter 16) or disease process (Box 24-3) causes loss of bone tissue.

TABLE 24-5

Definitions of Osteopenia and Osteoporosis

	Below Mean BMD of 20- to 29-Year-Olds
Osteopenia	1 to 2.5 Standard deviations
Osteoporosis	>2.5 Standard deviations

TABLE 24-6

Characteristics of Primary Osteoporosis

	Type 1	Type 2
Gender	Female; rare in males	Female and male
Age/period	Menopause ($\approx$50 Years)	After age 65
Bone tissue	Trabecular	Trabecular and cortical
Fracture sites	Lumbar vertebrae	Hips and vertebrae; other skeletal bones
Etiology	Loss of sex hormones	Aging

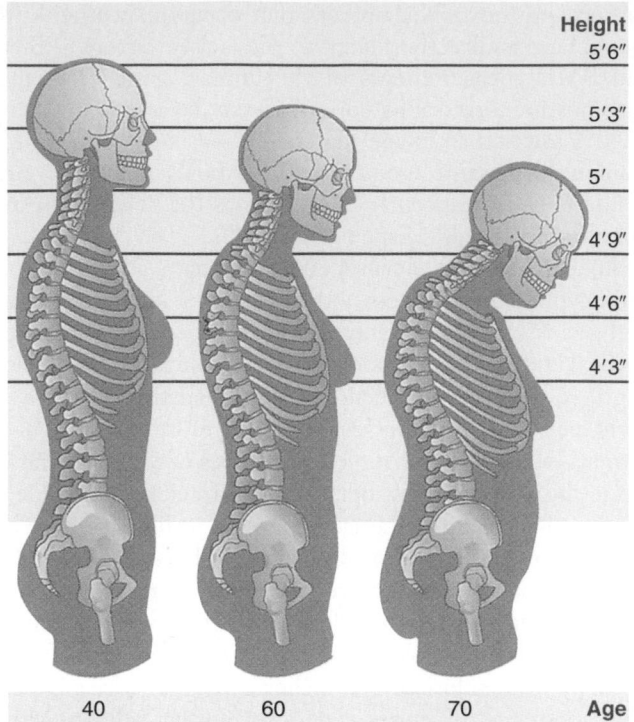

FIGURE 24-9 Normal spine at age 40 and osteoporotic changes at ages 60 and 70. These changes can cause a loss of as much as 6 to 9 in in height and result in the so-called dowager's hump (far right) in the upper thoracic vertebrae. *(From Ignatavicius D, Workman M: Medical-surgical nursing: critical thinking for collaborative care, ed 5, Philadelphia, 2006, Saunders).*

Etiology

Osteoporosis is a complex heterogeneous disorder of unknown etiology, but many risk factors contribute to this condition over a lifetime. Although the fracture-precipitating condition of low BMD is common to all types of osteoporosis, an imbalance between bone resorption and formation results from an array of etiologic factors characteristic of each form of this disease.

Loss of bone mass to a degree that produces fractures can result from: (1) an excessive acceleration of resorption, especially after the menopause; or (2) a suboptimal peak bone mass that results in bone after the menopause (or later in life in males) that becomes fragile and susceptible to fracture. The *Pathophysiology and Care Management Algorithm*, Parathyroid Hormone–Mediated Post-Menopausal Bone Osteoporosis, lists several risk factors and illustrates different scenarios of older or younger postmenopausal women that lead to osteoporotic fractures. Risk factors for osteoporosis include age, race, gender, and factors noted in Box 24-4.

Race and Ethnicity

Whites and Asians suffer more osteoporotic fractures than blacks and Hispanics, who have a greater bone density (Siris et al, 2001). Hypovitaminosis D with secondary hyperparathyroidism occur more often in the black population. Thin women, particularly of northern European extraction, are more at risk of osteoporosis than heavier women.

BOX 24-2

Common Medications That Increase Calcium Loss and Promote Risk of Osteoporosis

Phenytoin (Dilantin)
Phenobarbital
Thyroid hormone
Corticosteroids
Lasix and thiazide diuretics
Methotrexate
Cyclosporine
Lithium
Tetracycline
Aluminum-containing antacids
Heparin
Phenothiazine derivatives

BOX 24-3

Medical Conditions That Deplete Calcium and Promote Risk of Osteoporosis

Hyperthyroidism
Diabetes
Chronic renal failure
Scurvy
Chronic diarrhea or intestinal malabsorption
Hyperparathyroid disease
Chronic obstructive lung disease
Subtotal gastrectomy
Hemiplegia

Menstrual Status

Loss of menses at any age is a major determinant of osteoporosis risk in women. Acceleration of bone loss coincides with the menopause, either natural or surgical, at which time the ovaries stop producing estrogen. Estrogen replacement therapies have been shown to conserve BMD and reduce fracture risk within the first few years following the menopause, at least in short-term studies.

Any interruption of menstruation for an extended period results in bone loss. The amenorrhea that accompanies excessive weight loss seen in patients with anorexia nervosa or in individuals who participate in high-intensity sports, dance, or other forms of exercise has the same adverse effect on bones as the menopause. BMD in amenorrheic athletes has been measured at levels 25% to 40% below control levels. When menses were resumed in these athletes, bone mass increased, but eventually plateaued at a level lower than that of sedentary women. Young women with the "female athlete triad" of disordered eating, amenorrhea, and low BMD are at increased risk for hav-

PATHOPHYSIOLOGY AND CARE MANAGEMENT ALGORITHM

Parathyroid Hormone-Mediated Post-Menopausal Bone Osteoporosis

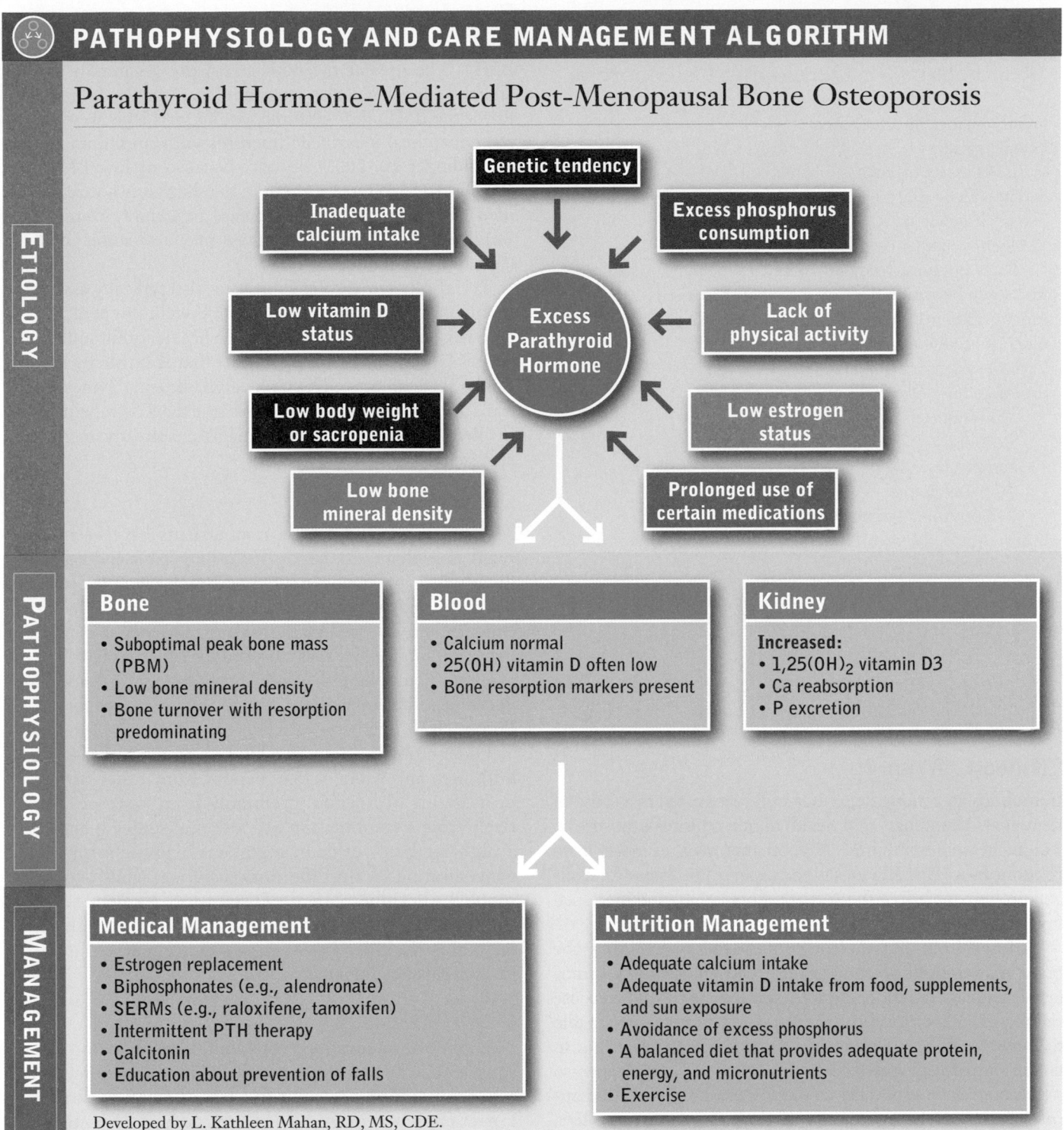

ETIOLOGY

- Genetic tendency
- Inadequate calcium intake
- Excess phosphorus consumption
- Low vitamin D status
- Excess Parathyroid Hormone
- Lack of physical activity
- Low body weight or sacropenia
- Low estrogen status
- Low bone mineral density
- Prolonged use of certain medications

PATHOPHYSIOLOGY

Bone
- Suboptimal peak bone mass (PBM)
- Low bone mineral density
- Bone turnover with resorption predominating

Blood
- Calcium normal
- 25(OH) vitamin D often low
- Bone resorption markers present

Kidney
Increased:
- 1,25(OH)$_2$ vitamin D3
- Ca reabsorption
- P excretion

MANAGEMENT

Medical Management
- Estrogen replacement
- Biphosphonates (e.g., alendronate)
- SERMs (e.g., raloxifene, tamoxifen)
- Intermittent PTH therapy
- Calcitonin
- Education about prevention of falls

Nutrition Management
- Adequate calcium intake
- Adequate vitamin D intake from food, supplements, and sun exposure
- Avoidance of excess phosphorus
- A balanced diet that provides adequate protein, energy, and micronutrients
- Exercise

Developed by L. Kathleen Mahan, RD, MS, CDE.

ing fractures while involved in athletics (Thrash and Anderson, 2000) (see Chapters 22 and 23). These young women may benefit from the use of oral contraceptive agents plus calcium and vitamin D supplements.

Lactations

A striking but transient bone loss occurs in women who breast-feed for 6 months or longer, especially from the femoral neck and lumbar spine. Sufficient calcium and vitamin D intake are essential during this time for the mother to replete her own serum and storage levels, but repletion typically does not occur until several months after peak lactation. Several successive pregnancies and lactations over a relatively few years may contribute to significant bone loss by the end of the period of childbearing if nutrition is not adequate.

BOX 24-4

Risk Factors for Developing Osteoporosis

Family history of osteoporosis
Female gender
White or Asian ethnicity
Sarcopenia or slight body build
Estrogen depletion
 Menopause
 Early oophorectomy in women
Androgen depletion with hypogonadism in men
Amenorrhea in women as a result of excessive exercise
Age, especially >age 60
Lack of exercise
Prolonged use of certain medications
 Aluminum-containing antacids
 Steroids
 Tetracyclines
 Anticonvulsants
 Use of exogenous thyroid
Diseases or conditions that affect calcium and bone metabolism (see Box 24-3)
 Underweight or low body fatness
 Cigarette smoking
 Excessive alcohol consumption
 Excessive fiber consumption
 Excessive caffeine consumption
 Inadequate calcium or vitamin D intake

Limited Exercise

Immobility in varying degrees is well recognized as a cause of bone loss. Maintenance of healthy bone requires exposure to weight-bearing pressures. A good diet plus exercise from roughly ages 10 to 20 years is particularly important for skeletal growth, including the accrual of bone mass and increased femoral bone dimensions (Iuliano-Burns et al., 2005).

Stresses from muscle contraction and maintaining the body in an upright position against the pull of gravity stimulate osteoblast function. Bones not subjected to normal use rapidly lose mass. Invalids confined to bed or persons unable to move freely are commonly affected. Astronauts living in conditions of zero gravity for only a few days experience so much bone loss, especially in the lower extremities, that appropriate exercise is a feature of their daily routines. To a lesser degree, lack of exercise and a sedentary mode of living that continue over a lifetime also contribute significantly to bone loss, although the most important influence is probably on inadequate accumulation of bone mass.

Physical activity, especially upper body activities, may also contribute to an increase in bone mass or density, although the evidence for skeletal benefit is limited (Chubak et al., 2006). But reduced activities in daily life may also contribute to bone loss. For example, Asian women who migrate to urban areas and change their lifestyles from more agrarian to less active ones also have increased risk of hip fractures (Lau et al., 2001).

Body Weight

Body weight is a very important factor that affects BMC and BMD. The greater the body mass, the greater the BMD; and the converse is also true, the lower the body mass, the lower the BMD. For example, young girls who are typically premenarcheal may incur fractures with minimum trauma (Gouldinget al., 2005), in part because of low BMC and BMD related to rapid growth in height that is not accompanied with a proportionate increase in weight. Young overweight males with low bone mass may also suffer fractures (Goulding et al., 2005).

Weight loss in dieting subjects is also typically associated with bone loss (Pluijm et al., 2001; Fogelholm et al., 2001). The reason for the greater BMD in heavier adult individuals relates largely to the load (weight) that is borne by the different skeletal sites. The nonweight-bearing bones of the arms are less affected by body weight than by repetitive use in physical activities. Sarcopenia is an already mentioned risk factor.

Dietary Factors

Many nutrients and several nonnutrients have been implicated as etiologic risk factors for osteoporosis and have been discussed in previous paragraphs. Frank vitamin deficiency has been widely reported at northerly latitudes in North America and Europe. Vitamin D insufficiency is considered more common at latitudes closer to the equator but still in the northern hemisphere than previously thought because of reduced exposure to sunlight during the year (Hypponen and Power, 2007; Lamberg-Allardt et al., 2001).

Older individuals in the United States and elsewhere, both men and women, may benefit from a diet with 1000 or more mg of calcium, preferably from foods or alternatively from a combination of foods and supplements. Such a high intake of calcium maintains a lower serum PTH concentration (within the normal range), and it may also support a healthier vitamin D status if the calcium is from vitamin D–fortified dairy products. Finally, such an intake maintains healthier bone tissue, and it may reduce fractures at all skeletal sites

Medications

A number of medications contribute adversely to osteoporosis, either by interfering with calcium absorption or by actively promoting calcium loss from bone (see Box 24-2). For example, corticosteroids affect vitamin D metabolism and can lead to bone loss. Excessive amounts of exogenous thyroid hormone can promote loss of bone mass over time.

Use of Alcohol and Cigarettes

Cigarette smoking and excessive alcohol consumption are risk factors for developing osteoporosis, probably because of toxic effects on osteoblasts. Alcohol at intakes of two drinks or more par day has been found to be a risk for bone fractures in an analysis of three large European studies (Kanis et al., 2005). Excesses should be avoided (see *Focus On: The Impact of Alcohol and Cigarette Smoking on the Skeleton—a Double Whammy!!*).

The Impact of Alcohol and Cigarette Smoking on the Skeleton—a Double Whammy!!

Cigarette smoking is a risk factor for vertebral, forearm, and hip fractures, especially in slender women. Women who smoke about one pack of cigarettes daily will have a deficit in bone density, which increases the risk of fracture. The strong correlation between reproductive function and bone mass and density appears to be affected by smoking through a decrease in estrogens. Alcohol, especially excessive consumption (more than two drinks a day) for an extended period of time, results in bone loss. The combination of smoking and alcohol, common among young women and men, places them at increased risk for osteoporosis.

Secondary Prevention and Treatment

Because virtually all elderly persons are affected by osteoporosis, the increasing longevity of the population emphasizes the need for prevention of osteoporosis. Secondary prevention is a form of treatment following the development of osteoporosis, either sex hormone–deficient or age-related onset. Primary prevention applies to individuals who have no osteoporotic disease, typically adults before age 50.

Because bone health of women especially is influenced by three major interacting factors—diet, exercise, and estrogen—it is never too early or too late to prevent or lessen the onset and severity of osteoporosis by ensuring adequate intakes of calcium from foods (and supplements); adequate intake of vitamin D either from sun exposure or foods or supplements; engaging in regular weight-bearing exercises; and, if necessary, taking bone-conserving drugs. Weight-bearing exercise may decrease the rate of loss of BMD of postmenopausal as well as older women if the activities are age appropriate.

All of the recommended bone-conserving drugs except intermittent PTH therapy have antiresorptive effects; only intermittent PTH is a practical bone-forming drug now being routinely used in the early prevention or later treatment of bone loss (see following paragraphs). All drugs are recommended to be taken along with calcium supplements (500 to 1000 mg of calcium per day) and vitamin D (approximately 400 to 800 IU per day) for the purpose of meeting the needs of calcium for bone formation.

Estrogen Replacement Therapy

Estrogen replacement therapy (ERT), or hormone-replacement therapy, a treatment previously used for reducing bone resorption and arresting early postmenopausal bone loss in women, is no longer recommended except for a period of a few years after the menopause. Concerns about the possible risks of breast and endometrial cancers in women, starting with a major report in 1995, have led to this change in the use of estrogens.

Other drugs have been used in place of estrogens for the prevention and treatment and osteoporosis. Also recently, many women have been exploring the use of **phytoestrogens** and other plant products as substitutes for estrogens, but these extracts of natural products have not been established as being effective in diminishing bone loss by randomized controlled trials.

Androgen Replacement Therapy

Testosterone replacement in elderly men may help to maintain bone mass and prevent fractures, but side effects, especially prostate growth, limit the use of testosterone and other androgens. New drugs on the horizon may be more effective.

Bisphosphonates

These drugs act as antiresorbers on osteoclasts to reduce their bone-degradative activities. They have been shown to be effective in reducing the incidence of new fractures (Epstein, 2006). Chemically, **bisphosphonates** resemble pyrophosphate, which is present at the surfaces of bone crystals. The bisphosphonates act by inhibiting osteoclast-mediated bone resorption. Examples include etidronate, a first generation drug little used today, and several second-generation bisphosphonates such as alendronate and pamidronate.

Etidronate

Cyclic administration of etidronate to women with postmenopausal osteoporosis resulted in greatly increased vertebral bone mineral content and reduced fractures.

Alendronate

The skeletal benefits of alendronate have been similar to those of etidronate, but alendronate has been more effective in fracture reduction (Black et al., 2000). Although this drug has become widely accepted in the United States and other nations, it may result in esophageal reflux, a side effect that makes it difficult for a small subset of the population to continue this oral therapy. Alendronate may be used in combination with a **selective estrogen receptor modulator (SERM)** (see paragraph that follows) or another bone-conserving drug in an effort to protect the skeleton.

Risedronate

This drug has effects similar to those of alendronate.

Pamidronate

This bisphosphonate has similar properties as the others, but it exerts its beneficial effects with fewer doses being required over a year.

Selective Estrogen Receptor Modulators

SERMs are able to stimulate **estrogen receptors (ER)** in bone tissue and yet have very little effect on the estrogen receptors of reproductive tissues (i.e., breast or uterus).

Two examples of these drugs in the marketplace are tamoxifen and raloxifene.

Tamoxifen

Tamoxifen was developed as an antiestrogen to help prevent breast cancer, and it was found by chance to conserve bone. However, it has not been prescribed for preventing bone loss.

Raloxifene

Raloxifene, a drug approved by the Food and Drug Administration (FDA) for the express purpose of maintaining bone and reducing fractures, has been found to be effective.

Intermittent Parathyroid Hormone Therapy

Intermittent parathyroid hormone (PTH) therapy uses low doses of a modified PTH (1-34) molecule to improve both bone mass and density. For example, BMD of the lumbar vertebrae may be increased by as much as 15% after 1 year of treatment, and total body BMD may be increased by 5% to 10%. Unfortunately BMD of the hip (proximal femur) does not increase much, although it does not decrease.

Reports of the few human investigations suggest that intermittent PTH therapy will be a boost to the therapeutic arsenal because it increases osteoblastic formation of new bone tissue, especially in trabecular bone, and reduces fractures (Thomas, 2006; Dempster et al., 2001; Neer et al., 2001). Calcium also needs to be taken along with this anabolic therapy. Now that this drug has been approved by the FDA for regular prescription use, it is the only practical agent that increases bone formation (i.e., it is anabolic) and thus bone mass. Although growth hormone, insulin-like growth factor-1, and a few other agents are anabolic, their use is not practical.

Other Drug Treatments

These treatment options are less used for the prevention or treatment of osteoporosis, but each one may be effective under special conditions or in certain individuals.

Calcitonin

Calcitonin, a hormone, is used as a drug to inhibit osteoclastic bone resorption by blocking the stimulatory effects of PTH on these cells. Calcitonin therapy decreases the rate of bone loss in osteoporotic women; however, it is most effective if given early after the menopause. Calcitonin can be administered by nasal spray. It improves BMD, especially of the lumbar spine, and it may reduce the recurrence of fractures in patients with osteoporosis.

Sodium Fluoride

Increases in bone mass, especially in trabecular bone, follow treatment with sodium fluoride, but the quality of the bone typically is not normal. Fluoride ions become incorporated at the surfaces of hydroxyapatite crystals; and the size and structure of the crystals become so altered that the mechanical competence of the bone declines. Fluoride therapy is not likely ever to be approved by the FDA because of these concerns; the use of fluoride must still be regarded as practical for dental applications but not for bone therapy (Palmer and Anderson, 2000).

Vitamin D

Maintenance of an adequate dietary intake of vitamin D (400 to 600 units or 20 to 30 mg of cholecalciferol) is important for healthy younger adults, but this dose may be inadequate for the many house-bound elderly who fail to get adequate exposure to sunlight. Supplements are most likely necessary because it is almost impossible for the elderly to consume enough from foods. Such individuals may need 800 to 1000 units of vitamin D, especially in winter months, but their serum 25-hydroxy vitamin D (calcidiol) concentrations need to be monitored periodically to avoid hypervitaminosis D and toxic reactions (see earlier discussion).

Calcitriol

Calcitriol or 1,25-dihyroxy vitamin D3, without calcium, has had little use in the treatment of osteoporosis because of its potential toxicity. Calcium plus calcitriol may be useful, however, in patients who are taking high-dose corticosteroid therapy, during which vertebral fractures are common.

Growth Hormone and Insulin-Like Growth Factors

Treatment with human growth hormone may improve bone through its anabolic effects (Rosen and Bilezekian, 2001). Similarly, insulin-like growth factor-1 (IGF-1) may improve bone BMC and BMD in human subjects by increasing bone formation (Rosen and Bilezekian, 2001).

Osteoprotegerin

This natural cytokine, osteoprotegerin (OPG), is secreted by osteoblasts as well as other cell types. OPG, which can be detected in human serum, acts by inactivating another cytokine that affects osteoclasts, thereby inhibiting osteoclast activation and bone resorption. Final results from clinical trials are anticipated.

Dietary Treatment

Calcium, vitamin D, and other micronutrients have been covered previously; combination supplementation of calcium and vitamin D has been found not to reduce fractures in postmenopausal women in the Women's Health Trial (Jackson et al., 2006). However, one approach to the dietary treatment of elderly patients who were recovering from hip fractures that has been shown to be effective is the provision of protein supplements coupled with adequate amounts of micronutrients. High-quality protein in supplements can increase serum IGF-1 concentrations and enhance new bone matrix formation.

Calcium (1000 mg/day) and vitamin D (800 to 1000 units/day) are typically recommended as supplements for patients being treated with one of the bone drugs, either antiresorptive or anabolic. The selection of these dose levels is not based on specific trial data using different doses of these two nutrients to test efficacy, but rather the doses have been chosen because these amounts are considered both sufficient for bone formation and safe. However, the question of safety has been raised because of concern about an increase of renal stone formation and arterial calcification in older subjects, as observed by x-rays or other types of scans, who have been taking these supplements of calcium and vitamin D as a preventive strategy against bone loss or as a treatment for osteopenia or osteoporosis for periods of as little as a few years. Although further investigation on the diet supplement–calcification linkage is clearly needed, caution is urged regarding the potential oversupplementation of these two nutrients.

Other Treatment Modalities

Several other approaches to prevent fractures have been demonstrated to have benefits in small study populations; they have not been adequately tested in the elderly. These approaches include exercise, strength activities, falls-prevention, UV lamps, and special hip padding.

Exercise

Physical activities such as regular walking and swimming appear to have minor skeletal benefits for older individuals, but more active participation such as weight-bearing exercises and intensive walking do have positive effects on BMD (Karlsson et al., 2001). Although most exercise studies have been conducted on healthy young adults, those that have been performed on older adult men and women have generated some impressive data (Wallace and Cumming, 2000). The difficulty with these studies is keeping up participation. Tai Chi may be modestly beneficial (Woo et al., 2007).

Strength Activities

Upper-body strength activities have been shown to improve bone measurements of the femur. In terms of prevention, these types of activities have been underused.

Prevention of Falls

Fractures of the humerus, wrist, pelvis, and hip are considered to be age related, resulting from a combination of osteoporosis and falling. Although only a small percentage of falls result in fractures, *preventing falls* through education and attention to the living environment of the very old is an important measure.

Hip-Protector Girdles

Wearing girdles with built-in pads to protect the hips during a fall has been demonstrated in some, but not all, studies to significantly reduce the rate of fractures in a well-controlled investigation.

Ultraviolet Lamps

The development of new UVB lamps with built-in safety against excessive skin damage may be a potential way to improve vitamin D status of elderly individuals, especially those living in northern latitudes or in nursing homes or similar institutions.

⚙ FOCAL POINTS

- Bone health depends on numerous factors, including genetics, dietary intake of specific nutrients, exposure to sunlight, exercise, management of chronic diseases, and use of medications.
- Whether young or old, any individual can make improvements in lifestyle, especially regular physical activity and dietary changes, which may protect and maintain skeletal tissues.
- Concern about excessive supplementation of calcium and vitamin D has arisen because of increasing recognition of arterial calcification in older individuals and in patients with or at risk of osteoporotic fractures but this is not the usual situation.

❋ CLINICAL SCENARIO

Annie B, a 70-year-old white woman of Northern European ancestry, developed lactose intolerance during her early '50s when she had a serious gastrointestinal infection. She currently is retired, lives alone, and stays indoors most of each day watching television. Approximately 3 years ago at age 67, she had dual-energy x-ray absorptiometry (DEXA) measurements that showed that she had low bone mineral density (BMD) values of her proximal femur and lumbar vertebrae (both values would be classified as osteoporotic according to World Health Organization definitions). Her physician recommended that she start taking supplements of calcium (1000 mg/day) and vitamin D (800 units/day) because of her lactose intolerance and her lack of consumption of all dairy products.

Annie took the supplements regularly for a year when a second set of DEXA measurements revealed that she had practically maintained her BMD values of 1 year earlier, with only a small decline in BMD. However, her continuing low measurements concerned her physician, and he ordered laboratory tests of calcium-regulatory hormones to see if she had any hormonal complications. These tests showed that her PTH and 25-hydroxy vitamin D concentrations fell in the upper half of the normal range for each variable. Other routine measurements such as serum calcium and phosphate were normal. After discussion of her high risk of an osteoporotic fracture, her physician decided to place Annie on a bisphosphonate drug in addition to calcium and vitamin D.

After 1 year on the new therapy plus continuing the calcium and vitamin D, her BMD values (her third set of DEXA measurements) actually increased a few percentage points, even though they remained within the classification of osteoporosis. She was then instructed by her physician to continue indefinitely on this therapeutic regimen.

Continued

✿ CLINICAL SCENARIO—cont'd

＊Nutrition Diagnosis: Inadequate calcium and vitamin D intake related to avoidance of dairy products as evidenced by diet history revealing less than 20% of estimated requirements. NOTE: This may be resolved once she starts taking supplements.

1. How would you classify Annie's calcium intake at the initial visit with her physician (who did not take a diet history or estimate her calcium intake)? Her vitamin D intake? Her exposure to sunlight?
2. What would you have recommended to improve her calcium intake from foods so that she could reduce her supplemental calcium to 500 mg/day? Why would you recommend foods to provide calcium rather than supplements? Could you make similar recommendations for improving her intake of vitamin D from foods?
3. Design a set (3 days' minimum) of daily menus that provide approximately 800 mg of calcium from foods alone, which, coupled with a 500-mg supplement, would provide a total of 1300 mg, the current adequate intake for calcium. Similarly, design these same meals to include 400 units of vitamin D, with another 400 units coming from supplements.

USEFUL WEBSITES

Consumer Lab calcium supplements
http://www.consumerlab.com/results/calcium.asp

Menopause
http://www.menopause.org/

National Osteoporosis Foundation
http://www.nof.org/

References

Abrams SA et al: Relationships among vitamin D levels, parathyroid hormone, and calcium absorption in young adolescents, *J Clin Endocrinol Metabol* 90:5576, 2005.

Alekel DL et al: Isoflavone-rich soy protein isolate attenuates bone loss in the lumbar spine of perimenopausal women, *Am J Clin Nutr* 72:844, 2000.

Alexy U et al: Long-term protein intake and dietary potential renal acid load are associated with bone modeling and remodeling at the proximal radius in healthy children, *Am J Clin Nutr* 82:1107, 2005.

Ammann P et al: Protein undernutrition-induced bone loss is associated with decreased IGF-1 levels and estrogen deficiency, *J Bone Miner Res* 15:683, 2000.

Anderson JJB: Oversupplementation of vitamin A and osteoporotic fractures in the elderly: to supplement or not to supplement with vitamin A (editorial), *J Bone Miner Res* 17:1359, 2002.

Anderson JJB et al: Soy isoflavones: no effects on bone mineral content and bone mineral density in healthy, menstruating young adult women after one year, *J Am Coll Nutr* 21:388, 2002.

Anderson JJB et al: Phosphorus. In Bowman B, Russell R, editors: *Present knowledge in nutrition*, ed 9, Washington, DC, 2006, ILSI Press.

Arjmandi BH et al: Soy protein has a greater effect on bone in postmenopausal women not on hormone replacement therapy as evidenced by reducing bone resorption and urinary calcium excretion, *J Clin Endocrinol Metabol* 88:1048, 2003.

Barker ME et al: Serum retinoids and β-carotene as predictors of hip and other fractures in elderly women, *J Bone Miner Res* 20:913, 2005.

Bischoff-Ferrari HA et al: Effect of vitamin D on falls: a meta-analysis, *JAMA* 291:199, 2004.

Bischoff-Ferrari HA et al: Fracture prevention with vitamin D supplementation, *JAMA* 293:2257, 2005.

Black DM et al: Fracture risk reduction with alendronate in women with osteoporosis: the fracture intervention trial, *J Clin Endocrinol Metabol* 85:4118, 2000.

Bonjour JP: Dietary protein: an essential nutrient for bone health, *J Am Coll Nutr* 24:5265, 2005.

Braam LA et al: Vitamin K_1 supplementation retards bone loss in postmenopausal women between 50 and 60 years of age, *Calcif Tissue Int* 73:21, 2003.

Chubak J et al: Effect of exercise on bone mineral density and lean mass in postmenopausal women, *Med Sci Sports Exerc* 38:1236, 2006.

Cummings SR, Melton LJ: Epidemiology and outcomes of osteopathic fractures, *Lancet* 359:1761, 2002.

Dempster DW et al: Effects of daily treatment with parathyroid hormone on bone microarchitecture and turnover in patients with osteoporosis: a paired biopsy study, *J Bone Miner Res* 16:1846, 2001.

Epstein S: Update of current therapeutic options for the treatment of postmenopausal osteoporosis, *Clin Ther* 28:151, 2006.

Feskanich D et al: Vitamin A intake and hip fractures among postmenopausal women, *JAMA* 287:47, 2002.

Fogelholm GM et al: Bone mineral density during reduction, maintenance and regain of body weight in premenopausal, obese women, *Osteoporos Int* 12:199, 2001.

Ford SK et al: Prospective study of supplemental vitamin K therapy in patients on oral anticoagulants with international normalized ratios, *J Thromb Thrombolysis*, February 24, 2007.

Goulding A et al: Bone and body composition of children and adolescents with repeated forearm fractures, *J Bone Miner Res* 20:2090, 2005.

Hathcock JN et al: Risk assessment for vitamin D, *Am J Clin Nutr* 85:6, 2007.

Heaney RP: Calcium, dairy products, and osteoporosis, *J Am Coll Nutr* 12:835, 2000.

Holick MF: The vitamin D epidemic and its health consequences, *Am J Clin Nutr* 135:2739S, 2005.

Hypponen E and Power C: Hypovitaminosis D in British adults at age 45 y: nationwide cohort study of dietary and lifestyle predictors, *Am J Clin Nutr* 85:860, 2007.

Ilich JZ, Kerstetter JE: Nutrition in bone health revisited: a story beyond calcium, *J Am Coll Nutr* 19:715, 2000.

Iuliano-Burns et al: Diet and exercise during growth have site-specific skeletal effects: a co-twin study, *Osteoporos Int* 16:1225, 2005.

Jackson RD et al: Calcium plus vitamin D supplementation and the risk of fractures, *N Engl J Med* 354:669, 2006.

Kanis JA et al: Alcohol intake as a risk factor for fracture, *Osteopros Int* 16:737, 2005.

Karlsson M et al: The evidence that exercise during growth or adulthood reduces the risk of fragility fractures is weak, *Best Practice Res Clin Rheumatol* 15:429, 2001.

Kerstetter JE et al: A threshold for low-protein-induced elevations in parathyroid hormone, *Am J Clin Nutr* 72:168, 2000.

Kerstetter JE et al: The impact of dietary protein on calcium absorption and kinetic measures of bone turnover in women, *J Clin Endocrinol Metabol* 90:26, 2005.

Lamberg-Allardt CJE et al: Vitamin D deficiency and bone health in healthy adults in Finland: Could this be a concern in other parts of Europe? *J Bone Miner Res* 16:2066, 2001.

Lau ERMC et al: The incidence of hip fractures in four Asian countries: the Asian Osteoporosis Study (AOS), *Osteoporos Int* 12:239, 2001.

Massey LK: Effect of dietary salt intake on circadian calcium metabolism, bone turnover, and calcium oxalate kidney stone risk in postmenopausal women, *Nutr Res* 25:891, 2005.

Michaelsson K et al: Serum retinol levels and the risk of fracture, *N Engl J Med* 348:287, 2003.

Neer RM et al: Effect of parathyroid hormone (1-34) on fractures and bone mineral density in postmenopausal women with osteoporosis, *N Engl J Med* 344:1434, 2001.

New SA et al: Dietary influence on bone mass and bone metabolism: further evidence of a positive link between fruit and vegetables consumption and bone health? *Am J Clin Nutr* 71:142, 2000.

NHANES: National Health and Nutrition Examination Survey, available at www.cdc.gov/nchs/nhanes.htm, accessed February 5, 2007.

Nieves JW: Osteoporosis: the role of micronutrients, *Am J Clin Nutr* 81:1232S, 2005.

Palacios C: The role of nutrients in bone health, from A to Z, *Crit Rev Food Sci Nutr* 46:621, 2006.

Palmer CA, Anderson JJB: Position of the American Dietetic Association: the impact of fluoride on health, *J Am Diet Assoc* 200:1208, 2000.

Pasco JA et al: Seasonal periodicity of serum vitamin D and parathyroid hormone, bone resorption, and fractures: the Geelong Osteoporosis Study, *J Bone Miner Res* 19:752, 2004.

Pluijm SMF et al: Determinants of bone mineral density in older men and women: body composition as a mediator, *J Bone Miner Res* 16:2142, 2001.

Porthouse J et al: Randomised controlled trial of calcium and supplementation with cholecalciferol (vitamin D_3) for prevention of fractures in primary care, *Br Med J* 330:1003, 2005.

Promislow JH et al: Retinol intake and bone mineral density in the elderly: the Rancho Bernardo Study, *J Bone Miner Res* 17:1349, 2002.

Rejnmark L et al: No effect of vitamin A intake on bone mineral density and fracture risk in perimenopausal women, *Osteoporos Int* 15:872, 2004.

Rosen CJ, Bilezekian JP: Anabolic therapy for osteoporosis, *J Clin Endocrinol Metabol* 86:957, 2001.

Ruffing J et al: Determinants of bone mass and bone size in a large cohort of physically active young adult men, *Nutr Metabol* 3:14, 2006.

Ryder KM et al: Magnesium intake from food and supplements is associated with bone mineral density in healthy older white subjects, *J Am Geriatr Soc* 53:1875, 2005.

Sebastian A: Dietary protein content and the diet's net acid load: opposing effects on bone health, *Am J Clin Nutr* 82:921, 2005.

Siris ES et al: Identification and fracture outcomes of undiagnosed low bone mineral density in postmenopausal women: results from the National Osteoporosis Risk Assessment, *JAMA* 286:2815, 2001.

Steingrimsdottir L et al: Relationship between serum parathyroid hormone levels, vitamin D sufficiency, and calcium intake, *JAMA* 294:2336, 2005.

Sullivan SS et al: Adolescent girls in Maine are risk for vitamin D deficiency, *J Am Diet Assoc* 105:971, 2005.

Surgeon General: Bone health and osteoporosis: A report of the Surgeon General, DHHS: Rockville, Md, 2004, website: www.surgeongeneral.gov/library/bonehealth/docs, accessed February 5, 2007.

Tfelt-Hansen J, Torring O: Calcium and vitamin D_3 supplements in calcium and vitamin D_3 sufficient early postmenopausal healthy women, *Eur J Clin Nutr* 58:1420, 2004.

Thomas T: Intermittent parathyroid hormone therapy to increase bone formation, *Join Bone Spine* 73:262, 2006.

Thrash LE, Anderson JJB: The female athlete triad, *Nutr Today* 35:168, 2000.

Tucker KL et al: The acid-base hypothesis: diet and bone in the Framingham Osteoporosis Study, *Eur J Nutr* 40:231, 2001.

Tucker KL et al: Colas, but not other carbonated beverages, are associated with low bone mineral density in older women: the Framingham Osteoporosis Study, *Am J Clin Nutr* 84(4):936, 2006.

Tylavsky FA et al: Vitamin D, parathyroid hormone, and bone mass in adolescents, *Am J Clin Nutr* 135:2735S, 2005.

Vieth R et al: The urgent need to recommend an intake of vitamin D that is effective (editorial), *Am J Clin Nutr* 85:649, 2007.

Vermeer C et al: Beyond deficiency: Potential benefits of increased intakes of vitamin K for bone and vascular health, *Eur J Nutr* 43:325, 2004.

Wallace BA, Cumming RG: Systematic review of randomized trials of the effect of exercise on bone mass in pre- and post-menopausal women, *Calcif Tissue Int* 67:10, 2000.

Walsh MC et al: Sarcopenia in premenopausal and postmenopausal women with osteopenia, osteoporosis and normal bone mineral density, *Osteoporos Int* 17:61, 2005.

Wengreen HJ et al: Dietary protein intake and risk of osteoporotic hip fracture in elderly residents in Utah, *J Bone Miner Res* 19:537, 2004.

Woo J et al: A randomized controlled trial of Tai Chi and resistance exercise on bone health, muscle strength, and balance in community-living elderly people, *Age Ageing*, March 13, 2007.

Wosje KS et al: High bone mass in Hutterite women, *J Bone Miner Res* 15:1429, 2000.

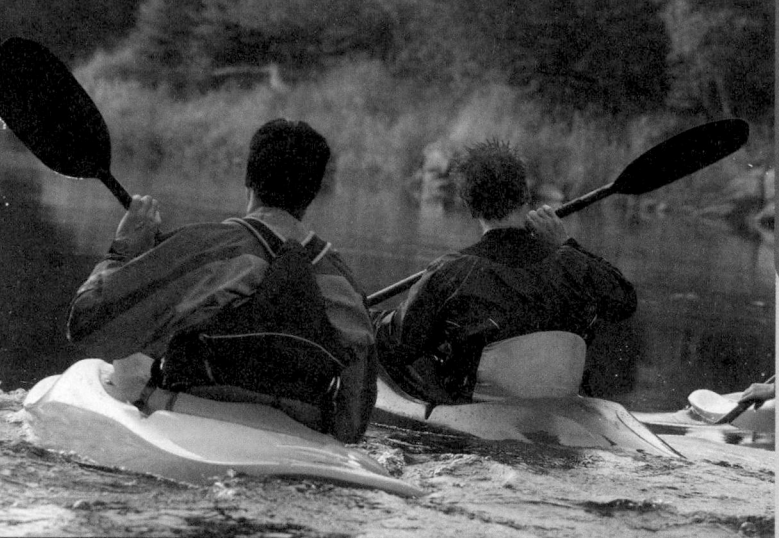

CHAPTER 25

Diane Rigassio Radler, PhD, RD
Riva Touger-Decker, PhD, RD, FADA

Nutrition for Oral and Dental Health

KEY TERMS

anticariogenic suppressing the development of caries by preventing plaque from recognizing an acidogenic food

calculus a hard, stone like concretion that forms on the teeth as a result of calcification of dental plaque

candidiasis an infection caused by the yeastlike fungus *Candida*, usually *Candida albicans*

cariogenic containing fermentable carbohydrates that can cause a decrease in salivary pH to less than 5.5 and demineralization when in contact with microorganisms in the mouth; promoting caries development

cariogenicity caries-promoting properties of a food

cariostatic having the characteristic of not being metabolized by microorganisms in plaque to cause a drop in salivary pH to less than 5.5

demineralization the dissolution of enamel or the loss of minerals from the hydroxyapatite, the principal component of the enamel

dental caries an oral infectious disease in which acid produced by bacterial metabolism of fermentable carbohydrates leads to bacterial invasion, causing demineralization of enamel and destruction of the tooth structure

dentin the chief organic tissue of the tooth that surrounds the pulp and is covered by enamel on the crown and cementum on the roots

early childhood caries (ECC) caries pattern in infants or children, also known as baby bottle tooth decay; generally caused by prolonged exposure of teeth to sweetened beverages

enamel an inorganic, white, crystalline, compact, and very hard substance that covers and protects the dentin of the tooth; the principal component is hydroxyapatite

fermentable carbohydrate any carbohydrate that is susceptible to the actions of salivary amylase

fluoroapatite the form in which the fluoride ion, along with calcium and phosphorus, is incorporated into dentin and enamel

fluorosis a condition of abnormal enamel caused by exposure of the tooth to excessive amounts of fluoride during enamel development before tooth eruption

gingiva the part of the oral mucosa overlying the crowns of unerupted teeth and encircling the necks of those that have erupted; the gums

gingival sulcus a shallow, V-shaped space around the tooth that is bounded by the tooth surface on one side and the epithelium lining the gingiva on the other

hydroxyapatite a naturally occurring form of calcium and phosphorus (apatite); the main mineral component of dental enamel and dentin

periodontal disease oral infectious disease characterized by inflammation and destruction of the attachment apparatus of the teeth, including the ligamentous attachment of the tooth to the surrounding alveolar bone

plaque a sticky, colorless film of microorganisms, salivary proteins, inorganic components, and polysaccharides that adheres to teeth and gums

remineralization the process of mineral restoration to the hydroxyapatite in the dental enamel

stomatitis inflammation of the oral mucosa

Streptococcus mutans an oral bacteria implicated in the formation of dental caries

xerostomia mouth dryness secondary to lack of or insufficient saliva

Diet and nutrition play key roles in tooth development, integrity of the **gingiva** (gums) and mucosa , bone strength, and the prevention and management of diseases of the oral cavity. Diet has a local effect on tooth integrity; that is, the type, form, and frequency of foods and beverages consumed have a direct effect on the oral pH and microbial activity, which may promote dental decay. By contrast, nutrition has a systemic effect. The impact of nutrient intake systemically affects the development, maintenance, and repair of the teeth and oral tissues. Deficiencies of several vitamins (riboflavin, folate, B_{12}, and C) and minerals (iron and zinc) may be first detected in the mouth because of the rapid tissue turnover rate of the oral mucosa.

Nutrition and diet affect the oral cavity, but the reverse also is true; that is, the status of the oral cavity may affect one's ability to consume an adequate diet and achieve nutrient balance. Oral diseases extend beyond dental caries. Partial or complete tooth loss (edentulism) is common in persons older than 65 years of age and can have a significant impact on dietary intake, especially fiber and protein. For the aging population in the United States, dietary intake, oral health and their influence on nutritional and overall well-being is paramount.. The following sections detail the known roles of nutrients in the growth, development, and maintenance of the oral cavity structure, bones, and tissues.

Periodontal disease is a local and systemic disease. Select nutrients, including vitamins A, C, E; folate; β-carotene; and the minerals calcium, phosphorus, and zinc play a role in this disease. Nutrition strategies and other strategies to modify risk factors for bone loss in osteoporosis also may contribute to reducing the risk of tooth loss.

Oral cancer, often a result of tobacco and alcohol abuse, can have a significant impact on eating ability and nutrition status. This problem is compounded by the increased caloric and nutrient needs of persons with oral carcinomas. In addition, surgery, radiation therapy, and chemotherapy are modalities used to treat oral cancer that also can affect dietary intake, appetite, and the integrity of the oral cavity.

Several chronic and acute diseases have oral consequences that affect eating ability. Poorly controlled diabetes can result in burning tongue syndrome, **candidiasis,** and xerostomia, which in turn compromise a person's eating ability and appetite and may exacerbate poor blood sugar control, leading to a cycle of debilitating health (see Chapter 30). Oral manifestations of immunosuppressive diseases such as human immunodeficiency virus (HIV)/ acquired immune deficiency syndrome (AIDS) also have an impact on appetite, dietary intake, and nutrient needs (Touger-Decker and Mobley, 2003) (see Chapter 38). Medications used to treat the diseases, either by prescription or over the counter, may have adverse effects, further compromising the ability to ingest an optimal diet (see Chapter 16).

NUTRITIONAL FACTORS IN TOOTH DEVELOPMENT

Primary tooth development begins at 2 to 3 months' gestation. Mineralization begins at about 4 months' gestation and continues through the preteen years. Therefore maternal nutrition must supply the preeruptive teeth with the appropriate building materials. Inadequate maternal nutrition will consequently impact tooth development; Table 25-1 details the effects of nutrient deficiencies and the presence of fluoride on tooth development; Figure 25-1 shows the parts of a tooth.

Teeth are formed by the mineralization of a protein matrix. In **dentin,** protein is present as collagen, which depends on vitamin C for normal synthesis. Vitamin D is essential to the process by which calcium and phosphorus are deposited in crystals of **hydroxyapatite,** a naturally occurring form of calcium and phosphorus that is the mineral component of dental **enamel** and dentin. Fluoride added to the hydroxyapatite provides unique caries-resistant properties to teeth in both prenatal and postnatal developmental periods.

Diet and nutrition are important in all phases of tooth development, eruption, and maintenance. Posteruption, diet and nutrient intake continue to affect tooth development and mineralization, enamel development and strength, and eruption patterns of the remaining teeth. The local effects of diet, particularly fermentable carbohydrates and eating frequency, affect the production of organic acids by oral bacteria and the rate of decay; the mechanism is

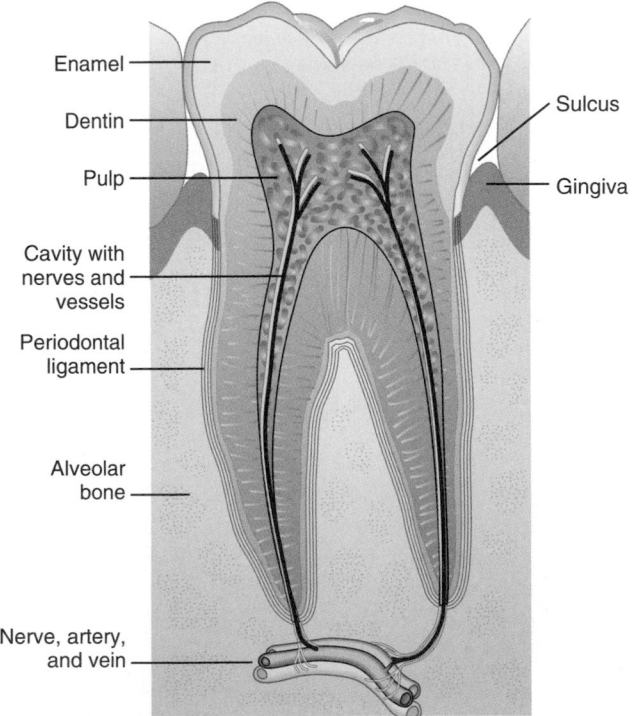

FIGURE 25-1 Anatomy of a tooth.

TABLE 25-1

Effects of Nutrients on Tooth Development

Nutrient	Effect On Tissue	Effect On Caries	Human Data
Protein/calorie malnutrition	Delayed tooth eruption Decreased tooth size Decreased enamel solubility Salivary gland dysfunction	Yes	Yes
Vitamin A deficiency	Decreased epithelial tissue development Tooth morphogenesis dysfunction Decreased odontoblast differentiation Increased enamel hypoplasia Hypomineralization (hypoplastic defects) Compromised tooth integrity (decreased mineral concentration) Delayed eruption patterns	Yes	Yes
Ascorbic acid deficiency	Dental pulpal alterations Odontoblastic degeneration Aberrant dentin	No	No
Fluoride presence	Increased stability of enamel crystal (enamel formation) Inhibition of demineralization Stimulation of remineralization Mottled enamel (excess) Inhibition of bacterial growth	Yes	Yes
Iodine deficiency	Delayed tooth eruption Altered growth patterns Malocclusions	No	Yes
Iron deficiency	Slow growth Salivary gland dysfunction	Yes	No

Modified from DePaola D et al: Nutrition in relation to dental medicine. In Shils ME, Olson JA, Shike M, editors: *Modern nutrition in health and disease*, vol 2, ed 8, Philadelphia, 1994, Lea & Febiger.

described later in the chapter in detail. Throughout the life span, diet and nutrition continue to affect tooth, bone, and oral mucosal integrity; resistance to infection; and tooth longevity.

DENTAL CARIES

Dental caries is one of the most common infectious diseases. According to the Surgeon General's 2000 Report on Oral Health, dental caries is seven times more common than hay fever and five times more common than asthma. Unfortunately differences are evident in caries prevalence; approximately 20% to 25% of U.S. children have 80% of the dental caries.

Trends in dental caries have demonstrated that children who come from homes in which parents have at least a college education have fewer caries than children from homes in which parents have less than a college education (USDHHS, 2000). These differences, or health dispari-

ties, may happen as a result of lack of access to care, cost of care not reimbursed by third-party payors (e.g., insurance, Medicaid), lack of knowledge of preventive dental care, or a combination of factors.

Pathophysiology

Dental caries is an oral infectious disease in which organic acid metabolites produced by the metabolism of oral microorganisms lead to gradual **demineralization** of tooth enamel, followed by rapid proteolytic destruction of the tooth structure. Caries can occur on any tooth surface.

The etiology of dental caries involves many factors. Four factors must be present simultaneously: (1) a susceptible host or tooth surface; (2) microorganisms such as *Streptococcus* or *Lactobacillus*, in the dental plaque or oral cavity; (3) fermentable carbohydrates in the diet, which serve as the substrate for bacteria; and (4) time (duration) in the mouth for bacteria to metabolize the fermentable carbohydrates, produce acids, and cause a drop in salivary pH to less than 5.5. Once the pH falls below 5.5, oral bacteria can initiate the demineralization process. Plaque pH can fall in as little as 5 minutes and take up to 2 hours to return to neutral levels if no oral hygiene measures are introduced. Figure 25-2 shows the formation of dental caries.

Susceptible Tooth

The development of dental caries requires the presence of a tooth that is vulnerable to attack. The composition of enamel and dentin, the location of teeth, the quality and quantity of saliva, and the presence and extent of pits and fissures in the tooth crown are some of the factors that govern susceptibility. The composition of the saliva also is important. Alkaline saliva may have a protective effect, whereas acidic saliva increases susceptibility to decay (see *Clinical Insight:* Acid Ash and Alkaline Ash Diets in Chapter 36).

Lifestyle, genetics, and oral hygiene also can affect caries risk. For example, a lifestyle with a diet regimen consisting of small frequent meals rather than two or three meals per day may expose the teeth more frequently to fermentable carbohydrates, increasing the risk of caries. Genetic variations of the type and quantity of bacteria present in the oral cavity may put someone at an increased risk for caries and periodontal disease, and the quantity and quality of oral hygiene certainly has a direct effect on the risk of oral infectious disease.

Microorganisms

Bacteria are an essential part of the decay process. Several microorganisms are capable of fermenting dietary carbohydrates. *Streptococcus mutans* is the most prevalent, followed by *Lactobacillus casein* and *Streptococcus sanguis*. All three contribute to the process because they metabolize carbohydrates in the mouth, producing acid as a by-product, which is sufficient to cause decay.

Substrate

Fermentable carbohydrates, those carbohydrates susceptible to the actions of salivary amylase, are the ideal substrate for bacterial metabolism. The acids produced by their metabolism cause a drop in salivary pH to less than 5.5, creating the environment for decay. In light of the Dietary Guidelines for Americans and the MyPyramid Food Guidance system, both of which support a diet high in carbohydrates, it is important to be aware of the cariogenicity of foods that can affect the potential for bacterial action on fermentable carbohydrates. Individuals should be aware of the form of food consumed and the frequency of intake in order to integrate positive diet and oral hygiene habits to help improve oral health status. Factors that affect the cariogenicity of substrates are listed in Box 25-1.

Fermentable carbohydrates are found in four of the six MyPyramid food groups: (1) grains, (2) fruits, (3) dairy products, and (4) added sugars in the category of fats and sweets. Although some vegetables may contain fermentable carbohydrates, little has been reported about the cariogenicity, or caries-promoting properties of vegetables. Examples of grains and starches that are cariogenic by nature of their fermentable carbohydrate composition, which can

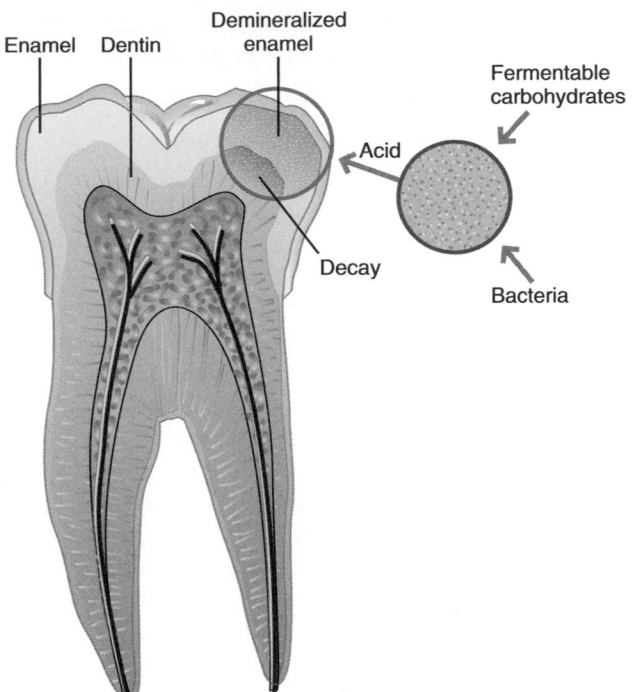

FIGURE 25-2 Formation of dental caries.

BOX 25-1

Factors Affecting Food Cariogenicity

Frequency of consumption of fermentable carbohydrates
Food form (e.g., liquid, solid, slowly dissolving)
Sequence of eating foods and beverages
Combination of foods
Nutrient composition of foods and beverages
Duration of exposure of teeth to foods and beverages

---

cause a decrease in salivary pH to less than 5.5, include crackers, chips, pretzels, hot and cold cereals, and breads.

All fruits (fresh, dried, and canned) and fruit juices may be cariogenic. Fruits with high water content such as melons have a lower cariogenicity than others such as bananas and dried fruits. Fruit drinks, sodas, ice teas, and other sugar-sweetened beverages; desserts; cookies; candies; and cake products may be cariogenic. Dairy products sweetened with fructose, sucrose, or other sugars can also be cariogenic because of the added sugars; however, dairy products are rich in calcium, and their alkaline nature may have a positive influence, reducing the cariogenic potential of the food.

Like other sugars (glucose, fructose, maltose, and lactose), sucrose stimulates bacterial activity. The causal relationship between sucrose and dental caries has been established (Lingstrom et al., 2000; Moynihan, 2005). All dietary forms of sugar, including honey, molasses, brown sugar, and corn syrup solids, have cariogenic potential and can be used by bacteria to produce organic acid by-products of metabolism. Maltose, found in candies, doughnuts, potato chips, crackers, and other snack foods, also contribute to the cariogenic potential of a food. Salivary amylase breaks down the dietary sugars over time.

Cariogenicity of Individual Foods

It is important to differentiate between cariogenic, cariostatic, and anticariogenic foods. Sophisticated testing methods have enabled an evaluation of the cariogenicity of specific foods. The amount of acid produced by bacteria when carbohydrates are present in the mouth is not proportional to the sugar content of the food; likewise the amount of tooth demineralization does not necessarily parallel the amount of acid produced from the food. Hence the formation of different types of fermentation products or the presence of substances in the food may reduce or enhance the caries-producing action of a sugar. Cariogenicity also is influenced by the volume and quality of saliva a person produces; the sequence, consistency, and nutrient composition of the foods eaten; plaque buildup; and the genetic predisposition of the host to decay. **Cariogenic** foods are those that contain fermentable carbohydrates, which, when in contact with microorganisms in the mouth, can cause a drop in salivary pH to 5.5 or less and stimulate the caries process.

Cariostatic foods, or foods that do not contribute to decay, are not metabolized by microorganisms in plaque and do not cause a drop in salivary pH to 5.5 or less within 30 minutes. Examples of cariostatic foods are protein foods such as eggs, fish, meat, and poultry; most vegetables; fats; and sugarless gums. Noncarbohydrate sweeteners such as saccharin, cyclamate, aspartame, and sucralose are cariostatic. Some evidence supports the idea that aspartame, saccharin, and sucralose may inhibit bacterial action because neither provides a usable substrate for streptococcus bacteria (Mandel and Grotz, 2002).

Anticariogenic foods are those that prevent plaque from recognizing an acidogenic food when it is eaten first. The five-carbon sugar alcohol, xylitol, is considered anticariogenic. It is not broken down by salivary amylase and is not subject to bacterial degradation. Its mechanisms of action include antimicrobial activity against *S. mutans* (Hildebrandt and Sparks, 2000) and the impact of gum chewing on salivary stimulation.

Salivary stimulation leads to increased buffering activity of the saliva and subsequent increased clearance of fermentable carbohydrates from tooth surfaces. Sugar-free chewing gum may help to reduce decay potential because of its ability to increase saliva flow and is recommended after meals and snacks to reduce the caries risk (Milgrom, 2006). **Remineralization** (mineral restoration to the hydroxyapatite in the dental enamel) capabilities are subsequently enhanced. Another anticariogenic mechanism of xylitol gum is that it replaces fermentable carbohydrates in the diet. *S. mutans* cannot metabolize xylitol; it actually inhibits the bacteria. Other anticariogenic foods are cheeses such as aged cheddar, Monterey jack, and Swiss because of the casein, calcium, and phosphate in the cheese. Recaldent, a substance derived from casein,

promotes remineralization of enamel surfaces. It is currently available as an ingredient in Trident brand chewing gums and is anticipated to be available in toothpastes and mouthwashes.

Factors Affecting Cariogenicity of Food

Foods contain fermentable carbohydrates, the basis for bacterial action, which, in turn, stimulates caries development. **Cariogenicity** refers to the caries-promoting properties of a diet or food, and the cariogenicity of a food varies, depending on the form in which it occurs, its nutrient composition, when it is eaten in relation to other foods and fluids, the duration of its exposure to the tooth, and the frequency with which it is eaten (see Box 25-1).

Form and Consistency

The form and consistency of a food have a significant impact on its cariogenic potential and pH-reducing or buffering capacity. Food form determines the duration of exposure or retention time of a food in the mouth, which, in turn, affects how long the decrease in pH or the acid-producing activity will last. Liquids are rapidly cleared from the mouth and have low adherence (or retentiveness) capabilities. Solid foods such as crackers, chips, pretzels, dry cereals, and cookies can stick between the teeth (referred to as the interproximal spaces) and have high adherence (or retention) capability. Consumption of hard candies, lollipops, and sugared breath mints result in prolonged sugar exposure in the mouth.

Consistency also affects adherence. Chewy foods such as gum drops and marshmallows although high in sugar content, stimulate saliva production and have a lower adherence potential than solid, sticky foods such as pretzels, bagels, or bananas. High-fiber foods with few or no fermentable carbohydrates, such as popcorn and raw vegetables, are cariostatic.

Exposure

The duration of exposure may be best explained with starchy foods, which are fermentable carbohydrates subject to the action of salivary amylase. The longer starches are retained in the mouth, the greater their cariogenicity (Lingstrom et al., 2000). Given sufficient time, such as when food particles become lodged between the teeth, salivary amylase makes additional substrate available as it hydrolyzes starch to simple sugars. Processing techniques make some starches rapidly fermentable, either by partial hydrolysis or by reducing particle size, thus increasing availability for enzyme action.

Although sugar-containing candies cause a rapid increase in the amount of sugars available in the oral cavity to be hydrolyzed by bacteria, their effect is short lived. By comparison, simple carbohydrate-based snacks and dessert foods (e.g., potato chips, pretzels, cookies, cakes, and doughnuts) provide gradually increasing oral sugar concentrations for a longer duration because these foods often adhere to the tooth surfaces and are retained for longer periods than candies (Lingstrom et al., 2000).

Nutrient Composition

Nutrient composition contributes to the ability of a substrate to produce acid and to the duration of acid exposure. Dairy products, by virtue of their calcium- and phosphorus-buffering potential, are considered to have low cariogenic potential. Studies have shown that cheese and milk, when consumed with cariogenic foods, help to buffer the acid pH produced by cariogenic foods (Marshall et al., 2003). Because of the anticariogenic properties of cheese, eating cheese with a fermentable carbohydrate, such as dessert at the end of a meal, may decrease the cariogenicity of the meal (Kashket and DePaola, 2002).

Nuts, which do not contain a significant amount of fermentable carbohydrates and are high in fat and dietary fiber, are cariostatic. Protein foods such as seafood, fish, meats, eggs, and poultry, along with other fats such as oils, margarine, butter, and seeds, are also cariostatic. Overall good dietary habits in children are associated with reduced caries experience (Dye et al., 2004).

Sequence and Frequency of Eating

Eating sequence and combination of foods also affect the caries potential of the substrate. Bananas, which are cariogenic because of their fermentable carbohydrate content and adherence capability, have less potential to contribute to decay when eaten with cereal and milk than when eaten alone as a snack. Milk, as a liquid, reduces the adherence capability of the fruit. Crackers eaten with cheese are less cariogenic than when eaten alone. The buffering capacity of cheese and milk makes them desirable foods to eat at the end of a meal or in combination with other fermentable carbohydrates to reduce potential cariogenicity.

The frequency with which a cariogenic food or beverage is consumed determines the number of opportunities for acid production. Every time a fermentable carbohydrate is consumed, a decline in pH is initiated within 5 to 15 minutes, causing caries-promoting activity. Small, frequent meals and snacks, often high in fermentable carbohydrate, increase the cariogenicity of a diet considerably more than a diet consisting of three meals and minimal snacks. Eating several cookies at once, followed by brushing the teeth or rinsing the mouth with water, is less cariogenic than eating a cookie at several times throughout a day. Table 25-2 lists messages that can be given to children to prevent caries.

The Decay Process

The carious process begins with the production of acids as a by-product of bacterial metabolism taking place in the dental plaque. Decalcification of the surface enamel continues until the buffering action of the saliva is able to raise the pH above the critical level.

TABLE 25-2

Oral Health and Nutrition Messages for 3- to 10-Year-Old Children and Their Caregivers

Message	Rationale
Starchy, sticky, or sugary foods should be eaten with nonsugary foods.	The pH will rise if a nonsugary item that stimulates saliva is eaten immediately before, during, or after a challenge.
Combine dairy products with a meal or snack.	Dairy products (nonfat milk, yogurt) enhance remineralization and contain calcium.
Combine chewy foods such as fresh fruits and vegetables with fermentable carbohydrates.	Chewy, fibrous foods induce saliva production and buffering capacity.
Space eating occasions at least 2 hours apart and limit snack time to 15-30 minutes.	Fermentable carbohydrates eaten sequentially one after another promote demineralization.
Limit bedtime snacks.	Saliva production declines during sleep.
Limit consumption of acidic foods such as sports drinks, juices, and sodas.	Acidic foods promote tooth erosion that increases risk for caries.
Combine proteins with carbohydrates in snacks: Examples: tuna and crackers, apples and cheese	Proteins act as buffers and are cariostatic.
Combine raw and cooked or processed foods in a snack.	Raw foods encourage mastication and saliva production, whereas cooked or processed foods may be more available for bacterial metabolism if eaten alone.
Encourage use of xylitol/sorbitol–based chewing gum and candies immediately following a meal or snack.*	Five minutes of exposure is effective in increasing saliva production and dental plaque pH.
Sugar-free chewable vitamin/mineral supplements and syrup-based medication should be recommended.	Sugar-free varieties are available and should be suggested for high–caries risk groups.
Encourage children with pediatric gastroesophageal reflux disease (GERD) to adhere to dietary guidelines.	GERD increases risk for dental erosion and thus increases risk for caries.

Modified from Mobley C: Frequent dietary intake and oral health in children 3 to 10 years of age, *Building Blocks* 25(1):17-20, 2001.

* Gum is not recommended for children under the age of 6.

Plaque Formation

Plaque is a sticky, colorless mass of microorganisms and polysaccharides that forms around the tooth and adheres to teeth and gums. It harbors acid-forming bacteria and keeps the organic products of their metabolism in close contact with the enamel surface. As a cavity develops, the plaque shields the tooth, to some extent, from the buffering and remineralization action of the saliva. In time the plaque combines with calcium and hardens to form **calculus.**

Acid Production

Several beverage categories such as soft drinks (diet and regular), sports beverages, citrus juices and "ades," and vitamin C supplements have high acid content and therefore can contribute to an acidic pH. Research using the National Health and Nutrition Examination Survey (NHANES) III data reported significantly more dental caries experience in children (ages 2 to 10 years) who consumed large amounts of carbonated soft drinks when compared to children who had high consumption of water or milk. Those children who consumed large amounts of juice showed a trend toward greater incidence of dental caries versus those who consumed milk or water (Sohn et al., 2006).

Foods and beverages may also contribute to dental erosion, a loss of minerals from tooth surfaces by a chemical process in the presence of acid (Wongkhantee et al., 2006). For example, diet soft drinks, which may not contain sugar, also are acidic by nature and therefore cause a drop in pH. Chewable vitamin C supplements provide an acidic substance that directly contacts tooth surfaces and causes a drop in pH of the oral cavity, making teeth susceptible to decay. Box 25-2 contains tips on reducing the likelihood of caries.

Saliva Function

Salivary flow clears food from around the teeth. By means of the bicarbonate-carbonic acid and phosphate buffer system, it also provides buffering action to neutralize bacterial acid metabolism. Chewing promotes saliva production and may account for the reduced cariogenicity of fermentable carbohydrates consumed with a meal.

BOX 25-2

Caries Prevention Guidelines

Brush at least twice daily, preferably after meals.
Rinse mouth after meals and snacks when brushing is not possible.
Chew sugarless gum for 15 to 20 min after meals and snacks.
Floss twice daily.
Use fluoridated toothpastes.
Pair cariogenic foods with cariostatic foods.
Snack on cariostatic and anticariogenic foods such as cheese, nuts, popcorn, and vegetables.
Limit between-meal eating and drinking of fermentable carbohydrates.

Saliva is supersaturated with calcium and phosphorus. Once buffering action has restored pH above the critical point, remineralization can occur. If fluoride is present in the saliva, the minerals are deposited in the form of fluoroapatite, which is resistant to erosion. It should be noted that salivary production decreases as a result of diseases affecting salivary gland function (e.g., Sjögren's syndrome), as a side effect of fasting, as a result of radiation therapy to the head and neck involving the parotid gland, normally during sleep, with the use of medications associated with reduced salivary flow, or with **xerostomia,** dry mouth due to inadequate saliva production (see Chapter 16). There are estimates that between 400 and 500 medications currently available by prescription or over the counter may cause dry mouth. The degree of xerostomia may vary but may be caused by medications such as those to treat depression, hypertension, anxiety, HIV, and allergies, to name a few.

Caries Patterns

Caries patterns describe the location and surfaces of the teeth affected. Although the overall incidence of decay in the United States has declined, as many as 17% of children between 2 and 4 years of age have tooth decay (Centers for Disease Control and Prevention, 2005). According to the National Health and Nutrition Examination Survey (NHANES) III, as many as 50% of children have experienced some decay by age 8 (USDHHS, 2000).

Root caries, occurring on the root surfaces of teeth secondary to gingival recession, affect a large portion of the older population. In a 2-year cohort study of people ages 45 and older, 36% of people had at least one new root decayed surface (Gilbert et al., 2001). A primary factor in the development of root decay is gingival recession, often secondary to periodontal disease, which results in exposure of root surfaces to the oral environment (Gilbert et al., 2001; Takano, 2003). These surfaces lack an enamel layer and therefore are more vulnerable to rapid decay.

Other factors related to the increased incidence of this decay pattern are age, lack of fluoridated water, poor oral hygiene practices, decreased saliva, and frequent eating of fermentable carbohydrates (Siukosaari et al., 2005). Root caries is a dental infectious disease that is increasing in older adults, partly because this population is retaining their natural teeth longer. The gums recede in older age, exposing the root surface. If fermentable carbohydrates are not cleared from the oral cavity, the decay process begins and can easily affect the roots of the teeth that are exposed due to the receding gum line. Management of root caries includes dental restoration and nutrition counseling.

Lingual caries, or caries on the lingual side (surface next to or toward the tongue) of the anterior teeth, are seen in persons with bulimia or anorexia-bulimia (see Chapter 22). Frequent intake of fermentable carbohydrates, combined with repeated episodes of induced vomiting of acidic stomach contents, results in a constant influx of acid into the oral cavity. The caries are the end result of tooth erosion characterized by erosion of the palatal and buccal surfaces of the maxillary anterior teeth and the lingual surfaces of the palatal surface of the maxillary posterior teeth (Little, 2002). Lingual caries may also be seen in persons with gastroesophageal reflux disease as a result of repeated episodes of acid regurgitation (Munoz et al., 2003).

Fluoride

Fluoride is a primary anticaries agent. Used systemically and locally, it is a safe, effective public health measure to reduce the incidence and prevalence of dental caries (Palmer and Wolfe, 2005). Water fluoridation began in 1940; by 1999 the Centers for Disease Control and Prevention listed water fluoridation as one of the top 10 greatest public health achievements of the 20th century because of its impact on decreasing the rate of dental caries (CDC, 2006).

The impact of fluoride on caries prevention continues with water fluoridation, fluoridated toothpastes, oral rinses, and dentifrices, as well as beverages made with fluoridated water. Fluoridation is "the adjustment of fluoride in the water supply to an optimal concentration of 0.7 to 1.2 ppm" (Palmer and Wolfe, 2005). Optimal water fluoridation concentrations (0.7 to 1.2 ppm) can provide protection against caries development without causing tooth staining.

Mechanism of Action

The three primary mechanisms of fluoride action on teeth are: (1) when incorporated into enamel and dentin along with calcium and phosphorus, it forms **fluoroapatite**, a compound more resistant to acid challenge than hydroxyapatite; (2) fluoride also promotes repair and remineralization of tooth surfaces with early signs of decay (incipient carious lesions); it helps to reverse the decay process while promoting the development of a tooth surface that has increased resistance to decay; and (3) fluoride also may help to deter the harmful effects of bacteria in the oral cavity by interfering with the formation and function of microorganisms.

Fluoride can be used topically and systemically. When consumed in food and drink, it enters the systemic circulation and is deposited in bones and teeth. Systemic sources have a topical benefit as well by providing fluoride to the saliva. A small amount of fluoride enters the soft tissues; the remainder is excreted. The primary source of systemic fluoride is fluoridated water; food and beverages supply a smaller amount. Table 25-3 contains a schedule of fluoride supplementation for the public through age 16.

Topical fluoride sources include toothpastes, gels, and rinses used by consumers daily, along with more concentrated forms applied by dental professionals in the form of gels, foams, and rinses. Frequent fluoride exposure via topical fluorides, fluoridated toothpastes, rinses, and fluoridated water is important in maintaining a high concentration of fluoride on the tooth enamel (see *Focus On:* Water Fluoridation).

Sources of Fluoride

Most foods, unless prepared with fluoridated water, contain minimal amounts of fluoride, except for brewed tea, with approximately 1.4 ppm (Morin, 2006). Fluoride may be unintentionally added to the diet in a number of ways, including the use of fluoridated water in the processing of foods and beverages. Fruit juices and drinks, particularly white grape juice produced in cities with fluoridated water, may have increased fluoride content; however, because of the wide variation in fluoride content, it is difficult to estimate amounts consumed.

It is prudent for health professionals to consider a child's fluid intake as well as food sources and the availability of fluoridated water in the community before prescribing fluoride supplements. Because bones are repositories of fluoride, bone meal, fish meal, and gelatin made from bones are potent sources of the mineral. In communities without fluoridated water, dietary fluoride supplements are recommended for children ages 6 months to 16 years (see

TABLE 25-3

Dietary Fluoride Supplement Schedule

	Fluoride Ion Level In Drinking Water (ppm)[*]		
Age	< 0.3 ppm	0.3-0.6 ppm	> 0.6 ppm
Birth-6 mo	None	None	None
6 mo-3 yr	0.25 mg/day[†]	None	None
3-6 yr	0.50 mg/day	0.25 mg/day	None
6-16 yr	1.0 mg/day	0.50 mg/day	None

From American Dietetic Association: Position of the American Dietetic Association: impact of fluoride on dental health, *J Am Diet Assoc* 100:128, 2000.

[*]1 part per million (ppm) = 1 mg/L.

[†]2.2 mg of sodium fluoride contains 1 mg of fluoride ion.

◎ FOCUS ON

Water Fluoridation

Fluoride supplementation has been endorsed as a public health measure by the American Dental Association and American Dietetic Association (Palmer and Wolfe, 2005). The U.S. Surgeon General's Report on Oral Health (USDHHS, 2000) also stresses the value of fluoridation in dental disease prevention and tooth protection. However, despite this support, the widespread use of fluoride has been challenged by "antifluoridationists" who claim that fluoridation restricts individual freedom of choice and increases the risk of acquired immune deficiency syndrome (AIDS) and cancer. Disease-associated risks of fluoride are unfounded. No epidemiologic studies have demonstrated any link between fluoride and cancer or AIDS. Fluoride has no adverse health effects, and the risk of toxicity is negligible (Palmer and Wolfe, 2005). The American Dietetic Association endorses the use of systemic and topical fluoride and water fluoridation as a vital public health measure (Palmer and Wolfe, 2005).

Table 25-3).

Causes of mild fluorosis from excessive fluoride intake include misuse of dietary fluoride supplements, ingestion of fluoridated toothpastes and rinses, or excessive fluoride intake secondary to fluoride in foods and beverages processed in fluoridated areas and transported to other areas (Palmer and Wolfe, 2005). It is now recommended that supplementation start at the age of 6 months if the level of fluoride in the water supply is less than 0.6 ppm (not 0.7 ppm as previously designated). Because there is a low level of fluoride in breast milk, other sources of fluoride in the diet of an infant should be assessed. Fluoride supplements are not recommended for breast-fed infants living in fluoridated communities if these infants receive drinking water between feedings. If the infant does not drink water between feedings and consumes only breast milk, he or she should be supplemented according to the fluoride supplement guidelines (see Table 25-3). Fluoride supplements must be prescribed by the child's doctor; they are not available as over-the-counter supplements.

Topical fluorides, available as fluoridated toothpaste and mouthwashes, are effective sources of fluoride that can be used in the home, school, or dental office. Caries prevention efforts in preschool children include diet modification, water fluoridation or supplements in nonfluoridated areas, and supervised toothbrushing with fluoridated toothpaste (Tinanoff, 2002).

Children younger than 6 years of age should not use fluoridated mouthwashes, and older children should be instructed to rinse, but not swallow, mouthwash. No more than a pea-size amount of toothpaste should be placed on a child's toothbrush to reduce the risk of accidental fluoride ingestion. Topical fluorides may be administered in the dental office.

Fluoride gels often are prescribed for adults and older adults. Such gels are effective in reducing the risk of coronal and root decay and tooth loss (Weintraub et al., 2006). Fluoride is most effective when given from birth through ages 12 to 13, the period when mineralization of unerupted permanent teeth occurs.

Fluorosis, or mottling of the tooth, can occur secondary to excessive fluoride intake from diet and supplements; excessive topical fluoride; or ingestion of fluoridated toothpastes, rinses, or dentifrices during the early years of tooth development. Excessive dietary intake of fluoride can occur as a result of long-term use of infant formulas in powder form that are reconstituted with fluoridated water. Mild fluorosis starts with white patchy spots. Fluorosis progresses to dark brown stains on the teeth as it becomes severe. Mottling occurs in severe fluorosis, which results in pitting in the enamel surface of the tooth, weakening it and making it susceptible to decay.

PREVENTIVE CARE

Caries prevention programs focus on a balanced diet, modification of the sources and quantities of fermentable carbohydrates, and the integration of oral hygiene prac-

tices into individual lifestyles (Tinanoff, 2005). Meals and snacks should be followed with brushing, rinsing the mouth vigorously with water, or chewing sugarless gum for 15 to 20 minutes. Positive habits should be encouraged, including snacking on anticariogenic or cariostatic foods, chewing sugarless gum after eating or drinking cariogenic items, and having sweets with meals rather than as snacks. Despite the potential for a diet that is based on the dietary guidelines to be cariogenic, with proper planning and good oral hygiene a balanced diet low in cariogenic risk can be planned. Figure 25-3 contains a sample diet plan that is low in cariogenic risk.

Practices to avoid include sipping carbonated beverages over extended periods; frequent snacking; and harboring candy, sugared breath mints, or hard candies in the mouth for extended periods. Over-the-counter chewable or liquid medications and vitamin preparations also may contain sugar. Chewable vitamin C is one example of a sugar-containing acid product that may contribute to tooth decay. Careful label reading is important to avoid or minimize the use of such products.

Fermentable carbohydrates such as candy, crackers, cookies, pastries, pretzels, snack crackers, chips, and even fruits should be eaten with meals. Notably, "fat-free" snack and dessert items and "baked" chips and snack crackers tend to have a higher simple sugar concentration than their higher fat-containing counterparts. A piece of cheese at the end of

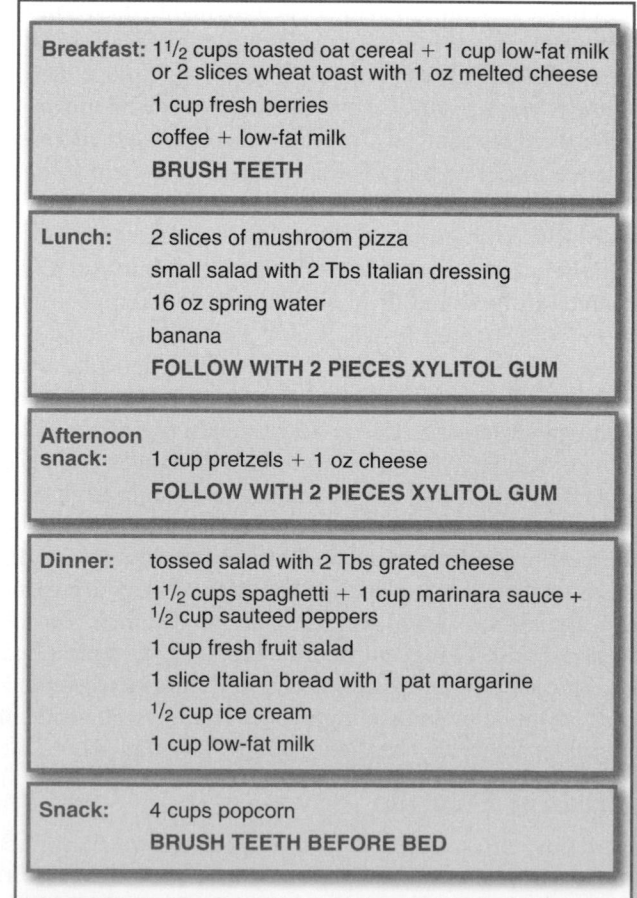

Breakfast: 1½ cups toasted oat cereal + 1 cup low-fat milk or 2 slices wheat toast with 1 oz melted cheese
1 cup fresh berries
coffee + low-fat milk
BRUSH TEETH

Lunch: 2 slices of mushroom pizza
small salad with 2 Tbs Italian dressing
16 oz spring water
banana
FOLLOW WITH 2 PIECES XYLITOL GUM

Afternoon snack: 1 cup pretzels + 1 oz cheese
FOLLOW WITH 2 PIECES XYLITOL GUM

Dinner: tossed salad with 2 Tbs grated cheese
1½ cups spaghetti + 1 cup marinara sauce + ½ cup sauteed peppers
1 cup fresh fruit salad
1 slice Italian bread with 1 pat margarine
½ cup ice cream
1 cup low-fat milk

Snack: 4 cups popcorn
BRUSH TEETH BEFORE BED

FIGURE 25-3 A balanced diet plan with low cariogenic risk.

a meal or with a snack is an example of a caries reduction strategy when consuming these foods.

Evidence supports the use of xylitol-sweetened gum as an anticaries agent after meals and snacks (Hildebrandt and Sparks, 2000; Milgrom, 2006). Xylitol is a five-carbon sugar that cannot be metabolized by oral bacteria. Research has documented its ability to reduce caries incidence by reducing the levels of *S. mutans* in saliva. The current recommended dose is two pieces after each meal or snack containing fermentable carbohydrates. Twenty minutes of chewing appears to cause a rise in salivary pH to a level greater than 5.5.

PERIODONTAL DISEASE

Pathophysiology

Periodontal disease is an inflammation of the gingiva with infection caused by oral bacteria and subsequent destruction of the tooth attachment apparatus. Untreated periodontitis results in a gradual loss of tooth attachment to the bone. Progression is influenced by the overall health of the host and the integrity of the immune system.

The primary etiologic factor in the development of periodontal disease is plaque. Plaque in the **gingival sulcus,** a shallow, V-shaped space around the tooth, produces toxins that destroy tissue and permit loosening of the teeth. Important factors in the defense of the gingiva to bacterial invasion are: (1) oral hygiene; (2) integrity of the immune system; and (3) optimal nutrition. The defense mechanisms of the gingival tissue, epithelial barrier, and saliva are affected by nutritional intake and status. Healthy epithelial tissue prevents the penetration of bacterial endotoxins into subgingival tissue.

Nutritional Care

Deficiencies of vitamin C, folate, and zinc increase the permeability of the gingival barrier at the gingival sulcus, increasing susceptibility to periodontal disease. Severe deterioration of the gingiva is seen in individuals with scurvy or vitamin C deficiency. Although other nutrients, including vitamins A, E, β-carotene, and protein, have a role in maintaining gingival and immune system integrity, there are no scientific data to support supplemental uses of any of these nutrients to treat periodontal disease.

Nutrient deficits have been implicated in the incidence and severity of periodontal disease. However, although optimal nutrition may play a role in positive outcomes of periodontal treatment, nutrients alone are not a cure for the disease (Schifferle, 2005). In societies where malnutrition and periodontal disease are prevalent, poor oral hygiene is also usually evident. In such instances it is difficult to determine whether malnutrition is the cause of the disease or one of many contributing factors, including poor oral hygiene, heavy plaque buildup, insufficient saliva, or coexisting illness. The roles of calcium and vitamin D relate to the link between osteoporosis and periodontal disease, in which bone loss is the common denominator. The association between periodontal disease and systemic osteopenia and osteoporosis has been documented (Gur et al., 2003; Jeffcoat, 2005), as has tooth loss and osteoporosis in postmenopausal women (Krall, 2001) (see Chapter 24). The inverse relationship between decreased calcium intake and increased risk of periodontal disease has also been demonstrated (Nishida, 2000). Since dairy foods are a rich source of calcium, researchers documented a similar inverse relationship between increased dairy food intake and decreased incidence of periodontal disease (Al-Zahrani, 2006). Although causal relationships have not been determined, the association of calcium and dairy foods with periodontal disease warrants advocating a sufficient intake of dairy foods such as that recommended by the MyPyramid Food Guidance system.

Beginning with a diet evaluation, including a several-day food diary or diet recall to determine eating frequency, food intake, and oral hygiene habits, a dental professional or registered dietitian can evaluate the overall eating pattern and nutritional adequacy of the diet. Individual dental nutrition risk factors that may contribute to oral disease are areas that can then be addressed in counseling the patient or client. Nutrition and dietary management of the patient or client with periodontal disease follows many of the same caries prevention guidelines listed in Box 25-2.

Severe periodontal disease may be treated surgically with periodontal surgery. Diet adequacy is particularly important both before and after periodontal surgery, when adequate nutrients are needed to regenerate tissue and maintain an immune response to prevent infection. Adequacy of calories, protein, and micronutrients should be ensured. If the ability to consume one's regular diet will be altered, a diet modified in consistency can be individually designed for the patient or client. Oral supplements can be used when necessary to attain nutrient adequacy.

EARLY CHILDHOOD CARIES

Early childhood caries (ECC), often called baby-bottle tooth decay (BBTD), is a term used to describe a caries pattern in the maxillary anterior teeth of infants and young children. Characteristics include rapidly developing carious lesions in the primary anterior teeth and the presence of lesions on tooth surfaces not usually associated with a high caries risk (Berkowitz, 2003). Because tooth decay remains a common oral disease of childhood, caries are a primary marker for children's oral health. Good behavioral habits and child nutrition patterns must be encouraged beginning in infancy.

Pathophysiology and Incidence

Often ECC occurs secondary to prolonged bottle-feeding, especially at night, of juice, milk, formula, or other sweetened beverages. The extended contact time with the fermentable carbohydrate–containing beverages, coupled with the position of the tongue against the nipple, which causes pooling of the liquid around the maxillary incisors, particularly during sleep, contributes to the decay process. The mandibular anterior teeth are usually spared (Figure 25-4)

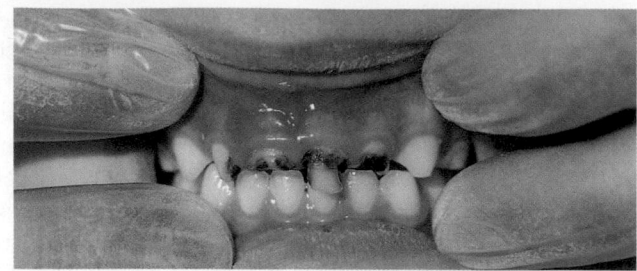

FIGURE 25-4 Early childhood caries. *(From Swartz MH: Textbook of physical diagnosis, history, and examination, ed 5, Philadelphia, 2006, Saunders.)*

because of the protective position of the lip and tongue and the presence of a salivary duct in the floor of the mouth.

Generally children in low-income, undereducated groups are at high risk for ECC and other dental diseases. In a study of the nutrition and oral health habits of infants and young children in Iowa, researchers noted a 23% incidence of decay (Levy et al., 2003). In a study of more than 1600 children in Manhattan, the level of untreated decay was 91%, significantly higher than the U.S. national population, which is 76% overall and 76% for blacks and Mexican-Americans within the population (Albert et al., 2002). In general, children from low-income families experience the greatest amount of oral disease, the most extensive disease, and the most frequent use of dental services for pain relief; yet these children have the fewest overall dental visits (Edelstein, 2002).

Psoter and colleagues (2006) have reported that income and education levels are inversely related with ECC. In addition, people belonging to minority races and ethnicities are among those with greater ECC prevalence. Shiboski and colleagues (2001) reported a high prevalence of ECC (30% to 33%) among Asian and Latino/Hispanic communities compared to their white counterparts. Not surprisingly the risk of ECC increased in those children who fell asleep while sucking on a bottle.

Nutrition Care

Management of ECC includes diet and oral hygiene education for parents, guardians, and caregivers (Albert et al., 2002). Messages should be targeted to counter the health habits that contribute to this problem, including poor oral hygiene, failure to brush a child's teeth at least daily, frequent use of bottles filled with sweetened beverages, and lack of fluoridated water (Levy et al., 2003). Dietary guidelines include removal of the bedtime bottle and modification of the frequency and content of the daytime bottles. Bottle contents should be limited to water, formula, or milk. Infants and young children should not be put to bed with a bottle. Teeth and gums should be cleaned with a gauze pad or washcloth after all bottle feedings. All efforts should be made to wean children from a bottle by 1 year of age. Juice can be provided in a diluted form in a cup (Bowen and Lawrence, 2005).

Educational efforts should be positive and simple, focusing on oral hygiene habits and promotion of a balanced, healthy diet. Between-meal snacks should include cariostatic foods or, when foods are cariogenic, they should be followed by toothbrushing or rinsing the mouth. Parents and caregivers need to understand the causes and consequences of ECC and how they can be avoided.

TOOTH LOSS AND DENTURES

Tooth loss (edentulism) and removable prostheses (dentures) can have a significant impact on dietary habits, masticatory function, olfaction, and nutritional adequacy. Compromised masticatory function, from partial or complete edentulism or complete dentures, may have a negative impact on food choices, resulting in decreased intake of whole grains, fruits, and vegetables (Nowjack-Raymer and Sheiham, 2003).

Increased tooth loss results in an inadequate intake of dietary fiber, vitamins, and minerals (Hung et al., 2003; Sheiham et al., 2001). As dentition status declines, masticatory performance is compromised. This problem is more pronounced in older adults, whose appetite and intake may be compromised further by chronic disease, social isolation, and the use of multiple medications (see Chapter 16).

Unfortunately dentures do not fully solve the problem. Full dentures replace missing teeth and are not a perfect substitute for natural dentition. Both before and after denture placement, many individuals may experience eating difficulty (biting and chewing) even after denture insertion (Morais et al., 2003). The foods found to cause the greatest difficulty for persons with complete dentures include fresh whole fruits and vegetables (e.g., apples and carrots), hard-crusted breads, and steak.

Dentures need to be checked periodically by a dental professional for appropriate fit. Changes in body weight or changes in alveolar bone over time possibly may alter the fit of the dentures. Counseling on appropriate food choices and textures is advocated.

Nutrition Care

Dietary assessment and counseling related to oral health should be provided to the denture wearer. Simple guidelines should be provided for cutting and preparing fruits and vegetables to minimize the need for biting and reduce the amount of chewing. The importance of positive eating habits needs to be stressed as a component of preventive health. Overall, health guidelines that reinforce the importance of a balanced diet based on the MyPyramid Food Guidance system should be part of the routine health counseling given to all patients.

Consumers can be guided to peel and chop fruits, vegetables, and other foods to reduce the need for biting and chewing. Foods can be cooked to a softer consistency, and meats and vegetables can be cut across the fibers into bite-size pieces to make eating easier. Sticky foods such as soft white breads, caramels, chewing gum, toffees, and chewy candies should be avoided. Patients can be encouraged to use their knife and fork as their "teeth" initially, cutting food into small pieces.

ORAL MANIFESTATIONS OF SYSTEMIC DISEASE

Acute systemic diseases such as cancer and infections, as well as chronic diseases such as diabetes mellitus, autoimmune diseases, and end-stage renal disease, are characterized by oral manifestations that may alter the diet and nutritional status. Cancer therapies, including irradiation of the head and neck region, chemotherapy, and surgeries to the oral cavity, have a significant impact on the integrity of the oral cavity and on an individual's eating ability, which may consequently affect nutrition status (see Chapter 37).

If the condition of the mouth adversely affects one's food choices, the person with chronic disease may not be able to follow the diet optimal for medical nutrition therapy. For example, poorly controlled diabetes may manifest in xerostomia or candidiasis, which may then impact the ability to consume a diet to appropriately control blood sugar, further deteriorating the glucose control.

Manifestations of HIV/AIDS

Viral and fungal infections, stomatitis, xerostomia, periodontal disease, and Kaposi's sarcoma are oral manifestations of HIV that can cause limitations in nutrient intake and result in weight loss and compromised nutrition status. These infections often are compounded by a compromised immune response, preexisting malnutrition, and gastrointestinal consequences of HIV infection (see Chapter 38). Viral diseases, including herpes simplex and cytomegalovirus, result in painful ulcerations of the mucosa. Candidiasis on the tongue, palate, or esophagus can make chewing, sucking, and swallowing painful (odynophagia), thus compromising intake. Table 25-4 outlines the impact of associated oral infections in the upper gastrointestinal tract.

Fungal Infections

Oropharyngeal fungal infections may cause a burning, painful mouth and dysphagia. The ulcers that accompany viral infections such as herpes simplex and cytomegalovirus cause pain and can lead to reduced oral intake. Very hot and cold foods or beverages, spices, and sour or tart foods also may cause pain and should be avoided. Consumption of temperate, moist foods without added spices should be encouraged. Small, frequent meals followed by rinsing with lukewarm water or brushing to reduce the risk of dental caries are helpful. Once the type and extent of oral manifestations are identified, a nutrition care plan can be developed. Oral high calorie–high protein supplements in liquid or pudding form may be needed to meet nutrient needs and optimize healing.

Other Painful Mouth Problems

Stomatitis, or inflammation of the oral mucosa, causes severe pain and ulceration of the gingiva, oral mucosa, and palate, which makes eating painful. Xerostomia, or dry mouth, is seen in poorly controlled diabetes mellitus, Sjögren's syndrome, and several autoimmune diseases and as a consequence of radiation therapy and certain medications (Box 25-3). Xerostomia from radiation therapy may be more permanent than that from other causes (Kielbassa et al., 2006). Radiation therapy procedures to spare the parotid gland should be implemented when possible to reduce the damage to the salivary gland. Efforts to stimulate saliva production using pilocarpine and citrus-flavored, sugar-free candies may ease eating difficulty.

Individuals without any saliva at all have the most difficulty eating; artificial salivary agents may not offer relief. Lack of saliva impedes all aspects of eating, including chewing, forming a bolus, swallowing, and sensing taste; causes pain; and increases the risk of dental caries and infections. Dietary guidelines focus on the use of moist foods without added spices, increased fluid consumption

TABLE 25-4

Impact of Oral Infections

Location	Problem	Effect	Diet Management
Oral cavity	Candidiasis, KS, herpes, stomatitis	Pain, infection, lesions, altered ability to eat, dysgeusia	Increase kilocalorie and protein intake; administer oral supplements; provide caries risk reduction education
	Xerostomia	Increased caries risk, pain, no moistening power, tendency of food to stick, dysgeusia	Moist, soft, nonspicy foods; "smooth" cool or warm foods and fluids; caries risk reduction education
Esophagus	Candidiasis, herpes, KS, cryptosporidiosis	Dysphagia, odynophagia	Try oral supplementation first; if that is unsuccessful, initiate NG feedings using silastic feeding tube or PEG
	CMV, with or without ulceration	Dysphagia, food accumulation	PEG

CMV, Cytomegalovirus; *KS,* Kaposi's sarcoma; *NG,* nasogastric; *PEG,* percutaneous endoscopic gastrostomy.

Medications That May Cause Xerostomia

Antianxiety agents
Anticonvulsants
Antidepressants
Antihistamines
Antihypertensives
Diuretics
Narcotics
Sedatives
Serotonin uptake inhibitors
Tranquilizers

with and between all meals and snacks, and judicious food choices.

Problems with chewy (steak), crumbly (cake, crackers, rice), dry (chips, crackers), and sticky (peanut butter) foods are common in persons with severe xerostomia; alternatives should be suggested, or the foods should be avoided to avert dysphagia risk. Drinking water with a lemon or lime twist or citrus-flavored seltzers or sucking on frozen tart grapes or berries or sugar-free candies may help. Good oral hygiene habits are important in reducing the risk of tooth decay and should be practiced after all meals and snacks. Xylitol-flavored gums and mints may help to reduce the risk of associated decay.

Diabetes Mellitus

Diabetes is associated with several oral manifestations, many of which occur only in periods of poor glucose control. These include burning mouth syndrome, periodontal disease, candidiasis, dental caries, and xerostomia (Mattson and Cerutis, 2001). The microangiopathies seen in diabetes, along with altered responses to infection, contribute to risk of periodontal disease in affected persons. Tooth infection, more common in those with diabetes, leads to deterioration of diabetes control (Bender and Bender, 2003). Besides blood glucose control, dietary management for people with diabetes after any oral surgery procedures and or placement of dentures should include modifications in the consistency, temperature, and texture of food to increase eating comfort, reduce oral pain, and prevent infections or decay while managing glucose control (see Chapter 30).

Head and Neck Cancers

Head, neck, and oral cancers can alter eating ability and nutrition status by virtue of the surgeries and therapies used to treat these cancers. Surgery, depending on the location and extent, may alter eating or swallowing ability, as well as the capacity to produce saliva. Radiation therapy of the head and neck area and chemotherapeutic agents can affect the quantity and quality of saliva and the integrity of the oral mucosa. Thick, ropey saliva is often the result of radiation therapy to the head and neck area, causing xerostomia. Dietary management focuses on the recommendations described earlier for xerostomia, along with modifications in food consistency following surgery (see Chapter 37).

POLYPHARMACY

Several categories of medications can alter the integrity of the oral mucosa, taste sensation, and salivary production (see Chapter 16). Phenytoin (Dilantin) may cause severe gingivitis. Many of the protease inhibitor drugs used to treat HIV/AIDS are associated with altered taste and dry mouth. Care should be taken to assess the effects of medication on the oral cavity and how these effects can be minimized by alterations in diet or drug therapy.

FOCAL POINTS

- As the gateway to the human body, the oral cavity can have a significant effect on nutrition and overall health and well-being.
- Diet and nutrition are important in the phases of managing oral health and disease.
- The integrity of the oral cavity and surrounding structures can affect functional and sensory components of normal dietary intake and subsequent nutritional status.
- Similarly, compromised nutrition status resulting from poor diet or disease can affect the integrity of the oral cavity.

- In planning nutrition care, the registered dietitian is encouraged to consider the status of the client's oral health as a component of nutritional screening and assessment, including problems with biting, chewing, or swallowing; dry mouth; or the presence of sores in the mouth that interfere with eating.
- Food and eating guidelines to facilitate biting and chewing for optimal intake can be integrated into the nutrition care process.

Shelly is a 51-year-old single mother of two teenage daughters who works full-time as a real estate agent. She goes to the dentist for the first time in 5 years because she just got dental insurance. Her chief complaint is, "All my teeth hurt." She further states that she spends 50% of her time in her car traveling between appointments. She has no significant medical history; her family history reveals that her mother has type 2 diabetes. She quit smoking 1 pack per day 6 months ago and at that time went on a diet. She is presently 5 ft 6 in. tall and weighs 135 lb. Six months ago she weighed 165 lb. Since then she has been on a fruit-based vegetarian diet. She has always chewed sugar gum but since quitting smoking has increased her gum chewing and reports chewing three jumbo packs (18 sticks per pack) of cinnamon-flavored sugar gum daily. On examination the dentist determines that she has periodontal disease, extensive dental caries, two broken teeth, and a broken three-unit bridge (a bridge that supports three teeth). She needs root canal surgery in three teeth. To restore her smile aesthetically, she will either need a removable partial denture or implants. Her food recall is as follows:

7:30 AM	1 banana
7:45 AM	½ large cantaloupe
8:00 AM	2 c watermelon
8:15 AM	1 banana and 1 apple
10:00 AM	2 bite-size chocolate mint patties

Noon sandwich:	2 slices wheat bread with 1 tsp mustard, ½ c alfalfa sprouts, 1 c sliced tomatoes and cucumbers, ¼ c avocado; 15 mini pretzels
12:45 PM	½ c vanilla custard
3 PM	1 each apple and banana, 2 chocolate mint patties
6:30 PM	3 c mixed salad, 1 c Japanese noodles
9:00 PM	4 bite-size chocolates

She drinks 2-3 L of water throughout the day.

✳**Nutrition Diagnosis 1:** Chewing difficulty related to avoidance of many foods and preference for soft fruits as evidenced by mouth pain

✳**Nutrition Diagnosis 2:** Inadequate protein intake related to fruit-based diet as evidenced by intake of less than 50% of estimated requirements

1. What are the social, lifestyle, and environmental influences that are affecting Shelly's dental and nutritional health?
2. What are her nutrition and dietary risk factors?
3. What are appropriate diet counseling recommendations for this patient?

Nathan, a 3-year-old black male, is brought to the local health clinic by his grandmother because his front teeth are "turning black." Nathan seems small for his age; his height is measured at 35.5 in., and his weight is 25 lb. According to the growth charts, he is in the 10th percentile for height, the 5th percentile for weight, and below the 5th percentile of weight for height.

On examination by the dentist, the child is found to have eight decayed surfaces on his four anterior teeth (the two central incisors and the two lateral incisors). The dentist recommends that Nathan have metal crowns put on the decayed teeth. She also recommends that the grandmother have the child's diet and nutritional status evaluated by the clinic's registered dietitian. The grandmother agrees, and the dietary history taken by the dietitian reveals the following:

- A diet high in simple sugar with small, frequent meals
- Continued use of a bottle filled with fruit drink, soda, or strawberry-flavored milk three times a day, including at nap time
- Suboptimal calorie and protein intake (70% and 75% of estimated needs, respectively)

- Lack of vitamin-mineral and fluoride supplements
- Nonrenewal of Women, Infants and Children (WIC) checks within the last 6 months because the grandmother does not like traveling to the area where the clinic is located
- Inconsistent toothbrushing (grandmother reports brushing the child's teeth three to four times per week. She does not think care of baby teeth is important because "they fall out anyway."

✳**Nutrition Diagnosis 1:** Underweight related to inadequate protein/energy intake as evidenced by diet history revealing 70% of energy needs and 75% of protein needs

✳**Nutrition Diagnosis 2:** Undesirable food choices related to high sugar intake as evidenced by high sugar beverages at least three times daily

Continued

⚜ CLINICAL SCENARIO 2—cont'd

✴Nutrition Diagnosis 3: Food- and nutrition-related knowledge deficit related to appropriate diet for toddler as evidenced by continued use of bottle containing high sugar beverages several times daily

1. What are the cultural, educational, and environmental influences affecting Nathan's dental and nutritional health?

2. What type of dental condition does Nathan have? What are the diet counseling recommendations for this condition?
3. What are the nutritional and dietary risk factors?
4. Design a nutrition care plan to improve this youngster's dental health and growth.

USEFUL WEBSITES

American Dental Association
http://www.ada.org/

American Dental Hygienists Association
http://www.adha.org/

American Academy of Periodontology
http://www.perio.org/

Colgate Kids
http://www.colgate.com/app/Colgate/US/OC/
Information/InteractiveGuides/EveryAge.cvsp

HIV Dent
http://www.hivdent.org/

Diabetes and Oral health
http://www.nidcr.nih.gov/HealthInformation/
DiseasesAndConditions/DiabetesAndOralHealth/
default.htm
http://www.diabetes.org/type-2-diabetes/mouth-care.jsp

**National Institute of Dental
and Craniofacial Research**
http://www.nidcr.nih.gov/

Surgeon General Report on Oral Health
http://www.surgeongeneral.gov/library/oralhealth/

Oral Health America
http://www.oralhealthamerica.org/

World Health Organization on Oral Health
http://www.who.int/oral_health/en/

References

Al-Zahrani MS: Increased intake of dairy products is related to lower periodontitis prevalence. *J Periodontol* 77:289, 2006.

Albert DA et al: Dental caries among disadvantaged 3- to 4-year-old children in northern Manhattan, *Pediatr Dent* 24:229, 2002.

Bender IB, Bender AB: Diabetes mellitus and the dental pulp, *J Endod* 29:383, 2003.

Berkowitz RJ: Causes, treatment and prevention of early childhood caries: a microbiologic perspective, *J Can Dent Assoc* 69:304, 2003.

Bowen WH, Lawrence RA: Comparison of the cariogenicity of cola, honey, cow milk, human milk, and sucrose, *Pediatrics* 116):921, 2005.

Centers for Disease Control and Prevention: *Improving oral health: preventing cavities, gum disease and tooth loss,* http://www.cdc.gov/nccdphp/aag/aag_oh.htm, accessed November 3, 2005.

Centers for Disease Control and Prevention: *Recommendations for using fluoride to prevent and control dental caries in the United States,* http://www.cdc.gov/mmwr/preview/mmwrhtml/rr5014a1.htm, accessed May 15, 2006.

Dye BA et al: The relationship between healthful eating practices and dental caries in children aged 2-5 years in the United States, 1988-1994, *J Am Dent Assoc* 135:55, 2004.

Edelstein BL: Disparities in oral health and access to care: findings of national surveys, *Ambul Pediatr* 2(2 Suppl):141, 2002.

Gilbert GH et al: Twenty-four month incidence of root caries among a diverse group of adults, *Caries Res* 35:366, 2001.

Gur A et al: The relation between tooth loss and bone mass in postmenopausal osteoporotic women in Turkey: a multicenter study, *J Bone Miner Metabol* 21:43, 2003.

Hildebrandt GH, Sparks BS: Maintaining mutans streptococci suppression with xylitol chewing gum, *J Am Dent Assoc* 131:909, 2000.

Hung HC et al: Tooth loss and dietary intake, *J Am Dent Assoc* 134:1185, 2003.

Jeffcoat M: The association between osteoporosis and oral bone loss, *J Periodontol* 76(11 suppl):2125, 2005.

Kashket S, DePaola DP: Cheese consumption and the development and progression of dental caries, *Nutr Rev* 60:97, 2002.

Kielbassa AM et al: Radiation-related damage to dentition, *Lancet Oncol* 7:326, 2006.

Krall EA: The periodontal-systemic connection: Implications for treatment of patients with osteoporosis and periodontal disease, *Ann Periodontol* 6:209, 2001.

Levy SM et al: Fluoride, beverages and dental caries in the primary dentition, *Caries Res* 37:157, 2003.

Lingstrom P et al: Food starches and dental caries, *Crit Rev Oral Biol Med* 11:366, 2000.

Little JW: Eating disorders: dental implications, *Oral Surg Oral Med Oral Pathol Oral Radiol Endodon* 93:138, 2002.

Mandel ID, Grotz VL: Dental considerations in sucralose use, *J Clin Dentistry* 13:116, 2002.

Marshall TA et al: Dental caries and beverage consumption in young children, *Pediatrics* 112(3 Pt 1):e184, 2003.

Mattson JS, Cerutis DR: Diabetes mellitus: a review of the literature and dental implications, *Compend Contin Educ Dentistry* 22):757, 2001.

Milgrom P: Mutans streptococci dose response to xylitol chewing gum, *J Dent Res* 85:177, 2006.

Morais JA et al: The effects of mandibular two-implant overdentures on nutrition in elderly edentulous individuals, *J Dent Res* 82:53, 2003.

Morin K: Fluoride: action and use, *MCN Am J Matern Child Nurs* 31:127, 2006.

Moynihan P: The interrelationship between diet and oral health, *Proc Nutr Soc* 64:571, 2005.

Munoz JV et al: Dental and periodontal lesions in patients with gastroesophageal reflux disease, *Dig Liver Dis* 35:461, 2003.

Nishida M: Calcium and the risk for periodontal disease, *J Periodontol* 71:1057, 2000.

Nowjack-Raymer RE, Sheiham A: Association of edentulism and diet and nutrition in U.S. adults, *J Dent Res* 82:123, 2003.

Palmer C, Wolfe SH: Position of the American Dietetic Association: the impact of fluoride on health, *J Am Diet Assoc* 105:1620, 2005.

Psoter WJ et al: Associations of ethnicity/race and socioeconomic status with early childhood caries patterns, *J Public Health Dentistry* 66:23, 2006.

Schifferle RE: Nutrition and periodontal disease, *Dent Clin North Am* 49:595, 2005.

Sheiham A et al: The relationship among dental status, nutrient intake, and nutritional status in older people, *J Dent Res* 80:408, 2001.

Shiboski CH et al: The association of early childhood caries and race/ethnicity among California preschool children, *J Public Health Dentistry* 63:38, 2001.

Siukosaari P: Level of education and incidence of caries in the elderly: a 5-year follow-up study, *Gerodontology* 22:130, 2005.

Sohn W et al: Carbonated soft drinks and dental caries in the primary dentition, *J Dent Res* 85:262, 2006.

Takano N: Factors associated with root caries incidence in an elderly population, *Community Dent Health* 20:217, 2003.

Tinanoff N: Association of diet with dental caries in preschool children, *Dent Clin North Am* 49:725, 2005.

Tinanoff N: Current understanding of the epidemiology mechanisms, and prevention of dental caries in preschool children, *Pediatr Dentistry* 24:543, 2002.

Touger-Decker R, Mobley CC: Position of the American Dietetic Association: oral health and nutrition, *J Am Diet Assoc* 103:615, 2003.

U.S. Department of Health and Human Services: *Oral health in America: a report of the Surgeon General*, Rockville, Md, 2000, U.S. Department of Health and Human Services, National Institute of Dental and Craniofacial Research, National Institutes of Health.

Weintraub JA et al: Fluoride varnish efficacy in preventing early childhood caries, *J Dent Res* 85:172, 2006.

Wongkhantee S et al: Effect of acidic food and drinks on surface hardness of enamel, dentine, and tooth-coloured filling materials, *J Dentistry* 34:214, 2006.

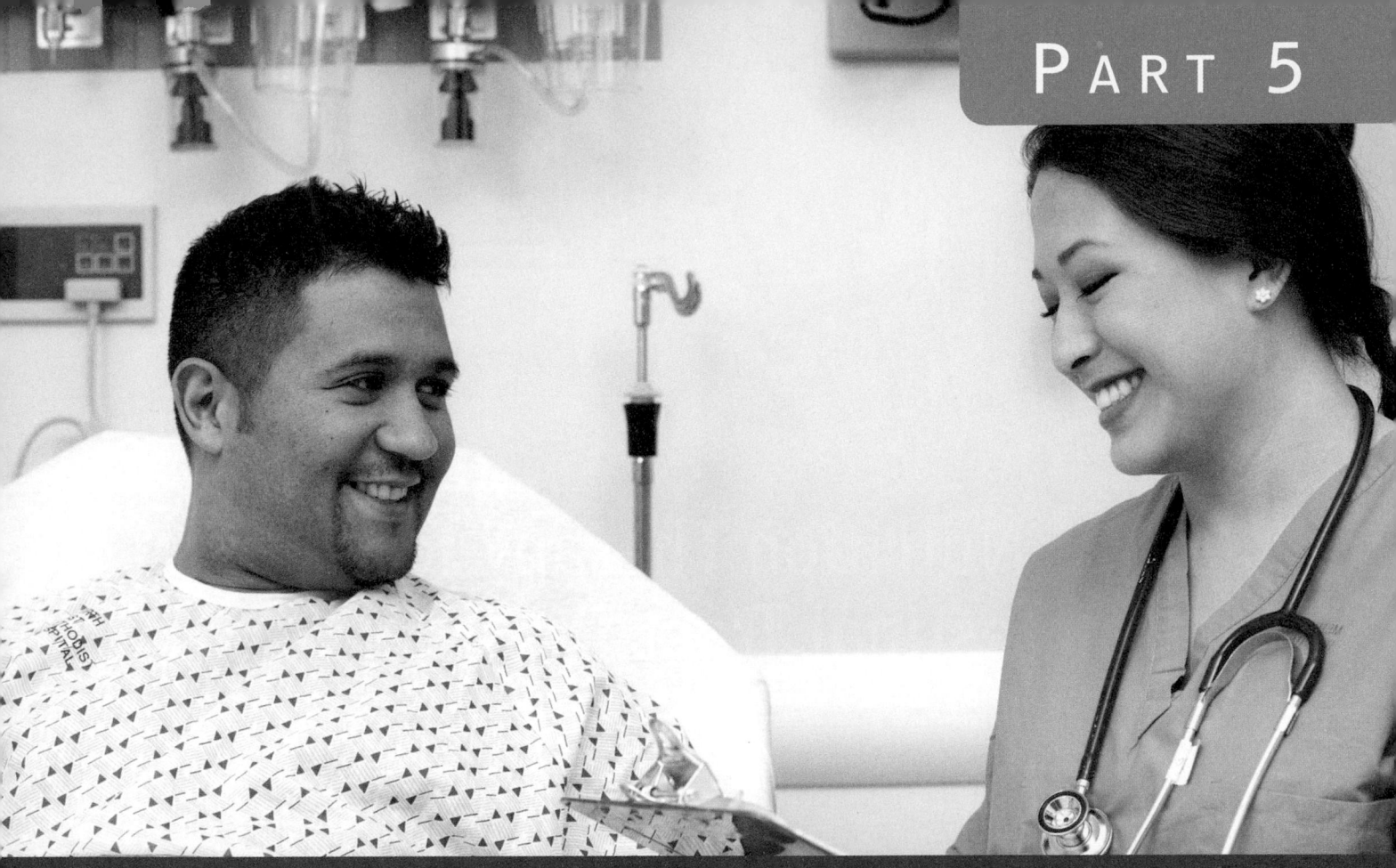

PART 5

Medical Nutrition Therapy

NUTRITION plays a primary role in growth, development, health, and fitness. Maintaining appropriate nutrition throughout life can also prevent or delay the onset of some nutrition-related diseases. This section clarifies the role of medical nutrition therapy (MNT) in the treatment of established disease.

As the knowledge base expands, the list of diseases amenable to nutrition intervention increases. Availability of sophisticated feeding and nourishment procedures places increased responsibility on those who provide nutrition care. Most of the nutrition-related disorders included here can be prevented or at least well-managed by changes in dietary practices based on current knowledge. Exceptions, such as some forms of cancer, are discussed in terms of both the evidence for prevention and the appropriate nutrition care in disease.

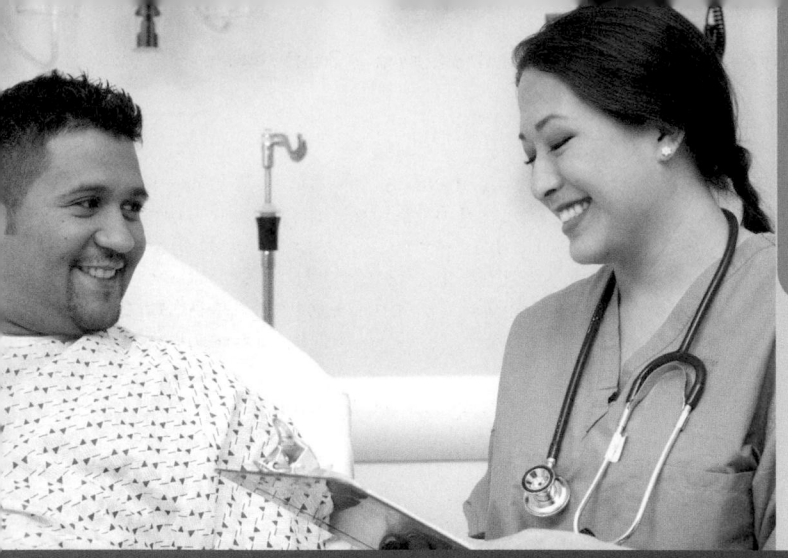

CHAPTER 26

Peter L. Beyer, MS, RD

Medical Nutrition Therapy for Upper Gastrointestinal Tract Disorders

KEY TERMS

achlorhydria absence of hydrochloric acid from maximally stimulated gastric secretions

achylia gastrica absence of hydrochloric acid and pepsin in the gastric juice

alimentary hypoglycemia low blood glucose manifesting as weakness, perspiration, hunger, nausea, anxiety, and tremors 1 to 2 hours after a meal

atrophic gastritis chronic inflammation of the stomach with deterioration of the mucous membrane and glands, resulting in achlorhydria and loss of intrinsic factor

Barrett's esophagus (BE) a condition in which cells lining the distal esophagus become abnormal and premalignant

dumping syndrome a complex physiologic response to the rapid emptying of hypertonic contents into the duodenum and jejunum

duodenal ulcer a peptic ulcer situated in the duodenum

dyspepsia (indigestion) a general term used to describe epigastric discomfort following meals

endoscopy a procedure used to view the esophagus, stomach, and upper part of the small intestine using a flexible tube with a camera

epigastric referring to the upper middle region of the abdomen

esophagitis inflammation of the esophagus

functional dyspepsia unexplained persistent or recurrent upper GI discomfort; symptoms may include vague abdominal discomfort, bloating, early satiety, nausea, and belching; underlying mechanisms are not entirely clear, but may include visceral hypersensitivity to acid or distention, impaired gastric accommodation, altered brain-gut axis, and abnormal gastric motility

fundoplication a surgical procedure for the treatment of reflux esophagitis in which the fundus of the stomach is wrapped around the lower end of the esophagus

gastrectomy removal of all (e.g., total gastrectomy) or part (hemi-gastrectomy) of the stomach

gastric ulcers lesions that are associated with disruption of the gastric mucosal barrier

gastritis inflammation of the stomach

gastroesophageal reflux disease (GERD) backward flow of the stomach or duodenal contents into the esophagus; may occur normally or as a chronic pathologic condition

heartburn a retrosternal burning related to reflux of gastric contents into the esophagus

Helicobacter pylori a type of bacteria that can chronically infect the stomach; known to be a primary contributor to the development of gastritis, peptic ulcers, and even gastric cancer

hiatal hernia an outpouching of a portion of the stomach into the chest through the esophageal hiatus of the diaphragm

lower esophageal sphincter (LES) the last few centimeters of the esophagus, which prevents reflux of gastric contents into the esophagus

melena black, tarry stools indicative of gastrointestinal bleeding

parietal cells large cells, located on the margin of the peptic glands of the stomach, which secrete hydrochloric acid and produce intrinsic factor

parietal cell vagotomy resection or removal of the portion of the vagus nerve innervating the parietal cells for the purpose of diminishing gastric acid secretion

peptic ulcer an eroded lesion in either the esophageal, gastric, or duodenal mucosa resulting from the action of gastric secretions and typically *H. pylori* bacterial inflammation

truncal vagotomy resection or removal of portions of the vagus nerve to decrease the cholinergic stimulation of parietal cells and reduce the cellular response to stimulants such as gastrin

vagus nerve the tenth cranial nerve, which has many branches that supply sensory fibers to the ear, tongue, pharynx, and larynx; motor fibers to the pharynx, larynx, and esophagus; and parasympathetic and visceral afferent fibers to the thoracic and abdominal viscera

Digestive disorders are among the most common problems in health care. About 30% to 40% of adults claim to have frequent indigestion, and over 50 million visits are made annually to ambulatory care facilities for symptoms related to the digestive system. Over 10 million endoscopies and surgical procedures involving the gastrointestinal (GI) tract are performed each year (Woodell and Cherry, 2004).

Dietary habits and specific food types can play a significant role in the onset, treatment, and prevention of many GI disorders. In many cases diet can also play a role in improving patients' sense of well-being and quality of life by decreasing pain, suffering, worry, health care visits, and the costs associated with GI disease. Table 26-1 lists disorders of the upper GI tract that are described in this chapter and the typical symptoms and nutritional consequences.

DISORDERS OF THE ESOPHAGUS

The entire esophagus functions as one tissue during swallowing. As a bolus of food is moved voluntarily from the mouth to the pharynx, the upper sphincter relaxes, the food moves into the esophagus, and peristaltic waves move the bolus down the esophagus; the **lower esophageal sphincter (LES)** relaxes to allow the food bolus to pass into the stomach (Figure 26-1).

Disorders of the esophagus may be caused by derangement of the swallowing mechanism, obstruction, inflammation, or abnormal sphincter function. Because difficulty in swallowing (dysphagia) is often the result of a neurologic problem, it is discussed in Chapter 41.

Gastroesophageal Reflux and Esophagitis

Prevalence and Pathophysiology

Reflux of gastric contents into the esophagus occurs occasionally in healthy individuals, and some even experience classic heartburn symptoms episodically. However, about 7% to 8% of the population experience daily **heartburn,** resulting from frequent reflux of gastric and sometimes duodenal contents into the esophagus. The prevalence of

TABLE 26-1

Upper Gastrointestinal Disorders and Nutritional Consequences

Gastrointestinal Condition	Common Symptoms	Possible Nutritional Consequences
Esophageal reflux or esophageal reflux disease (GERD)	Acid taste, increased belching, hoarseness, dry cough, burning sensation in upper middle of chest, sometimes spasm, difficulty swallowing, bloating	Altered food choices, not eating evening meals, avoidance of acid foods, reduced quality and quantity of dietary intake
Esophageal stricture or tumor	Asymptomatic, or difficulty swallowing foods; solids may especially cause discomfort	Reduced energy intake, diet not nutritionally complete, decreased fiber intake, weight loss
Hiatal hernia	Asymptomatic, or contributes to prolonged exposure of esophagus to gastric contents with reflux symptoms	May not have any consequence or may experience discomfort after meals and with position changes
Cancer of the oral cavity, esophagus, or stomach	Asymptomatic, or difficulty chewing, swallowing, epigastric discomfort, delayed gastric emptying	Anorexia, decreased amount or number of foods, weight loss, change in food textures; may require surgery, radiation, chemotherapy, enteral feeding
Dyspepsia	Upper abdominal discomfort, bloating, especially after meals	Increased concerns about diet, possible decreased intake of food in general or selected foods
Duodenal ulcer	Pain several hours after meals; may be relieved by eating	Perceived food intolerances, increased or decreased food intake
Gastric ulcer	Vague epigastric discomfort associated with eating	Decreased intake in general or of selected foods
Dumping syndrome after gastrectomy, pyloroplasty, fundoplication, Roux-en-Y gastric by-pass procedure	Early: satiety, bloating, nausea; weak, lightheaded, sweaty; later: symptoms such as reactive hypoglycemia and possibly cramping, diarrhea	Decreased intake, malabsorption of nutrients, weight loss, micronutrient deficiencies

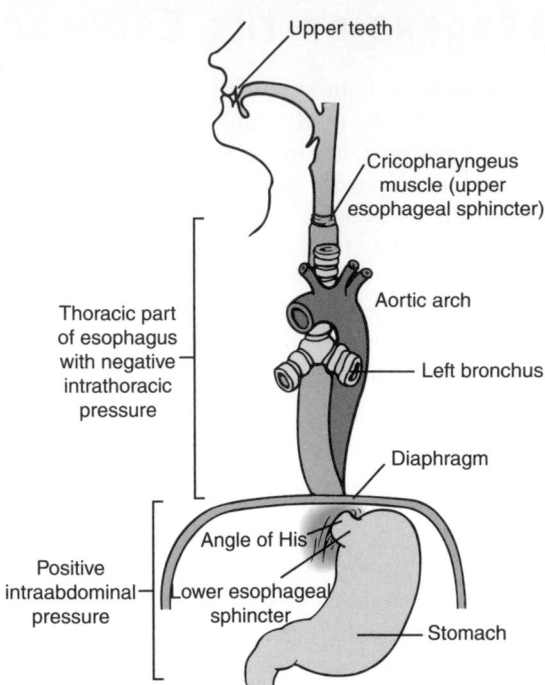

Upper teeth

Cricopharyngeus
muscle (upper
esophageal sphincter)

Thoracic part
of esophagus
with negative
intrathoracic
pressure

Aortic arch

Left bronchus

Diaphragm

Angle of His

Positive
intraabdominal
pressure

Lower esophageal
sphincter

Stomach

FIGURE 26-1 Normal esophagus. (*Modified from Price SA, Wilson LM: Pathophysiology: clinical concepts of disease processes, ed 6, St Louis, 2003, Mosby*).

esophageal reflux varies with the description of the symptoms, but about 20% to 40% of adults report symptoms of **gastroesophageal reflux disease (GERD)** at least one time per week (Talley and Wiklund, 2005). Regurgitation occurs in about half of infants in the first few months of life; most cases resolve after the first year. The prevalence of GERD in childhood is not entirely clear but may range from about 2% to 20% (Craig et al., 2004; Gold, 2004).

The presentation of symptoms varies but may include reflux of gastric secretions, heartburn with episodes of substernal pain, belching, and esophageal spasm. In children, vomiting, dysphagia, refusal to eat, or complaints of abdominal pain may be present (Hassall, 2005). Manifestations such as pharyngeal irritation, frequent throat clearing, hoarseness, and worsening of asthmatic symptoms may also occur with or without classic heartburn or noticeable acid reflux. The frequency and severity of symptoms do not always predict the severity or complications of the disease and may not correlate with endoscopic findings.

Some patients have few overt symptoms and relatively significant disease; others may have considerable discomfort without erosive and long-standing consequences. Regardless, reflux symptoms deserve appropriate evaluation and follow-up. Long-term studies imply that the disease waxes and wanes but appears not to be self-limiting. Patients who are treated and have a decrease in symptoms are not likely to be permanently "cured." Prolonged erosive disease can result in **esophagitis** (inflammation of the esophagus), esophageal erosions, ulceration, scarring, stricture, and, in some cases, dysphagia (see *Pathophysiology and Care Management Algorithm*: Esophagitis). Symptoms often interfere with sleep, work, social events, and the overall quality of life.

A major concern in persons with long-standing and more significant esophageal reflux is the development of **Barrett's esophagus (BE)**, a condition in which cells lining the distal esophagus become abnormal, even premalignant. Gastroesophageal reflux and BE are partly responsible for the rising incidence of adenocarcinoma of the esophagus, although esophageal cancer may develop in the absence of known reflux disease and BE (Chang and Katzka, 2004). Although 5% to 15% of persons with GERD will have BE, the incidence of esophageal adenocarcinoma is still less than 1% per year (Pera et al., 2005).

Acute esophagitis may be caused by ingestion of a corrosive agent, viral inflammation, or intubation. Risk of reflux is increased with hiatal hernia, reduced LES pressure, tobacco use, increased abdominal pressure (as in obstructive lung disease), delayed gastric emptying, recurrent vomiting, pregnancy, or other factors. The severity of the esophagitis resulting from gastroesophageal reflux is influenced by the composition, frequency, and volume of the gastric reflux; the health of the mucosal barrier; rate of clearance from the esophagus; and the rate of gastric emptying. Recently distinctions between erosive and nonerosive GERD and daytime and nighttime GERD have been described. Erosive and nighttime GERD are considered to be associated with more severe and prolonged symptoms. Nighttime GERD is related to altered physiology and anatomy during sleep from decreased salivary secretions and swallowing, decreased GI motility, prolonged exposure to acid, and the supine position (Brunton and McGuigan, 2005).

Competency of the LES is also important. The pressure of this sphincter is influenced by many factors, including scleroderma-like disorders, smoking, diet, and smooth-muscle relaxants. LES pressure also decreases during pregnancy, in women taking progesterone-containing oral contraceptives, and even in the late stage of a normal menstrual cycle. Although most cases of esophagitis are related to reflux of gastric contents, esophagitis may also be related to viral and bacterial infection, ingestion of corrosive agents, and radiation. Smoking, large doses or chronic use of aspirin or the nonsteroidal antiinflammatory drugs (NSAIDs), and several other oral medications can increase the risk of esophagitis in susceptible persons (Nilsson et al., 2004; Pera et al., 2005).

Medical and Surgical Management

Primary medical treatment of esophageal reflux is directed toward reduction of acid secretion. Proton pump inhibitors, which decrease acid production by the gastric parietal cell, are considered the most effective treatments (Holtman et al., 2004), but milder forms of reflux are sometimes managed by H_2 receptor antagonists and antacids. Prokinetic agents may be used in persons who have delayed gastric emptying. Activities that require frequent bending should be avoided, and raising the head of the bed 4 to 6 inches can reduce the likelihood of nocturnal reflux.

Five percent to 10% of patients with severe gastroesophageal reflux do not respond to medical therapy and repeatedly deal with symptoms and complications. They may be

PATHOPHYSIOLOGY AND CARE MANAGEMENT ALGORITHM

Esophagitis

ETIOLOGY

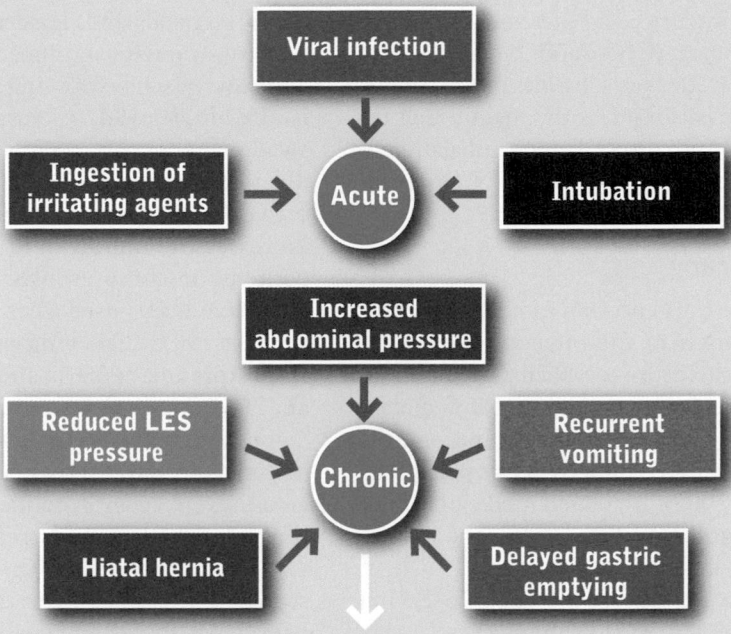

Viral infection

Ingestion of irritating agents → Acute ← Intubation

Increased abdominal pressure

Reduced LES pressure → Chronic ← Recurrent vomiting

Hiatal hernia → Chronic ← Delayed gastric emptying

PATHOPHYSIOLOGY

Reflux of gastric acid and/or intestinal contents through the lower esophageal sphincter (LES) and into the esophagus

MANAGEMENT

Behavioral Modification

Avoid:
- Eating within 3 hours of retiring
- Lying down after meals
- Tight-fitting garments
- Cigarette smoking

Medical/Surgical Management

- Protein pump inhibitors
- Histamine-2 receptor antagonists
- Antacids
- Prokinetic agents
- Fundoplication

Nutrition Management

Goal:
Decrease exposure to gastric contents
Avoid:
- Large meals
- Dietary fat
- Alcohol

Goal:
Decrease acidity of gastric secretions
Avoid:
- Coffee
- Fermented alcoholic beverages

Goal:
Prevent pain and irritation
Avoid:
- Acid pH foods
- Spices

Algorithm content developed by John J.B. Anderson, PhD, and Sanford C. Garner, PhD, 2000. Updated by Peter L. Beyer, MS, RD, LD, 2006.

treated surgically with **fundoplication**, a procedure in which the fundus of the stomach is wrapped around the lower esophagus to limit reflux (Urbach et al., 2004).

Use of tobacco products is contraindicated with reflux. Nicotine decreases LES pressure, and the use of tobacco products compromises GI integrity and increases the risk of esophageal and other cancers (Crew and Neugut, 2004; Nilsson et al., 2004). Cigarette smoking has been studied most thoroughly, primarily because it is the main use of tobacco, and the exposure from direct smoke inhalation is considered greater than with other forms (see *Clinical Insight: Smoking and Gastrointestinal Function*).

Medical Nutrition Therapy

The objectives of MNT are to (1) prevent esophageal reflux, (2) prevent pain and irritation of the inflamed esophageal mucosa, and (3) decrease the erosive capacity or acidity of gastric secretions. High fat, high protein, and low dietary fiber intake; obesity; and alcohol consumption increase the likelihood of reflux but may not be underlying or precipitating causes (El-Serag et al., 2005). Increased intake of certain foods may exacerbate or prolong reflux or alter the inflammatory or protective mechanisms.

Many measures help to manage reflux (Box 26-1), but probably the most effective is to avoid eating several hours before retiring. Large, high-fat meals lower LES pressure, delay gastric emptying, and increase latent acid production, all of which increase the risk of reflux while the person is reclined. Avoiding late evening meals might be difficult for many individuals, especially because in the United States and Latin America nighttime meals are often the largest meals of the day and are part of socialization or recreation. However, most affected individuals admit that avoiding foods in the evening reduces their symptoms.

Large meals and desserts that are high in fat or caloric density stimulate significant amounts of gastric secretions and slow gastric emptying. During sleep gastric emptying is already delayed, salivary secretions are decreased, and swallowing occurs less frequently. The combination of delayed emptying, decreased clearance of esophagus, increased digestive secretions, and the recumbent position increases the opportunity for prolonged reflux of gastric contents into the esophagus. In infants, thickened feedings have been used for a number of years, and evidence suggests that thickening may be helpful in the frequency of postprandial emesis and reflux (Hassel, 2005; Craig et al., 2004; Vanderhoof et al., 2003).

For a person who has severe esophagitis, a low-fat, liquid diet may be better tolerated initially because it does not increase esophageal distention and it may pass more easily through any strictured areas. Liquids also empty from the stomach more rapidly than solids. Foods with an acidic pH such as citrus juices, tomatoes, and soft drinks may cause pain when the esophagus is already inflamed. In rare circumstances harsh foods may cause perforation (e.g., chips, crisp crackers, and hulls).

The role of spices in the pathology of upper GI disorders is not clear, and one cannot generalize symptoms to all spices at all doses. In some of the published research, tests have been done with isolated tissues or in animals and humans with doses of spices far in excess of what people would consume in a normal meal. Some spices have been shown to increase GI permeability, and some may cause significant allergic reactions in some individuals; others may be viewed as beneficial because they increase GI secretions and im-

---

✳ CLINICAL INSIGHT

Smoking and Gastrointestinal Function

The gastrointestinal effects of smoking include the reduction of lower esophageal and pyloric sphincter pressure, increased reflux, alteration of the nature of the gastric contents, inhibition of pancreatic bicarbonate secretion, accelerated gastric emptying of liquids, and lower duodenal pH. The acid secretory response to gastrin or acetylcholine is increased considerably. Smoking also impairs the ability of cimetidine and other drugs to lower the overnight acid secretion that is thought to play a key role in ulcerogenesis. Nicotine is responsible for many of the effects of tobacco use; but increased exposure to hydrocarbons, oxygen radicals, and a number of other substances is thought to also contribute to the overall effects. Finally, smoking impairs spontaneous healing and increases the risk and rapidity of ulcer recurrence, as well as the likelihood that the ulcer will perforate and require surgery.

An interesting finding is the role of tobacco exposure in the development of inflammatory bowel disease (IBD). While smoking impairs the formation of granulomas in Crohn's disease (Leong et al., 2006), passive and active smoking exposure in childhood (by age 10 to 15) seems to be associated with the development of IBD (Mahid et al., 2006) (see Chapter 27).

BOX 26-1

Nutrition Care Guidelines for Reducing Gastroesophageal Reflux and Esophagitis

1. Avoid large, high-fat meals.
2. Avoid eating at least 3 to 4 hr before retiring.
3. Avoid smoking.
4. Avoid alcoholic beverages.
5. Avoid caffeine containing foods and beverages.
6. Stay upright and avoid vigorous activity soon after eating.
7. Avoid tight-fitting clothing, especially after a meal.
8. Consume a healthy, nutritionally complete diet with adequate fiber.
9. Avoid acidic and highly spiced foods when inflammation exists.
10. Lose weight if overweight.

Data from National Digestive Diseases Information Clearinghouse, http://digestive.niddk.nih.gov/, accessed February 17, 2006.

prove mucosal protective systems (Scholl and Jensen-Jarolim, 2004; Platel and Srinivasan, 2004).

In surveys of patients with GI lesions, the use of foods highly seasoned with chili powder and pepper are commonly but not universally incriminated in causing discomfort. The type of chili and amount of capsaicin consumed seem to make the difference (Milke et al., 2006).

Certain foods have been reported to lower LES pressure such as carminatives (peppermint and spearmint) and coffee, but little research has been done to establish their clinical significance in GERD symptoms or reflux or their complications when used in normal amounts. Peppermint oil has been studied and has been found to have strong antibacterial and antiviral benefits; however, its use in GERD should be limited (McKay and Blumberg, 2006).

Fermented alcoholic beverages (such as beer and wine) stimulate the secretion of gastric acid and may compromise GI protective mechanisms. Chewing gum has been shown to increase salivary secretions, which help to raise esophageal pH, but no studies have demonstrated its efficacy when compared with other lifestyle measures.

Obesity is a contributing factor to hiatal hernia and reflux because it increases intragastric pressure. Partial weight loss may reduce reflux symptoms (Nilsson et al., 2004). Use of loose-fitting garments by obese or normal-weight persons is also thought to decrease the risk of reflux.

Obesity, alcohol and its degradation into acetaldehyde, nitrites, a diet low in selenium, fruits and vegetables, and cereal fiber have been implicated in increasing the risk of esophageal cancer; therefore the same advice for maintaining good health is appropriate for persons with GERD. Finally, lifestyle modifications are the first-line of therapy for patients with GERD, including change in dietary practices, weight loss, smoking cessation, and elevation of the head of the bed (Kaltenbach et al., 2006).

Hiatal Hernia

Pathophysiology

A common contributor to gastroesophageal reflux and esophagitis is **hiatal hernia.** The presence of hiatal hernia is not synonymous with reflux, but it increases the likelihood of symptoms and complications. The esophagus passes through the diaphragm by way of the esophageal hiatus or ring. The attachment of the esophagus to the hiatal ring may become compromised, allowing the esophagus or a portion of the upper stomach to move above the diaphragm. The most common type of hiatal hernia is the sliding hernia, and the less common form is the paraesophageal hernia (Mittal and Balaban, 1997) (Figure 26-2).

When acid reflux occurs with a hiatal hernia, the gastric contents remain above the hiatus longer than if the canal were intact. The prolonged acid exposure increases the risk of developing more serious esophagitis (Kahrilas and Lee, 2005). Because increases in intragastric pressure force acidic stomach contents up into the esophagus, persons with hiatal hernia may experience difficulty when lying down or bending over and **epigastric** (the upper middle region of the abdomen) discomfort after large, energy-dense meals.

Medical Nutrition Therapy

Weight reduction and decreasing meal size decreases the impact of the hiatal hernia. Dietary recommendations are similar to those for GERD and esophagitis: avoidance of heavy meals, omitting snacks and meals before reclining (especially high in fat and calories), and minimizing alcohol consumption.

Oral Cavity Cancer and Surgery

Pathophysiology

The patient diagnosed with cancer of the oral cavity, pharynx, or esophagus may present with existing nutritional problems and eating difficulties caused by the tumor mass, obstruction, oral infection or ulceration. Nutritional deficits may be compounded by the treatment, which commonly involves surgical resection, regional irradiation, or chemotherapy. Chewing, swallowing, salivation, and taste acuity are often affected. Extensive dental decay, osteoradionecrosis, and infections may also occur. Chemotherapy can be expected to produce nausea, vomiting, and anorexia (see Chapter 37).

Surgery of the Mouth or Esophagus

After extensive surgery of the mouth or esophagus, it may be necessary to provide oral nutrition support in liquid form. Many nutritionally complete formulas are available (see Appendix 32). To add variety to the diet, ordinary foods such as fruits can be puréed and mixed with water until liquefied. With more extensive oral involvement, it may be necessary to use a gastrostomy or jejunostomy tube for administering the formula. Enteral tube feedings may involve the use of ready-to-feed formulas or table foods put in a blender. If the GI tract is not functioning, nutritional support can be provided parenterally (see Chapter 20).

Tonsils are lymphatic tissue and part of the immune system. Tonsillectomy is less common today than in the past because mild inflammation of the tonsils is considered a natural part of the efforts of the immune system to fight infection. When necessary, the doctor may remove the tonsils in an

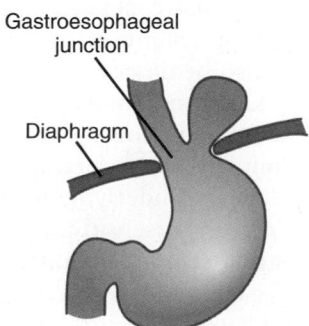

FIGURE 26-2 Hiatal hernia. (*Modified from Price SA, Wilson LM:* Pathophysiology: clinical concepts of disease processes, *ed 6, St. Louis, 2003, Mosby*).

attempt to reduce the number and frequency of ear infections, tonsillitis, and sinusitis. The convalescent period following a tonsillectomy is short. Cold, mild-flavored, soft, moist foods bring the most comfort to the patient and offer the most protection against unexpected bleeding from the surgical area. During the first 24 hours after surgery, foods that are best accepted are typically chilled or frozen dairy products or fruit slurries, and noncitrus juices. By the second day warm fluids and soft foods may be introduced; thereafter hot foods can be introduced cautiously as healing progresses and as these foods are tolerated. The patient can typically consume a normal diet within 3 to 5 days.

Medical Nutrition Therapy

If the patient with oral cancer is unable to eat for prolonged periods, nutritional support may be provided by tube feeding if the remainder of the GI tract is functional. Gastrostomy feedings can be used if long-term feeding by tube is necessary for total or supplemental support. If oral feeding is possible after surgery, general dietary recommendations include liquid or soft-textured, moist foods for easy mastication and swallowing and small, frequent meals of relatively high caloric density. Complex carbohydrates are preferred over simple sugars.

Periodic use of an artificial saliva solution is also helpful, as is the frequent consumption of fluids to prevent dry mouth. Normal saline rinses may ameliorate mucositis (see Figure 37-4 in Chapter 37), and topical anesthetics can be used to relieve pain. Necessary dental restorations, aggressive oral hygiene, and daily use of fluoride are recommended. Oral infections are usually fungal. Unfortunately some of the medications used in treatment may leave a metallic taste in the mouth that can further compromise the patient's desire to eat (see Chapters 16 and 37).

DISORDERS OF THE STOMACH

Indigestion and Dyspepsia

Pathophysiology

In its broadest sense **dyspepsia** refers to persistent upper abdominal discomfort or pain. The discomfort may be related to organic causes such as esophageal reflux, gastritis, or peptic ulcer, gallbladder disease, or other identifiable pathology. **Functional dyspepsia** is a term that describes unexplained persistent or recurrent upper GI discomfort. It may also be described as nonulcer dyspepsia. Symptoms of functional dyspepsia are reported in about 15% to 20% of adults over a year's time and may include vague abdominal discomfort, bloating, early satiety, nausea, and belching. Underlying mechanisms are not entirely clear; visceral hypersensitivity to acid or distention, impaired gastric accommodation, altered brain-gut axis, and abnormal gastric motility and emptying have all been considered (Fahardo et al., 2005; Smith, 2005). Because of the variety of presentations and symptoms, dyspepsia may overlap with other problems such as GERD or

irritable bowel syndrome, anxiety, and depression. Diet, stress, and other lifestyle factors may contribute to the symptoms of patients with functional dyspepsia.

Medical Nutrition Therapy

Dietary indulgences—excessive volumes of food or high intake of fat, sugar, caffeine, spices, or alcohol—are commonly implicated in dyspepsia. However, little research has been done in controlled settings with diet or specific foods in persons with dyspepsia. Because the symptoms and underlying mechanisms may be diverse, it is unlikely that dietary advice would be needed for all cases of dyspepsia. Delayed emptying and increased sensation of fullness are common features of the problem. Reduction of dietary fat intake, use of smaller meals, and diets of low caloric density may be helpful (Delgado-Aros et al., 2004; Feinle-Bisset and Horowitz, 2006). Because alcoholic beverages may alter GI functions in a number of ways, they are also normally limited. Mild exercise enhances movement of foodstuffs through the GI tract and increases one's sense of well-being. Reaction to life stresses may also contribute to abdominal distress, in which case behavioral management and emotional support may also help. If symptoms persist despite these strategies, further evaluation and diet therapy should be tailored to the underlying cause.

Gastritis and Peptic Ulcer Disease

Pathophysiology

Gastritis and peptic ulcers may result when infectious, chemical, or neural abnormalities disrupt mucosal integrity of the stomach. The most common cause of gastritis and peptic ulcer is now known to be **Helicobacter pylori** infection. *H. pylori* infection is responsible for most cases of chronic inflammation of the gastric mucosa, peptic ulcer, **atrophic gastritis** (chronic inflammation with deterioration of the mucous membrane and glands, resulting in achlorhydria and loss of intrinsic factor), and gastric cancer (Israel and Peek, 2006; Candelli et al., 2005; Bytzer and O'Morain, 2005). The infection does not resolve spontaneously, and risks of complications increase with duration of the infection. Other factors affect the risk of pathologic consequences, including the patient's age at onset of the initial infection, the specific strain and concentration of organism, genetic factors related to the host, and the lifestyle and overall health of the patient. The infection is typically confined to the mucosa of the stomach.

H. pylori organisms are gram-negative bacteria with flagella that facilitate mobility. The size and shape of these organisms range from spirals to coils to rods, depending on the culture media of the stomach. These organisms are somewhat resistant to the acidic medium of the stomach, but additional protection is provided by their colonization beneath the protective mucosal layer and by significant urease production. Urease allows the generation of ammonia to facilitate alkalinization of the immediate surroundings. The urease test is now used as one of the diagnostic tools for the presence of *H. pylori* infection.

The prevalence of *H. pylori* infection generally correlates with the socioeconomic status of the population. Among the adult population prevalence ranges from about 10% in countries that have the resources to identify, prevent, and treat the disease to 80% to 90% of the population in developing countries. Although gastritis is a characteristic observation, only 10% to 15% of those infected by the organism develop symptomatic ulceration, and approximately 1% develop gastric cancer. Although the exposure, prevalence, and complications related to *H. pylori* in the United States are declining, it is still a still a problem in the elderly and in populations with limited access to health care (Ernst et al., 2006; Fennerty, 2005).

Infection with the *H. pylori* organism results in a chronic inflammatory state. Infection induces inflammation from both humoral and systemic immune response, with damage resulting from cytotoxins produced by the organism during the inflammatory response by the host. Treatment of *H. pylori* ameliorates the gastritis, improves digestive function at least somewhat, and at least reduces the conditions that favor carcinogenesis.

Treatment typically involves the use of two or three antibiotics and acid-suppressing medications. The extent of microbial resistance to specific agents in different parts of the world and the varying strains of the organism may necessitate the use of different protocols and combinations of medications (Guzzo et al., 2005; Bytzer and O'Morain, 2005) (see *New Directions:* The Genome of *Helicobacter pylori*).

Other Forms of Gastritis

The mucosa of the stomach and duodenum is normally protected from the proteolytic actions of gastric acid and pepsin by a coating of mucus secreted by glands in the epithelial walls from the lower esophagus to the upper duodenum. The mucosal layer is also protected from bacterial invasion by the digestive actions of pepsin and hydrochloric acid and the mucus secretions. Hydrochloric acid is secreted by the parietal cells in response to stimuli by gastrin, acetylcholine, and histamine. The mucus contains acid-neutralizing bicarbonates, and additional bicarbonates are provided by the pancreatic juice secreted into the intestinal lumen. Production of mucus is stimulated by the action of prostaglandins.

Chronic use of aspirin or other NSAIDs, steroids, alcohol, erosive substances, tobacco, or any combination of these factors may also compromise mucosal integrity and increase the chance for acquiring acute or chronic gastritis. Autoimmune gastritis may also contribute to some cases of gastritis (Whittingham and Mackay, 2005). Poor nutrition and general poor health may contribute to the onset and severity of the symptoms and can delay the healing process.

Acute gastritis refers to rapid onset of inflammation and symptoms. Chronic gastritis may occur over a period of months to decades, with waxing and waning of symptoms. Gastritis may manifest by a number of symptoms, including nausea, vomiting, malaise, anorexia, hemorrhage, and epi-gastric pain. Prolonged gastritis may result in atrophy and loss of stomach parietal cells, with a loss of secretion of hydrochloric acid (**achlorhydria**) and intrinsic factor. Patients may have a low serum vitamin B_{12} level and elevated serum homocystine levels and may not process other nutrients efficiently (including iron or calcium) without normal acid production.

Medical Treatment

Endoscopy is a common procedure used to identify problems (see *Focus On:* Endoscopy and Capsules). Treatment of gastritis includes the eradication of pathogenic organisms (e.g., *H. pylori*) and withdrawal of any provoking agents. Antibiotics and proton pump inhibitors are the primary medical treatments.

Medical Nutrition Therapy

In persons with atrophic gastritis vitamin B_{12} status should be evaluated because a lack of intrinsic factor and acid results in malabsorption of this vitamin (see the discussion on vitamin status assessment in Chapters 3, 15, and 31). Reduced absorption of iron, calcium, and other nutrients occurs in chronic gastritis because of the role of gastric acid in increasing their bioavailability. In the case of iron, the underlying cause of anemia may be confounded by the use of powerful acid-suppressing medications and bleeding that may also impact anemia (Banerjee and Bishop, 2005; Sharma et al., 2004). See "Medical and Surgical Management of Ulcers" for peptic ulcers in the following paragraphs.)

⇄ NEW DIRECTION

The Genome of *Helicobacter pylori*

The ability of robotic analyzers to sequence long lengths of deoxyribonucleic acid automatically and the rapidity with which computers can scan gene data banks have spawned a new discipline in the biomedical sciences: genomics. Sequencing genomes for microbial conditions offers an expeditious means of searching for novel treatments for infectious disease. *H. pylori* genome studies are important in this realm. *H. pylori* organisms live only in the human stomach, and the enzymatic pathways they need for survival in this harsh milieu are continually switched on. A number of antigenic variations occur. Many genes have been found to code for iron-scavenging pathways, indicating a crucial role for iron in the survival of *H. pylori* in the stomach. The *H. pylori* gene causes the making of a protein that alters GI epithelial cells and T-lymphocytes, suggesting that bacterial, host genetic and environmental factors all play a role (Pritchard and Crabtree, 2006). The unlocking of the genome and the logical sequencing of key targets will allow the creation of novel inhibitory and bactericidal products against which no microbe has yet had the chance to become resistant (Fox and Wang, 2002).

◉ FOCUS ON

Endoscopy and Capsules

The mucosa of the upper gastrointestinal (GI) tract can be viewed, photographed, and biopsied by means of endoscopy, a procedure that involves passing a flexible tube into the esophagus that has a light and camera on the distal end. It can be passed through the esophagus and into the stomach or upper small bowel. Inflammation, erosions, ulcerations, changes in the blood vessels, and destruction of surface cells can be identified. These changes can then be correlated with chemical, histologic, and clinical findings to formulate a diagnosis. Endoscopy is also important in the long-term monitoring of patients with chronic esophagitis and gastritis because of the possibility that they will develop premalignant lesions or carcinoma. Recently small capsules can be swallowed with an attached line; or wireless type capsules can be used to view segments of the GI tract for abnormalities or bleeding, check pH, and measure the time it takes to pass through different segments of the GI tract. The wireless capsules transmit signals that send photographs and other information that are being used for diagnostic and research purposes. The procedure is less invasive than normal endoscopy and provides the advantage of being able to observe, record, and measure GI function as the patient is ambulatory (Selby, 2004).

Peptic Ulcers

Pathophysiology

Normal gastric and duodenal mucosa is protected from the digestive actions of acid and pepsin by the secretion of mucus, the production of bicarbonate, the removal of excess acid by normal blood flow, and the rapid renewal and repair of epithelial cell injury. **Peptic ulcer** refers to an ulcer that occurs as a result of the breakdown of these normal defense and repair mechanisms. Typically more than one of the mechanisms must be malfunctioning for symptomatic peptic ulcers to develop. Peptic ulcers typically show evidence of chronic inflammation and repair processes surrounding the lesion.

The primary causes of peptic ulcers are *H. pylori* infection, gastritis, the use of aspirin and other NSAIDs, corticosteroids (see *Pathophysiology and Care Management Algorithm:* Peptic Ulcer), and stress (so-called stress-induced ulcers). Excessive use or concentrated forms of ethanol can damage gastric mucosa, worsen symptoms of peptic ulcers, and interfere with ulcer healing. Modest doses of alcoholic beverages in otherwise healthy persons do not appear to cause peptic ulcers. Consumption of beer and wine increases gastric secretions, whereas low concentrations of ethanol may not (Bujanda, 2000). Use of tobacco products decreases bicarbonate secretion, decreases mucosal blood flow, exacerbates inflammation, and is associated with additional complications of *H. pylori* infection.

As a result of earlier screening for *H. pylori* and early recognition of the symptoms and risk factors associated with peptic ulcers, their incidence and prevalence and the number of surgical procedures related to them have decreased markedly in the last three decades. Other risk factors include gastrinoma; Zollinger-Ellison syndrome; and the use of tobacco products, alcohol, NSAIDs, and aspirin (Scheiman, 2005; Israel and Peek, 2006; Guzzo, 2005).

Peptic ulcers normally involve two major regions: gastric and duodenal. Uncomplicated peptic ulcers in either region may present with signs similar to those associated with dyspepsia and gastritis. Abdominal pain or discomfort is characteristic of both gastric and duodenal ulcers, although anorexia, weight loss, nausea and vomiting, and heartburn may occur slightly more often in persons with gastric ulcers. In some patients peptic ulcers are asymptomatic.

Complications of hemorrhage and perforation contribute significantly to the morbidity and mortality of peptic ulcers. Ulcers can perforate into the peritoneal cavity or penetrate into an adjacent organ (usually the pancreas), or they may erode an artery and cause massive hemorrhage. **Melena**, which refers to black, tarry stools, is a common finding associated with peptic ulcer disease in older adults. Melena may suggest either acute or chronic GI bleeding.

Characteristics of and Comparisons Between Gastric and Duodenal Ulcers

Although **gastric ulcers** can occur anywhere in the stomach, most occur along the lesser curvature of the stomach (Figure 26-3). Gastric ulcers typically are associated with widespread gastritis, inflammatory involvement of oxyntic (acid-producing) cells, and atrophy of acid- and pepsin-producing cells with advancing age. In some cases gastric ulceration develops despite relatively low acid output. Antral hypomotility, gastric stasis, and increased duodenal reflux are common in gastric ulcer and, when present, may increase the severity of the gastric injury. With a gastric ulcer, hemorrhage and overall mortality are higher than with a duodenal ulcer.

Duodenal ulcer is characterized by considerably increased acid secretion, nocturnal acid secretion, and decreased bicarbonate secretion. Most duodenal ulcers occur within the first few centimeters of the duodenal bulb, in an area immediately below the pylorus. Gastric outlet obstruction occurs more commonly with duodenal ulcers than with gastric ulcers, and gastric metaplasia may occur with duodenal ulcer related to *H. pylori* (i.e., replacement of duodenal villous cells with gastric-type mucosal cells).

Medical and Surgical Management of Ulcers

Peptic Ulcers. Because the primary cause of gastritis and peptic ulcers is *H. pylori* infection, the primary focus of treatment in most cases is the eradication of this organism. Because of the presence of different strains of this organism and the relative resistance of the organism throughout the world, the medication protocol usually involves the use of two or three antibiotics and acid-suppressing medications. In peptic ulcer disease independent of infection, suppression of acid with proton pump inhibitors or H_2-receptor blockers is the primary treatment.

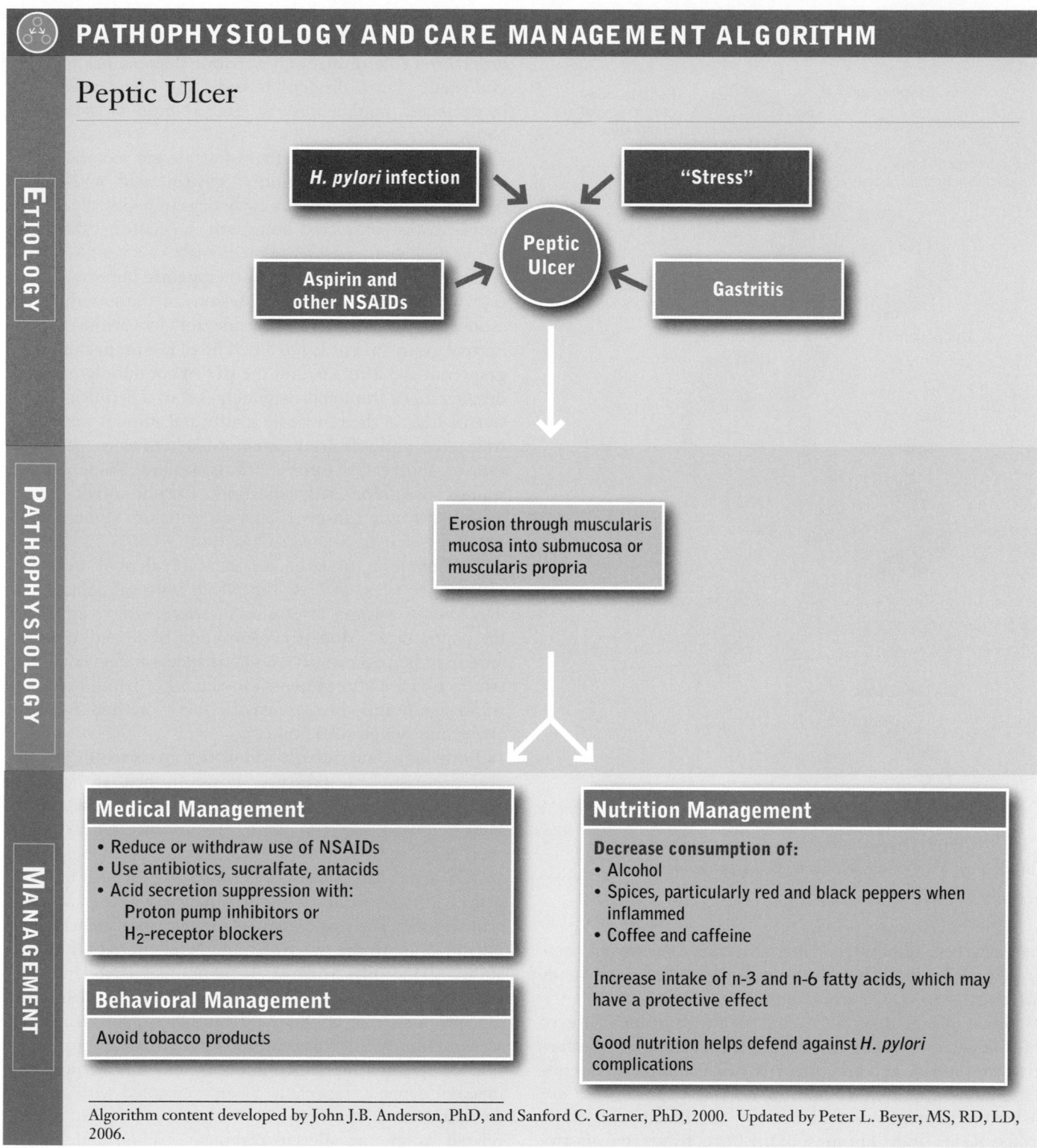

PATHOPHYSIOLOGY AND CARE MANAGEMENT ALGORITHM

Peptic Ulcer

ETIOLOGY

H. pylori infection → Peptic Ulcer ← "Stress"

Aspirin and other NSAIDs → Peptic Ulcer ← Gastritis

PATHOPHYSIOLOGY

Erosion through muscularis mucosa into submucosa or muscularis propria

MANAGEMENT

Medical Management

- Reduce or withdraw use of NSAIDs
- Use antibiotics, sucralfate, antacids
- Acid secretion suppression with:
  Proton pump inhibitors or
  H_2-receptor blockers

Behavioral Management

Avoid tobacco products

Nutrition Management

Decrease consumption of:
- Alcohol
- Spices, particularly red and black peppers when inflamed
- Coffee and caffeine

Increase intake of n-3 and n-6 fatty acids, which may have a protective effect

Good nutrition helps defend against *H. pylori* complications

Algorithm content developed by John J.B. Anderson, PhD, and Sanford C. Garner, PhD, 2000. Updated by Peter L. Beyer, MS, RD, LD, 2006.

As a result of the ability to recognize and eradicate *H. pylori*, surgical intervention for peptic ulcer management is less frequent, although emergent and elective surgeries are still needed for complications related to both *H. pylori* and other cases. Interventions may include endoscopic, open, and laparoscopic procedures to treat individual lesions to partial gastrectomy and selective vagotomies (Paimela et al., 2004). One measure includes regular use of protective foods that contain phenolic antioxidants such as cranber-ries, which may have the capacity to help eradicate *H. pylori* (Vattem et al., 2005).

Stress Ulcers. Stress ulcers may occur as a complication of severe burns, trauma, surgery, shock, renal failure, or radiation therapy. A primary concern with stress ulceration is the potential for significant hemorrhage. Gastric ischemia with GI hypoperfusion, oxidative injury, reflux of bile salts and pancreatic enzymes, microbial colonization, and mucosal barrier changes

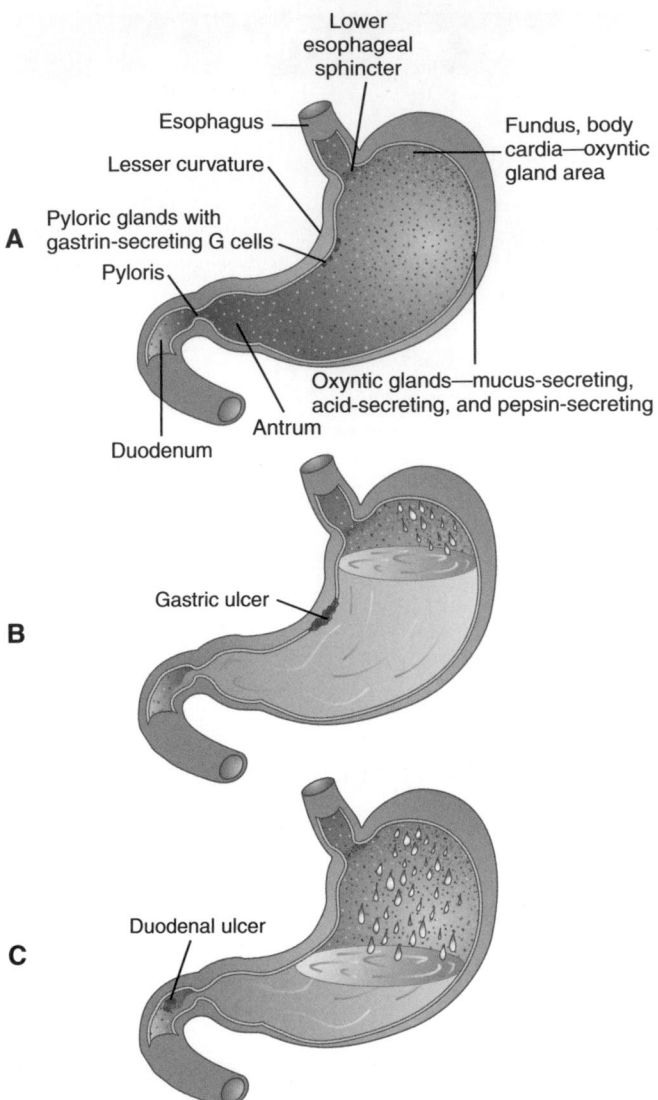

FIGURE 26-3 Diagram showing **A,** the stomach and duodenum with eroded lesions; **B,** a gastric ulcer; and **C,** a duodenal ulcer.

have also been implicated. The true mechanisms are not completely understood, but the use of antioxidant compounds shows promise (Doug and Kaunitz, 2006).

Stress ulcers that bleed can be a significant cause of morbidity in critically ill patients, but knowledge of effective prevention and treatment is still incomplete. Sucralfate, acid suppressives, and, as necessary, antibiotics are used for prophylaxis and therapy (Stollman and Metz, 2005; Kallet and Quinn, 2005). Efforts to prevent gastric ulcers in "stressed" patients have focused on preventing or limiting conditions leading to hypotension and ischemia and coagulopathies. Avoiding NSAIDs and large doses of corticosteroids is also beneficial. Providing oral or enteral feeding when possible increases GI vascular perfusion and stimulates secretion and motility.

Medical Nutrition Therapy for Ulcers

For several decades dietary factors have gained or lost favor as a significant component in the cause and treatment of

dyspepsia, gastritis, and peptic ulcer disease. Since the identification of *H. pylori* as the major contributor to these disorders, the role of diet and nutritional status has been re-evaluated. Few dietary factors can be consistently incriminated in the cause or exacerbation of gastritis or peptic ulcer disease.

Protein foods temporarily buffer gastric secretions, but they also stimulate secretion of gastrin, acid, and pepsin. Milk or cream, which in the early days of peptic ulcer management was considered important in "coating" the stomach, is no longer considered medicinal.

The pH of a food has little therapeutic importance, except for patients with existing lesions of the mouth or the esophagus. Most foods are considerably less acidic than the normal gastric pH of 1.0 to 3.0. The pH of orange juice and grapefruit is 3.2 to 3.6, and the pH of commonly used soft drinks ranges from approximately 2.8 to 3.5 (Flick, 1970). On the basis of their intrinsic acidity and amount consumed, fruit juices and soft drinks are not likely to cause peptic ulcers or appreciably interfere with healing. Some patients express discomfort with ingestion of acidic foods, but the response is not consistent among patients, and in some, symptoms may be related to heartburn.

Consumption of large amounts of alcohol from any source may cause at least superficial mucosal damage and may worsen existing disease or interfere with treatment of the peptic ulcer. Modest consumption of alcohol does not appear to be pathogenic for peptic ulcers unless coexisting risk factors are also present. On the other hand, beers and wines significantly increase gastric secretions and should be avoided in symptomatic disease.

Both coffee and caffeine stimulate acid secretion and may also decrease LES pressure; however, neither has been strongly implicated as a cause of peptic ulcers outside of the increased acid secretion and discomfort associated with their consumption.

When very large doses of certain spices are fed orally or placed intragastrically without other foods, they increase acid secretion and cause small, transient superficial erosions, inflammation of the mucosal lining, and altered GI permeability or motility. Most often incriminated are chili, cayenne, and black peppers (Milke et al., 2006). Small amounts of chili pepper or its pungent ingredient, capsicum, may serve to increase mucosal protection by increasing production of mucus; but large amounts may cause superficial mucosal damage, especially when consumed with alcohol. At least a small percentage of intolerances to spices may be related to specific allergic responses (Scholl and Jensen-Jarolim, 2004). Interestingly, turmeric may actually inhibit adhesion of *H. pylori* to the stomach wall (O'Mahony et al, 2005). The long-term use of spices, either as protective or harmful agents, requires further study.

The use of probiotics has been studied in the prevention, management, and eradication of *H. pylori*. In some of the studies their role as complementary therapy and to a lesser degree in eradication are promising (Hamilton-Miller, 2003). More controlled studies with different forms and combinations of probiotics are worthwhile.

Because prostaglandins from omega-3 and omega-6 fatty acids are involved in inflammatory, immune, and cytoprotective physiology of the GI mucosa, they have been considered for use in management of *H. pylori* infection and peptic damage. In vitro and animal and human studies are conflicting, with some showing protective and others reporting harmful effects of both omega-3 (n-3) and omega-6 fatty acids. When protected from lipid peroxidation, omega-3 fatty acids have shown antiinflammatory properties and have been shown to be protective against mucosal injury evoked from drugs and *H. pylori* (Shimizu et al., 2001). Long-term clinical trials have not been performed using specific fatty acids, and identification of the ideal dose or form of lipids to be used in the diet has not yet been established.

Good dietary practices with adequate nutrient, fruit and vegetable, and fiber intakes may decrease risk of complications from *H. pylori* infection. Malnutrition originating from either micronutrient deficiencies or generalized protein-calorie malnutrition affects rapidly dividing cells such as those of the GI tract, and deficiencies may compromise GI wound healing. Overall a high-quality diet and avoiding nutrient deficiencies may offer some protection from peptic ulcer disease and may play a role in healing. From a practical perspective, persons being treated for gastritis and peptic ulcer disease may be advised to avoid the excessive use of specific spices, alcohol, and coffee (both caffeinated and decaffeinated) and to consume a nutritionally complete diet with adequate dietary fiber from fruits and vegetables (Ryan-Harshman and Aldoori, 2004). It is also reasonable to use supplements to make up for dietary inadequacies as needed. Because some patients may have significant gastric outlet obstruction or bezoars, chewing thoroughly and avoiding foods with skins that are difficult to break down is advisable, especially in persons with dentures or missing teeth.

Meal frequency is a controversial issue in the management of peptic ulcer disease. Frequent, small meals may increase comfort, decrease the chance for acid reflux, and stimulate gastric blood flow; but they also may increase net acid output. There is broad agreement that affected persons should avoid consuming large meals, especially before retiring, to reduce latent increases in acid secretion. In the case of stress ulcers, continuous enteral feeding and early postoperative feeding may help maintain the mucosal barrier and GI circulation, thus reducing the risk of stress ulceration. Factors that increase or decrease gastric acidity are listed in Box 26-2.

Carcinoma of the Stomach

Pathophysiology

Malignant neoplasms of the stomach can lead to malnutrition as a result of excessive blood and protein losses or, more commonly, because of obstruction and mechanical interference with food intake. Most cancers of the stomach are treated by surgical resection; thus part of the nutritional considerations includes partial or total resection of the stomach, or **gastrectomy.**

BOX 26-2

Factors That Affect Gastric Acidity

Increase Gastric Acidity

Cephalic Phase of Digestion

Thought, taste, smell of food, and chewing and swallowing initiate vagal stimulation of the parietal cells in the fundic mucosa, resulting in secretion of gastric acid.

Gastric Phase of Digestion

Effect of food in the stomach:

- Distention of the fundus stimulates the parietal cells to produce acid.
- Increased alkalinity of antrum causes the release of gastrin, which stimulates gastric acid secretion.
- Distention of the antrum causes release of gastrin.
- Substances in certain foods and digestive products increase acidity (e.g., coffee, both with or without caffeine; alcohol; polypeptides and amino acids [products of protein digestion]).

Decrease Gastric Acidity

Gastric Phase of Digestion

Acidification of the antrum reduces gastrin release and thus gastric acid secretion.

Food, especially protein, has an initial buffering effect.

Intestinal Phase of Digestion

Fat, acid, and protein in the small intestine stimulate release of one or more gastrointestinal hormones that inhibit gastric acid secretion.

Because symptoms are slow to manifest themselves and the growth of the tumor is rapid, carcinoma of the stomach is frequently overlooked until it is too late for a cure. Loss of appetite, strength, and weight frequently precede other symptoms. In some cases **achylia gastrica** (absence of hydrochloric acid and pepsin) or achlorhydria may exist for years before the onset of gastric carcinoma.

Consumption of fruits, vegetables, and selenium appears to have a modest role in the prevention of GI cancers, whereas alcohol consumption and overweight increase the risk (van den Brandt and Goldbohm, 2006). Other factors include chronic infection with *H. pylori*, smoking, intake of highly salted or pickled foods, or inadequate amounts of micronutrients (Lynch et al., 2005).

Medical Nutrition Therapy

The dietary regimen for carcinoma of the stomach is determined by the location of the cancer, the nature of the functional disturbance, and the stage of the disease. Gastrectomy is one of the possible therapies, and some patients may experience difficulties with nutrition after surgery (see "Dumping Syndrome" later in this chapter).

The patient with advanced, inoperable cancer should receive a diet that is adjusted to his or her tolerances, preferences, and comfort. Anorexia is almost always present from the early stages. In the later stages of the disease, the patient may tolerate only a liquid diet, or it may be necessary to use parenteral nutrition. As long as other therapeutic procedures, such as surgery, radiation therapy, or chemotherapy, are being performed, the nutritional support for the patient should be equally aggressive (see Chapter 37 for further discussion of nutrition in cancer treatment).

Gastric Surgery

Historically gastric surgery played a more predominant role for treatment of ulcer disease and gastric cancer than it does today. Because the role impact of *H. pylori* was not understood until the early 1980s, gastric surgery was used not only for malignancies but also was a common surgical procedure for treatment of peptic ulcers and their complications. Partial and total gastrectomies were developed with many modifications to minimize the complications of resected gastric and duodenal structures. Vagotomy with and without gastric resection was later performed after it was demonstrated that the **vagus nerve** was not only responsible for motility of the stomach but also stimulated the parietal cells in the proximal stomach to secrete acid (Weil and Buchberger, 1999). Total vagal denervation **(truncal vagotomy)** decreased acid secretion by **parietal cells** in the stomach and decreased their response to gastrin, but it also decreased motor function of the stomach and delayed gastric emptying.

When truncal (more complete) vagototomy is performed, pyloroplasty or gastroenterostomy is normally performed to allow better gastric emptying of solids. A **parietal cell vagotomy** (partial or selective) may be performed because it affects only the proximal stomach where gastric acid secretion occurs. The antrum and pylorus remain innervated by the vagus nerve, and gastric emptying can proceed more normally.

Because of more effective medical treatment of *H. pylori* and acid secretion, gastric surgery and gastrectomy for peptic ulcer disease are performed less frequently. Partial or total gastrectomy may still be necessary with gastric cancer or when peptic ulcers are complicated by hemorrhage, perforation, intractability, or obstruction. Complications such as obstruction, dumping, abdominal discomfort, diarrhea, and weight loss may still occur, depending on the nature and extent of the disease and surgical interventions (Guzzo et al., 2005) (Figure 26-4).

Performed more frequently now are gastric banding, gastroplasty or gastric bypass surgeries for obesity treatment. See Figure 21-5 for diagrams of these surgeries, and Chapter 21.

Medical Nutrition Therapy After Gastric Surgery

After most types of gastric surgery, oral intake of foods and fluids is suspended until GI tract function returns. Once function is regained, small frequent feedings of liquid foods are initiated, after which the patient can progress to solids as tolerated based on volume and consistency. If the surgery requires an extended period for healing, the patient may be fed enterally through a tube, often placed as a jejunostomy. The use of total parenteral nutrition is usually reserved for patients with postoperative complications that delay enteral feeding for an extended period (see Chapter 20).

The first type of fluid allowed by mouth is usually ice, given in small amounts and allowed to melt in the mouth or frequent sips of water. Gastric surgeries vary in terms of the resultant risk for dysmotility (i.e., obstruction or rapid emptying and dumping), so foods may be altered somewhat, depending on the type of procedure performed. Generally all patients can tolerate dilute and isotonic liquids such as soups or cooked cereals rather than sweet, high-fat foods or solids. Later patients usually tolerate small solid meals made of foods that can easily be cut and masticated into small particles such as meats, starches, and cooked vegetables. Highly spiced, fatty, or hypertonic foods may not be well tolerated initially. When "full liquid" diets are high in sugars and lactose, they may not be well digested, and low-lactose and more isotonic liquids might be better tolerated.

Nutritional impairment occurs in some patients after gastrectomy, and some have difficulty regaining normal preoperative weight because of (1) inadequate food intake related to anorexia or to symptoms related to dumping syndrome, or (2) malabsorption of ingested food. Patients who have had total or almost total gastrectomy often have difficulty eating large amounts of food and may need to make a permanent habit of eating several small meals daily.

Dumping Syndrome

Pathophysiology

The **dumping syndrome** is a complex physiologic response to the presence of larger-than-normal quantities of hypertonic foods and liquids in the proximal small intestine. Dumping syndrome usually occurs as a result of surgical procedures that allow excessive amounts of liquid or solid foods to enter the small intestine in a concentrated form. Milder forms of dumping may rarely occur to varying degrees in persons without surgical procedures, and most of the symptoms can be reproduced in normal individuals by infusing a loading dose of glucose into the jejunum (Ukleja, 2005).

The syndrome may occur as a result of total or subtotal gastrectomy, manipulation of the pylorus, after fundoplication, and after some gastric bypass procedures for obesity (Ukleja, 2005; Bufler et al., 2001). As a result of better medical management of peptic ulcers, use of selective vagotomies, and newer surgical procedures to avoid complications, classic dumping is not as likely to be as severe or frequently encountered in clinical practice today as it once was.

Medical Management

The severity of symptoms ranges from mild to relatively debilitating, depending on the nature of the surgery and the individual's dietary practices. Short- and long-term implications are numerous, but dietary interventions can reduce or eliminate symptoms in most persons. Medications that slow motility may be advised for those whose symptoms persist after changing dietary habits.

Symptoms may occur in several stages; each is related to the "dumping" of foods and beverages into the small intes-

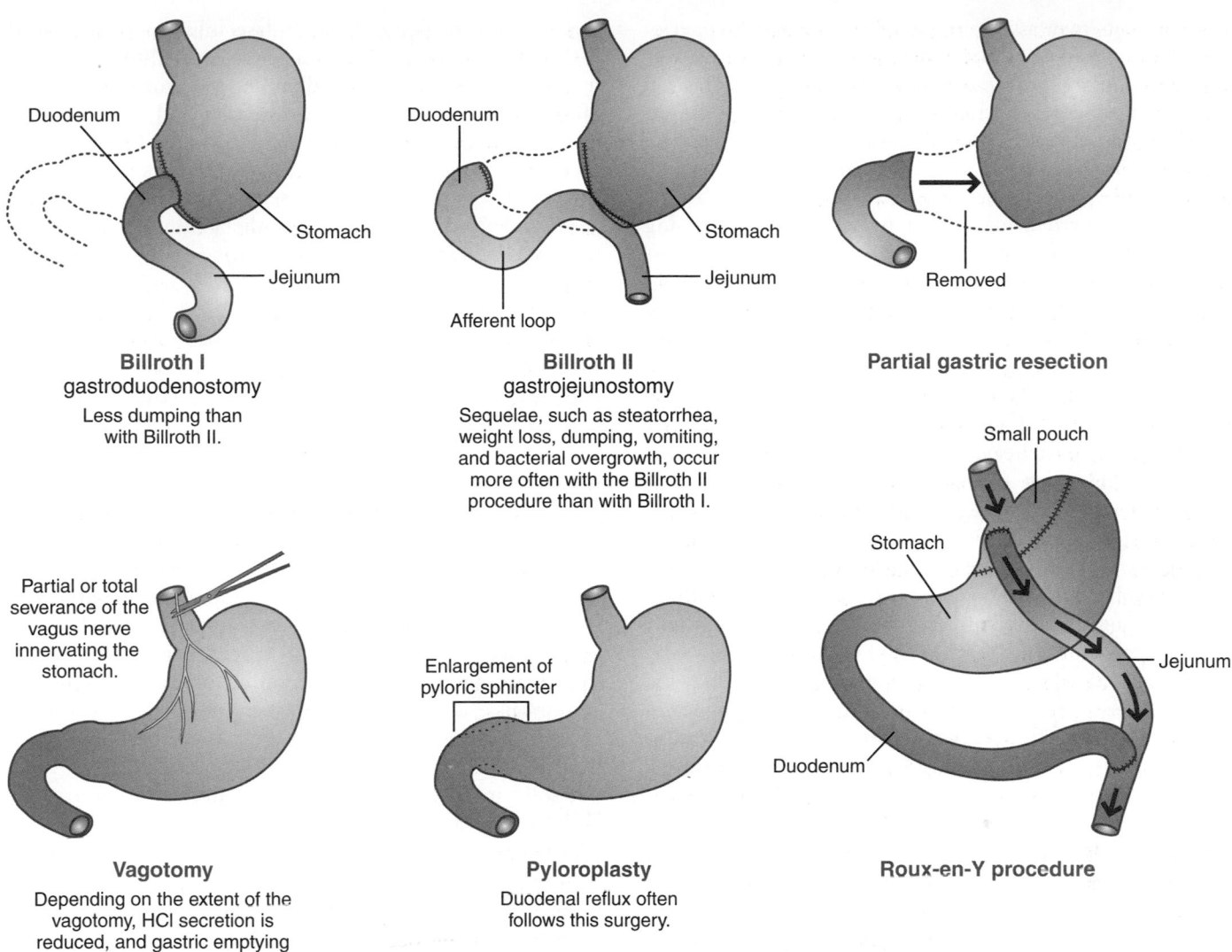

FIGURE 26-4 Gastric surgical procedures.

tine, but the mechanisms vary. Not all patients suffer all consequences or to the same degree. In the first stage (early dumping) patients may experience abdominal fullness and nausea within 10 to 20 minutes of eating a meal. This stage may be attributed to distention of the small bowel from foods and liquids plus a modest fluid shift from systemic circulation into the small intestine as a result of ingestion of sugars or foods that become hypertonic from the action of digestive enzymes. At the same time patients may experience flushing, rapid heartbeat, faintness, and sweating and feel the need to sit or lie down. This set of systemic symptoms was originally attributed to fluid loss from the vascular space into the mesenteric bed and GI tract. Fluid does shift from systemic circulation into the GI tract but the fluid shift may not be sufficient to account for the magnitude of vascular symptoms. It is now thought that patients with these early dumping symptoms are experiencing a decrease in peripheral vascular resistance and perhaps visceral pooling of blood.

In the intermediate stage, which can occur from 20 minutes to more than 1 hour after eating, patients may experience abdominal bloating, increased flatulence, crampy ab-

dominal pain, and diarrhea. The "colonic" symptoms are likely related to the increased malabsorption of carbohydrates and other foodstuffs and the subsequent fermentation of the substrates entering the colon (see Chapter 1).

The late stage, occurring from 1 to 3 hours after a meal, is related to reactive hypoglycemia, sometimes referred to as late effects of dumping or **alimentary hypoglycemia**. Patients may perspire; feel anxious, weak, shaky, or hungry; and have difficulty concentrating. Rapid delivery, as well as hydrolysis and absorption of carbohydrates, produces an exaggerated rise in insulin level with a subsequent decline in blood glucose level (see Chapter 30). The rapid changes in blood glucose and the secretion of gut peptides, glucose insulinotropic polypeptide, and glucagon-like polypeptide-1 appear to be at least partly responsible for the late symptoms (Ukleja, 2005).

Complications

Patients who are symptomatic after gastric surgery often lose weight. The weight loss may be attributable to inadequate intake resulting from the fear and anxiety that is often associated with the confusing and often distressing symptoms.

Some patients may associate the symptoms with the act of eating rather than attributing them to specific patterns, volumes, or types of foods consumed. Patients sometimes can correctly relate consumption of food types with distress, but rarely can they identify specific foods based on experience with foods or meals.

Following some forms of gastric surgery, malabsorption and steatorrhea may occur in addition to dumping and hypoglycemia. Approximately 10% of these patients have clinically significant steatorrhea secondary to rapid transit, loss of gastric lipase, or pancreatic or biliary insufficiency. Because of disturbances in the timing of entry of food into the small intestine and the release of intestinal hormones and enzymes, efficiency of digestion may be reduced. Patients who were lactose tolerant before gastric surgery may experience relative lactase deficiency, either because food enters the small intestine further downstream or because the rate of transit through the proximal small intestine is increased.

Over the long term, anemia, osteoporosis, and select vitamin and mineral deficiencies may occur as a result of malabsorption or limited dietary intake. Iron deficiency may be attributable to loss of acid secretion. Gastric acid normally facilitates the reduction of iron compounds, allowing their absorption. Rapid transit and diminished contact of dietary iron with sites of iron absorption can also lead to iron deficiency anemia. Vitamin B_{12} deficiency may cause a megaloblastic anemia. If the amount of gastric mucosa is reduced, intrinsic factor may not be produced in quantities adequate to allow for complete vitamin B_{12} absorption, and pernicious anemia may result (see Chapter 31). Bacterial overgrowth in the proximal small bowel or in the afferent loop contributes to vitamin B_{12} depletion because bacteria compete with the host for use of the vitamin. Therefore after gastrectomy patients generally receive prophylactic vitamin B_{12} injections. Because of the complications of reflux or dumping syndrome associated with traditional gastrectomies, other procedures are used, including truncal, selective, or parietal cell vagotomy, pyloromyotomy, antrectomy, Roux-en-Y esophagojejunostomy, loop esophagojejunostomy, and pouches or reservoirs made from jejunal or ileocecal segments (Tomita et al., 2001) (see Figure 26-4).

Somatostatin analogs are used to slow gastric emptying in patients with rapid emptying and dumping syndrome.

Acarbose, an α-glucoside hydrolase inhibitor that is normally used to manage type 2 diabetes mellitus, has been used in some persons with dumping syndrome (Ng et al., 2001). Acarbose inhibits the digestion and absorption of starch, sucrose, and maltose. Acarbose may blunt the alimentary hyperglycemia or hypoglycemia related to dumping but has the potential to worsen the colonic gas and diarrhea. Table 26-2 lists some of the other common medications used in GI disorders.

Medical Nutrition Therapy

Because of the problems that accompany eating, patients with dumping syndrome frequently do not eat enough; have diarrhea from the increased intestinal activity; and become underweight, malnourished, and frustrated. The prime objective of nutrition therapy is to restore nutrition status and quality of life.

Proteins and fats are better tolerated than carbohydrates because they are hydrolyzed more slowly into osmotically active substances. Simple carbohydrates such as lactose, sucrose, and dextrose are hydrolyzed rapidly; thus quantities should be limited, but complex carbohydrates (starches) can be included in the diet. Liquids enter the jejunum rapidly; thus some patients may have problems tolerating liquids with meals. Patients who have severe problems with dumping may fare better if they limit the amount of liquids taken with meals, or if they take liquids only between meals, without solid food. Lying down immediately after meals may also decrease the severity of symptoms.

The use of fiber supplements can be beneficial in managing dumping syndrome because they reduce upper GI transit time and decrease the rate of glucose absorption, thus decreasing the insulin response. Pectin, the dietary fiber contained in fruits and vegetables, or gums (e.g., guar) may be useful in treating dumping syndrome. However, caution must be exercised with the use of bulk fiber sources. Several cases of obstruction have been reported with the use of guar gum and other viscous substances when large amounts have been taken, especially without adequate water.

Basically a diet that aims to prevent symptoms of dumping syndrome is somewhat higher in fat content (35% to 45% of calories), low in simple carbohydrates, and high in protein (20% of energy intake). Such a diet helps the patient achieve and maintain optimal weight and nutrition status. Portion

TABLE 26-2

Common Medications Used in the Treatment of Gastrointestinal Disorders

Type of Medication	Example of Use/Application
Antibiotics	Eradicate *Helicobacter pylori*, prevent or treat infection after abdominal wounds or surgery
Antacids	Neutralize gastric acid in acid reflux, peptic ulcer
Proton pump inhibitors (omeprazole, lansoprazole)	Decrease gastric acid secretion
H_2 receptor antagonists (cimetidine, ranitidine)	Inhibit gastric acid secretion
Sucralfate (sulfated disaccharide)	Protects stomach lining and may increase mucosal resistance to acid or enzyme damage

sizes of foods, especially carbohydrate foods such as juices, soft drinks, desserts, and milk, have increased considerably; thus patients may need to learn new serving sizes using models or graphics. The exchange lists given in Appendix 34 can be used to calculate carbohydrate intake and teach the patient about carbohydrate control (see Chapter 30).

After gastrectomy patients often do not tolerate lactose, but small amounts (e.g., 6 g or less per meal) may be tolerated at one time. Because individual dairy drinks may be served in portions of 12 to 16 oz. instead of the old standard 8-oz size, patients may need to be made aware of serving sizes. Patients typically do better with cheeses or unsweetened yogurt than with fluid milk. Non-dairy milks are also useful. Vitamin D and calcium supplements may be needed when intake is inadequate. Commercial lactase products are available for those with significant lactose malabsorption (see Chapter 27).

When steatorrhea is a problem, formulas whose fat content is derived primarily from medium-chain triglycerides may be better tolerated. Box 26-3 provides general nutrition guidelines for patients with dumping syndrome after gastric surgery; however, each diet must be adjusted based on a careful dietary and social history from the patient.

BOX 26-3

Nutrition Care Guidelines for Patients With Dumping Syndrome and Alimentary Hypoglycemia

1. Small meals spread throughout the day are likely to result in improved net absorption and less dramatic fluid shifts.
2. High-protein, moderate-fat foods are recommended, with sufficient calories for weight maintenance or gain as needed. Complex carbohydrates are included as tolerated.
3. Intake of fibrous foods slows upper GI transit and increases viscosity. However, to avoid obstruction, caution should be used with large particles and fiber supplements, especially with esophageal or gastric outlet narrowing or dysmotility.
4. Lying down and avoiding activity an hour after eating may help slow gastric emptying.
5. Taking large amounts of liquids with meals is thought to hasten GI transit, but adequate amounts of liquid should be consumed throughout the day, small amounts at a time.
6. Only very small quantities of hypertonic, concentrated sweets should be ingested. These include soft drinks, juices, pies, cakes, cookies, and frozen desserts (unless made with sugar substitutes).
7. Lactose, especially in milk or ice cream, may be poorly tolerated because of rapid transit and thus may need to be avoided. Cheeses and yogurt are likely to be better tolerated.

◎ **FOCUS ON**

Milestones in Dietary Management of Upper GI Disorders

The treatment of peptic ulcer disease has involved attempts to control gastric acid secretion to heal and prevent recurrence of duodenal ulcers.

Before 1900: Surgeons began performing gastric resections. Early treatment attempted to heal by neutralizing gastric acid with diet modification and the milk and cream-based sippy diet.

1943: Dr. Lester Dragstedt performed the first truncal vagotomy to limit cholinergic stimulation of gastric acid secretion. This led to surgery that combined gastric resections with vagotomy.

1960s: The bland diet with four levels, starting with stage 1 as a sippy diet and progressing to stage 4, a liberal bland diet that omitted only chocolate, peppermint, black pepper, and alcoholic beverages, was used to address various levels of healing. Antacids to neutralize acid and anticholinergics to reduce the amount of acid produced were widely used.

1970: The first parietal cell vagotomy was performed to limit vagal initiation of acid secretion while minimizing the impact on other gastrointestinal functions.

1976: Introduction of the first H_2-receptor antagonist, cimetidine. Ranitidine, the second H_2-receptor antagonist, produced greater acid suppression in the morning and at night with twice daily dosing than cimetidine with four doses each day. The bland diet was refined to have just two levels: restricted and liberal.

1983: Barry Marshall and J. Robin Warren discovered that *H. pylori* was responsible for typical signs of gastritis and peptic ulcer disease. Later in 2005 they received the Nobel prize in Physiology or Medicine.

Currently: *H. pylori* can be eliminated with use of antibiotics, antacids, and proton pump inhibitors. Diet alterations are minimal and specific to the patient.

Modified from Warner CW, McIsaac RL: The evolution of peptic ulcer therapy: a role for temporal control of drug delivery, *Ann N Y Acad Sci* 618:504, 1991.

◉ **FOCAL POINTS**

- Treatment for disorders of the upper GI tract has changed drastically in the last century. For many years patients were given "sippy diets" with high amounts of milk and cream because it was thought that this would coat the stomach lining and reduce pain; however, it was later discovered that this diet was ineffective.
- Progress in the medical management of GI disorders has mostly eliminated the need for restrictions in MNT (see *Focus On:* Milestones in Dietary Management of Upper GI Disorders).

Continued

⊚ FOCAL POINTS—cont'd

- Today nutrition care for patients with upper GI disorders is specific, individualized, and far more effective than in the past because of increased knowledge of neuroendocrine mechanisms, pathogens, and environmental agents.

- The registered dietitian has many tools and food manipulations available that can enhance gastric surgery and overall treatment.

❄ CLINICAL SCENARIO 1

Jim, a 45-year-old man, is an executive who travels extensively in his work. He is 6 ft tall and weighs 186 lb. He recently visited his doctor complaining about upper gastrointestinal (GI) distress. He reports frequent bouts of heartburn in the middle of the night, and he has lost 15 lb over the last year without intentionally dieting. Jim also occasionally experiences heartburn soon after consumption of specific meals and foods. Jim's doctor diagnosed esophageal reflux, and x-ray studies revealed a hiatal hernia.

Jim has received a good deal of advice regarding specific foods and diets from a variety of sources, but he is confused about what he should eat. Jim is coming to you to discuss nutrition therapies.

✳**Nutrition Diagnosis 1:** Involuntary weight loss related to heartburn and GI pain after some meals and foods as evidenced by 15 lb weight loss in the absence of dieting.

✳**Nutrition Diagnosis 2:** Food- and nutrition-related knowledge deficit related to appropriate foods for reflux as evidenced by confusion related to multiple sources of information.

1. What is heartburn? Does hiatal hernia have anything to do with it?
2. Why might Jim experience heartburn in the middle of the night?
3. Why might Jim experience burning after consumption of certain foods or meals?
4. Why do you suppose Jim lost weight?
5. Do you recommend that he regain the weight?
6. What recommendations would you give for reducing or preventing Jim's symptoms and further complications?

❄ CLINICAL SCENARIO 2

Mr. Smith had his stomach removed as a result of gastric cancer and is having difficulty with bloating, nausea, and light-headedness soon after meals. Later, after the meal, he often experiences lower abdominal cramping and diarrhea.

✳**Nutrition Diagnosis:** Altered GI function related to dumping symptoms following meals as evidenced by history of gastric carcinoma requiring resection of stomach.

1. What do you think could be responsible for the different symptoms Mr. Smith is experiencing?
2. Are there dietary measures that would prevent the postprandial discomfort?

3. Are there any medications that could help his situation?
4. Are there any surgical procedures that could reduce the likelihood that these symptoms do not occur after gastrectomy?

USEFUL WEBSITES

American College of Gastroenterology
http://www.acg.gi.org/

American Gastrointestinal Association
www.gastro.org/

National Institute of Diabetes, Digestive Diseases, and Kidney Disorders
http://digestive.niddk.nih.gov/

References

Banerjee S, Bishop W: Effect of *Helicobacter pylori* infection on gastric acid secretion and iron absorption: can we iron out the issue? *J Pediatr Gastroenterol Nutr* 40:102, 2005.

Brunton S, McGuigan J: Diagnostic challenges: differentiating nighttime GERD, *J Fam Pract* 54:1073, 2005.

Bufler P et al: Dumping syndrome: a common problem following Nissen fundoplication in young children, *Pediatr Surg Int* 17:351, 2001.

Bujanda L: The effects of alcohol consumption upon the gastrointestinal tract, *Am J Gastroenterol* 95:3374, 2000.

Bytzer P, O'Morain C: Treatment of *Helicobacter pylori*, *Helicobacter* 10(1S):40, 2005.

Candelli M et al: Treatment of *H. pylori* infection: a review, *Curr Med Chem* 12:375, 2005.

Chang JT, Katzka DA: Gastroesophageal reflux disease, Barrett esophagus, and esophageal carcinoma, *Arch Intern Med* 164:1482, 2004.

Craig WR et al: Metoclopramide, thickened feedings, and positioning for gastro-oesophageal reflux in children under two years, *Cochrane Database Syst Rev* 4:CD003502, 2004.

Crew KD, Neugut AI: Epidemiology of upper gastrointestinal malignancies, *Semin Oncol* 31:450, 2004.

Delgado-Aros S et al: Contributions of gastric volumes and gastric emptying to meal size and postmeal symptoms in functional dyspepsia, *Gastroenterology* 127:1844, 2004.

Doug MH, Kaunitz JD: Gastroduodenal mucosal defense, *Curr Opin Gastroenterol* 22:599, 2006.

El-Serag HB et al: Dietary intake and the risk of gastroesophageal reflux disease: a cross sectional study in volunteers, *Gut* 54: 11, 2005.

Ernst PB et al: The translation of *Helicobacter pylori* Basic research to patient care, *Gastroenterology* 130:188, 2006.

Fahardo NR et al: Frontiers in functional dyspepsia, *Curr Gastroenterol Rep* 7:289, 2005.

Fennerty MB: *Helicobacter pylori:* why it still matters in 2005, *Cleve Clin J Med* 2S:1 2005.

Feinle-Bisset C, Horowitz M: Dietary factors in functional dyspepsia, *Neurogastroenterol Motil* 18:608, 2006.

Flick AL: Acid content of common beverages, *Am J Dig Dis* 15:317, 1970.

Fox JG, Wang TC: *Helicobacter pylori* infection: pathogenesis, *Curr Opin Gastroenterol* 18:15, 2002.

Gold BD: Gastroesophageal reflux disease: could intervention in childhood reduce the risk of later complications? *Am J Med* 117S:23 2004.

Guzzo JL et al: Severe and refractory peptic ulcer disease: the diagnostic dilemma, *Dig Dis Sci* 50:1999, 2005.

Hamilton-Miller JM: The role of probiotics in the treatment and prevention of *Helicobacter pylori* infection, *Int J Antimicrob Agents* 22:360, 2003.

Hassall E: Decisions in diagnosing and managing chronic gastroesophageal reflux disease in children, *J Pediatr* 146S:3, 2005.

Holtman G et al: Heartburn in primary care: problems below the surface, *J Gastroenterol* 39:1027, 2004.

Israel D, Peek RM: The role of persistence in *Helicobacter pylori* pathogenesis, *Curr Opin Gastroenterol* 22:3, 2006.

Kahrilas PJ, Lee TJ: Pathophysiology of gastroesophageal reflux disease, *Thorac Surg Clin* 15:323, 2005.

Kallet RH, Quinn TE: The gastrointestinal tract and ventilator-associated pneumonia, *Respir Care* 50:910, 2005.

Kaltenbach T et al: Are lifestyle measures effective in patients with gastroesophageal reflux disease? An evidence-based approach, *Arch Intern Med* 166:965, 2006.

Leong RW et al: Association of intestinal granulomas with smoking, phenotype and serology in Chinese patients with Crohn's disease, *Am J Gastroenterol* 101:1024, 2006.

Lynch HT et al: Gastric cancer: new genetic developments, *J Surg Oncol* 90:114, 2005.

Mahid SS et al: Active and passive smoking in childhood is related to the development of inflammatory bowel disease, *Inflamm Bowel Dis*, Dec. 19, 2006.

Mayne ST, Navarro SA: Diet, obesity and reflux in the etiology of adenocarcinomas of the esophagus and gastric cardia in humans, *J Nutr* 132:3467S, 2002.

McKay DL, Blumberg JB: A review of the bioactivity and potential health benefits of peppermint tea (Mentha piperita L), *Phytother Res* 20(8):619, 2006.

Milke P et al: Gastroesophageal reflux in healthy subjects induced by two different species of chili (*Capsicum annum*), *Dig Dis* 24(1-2):184, 2006.

Mittal RK, Balaban DH: The esophagogastric junction, *N Engl J Med* 336:924, 1997.

Ng DD et al: Acarbose treatment of postprandial hypoglycemia in children after Nissen fundoplication, *J Pediatr* 139:877, 2001.

Nilsson M et al: Lifestyle related risk factors in the aetiology of gastro-esophageal reflux, *Gut* 53:1730, 2004.

O'Mahony R et al: Bactericidal and anti-adhesive properties of culinary and medicinal plants against *Helicobacter pylori*, *World J Gastroenterol* 11:7499, 2005.

Paimela H et al: Surgery for peptic ulcer today, *Dig Surg* 21:185, 2004.

Pera M et al: Epidemiology of esophageal adenocarcinoma, *J Surg Oncol* 92:151 2005.

Platel K, Srinivasan K: Digestive stimulant action of spices: a myth or reality? *Indian J Med Res* 119:167, 2004.

Pritchard DM, Crabtree JE: *Helicobacter pylori* and gastric cancer, *Curr Opin Gastroenterol* 22:620, 2006.

Ryan-Harshman M, Aldoori W: How diet and lifestyle affect duodenal ulcers: review of the evidence, *Can Fam Physician* 50:727, 2004.

Scheiman JM: Nonsteroidal anti-inflammatory drugs, aspirin, and gastrointestinal prophylaxis: an ounce of prevention, *Rev Gastroenterol Disord* 2S:39, 2005.

Scholl I, Jensen-Jarolim E: Allergenic potency of spices: hot, medium hot, or very hot, *Int Arch Allergy Immunol* 135:247, 2004.

Selby W: Can clinical features predict the likelihood of finding abnormalities when using capsule endoscopy in patients with GI bleeding of obscure origin? *Gastrointest Endosc* 59:782, 2004.

Sharma VR et al: Effect of omeprazole on oral iron replacement with iron deficiency anemia, *South Med J* 97:887, 2004.

Shimizu T et al: Effects of n-3 fatty acids and vitamin E on colonic mucosal leukotriene generation, lipid peroxidation, and microcirculation in rats with experimental colitis, *Digestion* 63:49, 2001.

Smith ML: Functional dyspepsia pathogenesis and therapeutic options—implications for management, *Dig Liver Dis* 37:547, 2005.

Stollman N, Metz DC: Pathophysiology and prophylaxis of stress ulcer in intensive care unit patients, *J Crit Care* 20:35, 2005.

Talley NJ, Wicklund I: Patient-reported outcomes in gastroesophageal reflux disease: an overview of available measures, *Qual Life Res* 14:21, 2005.

Tomita R et al: Operative technique on nearly total gastrectomy reconstructed by interposition of a jejunal J pouch with preservation of vagal nerve, lower esophageal sphincter, and pyloric sphincter for early gastric cancer, *World J Surg* 25:1524, 2001.

Ukleja A: Dumping syndrome: pathophysiology and treatment, *Nutr Clin Pract* 20:517, 2005.

Urbach DR et al: Whither surgery in the treatment of gastroesophageal reflux disease (GERD)? *CMAJ* 170:219, 2004.

van den Brandt PA, Goldbohm RA: Nutrition in the prevention of gastrointestinal cancer, *Best Pract Res Clin Gastroenterol* 20(3):589, 2006.

Vanderhoof JA et al: Efficacy of a pre-thickened infant formula: a multicenter, double-blind, placebo controlled parallel group trial in 104 infants with symptomatic gastroesophageal reflux, *Clin Pediatr* 42:483, 2003.

Vattem DA et al: Enhancing health benefits of berries through phenolic antioxidant enrichment: focus on cranberry, *Asia Pac J Clin Nutr* 14 (2):120, 2005.

Weil PH, Buchberger R: From Billroth to PCV: a century of gastric surgery, *World J Surg* 23:736, 1999.

Wittingham S, Mackay IR: Autoimmune gastritis: historical antecedents, outstanding discoveries and unresolved problems, *Int Rev Immunol* 24:1, 2005.

Woodwell DA, Cherry DK: *National Ambulatory Medical Care Survey 2002: advance data from vital and health statistics: no. 346 2004*, Hyattsville, Md, 2004, National Center for Health Statistics.

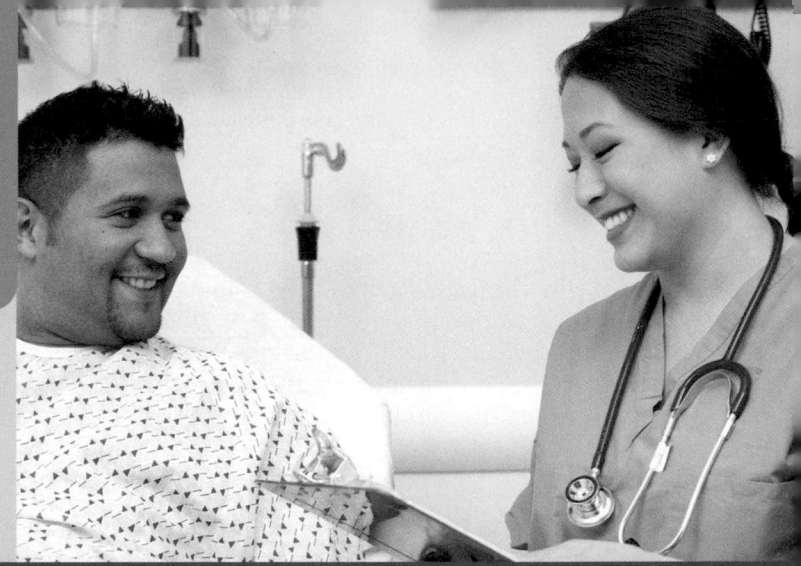

CHAPTER 27

Peter L. Beyer, MS, RD

Medical Nutrition Therapy for Lower Gastrointestinal Tract Disorders

KEY TERMS

aerophagia swallowing of air

blind loop syndrome a malabsorption syndrome resulting from bacterial overgrowth in a surgically created loop or dysfunctional segments of small intestine

borborygmus intestinal rumbling

celiac disease common term for gluten-sensitive enteropathy

colostomy surgically created colonic opening (stoma) through the abdominal wall to permit defecation

constipation a condition in which the frequency or quantity of stools is reduced

Crohn's disease a chronic, granulomatous inflammatory disease of unknown etiology involving the small or large intestine that can result in diarrhea, strictures, fistulas, and malabsorption

dermatitis herpetiformis a skin disorder that is a variant of celiac disease

diarrhea abnormal volume and liquidity of stools

dietary fiber edible plant materials not digested by the enzymes in the upper digestive tract of humans; consists of cellulose, hemicelluloses, pectins, gums, lignin, starchy materials, and oligosaccharides that are partially resistant to digestive enzymes

diverticulitis inflammation of diverticula

diverticulosis presence of herniations of the mucous membrane through the muscular layers of the colonic wall

fistula an abnormal passage between two internal organs or from an internal organ to the skin surface of the body

flatulence excessive collection and anal passage of gas from the gastrointestinal tract

flatus gas in the gastrointestinal tract that is expelled through the anus

glutamine an amino acid and the preferred fuel of the enterocyte

gluten-sensitive enteropathy (celiac disease) a syndrome precipitated by the immunologic interaction of gluten in the grains wheat, rye, barley and oats (by contamination) and intestinal cells; characterized by flattening of the villi of the small intestine

high-fiber diet a diet containing more than 25 to 38 g of dietary fiber per day

hypolactasia a decrease in the amount of the intestinal enzyme lactase

ileal pouch surgical creation of a small reservoir, using folds of the distal ileum, which is then attached to the rectum

ileostomy surgical creation of an opening (stoma) of the ileum through the abdominal wall

inflammatory bowel disease (IBD) a general term for inflammatory diseases of the bowel, including Crohn's disease and ulcerative colitis

irritable bowel syndrome (IBS) an abnormal stooling pattern associated with symptoms of intestinal dysfunction that persists for more than 3 months of the year

lactose maldigestion the inability to digest lactose to galactose and glucose because of a deficiency of the enzyme lactase with resulting intolerance to normal amounts of lactose

medium-chain triglycerides (MCTs) triacylglycerols with fatty acids of 8 and 10 carbons in length—short enough to be absorbed directly into the portal blood

phytobezoars stomach obstructions composed of partially digested plant foods

prebiotics dietary substrates used to promote the growth of beneficial intestinal bacteria

probiotics orally consumed sources of bacteria used to reestablish the presence of beneficial intestinal flora

refractory sprue celiac disease that persists even after adherence to a strict gluten-free diet

residue the fecal contents, including bacteria and any remaining gastrointestinal secretions and foods not digested or absorbed

short-bowel syndrome (SBS) a malabsorption syndrome resulting from major resections of the small bowel; characterized by diarrhea, steatorrhea, and malnutrition

steatorrhea excessive amounts of fat in the feces, as seen in malabsorption syndromes

tropical sprue a syndrome of unknown etiology that causes diarrhea and malabsorption but is not responsive to gluten-free diet therapy

ulcerative colitis an inflammatory disease of the colonic mucosa

Dietary modifications in disorders of the intestinal tract are designed to alleviate symptoms, correct nutrient deficiencies, and, when possible, address the primary cause of difficulty. Careful assessment of the nature and severity of the primary gastrointestinal (GI) problem is necessary to identify the nutrition diagnosis and lead to appropriate interventions. Assessment of GI patients may include evaluating the frequency and amount of nutrients consumed, learning about the patient's medical and surgical history, medications used, and the patient's subjective experiences with foods and understanding of the relationship between diet and the GI problem. In particular the GI assessment may include information on the duration and severity of the disorder; its impact on digestion, secretion, and absorption of nutrients; and its affect on symptoms and complications. Meal consistency, frequency, and size, as well as other characteristics of the diet, may be altered to better fit the patient's needs.

COMMON INTESTINAL PROBLEMS

Before starting to describe specific nutrition-related lower GI problems such as celiac disease and irritable bowel syndrome, it is important to discuss some of the most common GI symptoms that occur both in everyday life and in serious GI disorders (i.e., intestinal gas and flatulence, constipation, and diarrhea). Many of the dietary principles that can be applied to milder forms of these common complaints are used in the management of more serious GI disorders.

Intestinal Gas and Flatulence

Pathophysiology

Considerable amounts of gas may be swallowed or produced within the GI tract and may be absorbed across the alimentary tract into the bloodstream and expired through the lungs, expelled through belching (eructation) or passed rectally **(flatus).** Intestinal gases include nitrogen (N_2), oxygen (O_2), carbon dioxide (CO_2), hydrogen (H_2), and in some persons methane (CH_4).

Approximately 200 ml of gas is normally present in the GI tract. Humans excrete an average of 700 ml of gas each day but are capable of moving considerably more through the GI tract. The amount of intestinal gas varies greatly among individuals and from one day to the next (Strocchi and Levitt, 1998). When patients complain about "excessive gas," or **flatulence** they may be referring to increased volume or frequency of belching or passage of gas rectally. They may also be referring to abdominal distention or cramping pain associated with the accumulation of gases in the upper or lower GI tract. The association between the amount of gas in the GI tract perceived by an individual and the amount actually measured is not always accurate (Azpiroz, 2005). Inactivity, decreased GI motility, aerophagia, dietary components, and GI disorders can all contribute to the amount of intestinal gas and an individual's gas-related symptoms.

Gas in the upper intestinal tract results from **aerophagia** (the swallowing of air), and from chemical reactions that occur during digestion. Normally only small amounts of swallowed air or gases dissolved in foods make their way as far as the colon. High N_2 and O_2 concentrations in rectal gas, both of which are substances that are present in the atmosphere in high concentrations, may indicate aerophagia. Aerophagia can be avoided to some degree by eating slowly, chewing with the mouth closed, and refraining from drinking through straws. Movement of gas may be enhanced with upright stance and mild exercise.

Increased gas production may occur in the stomach and small intestine because of bacterial fermentation, particularly from carbohydrates, and can result in abdominal discomfort and distention. Bacterial overgrowth may occur in the stomach or small intestine with partial obstruction, with dysmotility, in immune disorders, or after some GI surgical procedures (Huesbye, 2005). Persons with small intestinal bacterial overgrowth may experience abdominal distress relatively soon after meals as a result of the fermentation of potentially large amounts of carbohydrate not yet absorbed from the small bowel (Lin, 2004; Nucera et al., 2005). The small intestine is less tolerant of gas than the colon, and distention may cause pain.

The movement of gas into the proximal small intestine and beyond may be slowed by high-calorie meals and meals high in lipid. Slowed excretion or retained gas may contribute to the perception of distention or bloating with large meals in normal circumstances and with the abdominal discomfort that is experienced in some functional GI disorders such as irritable bowel syndrome (Harder et al., 2006; Azpiroz, 2005).

Increased amounts of H_2 and CO_2—and sometimes, CH_4—in rectal gas with lowered fecal pH indicate excessive colonic bacterial fermentation and suggest malabsorption of a fermentable substrate. The amounts and types of gases produced may depend on the mix of microorganisms in the individual's colon. Consumption of large amounts of dietary fiber (especially soluble fiber), resistant starches, lactose in persons who are lactase deficient, or modest amounts of fructose or alcohol sugars (such as sorbitol) may result in increased gas production in the colon and increased flatulence (Beyer et al., 2005).

Consumption of fructose in the United States, especially from fruit juices, fruit drinks, and high-fructose corn syrup (HFCS) in soft drinks and confections, has increased significantly in recent years. Fructose is normally well absorbed when consumed in the form of sucrose or as small amounts of HFCS, but not as well as when consumed as the only or predominant sugar (see Chapter 1). A 10- to 20-g amount of fructose in children or 25 g in adults is sufficient to result in malabsorption symptoms. Sucrose is normally well tolerated; but if it is taken in large quantities, especially with GI dysfunction, it may also result in increased amounts of fecal substrate.

Medical Nutrition Therapy

In the assessment of the patient, one must ask whether the problem is increased production of gas or whether gas is not being passed. Inactivity, dysmotility, or partial obstruction may be contributing to the inability to move normal amounts of gas as produced. Consuming low-calorie or low-lipid meals may enhance the movement of gas from the upper GI tract, and movement or exercise may help expel gases through eructation or rectal passage. Patients with small intestinal bacterial overgrowth may benefit from limiting the amount of easily fermented, refined carbohydrates that could contribute to the gas and organic acids produced, at least until the overgrowth is treated medically.

The primary emphasis in dietary management of gas production in the colon is to reduce the intake of carbohydrates that are likely to be malabsorbed and fermented. Examples include legumes, soluble fiber, resistant starches, and simple sugars such as fructose and alcohol sugars. When undigested carbohydrates pass into the colon, they are fermented in varying degrees to short-chain fatty acids and gases. The primary gases include H_2, CO_2, and, in about one third of individuals, CH_4. The widely recognized propensity of legumes to produce flatus is related to the presence not only of ample amounts of fiber but also of stachyose and raffinose, carbohydrates that are only partially digested in the small intestine.

Excess production of gas may also be related to the dose of carbohydrate foods consumed at one time. Starches such as breads, baked goods, and starchy vegetables may be almost completely digested in normal portions but, when consumed in large quantities, may leave a considerable fraction of undigested or unabsorbed **residue** for bacterial action in the colon. The properties of some so-called gas-forming foods may be explained simply by the type and amount of sugar, starch, or fiber they contain.

Constipation

Pathophysiology

Constipation is one of the most common intestinal maladies in Western societies, and it occurs in from 5% to more than 25% of the population, depending on the definition of the disorder (Candelli et al., 2001; Higgins and Johanson, 2004). In children, as many as one third from ages 6 to 12 years complain of constipation in any given year (Biggs and Dery, 2006). Definitions of constipation tend to be highly subjective but usually include hard stools, straining with defecation, and infrequent large bowel movements. Children may also exhibit vomiting, abdominal pain, anorexia, or encopresis (i.e., involuntary passage of stool or *fecal soiling*) (Benniga et al., 2004). At least in older patients, hard stools, incomplete evacuation, and difficulty passing stools may be more troublesome than the infrequency of bowel movements.

In adults normal stool weight is about 100 to 200 g daily, and normal frequency may range from one stool every 3 days to three times per day. Normal transit time through the GI tract ranges approximately from 18 to 48 hours. Children normally have more frequent stools, ranging from an average of two to three stools daily for the first few months of life to approximately one and a half bowel movements daily at age 3. Individuals who consume a diet that contains the recommended amounts of dietary fiber in the form of fruits, vegetables, and whole-grain breads and cereals tend to have larger, softer stools that are relatively easy to pass.

The most common causes of constipation in otherwise healthy persons include repeated lack of response to the urge to defecate, lack of fiber in the diet, insufficient fluid intake, inactivity, and chronic use of laxatives. Nervous strain or anxiety may aggravate the condition. Chronic constipation may also result from a number of organic causes, as outlined in Box 27-1.

Most health practitioners have encountered individuals who believe that it is necessary to have scheduled and frequent bowel movements, yet they ignore dietary and other recommendations for maintaining laxation. When the desired stool frequency or timing of defecation does not occur, they may try to compensate with the use of medications and enemas.

Medical Treatment for Adults

The first approach to treatment of mild and functional constipation is to ensure adequate dietary fiber, fluid, and exercise and to advise the patient to heed the urge to defecate. Patients dependent on laxatives are usually encouraged to use milder products and reduce the dose until withdrawal is complete.

When the patient is unable to consume an adequate amount of fibrous foods or exercise, substances that promote regular evacuation of soft stools may be prescribed. Polyethylene glycol, tegaserod, psyllium seed, and lactulose have shown to be effective, but a number of other bulking and osmotic agents such as magnesium hydroxide and sorbitol have been used (Ramkumar and Rao, 2005). Impactions of stool require evacuation and a more stringent preventive and maintenance program, including combinations of medications, fluids, activity, and perhaps enemas (Candelli et al., 2001). In more extreme cases such as toxic megacolon, surgery may be advised.

Medical Treatment for Infants and Children

About 3% to 5% of all pediatric outpatient visits are related to chronic constipation. In the most severe cases of functional constipation with frequent stool retention, the rectum becomes insensitive to distention, and encopresis develops. After organic disease is ruled out, treatment includes laxatives and lubricants and ensuring adequate dietary fiber and fluid intake. A careful history and physical examination followed by parent and child education, behavioral intervention, and appropriate use of laxatives often leads to dramatic improvement (Biggs and Dery, 2006; Loening-Baucke, 2002) (see Chapter 7).

Medical Nutrition Therapy

Primary nutrition therapy for constipation is consumption of adequate amounts of both soluble and insoluble dietary fiber. Fiber increases colonic fecal fluid, microbial mass, stool weight and frequency, and the rate of colonic transit. Fiber also softens stools and makes them easier to pass.

Most adults and children in the United States chronically consume only about half the amount of fiber recommended (Institute of Medicine, 2002). The recommended amount of dietary fiber is about 14 g/1000 kcal. The diet of an adult woman should contain about 25 g of fiber daily; that of a man, about 38 g daily (Institute of Medicine, 2002). For children recommended fiber intake ranges from 19 to 25 g daily.

Fiber can be provided in the form of whole grains, fruits, vegetables, legumes, seeds, and nuts (Marlett et al., 2002). These foods are also high in nutrients, healthful phytochemicals and resistant starches, and may serve as **prebiotics** to maintain the desired colonic microflora. Bran and powdered fiber supplements may be helpful in persons who cannot or will not eat sufficient amounts of fibrous foods. When changes in diet and activity patterns do not improve constipation, further evaluation is warranted.

High-Fiber Diet

Dietary fiber refers primarily to edible plant materials not digested by the enzymes in the upper digestive tract of humans. It consists of cellulose, hemicelluloses, pectins, gums, lignin, starchy materials, and oligosaccharides that are partially resistant to digestive enzymes.

The term roughage tends to refer to vegetable matter, but it is not a quantitative term. **Residue** is not the same as fiber; this term refers to the end result of digestive, secretory, absorptive, and fermentative processes. Thus increasing dietary fiber may result in increased fecal output, but increasing dietary lactose (a fiber-free food) in a person who is a lactose malabsorber would also increase fecal weight (residue).

The **high-fiber diet** in Box 27-2 provides more than the amount of fiber recommended. Most individuals consume considerably less that the recommended amount; thus to many individuals it is a large departure from their normal intake. Reaching the recommended levels of fiber may be sufficient to achieve normal laxation in many individuals, but a high-fiber therapeutic diet may need to exceed 25 to 38 g. However, amounts greater than 50 g/day are not likely to be necessary and may increase abdominal distention and excessive flatulence in some persons. Appendix 41 provides a list of the fiber content of foods.

Ideally fiber in the diet should be ingested in the form of foods such as fruits, vegetables, whole-grain breads and cereals, legumes, nuts, and seeds. These foods are not only rich in fiber but are excellent sources of vitamins, minerals, trace elements, antioxidants, and numerous protective phytochemicals. Fibrous powders or bran concentrates may be necessary to obtain the desired fiber level in some persons. Several of these concentrates available on the market are palatable and can be added to cereals, yogurts, fruit sauces, juices, or soups. Cooking does not destroy fiber, although the structure may change. Consumption of at least eight 8-oz glasses (2 L) of fluids daily is recommended to facilitate the effectiveness of a high-fiber intake. Gastric obstruction and fecal impaction may occur when boluses of fibrous gels or bran are not consumed with sufficient fluid to disperse the fiber. Appropriate cautions are also warranted for persons with GI strictures or dysmotility syndromes. In these situations the fiber content of the diet should be increased slowly, taking almost a month to reach desired intakes of 25 to 38 g of fiber per day.

BOX 27-2

Guidelines for High-Fiber Diets

1. Increase consumption of whole grain breads and cereals and other whole grain products to 6-11 servings daily.
2. Increase consumption of vegetables, legumes, and fruits, nuts, and edible seeds to 5-8 servings daily.
3. Consume high-fiber cereals, granolas, and legumes as needed to bring fiber intake to 25 g in women or 38 g in men or more daily.
4. Increase consumption of fluids to at least 2 L (or about 2 qt) daily.

    Following these guidelines may cause an increase in stool weight, fecal water, and gas. The amount that causes clinical symptoms varies among individuals, depending on age and presence of gastrointestinal (GI) disease, malnutrition, or resection of the GI tract. These guidelines should be implemented slowly over a period of 1 to 2 weeks to give the GI tract time to adjust and thus minimize symptoms of discomfort or gas.

Gradual initiation of a high-fiber diet may help reduce unpleasant side effects such as increased flatulence, **borborygmus** (intestinal rumbling), cramps, or diarrhea. A gradual increase in fiber intake helps alleviate these symptoms. If fiber supplements are used, doses should be interspersed with meals, preferably in two or more small doses per day with increased fluid intake. GI disturbances associated with initial fiber ingestion usually decrease within 4 to 5 days, but some increase in flatulence is normal with a high-fiber intake. The high-fiber diet is most effective when consumed continuously for several months.

Diarrhea

Pathophysiology

Diarrhea is characterized by the frequent evacuation of liquid stools, usually exceeding 300 ml, accompanied by an excessive loss of fluid and electrolytes, especially sodium and potassium. It occurs when there is excessively rapid transit of intestinal contents through the small intestine, decreased enzymatic digestion of foodstuffs, decreased absorption of fluids and nutrients, increased secretion of fluids into the GI tract, or exudative losses. Causes may be related to inflammatory disease; infections with fungal, bacterial, or viral agents; medications; the overconsumption of sugars; an insufficient or damaged mucosal absorptive surface; or GI resections or malnutrition.

Osmotic diarrheas occur when osmotically active solutes are present in the intestinal tract and are poorly absorbed. Examples include the diarrhea that accompanies dumping syndrome and that which follows lactose ingestion in the person with a lactase deficiency.

Secretory diarrheas are the result of active intestinal secretion of electrolytes and water by the intestinal epithelium, resulting from bacterial exotoxins, viruses, and increased intestinal hormone secretion. Unlike osmotic diarrhea, fasting does not relieve secretory diarrhea.

Exudative diarrheas are always associated with mucosal damage, which leads to an outpouring of mucus, fluid, blood, and plasma proteins, with a net accumulation of electrolytes and water in the gut. Prostaglandin and cytokine release may be involved. The diarrheas associated with Crohn's disease, ulcerative colitis, and radiation enteritis are typically exudative, but secretory and osmotic diarrheas may also occur.

Medication-induced diarrheas may be caused by several medications, but especially antibiotics. Antibiotics can reduce the usual "salvage" by colonic bacteria of the small amounts of foodstuffs that escape digestion and absorption. Broad-spectrum antibiotics can greatly reduce the numbers of colonic bacteria that normally convert osmotically active molecules (carbohydrate and amino acids) to gases and short-chain fatty acids (SCFAs). The SCFAs are normally absorbed from the lumen of the colon as long as the amount produced is close to normal. Absorption of the SCFAs facilitates absorption of electrolytes and water from the colon. Eradication of the bacteria from the colon results in accumulation of osmotically active molecules and reduced absorption of electrolytes and water. If more substrates than usual are malabsorbed, as often occurs in acutely ill patients, the resulting rise in osmolality can cause considerable fluid loss.

Antibiotics can also have direct effects on GI function (see Chapter 16). For example, erythromycin increases GI motility; clarithromycin, and clindamycin may also increase GI secretions. Finally, some antibiotics allow opportunistic proliferation of pathogenic organisms normally suppressed by competitive organisms in the GI tract. The organisms or the toxins produce decrease absorption and increase secretion of fluid and electrolytes. *Clostridium difficile* is most commonly associated with antibiotic-related diarrhea and accounts for 15% to 25% of cases, but *C. perfringens, Salmonella, Shigella, Campylobacter, Yersinia enterocolitica,* and *Escherichia coli* organisms have also been implicated in antibiotic-associated diarrhea (Bartlett, 2002; Schroeder 2005). Clindamycin, penicillins, and cephalosporins are associated most often with the development of *C. difficile* infection, and its occurrence depends on the number of antibiotics used, the duration of exposure to antibiotics, and the patient's overall health.

With human immunodeficiency virus (HIV) and other immune deficiency states, several factors may contribute to the diarrhea, including the toxic effects of medications, proliferation of opportunistic organisms, and the GI manifestations of the disease itself (Mitra et al., 2001) (see Chapter 38). Increased risk of opportunistic infection is also associated with use of antineoplastic agents (Kornblau et al., 2000) and severe malnutrition. Antacids (especially magnesium salts), H_2-receptor blockers, and proton pump inhibitors have also been implicated in cases of diarrhea.

Malabsorptive diarrhea is often complicated by steatorrhea (lipid malabsorption) and maldigestion of other macronutrients or micronutrients. Malabsorptive diarrhea occurs when there is not enough healthy absorptive area or there is rapid transit of chyme, such as what might occur in inflammatory bowel disease or after extensive bowel resection.

Medical Treatment

Because diarrhea is a symptom of a disease state, the first step in medical treatment is to identify and treat the underlying problem. The next priority is to manage fluid and electrolyte replacement. Losses of electrolytes, especially potassium and sodium, should be corrected early by using oral glucose electrolyte solutions with added potassium. With intractable diarrhea, especially in an infant or young child, parenteral feeding may be required. Parenteral nutrition may even be necessary if exploratory surgery is anticipated or if the patient is not expected to resume full oral intake within 5 to 7 days (see Chapter 20).

Medical Nutrition Therapy

Replacement of necessary fluids and electrolytes is the first step in managing diarrhea, using electrolyte solutions, soups and broths, vegetable juices, and other isotonic liquids. Later, starchy carbohydrates such as cereals, breads, low-fat meats, and small amounts of vegetables and fruits can be added, followed by lipids. In most cases a minimum-residue diet similar to that outlined in Table 27-1 may be started as the acute episode resolves. The key objective is to limit large amounts of hyperosmotic carbohydrates that may be maldigested or malabsorbed, foods that stimulate secretion of fluids, and foods that speed the rate of GI transit.

Modest amounts of fat can be used if digestive mechanisms for lipid are intact. Sugar alcohols, lactose, fructose, and large amounts of sucrose may worsen osmotic diarrheas. Because the activity of the disaccharidases and transport mechanisms may be decreased during inflammatory and infectious intestinal disease, sugars may need to be limited, especially in children (Robayo-Torres et al., 2006).

Use of modest amounts of foods or dietary supplements containing prebiotic components such as pectin, fructose oligosaccharides, inulin, oats, banana flakes, and chicory may actually help to control or treat diarrhea. Prebiotics help because they favor the maintenance of "friendly" lactobacillus and bifidus microbes and may prevent the overgrowth of potentially pathogenic organisms (Broussard and Surawicz, 2004). SCFAs in physiologic quantities serve as substrate for colonocytes, facilitate the absorption of fluid and salts, and may help to regulate GI motility. Fibrous material and several types of prebiotic foods also tend to slow gastric emptying, moderate overall GI transit, and hold water.

Ingestion of some types of **probiotics** (sources of bacteria used to reestablish beneficial gut flora) in the form of cultured foods or supplements, with or without prebiotics, has been modestly successful in antibiotic-related diarrhea, traveler's diarrhea, bacterial overgrowth, and several types of pediatric diarrhea. The use of several probiotics was evaluated in preventing antibiotic-associated diarrhea (AAD) in children. Risk reduction for AAD ranged from 0.2 for *Saccharomyces boulardii*, 0.3 for *Lactobacillus GG* and 0.5 for *L. bifidus* and *Streptococcus thermophilus* (Szajewska et al., 2006). Additional study is needed to sort out which combination of probiotics alone, in combination with other probiotics and prebiotics, and antibiotics work most effectively in each situation (Teitelbaum, 2005; Madsen, 2001).

Severe and chronic diarrhea is accompanied by dehydration and electrolyte depletion. If also accompanied by prolonged infectious, immunodeficiency, or inflammatory disease, malabsorption of vitamins, minerals, and protein or lipid may also occur, and the nutrients may need to be re-

---

TABLE 27-1

Food to Limit in a Low- or Minimum-Residue Diet

Food	Comments
Lactose (in lactose malabsorbers)	6-12 g normally tolerated in healthy lactase-deficient individuals, but may not be in some individuals
Fiber (quantities >20 g)	Modest amounts (10-15 g) may help maintain normal consistency of gastrointestinal (GI) contents and normal colonic mucosa in healthy states and GI disease
Resistant starch (especially raffinose and stachyose found in legumes)	
Sorbitol, mannitol, and xylitol (excess, >10 g/day)	
Fructose (excess, 20-25 g/meal)	
Sucrose (excess, >25-50 g/meal)	Well tolerated in moderate amounts; large amounts may cause hyperosmolar diarrhea or decreased fecal pH with fermentation to short-chain fatty acids
Caffeine	Increases GI secretions, colonic motility
Alcoholic beverages (especially wine and beer)	Increase GI secretions

Data from Rummessen JJ, Gudman-Hoyer E: Functional bowel disease: malabsorption and abdominal distress after ingestion of fructose, sorbitol, and fructose-sorbitol mixtures, *Gastroenterology* 95:694, 1998; Gudmand-Hoyer E: The clinical significance of disaccharide maldigestion, *Am J Clin Nutr* 59:(suppl):735, 1994; Piche T et al: Colonic fermentation influences lower esophageal sphincter function in gastroesophageal reflux disease, *Gastroenterology* 124:894, 2003; and Rao SS et al: Is coffee a colonic stimulant? *Eur J Gastroenterol Hepatol* 10:113, 1998.

placed parenterally or enterally. In particular the loss of potassium alters bowel motility, encourages anorexia, and can introduce a cycle of bowel distress.

In some forms of infectious diarrheas loss of iron from GI bleeding may be severe enough to cause anemia. Nutrient deficiencies themselves cause mucosal changes such as decreased villi height and reduced enzyme secretion, further contributing to malabsorption. As the diarrhea begins to resolve, the addition of more normal amounts of fiber to the diet may help to restore normal mucosal function, increase electrolyte and water absorption, and increase the firmness of the stool.

Food in the lumen is needed to restore the compromised GI tract after disease and periods of fasting. Early refeeding after rehydration reduces stool output and shortens the duration of illness. Micronutrient replacement or supplementation may also be useful for acute diarrhea, probably because it accelerates the normal regeneration of damaged mucosal epithelial cells.

Treating Diarrhea in Infants and Children

Acute diarrhea is most dangerous in infants and small children, who are easily dehydrated by large fluid losses. In these cases replacement of fluid and electrolytes must be aggressive and immediate. Standard oral rehydration solutions recommended by the World Health Organization (WHO) since 1986 and the American Academy of Pediatrics (AAP) contain a 2% concentration of glucose (20 g/L), 45 to 90 mEq/L of sodium, 20 mEq/L of potassium, and a citrate base (Table 27-2).

Newer, reduced osmolarity solutions (≈130 to 200 mOsm/L) have been shown to be equally effective in treating persistent diarrhea in children (Hahn et al., 2002), and their use is being evaluated (Murphy et al., 2004). Commercial solutions such as Pedialyte, Infalyte, Lytren, Equalyte,

and Rehydralyte typically contain less glucose and slightly less salt and are available in pharmacies, often without prescription. Oral rehydration therapy is less invasive and less expensive than intravenous rehydration and, when used with children, allows parents to assist with their children's recovery (Sentongo, 2004).

A substantial proportion of children 9 to 20 months of age can maintain adequate intake when offered either a liquid or a semisolid diet continuously during bouts of acute diarrhea. Even during acute diarrhea, the intestine can absorb up to 60% of the food eaten. Some practitioners have been slow to adopt the practice of early refeeding after severe diarrhea in infants despite evidence that "resting the gut" is actually more damaging (Steffen and Gyr, 2004). A report from the working group of the World Congress of Pediatric Gastroenterology, Hepatology, and Nutrition suggests that strategies must be cohesive and uniform to address the problems of pediatric diarrhea and reduce the number of deaths worldwide (Davidson et al., 2002). Prescription of the typical hospital "full liquid" or "clear liquid" diet that is commonly high in fructose, lactose, and other sugars is inappropriate for recovery from diarrhea.

Steatorrhea

Pathophysiology

Steatorrhea, or excessive fat in the stool, is a consequence of disease or surgical resection of organs involved in the digestion and absorption of lipid. Normally 94% to 98% of ingested fat is absorbed; in steatorrhea the percent remaining in the stool may increase to 20% or more. Diagnosis is usually based on a ratio of fecal fat to ingested fat or a coefficient of absorption. A diet containing 75 to 100 g of fat is usually fed for 72 hours, the amount of fat actually consumed is recorded, and the fecal fat content is analyzed. The upper limit of normal fecal fat is usually in the range of 7%.

Steatorrhea may result from (1) pancreatic lipase insufficiency; (2) insufficient functional small surface area for absorption of lipids as in short-bowel syndrome, celiac disease, or inflammatory bowel disease; (3) inadequate bile secretion secondary to liver disease or biliary obstruction; (4) malabsorption of bile salts resulting from **blind loop syndrome** (resection or inflammation involving the distal ileum, the site of bile salt reabsorption); or (5) decreased reesterification of fatty acids with decreased formation and transport of chylomicrons, as seen in abetalipoproteinemia and intestinal lymphangiectasia. Box 27-3 lists disorders associated with malabsorption.

Medical Treatment

Because steatorrhea is a symptom and not a disease, the underlying cause of malabsorption must be determined and treated. With pancreatic insufficiency, oral pancreatic enzymes can be used to increase lipid digestion.

Medical Nutrition Therapy

Steatorrhea can result in chronic weight loss and may require compensatory increased energy intake, primarily in the form of dietary protein and complex carbohydrates.

TABLE 27-2

Oral Rehydration Solution: Composition and Recipe

Element	Composition
Glucose (g/100 ml)	20
Sodium (mEq/L)	90
Potassium (mEq/L)	20
Chloride (mEq/L)	80
Bicarbonate (mEq/L)	30
Osmolarity (mOsm/L)	330

Recipe*

To 1 L of water add the following:
  3.5 g sodium chloride
  2.5 g sodium bicarbonate
  1.5 g potassium chloride
  20 g glucose

Data from World Health Organization: Guidelines for cholera control, WHO/COD/Ser/80.4, Rev 1, Geneva, 1986.

*The solution should be made fresh every 24 hr.

BOX 27-3

Diseases and Conditions Associated With Malabsorption

Inadequate Digestion

Pancreatic insufficiency
Gastric acid hypersecretion
Gastric resection

Altered Bile Salt Metabolism With Impaired Micelle Formation

Hepatobiliary disease
Interrupted enterohepatic circulation of bile salts
Bacterial overgrowth
Drugs that precipitate bile salts

Abnormalities of Mucosal Cell Transport

Biochemical or genetic abnormalities
  Disaccharidase deficiency
  Monosaccharide malabsorption
  Specific disorders of amino acid malabsorption
  Abetalipoproteinemia
  Vitamin B_{12} malabsorption
  Celiac disease
Inflammatory or infiltrative disorders
  Crohn's disease
  Ulcerative colitis
  Amyloidosis

Inflammatory or infiltrative disorders—cont'd
  Scleroderma
  Tropical sprue
  Gastrointestinal allergy
  Infectious enteritis
  Whipple's disease
  Intestinal lymphoma
  Radiation enteritis
  Drug-induced enteritis
  Endocrine and metabolic disorders
  Short-bowel syndrome

Abnormalities of Intestinal Lymphatics and Vascular System

Intestinal lymphangiectasia
Mesenteric vascular insufficiency
Chronic congestive heart failure

Data from Beyer PL: Short bowel syndrome. In Coulston AM, Rock CL, Monson ER, editors: *Nutrition in the prevention and treatment of disease*, ed 1, San Diego, 2001, Academic Press; Sundarum A et al: Nutritional management of short bowel syndrome in adults, *J Clin Gastroenterol* 34:207, 2002; Podolsky DK: Inflammatory bowel disease, *N Engl J Med* 347:417, 2002; Mitra AD et al: Management of diarrhea in HIV-infected patients, *Int J STD AIDS* 12:630, 2001; Branski D et al: Chronic diarrhea and malabsorption, *Pediatr Clin North Am* 43:307, 1996; and Fine KD: Diarrhea. In Feldman M, Sleisenger MH, Scharschmidt BF, editors: *Gastrointestinal and liver disease*, ed 6, Philadelphia, 1998, Saunders.

Medium-chain triglycerides (MCTs) can be used in the diet because they have a short chain length, allowing easier absorption in the absence of bile acids. Medium-chain fatty acids and SCFAs are able to enter the portal venous blood for transport to the liver without requiring digestion by pancreatic lipase, micelle formation digestion, and resynthesis into triglycerides in the intestinal cell.

The MCTs are available in some enteral formulas and also as MCT oil (8.3 kcal/kg). The oil is best used when it is incorporated into foods rather than administered by the spoonful. MCTs can be used to make salad dressings, sandwich spreads, or confections; and they can be substituted for fats in most recipes. Normally divided doses of less than 15 g of oil per feeding are better tolerated and absorbed than larger quantities. When steatorrhea is present, vitamin deficiencies may occur, especially of fat-soluble vitamins; calcium, zinc, and magnesium losses are increased as a result of the formation of insoluble soaps.

Gastrointestinal Strictures and Obstruction

Pathophysiology

The presence of intestinal tumors or scarring from GI surgeries, inflammatory bowel disease, peptic ulcer, or radiation enteritis may partially or completely obstruct the GI tract or result in dysfunctional segments. When sections of the GI tract are partially obstructed or not moving appropriately, obstructions from foods may occur.

The most common foods that may cause obstructions are fibrous plant foods because the fiber in the foods may not be completely chewed or reduced in size enough to pass through abnormal or narrowed segments of the GI tract. Obstructions in the stomach that result from the ingestion of plant foods are called **phytobezoars.** They are more common in patients who have had the GI maladies mentioned previously or have gastroparesis from diabetes mellitus, have poor dentition, or use dentures. Foods most commonly incriminated in the formation of phytobezoars include potato skins, oranges, and grapefruit; but many foods that are consumed in large segments or that have skins that are difficult to chew may be problematic. When obstructions occur in the intestine, the patient usually experiences prolonged bloating, abdominal distention and pain, and sometimes nausea and vomiting.

Medical Nutrition Therapy

Because fiber is not digested to any significant degree (except by fermentation in the colon), and because chewing is not a reliable way of reducing the size of fibrous foods, both the amount and size of fibrous material usually must be controlled. A restricted-fiber diet typically limits fruits, vegetables, and coarse grains and provides less than 10 to 15 g of dietary fiber, usually in the form of small particulate matter such as vegetable and fruit juices, cereals, and breads. Particularly with distal obstructions or strictures, it may be beneficial to keep the stool soft by including modest amounts of fiber, but of small particle size, and adequate water.

Some intestinal obstruction cases may require clear liquids or total restriction of food, and parenteral nutrition and fluid may be needed. Working with the patient and physician is necessary to determine the nature, site, and duration of the obstruction so that nutrition therapy can be individualized.

DISEASES OF THE SMALL INTESTINE

Celiac Disease (Gluten-Sensitive Enteropathy)

Pathophysiology

Under normal conditions the GI tract is confronted with a tremendous number of antigens from the ingestion of food and from transient or established flora that pass through or reside in its lumen. The GI tract is protected by physical and chemical barriers and can digest potential antigens from bacteria and food using gastric acid and enzyme secretions. The GI immune system normally can recognize and tolerate proteins, peptides, and cellular components and mount both general and specific immune responses to foreign and potentially harmful antigens. In the case of celiac disease, some combination of genetic susceptibility and an unknown trigger allows the immune system to create an abnormal immune response when it is exposed to gluten (Seibold, 2005).

Celiac disease, or **gluten-sensitive enteropathy**, is an inflammatory small intestinal disorder that results from an inappropriate T cell–mediated autoimmune response to the ingestion of gluten by people who are genetically predisposed. Predisposed persons express the antigen-presenting molecules HLA-DQ$_2$ and HLA-DQ$_8$ haplotypes that bind gluten peptides. When T cells present the gluten peptide molecules, they produce cytokines that start the inflammatory and autoimmune reaction and stimulate plasma cells to produce antibodies to gliadin, transglutaminase, and endomysium (Chand and Mihas, 2006). The autoimmune inflammatory response leads to villous atrophy, malabsorption, malnutrition, and possibly malignancy.

The prevalence of the disease has been underestimated in the past and now is considered to be about 1 in 133 persons in the United States. Prevalence is higher in relatives of persons with celiac disease (Fasano et al., 2003). The onset and first occurrence of symptoms may appear any time from infancy to adulthood, but the peak in diagnosis occurs between the fourth and sixth decade. Approximately 20% of cases are diagnosed after the age of 60 years. Delay in diagnosis is attributed to the tremendous variety of presentations and silent forms of the disease (Farrell and Kelly, 2002).

Gluten refers to specific peptide fractions of proteins found in wheat, rye, and barley. In wheat the offending peptides are glutenins and gliadins; in rye, secalinus; and in barley, hordeins. These peptide molecules are resistant to complete digestion by GI enzymes, and their interaction with the immune system of the GI tract can trigger an inflammatory response against the small intestinal mucosa and a more general systemic immune response.

In untreated cases the overzealous immune and inflammatory response eventually results in enough damage to the intestinal mucosa to compromise normal secretory, digestive, and absorptive functions, especially in the proximal small intestine. Cells of the villi become deficient in the disaccharidases and peptidases needed for digestion and also in the carriers needed to transport nutrients into the bloodstream. The extent of the damage to the intestinal villi and surrounding structures varies greatly, but atrophy and flattening of the villi reduce absorption and eventually micronutrient and macronutrient absorption (Figure 27-1).

Decreased release of hormones from the small intestine results in reduced secretions from the gallbladder and pancreas, further contributing to maldigestion. The disease primarily affects the proximal and middle sections of the small bowel, although the more distal segments may also be involved. Because the presentation and onset of symptoms vary so greatly, celiac disease may be misdiagnosed for years as irritable bowel, lactase deficiency, gallbladder disease, or other disorders not necessarily involving the GI tract. Box 27-4 lists the extraintestinal manifestations.

The disease may also be associated with other inflammatory states such as **dermatitis herpetiformis** (a variant of celiac disease that involves the skin), muscle and joint pain, and other autoimmune diseases such as thyroiditis and type 1 diabetes. Celiac disease is normally considered chronic and requires lifelong omission of gluten from the diet. Morbidity and mortality rates may be increased in persons who are undiagnosed until late or in persons who are unable to comply with the diet (Seraphin and Mobarin, 2002). Those who continue to eat gluten-containing foods have an increased risk of lymphomas and other malignancies that influences overall morbidity.

The diagnosis of celiac disease is made by a combination of clinical, laboratory, and histologic evaluations, but small bowel biopsy serves as the final diagnostic confirmation (Chand and Mihas, 2006). The disease may become apparent when an infant begins eating gluten-containing cereals; it may not appear until adulthood, when it may be triggered or unmasked by GI surgery, stress, pregnancy, viral infection; or it may be discovered as a result of evaluation for other suspected problems. The presentation in young children is likely to include the more "classic" GI symptoms of diarrhea and steatorrhea, malodorous stools, abdominal bloating, apathy, and poor weight gain. With later onset the first manifestation is more varied and may include other inflammatory and autoimmune disorders; generalized fatigue; failure to gain or maintain weight; or the consequences of nutrient malabsorption, including anemias, osteoporosis, or vitamin K–related coagulopathy. However, 50% of celiac patients have few or no obvious symptoms, and some may be overweight at presentation (Fasano and Catassi, 2001).

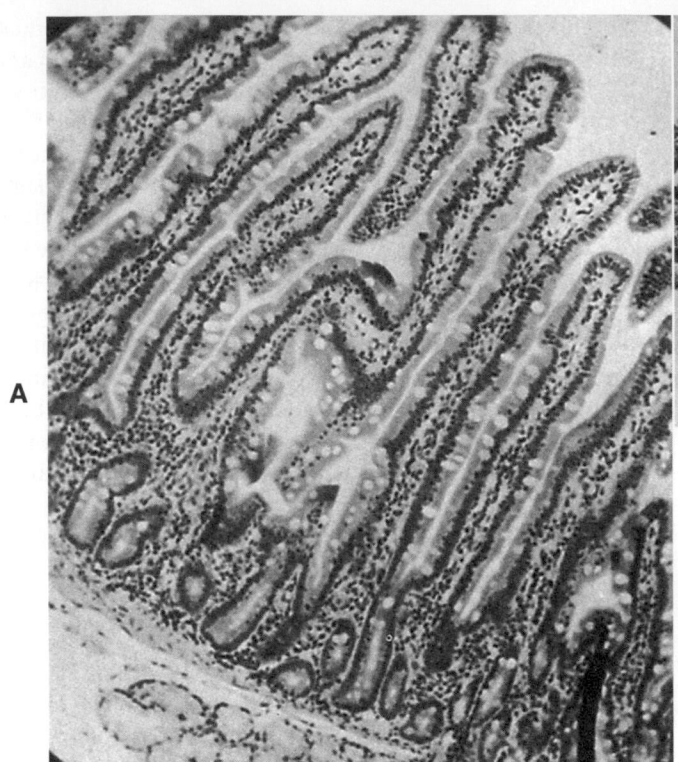

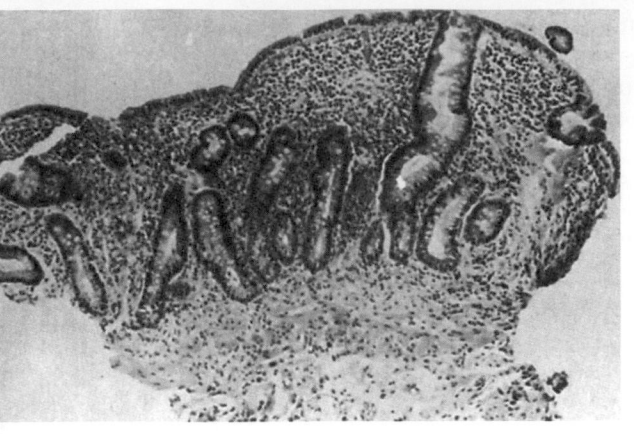

FIGURE 27-1 A, Low-power photomicrograph (×100) of a normal human duodenal mucosa. Note the long, thin villi. **B,** Low-power photomicrograph (×100) of a peroral small-bowel biopsy specimen from a patient with gluten enteropathy. Note the complete loss of villi and the heavy infiltrate of white blood cells in the lamina propria. *(From Floch MH:* Nutrition and diet therapy in gastrointestinal disease, *New York, 1981, Plenum Medical.)*

Persons suspected of having celiac disease should be evaluated for the overall pattern of symptoms and family history. Screening serologic tests include testing for the presence of immunoglobulin IgA and IgG antiendomysial antibodies (AEMAs) or the autoantigen that appears to trigger the immune response: IgA and IgG antitissue transglutaminase (ATTGA). IgA and IgG antigliadin antibodies (AGAs) have been used, but they are considered less sensitive than AEMAs or ATTGA (NIH Consensus Panel, 2006; Koning, 2005). Some persons thought to have celiac disease may be IgA deficient; thus IgG levels are tested. The serologic tests may also be used for monitoring the progress of persons with confirmed celiac disease.

The serologic tests are quite specific and sensitive for celiac disease, but not foolproof. The gold standard for final confirmation of the diagnosis is still the intestinal mucosal biopsy (Farrell and Kelly, 2002). Because intestinal biopsy is relatively expensive and must be performed by upper GI endoscopy, it is not usually used for initial screening. However, capsules are now available that when swallowed can send images of the entire intestinal mucosa and are bringing new technology to the diagnosis of celiac disease (Lee and Green, 2005). Because dietary change would alter the diagnostic results, initial diagnostic evaluation should be done before the person has eliminated gluten-containing foods from his or her diet.

Within 2 to 8 weeks of starting a gluten-free diet, most patients report that their clinical symptoms have abated, but for some it may take longer. Histologic, immunologic, and functional improvements may take months to years, depending on the duration of the disease, age of the subject, and degree of compliance. With strict dietary control, levels

of the specific antibodies usually become undetectable in 3 to 6 months in most persons, but in some the recovery may be slower or never completely occur (Farrell and Kelly, 2002). A small percentage of patients may be refractory to dietary therapy because of inadvertent gluten intake, pancreatic insufficiency, irritable bowel, bacterial overgrowth, fructose intolerance, other coexisting GI maladies, or unknown etiologies (Abdulkarim et al., 2002).

Medical Treatment

Institution of a gluten-free diet greatly diminishes the autoimmune process, and the intestinal mucosa usually reverts to normal or near normal. Some patients, however, may require months or even years of diet therapy for maximum recovery. The toxic peptide fractions of the respective cereals must be avoided for life.

Refractory celiac disease may not respond entirely to the removal of gluten, or it may respond only temporarily. However, many of these patients do show a response to steroids, azathioprine, cyclosporine, or other medications classically used to suppress inflammatory or immunologic reactions. For some, treatment of other underlying disease may further resolve the symptoms (see *Pathophysiology and Care Management Algorithm:* Celiac Disease [Gluten-Sensitive Enteropathy or Nontropical Sprue]).

A new approach to celiac disease is to digest the normally resistant gluten peptide, using an endopeptidase enzyme either in the diet or in the foods that contain gluten. Initial studies have shown that this enzyme works to some degree in that the digested product does not produce the same immunologic response, but it is not known to what degree the gluten peptides might escape digestion (Matysiak-Budnik et

BOX 27-4

Nutritional and Extraintestinal Manifestations of Celiac Disease and Associated Disorders

Nutritional

Anemia (iron or folate, B_{12}, rarely)

Osteomalacia, osteopenia, fractures (vitamin D deficiency, inadequate calcium absorption)

Coagulopathies (vitamin K deficiency)

Dental enamel hypoplasia

Delayed growth, delayed puberty, underweight

Lactase deficiency

Extraintestinal

Lassitude, malaise (sometimes despite lack of anemia)

Arthritis, arthralgia

Dermatitis herpetiformis

Infertility, increased risk of miscarriage, hepatic steatosis, hepatitis

Neurologic symptoms (ataxia, polyneuropathy, seizures); may be partly nutrition related

Psychiatric syndromes

Associated Disorders

Autoimmune diseases: type 1 diabetes, thyroiditis, hepatitis, collagen vascular disease

Malignancies

IgA deficiencies

Data from Hill ID et al: Celiac disease: working group report of the First World Congress of Pediatric Gastoenterology, Hepatology and Nutrition, *J Pediatr Gastroenterol Nutr* 35:785, 2002; Fasano A, Catassi C: Current approaches to diagnosis and treatment of celiac disease: an evolving spectrum, *Gastroenterology* 120:636, 2001.

IgA, Immunoglobulin.

al., 2005; Marti et al., 2004) (see *New Directions:* Bacterial Endopeptidase—A New Treatment for Celiac Disease?).

Medical Nutrition Therapy

The diet requires a major life change on the part of the patient if he or she is to adhere to it sufficiently to diminish the immune and inflammatory responses. Elimination of the peptides from the diet is the only treatment of celiac disease. Insofar as possible, the diet omits all dietary wheat (gliadin), rye (secalin), and barley (hordein), which are sources of the prolamin fractions (Thompson, 2001) (Box 27-5).

Initially the diet should be supplemented with vitamins, minerals, and extra protein to remedy deficiencies and replenish nutrient stores. Not all of the specialty gluten-free products are fortified like other grain products, so the diet may not be as complete without at least partial supplementation. Anemia should be treated with iron, folate, or vitamin B_{12}, depending on the nature of the anemia. Calcium and vitamin D administration may be necessary to correct osteoporosis or osteomalacia; and zinc, magnesium, and other mineral deficits

may need to be corrected. Vitamins A and E may be necessary to replenish stores depleted by steatorrhea. Vitamin K may be prescribed for purpura, bleeding, or prolonged prothrombin time. Electrolyte and fluid replacement is essential for those dehydrated from severe diarrhea.

Those who continue to have malabsorption should take vitamin and mineral supplements as appropriate to at least meet dietary reference intakes. MCT may help provide calories, especially in persons with steatorrhea. Lactose and fructose intolerance sometimes occur secondary to celiac disease, and polyol sugars are not well absorbed, even in a healthy gut. A low-lactose or low-fructose diet may be useful in controlling symptoms, at least initially. Once the GI tract returns to more normal function, lactase activity may also return, and the person can incorporate lactose and dairy products back into the diet.

In the traditional gluten-free diet, wheat, rye, barley, and oats are normally excluded. The need for exclusion of oats from the diet of persons with celiac disease and dermatitis herpetiformis has been challenged (Janatuinen et al., 2002). Clinical and GI manifestations of gluten sensitivity do not appear to recur in evaluations of oat intake lasting from 6 months to 5 years or longer. Oat products that are claimed to be gluten-free are beginning to appear throughout the world, but specific labeling policies and brand identities should be checked with local celiac organizations. However, until larger numbers of patients have been evaluated, some clinicians and patients may still be reluctant to recommend oat products. Many oat products may be contaminated with wheat or other grains, and contamination may not be easily detected. Long-term study in larger populations and strict guidelines regarding contamination with gluten-containing grains in oat products may help to resolve the issue in the future.

Products made from corn, potatoes, rice, soybean, tapioca, arrowroot, amaranth, quinoa, millet, and buckwheat can be substituted in food products. When using these flours, it is important that they also not be contaminated with gluten-containing flour during milling. Patients can expect differences in textures and flavors of common foods using the substitute flours, but new recipes can be quite acceptable once the adjustment is made.

In some countries specially processed wheat starch has been considered sufficiently low in gluten to be safe for consumption, but in other countries the protein fraction remaining after extraction may be expressed only as nitrogen or protein rather than the more specific gluten or gliadin. When reading the product label listing only nitrogen content, one would not know if the source of the remaining nitrogen or protein was gliadin or another protein (Thompson, 2001). Celiac organizations in North America do not yet recommend consumption of these wheat starch products or oat products. Box 27-6 provides suggestions for incorporating flour substitutions into recipes.

The diet for the person with celiac disease requires a major life change because of the drastic change from traditional grains in the diet. A tremendous number of foods made with wheat (in particular breads, cereals, pastas, and

PATHOPHYSIOLOGY AND CARE MANAGEMENT ALGORITHM

Celiac Disease (Gluten-Sensitive Enteropathy or Nontropical Sprue)

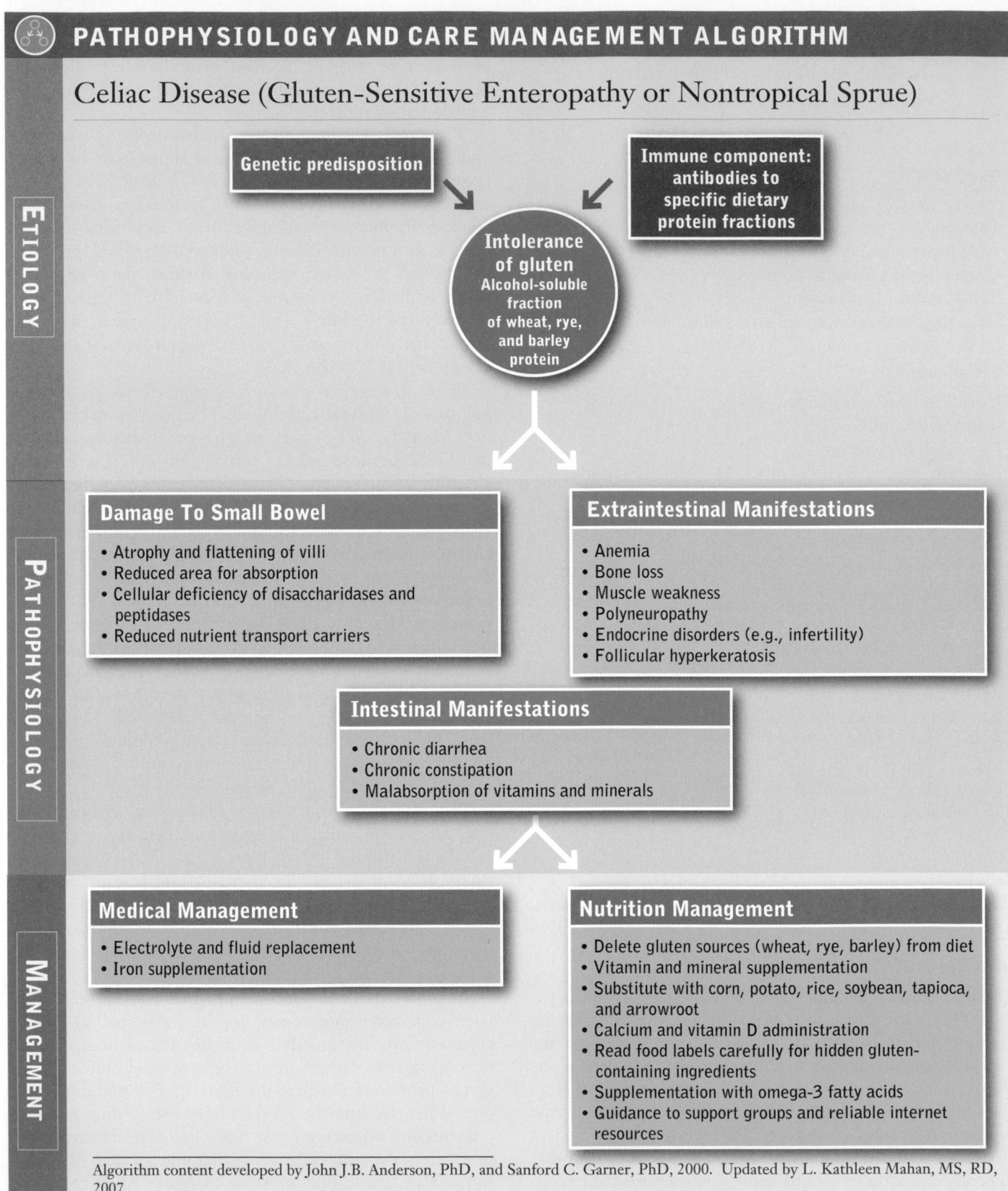

ETIOLOGY

Genetic predisposition

Immune component: antibodies to specific dietary protein fractions

Intolerance of gluten
Alcohol-soluble fraction of wheat, rye, and barley protein

PATHOPHYSIOLOGY

Damage To Small Bowel

- Atrophy and flattening of villi
- Reduced area for absorption
- Cellular deficiency of disaccharidases and peptidases
- Reduced nutrient transport carriers

Extraintestinal Manifestations

- Anemia
- Bone loss
- Muscle weakness
- Polyneuropathy
- Endocrine disorders (e.g., infertility)
- Follicular hyperkeratosis

Intestinal Manifestations

- Chronic diarrhea
- Chronic constipation
- Malabsorption of vitamins and minerals

MANAGEMENT

Medical Management

- Electrolyte and fluid replacement
- Iron supplementation

Nutrition Management

- Delete gluten sources (wheat, rye, barley) from diet
- Vitamin and mineral supplementation
- Substitute with corn, potato, rice, soybean, tapioca, and arrowroot
- Calcium and vitamin D administration
- Read food labels carefully for hidden gluten-containing ingredients
- Supplementation with omega-3 fatty acids
- Guidance to support groups and reliable internet resources

Algorithm content developed by John J.B. Anderson, PhD, and Sanford C. Garner, PhD, 2000. Updated by L. Kathleen Mahan, MS, RD, 2007.

baked goods), are consumed in the U.S. diet. The individual and family members must learn a great deal about food, food additives, recipes, food preparation, food terminology, and dietary requirements to be reasonably compliant. Eating in cafeterias, restaurants, vending outlets, street markets, at friends' homes, and at social events presents challenges, limitations, and frustrations.

A truly gluten-free diet requires careful scrutiny of the labels of all bakery products and packaged foods. Gluten-containing grains are not only used as a primary ingredient

BOX 27-5

The Basic Gluten-Free Diet

Milk Products

Milk, cream, most ice cream, buttermilk, plain yogurt, cheese, cream cheese, processed cheese, processed cheese foods, cottage cheese

Grain Products

Breads

Bread and baked products containing amaranth, arrowroot, buckwheat, corn bran, corn flour, cornmeal, cornstarch, flax, legume flours (bean, garbanzo or chickpea; garfava; lentil; pea), millet, Montina flour (Indian rice grass), potato flour, potato starch, quinoa, rice bran, rice flours (white, brown, sweet), sago, sorghum flour, soy flour, sweet potato flour, tapioca, and teff

Cereals

Hot: puffed amaranth, cornmeal, cream of buckwheat, cream of rice (brown, white), hominy grits, rice flakes, quinoa flakes, soy flakes, and soy grits

Cold: puffed amaranth, puffed buckwheat, puffed corn, puffed millet, puffed rice, rice flakes, and soy cereals

Pastas

Macaroni, spaghetti, and noodles made from beans, corn, pea, potato, quinoa, rice, soy and wild rice

Miscellaneous

Corn tacos, corn tortillas

Meats and Alternatives

Meat, Fish, Poultry
Fresh

Eggs

Others

Lentils, chickpeas (garbanzo beans) peas, beans, nuts, seeds, tofu

Fruits and Vegetables

Fruits

Fresh, frozen, and canned fruits and juices

Vegetables

Fresh, frozen, and canned vegetables and juices
Soups

Fats

Butter, margarine, lard, vegetable oil, cream, shortening, homemade salad dressing with allowed ingredients

Desserts

Ice cream, sherbet, whipped toppings, egg custards, gelatin desserts; cakes, cookies, pastries made with allowed ingredients, gluten-free ice cream cones, wafers, and waffles

Miscellaneous

Beverages

Tea, instant or ground coffee (regular or decaffeinated), cocoa, soft drinks, cider; distilled alcoholic beverages such as rum, gin, whiskey, vodka, wines, and pure liqueurs; some soy, rice and nut beverages

Sweets

Honey, jam, jelly, marmalade, corn syrup, maple syrup, molasses, sugar (brown and white), icing sugar (confectioner's)

Snack Foods

Plain popcorn, nuts, and soy nuts

Condiments

Plain pickles, relish, olives, ketchup, mustard, tomato paste, pure herbs and spices, pure black pepper, vinegars (apple or cider, distilled white, grape, or wine, spirit), gluten-free soy sauce

Other

Sauces and gravies made with ingredients allowed, pure cocoa, pure baking chocolate, carob chips and powder, chocolate chips, monosodium glutamate (MSG), cream of tartar, baking soda, yeast, brewer's yeast, aspartame, coconut, vanilla, and gluten-free communion wafers

Used with permission from Dennis M, Case S: Going gluten-free: a primer for clinicians, *Pract Gastroenterol* 28:90, 2004.

but may also be added during processing or preparation of foods. For example, hydrolyzed vegetable protein can be made from wheat, soy, corn, or mixtures of these grains (Box 27-7).

Typically clients should be started with "survival" guidelines that include foods they can rely on to be nutritious and gluten free, along with accessible resources for further guidance and support. Persons with celiac disease generally need several education or counseling sessions with registered dietitians knowledgeable in the disease management (Case, 2005; NIH Consensus Statement, 2006). After the

initial overview, patients will have the opportunity to ask specific questions; identify the need for specialty foods, food preparation techniques, and key nutrients; and learn more about expanding their dietary choices. Periodic evaluation of understanding, appropriateness, and completeness of the diet and nutrition status should be scheduled as part of the continuing medical nutrition therapy.

Freedom from symptoms after eating gluten does not necessarily mean that cells of the GI tract are undamaged. The precipitating condition usually continues to exist, and gluten

BOX 27-6

Thickener Tips and Substitutions for Wheat Flour

Bake gluten-free items in smaller sizes (e.g., cupcakes, muffins, and biscuits).

Bake quick breads in mini loaf pans for better texture.

Thicken sauces, gravies, and cream pies with rice flour. Use the same amount of rice flour as wheat flour. For a smoother mixture whisk rice flour and liquid together and heat over medium heat until bubbles first appear.

Substitute for 1 Tbsp of wheat flour:
1½ tsp amaranth starch
1½ tsp arrowroot starch
1½ tsp cornstarch
1½ tsp unflavored gelatin powder
1 Tbsp garbanzo or chickpea bean flour
1 Tbsp white or brown rice flour
1 Tbsp sweet rice flour
1 Tbsp tapioca flour
2 tsp quick-cooking tapioca

Generic gluten-free flour mixture:
4 cups white rice flour
1⅓ cup potato starch
1 cup tapioca flour
Sift ingredients together and store in plastic self-seal bags or containers. Refrigerate for longer storage periods. Makes 6⅓ cups.

Suitable thickeners:
Cream soups: amaranth starch, bean flour, rice flour (brown, sweet, white), tapioca flour
Fruit sauces: arrowroot starch, cornstarch, sweet rice flour
Fruit pies or cobbler: cornstarch, quick-cooking tapioca
Gravy: rice flour (brown, sweet, white) tapioca flour
Puddings: amaranth starch, cornstarch, gelatin, sweet rice flour
Savory sauces: amaranth starch, arrowroot starch, bean flour, corn starch, gelatin, sweet rice flour
Stews: bean flour, rice flour (brown, sweet, white), tapioca flour
Stir-fry dishes: arrowroot, cornstarch, tapioca flour

Adapted from Case S: *Gluten-free diet: a comprehensive resource guide*, expanded ed., Saskatchewan, Canada, 2006, Case Nutrition Consulting.

⇄ NEW DIRECTIONS

Bacterial Endopeptidase—A New Treatment for Celiac Disease?

Scientists identified a 33-amino acid peptide fraction from the 266-amino acid gliadin that triggers the destructive inflammatory response in celiac disease (Shan et al., 2002). The fragment appears to be the same one in other grains that contain gluten. It appears that this peptide fraction is resistant to digestion by normal human digestive enzymes, but it can be degraded by bacterial endopeptidases. In preliminary studies destruction of the peptide fragment by the addition of the endopeptidase enzyme prevented the typical immunologic response seen with celiac disease. The hope is that oral endopeptidase enzymes can be used as an oral supplement to digest and destroy the specific fragment of gliadin in the foods that contain gluten, thus allowing their consumption.

causes mucosal changes within hours; however, overt symptoms may take 8 weeks or longer to reappear, or they may remain latent. Adults who start and stop a gluten-free diet numerous times eventually may reach a state in which they do not respond to the diet. Complications of chronic ulcerative jejunoileitis and extraintestinal manifestations may develop, and the risk of malignant disease, especially lymphoma, is increased. Strict adherence to a gluten-free diet appears to reduce this risk.

Tropical Sprue

Pathophysiology

Tropical sprue is an acquired diarrheal syndrome with malabsorption that occurs in many tropical areas (Nath, 2005). Diarrhea appears to be an infectious type, although the sequence of pathogenic events is not clear. The syndrome may include bacterial overgrowth, changes in GI motility, and cellular changes in the GI tract. Identified intestinal organisms may differ from one region of the tropics to the next (Farthing, 1998). As in celiac disease, the intestinal villi may be abnormal, but the surface cell alterations are much less severe. The gastric mucosa may be atrophied and inflamed with diminished secretion of hydrochloric acid and intrinsic factor.

In addition to diarrhea and malabsorption, anorexia, abdominal distention, and nutritional deficiency as evidenced by night blindness, glossitis, stomatitis, cheilosis, pallor, and edema, can occur. Anemia may result from iron, folic acid, and vitamin B_{12} deficiencies.

Medical Treatment

Treatment of tropical sprue typically includes use of broad-spectrum antibiotics, folic acid, and restoration of fluid and electrolyte balance.

Medical Nutrition Therapy

Nutrition management includes restoration and maintenance of fluids and electrolytes, macronutrients and micronutrients, and introduction of a diet that is appropriate for the extent of malabsorption (see "Diarrhea" earlier in the

BOX 27-7

Allowed, Questionable, and Toxic Grains, Starches, and Flours

Allowed Grains, Starches, and Flours

Arrowroot
Amaranth
Buckwheat
Flax
Corn (maize)
Legume flours (garbanzo/chickpea, lentil, pea)
Millet
Montina (Indian rice grass)
Nut flours (almond, hazelnut, pecan)
Quinoa
Rice (e.g., brown, white, wild, Basmati)
Rice bran
Malt, malt extract, malt flavoring
Potato starch, potato flour, sweet potato flour
Sago
Seed flours (sesame)
Sorghum
Soy (soya)
Tapioca (also called cassava or manioc)
Teff (tef)

Questionable Ingredients

Dextrin—usually made from corn but may be made from
    wheat
Flavorings
Modified food starch/food starch
Seasonings
"Starch" in pharmaceuticals, vitamin/mineral and herbal
    supplements
Unidentified sources of hydrolyzed plant protein,
    hydrolyzed vegetable protein, textured
    vegetable protein

Toxic Grains, Starches, and Flours Not Allowed

Barley
Bran
Bulgar
Couscous
Durum flour
Einkorn*
Emmer*
Farina
Farro*
Gluten, gluten flour
Graham flour
Kamut*
Malt, malt extract, malt flavoring
Oats,† oat bran, or oat syrup†
Orzo
Rye
Semolina
Spelt
Triticale
Wheat germ, wheat starch, wheat bran, any word with
    wheat in its name

Used with permission from Dennis M, Case S: Going gluten-free: a primer for clinicians, *Pract Gastroenterol* 28:86, 2004.

*Types of wheat.

†Although many studies have indicated that a moderate amount of oats can safely be eaten by people with celiac disease, there is concern over the contamination of oats by wheat and/or barley. Currently oats are not recommended on the gluten-free diet in North America.

---

chapter). Along with other nutrients as needed, folate is given orally at 5 mg daily, along with intramuscular vitamin B_{12} (1000 mg/month) until symptoms subside. Nutritional deficiency may increase susceptibility to infectious agents, further aggravating the condition.

INTESTINAL BRUSH-BORDER ENZYME DEFICIENCIES

Intestinal enzyme deficiency states involve deficiencies of the brush-border disaccharidases that hydrolyze disaccharides at the mucosal cell membrane. Disaccharidase deficiencies may occur as (1) rare congenital defects such as the sucrase, isomaltase, or lactase deficiencies seen in the newborn; (2) generalized forms secondary to diseases that damage the intestinal epithelium (e.g., Crohn's disease or celiac disease); or, most commonly, (3) a genetically acquired form

(e.g., lactase deficiency) that usually appears after childhood but can appear as early as 2 years of age. For purposes of this chapter, only lactose maldigestion is described in detail (see Chapter 44 for a discussion of metabolic disorders).

Lactose Maldigestion or Lactose Intolerance

Pathophysiology

Lactose maldigestion or intolerance is the most common carbohydrate intolerance, and it can affect persons of all age-groups, although it occurs more often with advancing age. Lactose maldigestion and intolerance to lactose are caused by a deficiency of lactase, the enzyme that digests the sugar in milk. Lactose that is not hydrolyzed into galactose and glucose in the upper small intestine passes into the colon, where bacteria ferment the lactose to SCFAs and gases, carbon dioxide, and hydrogen gas. Consumption of small amounts should be of little consequence because the SCFAs

⊚ **FOCUS ON**

Lactose Tolerance—An Uncommon Anomaly?

When lactose intolerance was first described in 1963, it appeared to be an infrequent occurrence, arising only occasionally in the white population. Because the capacity to digest lactose was measured in people from a wide variety of ethnic and racial backgrounds, it soon became apparent that disappearance of the lactase enzyme shortly after weaning, or at least during early childhood, was actually the predominant (normal) condition in most of the world's population. With a few exceptions, the intestinal tracts of adult mammals produce little, if any, lactase after weaning. (The milk of pinnipeds— seals, walruses, and sea lions—does not contain lactose.)

The exception of lactose tolerance has attracted the interest of geographers and others concerned with the evolution of the world's population. A genetic mutation favoring lactose tolerance appears to have arisen around 10,000 years ago, when dairying was first introduced. Presumably, it would have occurred in places where milk consumption was encouraged because of some degree of dietary deprivation and in groups in which milk was not fermented before consumption. (Fermentation breaks down much of the lactose into monosaccharides.) The mutation would have selectively endured, because it would promote greater health, survival, and reproduction of those who carried the gene.

It is proposed that the mutation occurred in more than one location and then accompanied migrations of populations throughout the world. It continues primarily among whites from northern Europe and in ethnic groups in India, Africa, and Mongolia. The highest frequency (97%) of lactose tolerance occurs in Sweden and Denmark, suggesting an increased selective advantage in those able to tolerate lactose related to the limited exposure to ultraviolet light typical of northern latitudes. Lactose favors calcium absorption, which is limited in the absence of vitamin D produced by skin exposure to sunlight (see Chapter 3).

Dairying was unknown in North America until the arrival of Europeans. Thus Native Americans and all of the non-European immigrants are among the 90% of the world's population who tolerate milk poorly, if at all. This has practical implications with respect to group feeding programs such as school breakfasts and lunches. Fortunately, most lactose-intolerant people are able to digest milk in small-to-moderate amounts.

---

are readily absorbed and the gases can be absorbed or passed. Larger amounts, usually greater than 12 g, consumed in a single food (the amount typically found in 240 ml of milk), may result in more substrate entering the colon than can be disposed of by normal processes.

As is the case with any malabsorbed sugar, the lactose may act osmotically and increase fecal water, and rapid fermentation by intestinal bacteria may result in bloating, flatulence, and cramps. When large amounts of lactose are consumed, especially by persons who have little remaining lactase enzyme or with concurrent GI problems, loose stools or diarrhea can occur. Because serving sizes of milk drinks are increasing and more than one source of lactose might be consumed in the same meal, the amounts of lactose consumed may be more important than before.

Seventy percent of the adult worldwide population, especially blacks, Asians, and South Americans, are lactase deficient, which implies that decline of the lactase enzyme after early childhood is the more normal state and lactase sufficiency is abnormal. Although it has been suggested that lactase persistence is induced by the continuation of milk in the diet after weaning, no evidence has been found to support this theory. It is more likely that the maintenance of lactase throughout adulthood reflects the continuation of an ancient genetic mutation (see *Focus On:* Lactose Tolerance—An Uncommon Anomaly?).

Typically lactase activity declines exponentially at weaning to about 10% of the neonatal value. Even in adults who retain a high level of lactase levels (75% to 85% of white adults of Western European heritage), the quantity of lactase is about half that of other saccharidases such as sucrase, α-dextrinase, or glucoamylase. The decline of lactase is commonly known as **hypolactasia;** the adult form involves down-regulation after weaning (Jarvela, 2005) and may have a relationship to increased risk of colon cancer in some populations (Rasinpera et al., 2005).

Secondary lactose intolerance can also develop as a consequence of infection of the small intestine, inflammatory disorders, HIV, or malnutrition. In children it is typically secondary to viral or bacterial infections. Lactase activity may also be slow to return after prolonged parenteral nutrition. Lactose maldigestion with all its symptoms may also occur in adults with irritable bowel syndrome or in children with recurrent abdominal pain.

Lactase deficiency is typically diagnosed on the basis of (1) a history of GI symptoms occurring after milk ingestion, (2) a test for abnormal hydrogen levels in the breath, or (3) an abnormal lactose tolerance test. The lactose tolerance test was originally based on an oral dose of lactose equivalent to the amount in 1 quart of milk (50 g). Recently doses lower than 50 g of lactose have been used to approximate more closely the usual consumption of lactose from milk products.

If the patient has insufficient lactase enzyme, blood glucose produced from the lactose increases less than 25 mg/100 ml of serum above the fasting level, and GI symptoms may appear. Because hydrogen production in the colon increases significantly if lactose is not digested in the small intestine, hydrogen absorbed into the bloodstream and exhaled through the lungs can be used as another test of malabsorption. The breath hydrogen test shows increased levels 60 to 90 minutes after ingestion.

Medical Nutrition Therapy

Management of lactase insufficiency requires dietary change. The symptoms of lactose intolerance are alleviated by reduced consumption of lactose-containing foods. Persons who avoid dairy products should take calcium and probably vitamin D supplements and should read ingredient labels carefully. A completely lactose-free diet is not necessary in lactase-deficient persons. Most lactose maldigesters can consume some lactose (6 to 12 g/day) without major symptoms, especially when taken with meals or in the form of cheeses or cultured dairy products.

Many adults with intolerance to moderate amounts of milk can ultimately adapt to and tolerate 12 g or more of lactose in milk (equivalent to 240 ml of full-lactose milk) when introduced gradually, in increments, over several weeks (Byers and Savaiano, 2005). Incremental or continuous exposure to increasing quantities of fermentable sugar can lead to improved tolerance, not as a consequence of increased lactase enzyme production but perhaps by altered colonic flora. This has been shown with lactulose, a nonabsorbed carbohydrate that is biochemically similar to lactose (Bezkorovainy, 2001). Individual differences in tolerance may relate to the state of colonic adaptation. Regular consumption of milk by lactase-deficient persons may increase the threshold at which diarrhea occurs.

Lactase enzyme and milk products treated with lactase enzyme (e.g., Lactaid) are available for lactase maldigesters who have discomfort with milk ingestion. Commercial lactase preparations may differ in their effectiveness.

Often solid or semisolid milk products, such as aged cheeses, are well tolerated because gastric emptying of these foodstuffs is slower than for liquid milk beverages, and the lactose content is low. Tolerance of yogurt may be the result of a microbial galactosidase in the bacterial culture that facilitates lactose digestion in the intestine. The presence of galactosidase depends on the brand and processing method. Because this microbial enzyme is sensitive to freezing, frozen yogurt may not be as well tolerated, but the addition of probiotics may change this (Davidson et al., 2000).

INFLAMMATORY BOWEL DISEASES

The two major forms of **inflammatory bowel disease (IBD)** are Crohn's disease and ulcerative colitis. Both Crohn's disease and ulcerative colitis are relatively rare disorders, but because they may result in frequent use of health care resources, the prevalence may seem higher. The prevalence of Crohn's disease is approximately 130 cases per 100,000 persons and 100 per 100,000 for ulcerative colitis. The onset of IBD occurs most often in patients 15 to 30 years of age, but for some it occurs later in adulthood. Both sexes are equally affected.

Crohn's disease and **ulcerative colitis** share some clinical characteristics, including diarrhea, fever, weight loss, anemia, food intolerances, malnutrition, growth failure, and extraintestinal manifestations (arthritic, dermatologic, and hepatic). In both forms of IBD, the risk of malignancy increases with the duration of the disease. The reasons for the increased risk are not firmly established but are likely related to the increased inflammatory and proliferative state and nutritional factors. Although malnutrition can occur in both forms of IBD, it is more of a lifelong concern in patients with Crohn's disease. The features that distinguish the forms of the disease in terms of genetic characteristics, clinical presentation, and treatment are shown in Table 27-3 and discussed in the following paragraphs.

Crohn's Disease and Ulcerative Colitis

Crohn's disease may involve any part of the GI tract, but about 50% to 60% of cases involve both the distal ileum and the colon. Fifteen to 25% of cases involve only the small intestine or only the colon. In Crohn's disease segments of inflamed bowel may be separated by healthy segments, whereas in ulcerative colitis the disease process is continuous (Figure 27-2). Mucosal involvement in Crohn's disease is transmural in that it affects all layers of the mucosa; in ulcerative colitis the disease normally is limited to the mucosa. Crohn's disease is characterized by abscesses, fistulas, fibrosis, submucosal thickening, localized strictures, narrowed segments of bowel, and partial or complete obstruction of the intestinal lumen. Bleeding is more common in ulcerative colitis.

Pathophysiology

The cause of IBD is not completely understood, but it involves the interaction of the GI immunologic system and genetic and environmental factors. The genetic susceptibility is now recognized to be diverse, with a number of possible gene mutations that affect risk and characteristics of the disease. The diversity in the genetic alterations among individuals may help explain differences in the onset, aggressiveness, complications, location, and responsiveness to different therapies as seen in the clinical setting (Matthew and Lewis, 2004; Ahmad et al., 2004; MacDonald et al., 2005). The major environmental factors include resident and transient microorganisms in the GI tract and dietary components.

The genes affected (e.g., C677T mutation related to methylene-tetrahydrofolate reductase) normally play a role in the reactivity of the host GI immune system to luminal antigens such as those provided by intestinal flora and the diet. In animal models inflammatory disease does not occur without the intestinal flora. Normally, when an antigenic challenge or trauma occurs, the immune response rises to the occasion; it is then turned off and continues to be held in check after the challenge resolves. In IBD increased exposure, decreased defense mechanisms, or decreased tolerance to some component of the GI microflora may occur. Inappropriate inflammatory response and an inability to suppress the inflammatory response play primary roles in the disease. For example, one of the genes affected in

TABLE 27-3

Ulcerative Colitis vs. Crohn's Disease

Ulcerative Colitis	Crohn's Disease
Presentation	
Bloody diarrhea	Perianal disease
	Abdominal pain (65%)
	Mass in abdomen
Gross Pathology	
Rectum always involved	Rectum may not be involved
Moves continuously, proximally from rectum	Can occur anywhere along gastrointestinal tract
	Not continuous: "skip lesions"
Thin wall	Thick wall
Few strictures	Strictures common
Diffuse ulceration	Cobblestone appearance
Histopathology	
No granulomas	Granulomas
Low inflammation	More inflammation
Deeper ulcers (hence named ulcerative)	Shallow ulcers
Pseudopolyps	Fibrosis
Abscesses in crypts	
Extraintestinal Manifestations	
Sclerosing cholangitis	Erythema nodosum
Pyoderma gangrenosum	Migratory polyarthritis
	Gallstones
Complications	
Toxic megacolon	Fistulas
Cancer	Stricture
Strictures and fistulas are very rare	Malabsorption
	Perianal disease
	Cancer

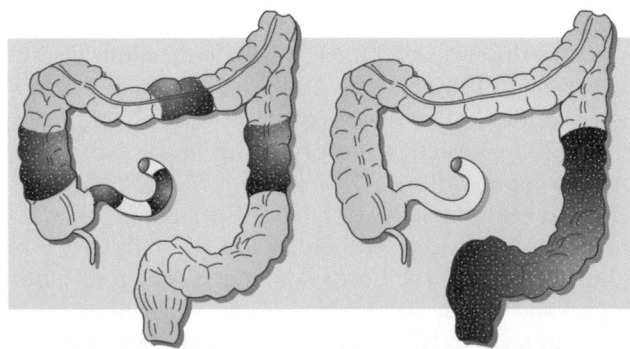

FIGURE 27-2 Crohn's disease *(left)* and ulcerative colitis *(right)*. Crohn's disease typically involves the small and large intestine in a segmental manner, with intervening "skip" areas; ulcerative colitis is generally a contiguous disease process that starts in the rectum and progresses in a retrograde fashion to involve varying lengths of the colon. *(Modified from Cotran KS, Kumar V, Robbins SI: Robbins and Cotran pathologic basis of disease, ed 7, Philadelphia, 2005, Saunders.)*

Crohn's disease is the $NOD_2/CARD_{15}$ gene, which codes for a small peptide that interacts with a host of GI bacteria. Failure to produce that peptide may result in abnormal immune responses (Mueller and Macpherson, 2006).

The inflammatory response (e.g., increased cytokines and acute phase proteins, increased GI permeability, increased proteases, and increased oxygen radicals and leukotrienes) is thought to be responsible for the resulting GI tissue damage (Sanders, 2005; Laroux and Grisham, 2001). In IBD either the regulatory mechanisms are defective or the factors perpetuating the immune and acute-phase responses are enhanced, leading to tissue fibrosis and destruction. The clinical course of the disease may be mild and episodic or severe and unremitting (see *Pathophysiology and Care Management Algorithm: Inflammatory Bowel Disease*).

Diet is one of the environmental factors that triggers relapses of IBD. Foods, microbes, individual nutrients, and incidental contaminants provide a huge number of potential antigens, especially considering the complexity and diversity of the modern diet. Malnutrition can affect the function and

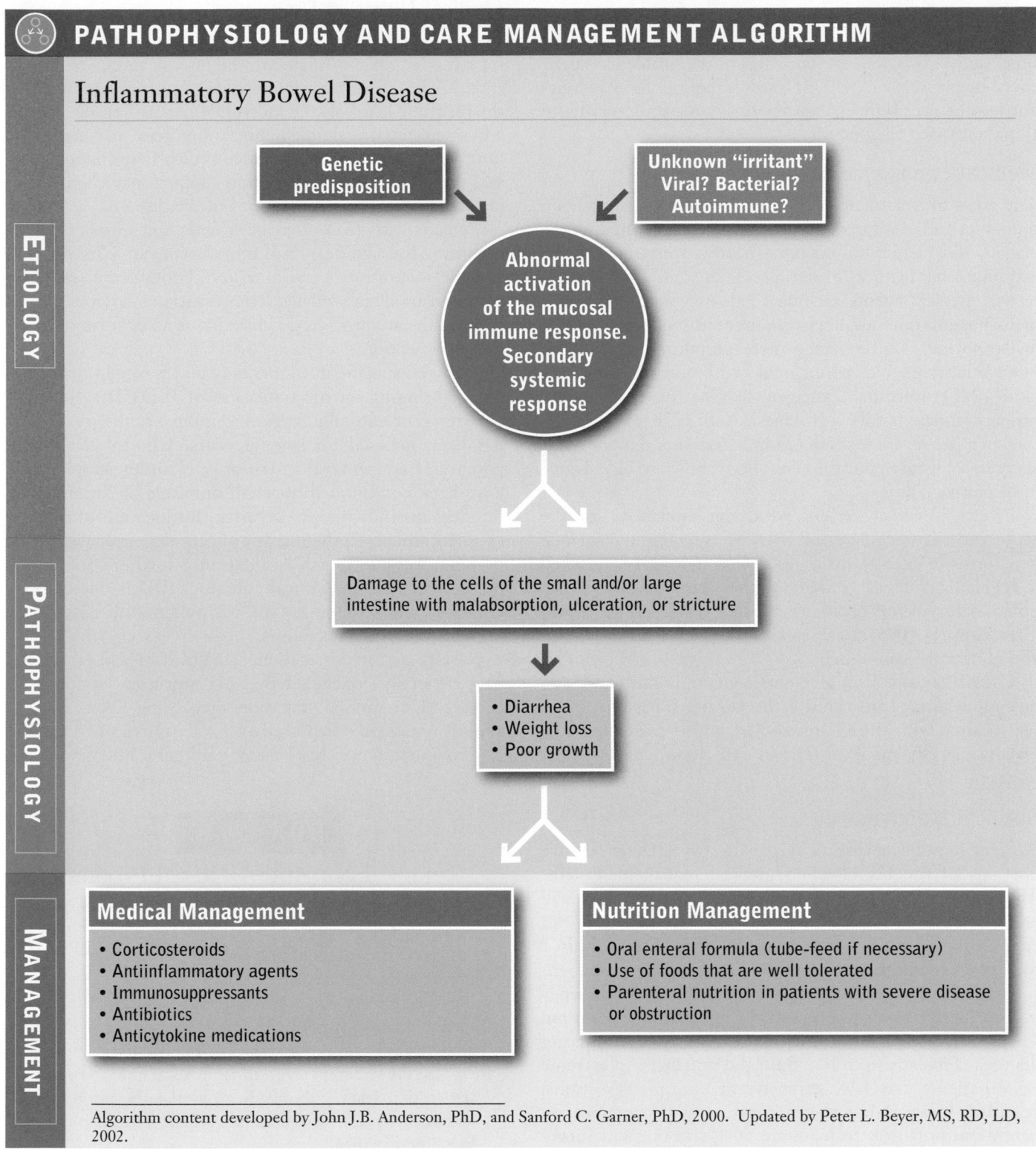

PATHOPHYSIOLOGY AND CARE MANAGEMENT ALGORITHM

Inflammatory Bowel Disease

ETIOLOGY

Genetic predisposition

Unknown "irritant" Viral? Bacterial? Autoimmune?

Abnormal activation of the mucosal immune response. Secondary systemic response

PATHOPHYSIOLOGY

Damage to the cells of the small and/or large intestine with malabsorption, ulceration, or stricture

- Diarrhea
- Weight loss
- Poor growth

MANAGEMENT

Medical Management

- Corticosteroids
- Antiinflammatory agents
- Immunosuppressants
- Antibiotics
- Anticytokine medications

Nutrition Management

- Oral enteral formula (tube-feed if necessary)
- Use of foods that are well tolerated
- Parenteral nutrition in patients with severe disease or obstruction

Algorithm content developed by John J.B. Anderson, PhD, and Sanford C. Garner, PhD, 2000. Updated by Peter L. Beyer, MS, RD, LD, 2002.

effectiveness of the mucosal, cellular, and immune barriers; diet can also affect the type and relative composition of the resident microflora. Several nutrients (e.g., dietary lipids) can affect the intensity of the inflammatory response.

Food allergies and other immunologic reactions to specific foods have been considered in the pathogenesis of IBD and its symptoms; however, the incidence of documented food allergies, compared with food intolerances, is relatively small. The permeability of the intestinal wall to molecules of food and cell fragments is likely increased in inflammatory states, allowing the potential for increased interaction of antigens with host immune systems (Seibold, 2005).

Food intolerances occur more often in persons with IBD than in the population at large, but the patterns are not consistent among individuals or even between exposures from one time to the next. Reasons for specific and nonspecific food intolerances are abundant and are related to the severity, location, and complications associated with the disease process. Partial GI obstructions, malabsorption, diarrhea, altered GI transit, increased secretions, food aversions, and associations are but a few of the problems experienced by persons with IBD. However, neither food allergies nor intolerances fully explain the onset or manifestations in all patients (see Chapter 29).

Medical Management

The goals of treatment in IBD are to induce and maintain remission and to improve nutrition status. Treatment of the primary GI manifestations appears to correct most of the extraintestinal features of the disease as well. The most effective medical agents include corticosteroids, antiinflammatory agents (aminosalicylates), immunosuppressive agents (cyclosporine, azathioprine, mercaptopurine), antibiotics (metronidazole), and monoclonal antitumor necrosis factor (anti-TNF) (infliximab), an agent that inactivates one of the primary inflammatory cytokines. Anti-TNF is normally used in more severe cases of Crohn's disease and in the management of fistulas, but it has not been shown to be effective in ulcerative colitis.

Investigations of various treatment modalities for the acute and chronic stages of IBD are ongoing and include new forms of existing drugs, as well as new agents targeted to regulate cytokines, eicosanoids, or other mediators of the inflammatory/acute-phase response (Travis et al., 2006; Caprilli et al., 2005). Each carries the potential for medical and nutritional consequences.

Use of foods and supplements containing prebiotics and probiotic cultures are plausible because each has the potential to alter both the GI microflora and the immunologic response at the gut level (Dotan and Rachmilewitz, 2005; Madsen, 2001).

Surgical Management

Surgery may be necessary to repair strictures or remove portions of the bowel when medical management fails. About 50% to 70% of persons with Crohn's disease will undergo surgery related to the disease. Surgery does not cure Crohn's disease, and recurrence often occurs within 1 to 3 years of surgery. The chance of needing subsequent surgery in the patient's life is about 30% to 70%, depending on the type of surgery and the age at first operation. Major resections of the intestine may result in varying degrees of malabsorption of fluid and nutrients. In extreme cases patients may have extensive or multiple resections, resulting in short-bowel syndrome, and dependence on parenteral nutrition to maintain adequate nutrient intake and hydration.

With ulcerative colitis, approximately 20% of patients have a colectomy and removal of the colon, and this resolves the disease. Inflammation does not occur in the remaining GI tract. Whether a colectomy is necessary depends on the severity of the disease and indicators of increased cancer risk. After a colectomy for ulcerative colitis, surgeons may create an ileostomy with an external collection pouch and an internal abdominal reservoir fashioned with a segment of ileum or an ileoanal pouch to serve as a reservoir for stool.

Medical Nutrition Therapy

Persons with IBD are at increased risk of nutrition problems for a host of reasons related to the disease and its treatment (Box 27-8); thus the primary goal is to restore and maintain the nutrition status of the individual patient. Foods, dietary and micronutrient supplements, and enteral and parenteral nutrition may all be used to accomplish that mission. Diet and the other means of nutrition support may change during remissions and exacerbations of the disease.

Persons with IBD often have fears and misconceptions regarding the significance of minor or major GI symptoms and the role of foods and nutrition. Patients are also often confused by dietary advice from associates, various media, and health care providers. Education is a key form of nutrition intervention.

Diet and specific nutrients may play a role in maintaining or bringing on the remission of IBD. The ability of parenteral or enteral nutrition to induce remission of IBD has been debated for several years. Clinical trials with parenteral and enteral nutrition and other supplements have been confounded by small numbers of patients, differences in study design, severity and location of the disease, differences in the nutrition formulas, and whether an oral diet was continued. Evaluation is further confounded by the fact that the natural course of IBD is one of exacerbations and remissions, and the genetic diversity of the patients may alter responses.

Results of reviews and metaanalyses of several studies have generally concluded that (1) nutrition support with parenteral or enteral nutrition may bring about at least clinical remission when used as a sole source of treatment; (2) "complete bowel rest" using parenteral nutrition is not

---

BOX 27-8

Potential Nutrition-Related Problems With Inflammatory Bowel Disease

Anemias related to blood loss and poor food intake

Gastrointestinal (GI) narrowing and strictures leading to bloating, nausea, bacterial overgrowth, and diarrhea

Inflammation and surgical resections resulting in diarrhea and malabsorption of bile salts and nutrients

Increased GI secretions with inflammation and decreased transit time leading to diarrhea and malabsorption

Malabsorption related to abdominal pain, nausea, vomiting, bloating, diarrhea

Food aversions or associations, anxiety, and fear of eating related to abdominal pain, bloating, nausea, or diarrhea

Drug-nutrient interactions

True and perceived food allergies

Dietary restrictions, both iatrogenic and self-imposed

Growth failure, weight loss, micronutrient deficiencies, and protein-calorie malnutrition

Elevated serum homocysteine levels, representing depletion of B-complex vitamins, especially folate (Nakano et al., 2003)

necessarily required to achieve remission; (3) enteral nutrition, because it has the potential to feed the intestinal epithelium and alter GI flora, may be the preferred means of nutritional support; (4) enteral nutrition may temper some elements of the inflammatory process, serve as a valuable source of nutrients needed for restoration of GI defects, and

be steroid sparing; (5) children benefit from the use of enteral nutrition to maintain growth and reduce the dependence on steroids that may affect growth and bone disease (Lochs 2006; Sanderson and Croft, 2005; Griffiths, 2005). Figure 27-3 shows an algorithm for reversing growth failure. Patients and caretakers must be very committed when

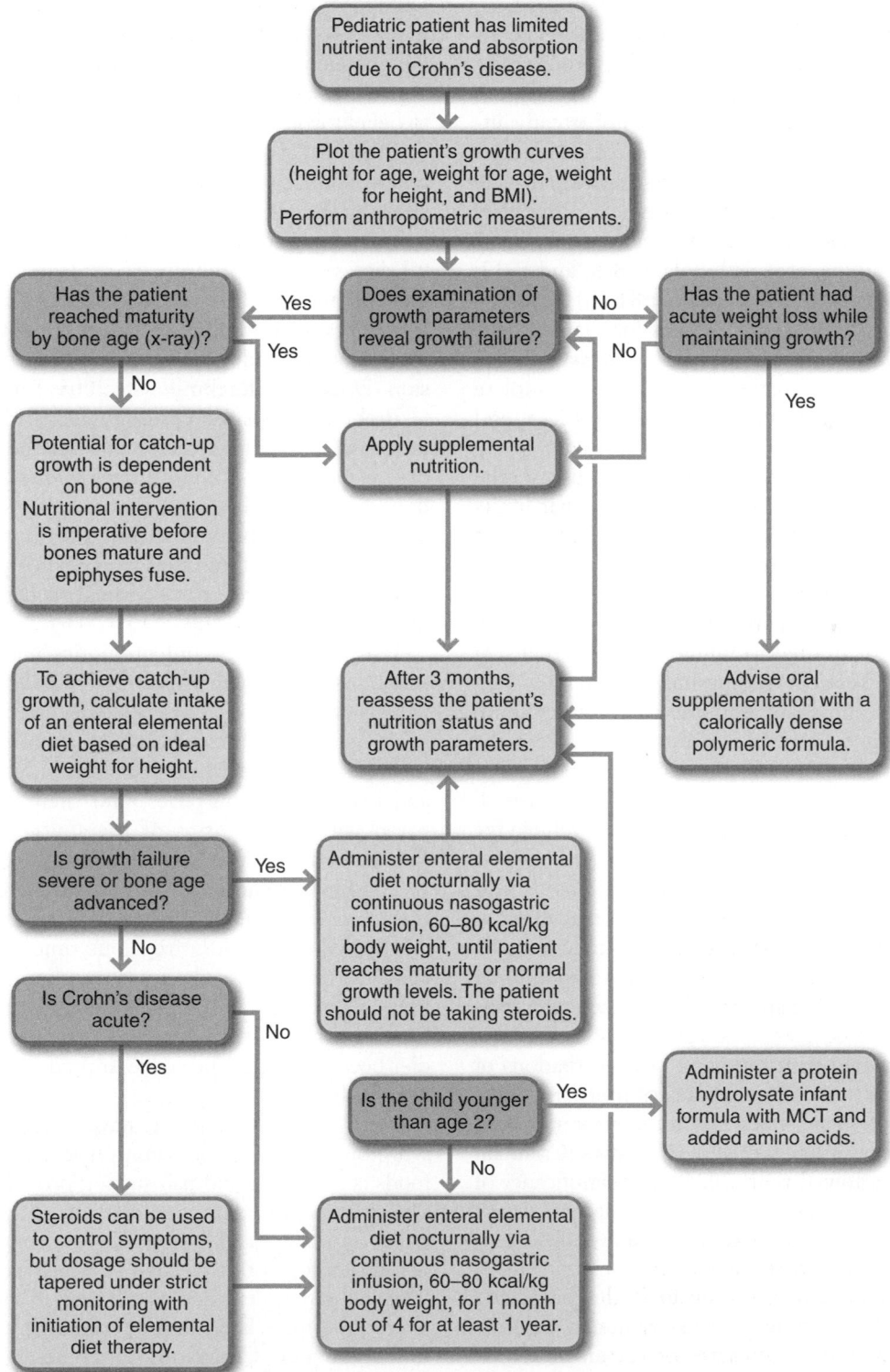

FIGURE 27-3 Algorithm for reversing growth failure in pediatric patients with Crohn's disease. *MCT*, Medium-chain triglyceride. (*Modified from RD 11:5, 1991, Norwich-Eaton Pharmaceuticals, New York, N.Y.*)

using enteral nutrition formulas or tube feeding because it takes 4 to 8 weeks before one sees the clinical effects.

Timely nutritional support is a vital component of therapy to restore and maintain nutritional health. Malnutrition itself compromises digestive and absorptive function and may increase the permeability of the GI tract to potential inflammatory agents. Parenteral solutions currently available are not as complete or well suited as enteral nutrition, but parenteral nutrition may be required to restore nutrition in patients with obstructions, fistulas, severe disease, and major GI resections.

Energy needs of patients with IBD are not greatly increased (unless weight gain is desired), but protein requirements may be increased, depending on the severity and stage of the disease and the restoration requirements. Requirements rarely are more than 50% greater than normal needs.

Supplemental vitamins, especially folate, B-6, and B-12, may be needed (Zezos et al., 2005). Minerals and trace elements may be needed to replace stores or for maintenance because of maldigestion, malabsorption or drug-nutrient interactions or because the patient cannot eat a complete diet. Diarrhea can aggravate losses of zinc, potassium, and selenium.

During acute and severe exacerbations of the disease, the diet is tailored to the individual patient. A diet that limits poorly absorbed or hyperosmolar sugars and caffeine might be used initially to reduce diarrhea. During either acute or chronic stages, inflammation or scarring may result in a partially obstructed bowel; in that case dietary fiber may have to be reduced or limited to minute particles that will pass through. Small, frequent feedings may be tolerated better than large meals; and small amounts of isotonic, liquid, oral supplements may be valuable in restoring intake without provoking symptoms. In cases in which fat malabsorption is likely, supplementation with foods made with MCT may be useful in adding calories and serving as a vehicle for fat-soluble nutrients.

Whether dietary factors trigger exacerbations is not clear, but they certainly can aggravate symptoms. Because absorption may not be as complete as normal, excess intake of lactose, fructose, or sorbitol may contribute to abdominal cramping, gas, and diarrhea; and high fat intake may result in steatorrhea.

Risk factors associated with the onset of exacerbations of IBD include increased sucrose intake, lack of fruits and vegetables, a low intake of dietary fiber, use of red meat and alcohol, and altered omega-6/omega-3 fatty acid ratios (Cashman and Shanahan, 2003; Jowett et al., 2004). The significance of these factors is not clear, but they may simply reflect an overall poor-quality diet that results in increase of the overall susceptibility of the GI tract to the disease process.

In some patients there may be specific food allergies related to increased permeability of the mucosa or altered immune sensitivity during the disease, or there may be an incidental relationship that serves as a trigger (Seibold, 2005). Enhancement of oral diets and nutritional formulas with omega-3 fatty acids, specific amino acids (e.g., glutamine), and antioxidants and the use of fermentable fibers (prebiotics) or probiotics are

therapeutic strategies being evaluated for management of IBD (Penner et al., 2005; Madsen, 2001).

In daily life people with IBD may have intermittent "flares" of the disease characterized by partial obstructions, nausea, abdominal pain, bloating, or diarrhea. They can be taught to manage at least some of the symptoms of their disease by selecting appropriate foods and beverages. For example, patients might be taught to restrict foods during bouts of diarrhea (see Table 27-1) or to limit fiber (especially large particles) if partial obstruction is suspected. They can also be shown how to increase omega-3 fats with food choices and supplements so as to benefit from their anti-inflammatory effect.

Probiotic foods and supplements hold promise by modifying the microbial flora, especially if they can be shown to alter the flora that is incriminated in IBD or to suppress the inflammatory response. In animal models of inflammatory GI disease and in preliminary studies of humans with IBD, ingestion of specific strains or mixtures of probiotic organisms alters the GI flora, decreases elements of the inflammatory response, and in some cases prolongs periods of remission (Dotan and Rachmilewitz 2005; Linskens et al., 2001).

Prebiotic foods such as oligosaccharides, fermentable fibers, and resistant starches may alter the mixture of microorganisms in the colonic flora, favoring lactobacillus and bifidobacteria and at least theoretically suppressing pathogenic or opportunistic microflora and increased production of SCFAs. The altered flora and SCFAs produced may also serve to attenuate the inflammatory process, especially in ulcerative colitis.

Use of probiotics and prebiotics may serve to prevent small intestine bacterial overgrowth in predisposed individuals and to treat diarrhea. Additional study continues to identify the dose and most effective prebiotic and probiotic foods, the form in which they can be used for therapeutic and maintenance purposes, and their relative value compared with other forms of therapy (Penner et al., 2005; Fukuda et al., 2002).

Food intolerances are common in patients with IBD, but the foods are variable among patients and may not be incriminated consistently from one time to the next. Patients are sometimes advised simply to eliminate the foods that they suspect are responsible for the intolerance. Often, however, the patient becomes increasingly frustrated as the diet becomes more and more limited and symptoms still do not resolve.

Food allergies certainly have the potential to worsen symptoms of IBD. Confirming true allergic GI reactions to foods is a difficult and painstaking process (see Chapter 29). One method to attempt to confirm allergies is to consume either an amino acid–based diet or a very limited diet composed of a few foods and add suspected foods one at a time. The allergen is identified on the basis of subjective and objective symptoms related to the repeated addition and elimination of the food. Circulating antibodies to food proteins have been considered a sign of allergy but may in fact be a sign of increased permeability rather than local GI allergy.

The same foods that are usually responsible for GI symptoms (gas, bloating, and diarrhea) in a normal healthy population are likely to be the triggers for the same symptoms in patients with mild stages of IBD or those in remission. Patients receive nutritional information from a variety of sources, including support groups, Internet news groups, the audio and printed media, well-meaning friends, and food supplement salespersons. The information is sometimes inaccurate or exaggerated, or it may pertain only to one individual's situation. The health care provider can help patients sort out the role of foods in normal everyday GI disturbances and in IBD and teach them how to evaluate valid nutrition information from unproved or exaggerated claims. Patients' participation in the management of their disease may help to reduce not only the symptoms of the disease but the associated anxiety level as well.

OTHER DISORDERS OF THE LARGE INTESTINE

Irritable Bowel Syndrome

Prevalence and Characteristics

Irritable bowel syndrome (IBS) is one of the most common reasons for primary care visits and consultations with gastroenterologists. Typically symptoms first occur between adolescence and the fourth decade of life, but many persons do not bring the problem to the attention of a physician. In the United States, IBS occurs in about 15% of women and 10% of men. Persons with IBD often have increased absenteeism from school and work, decreased productivity, increased health care costs, and decreased quality of life as a result of their symptoms.

Irritable bowel syndrome is characterized by chronically recurring symptoms, including abdominal discomfort and altered intestinal motility. Also commonly included are bloating, feelings of incomplete evacuation, presence of mucus in the stool, straining or increased urgency (depending on the type of presentation), and increased GI distress associated with psychosocial distress.

Diagnosis is based on international consensus criteria (ROME I or II criteria) and diagnostic algorithms that help separate other medical or surgical disorders that manifest with similar symptoms (Malagelada, 2006; Silk, 2003). According to the criteria, symptoms of abdominal discomfort must be present for at least 12 weeks of the past year and include at least two of three features: discomfort relieved by defecation, onset associated with a change in frequency of stool, and onset associated with a change in form of the stool. Diagnosis further categorizes the syndrome into subtypes, such as predominant patterns of diarrhea, constipation, or alternating constipation and diarrhea.

Pathophysiology

The normal enteric nervous system is sensitive to the presence, chemical composition, and volume of foods and also responds to a variety of inputs from the central nervous system (see Chapter 1). Increased awareness and sensitivity of the GI tract to internal and external stimuli and altered motility appear to be primary features of IBS (Malagelada, 2006; Silk, 2003). Persons with IBS have heightened enteric sensitivity and motility in response to usual GI and environmental stimuli. They react more significantly than normal persons to intestinal distention, dietary indiscretions, and psychosocial factors. People without IBS may experience GI disturbances in response to all the situations mentioned, but they will be milder. Life stressors such as employment changes, travel, relocation, or uncomfortable social situations may trigger the onset or worsen symptoms and may override many therapeutic efforts. A history of psychosocial trauma such as physical or sexual abuse has been reported in some cases.

The mediators of GI responses may be abnormal secretion of peptide hormones or signaling agents (e.g., neurotransmitters secreted in response to the hormones); but altered handling of intestinal gas, microbial flora, small intestinal bacterial overgrowth and other contributors affect some forms of IBS. A syndrome that mimics IBS is post-infectious IBS; it typically appears abruptly after gastroenteritis and is essentially managed with the same approach as other forms (Parry and Forgacs, 2005).

In addition to stress and dietary patterns, factors that may worsen symptoms include (1) excess use of laxatives and other over-the-counter medications; (2) antibiotics; (3) caffeine; (4) previous GI illness; and (5) lack of regularity in sleep, rest, and fluid intake. In patients with a strong family history of allergy, hypersensitivity to certain foods may aggravate IBS, and a trial of food elimination and challenge may be justified (see Chapter 29).

Medical Management

Management of IBS includes approaches to deal with the symptoms and the factors that may trigger them. Education, medications, counseling, and diet all play a role in the care. Depending on the predominant pattern and severity of the symptoms, medications may include those that affect GI motility, visceral hypersensitivity, or psychological symptoms. Relaxation and stress reduction techniques may also be useful. Newer agents that continue to be used and evaluated include those that affect how the GI tract responds to serotonin. Serotonin, or 5-hydroxytryptamine (5-HT) is a major mediator in the sensory functions of the enteric nervous system.

Two major 5-hydroxytryptamine receptors, $5-HT_3$ antagonists, and $5-HT_4$ agonists have been targeted for use in treating patients with different forms of IBS. $5-HT_3$ antagonists have shown some success in females with diarrhea-predominant IBS, whereas $5-HT_4$ agonists serve as prokinetic agents that stimulate peristalsis of the small and large intestine and are used in the management of constipation-predominant IBS. A number of other agents are being evaluated (Bueno, 2005).

Small intestinal bacterial overgrowth (SIBO) has been described in a significant number of patients with IBS (Lin,

2004). Diagnosis is more commonly made by the normal criteria for IBS plus evidence of increased breath hydrogen after a dose of glucose, lactulose, or other sugar. If the breath hydrogen peaks early and at sufficient levels, it indicates fermentation of the carbohydrate soon after leaving the stomach, and it reflects the probability of increased concentrations of microbes in the small bowel. Eradication of the microbes by antibiotics may eradicate the microbial population, normalize the breath hydrogen test, and at least reduce the symptoms of IBS. The prevalence of SIBO, its diagnosis, and clinical significance are still being evaluated (Quigley and Quera, 2006; Lapascu et al., 2005).

Medical Nutrition Therapy

The goals of nutrition therapy for IBS are to ensure adequate nutrient intake, tailor the diet for the specific GI pattern of IBS, and explain the potential roles of foods in the management of symptoms. The recommendations made for all persons for a good-quality diet are probably even more important for those with IBS. Large meals, excess quantities of dietary fat, caffeine, sugars (e.g., lactose, fructose, and sorbitol) and alcohol are likely to be more poorly tolerated in IBS (Rumessen and Gudmand-Hoyer, 1998). This is especially true in persons with diarrhea-predominant IBS and those with alternating constipation and diarrhea.

Dietary fiber intake in adolescents and adults is in the United States is typically about half that recommended; increasing dietary fiber to recommended levels is likely to help normalize GI function in those with all types of IBS. However, large doses of wheat bran are no longer recommended and may exacerbate symptoms in some persons with IBS. If the patient is not able to consume fiber from food sources or does not respond adequately, fiber in the form of bulk laxatives (e.g., psyllium) may be helpful. Consumption of adequate fluid is recommended, especially when powdered fiber supplements are used.

Food allergies or food hypersensitivities may be common (Kalliomaki, 2005; Seibold, 2005). Food intolerances and allergies should be evaluated as objectively as possible because patients may unnecessarily limit large groups of foods, resulting in frustration and an incomplete diet. Food elimination based on IgG antibodies may be useful (Atkinson et al., 2004) (see Chapter 29).

Foods with fiber, resistant starches, and oligosaccharides may serve as prebiotic foods, which favor the maintenance of "healthy" microflora and resistance to pathogenic infections (Nobaek et al., 2000; Broussard and Surawicz, 2004). Results of initial studies on the use of prebiotic and probiotic supplements have been mixed (Barbera et al., 2005); additional studies with different products, doses, and subtypes of IBS are needed.

The nutrition practitioner can work with the person with IBS to identify his or her concerns and perceptions, review the characteristics of the disease and the potential role of various foods, and teach the client how to reduce the food-related symptoms associated with the syndrome. Sometimes clients become trapped in a vicious cycle in which anxiety about food, GI distress, and social embarrassment leave them with an unnecessarily restrictive diet, declining nutrition status, increasing anxiety, and worsening symptoms. Calming reassurance and gradual return to a good diet with limitations of only items that may exacerbate symptoms often greatly improve the patient's quality of life.

Diverticular Disease

Pathophysiology

Diverticulosis is a situation of saclike herniations (diverticula) of the colonic wall, thought to result from long-term constipation and increased colonic pressures. The incidence of diverticulosis increases with age. Sigmoid involvement occurs in almost all cases; right-sided colonic involvement occurs in Asians, but it is rare in whites. Most persons are asymptomatic, but 15% to 20 % of persons with diverticulosis may experience colicky pain, and approximately 5% may experience inflammation and diverticulitis.

The cause is not known for certain, but studies in animals and humans attribute the disorder to a mixture of colonic structure, motility, genetics, and a lifelong diet low in fiber, resulting in increased intracolonic pressures (Salzman and Lillie, 2005; Parra-Blanco, 2006). The pressures result from attempts to propel small, dry, hard fecal material through the lumen of the bowel. Theoretically circular muscles completely close around the fecal material when the stools are small and longitudinal muscles contract, attempting to push the contents distally. Increased pressures result in the opportunity for herniations of the mucosal wall to develop through weaker segments of the colon (Figures 27-4 and 27-5). This theory is supported by epidemiologic studies of populations consuming high- and low-fiber diets, prospective cohort studies, and experimental studies in animals fed low-fiber diets throughout their lifetimes (Scheppach et al., 2001). An abnormal pattern of excitatory innervation of the colon

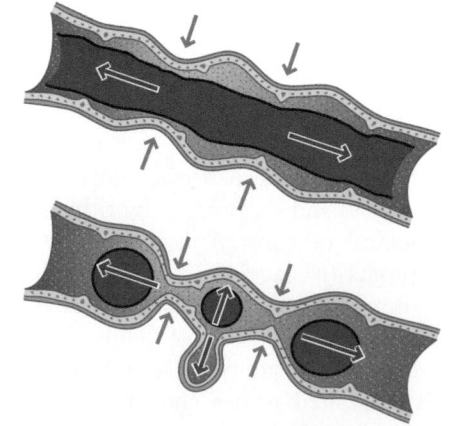

FIGURE 27-4 Mechanism by which low-fiber, low-bulk diets might generate diverticula. Where the colon contents are bulky *(top)*, muscular contractions exert pressure longitudinally. If the fecal contents are small in diameter *(bottom)*, contractions can produce occlusion and exert pressure against the colon wall, which may produce a diverticular hernia.

has been associated with intraluminal pressures and the presence of diverticulosis, but it is not known whether the pattern is a consequence of the disorder or related to the cause (Tomita et al., 1999).

In general, diverticular disease is (1) relatively rare in countries where a high-fiber diet is part of the lifelong pattern, and (2) increasing where there is "westernization" of the diet and increased intake of refined foods (Salzman and Lillie, 2005; Scheppach et al., 2001). Lack of exercise may also contribute to the development of diverticular disease, presumably because of the more sluggish movement of GI contents (Peters et al., 2001).

Medical and Surgical Treatment

Complications of diverticular disease range from painless, mild bleeding and altered bowel habits to diverticulitis. **Diverticulitis** may include its own clinical spectrum of inflammation, abscess formation, acute perforation, acute bleeding, obstruction, and sepsis. Treatment typically includes antibiotics, a modified diet, or bowel rest (Salzman and Lillie, 2005; Steel, 2004). Colon cleansers that cause hard stools, constipation, and straining are not recommended. About 10% to 25% of patients with diverticulosis develop diverticulitis, and about one forth to one third of those admitted to hospitals for diverticular disease require surgery.

Medical Nutrition Therapy

At one time it was thought that "roughage" (dietary fiber) aggravated diverticular disease; thus the classic diet therapy was one that was low in fiber. It is now recognized that a high-fiber diet promotes soft, bulky stools that pass more swiftly, require less straining with defecation, and result in lower intracolonic pressures (Scheppach et al., 2001). High-fiber intakes have been found to relieve symptoms for most patients, and exercise appears to aid in preventing constipation and thus diverticular disease (Cheek and Radley, 1999; Peters, 2001; Sheppach et al., 2001).

Patients who have followed a low-fiber diet for years may require extensive encouragement to adopt the high-fiber approach. Fiber intake should be increased gradually because it may cause bloating or gas; however, these side effects usually disappear within 2 to 3 weeks. Recommend

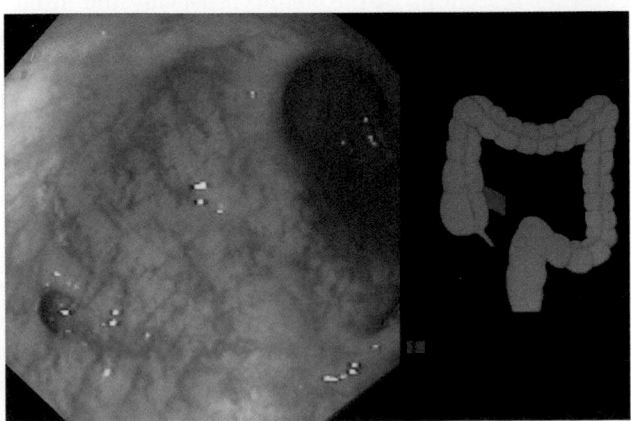

FIGURE 27-5 Internal photograph of diverticular pouch. *(Courtesy Pitt County Memorial Hospital, Greenville, N.C.)*

intakes of dietary fiber, preferably from foods, are 25 g/day for adult females and 38 g/day for males. If an individual cannot or will not consume the necessary amount of fiber, methylcellulose and psyllium fiber supplements have been used with good results. Adequate fluid intake (e.g., 2 to 3 L daily) should accompany the high-fiber intake.

For patients with an acute flare of diverticulitis, a low-residue diet, elemental diet, or, in complicated cases, total parenteral nutrition may be required initially, followed by a gradual return to a high-fiber diet. Colonic smooth-muscle contractions, which intensify after a high-fat meal, may contribute to the discomfort felt by persons with diverticular disease. Therefore it may be reasonable to suggest a low-fat diet for these patients, at least initially.

The question of whether the consumption of seeds, nuts, or skins of plant matter should be avoided to prevent complications of diverticular disease or after bouts of diverticulitis remains unresolved. Common sense tends to favor avoiding consumption of very coarse materials such as husks (not necessarily seeds) like those surrounding sunflower seeds and peanuts.

Whether seeds or normal fibrous materials play any role in the onset of symptoms or actually harm the diverticula has not been determined. In general, foods such as nuts, popcorn hulls, sunflower seeds, pumpkin seeds, caraway seeds, and sesame seeds may be limited. The seeds in tomatoes, zucchini, cucumbers, strawberries, raspberries, and poppy seeds are not problematic. In patients with perforation or obstruction, large pieces of coarse plant matter might be restricted, and patients should be encouraged to chew fibrous foods thoroughly.

Intestinal Polyps and Colon Cancer

Pathophysiology

In the United States and worldwide colorectal cancer is the third most common cancer in adults and is also the second most common cause of cancer death. The number of new cases of colorectal cancer is estimated to be about 150,000 per year, and the incidence is higher in men than women at about 59 and 44 cases respectively per 100,000 population (NIH, NCI, 2006). The highest rates are seen in whites of northern European origin. Rates in Africa and Asia are lower, but they tend to rise with migration and westernization. Polyps are considered precursors of colon cancers (see Chapter 37 for more details).

Factors that increase the risk of colorectal cancer include family history, occurrence of IBD, familial polyposis, adenomatous polyps, and several dietary components. Use of aspirin and nonsteroidal antiinflammatory agents and exercise appear to be protective (Raju and Cruz-Correa, 2006; Peters et al., 2001). Dietary risk factors may include increased meat, fat, or alcohol intake; obesity; and inadequate intake of several micronutrients. Micronutrients considered protective in animal and some epidemiologic and cohort studies include vitamin D, folate, calcium, and selenium. There have been several types of supportive studies regarding the protective role of fruits and vegetables as a group, individual plant foods, high-fiber grains, omega-3 fatty acids, several antioxidants, and phytochemicals; but the data are not always consistent.

Patterns of dietary practices rather than specific nutrients may be more predictive of the risk of developing colorectal cancer. Diets high in calories, fat, and animal protein and inadequate in fruits, vegetables, and grains tend to be associated with increased risk. Food preparation methods may also influence the carcinogenic potential of meats and fatty foods (Raju and Cruz-Correa, 2006; McGarr et al., 2005) (see Chapter 37).

The use of prebiotics and probiotics alters colonic microflora, induces glutathione transferase, increases butyrate content of the stool, reduces toxic and genotoxic compounds, and in animal models reduces the development of some precancerous lesions (McGarr et al., 2005; Brady et al., 2000; Wollowske et al., 2001).

Medical Management

Patients diagnosed with colorectal polyps or cancer may require moderate to significant interventions, including medications, radiation therapy, chemotherapy, colonic surgery, and parenteral nutrition support.

Medical Nutrition Therapy

Generally Americans consume a diet that fits the pattern for increased risk of colon cancer, and they lead sedentary lifestyles. Current recommendations from health organizations that publish public health messages or consensus statements (e.g., National Cancer Institute, American Cancer Society) include notations that specifically target colon cancer. These recommendations typically include sufficient exercise; weight maintenance or reduction; modest and balanced intake of lipids; adequate intake of micronutrients from fruits, vegetables, legumes, whole grains, and dairy products; and limited use of alcohol. Supplements are normally encouraged if the diet is not adequate. The diet for cancer survivors typically follows these prevention guidelines (see Chapter 37).

INTESTINAL SURGERY

Small-Bowel Resections and Short-Bowel Syndrome

Short-bowel syndrome (SBS) refers to nutritional and medical consequences resulting from major resections of the small intestine. The amount of remaining GI tract required to maintain acceptable digestive and absorptive capacity depends on a number of factors, including the age of individual, the original reason for the resection, which portions of the GI tract remain, and the health of the remaining GI tract.

The most common reasons for major resections of the intestine in adults include Crohn's disease, radiation enteritis, mesenteric infarct, malignant disease, and volvulus (Beyer, 2001). In the pediatric population most cases of SBS result from congenital anomalies of the GI tract, atresia, volvulus, or necrotizing enterocolitis (Sigalet, 2001).

Consequences of SBS include malabsorption of micronutrients and macronutrients, frequent diarrhea, steatorrhea, dehydration, electrolyte imbalances, weight loss, and growth failure in children. Other complications include gastric hypersecretion, oxalate renal stones, cholesterol gallstones, and, rarely, d-lactic acidosis (Sundarum et al., 2002). Individuals who eventually need long-term parenteral nutrition have increased risk of catheter infection, sepsis, cholestasis, and liver disease and reduced quality of life associated with chronic intravenous nutrition support (Gupte et al., 2006).

Essentially all patients who have bowel resections that result in removal of greater than 70% to 80% of small intestine suffer some initial and chronic problems related to malabsorption of nutrients, fluids, and electrolytes. Bowel adaptation can occur to varying degrees, and absorption improves. Frequent feeding with small amounts of simple foods, use of dilute enteral feedings, and the addition of a number of enteral growth factors may enhance absorption. Individuals at increased risk of intestinal failure and dependence on parenteral nutrition include the elderly; those who have had distal ileal resections, resection of the ileocecal valve, or colonic resection in addition to small bowel; and those whose reason for bowel resection included radiation enteritis or mesenteric infarct (Beyer, 2001; Parekh et al., 2005; Wilmore et al., 1997) (Box 27-9).

Jejunal Resections

Normally most digestion and absorption of food and nutrients occurs in the first 100 cm of small intestine. What remains to be digested or fermented and absorbed are small amounts of sugars, resistant starch, fiber, lipids, dietary fiber, and fluids. After jejunal resections, the ileum is able to perform the functions of the jejunum, especially after a period of adaptation. The motility of the ileum is comparatively slow, and hormones secreted in the ileum and colon help to slow gastric emptying and secretions. Because jejunal resections result in reduced surface area and shorter intestinal transit than normal, the functional reserve for absorption of micronutrients, excess amounts of sugars (especially lactose), and lipids is reduced.

Ileal Resections

Significant resections of the ileum, especially the distal ileum, generally produce major nutritional and medical complications. The distal ileum is the only site for absorption of the vitamin B_{12} and intrinsic factor complex and bile salts, and the ileum normally absorbs a major portion of the several liters of fluid ingested and secreted into the GI tract (see Chapter 1). Although malabsorption of bile salts may appear to be a rather benign problem, it creates a potentially serious cascade of consequences (Beyer, 2001) (Box 27-10).

If the ileum cannot "recycle" bile salts secreted into the GI tract, hepatic production cannot maintain a sufficient bile salt pool or the secretions to emulsify lipids. The gastric and pancreatic lipases are capable of digesting some triglycerides to fatty acids and monoglycerides, but, without adequate micelle formation facilitated by bile salts, lipids are poorly absorbed. This can result in significant malabsorp-

BOX 27-9

Factors Affecting the Course of Short-Bowel Syndrome

Length of remaining small intestine
Loss of ileum, especially distal one third
Loss of ileocecal valve
Loss of colon
Disease in remaining segment(s) of gastrointestinal tract
Radiation enteritis
Coexisting malnutrition
Older age at surgery

BOX 27-10

Consequences of Ileal Resection

Rapid transit of intestinal contents
Decreased fluid absorptive area
Malabsorption of vitamin B_{12}/intrinsic factor complex
Malabsorption of bile salts
Inadequate bile salts for lipid solubilization, digestion, and absorption, leading to loss of fat and fat-soluble nutrients
Loss of secreted bile salts into colon because of decreased reabsorption
Formation of hydroxy fatty acids by colonic bacteria from malabsorbed fat, resulting in decreased fluid and electrolyte absorption
Malabsorption of Ca^{2+}, Mg^{2+}, and Zn^{2+} because of formation of insoluble "soaps" with malabsorbed free fatty acids
Increased risk of oxalate stones because of increased colonic absorption of oxalate, which normally binds to Ca^{2+}, Zn^{2+}, and Mg^{2+}

tion of fats and fat-soluble vitamins A, D, and E. In addition, malabsorption of fatty acids results in their combination with divalent cations such as calcium, zinc, and magnesium to form fatty acid–mineral soaps. This results in malabsorption of these nutrients. To compound matters, colonic absorption of oxalate, which normally is bound to the divalent cations, is increased, leading to hyperoxaluria and increased renal oxalate stones. Relative dehydration and concentrated urine, which are common with ileal resections, may further increase the risk of stone formation (see Chapter 36).

If the patient has any colon left, malabsorption of what bile salts are secreted can act as irritants to the mucosa, resulting in increased fluid and electrolyte secretion and increased colonic motility rather than absorption. Consumption of high-fat diets with ileal resections and retained colon may also result in the formation of hydroxy fatty acids, which also can increase fluid secretion. Cholesterol gallstones may occur because the ratio of bile acid, phospholipid, and cholesterol in biliary secretions is altered. Dependence on parenteral nutrition may further increase the risk of biliary "sludge" secondary to decreased stimulus for evacuation of the biliary tract (see Chapter 28).

Lactic acidosis is a relatively rare complication that occurs only with severe SBS and remaining colon. The problem results from excessive intake and malabsorption of carbohydrate. Metabolic acidosis and production of d-lactate result from fermentation of carbohydrate, production of SCFAs, reduced colonic pH, and proliferation of acid-resistant colonic microbes that produce d-lactate (Bongaerts et al., 1997). The problem is resolved by treating the metabolic acidosis and reducing the intake of sugars and total carbohydrates.

Medical and Surgical Management of Resections

Medications are prescribed to retard gastric emptying, decrease secretions, slow GI motility, and treat bacterial overgrowth. Recently somatostatin and somatostatin analogs; glucagon-like polypeptide 2; growth hormone; and other hormones with antisecretory, antimotility, or trophic actions have been used to retard both motility and secretions (Thompson et al., 2003; Drucker, 2002; Sundarum et al., 2002). Surgical procedures, including reversal of segments of bowel to

slow transit of GI contents, creation of reservoirs ("pouches") to serve as a form of colon, intestinal lengthening, and intestinal transplant, have been performed to help patients with major GI resections (Pirenne et al., 2001). Intestinal transplant is still one of the most difficult organ transplants and is typically reserved for gut failure and when patients develop significant complications from total parenteral nutrition (Weseman and Gilroy, 2005; Gupte et al., 2006).

Medical Nutrition Therapy

Most patients who have significant bowel resections require total parenteral nutrition initially to restore and maintain nutrition status (Sundaram et al., 2002). The duration of total parenteral nutrition and subsequent nutrition therapy is based on the extent of the bowel resection, the health of the patient, and the condition of the remaining GI tract. In general, older patients with major ileal resections, patients who have lost the ileocecal valve, and patients with residual disease in the remaining GI tract do not fare as well. Some may require lifetime supplementation with parenteral nutrition to maintain adequate fluid and nutrition status.

The two general principles for resuming enteral nutrition after small-bowel resections are (1) to start enteral feedings early, and (2) to increase feeding concentration and volume gradually over time (Beyer, 2001; Vanderhoof and Young, 2001). The role of enteral feedings is to provide a trophic stimulus to the GI tract; parenteral nutrition is used to restore and maintain nutrient status. The more extreme and severe the problem, the slower the progression. Small, frequent, mini meals (6 to 10 per day) are likely to be better tolerated than larger feedings (Matarese et al., 2005; Beyer, 2001).

If enteral feedings are used, gradual introduction of feedings stimulates GI adaptation; total parenteral nutrition provides the major source of fluid and nutrients.

More nutrients are gradually added enterally, and the volume or concentration of total parenteral nutrition decreases accordingly. Because of malnutrition and disuse of the GI tract, the digestive and absorptive functions of the remaining GI tract may be compromised, and malnutrition itself will delay adaptation (Cronk et al., 2000). The transition to more normal foods may take weeks to months, and some patients may never tolerate normal concentrations or volumes of foods.

Maximum adaptation of the GI tract may take up to a year after surgery. Adaptation improves function, but it does not restore the intestine to normal length or capacity. Whole foods are some of the most important stimuli to the GI tract, but other nutritional measures have been considered as a means of hastening the adaptive process and decreasing malabsorption. For example, **glutamine** is the preferred fuel for small intestinal enterocytes and thus may be valuable in enhancing adaptation. Nucleotides (in the form of purines, pyrimidine, ribonucleic acid) may also enhance mucosal adaptation, but unfortunately they are often lacking in parenteral and enteral nutritional products. SCFAs (e.g., butyrate, propionate, acetate) produced from microbial fermentation of carbohydrate and fibers, are major fuels of the colonic epithelium.

Patients with jejunal resections and an intact ileum and colon will likely adapt quickly to normal diets. A normal balance of protein, fat, and carbohydrate sources is satisfactory. Six small feedings with avoidance of lactose, large amounts of concentrated sweets, and caffeine may help to reduce the risk of bloating, abdominal pain, and diarrhea. Because the typical American diet may be nutritionally lacking and use of some micronutrients may be marginal, patients should be advised that the quality of their diet is of utmost importance. A multivitamin and mineral supplement may be required to meet all their nutritional needs.

Patients with ileal resections require increased time and patience in the advancement from parenteral to enteral nutrition. Because of losses, fat-soluble vitamins, calcium, magnesium, and zinc may need to be supplemented. Dietary fat may need to be limited, especially in those with remaining colon. Small amounts at each feeding are more likely to be tolerated and absorbed.

MCT products add to the caloric intake and serve as a vehicle for lipid-soluble nutrients. Because boluses of MCT oil (e.g., taken as a medication in tablespoon amounts) may add to the patient's diarrhea, it is best to divide the doses equally in feedings throughout the day. Fluid and electrolytes, especially sodium, should be provided in small amounts and frequently.

In patients with massive resections (e.g., when the duodenum and a few inches of jejunum are anastomosed to segments of colon), an oral diet will be able to nourish only partially. In some cases overfeeding in an attempt to compensate for malabsorption results in further malabsorption, not only of ingested foods and liquids but also of the significant amounts of GI fluids secreted in response to food ingestion. Patients with an extremely short bowel are typically nutritionally dependent on parenteral solutions for at least part of their nutrient and fluid supply. Small, frequent snacks provide some oral gratification for these patients, but typically they can supply only a portion of their fluid and nutrient needs.

Blind Loop Syndrome (Small Intestine Bacterial Overgrowth)

Pathophysiology

Blind loop syndrome is a disorder characterized by bacterial overgrowth resulting from stasis of the intestinal tract as an outcome of obstructive disease, radiation enteritis, fistula formation, or surgical repair of the intestine. Bacteria deconjugate bile salts; deconjugated bile salts are cytotoxic, and they are also less effective as micelle formers. Poor fat absorption and steatorrhea result. Carbohydrate malabsorption occurs because of injury to the brush border secondary to the toxic effects of the products of bacterial catabolism and consequent enzyme loss. The expanding numbers of bacteria use the available vitamin B_{12} and other nutrients for their own growth; and the host becomes deficient.

Medical Treatment

Treatment is directed toward control of the bacterial growth with antibiotics, probiotics, prebiotics, and in some cases surgical modification of the blind loop.

Medical Nutrition Therapy

Part of the problem with bacterial overgrowth in the small intestine is that carbohydrates reaching the site where microbes are harbored serve as fuel for their proliferation, with subsequent increased production of gases and organic acids. At least theoretically a diet that limits refined carbohydrates that are readily fermented such as refined starches and sugars (e.g., lactose, fructose, alcohol sugars) and substitutes whole grains, vegetables and oligosaccharides can limit the proliferation and increase motility.

Limited studies are available as to the effectiveness of diets and probiotic and prebiotic materials in the prevention and treatment of altered GI motility, strictures, abnormal anatomy of the GI tract, and the presence of opportunistic organisms in the colon (*C. difficile* and other organisms). Because vitamin B_{12} may be lost in fermentation and some dietary nutrients may be lacking, an assessment of the medical problem and the patient's dietary intake is in order. If bile salts are being degraded, as in the case of blind loop syndrome, MCTs may be helpful if they provide a source of lipid and energy.

Fistula Repair

Pathophysiology

Fistulas occur as a result of prenatal developmental error, trauma, or inflammatory or malignant disease processes. Fistulas of the intestinal tract can be serious threats to nutrition status because large amounts of fluid and electrolytes are lost and malabsorption and infection can occur.

Medical Treatment

Fluid and electrolyte balance must be restored, infection must be brought under control, and aggressive nutrition support is mandatory to permit spontaneous or surgical closure of the fistula and wound.

Medical Nutrition Therapy

Either total parenteral nutrition or defined liquid formula diets are used successfully in patients with fistulas (see Chapter 20). The success rate of either method depends on the location and cause of the fistula and the patient's overall condition.

Ileostomy or Colostomy

Pathophysiology

Patients with severe ulcerative colitis, Crohn's disease, colon cancer, or intestinal trauma frequently require the surgical creation of an opening from the body surface to the intestinal tract to permit defecation from the intact portion of the intestine. When the entire colon, rectum, and anus must be removed, an **ileostomy**, or opening into the ileum, is performed. If only the rectum and anus are removed, a **colostomy** can provide entrance to the colon. In some cases a temporary opening may be made to allow surgery and healing of more distal parts of the intestinal tract.

The opening, or stoma, eventually shrinks to the size of a nickel. The output from the stoma depends on its location, as shown in Figure 27-6. The consistency of the stool from an ileostomy is liquid, whereas that from a colostomy ranges from mushy to fairly well formed. Stool from a colostomy on the left side of the colon is firmer than that from a colostomy on the right side. Odor is a major concern of the patient with an ileostomy or colostomy; however, an ileostomy stool usually has a weakly acidic odor that is not unpleasant.

Medical Treatment

Patients with a permanent colostomy or ileostomy require sympathetic understanding from the entire health care team. Acceptance of the condition and the problems involved in maintaining bowel regularity is usually difficult. Nursing personnel, especially enterostomal therapists, play a major role in supporting and teaching patients with ostomies. Having these patients meet other people who have undergone similar surgery may help with the adjustment. Eventually they may be encouraged by the realization that in the future they will not have the multiple hospitalizations or chronic disabilities that accompanied their intestinal disease.

Medical Nutrition Therapy

Malodorous stools may be caused by steatorrhea or partial digestion or bacterial fermentation of foodstuffs. SCFAs, sulfur-containing compounds, ammonia, methane, and other end products can produce odors. Because an individual patient may have different flora, types and amounts of gases and odors may differ among patients and with different dietary practices. Patients learn to observe their stools to determine which foods to eliminate; this differs from one patient to the next.

Foods that tend to cause odor from a colostomy are legumes, onions, garlic, cabbage, eggs, fish, some medications, and some vitamin and mineral supplements. Persistent odor may be attributable to poor stoma hygiene or to an ileostomy complication that allows bacterial overgrowth in the ileum. Deodorants are available, and modern pouch appliances are odor proof. Gas production may cause the pouch to become tense and distended, and accidental dislodgment is likely. The nutritional recommendations for reducing flatulence, presented at the beginning of this chapter, may be helpful for patients with colostomies.

The normal output from the ileum to the colon is in the range of 750 ml to 1.5 L in the intact GI tract. After a colectomy and creation of an ileostomy, adaptation occurs within 1 to 2 weeks. Fecal output will lessen, and stools will become less liquid. Reduction in stool volume may not occur to the same extent in patients who have had an ileal resection in addition to a colectomy. Depending on the amount of ileum resected, the ileal output may be 1.5 to 5 times greater than that of the patient who has had only a colectomy. Patients with ileostomies have an above-average need for salt and water to compensate for excessive losses in stool. Inadequate water intake can result in small urine volumes and a predisposition for renal calculi. A normal diet provides adequate sodium, and patients should be instructed to drink at least 1 L more than their ostomy output daily.

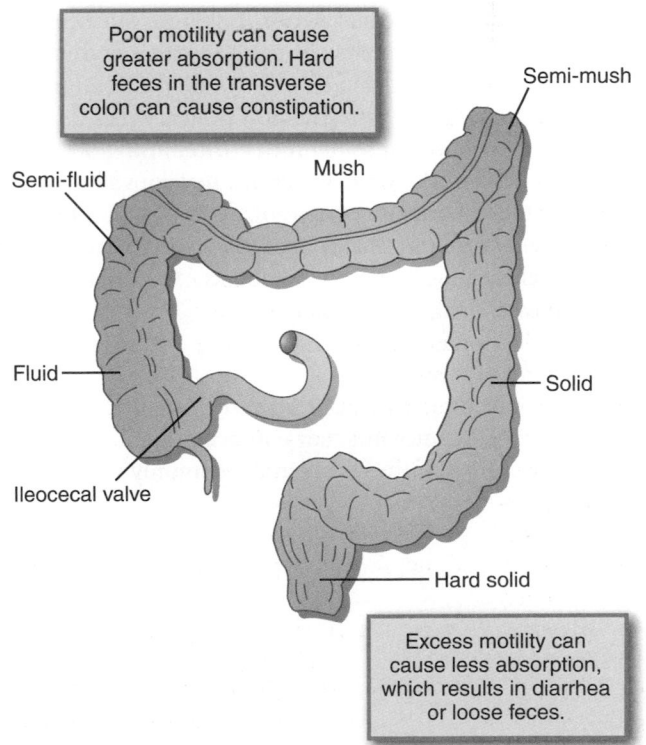

Poor motility can cause greater absorption. Hard feces in the transverse colon can cause constipation.

Semi-mush

Semi-fluid

Mush

Fluid

Solid

Ileocecal valve

Hard solid

Excess motility can cause less absorption, which results in diarrhea or loose feces.

FIGURE 27-6 As the feces move from the ileocecal valve to the anus, water is absorbed, and the feces become more solid. The characteristics of the output from a colostomy depend on its location in the colon.

The patient with a normal, functional ileostomy usually does not become nutritionally depleted. Surgical procedures such as ileostomy may require specific dietary changes but no greater energy intake; caloric expenditures in these patients are similar to those of normal subjects. Those who also undergo resection of the terminal ileum need vitamin B_{12} supplementation or intravenous injections. Patients with an ileostomy may have low vitamin C and folate intakes because of low fresh vegetable and fruit intakes, and they require supplementation.

Patients with ileostomies should be guided by physiologic reasons for intolerance of foods and not by anecdotal reports. Because gastric emptying may be more rapid and foodstuffs are not fermented to the same degree after colostomy, absorption of nutrients may be somewhat better from cooked, shredded, or pureed fruits and vegetables (Robertson and Mathers, 2000; Livny et al., 2003). Because it is possible for a food bolus to get caught at the point where the ileum narrows as it enters the abdominal wall, it is important to warn the patient to avoid very fibrous vegetables and to chew all food well. Other than this, patients with either an ileostomy or a colostomy should be encouraged to follow their normal diet, omitting only foods known to cause problems.

Ileal Pouch after Colectomy

Pathophysiology

As an alternative to creation of an ileostomy for persons who have had their colons removed, surgeons can create a reservoir using a portion of the distal ileum. Folds of the ileum are joined together to create a small pouch, which is then connected to the rectum and ileum. This is called an **ileal pouch**–anal anastomosis. The most common pouch is the J pouch, but S and W pouches are sometimes created using additional folds of ileum. Like the colon, the pouch develops a microflora capable of at least partially fermenting fiber and carbohydrate. Because the reservoir is smaller than the colon, bowel movements are likely to occur more frequently than normal (i.e., between four and eight times daily).

Medical Treatment

Vitamin B_{12} injections are usually required because, as in blind loop syndrome, the microbes may compete for and bind intraluminal vitamin B_{12}. Other problems commonly reported include obstruction; "pouchitis"; and increased stool output, frequency, and gas (Thompson-Fawcett et al., 1997).

The incidence of obstruction may be lessened with attention to particle size of fibrous foods, chewing thoroughly, and consuming small meals frequently throughout the day. Stool frequency and volume do not return to normal, however. The normal, intact colon absorbs 80% to 90% of the liter or so of fluid entering from the ileum, leaving only 100 to 200 ml. After surgery the remaining ileum does adapt to a small degree by increasing efficiency of fluid absorption, but even after adaptation, fluid output is always in the range of 300 to 600 ml.

Pouchitis, as implied by the name, is an inflammation of the mucosal tissue forming the pouch. The associated pathologic changes have been described as being somewhat similar to that of IBD (e.g., ulcerative colitis). The cause of pouchitis is not entirely clear, but it may be related to selected bacterial overgrowth, bile salt malabsorption, or insufficient SCFA production. Antibiotics are the primary form of therapy, but experiments with different types of dietary fiber, prebiotics and probiotics, and other nutrient components have been used successfully to reduce the incidence of pouchitis (Meier and Steuerwald, 2005; Guarner, 2005).

Medical Nutrition Therapy

The same dietary measures that are used by others to reduce excessive stool output (reduced caffeine, lactose avoidance in lactase-deficient persons, limitation of fructose and sorbitol) will likely reduce stool volume and frequency in persons with pouches. Adequate fluid and electrolyte intake are especially important because of the increase in intestinal losses.

Rectal Surgery

Nutrition care after rectal surgery such as hemorrhoidectomy should be directed toward maintaining an intake that will allow wound repair and prevent infection of the wound by feces. The frequency of stools is minimized by the use of constipating drugs and a minimum-residue diet (see Table 27-1). Chemically defined diets are low in residue, and their use can reduce stool volume and frequency to as little as 50 g every 6 days, making the surgical construction of a temporary colostomy unnecessary. A normal diet is resumed after healing is complete, and the patient is instructed about the benefits of eating a high-fiber diet to avoid constipation in the future.

- The GI tract has the largest surface area of any tissue, and 70% of the body's immune cells, contains more bacterial than somatic cells in the body, and has the greatest exposure to elements of the environment.
- The function of the GI tract in preventing inappropriate interaction with the environment (primarily food, beverages, contaminants, endogenous ingested microbes), known as the gut barrier, plays a primary role in health maintenance.

- Disruptions in the gut barrier following injury from drugs, toxins, infection, malnutrition, allergic responses, bacterial overgrowth, and oxidative stress have been linked to immune dysregulation and a number of GI disorders, including inflammatory bowel disease, celiac disease, food allergy, and multi-organ system failure.
- New medical and nutritional approaches are being evaluated to improve gut barrier function and tolerance between the GI luminal environment and host tissues and to treat lower intestine disease.

⊛ **CLINICAL SCENARIO 1**

Suzanne is a 33-year-old teacher with Crohn's disease who has been referred for evaluation because of abdominal pain, bloating, and occasional nausea and diarrhea. The physician suspects a distal small-bowel stricture. Suzanne is seeking information about what to eat to prevent the problem from worsening during the 3-day period before her appointment at the clinic.

✳**Nutrition Diagnosis:** Altered GI function related to pain, bloating, nausea, and diarrhea following meals as evidenced by history of Crohn's disease

1. What information would be appropriate to gather about this patient before you advise her about a nutrition plan?
2. What, in terms of Suzanne's symptoms, makes the physician suspect a stricture?
3. What kind of dietary advice, based solely on her presumed problem, might be warranted?

⊛ **CLINICAL SCENARIO 2**

Mrs. Smith has irritable bowel syndrome with a pattern of alternating constipation and diarrhea. She comes to you requesting dietary advice for (1) day-to-day management, and (2) what might be "safest" to eat when she is getting ready to present weekly to biweekly reports to the executives in her large consulting company.

✳**Nutrition Diagnosis:** Food- and nutrition-related knowledge deficit related to management of irritable bowel syndrome as evidenced by questions regarding management of symptoms.

1. What do you want to know about Mrs. Smith's diet, perspectives, and lifestyle?
2. What foods or eating patterns would be best (or best to avoid) for Mrs. Smith for her day-to-day activities?
3. Why might she be asking for advice during stressful periods?

USEFUL WEBSITES

Celiac disease and gluten enteropathy resources
www.gluten.net
www.glutenfreediet.com
www.niddk.nih.gov/health/digest/pubs/celiac/
www.niddk.nih.gov/health/digest/pubs/celiac/

Crohn's and Colitis Foundation
www.ccfa.org/

Gastrointestinal disorders and treatment
www.niddk.nih.gov/health/digest/digest.htm

Ileostomy, colostomy, pouches
http://digestive.niddk.nih.gov/ddiseases/pubs/ileostomy/index.htm
http://www.nlm.nih.gov/medlineplus/tutorials/colostomy/htm/index.htm

References

Abdulkarim AS et al: Etiology of nonresponsive celiac disease: results of a systematic approach, *Am J Gastroenterol* 97:2016, 2002.

Ahmad T et al: Clinical relevance of advances in genetics and pharmacogenetics of IBD, *Gastroenterology* 126:1533, 2004.

Atkinson W et al: Food elimination based on IgG antibodies in irritable bowel syndrome: a randomized controlled trial, *Gut* 53:1459, 2004.

Azpiroz F: Intestinal gas dynamics: mechanisms and clinical relevance, *Gut* 54:893, 2005.

Barbera G et al: Interactions between commensal bacteria and gut sensorimotor function in health and disease, *Am J Gastroenterol* 100:2560, 2005.

Bartlett JG: Antibiotic-associated diarrhea, *N Engl J Med* 346:334, 2002.

Benninga MA et al: Childhood constipation: is there new light in the tunnel? *J Pediatr Gastroenterol Nutr* 39:448, 2004.

Beyer PL: Short bowel syndrome. In Coulston AM, Rock CL, Monson ER, editors: *Nutrition in the prevention and treatment of disease*, ed 1, San Diego, 2001, Academic Press.

Beyer PL et al: Fructose intake at current levels in the United States may cause gastrointestinal distress in normal adults, *J Am Diet Assoc* 105:1559, 2005.

Bezkorovainy A: Probiotics: determinants of survival and growth in the gut, *Am J Clin Nutr* 73:399S, 2001.

Biggs WS, Dery WH: Evaluation and treatment of constipation in infants and children, *Am Fam Phys* 73:469, 2006.

Bongaerts GP et al: Role of bacteria in the pathogenesis of short bowel syndrome associated *d*-lactic acidemia, *Microb Pathog* 22:285, 1997.

Brady LJ et al: The role of probiotic cultures in the prevention of colon cancer, *J Nutr* 130S:410, 2000.

Broussard EK, Surawicz CM: Probiotics and prebiotics in clinical practice, *Nutr Clin Care* 7:104, 2004.

Bueno L: Gastrointestinal pharmacology: irritable bowel syndrome, *Curr Opin Pharmacol* 5:583, 2005.

Byers KG, Savaiano DA: The myth of increased lactose intolerance in African-Americans, *J Am Coll Nutr* 24:569S, 2005.

Candelli M et al: Idiopathic chronic constipation: pathophysiology, diagnosis and treatment, *Hepatogastroenterology* 48:1050, 2001.

Caprilli R et al: European evidence-based consensus on the diagnosis and management of Crohn's disease: special situations, *Gut* 55:36, 2005.

Case S: The gluten-free diet: how to provide effective education and resources, *Gastroenterology* 128:S128, 2005.

Cashman KD, Shanahan F: Is nutrition an aetiological factor for inflammatory bowel disease? *Eur J Gastroenterol Hepatol* 15:607, 2003.

Chand N, Mihas AA: Celiac disease: current concepts in diagnosis and treatment, *J Clin Gastroenterol* 40:3, 2006.

Cheek C, Radley S: Diverticulosis: fiber is the key, *Practitioner* 243:321, 1999.

Cronk DR et al: Malnutrition impairs postresection intestinal adaptation, *JPEN Parenter Enteral Nutr* 24:76, 2000.

Davidson G et al: Infectious diarrhea in children: working group report of the first world congress of pediatric gastroenterology, hepatology, and nutrition, *J Pediatr Gastroenterol Nutr* 35:143S, 2002.

Davidson RH et al: Probiotic culture survival and implications in fermented frozen yogurt characteristics, *J Dairy Sci* 83:666, 2000.

Dotan I, Rachmilewitz: Probiotics in inflammatory bowel disease: possible mechanisms of action, *Curr Opin Gastroenterol* 21:426, 2005.

Drucker DJ: Gut adaptation and the glucagon-like peptides, *Gut* 59:428, 2002.

Farrell RJ, Kelly CP: Celiac sprue, *N Engl J Med* 346:180, 2002.

Farthing MJG: Tropical malabsorption and tropical diarrhea. In Feldman M, Sleisenger MH, Scharschmidt BF, editors: *Gastrointestinal and liver disease*, ed 6, Philadelphia, 1998, Saunders.

Fasano A, Catassi C: Current approaches to diagnosis and treatment of celiac disease: an evolving spectrum, *Gastroenterology* 120:636, 2001.

Fasano A et al: Prevalence of celiac disease in at-risk and not at-risk groups in the United States: a large multicenter study, *Arch Intern Med* 163:286, 2003.

Fukuda M et al: Prebiotic treatment of experimental colitis with germinated barley foodstuff: a comparison with probiotic or antibiotic treatment, *Int J Mol Med* 9:65, 2002.

Griffiths AM: Enteral nutrition in the management of Crohn's disease, *JPEN J Parenter Enteral Nutr* 29S:108, 2005.

Guarner F: Inulin and oligofructose: impact on intestinal diseases and disorders, *Br J Nutr* 93S:S61, 2005.

Gupte GL, et al: Current issues in the management of intestinal failure, *Arch Dis Child* 91:259, 2006.

Hahn S et al: Reduced osmolarity oral rehydration solution for treating dehydration caused by acute diarrhoea in children, *Cochrane Database Syst Rev* 1:CD002847, 2002.

Harder H, et al: Effect of high- and low-caloric mixed liquid meals on intestinal gas dynamics, *Dig Dis Sci* 51:140, 2006.

Higgins PD, Johanson JF: Epidemiology of constipation in North America: a systematic review, *Am J Gastroenterol* 99:750, 2004.

Huesbye E: The pathogenesis of gastrointestinal bacterial overgrowth, *Chemotherapy* 51S:1, 2005.

Institute of Medicine: *Dietary reference intakes for energy, carbohydrate, fiber, fatty acids, cholesterol, protein and amino acids*, Washington, DC, 2002, National Academies Press.

Janatuinen EK et al: No harm from five-year ingestion of oats in coeliac disease, *Gut* 50:332, 2002.

Jarvela IE: Molecular genetics of adult-type hypolactasia, *Ann Med* 37:179, 2005.

Jowett SL et al: Influence of dietary factors on the clinical course of ulcerative colitis: a prospective cohort study, *Gut* 53:1479 2004.

Kalliomaki MA: Food allergy and irritable bowel syndrome, *Curr Opin Gastroenterol* 21:708, 2005.

Koning F: Celiac disease: caught between a rock and a hard place, *Gastroenterology* 129:1294, 2005.

Kornblau S et al: Management of cancer treatment–related diarrhea: issues and therapeutic strategies, *J Pain Symptom Manage* 19:118, 2000.

Lapascu et al: Hydrogen breath test to detect small intestinal bacterial overgrowth: a prevalence case-control study in irritable bowel syndrome, *Aliment Pharmacol Ther* 22:1157, 2005.

Laroux FS, Grisham MB: Immunological basis of inflammatory bowel disease: role of microcirculation, *Microcirculation* 8:283, 2001.

Lee SL, Green PH: Endoscopy in celiac disease, *Curr Opin Gastroenterol* 21:589, 2005.

Lin HC: Small intestinal bacterial overgrowth: a framework for understanding irritable bowel syndrome, *JAMA* 292:852, 2004.

Linskens RK et al: The bacterial flora in inflammatory bowel disease: current insights in pathogenesis and the influence of antibiotics and probiotics, *Scand J Gastroenterol* 234S:29, 2001.

Livny O et al: Beta-carotene bioavailability from differently processed carrot meals in human ileostomy volunteers, *Eur J Nutr* 42:338, 2003.

Lochs H: To feed or not to feed? Are nutritional supplements worthwhile in active Crohn's disease? *Gut* 55:306, 2006.

Loening-Baucke V: Encopresis, *Curr Opin Pediatr* 14:570, 2002.

MacDonald TT et al: Immunopathogenesis of Crohn's disease, *JPEN J Parenter Enteral Nutr* 29:S118, 2005.

Madsen KL: Use of probiotics in gastrointestinal disease, *Can J Gastroenterol* 15:817, 2001.

Malagelada JR: A symptom-based approach to making a positive diagnosis of irritable bowel syndrome with constipation, *Int J Clin Pract* 60:57, 2006.

Marlett JA et al: Position of the American Dietetic Association: health implications of dietary fiber, *J Am Diet Assoc* 102:993, 2002.

Marti T et al: Prolyl endopeptidase-mediated destructions of T cell epitopes in whole gluten: chemical and immunological characterization, *J Pharmacol Exp Ther* 12:19, 2004.

Matarese LE et al: Short bowel syndrome: Clinical guidelines for nutritional management, *Nutr Clin Pract* 20:493, 2005.

Matthew CG, Lewis CM: Genetics of inflammatory bowel disease: progress and prospects, *Hum Mol Genet* 13:161, 2004.

Matysiak-Budnik T et al: Limited efficiency of prolyl-endopeptidase in the detoxification of gliadin peptides in celiac disease, *Gastroenterology* 129:786, 2005.

McGarr SE et al: Diet, anaerobic bacterial metabolism, and colon cancer: a review of the literature, *J Clin Gastroenterol* 39:98, 2005.

Meier R, Steuerwald M: Place of probiotics, *Curr Opin Crit Care* 11:318 2005.

Mitra AD et al: Management of diarrhea in HIV-infected patients, *Int J STD AIDS* 12:630, 2001.

Mueller C, Macpherson AJ: Layers of mutualism with commensal bacteria protect us from intestinal inflammation, *Gut* 55:276, 2006.

Murphy C et al: Reduced osmolarity oral rehydration solution for treating cholera, *Cochrane Database Syst Rev* 4:CD003754, 2004.

Nakano E et al: Hyperhomocystinemia in children with inflammatory bowel disease, *J Pediatr Gastroenterol Nutr* 37:586, 2003.

Nath SK: Tropical sprue, *Curr Gastroenterol Rep* 7:343, 2005.

NIH Consensus development Conference on Celiac Disease, http://consensus.nih.gov/2004/2004CeliacDisease118html.htm, accessed April 12, 2006.

National Institutes of Health, National Cancer Institute: Table 53: Age-adjusted cancer incidence rates for selected cancer sites, http://www.cancer.org/downloads/STT/CAFF2005f4Pwsecured.pdf, accessed October 1, 2006.

Nobaek S et al: Alteration of intestinal microflora is associated with reduction in abdominal bloating and pain in patients with irritable bowel syndrome, *Am J Gastroenterol* 95:1231, 2000.

Nucera G et al: Abnormal breaths to lactose, fructose and sorbitol in irritable bowel syndrome may be explained by small intestinal bacterial overgrowth, *Aliment Pharmacol Ther* 21:1391, 2005.

Parekh N et al: Managing short bowel syndrome: making the most of what the patient still has, *Cleve Clin J Med* 72:833, 2005.

Parra-Blanco A: Colonic diverticular disease: pathophysiology and clinical picture, *Digestion* 73S:47, 2006.

Parry S, Forgacs I: Intestinal infection and irritable bowel syndrome, *Eur J Gastroenterol Hepatol* 17:5, 2005.

Penner R et al: Probiotics and nutraceuticals: non-medical treatments of gastrointestinal diseases, *Curr Opin Pharmacol* 5:596, 2005.

Peters HP et al: Potential benefits and hazards of physical activity and exercise on the gastrointestinal tract, *Gut* 48:435, 2001.

Pirenne J et al: Recent advances and future prospects in intestinal and multivisceral transplantation, *Pediatr Transplant* 5:452, 2001.

Quigley EM, Quera R: Small intestinal bacterial overgrowth: riles of antibiotics, prebiotics and probiotics, *Gastroenterology* 130S:S67, 2006.

Raju R, Cruz-Correa M: Chemoprevention of colorectal cancer, *Dis Colon Rectum* 49:113, 2006.

Ramkumar D, Rao SSC: Efficacy and safety of traditional medical therapies for chronic constipation: systematic review, *Am J Gastroenterol* 100:936 2005.

Rasinpera H et al: The C/C-13910 genotype of adult-type hypolactasia is associated with an increased risk of colorectal cancer in the Finnish population, *Gut* 54:643, 2005.

Robayo-Torres CC et al: Disaccharide digestion: clinical and molecular aspects, *Clin Gastroenterol Hepatol* 4:276, 2006.

Robertson MD, Mathers JC: Gastric emptying rate of solids is reduced in a group of ileostomy patients, *Dig Dis Sci* 45:1285, 2000.

Rumessen JJ, Gudmand-Hoyer E: Functional bowel disease: malabsorption and abdominal distress after ingestion of fructose, sorbitol, and fructose-sorbitol mixtures, *Gastroenterology* 95:694, 1998.

Salzman H, Lillie D: Diverticular disease: diagnosis and treatment, *Am Fam Physician* 72:1229, 2005.

Sanders DSA: Mucosal integrity and barrier function in the pathogenesis of early lesions in Crohn's disease, *J Clin Pathol* 58:568, 2005.

Sanderson IR, Croft NM: The anti-inflammatory effects of enteral nutrition, *JPEN J Parenter Enteral Nutr* 29S:134, 2005.

Scheppach W et al: Beneficial health effects of low-digestible carbohydrate consumption, *Br J Nutr* 1S:23, 2001.

Schroeder MS: *Clostridium difficile*-associated diarrhea, *Am Fam Physician* 71:921, 2005.

Seibold F: Food-induced immune responses as origin of bowel disease, *Digestion* 71:251, 2005.

Sentongo TA: The use of oral rehydration solutions in children and adults, *Curr Gastroenterol Rep* 6:307, 2004.

Seraphin P, Mobarin S: Mortality in patients with celiac disease, *Nutr Rev* 60:116, 2002.

Shan L et al: Structural basis for gluten intolerance in celiac sprue, *Science* 297:2275, 2002.

Sigalet DL: Short-bowel syndrome in infants and children: an overview, *Semin Pediatr Surg* 10:49, 2001.

Silk DBA: Management of irritable bowel syndrome: start of a new era? *Eur J Gastroenterol Hepatol* 15:679, 2003.

Steel M: Colonic diverticular disease, *Aust Fam Physician* 23:1, 2004.

Steffen R, Gyr K: Diet in the treatment of diarrhea: from tradition to evidence, *Clin Infect Dis* 39:472, 2004.

Strocchi A, Levitt MD: Intestinal gas. In Feldman M, Sleisenger MH, Scharschmidt BF, editors: *Gastrointestinal and liver disease*, ed 6, Philadelphia, 1998, Saunders.

Sundarum A et al: Nutritional management of short bowel syndrome in adults, *J Clin Gastroenterol* 34:207, 2002.

Szajewska H et al: Probiotics in the prevention of antibiotic-associated diarrhea in children: a meta-analysis of randomized controlled trials, *J Pediatr* 149:367, 2006.

Teitelbaum JE: Probiotics and the treatment of infectious diarrhea, *Pediatr Infect Dis J* 25:267, 2005.

Thompson ABR et al: Small bowel review: diseases of the small intestine, *Dig Dis Sci* 48:1582, 2003.

Thompson T: Wheat starch, gliadin and the gluten-free diet, *J Am Diet Assoc* 101:1456, 2001.

Thompson-Fawcett MW et al: Ileoanal reservoir dysfunction: a problem-solving approach, *Br J Surg* 84:1351, 1997.

Tomita R et al: Physiological studies on nitric oxide in the right sided colon of patients with diverticular disease, *Hepatogastroenterology* 46:2839, 1999.

Travis SPL et al: European evidence-based consensus on the diagnosis and management of Crohn's disease: current management, *Gut* 55S:16, 2006.

Vanderhoof JA, Young RJ: Enteral nutrition in short-bowel syndrome, *Semin Pediatr Surg* 10:65, 2001.

Weseman RA, Gilroy R: Nutritional management of small bowel transplant patients, *Nutr Clin Pract* 20:509, 2005.

Wilmore DW et al: Factors predicting a successful outcome after pharmacological bowel compensation, *Ann Surg* 226:288, 1997.

Wollowske et al: Protective role of probiotics and prebiotics in colon cancer, *Am J Clin Nutr* 73S:451, 2001.

Zezos P et al: Hyperhomocystinemia in ulcerative colitis is related to folate levels, *World J Gastroenterol* 11:6038, 2005.

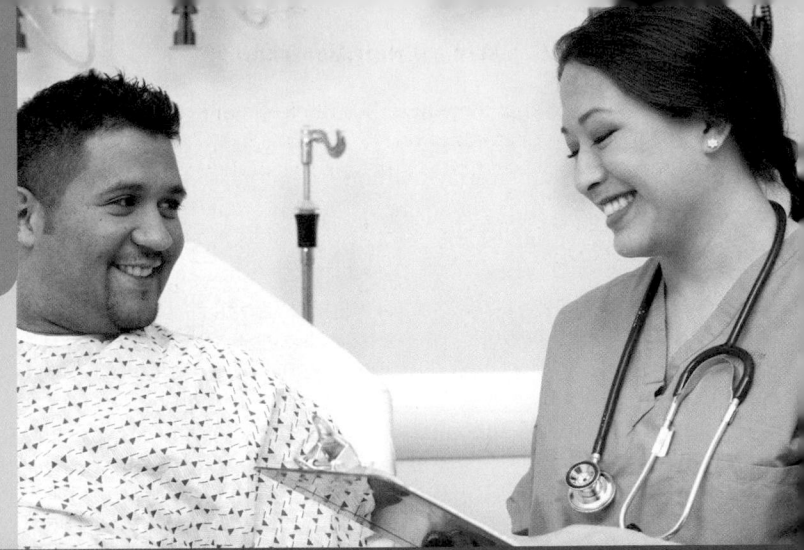

CHAPTER **28**

Jeanette M. Hasse,
PhD, RD, LD, CNSD, FADA
Laura E. Matarese,
MS, RD, LDN, CNSD, FADA

Medical Nutrition Therapy for Liver, Biliary System, and Exocrine Pancreas Disorders

KEY TERMS

alcoholic liver disease disease resulting from excessive alcohol ingestion, characterized by fatty liver (hepatic steatosis), hepatitis, or cirrhosis

aromatic amino acids (AAAs) the amino acids phenylalanine, tryptophan, and tyrosine

ascites accumulation of fluid, serum protein, and electrolytes within the peritoneal cavity caused by increased pressure from portal hypertension and decreased production of albumin (which maintains serum colloidal osmotic pressure)

bile thick, viscous fluid secreted from the liver, stored in the gallbladder, and released into the duodenum when fatty foods enter the duodenum; emulsifies fats in the intestine and forms compounds with fatty acids to facilitate their absorption

branched-chain amino acids (BCAAs) the amino acids valine, isoleucine, and leucine

cholangitis inflammation in the bile ducts; may be acute or sclerosing

cholecystectomy removal of the gallbladder

cholecystitis inflammation of the gallbladder

choledocholithiasis presence of gallstones in the common bile duct

cholelithiasis presence or formation of gallstones

cholestasis suppression of biliary flow

cirrhosis chronic liver disease caused by diffuse necrosis and regeneration, leading to an increase in fibrous tissue formation disrupting the normal liver structure

fasting hypoglycemia low blood glucose caused by decreased availability of glucose from glycogen as a result of depressed liver function

fatty liver a condition (hepatic steatosis) characterized by the accumulation of excess fat in the liver commonly caused by alcohol abuse but also associated with obesity, starvation, intestinal bypass, parenteral alimentation, and insulin resistance

fulminant liver disease absence of preexisting liver disease and development of liver disease with hepatic encephalopathy within 2 months of onset of illness

hepatic encephalopathy a clinical syndrome characterized by impaired mentation, neuromuscular disturbances, and altered consciousness; four stages of progression

hepatic failure condition in which liver function is diminished to 25% or less

hepatic osteodystrophy a complication of chronic liver disease in which bone mass declines

hepatic steatosis fatty liver

hepatitis widespread inflammation of the liver; usually viral in origin

hepatorenal syndrome functional renal failure without anatomic or histopathologic renal changes; associated with cirrhosis and ascites or with obstructive jaundice

jaundice (icterus) a syndrome characterized by hyperbilirubinemia and deposition of bile pigment, resulting in yellowing of skin, mucous membranes, and sclera

Kayser-Fleischer ring greenish yellow pigmented ring encircling the cornea just within the corneoscleral margin; formed by copper deposits in Descemet's membrane of the cornea; occurs in patients with Wilson's disease

Kupffer cells fixed phagocytes in the sinusoids of the liver

nonalcoholic steatohepatitis (NASH) an intermediate stage in fatty liver disease characterized by the accumulation of fat droplets in the hepatocytes and the presence of fibrous tissue and acute and chronic inflammatory cells

pancreaticoduodenectomy (Whipple procedure) excision of the head of the pancreas along with the encircling loop of the duodenum; may include partial gastrectomy

pancreatitis inflammation of the pancreas caused by auto-digestion of pancreatic tissue by its own enzymes

paracentesis a procedure during which fluid from the abdomen (ascites) is removed through a needle

portal hypertension abnormally increased blood pressure in the portal venous system due to the obstruction of blood flow through the liver

portal systemic encephalopathy hepatic encephalopathy

primary biliary cirrhosis (PBC) an immune-mediated chronic cirrhosis of the liver caused by obstruction or infection of the small and intermediate-size intrahepatic bile ducts; the extrahepatic biliary tree and larger intrahepatic ducts are normal; 90% of patients are women

secondary biliary cirrhosis liver damage that results from bile backup as a result of gallbladder disease

steatorrhea presence of excess fat in the stool

varices low-pressure veins that become distended from increased pressure; most commonly develop in the lower esophagus and upper stomach

Wernicke's encephalopathy condition of damage to the central nervous system from thiamin deficiency; common with alcoholism

Wilson's disease autosomal-recessive disorder of copper metabolism in which excessive accumulation of copper occurs in the liver, central nervous system, and kidney

The liver is an organ of primary importance to the body. One cannot survive without a liver. The pancreas and liver are essential to digestion and metabolism. Although it is important, the gallbladder can be removed, and the body will adapt comfortably to its absence. Knowledge of the structure and functions of these organs is vital, and, when they are diseased, the necessary medical nutrition therapy (MNT) is complex.

PHYSIOLOGY AND FUNCTIONS OF THE LIVER

Structure

The liver is the largest gland in the body, weighing about 1500 g. The liver has two main lobes: the right and left. The right lobe is further divided into the anterior and posterior segments; the right segmental fissure, which cannot be seen externally, separates the segments. The externally visible falciform ligament divides the left lobe into the medial and lateral segments. The liver is supplied with blood from two sources: the hepatic artery, which supplies about one third of the blood from the aorta; and the portal vein, which supplies the other two thirds and collects blood drained from the digestive tract.

About 1500 ml of blood per minute circulates through the liver and exits via the right and left hepatic veins into the inferior vena cava. Just as there is a system of blood vessels throughout the liver, there also exists a series of bile ducts. **Bile,** which is formed in the liver cells, exits the liver through a series of bile ducts that increase in size as they approach the common bile duct. It is a thick, viscous fluid secreted from the liver, stored in the gallbladder, and released into duodenum when fatty foods enter the duodenum. It emulsifies fats in the intestine and forms compounds with fatty acids to facilitate their absorption.

Functions

The liver has the ability to regenerate itself. Only 10% to 20% of functioning liver is required to sustain life, although removal of the liver will result in death within 24 hours. The liver is integral to most metabolic functions of the body and performs more than 500 tasks. The main functions of the liver include metabolism of carbohydrate, protein, and fat; storage and activation of vitamins and minerals; formation and excretion of bile; conversion of ammonia to urea; metabolism of steroids; and action as a filter and flood chamber.

The liver plays a major role in carbohydrate metabolism. Galactose and fructose, products of carbohydrate digestion, are converted into glucose in the hepatocyte or liver cell. The liver stores glucose as glycogen (glycogenesis) and then returns it to the blood when glucose levels become low (glycogenolysis). The liver also produces "new" glucose (gluconeogenesis) from precursors such as lactic acid, glycogenic amino acids, and intermediates of the tricarboxylic acid cycle (see Chapter 3).

Important protein metabolic pathways occur in the liver. Transamination and oxidative deamination are two such pathways that convert amino acids to substrates that are used in energy and glucose production as well as in the synthesis of nonessential amino acids. Blood-clotting factors such as fibrinogen; prothrombin; and serum proteins, including albumin, α-globulin, β-globulin, transferrin, ceruloplasmin, and lipoproteins are formed by the liver.

Fatty acids from the diet and adipose tissue are converted in the liver to acetyl-coenzyme A (CoA) by the process of β-oxidation to produce energy. Ketone bodies are also produced. The liver synthesizes and hydrolyzes triglycerides, phospholipids, cholesterol, and lipoproteins as well.

The liver is involved in the storage, activation, and transport of many vitamins and minerals. It stores all the fat-soluble vitamins in addition to vitamin B_{12} and the minerals zinc, iron, copper and magnesium. Hepatically synthesized proteins transport vitamin A, iron, zinc, and copper in the bloodstream. Carotene is converted to vitamin A, folate to 5-methyl tetrahydrofolic acid, and vitamin D to an active form (25-hydroxycholecalciferol) by the liver.

In addition to functions of nutrient metabolism and storage, the liver forms and excretes bile. Bile salts are metabolized and used for the digestion and absorption of fats and fat-soluble vitamins. Bilirubin is a metabolic end product from red blood cell destruction; it is conjugated and excreted in the bile.

Hepatocytes detoxify ammonia by converting it to urea, 75% of which is excreted by the kidneys. The remaining urea finds its way back to the gastrointestinal tract.

The liver also metabolizes steroids. It inactivates and excretes aldosterone, glucocorticoids, estrogen, progesterone, and testosterone. It is responsible for the detoxification of substances, including drugs and alcohol.

Finally, the liver acts as a filter and flood chamber by removing bacteria and debris from blood through the phagocytic action of **Kupffer cells** located in the sinusoids and by storing blood backed up from the vena cava as in right heart failure.

LABORATORY ASSESSMENT OF LIVER FUNCTION

Biochemical markers are used to evaluate and monitor patients having or suspected of having liver disease. Enzyme assays measure the release of liver enzymes, and other tests measure liver function. Screening tests for hepatobiliary disease include serum levels of bilirubin, alkaline phosphatase, aspartate amino transferase, and alanine aminotransferase. Table 28-1 elaborates common laboratory tests for liver disorders (see also Appendix 30).

TABLE 28-1

Common Laboratory Tests Used To Test Liver Function

Laboratory Test	Comment
Hepatic Excretion	
Total serum bilirubin	When increased, may indicate bilirubin overproduction or defect in hepatic uptake or conjugation
Indirect serum bilirubin	Unconjugated bilirubin; increased with excessive bilirubin production (hemolysis), immaturity of enzyme systems, inherited defects, drug effects
Direct serum bilirubin	Conjugated bilirubin; increased with depressed bilirubin excretion, hepatobiliary disease, intrahepatic or extrahepatic cholestasis, benign postoperative jaundice and sepsis, and congenital conjugated hyperbilirubinemia
Urine bilirubin	More sensitive than total serum bilirubin; confirms if liver disease is cause of jaundice
Urine urobilinogen	Used when obstructive jaundice is expected; rarely used
Serum bile acids	Reflects efficacy of ileal resorption and hepatic extraction of bile acids from portal circulation; levels increase with liver disease; little clinical use
Cholestasis	
Serum alkaline phosphatase	Enzyme widely distributed in liver, bone, placenta, intestine, kidney, leukocytes; mainly bound to canalicular membranes in liver; increased levels suggest cholestasis but can be increased with bone disorders, pregnancy, normal growth, and some malignancies
5′-Nucleotidase (5′ NT)	Enzyme present in canalicular and plasma membranes of hepatocytes; also in heart and pancreas; increases with liver disease
Leucine aminopeptidase (LAP)	Cellular peptidase; usually increased in cholestasis and suggests hepatobiliary origin of elevation of alkaline phosphatase; may also increase with pregnancy
γ-Glutamyl transpeptidase (GGT)	Enzyme associated with microsomes and plasma membranes in hepatocytes; also present in kidney, pancreas, heart, brain; increased with liver disease, but also after myocardial infarction, in neuromuscular disease, pancreatic disease, pulmonary disease, diabetes mellitus, and during alcohol ingestion
Hepatic Enzymes	
Alanine aminotransferase (ALT, formerly SGPT)	Located in cytosol of hepatocyte; found in several other body tissues but highest in liver; increased with liver cell damage
Aspartate aminotransferase (AST, formerly SGOT)	Located in cytosol and mitochondria of hepatocyte; also in cardiac and skeletal muscle, brain, pancreas, kidney, and leukocytes; increased with liver cell damage
Serum lactic dehydrogenase	Located in liver, red blood cells, cardiac muscle, kidney; increased with liver disease but lacks sensitivity and specificity because it is found in most other body tissues

Data from Baker AL: Liver chemistry tests. In Kaplowitz N, editor: *Liver and biliary diseases*, ed 2, Baltimore, 1996, Williams & Wilkins; Hoofnagle JH, Lindsay KL: Acute viral hepatitis. In Goldman L, Bennett JC, editors: *Cecil textbook of medicine*, ed 21, Philadelphia, 2000, Saunders; Kamath PS: Clinical approach to the patient with abnormal liver test results, *Mayo Clin Proc* 71:1089, 1996; Lindsay KL, Hoofnagle JH: Serologic tests for viral hepatitis. In Kaplowitz N, editor: *Liver and biliary diseases*, ed 2, Baltimore, 1996, Williams & Wilkins; Weisiger RA: Laboratory tests in liver disease. In Goldman L, Bennett JC, editors: *Cecil textbook of medicine*, ed 21, Philadelphia, 2000, Saunders.

HAV, Hepatic A virus; *HBc*, hepatitis B core; *HbeAG*, hepatitis B antigen; *HbsAG*, hepatitis B surface antigen; *HCV*, hepatitis C virus; *HDV*, hepatitis D virus; *HEV*, hepatitis E virus; *IgG*, immunoglobin G; *IgM*, immunoglobulin M; *PBC*, primary biliary cirrhosis.

Continued

TABLE 28-1

Common Laboratory Tests Used To Test Liver Function—cont'd

Laboratory Test	Comment
Serum Proteins	
Prothrombin time (PT)	Most blood coagulation factors are synthesized in the liver; vitamin K deficiency and decreased synthesis of clotting factors increase prothrombin time and risk of bleeding
Partial thromboplastin time (PTT)	Assesses the "intrinsic" clotting mechanism; reflects activity of all clotting factors except platelet factor E, factors VII and XII; complementary to PT
Serum albumin	Main export protein synthesized in the liver and most important factor in maintaining plasma oncotic pressure; decreased synthesis occurs with liver dysfunction, thyroid and glucocorticoid hormone dysfunction, abnormal plasma colloid osmotic pressure, and toxins; increased losses occur with protein-losing enteropathy, nephrotic syndrome, burns, gastrointestinal bleeding, exfoliative dermatitis
Serum globulin	α_1 and α_2-globulins are synthesized in the liver; levels increase with chronic liver disease; limited diagnostic use in hepatobiliary disease
Mitochondrial antibody	90% of patients with PBC have antibodies in their serum against a lipoprotein component of the inner mitochondrial membrane; also present in 25% of patients with chronic active hepatitis and postnecrotic cirrhosis
Antinuclear and smooth-muscle antibodies	May be positive in patients with chronic active hepatitis (usually not associated with hepatitis B or C virus) and in a minority of patients with PBC; not organ or species specific
Markers of Specific Liver Diseases	
Serum ferritin	Major iron storage protein; increased level sensitive indicator of genetic hemochromatosis
Ceruloplasmin	Major copper-binding protein synthesized by liver; decreased in Wilson's disease
α-Fetoprotein	Major circulating plasma protein; increased with hepatocellular carcinoma
α_1-Antitrypsin	Main function is to inhibit serum trypsin activity; decreased levels indicate α_1-antitrypsin deficiency, which can cause liver and lung damage
Markers for Viral Hepatitis	
IgM anti-HAV	Marker for hepatitis A; indicates current or recent infection or convalescence
IgG anti-HAV	Marker for hepatitis A; indicates current or previous infection and immunity
HbsAG	Marker for hepatitis B; positive in most cases of acute or chronic infection
HbeAG	Marker for hepatitis B; transiently positive during active virus replication; reflects concentration and infectivity of virus
IgM or IgG anti-HBc	Marker for hepatitis B; positive in all acute and chronic cases; positive in carriers; not protective
Anti-Hbe	Marker for hepatitis B; transiently positive during convalescence and in some chronic cases and carriers; not protective; reflects low infectivity
Anti-HBs	Marker for hepatitis B; positive late in convalescence; protective
Anti-HCV	Marker for hepatitis C; positive 5-6 weeks after onset of hepatitis C virus; not protective; reflects infectious state
HCV-RNA	Marker for hepatitis C
IgM or IgG anti-HDV	Marker for hepatitis D; indicates infection; not protective
IgM anti-HEV	Marker for hepatitis E; indicates current or recent infection; not protective
IgG anti-HEV	Marker for hepatitis E; indicates current or previous infection and immunity
Miscellaneous	
Ammonia	Liver converts ammonia to urea; may increase with hepatic failure and portal-systemic shunts

DISEASES OF THE LIVER

Diseases of the liver can be acute or chronic, inherited or acquired. Liver disease is classified in various ways: acute viral hepatitis, fulminant hepatitis, chronic hepatitis, non-alcoholic steatohepatitis (NASH), alcoholic hepatitis and **cirrhosis**, cholestatic liver diseases, inherited disorders, and other liver diseases.

Acute Viral Hepatitis

Acute viral **hepatitis** is a widespread inflammation of the liver and is caused by hepatitis viruses A, B, C, D, and E (Figure 28-1). Hepatitis A and E are the infectious forms (mainly spread by fecal-oral route) and hepatitis B, C, and D are the serum forms (spread by blood and body fluids) (Hoofnagle and Lindsay, 2004). Minor agents such as Epstein-Barr virus, cytomegalovirus, herpes simplex, yellow fever, and rubella can also cause an acute hepatitis.

Hepatitis A

Hepatitis A (HAV) is transmitted by the fecal-oral route and is contracted through contaminated drinking water, food, and sewage. Anorexia is the most frequent symptom, and it can be severe. Other common symptoms include nausea,

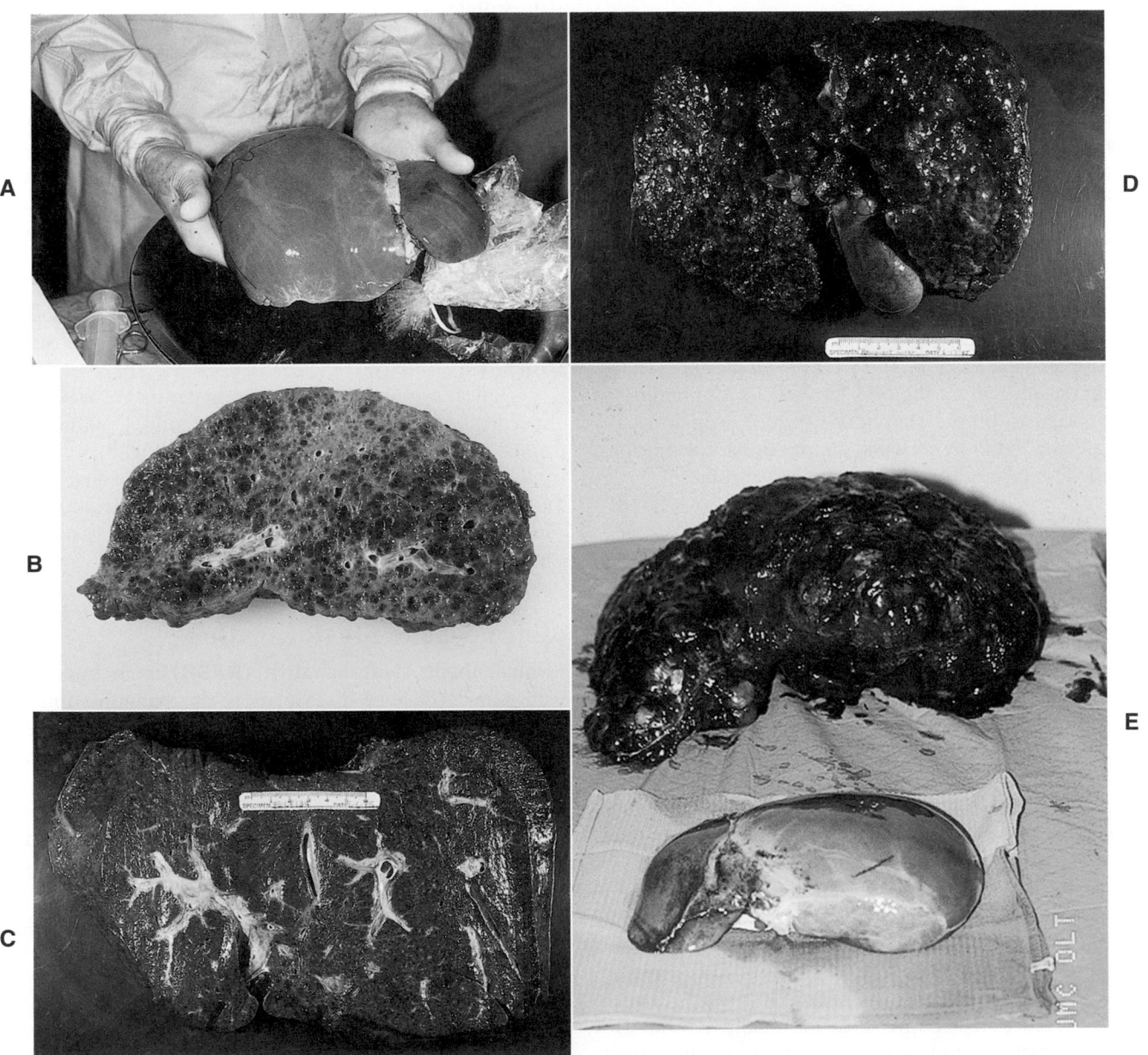

FIGURE 28-1 A, Normal liver. **B,** Liver with damage from chronic active hepatitis. **C,** Liver with damage from sclerosing cholangitis. **D,** Liver with damage from primary biliary cirrhosis. **E,** Liver with damage from polycystic liver disease *(background)* and normal liver *(foreground)*. *(Courtesy Baylor Regional Transplant Institute, Baylor University Medical Center, Dallas, Tex.)*

vomiting, right upper quadrant abdominal pain, dark urine, and **jaundice (icterus).** Recovery is usually complete, and long-term consequences are rare. Serious complications may occur in high-risk patients; subsequently, great attention must be given to adequate nutritional intake.

Hepatitis B and C

Hepatitis B (HBV) and hepatitis C (HCV) can lead to chronic and carrier states. HBV and HCV are transmitted via blood, blood products, semen, and saliva. For example, they can be spread from contaminated needles, blood transfusions, open cuts or wounds, splashes of blood into the mouth or eyes, or sexual contact. Chronic active hepatitis can also develop, leading to cirrhosis and liver failure.

Hepatitis D

The hepatitis D virus (HDV) is rare in the United States and depends on the HBV for survival and propagation in humans. HDV may be a coinfection (occurring at the same time as HBV) or a superinfection (superimposing itself on the HBV carrier state) (Hoofnagle and Lindsay, 2004). This form of hepatitis usually becomes chronic.

Hepatitis E

Hepatitis E virus (HEV) is rare in the United States (typically only occurs when imported), but it is reported more frequently in many countries of southern, eastern, and central Asia; northern, eastern, and western Africa; and Mexico. HEV is transmitted via the oral-fecal route. Contaminated water appears to be the source of infection, which usually afflicts people living in crowded and unsanitary conditions. Hepatitis E is generally acute rather than chronic.

Hepatitis G/GB

Hepatitis G virus (HGV) and a virus labeled GB-C (GBV-C) appear to be variants of the same virus. Although HGV infection is present in a significant proportion of blood donors and is transmitted through blood transfusions, it does not appear to cause liver disease (Berenguer et al., 2002).

The general symptoms of acute viral hepatitis are divided into four phases. The first phase, the early *prodromal* phase, affects about 25% of patients, causing fever, arthralgia, arthritis, rash, and angioedema. This is followed by the *preicteric* phase, in which malaise, fatigue, myalgia, anorexia, nausea, and vomiting occur. Some patients complain of epigastric or right upper quadrant pain. The third phase is the *icteric* phase, in which jaundice appears. Finally, during the *convalescent* phase, jaundice and other symptoms begin to subside.

Complete recovery is expected in 95% of HAV cases, in 90% of acute HBV cases, but in only 15% to 45% of acute HCV cases. Chronic hepatitis does not usually develop with HEV, and symptoms and liver function tests usually normalize within 6 weeks (Hoofnagle and Lindsay, 2004).

Fulminant Hepatitis

Fulminant hepatitis is a syndrome in which severe liver dysfunction is accompanied by **hepatic encephalopathy,** a clinical syndrome characterized by impaired mentation, neuromuscular disturbances, and altered consciousness. **Fulminant liver disease** is defined by the absence of pre-existing liver disease and the development of hepatic encephalopathy within 2 to 8 weeks of the onset of illness (Keefe, 2004). The causes of fulminant hepatitis include viral hepatitis (about 75% of cases), chemical toxicity (e.g., acetaminophen, drug reactions, poisonous mushrooms, industrial poisons), and other causes (e.g., Wilson's disease, fatty liver of pregnancy, Reye's syndrome, hepatic ischemia, hepatic vein obstruction, and disseminated malignancies). Extrahepatic complications of fulminant hepatitis are cerebral edema, coagulopathy and bleeding, cardiovascular abnormalities, renal failure, pulmonary complications, acid-base disturbances, electrolyte imbalances, sepsis, and pancreatitis.

Chronic Hepatitis

To be defined as chronic hepatitis, a patient must have at least a 6-month course of hepatitis or biochemical and clinical evidence of liver disease with confirmatory biopsy findings of unresolving hepatic inflammation (Lindsay and Hoofnagle, 2004). Chronic hepatitis can have autoimmune, viral, metabolic, or medicine or toxin etiologies. The most common causes of chronic hepatitis are hepatitis B, hepatitis C, and autoimmune hepatitis. Other common causes are drug-induced liver disease, metabolic diseases, and NASH. Cryptogenic cirrhosis is cirrhosis of an unknown etiology.

Clinical symptoms of chronic hepatitis are usually nonspecific, occur intermittently, and are mild. Common symptoms include fatigue, sleep disorders, difficulty concentrating, and mild right upper quadrant pain. Severe advanced disease can lead to jaundice, muscle wasting, tea-colored urine, ascites, edema, hepatic encephalopathy, gastrointestinal bleeding, splenomegaly, palmar erythema, and spider angiomata.

Nonalcoholic Steatohepatitis

Nonalcoholic steatohepatitis (NASH) is an intermediate stage in fatty liver disease. It is the accumulation of fat droplets in the hepatocytes, which are surrounded by acute and chronic inflammatory cells. Steatohepatitis is associated with accumulation of fibrous tissue in the liver. Nonalcoholic causes include drugs, inborn errors of metabolism, and acquired metabolic disorders (type 2 diabetes mellitus, lipodystrophy, jejunal ileal bypass, obesity, malnutrition) (Diehl, 2004).

Patients with NASH may be asymptomatic but can experience malaise, weakness, or hepatomegaly. The treatment is often weight loss (although extreme, rapid weight loss can accelerate NASH developing into cirrhosis and increase the chance of gallstone development), the use of insulin-sensitizing drugs, treatment of the dyslipidemia, and administration of ursodeoxycholic acid. Chronic liver disease and cirrhosis can develop in patients with NASH, and the progression to cirrhosis is variable, depending on age and the presence of obesity and type 2 diabetes, which contribute to a worsening prognosis (Diehl, 2004).

Alcoholic Liver Disease

Alcoholic liver disease is the most common liver disease in the United States accounting for 50% of all chronic liver disease (Kim et al., 2002). According to the National Institute on Alcohol and Alcohol Abuse, 4.65% of adults in the United States abuse alcohol or are alcoholics. Alcohol problems are highest among young adults 18 to 29 years of age and lowest among adults ages 65 and older (www.niaaa.nih.gov). Acetaldehyde, a toxic by-product of alcohol metabolism, causes damage to mitochondrial membrane structure and function. Acetaldehyde is produced by multiple metabolic pathways, one of which involves alcohol dehydrogenase (see *Focus On:* Metabolic Consequences of Alcohol Consumption).

Several variables predispose some people to alcoholic liver disease. These include genetic polymorphisms of alcohol-metabolizing enzymes, gender (female more than male), simultaneous exposure to other drugs, infections with hepatotropic viruses, immunologic factors, and poor nutrition status. The pathogenesis of alcoholic liver disease progresses in three stages (Figure 28-2): hepatic steatosis (Figure 28-3), alcoholic hepatitis, and finally cirrhosis.

Hepatic Steatosis

Fatty infiltration or **hepatic steatosis** or **fatty liver** is caused by a culmination of these metabolic disturbances: (1) an increase in the mobilization of fatty acids from adipose tissue; (2) an increase in hepatic synthesis of fatty acids; (3) a decrease in fatty acid oxidation; (4) an increase in triglyceride production; and (5) a trapping of triglycerides in the liver. Hepatic steatosis is reversible with abstinence from alcohol. Conversely, if alcohol abuse continues, cirrhosis can develop.

Alcoholic Hepatitis

Alcoholic hepatitis is generally characterized by hepatomegaly, modest elevation of transaminase levels, increased serum bilirubin concentrations, normal or depressed serum albumin concentrations, or anemia. Patients may also have abdominal pain, anorexia, nausea, vomiting, weakness, diarrhea, weight loss, or fever. If patients discontinue alcohol intake, hepatitis may resolve; however, the condition often progresses to the third stage. Nutrition support is the main treatment in addition to counseling or support to continue avoidance of alcohol. Molecular genetics may lead to new therapies in the future (Willner and Reuben, 2005).

Alcoholic Cirrhosis

Clinical features of the third stage, alcoholic **cirrhosis** vary. Symptoms can mimic those of alcoholic hepatitis; or patients can develop gastrointestinal bleeding, hepatic encephalopathy, or **portal hypertension** (i.e., elevated blood pressure in the portal venous system caused by the obstruction of blood flow through the liver) and other symptoms of liver disease. They can also develop **ascites,** the accumulation of fluid, serum protein, and electrolytes within the peritoneal cavity caused by increased pressure from portal hypertension and decreased production of albumin (which maintains serum colloidal osmotic pressure). A liver biopsy usually reveals micronodular cirrhosis, but it can be macronodular or mixed. Prognosis depends on abstinence from alcohol and the degree of complications already developed. Ethanol ingestion creates specific and severe nutritional abnormalities (see *Clinical Insight:* Malnutrition in the Alcoholic).

Cholestatic Liver Diseases

Primary Biliary Cirrhosis

Primary biliary cirrhosis (PBC) is a chronic cholestatic disease caused by progressive destruction of small and intermediate-size intrahepatic bile ducts. The extrahepatic biliary tree and larger intrahepatic ducts are normal. Ninety percent of patients with PBC are women; this disease progresses slowly, eventually resulting in cirrhosis and portal hypertension and liver transplantation or death.

PBC is an immune-mediated disease in which serum autoantibodies, elevated immunoglobulin levels, circulating immune complexes, and depressed cell-mediated immune response are present. PBC typically presents with a mild elevation of liver enzymes with physical symptoms of pruri-

© **FOCUS ON**

Metabolic Consequences of Alcohol Consumption

Ethanol is metabolized primarily in the liver by alcohol dehydrogenase. This results in acetaldehyde production with the transfer of hydrogen to nicotinamide adenine dinucleotide (NAD), reducing it to NADH. The acetaldehyde then loses hydrogen and is converted to acetate, most of which is released into the blood.

Many metabolic disturbances occur because of the excess of NADH, which overrides the ability of the cell to maintain a normal redox state. These include hyperlacticacidemia, acidosis, hyperuricemia, ketonemia, and hyperlipemia. The tricarboxylic acid (TCA) cycle is depressed because it requires NAD. The mitochondria, in turn, use hydrogen from ethanol rather than from the oxidation of fatty acids to produce energy via the TCA cycle, which leads to a decreased fatty acid oxidation and accumulation of triglycerides. In addition, NADH may actually promote fatty acid synthesis. Hypoglycemia can also occur in early alcoholic liver disease secondary to the suppression of the TCA cycle, coupled with decreased gluconeogenesis due to ethanol.

$$C_2H_2OH + NAD \xrightarrow{\text{alcohol dehydrogenase}} $$
$$\text{ethanol}$$

$$NADH + CH_3—CHO$$
$$\text{acetaldehyde}$$

$$CH_3\text{-}CHO + NADH + H_2O \xrightarrow{\text{alcohol dehydrogenase}} :$$
$$\text{acetaldehyde}$$

$$NAD + H^+ + CH_3\text{-}CHOOH$$
$$\text{acetate}$$

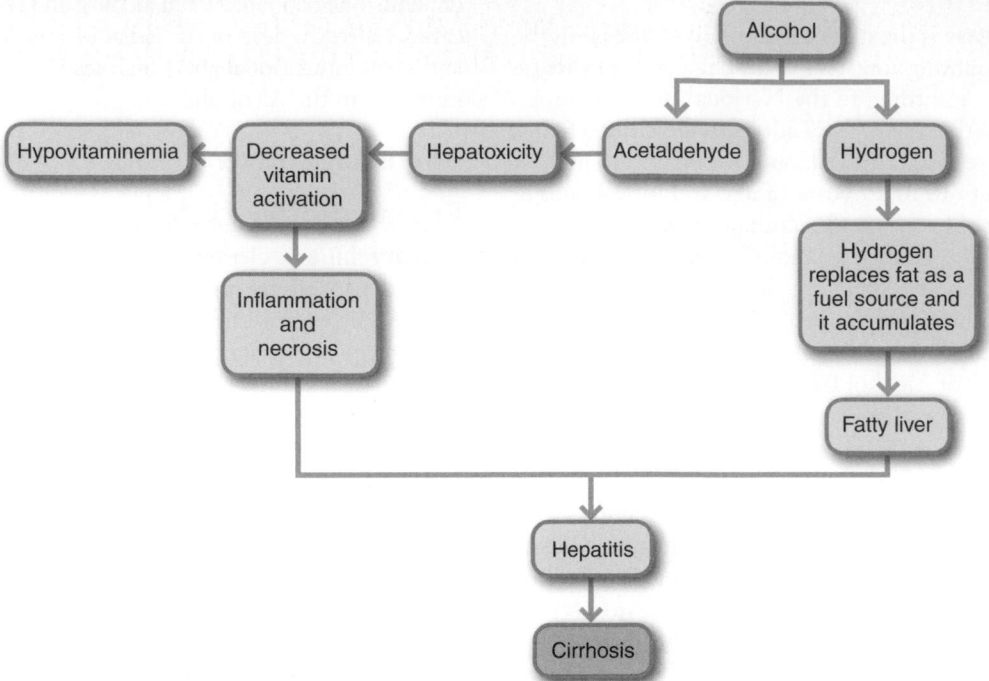

FIGURE 28-2 Complications of excessive alcohol consumption stem largely from excess hydrogen and from acetaldehyde. Hydrogen produces fatty liver and hyperlipemia, high blood lactic acid, and low blood sugar. The accumulation of fat, the effect of acetaldehyde on liver cells, and other factors as yet unknown lead to alcoholic hepatitis. The next step is cirrhosis. The consequent impairment of liver function disturbs blood chemistry, notably causing a high ammonia level that can lead to coma and death. Cirrhosis also distorts liver structure, inhibiting blood flow. High pressure in vessels supplying the liver may cause ruptured varices and accumulation of fluid in the abdominal cavity. Response to alcohol differs among individuals; in particular, not all heavy drinkers develop hepatitis and cirrhosis.

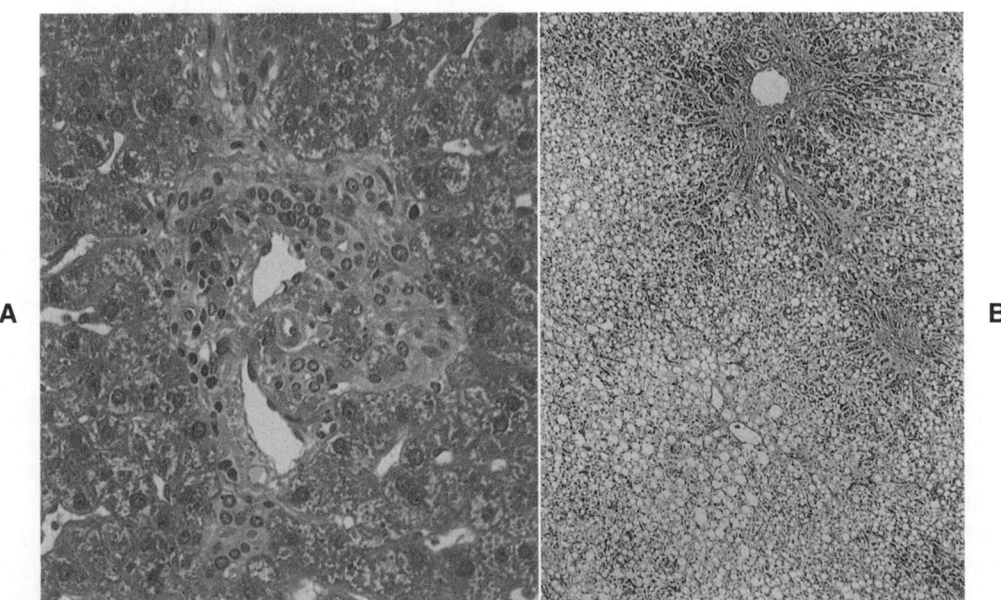

FIGURE 28-3 A, Microscopic appearance of a normal liver. A normal portal tract consists of the portal vein, hepatic arteriole, one to two interlobular bile ducts, and occasional peripherally located ductules. **B,** Acute fatty liver. This photomicrograph on low power exhibits fatty change involving virtually all the hepatocytes, with slight sparing of the liver cells immediately adjacent to the portal tract *(top)*. *(From Kanel G, Korula J:* Atlas of liver pathology, *Philadelphia, 1992, Saunders.)*

Malnutrition in the Alcoholic

Several factors contribute to the malnutrition that is common in chronic alcoholics with liver disease:

1. Alcohol can replace food in the diet of moderate and heavy drinkers, displacing the intake of adequate calories and nutrients. In light drinkers it is usually an additional energy source (Stickel et al., 2003), also called *empty calories*. Although alcohol yields 7.1 kcal/g, when it is consumed in large amounts it is not used efficiently as a fuel source. When individuals consume alcohol on a regular basis but do not fulfill criteria for alcohol abuse, they are often overweight because of increase in calories from alcohol (so-called *alcohol addition*). This is different from the heavy drinker who replaces calories with alcohol (alcohol substitution) (Stickel et al., 2003).

2. In the alcoholic impaired, digestion and absorption are related to pancreatic insufficiency, as well as morphologic and functional alterations of the intestinal mucosa (Stickel et al., 2003). Acute and chronic alcohol intake impairs hepatic amino acid uptake and synthesis into proteins, reduces protein synthesis and secretion from the liver, and increases catabolism in the gut (Stickel et al., 2003).

3. Use of lipids and carbohydrates is compromised. An excess of reduction equivalents (e.g., NADPH) and impaired oxidation of triglycerides result in fat deposition in the hepatocytes and an increase in circulating triglycerides (Stickel et al., 2003). Insulin resistance is also common among alcoholics.

4. Vitamin and mineral deficiencies occur in alcoholic liver disease as a result of reduced intake and alterations in absorption, storage, and ability to convert the nutrients to their active forms (Leevy and Moroianu, 2005). Steatorrhea resulting from bile acid deficiency is also common in alcoholic liver disease affecting fat-soluble vitamin absorption. Vitamin A deficiency can lead to night blindness (Leevy and Moroianu, 2005; Stickel et al., 2003). Thiamin deficiency is the most common vitamin deficiency in alcoholics and is responsible for Wernicke's encephalopathy (Leevy and Moroianu, 2005). Folate deficiency can occur as a result of poor intake, impaired absorption, accelerated excretion, and altered storage and metabolism. Inadequate dietary intake and interactions between pyridoxal-5'-phosphate (active coenzyme of vitamin B_6) and alcohol reduce vitamin B_6 nutriture (Stickel et al., 2003). Deficiency of all B vitamins and vitamins C, D, E, and K is also common (Leevy and Moroianu, 2005). Hypocalcemia, hypomagnesemia, and hypophosphatemia are not uncommon among alcoholics; furthermore, zinc deficiency and alterations in other micronutrients can accompany chronic alcohol intake (Leevy and Moroianu, 2005).

---

tus and fatigue. Treatment with ursodeoxycholic acid can slow progression of the disease. Several nutritional complications from cholestasis can occur with PBC, including osteopenia, hypercholesterolemia, and fat-soluble vitamin deficiencies (Friedman and Schiano, 2004).

Sclerosing Cholangitis

Sclerosing cholangitis is another chronic cholestatic liver disease. Fibrosing inflammation of segments of extrahepatic bile ducts, with or without involvement of intrahepatic ducts, characterizes the disease. Progression of the disease leads to complications of portal hypertension, **hepatic failure** (liver function diminished to 25% or less), and cholangiocarcinoma. Primary sclerosing cholangitis (PSC) is the most common type of sclerosing cholangitis.

In general, PSC lacks any apparent etiology and usually occurs in association with inflammatory bowel disease (Mahadevan et al., 2002). Like PBC, PSC may be an immune disorder because of its strong association with human leukocyte antigen haplotypes, autoantibodies, and multiple immunologic abnormalities. Seventy to 90% of patients with PSC also have inflammatory bowel disease (especially ulcerative colitis), and men are more likely than women (2.3:1) to have PSC (Afdhal, 2004). Patients with PSC are also at increased risk of fat-soluble vitamin deficiencies resulting from steatorrhea associated with this disease.

Hepatic osteodystrophy may occur from vitamin D and calcium malabsorption, resulting in secondary hyperparathyroidism and osteomalacia or rickets (Klein et al., 2002). No treatment slows progression of the disease or improves survival. Ursodeoxycholic acid may improve laboratory values (serum bilirubin, alkaline phosphatase, and albumin) but has no effect on survival (Afdhal, 2004).

Inherited Disorders

Inherited disorders of the liver include hemochromatosis, Wilson's disease, α_1-antitrypsin deficiency, protoporphyria, cystic fibrosis, glycogen storage disease, amyloidosis, and sarcoidosis. The first three disorders are the most commonly inherited disorders resulting in liver failure. Hemochromatosis is an inherited disease of iron overload. Patients with hereditary hemochromatosis absorb excessive iron from the gut and may store 20 to 40 g of iron compared with 0.3 to 0.8 g in normal persons (see Chapter 31).

A gene, HFE, is associated with hereditary hemochromatosis (Maher, 2004). Hepatomegaly, esophageal **varices,** ascites, impaired hepatic synthetic function, abnormal skin pigmentation, glucose intolerance, cardiac involvement, hypogonadism, arthropathy, and hepatocellular carcinoma may develop. Early diagnosis includes clinical, laboratory, and pathologic testing, including elevated serum transferrin levels. Increased transferrin saturation ($\geq$45%) and ferritin (more than two times normal) are suggestive of hemochromatosis (Maher, 2004) (see Chapter 15). Life expectancy is normal if phlebotomy is initiated before the development of cirrhosis or diabetes mellitus (Brandhagen et al., 2002).

Wilson's disease is an autosomal-recessive disorder associated with impaired biliary copper excretion. Copper accumulates in various tissues, including the liver, brain, cornea, and kidneys. Low serum ceruloplasmin levels and the presence of **Kayser-Fleischer rings,** (greenish yellow pigmented rings encircling the cornea just within the corneoscleral margin, formed by copper deposits) confirm the diagnosis, although patients with this disease may consult a physician before these confirming symptoms develop. Patients can present with acute, fulminant, or chronic active hepatitis. Liver and neurologic signs may be the first signs of illness (Medici et al., 2006).

Copper-chelating agents and possibly zinc supplementation (to inhibit intestinal copper absorption and binding in the liver) are used to treat Wilson's disease once it is diagnosed. Copper chelation improves survival but does not prevent cirrhosis; transplantation corrects the meta-

TABLE 28-2

Copper Content of Commonly Used Foods*

Food Groups	High (>0.2 mg/Portion Commonly Used†) (Avoid)	Moderate (0.1-0.2 mg/Portion) (No More Than 6 Servings/Day)	Low (< 0.1 mg/ Portion Commonly Used†) (May Be Eaten As Desired)
Meat and meat substitutes	Lamb; pork; pheasant; quail; duck; goose; squid; salmon; all organ meats including liver, heart, kidney, brain; all shellfish, including oysters, scallops, shrimp, lobster, clams, and crab; meat gelatin; soy protein meat substitutes; tofu; all nuts and seeds	All other fish (3 oz), dark meat turkey (3 oz), peanut butter (2 tbsp)	Beef, cheese, cottage cheese, eggs, light meat turkey; cold cuts and frankfurters that do not contain pork, dark turkey or organ meats, all others not listed on high or moderate list
Fats and oil	Avocado	Olives (2 medium); cream (½ c)	Butter, cream, margarine, mayonnaise, nondairy cream substitutes, oils, sour cream, salad dressings (made from allowed ingredients), all others not listed on high or moderate list
Milk	Chocolate, cocoa, soy milk		All other daily products, milk flavored with carob

From Pemberton CM et al: *Mayo Clinic diet manual: a handbook of nutrition practices,* ed 7, St. Louis, 1994, Mosby.

*Data that are available on the average copper content of foods vary greatly. There is disagreement on the copper content of the usual American diet, with estimates that range from 1 mg of copper a day to 5 mg/day. The concentration of copper in foods is affected by many factors, including soil conditions, geographic location, species, diet, processing method, and contamination in processing. The exact copper content of foods is difficult to verify. It is estimated that avoiding high-copper foods and restricting moderate-copper foods result in a diet of approximately 1 mg/day. For practical purposes, diets are designed to limit foods with higher copper content rather than to achieve a specific level of copper in the diet.

†Portions commonly used are those generally accepted as typical portion sizes in various nutrient data source manuals.

‡A water sample from the patient's home water supply should be analyzed for copper content. Demineralized water should be used if the water contains more than 100 mcg/L.

§Although not necessarily high in copper, alcohol is discouraged because of its action as a hepatotoxin.

bolic defect (Maher, 2004). A low-copper diet is implemented if other therapies are unsuccessful (Table 28-2). If this disease is not diagnosed until onset of fulminant failure, survival is not possible without transplantation (Kayler et al., 2002).

α_1-Antitrypsin deficiency is another inherited disorder, and it can cause both liver and lung disease. α_1-Antitrypsin is a glycoprotein found in serum and body fluids; it inhibits neutrophil proteinases. Cholestasis or cirrhosis is caused by this deficiency and there is no treatment except liver transplantation (Maher, 2004).

Other Liver Diseases

Liver disease has several other causes. Liver tumors can be primary or metastatic, benign or malignant. Hepatocellular carcinoma usually develops in cirrhotic livers. The highest risk occurs in those with HBV, HCV, and hereditary hemochromatosis (Fallon, 2004). The liver can be affected when there is systemic disease such as rheumatoid arthritis, systemic lupus erythematosus, polymyalgia, rheumatic or temporal arteritis, polyarteritis nodosa, systemic sclerosis, and Sjögren's syndrome.

When hepatic blood flow is altered as in acute ischemic and chronic congestive hepatopathy, Budd-Chiari syndrome, and hepatic venoocclusive disease, hepatic dysfunction occurs. Individuals with hepatic or portal vein thromboses should be evaluated for a myeloproliferative disorder. Parasitic, bacterial, fungal, and granulomatous liver diseases also occur. Finally, cryptogenic cirrhosis is any cirrhosis for which the etiology is unknown.

TABLE 28-2

Copper Content of Commonly Used Foods*—cont'd

Food Groups	High (>0.2 mg/Portion Commonly Used†) (Avoid)	Moderate (0.1-0.2 mg/Portion) (No More Than 6 Servings/Day)	Low (< 0.1 mg/Portion Commonly Used†) (May Be Eaten As Desired)
Starch	Dried beans, including soybeans, lima beans, baked beans, garbanzo beans, pinto beans; dried peas; lentils; millet; barley; wheat germ; bran breads and cereals; cereals with >0.2 mg of copper per serving (check label); soy flour; soy grits; sweet potatoes (fresh)	Whole-wheat bread (1 slice), potatoes in any form (½ c or 1 small), pumpkin (¾ c), melba toast (4), whole-wheat crackers (6), parsnips (⅔ c), winter squash (½ c), green peas (½ c), instant oatmeal (½ c), instant Ralston (½ c), cereals with 0.1-0.2 mg of copper per serving (check labels), dehydrated and canned soups (1 c)	Breads and pasta from refined flour, canned sweet potatoes, rice, regular oatmeal, cereals with <0.1 mg of copper per serving (check label), all others not listed on high or moderate list
Vegetables	Mushrooms, vegetable juice cocktail	Bean sprouts (1 c), beets (½ c), spinach (½ c cooked, 1 c raw), tomato juice and other tomato products (½ c), broccoli (½ c), asparagus (½ c)	All others, including fresh tomatoes
Fruits	Nectarines; dried fruits, including raisins, dates, and prunes (dried fruits are permitted if dried at home)	Mango (½ c), pears (1 medium), pineapple (½ c), papaya ¼ average)	All others
Desserts	Desserts that contain significant amounts of any foods high in copper		All others
Sugar and sweets	Chocolate, cocoa	Licorice (1 oz), syrups (1 oz)	All others including jams, jellies, and candies made with allowed fruits; carob; flavoring extracts
Miscellaneous	Brewer's yeast	Ketchup	
Beverages‡	Instant breakfast beverages, mineral water, alcohol§	Postum and other cereal beverages	All others, including fruit-flavored beverages; lemonade

TREATMENT OF CIRRHOSIS AND ITS COMPLICATIONS

Cirrhosis has many clinical manifestations, as illustrated in Figure 28-4. Several major complications of cirrhosis and end-stage liver disease (ESLD), including malnutrition, ascites, hyponatremia, hepatic encephalopathy, glucose alterations, fat malabsorption, hepatorenal syndrome, and osteopenia have nutritional implications. When appropriate nutrition therapy is provided to patients with liver disease, malnutrition can be reversed, and clinical outcomes improved. Studies to date have been able to show positive outcomes with oral and enteral nutrition (EN) in malnourished patients with cirrhosis, including improvement in nutrition status and clinical complications of cirrhosis such as ascites, encephalopathy, and infection (Campillo et al., 2005; Cuhna et al., 2004).

Nutrition Assessment

Before appropriate nutrition therapy can be implemented, a nutrition assessment must be performed to determine the extent and cause of malnutrition. Many traditional markers of nutrition status are affected by liver disease and its consequences, making assessment difficult. Table 28-3 summarizes the factors that affect interpretation of nutrition assessment parameters in patients with liver dysfunction.

Objective parameters that may be helpful when monitored serially include anthropometric measurements and dietary intake evaluation (Hasse, 2001; McCullough, 2000) (see Chapter 14). The best way to perform a nutrition assessment may be to combine these parameters with the subjective global assessment (SGA) approach. The SGA has been used to evaluate patients with liver disease and transplantation and has demonstrated an acceptable level of reliability and validity (Detsky et al., 1987; Hasse et al., 1993; Stephenson et al., 2001). This method uses a few readily available parameters obtained by an experienced clinician. The SGA gives a broad perspective, but it is not sensitive to changes in nutrition status. Other available parameters should also be reviewed for their impact on the patient's overall health status. The elements of SGA in evaluating nutrition status are summarized in Box 28-1.

Malnutrition

Moderate-to-severe malnutrition is a common finding in patients with advanced liver disease (Figure 28-5). This is extremely significant, considering that malnutrition plays a major role in the pathogenesis of liver injury and has a profound negative impact on prognosis (Donaghy, 2002). The prevalence of malnutrition depends on nutrition assessment parameters used, type of liver disease, degree of liver disease, and socioeconomic status (Alberino et al., 2001; Alvares-da-Silva and Reverbel da Silveira T, 2005;

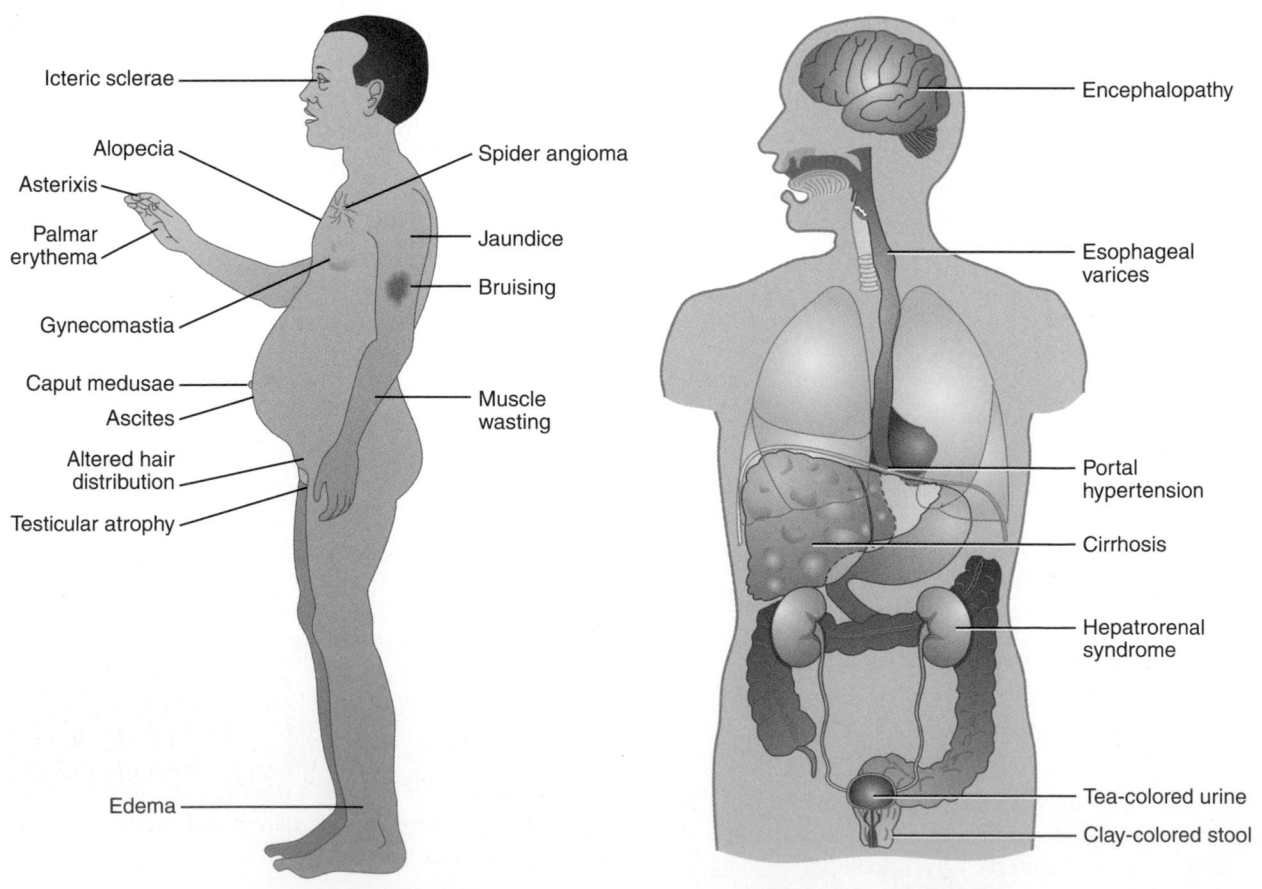

EXTERNAL SYMPTOMS **INTERNAL SYMPTOMS**

FIGURE 28-4 Clinical manifestations of cirrhosis.

TABLE 28-3

Factors That Affect Interpretation of Objective Nutrition Assessment Tests in Patients With End-Stage Liver Disease

Parameter	Factors Affecting Interpretation
Body weight	Affected by edema, ascites, and diuretic use
Anthropometric measurements	Questionable sensitivity, specificity, and reliability
	Multiple sources of error
	Unknown if skinfold measurements reflect total body fat
	References do not account for variation in hydration status and skin compressibility
Creatinine-height index	Affected by malnutrition, aging, decreased body mass, and protein intake
	Affected by renal function
	Creatinine is a metabolic end product of creatine synthesized in the liver; therefore severe liver disease alters creatinine synthesis rates
Nitrogen balance studies	Nitrogen is retained in the body in the form of ammonia
	Hepatorenal syndrome can affect the excretion of nitrogen
3-Methyl histidine excretion	Affected by dietary intake, trauma, infection, and renal function
Visceral protein levels	Synthesis of visceral proteins is decreased
Immune function tests	Affected by hydration status, malabsorption, and renal insufficiency
	Affected by hepatic failure, electrolyte imbalances, infection, and renal insufficiency
Bioelectrical impedance	Invalid with ascites and/or edema

Modified from Hasse J: Nutritional aspects of adult liver transplantation. In Busuttil RW, Klintmalm GB, editors: *Transplantation of the liver*, ed 2, Philadelphia, 2005, Saunders.

BOX 28-1

Subjective Global Assessment Parameters for Nutrition Evaluation of Liver Disease Patients

History

Weight change (consider fluctuations resulting from ascites and edema)
Appetite
Taste changes and early satiety
Dietary recall (calories, protein, sodium)
Persistent gastrointestinal problems (nausea, vomiting, diarrhea, constipation, difficulty chewing or swallowing)

Physical

Muscle wasting
Fat stores
Ascites or edema

Existing Conditions

Disease state and other problems that could influence nutrition status such as hepatic encephalopathy, gastrointestinal bleeding, renal insufficiency, infection

Nutritional Rating (based on results of parameters)

Well nourished
Moderately (or suspected of being) malnourished
Severely malnourished

From Hasse J: Nutritional aspects of adult liver transplantation. In Busuttil RW, Klintmalm GB, editors: *Transplantation of the liver*, ed 2, Philadelphia, 2005, Saunders.

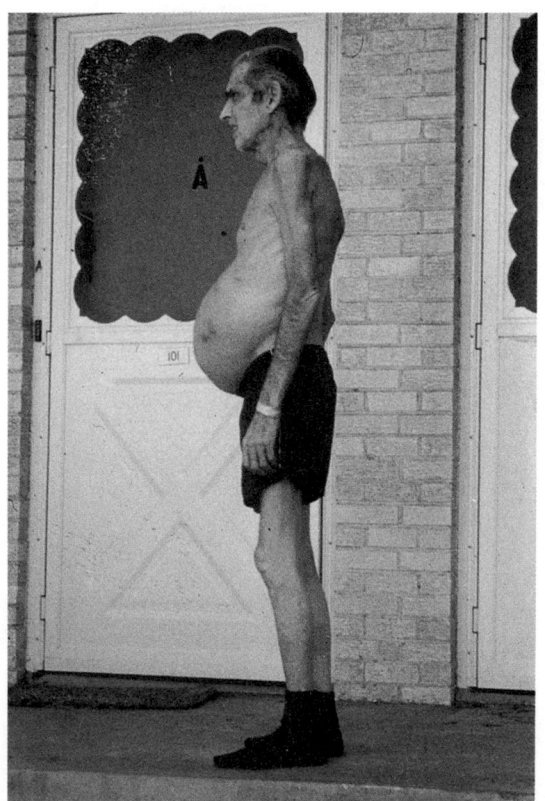

FIGURE 28-5 Severe malnutrition and ascites in a man with end-stage liver disease.

Campillo et al., 2003; Figueiredo et al., 2005; Zaina et al., 2004).

Numerous coexisting factors are involved in the development of malnutrition in liver disease (see *Pathophysiology and Care Management Algorithm:* Malnutrition in Liver Disease). Inadequate oral intake, a major contributor, is caused by anorexia, dysgeusia, early satiety, and nausea and vomiting associated with liver disease and the drugs used to treat it.

Other causes of inadequate intake are related to dietary restrictions and unpalatable hospital diets.

Maldigestion and malabsorption also play a role in the malnutrition of liver disease. **Steatorrhea,** or the presence of fat in the stool, is common in cirrhosis, especially if there is disease involving bile duct injury and obstruction. The medications previously mentioned may also cause specific malabsorptive losses. In addition, altered metabolism sec-

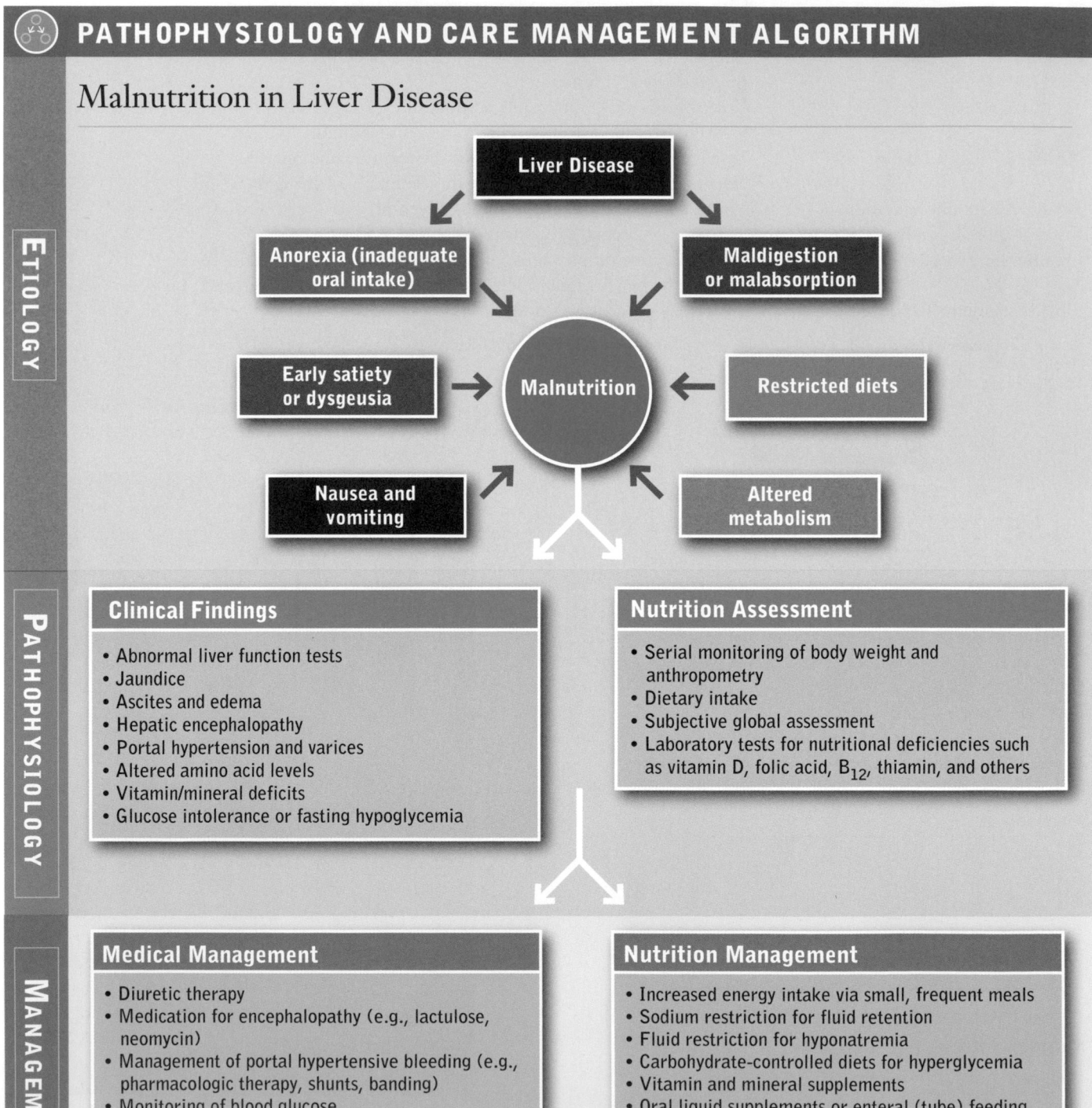

PATHOPHYSIOLOGY AND CARE MANAGEMENT ALGORITHM

Malnutrition in Liver Disease

ETIOLOGY

Liver Disease
→ Anorexia (inadequate oral intake)
→ Maldigestion or malabsorption
Early satiety or dysgeusia →
← Restricted diets
Nausea and vomiting →
← Altered metabolism
→ Malnutrition

PATHOPHYSIOLOGY

Clinical Findings
- Abnormal liver function tests
- Jaundice
- Ascites and edema
- Hepatic encephalopathy
- Portal hypertension and varices
- Altered amino acid levels
- Vitamin/mineral deficits
- Glucose intolerance or fasting hypoglycemia

Nutrition Assessment
- Serial monitoring of body weight and anthropometry
- Dietary intake
- Subjective global assessment
- Laboratory tests for nutritional deficiencies such as vitamin D, folic acid, B_{12}, thiamin, and others

MANAGEMENT

Medical Management
- Diuretic therapy
- Medication for encephalopathy (e.g., lactulose, neomycin)
- Management of portal hypertensive bleeding (e.g., pharmacologic therapy, shunts, banding)
- Monitoring of blood glucose

Nutrition Management
- Increased energy intake via small, frequent meals
- Sodium restriction for fluid retention
- Fluid restriction for hyponatremia
- Carbohydrate-controlled diets for hyperglycemia
- Vitamin and mineral supplements
- Oral liquid supplements or enteral (tube) feeding

Algorithm content developed by John J.B. Anderson, PhD, and Sanford C. Garner, PhD, 2000. Updated by Jeanette Hasse, PhD, RD, LD, CNSD, FADA, and Laura E. Matarese, MS, RD, LD, CNSD, FADA, 2006.

ondary to liver dysfunction causes malnutrition in various ways. Micronutrient function is affected by altered storage in the liver, decreased transport by liver-synthesized proteins, and renal losses associated with alcoholic and advanced liver disease. Abnormal macronutrient metabolism and increased energy expenditure can also contribute to malnutrition. Finally, protein losses can occur from large-volume **paracentesis** when fluid from the abdomen (ascites) is removed through a needle.

Problems in Feeding

Because anorexia, nausea, dysgeusia, and other gastrointestinal symptoms are common, adequate nutrition intake is difficult to achieve. With ascites, early satiety is also a frequent complaint. Smaller, more frequent meals are better tolerated than three traditional meals. In addition, evidence suggests that frequent feedings also improve nitrogen balance and prevent hypoglycemia. Oral liquid supplements should be encouraged, and, when necessary, enteral tube feedings used. Adjunctive nutrition support should be given to malnourished patients with liver disease if their intake is less than DRI levels of 0.8 g of protein and 30 calories per kilogram of body weight daily and if they are at risk for fatal complications from the disease. Esophageal varices are usually not a contraindication for tube feeding (Crippin, 2006).

Nutrient Requirements

Energy

Energy requirements vary among patients with cirrhosis. Several studies have measured resting energy expenditure (REE) in patients with liver disease to determine energy requirements. Some found that patients with ESLD had normal metabolism and that others had hypometabolic or hypermetabolic metabolism. Although several studies concluded that patients with cirrhosis did not require any more calories than did healthy controls, Dolz and colleagues (1991) determined that ascites increases energy expenditure slightly. On the other hand, two studies found REE increased at 3 or 6 months and again at 12 months after placement of a shunt (Allard et al., 2001; Plauth et al., 2004). However, this increase may be the result of the fact that dry body weight increased after the shunt placement.

In general, energy requirements for patients with ESLD and without ascites are about 120% to 140% of the REE. Requirements increase to 150% to 175% of REE if ascites, infection, or malabsorption is present or if nutritional repletion is necessary. This equates to about 25 to 35 calories per kilogram body weight; estimated dry body weight should be used in calculations to prevent overfeeding. Oral nutritional supplements or tube feeding can be effective in increasing or ensuring optimal intake in malnourished patients and reducing complications and prolonging survival (Plauth et al., 2006).

Carbohydrates

Determining carbohydrate needs is often challenging in liver failure because of the primary role of the liver in car-

bohydrate metabolism. Liver failure reduces glucose production and peripheral glucose use. The rate of gluconeogenesis is decreased, with preference for lipids and amino acids for energy. Alterations in the hormones insulin, glucagon, cortisol, and epinephrine are responsible in part for the preference for alternative fuels.

Lipid

In cirrhosis, plasma free fatty acids, glycerol, and ketone bodies are increased in the fasting state. The body prefers lipids as an energy substrate, and lipolysis is increased with active mobilization of lipid deposits, but the net capacity to store exogenous lipid is not impaired. A range of 25% to 40% of calories as fat is generally recommended.

Protein

Protein is by far the most controversial nutrient in liver failure, and its management is also the most complex. Cirrhosis has long been thought of as a catabolic disease with increased protein breakdown and inadequate resynthesis, resulting in depletion of visceral protein stores and muscle wasting. Protein kinetic studies have been able to demonstrate increased nitrogen losses only in patients with fulminant hepatic failure or decompensated disease but not in patients with stable cirrhosis (McCullough and Tavill, 1991).

Patients with cirrhosis also have increased protein use. At least one study (Nielsen et al., 1995) suggests that 0.8 g of protein per kilogram per day is the mean protein requirement to achieve nitrogen balance in patients with stable cirrhosis. Therefore, in uncomplicated hepatitis or cirrhosis without encephalopathy, protein requirements range from 0.8 to 1 g/kg of dry weight per day to achieve nitrogen balance.

To promote nitrogen accumulation or positive balance, at least 1.2 to 1.3 g/kg daily is needed (Nielsen et al., 1995). In situations of stress such as alcoholic hepatitis or decompensated disease (sepsis, infection, gastrointestinal bleeding, severe ascites), at least 1.5 g of protein per kilogram per day should be provided.

Vitamins and Minerals

Vitamin and mineral supplementation is needed in all patients with ESLD because of the intimate role of the liver in nutrient transport, storage, and metabolism, in addition to the side effects of drugs (Table 28-4). Vitamin deficiencies can contribute to complications. For example, folate and vitamin B_{12} deficiencies can lead to macrocytic anemia. Deficiency of pyridoxine, thiamin, or vitamin B_{12} can result in neuropathy. Confusion, ataxia, and ocular disturbances can result from a thiamin deficiency; impaired dark adaptation can occur from vitamin A deficiency; and hepatic osteodystrophy or osteopenia can develop from vitamin D deficiency (Stickel et al., 2003).

Deficiencies of fat-soluble vitamins have been found in all types of liver failure, especially in cholestatic diseases in which malabsorption and steatorrhea occur. Therefore supplementation is necessary, using water-soluble forms. Intravenous or intramuscular vitamin K is often given for 3 days to rule out vitamin K deficiency as the cause of a prolonged prothrombin times. Water-soluble vitamin deficiencies associated with alcoholic liver disease include thiamin (which can lead to **Wernicke's encephalopathy**), pyridoxine (B_6), cyanocobalamin (B_{12}), folate, and niacin (B_3). Large doses (100 mg) of thiamin are given daily for a limited time if deficiency is suspected.

Mineral nutriture is also altered in liver disease. Iron stores may be depleted in patients experiencing gastrointestinal bleeding; however, iron supplementation should be avoided by persons with hemochromatosis or hemosiderosis (see Chapter 31). Elevated serum copper levels are found in cholestatic liver diseases (i.e., PBC and PSC). Because copper and manganese are excreted primarily via bile, supplements should not contain these minerals.

Wilson's disease is a disorder of abnormal copper metabolism in which urinary excretion is high, serum levels are low, and excess copper in various organs causes severe damage. Oral chelating agents such as zinc acetate or *d*-penicillamine are the primary treatment. A vegetarian diet may be useful as adjunctive therapy because copper is less available (Brewer et al., 1993). Dietary copper restriction (see Table 28-2) is not routinely prescribed unless other therapies are unsuccessful.

Zinc and magnesium levels are low in liver disease related to alcoholism, in part because of diuretic therapy. Calcium, as well as magnesium and zinc, may be malabsorbed with steatorrhea. Therefore the patient should take supplements of these minerals at least at the level of the DRI.

Herbal Supplements

Two herbal supplements have become popular in the treatment of liver disease. Milk thistle is popular among those suffering from viral hepatitis or alcoholic liver disease. The active component in milk thistle is silymarin. It is proposed to reduce free radical production and lipid peroxidation associated with hepatotoxicity and act as an antifibrotic agent (Jacobs et al., 2002). However, a metaanalysis (Jacobs et al., 2002) and a Cochrane review (Rambaldi et al., 2005) have not shown benefit from milk thistle in the treatment of liver disease.

S-adenosyl-*L*-methionine (SAMe) is another popular complementary medicine product purported to act as a methyl donor for methylation reactions and participate in glutathione (an antioxidant) synthesis. A Cochrane review did not show any beneficial effect of SAMe in patients with alcoholic liver disease (Rambaldi and Gluud, 2006). Further discussion on complementary medicine and supplements and liver disease is available in a recent review (Hanje et al., 2006).

Portal Hypertension

Pathophysiology and Medical Treatment

Portal hypertension increases collateral blood flow and can result in varices in the gastrointestinal tract. These varices often bleed, causing a medical emergency. Treatment includes administration of α-adrenergic blockers to decrease heart rate, endoscopic banding or variceal ligation, and radiologic or surgical placement of shunts. During an acute

---

TABLE 28-4

Vitamin and Mineral Deficits in Severe Hepatic Failure

Vitamin or Mineral	Predisposing Factors	Signs of Deficiency
Vitamin A	Steatorrhea, neomycin, cholestyramine, alcoholism	Dermatitis, night-blindness
Vitamin D	Steatorrhea, glucocorticoids, cholestyramine	Osteomalacia
Vitamin E	Steatorrhea, cholestyramine	Edema, peripheral neuropathy
Vitamin K	Steatorrhea, antibiotics, cholestyramine	Excessive bleeding; bruising
Vitamin B_6	Alcoholism	Mucous membrane lesions, dermatitis
Vitamin B_{12}	Alcoholism, cholestyramine	Megaloblastic anemia, glossitis, CNS dysfunction
Folate	Alcoholism	Megaloblastic anemia, glossitis, irritability
Niacin	Alcoholism	Dermatitis, dementia, diarrhea, inflammation of mucous membranes
Thiamin	Alcoholism, high CHO diet	Neuropathy, ascites, edema, CNS dysfunction
Zinc	Diarrhea, diuretics, alcoholism	Immunodeficiency, impaired taste acuity, wound healing, protein synthesis
Magnesium	Alcoholism, diuretics	Neuromuscular irritability, hypokalemia, hypocalcemia
Iron	Chronic bleeding	Stomatitis, microcytic anemia, malaise
Potassium	Diuretics, anabolism, insulin use	Muscular weakness, malaise, respiratory or cardiac arrest
Phosphorus	Anabolism, alcoholism	Anorexia, weakness, cardiac failure, glucose intolerance

Modified from Shronts EP: Nutritional assessment of adults with end-stage hepatic failure, *Nutr Clin Pract* 3:113, 1988.

CHO, Carbohydrate; *CNS*, central nervous system.

bleeding episode, somatostatin analog may be administered to decrease bleeding, or a nasogastric tube equipped with an inflatable balloon is placed to tamponade bleeding vessels (Sharma et al., 2005).

Medical Nutrition Therapy

During acute bleeding episodes, nutrition cannot be administered enterally. Parenteral nutrition (PN) is indicated if a patient will be taking nothing orally for at least 5 days. Repeated endoscopic therapies may cause esophageal strictures or impair a patient's swallowing. Finally, surgically or radiologically placed shunts may increase the incidence of encephalopathy and reduce nutrient metabolism because blood is shunted past the liver cells.

Ascites

Pathophysiology and Medical Treatment

Fluid retention is common, and ascites (accumulation of fluid in the abdominal cavity) is a serious consequence of liver disease. Portal hypertension, hypoalbuminemia, lymphatic obstruction, and renal retention of sodium and fluid contribute to fluid retention. Increased release of catecholamines, renin, angiotensin, aldosterone, and antidiuretic hormone secondary to peripheral arterial vasodilation causes renal retention of sodium and water.

Large-volume paracentesis may be used to relieve ascites. Diuretic therapy is often used and includes spironolactone and furosemide (Sharma et al., 2005). These drugs are often used in combination for best effect. Major side effects of loop diuretics such as furosemide include hyponatremia, hypokalemia, hypomagnesemia, hypocalcemia, and hypochloremic acidosis. Conversely, spironolactone is potassium sparing. Therefore serum potassium levels must be monitored carefully and supplemented or restricted if necessary because deficiency or excess can contribute to metabolic abnormalities. Weight; abdominal girth; urinary sodium concentration; and serum levels of urea nitrogen, creatinine, albumin, uric acid, and electrolytes should be monitored during diuretic therapy.

Medical Nutrition Therapy

Dietary treatment for ascites includes sodium restriction in addition to diuretic therapy. Sodium is commonly restricted to 2 g/day (see Chapters 33 and 34, and Appendix 37 for discussion of low-sodium diets). More severe limitations may be imposed; however, caution is warranted because of the limited palatability of these diets. Adequate protein intake is also important when a patient undergoes frequent paracentesis.

Hyponatremia

Pathophysiology

Hyponatremia often occurs because of decreased ability to excrete water resulting from the persistent release of antidiuretic hormone, sodium losses via paracentesis, excessive diuretic use, or overly aggressive sodium restriction.

Medical Nutrition Therapy

Fluid intake is usually restricted to 1 to 1.5 L/day, depending on the severity of the edema and ascites. A moderate sodium intake should be continued because excessive sodium intake will worsen fluid retention and the dilution of serum sodium levels.

Hepatic Encephalopathy

Pathophysiology and Medical Treatment

Many conditions can cause **hepatic encephalopathy,** a syndrome characterized by impaired mentation, neuromuscular disturbances, and altered consciousness. Gastrointestinal bleeding, fluid and electrolyte abnormalities, uremia, infection, use of sedatives, hyperglycemia or hypoglycemia, alcohol withdrawal, constipation, azotemia, dehydration, portosystemic shunts, and acidosis can precipitate hepatic encephalopathy.

Subclinical hepatic encephalopathy occurs in 50% to 80% of patients with chronic hepatic failure (Friedman and Schiano, 2004), but it is precipitated by excessive dietary protein intake in only about 7% to 9% of patients with liver failure (Leevy and Davison, 1967). Hepatic or **portal systemic encephalopathy** results in neuromuscular and behavioral alterations. Box 28-2 describes the four stages of hepatic encephalopathy.

Just as there are multiple causes of hepatic encephalopathy, there are multiple theories as to the mechanism by which hepatic encephalopathy occurs. Ammonia is considered an important etiologic factor in the development of encephalopathy (Friedman and Schiano, 2004). When the liver fails, it is unable to detoxify ammonia to urea, and ammonia is a direct cerebral toxin. Although serum and cerebrospinal fluid ammonia levels do not correlate well with the degree of hepatic encephalopathy, treatment is based on lowering these levels. However, ammonia metabolites such as glutamine and α-ketoglutarate in cerebrospinal fluid have correlated more closely with the severity of encephalopathy.

The main source of ammonia is its endogenous production by the gastrointestinal tract from the metabolism of protein and from the degradation of bacteria and blood

---

BOX 28-2

Four Stages of Hepatic Encephalopathy

Stage	Symptoms
I	Mild confusion, agitation, irritability, sleep disturbance, decreased attention
II	Lethargy, disorientation, inappropriate behavior, drowsiness
III	Somnolent but arousable, incomprehensible speech, confused, aggressive behavior when awake
IV	Coma

from gastrointestinal bleeding. Therefore drugs such as lactulose and neomycin are given. Lactulose is a nonabsorbable disaccharide. It acidifies the colonic contents, retaining ammonia as the ammonium ion. It also acts as an osmotic laxative to remove the ammonia. Neomycin is a nonabsorbable antibiotic that helps decrease colonic ammonia production.

Exogenous protein is also a source of ammonia. Some clinicians suggest that dietary protein causes an increase in ammonia levels and subsequently hepatic encephalopathy, but this has not been proven in studies. One study even showed that patients with worsening hepatic encephalopathy often have decreased protein intakes and increased blood urea nitrogen and creatinine levels. Patients with improved encephalopathy had higher protein intakes and lower blood urea nitrogen and creatinine levels (Morgan et al., 1995).

Another major hypothesis for the pathogenesis of portal systemic encephalopathy has been termed the altered neurotransmitter theory. A plasma amino acid imbalance exists in ESLD in which the **branched-chain amino acids (BCAAs)** valine, leucine, and isoleucine are decreased, and **aromatic amino acids (AAAs)** tryptophan, phenylalanine, and tyrosine, plus methionine, glutamine, asparagine, and histidine are increased (Box 28-3).

The BCAAs furnish as much as 30% of energy requirements for skeletal muscle, heart, and brain when gluconeogenesis and ketogenesis are depressed (Latifi et al., 1991). This causes serum BCAA levels to fall. At the same time, plasma AAAs and methionine are released into circulation by muscle proteolysis, but the synthesis into protein and liver clearance of AAAs is depressed (Hiyama and Fischer, 1988). This changes the plasma molar ratio of BCAAs to AAAs and may contribute to the development of hepatic encephalopathy; AAAs may limit the cerebral uptake of BCAAs because they compete for carrier-mediated transport at the blood-brain barrier (Latifi et al., 1991).

Several other substances have been implicated in the development of hepatic encephalopathy, such as short-chain fatty acids, mercaptans, phenols, and α-aminobutyric acid (Diehl, 2000). Another final dietary theory implicates zinc deficiency, types of fatty acids, or the amino acid tryptophan in the development of hepatic encephalopathy (Mullen and Weber, 1991).

Medical Nutrition Therapy

The practice of protein restriction in patients with low-grade hepatic encephalopathy is based on empiric evidence that protein intolerance causes hepatic encephalopathy, but it has never been proven in a study. Unnecessary protein restriction may only worsen body protein losses and therefore must be avoided. Patients with encephalopathy often do not receive adequate protein. More than 95% of patients with cirrhosis can tolerate mixed-protein diets up to 1.5 g/kg of body weight. True dietary protein intolerance is rare except in fulminant hepatic failure, or in a rare patient with chronic endogenous hepatic encephalopathy.

A study evaluated the outcomes in patients with encephalopathy who were admitted to the hospital and randomized to receive 1.2 g of protein per kilogram at admission versus a low-protein diet (with protein intake advancing gradually). The low-protein diet exacerbated protein breakdown, and there was no benefit of a low-protein diet in management of hepatic encephalopathy or serum ammonia levels (Cordoba, 2004).

Studies evaluating the benefit of supplements enriched with BCAAs and restricted in AAAs have varied in study design, sample size, composition of BCAA-enriched formulas, level of encephalopathy, type of liver disease, duration of therapy, and control groups. A Cochrane Review published in 2003 evaluated the literature with regard to effectiveness of BCAAs on outcomes in liver failure (Als-Nielson et al., 2003). The conclusions of the study were that, when high methodologic quality studies were evaluated, there were no significant improvements associated with giving BCAA to patients. In addition, BCAAs did not confer a survival benefit. Marchesini (2003) conducted a randomized, controlled trial of 174 patients with liver disease and also found that a BCAA formula did not have a significant effect on hepatic encephalopathy. However, nutrition status was improved with BCAAs.

Other theories postulate that vegetable proteins and casein may improve mental status compared with meat protein (Bianchi et al., 1993). Casein-based diets are lower in AAAs and higher in BCAAs than meat-based diets. The potential advantage of vegetable protein is that it is low in methionine and ammoniagenic amino acids and it is BCAA rich. The high-fiber content of a vegetable-protein diet may also play a role in the excretion of nitrogenous compounds.

BOX 28-3

Amino Acids Commonly Altered in Liver Disease

Aromatic Amino Acids

Tyrosine
Phenylalanine*
Free tryptophan*

Branched-Chain Amino Acids

Valine*
Leucine*
Isoleucine*

Ammoniogenic Amino Acids

Glycine
Serine
Threonine*
Glutamine
Histidine*
Lysine*
Asparagine
Methionine*

*Denotes essential amino acids.

Finally, it has been proposed that probiotics and synbiotics (sources of friendly bacteria and fermentable fibers) can be used to treat hepatic encephalopathy (Solga, 2003; Liu et al., 2004). Probiotics (see Chapters 1 and 27) may improve hepatic encephalopathy by reducing ammonia in portal blood, decreasing inflammation and oxidative stress in the hepatocyte (thus increasing hepatic clearance of toxins including ammonia), and minimizing uptake of other toxins (Solga, 2003).

Glucose Alterations

Pathophysiology

Glucose intolerance occurs in almost two thirds of patients with cirrhosis, and 10% to 37% of patients will develop overt diabetes. Glucose intolerance in patients with liver disease occurs because of insulin resistance in peripheral tissues. Hyperinsulinism also occurs in patients with cirrhosis, possibly because insulin production is increased, hepatic clearance is decreased, portal systemic shunting occurs, there is a defect in the insulin-binding action at the receptor site, or there is a postreceptor defect.

Fasting hypoglycemia, or *low blood glucose,* can occur because of the decreased availability of glucose from glycogen in addition to the failing gluconeogenic capacity of the liver when the patient is in ESLD. Hypoglycemia occurs more often in acute or fulminant liver failure than in chronic liver disease. Hypoglycemia may also occur after alcohol consumption in patients whose glycogen stores are depleted by starvation because of the block of hepatic gluconeogenesis by ethanol.

Medical Nutrition Therapy

Patients with diabetes should receive standard medical and nutrition therapy to achieve normoglycemia (see Chapter 30). Patients with hypoglycemia should eat frequently to prevent this condition (see *Clinical Insight:* Fasting Hypoglycemia).

Fat Malabsorption

Pathophysiology

Fat absorption may be impaired in liver disease. Possible causes include decreased bile salt secretion (as in PBC, sclerosing cholangitis, and biliary strictures), administration of neomycin or cholestyramine, and pancreatic enzyme insufficiency. Stools may be greasy, floating, or light or clay colored, signifying malabsorption, which can be verified by a 72-hour fecal fat study (see Chapter 27 and Appendix 30).

Medical Nutrition Therapy

If significant steatorrhea is present, replacement of some of the long-chain triglycerides (LCTs) or dietary fat with medium-chain triglycerides (MCTs) may be useful. Because MCTs do not require bile salts and micelle formation for absorption, they are readily taken up via the portal route (see Chapter 27). Some nutrition supplements contain MCTs, which can be used in addition to liquid MCT oil (see Appendix 32).

Significant stool fat losses may warrant a trial of a low-fat (40 g/day) diet. If diarrhea does not resolve, fat restriction should be discontinued because it decreases the palatability of the diet and severely hampers adequate calorie intake.

Renal Insufficiency and Hepatorenal Syndrome

Pathophysiology, Medical and Nutrition Therapy

Hepatorenal syndrome is renal failure associated with severe liver disease without intrinsic kidney abnormalities. Hepatorenal syndrome is diagnosed when the urine sodium level is less than 10 mEq/L and oliguria persists in the absence of intravascular volume depletion (Friedman and Schiano, 2004). If conservative therapies, including discontinuation of nephrotoxic drugs, optimization of intravascular volume status, treatment of underlying infection, and monitoring of fluid intake and output fail, dialysis may be required. In any case, renal insufficiency and failure may necessitate alteration in fluid, sodium, potassium, and phosphorus intake (see Chapter 36).

Osteopenia

Pathophysiology

Osteopenia often exists in patients with PBC, sclerosing cholangitis, and alcoholic liver disease. Depressed osteoblastic function and osteoporosis also can occur in patients with hemochromatosis, and osteoporosis is prevalent in

---

✳ CLINICAL INSIGHT

Fasting Hypoglycemia

Two thirds of the glucose requirement in an adult is used by the central nervous system. During fasting, plasma glucose concentrations are maintained for use by the nervous system and the brain because liver glycogen is broken down, or new glucose is made from nonglucose precursors such as alanine (Polonsky, 1992). Fasting hypoglycemia occurs when there is reduced synthesis of new glucose or reduced liver glycogen breakdown.

Causes of fasting hypoglycemia include cirrhosis, consumption of alcohol, extensive intrahepatic cancer, deficiency of the hormones cortisol and growth hormone, or non–β cell tumors of the pancreas. The method for detecting it involves measuring plasma insulin when plasma glucose is low. The diagnostic hallmark of an insulinoma is altered insulin secretion in the presence of hypoglycemia. Fasting hypoglycemia may also be caused by spontaneously produced antibodies. All patients with liver or pancreatic disease should be monitored for fasting hypoglycemia. Nutrition therapy involves balanced meals with small, frequent snacks to avoid periods of fasting. Monitoring of blood glucose and insulin levels is required.

patients who have had long-term treatment with corticosteroids. Corticosteroids increase bone resorption; suppress osteoblastic function; and affect sex hormone secretion, intestinal absorption of dietary calcium, renal excretion of calcium and phosphorus, and the vitamin D system (Hay et al., 2001; Isoniemi et al., 2001; Trautwein et al., 2000).

Medical Nutrition Therapy

Prevention or treatment options for osteopenia include weight maintenance, ingestion of a well-balanced diet, adequate protein to maintain muscle mass, 1500 mg of calcium per day, adequate vitamin D from the diet or supplements (400 to 800 units or more per day), avoidance of alcohol, and monitoring for steatorrhea, with diet adjustments as needed to minimize nutrient losses.

LIVER RESECTION AND TRANSPLANTATION

Liver resection and thermal ablation are fairly common now that problem areas can be located by means of tomography and arteriography. As with any major surgery, protein and energy needs increase after liver resection. Needs are also increased for liver cell regeneration. EN is vital because of the role of portal hepatotropic factors necessary for liver cell proliferation. Optimal nutrition is most important for patients with poor nutrition status before hepatectomy (e.g., patients with hepatocellular carcinoma or cholangiocarcinoma).

Liver transplantation has become an established treatment for ESLD. Malnutrition is common in liver transplant candidates. Dietary intake can often be enhanced if patients eat small, frequent, nutrient-dense meals; oral nutritional supplements may also be well tolerated. Enteral tube feeding is indicated when oral intake is inadequate or contraindicated. Varices are not an absolute contraindication for placement of a feeding tube (Crippin, 2006). PN is reserved for patients without adequate gut function. Because PN can adversely affect liver function, EN is preferred (Hasse, 2005).

In the acute posttransplant phase, nutrient needs are increased to promote healing, deter infection, provide energy for recovery, and replenish depleted body stores. Nitrogen requirements are elevated in the acute posttransplant phase and can be met with early postoperative tube feeding (Hasse et al., 1995). Two studies have shown that probiotics and fiber added to tube feeding can reduce postoperative infection rate better than tube feeding or fiber alone (Rayes et al., 2002; Rayes et al., 2005).

Multiple medications used after transplant have nutritional side effects such as anorexia, gastrointestinal upset, hypercatabolism, diarrhea, hyperglycemia, hyperlipidemia, sodium retention, hypertension, hyperkalemia, and hypercalciuria (see Chapter 16). Therefore dietary modification is based on the specific side effects of drug therapy (Table 28-5). During the posttransplant phase, nutrient requirements are adjusted to prevent or treat problems of obesity, hyperlipidemia, hypertension, diabetes mellitus, and osteopenia (Davidson et al., 2003; Heisel et al., 2004; Marchetti et al., 2005). Table 28-6 summarizes nutrient needs following liver transplantation.

TABLE 28-5

Drugs Commonly Used After Liver Transplantation

Immunosuppressant Drug	Possible Nutritional Side Effects	Proposed Nutrition Therapy
Azathioprine	Macrocytic anemia	Give folate supplements
	Mouth sores	Adjust food and meals as needed; monitor intake
	Nausea, vomiting, diarrhea, anorexia, sore throat, stomach pain, decreased taste acuity	
Antithymocyte globulin	Nausea, vomiting	Adjust food and meals as needed; monitor intake
Basiliximab	None reported	
Cyclosporine	Sodium retention	Decrease sodium intake
	Hyperkalemia	Decrease potassium intake
	Hyperlipidemia	Limit fat and simple carbohydrate intake
	Hyperglycemia	Decrease simple carbohydrate intake
	Decreased serum magnesium level	Increase magnesium intake; give supplements
	Hypertension	Limit sodium intake
	Nausea, vomiting	Adjust food and meals as needed; monitor intake

Modified from Hasse J: Role of the dietitian in the nutrition management of adults after liver transplantation, *J Am Diet Assoc* 91:473, 1991.

TABLE 28-5

Drugs Commonly Used After Liver Transplantation—cont'd

Immunosuppressant Drug	Possible Nutritional Side Effects	Proposed Nutrition Therapy
Daclizumab	None reported	
Glucocorticoids	Sodium retention	Decrease sodium intake
	Hyperglycemia	Decrease simple carbohydrate intake
	Hyperlipidemia	Limit fat and simple carbohydrate intake
	False hunger	Avoid overeating
	Protein wasting with high doses	Increase protein intake
	Decreased absorption of calcium and phosphorus	Increase calcium and phosphorus intake; give supplements as needed
Muromonab-CD3	Nausea, vomiting, anorexia	Adjust food and meals as needed; monitor intake
Mycophenolate mofetil	Nausea, vomiting, diarrhea	Adjust food and meals as needed; monitor intake
Sirolimus	Possible hyperglycemia	Decrease simple carbohydrate intake
	Possible GI symptoms	Adjust food and meals as needed; monitor intake
	Hyperlipidemia	Limit fat and simple carbohydrate intake
Tacrolimus	Hyperglycemia	Decrease simple carbohydrate intake
	Hyperkalemia	Decrease potassium intake
	Nausea, vomiting	Adjust food and meals as needed; monitor intake
15-Deoxyspergualin	GI symptoms	Adjust food and meals as needed; monitor intake

TABLE 28-6

Nutrition Care Guidelines for Liver Transplant Patient

	Pretransplantation	Immediate Posttransplantation (First 2 Posttransplant Months)	Long-Term Post-transplantation
Calories protein*	High calorie (basal + 20% or more)	Moderate calorie (basal + 15%-30%)	Weight maintenance (basal + 10%-20%)
	Moderate protein (1-1.5 g/kg: minimize need for restriction)	High protein (1.2-1.75 g/kg)	Moderate protein (1 g/kg)
Fat	As needed	20%-30% of calories	Low fat (≤30% of calories)
Carbohydrate	High carbohydrate (complex and simple)	70% of calories	Reduced simple carbohydrate
Sodium	2-4 g/d (as indicated)	2-4 g/d (as indicated)	2-4 g/d (as indicated)
Fluid	Restrict to 1000-1500 ml/d (as indicated)	As needed	As needed
Calcium	800-1200 mg/d	800-1200 mg/d	1200-1500 mg/d
Vitamins	Multivitamin/mineral supplementation to DRI levels; additional water- and fat-soluble vitamins as indicated	Multivitamin/mineral supplementation to DRI levels; additional water- and fat-soluble vitamins as indicated	Multivitamin/mineral supplementation to DRI levels for first post-transplant year

Modified from Porayko MK et al: Impact of malnutrition and its therapy on liver transplantation, *Semin Liv Dis* 11(4):305, 1991.

*Use estimated dry or ideal weight.

RDA, Recommended dietary allowance.

PHYSIOLOGY AND FUNCTIONS OF THE GALLBLADDER

The gallbladder lies on the undersurface of the right lobe of the liver (Figure 28-6). The main function of the gallbladder is to concentrate, store, and excrete bile, which is produced by the liver. During the concentration process, water and electrolytes are resorbed by the gallbladder mucosa. The chief constituents of bile are cholesterol, bilirubin, and bile salts. Bilirubin, the main bile pigment, is derived from the release of hemoglobin from red blood cell destruction. It is transported to the liver, where it is conjugated and excreted via bile.

Bile salts, made by liver cells from cholesterol, are essential for the digestion and absorption of fats, fat-soluble vitamins, and some minerals (see Chapter 1). Excreted into the small intestine via bile, bile salts are then resorbed into the portal system (enterohepatic circulation). Bile also contains immunoglobulins that support the integrity of the intestinal mucosa. In addition, it is the primary excretory pathway for the minerals copper and manganese.

Bile is removed by the liver via bile canaliculi that drain into intrahepatic bile ducts. The ducts lead to the left and right hepatic ducts, which leave the liver and join to become the common hepatic duct. The bile is directed to the gallbladder via the cystic duct for concentration and storage. The cystic duct joins the common hepatic duct to form the common bile duct. The bile duct then joins the pancreatic duct, which carries digestive enzymes.

During the course of digestion, food reaches the duodenum, causing the release of intestinal hormones such as cholecystokinin and secretin. This stimulates the gallbladder and pancreas and causes the sphincter of Oddi to relax, allowing pancreatic juice and bile to flow into the duode-

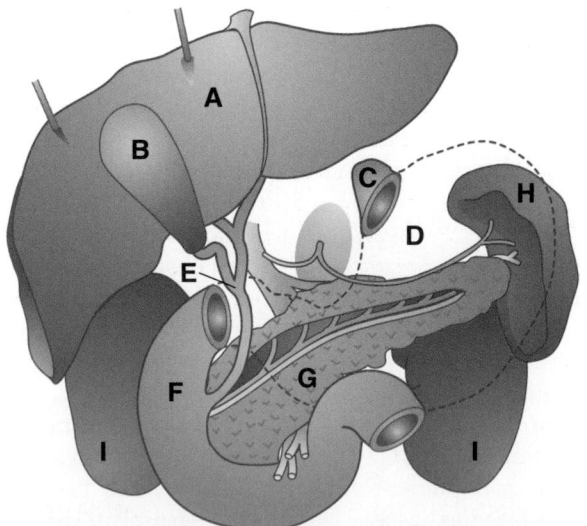

FIGURE 28-6 Schematic drawing showing relationship of organs of the upper abdomen. *A*, Liver (retracted upward); *B*, gallbladder; *C*, esophageal opening of stomach; *D*, stomach *(shown in dotted outline)*; *E*, common bile duct; *F*, duodenum; *G*, pancreas and pancreatic duct; *H*, spleen; *I*, kidneys. *(Courtesy the Cleveland Clinic Foundation, Cleveland, Ohio, 2002.)*

num at the ampulla of Vater to assist in fat digestion. For this reason diseases of the gallbladder, liver, and pancreas are often interrelated.

DISEASES OF THE GALLBLADDER

Disorders of the biliary tract affect millions of people each year, causing significant suffering and even death by precipitating pancreatitis and sepsis. A diverse spectrum of disease affects the biliary system, often presenting with similar clinical signs and symptoms. Treatment may involve diet, medication, or surgery.

Cholelithiasis

Pathophysiology

The formation of gallstones (calculi) in the absence of infection of the gallbladder is called **cholelithiasis.** Virtually all gallstones form within the gallbladder. With rare exceptions, stones form behind biliary duct strictures as a result of stasis in bile ducts after **cholecystectomy** (surgical removal of the gallbladder). Gallstone disease affects millions of Americans each year and causes significant morbidity. In most cases gallstones are asymptomatic; however, symptomatic gallstone disease can have serious complications.

Gallstones that pass from the gallbladder into the common bile duct may remain there indefinitely without causing symptoms, or they may pass into the duodenum with or without symptoms. **Choledocholithiasis** develops when stones slip into the bile ducts, producing obstruction, pain, and cramps. If passage of bile into the duodenum is interrupted, cholecystitis can develop. In the absence of bile in the intestine, lipid absorption is impaired, and without bile pigments, stools become light in color (acholic). If uncorrected, bile backup can result in jaundice and liver damage **(secondary biliary cirrhosis).** Obstruction of the distal common bile duct can lead to pancreatitis if the pancreatic duct is blocked (see "Cholecystitis" in the following paragraphs).

Most gallstones in people in the United States are unpigmented cholesterol stones composed primarily of cholesterol, bilirubin, and calcium salts. Risk factors for cholesterol stone formation include female gender, pregnancy, older age, family history, obesity and truncal body fat distribution, diabetes mellitus, inflammatory bowel disease, and drugs (lipid-lowering medications, oral contraceptives, and estrogens). Certain ethnic groups are at greater risk of stone formation, including Pima Indians, Scandinavians, and Mexican-Americans. Rapid weight loss (as with jejunoileal and gastric bypass and fasting or severe calorie restriction) is associated with a high incidence of biliary sludge and gallstone formation (Al-Jiffry et al., 2003; Iglezias et al., 2003).

Bacteria may also play a role in gallstone formation. Low-grade chronic infections produce changes in the gallbladder mucosa, which affect its absorptive capabilities. Excess water or bile acid may be absorbed as a result. Cholesterol may then precipitate out and cause gallstone formation (Volzke et al., 2005). High dietary fat intake over a prolonged period may predispose a person to gallstone formation because of the constant stimulus to produce more cholesterol for bile synthesis required in fat digestion.

Pigmented stones typically consist of bilirubin polymers or calcium salts. They are associated with chronic hemolysis. Risk factors associated with these stones are age, sickle cell anemia and thalassemia, biliary tract infection, cirrhosis, alcoholism, and long-term PN (Abayli et al., 2005).

Medical Management

Treatment of gallstone disease includes cholecystectomy, especially if the stones are numerous, large, or calcified. The cholecystectomy may be done as a traditional open laparotomy or as a less invasive laparoscopic procedure. Chemical dissolution with the administration of bile salts, chenodeoxycholic acid, and ursodeoxycholic acid (litholytic therapy) or dissolution by extracorporeal shock-wave lithotripsy may also be used; but these are much less common than surgical techniques. Patients with gallstones that have migrated into the bile ducts may be candidates for endoscopic retrograde cholangiopancreatography techniques (Adler et al., 2005).

Medical Nutrition Therapy

No specific dietary treatment is available to prevent cholelithiasis in susceptible persons. Nutrition-related factors include obesity and severe fasting, and these should be corrected when possible. In cholecystitis, dietary treatment includes a low-fat diet to prevent gallbladder contractions. Data are conflicting as to whether intravenous lipids stimulate gallbladder contraction (Priori et al., 1997).

After surgical removal of the gallbladder, oral feedings are usually resumed with the return of bowel sounds and after the patient can tolerate removal of the nasogastric drainage tube. The diet can be advanced to a regular diet as tolerated. In the absence of the gallbladder, bile is secreted directly by the liver into the intestine. The biliary tract dilates, forming a "simulated pouch" over time, to allow bile to be held in a manner similar to the original gallbladder.

Cholecystitis

Pathophysiology

Inflammation of the gallbladder is known as **cholecystitis**, and it may be chronic or acute. It is usually caused by gallstones obstructing the bile ducts (calculous cholecystitis), leading to the backup of bile. Bilirubin, the main bile pigment, gives bile its greenish color. When biliary tract obstruction prevents bile from reaching the intestine, it backs up and returns to the circulation. Bilirubin has an affinity for elastic tissues; therefore, when it overflows into the general circulation, it causes the yellow skin pigmentation and eye discoloration typical of jaundice.

Acute cholecystitis without stones (acalculous cholecystitis) may occur in critically ill patients or when the gallbladder and its bile are stagnant. Impaired gallbladder emptying in chronic acalculous cholecystitis appears to be due to diminished spontaneous contractile activity and decreased contractile responsiveness to the hormone cholecystokinin (Merg et al., 2002). The walls of the gallbladder become inflamed and distended, and infection can occur. During such episodes, the patient experiences upper quadrant abdominal pain accompanied by nausea, vomiting, and flatulence.

Chronic cholecystitis is long-standing inflammation of the gallbladder. It is caused by repeated mild attacks of acute cholecystitis. This leads to thickening of the walls of the gallbladder. The gallbladder begins to shrink and eventually loses the ability to perform its function: concentrating and storing bile. Eating foods that are high in fat may aggravate the symptoms of cholecystitis, because bile is needed to digest such foods. Chronic cholecystitis occurs more often in women than in men, and the incidence increases after the age of 40. Risk factors include the presence of gallstones and a history of acute cholecystitis.

Medical Management

Acute cholecystitis requires surgical intervention unless medically contraindicated. Without surgery, the condition may either subside or progress to gangrene.

Medical Nutrition Therapy

Acute Cholecystitis. In an acute attack, oral feedings are discontinued. PN may be indicated if the patient is malnourished and it is anticipated that he or she will not be taking anything orally for a prolonged period. When feedings are resumed, a low-fat diet is recommended to decrease gallbladder stimulation. A hydrolyzed low-fat formula (see Appendix 32), or an oral low-fat diet consisting of 30 to 45 g of fat per day can be given. Studies have failed to show a relationship between dietary cholesterol and gallstone formation. Table 28-7 shows a fat-restricted diet.

Chronic Cholecystitis. Patients with chronic conditions may require a long-term low-fat diet that contains 25% to 30% of total kilocalories as fat. Stricter limitation is undesirable because fat in the intestine is important for some stimulation and drainage of the biliary tract. The degree of food intolerance varies widely among persons with gallbladder disorders; many complain of foods that cause flatulence and bloating. For this reason it is best to determine with the patient which foods should be eliminated. See Chapter 27 for a discussion of potential gas-forming foods. Administration of water-soluble forms of fat-soluble vitamins may be of benefit in patients with chronic gallbladder conditions or in those in whom fat malabsorption is suspected.

Acute Cholangitis

Pathophysiology and Medical Management

Inflammation of the bile ducts is known as **cholangitis.** Patients with acute cholangitis need resuscitation with fluids and broad-spectrum antibiotics. If the patient does not improve with conservative treatment, placement of a percutaneous biliary stent or cholecystectomy may be needed (Lee et al., 2002).

TABLE 28-7

Fat-Restricted Diet*

Food Allowed	Food Excluded
Beverages	
Skim milk or buttermilk made with skim milk; coffee, tea, Postum, fruit juice, soft drinks, cocoa made with cocoa powder and skim milk	Whole milk, buttermilk made with whole milk, chocolate milk, cream in excess of amounts allowed under fats
Bread and Cereal Products	
Plain, nonfat cereals; spaghetti, noodles, rice, macaroni; plain whole grain or enriched breads, air-popped popcorn, bagels, English muffins	Biscuits, breads, egg or cheese bread, sweet rolls made with fat, pancakes, doughnuts, waffles, fritters, popcorn prepared with fat, muffins, natural cereals and breads to which extra fat is added
Cheese	
Cottage cheese, ¼ c to be used as substitute for 1 oz of cheese, or low-fat cheeses containing less than 5% butterfat	Whole-milk cheeses
Desserts	
Sherbet made with skim milk; nonfat frozen yogurt; nonfat frozen nondairy desserts; fruit ice; sorbet; gelatin; rice, bread, cornstarch, tapioca, or pudding made with skim milk; fruit whips with gelatin, sugar, and egg white; fruit; angel food cake; graham crackers; vanilla wafers; meringues	Cake, pie, pastry, ice cream, or any dessert containing shortening, chocolate, or fats of any kind, unless especially prepared using part of fat allowance
Eggs	
Three per week prepared only with fat from fat allowance; egg whites as desired; low-fat egg substitutes	More than one/day unless substituted for part of the meat allowed
Fats	
Choose up to the limit allowed among the following (1 serving in the amount listed equals 1 fat choice): 1 tsp butter or margarine 1 Tbsp reduced-fat margarine 1 tsp shortening or oil 1 tsp mayonnaise 2 tsp Italian or French dressing 1 Tbsp reduced-fat salad dressing 1 strip crisp bacon ⅛ avocado (4-inch diameter) 2 Tbsp light cream 1 Tbsp heavy cream 6 small nuts 5 small olives	Any in excess of amount prescribed on diet; all others
Fruits	
As desired	Avocado in excess of amount allowed on fat list
Lean Meat, Fish, Poultry, and Meat Substitutes	
Choose up to the limit allowed among the following: poultry without skin, fish, veal (all cuts), liver, lean beef, pork, and lamb, all with visible fat removed—1 oz cooked weight equals 1 equivalent; ¼ c water packed tuna or salmon equals 1 equivalent; tofu or tempeh—3 oz equals 1 equivalent	Fried or fatty meats, sausage, scrapple, frankfurters, poultry skins, stewing hens, spareribs, salt pork, beef unless lean, duck, goose, ham hocks, pig's feet, luncheon meats (unless reduced fat), gravies unless fat-free, tuna and salmon packed in oil, peanut butter

*Fat content can be reduced further by reducing the fat exchanges. 1 Fat exchange = 5 g of fat.

TABLE 28-7	

Fat-Restricted Diet*—cont'd

Food Allowed	Food Excluded
Milk	
Skim, buttermilk, or yogurt made from skim milk	Whole, 2%, 1%, chocolate, buttermilk made with whole milk
Seasonings	
As desired	None
Soups	
Bouillon, clear broth, fat-free vegetable soup, cream soup made with skimmed milk, packaged dehydrated soups	All others
Sweets	
Jelly, jam, marmalade, honey, syrup, molasses, sugar, hard sugar candies, fondant, gumdrops, jelly beans, marshmallows, cocoa powder, fat-free chocolate sauce, red and black licorice	Any candy made with chocolate, nuts, butter, cream, or fat of any kind
Vegetables	
All plainly prepared vegetables	Potato chips; buttered, au gratin, creamed, or fried potatoes and other vegetables unless made with allowed fat; casseroles or frozen vegetables in butter sauce

Daily Food Allowances for 40-g–Fat Diet

Food	Amount	Approximate Fat Content (g)
Skim milk	2 c or more	0
Lean meat, fish, poultry	6 oz or 6 equivalents	18
Whole egg or egg yolks	3 per week	2
Vegetables	3 servings or more, at least 1 or more dark green or deep yellow	0
Fruits	3 or more servings, at least 1 citrus	0
Breads, cereals	As desired, fat-free	0
Fat exchanges*	4-5 exchanges daily	20-25
Desserts and sweets	As desired from permitted list	0
	TOTAL FAT	38-43

Sclerosing Cholangitis

Pathophysiology and Medical Management

Sclerosing cholangitis can result in sepsis and liver failure. Most patients have multiple intrahepatic strictures, which makes surgical intervention difficult, if not impossible. Patients are generally on broad-spectrum antibiotics. Percutaneous ductal dilation may provide short-term bile duct patency in some patients. When sepsis is recurrent, patients may require chronic antibiotic therapy. See the section on sclerosing cholangitis in the liver disease section for more information and nutrition therapy.

Cholestasis

Pathophysiology and Medical Management

Cholestasis is a condition in which little or no bile is secreted or the flow of bile into the digestive tract is ob-structed. This can occur in patients without oral or enteral feeding for a prolonged period, such as those requiring PN, and can predispose to acalculous cholesystitis. Prevention includes stimulation of intestinal and biliary motility and secretions by at least minimum enteral feedings (Hager, 1994). If this is not possible, drug therapy is used.

PHYSIOLOGY AND FUNCTIONS OF THE EXOCRINE PANCREAS

The pancreas is an elongated, flattened gland that lies in the upper abdomen behind the stomach. The head of the pancreas is in the right upper quadrant below the liver within the curvature of the duodenum, and the tapering tail slants upward to the hilum of the spleen. This glandular organ has both an endocrine and exocrine function. Pancreatic cells manufacture glucagon, insulin, and somatostatin for absorption into the bloodstream (endocrine function) for regulation of glucose homeostasis (see Chapter 30). Other cells secrete enzymes and other substances directly into the intestinal lumen, where they aid in digesting proteins, fats, and carbohydrates (exocrine function).

In most people the pancreatic duct, which carries the exocrine pancreatic secretions, merges with the common bile duct into a unified opening through which bile and pancreatic juices drain into the duodenum at the ampulla of Vater. Many factors regulate exocrine secretion from the pancreas. Neural and hormonal responses play a role, with the presence and composition of ingested foods being a large contributor. The two primary hormonal stimuli for pancreatic secretion are secretin and cholecystokinin (see Chapter 1).

Factors that influence pancreatic secretions during a meal can be divided into three phases: (1) the cephalic phase is mediated through the vagus nerve and initiated by the sight, smell, taste, and anticipation of food; it leads to the secretion of bicarbonate and pancreatic enzymes; (2) gastric distention with food initiates the gastric phase of pancreatic secretion, which stimulates enzyme secretion; and (3) the intestinal phase has the most potent effect on pancreatic secretions and is mediated by the release of cholecystokinin.

DISEASES OF THE
EXOCRINE PANCREAS

Pancreatitis

Pathophysiology and Medical Management

Pancreatitis is an inflammation of the pancreas and is characterized by edema, cellular exudate, and fat necrosis. The disease can range from mild and self-limiting to severe, with autodigestion, necrosis, and hemorrhage of pancreatic tissue. Ranson and colleagues (1974) identified 11 signs that could be measured during the first 48 hours of admission and that have prognostic significance (Box 28-4). By using these observations, one can determine the likely outcome of hospitalization. Surgical intervention may be necessary. Pancreatitis is classified as either acute or chronic, the latter with pancreatic destruction so extensive that exocrine and endocrine function are severely diminished and maldigestion and diabetes may result.

The symptoms of pancreatitis can range from continuous or intermittent pain of varying intensity to severe upper abdominal pain, which may radiate to the back. Symptoms may worsen with the ingestion of food. Clinical presentation may also include nausea, vomiting, abdominal distention, and steatorrhea. Severe cases are complicated by hypotension, oliguria, and dyspnea. There is extensive destruction of pancreatic tissue with subsequent fibrosis, enzyme production is diminished, and serum amylase and lipase may

---

BOX 28-4

Ranson's Criteria to Classify the Severity of Pancreatitis

At Admission or Diagnosis

Age >55 yr
White blood cell count >16,000 m³
Blood glucose level >200 mg/100 ml
Lactic dehydrogenase >350 units/L
Aspartate transaminase >250 units/L

During the Initial 48 Hours

Hematocrit decrease of >10 mg/dl
Blood urea nitrogen increase of >5 mg/dl
Arterial PO_2 <60 mm Hg
Base deficit >4 mEq/L
Fluid sequestration >6000 ml
Serum calcium level <8 mg/ml

Modified from Ranson JH et al: Prognostic signs and the role of operative management in acute pancreatitis, *Surg Gynecol Obstet* 139:69, 1974.

---

appear normal. However, absence of enzymes to aid in the digestion of food leads to steatorrhea and malabsorption. Table 28-8 describes several tests used to determine the extent of pancreatic destruction.

Medical Nutrition Therapy

Acute Pancreatitis. Pain associated with pancreatitis is partially related to the secretory mechanisms of pancreatic enzymes and bile. Therefore nutrition therapy is adjusted to provide minimum stimulation of these systems (see *Pathophysiology and Care Management Algorithm: Pancreatitis*).

In the past the pancreas was put "at rest." During acute attacks all oral feeding is withheld, and hydration maintained intravenously. In less severe attacks a clear liquid diet with negligible fat may be given in a few days. The patient should be monitored for any symptoms of pain, nausea, or vomiting. The diet should be progressed as tolerated to easily digested foods with a low fat content and then advanced as tolerated. Foods may be better tolerated if they are divided into six small meals. The low-fat diet described in Table 28-7 can be used.

Severe acute pancreatitis results in a hypermetabolic and catabolic state. Induction of severe acute pancreatitis results in immediate metabolic alterations in the pancreas, with rapid onset of metabolic disturbances, not only in the local, challenged organ (pancreas) but also in remote organs (Ederoth et al., 2002). Metabolic demands have been compared with those of a patient with sepsis. Amino acids are released from muscle and used for gluconeogenesis. These patients often exhibit signs of malnutrition such as decreased serum levels of albumin, transferrin, and lymphocytes. Attention should be given to a nutrition regimen with adequate protein in an effort to achieve positive nitrogen balance.

TABLE 28-8	
Some Tests of Pancreatic Function	
Test	**Significance**
Secretin stimulation test	Measures pancreatic secretion, particularly bicarbonate, in response to secretin stimulation
Glucose tolerance test	Assesses endocrine function of the pancreas by measuring insulin response to a glucose load
72-hr stool fat test	Assesses exocrine function of the pancreas by measuring fat absorption that reflects pancreatic lipase secretion

Oral nutrition must be further delayed when the acute illness persists longer than a few days as evidenced by persistent or recurrent elevation of serum amylase, continued abdominal pain, and ileus; or when cessation of nasogastric suction is followed by return of symptoms, the presence of a complication such as pancreatic abscess or pseudocyst, or a suspected obstruction to the main pancreatic ducts. In these severe, prolonged cases, PN may be necessary. Patients with mild-to-moderate stress can tolerate dextrose-based solutions, whereas patients with more severe stress require a mixed fuel system of dextrose and lipid to avoid complications of glucose intolerance.

Lipid emulsion should not be included in a PN regimen if hypertriglyceridemia is the cause of the pancreatitis. A serum triglyceride level should be obtained before PN with lipids is initiated. Lipids may be given to patients with triglyceride values less than 400 mg/dl. Because of the possibility of pancreatic endocrine abnormalities and a relative insulin resistance, close glucose monitoring is also warranted. H_2-receptor antagonists may be prescribed to decrease hydrochloric acid production, which will reduce stimulation of the pancreas. Somatostatin is considered the best inhibitor of pancreatic secretion and may be added to the PN solution.

The optimal route of nutrition in acute pancreatitis has been the subject of much controversy over the years. To summarize, studies have shown equal effectiveness of PN or EN in terms of days to normalization of serum amylase, days to resumption of oral feeding, serum albumin levels, nosocomial infections, and clinical outcome. But there is a substantial cost savings with EN and fewer septic complications. In some cases clinical outcome measures improve in enterally fed patients as compared to the parenterally fed patients. EN shows a trend toward faster attenuation of inflammation, with fewer septic complications (Louie et al., 2005).

Depressed serum calcium levels are often identified in patients with acute pancreatitis. Possible causes include hypoalbuminemia with subsequent third spacing of fluid. The calcium, which is bound to the albumin, is thus affected and may appear artificially low. Another possible explanation is a "soap" formation in the gut by the calcium and fatty acids created by the fat necrosis that results in less calcium absorption. Checking an ionized calcium level is a method of determining available calcium.

Aggressive nutrition support may also include attempts to use the gastrointestinal tract. The location of the feeding and the composition of the formula determine the degree of pancreatic stimulation. Intraduodenal infusion of the same formula increased the volume of secretions, whereas infusion into the jejunum did not change basal pancreatic output. By feeding into the jejunum in patients, the cephalic and gastric phases of exocrine pancreatic stimulation are eliminated (Stanga et al., 2005).

Various formulations have been used in pancreatitis, but no comparative studies exist to determine the relative merits of standard, partially digested, elemental, or "immune-enhanced" formulations. Polymeric formulas infused at various sections of the gut stimulate the pancreas more than elemental and hydrolyzed formulas. Close observation for patient tolerance is important. Chapter 20 discusses jejunal feedings in detail. When the patient is allowed to eat, supplemental pancreatic enzymes may be needed to treat steatorrhea.

Chronic Pancreatitis. In contrast to acute pancreatitis, chronic pancreatitis usually evolves insidiously over many years. Chronic pancreatitis is characterized by recurrent attacks of epigastric pain of long duration that may radiate into the back. The pain can be precipitated by meals. Associated nausea, vomiting, or diarrhea makes it difficult to maintain adequate nutrition status. Patients with chronic pancreatitis are at increased risk of developing protein-calorie malnutrition because of pancreatic insufficiency and inadequate oral intake resulting from postprandial pain. In one study patients with chronic pancreatitis admitted to a tertiary care center were found to have a 90% incidence of malnutrition, including weight loss, deficits of lean muscle and adipose tissue, visceral protein depletion, and impaired immune function (Matarese et al., 2000). There is also an increase in energy requirements, and weight loss may result.

The objective of therapy for patients with chronic pancreatitis is to prevent further damage to the pancreas, decrease the number of attacks of acute inflammation, alleviate pain, decrease steatorrhea, and correct malnutrition. Dietary intake should be as liberal as possible, but modifications may be necessary to minimize symptoms (see *Clinical Insight:* Nutrition for Chronic Pancreatitis).

Substitution of dietary fat with MCT oil may relieve steatorrhea and lead to weight gain. Malabsorption of the

Pancreatitis

ETIOLOGY

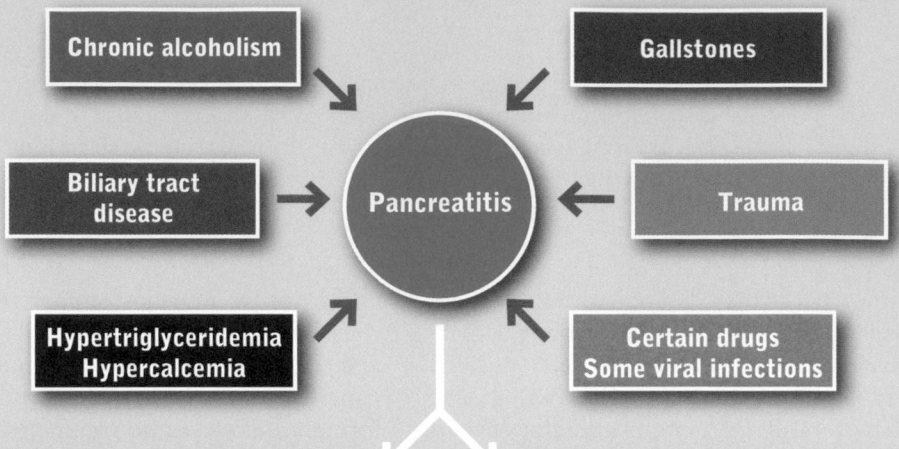

PATHOPHYSIOLOGY

Diagnosis

I: Apply Ranson's criteria
II: Tests of pancreatic function
  Secretin stimulation test
  Glucose tolerance test
  72-hour stool fat test

Clinical Findings

Symptoms:
• Abdominal pain and distention
• Nausea
• Vomiting
• Steatorrhea
In severe form:
• Hypotension
• Oliguria
• Dyspnea

MANAGEMENT

Medical Management

Acute:
• Withhold oral feeding
• Give IV fluids
• Administer H$_2$-receptor antagonists, somatostatin
Chronic:
• Manage intestinal pH with:
  • Antacids
  • H$_2$-receptor antagonists
  • Proton pump inhibitors
• Administer insulin for glucose intolerance

Nutrition Management

Acute:
• Withhold oral and enteral feeding
• Support with IV fluids
• If oral nutrition cannot be initiated in 5 to 7 days, start nutrition support
• For less severe cases of prolonged acute pancreatitis, TF can be initiated beyond the ligament of Treitz using a polymeric formula
• For severe acute pancreatitis, PN should be initiated
  • If TGs are <400 mg/dl before PN initiation, use a 3-in-1 solution and monitor TG levels
  • If TGs are elevated (≥400 mg/dl), use a dextrose-based solution, monitor serum glucose frequently, and treat as needed with insulin
• Once oral nutrition is started, provide
  • Easily digestible foods
  • Low-fat diet
  • 6 small meals
  • Adequate protein intake
  • Increased calories
Chronic:
• Provide oral diet as in acute phase
• TF can be used when oral diet is inadequate
• Supplement pancreatic enzymes
• Supplement fat-soluble vitamins and vitamin B$_{12}$

Algorithm content developed by John J.B. Anderson, PhD, and Sanford C. Garner, PhD, 2000. Updated by Jeanette Hasse, PhD, RD, LD, CNSD, FADA, and Laura E. Matarese, MS, RD, LD, CNSD, FADA, 2006.

Nutrition for Chronic Pancreatitis

The first goal of medical nutrition therapy is to provide optimal nutrition support, and the second is to decrease pain by minimizing stimulation of the exocrine pancreas. Because cholecystokinin (CCK) stimulates secretion from the exocrine pancreas, one approach is to decrease CCK levels. If postprandial pain is a limiting factor, alternative enteral therapies that minimally stimulate the pancreas are warranted. Nutrition counseling, antioxidants, and pancreatic enzymes may play a role in effective management of chronic pancreatitis (CP) as well (Shea et al., 2000).

Idiopathic CP is often associated with a cystic fibrosis gene mutation, and therapies directed toward cystic fibrosis may benefit these patients (Shea et al., 2000). When pancreatic function is diminished by about 90%, enzyme production and secretion are insufficient; maldigestion and malabsorption of protein and fat thus become a problem. Large meals with high-fat foods and alcohol should be avoided. The patient may present with weight loss despite adequate energy intake and will complain of bulky, greasy stools. Pancreatic enzyme replacement is mandatory at this time.

Pancreatic enzyme replacements are given orally with meals; the dosage should be at least 30,000 units of lipase with each meal. To promote weight gain, the level of fat in the diet should be the maximum a patient can tolerate without increased steatorrhea or pain. Additional therapies that may be tried to maintain nutrition status and minimize symptoms in patients with maximum enzyme supplementation include a lower-fat diet (40 to 60 g/day) or substitution of some dietary fat with medium-chain triglyceride oil to improve fat absorption and weight gain. Meals should be small and frequent.

---

fat-soluble vitamins may occur in patients with significant steatorrhea. Also, deficiency of pancreatic protease, necessary to cleave vitamin B_{12} from its carrier protein, could potentially lead to vitamin B_{12} deficiency. With appropriate supplemental enzyme therapy, vitamin absorption should be improved; however, the patient should still be monitored periodically for vitamin deficiencies. Water-soluble forms of the fat-soluble vitamins or parenteral administration of vitamin B_{12} may be necessary (see Chapter 31 for a discussion of B_{12} administration).

Because pancreatic bicarbonate secretion is frequently defective, medical management may also include maintenance of an optimal intestinal pH to facilitate enzyme activation. Antacids, H_2-receptor antagonists, or proton pump inhibitors that reduce gastric acid secretion may be used to achieve this effect.

In chronic cases with extensive pancreatic destruction, the insulin-secreting capacity of the pancreas decreases, and glucose intolerance develops. Treatment with insulin and nutrition care similar to that used for a patient with diabetes mellitus is then required (see Chapter 30). Management is delicate and should focus on control of symptoms rather than normoglycemia as the goal (see *Clinical Insight:* Fasting Hypoglycemia).

Effort should be made to cater to the patient's tolerances and preferences for nutritional management; however, alcohol is prohibited because of the possibility of exacerbating the pancreatic disease. There is evidence that the progressive destruction of the pancreas will be slowed in the alcoholic patient who abstains from alcohol.

Pancreatic Surgery

A surgical procedure often used for pancreatic carcinoma is a **pancreaticoduodenectomy (Whipple procedure).** A cholecystectomy, vagotomy, or a partial gastrectomy may also be done during the surgery. The pancreatic duct is reanastomosed to the jejunum. Partial or complete pancreatic insufficiency can result, depending on the extent of the pancreatic resection. Most patients who have undergone pancreatic resection are at risk for vitamin and mineral deficiencies and will benefit from vitamin and mineral supplementation. Nutrition care is similar to that for chronic pancreatitis.

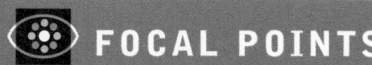

FOCAL POINTS

- The goals of nutrition care in diseases of the liver, biliary system, and exocrine pancreas are to improve nutrition status and to support the patient during the acute phases of illness.
- Understanding the physiology and function of these vital organs along with the pathology that results from disease will decrease patient morbidity and lead to more specific and complete nutrition care and better treatment and outcomes.

CLINICAL SCENARIO 1

Frank is a 40-year-old man admitted to the hospital with chief complaints of right upper quadrant pain, anorexia, nausea, dysgeusia, and frequent loose stools. On physical examination he has mild peripheral edema with a slightly jaundiced appearance. No asterixis is noted. The patient's mental status is clear, but he appears lethargic. He reports no history of portal hypertension, ascites, or gastrointestinal bleeding. Muscle wasting is noted along with stomatitis. The patient has a significant alcohol abuse history spanning 15 years.

Abnormal laboratory values include elevated liver enzymes and total bilirubin; serum albumin, 2.5 g/dl; transferrin, 150 mg/dl; megaloblastic anemia profile; $NH_3 = 75$ mmol/L. A preliminary diagnosis of alcoholic hepatitis with possible mild pancreatic insufficiency is made. On biopsy steatosis and fibrosis are found. Nutritional data include height, 177.8 cm; weight, 67 kg; ideal body weight, 75 kg ± 10%; usual body weight, 82 kg (5 years ago), 73 kg (6 months ago).

✳**Nutrition Diagnosis:** Excessive alcohol consumption as evidenced by patient history and physical examination findings

✳**Nutrition Diagnosis:** Evident protein-calorie malnutrition related to inadequate protein-calorie intake as evidenced by 82% usual weight, and physical examination findings of muscle wasting

1. Based on available data, what vitamin or mineral deficiencies may exist?
2. What nutrition therapy would you prescribe?
3. What nutrition parameters are affected by the patient's liver dysfunction?
4. What is Frank's overall nutrition status?
5. What conditions may be leading to his frequent loose stools?
6. What further information would you require or obtain to complete your assessment?

✳ **CLINICAL SCENARIO 2**

Michael is a 25-year-old white college student who was struck by a car 3 years ago. After the accident his spleen was removed, and recovery seemed to be unremarkable; however, for about 6 months Michael has been unable to eat meals with his friends and has noticed a weight loss of 25 lb. He is 6 ft tall and weighs 160 lb; previously his usual weight was 185 lb. His physicians are puzzled but have identified chronic pancreatitis as a result of the injuries to his internal organs. Michael complains of postprandial pain and steatorrhea with every meal.

✳**Nutrition Diagnosis:** Involuntary weight loss related to postprandial pain as evidenced by 25 lb weight loss

1. What dietary changes might be helpful?
2. If Michael was to try using pancreatic enzymes, what modifications in fat intake would you recommend?
3. Does Michael need nutrition support? If yes, what do you recommend?

USEFUL WEBSITES

National Institute on Alcohol Abuse and Alcoholism
www.niaaa.nih.gov

American Liver Foundation
www.liverfoundation.org

Euroliver Foundation
www.liver.org

Transplant Living
http://www.transplantliving.org/OrganFacts/liver.aspx

References

Abayli B et al: Helicobacter pylori in the etiology of cholesterol gallstones, *J Clin Gastroenterol* 39(2):134, 2005.
Adler DG et al: Standards of Practice Committee of American Society for Gastrointestinal Endoscopy: ASGE guideline: the role of ERCP in diseases of the biliary tract and the pancreas, *Gastrointest Endosc* 62(1):1, 2005.
Afdhal NH: Diseases of the gallbladder and bile ducts. In Goldman L, Ausiello D, editors: *Cecil textbook of medicine*, ed 22, Philadelphia, 2004, Saunders.
Alberino F et al: Nutrition and survival in patients with liver cirrhosis, *Nutrition* 17:445, 2001.

Al-Jiffry BO et al: Changes in gallbladder motility and gallstone formation following laparoscopic gastric banding for morbid obesity, *Can J Gastroenter* 17(3):169, 2003.

Allard JP et al: Effects of ascites resolution after successful TIPS on nutrition in cirrhotic patients with refractory ascites, *Am J Gastroenterol* 96(8):2442, 2001.

Als-Nielsen B et al: Branched-chain amino acids for hepatic encephalopathy, *Cochrane Database Syst Rev* 1:CD001939, 2003.

Alvares-da-Silva MR, Reverbel da Silveira T: Comparison between handgrip strength, subjective global assessment, and prognostic nutritional index in assessing malnutrition and predicting clinical outcome in cirrhotic outpatients, *Nutrition* 21:113, 2005.

Berenguer M et al: Viral hepatitis. In Feldman M et al, editors: *Sleisenger and Fordtrans' gastrointestinal and liver disease*, ed 7, Philadelphia, 2002, Saunders.

Bianchi GP et al: Vegetable versus animal protein diet in cirrhotic patients with chronic encephalopathy: a randomized crossover comparison, *J Intern Med* 233:385, 1993.

Brandhagen DJ et al: Recognition and management of hereditary hemochromatosis, *Am Fam Physician* 65:853, 2002.

Brewer G et al: Does a vegetarian diet control Wilson's disease? *J Am Coll Nutr* 12:527, 1993.

Campillo B et al: Evaluation of nutritional practice in hospitalized cirrhotic patients: results of a prospective study, *Nutrition* 19:515, 2003.

Campillo B et al: Enteral nutrition in severely malnourished and anorectic cirrhotic patients in clinical practice, *Gastroenterol Clin Biol* 29(6):645, 2005.

Cordoba J: Normal protein diet for episodic hepatic encephalopathy: results of a randomized study, *J Hepatol* 41:38, 2004.

Crippin JS: Is tube feeding an option in patients with liver disease? *Nutr Clin Pract* 21:296, 2006.

Cuhna L et al: Effects of prolonged oral nutritional support in malnourished cirrhotic patients: results of a pilot study, *Gastroenterol Clin Biol* 28:36, 2004.

Davidson J et al: New-onset diabetes after transplantation: 2003 international consensus guidelines, *Transplantation* 75(suppl): SS3, 2003.

Detsky AS et al: What is subjective global assessment? *JPEN J Parenter Enteral Nutr* 11:8, 1987.

Diehl AM: Acute and chronic liver failure and hepatic encephalopathy. In Goldman L, Bennett JC, editors: *Cecil textbook of medicine*, ed 21, Philadelphia, 2000, Saunders.

Diehl AM: Alcoholic and nonalcoholic steatohepatitis. In Goldman L, Ausiello D, editors: *Cecil textbook of medicine*, ed 22, Philadelphia, 2004, Saunders.

Dolz C et al: Ascites increases the resting energy expenditure in liver cirrhosis, *Gastroenterology* 100:738, 1991.

Donaghy A: Issues of malnutrition and bone disease in patients with cirrhosis, *J Gastroenterol Hepatol* 17:462, 2002.

Ederoth P et al: Experimental pancreatitis causes acute perturbation of energy metabolism in the intestinal wall, *Pancreas* 25:270, 2002.

Fallon M: Hepatic tumors. In Goldman L, Ausiello D, editors: *Cecil textbook of medicine*, ed 22, Philadelphia, 2004, Saunders.

Figueiredo F et al: Effect of liver cirrhosis on body composition: evidence of significant depletion even in mild disease, *J Gastroenterol Hepatol* 20:209, 2005.

Friedman SL, Schiano TD: Cirrhosis and its sequelae. In Goldman L, Ausiello D, editors: *Cecil textbook of medicine*, ed 22, Philadelphia, 2004, Saunders.

Hager LA: Hepatic complications associated with total parenteral nutrition, *Support Line* 16(3):1, 1994.

Hanje AJ et al: The use of selected nutritional supplements and complementary and alternative medicine in liver disease, *Nutr Clin Pract* 21:255, 2006.

Hasse J: Nutritional aspects of adult liver transplantation. In Busuttil RW, Klintmalm GB, editors: *Transplantation of the liver* ed 2, Philadelphia, 2005, Saunders.

Hasse J et al: Subjective global assessment—alternative nutritional assessment technique for adult liver transplant candidates, *Nutrition* 9:330, 1993.

Hasse JM: Nutrition assessment and support of organ transplant recipients, *JPEN J Parenter Enteral Nutr* 25:120, 2001.

Hasse JM et al: Early enteral nutrition support in patients undergoing liver transplantation, *JPEN J Parenter Enteral Nutr* 19:437, 1995.

Hay JE et al: A controlled trial of calcitonin therapy for the prevention of postliver transplantation atraumatic fractures in patients with primary biliary cirrhosis and primary sclerosing cholangitis, *J Hepatol* 34:292, 2001.

Heisel O et al: New onset diabetes mellitus in patients receiving calcineurin inhibitors: a systematic review and meta-analysis, *Am J Transplant* 4:583, 2004.

Hiyama DT, Fischer JE: Nutritional support in hepatic failure, *Nutr Clin Pract* 3:96, 1988.

Hoofnagle JH, Lindsay KL: Acute viral hepatitis. In Goldman L, Ausiello D, editors: *Cecil textbook of medicine*, ed 22, Philadelphia, 2004, Saunders.

Iglezias Brandao de Oliveira C et al: Impact of rapid weight reduction on risk of cholelithiasis after bariatric surgery, *Obes Surg* 13:625, 2003.

Isoniemi H et al: Transdermal oestrogen therapy protects postmenopausal liver transplant women from osteoporosis: a 2-year follow-up study, *J Hepatol* 34:299, 2001.

Jacobs BP et al: Milk thistle for the treatment of liver disease: a systematic review and meta-analysis, *Am J Med* 113:506, 2002.

Kayler LK et al: Long-term survival after liver transplantation in children with metabolic disorders, *Pediatr Transplant* 6:295, 2002.

Keefe EB: Hepatic failure and liver transplantation. In Goldman L, Ausiello D, editors: *Cecil textbook of medicine*, ed 22, Philadelphia, 2004, Saunders.

Kim WR et al: Burden of liver disease in the United States: summary of a workshop, *Hepatology* 36:227, 2002.

Klein GL et al: Hepatic osteodystrophy in chronic cholestasis: evidence for a multifactorial etiology, *Pediatr Transplant* 6:136, 2002.

Latifi R et al: Nutritional support in liver failure, *Surg Clin North Am* 71:567, 1991.

Lee DW et al: Biliary decompression by nasobiliary catheter or biliary stent in acute suppurative cholangitis: a prospective randomized trial, *Gastrointest Endosc* 56:361, 2002.

Leevy CM, Davison E: Portal hypertension and hepatic coma, *Postgrad Med J* 41:84, 1967.

Leevy CM, Moroianu SA: Nutritional aspects of alcoholic liver disease, *Clin Liver Dis* 9:67, 2005.

Liu Q et al: Synbiotic modulation of gut flora: effect on minimal hepatic encephalopathy in patients with cirrhosis, *Hepatology* 39:1441, 2004.

Louie BE et al: 2004 MacLean-Mueller prize enteral or parenteral nutrition for severe pancreatitis: a randomized controlled trial and health technology assessment, *Can J Surg* 48(4):298, 2005.

Mahadevan U et al: Sclerosing cholangitis and recurrent pyogenic cholangitis. In Feldman M et al, editors: *Sleisenger and Fordtrans' gastrointestinal and liver disease*, ed 7, Philadelphia, 2002, Saunders.

Maher JJ: Inherited, infiltrative, and metabolic disorders involving the liver. In Goldman L, Ausiello D, editors: *Cecil textbook of medicine*, ed 22, Philadelphia, 2004, Saunders.

Marchesini G: Nutritional supplementation with branched-chain amino acids in advanced cirrhosis: a double-blind, randomized trial, *Gastroenterology* 124(7):1792, 2003.

Marchetti P: New-onset diabetes after liver transplantation: from pathogenesis to management, *Liver Transplant* 11:612, 2005.

Matarese LE et al: Nutritional status of patients with chronic pancreatitis admitted to a tertiary care center, *Am J Gastroenterol* 95:A2481, 2000.

McCullough AJ: Malnutrition in liver disease, *Liver Transplant* 6(4):S85, 2000.

McCullough AJ, Tavill AS: Disordered energy and protein metabolism in liver disease, *Semin Liver Dis* 11:265, 1991.

Medici V et al: Diagnosis and management of Wilson's disease: results of a single center experience, *J Clin Gastroenterol* 40(10):936, 2006.

Merg AR et al: Mechanisms of impaired gallbladder contractile response in chronic acalculous cholecystitis, *J Gastrointest Surg* 6:432, 2002.

Morgan TR et al: Protein consumption and hepatic encephalopathy in alcoholic hepatitis, *J Am Coll Nutr* 14:152, 1995.

Mullen KD, Weber FL: Role of nutrition in hepatic encephalopathy, *Semin Liver Dis* 11(4):292, 1991.

Nielsen K et al: Long-term oral refeeding of patients with cirrhosis of the liver, *Br J Nutr* 74:557, 1995.

Plauth M et al: Weight gain after transjugular intrahepatic protosystemic shunt is associated with improvement in body composition in malnourished patients with cirrhosis and hypermetabolism, *J Hepatol* 24:228, 2004.

Polonsky K: A practical approach to fasting hypoglycemia, *N Engl J Med* 326:1020, 1992.

Priori P et al: Stimulation of gallbladder emptying by intravenous lipids, *JPEN J Parenter Enteral Nutr* 21(6):350, 1997.

Rambaldi A, Gluud C: S-adenosyl-L-methionine for alcoholic liver diseases, *Cochrane Database Syst Rev* April 19(2): CD002235, 2006.

Ranson JH et al: Prognostic signs and the role of operative management in acute pancreatitis, *Surg Gynecol Obstet* 139:69, 1974.

Rayes N et al: Early enteral supply of lactobacillus and fiber versus selective bowel decontamination: a controlled trial in liver transplant recipients, *Transplantation* 74(1):123, 2002.

Rayes N et al: Supply of pre- and probiotics reduces bacterial infection rates after liver transplantation—a randomized, double-blind trial, *Am J Transplant* 5(1):125, 2005.

Sharma P et al: Monitoring and care of the patient before liver transplantation. In Busuttil RW, Klintmalm GB, editors: *Transplantation of the liver*, ed 2, Philadelphia, 2005, Saunders.

Shea JC et al: Advances in nutritional management of chronic pancreatitis, *Curr Gastroenterol Rep* 2:323, 2000.

Solga SF: Probiotics can treat hepatic encephalopathy, *Med Hypotheses* 561:307, 2003.

Stanga Z et al: Effect of jejunal long-term feeding in chronic pancreatitis, *JPEN J Parenter Enteral Nutr* 29(1):12, 2005.

Stickel F et al: Review article: nutritional therapy in alcoholic liver disease, *Aliment Pharmacol Ther* 18:357, 2003.

Trautwein C et al: Bone density and metabolism in patients with viral hepatitis and cholestatic liver diseases before and after liver transplantation, *Am J Gastroenterol* 95:2343, 2000.

Volzke H et al: Independent risk factors for gallstone formation in a region with high cholelithiasis prevalence, *Digestion* 71(2):97, 2005.

Willner IR, Reuben A: Alcohol and the liver, *Curr Opin Gastroenterol* 21:323, 2005.

Zaina FE et al: Prevalence of malnutrition in liver transplant candidates, *Transplant Proc* 36:923, 2004.

CHAPTER 29

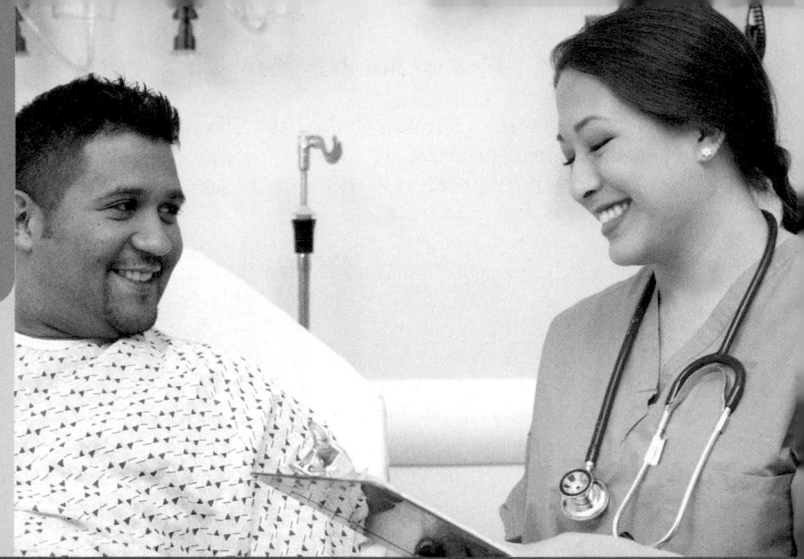

Sherry K. Hubbard, RD, LD

Medical Nutrition Therapy for Food Allergy and Food Intolerance

KEY TERMS

adverse food reaction any undesired response to a food regardless of mechanism

allergen a substance foreign to the body that, on interaction with the immune system, causes an allergic reaction

anaphylaxis an acute, often severe, and sometimes fatal immune response that can affect one or more organ systems

antibodies immunoglobulins produced in response to an antigen or allergen

antigen a foreign substance (e.g., protein, cells, bacteria, polysaccharides) that stimulates antibody production

atopic dermatitis (eczema) a skin rash characterized by an itchy inflammation with small red and white bumps that itch; often a symptom of allergy

atopic march the presence of atopic characteristics, events, or conditions that develop into more permanent disease

atopy tendency toward allergies; determined genetically

cap-FEIA (fluorescein-enzyme immunoassay) a blood test, more sensitive than the radioallergosorbent test (RAST), that provides quantitative assessment of food-specific IgE antibodies

cell-mediated immunity immunity that is mediated by T lymphocytes, either through the release of lymphokines or by direct cytotoxicity

cross-reactivity an allergic response to a food or substance either within a given group (e.g., Crustacea, legumes) or with unrelated substances (e.g., banana, kiwi, or chestnuts with latex)

double-blind, placebo-controlled food challenge (DBPCFC) a food test in which the suspect food is disguised such that neither the patient nor the researcher knows when it is being given; the gold standard for establishing food allergy

elimination diet an investigational short-term or possible life-long eating plan that omits one or more foods suspected or known to cause an adverse food reaction or allergic response

eosinophilic esophagitis abnormal presence of a high number of eosinophils in the mucosa and submucosa; may or may not be food allergy associated

eosinophilic gastroenteritis abnormal presence of a high number of eosinophils in the mucosal surface, muscularis or subserosa; may or may not be food allergy associated

food allergen families cupin superfamily, prolamin superfamily, protein of the plant defense system pathogenesis-related proteins and profilins

food allergy (hypersensitivity) an adverse food reaction that is mediated by an immunoglobulin E (IgE) immunologic mechanism; induced by cell-mediated or immune-complex disease; reaction occurs consistently after ingestion, inhalation, or touch of a particular food, causing functional changes in target organs

food and symptom diary a subjective tool for recording food and drink consumed and onset, intensity, and duration of symptoms

food challenge presenting a food to a patient with or without knowledge of when the food is being ingested using tolerated food vehicles to hide the food as necessary to prove or disprove a food-symptom relationship (open-, single-blind placebo-controlled, and double-blind placebo-controlled food challenges)

food immunotherapy vaccine future treatment designed to prevent an allergic reaction, reduce its severity, and prevent death in the event of accidental exposure

food intolerance an adverse reaction to a food caused by toxic, pharmacologic, metabolic, or idiosyncratic reactions to the food or chemical substances in the food

humoral immunity immunity mediated by antibodies produced by B lymphocytes

immunoglobulin E (IgE) mediated reaction rapid onset of symptoms occurring after ingestion of a specific allergen that cross-links the antigen-specific IgE molecule to mast cells and basophils

immunoglobulin G (IgG) indicates previous food exposure; used mainly for research

mast cells tissue cells that release histamine or other substances, causing allergic symptoms

oral allergy syndrome (OAS)/pollen-food syndrome (PFS) a mild-to-severe itch, tingle, or burning sensation affecting the mouth, tongue, or throat; throat tightness or lip swelling after ingesting a food protein (e.g., melons) known to cross-react with a pollen (e.g., ragweed)

oral tolerance an inhibited immune response associated with prior exposures to food antigen or bacteria by the oral route

probiotics a microbial dietary supplement affecting the intestinal tract that may modify immune response

radioallergosorbent test (RAST) a test that measures specific IgE antibodies in serum; used as an alternative to skin tests

sensitization exposure to an antigen or allergen that results in the development of hypersensitivity

skin test a test in which an antigen is applied directly to the skin and then pricked or scratched through with a needle or a specifically designed prick or scratch implement to observe the histamine response

thymus and tonsils tissues of lymphoid material that contribute to immunity

Food allergy prevalence has almost doubled during the past 20 years, with a defined increase in severity and scope. Approximately 20% of the population believes any adverse reaction to a food is a food allergy. Food allergy evaluation requests increase with public awareness (Nowak-Wegrzyn and Sampson, 2006). This does not dissolve the frequent misconception that all reactions to food are allergy based. Until actual food allergy is properly diagnosed, the term **adverse food reaction,** an umbrella term used for any undesired food reaction, should be emphasized.

IMMUNOLOGIC BASIS

Definitions

The term *adverse food reaction* encompasses food intolerance and food hypersensitivity. **Food intolerance** is an adverse reaction to a food caused by toxic, pharmacologic, metabolic, idiosyncratic, or nonimmunoglobulin E (IgE) reactions to food or chemical substances in the food. **Food allergy (hypersensitivity)** is an IgE-mediated reaction that occurs when the immune system reacts to a normally harmless food protein that the body has erroneously identified as harmful. This immunopathologic IgE-mediated process is reproducible through a "cause-and-effect relationship." IgE reactions usually occur instantly or within 2 hours of exposure, with severity ranging from mild to life threatening. Exposure includes inhalation, ingestion, and skin contact. Reactions to foods are not limited to ingestion reactions (Bahna, 2001).

Any person, especially a child, who has a genetic predisposition to atopic disease, or **atopy,** has an increased probability of developing food allergies. Allergic disease includes allergies to airborne particles (pollen, molds, grasses, weeds), food allergy, **atopic dermatitis (eczema),** and atopic-induced asthma. Children with atopic dermatitis are 35% more likely to develop food allergies than other atopic children with approximately 6% to 8% asthmatic children experiencing food-induced wheezing (Sampson, 2004).

The incidence of food allergy appears to decrease with age. Infants younger than 2 years of age are more likely to develop food allergies than are older children or adults. Older children and adults are more likely to develop inhalant allergies than food allergies. Incidence estimates of food allergy indicate population ranges from 6% to 8% in children to 3% to 4% in adults (Sicherer and Sampson, 2006; Nowak-Wegrzyn and Sampson, 2006).

Immune System

The immune system functions to clear the body of foreign substances or **antigens** such as viruses, bacteria, blood cells, and tissue cells. Normally, when antigens interact with cells of the immune system, they are cleared from the body without an adverse reaction. Allergy is different in that **sensitization** occurs. This happens on the first exposure of the immune cells to the allergen, when the immune cells are changed so that they subsequently recognize the allergen at the next exposure to it. Three types of cells respond to antigens presented: B lymphocytes, T lymphocytes, and macrophages. The lymphocytes arising from stem cells in the bone marrow, along with T cells originating from stem cells in the thymus, function as the basis for the two branches of the immune system: the humoral pathway and the cell-mediated pathway.

Humoral immunity involves **antibodies** (immunoglobulins) and has an important role in food allergy. Antigen-specific antibodies are produced by the B lymphocytes (B cells) in response to the antigen presented. The union of an antigen and its antibody results in the production of chemical mediators by the mast cells or direct cellular damage, which, in turn, causes symptoms. Five classes of antibodies have been identified: IgA, IgD, IgE, IgG, and IgM; they protect the body against bacteria and viruses. Secretory IgA antibodies in breast milk provide breast-fed infants with local intestinal protection against viruses and bacteria. IgA antibodies, present in saliva and intestinal secretions, block the absorption of antigens. IgE antibodies help to eliminate parasites from the body and are also responsible for classic allergic reactions: the **immunoglobulin E (IgE)-mediated**

reactions. IgD is involved in immunoglobulin class switching, but its other functions remain elusive. Many attempts have been made to suggest that **immunoglobulin G (IgG)** is an important indicator of allergy, especially food allergy. According to the World Allergy Organization Nomenclature Review Committee in October 2003, "food-specific IgG antibodies in serum are not of clinical importance but merely indicate previous exposure to the food." Researchers continue to use IgG and IgG4 levels as a tool, attempting to find a clinical usefulness (Johansson et al., 2004; Hamilton and Adkinson, 2004; Akdis et al., 2006).

Cellular or **cell-mediated immunity** involves the action of T lymphocytes (T cells). T cells do not produce antibodies, but they do recognize antigens. When an antigen stimulates T-cell growth, the T cells produce lymphokines and cytokines, substances that help regulate the activities of the B cells or that cause direct cellular damage to target cells, resulting in the destruction of antigens. Cellular immunity has an important role in resistance to viruses, fungi, tumor cells, and other foreign cells through its production of the controller lymphocytes identified as Th1 and Th2 cells. Both Th1 and Th2 cells may work together.

Cell-mediated immunity is stimulated by Th1-like cells linked to specific lymphokine profiles. IgE antibody formation is associated with Th2 type cells. Th2 stimulation produces eosinophils and mast cells, and the result is atopic disease. The Th1 cells linked to lymphokines stimulate cell-mediated immunity, and yet they suppress IgE antibody formation (Kay, 2001). The balance between antigen-specific Th1 and Th2 cells may have a significant effect on the antigen-specific IgE immune response. Future allergy prevention using probiotic supplementation in high-risk or normal newborns includes manipulating the Th1 and Th2 immune response and thus possibly protecting against Th1 type autoimmune disease and Th2-mediated atopic disease (Isolauri and Salminen, 2005). Tissue macrophages, derived from monocytes in the blood, also have important roles in the recognition, clearance, and presentation of antigens. Through the process of phagocytosis, the macrophage engulfs and destroys antigens. B cells, T cells, mast cells, and macrophages are all thought to interact (Figure 29-1).

The **thymus and tonsils** also play a role in immunity. The thymus is a ductless, glandlike organ that, because of its T-cell production, is essential to the development of peripheral lymphoid tissue. Although the thymus is largest and most active before puberty, the mature T cells it exports exert their effect into adulthood. Removal of the thymus during adulthood has little effect on a person's resistance to disease.

The tonsils consist of two small, rounded masses of lymphoid tissue that lie in the path of inspired air and all ingested food and liquids. Foreign material that is inspired into the airways and becomes trapped in the tonsillar crypts comes in contact with antigen-processing cells. Tonsils are particularly useful to children under the age of 8, protecting them against respiratory infections. With increased age or surgical removal of the tonsils lymphatic tissues help cover the immunologic function of the tonsils.

Allergic Reactions

Allergic reactions are unusual responses of the immune system and represent altered reactivity to an antigen. The antigens involved in allergic reactions are called **allergens.** Immune reactions are classified into four types: types I, II, and III, which are antibody-dependent; and type IV, which is T cell–dependent (Table 29-1).

Immediate hypersensitivity (type I), involving IgE, is the most common allergic reaction and has the most clearly understood mechanism. The combination of an allergen with allergen-specific IgE fixed to tissue **mast cells** or circulating basophils causes the release of chemical mediators, including histamine, cytokines, lipid-derived prostaglandins, interleukins, and others. When released, these inflammatory mediators can cause itching, contraction of smooth muscle, vasodilation, and secretion of mucus. Manifestations, which are most often systemic, may involve the skin, gastrointestinal tract, or respiratory system (see Figure 29-1).

The gastrointestinal tract is the most frequent means of food allergy development. A lack of **oral tolerance** is the current focus in food allergy development. The gastrointestinal tract determines how to consider each food protein with every exposure. The potential to develop food allergies is great, yet comparatively few people do. Basically the body inhibits immune responses by prior exposure via the T regulatory cells. Food allergy is believed to occur when oral tolerance fails (Chehade and Mayer, 2005; Akdis et al., 2005).

Researchers are now focusing on what goes on with oral tolerance and how this relates to **food allergen families.** In recent years common plant food allergens have been identified with a limited number of protein families. There appears to be significant cross-reactivity of most food allergens with specific proteins causing the majority of allergic reactions. The families are characterized by biochemical and physicochemical properties. Surprisingly, food allergens of animal origin share many of the same properties as plant allergens. The families identified are the cupin superfamily, prolamin superfamily, protein of the plant defense system pathogenesis-related proteins, and profilins (Chapman et al., 2007; Breiteneder and Mills, 2005; Jenkins et al., 2005).

The contribution of non–IgE-mediated immunologic reactions to food hypersensitivity is not as clear. Circulating food-specific antibodies (IgA, IgG, and IgM) are common. IgG specifically indicates that a person has been exposed to a food, but it continues to be considered clinically irrelevant. Yet IgG blood testing for food allergies is touted as valid. Hopefully in years to come IgG will be a more useful test (Johansson, 2004). Defined, carefully orchestrated research needs to better define the clinical relevance of IgG in food-related issues.

It has also been postulated that antigen-antibody complexes (non-IgE mediated reactions) may have a role in food-related inflammatory diseases. These include various forms of colitis, enteritis with bleeding, malabsorptive disorders, ulceration, and chronic pneumonitis (Heiner's syndrome). Cell-mediated hypersensitivity may have a role in celiac disease, protein-losing enteropathies, eosinophilic gastroenteritis, and inflammatory bowel disorders such as ulcerative colitis (Table 29-2).

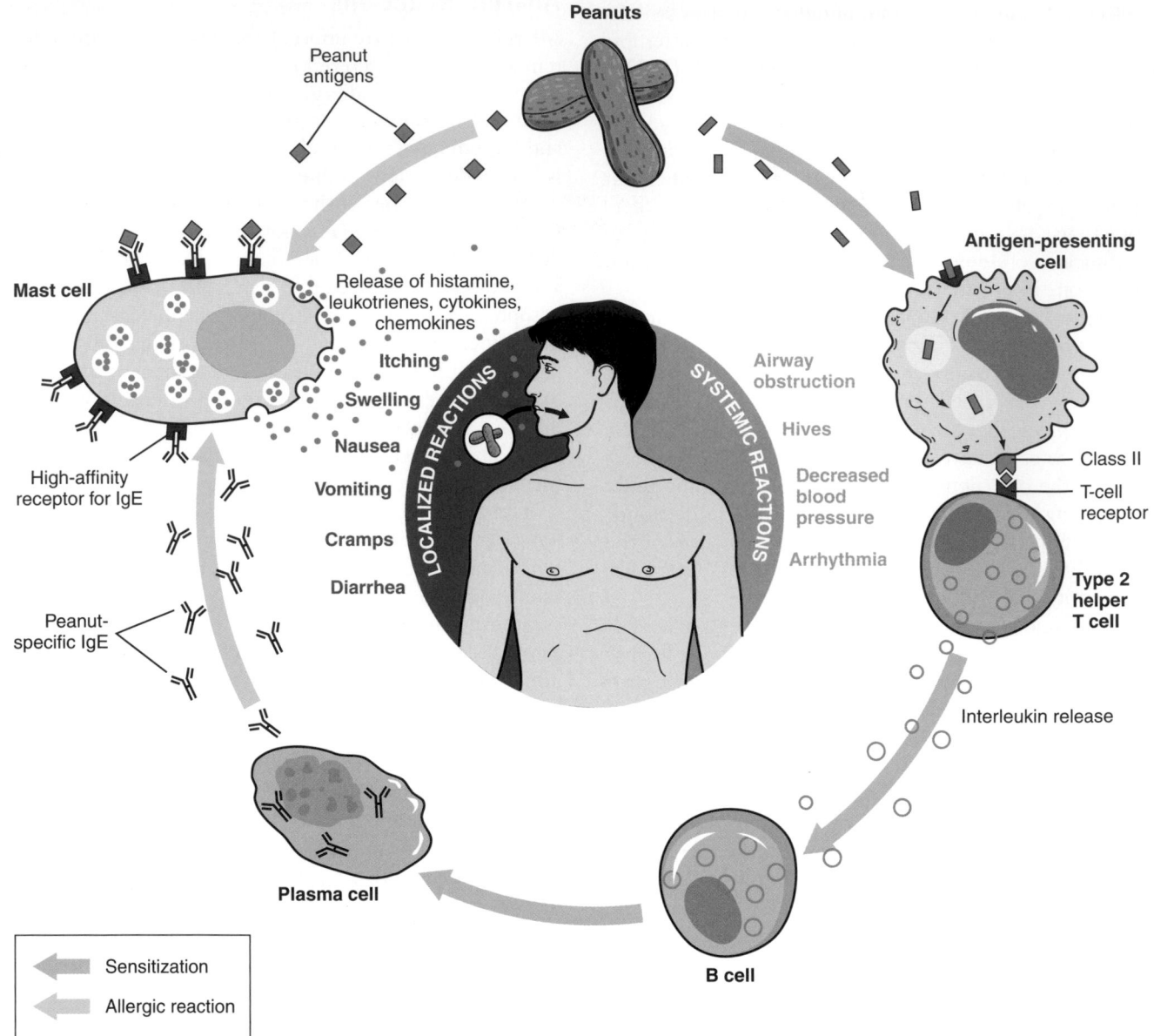

FIGURE 29-1 Sensitization process and allergic reaction.

TABLE 29-1

Types of Allergic Reactions

Reaction/Classification	Mechanism	Comments
Type 1		
Immediate hypersensitivity, anaphylactic IgE-mediated, or reaginic reaction	The allergen binds with sensitized IgE antibody on mast cells (specialized granular cells in the intestines, skin, and respiratory tract) or basophils (similar cells in blood). This results in release of mediators (e.g., histamine, eosinophilic chemotactic factor, bradykinin). IgG has also been identified as being involved in this type of reaction.	Applies to hay fever, anaphylaxis, most food allergies, atopic dermatitis, and asthma. Symptoms occur within seconds or up to 2 hr. Symptoms of food reactions may include laryngeal edema, nausea, vomiting, severe abdominal pain, bloating, diarrhea, angioedema, eczema, erythema, itching, hoarseness, wheezing, cough, chest tightness, hypotension, bronchospasm, and shock.

Modified from Butkus SN, Mahan LK: Food allergies: immunological reactions to foods, *J Am Diet Assoc* 86:601, 1986.

IgE, Immunoglobulin E; *IgG,* immunoglobulin G.

TABLE 29-1

Types of Allergic Reactions—cont'd

Reaction/Classification	Mechanism	Comments
Type II		
Cytotoxic	IgG antibody reacts with the cell membrane or an antigen associated with the cell membrane.	Results from transfusion of incompatible blood types. No food reactions have been demonstrated.
Type III		
Antigen-antibody complex Arthus reaction	Antigen and antibodies (IgG and IgM) form a complex called a "precipitating antibody." The antigen-antibody complex is known as an Arthus reaction when it occurs in soft tissues such as blood vessels, lungs, or kidneys and as serum sickness when the complex circulates. Complement is also activated in some cases.	Occurs in some food reactions. Milk precipitins have been found in the lungs of some children with chronic respiratory infection and in the gastrointestinal tract of those with gastroenteropathy. Reactions usually take 6 hr or more to appear and may take several days to become clinically apparent.
Type IV		
Delayed or cell-mediated hypersensitivity	T cells interact directly with antigen.	Usual mechanism of graft rejection. Possibly involved in some food allergies such as protein-losing enteropathies.

TABLE 29-2

Food Allergy Disorders

Disorder	IgE-Mediated	Mixed Mechanism: IgE and Cell-Mediated	Non-IgE or Cell-Mediated
Timing	Within minutes to 1 hour	Delayed onset >2 hr; chronic, relapsing	Delayed onset >2 hr; chronic, relapsing
Generalized	Anaphylactic shock, food-dependent exercised-induced anaphylaxis		
Cutaneous	Urticaria, angioedema, flushing, morbilliform rash, acute contact urticaria	Atopic dermatitis, contact dermatitis	Dermatitis herpetiformis
Gastrointestinal	Oral allergy syndrome, immediate gastrointestinal food allergy	Allergic eosinophilic esophagitis, allergic eosinophilic gastroenteritis	Allergic proctocolitis, food protein-induced enterocolitis syndrome, celiac disease, infantile colic
Respiratory	Acute rhinoconjunctivitis; bronchospasm	Asthma	Pulmonary hemosiderosis (Heiner's syndrome)

From: Nowak-Wegrzyn A, Sampson HA: Adverse reactions to foods, *Med Clin North Am* 90(1):97, 2006.

SYMPTOMS

A wide range of symptoms has been attributed to food allergy (Box 29-1). Skin, respiratory, cardiovascular, and gastrointestinal symptoms may express during an allergic reaction. Most frequently affected are the skin and respiratory systems (Nowak-Wegrzyn and Sampson, 2006) (Figure 29-2).

Food-induced **anaphylaxis** is an acute, often severe, and sometimes fatal immune response that usually occurs within a limited time following exposure to an antigen. Systemic anaphylaxis is the most dangerous allergic reaction and can include abdominal pain, nausea, vomiting, cyanosis, a drop in blood pressure, angioedema, chest pain, urticaria, diarrhea, shock, and death. A review of 32 fatal anaphylactic reactions to foods identified peanuts and tree nuts as causing the majority of deaths. Milk and fish were identified as causing 2 of the 32 deaths (Bock et al., 2001). People with known anaphylactic reactions to any food allergen should carry and be prepared to use epinephrine (such as an Epi-Pen), the drug of choice to reverse an allergic reaction, at all times (Simons, 2006). Food-dependent, exercise-induced anaphylaxis (FEIAn) is a distinct form of physical allergy. FEIAn may occur within 2 hours after rigorous activ-

ity when it is followed by the ingestion of one or more specific foods that are normally well tolerated. The pathophysiology is unknown (Nowak-Wegrzyn and Sampson, 2006).

Unclear or Unproven Relationships

The role of food allergy in behavioral, psychological, neurologic, and musculoskeletal disorders remains largely unproven. When suspect symptoms not normally considered IgE mediated can be objectively measured without relying on the report of subjective symptoms, a double-blind, placebo-controlled food challenge can help to determine whether a food-symptom relationship exists. This could apply to hyperactivity, tension fatigue syndrome, and migraine headaches. Measuring identifiable objective symptoms may require several disciplines and specialists, depending on the equipment needed to prove or disprove a food-symptom relationship. Even if a food-symptom relationship is not proven but food avoidance is perceived as necessary for an investigation or because of personal choice, appropriate nutrition intervention may prevent or reduce nutritional risk.

BOX 29-1

Symptoms of Food Allergy

Gastrointestinal Manifestations

Abdominal pain
Nausea
Vomiting
Diarrhea
Gastrointestinal bleeding
Protein-losing enteropathy
Oral and pharyngeal pruritus

Cutaneous Manifestations

Urticaria (hives)
Angioedema
Eczema
Erythema (skin inflammation)
Itching
Flushing

Respiratory Manifestations

Rhinitis
Asthma
Cough
Laryngeal edema
Milk-induced syndrome with respiratory disease
  (Heiner's syndrome)
Airway tightening

Systemic Manifestations

Anaphylaxis
Hypotension
Dysrhythmias

Controversial or Unproven Manifestations

Behavioral disorders
Tension-fatigue syndrome
Attention-deficit and hyperactivity disorder
Otitis media
Psychiatric disorders
Neurologic disorders
Musculoskeletal disorders
Migraine headache

RISK FACTORS FOR THE DEVELOPMENT OF FOOD ALLERGY

The risk of developing food allergy depends on heredity, exposure to a food (antigen), gastrointestinal permeability, and environmental factors such as microbial exposure. Heredity is thought to play a major role in the development of atopic disease. Ironically, reduced childhood infections and exposures to microbes are perceived as a cause for the increased incidence of atopic disease in the population, thus initiating the **atopic march,** a collection of conditions, events, and characteristics preceding development of permanent atopic (allergic) disorders (Hahn et al., 2005). Infants who develop food allergies and atopic dermatitis are considered at risk for developing allergic rhinitis and asthma.

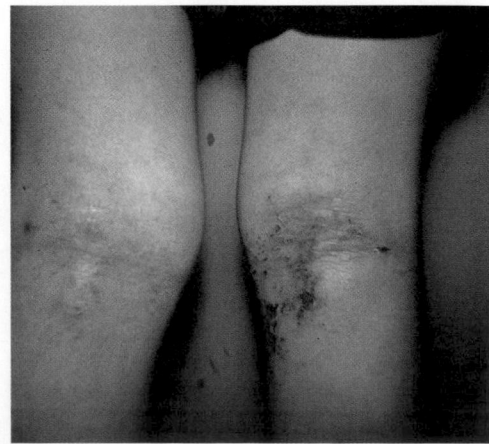

FIGURE 29-2 Atopic eczema—an immunoglobulin E (IgE)–mediated skin reaction to a food allergen. Commonly seen on the back of knees and the inside of elbows.

Exposure to an antigen is a prerequisite for the development of food allergy. The initial exposure can occur prenatally or postnatally. Postnatal sensitization may occur with exposure to food allergens by inhalation, skin contact, or ingestion. Food allergen sensitization can happen with a food antigen in breast milk. Remembering this when taking a medical nutrition history can be very useful and may explain an allergic reaction that occurs at what appears to be the first time an infant eats the antigen in food (Friedman and Zeiger, 2005). Gastrointestinal permeability may allow antigen penetration and presentation to the lymphocytes. Gastrointestinal permeability is thought to be greatest in early infancy and to decline with intestinal maturation. Other conditions such as gastrointestinal disease, malnutrition, prematurity, and immunodeficiency states may also be associated with increased permeability and risk of developing food allergy (see *Pathophysiology and Care Management Algorithm:* Food Allergies).

The amount of antigen present and environmental factors can also influence the development of food allergy. The effects of foods and other antigens may be additive. Clinical symptoms of food allergy may increase when inhalant allergies are exacerbated by seasonal or environmental changes. Similarly, the effects of environmental factors, such as early exposure to microbes, tobacco smoke, stress, exercise, and cold, may enhance the clinical symptoms of food allergy.

FOOD INTOLERANCES

Food intolerances are adverse reactions to foods caused by nonimmunologic or non-IgE mechanisms, including toxic, pharmacologic, metabolic, or idiosyncratic reactions (Table 29-3). Symptoms caused by food intolerances include gastrointestinal, cutaneous, and respiratory disorders and are often similar to those of food allergy. Therefore food intolerances must be considered in the differential diagnosis of food allergy. Although symptoms of food intolerance may be similar to those of food allergy, treatment may be different, depending on the mechanism involved. Allergy skin or blood testing is not useful in the diagnosis and treatment of these conditions.

Food Additives

Historically, food additives such as preservatives, flavor enhancers, and coloring agents have been linked to adverse reactions. Additives implicated include tartrazine (FD&C no. 5), carmine, azo dyes and other coloring agents, benzoic acid, sodium nitrate, butylated hydroxyanisole (BHA), butylated hydroxytoluene (BHT), monosodium glutamate (MSG), and sulfites (see Table 29-3).

A study attempting to confirm symptoms perceived to be associated with food additives, including azo-dyes, benzoates, MSG, sorbates, BHT/BHA, and sulfites, found only

---

TABLE 29-3

Representative Nonimmunologic Reactions to Food

Cause	Associated Food	Symptoms
Gastrointestinal Disorders		
Enzyme deficiency		
Lactase	Foods containing lactose and mammalian milk	Bloating, flatulence, diarrhea, abdominal pain
Glucose-6 phosphate dehydrogenase	Fava or broad beans	Hemolytic anemia
Fructase	Foods containing sucrose or fructose	Bloating, flatulence, diarrhea, abdominal pain
Disease		
Cystic fibrosis	Symptoms may be precipitated by many foods, especially high-fat foods or certain proteins	Bloating, loose stools, abdominal pain
Gallbladder disease		
Enteropathies		
Inborn Errors of Metabolism		
Phenylketonuria	Foods containing phenylalanine	Elevated serum phenylalanine levels, mental retardation
Galactosemia	Foods containing lactose or galactose	Vomiting, lethargy, failure to thrive
Psychological reactions	Symptoms may be precipitated by any food	Wide variety of symptoms involving any system
Reactions to Pharmacologic Agents in Foods		
Phenylethylamine	Chocolate, aged cheese, red wine	Migraine headaches

Continued

TABLE 29-3

Representative Nonimmunologic Reactions to Food—cont'd

Cause	Associated Food	Symptoms
Reactions to Pharmacologic Agents in Foods—cont'd		
Vasoactive amines		
Tyramine	Cheddar cheese, French cheeses, brewers' yeast, Chianti wine, canned fish	Migraine headaches, cutaneous erythema, urticaria and hypertensive crisis in patients taking monoamine oxidase inhibitors
Histamine	Fermented cheeses, fermented foods (e.g., sauerkraut, pork sausages, canned tuna, anchovies, sardines)	Erythema, headaches, decreased blood pressure
Histamine-releasing agents	Shellfish, chocolate, strawberries, tomatoes, peanuts, pork, wine, pineapple	Urticaria, eczema, pruritus
Reactions to Food Additives		
Tartrazine or FD&C yellow no. 5	Yellow- or yellow-orange–colored foods, soft drinks, medicine	Hives, rash, asthma
Benzoic acid or sodium benzoate	Soft drinks and some cheeses, salt-free margarines, and processed potato products	Hives, rash, asthma
Sulfites		
Sodium sulfite, potassium sulfite, sodium metabisulfite, potassium metabisulfite, sodium bisulfite, potassium bisulfite, sulfur dioxide	Shrimp, many processed foods, avocado, instant potatoes, dried fruits and vegetables and fresh fruits and vegetables treated with sulfites to prevent browning, acidic juices, wine, beer	Acute asthma and anaphylaxis, loss of consciousness
Reactions to Microbial Contamination of Foods		
Proteus causes histidine to break down to a histamine-like substance (anaphylactic type reaction)	Unrefrigerated scombroid fish (tuna, bonita, mackerel); heat-stable toxin produced	Scombroid fish poisoning (itching, rash, vomiting, diarrhea)
Gonyaulax catenella (red tide)	Mussels and clams that ingest the organism that produces saxitoxin, a heat-stable neurotoxin	Paralytic shellfish poisoning (progressive numbness from head to arms); frequently fatal

sulfites to cause asthma and anaphylaxis (Reus et al., 2000). However, a case of nitrate causing anaphylaxis (Hawkins and Katelaris, 2000), an anaphylactic-asthmatic reaction to the color carmine (Spergel and Fiedler, 2005), and hives after ingestion of ice cream that contained acetylsalicylic acid (Bahna, 2001) have been documented. Reactions to sulfites are rare but still occur. Sensitive asthmatics are the most likely to react to sulfites.

Adverse reactions to MSG are reported to include headache, nausea, flushing, abdominal pain, and asthma occurring several hours after ingestion. The results from a study using double-blind, placebo-controlled food challenges (DBP-CFCs) found symptoms perceived to be caused by MSG to be "neither persistent nor serious effects from MSG ingestion" (Geha et al., 2000). MSG is thought to be safe for most people. It is found naturally in tomatoes, Parmesan cheese, and mushrooms. Restaurant meals prepared with limited amounts or without MSG are usually available.

Multiple conditions have been "blamed" on foods and environment without properly controlled studies and in-

PATHOPHYSIOLOGY AND CARE MANAGEMENT ALGORITHM

Food Allergies

ETIOLOGY

Common food allergens
Foods with high protein content, usually of plant or marine origin

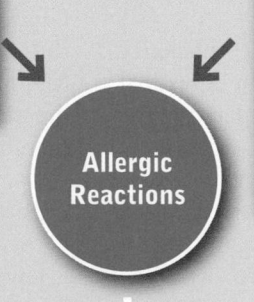

Allergic Reactions

Risk factors
- Heredity
- Atopy
- Antigen exposure
- GI permeability
- Amount of antigen presented
- Environmental factors

PATHOPHYSIOLOGY

IgE-mediated
Immediate hypersensitivity

IgE- and cell-mediated
Hypersensitivity

Cell mediated
Delayed hypersensitivity

GI, Cutaneous, and Respiratory Symptoms
Anaphylaxis

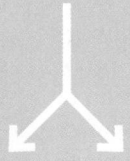

MANAGEMENT

Medical Management

Diagnosis
- History
- Physical examination
- Food and symptom diaries
- Biochemical and immunologic testing
- Food elimination

Reintroduction of foods by food challenge (DBPCFC) to test for resolution of allergy (with treatment for anaphylaxis available)

Epinephrine for management of acute reactions and anaphylaxis

Nutrition Management

- Total avoidance of food allergens
- Provide alternative nutrient sources

Algorithm content developed by John J.B. Anderson, PhD, and Sanford C. Garner, PhD, 2000.

clude behavior disorders, learning disabilities, depression, chronic fatigue, arthritis, and others. It is possible for symptoms to improve with diet manipulation without defined cause and effect. This is an exciting new area of research (see Chapter 42). When patients or their families choose to pursue an altered diet instead of or in conjunction with recommended therapy, advice on implementing a nutritionally adequate and safe diet should be provided.

Carbohydrate Intolerance

Lactase deficiency is the most common enzyme deficiency worldwide. Persons who have a deficiency of the intestinal enzyme lactase have a decreased ability to digest lactose, the sugar in milk, and experience symptoms of abdominal cramping, flatulence, and diarrhea after its ingestion. Because the symptoms are similar, lactose intolerance is often confused with allergy to cow's milk. Deficiencies of lactase and other carbohydrate-digesting enzymes are discussed further in Chapter 27.

Gastrointestinal symptoms after the ingestion of fruit juice are commonly reported in infants and children, and they may be related to carbohydrate intolerance (particularly sorbitol, maltitol, or other sugar alcohols) rather than to food allergy. Carbohydrate malabsorption has been documented following ingestion of pear, apple, and grape juices. A brief restriction of fruit juices may be useful in the evaluation of infants and children with chronic, nonspecific diarrhea (see Chapters 7 and 27).

DIAGNOSIS

No simple test can be used to diagnose food allergy. Diagnosis requires identification of the suspected food, proof that the food causes an adverse response, and verification of immunologic involvement. Nonallergic mechanisms must be ruled out. The omission of foods from the diet on the basis of proper or improper diagnosis can and has threatened the nutritional status of the affected individual (Nowak-Wegrzyn and Sampson, 2006).

The first diagnostic tool is the clinical history. Gathered information should include a description of symptoms, the time of food ingestion relative to the onset of symptoms, a description of the most recent reactions, a list of suspected foods, and an estimate of the quantity of food required to cause a reaction. Food allergy may be linked to prenatal and postnatal exposures.

The first exposure to suspect food allergens may occur during pregnancy or lactation or in early childhood. The food does not have to be ingested by the infant directly. Introduction of highly allergenic foods (e.g., peanuts or other nuts) to the fetus during pregnancy or nursing can increase the likelihood of food allergy development (Norwak-Wegrzyn and Sampson, 2006). Eating peanuts more than once a week during pregnancy may increase peanut allergy risk. If peanut allergy already exists, there is a risk of the infant developing more food allergies (Sampson,

2002). Family history of atopic disease should be reviewed with both parents.

Physical examination includes measurements of weight, height, and body mass index (and head circumference for an infant) plotted on a growth chart and evaluated in relationship to earlier measurements. Decreased weight for height measurements may be related to malabsorption and potential food allergy. Therefore, patterns of growth and their relationship to the onset of symptoms should be explored. Clinical signs of malnutrition should be assessed, including the evaluation of fat and muscle stores (see Chapter 14). Malnutrition can affect skin test results and should be addressed before testing when possible. Evidence of atopic march that includes atopic dermatitis or eczema (itchy rash with red and white bumps), allergic rhinitis, and asthma must be evaluated.

A 7- to 14-day **food and symptom diary** is useful if there is a perceived general food reaction with chronic symptoms but no specific suspect food(s) (Figure 29-3). This diary can also be used to identify possible nutrient deficiencies. A 24-hour recall is helpful when reactions occur less frequently. Both the food diary and the 24-hour recall should include the time the food is eaten, the quantity and type of food, all food ingredients identifiable, the time symptoms appear relative to the time of food ingestion, and any medications taken before or after the onset of symptoms because medications may alter the symptoms observed.

The location where the reaction occurred can be informative, providing unexpected insights into possible food sources of allergen exposure. Sometimes the information obtained indicates something other than a food reaction. A reaction that appears to be caused by a food allergen when the food allergen cannot be found may be caused by a nonfood allergy source such as a cat or dog. The more information obtained when a reaction occurs, the more useful the diary or recall. The 1- to 2-week diary record also can serve as a baseline for future intervention. It is especially useful when reactions to food preservatives or additives are suspected.

Biochemical testing can rule out nonallergenic causes of symptoms. A complete blood count and differential; tests of stool for reducing substances, ova, parasites, or occult blood; and a sweat chloride test for the exclusion of cystic fibrosis are examples of tests that may be useful (see Chapter 15).

Immunologic testing is useful for screening patients and as a diagnostic tool. The **radioallergosorbent test (RAST)** and the enzyme-linked immunosorbent assay (ELISA) are diagnostic tools being replaced by the CAP-FEIA blood test. The Pharmacia **CAP-FEIA (fluorescein-enzyme immunoassay)** blood test appears promising in the food allergy diagnostic process because it provides a quantitative assessment of allergen-specific IgE antibodies and higher levels of antibodies are predictors of clinical symptoms. The blood test is specific, with 96% to 100% accuracy, in identifying children with milk, egg, fish, wheat, and peanut allergy; but identification of soy allergy is still only 86% accurate. It is effective as shown by testing known food-allergic children whose food allergies had been previously proven with

Name _____

	DAY 1 DATE __	DAY 2 DATE __	DAY 3 DATE __	DAY 4 DATE __	DAY 5 DATE __	DAY 6 DATE __	DAY 7 DATE __
SYMPTOMS							
B R E A K F A S T							
SNACK SUPPLEMENTS							
SYMPTOMS							
L U N C H							
SNACK SUPPLEMENTS							
SYMPTOMS							
D I N N E R							
SNACK							
SYMPTOMS							
MEDICATION							

FIGURE 29-3 Food and symptom diary.

DBPCFCs (Sampson, 2001). However, until test results are more accurate for more foods, skin testing and DBPCFCs will need to be used in the diagnostic process. The DBPCFC remains the "gold standard" for identifying food-induced symptoms (Sampson, 2004) (Table 29-4). The CAP-FEIA test has been approved for only six foods: egg, milk, peanut, fish, wheat, and soy, even though soy is still not as predictive (Sampson, 2004).

Skin tests are the most economic and provide results within 15 to 30 minutes. Control comparisons using histamine skin-prick test results provide both positive and negative wheal diameters necessary for accurate readings (Figure 29-4). All skin-prick tests are compared with the control wheal. Test wheals that are 3 mm greater than the negative control indicate a positive result. Negative skin-prick tests have excellent negative predictive accuracy and suggest the absence of an IgE-mediated reaction. For children younger than 2 years of age, the skin test is reserved to confirm immunologic mechanisms after symptoms have been confirmed by a positive test result from a food challenge or when the history of the reaction is impressive.

Many children with atopic dermatitis have a food allergy that can be diagnosed using a skin-prick test for the most common food allergens (milk, egg, peanut, soy, wheat, fish, and tree nuts) because these foods account for most of the positive food challenge tests (Nowak-Wegrzyn and Sampson, 2006). All foods that test positive must correlate with a strong exposure history (e.g., anaphylaxis) or be proven to cause allergic reactions through food challenges before they can be considered allergenic.

Specific IgG, IgM, and IgA antibody assays should be used for research purposes only (Bahna, 2001) (see Table 29-4). Sometimes laboratories that provide unproven or unreliable "diagnostic tests" are not appropriately regulated or are connected to products directed for the food allergic person's purchase. Several food allergy in vitro "diagnostic tests" are considered unproven or unreliable and have no diagnostic validity (Table 29-5).

Food Elimination Diet

Food elimination is another tool in the diagnosis process used for chronic symptoms such as hives, angioedema, and eczema. With an **elimination diet,** all forms (i.e., cooked, raw, and protein derivatives) of that food must be removed from the diet. A food record is kept during the elimination phase (see Figure 29-3). This record is used to ensure that all forms of suspected foods have been eliminated from the diet and to evaluate the nutritional adequacy of the diet.

TABLE 29-4

Diagnostic Tests

Type	Description	Comments
Skin testing (scratch, prick, or puncture)	A drop of antigen is placed on the skin, and the skin is then scratched or punctured to allow penetration	Screening test; cannot be relied on as sole diagnostic tool; a history of food-symptom relationship also important
Radioallergosorbent test (RAST)	Serum is mixed with food on a paper disk and then washed with radioactively labeled IgE	No more accurate than the skin test, but more costly; useful in people who have skin disease
Enzyme-linked immunosorbent assay (ELISA)	Much like RAST, except that no radioactive material is used	Same as for RAST
CAP-RAST fluroscein-enzyme immunoassay (FEIA)	Compared to RAST, this test binds more allergen	Reliable for only six foods
Double-blind, placebo-controlled food challenge (DBPCFC)	Allergen is disguised and given orally and patient monitored for reaction; patient and MD blinded; also tested with placebo	"Gold standard" for allergy testing
Specific IgG, IgM, IgA antibody assays	Techniques of precipitation hemagglutination, complement fixation; requires special expertise	Best used in research only
IgG4	Blood testing for food-specific IgG4	Not widely validated for diagnostic use

Vitamin and mineral supplementation should be considered when a severely limited diet continues for more than 7 to 14 days. When possible, a temporary elimination diet should be personalized, eliminating only one or two suspect foods at a time for each 2-week period. If multiple foods are suspected, a variation of the "strict" elimination diet shown in

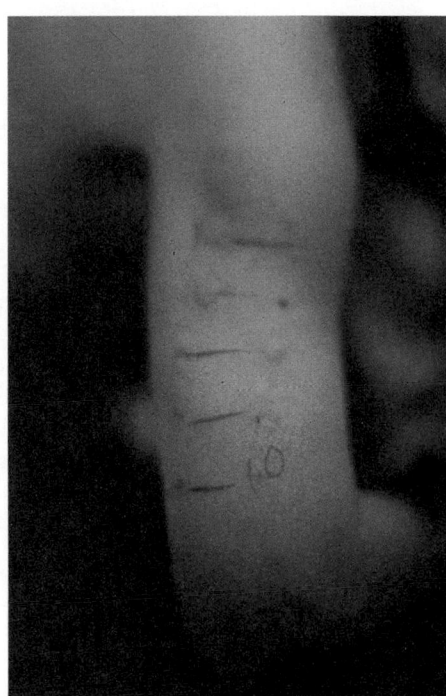

FIGURE 29-4 A skin-prick test showing the wheal and flare of the reaction to the allergen as compared with the reaction to the histamine control at the bottom.

Table 29-6 should be used. Any food on the list that is suspect or that is eaten more often than once every 4 months should be substituted with a food that is rarely or almost never eaten.

If the individual or the health care provider continues to suspect foods or is given a diagnosis of **eosinophilic gastroenteritis** or **eosinophilic esophagitis,** an elemental diet, the most severe form of elimination diet, may be considered. An elemental diet prevents malnutrition but is expensive, not well accepted, and should be reserved for the most restrictive cases. Products such as EleCare, Neocate (infants), or Neocate One Plus and Ultracare Kids for infants and young children; and Tolerex, L-Emental, Ultraclear, and EO28 formulas for teenagers and adults are examples of formulas that can be used. Foods are returned to the diet one at a time while the patient is receiving the formula. Anyone on an elemental diet must be carefully monitored (Nowak-Wegrzyn and Sampson, 2006).

The elimination process will determine whether symptoms improve or resolve with avoidance. If symptoms persist with careful avoidance of suspect foods, other causes for the symptoms should be considered. If a positive result has been obtained on a skin test and symptoms improve unequivocally with the elimination of the food, that food should be eliminated from the diet until an oral food challenge is appropriate. The oral food challenge will prove or disprove a food symptom relationship. If symptoms improve with only the elimination of multiple foods, multiple food challenges are necessary.

Food Challenge

A **food challenge** is conducted once symptoms have resolved and all antihistamines are stopped. Foods are challenged one at a time on different days, thus eliminating confusion while the person is carefully observed in a medical setting

TABLE 29-5

Unreliable Food Allergy Tests

Type Of Test	Description
Cytotoxic testing	Allergen is mixed with whole blood or serum leukocyte suspension; lysed leukocytes are then counted.
Sublingual testing	Drops of allergen extract are placed under the tongue, and symptoms are recorded.
Provocation testing and neutralization	Subcutaneous injection of allergen extract elicits symptoms; this is then followed by injection of a weaker or stronger preparation to neutralize symptom.
Kinesiologic testing	Subject's arm is extended and foods to be tested are placed in the hand; test is considered to yield positive results if the arm moves more easily after the food has been placed in hand.
Change in leukocyte size Antigen leukocyte cellular antibody test (ALCAT)	Exposure to food allergen supposedly increases leukocyte diameter.

TABLE 29-6

Three Stages of Elimination Diets

	Foods Allowed	Foods To Avoid
Elimination Diet Level I: Milk-, Egg-, and Wheat-Free		
Animal protein sources	Lamb, chicken, turkey, beef, pork	Cow's milk, chicken eggs
Vegetable protein sources	Soy milk, soybeans, other beans, lentils	
Grains or alternative starches	White potato, sweet potato, yams, rice, tapioca, arrowroot, buckwheat, corn, barley, rye, millet, oats	Wheat
Vegetables	All vegetables	
Fruits	All fruits and juices	
Sweeteners	Cane or beet sugar, maple syrup, corn syrup	
Oils	Soy oil, corn oil, safflower oil, coconut oil, vegetable oil, olive oil, peanut oil, milk-free margarines	Butter and margarines that include milk
Other	Salt, all spices	
Elimination Diet Level 2: Stricter		
Animal protein sources	Lamb	All other animal proteins, including meat, fish, poultry, eggs, and milk
Vegetable protein sources	None	Soy milk, soybeans, peas, other beans, lentils, peanuts, bean sprouts, all nuts
Grains or alternative starches	White potato, sweet potato, yams, rice, tapioca, buckwheat, arrowroot, corn	Wheat, oats, barley, millet, rye
Vegetables	Most vegetables	Peas, tomatoes
Fruits	Most fruits and juices	Citrus fruits, strawberries
Sweeteners	Cane or beet sugar, maple syrup, corn syrup	
Oils	Safflower oil, coconut oil, olive oil, sesame oil	Butter, margarine, vegetable oils, soy oil, corn oil, peanut oil, nonspecific shortening, or fats of animal origin
Other	Salt, pepper, all spices,* vanilla or lemon extract, baking soda, cream of tartar	Chocolate, coffee, tea, colas and other soft drinks; alcoholic beverages
Elimination Diet Level 3: Severe†		
	Rice in any form (rice cakes and rice cereal being especially helpful) Pineapple Apricots Cranberries Peaches Pears Apples including canned fruit and juices of these Lamb Chicken	Asparagus Beets Carrots Lettuce Sweet potatoes White vinegar Olive oil Honey Cane or beet sugar Salt Safflower oil	All other foods

Modified from Bock SA: *Food allergy: a primer for people*, New York, 1988, Vantage Press.

*Suggest limiting number to five to minimize dietary variables.

†This is not a nutritionally complete diet and must only be used with the advice of a physician or nutritionist for short periods (2 weeks or less).

for the recurrence of symptoms. The three types of food challenges are as follows: open food challenge, which allows the food to be given openly; single-blind, placebo-controlled food challenge, in which the food is hidden from the patient with at least one placebo; and **double-blind, placebo-controlled food challenge (DBPCFC)**, in which the food is hidden from the patient and the health practitioner and is presented with at least one to three placebos. Increasing amounts of the offending food should be given every 15 to 60 minutes until there is a convincing but not life-threatening response. The goal is to ingest 6 g to 10 g of dry food or 80 ml of liquid food mixed in a masking food the patient tolerates (Nowak-Wegrzyn and Sampson, 2006).

A person with a positive challenge response must be given appropriate medications to stop symptoms and be observed for an additional 1 to 2 hours. Those who are observed to have a negative challenge response should also be observed for an additional 1 to 2 hours. Occasionally a reaction may occur later than expected. The amount of food tolerated under observation can then be offered at home.

The DBPCFC, which provides objective results by eliminating outside influences, is considered the gold standard when attempting to establish a food and symptom relationship, and it is used to confirm a food allergy. Each DBPCFC must be personalized. Single foods (e.g., applesauce, grape juice) or tolerated food combinations can "hide" a suspect food. The product must mask any hint of the flavor, color, or texture of the suspect food or allergen. The patient should not be able to detect the differences between the "active" food and the placebo food. Because severe reactions can occur during a challenge, a physician must be in attendance with emergency supplies measured and ready to be administered.

After a negative DBPCFC, an open challenge should be given. In this challenge the patient is given a serving of the suspect food. Interestingly, reactions have occurred during the open challenge that did not occur in the blind challenge. Occasionally symptoms may accompany the last presentation if the threshold is greater than indicated by the history. Most allergic reactions occur within 2 hours of the challenge. Non–IgE-mediated reactions may occur more than 24 hours after challenge. Monitoring of the patient should continue during this time.

Although most food allergy reactions are not fatal, about 30,000 anaphylactic reactions, 2000 hospitalizations, and 200 deaths occur in the United States each year; peanuts and tree nuts are believed to cause most of these near-fatal and fatal anaphylactic reactions (Sampson, 2002). If there is a clear history of a life-threatening anaphylactic reaction after eating a specific food, that food should not be challenged unless there is sufficient evidence that the person is no longer reacting to the allergen and skin test results are negative.

A single-blind food challenge, in which the person receiving the challenge does not know what has been offered, may be useful in similar situations and is easier to implement; however, challenges carried out for research purposes should be DBPCFCs.

TREATMENT

Total avoidance of a food allergen is the only proven treatment for food allergy (Nowak-Wegrzyn and Sampson, 2006; Sicherer and Sampson, 2006). **Food immunotherapy vaccine** is a possible future treatment meant to complement food allergen avoidance, but these vaccines are still considered experimental. Although many food intolerances may allow some ingestion of the offending food, food hypersensitivities or allergies do not. Families and individuals need guidelines and suggestions for avoiding allergenic foods, substituting permissible foods for restricted foods in meal planning and preparation, and selecting nutritionally adequate replacement foods.

To help identify and avoid offending foods, allergy-specific lists that describe foods to avoid, state key words for ingredient identification, and present acceptable substitutes may be useful (see Boxes 29-2 through 29-6). Caretakers and school personnel working with the food-allergic child should be cautioned to read labels carefully before purchasing or serving food. The Food Allergy and Anaphylaxis Network (FAAN), a nonprofit organization created to support the food-allergic child, has developed through work with board-certified allergists and dietitians an excellent education program for day-care or school programs. Food substitutions can be challenging when working to stay within U.S. Department of Agriculture Child Nutrition Program Guidelines, and state education departments should be contacted for specific information.

Foods to be avoided may be hidden in the diet in unfamiliar forms. When a food-sensitive person ingests a hidden allergen, the most common reason is that the "safe" food was contaminated. This may happen as a result of using common serving utensils such as at an ice cream parlor, salad bar, or deli (where the meat slicer may be used to slice both meat and cheese). Manufacturing plants or restaurants may use the same equipment to produce two different products (e.g., peanut butter and almond butter); and, despite cleaning, traces of an allergen may remain on the equipment between uses. Alternatively, a restaurant may use the same oil to fry both potatoes and fish (Box 29-7 and *Clinical Insight:* Does "Pareve" Really Mean Milk Free?).

Another situation that may lead to the unknowing ingestion of an allergenic food occurs when one product is used to make a second product, and only the ingredients of the second product are listed on the food label. An example would be the listing of mayonnaise as an ingredient in a salad dressing without specifically listing egg as an ingredient of the mayonnaise. Labels must be read often to ensure that ingredients have not changed in the processing of the food.

BOX 29-2
Egg Allergy

Foods and Ingredients to Avoid*

Albumin	Egg substitutes	Imitation egg product	Ovoglycoprotein
Apovitellin	Egg white	Livetin	Ovomucin
Avidin	Egg yolk	Lysozyme	Ovomucoid
Bernaise sauce	Flavoprotein	Mayonnaise	Ovomuxoid
Dried eggs	Frozen eggs	Meringue	Powdered egg
Eggnog	Globulin	Ovalbumin	Simplesse
Egg solids	Hollandaise sauce	Ovoglobulin	Vitellin

Egg Substitutes (Equivalent to 1 Egg)

Ener G Egg Replacer (ENERG-G Foods, Inc.)—1½ tsp + 1 Tbsp of water

1 packet plain gelatin + 1 c boiling water—3 Tbsp of this mixture

½ tsp baking powder + 1 Tbsp liquid + 1 Tbsp vinegar

3 Tbsp puréed apple

¼ cup pureed prunes

1 tbsp ground flaxseed mixed with 3 Tbsp of water

1 tsp yeast dissolved in ¼ c warm water

1 medium banana

1 Tbsp fruit purée

1½ Tbsp water + 1½ Tbsp oil + 1 tsp baking powder

2 Tbsp fruit juice, milk, milk substitute, or water

¼ cup soft tofu, beaten

Modified from Burns-Ogle G, Doerr J, Martin B, editors: *Manual of medical nutrition therapy*, ed 3, Oklahoma City, 1996, Oklahoma Dietetic Association.

*Eliminate the following foods, as well as any foods containing any of these ingredients.

BOX 29-3
Cow's Milk Allergy

Foods and Ingredients to Avoid*†

Acidophilus milk	Chocolate milk	Lactulose
Ammonium caseinate	Creamed candies	Low-fat ice cream
Artificial butter flavor	Cultured buttermilk	Magnesium caseinate
Butter	Curds	Malted milk
Butter fat	Custard	Milk chocolate
Butter oil	Delactosed whey	Milk (whole, 2%, 1½%, 1%, ½%,
Calcium caseinate	Dry milk (whole, low-fat, nonfat)	skim, nonfat condensed milk)
Caramel candy	Eggnog	Milk protein
Carob candies	Evaporated milk	Milk protein hydrolysates
Casein	Goat's milk‡	Nougat
Casein hydrolysate	Half & half cream	Potassium caseinate
Cheese (e.g., cheddar, Colby, cream, Edam,	Ice cream	Protein hydrolysate
Gouda, Monterey Jack, mozzarella,	Lactalbumin	Pudding
Muenster, Neufchâtel, parmesan,	Lactalbumin phosphate	Rennet casein
provolone, ricotta, Romano, Swiss,	Lactoglobulin	Semisweet chocolate
cottage)	Lactose	Sherbet, most types

Modified from Burns-Ogle G, Doerr J, Martin B, editors: *Manual of medical nutrition therapy*, ed 3, Oklahoma City, 1996, Oklahoma Dietetic Association.

*Eliminate the following foods, as well as any foods containing any of these ingredients.

†Individuals who must avoid all cow's milk sources frequently need a calcium supplement.

‡Goat's milk protein is similar to cow's milk protein. Those with cow's milk allergy may experience similar symptoms with goat's milk ingestion. Goat's milk is not recommended as a cow's milk substitute.

§Protein hydrolysate–containing formulas may cause symptoms in some infants.

Cow's Milk Allergy—cont'd

Foods and Ingredients to Avoid*†—cont'd

Sodium caseinate	Sweet whey	Whipping cream
Sour cream	Sweetened condensed milk	Yogurt, frozen
Sour cream dressings	Whey	Yogurt, regular
Sour cream solids	Whey protein concentrate	
Sour milk solids	Whey protein hydrolysate	

Ingredients Potentially Made With Cow's Milk Products

Bavarian cream flavoring	Caramel flavoring	Natural flavoring
Brown sugar flavoring	Coconut cream flavoring	Simplesse
Butter flavoring		

Milk Substitutes to Use in Recipes (Use to Replace 1 c of Cow's Milk)

1 c light-colored fruit juice (e.g., apple, orange, white grape)
1 c soy-based infant formula
1 c soy milk (e.g., Edensoy, Westsoy, Vitasoy, Silk)
1 c water
Milk-free infant formulas

Elemental

Neocate (Scientific Hospital Supplies International, Ltd.)
Neocate One + (Scientific Hospital Supplies International, Ltd.)

Protein Hydrolysates§

Alimentum (Ross Laboratories)
EleCare (Ross Laboratories)
Nutramigen (Mead Johnson)
Ultracare for Kids (Metagenics)

Peanut Allergy

Foods and Ingredients to Avoid*

Arachis oil	Expelled or expressed	Hydrolyzed vegetable protein	Peanut flakes
Artificial tree nuts	peanut oil	Marzipan	Peanut flour
Beer nuts	Fresh peanuts	Mixed nuts	Peanut meal
Chopped peanuts	Granulated peanuts	Nougat	Peanut oil
Cold-pressed peanut oil	Ground nuts	Peanuts, whole, roasted	Peanut soup
Defattened peanuts	High-protein food	in-shell	Peanuts, roasted
Egg rolls	Hydrolyzed plant protein	Peanut butter	Peanuts, shelled

Additional Products That May Contain Peanuts

Baked goods	Chili	Ice cream	Salad dressing
Candy	Chocolate candy	Livestock feed	Sauces
Cashew butter	Frozen desserts	Pie crusts	Sunflower seeds
Cheesecake crusts	Hamster feed		

Modified from Fenster C: Special diet solutions: healthy cooking without wheat, gluten, dairy, eggs, yeast, or refined sugar, ed 3, Centennial, CO, 1997, Savory Palate, Inc.

*Eliminate all sources of peanuts from diet. DO NOT eat any food that has touched peanuts or use any utensils used in preparing peanut-containing dishes. Remember that peanut powder, peanut butter, and peanuts may be used in casseroles, sprinkled on top of dishes, or used as an ingredient (e.g., in vegetable dishes, fruit dishes, cookies, cakes, pastries, desserts, chili, soups, stews, egg rolls). Be careful when eating at social functions or when dining out! Take extra precautions when dining at Asian, Chinese, Mexican, Thai, Mediterranean, and Indian restaurants. When possible call the manager of a restaurant 2 or 3 days before dining out. Explain why peanuts must be avoided and find out if any form of peanuts is used as a recipe ingredient or as garnish or if the food is cooked in peanut oil. Explain the severe reactions to peanuts. NEVER, NEVER assume that a dish is peanut free just because the menu description does not mention peanuts. Many restaurant dishes are purchased prepared to heat and serve.

BOX 29-5

Soy Allergy

Foods and Ingredients to Avoid*

Chee-fan	Miso	Soybean curd	Tao-si
Deep-fried mature soy seed	Natto	Soybean hydrolysates	Taotjo
Fermented soybean paste	Soy flour	Soybean milk	Tempeh
Fermented soybeans	Soy grits	Soybean oil	Textured soy protein
Hamanatto	Soy protein concentrates	Soybean or soy lecithin†	Textured vegetable
Immature green soy seed	Soy protein isolates	Soybean sprouts	protein
Ketjap	Soy protein shakes	Sufu	Tofu
Metiauza	Soy sauce	Tao-cho	Whey-soy drink

Ingredients Potentially Made From Soybean Products

Hydrolyzed plant protein   Vegetable broth
Hydrolyzed soy protein   Vegetable gum
Hydrolyzed vegetable protein   Vegetable starch
Natural flavoring

Soy and Milk Substitutes

Fruit juices
Rice milk or nut or grain milks

Infant Formulas

Elemental
Neocate (Scientific Hospital Supplies International, Ltd.)
Neocate One+ (Scientific Hospital Supplies International, Ltd.)

Protein Hydrolysates‡
Alimentum (Ross Laboratories)
EleCare (Ross Laboratories)
Nutramigen (Mead Johnson)

Modified from Burns-Ogle G, Doerr J, Martin B, editors: *Manual of medical nutrition therapy*, ed 3, Oklahoma City, 1996, Oklahoma Dietetic Association.

*Eliminate the following foods, as well as any foods containing any of these ingredients, from your diet.

†Several studies indicate that soybean lecithin and soy oil are frequently tolerated by individuals who are soy allergic.

‡Note: Protein hydrolysate–containing formulas may cause symptoms in some infants. Ask your allergist, physician, or dietitian to recommend the best formula for your infant.

BOX 29-6

Wheat Allergy

Foods and Ingredients to Avoid*

Acker meal	Cracked wheat	Malted cereals	Spelt	Wheat protein
Atta	Doughnuts	Minchin	Superamine	beverage
Bal ahar	Durum flour	Multi-grain breads	Tortillas	Wheat protein
Bran	Durum	Multi-grain flours	Triticale	powder
Bread	Enriched flour	Pasta	Wheat bran	Wheat starch
Bread crumbs	Farina	Pastries	Wheat bread	Wheat tempeh
Bread flour	Gluten	Pies	Wheat bread crumbs	White flour
Bulgar	Graham flour	Puffed wheat	Wheat flakes	Whole-wheat
Cake flour	High-gluten flour	Red wheat flakes	Wheat germ	berries
Cakes	High-protein flour	Rolled wheat	Wheat gluten	Whole-wheat flour
Cereal extract	Kamut flour	Semolina	Wheat malt	Vital gluten
Cookies	Laubina	Shredded wheat	Wheat meal	Winter wheat flour
Couscous	Leche alim	Soft wheat flour	Wheat pasta	Vitalia macaroni

Modified from Burns-Ogle G et al., editors: Manual of medical nutrition therapy, ed 3, Oklahoma City, 1996, Oklahoma Dietetic Association.
Updated from: www.foodallergyinitiative.org

*Eliminate the following foods, as well as any foods containing any of these ingredients, from the diet.

BOX 29-6

Wheat Allergy—cont'd

Ingredients Potentially Made from Wheat Products

Gelatinized starch
Hydrolyzed vegetable protein
Modified food starch
Modified starch
Starch
Vegetable gum
Vegetable starch

Substitutions

When substituting any flour, either nongluten or low gluten–containing flour, use a recipe developed specifically for that flour. No nonwheat flour will produce an acceptable end product when substituted for wheat flour in a wheat flour–based recipe. A variety of recipes have been developed specifically for these particular grains as a replacement for wheat-containing products. More leavening is required in nongluten and low gluten–containing flours. Try adding 2 to 2½ tbsp baking powder per cup of nongluten or low-gluten flours.

Alternatives

Amaranth	Millet
Barley (if not intolerant of gluten)	Oats (if not intolerant of gluten)
Buckwheat	Quinoa
Chickpea	Rice
Corn	Rye (if not intolerant of gluten)
Lentil	Tapioca

When foods are removed from the diet, alternative nutrient sources must be provided. Table 29-7 defines the levels of nutritional risk based on the types of food removed from the diet. For example, when dairy products are omitted, other foods must provide calcium, vitamin D, protein, riboflavin, and energy.

The nutritional adequacy of the diet should be monitored on a regular basis by conducting an ongoing evaluation of the patient's growth, nutrition status, and food records. Malnutrition and poor growth may occur in children who consume inadequate elimination diets. Vitamin and mineral supplementation is needed, especially when multiple foods are omitted.

Unless a clear diagnosis of food allergy is established, the patient may be well advised to return to a normal diet as tolerated. If symptoms persist or reappear, a review of intake will determine whether all forms of suspected foods have been omitted from the diet. If symptoms persist even with adherence to the diet, other causes for the allergy or other nonallergic causes for the symptoms should be investigated. Because food is an important part of a person's culture, the social aspects of eating can make adherence difficult. Continued support from health care providers is needed to minimize the impact of dietary changes on family and social life. The strategies listed in Box 29-8 can help families and individuals cope with food allergies.

BOX 29-7

Reasons Why Allergens May Contaminate a Food

- Common serving utensils used to serve different foods
- Manufacture of two different food products using the same equipment without proper cleansing in between
- Misleading labels (e.g., nondairy creamers that contain sodium caseinate)
- Ingredients added for a specific purpose are listed on the label only in general terms of their purpose rather than as a specific ingredient (e.g., egg white that is simply listed as an "emulsifier")
- Addition of an allergenic product to a second product that bears a label listing only the ingredients of the second product (e.g., mayonnaise, without noting eggs)
- Switching of ingredients by food manufacturers (e.g., a shortage of one vegetable oil prompting substitution with another)
- An ingredient that is present in a food but in such a low percentage that it does not have to be listed on a label

Modified from Steinman HA: Hidden allergens in foods, *J Allergy Clin Immunol* 98:241, 1996.

✴ CLINICAL INSIGHT

Does "Pareve" Really Mean Milk Free?

For many years, milk-allergic persons have used the kosher designation "pareve" or "parvre" to mean that the food is milk free and therefore "safe."

Pareve products are considered milk free from a religious standpoint and meet Jewish Dietary Law requirements; however, from a food allergy standpoint, pareve may NOT be 100% milk free. Equipment that has been cleaned to the Kosher Dietary Law specifications may contain trace amounts of milk or trace contamination from airborne dust in a food plant. These trace amounts of milk in products labeled "pareve" do not violate religious law, and these products can still be labeled as such; however, these products could present a problem to a milk-allergic person. Kosher labeling does help identify products that do have milk, such as kosher dairy (D) and dairy equipment (DE), but relying on pareve-labeled products as 100% milk free is not recommended.

The Food Allergy Network no longer recommends relying on pareve-labeled products for milk-free diets (Regenstein, 1998).

Content developed by Leila Beker, PhD, RD.

BOX 29-8

Strategies for Coping With Food Allergy

Food Substitutions

Try to substitute item-for-item at meals. For example, if the family is eating ice cream for dessert, substitution of another type of frozen dessert may be better accepted than a dissimilar dessert such as cookies.

Dining Out and Eating Away From Home

Eating meals away from home can be risky for individuals with food allergies. Whether at a fancy restaurant or a fast-food establishment, inadvertent exposure to an allergen can occur, even among the most knowledgeable individuals. Here are some precautions to take:

- Bring "safe" foods along to make eating out easier. For breakfast, bring along soy milk if others will be having cereal with milk.
- Alert the wait staff to the potential severity of your food allergy or allergies.
- Question the wait staff carefully about ingredients.
- Always carry medications.

Special Occasions

Call the host family in advance to determine what foods will be served. Offer to provide an acceptable dish that all can enjoy.

Grocery Shopping

Be informed about what foods are acceptable, and read labels carefully. Product ingredients change over time; continue to read the labels on foods, even if they were previously determined to be "safe" foods. Allow for the fact that shopping will take extra time.

Label Reading

New labeling legislation makes it easier for individuals with food allergies to identify certain potential allergens from the ingredient list on food labels. For example, when food manufacturers use protein hydrolysates or hydrolyzed vegetable protein, they must now specify the source of protein used (e.g., hydrolyzed soy or hydrolyzed corn). Although reactions to food colors or food dyes are rare, individuals who suspect an intolerance will find them listed separately on the food label, rather than categorized simply as "food color."

Substitutions in Cooking

Milk: Use soy or rice milk or fruit juice in recipes calling for milk. Use soy or rice milk for milk replacement. Use a 1:1 replacement ratio. Infant formulas such as Neocate, Neocate One Plus, Nutramigen, or Alimentum can also be used.

Egg: In baking, achieve the emulsifying effect of one egg by combining 2 Tbsp whole-wheat flour, ½ tsp oil, ½ tsp baking powder, and 2 Tbsp milk, water, or fruit juice. Egg-free substitutes are also available (see Box 29-2).

Chocolate: Use carob powder, measure for measure, when substituting for cocoa. As a substitute for one square of chocolate, use 3 Tbsp carob powder plus 2 Tbsp milk, water, butter, or margarine.

Wheat: Wheat flour replacements and tips for cooking without wheat are available from many sources.

TABLE 29-7

Nutritional Risk in Food Allergy Management

Level of Risk	Food Characteristics/Examples
Low risk	Any food that can easily be eliminated with minimum or no nutritional risk to the patient; protein, calorie, and nutrient consumption is adequate *Example:* Avoidance of a specific fruit or vegetable
Moderate risk	Any food that may be encountered frequently throughout the food supply yet whose elimination does not significantly limit food choices or vital nutrient sources; questionable adequacy of protein, calorie, and nutrient consumption *Example:* Avoidance of fish, crustaceans, and tree nuts
Complex risk	Any food that permeates the food supply, providing a significant source of specific nutrients that are not readily available through other foods that are a part of the normal diet, whose elimination results in a significant lifestyle and dietary change because of the difficulty of avoiding that food and products containing that food; adequate protein, calorie, and nutrient consumption unlikely *Example:* Avoidance of wheat, soy, egg, milk, peanuts, or multiple foods

NATURAL HISTORY OF FOOD ALLERGY

Food allergy, asthma, and atopic dermatitis (eczema) are atopic diseases that produce specific IgE antibodies; however, test results that indicate high IgE levels (skin or blood) do not automatically point to allergy. Clinical symptoms occur in only 30% to 40% of those testing positive to a food. The development of food allergy may precede the development of the other atopic diseases such as atopic dermatitis (AD) and asthma. Infant gastroesophageal reflux may complicate asthma and food allergy symptoms. The process of developing any atopic disease is called the atopic march (Sicherer, 2002) and possibly has beginnings before birth (Jones et al., 2001).

There is indication that the improved hygiene of our society has caused changes in the neonatal gastrointestinal microflora, which directly affects the maturation process of the immune system (Kalliomaki and Isolauri 2004). The result is that with the greater cleanliness there is greater incidence of atopic disease, including food allergy.

Probiotics are microbial dietary supplements that directly affect the intestinal tract by changing and adding to the gut flora, and their use may prevent food allergy development (see Chapters 1 and 27). *Lactobacillus GG*, a probiotic supplement, has been found to improve gastrointestinal microflora, thus reducing the incidence of atopic march from AD to food allergy and asthma (Neu, 2005; Del Giudice et al., 2006; Schneider, 2002; Rautava et al., 2005; Kalliomaki and Isolauri, 2004). Currently it is suspected that by supplementing the pregnant woman 1 month before delivery, or providing the infant with 6 months' treatment of probiotic therapy either from the nursing mother or with direct supplementation, that infant food allergy–related atopic eczema can be reduced (Schneider, 2002; Rautava et al., 2005).

Breast-feeding continues to be the infant's best nutrition and protection against food allergy disease, but it does not eliminate the risk of developing food allergies (Friedman and Zeiger, 2005). When possible, nursing the infant exclusively for the first 3 months should be encouraged. Even as little as 3 months of exclusive breast-feeding reduces the potentially atopic infant's risk of food allergy development (Gdalevich et al., 2001; Friedman and Zeiger, 2005). If the mother chooses to nurse her infant, she should be encouraged to not eat peanuts while nursing because of the increased risk of developing peanut allergy on the part of the infant (Sampson, 2002). Once food allergy has developed, the only treatment continues to be total avoidance of the food allergen and its protein sources.

Hypersensitivity to foods is most common in the first 1 to 2 years of life, and most infants outgrow their sensitivities by the age of 3 years. Because symptoms of food allergy tend to resolve with age, nutrient-dense allergenic foods such as wheat, soy, eggs, and cow's milk should be reintroduced by food challenge every 6 to 12 months to ensure that they are not being restricted unnecessarily. After two to three negative open challenges, blind challenges may be useful in overcoming any bias that has developed. It should be noted that CAP-FEIA or skin testing results for IgE sensitization may remain positive even after the food can be eaten without symptoms.

FOOD ALLERGY IN INFANCY

Cow's milk protein (CMP) is one of the most common allergens for infants. Prevalence of this allergy is about 2.5% in the first 3 years of life (Tiemessen et al., 2004). Studies suggest that some cases of constipation among infants and children may be related to cow's milk allergy (Turunen et al, 2004). Hypersensitivity and constipation may have an allergenic pathogenesis in this population (Turunen et al., 2004). Fortunately, most but not all CMP-allergic patients will outgrow their allergy by age 3 (Tiemessen et al., 2004).

Recommendations for Infant Feeding

Human milk, the infant's best source of nutrition and protection against atopic disease, is the preferred food for all infants. When the use of human milk is not possible, extensively hydrolysated cow's milk formulas are preferred alternatives to standard cow's milk formulas (Sicherer and Sampson, 2006). If symptoms continue, an amino-based formula may be offered. The American Academy of Pediatrics recommends the use of human milk or casein or whey protein hydrolysates with peptides having a molecular weight of less than 1200 daltons for infants with clinical symptoms of cow's milk or soy allergy. Commercially available casein protein hydrolysate formulas (Nutramigen, Pregestimil, and Alimentum) that meet this criterion have been used routinely to feed infants who are allergic to cow's milk protein, and adverse reactions have only rarely been reported. However, some partially hydrolysate whey proteins contain larger peptides and are not acceptable alternatives for these infants (Simpson and Hanifin, 2006).

The use of goat's milk as an alternative to cow's milk is not recommended because of the potential cross-reactivity with β-lactoglobulin in cow's milk (Pina et al., 2003; Pessler and Nejat, 2004). In addition, goat's milk is deficient in several nutrients and has a high renal solute load. It is especially low in folic acid, containing about one tenth the level present in whole cow's milk or human milk. Infants receiving goat's milk instead of infant formula require supplements of iron; folacin; and vitamins A, C, and D. Goat's milk must be diluted to three-quarter strength, and carbohydrate must be added to decrease the renal solute load.

Sensitivity to breast milk has been reported. Allergens in the mother's diet such as cow's milk, eggs, and peanuts can pass into the breast milk and cause sensitization and then an allergic reaction in the exclusively breast-fed infant (Vadas et al., 2001). Sometimes the reaction does not occur until the allergenic food is actually eaten by the infant. Infants with atopic dermatitis should be evaluated for possible food allergies. If the infant is still nursing, the mother should be placed on a 2-week diet free of milk, eggs, peanut, and soy to see whether her infant's symptoms improve.

Food challenges to each food will determine food symptom relationships. The mother eats a suspect food before nursing, and the infant is observed for symptoms. If a food is judged to yield a positive test result through challenge, that food is eliminated from the mother's diet until the infant is weaned. If the mother is willing, continued breast-feeding is preferred while the offending food allergen is removed from her diet until the infant is weaned. The nutritional adequacy of the mother's diet should be monitored when foods, especially cow's milk, are omitted from her diet. A calcium supplement with vitamin D can help meet the requirements for calcium and vitamin D during lactation (see Chapter 5).

Foods in the mother's diet may also be associated with nonallergic reactions, usually gastrointestinal upset. Implicated foods include caffeinated beverages, chocolate, some herbal teas, cabbage, onions, turnips, garlic, radishes, rhubarb, spinach, and spices. Avoidance of the problem food by the mother may alleviate her infant's symptoms, which is preferable to discontinuing breast-feeding; but in some cases the infant may need to be weaned from the breast.

Colic

The association between colic and food allergy remains controversial, but it appears that it is a non-IgE- or cell-mediated reaction. Persistent colic may warrant trial of an elimination diet for the breast-feeding mother, a trial of a fiber-enriched casein hydrolysate formula for the infant receiving formula based on cow's milk or soy protein, or a trial of an amino acid–based formula such as Neocate.

DIET AND PREVENTION OF ALLERGIC DISEASE

Early feeding of foods other than breast milk is believed to contribute to the increase in food allergy development among infants. Breast-feeding, together with maternal avoidance of allergens, may delay the development of allergic disease in high-risk infants. Reduced exposure to allergenic foods during infancy has been associated with a decreased prevalence of food allergy during the first year and a delay in the onset of atopic dermatitis (Sicherer and Sampson, 2006).

Breast-feeding the infant is strongly encouraged, even if only for the first few days of life. Breast milk is always best, but an extensively hydrolysated casein formula or an amino acid–based formula can be used for infants at risk for atopic disease. When possible, the infant should be exclusively breast-fed for the first 6 months of life. A protein hydrolysate or amino acid–based formula can be used to supplement as necessary. Withholding highly allergenic foods such as peanuts, tree nuts, and fish from children at high risk for allergy for the first 2 to 3 years of life is recommended (Sicherer and Sampson, 2006).

Oral Allergy Syndrome

Individuals with pollen allergy may experience a rapid onset of pruritus (itch) or angioedema (swelling) involving the lips, tongue, throat, and palate within moments of eating fresh fruits or vegetables. About 50% of pollen-allergic adults experience **oral allergy syndrome (OAS)/food-pollen syndrome (FPS).** Symptom intensity varies with patients, and the symptoms usually are not life threatening but may precede anaphylactic reactions. The cooked fruit or vegetable is usually tolerated. The response is believed to be a cross-reaction between common pollen allergens and fresh fruits or vegetables. Patients with birch pollinosis may experience OAS/FPS symptoms with apples, carrots, celery, potatoes, and hazelnuts; ragweed pollinosis with melons and bananas; and brazil nut allergy with cherry, apricot, plum, and peach (Nowak-Wegrzyn and Sampson, 2006).

Latex Allergy

Repeated exposure to latex is considered the most potent cause of natural latex rubber (NRL) allergy. Occupational exposure provides the greatest risk for developing latex allergy. Symptoms include contact dermatitis and immediate allergic reactions, as manifested by rhinitis, asthma, conjunctivitis, angioedema, urticaria, anaphylaxis, and death. The recommendation is to reduce latex glove use and thus reduce latex exposure by reducing latex aeroallergens in the air. Food handling by workers wearing latex gloves is a source of oral ingestion of latex molecules, and latex gloves should not be worn while preparing foods to reduce allergic and nonlatex allergic exposures.

Cross-reactivity between latex and one or more foods is now estimated to be at least 50% (Yagami et al., 2000). It should also be noted that persons with latex allergy could also have food allergies. Latex allergy may develop before food allergy, or food allergy may develop before latex allergy. Sometimes food allergy appears probable when actually latex has contaminated the food. When working with either the latex- or food-allergic patient, a careful history is critical. Research continues to try to define this cross-reactivity and to identify whether foods should be avoided and, if so, which ones. The most frequent related latex-fruit dual allergies are banana, avocado, chestnut, and kiwi (Condemi, 2002) (Box 29-9).

Interesting studies suggest that herbal therapies may be beneficial. Curcumin has strong potential for controlling allergic responses (Kurup et al., 2007).

Genetic Engineering

Genetic engineering can transfer a protein from one plant to another (see Chapter 13). The potential benefits are many to the consumer and food producer. Plants can be made more insect and disease resistant and climate tolerant with improved taste, texture, and appearance. Once a protein has been transferred, the allergenicity potential must be evaluated. The evaluation should include the gene source, how closely the new protein resembles known allergens, and how persons with known allergy to the protein transferred might react, if exposed. In addition, the food industry must consider the effect the new protein has on the growth of the plant, functions within the plant, and physiochemical properties such as heat and digestion stability. Current potential transfer proteins will probably come from known allergenic sources (Taylor et al., 2001). Further engineering may someday be available to reduce levels of specific antigens in the food supply.

BOX 29-9

Foods Known to Cross-React in Latex Allergy

Apple	Coconut	Nectarine	Potato
Apricot	Fig	Papaya	Rye
Avocado*	Fish	Passion	Shellfish
Banana*	Grape	fruit	Strawberry
Carrot	Hazelnut	Pear	Tomato
Celery	Kiwi*	Pineapple	Wheat
Cherry	Mango	Plum	Peach
Chestnut*	Melon		

*Most frequent.

FOCAL POINTS

- Adverse reactions to foods are associated with different physical response mechanisms; allergy is just one of these mechanisms.
- The incidence of food allergy appears to decrease with age; infants younger than 2 years of age are more likely to develop food allergies than are older children or adults.
- The allergic response varies, usually affecting the gastrointestinal tract, the skin, the pulmonary system, and sometimes other systems.
- The only therapy for food allergies is nutritional with the avoidance of the allergenic foods and molecules and the supplementation of the diet with probiotics and phytonutrients that may reduce the severity and frequency of reactions.
- It is important for food and nutrition professionals to understand the differences between allergies and intolerances and the ingredient and nutrient content of food so that nutrient deficiencies are less likely as a result of foods being omitted.

CLINICAL SCENARIO 1

Sally is 18 months old. At birth she was unable to tolerate cow's milk–based formulas. Each feeding brought diarrhea and vomiting. The pediatrician recommended that her mother switch to a casein hydrolysate formula, which Sally tolerated well. Within 2 months she developed eczema that was treated with steroid creams. Cow's milk was introduced when Sally was 12 months of age. Skin symptoms increased remarkably. When eggs and later peanut butter were introduced, she experienced immediate wheezing, watery swelling eyes, hives, increased skin itch, and diarrhea. Sally's parents are unaware of how to look for egg or peanut sources; thus Sally experienced several trips to the emergency room. The last reaction was much more intense. Her family physician suspects egg and peanut allergies and has sent her to see a board-certified allergist and a nutritionist.

Continued

CLINICAL SCENARIO 1—cont'd

∗Nutrition Diagnosis 1:   Food and nutrition-related knowledge deficit on the part of the parents related to food sources of eggs and peanuts as evidenced by serious reactions in their daughter following ingestion

∗Nutrition Diagnosis 2:   Intake of unsafe foods related to ingestion of egg- and peanut-containing foods as evidenced by serious reactions to foods

1. How many food allergen suspects are there, and what are they? Why?
2. What measures will her mother need to take if Sally is to lose sensitivity to any of the food allergens?
3. What other circumstances may arise that may warrant special instructions to caregivers?
4. How often should Sally be checked for sensitivity changes?
5. What would you tell Sally's parents to look for on food labels?
6. What nutrient substitutions must be considered?

CLINICAL SCENARIO 2

Mrs. L. was recently diagnosed with diabetes. She is coming to see you, the nutritionist, for a medical nutrition assessment and evaluation to assist her with the multiple nutrition changes she knows she will have to make. She wishes to continue nursing Levi, her 6-month-old son. In the process of doing a history, you learn that Levi has several problems, including severe eczema since birth. He has had episodes of turning bright red head to toe and clawing at his skin, followed by intense sneezing and coughing. Symptoms have occurred on 6 different days, 30 minutes after either his 2:00 PM or 6:00 PM feeding, except that the last episode occurred after his 10:00 am feeding. Each episode lasts 12 hours and then begins to resolve. His pediatrician instructed the parents to give Levi ¼ teaspoon of Triaminic cough syrup every 4 to 6 hours for 48 hours once symptoms begin. Mom says that this helps his cough a little but it does not relieve the other symptoms. With the most recent episode, a family friend suggested that the parents give Benadryl to Levi. Skin and respiratory symptoms improved within the hour. Mrs. L. has no idea what causes these dramatic, frightening episodes.

∗Nutrition Diagnosis 1:   Intake of unsafe food related to symptoms occurring following feedings of infant as evidenced by coughing, sneezing, and rash

∗Nutrition Diagnosis 2:   Food- and nutrition-related knowledge deficit related to potential sources of food allergies as evidenced by mom's statement that she isn't aware of links to foods

1. Do you suspect food allergies? More than one?
2. What are the most likely food allergen suspects without knowing exactly what Mrs. L. ate before nursing?
3. Would you consider putting Mrs. L. on an elimination diet or switching Levi to infant formula?
4. How would you personalize an elimination diet without confusing the end results?
5. How would you help Mrs. L. integrate the eating plan for managing her diabetes with what you would recommend for her to do to solve Levi's problem?
6. What recommendations are you going to make to the infant's pediatrician?

USEFUL WEBSITES

Food Allergy and Anaphylaxis Network (FAAN)
www.foodallergy.org

Latex Allergy—Latex Education and Resource Team, Inc.
www.execpc.com/~alert

American Academy of Allergy, Asthma, and Immunology
www.aaaai.org

American College of Allergy, Asthma, and Immunology
www.allergy.mcg.edu

The Asthma and Allergy Foundation of America
www.aafa.org

References

Akdis CA et al: Diagnosis and treatment of atopic dermatitis in children and adults: European Academy of Allergology and Clinical Immunology/American Academy of Allergy, Asthma and Immunology/PRACTALL Consensus Report, *J Allergy Clin Immunol* 118:1, 2006.

Akdis M et al: T regulatory cells in allergy: Novel concepts in the pathogeneses, prevention, and treatment of allergic diseases, *J Allergy Clin Immunol* 116:5, 2005.

Arshad, SH: Primary prevention of asthma and allergy, *J Allergy Clin Immunol* 116:1, 2005.

Bahna SL: In vitro food allergy tests: the good, the bad and the worst, San Antonio, Tex, November 19, 2001, American College of Allergy, Asthma and Immunology, Sixtieth Annual Meeting.

Bock S et al: Fatalities due to anaphylactic reactions to foods, *J Allergy Clin Immunol* 107:191, 2001.

Breiteneder H, Mills C: Molecular properties of food allergens, *J Allergy Clin Immunol* 115:1, 2005.

Chapman MD et al: Nomenclature and structural biology of allergens, *J Allergy Clin Immunol* 119:414, 2007.

Chehade M, Mayer L: Oral tolerance and its relation to food hypersensitivities, *J Allergy Clin Immunol* 115:1, 2005.

Condemi J: Allergic reactions to natural rubber latex at home, to rubber products, and to cross-reacting foods, *J Allergy Clin Immunol* 110:S107, 2002.

Del Giudice MM et al: Probiotics in the atopic march: highlights and new insights, *Dig Liver Dis* 38:2885, 2006.

Friedman N, Zeiger R: The role of breast-feeding in the development of allergies and asthma, *J Allergy Clin Immunol* 115:1238, 2005.

Gdalevich M et al: Breast-feeding and the onset of atopic dermatitis in childhood: a systematic review and metaanalysis of prospective studies, *J Am Acad Dermatol* 45:520, 2001.

Geha R et al: Multicenter, double-blind, placebo-controlled, multiple-challenge evaluation of reported reactions to monosodium glutamate, *J Allergy Clin Immunol* 106:973, 2000.

Hahn E et al: The atopic march: The pattern of allergic disease development in childhood, *Immunol Allergy Clin North Am* 25:2, 2005.

Hamilton R, Adkinson NF: In vitro assays for the diagnosis of IgE-mediated disorders, *J Allergy Clin Immunol* 114:2, 2004.

Hawkins C, Katelaris C: Nitrate anaphylaxis, *Ann Allergy Asthma Immunol* 85:74, 2000.

Isolauri E, Salminen S: Probiotics, gut inflammation and barrier function, *Gastroenterol Clin* 34:3, 2005.

Jenkins A et al: Structural relatedness of plant food allergens with specific reference to cross-reactive allergens: an in silico analysis, *J Allergy Clin Immunol* 115:1, 2005.

Johansson SGO et al: Revised nomenclature for allergy for global use: report of Nomenclature Review Committee of the World Allergy Organization, October 2003, *J Allergy Clin Immunol* 113:5, 2004.

Jones CA et al: Costimulatory molecules in the developing human gastrointestinal tract: a pathway for fetal allergen priming, *J Allergy Clin Immunol* 108:235, 2001.

Kalliomaki MA, Isolauri E: Probiotics and down-regulation of allergic response, *J Allergy Clin Immunol* 24:4, 2004.

Kay AB: Allergy and allergic diseases, Part 1, *N Engl J Med* 344:30, 2001.

Kumar A et al: Why do people die of anaphylaxis: a clinical review, *Clin Dev Immunol* 12:281, 2005.

Kurup VP et al: Immune response modulation by curcumin in a latex allergy model, *Clin Mol Allergy* 5:1, 2007.

Neu J: Probiotics: protecting the intestinal ecosystem? *J Pediatr* 147:2, 2005.

Nowak-Wegrzyn A, Sampson H: Adverse reactions to foods, *Medical Clin North Am* 90:1, 2006.

Pina I et al: Use of goat's milk in patients with cow's milk allergy, *An Pediatr (Barc)* 59(2): 138, 2003.

Rautava S et al: New therapeutic strategy for combating the increasing burden of allergic disease: probiotics—a Nutrition, Allergy, Mucosal immunology and Intestinal Microbiota (NAMI) Research Group report, *J Allergy Clin Immunol* 116:1, 2005.

Regenstein JM: Are "Pareve" products really milk-free? *Food Allergy News* 17(6):1, 1998.

Reus K et al: Food additives as a cause of medical symptoms: relationship shown between sulfites and asthma and anaphylaxis: results of a literature review, *Nederlans Tijdschrift voor Geneeskunde* 144:38, 2000.

Sampson H: Peanut allergy, *N Engl J Med* 346:17, 2002.

Sampson H: Update on food allergy, *J Allergy Clin Immunol* 113:5, 2004.

Sampson H: Utility of food-specific IgE concentrations in predicting symptomatic food allergy, *J Allergy Clin Immunol* 107:5, 2001.

Schneider LC: New treatment for atopic dermatitis, *Immunol Allergy Clin North Am* 22(1):141, 2002.

Sicherer S: The genetics of food allergy, *Immunol Allergy Clin North Am* 22:2, 2002.

Sicherer S, Sampson H: Food allergy, *J Allergy Clin Immunol* 117:2, 2006.

Simons FER: Anaphylaxis, killer allergy: long-term management in the community, *J Allergy Clin Immunol* 117:2, 2006.

Simpson E, Hanifin J: Atopic dermatitis, *Med Clin North Am* 90:1, 2006.

Spergel J, Fiedler J: Food allergy and additives: triggers in asthma, *J Allergy Clin Immunol* 25:1, 2005.

Taylor SL et al: Will genetically modified foods be allergenic? *J Allergy Clin Immunol* 107:765, 2001.

Tiemessen M et al: Cow's milk–specific T-cell reactivity of children with and without persistent cow's milk allergy: key role for IL-10, *J Allergy Clin Immunol* 113:5, 2004.

Turunen S et al: Lymphoid nodular hyperplasia and cow's milk hypersensitivity in children with chronic constipation, *J Pediatr* 145:5, 2004.

Vadas P et al: Detection of peanut allergens in breast milk of lactating women, *JAMA* 285:1746, 2001.

Yagami T et al: Digestibility of allergens extracted from natural rubber latex and vegetable foods, *J Allergy Clin Immunol* 106:752, 2000.

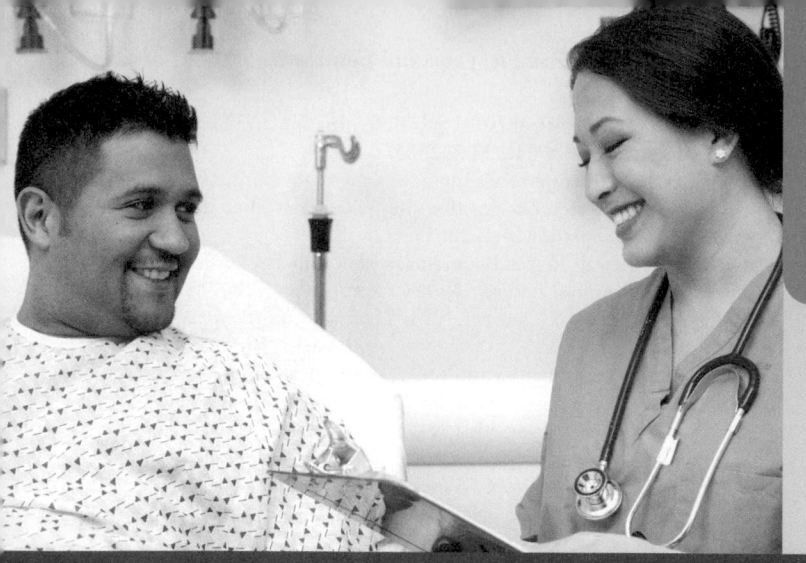

Medical Nutrition Therapy for Diabetes Mellitus and Hypoglycemia of Nondiabetic Origin

KEY TERMS

A1C an evaluation of a combination of all fractions of the hemoglobin molecule; a measurement of the glycosylation of the "c" fraction and the recommended assay method (simplified to A1C). An A1C of 6% reflects an average plasma glucose level of ≈120 mg/dl. In general, each 1% increase in A1C is a reflection of an increase in average glucose levels of ≈30 mg/dl

autonomic symptoms symptoms of hypoglycemia that are adrenergically based and that arise from the action of the autonomic nervous system

carbohydrate counting a commonly used method for diabetes food and meal planning based on research showing that carbohydrate is the primary nutrient affecting postprandial blood glucose and insulin levels and that all carbohydrates affect blood glucose levels approximately the same when eaten in similar gram amounts; carbohydrates can be measured in grams or carbohydrate servings—one carbohydrate serving is a portion of food that contains 15 g of carbohydrate

combination therapy a form of therapy for diabetes using combinations of oral glucose-lowering medications or a combination of oral glucose-lowering medication(s) and insulin(s) or other injectable medications

correction factor (CF) a factor determined from the "1700 rule," which defines how many milligrams per deciliter a unit of rapid-acting or short-acting insulin will lower blood glucose levels over a 2- to 4-hr period in an individual

counterregulatory (stress) hormones hormones, including glucagon, epinephrine (adrenaline), norepinephrine, cortisol, and growth hormone, released during stressful situations, that have the opposite effect of insulin and cause the liver to release glucose from stored glycogen (glycogenolysis) and the adipose cells to release fatty acids (lipolysis); these hormones also counterbalance declining glucose levels

dawn phenomenon a natural increase in morning blood glucose levels and insulin requirements that occurs in people with and without diabetes but tends to be more marked in people with diabetes; possibly caused by a diurnal variation in growth hormone, cortisol, or catecholamines

Diabetes Control and Complications Trial (DCCT) a 10-year study in people with type 1 diabetes who were treated with either conventional or intensive therapy; follow-up evaluations proved that intensive blood glucose control reduces the risk of diabetic microvascular and macrovascular complications

diabetic ketoacidosis (DKA) severe, uncontrolled diabetes resulting from insufficient insulin, in which ketone bodies (acids) build up in the blood; if left untreated (with immediate administration of insulin and fluids), DKA can lead to coma and even death

exchange lists foods grouped into six lists: starch, fruit, milk, vegetables, meat and meat substitutes, and fat; each list is a group of measured foods of approximately the same nutritional value; therefore foods on the same list can be "exchanged" or substituted for one another

fasting (food-deprived) hypoglycemia low blood glucose concentrations in response to no food intake for 8 hours or longer

gastroparesis impaired gastric motility; results in delayed or irregular contractions of the stomach, leading to various gastrointestinal symptoms such as feelings of fullness, bloating, nausea, vomiting, diarrhea, or constipation

gestational diabetes mellitus (GDM) glucose intolerance, the onset or first recognition of which occurs during pregnancy

glycemic index (GI) a measurement of the relative area under the postprandial glucose curve of 50 g of digestible carbohydrates compared with 50 g of a standard food, either glucose or white bread

glycemic load (GL) the estimated GL of foods, meals and dietary patterns is calculated by multiplying the glycemic index by the amount of carbohydrate in each food and then totaling the values for all foods in a meal or dietary pattern

glucagon a hormone produced by the α-cells of the pancreas that causes an increase in blood glucose levels by stimulating the release of glucose from liver glycogen stores

glucose-lowering medications drugs administered orally that are used to control or lower blood glucose levels, including first- and second-generation sulfonylureas, nonsulfonylureas, secretagogues, biguanides, α-glucosidase inhibitors, and thiazolidinediones

glucotoxicity β-cells chronically exposed to hyperglycemia become progressively less efficient in responding to a glucose challenge

glycosylated hemoglobin a blood test that reflects the blood glucose concentration over the life span of red blood cells (≈120 days), expressed as a percentage of total hemoglobin with glucose attached; also may be called glycated hemoglobin or glycohemoglobin

honeymoon phase the period after the initial diagnosis of type 1 diabetes when there may be some recovery of β-cell function and a temporary decrease in exogenous insulin requirement

hyperglycemia excessive glucose in the blood (generally 180 mg/dl or above) caused by too little insulin, insulin resistance, or increased food intake; symptoms include frequent urination, increased thirst, weight loss, and often tiredness or fatigue

hyperglycemic hyperosmolar state (HHS) extremely high blood glucose levels with an absence of or only slight ketosis and profound dehydration

hypoglycemia (or insulin reaction) low blood glucose level (70 mg/dl or less) caused by the administration of excessive insulin or insulin secretagogues, too little food, delayed or missed meals or snacks, increased exercise or other physical activity, or alcohol intake without food

hypoglycemia of nondiabetic origin low levels of blood glucose that lead to neuroglycopenia symptoms that are ameliorated by the ingestion of carbohydrate

immune-mediated diabetes mellitus a form of type 1 diabetes resulting from autoimmune destruction of the β-cells of the pancreas

incretins hormones released during nutrient absorption, which increase glucose-dependent insulin secretion

injectable glucose-lowering medications drugs administered by injection that are used to control or lower blood glucose levels; incretin mimetics that have the same glucose-lowering effects as the body's naturally occurring incretins; synthetic amylin—a polypeptide hormone normally co-secreted with insulin by the β-cells of the pancreas in response to food intake

insulin a hormone released from the β-cells of the pancreas that enables cells to metabolize and store glucose and other fuels

insulin resistance an impaired biologic response (sensitivity) to either exogenous or endogenous insulin; involved in the etiology of type 2 diabetes

insulin secretagogues oral medications that stimulate insulin release from the β-cell of the pancreas, such as sulfonylureas and nonsulfonylurea secretagogues (i.e., repaglinide and nateglinide)

insulin sensitizers oral medications that enhance insulin action and include biguanides (metformin) and thiazolidinediones

macrovascular diseases diseases of the large blood vessels, including coronary artery disease, cardiovascular disease, and peripheral vascular disease

metabolic syndrome characterized by central obesity and insulin resistance with increased risk for cardiovascular disease and type 2 diabetes; associated risk factors include dyslipidemia hypertension, presence of prothrombotic factors, and impaired glucose tolerance

microvascular diseases diseases of the small blood vessels, including retinopathy and nephropathy

neuroglycopenic symptoms neurologic symptoms of hypoglycemia that are related to an insufficient supply of glucose to the brain

polydipsia excessive thirst

polyuria excessive urination

postprandial (after a meal) blood glucose blood glucose level 1 to 2 hours after eating

postprandial (reactive) hypoglycemia low blood glucose within 2 to 5 hours after eating

pre-diabetes (impaired glucose homeostasis) blood glucose concentrations that are higher than normal but not yet high enough to be diagnosed as diabetes; sometimes referred to as impaired glucose tolerance (IGT) or impaired fasting glucose (IFG); risk factor for future diabetes and cardiovascular disease

preprandial (fasting) blood glucose blood glucose level before eating

self-monitoring of blood glucose (SMBG) individuals testing their own blood glucose levels using a chemically treated strip and visually comparing the strip to a color chart or by inserting the strip into a meter that measures the glucose level

Somogyi effect hypoglycemia followed by "rebound" hyperglycemia; originates during hypoglycemia with the secretion of counterregulatory hormones (glucagon, epinephrine, growth hormone, and cortisol) and is usually caused by excessive exogenous insulin doses

target blood glucose goals levels for capillary blood glucose tests that are as near normal as possible and that can be achieved without risk of serious hypoglycemia

type 1 diabetes a type of diabetes that usually occurs in persons younger than 30 years of age but can occur at any age; previously known as insulin-dependent diabetes mellitus (IDDM) or juvenile-onset diabetes

type 2 diabetes a type of diabetes usually occurring in persons older than 30 years of age, previously known as noninsulin-dependent diabetes mellitus (NIDDM) or maturity-onset diabetes; now also frequently diagnosed in youth and young adults

Continued

United Kingdom Prospective Diabetes Study (UKPDS) a 20-year multicenter trial of subjects with type 2 diabetes during which lowering of A1C and aggressive treatment of hypertension significantly reduced the development of microvascular complications and lowered the risk for macrovascular complications

Whipple's triad a triad of clinical features that includes (1) low blood glucose levels (2) accompanied by symptoms that are (3) relieved by administration of glucose

Diabetes mellitus is a group of diseases characterized by high blood glucose concentrations resulting from defects in insulin secretion, insulin action, or both. Abnormalities in the metabolism of carbohydrate, protein, and fat are also present. Persons with diabetes have bodies that do not produce or respond to **insulin,** a hormone produced by the β-cells of the pancreas that is necessary for the use or storage of body fuels. Without effective insulin, **hyperglycemia** (elevated blood glucose) occurs, which can lead to serious complications and premature death; but, people with diabetes can take steps to control the disease and lower the risk of complications.

In 2005 total prevalence of diabetes in the United States, all ages, was 20.8 million people or 7% of the population. Of these, 14.6 million are diagnosed, and 6.2 million undiagnosed. About 10.9 million men and 9.7 million women 20 years of age or older had diagnosed diabetes, or 9.6% of all people in this age-group, representing an increase from 4.9% of the adult population in 1990 and 7.3% in 2000. Diabetes prevalence increases with age, affecting 10.3 million people age 60 years or older, or 21% of all people in this age-group. Furthermore, in 2005 1.5 million people age 20 years or older were newly diagnosed with diabetes (Centers for Disease Control and Prevention, 2005).

Much of the increase is because type 2 diabetes is no longer a disease that affects mainly older adults. Between 1990 and 1998 the prevalence of diabetes increased by 76% among people in their thirties (Mokdad et al., 2001). Among children with newly diagnosed diabetes, the prevalence of type 2 diabetes also increased dramatically in the past decade, growing from less than 4% in the years preceding 1990 to as high as 45% in certain racial and ethnic groups in recent years (American Diabetes Association [ADA], 2000).

The prevalence of type 2 diabetes is highest in ethnic groups in the United States. Non-Hispanic blacks are 1.8 times as likely to have diabetes as non-Hispanic whites; Hispanic Latinos, 1.7 times; American Indians and Alaska Natives, 2.2 times, and Asian-Americans and Pacific Islanders 1.5 times (Centers for Disease Control and Prevention, 2005) (see *Focus On:* Diabetes Does Discriminate!)

In addition, another 41 million people are estimated to have pre-diabetes, which includes impaired glucose tolerance (IGT) (2-hour postchallenge glucose of 140-199 mg/dl) and impaired fasting glucose (IFG) (fasting plasma glucose 100 to 125 mg/dl) (Centers for Disease Control and Prevention,

2005). Persons with pre-diabetes are at high risk for conversion to type 2 diabetes and cardiovascular disease (CVD) if lifestyle prevention strategies are not implemented.

Diabetes mellitus contributes to a considerable increase in morbidity and mortality rates, which can be reduced by early diagnosis and treatment. In 2002 diabetes costs in the United States were $132 billion. Direct medical expenditures such as inpatient care, outpatient services, and nursing home care totaled $92 billion, or an average annual total direct cost of medical care of $13,243 per person with diabetes compared with $2560 per person without diabetes. Indirect costs, totaling $40 billion, were associated with lost productivity, including premature death and disability (ADA, 2003a).

PATHOPHYSIOLOGY

Assigning a type of diabetes to an individual often depends on the circumstances present at the time of diagnosis, and many individuals do not easily fit into a single category. Thus it is less important to label the particular type of diabetes than it is to understand the pathogenesis of the hyperglycemia and to treat it effectively (ADA, 2006a). What is clear, however, is the need to intervene early with lifestyle interventions, beginning with pre-diabetes and continuing through the disease process. In 1997 recommendations were made to eliminate the terms *insulin-dependent diabetes mellitus (IDDM)* and *noninsulin-dependent diabetes mellitus (NIDDM)* and to keep the terms *type 1* and *type 2 diabetes* and to use Arabic rather than Roman numerals (Table 30-1).

Pre-diabetes

A stage of impaired glucose homeostasis that includes IFG and GT is called **pre-diabetes.** People with pre-diabetes have IFG, IGT, or both. Individuals with pre-diabetes are at high risk for future diabetes and CVD.

Type 1 Diabetes

At diagnosis, people with **type 1 diabetes** are often lean and experience excessive thirst, frequent urination, and significant weight loss. The primary defect is pancreatic β-cell destruction, usually leading to absolute insulin deficiency and resulting in hyperglycemia, **polyuria** (excessive urination), **polydipsia** (excessive thirst), weight loss, dehydration, electrolyte disturbance, and ketoacidosis. The rate of β-cell destruction is quite variable, proceeding rapidly in some persons (mainly infants and children) and slowly in others (mainly adults). The capacity of a healthy pancreas to secrete insulin is far in excess of what is needed normally; therefore, the clinical onset of diabetes may be preceded by an extensive asymptomatic period of months to years, during which β-cells are undergoing gradual destruction (see *Pathophysiology and Care Management Algorithm:* Type 1 Diabetes Mellitus).

Type 1 diabetes accounts for 5% to 10% of all diagnosed cases of diabetes. Persons with type 1 diabetes are dependent on exogenous insulin to prevent ketoacidosis and

Diabetes Does Discriminate!

Diabetes strikes particularly hard in certain ethnic populations. Certain environmental or lifestyle factors may increase the risk of developing type 2 diabetes in susceptible populations. For example, an increase in the prevalence is observed in populations who have migrated to more urbanized locations compared with people of the same group who remained in their traditional home. Urbanization is usually related to major changes in diet, physical activity, and socioeconomic status, as well as increased obesity.

One theory that might explain the increased prevalence of diabetes and insulin resistance among Native people is the "thrifty" gene. Years of subsistence living have created a thrifty genotype that allows Native people to extract a lot of energy and fat from small amounts of food. In an era of store-bought processed food, that gene backfires to induce obesity and diabetes. Adoption of a "Western" lifestyle (which may include a diet high in fat and a sedentary way of life) has been associated with a dramatically increased rate of type 2 diabetes in the Pima Indians of Arizona (ADA, 2001). Among the Pima Indians of Arizona, about 55% of adults older than 35 years of age have type 2 diabetes. This disease is increasingly being diagnosed in Native Americans younger than 30 years of age and has been diagnosed in some as young as 7 years.

Ravussin and colleagues (1994) surveyed a closely related population of Pima Indians living in Maycoba, a small village in a remote, mountainous region of northwestern Mexico. They found that individuals in this community ate a diet lower in fat than is typically consumed in Arizona, and both men and women were very physically active. The men and women of Maycoba weighed, on average, 50 lb less than a comparable group of Pimas from the Phoenix area. More importantly, diabetes was diagnosed in about 10% of the Maycoba Pimas compared with almost 50% of the Arizona Pimas.

The main staples of the Maycoba Pimas' diet are beans, corn (as tortillas), and potatoes. Several essential nutrients are lacking because of the relative absence of fruits and vegetables. Diet analysis reveals a diet composed of 13% protein, 23% fat, 63% carbohydrate, and less than 1% alcohol and containing more than 50 g of fiber. This is in sharp contrast to the present diet of the Arizona Pimas. Even more striking than the low-fat diet of the Maycoba population, however, was the high level of physical activity in this population; more than 40 hours a week were spent engaged in hard physical work (Ravussin et al., 1994).

Interventions involving increased physical activity and a reduced fat and energy diet slowed the progression to type 2 diabetes in high-risk populations (Diabetes Prevention Program Research Group, 2002). Health promotion activities through community-based exercise programs and a return to more traditional diets also may help to reduce the diabetes epidemic that affects many developing countries and ethnic groups in industrialized nations.

TABLE 30-1

Types of Diabetes and Pre-Diabetes

Classification	Distinguishing Characteristics
Type 1 diabetes	Affected persons are usually children and young adults, although it can occur at any age, and are dependent on exogenous insulin to prevent ketoacidosis and death. Type 1 diabetes accounts for 5% to 10% of all diagnosed cases of diabetes.
Type 2 diabetes	Affected persons are often older than 30 yr at diagnosis, although it is now occurring frequently in young adults and children. The disease is slowly progressive, and treatment necessary to control hyperglycemia varies over time. Individuals are not dependent on exogenous insulin for survival but often require it for adequate glycemic control. Complications of diabetes may be present at diagnosis.
Gestational diabetes	Diabetes diagnosed in some women during pregnancy.
Other specific types	Diabetes that results from specific genetic syndromes, surgery, drugs, malnutrition, infections, or other illnesses.
Pre-diabetes	Fasting or glucose tolerance test results above normal, but not diagnostic of diabetes. These persons should be monitored closely because they have an increased risk of developing diabetes.

Modified from American Diabetes Association: Diagnosis and classification of diabetes mellitus (Position Statement), *Diabetes Care* 30:S48, 2007.

PATHOPHYSIOLOGY AND CARE MANAGEMENT ALGORITHM

Type 1 Diabetes Mellitus

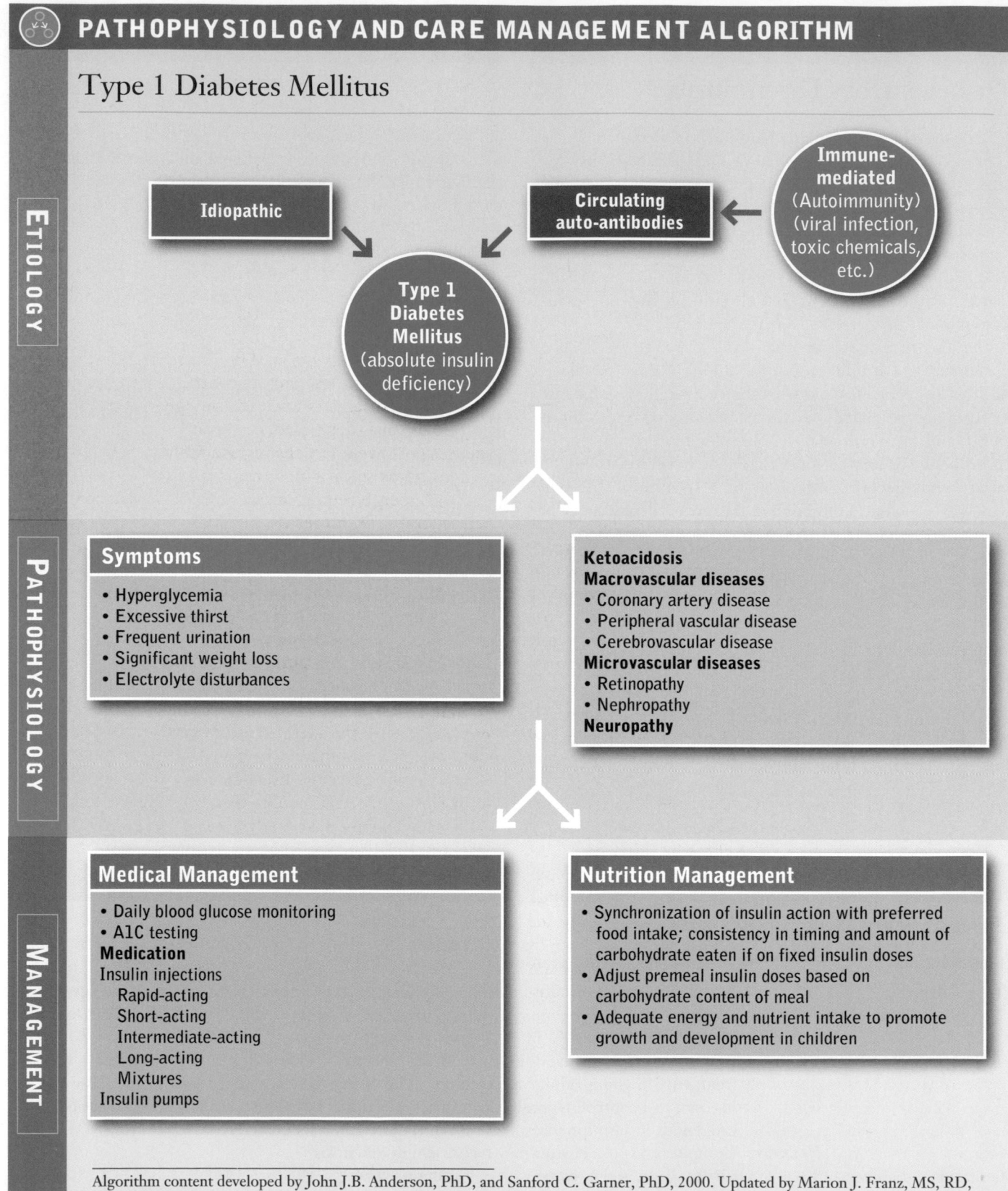

Algorithm content developed by John J.B. Anderson, PhD, and Sanford C. Garner, PhD, 2000. Updated by Marion J. Franz, MS, RD, LD, CDE, 2006.

death. Although it may occur at any age, even in the eighth and ninth decades of life, most cases are diagnosed in people younger than 30 years of age, with a peak incidence at around ages 10 to 12 years in girls and ages 12 to 14 years in boys.

Type 1 diabetes has two forms: immune-mediated diabetes mellitus and idiopathic diabetes mellitus. **Immune-mediated diabetes mellitus** results from an autoimmune destruction of the β-cells of the pancreas, the only cells in the body that make the hormone insulin that regulates blood glucose. Idiopathic type 1 diabetes mellitus refers to forms of the disease that have no known etiology. Although only a minority of persons with type 1 diabetes fall into this category, of those who do, most are of African or Asian origin (ADA, 2006a).

Risk factors for type 1 diabetes may be genetic, autoimmune, or environmental. The genetic predisposition to type 1 diabetes is the result of the combination of HLA-DQ coded genes for disease susceptibility offset by genes that are related to disease resistance (ADA, 2006a). However, the genetic factors that confer susceptibility or protection remain unclear. A 50% discordance rate of type 1 diabetes exists between identical twins, suggesting that specific genes are necessary but not sufficient for its development. A trigger, likely environmental, is necessary for the expression of the genetic propensity. There are no known means to prevent type 1 diabetes.

Regardless of the trigger, early type 1 diabetes is first identified by the appearance of active autoimmunity directed against pancreatic β-cells and their products. At diagnosis, 85% to 90% of patients with type 1 diabetes have one or more circulating autoantibodies to islet cells, endogenous insulin, or other antigens that are constituents of islet cells. Antibodies identified as contributing to the destruction of β-cells are (1) islet cell autoantibodies; (2) insulin autoantibodies, which may occur in persons who have never received insulin therapy; (3) antibodies against islet tyrosine phosphatase (known as IA2 and IA2); and (4) autoantibodies to glutamic acid decarboxylase (GAD), a protein on the surface of β-cells. GAD autoantibodies appear to provoke an attack by the T cells (killer T lymphocytes), which may be what destroys the β-cells in diabetes. The clinical onset of diabetes may be abrupt, but the pathophysiologic insult is a slow, progressive process. Hyperglycemia and symptoms develop only after greater than 90% of the secretory capacity of the β-cell mass has been destroyed.

Frequently, after diagnosis and the correction of hyperglycemia, metabolic acidosis, and ketoacidosis, endogenous insulin secretion recovers. During this **honeymoon phase** exogenous insulin requirements decrease dramatically for up to 1 year; however, the need for increasing exogenous insulin replacement is inevitable, and within 5 to 10 years after clinical onset, β-cell loss is complete, and circulating islet cell antibodies can no longer be detected.

Type 2 Diabetes

Type 2 diabetes may account for 90% to 95% of all diagnosed cases of diabetes and is a progressive disease that, in many cases, is present long before it is diagnosed. Hyperglycemia develops gradually and is often not severe enough in the early states for the patient to notice any of the classic symptoms of diabetes. Although undiagnosed, these individuals are at increased risk of developing macrovascular and microvascular complications.

Risk factors for type 2 diabetes include genetic and environmental factors, including a family history of diabetes, older age, obesity, particularly intraabdominal obesity, physical inactivity, a prior history of gestational diabetes, pre-

diabetes, and race or ethnicity. Adiposity and a longer duration of obesity are powerful risks factors for type 2 diabetes, and even small weight losses are associated with a change in glucose levels toward normal in persons with pre-diabetes. Nevertheless, type 2 diabetes is found in persons who are not obese, and many obese persons never develop type 2 diabetes. Obesity combined with a genetic predisposition may be necessary for type 2 diabetes to occur. Another possibility is that a similar genetic predisposition leads independently to both obesity and insulin resistance, which increases the risk for type 2 diabetes (ADA, 2001). A sedentary lifestyle has also been linked to an increased propensity to develop type 2 diabetes (see *Pathophysiology and Care Management Algorithm: Type 2 Diabetes Mellitus*).

In most cases type 2 diabetes results from a combination of insulin resistance and β-cell failure, but the extent to which each of these factors contributes to the development of the disease is unclear. Endogenous insulin levels may be normal, depressed, or elevated; but they are inadequate to overcome concomitant **insulin resistance** (decreased tissue sensitivity or responsiveness to insulin); as a result, hyperglycemia ensues. Insulin resistance is first demonstrated in target tissues, mainly muscle, liver, and adipose cells. Initially there is a compensatory increase in insulin secretion, which maintains normal glucose concentrations; but, as the disease progresses, insulin production gradually decreases. Hyperglycemia is first exhibited as an elevation of **postprandial (after a meal) blood glucose** caused by insulin resistance at the cellular level and is followed by an elevation in fasting glucose concentrations. As insulin secretion decreases, hepatic glucose production increases, causing the increase in **preprandial (fasting) blood glucose** levels. Compounding the problem is the deleterious effect of hyperglycemia itself—**glucotoxicity**—on both insulin sensitivity and insulin secretion; hence the importance of achieving near-euglycemia in persons with type 2 diabetes.

Insulin resistance is also demonstrated at the adipocyte level, leading to lipolysis and an elevation in circulating free fatty acids. In particular, excess intraabdominal obesity, characterized by an excess accumulation of visceral fat around and inside abdominal organs, results in an increased flux of free fatty acids to the liver, leading to an increase in insulin resistance. Increased fatty acids also cause a further decrease in insulin sensitivity at the cellular level, impair pancreatic insulin secretion, and augment hepatic glucose production (lipotoxicity) (Bergman and Adler, 2000). The above defects contribute to the development and progression of type 2 diabetes and are also primary targets for pharmacologic therapy.

Persons with type 2 diabetes may or may not experience the classic symptoms of uncontrolled diabetes, and they are not prone to develop ketoacidosis. Although persons with type 2 diabetes do not require exogenous insulin for survival, about 40% or more will eventually require exogenous insulin for adequate blood glucose control. Insulin may also be required for control during periods of stress-induced hyperglycemia, such as during illness or surgery.

PATHOPHYSIOLOGY AND CARE MANAGEMENT ALGORITHM

Type 2 Diabetes Mellitus

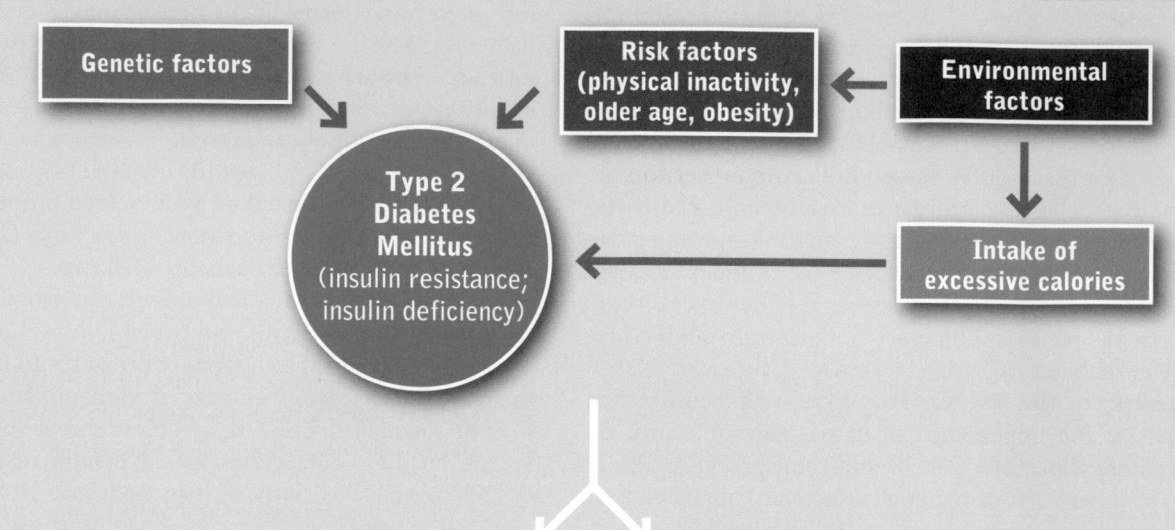

ETIOLOGY

Genetic factors

Risk factors (physical inactivity, older age, obesity)

Environmental factors

Intake of excessive calories

Type 2 Diabetes Mellitus (insulin resistance; insulin deficiency)

PATHOPHYSIOLOGY

Clinical Findings

- Abnormal pattern of insulin secretion and action
- Decreased cellular uptake of glucose and increased postprandial glucose
- Increased release of glucose by liver (gluconeogenesis) in early morning hours

Symptoms (variable)

- Hyperglycemia
- Excessive thirst
- Frequent urination
- Polyphagia
- Weight loss

MANAGEMENT

Medical Management

Diagnosis
- FBG >126 mg/dl
- Nonfasting glucose >200 mg/dl (with symptoms)
- Oral GTT >200 mg/dl

Monitoring
- Blood glucose
- A1C testing

Medication
- Sulfonylureas
- Non-sulfonylurea secretagogues
- Biguanides
- α-Glucosidase inhibitors
- Thiazolidinediones
- Incretins

Nutrition Management

- Lifestyle strategies (food/eating and physical activity) that improve glycemia, dyslipidemia, and blood pressure
- Nutrition education (carbohydrate counting and fat modification)
- Energy restriction to promote 5%–10% weight loss
- Blood glucose monitoring to determine adjustments in food or medications

Algorithm content developed by John J.B. Anderson, PhD, and Sanford C. Garner, PhD, 2000. Updated by Marion J. Franz, MS, RD, LD, CDE, 2006.

Gestational Diabetes Mellitus

Gestational diabetes mellitus (GDM) is defined as any degree of glucose intolerance with onset or first recognition during pregnancy. It occurs in about 7% of all pregnancies, resulting in more than 200,000 cases annually (ADA, 2001). Women with known diabetes mellitus before pregnancy are not classified as having GDM. GDM is usually diagnosed during the second or third trimester of pregnancy. At this point, insulin-antagonist hormone levels increase, and insulin resistance normally occurs. During pregnancy gestational diabetes requires treatment to normalize maternal blood glucose levels to avoid complications in the infant.

Other Types of Diabetes

This category includes diabetes associated with specific genetic syndromes (such as maturity-onset diabetes of youth), surgery, drugs, malnutrition, infections, and other illnesses. Such types of diabetes may account for 1% to 5% of all diagnosed cases of diabetes.

DIAGNOSTIC AND SCREENING CRITERIA

Diagnostic criteria for diabetes are summarized in Table 30-2. Three diagnostic methods may be used to diagnose diabetes and each, in the absence of unequivocal hyperglycemia, must be confirmed, on a subsequent day, by any of the following three methods (ADA, 2006a). At this time, hemoglobin A1C (A1C) is not recommended for diagnosis. In pregnant women different criteria are applied in establishing the diagnosis of gestational diabetes.

- Symptoms of diabetes plus a casual plasma glucose value of ≥200 mg/dl (11.1 mmol/l). *Casual* is defined to any time of the day without regard to time since last meal. The classic symptoms of diabetes include polyuria, polydipsia, and unexplained weight loss.

- A fasting plasma glucose (FPG) value ≥126 mg/dl (7 mmol/L). Fasting is defined as no caloric intake for at least 8 hr.
- A 2-hour postload glucose ≥200 mg/dl (11.1 mmol/L) during an oral glucose tolerance (OGT) test involving administration of 75 g of glucose

Testing or screening for diabetes should be considered in all individuals at age 45 years and above, particularly in those with a body mass index (BMI) of 25 kg/m² or more, and, if normal, should be repeated at 3-year intervals (ADA, 2006b). Testing should be considered at a younger age or be carried out more frequently in individuals who are overweight (BMI (>25 kg/m²) and have additional risk factors:

- Are habitually physically inactive
- Have a first-degree relative with diabetes
- Are members of a high-risk ethnic population (e.g., black, Latino, Native American, Asian-American, and Pacific Islander)
- Have delivered a baby weighing more than 9 lb or have been diagnosed with gestational diabetes
- Are hypertensive (blood pressure ≥140/90 mm Hg)
- Have a high-density lipoprotein (HDL) cholesterol level <35 mg/dl (0.9 mmol/L) and/or a triglyceride level >250 mg/dl (2.82 mmol/L)
- Have polycystic ovary syndrome (PCOS)
- On previous testing, had IGT or IFG
- Have other clinical conditions associated with insulin resistance (e.g., PCOS or acanthosis nigricans [i.e., gray-brown skin pigmentations])
- Have a history of vascular disease

The incidence of type 2 diabetes in children and adolescents is increasing dramatically and is consistent with screening recommendations for adults: children and youth at increased risk for type 2 diabetes should be tested. Youth who are overweight (BMI >85th percentile for age and sex) and have any two of the following risk factors should be screened: family history of type 2 diabetes, members of high-risk

---

TABLE 30-2

Diagnosis of Diabetes Mellitus and Impaired Glucose Homeostasis

Diagnosis	Criteria
Diabetes	FPG ≥126 mg/dl (≥7.0 mmol/L)
	CPG ≥200 mg/dl (≥11.1 mmol/L) plus symptoms
	2hPG ≥200 mg/dl (≥11.1 mmol/L)
Pre-diabetes	
Impaired fasting glucose	FPG 100-125 mg/dl (5.6-7.0 mmol/L)
Impaired glucose tolerance	2hPG 140-199 mg/dl (7.8-11.0 mmol/L)
Normal	FPG <100 mg/dl (<5.6 mmol/L)
	2hPG <140 mg/dl (<7.8 mmol/L)

Modified from American Diabetes Association: Diagnosis and classification of diabetes mellitus (Position Statement), *Diabetes Care* 30:S48, 2007.

CPG, Casual plasma glucose; *FPG,* fasting plasma glucose; *2hPG,* 2-hour plasma glucose level (measured 2 hours after an oral glucose tolerance test with administration of 75 g of glucose).

ethnic populations, signs of insulin resistance (acanthosis nigricans, hypertension, dyslipidemia, or PCOS [see *Focus On:* Polycystic Ovary Syndrome in Chapter 21]), or maternal history of diabetes or gestational diabetes. The age of initiation of screening is age 10 years or onset of puberty, and the frequency is every 2 years (ADA, 2006b).

Screening and diagnosis for GDM are discussed later in this chapter.

MANAGEMENT OF PRE-DIABETES

Based on early observational and intervention studies, the Finnish Diabetes Prevention Study (Tuomilehto et al., 2001) and the Diabetes Prevention Program (DPP) (DPP Research Group, 2002) were designed to investigate the effects of lifestyle interventions on prevention of diabetes in those at high risk (presence of IGT).The development of type 2 diabetes is strongly related to lifestyle factors, thus suggesting to researchers that it might be a preventable disease. Observational studies, as well as early intervention trials addressing physical activity, weight loss, and dietary intake, including whole grains and fiber and dietary fat, provided evidence for factors that might delay or prevent type 2 diabetes, but all had methodologic limitations.

In the Finnish study 522 middle-age, overweight subjects with IGT were randomized to receive either brief diet and exercise counseling (control group) or intensive individualized instruction on how to reduce weight (goal of 5% weight reduction), reduce total intake of fat (goal of <30% of energy intake) and saturated fat (goal of <10% of energy intake), and increase fiber intake (goal of 15 g/1000 kcal) and physical activity (goal of >150 minutes weekly). After an average follow-up of 3.2 years, there was a 58% reduction in the incidence of type 2 diabetes in the intervention group compared with the control group. The reduction in the incidence of diabetes was directly associated with the ability of the subjects to achieve one or more of the lifestyle strategies.

The Diabetes Prevention Program (DPP) randomized 3234 persons (45% from minority groups) with IGT to placebo, metformin, or lifestyle intervention. Subjects in the placebo and medication arms received standard lifestyle recommendations that included written information and an annual 20- to 30-minute individual session. Subjects in the lifestyle arm were expected to achieve and maintain a weight loss of at least 7% and to perform 150 minutes of physical activity per week. Subjects were seen weekly for the first 24 weeks, followed by monthly sessions. After an average follow-up of 2.8 years, a 58% decrease in the progression to diabetes was observed in the lifestyle group, and a 31% relative reduction was observed in the metformin group. On average, 59% of the lifestyle group achieved the goal of 7% or greater weight reduction, and 74% maintained at least 150 minutes per week of moderately intense activity (Fujimoto et al., 2007).

Three diabetes prevention trials in individuals with IGT using pharmacologic therapy also reported a lowering of the incidence of diabetes. Metformin reduced the risk of diabetes by 31% (DPP Research Group, 2002), the α-glucosidase inhibitor acarbose reduced risk by 32% (Chiasson et al., 2002), and the thiazolidinedione troglitazone reduced risk by 56% (Buchanan et al., 2002). In a group of obese individuals with or without IGT, orlistat added to lifestyle delayed the risk of diabetes by 45% in subjects with IGT but had no effect in those without IGT (Torgerson et al., 2004). Studies comparing lifestyle modifications to medication strongly provide support for the greater benefit of weight loss and physical activity as the first choice to prevent or delay diabetes. Modest weight loss (5% to 10% of body weight) and modest physical activity (30 minutes daily) are the recommended goals. Follow-up counseling is necessary to accomplish these objectives. There is insufficient evidence to support the use of drug therapy as a substitute for lifestyle modifications (ADA).

Medical Nutrition Therapy for Pre-Diabetes

Over the next decade the number of persons with diabetes and at risk for diabetes and CVD is expected to grow by 25%, largely driven by the rising prevalence of obesity and inactivity. Unless action is taken to change the predicted estimates of diabetes, the disease will also become a huge economic burden because of both direct health care costs and indirect costs resulting from a decline in workplace productivity. It is essential that individuals at risk for diabetes be identified and treatment interventions implemented. In no other disease does the role of lifestyle—healthy and appropriate food choices and physical activity—play a more important role in both prevention and treatment than in diabetes.

Goals of medical nutrition therapy (MNT) for pre-diabetes emphasize the importance of lifestyle in decreasing the risk of type 2 diabetes by increasing physical activity and promoting food choices that facilitate moderate weight loss (Box 30-1). Because of the effects of obesity on insulin resistance, weight loss is an important goal for persons with pre-diabetes or metabolic syndrome. Structured programs that emphasize lifestyle changes, including education, reduced fat (≈30% of total energy) and energy intake, regular physical activity, and regular participant contact have been shown to result in long-term weight loss of 5% to 7% of starting weight. In the DPP, weight loss of 3 kg from baseline was also associated with an improved lipid profile (Ratner et al., 2005).

Although desired by the public, there is no "miracle diet" for weight loss. Low-carbohydrate and low-fat, energy-restricted diets both result in weight loss for up to 1 year. The low-carbohydrate diets have potential favorable effects on triglyceride and HDL cholesterol values; however, this should be weighed against potential unfavorable effects in low-density lipoprotein (LDL) cholesterol values from low-carbohydrate diets (Nordmann et al., 2006). Of prime importance is a reduced-energy diet that an individual can follow long term. Lifestyle modifications are reported to produce weight loss of approximately 10%, or 10 to 12 kg, over 3 to 6 months (Douketis et al., 2005) and can maintain

Goals of Medical Nutrition Therapy for Diabetes Mellitus

Goals of Medical Nutrition Therapy That Apply to Persons at Risk for Diabetes or With Pre-Diabetes:

1. To decrease risk of diabetes and cardiovascular disease by promoting healthy food choices and physical activity leading to moderate weight loss that is maintained

Goals of Medical Nutrition Therapy for Persons With Diabetes

1. To the extent possible, achieve and maintain:
   - Blood glucose levels in the normal range or as close to normal as is safely possible
   - A lipid and lipoprotein profile that reduces the risk for vascular disease
   - Blood pressure levels that reduce the risk for vascular disease
2. To prevent, or at least slow the rate of development of, the chronic complications of diabetes by modifying nutrient intake and lifestyle as appropriate
3. To address individual nutrition needs, taking into account personal and cultural preferences and willingness to change
4. To limit food choices based only on evidence and to maintain the pleasure of eating

Goals of Nutrition Therapy That Apply to Specific Situations

1. For youth with type 1 diabetes, youth with type 2 diabetes, pregnant and lactating women, and older adults with diabetes, to meet the nutritional needs of these unique times in the life cycle
2. For individuals treated with insulin or insulin secretagogues, to provide self-management training for safe conduct of exercise, prevention and treatment of hypoglycemia, and treatment of acute illness

Adapted from American Diabetes Association: Nutrition recommendations and interventions for diabetes (Position Statement) *Diabetes Care* 30:S48 2007.

weight loss of 4.5 kg after 2 to 4 years (Curioni et al., 2005). Support from family, peers, or health care professionals; setting realistic weight loss goals (Grave et al., 2005); and monitoring food intake (Wadden et al., 2005) have been shown to assist in accomplishing required lifestyle modifications (see Chapter 21).

Physical activity is important to prevent weight gain and maintain weight loss. For cardiovascular fitness and to reduce risk of chronic health problems, including type 2 diabetes, 30 min/day of moderate physical activity is recommended. Sixty minutes per day is recommended to prevent weight gain, whereas 60 to 90 minutes may be required to avoid regain after weight loss (Dietary Guidelines Advisory Committee, 2005). Furthermore, physical activity independent of weight loss also improves insulin sensitivity (Duncan et al., 2003).

Whole grains and dietary fiber are associated with reduced risk of diabetes. Increased intake of whole grain–containing foods has been associated with improved insulin sensitivity independent of body weight (Liese et al., 2003), and increased intake of dietary fiber has been associated with improved insulin sensitivity and improved ability to secrete insulin adequately to overcome insulin resistance (Mayer-Davis et al., 2006a).

Observational studies suggest an association between moderate consumption of alcohol (1 to 3 drinks per day [15 to 45 g alcohol]) and decreased risk of type 2 diabetes, coronary heart disease, and stroke (Howard et al., 2004). But the data do not support recommending alcohol consumption to persons at risk for diabetes who do not already drink alcoholic beverages (ADA, 2007).

MANAGEMENT OF DIABETES

Two classic clinical trials have demonstrated beyond a doubt the clear link between glycemic control and the development of complications in persons with type 1 and type 2 diabetes, as well as the importance of nutrition therapy in achieving control. The **Diabetes Control and Complications Trial (DCCT)** was a long-term, prospective, randomized, controlled, multicenter trial that studied approximately 1400 young adults (ages 13 to 39 years) with type 1 diabetes who were treated with either intensive therapeutic regimens (multiple injections of insulin or use of insulin infusion pumps guided by blood glucose monitoring results) or conventional regimens (one or two insulin injections per day). Intensively treated patients experienced a 50% to 75% reduction in the risk of progression to retinopathy, nephropathy, and neuropathy after 8 to 9 years (DCCT Research Group, 1993). Furthermore, average A1C values in patients who adhered to the prescribed meal plan and adjusted food and insulin in response to hyperglycemia were 0.25% to 1% lower than among patients who did not follow these behaviors (Delahanty and Halford, 1993).

After a mean 17 years of follow-up, intensive diabetes therapy implemented during the trial was shown to reduce the risk of any CVD event by 42% and the risk of nonfatal myocardial infarction, stroke, or death from CVD by 57% (DCCT, 2005). Thus, in persons with type 1 diabetes, intensive therapy not only reduces the risk of microvascular complications, but also reduces the risk of macrovascular complications.

The reports of the **United Kingdom Prospective Diabetes Study (UKPDS)** demonstrated conclusively that elevated blood glucose levels cause long-term complications in type 2 diabetes, just as in type 1 diabetes (United Kingdom Prospective Diabetes Study Group [UKPDS], 1998a). The UKPDS recruited and followed up on 5102 newly diagnosed type 2 diabetic patients for an average of 10 to 11 years. Subjects were randomized into a group treated conventionally, primarily with nutrition therapy, and compared with subjects randomized into an intensively treated group, initially treated with sulfonylureas. In the intensive therapy group the microvascular complication rate decreased significantly by 25%, and the risk of macrovascular disease decreased by 16%. Combination therapy (combining insulin or metformin with sulfonylureas) was needed in both groups to meet glycemic goals as loss of glycemic control was noted over the 10-year trial. Aggressive treatment of even mild-to-moderate hypertension was also beneficial in both groups (UKPDS, 1998b).

The importance of implementing nutrition therapy at diagnosis was clearly demonstrated. Before randomization into intensive or conventional treatment, subjects received individualized intensive nutrition therapy for 3 months. During this period the mean A1C decreased by 1.9% (≈9% to ≈7%) (the greatest reduction in A1C during the trial) with only a modest average weight loss of 3.5 kg (8 lb). UKPDS researchers concluded that in determining FPG, the reduction of energy intake was at least as important, if not more important, than the actual weight lost.

This study illustrates the progressive nature of type 2 diabetes. An important lesson learned from the UKPDS is that therapy needs to be intensified over time and that, as the disease progresses, MNT alone is not enough to keep most patients' A1C level at 7% or less. Medication(s), and for many patients, eventually insulin, needs to be combined with nutrition therapy. The "diet" doesn't fail; the pancreas fails to secrete enough insulin to maintain adequate glucose control.

The management of diabetes includes MNT, physical activity, monitoring, medications, and self-management education. An important goal of treatment is to provide the patient with the necessary tools to achieve the best possible control of glycemia, lipidemia, and blood pressure to prevent, delay, or arrest the microvascular and macrovascular complications while minimizing hypoglycemia and excess weight gain (ADA, 2006b). Optimal control of diabetes also requires the restoration of normal carbohydrate, protein, and fat metabolism. Insulin is both anticatabolic and anabolic and facilitates cellular transport (Table 30-3). In general, the **counterregulatory (stress) hormones** (glucagon, growth hormone, cortisol, epinephrine, and norepinephrine) have the opposite effect of insulin.

Glycemic treatment goals for persons with diabetes are listed in Table 30-4. Achieving goals requires open communication and appropriate self-management education. Patients can assess day-to-day glycemic control by self-monitoring of blood glucose (SMBG) and measurement of urine or blood ketones. Longer-term glycemic control is assessed from the results of **glycosylated hemoglobin** (simplified as **A1C**) tests. When hemoglobin and other proteins are exposed to glucose, the glucose becomes attached to the protein in a slow, nonenzymatic, and concentration-dependent fashion. Measurements of A1C reflect a weighted average of plasma glucose concentration over the preceding weeks, thereby complementing day-to-day testing. In nondiabetic persons A1C values are 4%

TABLE 30-3

Action of Insulin on Carbohydrate, Protein, and Fat Metabolism

Effect	Carbohydrates	Protein	Fat
Anticatabolic (prevents breakdown)	Decreases breakdown and release of glucose from glycogen in the liver	Inhibits protein degradation, diminishes gluconeogenesis	Inhibits lipolysis, prevents excessive production of ketones and ketoacidosis
Anabolic (promotes storage)	Facilitates conversion of glucose to glycogen for storage in liver and muscle	Stimulates protein synthesis	Facilitates conversion of pyruvate to free fatty acids, stimulating lipogenesis
Transport	Activates the transport system of glucose into muscle and adipose cells	Lowers blood amino acids in parallel with blood glucose levels	Activates lipoprotein lipase, facilitating transport of triglycerides into adipose tissue

---

TABLE 30-4

Recommendations for Glycemic Control for Adults With Diabetes

Glycemic Control

A1C	<7.0%*
Preprandial capillary plasma glucose	90-130 mg/dl (5.0-7.2 mmol/l)
Peak postprandial capillary plasma glucose†	<180 mg/dl (<10.0 mmol/l)

Modified from American Diabetes Association: Standards of medical care in diabetes—2007, *Diabetes Care* 30:54, 2007.

*Referenced to a nondiabetic range of 4%-6% using a DCCT-based assay.

†Peak levels in patients with diabetes.

to 6%; these values correspond to mean blood glucose levels of about 90 mg/dl (or about 5 mmol/L). An A1C of 6% reflects an average plasma glucose level of ≈120 mg/dl. In general, each 1% increase in A1C is a reflection of an increase in average glucose levels of ≈30 mg/dl.

Lipid levels and blood pressure must also be monitored (Table 30-5). Lipids should be measured annually, and blood pressure at every diabetes management visit (ADA, 2006b).

Medical Nutrition Therapy for Diabetes

MNT is integral to total diabetes care and management. To integrate MNT effectively into the overall management of diabetes requires a coordinated team effort, including a registered dietitian (RD) who is knowledgeable and skilled in implementing current principles and recommendations for diabetes. MNT requires an individualized approach and effective nutrition self-management education and counseling. Monitoring glucose, A1C and lipid levels, blood pressure, weight, and quality-of-life issues is essential in evaluating the success of nutrition-related recommendations. If desired outcomes from MNT are not met, changes in overall diabetes care and management should be recommended (ADA, 2007).

The ADA's nutrition guidelines underscore the importance of individualizing nutrition care. Before 1994 nutrition recommendations attempted to define optimal percentages for macronutrient intake. Then, by determining a person's energy needs based on theoretic calorie requirements and using the ideal percentages for carbohydrate, protein, and fat, a nutrition prescription was developed (e.g., 1800 calories, 225 g of carbohydrate [50%], 90 g of protein [20%], and 60 g of fat [30%]). The problem with this approach is that the prescribed "diet" cannot really be individualized; and it often lacks relevance to the patient's personal lifestyle, culture, or socioeconomic status. Furthermore, this approach is not supported by scientific evidence and usually does not produce successful outcomes. Beginning in 1994 the ADA recommended that an individualized

nutrition prescription be based on metabolic profiles, treatment goals, and changes that the person with diabetes is willing and able to make and not on rigid, predetermined calorie levels and macronutrient percentages (Franz et al., 1994). This approach continues with the 2002 and 2007 ADA nutrition recommendations for persons with diabetes (ADA, 2007; Franz, 2002).

Although numerous studies have attempted to identify the optimal percentages of macronutrients for the diet of persons with diabetes, it is unlikely that one such combination of macronutrients exists. The best mix appears to vary, depending on individual circumstances. If guidance is needed, the dietary reference intakes (DRIs) may be helpful to meet the body's daily nutritional needs while at the same time minimizing risk for chronic diseases (ADA, 2007). The DRIs recommend that adults should consume 45% to 65% of total energy from carbohydrate, 20% to 35% from fat, and 10% to 35% from protein (Institute of Medicine, 2002).

Goals and Outcomes of Medical Nutrition Therapy for Diabetes

The goals for MNT for diabetes emphasize the role of lifestyle in improving glucose control, lipid and lipoprotein profiles, and blood pressure. Improving health through food choices and physical activity is the basis of all nutrition recommendations for the treatment of diabetes (see Box 30-1).

Besides being skilled and knowledgeable in assessing and implementing MNT, RDs must also be aware of expected outcomes from nutrition therapy, when to assess outcomes, and what feedback, including recommendations, should be given to referral sources. Research supports MNT as an effective therapy in reaching diabetes treatment goals. Outcomes studies demonstrate that MNT provided by an RD as MNT alone or as MNT in combination with diabetes self-management training is associated with a decrease in A1C of approximately 1% in patients with type 1 diabetes and 1% to 2% in type 2 diabetes, depending on the duration of diabetes (Pastors et al., 2003; DAFNE Study Group, 2002; Lemon et al., 2004). These outcomes are similar to those from oral glucose-lowering medications. Interventions include reduced energy or reduced carbohydrate or fat intake, basic nutrition education with healthy food choices for improved glycemia, and matching insulin doses to carbohydrate intake. Furthermore, the effect of MNT on A1C will be known by 6 weeks to 3 months, at which time the RD must assess whether the goals of therapy have been met by changes in lifestyle or whether changes or additions of medications are needed (Franz et al., 1995).

Metaanalysis of studies in nondiabetic free-living subjects and expert committees report that MNT reduces LDL cholesterol by 15 to 25 mg/dl (Yu-Poth et al., 1999, NCEP, 2001). After initiation of MNT, improvements were apparent in 3 to 6 months. Metaanalysis and expert committees also support the role of lifestyle modifications in treatment of hypertension (Chobanian et al., 2003) (see Chapter 33).

TABLE 30-5

Recommendations for Lipid and Blood Pressure for Adults With Diabetes

Lipids

LDL cholesterol	<100 mg/dl (<2.6 mmol/l)
HDL cholesterol	
Men	>40 mg/dl (>1.1 mmol/l)
Women	>50 mg/dl (>1.4 mmol/l)
Triglycerides	<150 mg/dl (<1.7 mmol/l)
Blood Pressure	<130/80 mm Hg

Modified from American Diabetes Association: Standards of medical care in diabetes—2007, *Diabetes Care* 30:54, 2007.

HDL, High-density lipoprotein; *LDL*, low-density lipoprotein.

Carbohydrates and Diabetes

Sugars, starch, and *fiber* are the preferred terms for carbohydrates. Foods that contain carbohydrates from whole grains, fruits, vegetables, and low-fat milk are excellent sources of vitamins, minerals, dietary fiber, and energy; therefore these foods are important components of a healthy diet for all Americans, including those with diabetes. Although low-carbohydrate diets might seem to be a logical approach to lowering postprandial glucose, the ADA specifically states that "low-carbohydrate diets (restricting total carbohydrate to <130 g/day) are not recommended in the management of diabetes" (ADA, 2006b).

Historically it was a long-held belief that sucrose must be restricted based on the assumption that sugars such as sucrose (see Chapter 3) are more rapidly digested and absorbed than starches and thus aggravate hyperglycemia; however, scientific evidence does not justify restricting sugars or sucrose based on this belief. In approximately 20 studies in which sucrose was substituted for other carbohydrates, sucrose did not increase glycemia to a greater extent than isocaloric amounts of starch (ADA, 2007; Franz et al., 2002a). The glycemic effect of carbohydrate foods cannot be predicted based on their structure (i.e., starch versus sugar) owing to the efficiency of the human digestive tract in reducing starch polymers to glucose. Starches are rapidly metabolized into 100% glucose during digestion, in contrast to sucrose, which is metabolized into glucose and fructose. Fructose has a lower glycemic index (GI), which has been attributed to its slow rate of absorption and its storage in the liver as glycogen (see Chapters 3 and 9, and Appendix 43).

Numerous factors influence glycemic responses to foods, including the amount of carbohydrates, type of sugar (glucose, fructose, sucrose, lactose), nature of the starch (amylose, amylopectin, resistant starch), cooking and food processing, particle size, and food form, as well as the fasting and preprandial glucose concentrations, severity of the glucose intolerance, and the second meal or lente effect of carbohydrates. Although both the amount (grams) and type of carbohydrates in a food influence the blood glucose levels, monitoring total grams of carbohydrates, whether by use of carbohydrate counting or exchanges, remains a key strategy in achieving glycemic control (ADA, 2007). Numerous studies have reported that, when subjects are allowed to choose from a variety of starches and sugars, the glycemic response is identical if the total amount of carbohydrate is similar (Franz, 2002). In studies comparing low– and high–GI diets, total carbohydrate is first of all kept consistent (Rizkalla et al., 2004). However, some individuals may note improvements in postprandial glucose responses with use of the GI or glycemic load (GL) factors when choosing foods or meals.

An important priority for food and meal planning is the total amount of carbohydrates that the person with diabetes chooses to have for meals or snacks. A variety of methods can be used to estimate the nutrient content of meals, including carbohydrate counting, exchange lists, and experience-based estimation (ADA, 2007). In **carbohydrate counting** food portions contributing 15 g of carbohydrates (regardless of the source) are considered to be one carbohydrate serving.

Testing premeal and postmeal glucose levels is important for making adjustments in either food intake or medication to achieve glucose goals. In using **exchange lists** foods are grouped into six lists—starch, fruit, milk, vegetables, meat and meat substitutes, and fat—and each list is a group of measured foods of approximately the same nutritional value. Therefore foods on the same list can be "exchanged" or substituted for one another. In addition, the exchange lists have an "other carbohydrates" list of sweets and snack foods and identify foods that are good sources of fiber; high in sodium; and combination foods such as casseroles, pizza, and soups, which fit into more than one exchange group.

Glycemic Index and Glycemic Load

Glycemic indexing of food was developed to compare the physiologic effects of carbohydrates on glucose. The **glycemic index (GI)** measures the relative area under the postprandial glucose curve of 50 g of digestible carbohydrates compared with 50 g of a standard food, either glucose or white bread. When bread is the reference food, the GI value for the food is multiplied by 0.7 to obtain the GI value that is comparable to glucose being used as the reference food (GI of glucose = 100; GI of white bread = 70). The GI does not measure how rapidly blood glucose levels increase. When reported, the peak glucose response for individual foods (Crapo et al., 1977) and meals, either high or low GI (Rizkalla et al., 2004), occurs at approximately the same time. Low-GI foods are usually defined as having a GI less than 55, moderate as GI 55 to 70, and high as GI more than 70. Refined starches often have a high GI; sugars such as fructose, lactose, and sucrose and fats a moderate to low GI (Foster-Powell et al., 2002).

The estimated **glycemic load (GL)** of foods, meals, and dietary patterns is calculated by multiplying the GI by the amount of carbohydrates in each food and then totaling the values for all foods in a meal or dietary pattern.

Low GI diets have been reported to improve glycemic control compared with high GI diets in persons with diabetes (Brand-Miller et al., 2003). However, there are substantial inconsistencies in study outcomes (Pi-Sunyer, 2002; Franz, 2003). Most people likely already consume a moderate GI diet (Rizkalla et al., 2004), and it is unknown whether further lowering of the dietary GI can be achieved long term.

A major problem with the GI is the variability of response to a specific carbohydrate food. For example, Australian potatoes are reported to have a high GI, whereas potatoes in the United States and Canada have moderate GIs (Fernandes et al., 2005). The concept of the GI can be best used for fine-tuning postprandial responses after focusing on total carbohydrate. See Appendix 43 for GI and GL factors for foods.

Fiber

Early short-term studies using large amounts of fiber (>30 g daily) in small numbers of subjects suggested a positive effect on glycemia; however, results from later studies have shown mixed effects. In subjects with type 1 diabetes, a high-fiber diet (56 g daily) had no beneficial effects on glycemic control (Lafrance et al., 1998). Another study of subjects with type 1 diabetes showed positive effects from 50 g of fiber on glucose concentrations but no beneficial effects on lipids (Giacco et al., 2000). In persons with type 2 diabetes, increasing fiber from 11 to 27 g/1000 kcal did not improve glycemia, insulinemia, or lipemia (Hollenbeck et al., 1986); whereas another study comparing 24 g of fiber per day with 50 g of fiber reported improved glycemic control, reduced hyperinsulinemia, and decreased plasma lipids (Chandalia et al., 2000). Therefore it appears that ingestion of large amounts of fiber (≈50 g/day) is necessary to have beneficial effects.

It is unknown whether free-living individuals can maintain such high levels of fiber and whether this amount would be acceptable to most people. As for the general public, people with diabetes are encouraged to choose a variety of fiber-containing foods such as legumes, fiber-rich cereals (≥5 g of fiber per serving), fruits, vegetables, and whole grain products. However, evidence is lacking to recommend a higher fiber intake for people with diabetes than for the population as a whole (ADA, 2007).

Sweeteners

Even though sucrose restriction cannot be justified on the basis of its glycemic effect, it is still good advice to suggest that persons with diabetes be careful in their consumption of foods containing large amounts of sucrose. Besides often being high in total carbohydrate content, these foods may also contain significant amounts of fat. If sucrose is included in the food and meal plan, it should be substituted for other carbohydrate sources or, if added, be adequately covered with insulin or other glucose-lowering medications. Sucrose and sucrose-containing foods also should be eaten in the context of a healthy diet, and care taken to avoid excess energy intake (ADA, 2007).

There appears to be no significant advantage of alternative nutritive sweeteners such as fructose over sucrose. Fructose provides 4 kcal/g, as do other carbohydrates, and even though it does have a lower glycemic response than sucrose and other starches, large amounts (15% to 20% of daily energy intake) of fructose have an adverse effect on plasma lipids (Bantle et al., 2000). However, there is no reason to recommend that persons with diabetes avoid fructose, which occurs naturally in fruits and vegetables as well as in foods sweetened with fructose (ADA, 2007).

Reduced calorie sweeteners approved by the U.S. Food and Drug Administration (FDA) include sugar alcohols (erythritol, sorbitol, mannitol, xylitol, isomalt, lactitol, and hydrogenated starch hydrolysates) and tagatose. They produce a lower glycemic response and have a lower caloric content than sucrose and other carbohydrates. Sugar alcohols contain, on average, approximately 2 calories per gram. With foods containing sugar alcohols, one half of sugar alcohol grams can be subtracted from total carbohydrate grams, particularly when using carbohydrate counting for meal planning. Although their use appears to be safe, it is unlikely that sugar alcohols in the amounts likely to be in-

gested in individual food servings or meals will contribute to significant reduction in total energy or improvement in glycemia (ADA, 2007). Some people report gastric discomfort after eating foods sweetened with these products, and consuming large quantities may cause diarrhea, especially in children.

Saccharin, aspartame, neotame, acesulfame potassium, and sucralose are nonnutritive sweeteners currently approved for use by the FDA. All such products must undergo rigorous testing by the manufacturer and scrutiny from the FDA before they are approved and marketed to the public. For all food additives, including nonnutritive sweeteners, the FDA determines an acceptable daily intake (ADI), defined as the amount of a food additive that can be safely consumed on a daily basis over a person's lifetime without risk (see Chapter 11). The ADI includes a 100-fold safety factor and greatly exceeds average consumption levels. For example, aspartame actual daily intake in persons with diabetes is 2 to 4 mg/kg of body weight daily, well below the ADI of 50 mg/kg daily (Butchko and Stargel, 2001). All FDA-approved nonnutritive sweeteners, when consumed within the established daily intake levels, can be used by persons with diabetes, including pregnant women (ADA, 2007). However, clinical studies in subjects without diabetes provide no evidence that nonnutritive sweeteners in foods cause weight loss or gain (Raben et al., 2002).

Protein

The rate of protein degradation and conversion of protein to glucose in type 1 diabetes depends on the state of insulinization and the degree of glycemic control. With less than optimal insulinization, conversion of protein to glucose can occur rapidly, adversely influencing glycemic control. In poorly controlled type 2 diabetes, gluconeogenesis is also accelerated and may account for most of the increased glucose production in the postabsorptive state. However, in those with controlled type 2 diabetes (Gannon et al., 2001; Nuttall et al., 1984) and well-controlled type 1 diabetes (Peters and Davidson, 1993), ingested protein did not increase plasma glucose concentrations. Although nonessential amino acids undergo gluconeogenesis, it is unclear why the glucose produced does not appear in the general circulation after ingestion of protein. Furthermore, protein does not slow the absorption of carbohydrates (Nuttall et al., 1984), and adding protein to the treatment of hypoglycemia does not prevent subsequent hypoglycemia (Gray et al., 1996). In patients with type 2 diabetes who are still able to produce insulin, ingested protein is just as potent a stimulant of insulin secretion as carbohydrate (Gannon et al., 2001; Nuttall et al., 1984).

For persons with diabetes and normal renal function, there is insufficient evidence to suggest that usual protein intake (10% to 20% of energy) should be modified (ADA, 2007). Intake of protein in this range does not appear to be associated with the development of diabetic nephropathy; however, the long-term effects of consuming more than 20% of energy as protein on the development of nephropathy has not been adequately studied.

Short-term studies with small numbers of subjects with diabetes suggest that diets with protein contents greater than 20% of total energy may improve glucose and insulin concentrations, reduce appetite, and improve satiety (Gannon et al., 2003; Gannon et al., 2004). However, such diets appear to be difficult to follow outside of a research setting (Brinkworth et al., 2004). The effects of protein on regulation of energy intake, satiety, and long-term weight loss have not been adequately studied.

Dietary Fat

Studies in persons with diabetes demonstrating the effects of specific percentages of dietary saturated and *trans*-fatty acids and specific amounts of cholesterol on CVD risk are not available. However, those with diabetes are considered to be at risk similar to those with a past history of CVD. Therefore, because of a lack of specific information, the goal for dietary fat intake (amount and type) for persons with diabetes is the same as for those without diabetes with a history of CVD. It is recommended that total fat be 25% to 35% of total energy, and saturated fatty acids less than 7%. Intake of *trans*-fat should be minimized or eliminated (ADA, 2007). Diets high in polyunsaturated fatty acids appear to have effects on lipids similar to those from diets high in monounsaturated fatty acids (Summer et al., 2002). Therefore, to lower LDL cholesterol, energy derived from saturated fatty acids should be replaced with either monounsaturated or polyunsaturated fatty acids. In persons without diabetes, reducing saturated and *trans*-fatty acids decreases total and LDL cholesterol but may also reduce HDL cholesterol. However, importantly, the ratio of LDL to HDL cholesterol is not adversely affected.

In metabolic studies in which energy intake is maintained so that subjects do not lose weight, diets high in either carbohydrates or monounsaturated fat lower LDL cholesterol equivalently, but the concern has been the potential of a high-carbohydrate diet (greater than 55% of energy intake) to increase triglycerides and postprandial glucose compared with a high–monounsaturated fat diet (Garg et al., 1994). However, in other studies when energy intake is reduced, the adverse effects of high-carbohydrate diets are not observed (Heilbronn et al., 1999; Parker et al., 2002). Therefore energy intake appears to a factor in determining the effects of a high-carbohydrate versus a high–monounsaturated fat diet.

There is evidence from the general population that foods containing very long omega-3 polyunsaturated fatty acids are beneficial, and two to three servings of fish per week are recommended. Although most studies in persons with diabetes have used omega-3 supplements and show beneficial lowering of triglycerides, an accompanying rise in LDL cholesterol also has been noted (Montori et al., 2000). If supplements are used, the effects on LDL cholesterol should be monitored. The omega-3 supplements may be most beneficial in the treatment of severe hypertriglyceridemia (Patti et al., 1999). In addition, two or more servings of fish per week (with the exception of commercially fried fish filets) can be recommended (ADA, 2007).

Plant sterol and stanol esters block the intestinal absorption of dietary and biliary cholesterol. In the general public (Hallikainen et al., 1999) and in persons with type 2 diabetes (Lee et al., 2000), intake of 2 to 3 g of plant stanols or sterols per day is reported to decrease total and LDL cholesterol levels by 9% to 20% (see Chapter 32).

Alcohol

The same precautions that apply to alcohol consumption for the general population apply to persons with diabetes. Abstention from alcohol should be advised for people with a history of alcohol abuse or dependence; for women during pregnancy; and for people with medical problems such as liver disease, pancreatitis, or advanced neuropathy. If individuals choose to drink alcohol, daily intake should be limited to one drink or less for adult women and two drinks or less for adult men (1 drink = 12 oz beer, 5 oz of wine, or 1½ oz of distilled spirits). Each drink contains ≈15 g alcohol. The type of alcoholic beverage consumed does not make a difference (ADA, 2007).

Moderate amounts of alcohol ingested with food have minimum, if any, acute effect on glucose and insulin levels (Howard et al., 2004). However, alcoholic beverages should be considered an addition to the regular food and meal plan for all persons with diabetes. No food should be omitted, given the possibility of alcohol-induced hypoglycemia and the fact that alcohol does not require insulin to be metabolized. Excessive amounts of alcohol (three or more drinks per day) on a consistent basis, contribute to hyperglycemia. This hyperglycemia improves as soon as alcohol use is discontinued (Howard et al., 2004).

In persons with diabetes, light-to-moderate amounts of alcohol (1 to 2 drinks per day; 15 to 30 g of alcohol) are associated with a decreased risk of coronary heart disease (Howard et al., 2004), perhaps because of the concomitant increase in HDL cholesterol and improved insulin sensitivity associated with alcohol consumption. Long-term, prospective studies are needed to confirm these observations (ADA, 2007) (see Chapter 32). In observational studies and in short-term studies, moderate amounts of alcohol did not increase triglyceride levels in hypertriglyceridemic individuals (Pownall et al., 1999) and had beneficial effects on blood pressure and triglyceride levels in postmenopausal women (Davies et al., 2002). Ingestion of light-to-moderate amounts of alcohol does not raise blood pressure; whereas excessive, chronic ingestion of alcohol does raise blood pressure and may be a risk factor for stroke (Chobanian et al., 2003). The contribution of alcohol to excessive energy intake in the overweight individual always has to be considered.

Micronutrients

No clear evidence has been established for benefits from routine vitamin or mineral supplements in persons with diabetes who do not have underlying deficiencies. Exceptions include folate for the prevention of birth defects (ADA, 2007). Since diabetes may be a state of increased oxidative stress, there has been interest in prescribing antioxidant vitamins in people with diabetes. Large observational studies and several placebo-controlled clinical trials with small subject numbers have found beneficial effects of antioxidants, especially vitamin E, on physiologic and biochemical end points. However, large placebo-controlled clinical trials have failed to show benefit from antioxidants and in some instances have suggested adverse effects (Hasanain et al., 2002). Of interest is the Heart Outcomes Prevention Evaluation Trial, which included 9541 subjects, 38% of whom had diabetes (Yusuf et al., 2000). Supplementation with 400 units daily of vitamin E for 4.5 years did not result in any significant benefit on cardiovascular outcomes. Routine supplementation with antioxidants such as vitamins E and C and β-carotene is not advised because of lack of evidence of effectiveness and concern related to long-term safety (ADA, 2007).

Because the response to supplements is determined largely by a person's nutrition status, persons with micronutrient deficiencies are most likely to respond favorably. Although difficult to ascertain, if deficiencies of vitamins or minerals are identified, supplementation can be beneficial. Those at greatest risk of deficiency who may benefit from prescription of vitamin and mineral supplements include patients who consume obviously poor diets or extreme calorie-restricted diets, strict vegetarians, older adults, pregnant or lactating women, those taking medication known to alter micronutrient metabolism (see Chapter 16), patients in poor metabolic control (glycosuria), and patients in critical care environments.

Several small studies have suggested a role for chromium supplementation in the management of glucose intolerance, gestational diabetes, body weight, and corticosteroid-induced diabetes In two randomized, placebo-controlled studies in Chinese subjects with diabetes, chromium supplementation did have beneficial effects on glycemia (Anderson et al., 1997; Cheng et al., 1999); however, the study population may have had marginal baseline chromium status because the chromium status was not evaluated either at baseline or after supplementation. According to a recent FDA statement there is insufficient evidence to support any of the proposed health claims of chromium supplementation. The FDA concluded that, although a small study suggested that chromium picolinate may reduce the risk of insulin resistance, the existence of such a relationship between chromium picolinate and either insulin resistance or type 2 diabetes is highly uncertain. In addition, a metaanalysis of randomized controlled trials suggests no benefit of chromium picolinate supplementation in reducing body weight (Pittler et al., 2003). Therefore chromium supplementation is not recommended unless the individual's intake of chromium does not meet the DRI of 20 to 25 mcg/day (ADA, 2006b).

Physical Activity/Exercise

Physical activity involves bodily movement produced by the contraction of skeletal muscles that requires energy expenditure in excess of resting energy expenditure Exercise is a subset of physical activity: planned, structured, and repetitive bodily movement performed to improve or maintain one or more components of physical fitness. Aerobic exercise consists of rhythmic, repeated, and continuous move-

ments of the same large muscle groups for at least 10 minutes at a time. Examples include walking, bicycling, jogging, swimming, and many sports. Resistance exercise consists of activities that use muscular strength to move a weight or work against a resistive load. Examples include weight lifting and exercises using resistance-providing machines.

Physical activity should be an integral part of the treatment plan for persons with diabetes. Exercise helps all persons with diabetes improve insulin sensitivity, reduce cardiovascular risk factors, control weight, and improve well-being (ADA, 2004a). Furthermore, regular exercise may prevent type 2 diabetes in high-risk individuals. Given appropriate guidelines, the majority of people with diabetes can exercise safely. The exercise plan will vary, depending on interest, age, general health, and level of physical fitness. Despite the increase in glucose uptake by muscles during exercise, glucose levels change little in individuals without diabetes. Muscular work causes insulin levels to decline while counterregulatory hormones (primarily glucagon) rise. In this way, increased glucose use by the exercising muscle is matched precisely with increased glucose production by the liver. This balance between insulin and counterregulatory hormones is the major determinant of hepatic glucose production, underscoring the need for insulin adjustments in addition to adequate carbohydrate intake during exercise for people with diabetes.

In persons with type 1 diabetes, the glycemic response to exercise varies, depending on overall diabetes control, plasma glucose, and insulin levels at the start of exercise; timing, intensity and duration of the exercise; previous food intake; and previous conditioning. An important variable is the level of plasma insulin during and after exercise. Hypoglycemia can occur because of insulin-enhanced muscle glucose uptake by the exercising muscle. In contrast, insulin deficiency in a poorly controlled (underinsulinized) exerciser results in increases in glucose concentrations, and free fatty acid release continues with minimum uptake. This can result in large increases in plasma glucose and ketone levels (Wasserman and Zinman, 1994).

In persons with type 2 diabetes, blood glucose control can improve with exercise, largely because of decreased insulin resistance and increased insulin sensitivity, which results in increased peripheral use of glucose not only during but also after the activity. This exercise-induced enhanced insulin sensitivity occurs independent of any effect on body weight (Boulé et al., 2001). Exercise also decreases the effects of counterregulatory hormones; this, in turn, reduces the hepatic glucose output, contributing to improved glucose control.

Exercise regimens at an intensity of 50% to 80% Vo_{2max} three to four times a week for 30 to 60 minutes a session can result in a 10% to 20% baseline improvement in A1C and are most beneficial in persons with mild type 2 diabetes and in those who are likely to be the most insulin resistant. Regular exercise also has consistently been shown to be effective in reducing triglyceride levels in persons with type 2 diabetes; however, the effect of exercise on HDL cholesterol levels is unclear. Reductions in blood pressure and improvements in impaired fibrinolysis have also been noted (Sigal et al., 2004).

Potential Problems With Exercise

Hypoglycemia is a potential problem associated with exercise in persons taking insulin or insulin secretagogues. Hypoglycemia can occur during, immediately after, or many hours after exercise. Hypoglycemia has been reported to be more common after exercise, especially exercise of long duration, strenuous activity or play, or sporadic exercise, than during exercise (MacDonald et al., 1987). This is because of increased insulin sensitivity after exercise and the need to replete liver and muscle glycogen, which can take up to 24 to 30 hours (see Chapter 23). Hypoglycemia can also occur during or immediately after exercise. Blood glucose levels before exercise reflect only the value at that time, and it is unknown if this is a stable blood glucose level or a blood glucose level that is dropping. If blood glucose levels are dropping before exercise, adding exercise can contribute to hypoglycemia during exercise. Furthermore, hypoglycemia on the day before exercise is reported to increase the risk of hypoglycemia on the day of exercise as well (Davis et al., 2000).

Hyperglycemia can also result from exercise. When a person exercises at what for him or her is a high level of exercise intensity, there is a greater-than-normal increase in counterregulatory hormones. As a result, hepatic glucose release exceeds the rise in glucose use. The elevated glucose levels may also extend into the postexercise state (Purdon et al., 1993). Hyperglycemia and worsening ketosis can also result in persons with type 1 diabetes who are deprived of insulin for 12 to 48 hours and are ketotic. Vigorous activity should probably be avoided in the presence of ketosis (ADA, 2006b). The latter cause of hyperglycemia is not as likely to occur as the first.

Exercise Guidelines

The variability of glucose responses to exercise contributes to the difficulty in giving precise nutrition (and insulin) guidelines. Frequent blood glucose monitoring before, during, and after exercise helps individuals identify their response to physical activities. To meet their individual needs, patients must modify general guidelines to reduce insulin doses before (or after) or ingest carbohydrates after (or before) exercise.

Carbohydrate for Insulin or Insulin Secretagogue Users

During moderate-intensity exercise, glucose uptake is increased by 8 to 13 g/hr (Wasserman and Zinman, 1994), and this is the basis for the recommendation to add 15 g carbohydrate for every 30 to 60 minutes of activity (depending on the intensity) over and above normal routines. Moderate exercise for less than 30 minutes usually does not require any additional carbohydrate or insulin adjustment. Added carbohydrates should be ingested if preexercise glucose levels are less than 100 mg/dl (5.6 mmol/L). Supplementary carbohydrate is generally not needed in individuals who are not treated with insulin or insulin secretagogues (ADA, 2006b).

In all persons, blood glucose levels decline gradually during exercise, and ingesting a carbohydrate feeding during prolonged exercise can improve performance by maintaining the availability and oxidation of blood glucose. For the exerciser with diabetes whose blood glucose levels may drop sooner and lower than the exerciser without diabetes, ingesting carbohydrate after 40 to 60 minutes of exercise is important and may also assist in preventing hypoglycemia. Drinks containing 6% or less of carbohydrates empty from the stomach as quickly as water and have the advantage of providing both needed fluids and carbohydrates (see Chapter 23). Consuming carbohydrates immediately after exercise optimizes repletion of muscle and liver glycogen stores. For the exerciser with diabetes, this takes on added importance because of increased risk for late-onset hypoglycemia (Franz, 2002).

Insulin Guidelines

It is often necessary to adjust the insulin dosage to prevent hypoglycemia. This occurs most often with moderate to strenuous activity lasting more than 45 to 60 minutes. For most persons a modest decrease (of about 1 to 2 units) in the rapid- or short-acting insulin during the period of exercise is a good starting point. For prolonged vigorous exercise, a larger decrease in the total daily insulin dosage may be necessary. After exercise insulin may also need to be decreased. In addition to these acute reductions in insulin dosages, individuals who participate in a regular, long-term fitness program often find their usual total dosage of insulin decreasing by as much as 15% to 20% (Wasserman and Zinman, 1994).

Insulin doses should be reduced in anticipation of exercise after a meal, depending on the duration and intensity of the exercise. In persons with type 1 diabetes, Rabasa-Lhoret and colleagues (2001) validated that exercise at 25% Vo_{2max} for 60 minutes required a 50% reduction in mealtime rapid-acting insulin and exercise at 50% Vo_{2max} for 30 and 60 minutes required a 50% and 75% reduction in mealtime rapid-acting insulin, respectively. Such reductions in mealtime rapid-acting insulin for postprandial exercise resulted in a 75% decrease in exercise-induced hypoglycemia.

Precautions for Persons With Type 2 Diabetes

Persons with type 2 diabetes may have a lower Vo_{2max} and therefore need a more gradual training program. Rest periods may be needed; this does not impair the training effect from physical activity. Autonomic neuropathy or medications, such as for blood pressure, may not allow for increased heart rate, and individuals must learn to use perceived exertion as a means of determining exercise intensity. Blood pressure may also increase more in persons with diabetes than in those who do not have diabetes, and exercise should not be undertaken if systolic blood pressure is greater than 180 to 200 mm Hg.

Exercise Prescription

The ADA recommends that a graded exercise test with electrocardiogram should seriously be considered before undertaking aerobic physical activity with intensity exceeding the demands of everyday living (more intense than brisk walking) in previously sedentary individuals with diabetes whose 10-year risk of a coronary is likely to be higher (ADA, 2006b). However, there is no evidence that such testing is routinely necessary for those planning moderately intense activity such as walking.

The ADA also recommends that, to improve glycemic control, assist with weight maintenance, and reduce risk of CVD, at least 150 min/week of moderate-intensity aerobic physical activity (50% to 70% of maximum heart rate) or at least 90 min/week of vigorous aerobic exercise (>70% of maximum heart rate) is recommended. The physical activity should be distributed over at least 3 days/week and with no more than 2 consecutive days without physical activity. In the absence of contraindications, people with type 2 diabetes should be encouraged to perform resistance exercise three times a week, targeting all major muscle groups, progressing to three sets of 8 to 10 repetitions at a weight that cannot be lifted more than eight to ten times (ADA, 2006b).

Medications

Glucose-Lowering Medications

The use of the newer **glucose-lowering medications,** alone or in combination, provides numerous options for achieving euglycemia in persons with type 2 diabetes. Some persons with hyperglycemia that is not adequately controlled by MNT alone can be treated with MNT and glucose-lowering medications—frequently **combination therapy** using two, and occasionally even three, medications. If glycemic control cannot be attained with MNT and glucose-lowering medications, insulin, either alone or in combination with other medications, is required.

The transition to insulin often begins with a long-acting or premixed insulin given at bedtime to control fasting glucose levels. However, eventually many patients with type 2 diabetes will require a more physiologic insulin regimen to achieve control. If large doses of insulin are required, oral medications such as insulin sensitizers are often combined with the insulin regimen. Recently two new injectable medications—exenatide and pramlintide—have become available for use in combination therapies. Although these two drugs have some similarities in action, they are recommended for use in different populations.

Currently four classes of oral medications exist: (1) insulin secretagogues, which include the sulfonylureas (first- and second-generation) and the meglitinides (repaglinide and nateglinide); (2) biguanides (metformin); (3) thiazolidinediones (TZDs) (e.g., pioglitazone, rosiglitazone); and (4) α-glucosidase inhibitors (acarbose, miglitol). Each class has a different mechanism of action: in the pancreas insulin secretion is stimulated; at the cellular level (muscle and adipose tissue) insulin resistance is decreased, and glucose uptake enhanced; in the liver hepatic glucose output is decreased, especially overnight, improving fasting glucose levels; or in the intestine glucose absorption is slowed, improving postprandial glucose concentrations. Because of the different sites of action, the medications can be used alone or in combination. Because combination therapy is so common, drug companies now market combination pills (Table 30-6).

Insulin secretagogues (sulfonylureas and meglitinides) promote insulin secretion by the β-cells of the pancreas. First- and second-generation sulfonylurea drugs differ from one another in their potency, pharmacokinetics, and metabolism. Disadvantages of their use include weight gain and the potential to cause hypoglycemia. The meglitinides differ from the sulfonylureas in that they have short metabolic half-lives, which result in brief episodic stimulation of insulin secretion. As a result, a frequent dosing schedule is required with meals, postprandial glucose excursions are less, and because less insulin is secreted several hours after a meal, there is a decreased risk of hypoglycemia between meals and overnight. Nateglinide only works in the presence of glucose and is a somewhat less potent secretagogue (Inzucchi, 2002).

Insulin sensitizers enhance insulin action and include biguanides (metformin) and TZDs. Both classes require the presence of insulin, exogenous or endogenous, to be effective. Metformin (Glucophage) suppresses hepatic glucose production and lowers insulin resistance, but it does not stimulate insulin secretion. It is not associated with hypoglycemia, may cause small weight losses when therapy begins, and improves lipid levels. Adverse effects include gastrointestinal distress such as abdominal pain, nausea, and diarrhea in up to 50% of patients. The frequency of these adverse effects can be minimized with food consumption and slow titration of dose. A rare side effect is severe lactic acidosis, which can be fatal. Acidosis usually occurs in patients who use alcohol excessively, have renal dysfunction, or have liver impairments (Inzucchi, 2002). Biguanides can be used alone or in combination with other diabetes medications. Other available agents include metformin extended release (Glucophage XR); a liquid metformin (Riomet); and metformin combined with the sulfonylurea glyburide (Glucovance), with the sulfonylurea glipizide (Metaglip), and with the TZD rosiglitazone (Avandamet).

The TZDs decrease insulin resistance in peripheral tissues and thus enhance the ability of muscle and adipose cells to take up glucose. TZDs also have certain lipid benefits. HDL cholesterol increases, and triglycerides frequently decrease with TZD therapy. Although LDL cholesterol may increase because of a shift from small and dense to large and buoyant LDL particles, these types of particles are less atherogenic; thus the increase in LDL cholesterol may not be a concern (Inzucchi, 2002). Adverse effects include weight gain and edema, and these effects are more common in patients who receive TZDs along with insulin. Patients with advanced forms of congestive heart disease or hepatic impairment should not receive TZDs. Troglitazone (Rezulin), the first approved TZD, was removed from the market because of hepatocellular injury. Rosiglitazone (Avandia) and pioglitazone (Actos) are the two TZD drugs currently available and have not been associated with liver injury. However, a recent meta-analysis suggests that rosiglitazone may be associated with an increased risk of myocardial infarction in those who use it (Nissen and Wolski, 2007). This medication may become unavailable as further inquiry into its side effects is carried out. Also available is rosiglitazone combined with glimepiride (Avandaryl).

α-Glucosidase inhibitors work in the small intestine to inhibit enzymes that digest carbohydrates, thereby delaying carbohydrate absorption and lowering postprandial glycemia. Acarbose (Precose) and miglitol (Glyset) are competitive inhibitors of intestinal brush-border α-glucosidases required for the breakdown of starches, dextrins, maltose, and sucrose to absorbable monosaccharides. They do not cause hypoglycemia or weight gain when used alone, but they can frequently cause flatulence, diarrhea, cramping, or abdominal pain. Symptoms may be alleviated by initiating therapy at a low dose and gradually increasing the dose to therapeutic levels (van de Laar, 2005).

Injectables

There are two new **injectable glucose-lowering medications.** Exenatide (Byetta) is an incretin mimetic or incretin-like agent. **Incretins** are hormones (glucagon-like peptide-1 [GLP-1]) released during nutrient absorption from the cells of the gut and from pancreatic islet cells, which increase glucose-dependent insulin secretion, slow gastric emptying, decrease glucagon production, and decrease appetite. Exenatide is associated with reduction in A1C and modest weight loss (Kendall et al., 2005). It is approved for use in people with type 2 diabetes not achieving optimal glucose control with a sulfonylurea and/or metformin. Typically exenatide is injected twice a day, at breakfast and at the evening meal.

Pramlintide (Symlin) is a synthetic form of amylin, a hormone normally co-secreted with insulin by the β-cells in response to food intake and deficient in people with type 1 and type 2 diabetes. Pramlintide was developed to counter the effects of amylin deficiency and is given at each meal in addition to an insulin bolus. It is approved for use in adults with type 1 or type 2 diabetes who have not achieved optimal glucose control (Buse et al., 2002).

Insulin

Persons with type 1 diabetes depend on insulin to survive. In persons with type 2 diabetes, insulin may be needed to restore glycemia to near normal. Circumstances that require the use of insulin in type 2 diabetes include the failure to achieve adequate control with administration of oral medications; periods of acute injury, infection, or surgery; pregnancy; and allergy or serious reactions to sulfonylurea agents.

Insulin has three characteristics: onset, peak, and duration (Table 30-7). U-100 is the concentration of insulin available in the United States. This means it has 100 units of insulin per milliliter of fluid (100 units/ml). U-100 syringes deliver

---

TABLE 30-6

Glucose-Lowering Medications for Type 2 Diabetes

Class and Generic Names	Recommended Dose	Principal Action	Mean Decrease in A1C
Sulfonylureas **(Second-generation)** Glipizide (Glucotrol) Glipizide (Glucotrol XL) Glyburide (Glynase Prestabs) Glimepiride (Amaryl)	2.5-20 mg single or divided dose; single dose for XL 12 mg daily 4-8 mg daily	Stimulate insulin secretion from the β-cells	1% to 2%
Meglitinide Repaglinide (Prandin) Nateglinide (Starlix)	0.5-4 mg before meals 120 mg before meals	Stimulate insulin secretion from β-cells	1% to 2%
Biguanide Metformin (Glucophage) Metformin Extended Release (Glucophage XR)	500-850 mg tid or 1000 mg bid 500-2000 mg once daily	Decrease hepatic glucose production	1.5% to 2%
Thiazolidinediones Pioglitazone (Actos) Rosiglitazone (Avandia)	15-45 mg daily 2-8 mg daily	Improve peripheral insulin sensitivity	1% to 2%
Alpha Glucosidase Inhibitors Acarbose (Precose) Miglitol (Glyset)	25-100 mg three times daily with meals 25-100 mg three times daily with meals	Delay carbohydrate absorption	0.5% to 1%

TABLE 30-6

Glucose-Lowering Medications for Type 2 Diabetes—cont'd

Class and Generic Names	Recommended Dose	Principal Action	Mean Decrease in A1C
Incretin Mimetics Exenatide (Byetta)	Initially dosed at 5 mcg twice a day—at breakfast and lunch; increased to 10 mcg twice a day	Enhances glucose-dependent insulin secretion and suppresses postprandial glucagon secretion	0.5% to 0.9%
Amylinomimetic Pramlintide (Smylin)	Initially dosed at 60 mcg before meals; dose increased directly to 120 mcg if no clinically significant nausea occurs after 3-7 days	Decreases glucagon production, which decreases mealtime hepatic glucose release and prevents postprandial hyperglycemia	0.4% to 0.7%
Combination Medications		Combined action of each medication	
Glyburide/metformin (Glucovance) (1.25 mg/250 mg)	2.5/500 mg to 5/500 mg daily		≈2%
Glipizide/metformin (Metaglip) (2.5 mg/250 mg)	2.5 mg/500 mg to 4 mg/500 mg daily		≈2%
Rosiglitazone/metformin (Avandament) (1 mg/500 mg)	1 mg/500 mg to 4 mg/500 mg daily		≈2%
Rosiglitazone/glimepiride (Avandaryl) (4 mg/1, 2, or 4 mg)	4 mg/1.0 mg to 4 mg/4.0 mg daily		Unknown

Adapted from Franz MJ et al: *Implementing group and individual medical nutrition therapy for diabetes.* Alexandria, Va, 2002, American Diabetes Association, p 66.
bid, Twice daily; *tid,* three times daily.

TABLE 30-7

Action Times of Human Insulin Preparations

Type of Insulin	Onset of Action	Peak Action	Usual Effective Duration	Monitor Effect In
Rapid-Acting Insulin lispro (Humalog) Insulin aspart (NovoLog) Insulin glulisine (Apidra)	<15 min	1-2 hr	3-4 hr	2 hr
Short-Acting Regular	0.5-1 hr	2-3 hr	3-6 hr	≈4 hr
Intermediate-Acting NPH	2-4 hr	4-10 hr	10-16 hr	8-12 hr
Long-Acting Insulin glargine (Lantus)	2-4 hr	Peakless	20-24 hr	10-12 hr
Insulin determir (Levemir)	2-4 hr	Peakless	18-24 hr	10-12 hr
Mixtures 70/30 (70% NPH, 30% regular) 75/25 (75% neutral protamine lispro [NPL], 25% lispro) 70/30 (70% neutral protamine aspart [NPA], 30% aspart)	0.5 to 1 hr	Dual	10 to 16 hr	

Adapted from Bode BW: *Medical management of type 1 diabetes,* ed 4, Alexandria, Va, 2004, American Diabetes Association.

U-100 insulin; however, insulin pens are now being used more frequently as an alternative to the traditional syringe-needle units.

Rapid-acting insulins include insulin lispro (Humalog), insulin aspart (Novolog), and insulin glulisine (Apidra) and are used as bolus (mealtime) insulins. They are insulin analogs that differ from human insulin in amino acid sequence but bind to insulin receptors and thus function in a manner similar to human insulin. All have an onset of action within 15 minutes, a peak in activity at 60 to 90 min, and a duration of action of 3 to 5 hours. They result in fewer hypoglycemic episodes compared with regular insulin.

Regular is a short-acting insulin with an onset of action 15 to 60 minutes after injection and a duration of action ranging from 5 to 8 hours. For best results the slow onset of regular insulin requires it to be taken 30 to 60 minutes before meals. NPH is the only available *intermediate-acting insulin* (Lente insulin has been discontinued). Its appearance is cloudy, and its onset of action is about 2 hours after injection, with a peak effect from 6 to 10 hours.

Long-acting insulins are insulin glargine (Lantus) and insulin determir (Levemir) (Ultralente has been discontinued). Insulin glargine is an insulin analog that because of its slow dissolution at the injection site results in a relatively constant and peakless delivery over 24 hours. Because of its acidic pH, it cannot be mixed with any other insulin in the same syringe before injection and is usually given at bedtime. However, glargine can be given before any meal, but, whichever time is chosen, it must be given consistently at that time. Insulin determir is absorbed from the subcutaneous tissue relatively quickly but then binds to albumin in the bloodstream, resulting in a prolonged action time of approximately 17 hours. Therefore it may need to be given twice a day. Basal insulin analogs decrease the chances of hypoglycemia, especially nocturnal hypoglycemia (Rosenstock et al., 2005).

Premixed insulins are also available: 70% NPH/30% regular, 75% lispro protamine (NPL [addition of neutral protamine to lispro to create an intermediate-acting insulin])/25% lispro, and 70% protamine (addition of neutral protamine to aspart to create an immediate-acting insulin)/30% aspart. Persons using premixed insulins must eat at specific times and be consistent in carbohydrate intake to prevent hypoglycemia.

Insulin administered via the pulmonary route (*inhaled insulin*) has been approved by the FDA and also may be used as bolus insulin. The very thin alveolar-capillary barrier in the lungs allows for rapid uptake of insulin into the bloodstream after inhalation, similar to rapid-acting analogs or even faster (Rave et al., 2005). The overall bioavailability of inhaled insulin is generally 10% to 15% of the total dose used. Exubera, involving a spray-dried insulin powder contained in a blister packet and a simple inhalation device, is currently approved, but other inhaled insulin systems are under development (Patton et al., 2004). Inhaled insulin may facilitate early introduction of insulin therapy to people who need it but are averse to insulin injections.

All persons with type 1 diabetes and those with type 2 diabetes who no longer produce adequate endogenous insulin need replacement of insulin that mimics normal insulin action. After individuals without diabetes eat, their plasma glucose and insulin concentrations increase rapidly, peak in 30 to 60 minutes, and return to basal concentrations within 2 to 3 hours. To mimic this, rapid-acting (or short-acting) insulin is given before meals, and this is referred to as bolus or mealtime insulin. Mealtime insulin doses are adjusted based on the amount of carbohydrate in the meal. An insulin-to-carbohydrate ratio can be established for an individual that will guide decisions on the amount of mealtime insulin to inject. Basal or background insulin dose is that amount of insulin required in the postabsorptive state to restrain endogenous glucose output primarily from the liver. Basal insulin also limits lipolysis and excess flux of free fatty acids to the liver. Long-acting insulins are used for basal insulin.

The type and timing of insulin regimens should be individualized, based on eating and exercise habits and blood glucose concentrations. For persons with type 2 diabetes, there are three primary insulin regimens: (1) long-acting insulin and oral glucose-lowering agents; (2) premixed insulin; and (3) a basal long-acting insulin with rapid-acting insulin for meals (Raskin et al., 2005). Options one and two may suffice for persons with type 2 diabetes who still have significant endogenous insulin production. However, for persons with type 1 diabetes and many patients with type 2 diabetes, a more physiologic insulin regimen such as option three is preferred (Figure 30-1).

These types of insulin regimens allow increased flexibility in the type and timing of meals. For normal-weight persons with type 1 diabetes, the required insulin dosage is about 0.5 to 1 unit/kg of body weight per day. About 50% of the total daily insulin dose is used to provide for basal or background insulin needs. The remainder (rapid-acting insulin) is divided among the meals either proportionately to the carbohydrate content or by giving about 1 to 1.5 units of insulin per 10 to 15 g of carbohydrates consumed. The larger amount is usually needed to cover breakfast carbohydrates as a result of the presence in the morning of higher levels of counterregulatory hormones (Rabasa-Lhoret et al., 1999). Persons with type 2 diabetes may require insulin doses in the range of 0.5 to 1.2 units/kg of body weight daily. Large doses, even more than 1.5 units/kg of body weight daily, may be required at least initially to overcome prevailing insulin resistance.

Insulin pump therapy provides basal rapid-acting or short-acting insulin pumped continuously by a mechanical device in micro amounts through a subcutaneous catheter that is monitored 24 hours a day. Both lispro and aspart work well in insulin pumps, resulting in improved glycemia and less hypoglycemia than with regular insulin (Bode and Strange, 2001). Boluses of the insulin are given before meals. Pump therapy requires a committed and motivated person who is willing to do a minimum of four blood glucose tests per day, keep blood glucose and food records, and learn the technical features of pump use.

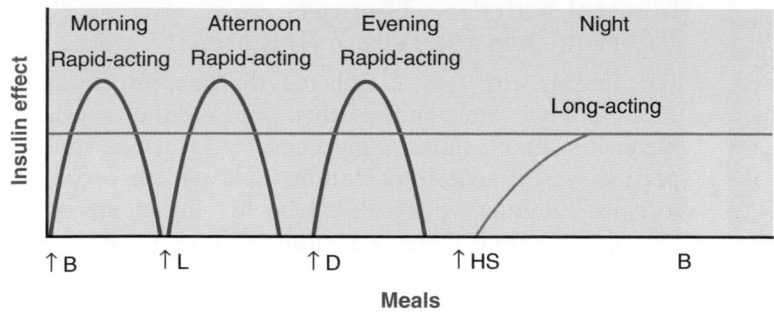

FIGURE 30-1 Time actions of flexible insulin regimens. *(Modified from Bode BW: Medical management of type 1 diabetes, ed 4, Alexandria, Va, 2004, American Diabetes Association.)*

B, Breakfast; *L,* lunch; *D,* dinner; *HS,* bedtime snack; *arrow,* time of insulin injection
Schematic representation only

Monitoring

Self-monitoring of blood glucose (SMBG) is used on a day-to-day basis to manage diabetes effectively and safely; however, laboratory measurement of glycated hemoglobin provides the best available index of overall diabetes control. The health care team, including the individual with diabetes, should work together to implement blood glucose monitoring and establish individual **target blood glucose goals** (see Table 30-4 for a listing of these goals). The frequency of monitoring depends on the type of diabetes and overall therapy.

Patients can perform SMBG up to eight times per day—before breakfast, lunch, and dinner; at bedtime; 1 to 2 hours after meals; and during the night or whenever needed to determine causes of hypoglycemia or hyperglycemia. For most patients with type 1 diabetes, SMBG is recommended four or more times a day, before each meal and at bedtime. SMBG in patients with type 2 diabetes should be sufficient to facilitate reaching glucose goals and is often performed one to four times a day, often before breakfast and before and 2 hours after the largest meal but only 3 or 4 days per week. When adding to or modifying therapy, type 1 and type 2 patients with diabetes should test more often than usual especially 2 hours after meals (ADA, 2004b).

Because the accuracy of SMBG is instrument and user dependent, it is important for health care providers to evaluate each patient's monitoring techniques, both initially and at regular intervals thereafter. Comparisons between results from patient self-testing in the clinic and simultaneous laboratory testing are useful to assess the accuracy of patient results. Meters now automatically convert the capillary whole-blood test to plasma glucose values so comparisons can readily be made with laboratory values.

It is important that the results of SMBG be written in a record book and that patients be taught how to adjust their management program based on these results. The first step in using such records is to learn how to identify patterns in blood glucose levels and how to adjust basic insulin doses. For example, if blood glucose levels are consistently (generally 3 days in a row) elevated at a specific testing time, adjustments are made in the insulin or medication acting at that time. Algorithms for insulin dose changes to compensate for an elevated or low glucose value also can be used. A commonly used formula determines the insulin sensitivity, or **correction factor (CF),** which defines how many milligrams per deciliter a unit of rapid- or short-acting insulin will lower blood glucose levels over a 2- to 4-hr period (Bode, 2004). The CF is determined by using the "1700 rule," in which 1700 is divided by the total daily dose (TDD) of insulin. For example, if the TDD is 50 units of insulin, the CF = 1700/50 = 35. In this case, 1 unit of insulin should lower the patient's blood glucose level by 35 mg/dl (2 mmol/L).

In using blood glucose monitoring records, it should be remembered that factors other than food affect blood glucose concentrations. An increase in blood glucose can be the result of insufficient insulin or insulin secretagogue; too much food; or increases in glucagon and other counterregulatory hormones as a result of stress, illness, or infection. Factors that contribute to hypoglycemia include too much insulin or insulin secretagogue, not enough food, unusual amounts of exercise, and skipped or delayed meals. Urine glucose testing, frequently used in the past, has so many limitations that it should not be used.

It is now possible to do continuous ambulatory blood glucose monitoring to determine 24-hour blood glucose patterns and to detect unrecognized hypoglycemia. One such system consists of a subcutaneous sensor that monitors interstitial glucose levels for up to 72 hours. Data can be downloaded in the physician's office after completion of the prescribed cycle. Another device is worn on the wrist and can provide up to three glucose readings each hour for a maximum of 12 hours. It works through a process called reverse iontophoresis, in which a low-level electric current passes through intact skin and extracts glucose molecules.

Urine or blood testing can be used to detect ketones. Testing for ketonuria or ketonemia should be performed regularly during periods of illness and when blood glucose levels consistently exceed 240 mg/dl (13.3 mmol/L). The presence of persistent, moderate, or large amounts of ke-tones, along with elevated blood glucose levels, requires insulin adjustments. Persons with type 2 diabetes rarely have ketosis; however, ketone testing should be done when the person is seriously ill.

Self-Management Education

Diabetes management is a team effort. Persons with diabetes must be at the center of the team because they have the responsibility for day-to-day management. RDs, nurses, physicians, and other health care providers contribute their expertise to developing therapeutic regimens that help the person with diabetes achieve the best metabolic control possible. The goal is to provide patients with the knowledge, skills, and motivation to incorporate self-management into their daily lifestyles.

NUTRITION THERAPY INTERVENTIONS FOR SPECIFIC POPULATIONS

Medical Nutrition Therapy Interventions for Type 1 Diabetes

For persons requiring insulin therapy, the first priority is to integrate an insulin regimen into their usual eating habits and physical activity schedule. With the many insulin options now available (rapid- and long-acting insulins), an insulin regimen usually can be planned that will conform to an individual's preferred meal routines and food choices (ADA, 2007; Franz et al., 2002a). It is no longer necessary to create unnatural or artificial divisions of meals and snacks.

Physiologic insulin regimens involve multiple injections (three or more insulin injections per day) or use of an insulin infusion pump and mimic natural insulin secretion. Approximately half of the required insulin dose is given as a basal or background insulin, and the other half is divided and given before meals (bolus or mealtime insulin). These types of insulin regimens allow increased flexibility in choosing when and what to eat. The total carbohydrate content of meals is the major determinant of the mealtime rapid-acting insulin dose and postprandial glucose response (Rabasa-Lhoret et al., 1999, DAFNE Study Group, 2002). Thus individuals can be taught how to adjust mealtime insulin doses based on the carbohydrate content of the meal. For persons who receive fixed insulin regimens such as with the use of premixed insulins or those who do not adjust their mealtime insulin doses, day-to-day consistency in the timing and amount of carbohydrates eaten is recommended.

Attention must also be paid to total energy intake as well as carbohydrate intake. Weight gain has the potential to adversely affect glycemia, lipids, blood pressure, and general health; thus prevention of weight gain is desirable.

Medical Nutrition Therapy Interventions for Type 2 Diabetes

For persons with type 2 diabetes, the first priority is to adopt lifestyle interventions that improve the associated metabolic abnormalities of glycemia, dyslipidemia, and hypertension. Lifestyle interventions independent of weight loss that can improve glycemia include reduced energy intake and increased energy expenditure through physical activity. Because many persons also have dyslipidemia and hypertension, limited consumption of saturated and trans-fatty acids, cholesterol, and sodium is recommended. These interventions should be implemented as soon as the diagnosis of diabetes is made.

MNT interventions for established type 2 diabetes differ in several aspects from interventions for prevention. Because of the progressive nature of type 2 diabetes, MNT interventions progress from prevention of obesity, to the prevention or delay of type 2 diabetes, to strategies for improved metabolic control. Modest weight loss is beneficial in persons with insulin resistance, but, as the disease progresses to insulin deficiency, medications usually need to be combined with MNT. Emphasis should be on blood glucose control, improved food choices, increased physical activity, and moderate energy restriction rather than weight loss alone.

Teaching which foods are carbohydrates (fruits, grains, starchy vegetables, milk, sweets), average portion sizes, and how many servings to select at meals (and snacks, if desired) is the first step in food and meal planning. Limiting fats, especially saturated and trans-fats, encouraging physical activity, and using blood glucose monitoring to adjust food and eating patterns and medications are also important components of successful MNT for type 2 diabetes. Frequent follow-up with an RD can provide the problem-solving techniques, encouragement, and support that lifestyle changes require.

Physical activity improves insulin sensitivity, acutely lowers blood glucose in persons with diabetes and may also improve cardiovascular status; but by itself it has only a modest effect on weight. However, it is essential for long-term weight maintenance. Cardiorespiratory fitness in persons with diabetes appears to be more important than thinness in relation to all-cause and cardiovascular mortality (Church, 2004). During an average 14-year follow-up of about 2000 men with diabetes, fit men had greater longevity than unfit men, regardless of their body composition or risk factor status. Fitness had a strong and independent inverse association with mortality, independent of BMI and percentage of body fat. This again highlights the importance of counseling persons with diabetes to increase physical activity and fitness levels.

Weight-loss drugs may be beneficial in the treatment of overweight persons with type 2 diabetes and can help achieve a 5% to 10% weight loss when combined with lifestyle modifications. They should be used only in people with a BMI greater than 27. Gastric reduction surgery can be an effective weight-loss treatment for severely obese patients with type 2 diabetes and can result in marked improvements in glycemia. However, it should be considered only in patients with a BMI greater than 35 because long-term benefits and risks of bariatric surgery in persons with diabetes have not been adequately studies (ADA, 2007) (see Chapter 21).

Medical Nutrition Therapy Interventions for Children and Adolescents with Diabetes

Involvement of a multidisciplinary team, including a physician, RD, nurse, and behavioral specialist, all trained in pediatric diabetes, is the best means of achieving optimal diabetes management in youth. However, the most important team members are the child or adolescent and his or her family.

Type 1 Diabetes in Youth

A major nutrition goal for children and adolescents with type 1 diabetes is maintenance of normal growth and development. Possible causes of poor weight gain and linear growth include poor glycemic control, inadequate insulin, and overrestriction of calories. The last may be a consequence of the common erroneous belief that restricting food, rather than adjusting insulin, is the way to control blood glucose. Other reasons unrelated to diabetes management include thyroid abnormalities and malabsorption syndromes. Excessive weight gain can be caused by excessive caloric intake, overtreatment of hypoglycemia, or overinsulinization. Other causes include low physical activity levels and hypothyroidism (accompanied by poor linear growth) (Silverstein et al., 2005).

The nutrition prescription is based on the nutrition assessment. Newly diagnosed children often present with weight loss and hunger; as a result, the initial meal plan must be based on adequate calories to restore and maintain appropriate body weight. In about 4 to 6 weeks the initial caloric level may need to be modified to meet more usual caloric requirements. Nutrient requirements for children and adolescents with diabetes appear to be similar to those of children and adolescents without diabetes. The DRIs can be used to determine energy requirements (Institute of Medicine, 2002). However, it may be preferable to use a food and nutrition history of typical daily intake, providing that growth and development are normal, to determine an individual child's or adolescent's energy needs. Since energy requirements change with age, physical activity, and growth rate, an evaluation of height, weight, BMI, and the nutrition plan is recommended at least every year. Good metabolic control is essential for normal growth and development (for growth charts see Appendixes 9 through 16). However, withholding food or having the child eat consistently without an appetite for food in an effort to control blood glucose should be discouraged. Calories should be adequate for growth and restricted if the child becomes overweight. Consultation with an RD to develop and discuss the medical nutrition plan is encouraged (Silverstein et al., 2005).

Individualized food and meal plans, insulin regimens using basal (background) and bolus (mealtime) insulins, and insulin algorithms or insulin pumps can provide flexibility for children with type 1 diabetes and their families. This approach accommodates irregular meal times and schedules and varying appetites and activity levels (ADA, 2007). Daily eating patterns in young children generally include three meals and two or three snacks, depending on the length of time between meals and the child's physical activity level. Children often prefer smaller meals and snacks. Snacks can prevent hypoglycemia between meals and provide adequate calories. Older children and teens may prefer only three meals. Blood glucose monitoring data are then used to integrate an insulin regimen into the meal, snack, and exercise schedules.

Realistic blood glucose goals should be determined and discussed with the youth and family. Youth with diabetes are also more likely than their age- and sex-matched nondiabetic peers to be at risk for CVD. Therefore it is essential to reduce the risk factors in youth with type 1 diabetes. Lipid levels should be monitored regularly, and National Cholesterol Education Program treatment guidelines for children and adolescents should be followed (ADA, 2003b) (see Chapter 32).

After the appropriate nutrition prescription has been determined, the meal planning approach can be selected. A number of meal planning approaches can be used. Carbohydrate counting for food planning provides youth and their families with guidelines that facilitate glycemic control while still allowing the choice of many common foods that children and adolescents enjoy. However, whatever approach to food planning is used, the youth and family must find it understandable and applicable to their lifestyle. Blood glucose records are essential to assist the RD and other team members in making appropriate changes in insulin regimens.

Type 2 Diabetes in Youth

Childhood obesity has been accompanied by an increase in the prevalence of type 2 diabetes among children and adolescents. IGT has been shown to be highly prevalent in obese youth, irrespective of ethnic group, and is associated with insulin resistance. Once type 2 diabetes develops, β-cell failure is also a factor (Sinha et al., 2002). Thus type 2 diabetes in youth appears to follow a progressive pattern similar to type 2 diabetes in adults.

Successful lifestyle treatment of type 2 diabetes in children and adolescents involves cessation of excessive weight gain, promotion of normal growth and development, and the achievement of blood glucose and A1C goals (ADA, 2000). Nutrition guidelines should also address comorbidities such as hypertension and dyslipidemia. Behavior modification strategies to decrease intake of high-caloric, high-fat, and high-carbohydrate foods (e.g., extra-large desserts) and drinks (e.g., regular soda and other high sugar beverages) while encouraging healthy eating habits and regular physical activity for the entire family should be considered. Unfortunately successful lifestyle treatment regimens for youth with type 2 diabetes have not been defined (ADA, 2007). Dietary intake in a large cohort of youth with diabetes substantially failed to meet current recommendations. Less than 50% met recommendations for total fat, fiber, fruits, vegetables, and grains (Mayer-Davis et al., 2006b). A multivitamin/mineral supplement with DRI amounts of chromium, magnesium, zinc and especially of vitamin D may be warranted.

Metformin is often used when lifestyle strategies alone have not achieved target glucose goals and has been shown to be safe and effective for the treatment of pediatric type 2 diabetes (Jones et al., 2002). Youth with type 2 diabetes may also require insulin therapy to achieve adequate glycemic control.

Medical Nutrition Therapy Interventions for Pregnancy and Diabetes

Normalization of blood glucose levels during pregnancy is very important for women who have preexisting diabetes or who develop GDM. MNT goals are to assist in achieving and maintaining optimal blood glucose control and to provide adequate maternal and fetal nutrition throughout pregnancy, energy intake for appropriate maternal weight gain, and necessary vitamins and minerals (ADA, 2007). Nutrition recommendations during pregnancy and lactation appear to be similar for women with and without diabetes; therefore the DRIs can be used to determine energy and nutrient requirements during pregnancy and for lactation (Institute of Medicine, 2002). Table 30-8 outlines blood glucose goals during pregnancy for preexisting diabetes and for GDM (ADA, 2006b; Jovanovic, 2000).

Preexisting Diabetes and Pregnancy

Preconception counseling and the ability to achieve near-normal blood glucose levels before pregnancy have been shown to be effective in reducing the incidence of anomalies in infants born to women with preexisting diabetes to nearly that of the general population.

As a result of hormonal changes during the first trimester, blood glucose levels are often erratic. Although caloric needs do not differ from those preceding pregnancy,

TABLE 30-8

Plasma Glucose Goals During Pregnancy

Test	Preexisting Diabetes (mg/dl)	Gestational Diabetes (mg/dl)
Fasting plasma glucose	65-100	65-95
Premeal	65-110	
1 hr postprandial	<145	≤140
2 hr postprandial	<135	≤120
2 to 6 hr postprandial	65-135	

Modified from Jovanovic L, editor: *Medical management of pregnancy complicated by diabetes*, ed 3, Alexandria, Va, 2000, American Diabetes Association; and American Diabetes Association: Gestational diabetes mellitus (Position Statement), *Diabetes Care* 27(suppl 1):S88, 2004c.

the meal plan may need to be adjusted to accommodate the metabolic changes. Women should be educated about the increased risk of hypoglycemia during pregnancy and cautioned against overtreatment.

The need for insulin increases during the second and third trimesters of pregnancy. (This is why screening for GDM is done between weeks 24 and 28 of pregnancy.) At 38 to 40 weeks' postconception, insulin needs and levels peak at two to three times prepregnancy levels. Pregnancy-associated hormones that are antagonistic to the action of insulin lead to an elevation of blood glucose levels. For women with preexisting diabetes, this increased insulin need must be met with increased exogenous insulin.

Meal plan adjustments are necessary to provide the additional calories required to support fetal growth, and weight should be monitored. During pregnancy the distribution of energy and carbohydrate intake should be based on the woman's food and eating habits and blood glucose responses. Insulin regimens can be matched to food intake, but maintaining consistency of times and amounts of food eaten are essential to avoid hypoglycemia caused by the continuous fetal draw of glucose from the mother. Smaller meals and more frequent snacks are often needed. A late-evening snack is often necessary to decrease the likelihood of overnight hypoglycemia and fasting ketosis. Records of food intake and blood glucose values are essential for determining whether glycemic goals are being met and for preventing and correcting ketosis.

Regular follow-up visits are needed to also monitor caloric and nutrient intake, blood glucose control, and whether there is starvation ketosis. Urine or blood ketones during pregnancy may signal starvation ketosis that can be caused by inadequate energy or carbohydrate intake, omission of meals or snacks, or prolonged intervals between meals (e.g., more than 10 hours between the bedtime snack and breakfast). Ketonemia during pregnancy has been associated with reduced IQ scores in children, and women should be instructed to test for ketones periodically before breakfast.

Gestational Diabetes Mellitus

About 7% of all pregnancies are complicated by GDM, resulting in more than 200,000 cases annually (ADA, 2004c). After delivery about 90% of all women with GDM become normoglycemic but are at increased risk of developing GDM earlier in subsequent pregnancies and for developing type 2 diabetes. After pregnancy, 5% to 10% of women with gestational diabetes are found to have type 2 diabetes. Women who have had gestational diabetes have a 20% to 50% chance of developing diabetes in the next 5 to 10 years (Centers for Disease Control and Prevention, 2005). Lifestyle modifications aimed at reducing or preventing weight gain and increasing physical activity after pregnancy are recommended and can reduce the risk of subsequent diabetes.

Because fetal morbidity may be increased, a risk assessment for GDM should be done at the first prenatal visit, and women at high risk (those with marked obesity, previous history of GDM, glycosuria, or a strong family history of diabetes) should be tested as soon as possible. An FPG of 126 mg/dl (7 mmol/L) or higher or a casual plasma glucose (CPG) of 200 mg/dl (11 mmol/L) meets the threshold for the diagnosis of diabetes and, if confirmed on a second day, requires no further testing (ADA, 2006b). High-risk women not found to have GDM at the initial screening and average risk women (a few women can be classified as low risk) should be tested between 24 to 28 weeks of gestation. An oral glucose challenge (which does not have to be preceded by fasting) with 50g glucose is performed, and an elevated plasma glucose level (>140 mg/dl [7.8 mmol/L]) 1 hour later is considered an indication of the need for diagnostic testing. The criteria for the diagnosis of GDM based on a 100-g OGT test are listed in Table 30-9. Low-risk women who do not need to be screened must meet all the following criteria: younger than 25 years of age; normal body weight; no family history of diabetes; no history of abnormal glucose tolerance; and not a member of an ethnic or racial group with a high prevalence of diabetes (ADA, 2006b).

MNT for GDM primarily involves a carbohydrate-controlled meal plan that promotes optimal nutrition for maternal and fetal health with adequate energy for appropriate gestational weight gain, achievement and maintenance of normoglycemia, and absence of ketosis. Specific nutrition and food recommendations are determined and modified based on individual assessment and blood glucose records. Monitoring blood glucose, fasting ketones, appetite, and weight gain can aid in developing an appropriate, individualized meal plan and in adjusting the meal plan throughout pregnancy.

Nutrition practice guidelines for gestational diabetes have been developed and field-tested (Reader et al., 2006). All women with GDM should receive MNT at diagnosis of GDM. Monitoring records guide nutrition therapy and are used to determine if insulin therapy is needed. Insulin therapy is added if glucose goals exceed target range (see Table 30-8) on two or more occasions in a 1- to 2-week period without some obvious explanation from food records or if glucose levels are consistently elevated because of patient's dietary indiscretions after MNT intervention. Weight gain or lack of

weight gain and ketone testing can be useful in determining whether women are undereating to keep glucose levels within target range to avoid insulin therapy.

Carbohydrates should be distributed throughout the day into three small-to-moderate size meals and two to four snacks. All women require a minimum of 175 g of carbohydrates daily (Institute of Medicine, 2002). An evening snack is usually needed to prevent accelerated ketosis overnight. Carbohydrates are not as well tolerated at breakfast as they are at other meals because of increased levels of cortisol and growth hormones. To compensate for this, the initial food plan may have approximately 30 g of carbohydrate at breakfast. To satisfy hunger, protein foods, because they do not affect blood glucose levels as much, can be added.

Although caloric restriction must be viewed with caution, in obese women with GDM a 30% caloric restriction (an intake of about 1700 to 1800 kcal daily) may reduce hyperglycemia without ketonemia and reduce the rate of maternal weight gain. Intake below these levels is not advised. The pattern of weight gain during pregnancy for women with GDM should be similar to that of women without diabetes. Weight loss is not recommended for overweight and obese women with GDM; however, modest energy and carbohydrate restriction may be appropriate (ADA, 2007).

Exercise can also assist in overcoming peripheral resistance to insulin and in controlling fasting and postprandial hyperglycemia. It may be used as an adjunct to nutrition therapy to improve maternal glycemia. The ideal form of exercise is unknown, but a brisk walk after meals is often recommended.

Women with GDM should be encouraged to breast-feed because even a short duration of breast-feeding may retard the future onset of diabetes (McManus, 2001).

Medical Nutrition Therapy Interventions for Older Adults

The prevalence of diabetes and IGT increases dramatically as people age. Many factors predispose older adults to diabetes: age-related decreases in insulin production and

TABLE 30-9	
Diagnosis of Gestational Diabetes Mellitus	
Type of Test	**Results**
Screening during pregnancy—a 50-g oral glucose challenge (does not have to be fasting) at 24- to 28-weeks' gestation	A plasma glucose level of 140 mg/dl (7.8 mmol/L) 1 hr later indicates the need for further diagnostic testing
Oral glucose tolerance test with an abnormal screen	After a 100-g oral glucose load, GDM may be diagnosed if two plasma glucose values equal or exceed: **Fasting**: ≥95 mg/dl **1 hr**: ≥180 mg/dl **2 hr**: ≥155 mg/dl **3 hr**: ≥140 mg/dl

Modified from American Diabetes Association: Standards of medical care in diabetes—2007, *Diabetes Care* 30:54, 2007.

increases in insulin resistance, adiposity, decreased physical activity, multiple prescription medications, genetics, and coexisting illnesses. A major factor appears to be insulin resistance. Controversy persists as to whether the insulin resistance is itself a primary change or whether it is attributable to reduced physical activity, decreased lean body mass (sarcopenia), and increased adipose tissue, which are all frequently seen in older adults. Furthermore, medications used to treat coexisting diseases may complicate diabetes therapy in older persons.

Despite the increase in glucose intolerance with age, aging per se should not be a reason for suboptimal control of blood glucose. Even if it is incorrectly assumed that preventing long-term diabetic complications is not relevant to the care of older adults, persistent hyperglycemia has deleterious effects on the body's defense mechanisms against infection. It also increases the pain threshold by exacerbating neuropathic pain, and it has a detrimental effect on the outcome of cerebrovascular accidents.

Nutrition recommendations for older adults with diabetes must be extrapolated from what is known from the general population and should address nutrition-related cardiovascular risk factors common in older adults and encourage consumption of a variety of foods. Because of changes in body composition (loss of lean body mass) and exercise patterns, the energy requirements of older adults are 20% to 30% lower than those of younger adults (ADA, 2007). Physical activity can significantly reduce the decline in aerobic capacity that occurs with age, improve risk factors for atherosclerosis, slow the decline in age-related lean body mass, decrease central adiposity, and improve insulin sensitivity; thus it should be encouraged.

Malnutrition, not obesity, is often the more prevalent nutrition-related problem of older adults. It often remains subclinical or unrecognized because the result of malnutrition—excessive loss of lean body mass—resembles the signs and symptoms of the aging process. Until a primary disease develops or chronic problems are exacerbated by illness or some other stress, malnutrition may remain unrecognized. Both malnutrition and diabetes adversely affect wound healing and defense against infection, and malnutrition is associated with depression and cognitive deficits. The most reliable indicator of poor nutrition status in older adults is probably a change in body weight. In general, involuntary weight gain or loss of more than 10 pounds or 10% of body weight in less than 6 months indicates a need to evaluate whether the reason is nutrition related.

Because of concern over malnutrition, it is essential that older adults, especially those in long-term care settings, be provided a diet that meets their nutritional needs, enables them to attain or maintain a reasonable body weight, helps control blood glucose, and is palatable. The imposition of dietary restriction on older residents in long-term health facilities is not warranted. Residents should be served the regular (unrestricted) menu with consistency in the amount and timing of carbohydrates (ADA, 2007). A multivitamin/mineral supplement to meet the DRIs may be necessary.

In older adults acute hyperglycemia and dehydration can lead to a serious complication of diabetes: the **hyperglycemic hyperosmolar state (HHS)**. Patients with HHS have a very high blood glucose level (ranging from 400 to 2800 mg/dl, [22.2-155.6 mmol/L] with an average of 1000 mg/dl [55.6 mmol/L]) without ketones. Patients are markedly dehydrated, and mental status often ranges from mild confusion to hallucinations or coma. Patients who have HHS have sufficient insulin to prevent lipolysis and ketosis. Treatment consists of hydration and small doses of insulin to control hyperglycemia.

THE NUTRITION CARE PROCESS

The nutrition care process (NCP) articulates the consistent and specific steps used to deliver MNT for diabetes. It is used to deliver MNT for some individuals in individual sessions and for others in group sessions. The NCP begins with developing rapport with the patient, and, whether provided individually or in groups, it involves a common process: nutrition assessment, nutrition diagnosis, nutrition intervention, and nutrition monitoring and evaluation (Lacey and Pritchett, 2003). When MNT is implemented individually, the intervention is individualized based on the needs of the patient and whether the intervention is for initial, continuing, or intensive care (see Chapter 17).

Providing nutrition interventions in groups is becoming increasingly more important, since reimbursement criteria for diabetes self-management education and for MNT recommend that, when possible, group sessions are preferable. It is helpful if the group participants are similar in their stage of diabetes management and if they all speak and understand the same language. Group education shifts more responsibility to the patient to provide the needed initial assessment information, to evaluate outcomes, and to decide about therapy changes (Franz et al, 2002b). However, group interventions must also allow for individualization of MNT and evaluation of outcomes. When compared with individual interventions, group interventions for diabetes self-management education have produced similar positive outcomes (Rickheim et al., 2002).

Nutrition Assessment

The nutrition assessment involves obtaining information before and during the encounter needed to identify nutrition-related problems. Within 30 days before the first encounter, the RD should obtain pertinent clinical data from the referral source or patient record or information system. Box 30-2 provides a summary of assessment data—minimum referral data and parameters to be assessed to develop an individualized nutrition care plan. Some of this information can be gathered from a patient questionnaire. By collecting the data before the first session, completion of the assessment and implementation of interventions can begin efficiently.

It is essential to learn about the patient's lifestyle and eating habits. Food and eating histories can be done several ways, with the objective being to determine a schedule and

BOX 30-2

Nutrition Assessment

Minimum Referral Data Needed Before First Encounter

- *Diabetes treatment regimen:* nutrition therapy alone; nutrition therapy and glucose-lowering medications; nutrition therapy and insulin (physiologic or fixed regimen); nutrition therapy and combination medications (type[s])
- *Laboratory data:* A1C, date of test; fasting or nonfasting plasma glucose; lipid fractionation (cholesterol, low-density lipoprotein and high-density lipoprotein cholesterol, triglycerides); urinary microalbumin (albumin-to-creatinine ratio); blood pressure
- *Goals for patient care:* target blood glucose levels (premeal and postmeal); target A1C; method and frequency of self-monitoring of blood glucose; plans for instruction and evaluation of glucose monitoring
- *Medical history:* other pertinent diagnoses—cardiovascular disease, hypertension, renal disease, autonomic neuropathy, especially gastrointestinal
- *Medications:* dose and frequency; dietary supplements
- *Guidelines for exercise:* medical clearance for exercise; exercise limitation, if any

Data to Be Obtained From a Food and Nutrition Assessment

- *Anthropometric measures:* weight; height (for adults at initial visit and for youth at every visit); body mass index; waist circumference
- *Diabetes history:* previous diabetes education, use of blood glucose monitoring, diabetes problems/concerns (hypoglycemia, hyperglycemia, fear of insulin)
- *Food and/nutrition history:* 24-hr recall or typical day's intake; meal and snack eating times; schedule changes; travel frequency; exercise routine/sports (type, amount, and time of exercise); usual sleep habits; appetite/gastrointestinal issues; food allergies/food intolerance; alcohol use; weight history, weight goals
- *Social history:* occupation, hours worked away from home, living situation, financial issues
- *Medications/supplements:* medications taken, vitamin/mineral/supplement use, herbal supplements
- *Knowledge base:* motivation to change; readiness to change

Modified from Franz MJ et al: *Implementing group and individual medical nutrition therapy for diabetes,* Alexandria, Va, 2002, American Diabetes Association.

---

pattern of eating that will be the least disruptive to the lifestyle of the individual with diabetes and, at the same time, will facilitate improved metabolic control. With this objective in mind, asking the individual either to record or report what, how much, and when he or she typically eats during a 24-hour period may be the most useful.

Another approach is to ask the patient to keep and bring a 3-day or 1-week food intake record. This request can be made when an appointment with the RD is scheduled. Assessment of the most typical daily pattern can then be made. The history can also reveal other useful information, including (1) usual caloric intake; (2) quality of the usual diet; (3) times, sizes, and contents of meals and snacks; (4) food idiosyncrasies; (5) frequency with which meals are eaten in restaurants; (6) who usually prepares food; (7) eating problems (e.g., as related to dental, gastrointestinal or other problems); (8) alcoholic beverage intake; and (9) supplements used (see Chapter 18). It is also essential to learn about the patient's daily routine and schedule. The following information is needed: (1) time of waking; (2) usual meal and eating times; (3) work schedule or school hours; (4) type, amount, and timing of exercise; and (5) usual sleep habits.

Nutrition Diagnosis

The nutrition diagnosis describes factors in the patients' nutrition status that RDs are responsible for treating independently (see Chapter 17). A nutrition diagnosis is written in the PES format that states the *problem* (P), the *etiology* (E), and *signs and symptoms* (S). Examples of P related to diabetes

are listed in Box 30-3. The following are examples of nutrition diagnosis statements:

- Altered blood glucose values (P) related to insufficient insulin (E) as evidenced by hyperglycemia despite excellent eating habits (S)
- Inconsistent carbohydrate intake (P) related to inconsistent timing of meals (E) as evidenced by wide fluctuations in blood glucose levels (S)
- Inappropriate intake of food fats (P) related to inadequate knowledge (E) as evidenced by high intake of foods containing saturated fats (S)

Nutrition Intervention

Nutrition interventions include two distinct processes: planning nutrition interventions and implementing the nutrition intervention. An individualized food and meal plan and behavioral goals focused on the etiology of the problem are developed, along with a statement of specific expected outcomes and timeline for each. A list of materials is provided with referrals or resources used and recommendations to other health care team members to reinforce nutrition and physical activity goals, recheck laboratory data, and reevaluate medications and/or doses.

Developing a Food/Meal Plan

Using the assessment data and food and nutrition history information, a preliminary food and meal plan can then be designed, and, if the patient desires, sample menus provided.

Developing a food and meal plan does not begin with a set calorie or macronutrient prescription; instead, it is determined by modifying the patient's usual food intake as necessary. The worksheet in Figure 30-2 can be used to record the usual foods eaten and to modify the usual diet as necessary. The macronutrient and caloric values for the exchange lists are listed on the form and in Table 30-10.

See Appendix 34 for portion sizes of the foods on the exchange lists. These tools are useful in evaluating nutrition assessments. Using the form in Figure 30-2, the RD begins by totaling the number of exchanges from each list and multiplying this number by the grams of carbohydrate, protein, and fat contributed by each. Next the grams of carbohydrate, protein, and fat are totaled from

---

BOX 30-3

Examples of Nutrition Diagnoses (Problems) Related to Diabetes Mellitus

√

NI-1.4 Inadequate energy intake
NI-1.5 Excessive energy intake
NI-4.3 Excessive alcohol intake
NI-51.2 Excessive fat intake
NI-51.3 Inappropriate intake of food fats—specify
NI-52.1 Excessive protein intake
NI-53.1 Inadequate carbohydrate intake
NI-53.2 Excessive carbohydrate intake
NI-53.3 Inappropriate intake of types of carbohydrate—specify
NI-53.4 Inconsistent carbohydrate intake
NI-53.5 Inadequate fiber intake
NC-1.4 Altered GI function
NC-2.2 Altered nutrition-related laboratory value (i.e., glucose)

√

NC-2.3 Food medication interaction
NC-3.1 Underweight
NC-3.2 Involuntary weight loss
NC-3.3 Overweight/obesity
NC-3.4 Involuntary weight gain
NB-1.1 Food- and nutrition-related knowledge deficit
NB-1.3 Not ready for diet/lifestyle change
NB-1.5 Disordered eating pattern
NB-1.6 Limited adherence to nutrition-related recommendations
NB-2.1 Physical inactivity
NB-2.3 Inability or lack of desire to manage self-care
NB-2.4 Impaired ability to prepare foods/meals

Modified from American Dietetic Association: *Nutrition diagnosis: a critical step in the nutrition care process*, Chicago, Ill, 2005, American Dietetic Association.

TABLE 30-10

Macronutrient and Caloric Values for Exchange Lists*

Groups/Lists	Carbohydrate (g)	Protein (g)	Fat (g)	Calories
Carbohydrate Group				
Starch	15	3	0-1	80
Fruit	15	—	—	60
Milk				
Skim	12	8	0-3	90
Reduced-fat	12	8	5	120
Whole	12	8	8	150
Other carbohydrates	15	Varies	Varies	Varies
Vegetables	5	2	—	25
Meat and Meat Substitute Group				
Very lean	—	7	0-1	35
Lean	—	7	3	55
Medium-fat	—	7	5	75
High-fat	—	7	8	100
Fat Group	—	—	5	45

From American Diabetes Association and American Dietetic Association: *Exchange lists for meal planning*, Alexandria, Va, 1995, American Diabetes Association.

*See Appendix 34.

each column; the grams of carbohydrates and protein are then multiplied by 4 (4 kcal/g of carbohydrates and protein), and the grams of fat are multiplied by 9 (9 kcal/g of fat). Total calories and percentage of calories from each macronutrient can then be determined. Numbers derived from these calculations are then rounded off. Figure 30-3 provides an example of a preliminary food and meal plan. In this example the nutrition prescription would be the following: 1900 to 2000 calories, 230 g of carbohydrates (50%), 90 g of protein (20%), 65 g of fat (30%).

The number of carbohydrate choices for each meal and snack is the total of the starch, fruit, and milk servings. Vegetables, unless starchy or eaten in very large amounts (three or more servings per meal), are generally considered "free foods." The carbohydrate choices are circled under each meal and snack column. Table 30-11 is an example of a sample meal plan and menu based on Figure 30-3.

The next step is to evaluate the preliminary meal plan. First and foremost, does the patient think it is feasible to implement the meal plan into his or her lifestyle? Second, is it appropriate for diabetes management? Third, does it encourage healthful eating?

To answer the first question concerning the feasibility of the food plan, the food and meal plan is reviewed with the patient in terms of general food intake. Timing of meals and snacks and approximate portion sizes and types of foods are discussed. Later a meal-planning approach can be selected that will assist the patient in making his or her own food choices. At this point it needs to be determined whether this meal plan is reasonable for the patient with diabetes. To determine the appropriateness of the meal plan for diabetes management involves assessing if the distribution of the meals (and snacks, if desired) is appropriate based on the types of medications prescribed and treatment goals. Methods for determining caloric requirements are only approximate. Adjustments in calories can be made during follow-up visits. Parameters that should be taken into consideration are weight changes, feelings of satiety and hunger, and concerns about palatability.

For patients with type 2 diabetes receiving MNT alone, often the food and meal plan begins with three or four carbohydrate servings per meal for adult women and four or five for adult men and, if desired, one or two for a snack. Blood glucose monitoring before the meal and 2 hours after the meal is recommended. Results of the blood glucose monitoring and feedback from the patient are used to assess if these recommendations are feasible and realistic and to determine if target glucose goals are being achieved.

For patients who require insulin, the timing of eating is extremely important. Food consumption must be synchronized with the time actions of insulin (see "Medications" earlier in the chapter). If the eating pattern is determined

Food Group	Meal/Snack/Time						Total servings/ day	CHO (g)	Protein (g)	Fat (g)	Calories
	Breakfast	Snack	Lunch	Snack	Dinner	Snack					
Starches								15	3	1	80
Fruit								15			60
Milk								12	8	1	90
Vegetables								5	2		25
Meats/ Substitutes									7	5(3)	75(55)
Fats										5	45
CHO Choices								Total grams			
							Calories/ gram	X4=	X4=	X9=	Total calories
							Percent calories				

Calculations are based on medium-fat meats and skim/very low-fat milk. If diet consists predominantly of low-fat meats, use the factor 3 g instead of 5 g fat; if predominantly high-fat meats, use 8 g fat. If low-fat (2%) milk is used, use 5 g fat; if whole milk is used, use 8 g fat.

FIGURE 30-2 Worksheet for assessment and design of a meal or food plan. *CHO*, Carbohydrate.

Food Group	Breakfast 7:30 AM	Snack 10:00	Lunch 12:00	Snack 3:00	Dinner 6:30	Snack 10:00	Total servings/day	CHO (g)	Protein (g)	Fat (g)	Calories
								15	3	1	80
Starches	2	1	2–3	1	2–3	1–2	10	150	30	10	
								15			60
Fruit	1		1		1	0–1	3	45			
								12	8	1	90
Milk	1				1		2	24	16	2	
								5	2		25
Vegetables			✓		✓			10	4		
									7	5(3)	75(55)
Meats/Substitutes			2–3		3–4		6		42	30	
										5	45
Fats	1	0–1	1–2	0–1	1–2	0–1	5			25	
CHO Choices	3–4 CHO	1 CHO	3–4 CHO	1 CHO	4–5 CHO	1–2 CHO	Total grams	229	92	67	
1900–2000 calories							Calories/gram	X4= 916	X4= 368	X9= 603	Total calories
230 g CHO-50% 90 g protein-20% 65 g fat-30%							Percent calories	50	19	30	1900–2000

Calculations are based on medium-fat meats and skim/very low-fat milk. If diet consists predominantly of low-fat meats, use the factor 3 g, instead of 5 g fat; if predominantly high-fat meats, use 8 g fat. If low-fat (2%) milk is used, use 5 g fat; if whole milk is used, use 8 g fat.

FIGURE 30-3 An example of a completed worksheet from the assessment, the nutrition prescription, and a sample 1900- to 2000-calorie meal plan. *CHO,* Carbohydrate.

first, an insulin regimen can be selected that will fit with it. To prevent overnight hypoglycemia, some patients may require a bedtime snack.

The best way to ensure that the meal plan encourages healthful eating is to encourage patients to eat a variety of foods from all the food groups. The Dietary Guidelines for Americans, with its suggested number of servings from each food group, can be used to compare the patient's meal plan with the nutrition recommendations for all Americans (see Chapter 12).

Self-Management Training

This step involves selecting an appropriate meal-planning approach and identifying strategies for behavioral change that enhance motivation and adherence to necessary lifestyle changes. A number of meal-planning approaches are available, ranging from simple guidelines or menus to more complex counting methods (Table 30-12). No single meal-planning approach has been shown to be more effective than any other, and the meal-planning approach selected should allow individuals with diabetes to select appropriate foods for meals and snacks.

A popular approach to meal planning is carbohydrate counting. It can be used as a basic meal-planning approach or for more intensive management. Carbohydrate-counting educational tools are based on the concept that, after eating it is the carbohydrate in foods that is the ma-

jor predictor of postprandial blood glucose levels. One carbohydrate serving contributes 15 g of carbohydrates. Basic carbohydrate counting emphasizes the following topics: basic facts about carbohydrates, primary food sources of carbohydrate, average portion sizes and the importance of consistency and measuring portions, amount of carbohydrates they should be eating, and label reading. Advanced carbohydrate counting emphasizes the importance of record keeping, pattern management, and calculating insulin-to-carbohydrate ratios.

Facilitating Behavioral Changes and Goal Setting

Optimal self-management of diabetes requires changes in existing behaviors in addition to the adoption of new ones. Successful behavioral change requires comprehensive education, skill development, and motivation. The transtheoretical model was proposed by Prochaska as a general model of intentional behavior change (Prochaska et al., 1994). It includes a sequence of stages along a continuum of behavioral change. Different intervention strategies may be needed for individuals at different stages of the change process. Motivational interventions may work best with patients in the earlier contemplative stages, whereas specific skill-training interventions may be most appropriate for persons who have decided to change. Relapse and recycling through the stages occur quite frequently as patients attempt to modify behaviors (see Chapter 19).

Short-term goals (days or weeks) are often behavioral goals and relate to lifestyle changes. Common self-management behavioral goals are consistent and appropriate carbohydrate servings, regular physical activity, correct medication dosage (if needed), and blood glucose monitoring as determined to be needed. Goals should be specific, realistic for the patient, and written in behavioral language.

Nutrition Monitoring and Evaluation

Before the patient leaves the session, plans for the next appointment should be identified. A timeline should be established for follow-up visits to monitor and evaluate responses to nutrition interventions. The patient is also given information on how to call or e-mail with questions and concerns. In making plans for the next encounter, the patient is asked to keep a 3-day or weekly food record with blood glucose–monitoring data.

Medical and clinical outcomes should be monitored after the second or third visit to determine whether the patient is making progress toward established goals. If no progress is evident, the individual and RD need to reassess and perhaps revise the nutrition care plan. If altering food intake alone is not achieving metabolic target ranges, the RD should recommend that medications be added or adjusted.

Documentation is essential for communication and reimbursement. An initial progress note is documented in the patient's medical record and information system according to the organization's policy, and a copy of the progress note is sent to the referral source. Box 30-4 lists some of the areas of the nutrition intervention that require documentation (see Chapter 17).

Follow-Up Encounters

Successful nutrition therapy involves a process of assessment, problem solving, adjustment, and readjustment. Food records can be compared with the meal plan, which will help to determine whether the initial meal plan needs changing, and can be integrated with the blood glucose–monitoring records to determine changes that can lead to improved glycemic control. For patients receiving oral medications or insulin, it can then be determined whether blood glucose values that are outside target ranges can be corrected with adjustments in the meal plan or whether adjustments in medications are needed.

The knowledge and skills needed to implement nutritional recommendations cannot be acquired in one session; therefore continued nutrition education is essential and must be an ongoing component of diabetes care. After the basic food and nutrition interventions have been mastered, other aspects of nutrition education should be presented to increase flexibility in food choices and lifestyle while still maintaining glucose control (Box 30-5). Of particular importance is information about eating out and the use of information from food labels. Persons using insulin also need information about how to make adjustments in food intake or insulin when schedules are disrupted.

Nutrition follow-up visits should provide encouragement and ensure realistic expectations for the patient.

TABLE 30-11	
Sample Menu for 1900-2000 Kilocalorie Meal Plan	
Meal/Timing	**Food Selections**
Breakfast—7:30 AM	
3–4 Carbohydrate choices (i.e., 2 starch, 1 fruit, 1 milk)	Raisin bran cereal, ½ c
	Bagel, ¼ (1 oz)
	Cantaloupe (5-inch), ⅓
	Skim milk, 1 c
1 Fat	Reduced-fat cream cheese, 1 Tbsp
Snack—10.00 AM	
1 Carbohydrate choice (i.e., 1 starch or fruit)	Bagel, ¼ (1 oz)
0-1 Fat	Reduced-fat cream cheese, 1 Tbsp
Lunch—Noon	
3-4 Carbohydrate choices (i.e., 2-3 starches, 1 fruit)	Whole-wheat bread, 2 slices
	Vegetable-beef soup, 1 c
	Apple, 1 small
Vegetable	Lettuce and tomato slices
2-3 Meats	Turkey, 2 oz
1-2 Fats	Reduced-fat mayonnaise, 1 Tbsp
Snack—3:00 PM	
1 Carbohydrate choice (i.e., 1 starch or fruit)	Pretzels, ¾ oz
0-1 Fat	
Dinner—6:30 PM	
4-5 Carbohydrate choices (i.e., 2-3 starch, 1 fruit, 1 milk)	Baked potato, 1 medium
	Dinner roll, 1
	Mandarin oranges, ¾ c
	Skim milk, 1 c
Vegetables	Broccoli spears, ½ c
	Dinner salad, 1 small
3-4 Meats	Chicken breast, baked, 3 oz
1-2 Fats	Sour cream, regular, 2 Tbsp
	Reduced-fat salad dressing, 2 Tbsp
Snack—10:00 PM	
1-2 Carbohydrate choices (i.e., 1-2 starches, 0-1 fruit)	Ice cream, light ½ c
	Strawberries, 1¼ c
0-1 Fat	

TABLE 30-12

Food-Planning Approaches for Diabetes

Approach	Publication	Description
Diabetes nutrition guidelines	*The First Step in Diabetes Meal Planning* (American Diabetes Association and American Dietetic Association)	A pamphlet that provides general guidelines for meal planning based on MyPyramid. Designed to be given to patients to use until an individualized meal plan can be implemented; however, for some individuals there may be no need to advance to more complex meal-planning approaches.
	Healthy Food Choices (American Diabetes Association and American Dietetic Association)	A pamphlet that promotes healthy eating. It is divided into two sections: (1) guidelines for making healthy food choices, and (2) simplified exchanges lists.
	Healthy Eating for People With Diabetes (International Diabetes Center, Minneapolis, Minn)	Based on the *plate method*, which visualizes kinds and amounts of food and is used to illustrate portions of common foods in relation to plate size. General guidelines for choosing healthy foods, lowering fat intake, and timing of meals and snacks are included.
	Eating Healthy With Diabetes Easy Reading Guide (American Diabetes Association and American Dietetic Association)	A booklet designed specifically for persons with minimum reading skills. The amount of text is limited, symbols and color codes are used, and concepts and foods are presented visually.
Menu approaches	*Month of Meals: Classic Cooking, Old-Time Favorites, Meals in Minutes, Vegetarian Pleasures, and Ethnic Delights* (American Diabetes Association)	Separate books, with each book containing 28 days of complete menus for breakfast, lunch, dinner, and snacks. Designed to help patients who need help in planning basic menus for their diabetes.
Carbohydrate counting	*Basic Carbohydrate Counting* (American Diabetes Association and American Dietetic Association)	A pamphlet that outlines which foods are carbohydrates and average portions sizes. It can be used as a basic meal-planning approach for anyone with diabetes and is based on the concept that, after eating, carbohydrate in foods has the major impact on blood glucose levels. One carbohydrate serving = 15 g of carbohydrates.
	Advanced Carbohydrate Counting (American Diabetes Association and American Dietetic Association)	A booklet for individuals who have chosen flexible insulin regimens or an insulin pump. The relationship between carbohydrates eaten and insulin injected can be shown as an insulin-to-carbohydrate ratio. This ratio gives the individual a good guide to how much bolus rapid-acting insulin is needed when eating more or less carbohydrates than usual; however, before insulin ratios can be established, blood glucose levels must be under control, and the usual dose of both the basal and rapid-acting (bolus) insulin determined. The grams of carbohydrates consumed at a meal are divided by the number of units of insulin needed to maintain target glucose goals. This is called an *insulin-to-carbohydrate ratio*. For example, 75 g of carbohydrates may require 8 units of rapid-acting insulin, and the insulin-to-carbohydrate ratio would be 1:10. Therefore, for each anticipated addition of 10 g of carbohydrates, an additional 1 unit of rapid-acting insulin is needed (or for 10 g less of carbohydrates, 1 less unit of rapid-acting insulin is needed).
	My Food Plan (International Diabetes Center, Minneapolis, Minn)	A pamphlet that combines both carbohydrate counting and calorie control in a simplified approach. It groups carbohydrate, meat, and fat choices by approximate portion sizes. A form for filling in an individualized meal plan is included.
Exchange list approaches	*Exchange Lists for Meal Planning* (American Diabetes Association and American Dietetic Association) (see Appendix 34).	A booklet that contains lists that group foods in measures that contribute approximately the same number of calories, carbohydrates, protein, and fat. Foods are divided into three basic lists: carbohydrates, meat and meat substitutes, and fat. An individualized food plan that outlines the number of servings from each list for each meal and for snacks is included.

Modified from Franz MJ et al: *Implementing group and individual medical nutrition therapy for diabetes*, Alexandria, Va, 2002, American Diabetes Association.

BOX 30-4

Nutrition Care Documentation

Documentation of each medical nutrition therapy (MNT) visit must include:

> Patient name and identification information
> Date of MNT visit and amount of time spent with patient
> Reason for visit
> Patient's current diagnosis (and relevant past diagnoses)
> Pertinent test results and current medications (name, dose)
> Names of others present during MNT
> Physician's referral for MNT (if billing Medicare)

Summaries of:

> **Nutrition assessment**
> - Histories: nutrition, medical, social, and family
> - Baseline for outcomes monitoring
> **Nutrition diagnoses**
> - Problem, etiology, symptoms (PES) format
> **Nutrition interventions**
> - Food and meal plan
> - Short- and long-term goals
> - Educational topics covered and materials provided
> **Nutrition monitoring and evaluation**
> - Registered dietitian's impressions related to patient's acceptance and understanding
> - Anticipated compliance
> - Successful behavior changes
> - Additional needed skills or information
> - Additional recommendations
> - Plans for ongoing care

Adapted from Franz MJ et al: *Implementing group and individual medical nutrition therapy for diabetes*, Alexandria, Va, 2002, American Diabetes Association.

BOX 30-5

Essential Self-Management Nutrition Education Skills*

- Sources of carbohydrates, protein, fat
- Understanding nutrition labels
- Modification of fat intake
- Alcohol consumption guidelines
- Use of blood glucose monitoring data for problem solving related to food choices and physical activity options
- Use of blood glucose monitoring data to identify blood glucose patterns and need for medication changes
- Adjustments in carbohydrates or insulin for exercise
- Grocery shopping guidelines
- Guidelines for eating out: restaurant, cafeteria, school lunch
- Snack choices
- Mealtime adjustments
- Use of sugar-containing foods and nonnutritive sweeteners
- Recipes, menu ideas, cookbooks
- Behavior modification techniques
- Problem-solving tips for birthdays, special occasions, holidays
- Travel, schedule changes
- Vitamin, mineral, and botanical supplements
- Work shift rotation, if needed

Modified from American Dietetic Association: *Medical nutrition therapy evidence-based guides for practice: nutrition practice guidelines for type 1 and type 2 diabetes [CD-ROM]*, Chicago, Ill, 2001, American Dietetic Association.

*Topics emphasized based on patient's lifestyle, level of nutrition knowledge, and experiences in planning, purchasing, and preparing food and meals.

A change in eating habits is not easy for most people, and they become discouraged without appropriate recognition of their efforts. Patients should be encouraged to speak freely about problems they are having with food and eating patterns. Furthermore, there may be major life changes that require changes in the meal plan. Job and schedule changes, travel, illness, and other factors all have an impact on the meal plan.

ACUTE COMPLICATIONS

Hypoglycemia and diabetic ketoacidosis are the two most common acute complications related to diabetes.

Hypoglycemia

A low blood glucose, or **hypoglycemia** (or **insulin reaction**), is a common side effect of insulin therapy, although patients taking insulin secretagogues can also be affected. **Autonomic**

symptoms arise from the action of the autonomic nervous system and are often the first signs of mild hypoglycemia. Adrenergic symptoms include shakiness, sweating, palpitations, anxiety, and hunger. **Neuroglycopenic symptoms,** related to an insufficient supply of glucose to the brain, can also occur at similar glucose levels as autonomic symptoms but with different manifestations. The earliest signs of neuroglycopenia include a slowing down in performance and difficulty concentrating and reading. As blood glucose levels drop further, the following symptoms occur: frank mental confusion and disorientation, slurred or rambling speech, irrational or unusual behaviors, extreme fatigue and lethargy, seizures, and unconsciousness. Symptoms differ for different people but tend to be consistent from episode to episode for any one person.

Several common causes of hypoglycemia are listed in Box 30-6. In general, glucose of 70 mg/dl or lower should be treated immediately (Cryer et al., 2003). Treatment of hypoglycemia requires ingestion of glucose or carbohydrate-containing food. Although any carbohydrate will raise glucose levels, glucose is the preferred treatment. Commercially

---

BOX 30-6

Common Causes of Hypoglycemia

Inadvertent or deliberate errors in insulin doses
Excessive insulin or oral secretagogue medications
Improper timing of insulin in relation to food intake
Intensive insulin therapy
Inadequate food intake
Omitted or inadequate meals or snacks
Delayed meals or snacks
Unplanned or increased physical activities or exercise
Prolonged duration or increased intensity of exercise
Alcohol intake without food

Modified from American Diabetes Association: *Medical management of type 1 diabetes*, ed 4, Alexandria, Va, 2004, American Diabetes Association.

BOX 30-7

Treatment of Hypoglycemia

- Immediate treatment with carbohydrates is essential.
  If the blood glucose level falls below 70 mg/dl (3.9 mmol/L), treat with 15 g of carbohydrates, which is equivalent to:
    3 glucose tablets
    Fruit juice or regular soft drinks, ½ c
    Saltine crackers, 6
    Syrup or honey, 1 Tbsp
- Wait 15 minutes and retest. If the blood glucose level remains <70 mg/dl (<3.9 mmol/L), treat with another 15 g of carbohydrates.
- Repeat testing and treatment until the blood glucose level returns to within normal range.
- Evaluate the time to the next meal or snack to determine the need for additional food. If it is more than an hour to the next meal, test again 60 minutes after treatment to see if additional carbohydrates are needed.

Modified from American Diabetes Association: *Medical management of type 1 diabetes*, ed 4, Alexandria, Va, 2004, American Diabetes Association.

---

available glucose tablets have the advantage of being premeasured to help prevent overtreatment. Ingestion of 15 to 20 g of glucose is an effective but temporary treatment. Initial response to treatment should be seen in about 10 to 20 minutes; however, blood glucose should be evaluated again in about 60 minutes because additional treatment may be necessary (Box 30-7). The form of carbohydrates (i.e., liquid or solid) used to treat does not make a difference. If patients are unable to swallow, administration of subcutaneous or intramuscular glucagon may be needed. Parents, roommates, and spouses should be taught how to mix, draw up, and administer glucagon so that they are properly prepared for emergency situations. Kits that include a syringe prefilled with diluting fluid are available.

Self-monitoring of blood glucose is essential for prevention and treatment of hypoglycemia. Changes in insulin injections, eating, exercise schedules, and travel routines warrant increased frequency of monitoring. Some patients experience hypoglycemia unawareness, which means that they do not experience the usual symptoms. Patients need to be reminded of the need to treat hypoglycemia, even in the absence of symptoms.

Hyperglycemia and Diabetic Ketoacidosis

Hyperglycemia can lead to **diabetic ketoacidosis (DKA)**, a life-threatening but reversible complication characterized by severe disturbances in carbohydrate, protein, and fat metabolism. DKA is always the result of inadequate insulin for glucose use. As a result, the body depends on fat for energy, and ketones are formed. Acidosis results from increased production and decreased use of acetoacetic acid and 3-β-hydroxybutyric acid from fatty acids. These ketones spill into the urine; hence the reliance on testing for ketones.

DKA is characterized by elevated blood glucose levels (>250 mg/dl but generally <600 mg/dl) and the presence of ketones in the blood and urine. Symptoms include polyuria, polydipsia, hyperventilation, dehydration, the fruity odor of ketones, and fatigue. SMBG, testing for ketones, and medical intervention can all help prevent DKA. If left untreated, DKA can lead to coma and death. Treatment

includes supplemental insulin, fluid and electrolyte replacement, and medical monitoring. Acute illnesses such as flu, colds, vomiting, and diarrhea, if not managed appropriately, can lead to the development of DKA. Patients need to know the steps to take during acute illness to prevent DKA (Box 30-8). During acute illness, oral ingestion of about 150 to 200 g of carbohydrates per day (45 to 50 g every 3 to 4 hr) should be sufficient, along with medication adjustments, to keep glucose in the goal range and to prevent starvation ketosis (ADA, 2007).

Fasting hyperglycemia is a common finding in persons with diabetes. The amount of insulin required to normalize blood glucose levels during the night is less in the predawn period (from 1:00 to 3:00 AM) than at dawn (4:00 to 8:00 AM). The increased need for insulin at dawn causes a rise in fasting blood glucose levels and is referred to as the **dawn phenomenon**. It may result if insulin levels decline between predawn and dawn or if overnight hepatic glucose output becomes excessive as is common in type 2 diabetes. To identify the dawn phenomenon, blood glucose levels are monitored at bedtime and at 2:00 to 3:00 AM. With the dawn phenomenon, predawn blood glucose levels will be in the low range of normal but not in the hypoglycemic range. For patients with type 2 diabetes, metformin is often used because of its effect on hepatic glucose output. For persons with type 1 diabetes, administering insulin that does not peak at 1:00 to 3:00 AM such as a long-acting insulin should be considered.

Hypoglycemia followed by "rebound" hyperglycemia is called the **Somogyi effect**. This phenomenon originates during hypoglycemia with the secretion of counterregulatory hormones (glucagon, epinephrine, growth hormone, and cortisol) and is usually caused by excessive exogenous

Sick-Day Guidelines for Persons with Diabetes

1. During acute illnesses, usual doses of insulin and other glucose-lowering medications are required. The need for insulin continues, or may even increase, during periods of illness. Fever, dehydration, infection, or the stress of illness can trigger the release of counterregulatory or "stress" hormones, causing blood glucose levels to become elevated.

2. Blood glucose levels and urine or blood testing for ketones should be monitored at least four times daily (before each meal and at bedtime). Blood glucose readings exceeding 250 mg/dl and the presence of ketones are danger signals indicating that additional insulin is needed.

3. Ample amounts of liquid need to be consumed every hour. If vomiting, diarrhea, or fever is present, small sips—1 or 2 Tbsp every 15 to 30 min—can usually be consumed. If vomiting continues and the individual is unable to take fluids for longer than 4 hr, the health care team should be notified.

4. If regular foods are not tolerated, liquid or soft carbohydrate-containing foods (such as regular soft drinks, soup, juices, and ice cream) should be eaten. Eating about 10 to 15 g of carbohydrate every 1-2 hr is usually sufficient.

5. The health care team should be called if illness continues for more than 1 day.

Modified from American Diabetes Association: *Medical management of type 1 diabetes*, ed 4, Alexandria, Va, 2004, American Diabetes Association.

insulin doses. Hepatic glucose production is stimulated, thus raising blood glucose levels. If rebound hyperglycemia goes unrecognized and insulin doses are increased, a cycle of overinsulinization may result. Decreasing evening insulin doses or, as for the dawn phenomenon, taking a long-acting insulin should be considered.

LONG-TERM COMPLICATIONS

Long-term complications of diabetes include macrovascular diseases, microvascular diseases, and neuropathy. **Macrovascular diseases** involve diseases of large blood vessels; **microvascular diseases** associated with diabetes involve the small blood vessels and include nephropathy and retinopathy. In contrast, diabetic neuropathy is a condition characterized by damage to the nerves.

MNT is important in managing several long-term complications of diabetes. Nutrition therapy is also a major component in reducing risk factors for chronic complications, especially those related to macrovascular disease. The DCCT and the UKPDS provided convincing evidence for the relationship between glycemic control and decreased risk of microvascular complications (DCCT Research Group, 1993; UKPDSG, 1998a), and between type 1 diabetes, and macrovascular disease (DCCT Research Group, 2005). Blood pressure control also benefited.

Macrovascular Diseases

Insulin resistance, which may precede the development of type 2 diabetes and macrovascular disease by many years, induces numerous metabolic changes known as the **metabolic syndrome** or the insulin resistance syndrome (see Chapters 9 and 32). It is characterized by intraabdominal obesity or the android distribution of adipose tissue (waist circumference greater than 102 cm [>40 in] in men and greater than 88 cm [>35 in] in women) and is associated with dyslipidemia, hypertension, glucose intolerance, and increased prevalence of macrovascular complications. Other risk factors include genetics, smoking, sedentary lifestyle, high-fat diet, renal failure, and microalbuminuria.

Macrovascular diseases, including coronary heart disease (CHD), peripheral vascular disease (PVD), and cerebrovascular disease are more common, tend to occur at an earlier age, and are more extensive and severe in people with diabetes. Furthermore, in women with diabetes the increased risk of mortality from heart disease is greater than in men, in contrast to the nondiabetic population, in which heart disease mortality is greater in men than in women (ADA, 2001). Diabetes itself has been elevated from a risk factor for cerebrovascular disease to a CHD risk equivalent in the National Cholesterol Education Panel Adult Treatment Program III (NCEP ATP III, 2001).

Dyslipidemia

Patients with diabetes have an increased prevalence of lipid abnormalities that contributes to higher rates of CVD. In type 2 diabetes the prevalence of an elevated cholesterol level is about 28% to 34%, and about 5% to 14% of patients with type 2 diabetes have high triglyceride levels; also, lower HDL cholesterol levels are common. Furthermore, patients with type 2 diabetes typically have smaller, denser LDL particles, which increase atherogenicity even if the total LDL cholesterol level is not significantly elevated. Lifestyle intervention, including MNT, increased physical activity, weight loss, and smoking cessation should always be implemented. MNT should focus on the reduction of saturated and *trans*-fatty acids and cholesterol.

Primary therapy is directed first at lowering LDL cholesterol levels with the goal in individuals without overt CVD of reducing LDL cholesterol concentrations to less than 100 mg/dl (2.6 mmol/L). In individuals with overt CVD a lower LDL cholesterol goal of less than 70 mg/dl (1.8 mmol/L) is suggested (ADA, 2006b). Pharmacologic therapy with a statin (HMG-CoA reductase inhibitors) is indicated if there is an inadequate response to lifestyle modifications and improved glucose control. For LDL lowering, statins are the drugs of choice with the goal being to achieve an LDL reduction of 30% to 40%. In addition, if the HDL cholesterol is less than 40 mg/dl, a fibric acid derivative or niacin might be used (ADA, 2006b). Combination therapy using statins and other lipid-lowering agents may be necessary to achieve lipid targets. Aspirin therapy should be used in all adult patients with diabetes and macrovascular disease and for primary prevention in patients 40 years of age or older with diabetes and one or more cardiovascular risk factors (ADA, 2006b) (see Chapter 32).

Medical Nutrition Therapy for Dyslipidemia. Studies in persons with diabetes demonstrating the effects of specific percentages of dietary saturated and *trans*-fatty acids and specific amounts of dietary cholesterol at risk for coronary heart disease are not available. In nondiabetic individuals, reducing saturated and *trans*-fatty acids and cholesterol intake decreases total and LDL cholesterol but may also reduce HDL cholesterol. However, importantly, the ratio of LDL to HDL cholesterol is not adversely affected. The most recent guidelines from the National Cholesterol Education Program recommend that total fat be 25% to 35% of total calories and saturated fat less than 7%. Intake of *trans*-fat should be minimized (NCEP ATP III, 2001). Either monounsaturated or polyunsaturated fats may be substituted for saturated fats.

Individuals with triglyceride measurements of 1000 mg/dl should restrict all types of dietary fat (except omega-3 fatty acids) and be treated with medication to reduce triglycerides. Supplementation with omega-3 fatty acids may benefit those with resistant hypertriglyceridemia (ADA, 2007).

Hypertension

Hypertension is a common comorbidity of diabetes, with about 73% of adults with diabetes having blood pressure of 130/80 mm Hg or higher or using prescription medications for hypertension (Centers for Disease Control and Prevention, 2005). Treatment of hypertension in persons with diabetes should also be vigorous to reduce the risk of macrovascular and microvascular disease. Blood pressure should be measured at every routine visit with a goal for blood pressure control of less than 130/80 mm Hg. Patients with systolic blood pressure of 130 to 139 mm Hg or a diastolic blood pressure of 80 to 89 mm Hg should be given MNT for hypertension (see Chapter 33) for a maximum of 3 months. If targets are not achieved, they should also be treated with pharmacologic agents that block the renin-angiotensin system. Patients with a systolic blood pressure of 140 mm Hg or greater or a diastolic pressure of 90 mm Hg or greater should receive drug therapy in addition to MNT. Lowering of blood pressure with antihypertensive drugs, including angiotensin-converting enzyme (ACE) inhibition, angiotensin receptor blockers (ARBs), β-blockers, diuretics, and calcium channel blockers, has been shown to be effective in reducing the number of cardiovascular events. Multiple drug therapy (two or more agents at proper doses) is generally needed to achieve blood pressure targets (ADA, 2006b). See Chapter 33 for MNT for hypertension.

Microvascular Diseases

Nephropathy

In the United States and Europe diabetic nephropathy has become the most common single cause of end-stage renal disease (ESRD) and accounts for about 40% of new cases of ESRD. About 20% to 40% of patients with diabetes develop evidence of nephropathy, but in type 2 diabetes a considerably smaller number progress to ESRD. However, because of the much greater prevalence of type 2 diabetes, such patients constitute over half of the patients with diabetes currently starting on dialysis (ADA, 2004d).

The earliest clinical evidence of nephropathy is the appearance of low but abnormal urine albumin levels (30 to 299 mg/24 hr), referred to as *microalbuminuria* or *incipient nephropathy*. Microalbuminuria is also a marker of increased cardiovascular disease risk. Without specific interventions, progression to overt nephropathy or clinical albuminuria (≥300 mg/24 hr) occurs over a period of years. An annual screening for microalbuminuria should be performed in patients who have had type 1 diabetes for more than 5 years and in all patients with type 2 diabetes starting at diagnosis and during pregnancy (ADA, 2006b). An analysis of a spot urine sample for the albumin-to-creatinine ratio is the preferred method. Two of three tests within a 6-month period should be abnormal before a patient is designated as having microalbuminuria. Table 30-13 defines abnormalities in albumin excretion based on spot urine collections.

Although diabetic nephropathy cannot be cured, persuasive data indicate that the clinical course of the disease can be modified. To reduce the risk or slow the progression of nephropathy, glucose and blood pressure control should be optimized. In the treatment of both microalbuminuria and macroalbuminuria, either ACE inhibitors or ARBs should be used except during pregnancy. Although there are no adequate head-to-head comparisons of the two drugs, evidence supports the following. In patients with type 1 diabetes, with hypertension and any degree of albuminuria, ACE

TABLE 30-13

Definitions of Abnormalities in Urine Albumin Excretion

Category	Spot Collection (mcg/mg Creatinine)
Normal	<30
Microalbuminuria	30–299
Macroalbuminuria	≥300

Exercise within 24 hr, infection, fever, coronary heart failure, marked hyperglycemia, and marked hypertension may elevate urinary albumin excretion over baseline values.

Modified from American Diabetes Association: Standards of medical care in diabetes—2007, *Diabetes Care* 30:54, 2007.

inhibitors delay the progression of nephropathy. In patients with type 2 diabetes, hypertension, microalbuminuria, and renal insufficiency, ARBs delay the progression of nephropathy. If one class is not tolerated, the other should be substituted, and their combination will decrease albuminuria more than use of either agent alone (ADA, 2006b).

Medical Nutrition Therapy for Nephropathy. Research on low-protein diets delaying the progression of renal disease has been controversial. The role of MNT in glucose and blood pressure control is clearly the first priority. However, there is some evidence that, once albuminuria is present, there may be beneficial effects for renal function with a reduction of protein to 0.8 to 1 g/kg of body weight per day (Franz and Wheeler, 2003). Several studies that attempted to reduce protein intake in persons with type 1 or type 2 diabetes and microalbuminuria achieved a protein reduction to about 1 g/kg of body weight. In a dose-response analysis (Pijls et al., 1999), a 0.1 g/kg of body weight per day decrease in the intake of protein was related to an improvement of 11.1% in albuminuria. In studies conducted in subjects with type 1 diabetes and macroalbuminuria (overt nephropathy), the achieved protein restriction ranged from 0.7 g/kg to 0.9 g/kg body weight daily, and slowed the rate of decline in the GFR significantly over 32 to 35 months (Zeller et al., 1991). However, one study raised concern that too low a protein intake may cause malnutrition (Meloni et al., 2002). Therefore protein must be reduced in the context of overall adequate energy and nutrient intake. In microalbuminuria there may be additional benefits in lowering phosphorus to 500 to 1000 mg/day along with the low-protein diet (Zeller et al., 1991). Although several studies have explored the potential of plant versus animal protein, the data are inconclusive (Wheeler et al., 2002). Despite the controversy, reduction of protein intake to 0.8 to 1 g/kg of body weight per day in individuals with diabetes and the earlier stages of chronic kidney disease (CKD) and to 0.8 g/kg of body weight per day in the later stages of CKD may improve measures of renal function such as urine albumin excretion rate and glomerular filtration rate (ADA, 2007) (see Chapter 36).

Retinopathy

Diabetic retinopathy is estimated to be the most frequent cause of new cases of blindness among adults 20 to 74 years of age. After 20 years of diabetes, nearly all patients with type 1 diabetes and more than 60% of patients with type 2 diabetes have some degree of retinopathy (ADA, 2004e). Laser photocoagulation surgery can reduce the risk of further vision loss but usually does not restore lost vision—thus the importance for a screening program to detect diabetic retinopathy. Adults and adolescents with type 1 diabetes should have an initial dilated and comprehensive eye examination by an ophthalmologist or optometrist within 3 to 5 years after the onset of diabetes and patients with type 2 diabetes should be examined shortly after the diagnosis of diabetes. Subsequent examinations for both groups should be done annually. Less frequent examinations may be considered (every 2 to 3 years) if the eye examination is normal (ADA, 2006b).

There are three stages of diabetic retinopathy. The early stage of nonproliferative diabetic retinopathy (NPDR) is characterized by microaneurysms, a pouchlike dilation of a terminal capillary, lesions that include cotton-wool spots (also referred to as soft exudates), and the formation of new blood vessels as a result of the great metabolic need of the retina for oxygen and other nutrients supplied by the bloodstream. As the disease progresses to the middle stages of moderate, severe, and very severe NPDR, gradual loss of the retinal microvasculature occurs, resulting in retinal ischemia. Extensive intraretinal hemorrhages and microaneurysms are common reflections of increasing retinal nonperfusion.

The most advanced stage, termed *proliferative diabetic retinopathy (PDR)*, is the final and most vision-threatening stage of diabetic retinopathy. It is characterized by the onset of ischemia-induced new vessel proliferation at the optic disk or elsewhere in the retina. The new vessels are fragile and prone to bleeding, resulting in vitreous hemorrhage. With time the neovascularization tends to undergo fibrosis and contraction, resulting in retinal traction, retinal tears, vitreous hemorrhage, and retinal detachment. Diabetic macular edema, which involves thickening of the central (macular) portion of the retina, and glaucoma, in which fibrous scar tissue increases intraocular pressure, are other clinical findings in retinopathy.

Neuropathy

Chronic high levels of blood glucose are also associated with nerve damage and affect 60% to 70% of patients with both type 1 and type 2 diabetes (ADA, 2001). Peripheral neuropathy usually affects the nerves that control sensation in the feet and hands. Autonomic neuropathy affects nerve function controlling various organ systems. Cardiovascular effects include postural hypotension and decreased responsiveness to cardiac nerve impulses, leading to painless or silent ischemic heart disease. Sexual function may be affected, with impotence the most common manifestation. Damage to nerves innervating the gastrointestinal tract can cause a variety of problems. Neuropathy can be manifested in the esophagus as nausea and esophagitis, in the stomach as unpredictable emptying, in the small bowel as loss of nutrients, and in the large bowel as diarrhea or constipation. Intensive treatment of hyperglycemia reduces the risk of developing diabetic neuropathy.

Medical Nutrition Therapy for Gastroparesis. **Gastroparesis** (impaired gastric motility) affects about 25% of this population and is perhaps the most frustrating condition that patients and RDs experience. It results in delayed or irregular contractions of the stomach, leading to various gastrointestinal symptoms such as feelings of fullness, bloating, nausea, vomiting, diarrhea, or constipation. Gastroparesis should be suspected in individuals with erratic glucose control. The first step in management of patients with neuropathy should be to aim for stable and optimal glycemic control.

Treatment involves minimizing abdominal stress. Small, frequent meals may be better tolerated than three full meals a day; and these meals should be low in fiber and fat. If solid foods are not well tolerated, liquid meals may need to be recommended. As much as possible, the timing of insulin administration should be adjusted to match the usually delayed nutrient absorption. Insulin injections may even be required after eating. Frequent blood glucose monitoring is important to determine appropriate insulin therapy.

HYPOGLYCEMIA OF NONDIABETIC ORIGIN

Hypoglycemia of nondiabetic origin has been defined as a clinical syndrome with diverse causes in which low levels of plasma glucose eventually lead to neuroglycopenia (Service, 1995). Hypoglycemia literally means low (hypo) blood glucose (glycemia). Normally the body is remarkably adept at maintaining fairly steady blood glucose levels—usually between 60 and 100 mg/dl (3.3 to 5.6 mmol/L), despite the intermittent ingestion of food. Maintaining normal levels of glucose is important because body cells, especially the brain and central nervous system, must have a steady and consistent supply of glucose to function properly. Under physiologic conditions the brain depends almost exclusively on glucose for its energy needs. Even with hunger, either because it is many hours since food was eaten or because the last meal was small, blood glucose levels remain fairly consistent.

Pathophysiology

However, in a small number of people blood glucose levels become too low. Symptoms of hypoglycemia are often felt when blood glucose is below 65 mg/dl (3.6 mmol/L). If the brain and nervous system are deprived of the glucose they need to function, symptoms such as sweating, shaking, weakness, hunger, headaches, and irritability can develop. Hypoglycemia can be difficult to diagnose because these typical symptoms can be caused by many different health problems besides hypoglycemia. For example, adrenaline (epinephrine) released as a result of anxiety and stress can trigger the symptoms of hypoglycemia.

The only way to determine whether hypoglycemia is causing these symptoms is to measure blood glucose levels while an individual is experiencing the symptoms (Brun et al., 2000). Therefore hypoglycemia can best be defined by the presence of three features known as **Whipple's triad:** (1) a low plasma or blood glucose level; (2) symptoms of hypoglycemia at the same time as the low blood glucose values; and (3) amelioration of the symptoms by correction of the hypoglycemia (Prince, 1997).

A fairly steady blood glucose level is maintained by the interaction of several mechanisms. After eating, food is broken down into glucose and enters the bloodstream. As blood glucose levels rise, the pancreas responds by releasing the hormone insulin, which allows glucose to leave the bloodstream and enter various body cells, where it fuels the body's activities. Glucose is also taken up by the liver and stored as glycogen for later use. When glucose concentrations from the last meal decline, the body goes from a "fed" to a "fasting" state. Insulin levels decrease, which keeps the blood glucose levels from falling too low. In addition, stored glucose is released from the liver back into the bloodstream with the help of **glucagon,** a hormone that is also released from the pancreas. Normally the body's ability to balance glucose, insulin, and glucagon (and other counterregulatory hormones) keeps glucose levels within the normal range. Glucagon provides the primary defense against hypoglycemia; without it full recovery does not occur. Epinephrine is not necessary for counterregulation when glucagon is present. However, in the absence of glucagon, epinephrine has an important role. Symptoms of hypoglycemia have been recognized at plasma glucose levels of about 60 mg/dl, and impaired brain function has occurred at levels of about 50 mg/dl (Cryer, 2003).

Types of Hypoglycemia

If blood glucose levels fall below normal limits within 2 to 5 hours after eating, this is often referred to as reactive hypoglycemia (named because the body is reacting to food) or **postprandial (reactive) hypoglycemia.** Postprandial hypoglycemia can be caused by an exaggerated or late insulin response caused by either insulin resistance or elevated GLP-1; alimentary hyperinsulinism; renal glycosuria; defects in glucagon response; high insulin sensitivity; rare syndromes such as hereditary fructose intolerance, galactosemia, leucine sensitivity; or a rare β-cell pancreatic tumor (insulinoma), causing blood glucose levels to drop too low (Brun et al., 2000).

Alimentary hyperinsulinism is the most common type of documented postprandial hypoglycemia and is seen in patients who have undergone gastric surgery or some other type of gastric surgery (Gebhard et al., 2001) (see Chapter 26). These procedures are associated with rapid delivery of food to the small intestine, rapid absorption of glucose, and exaggerated insulin response. These patients respond best to multiple, frequent feedings (Prince, 1997). α-Glucosidase inhibitors such as acarbose may also be helpful because they decrease the absorption of carbohydrates (Hasler, 2002).

The ingestion of alcohol after a prolonged fast or the ingestion of large amounts of alcohol and carbohydrates on an empty stomach ("gin-and-tonic" syndrome) may also cause hypoglycemia within 3 to 4 hours in some healthy persons.

Idiopathic reactive hypoglycemia is characterized by normal insulin secretion but increased insulin sensitivity and, to some extent, reduced response of glucagon to acute hypoglycemia symptoms (Brun et al., 2000). The increase in insulin sensitivity associated with a deficiency of glucagon secretion leads to hypoglycemia late postprandially (Leonetti et al., 1996). Idiopathic reactive hypoglycemia has been inappropriately overdiagnosed by both physicians and patients, to the point that some physicians doubt its existence. Although rare, it does exist but can be documented only in persons with hypoglycemia that occurs spontaneously and who meet the criteria of Whipple's triad.

Fasting (food-deprived) hypoglycemia may occur in response to having gone without food for 8 hours or longer and can be caused by certain conditions that upset the body's ability to balance blood glucose. These include eating disorders and other serious underlying medical conditions, including hormone deficiency states (e.g., hypopituitarism, adrenal insufficiency, catecholamine or glucagon deficiency), acquired liver disease, renal disease, certain drugs (e.g., alcohol, propranolol, salicylate), insulinoma (of which most are benign, but 6% to 10% can be malignant), and other nonpancreatic tumors. Taking high doses of aspirin may also lead to fasting hypoglycemia. Factitious hypoglycemia, or self-administration of insulin or sulfonylurea in persons who do not have diabetes, is a common cause as well (Prince, 1997). Symptoms related to fasting hypoglycemia tend to be particularly severe and can include a loss of mental acuity, seizures, and unconsciousness. If the underlying problem can be resolved, hypoglycemia is no longer a problem.

Diagnostic Criteria

One of the criteria used to confirm the presence of hypoglycemia is a blood glucose level of less than 50 mg/dl (<2.8 mmol/L). Previously the OGT test was the standard test for this condition; however, this test is not helpful because it involves a nonphysiologic stimulus and because results show little correlation with persons who later are documented to have hypoglycemia. Recording finger stick blood glucose measurements during spontaneously occurring symptomatic episodes at home is a method that is often used to establish the diagnosis. An alternative method is to perform a glucose test in a medical office setting, in which case the patient is given a typical meal that has been documented in the past to lead to symptomatic episodes; Whipple's triad can be confirmed if symptoms occur. If blood glucose levels are low during the symptomatic period and if the symptoms disappear on eating, hypoglycemia is probably responsible. It is essential to make a correct diagnosis in patients with fasting hypoglycemia because the implications for therapy are serious.

Management of Hypoglycemia

The management of hypoglycemic disorders involves two distinct components: (1) relief of neuroglycopenic symptoms by restoring blood glucose concentrations to the normal range, and (2) correction of the underlying cause. The immediate treatment is to eat foods or beverages containing carbohydrates. As the glucose from the breakdown of carbohydrates is absorbed into the bloodstream, it increases the level of glucose in the blood and relieves the symptoms. If an underlying problem is causing hypoglycemia, appropriate treatment of this disease or disorder is essential.

Almost no research has been done to determine what type of food-related treatment is best for the prevention of hypoglycemia. Traditional advice has been to avoid foods containing sugars and to eat protein- and fat-containing foods. Recent research on the GI and sugars has raised ques-

tions about the appropriateness of restricting only sugars because these foods have been reported to have a lower GI than many of the starches that were encouraged in the past. Restriction of sugars may contribute to a decreased intake in total carbohydrates, which may be more important than the source of the carbohydrates.

Guidelines for the prevention of hypoglycemia have been published (International Diabetes Center, 2004). The goal of treatment is to adopt eating habits that will keep blood glucose levels as static as possible. To stay symptom free, it is important for individuals to eat five to six small meals or snacks per day. Doing this provides manageable amounts of glucose to the body. Spreading carbohydrates throughout the day; eating consistent amounts of carbohydrates, particularly high-fiber carbohydrates, at meals and snacks from day to day; and avoiding skipping meals can also be helpful. Recommended guidelines are listed in Box 30-9.

BOX 30-9

Guidelines for Preventing Hypoglycemic Symptoms

1. Eat small meals, with snacks interspersed between meals and at bedtime. This means eating five to six small meals rather than two to three large meals to steady the release of glucose into the bloodstream.
2. Spread the intake of carbohydrate foods throughout the day. Eating large amounts of carbohydrates at one time produces increased amounts of glucose and stimulates the release of increased amounts of insulin, which can cause blood glucose levels to drop. Most individuals can eat two to four servings of carbohydrate foods at each meal and one to two servings at each snack. If carbohydrates are removed from the diet completely, the body loses its ability to handle carbohydrates properly, so this is not recommended. Carbohydrate foods include starches, fruits and fruit juices, milk and yogurt, and foods containing sugar.
3. Avoid foods that contain large amounts of carbohydrates. Examples of these foods are regular soft drinks, syrups, candy, fruit juices, regular fruited yogurts, pies, and cakes.
4. Avoid beverages and foods containing caffeine. Caffeine can cause the same symptoms as hypoglycemia and make the individual feel worse.
5. Limit or avoid alcoholic beverages. Drinking alcohol on an empty stomach and without food can lower blood glucose levels by interfering with the liver's ability to release stored glucose (gluconeogenesis). If an individual chooses to drink alcohol, it should be done in moderation (one or two drinks no more than twice a week), and food should always be eaten along with the alcoholic beverage.

Modified from International Diabetes Center: *Reactive and fasting hypoglycemia*, Minneapolis, 2004, International Diabetes Center.

Patients with hypoglycemia may also benefit from learning carbohydrate counting and, to prevent hypoglycemia, eating three to four carbohydrate servings (15 g of carbohydrate per serving) at meals and one to two for snacks (see Appendix 34). Foods containing protein that are also low in saturated fat can be eaten at meals or with snacks. These foods would be expected to have minimum effect on blood glucose levels and can add extra food for satiety and calories. However, because both protein and carbohydrate stimulate insulin release, a moderate intake may be advisable.

⊛ FOCAL POINTS

- Nutrition therapy is a challenging but essential aspect of the management of diabetes and hypoglycemia of nondiabetic origin.
- Attention to nutrition and food and meal-planning principles is essential for metabolic (glucose, lipids, and blood pressure) control and overall good health.
- An RD who is knowledgeable and skilled in implementing current nutrition principles and making recommendations for diabetes or hypoglycemia of nondiabetic origin is the medical team member who should plan, implement, and evaluate MNT and the nutrition care process.
- Effective education and counseling of the person with diabetes will lead to his or her becoming a team player in management of his or her blood glucose.
- The effectiveness of nutrition interventions need to be continually monitored and documented to promote the best possible outcomes.

⊛ CLINICAL SCENARIO 1

Type 1 Diabetes

Ellen is a 15-year-old girl with newly diagnosed type 1 diabetes referred for diabetes nutrition education. She is 5 ft 2 in tall, weighs 115 lb, and is active in cheerleading and basketball in high school. Her physician will be regulating the dosage and timing of her insulin regimen. Her grandmother has diabetes and is supportive of Ellen's need for education. Ellen's parents are divorced, and she now lives with her grandmother.

***Nutrition Diagnosis:** Food- and nutrition-related knowledge deficit related to adjustment of meals and insulin as evidenced by new diagnosis of type 1 diabetes mellitus

1. What assessment information do you need to determine a nutrition diagnosis?
2. Write a nutrition diagnosis for Ellen.
3. What meal planning system would be helpful for Ellen?
4. What guidance should you offer regarding Ellen's sports activities?
5. What signs and symptoms of lack of diabetes control must Ellen understand to manage her disease? Which problem is she more likely to experience—hyperglycemia or hypoglycemia?
6. What food- and meal-planning information needs to be shared with the health care team as insulin therapy is integrated into Ellen's normal eating and exercise habits?
7. How will you monitor and evaluate Ellen's progress?

✵ CLINICAL SCENARIO 2

Debra is a 45-year-old woman with a known diagnosis of type 2 diabetes for 3 years referred for nutrition counseling. She has not had a medical check-up for 2 years. She returns at this time with a primary complaint of chronic fatigue. Her laboratory test results show the following: A1C 8.3%; serum cholesterol 214 mg/dl; triglycerides 275 mg/dl. Her current weight is 175 lb, and her height is 64 in (BMI = 30). She states she hasn't returned for any follow-up visits because the only advice she gets is to lose weight and not to eat sugar, neither of which she is able to do.

✳**Nutrition Diagnosis 1:**   Not ready for diet/lifestyle change related to no change in weight or laboratory values as evidenced by patient statements that she cannot lose weight or refrain from eating sugar

✳**Nutrition Diagnosis 2:**   Overweight/obesity related to no change in diet habits as evidenced by BMI of 30 for past 3 years

1. What assessment information do you need to determine a nutrition diagnosis?
2. Write a nutrition diagnosis for Debra.
3. What advice will you offer to improve Debra's metabolic parameters and, in particular, to improve her blood glucose control?
4. What meal-planning method do you suggest for her?
5. What guidelines for carbohydrate intake can help Debra improve her glycemia?
6. What suggestions will you have about fat intake?
7. What information will you share about exercise?
8. What will you recommend regarding her sugar intake?
9. How will you monitor and evaluate Debra's progress?

✵ CLINICAL SCENARIO 3

John is a moderately obese (BMI = 29) 49-year-old man who complains of increased thirst, polyuria, and fatigue referred for nutrition counseling. His family history includes his mother and an older brother with type 2 diabetes. A random (casual) plasma glucose test shows a level of 480 mg/dl. His serum electrolyte level and anion gap are normal.

He reports finding it difficult to control his eating during the evening and, because of his long working hours, finds it difficult to work in an hour for exercise most days. When asked what he is interested in learning about, he replies that he would like to learn how to control his eating because he is always hungry.

✳**Nutrition Diagnosis 1:**   Food- and nutrition-related knowledge deficit related to appropriate diet for management of type 2 diabetes mellitus and moderate obesity as evidenced by self-reports of "constant hunger"

✳**Nutrition Diagnosis 2:**   Physical inactivity related to perceived lack of time to exercise as evidenced by patient reports

1. What assessment data do you need to determine a nutrition diagnosis?
2. Write a nutrition diagnosis for John.
3. What type of diabetes does John likely have? Is it likely to be controlled by nutrition therapy alone?
3. Given his degree of hyperglycemia, is it more likely that an oral agent or insulin therapy will be recommended?
4. What meal planning approach would be helpful for John?
5. What advice can you give to John to help him with his eating problems?
6. What other lifestyle strategies will be helpful?
7. How will you monitor and evaluate John's progress?

USEFUL WEBSITES

American Association of Diabetes Educators
www.aadenet.org

American Diabetes Association
www.diabetes.org (patient information, programs, and professional education)
www.diabetes.org/cpr (ADA clinical practice guidelines)
www.diabetes.org/recognition/education (Nationwide ADA-recognized patient education programs)
www.diabetes.org/MakeTheLink (Diabetes-Cardiovascular Disease Toolkit)

American Dietetic Association, Diabetes Care and Education Practice Group
www.dce.org

Children With Diabetes
www.childrenwithdiabetes.com

Coverage for Medical Nutrition Therapy
www.eatright.org/gov/reimbursement.html

International Diabetes Center, Minneapolis, Minnesota
www.idcdiabetes.org

Joslin Diabetes Center
www.joslin.harvard.edu

Lifestyle Manuals Used in the Diabetes Prevention Program
www.bsc.gwu.edu/dpp

National Diabetes Education Program
www.ndep.nih.gov

National Institute of Diabetes and Digestive Kidney Diseases
www.niddk.nih.gov

References

American Diabetes Association: Type 2 diabetes in children and adolescents (Consensus Statement), *Diabetes Care* 23:381, 2000.

American Diabetes Association: *Diabetes 2001 vital statistics*, Alexandria, Va, 2001, American Diabetes Association.

American Diabetes Association: Economic costs of diabetes in the U.S. in 2002, *Diabetes Care* 26:917, 2003a.

American Diabetes Association: Management of dyslipidemia in children and adolescents with diabetes (Consensus Statement), *Diabetes Care* 26:2194, 2003b.

American Diabetes Association: Physical activity/exercise (Position Statement), *Diabetes Care* 27(suppl 1):S58, 2004a.

American Diabetes Association: Tests of glycemia in diabetes (Position Statement), *Diabetes Care* 27(suppl 1):S91, 2004b.

American Diabetes Association: Gestational diabetes mellitus (Position Statement), *Diabetes Care* 27(suppl 1):S88, 2004c.

American Diabetes Association: Diabetic nephropathy (Position Statement), *Diabetes Care* 27(suppl 1):S79, 2004d.

American Diabetes Association: Diabetic retinopathy (Position Statement), *Diabetes Care* 27(suppl 1):S84, 2004e.

American Diabetes Association: Diagnosis and classification of diabetes mellitus (Position Statement), *Diabetes Care* 29(suppl 1):S43, 2006a.

American Diabetes Association: Standards of medical care in diabetes—2006 (Position Statement), *Diabetes Care* 29(suppl 1): S4, 2006b.

American Diabetes Association: Nutrition recommendations and interventions for diabetes (Position Statement), *Diabetes Care* 30:S48, 2007.

Anderson RA et al: Beneficial effects of chromium for people with diabetes, *Diabetes* 46:1786, 1997.

Bantle JP et al: Effects of dietary fructose on plasma lipids in healthy subjects, *Am J Clin Nutr* 72:1128, 2000.

Bergman RN, Adler M: Free fatty acids and pathogenesis of type 2 diabetes mellitus, *Trends Endocrinol Metabol* 11:351, 2000.

Bode BW, editor: *Medical management of type 1 diabetes*, ed 4, Alexandria, Va, 2004, American Diabetes Association.

Bode BW, Strange P: Efficacy, safety, and pump compatibility of insulin aspart use in continuous subcutaneous insulin infusion therapy in patients with type 1 diabetes, *Diabetes Care* 24:69, 2001.

Boulé NG et al: Effects of exercise on glycemic control and body mass index in type 2 diabetes: a meta-analysis of controlled clinical trials, *JAMA* 286:1218, 2001.

Brand-Miller J et al: Low-glycemic index diets in the management of diabetes: a meta-analysis of randomized controlled trials, *Diabetes Care* 26:2261, 2003.

Brinkworth GE et al: Long-term effects of a high-protein, low-carbohydrate diet on weight control and cardiovascular risk markers in obese hyperinsulinemic subjects, *Int J Obes* 28:661, 2004.

Brun JF et al: Postprandial reactive hypoglycemia, *Diabetes Metabol* 26:337, 2000.

Buchanan TA et al: Preservation of pancreatic beta-cell function and prevention of type 2 diabetes by pharmacological treatment of insulin resistance in high-risk Hispanic women, *Diabetes Care* 51:2796, 2002.

Buse JB et al: Amylin replacement with pramlintide in type 1 and type 2 diabetes: a physiologic approach to overcome barriers with insulin therapy, *Clin Diabetes* 20:137, 2002.

Butchko HH, Stargel WW: Aspartame: scientific evaluation in the postmarketing period, *Regul Toxicol Pharmacol* 34:221, 2001.

Centers for Disease Control and Prevention: *National diabetes fact sheet: general information and national estimates on diabetes in the United States, 2005*, Atlanta, Ga, 2005, U.S. Department of Health and Human Services, Centers for Disease Control and Prevention.

Chandalia M et al: Beneficial effects of a high dietary fiber intake in patients with type 2 diabetes, *N Engl J Med* 342:1392, 2000.

Cheng N et al: Follow-up survey of people in China with type 2 diabetes mellitus consuming supplemental chromium, *J Trace Elem Exp Med Biol* 12:55, 1999.

Chiasson J-L et al: Acarbose for prevention of type 2 diabetes: the STOP-NIDDM randomized trial, *Lancet* 359:2072, 2002.

Chobanian AV et al: Seventh Report of the Joint National Committee on Prevention, Detection, Evaluation, and Treatment of High Blood Pressure: the JNC 7 report, *JAMA* 289:2560, 2003.

Church TS et al: Exercise capacity and body composition as predictors of mortality among men with diabetes, *Diabetes Care* 27:83, 2004.

Crapo PA et al: Postprandial glucose and insulin responses to different complex carbohydrates, *Diabetes* 26:1178, 1977.

Cryer PE et al: Hypoglycemia in diabetes (technical review), *Diabetes Care* 26:1902, 2003.

Curioni CC et al: Long-term weight loss after diet and exercise: a systematic review, *Int J Obes* 29:1153, 2005.

Davies MJ et al: Effects of moderate alcohol intake on fasting insulin and glucose concentrations and insulin sensitivity in postmenopausal women: a randomized controlled trial, *JAMA* 287:2559, 2002.

DAFNE Study Group: Training in flexible, intensive insulin management to enable dietary freedom in people with type 1 diabetes: dose adjusted for normal eating (DAFNE) randomized controlled trial, *Br Med J* 325:746, 2002.

Davis SN et al: Effects of antecedent hypoglycemia on subsequent counterregulatory responses to exercise, *Diabetes* 49:73, 2000.

Delahanty LM, Halford BN: The role of diet behaviors in achieving improved glycemic control in intensively treated patients in the Diabetes Control and Complications Trial, *Diabetes Care* 16:1453, 1993.

Diabetes Control and Complications Trial Research Group: The effect of intensive treatment of diabetes on the development and progression of long-term complications in insulin-dependent diabetes mellitus, *N Engl J Med* 339:977, 1993.

Diabetes Control and Complications Trial/Epidemiology of Diabetes Interventions and Complications (DCCT/EDIC) Study Research Group: Intensive diabetes treatment and cardiovascular disease in patients with type 1 diabetes, *N Engl J Med* 353:2643, 2005.

Diabetes Prevention Program Research Group: Reduction in the incidence of type 2 diabetes with lifestyle intervention or metformin, *N Engl J Med* 346:393, 2002.

Dietary Guidelines Advisory Committee: *Dietary guidelines for Americans 2005*, www.health.gov/dietaryguidelines, accessed September 2005.

Douketis JD et al: Systematic review of long-term weight loss studies in obese adults: clinical significance and applicability to clinical practice, *Int J Obes* 29:1168, 2005.

Duncan GE et al: Exercise training without weight loss increases insulin sensitivity and postheparin plasma lipase activity in previously sedentary adults, *Diabetes Care* 26:557, 2003.

Fernandes G et al: Glycemic index of potatoes commonly consumed in North America, *J Am Diet Assoc* 105:557, 2005.

Foster-Powell K et al: International table of glycemic index and glycemic load values: 2002, *Am J Clin Nutr* 76:5, 2002.

Franz MJ: Nutrition, physical activity, and diabetes. In Ruderman N, editor: *Handbook of exercise in diabetes*, Alexandria, Va, 2002, American Diabetes Association.

Franz MJ: The glycemic index: not the most effective nutrition therapy intervention, *Diabetes Care* 26:2466, 2003.

Franz MJ and Wheeler ML: Nutrition therapy for diabetic nephropathy, *Curr Diab Rep* 3:412, 2003.

Franz MJ et al: Nutrition practice guidelines and basic care by dietitians for persons with noninsulin-dependent diabetes mellitus: medical and clinical outcomes, *J Am Diet Assoc* 95:1009, 1995.

Franz MJ et al: Nutrition principles for the management of diabetes and related complications (technical review), *Diabetes Care* 17:490, 1994.

Franz MJ et al: Evidence-based nutrition principles and recommendations for treatment and prevention of diabetes and related complications (technical review), *Diabetes Care* 25:148, 2002a.

Franz MJ et al: *Implementing group and individual medical nutrition therapy for diabetes*, Alexandria, Va, 2002b, American Diabetes Association.

Fujimoto WY et al: Body size and shape changes and the risk of diabetes in the Diabetes Prevention Program (DPP), *Diabetes*, March 30, 2007 (epub ahead of print).

Gannon MC et al: Effect of protein ingestion on the glucose appearance rate in people with type 2 diabetes, *J Clin Endocrinol Metabol* 86:1040, 2001.

Gannon MC et al: An increase in protein improves the glucose response in persons with type 2 diabetes, *Am J Clin Nutr* 78:734, 2003.

Gannon MC et al: Effect of a high protein, low carbohydrate diet on blood glucose control in people with type 2 diabetes, *Diabetes* 53:2375, 2004.

Garg A et al: Effects of varying carbohydrate content of diet in patients with non–insulin-dependent diabetes mellitus, *JAMA* 271:1421, 1994.

Gebhard B et al: Postprandial GLP-1, norepinephrine, and reactive hypoglycemia in dumping syndrome, *Dig Dis Sci* 46:1915, 2001.

Giacco R et al: Long-term dietary treatment with increased amounts of fiber-rich low-glycemic index natural food improves blood glucose control and reduces the number of hypoglycemic events in patients with type 1 diabetes, *Diabetes Care* 23:1451, 2000.

Grave RD et al: Weight loss expectations in obese patients and treatment attrition: an observational multicenter study, *Obes Res* l13:1961. 2005.

Gray RO et al: Comparison of the ability of bread versus bread plus meat to treat and prevent subsequent hypoglycemia in patients with insulin-dependent diabetes, *J Clin Endocrinol Metabol* 81:1508, 1996.

Hallikainen MA et al: Effects of 2 low-fat stanols ester-containing margarines on serum cholesterol concentrations as part of a low-fat diet in hypercholesterolemic subjects, *Am J Clin Nutr* 69:403, 1999.

Hasanain B et al: Antioxidant vitamins and their influence in diabetes mellitus, *Curr Diab Rep* 2:448, 2002.

Hasler WL: Dumping syndrome, *Curr Treat Options Gastroenterol* 5 (2):139, 2002.

Heilbronn L et al: Effect of energy restriction, weight loss, and diet composition on plasma lipids and glucose in patients with type 2 diabetes, *Diabetes Care* 22:889, 1999.

Hollenbeck CG et al: To what extent does increased dietary fiber improve glucose and lipid metabolism in patients with noninsulin-dependent diabetes mellitus (NIDDM)? *Am J Clin Nutr* 43:16, 1986.

Howard AA et al: Effect of alcohol consumption on diabetes mellitus: a systematic review, *Ann Intern Med* 140:211, 2004.

Institute of Medicine: *Dietary reference intakes: energy, carbohydrate, fiber, fat, fatty acids, cholesterol, protein, and amino acids*, Washington, DC, 2002, National Academies Press.

International Diabetes Center: *Reactive and fasting hypoglycemia*, Minneapolis, 2004, International Diabetes Center.

Inzucchi SE: Oral antihyperglycemic therapy for type 2 diabetes (scientific review), *JAMA* 287:360, 2002.

Jones KL et al: Effect of metformin in pediatric patients with type 2 diabetes: a randomized controlled trial, *Diabetes Care* 25:89, 2002.

Jovanovic L, editor: *Medical management of pregnancy complicated by diabetes*, ed 3, Alexandria, Va, 2000, American Diabetes Association.

Kendall DM et al: Effects of exenatide (exendin-4) on glycemic control over 30 weeks in patients with type 2 diabetes treated with metformin and a sulfonylurea, *Diabetes Care* 28:1083, 2005.

Lacey K, Pritchett E: Nutrition care process and model: ADA adopts road map to quality care and outcomes management, *J Am Diet Assoc*103:1061, 2003.

Lafrance L et al: The effects of different glycaemic index food and dietary fibre intakes on glycaemic control in type 1 patients with diabetes on intensive insulin therapy, *Diabet Med* 15:972, 1998.

Lee YM et al: A phytosterol-enriched spread improves the lipid profile of subjects with type 2 diabetes—a randomized controlled trial under free-living condition, *Eur J Nutr* 43:111, 2000.

Lemon CC et al: Outcomes monitoring of health, behavior, and quality of life after nutrition intervention in adults with type 2 diabetes, *J Am Diet Assoc* 104:1805, 2004.

Leonetti F et al: Increased nonoxidative glucose metabolism in idiopathic reactive hypoglycemia, *Metabolism* 45:606, 1996.

Liese AD et al: Whole-grain intake and insulin sensitivity; the Insulin Resistance Atherosclerosis Study, *Am J Clin Nutr* 78:965, 2003.

MacDonald MJ: Postexercise late-onset hypoglycemia in insulin-dependent diabetic patients, *Diabetes Care* 10:584, 1987.

Mayer-Davis EJ et al: Towards understanding of glycemic index and glycemic load in habitual diet: associations with glycemia in the Insulin Resistance Study, *Br J Nutr* 95:397, 2006a.

Mayer-Davis EJ et al: Dietary intake among youth with diabetes: the SEARCH for Diabetes in Youth study, *J Am Diet Assoc* 106:689, 2006b.

McManus RM et al: Beta-cell function and visceral fat in lactating women with a history of gestational diabetes, *Metabolism* 50:715, 2001.

Meloni C et al: Severe protein restriction in overt diabetic nephropathy: benefits or risks? *J Ren Nutr* 12:96, 2002.

Mokdad AH et al: The continuing epidemics of obesity and diabetes in the United States, *JAMA* 286:1195, 2001.

Montori VM et al: Fish oil supplementation in type 2 diabetes: a quantitative systematic review, *Diabetes Care* 23:1407, 2000.

NCEP: Executive Summary of The Third Report of The National Cholesterol Education Program (NCEP) Expert Panel on Detection, Evaluation, and Treatment of High Blood Cholesterol in Adults (Adult Treatment Panel III), *JAMA* 285:2486, 2001.

Nissen SE, Wolski K: The effect of rosiglitazone on the risk of myocardial infarction and death from cardiovascular causes, *N Engl J Med*, www.nejm.org, May 21, 2007 (epub before print).

Nordmann AJ et al: Effects of low-carbohydrate vs low-fat diets on weight loss and cardiovascular risk factors: a meta-analysis of randomized controlled trials, *Arch Intern Med* 166:285, 2006.

Nuttall FQ et al: Effect of protein ingestion on the glucose and insulin response to a standardized oral glucose load, *Diabetes Care* 7:465, 1984.

Parker B et al: Effect of a high-protein, high-monounsaturated fat weight loss diet on glycemic control and lipid levels in type 2 diabetes, *Diabetes Care* 25:425, 2002.

Pastors JG et al: How effective is medical nutrition therapy in diabetes care? *J Am Diet Assoc* 103:827, 2003

Patti L et al: Long-term effects of fish oil on lipoprotein subfractions and low-density lipoprotein size in noninsulin-dependent diabetic patients with hypertriglyceridemia, *Atherosclerosis* 146:361, 1999.

Patton JS et al: Clinical pharmacokinetics and pharmacodynamics of inhaled insulin, *Clin Pharmacokinet* 43:781, 2004.

Peters AL, Davidson MB: Protein and fat effects on glucose response and insulin requirements in subjects with insulin-dependent diabetes mellitus, *Am J Clin Nutr* 58:555, 1993.

Pi-Sunyer FX: Glycemic index and disease, *Am J Clin Nutr* 76:290S, 2002.

Pijls LTJ et al: The effect of protein restriction on albuminuria in patients with type 2 diabetes mellitus: a randomized trial, *Nephrol Dial Transplant* 14:1445, 1999.

Pittler MH et al: Chromium picolinate for reducing body weight: meta-analysis of randomized trials, *Int J Obes Relat Metab Disord* 27:522, 2003.

Pownall HJ et al: Effect of moderate alcohol consumption on hypertriglyceridemia: a study in the fasting state, *Arch Intern Med* 159:981, 1999.

Prince MJ: Hypoglycemia of nondiabetic origin, *Curr Ther Endocrinol Metabol* 6:454, 1997.

Prochaska JO et al: Stages of change and decisional balance for 12 problem behaviors, *Health Psychol* 13:39, 1994.

Purdon C et al: The roles of insulin and catecholamines in the glucoregulatory response during intense exercise and early recovery in insulin-dependent diabetic and control subjects, *J Clin Endocrinol Metabol* 76:566, 1993.

Rabasa-Lhoret R et al: The effects of meal carbohydrate content on insulin requirements in type 1 diabetic patients treated intensively with the basal bolus (Ultralente-regular) insulin regimen, *Diabetes Care* 22:667, 1999.

Rabasa-Lhoret R et al: Guidelines for premeal insulin dose reduction for postprandial exercise of different intensities and durations in type 1 diabetic subjects treated intensively with a basal-bolus insulin regimen (Ultralente-lispro), *Diabetes Care* 24:625, 2001.

Raben A et al: Sucrose compared with artificial sweeteners: different effects on ad libitum food intake and body weight after 10 wk of supplementation in overweight subjects, *Am J Clin Nutr* 76:721, 2002.

Raskin P et al: Initiating insulin therapy in type 2 diabetes: a comparison of biphasic and basal insulin analogs, *Diabetes Care* 28:260, 2005.

Ratner R et al: Impact of intensive lifestyle and metformin therapy on cardiovascular disease risk factors in the diabetes prevention program, *Diabetes Care* 28:888, 2005.

Rave K et al: Time-action profile of inhaled insulin in comparison with subcutaneously injected insulin lispro and regular human insulin, *Diabetes Care* 2:400, 2005.

Ravussin E et al: Effects of a traditional lifestyle on obesity in Pima Indians, *Diabetes Care* 17:1067, 1994.

Reader D et al: Impact of gestational diabetes mellitus nutrition practice guidelines implemented by registered dietitians on pregnancy outcomes, *J Am Diet Assoc* 106:1426, 2006.

Rickheim P et al: Assessment of group versus individual diabetes education: a randomized study, *Diabetes Care* 25:269, 2002.

Rizkalla SW et al: Improved plasma glucose control, whole-body glucose utilization, and lipid profile on a low-glycemic index diet in type 2 diabetic men, *Diabetes Care* 27:1866, 2004.

Rosenstock J et al: Reduced hypoglycemia risk with insulin glargine: a meta-analysis comparing insulin glargine with human NPH insulin in type 2 diabetes, *Diabetes Care* 28:950, 2005.

Service FJ: Hypoglycemic disorders, *N Engl J Med* 17:1144, 1995.

Sigal RJ et al: Physical activity/exercise and type 2 diabetes, *Diabetes Care* 27:2518, 2004.

Silverstein J et al: Care of children and adolescents with type 1 diabetes: a statement of the American Diabetes Association, *Diabetes Care* 28:186, 2005.

Sinha R et al: Prevalence of impaired glucose tolerance among children and adolescents with marked obesity, *N Engl J Med* 346:802, 2002.

Summer LK et al: Substituting dietary saturated fat with polyunsaturated fat changes abdominal fat distribution and improves insulin sensitivity, *Diabetologia* 45:369, 2002.

Torgerstein JS et al: Xenical in the prevention of diabetes in obese subjects (XENDOS) study: a randomized study of orlistat as an adjunct to lifestyle changes for the prevention of type 2 diabetes in obese patients, *Diabetes Care* 27:155, 2004.

Tuomilehto J et al: Prevention of type 2 diabetes mellitus by changes in lifestyle among subjects with impaired glucose tolerance, *N Engl J Med* 344:1390, 2001.

United Kingdom Prospective Diabetes Study Group: Intensive blood-glucose control with sulphonylureas or insulin compared with conventional treatment and risk of complications in patients with type 2 diabetes (UKPDS 34), *Lancet* 352:854, 1998a.

United Kingdom Prospective Diabetes Study Group: Tight blood pressure control and risk of macrovascular and microvascular complications in type 2 diabetes (UKPDS 38), *Br Med J* 317:703, 1998b.

U.S. Food and Drug Administration: CFSAN/Office of Nutrition Products, Labeling, and Dietary Supplements, http://www.cfsan.fda.gov/~dms/onplds.html, accessed February 13, 2007.

van de Laar et al: α-Glucosidase inhibitors for patients with type 2 diabetes, *Diabetes Care* 28:166, 2005.

Wasserman DH, Zinman B: Exercise in individuals with IDDM (technical review), *Diabetes Care* 17:924, 1994.

Wadden et al: Randomized trial of lifestyle modification and pharmacotherapy for obesity, *N Engl J Med* 353:2111, 2005.

Wheeler ML et al: Animal versus plant protein meals in individuals with type 2 diabetes and microalbuminuria, *Diabetes Care* 25:1277, 2002.

Yu-Poth S et al: Effects of the National Cholesterol Education Program's Step I and Step II dietary intervention programs on cardiovascular disease risk factors: a meta-analysis, *Am J Clin Nutr* 69:632, 1999.

Yusuf S et al: Vitamin E supplementation and cardiovascular events in high-risk patients: the Heart Outcomes Prevention Evaluation Study Investigators, *N Engl J Med* 342:154, 2000.

Zeller K et al: Effect of restricting dietary protein and progression of renal failure in patients with insulin-dependent diabetes mellitus, *N Engl J Med* 324:778, 1991.

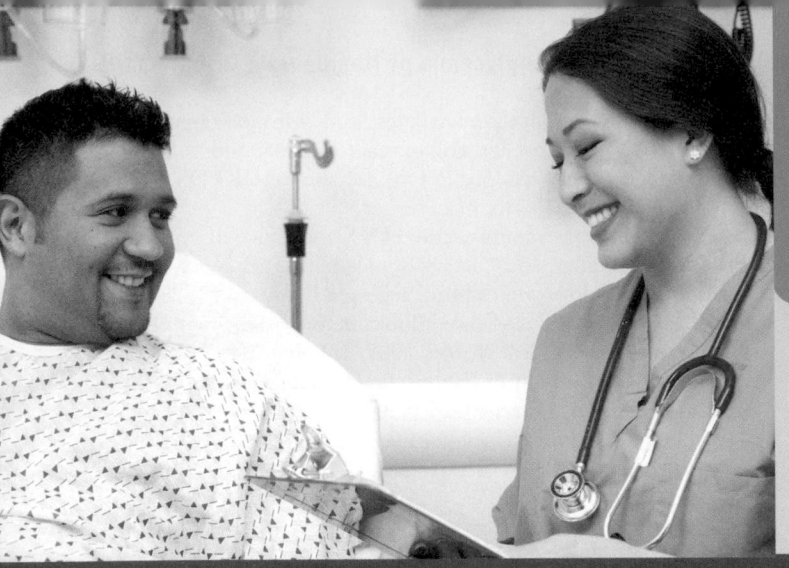

CHAPTER 31

Tracy Stopler, MS, RD

Medical Nutrition Therapy for Anemia

KEY TERMS

anemia a deficiency in the size or number of red blood cells or the amount of hemoglobin they contain that limits the exchange of oxygen and carbon dioxide between the blood and the tissue cells

aplastic anemia a normochromic-normocytic anemia accompanied by a deficiency of all the formed elements in the blood; can be caused by exposure to toxic chemicals, ionizing radiation, medications, although the cause is often unknown

ferritin an iron apoferritin complex; one of the chief storage forms of iron

hematocrit the volume percentage of erythrocytes in the blood

heme iron the organic form in which iron occurs in meat, fish, and poultry

hemochromatosis a genetically determined form of iron overload that results in progressive hepatic, pancreatic, cardiac, and other organ damage

hemoglobin a conjugated protein containing four heme groups and globin; the oxygen-carrying pigment of the erythrocytes

hemolytic anemia anemia caused by shortened survival of mature red blood cells

hepcidin a peptide hormone made in the liver; principal regulator of systemic iron homeostasis; controls plasma iron concentration and tissue distribution of iron by inhibiting intestinal iron absorption, iron recycling by macrophages, and iron mobilization from hepatic stores

holotranscobalamin II (holo TCII) vitamin B_{12} attached to the β-globulin, the major circulating vitamin B_{12} delivery protein

hypochromic characterized by deficient hemoglobin content of red blood cells

intrinsic factor (IF) a glycoprotein secreted by the gastric glands that is necessary for the absorption of exogenous vitamin B_{12} by ileal cell surface receptors for IF-B_{12} complexes

iron deficiency anemia characterized by the production of small (microcytic) erythrocytes and a diminished level of circulating hemoglobin; the last stage of iron deficiency, which represents the end point of a long period of iron deprivation

macrocytic anemia a form of anemia characterized by larger-than-normal red blood cells and increased mean corpuscular volume and mean corpuscular hemoglobin

meat, fish, and poultry (MFP factor) good sources of well-absorbed heme iron

megaloblastic anemia a form of anemia characterized by the presence of large, immature, abnormal, red blood cell progenitors in the bone marrow; 95% of cases are attributable to folic acid or vitamin B_{12} deficiency

microcytic anemia characterized by smaller-than-normal erythrocytes and less circulating hemoglobin; characteristic of iron deficiency and thalassemia

negative vitamin B_{12} balance a vitamin B_{12} pre-deficiency stage

non-heme iron iron that is not a part of the heme complex and that is present in foods such as eggs, grains, vegetables, and fruits; also present in small amounts in meat, fish, and poultry

pernicious anemia a macrocytic, megaloblastic anemia caused by a deficiency of vitamin B_{12}, secondary to lack of intrinsic factor

plasma liquid portion of whole blood that includes coagulation factors

protoporphyrin an iron-containing portion of the respiratory pigments that, when combined with protein, forms hemoglobin or myoglobin

serum liquid portion of whole blood without coagulation factors

sickle cell anemia a chronic hemolytic anemia, occurring most commonly in blacks, that is caused by homozygous inheritance of hemoglobin S, resulting in a defective hemoglobin synthesis that causes the red blood cells to become sickle shaped

sideroblastic anemia a microcytic, hypochromic anemia characterized by a derangement in the final pathway of heme synthesis, leading to a buildup of iron-containing immature red blood cells; responsive to pharmacologic doses of vitamin B_6

soluble serum transferrin receptors (SFTRs) molecules generated on the surface of a red blood cell in response to the need for iron that have broken away from red blood cells and are in the serum; measure of early iron deficiency

thalassemia anemia secondary to defective synthesis of the globin part of hemoglobin

total iron-binding capacity (TIBC) the capacity of transferrin to take on or become saturated with iron

transferrin globulin that binds and transports iron from the gut wall to the tissue cells

transferrin receptor molecule on the surface of the red blood cell that binds transferrin, the transport form of iron

transferrin saturation a measure of the amount of iron bound to transferrin; a gauge of iron supply to the tissues; percent saturation 5 serum iron/TIBC × 100

Anemia is a condition in which a deficiency in the size or number of erythrocytes or the amount of **hemoglobin** (composed of *heme*) limits the exchange of oxygen and carbon dioxide between the blood and the tissue cells. Classification is based on cell size—*macrocytic* (large), *normocytic* (normal), and *microcytic* (small)—and on hemoglobin content—*hypochromic* (pale color) and *normochromic* (normal color) (Table 31-1). Most anemias are caused by a lack of nutrients required for normal erythrocyte synthesis, principally iron, vitamin B_{12}, and folic acid. Others result from a variety of conditions such as hemorrhage, genetic abnormalities, chronic disease states, or drug toxicity. The anemias that result from an inadequate intake of iron, protein, certain vitamins (B_{12}, folic acid, pyridoxine, and ascorbic acid), copper, and other heavy metals are frequently called nutritional anemias. The most common nutritional anemias in the United States result from iron or folic acid deficiency.

IRON-RELATED BLOOD DISORDERS

Iron Deficiency Anemia

Iron deficiency anemia is characterized by the production of small (microcytic) erythrocytes and a diminished level of circulating hemoglobin. This **microcytic anemia** is actually the last stage of iron deficiency, and it represents the end point of a long period of iron deprivation.

Pathophysiology

There are many possible causes of iron deficiency anemia (see *Pathophysiology and Care Management Algorithm:* Iron Deficiency Anemia). The condition can arise from (1) inadequate iron intake secondary to a poor diet (such as a vegetarian lifestyle with insufficient heme iron); (2) inadequate absorption resulting from diarrhea, achlorhydria, intestinal disease such as celiac disease, atrophic gastritis, partial or total gastrectomy, or drug interference (antacids, cholestyramine, cimetidine [Tagamet], pancreatin, ranitidine [Zantac], tetracycline, and antiretroviral medications [especially the nucleoside reverse transcriptase inhibitors, Combivir, Epivir, Retrovir, Zerit and the protease inhibitor Crixivan]); (3) inadequate use secondary to chronic gastrointestinal disturbances; (4) increased iron requirement for growth of blood volume, which occurs during infancy, adolescence, pregnancy, and lactation; (5) increased excretion because of excessive menstrual blood (in females); hemorrhage from injury; or chronic blood loss from a bleeding ulcer, bleeding hemorrhoids, esophageal varices, regional enteritis, ulcerative colitis, parasites (hookworm disease), or malignant disease; or (6) defective release of iron from iron stores into the plasma and defective iron use owing to a chronic inflammation or other chronic disorder. With few exceptions iron deficiency anemia in male adults is the result of blood loss. Large losses of menstrual blood can cause iron deficiency in women, many of whom are unaware that their menses are unusually heavy.

Stages of Deficiency

One's iron status can range from iron overload to iron deficiency anemia. Routine measurement of iron status is necessary because about 6% of Americans have a negative iron balance, about 10% have a gene for positive balance, and about 1% have iron overload. Deviations from normal iron status are summarized as stages:

Stages I and II negative iron balance (i.e., iron depletion)—In these stages iron stores are low, and there is no dysfunction. In stage I negative iron balance, reduced iron absorption produces moderately depleted iron stores. Stage II negative iron balance is characterized by severely depleted iron stores. More than 50% of all cases of negative iron balance fall into these two stages. When persons in these two stages are treated with iron, they never develop dysfunction or disease.

Stages III and IV negative iron balance (i.e., iron deficiency)—Iron deficiency is characterized by inadequate body iron, causing dysfunction and disease. In stage III negative iron balance, dysfunction is not accompanied by anemia; however, anemia does occur in stage IV negative iron balance.

Stages I and II positive iron balance—Stage I positive iron balance usually lasts for several years with no accompanying dysfunction. Supplements of iron or vitamin C promote progression to dysfunction or

TABLE 31-1

Morphologic Classification of Anemia

Morphologic Type of Anemia	Underlying Abnormality	Clinical Syndromes/Causes	Treatment
Macrocytic (MCV >94; MCHC >31)			
Megaloblastic	Vitamin B_{12} deficiency	Pernicious anemia	Vitamin B_{12}
	Folic acid deficiency	Nutritional megaloblastic anemias, sprue, and other malabsorption syndromes	Folic acid
	Inherited disorders of deoxyribonucleic acid (DNA) synthesis	Orotic aciduria	Treatment based on the nature of the disorder
	Drug-induced disorders of DNA synthesis	Chemotherapeutic agents, anticonvulsants, oral contraceptives	Discontinue offending drug and administer folic acid
Nonmegaloblastic	Accelerated erythropoiesis	Hemolytic anemia	Treatment of underlying disease
	Increased membrane surface area		Treatment of underlying disease
Hypochromic Microcytic (MCV <80; MCHC <31)			
	Iron deficiency	Chronic loss of blood, inadequate diet, impaired absorption, increased demands	Ferrous sulfate and correction of underlying cause
	Disorders of globin synthesis	Thalassemia	Nonspecific
	Disorders of porphyrin and heme synthesis	Pyridoxine-responsive anemia	Pyridoxine
	Other disorders of iron metabolism		Treatment based on nature of disorder
Normochromic Normocytic (MCV 82-92; MCHC >30)			
	Recent blood loss	Various	Transfusion, iron Correction of underlying condition
	Overexpansion of plasma volume	Pregnancy	Restore homeostasis
	Hemolytic diseases	Overhydration	Treatment based on the nature of the disorder
	Hypoplastic bone marrow	Aplastic anemia	Transfusion
		Pure red blood cell aplasia	Androgens
	Infiltrated bone marrow	Leukemia, multiple myeloma, myelofibrosis	Chemotherapy
	Endocrine abnormality	Hypothyroidism, adrenal insufficiency	Treatment of underlying disease
	Chronic disorders		Treatment of underlying disease
	Renal disease	Renal disease	Treatment of underlying disease
	Liver disease	Cirrhosis	Treatment of underlying disease

Modified from Wintrobe MM et al: *Clinical hematology*, ed 8, Philadelphia, 1981, Lea & Febiger.

MCHC, Mean corpuscular hemoglobin concentration − concentration of hemoglobin expressed in grams per deciliter (g/dl); *MCV*, mean corpuscular volume = volume of one red blood cell expressed in femtoliters (fl).

PATHOPHYSIOLOGY AND CARE MANAGEMENT ALGORITHM

Iron Deficiency Anemia

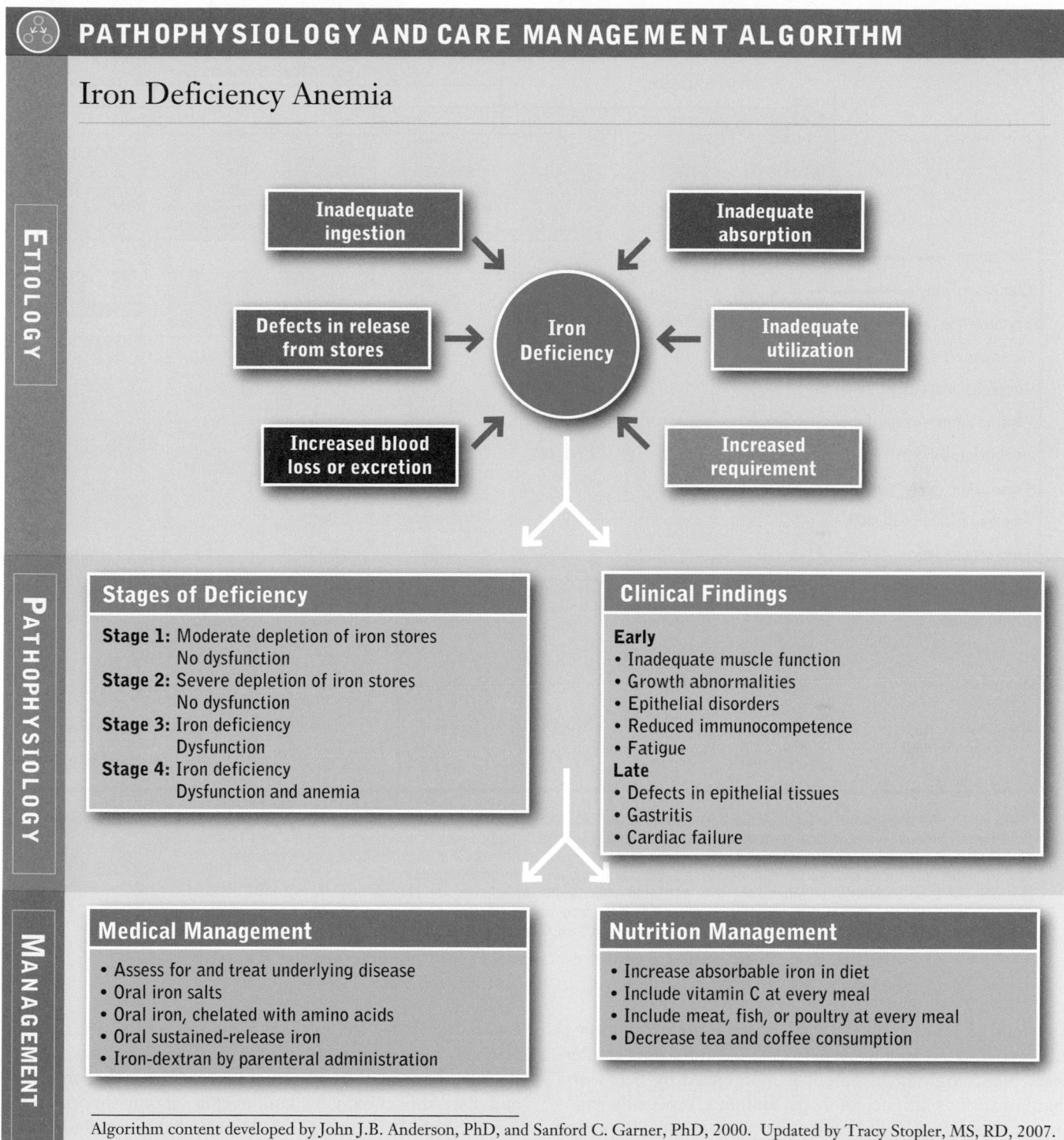

ETIOLOGY

Inadequate ingestion

Inadequate absorption

Defects in release from stores

Iron Deficiency

Inadequate utilization

Increased blood loss or excretion

Increased requirement

PATHOPHYSIOLOGY

Stages of Deficiency

Stage 1: Moderate depletion of iron stores
No dysfunction
Stage 2: Severe depletion of iron stores
No dysfunction
Stage 3: Iron deficiency
Dysfunction
Stage 4: Iron deficiency
Dysfunction and anemia

Clinical Findings

Early
• Inadequate muscle function
• Growth abnormalities
• Epithelial disorders
• Reduced immunocompetence
• Fatigue
Late
• Defects in epithelial tissues
• Gastritis
• Cardiac failure

MANAGEMENT

Medical Management

• Assess for and treat underlying disease
• Oral iron salts
• Oral iron, chelated with amino acids
• Oral sustained-release iron
• Iron-dextran by parenteral administration

Nutrition Management

• Increase absorbable iron in diet
• Include vitamin C at every meal
• Include meat, fish, or poultry at every meal
• Decrease tea and coffee consumption

Algorithm content developed by John J.B. Anderson, PhD, and Sanford C. Garner, PhD, 2000. Updated by Tracy Stopler, MS, RD, 2007.

disease, whereas iron removal prevents progression to disease. Iron overload disease develops in persons with stage II positive balance after years of iron overload have caused progressive damage to tissues and organs. Again, iron removal stops disease progression (Figure 31-1).

Iron status has a variety of indicators. **Serum** (whole blood without coagulation factors) ferritin levels are in equilibrium with body iron stores. Very early (stage I) positive iron balance may best be recognized by measuring **total iron-binding capacity (TIBC).** Conversely, measurement of serum or **plasma** (whole blood that includes coagulation factors) ferritin levels may best reveal early (stages I and II) negative iron balance, although serum TIBC may be as good an indicator (see Chapter 15).

Clinical Findings

Because anemia is the last manifestation of chronic, long-term iron deficiency, the symptoms reflect a malfunction of

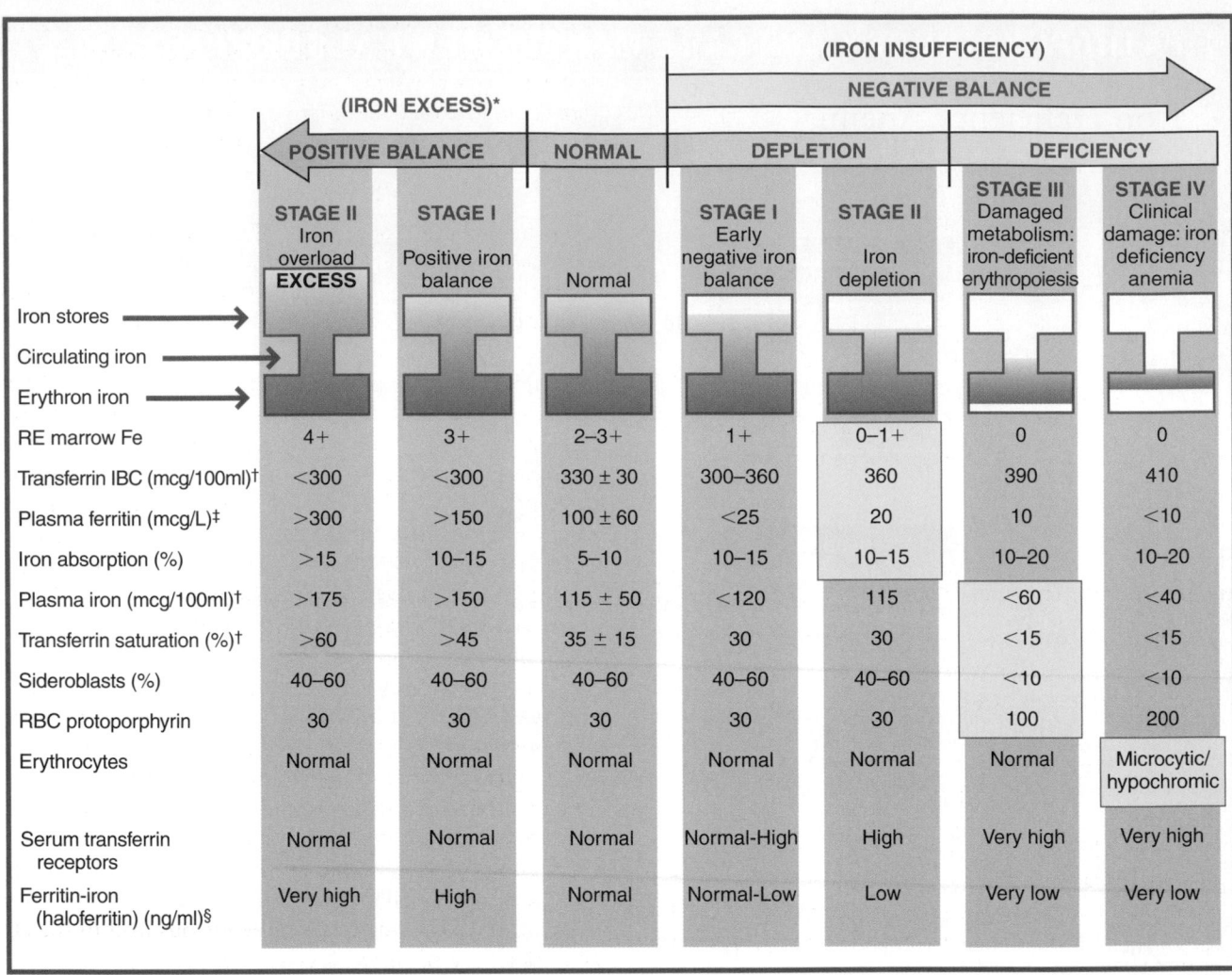

	STAGE II Iron overload **EXCESS**	**STAGE I** Positive iron balance	Normal	**STAGE I** Early negative iron balance	**STAGE II** Iron depletion	**STAGE III** Damaged metabolism: iron-deficient erythropoiesis	**STAGE IV** Clinical damage: iron deficiency anemia
RE marrow Fe	4+	3+	2–3+	1+	0–1+	0	0
Transferrin IBC (mcg/100ml)[†]	<300	<300	330 ± 30	300–360	360	390	410
Plasma ferritin (mcg/L)[‡]	>300	>150	100 ± 60	<25	20	10	<10
Iron absorption (%)	>15	10–15	5–10	10–15	10–15	10–20	10–20
Plasma iron (mcg/100ml)[†]	>175	>150	115 ± 50	<120	115	<60	<40
Transferrin saturation (%)[†]	>60	>45	35 ± 15	30	30	<15	<15
Sideroblasts (%)	40–60	40–60	40–60	40–60	40–60	<10	<10
RBC protoporphyrin	30	30	30	30	30	100	200
Erythrocytes	Normal	Normal	Normal	Normal	Normal	Normal	Microcytic/ hypochromic
Serum transferrin receptors	Normal	Normal	Normal	Normal-High	High	Very high	Very high
Ferritin-iron (haloferritin) (ng/ml)[§]	Very high	High	Normal	Normal-Low	Low	Very low	Very low

[*]Randall Lauffer of Harvard and Joe McCord of University of Colorado–Denver hold that *any* storage iron is excessive because of its potential to promote excessive free radical generation. (Herbert V et al: Most free radical injury is iron related, *Stem Cells* 12:289, 1994.)
[†]Inflammation reduces transferrin (and the plasma iron on it), because transferrin is a reverse acute-phase reactant.
[‡]Inflammation produces elevated ferritin, because ferritin protein is an acute-phase reactant.
[§]Ferritin-iron is unaffected by inflammation, so it is reliable when ferritin, transferrin, and plasma iron are not.
Dallman (pediatrician) definition of negative balance: less absorbed than *excreted.*
Herbert (internist) definition of negative balance: less absorbed than *needed.*

FIGURE 31-1 Sequential stages of iron status. *IBC,* Iron-binding capacity; *RBC,* red blood cell; *RE,* reticuloendothelial cells. *(Copyright Victor Herbert, 1995.)*

a variety of body systems. Inadequate muscle function is reflected in decreased work performance and exercise tolerance. Neurologic involvement is manifested by behavioral changes such as fatigue, anorexia, and pica, especially pagophagia (ice eating). Nokes and colleagues, in their Report of the International Nutritional Anemia Consultative Group (1998), supported earlier work by Pollitt and colleagues (1986) that abnormal cognitive development in children suggests the presence of iron deficiency before it has developed into overt anemia. Growth abnormalities, epithelial disorders, and a reduction in gastric acidity are common. A possible sign of early iron deficiency is reduced immunocompetence, particularly defects in cell-mediated immunity and the phagocytic activity of neutrophils, which may lead to an increased propensity for infection.

As iron deficiency anemia becomes more severe, defects arise in the structure and function of the epithelial tissues,

especially of the tongue, nails, mouth, and stomach. The skin may appear pale, and the inside of the lower eyelid may be light pink instead of red. Fingernails can become thin and flat, and eventually koilonychia (spoon-shaped nails) may be noted (Figure 31-2). Mouth changes include atrophy of the lingual papillae, burning, redness, and in severe cases a completely smooth, waxy, and glistening appearance to the tongue (glossitis). Angular stomatitis may also occur, as may a form of dysphagia (difficulty in swallowing). Gastritis occurs frequently and may result in achlorhydria. Progressive, untreated anemia results in cardiovascular and respiratory changes that can eventually lead to cardiac failure. Some behavioral symptoms of iron deficiency seem to respond to iron therapy before the anemia is cured, suggesting they may be the result of tissue depletion of iron-containing enzymes rather than from a decreased level of hemoglobin (see Chapters 3 and 15).

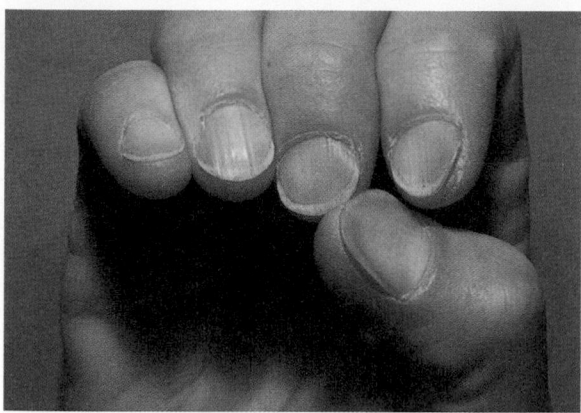

FIGURE 31-2 Fingernails with cuplike depressions (koilonychia) are a sign of iron deficiency in adults. *(From Callen JP et al: Color atlas of dermatology, Philadelphia, 1993, Saunders.)*

Diagnosis

Progressive stages of iron deficiency can be evaluated by six different measurements:

1. Quantity of serum or plasma ferritin
2. Quantity of serum or plasma iron
3. Quantity of total circulating transferrin
4. Percent saturation of circulating transferrin, which measures the iron supply to the tissues; it is calculated by dividing serum iron by the TIBC; levels less than 16% are considered inadequate for erythropoiesis
5. Percent saturation of ferritin with iron
6. Quantity of **soluble serum transferrin receptors (SFTR):** Transferrin molecules are generated on the surface of red blood cells in response to the need for iron. With iron deficiency, so many **transferrin receptors** are on the cell surface looking for iron that some of them break off and float in the blood (serum). Their presence is an early measurement of developing iron deficiency, with a higher quantity meaning greater deficiency of iron.

A definitive diagnosis of iron deficiency anemia requires more than one method of iron evaluation and preferably includes the first three of the measurements just listed. The evaluation should also include an assessment of cell morphology. The serum or plasma **ferritin** level is the most sensitive parameter of negative iron balance because it decreases only in the presence of true iron deficiency, as with **transferrin saturation.**

Protoporphyrin, the iron-containing portion of the respiratory pigments that combine with protein to form hemoglobin or myoglobin, can be used to assess iron deficiency. The zinc protoporphyrin (ZnPP)/heme ratio is measured. However, this ZnPP/heme ratio and hemoglobin levels are affected by chronic infection and other factors that can produce a condition that mimics iron deficiency anemia when, in fact, iron is adequate (Herbert et al., 1997).

The TIBC declines, and serum ferritin levels rise in chronic disease unrelated to iron metabolism (see Table 31-1). By it-

self, hemoglobin concentration is unsuitable as a diagnostic tool in cases of suspected iron deficiency anemia for three reasons: (1) it is affected only late in the disease; (2) it cannot distinguish iron deficiency from other anemias; (3) hemoglobin values in normal individuals vary widely.

Medical Management

Treatment should focus primarily on the underlying disease or situation leading to the anemia, although this is often difficult to determine. Repletion of iron stores, not merely alleviation of the anemia, should be the goal.

Supplementation. The chief treatment for iron deficiency anemia involves oral administration of inorganic iron in the ferrous form. At a dose of 30 mg, absorption of ferrous iron is three times greater than if the same amount were given in the ferric form. At larger doses the difference is even more marked. The most widely used preparation is ferrous sulfate, and the dose is calculated in terms of the amount of elemental iron provided. Other salts absorbed to about the same degree are the ferrous forms of lactate, fumarate, glycine sulfate, glutamate, and gluconate.

Iron is best absorbed when the stomach is empty; however, under these conditions it tends to cause gastric irritation. Gastrointestinal side effects can include nausea, epigastric discomfort and distention, heartburn, diarrhea, or constipation. If these side effects occur, the patient is told to take the iron with meals (breakfast, lunch, and dinner) instead of on an empty stomach; however, this sharply reduces the absorbability of the iron. Gastric irritation is a direct result of the high quantity of free ferrous iron in the stomach. Health professionals generally prescribe oral iron for iron deficiency for 3 months (three times daily).

Depending on the severity of the anemia and the patient's tolerance of iron supplementation, the daily dose of elemental iron should be 50 to 200 mg for adults and 6 mg/kg of body weight for children. Ascorbic acid greatly increases both iron absorption and iron gastric irritation through its capacity to maintain iron in the reduced state.

Absorption of 10 to 20 mg of iron per day permits red blood cell production to increase to about three times the normal rate and, in the absence of blood loss, hemoglobin concentration to rise at a rate of 0.2 g/dL daily. Increased reticulocytosis (an increase in the number of young red blood cells) is seen within 2 to 3 days after iron administration, but affected persons may report subjective improvements in mood and appetite even sooner. The hemoglobin level will begin to increase by day 4 of treatment. Iron therapy should be continued for 4 to 5 months, even after restoration of normal hemoglobin levels, to allow for repletion of body iron reserves.

If iron supplementation fails to correct the anemia, it is necessary to consider the following possibilities: (1) the patient may not be taking the medication as prescribed, most likely because of unpleasant side effects; (2) bleeding may be continuing at a rate faster than the erythroid marrow can replace blood cells; or (3) the supplemental iron is not being absorbed, possibly as a result of malabsorption secondary to steatorrhea, celiac disease, or hemodialysis. In these circumstances parenteral administration of iron in the form of iron-dextran may be necessary (see *Pathophysiology and Care Management Algorithm:* Iron Deficiency Anemia). Although replenishment of iron stores by this route is faster, it is more expensive than and not as safe as oral administration.

Medical Nutrition Therapy

In addition to iron supplementation, attention should be given to the amount of absorbable dietary iron consumed. A good source of iron contains a substantial amount of iron in relation to its calorie content (high nutrient density) and contributes at least 10% of the U.S. recommended dietary allowance (RDA) for iron. Liver; kidney; beef; dried fruits; dried peas and beans; nuts; green leafy vegetables; and fortified whole-grain breads, muffins, cereals, and nutrition bars are among the foods that rank highest in iron content (Table 31-2).

It is estimated that 1.8 mg of iron must be absorbed daily to meet the needs of 80% to 90% of adult women and adolescent males and females. Because typical Western diets generally contain 6 mg/1000 kcal of iron, the bioavailability of iron in the diet is clearly more important in correcting or preventing iron deficiency than the total amount of dietary iron consumed.

Bioavailability of Dietary Iron. Several factors influence the bioavailability of dietary iron. The rate of absorption depends on the iron status of the individual, as reflected in the level of iron stores. The lower the iron stores, the greater will be the rate of iron absorption. Individuals with iron deficiency anemia absorb about 20% to 30% of dietary iron compared with the 5% to 10% absorbed by those without iron deficiency.

The form of iron in the diet also influences absorption. **Heme iron** (about 15% absorbable), present in **meat, fish, and poultry (MFP factor),** is much better absorbed than **nonheme iron,** which can also be found in MFP, as well as in eggs, grains, vegetables, and fruits. The absorption rate of nonheme iron varies between 3% and 8%, depending on the presence of dietary enhancing factors, specifically ascorbic acid and MFP. Ascorbic acid is not only a powerful reducing agent, but it also binds iron to form a readily absorbed complex. The mechanism by which MFP potentiates the absorption of nonheme iron in other foodstuffs is unknown. MFP digestion may lead to the release of amino acids (particularly cysteine) and polypeptides in the upper small bowel, which then chelate with nonheme iron to form soluble, absorbable complexes (Mulvihill et al., 1998) (see Chapter 3).

Iron absorption can be inhibited to varying degrees by a number of factors that chelate iron, including carbonates, oxalates, phosphates, and phytates (unleavened bread, unrefined cereals, and soybeans). Factors in vegetable fiber may inhibit nonheme iron absorption. Taken with meals, tea, and coffee can reduce iron absorption by 50% through the formation of insoluble iron compounds with tannin. Iron in egg yolk is poorly absorbed because of the presence of phosvitin.

In summary, to maximize iron absorption and prevent iron deficiency anemia, one should (1) improve food choices to increase total dietary iron intake; (2) include a source of vitamin C at every meal; (3) include heme-containing MFP at every meal, if possible; and (4) avoid drinking large amounts of tea or coffee with meals. The Dietary Guidelines for Americans, 2005, recommend that women of childbearing age who may become pregnant eat foods high in heme-iron and consume iron-rich plant foods or iron-fortified foods with an enhancer of iron absorption (i.e., vitamin C–rich foods).

Hemochromatosis

Hemochromatosis is a genetically determined form of iron overload that results in progressive hepatic, pancreatic, cardiac, and other organ damage, which results in people absorbing three times more iron from their food than those without hemochromatosis. International scientists studying iron overload disorders at the University of Alabama discovered that Asians and Pacific Islanders have the highest levels of iron in their blood of all racial and ethnic groups who were screened, but they have the lowest prevalence of the particular gene mutation that is found in whites with the typical form of hemochromatosis (Adams et al., 2005).

Homozygotes (two genes) will die of iron overload unless they donate blood frequently. The Hemochromatosis and Iron Overload Screening Study concluded the following: Non-Hispanic whites have the highest prevalence of persons who have two copies of the C282Y mutation of the hereditary iron (HFE) gene (0.44%), followed by Native Americans (0.11 %), Hispanics (0.027 %), Blacks (0.014 %), and Pacific Islanders (0.012 %, or Asians (0.000039%). In women monthly menses slow the associated organ damage until after menopause (Adams et al., 2005).

Pathophysiology

Men are particularly susceptible to hemochromatosis because they have no physiologic mechanisms for losing iron such as menstruation, pregnancy, or lactation. Excessive iron intake usually stems from accidental incorporation of iron into the diet from environmental sources. In developing countries the iron overload can result from eating foods cooked in cast-iron cooking vessels or contaminated by iron-containing soils. In developed countries it likely results from excessive intake of iron-supplemented foods or inappropriate multivitamin/mineral supplementation.

After absorption, iron is transported by plasma **transferrin,** a β1-globulin (protein) that binds iron derived from the gastrointestinal tract, iron storage sites, or hemoglobin breakdown, to the bone marrow (hemoglobin synthesis), endothelial cells (storage), or placenta (fetal needs). The peptide **hepcidin** is synthesized in the liver and functions as a systemic iron-regulating hormone by regulating iron transport from iron-exporting tissues into plasma. Hepcidin inhibits the cellular efflux of iron by binding to, and inducing the degradation of ferroprotein, the sole iron exporter in iron-transporting cells. Hepcidin controls plasma iron concentration and tissue distribution of iron

TABLE 31-2

Iron Content of Some Common Foods

Food	Portion Size	Iron (mg)*	Food	Portion Size	Iron (mg)*
Protein Group			**Vegetable Group**		
Chicken, light meat	3 oz	0.9	Artichoke, cooked	1 c	5.1
Chicken, dark meat	3 oz	1.2	Baked potato	1 medium	2.7
Turkey, dark meat	3 oz	2.0	Broccoli	1 medium stalk	2.1
Pork chop	3 oz	0.7	Lima beans	½ c	2.1
Tenderloin steak	3 oz	1.3	Spinach	1 c	1.5
Venison, roasted	3 oz	3.0	**Grain Group**		
Liver, beef	3 oz	5.8	Pasta (enriched)	1 c (cooked)	2.0
Liver, chicken	3 oz	7.2	Rice (enriched)	1 c (cooked)	1.8
Liver, pork	3 oz	15.2	Whole-wheat bread	1 slice	1.0
Tuna fish	3 oz	0.6	CousCous (cooked)	⅓ c	0.9
Swordfish	3 oz	1.1	Matzo	1 board	0.9
Oysters, raw	3 oz	5.5	Pasta (enriched/cooked)	1 c	2.0
Tofu, raw	½ c	4.0	Quinoa (cooked)	1/4 c	1.5
Black beans	½ c	1.8	Rice (enriched/cooked)	1 c	1.8
Chickpeas	½ c	2.4	Vitalicious muffin	2 oz	9 mg
Kidney beans	½ c	2.6	Whole wheat bread	1 slice	1.0
Lentil beans	½ c	3.3	**Cereals**		
Egg	1 whole	0.6	Grapenuts	½ c	18.0
Cashew nuts	1 oz	1.7	Product 19	¾ c	18.0
Pistachio nuts	1 oz	1.9	Total	1 c	18.0
Sunflower seeds	2 Tbsp (1 oz)	1.9	Wheat germ	1 oz (¼ c)	2.6
Peanut butter (Jif)	2 Tbsp	0.6	Cream of Wheat, instant	¾ c	8.2
Peanut butter (Skippy)		0.3	Oatmeal, plain, instant	1 packet	6.7
Peanut butter (Peter Pan Plus)		3.75	Cornflakes	1 c	4.5
Soybeans (cooked)	½ c	4.4	Rice Krispies	1 c	0.9
Sesame seeds	2 Tbsp	1.2	Special K	1 c	2.5
Tempeh (cooked)	1 c	3.8	**Energy or Sports Bars**		
Dairy Group			Balance	1 bar, 1.76 oz	4.5
Milk	1 c	0.1	Clif	1 bar, 2.4 oz	4.5
Ricotta, part-skim	½ c	0.6	Genisoy	1 bar, 1.58 or 2.2 oz	4.5
Soy milk	1 c	1.8	Kashi Go Lean	1 bar, 2.75 oz	<1.0
Fruit Group			Luna	1 bar, 1.69 oz	6.3
Apricots	3 raw	0.6	Met Rx (Big 100)	1 bar, 3.5 oz	8.1
Apple, dried	10 rings	0.9	Power	1 bar, 2.29 oz	6.3
Figs, dried	1	0.4	Pria	1 bar, .98 oz	3.6
Peaches, dried	5 halves	2.6	Promax	1 bar, 2.7 oz	4.5
Raisins	½ c	1.5	Zone	1 bar, 1.76 oz	1.4
Strawberries	1 c, frozen	1.2	Myoplex Carb Sense	11 oz	1.8
Prune juice	1 c	3.0	WorldWide Pure Protein	11 oz	0.36 – 1.1

Copyright 2005 Tracy Stopler, MS, RD.

*Absorbability of iron from animal foods averages 15%; from plant foods, it averages only 3%.

by inhibiting intestinal iron absorption, iron recycling by macrophages, and iron mobilization from hepatic stores. Hepcidin synthesis is increased by iron loading and decreased by anemia and hypoxia. In addition, hepcidin synthesis is greatly increased during inflammation, trapping iron in macrophages, decreasing plasma iron concentrations and causing iron-restricted erythropoiesis characteristic of anemia of inflammation (anemia of chronic disease). Recent studies indicate that hepcidin deficiency underlies most known forms of hereditary hemochromatosis; thus iron absorption is excessive and uncontrolled (Nemeth and Ganz, 2006).

There is evidence that the mutation of the HFE gene leading to hemochromatosis is also associated with increased levels of gastrin in the stomach, leading to increased levels of gastric acid and thus increased absorption of iron (Smith et al., 2006).

Excess iron is stored as ferritin and hemosiderin in the macrophages of the liver, spleen, and bone marrow. The body has a limited capacity to excrete iron. About 1 mg of iron is excreted daily through the gastrointestinal tract, urinary tract, and skin. To maintain a normal iron balance, the daily obligatory loss must be replaced by the absorption of heme and nonheme food iron. Persons with iron overload excrete increased amounts of iron, especially in the feces, to compensate partially for the increased absorption and higher stores.

Clinical Findings

In hemochromatosis iron absorption is enhanced, resulting in a gradual, progressive accumulation of iron. This disease, associated with the HFE gene, is often underdiagnosed. Most affected persons do not know they have it. In its early stages iron overload may result in symptoms similar to iron deficiency such as fatigue and weakness; later it can cause chronic abdominal pain, aching joints, impotence, and menstrual irregularities.

A progressive positive iron balance may result in a variety of serious problems, including hepatomegaly, skin pigmentation, arthritis, heart disease, hypogonadism, diabetes mellitus, and cancer. The Nurse's Health Study concluded that higher iron stores (reflected by an elevated ferritin concentration and a lower ratio of transferrin receptors to ferritin) were found to be associated with an increased risk of type 2 diabetes in healthy women (Jiang et al., 2004).

Shaheen and associates (2003) found that individuals with abnormally high iron levels are 40% more likely to develop cancer of the colon. The authors state, "Iron is a pro-oxidant; thus high iron levels can lead to free radical formation and DNA damage . . . iron is an essential element for tumor cell growth and proliferation." There also seems to be increased risk for age-related macular degeneration and Alzheimer's disease because of the oxidant effect of iron overload (Dunaief, 2006; Connor and Lee, 2006). Mortality from hemochromatosis is preventable if excess body iron is removed by phlebotomy therapy before hepatic cirrhosis develops.

Diagnosis

If an iron overload is suspected, the following screening tests should be performed: serum ferritin level (storage iron), serum iron concentration, TIBC, and percent of transferrin saturation ([serum iron/TIBC] × 100). Iron overload may be present if the percent of transferrin saturation is greater than 50 in women and 60 in men and if the serum iron level is greater than 180 mg/dl. Deoxyribonucleic acid (DNA) testing, using blood or cheek cell samples, is also available for early detection of hemochromatosis.

Liver biopsy is the gold standard for the diagnosis of iron overload.

The patient with iron overload may simultaneously be anemic as a result of damage to the bone marrow or an inflammatory disorder (i.e., arthritis), cancer, internal bleeding, or chronic infection. Iron supplements should not be taken until the cause of the anemia is known.

Medical Management

For patients with significant iron overload, weekly phlebotomy for 2 to 3 years may be required to eliminate all excess iron. Treatment for iron overload may also involve iron depletion with intravenous desferrioxamine-B, a chelating agent that is excreted by the kidneys. Calcium disodium ethylenediaminetetraacetic acid (EDTA) can also be used. Patients diagnosed as having hemochromatosis should inform all blood relatives so that they too can be evaluated.

Medical Nutrition Therapy

Individuals with iron overload should ingest less heme iron (i.e., from MFP) compared with nonheme iron (plant groups). Persons with iron overload should also avoid alcohol and vitamin C supplements because both enhance iron absorption. However, some evidence shows that even though vitamin C enhances iron absorption at a meal, when it is given daily in increased amounts from food or supplements as part of the complete diet over the long-term, the facilitating effect on iron absorption is far less (Cook and Reddy, 2001). In addition, vitamin C supplements may cause release of harmful free radical–generating excess iron from body stores.

Affected persons should avoid foods that are highly fortified with iron (i.e., foods such as many breakfast cereals, fortified "energy" or sports bars and many meal-replacement drinks or shakes that are fortified with vitamins and minerals). They should also avoid iron supplements or multiple vitamin/mineral supplements that contain iron. The dietary requirement for iron should not be exceeded, and perhaps the intake of iron should be less in some persons. The new dietary reference intakes (DRIs) for iron are summarized on the inside front cover. The RDA for women in their childbearing years is 18 mg; for pregnant women, 27 mg; and the RDA for adult men and women 51 years of age and older is 8 mg (Institute of Medicine, 2001).

Iron Toxicity

Other disorders associated with iron overload include thalassemias, sideroblastic anemia, chronic hemolytic anemia, **aplastic anemia** (a normochromic-normocytic anemia), ineffective erythropoiesis, transfusional iron overload (secondary to multiple blood transfusions), porphyria cutanea tarda, and alcoholic cirrhosis. Excess dietary iron intake (as occurs in Bantu individuals [i.e., South African blacks who absorb excess dietary iron from alcoholic beverages fermented in iron stills and food cooked in iron pots]) or an overdose of iron medication (as may occasionally occur in children who mistake iron tablets for candy) can be fatal in doses of 3 to 10 g. Excessive iron can cause irritation of the mucosa as well as ulceration and bleeding, hypoxia, metabolic acidosis, alveolar and hepatic damage, and renal failure. Death can occur in 12 to 48 hours.

MEGALOBLASTIC ANEMIAS

Megaloblastic anemia reflects a disturbed synthesis of DNA, which results in morphologic and functional changes in erythrocytes, leukocytes, platelets, and their precursors in the blood and bone marrow. Megaloblastic anemia is usually caused by a deficiency of vitamin B_{12} or folic acid, both of which are essential to the synthesis of nucleoproteins. Hematologic changes are the same for both; however, the folic acid deficiency is the first to appear. Normal body folate stores are depleted within 2 to 4 months in individuals consuming folate-deficient diets; by contrast, vitamin B_{12} stores are depleted only after several years of a vitamin B_{12}–deficient diet. In persons with vitamin B_{12} deficiency, folic acid supplementation can mask B_{12} deficiency. In correcting the anemia, the vitamin B_{12} deficiency may remain undetected, leading to the irreversible neuropsychiatric damage that is only prevented with B_{12} supplementation (see Chapter 3).

Pernicious and Other Vitamin B_{12} Deficiency Anemias

Pathophysiology

Pernicious anemia is a megaloblastic **macrocytic anemia** caused by a deficiency of vitamin B_{12}. Most commonly the vitamin deficiency is secondary to a lack of **intrinsic factor (IF),** a glycoprotein in the gastric juice that is necessary for the absorption of dietary vitamin B_{12}. Rarely vitamin B_{12} deficiency anemia occurs in strict vegetarians whose diet contains no vitamin B_{12} except for traces found in plants contaminated by microorganisms capable of synthesizing vitamin B_{12}. Other causes are shown in Box 31-1.

Ingested vitamin B_{12} is freed from protein by gastric acid and gastric and intestinal enzymes. The free vitamin B_{12} attaches to salivary R-binder, which, at an acid pH (2.3) such as that found in the stomach, has a higher affinity for the vitamin than does IF. Secreted by parietal cells of the gastric mucosa, IF is necessary for the absorption of exogenous vitamin B_{12}. The release of pancreatic trypsin into the proximal small intestine destroys R-binder and releases vitamin B_{12} from its complex with R-protein. At an alkaline pH (6.8), as may be found in the intestine, IF then binds the vitamin B_{12}. The vitamin B_{12}–IF complex is then carried to the ileum, where in the presence of ionic calcium (Ca^{2+}) and a pH of greater than 6, it attaches to the surface vitamin B_{12}–IF receptors on the ileal cell brush border.

At the brush border the vitamin B_{12}–IF complex enters the ileal cell, where the vitamin B_{12} is released, attaching to **holotranscobalamin II (holo TCII).** Like IF, holo TCII plays an active role in binding and transporting vitamin B_{12}. The TCII–vitamin B_{12} complex then enters the portal venous blood. Other binding proteins in the blood include haptocorrin, also known as transcobalamin I (TCI), and transcobalamin III (TCIII). These are α-globulins—larger-macromolecular-weight glycoproteins—that make up the R-binder component of the blood. Unlike IF, the R-proteins are capable of binding not only vitamin B_{12} itself but also many of its biologically inactive analogs.

Although about 75% of the vitamin B_{12} in human serum is bound to haptocorrin and roughly 25% is bound to TCII, only TCII is important in delivering vitamin B_{12} to all the cells that need it. After transport through the bloodstream, TCII is recognized by receptors on cell surfaces. Patients with haptocorrin abnormalities have no symptoms of vitamin B_{12} deficiency. Those lacking TCII rapidly develop megaloblastic anemia (Herbert, 2001b).

As a result of normal enterohepatic circulation (i.e., excretion of vitamin B_{12} and analogs in bile and resorption of mainly vitamin B_{12} in the ileum), it generally takes decades for strict vegetarians who are not receiving vitamin B_{12} supplementation to develop a vitamin B_{12} deficiency. Vitamin B_{12} is also excreted in urine.

Stages of Deficiency

Figure 31-3 shows the sequential biochemical and hematologic stages of vitamin B_{12} deficiency. The sequence of events involves four stages of depletion.

Stage 1—Early **negative vitamin B_{12} balance;** begins when vitamin B_{12} intake is low or absorption is poor, depleting TCII, the primary delivery protein, resulting in a low TCII level. A low TCII (<40 pg/ml) may be the earliest detectable sign of a vitamin B_{12} deficiency (Herbert et al., 1990).

Stage 2—Vitamin B_{12} depletion. Besides the low B_{12} on TCII, there is also a gradual lowering of B_{12} on haptocorrin (holohap <150 pg/ml), the storage protein.

Stage 3—Damaged metabolism or vitamin B_{12}–deficient erythropoiesis; includes an abnormal deoxyuridine (dU) suppression, hypersegmentation, a decreased TIBC and holohap percent saturation, a low red blood cell folate level (<140 ng/ml), and subtle neuropsychiatric damage (impaired short-term and recent memory) (Herbert, 2001a).

Stage 4—Clinical damage, including vitamin B_{12} deficiency anemia; includes all preceding stages, including macroovalocytic erythrocytes, elevated mean corpuscular volume (MCV), elevated TCII levels, increased homocysteine (see Chapter 32) and methylmalonic acid levels, and myelin damage.

Clinical Findings

Pernicious anemia affects not only the blood but also the gastrointestinal tract and the peripheral and central nervous systems. This distinguishes it from folic acid deficiency anemia. The overt symptoms, which are caused by inadequate myelinization of the nerves, include paresthesia (especially numbness and tingling in the hands and feet), diminution of the senses of vibration and position, poor muscular coordination, poor

BOX 31-1

Causes of Vitamin B$_{12}$ Deficiency

I. Inadequate ingestion

A. Poor diet (lacking microorganisms and animal foods, which are the sole sources of vitamin B$_{12}$)

1. Strict vegetarianism (eating no meat, fowl, seafood, eggs, milk, or any products thereof)
2. Chronic alcoholism (no vitamin B$_{12}$ or folate in hard liquor; folate deficiency occurs first and is more common, partly because body stores of vitamin B$_{12}$ last much longer than those of folate)
3. Poverty, religious tenets (Hinduism, Seventh Day Adventism, certain Catholic orders), dietary faddism

II. Inadequate absorption

A. Gastric disorder producing inadequate or absent secretion by gastric acid and enzymes, reducing ability to split B$_{12}$ from food, followed in several years by loss of intrinsic factor secretion

1. Addisonian pernicious anemia (PA): The form of vitamin B$_{12}$ deficiency disease that is attributable to inadequate intrinsic factor secretion of uncertain cause
   a. Hereditary absence of normal intrinsic factor secretion: Absent secretion at birth (circulating antibody to intrinsic factor never present) supports the theory that antibody occurs only when antigenic stimulus is produced by intrinsic factor, which enters blood from damaged parietal cells and is recognized as foreign by the immunologic surveillance system; rare
   b. Congenital production of defective intrinsic factor molecule (three published cases)
   c. Autoimmunity-associated gastric atrophy: Affected patients usually have nondiagnostic-for-PA circulating parietal cell antibody, which is an index only of past or present gastric damage and not of the amount of intrinsic factor secretion (circulating diagnostic-for-PA antibody to intrinsic factor is always present in individuals younger than 21 years of age; however, there is a gradual decrease in measurable antibody so that, by the age of 65 years, only two thirds of patients present with measurable circulating antibody to intrinsic factor)
      (1) Juvenile pernicious anemia (usually presents between the ages of 3 and 14 years)
      (2) Hereditarily determined degenerative gastric atrophy (gradually progresses with increasing age; almost 50% of all adult PA cases fall into this category)
      (3) Acquired gastric atrophy as the end result of superficial inflammatory gastritis such as that produced by *Helicobacter pylori (H. pylori);* superficial gastritis with atrophy (almost 50% of all adult PA cases fall into this category, which includes acquired gastric damage related to iron deficiency or alcohol)
      (4) Endocrine disorders (hypothyroidism, polyendocrinopathy) associated with gastric damage

2. Gastrectomy
   a. Total
   b. Subtotal (approximately 20% develop PA within 10 years after surgery; associated with atrophy of remaining parietal cells)
      (1) Proximal
      (2) Distal
      (3) Lesions that destroy the gastric mucosa (ingested corrosives, linitis plastica)
      (4) Intrinsic factor inhibitor in gastric section

3. Antibody to intrinsic factor (in saliva or gastric juice)
   a. "Blocking" antibody (attaches to intrinsic factor to block ability of intrinsic factor to take up vitamin B$_{12}$)
   b. "Binding" antibody (attaches to intrinsic factor at a site distal to the site of vitamin B$_{12}$ attachment)

B. Small intestinal disorder (affecting ileum, which is the main site of vitamin B$_{12}$ absorption)

1. Gluten-induced enteropathy (childhood and adult celiac disease); idiopathic steatorrhea; nontropical sprue
2. Tropical sprue (vitamin B$_{12}$ is often the first nutrient to be subnormally absorbed and the last to return to normal absorption)
3. Regional enteritis
4. Strictures or anastomoses of the small bowel; other "stagnant bowel" syndromes
5. Intestinal resection
6. Cancers and granulomatous lesions involving the small intestine
7. Other conditions characterized by chronically disturbed intestinal function
8. Drugs inhibiting or preventing vitamin B$_{12}$ absorption
   a. Paraaminosalicylic acid
   b. Colchicine

Modified from Herbert V, Das KC: Folic acid and vitamin B$_{12}$. In Shils ME et al., editors: *Modern nutrition in health and disease*, ed 8, vol 1, Philadelphia, 1994, Lea & Febiger.

BOX 31-1

Causes of Vitamin B$_{12}$ Deficiency—cont'd

      c. Neomycin

      d. Ethanol

      e. Metformin (and possibly other biguanide agents)

      f. Antiretrovirals (see Chapter 38)

    9. Specific malabsorption for vitamin B$_{12}$

      a. Long-term ingestion of calcium-chelating agents

  10. Inadequately alkaline pH in ileum (Zollinger-Ellison syndrome, pancreatic disease)

  11. Unknown causes

      a. Congenital disorder

      b. Acquired disorder

  C. Competition for vitamin B$_{12}$ by intestinal parasites or bacteria

    1. Fish tapeworm (Diphyllobothrium latum)

    2. Bacteria: the blind loop syndrome

    3. *H. pylori*

  D. Pancreatic disease (normal pancreatic exocrine secretion of trypsin and bicarbonate required for normal vitamin B$_{12}$ absorption)

  E. Human immunodeficiency virus (HIV) infection (acquired immune deficiency syndrome [AIDS]) leading to gastrointestinal dysfunction and malabsorption

III. Inadequate use

  A. Vitamin B$_{12}$ antagonists

    1. Substituted vitamin B$_{12}$ amides and anilides (experimental agents)

    2. Cobaloximes (experimental agents)

  B. Congenital or acquired enzyme deficiency or deletion

    1. Methylmalonyl-CoA mutase

    2. Methyltetrahydrofolate-homocysteine methyltransferase

    3. Vitamin B$_{12a}$ reductase

    4. Vitamin B$_{12r}$ reductase

    5. Deoxyadenoxyltransferase

    6. Other enzyme reduction or deletion

  C. Abnormal vitamin B$_{12}$–binding protein in serum that irreversibly binds vitamin B$_{12}$, making it unavailable to tissues

    1. Increased TCI or TCIII glycoprotein (myeloproliferative disorders; "granulocyte-related" vitamin B$_{12}$ binders)

    2. Increased TCII protein (liver disease; "liver-related" vitamin B$_{12}$ binders)

    3. Other abnormal vitamin B$_{12}$ binding (a glycoprotein in some cases of hepatoma)

  D. Inadequate serum vitamin B$_{12}$–binding protein (congenital or acquired)

    1. TCII protein (the lack of which produces megaloblastic anemia; it delivers vitamin B$_{12}$ to blood cells as transferrin delivers iron)

    2. TCI glycoprotein (the lack of which is not known to produce megaloblastic anemia; it is mainly a storage protein for vitamin B$_{12}$, somewhat akin to ceruloplasmin for copper)

    3. TCIII (increasing amounts produced in vitro by granulocytes)

IV. Increased requirement (normal adult daily requirement from exogenous sources is 0.1 mcg [0.073 nmol])

  A. Hyperthyroidism

  B. Increased hematopoiesis

  C. Infancy

  D. Parasitization

    1. By fetus

V. Increased excretion

  A Inadequate vitamin B$_{12}$—binding protein in serum

  B. Liver disease (inadequate storage capacity for vitamin B$_{12}$)

  C. Renal disease

VI. Increased destruction by antioxidants

  A. Pharmacologic doses of ascorbic acid

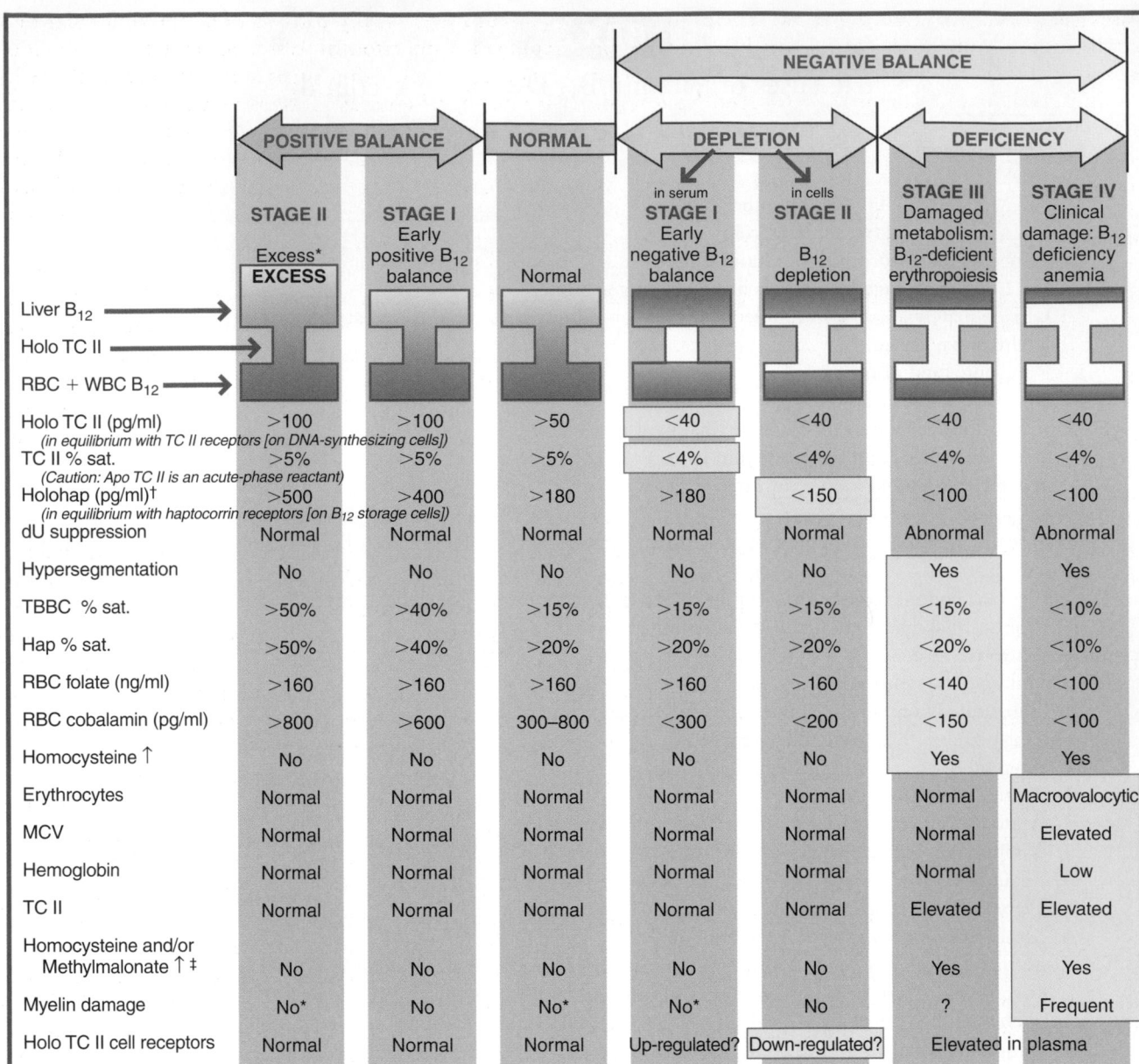

FIGURE 31-3 Sequential stages of vitamin B$_{12}$ status. *(From Herbert V: Staging vitamin B$_{12}$. In Ziegler EE, Filer LJ, editors:* Present knowledge in nutrition, *ed 7, Washington, DC, 1996, International Life Sciences Institute Press.)*

memory, and hallucinations. If the deficiency is prolonged, the nervous system damage may be irreversible, even with initiation of vitamin B$_{12}$ treatment.

A link between vitamin B$_{12}$ deficiency (which affects about 10% to 15% of men and women over 60 years of age) and *Helicobacter pylori* bacterium has been found. Researchers at the Turkish Military Medical Academy studied 138 patients with vitamin B$_{12}$ deficiency anemia and

found that 77 (58%) had *H. pylori* infection (Kaptan et al., 2000; Stopeck, 2000). Treating the infection corrected the anemia and normalized the serum B$_{12}$ levels in 31 (40%) of the 77 infected patients. The researchers concluded that *H. pylori* infection can cause a vitamin B$_{12}$ deficiency, which can be reversed by eradicating the infection.

Atrophic gastritis (inflammation of the stomach) affects up to 30% of people 50 years old and over. This condition decreases gastric acid secretion. Gastric acid helps to release vitamin B_{12} from the protein in food before it is bound to IF and absorbed in the intestines. Not only does the lower gastric acid decrease the vitamin B_{12} absorbed from food, but it also results in overgrowth of normal bacterial flora in the small intestines This bacterial flora is likely to take up the vitamin B_{12} for its own use, further contributing to a vitamin B_{12} deficiency (Suter et al., 1991).

Vitamin B_{12} deficiency may be an important modifiable risk factor for osteoporosis in both men and women. Tucker and Mayer (2005) reported that both men and women with vitamin B_{12} levels below 148 pg/ml had a lower average bone mineral density, putting them at greater risk of osteoporosis.

Diagnosis

Vitamin B_{12} stores are depleted after several years without vitamin B_{12} intake. Time-consuming microbiologic assays have largely been replaced by the less time-consuming, although still precise, simultaneous radioassays. Radioassays measure more than one component within the same biologic medium (i.e., the Becton-Dickinson SimulTRAC Radioassay Kit measures the levels of serum vitamin B_{12} and serum folate simultaneously in a single test tube). Other laboratory tests that may be helpful in diagnosing a vitamin B_{12} deficiency and determining its cause include measurements of unsaturated B_{12} binding capacity, IF antibody (IFAB), the Schilling test, the dU suppression test, and tests to determine serum homocysteine and serum methionine levels (see Chapter 15).

The IFAB and Schilling urinary excretion tests can determine whether the deficiency is caused by a lack of IF. The IFAB assay is performed on a patient's serum, whereas the Schilling test requires that the patient first swallow radioactive B_{12} alone and then a second time with IF.

The vitamin B_{12} assay is performed on the patient's urine after both steps of the Schilling test are completed. Patients with pernicious anemia excrete very little vitamin B_{12} during the first step because little or no vitamin B_{12} is absorbed; however, during the second step the urinary excretion becomes almost normal because more vitamin B_{12} is absorbed with the addition of the IF. Vitamin B_{12} deficiency secondary to malabsorption syndrome is manifested by a decrease in urinary excretion of B_{12} that remains unchanged with IF administration. A low holo-TCII value (<40 pg/ml) is a sign of early B_{12} deficiency.

Medical Management

Before 1926 pernicious anemia was incurable, and the diagnosis invariably meant death in a relatively short time. In 1926 Minot and Murphy reported on the effectiveness of liver therapy, and active concentrates of liver suitable for oral use were soon developed (Minot and Murphy, 1926). By 1936 relatively purified extracts of liver were available for intramuscular injection. In 1948 vitamin B_{12} was determined to be the active agent in liver, and it is now available for either oral or parenteral administration.

Treatment usually consists of an intramuscular or subcutaneous injection of 100 mcg or more of vitamin B_{12} once per week. After an initial response is elicited, the frequency of administration is reduced until remission can be maintained indefinitely with monthly injections of 100 mcg. Very large oral doses of vitamin B_{12} (1000 mcg daily) are also effective, even in the absence of IF, because about 1% of vitamin B_{12} will be absorbed by diffusion. A nasal gel and sublingual tablets are also available and are well absorbed. Initial doses should be increased when vitamin B_{12} deficiency is complicated by debilitating illness such as infection, hepatic disease, uremia, coma, severe disorientation, or marked neurologic damage. A response to treatment is evidenced by improved appetite, alertness, and cooperation, followed by improved hematologic results, as manifested by marked reticulocytosis within hours of an injection.

Medical Nutrition Therapy

A high-protein diet (1.5 g/kg of body weight) is desirable both for liver function and for blood regeneration. Because green leafy vegetables contain both iron and folic acid, the diet should contain increased amounts of these foods. Liver should be included frequently because it carries a good supply of iron, vitamin B_{12}, folic acid, and other important nutrients. Meats (especially beef and pork), eggs, milk, and milk products are particularly rich in vitamin B_{12} (Table 31-3).

For those individuals prescribed metformin for treatment of diabetes, 10% to 30% have reduced vitamin B_{12} absorption. Metformin negatively affects the calcium-dependent membrane and the B_{12}-intrinsic factor complex by decreasing the absorbability by the ileal cell surface receptors. Increased intake of calcium has been shown to reverse vitamin B_{12} malabsorption (Bauman et al., 2000) (see Chapter 16).

The Dietary Guidelines for Americans, 2005, recommend that people over age 50 consume vitamin B_{12} in its crystalline form (i.e., fortified cereals or supplements) to overcome the effects of atrophic gastritis. The DRIs for B_{12} are RDAs and are summarized on the inside front cover. The RDA for adult men and women is 2.4 mcg daily (IOM, 1998).

Folic Acid Deficiency Anemia

Pathophysiology

Folic acid deficiency anemia is associated with tropical sprue, can affect pregnant women, and occurs in infants born to mothers with folic acid deficiency. Folic acid deficiency in early pregnancy can also result in an infant with a neural tube defect (see Chapter 5). Prolonged inadequate diets, faulty absorption and use of folic acid, and increased requirements resulting from growth are believed to be the most frequent causes (Box 31-2). Because alcohol interferes with the folate enterohepatic cycle, most alcoholics have a negative folate balance, and most are folate deficient. Alcoholics constitute the only group that generally has all six causes of folic acid deficiency simultaneously: inadequate

Vitamin B₁₂ Content of Some Common Foods*

Food	Portion Size	Vitamin B₁₂ (mcg)
Mollusks	3 oz	84
Protein Group		
Chicken/turkey	3 oz	0.3
Hamburger	3 oz	8.0
Pork chop	3 oz	0.9
Tenderloin steak	3 oz	0.5
Liver, chicken	3 oz	16.5
Liver, pork	3 oz	15.8
Kidney, pork	3 oz	6.6
Swordfish	3 oz	1.7
Sardines (tomato sauce)	3 oz	7.7
Salmon	3 oz	5.8
Egg	1 whole	0.5
Dairy Group		
Milk (all varieties)	1 c	0.9
Yogurt	1 c	1.4
Cottage cheese	½ c	0.6
Cheese	1 oz	
Mozzarella/American		0.2
Ricotta/provolone		0.4
Swiss		0.5
Grain Group		
Fortified breakfast cereals (100% fortified)	¾ c	6

Copyright 2005 Tracy Stopler, MS, RD.

*Essentially, vitamin B₁₂ is in everything that walks, swims, and flies, and is not in anything that grows in the ground.

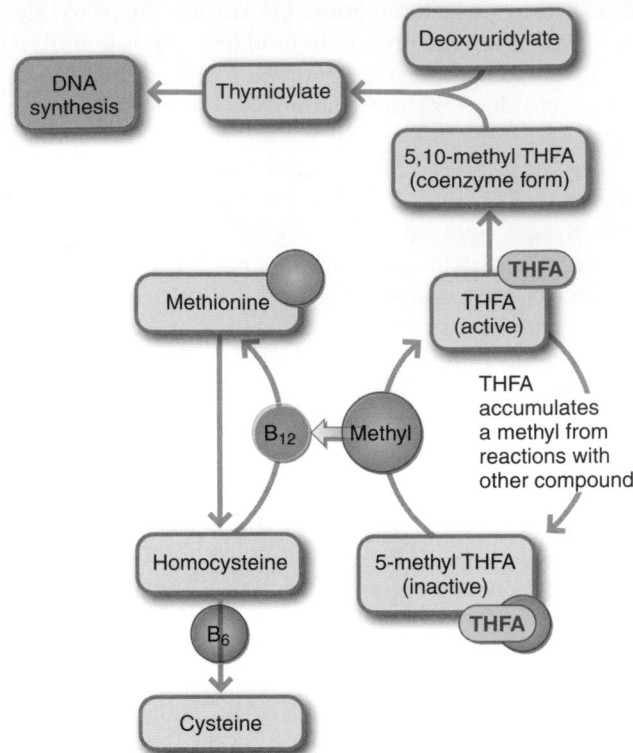

FIGURE 31-4 Methylfolate trap. A deficiency of vitamin B₁₂ can result in a deficiency of folic acid because folate is trapped in the form of 5-methyltetrahydrofolate (5-methyl THFA), which cannot be converted to THFA and methyl groups donated by the vitamin B₁₂–dependent pathway. *DNA,* Deoxyribonucleic acid.

ingestion; absorption; and use and increased excretion, requirement, and destruction of folic acid.

Folate absorption takes place in the small intestine. Enzyme conjugases (e.g., pteroylpolyglutamate hydrolase, commonly called folate conjugase), found in the brush border of the small intestine, hydrolyze the polyglutamates to monoglutamates and reduce them to dihydrofolate and tetrahydrofolate (THFA) in the small intestine epithelial cells (enterocytes). From the enterocytes these forms are transported to the circulation, where they are bound to protein and transported as methyl THFA into the cells of the body.

In the absence of vitamin B₁₂, 5-methyl THFA, the major circulating and storage form of folic acid, is metabolically inactive. To be activated the 5-methyl group is removed, and THFA is cycled back into the folate pool, where it functions as the main 1-carbon-unit acceptor in mammalian biochemical reactions. THFA may then be converted to the coenzyme form of folate required to convert deoxyuridylate to thymidylate, which is necessary for DNA synthesis.

Methylfolate Trap. Vitamin B₁₂ deficiency can result in a folic acid deficiency by causing folate entrapment in the metabolically useless form of 5-methyl THFA (Figure 31-4). The lack of vitamin B₁₂ to remove the 5-methyl unit means that metabolically inactive methyl THFA is trapped. It cannot release its 1-carbon methyl group to become THFA, the basic 1-carbon carrier that picks up 1-carbon units from one molecule and delivers them to another. Hence a functional folic acid deficiency results.

Stages of Deficiency

Folate deficiency develops in four stages: two that involve depletion, followed by two marked by deficiency (Figure 31-5) (Herbert, 1999).

Stage 1—Early negative folate balance (serum depletion). This stage is characterized by a reduction in serum folate levels to less than 3 ng/ml.

Stage 2—Negative folate balance (cell depletion). Folate depletion is characterized by a decrease in erythrocyte folate levels to less than 160 ng/ml.

Stage 3—Damaged folate metabolism, with folate-deficient erythropoiesis. This stage is characterized by slowed DNA synthesis, manifested by an abnormal diagnostic dU suppression test correctable

BOX 31-2

Causes of Folate Deficiency

I. Inadequate ingestion
 A. Poor diet (lack of unprocessed, fresh, uncooked, or slightly cooked food or fruit juices [folates are heat labile])
  1. Nutritional megaloblastic anemia
   a. Tropical
   b. Nontropical
   c. Scurvy (diets low in vitamin C are also low in folate)
  2. Chronic alcoholism, with or without cirrhosis

II. Inadequate absorption (affecting the upper third of the small intestine, which is the main site of folate absorption. Because most food folates are in polyglutamate forms, biliary and intestinal γ-glutamyl conjugases are necessary to split off excess glutamates to make folates absorbable)
 A. Malabsorption syndromes
  1. Gluten-induced enteropathy (childhood and adult celiac disease; idiopathic steatorrhea; nontropical sprue; coincident vitamin B$_{12}$ malabsorption only in rare cases)
  2. Any other chronic functional or structural disorder involving the upper small intestine
   a. Tropical sprue (coincident vitamin B$_{12}$ malabsorption almost invariably present)
   b. Associated with herpetic and other skin disorders
  3. Drugs
   a. Anticonvulsants (e.g., phenytoin, primidone)
   b. Barbiturates
   c. Cycloserine
   d. Ethanol
   e. Metformin
   f. Amino acid excess (glycine or methionine)
   g. Cholestyramine
   h. Sulfasalazine (Azulfidine)
 B. Specific malabsorption for folate
  1. Congenital nonconjugase defects (four cases published)
  2. Acquired nonconjugase defects
  3. Inadequate biliary or intestinal conjugases
  4. Conjugase inhibitors (e.g., such as those contained in some beans)
 C. Blind loop syndrome (More commonly, bacteria make folate and actually raise the serum folate level of the host.)

III. Inadequate use (metabolic block)
 A. Folic acid antagonists (dihydrofolate reductase inhibitors)
  1. 4-Amino-4-deoxyfolates (e.g., methotrexate [chemotherapy, immunosuppression, psoriasis])
  2. 2-4-Diaminopyrimidine (e.g., pyrimethamine, trimethoprim [malaria, toxoplasmosis, antibacterial])
  3. Triamterene (diuretic)
  4. Diamidine compounds (e.g., pentamidine, isethionate [*Pneumocystis carinii*, protozocidal])
 B. Diphenylhydantoin and possibly other anticonvulsants, which may block cell uptake or use folate
 C. Enzyme deficiency
  1. Congenital
   a. Formiminotransferase
   b. Dihydrofolate reductase
   c. Methyltetrahydrofolate transmethylase
   d. Other enzymes (some of which affect folate secondarily)
  2. Acquired due to liver disease
   a. Formiminotransferase
   b. Other enzymes
 D. Vitamin B$_{12}$ deficiency (reduced folate uptake and retention)
 E. Alcohol (both specific and nonspecific damage)
 F. Ascorbic acid deficiency
 G. Dietary amino acid excess (glycine, methionine)

IV. Increased requirement
 A. Extra tissue demand
  1. Pregnancy
  2. Lactation
  3. By malignant tissue (especially in lymphoproliferative disorders)
 B. Infancy
 C. Increased hematopoiesis
 D. Increased metabolic activity
 E. Lesch-Nyhan syndrome
 F. Drugs

V. Increased excretion
 A. Vitamin B$_{12}$ deficiency (possible obligatory excretion of folate in urine and bile)
 B. Liver disease
 C. Kidney dialysis
 D. Chronic exfoliative dermatitis

VI. Increased destruction
 A. Oxidants in diet

Modified from Herbert V, Das KC: Folic acid and vitamin B$_{12}$. In Shils ME et al., editors: *Modern nutrition in health and disease*, ed 8, vol 1, Philadelphia, 1994, Lea & Febiger.

in vitro by folates, granulocyte nuclear hypersegmentation, and macroovalocytic red cells.

Stage 4—Clinical folate deficiency anemia. This stage is manifested by an elevated MCV and anemia.

Clinical Findings

Because of their interrelated roles in the synthesis of thymidylate in DNA formation, a deficiency of either vitamin B_{12} or folic acid will result in the same clinical sign (i.e., a megaloblastic anemia). The immature nuclei do not mature properly in the deficient state; and large (macrocytic), immature (megaloblastic) red blood cells are the result. The common clinical signs of folic acid deficiency include fatigue, dyspnea, sore tongue, diarrhea, irritability, forgetfulness, anorexia, glossitis, and weight loss.

Diagnosis

Normal body folate stores are depleted within 2 to 4 months on a folate-deficient diet, resulting in a macrocytic, megaloblastic anemia. This state is also characterized by a decreased number of erythrocytes, leukocytes, and platelets. Folate deficiency anemia is manifested by very low serum folate (<3 ng/ml) and red blood cell (RBC) folate levels <140-160 ng/ml. Whereas a low serum folate level merely diagnoses a negative balance at the time the blood is drawn, an RCF level measures actual body folate stores and thus is the superior measurement for determining folate nutriture. To differentiate folate deficiency from vitamin B_{12} deficiency, levels of serum folate, RCF, serum vitamin B_{12}, and vitamin B_{12} bound to TCII can be measured simultaneously using a radioassay kit. Also diagnostic for folate deficiency is an elevated level of formiminoglutamic acid in the urine, as well as the dU suppression test in bone marrow cells or peripheral blood lymphocytes.

Medical Management

Before treatment is initiated, it is important to diagnose the cause of the megaloblastosis correctly. Administration of folate will correct megaloblastosis from either folate or vitamin B_{12} deficiency, but it can mask the neurologic damage of vitamin B_{12} deficiency, allowing the nerve damage to progress to the point of irreversibility.

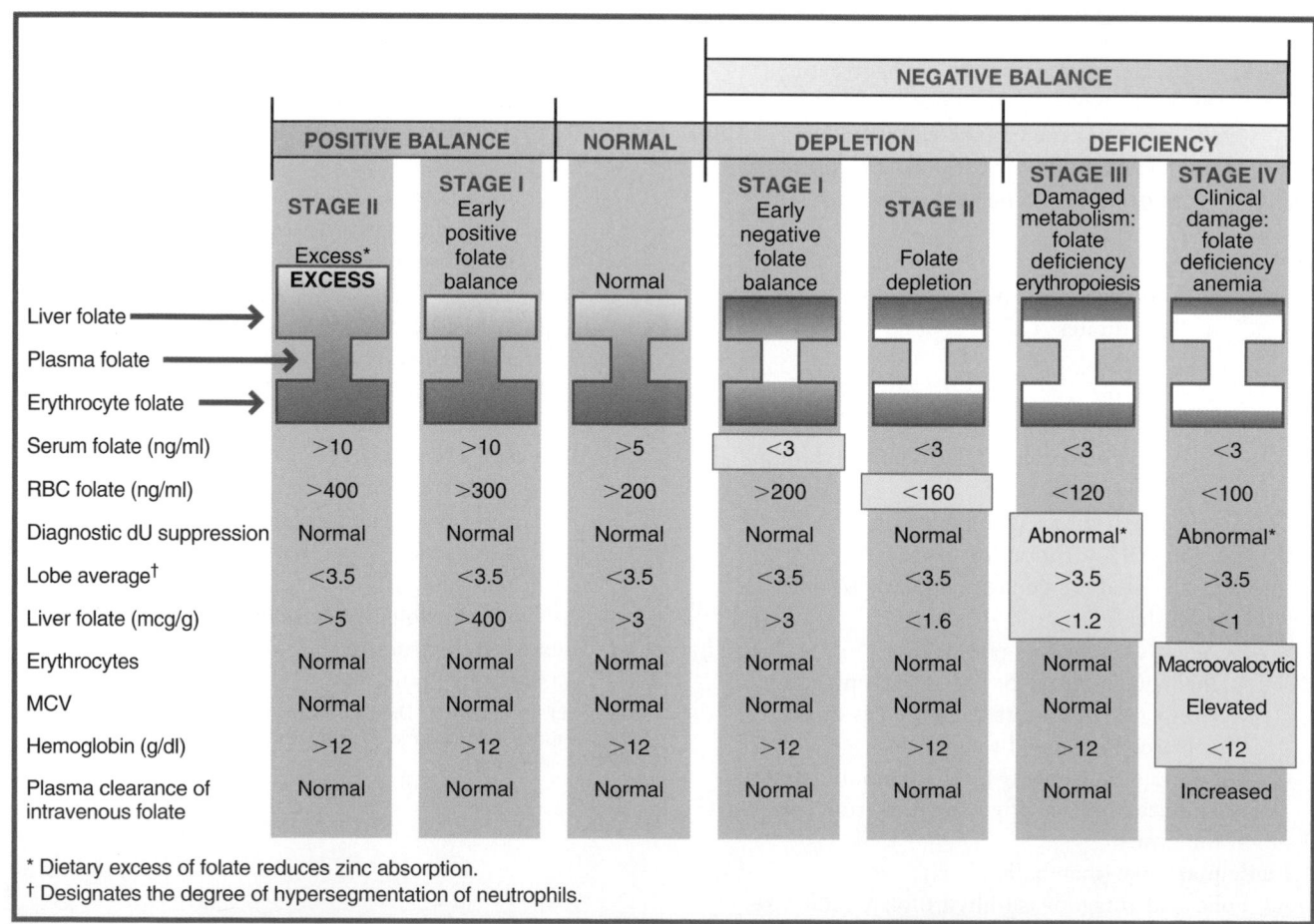

	POSITIVE BALANCE		NORMAL	NEGATIVE BALANCE			
				DEPLETION		DEFICIENCY	
	STAGE II	STAGE I Early positive folate balance		STAGE I Early negative folate balance	STAGE II	STAGE III Damaged metabolism: folate deficiency erythropoiesis	STAGE IV Clinical damage: folate deficiency anemia
	Excess* EXCESS		Normal		Folate depletion		
Serum folate (ng/ml)	>10	>10	>5	<3	<3	<3	<3
RBC folate (ng/ml)	>400	>300	>200	>200	<160	<120	<100
Diagnostic dU suppression	Normal	Normal	Normal	Normal	Normal	Abnormal*	Abnormal*
Lobe average†	<3.5	<3.5	<3.5	<3.5	<3.5	>3.5	>3.5
Liver folate (mcg/g)	>5	>400	>3	>3	<1.6	<1.2	<1
Erythrocytes	Normal	Normal	Normal	Normal	Normal	Normal	Macroovalocytic
MCV	Normal	Normal	Normal	Normal	Normal	Normal	Elevated
Hemoglobin (g/dl)	>12	>12	>12	>12	>12	>12	<12
Plasma clearance of intravenous folate	Normal	Normal	Normal	Normal	Normal	Normal	Increased

* Dietary excess of folate reduces zinc absorption.
† Designates the degree of hypersegmentation of neutrophils.

FIGURE 31-5 Sequential stages of folate status. *dU,* Deoxyuridine; *MCV,* mean corpuscular volume; *RBC,* red blood cell. (*From Herbert V: Folic acid. In Shils ME, Olson JA, Shike M, editors:* Modern nutrition in health and disease, *ed 9, Philadelphia 1998, Lea & Febiger.*)

A dosage of 1 mg of folate taken orally every day for 2 to 3 weeks will replenish folate stores. Maintaining repleted stores requires an absolute minimum oral intake of 50 to 100 mcg of folic acid daily. When folate deficiency is complicated by alcoholism or other conditions that suppress hematopoiesis, increase folate requirements, or reduce folate absorption, therapy should remain at 500 to 1000 mcg daily. Symptomatic improvement, as evidenced by increased alertness, cooperation, and appetite, may be apparent within 24 to 48 hours, long before hematologic values revert to normal, a gradual process that takes about a month.

Medical Nutrition Therapy

After the anemia is corrected, the patient should be instructed to eat at least one fresh, uncooked fruit or vegetable or to drink a glass of fruit juice daily. One cup of orange juice supplies about 135 mcg of folic acid (see Table 31-4 for a list of foods). Fresh, uncooked fruits and vegetables are good sources of folate because folate can easily be destroyed by heat.

Fortification of grains with folic acid, required by the Food and Drug Administration in January 1998, is an important addition of folate to the American diet (see *Focus On: Popular Low Carbohydrate Diets Increase the Risk of Birth Defects and Heart Disease*).

The Dietary Guidelines for Americans, 2005, recommend that women of childbearing age who may become pregnant and those in their first trimester of pregnancy consume adequate synthetic folic acid (from fortified foods and supplements) in addition to consuming a variety of foods containing folate. The DRIs for folate are RDAs and are summarized on the inside front cover of this text. The RDA for adults is 400 mcg daily (IOM, 1998).

TABLE 31-4

Folic Acid Content of Some Common Foods

Food	Portion Size	Folate (mcg)	Food	Portion Size	Folate (mcg)
Protein Group			**Vegetable Group**		
Chicken, light meat	3 oz	3.0	Baked potato	1 medium	22.0
Chicken, dark meat	3 oz	7.2	Sweet potato	1 medium	26.0
Turkey, dark meat	3 oz	7.9	Broccoli	1 c	62.0
Pork chop	3 oz	5.2	Brussels sprouts	½ c	47.0
Tenderloin steak	3 oz	5.0	Endive	½ c	36.0
Liver, chicken	3 oz	654.0	Spinach	½ c	108.0
Liver, pork	3 oz	139.0	**Grain Group**		
Tuna fish	3 oz	3.5	Barley	½ c	13.0
Sardines (tomato sauce)	3 oz	21.0	Whole-wheat bread	1 slice	14.0
Salmon	3 oz	13.0	Wheat germ	¼ c	99.0
Tofu, raw	½ c	37.0	Grapenuts cereal	¼ c	101.0
Egg	1	23.0	Fortified cereals (100% fortified)	Varies	400.0
Black beans	½ c	128.0			
Kidney beans	½ c	18.0			
Lentil beans	½ c	36.0			
Soybean nuts	½ c	122.0			
Cashew nuts	1 oz	19.6			
Dairy Group					
Milk (all varieties)	1 c	13.0			
Yogurt	1 c	28.0			
Cottage cheese	½ c	10.5			
Fruit Group					
Apricots	3 raw	9.1			
Orange	1	40.0			
Orange juice	1 c	136.0			
Strawberries, frozen	1 c	9.7			
Banana	1	22.0			

Copyright 2005 Tracy Stopler, MS, RD.

◎ **FOCUS ON**

Popular Low Carbohydrate Diets Increase the Risk of Birth Defects and Heart Disease

What do Atkins, South Beach, Carbohydrate Addicts, and Protein Power diets have in common? They all ignore the important role that folate plays in reducing the rate of neural tube defects, elevated homocysteine levels, and hypertension. Folate is so important that in January 1998, the Food and Drug Administration required the enrichment of breads, cereals, flours, pasta, rice and other grain products with at least 20% of the recommended dietary allowance of folic acid per serving. The widespread impact of low-carbohydrate diets, in which these grains are minimized or eliminated, increases the possibility of inadequate folic acid intake and risk for these disease states:

Neural Tube Defects: The role that folate plays in the development of the fetus' spinal cord and brain to prevent neural tube defects is well documented (see Chapter 5). Following a low-carbohydrate diet goes against the mother and her unborn child's best interest. Women should begin eating foods and supplements containing folic acid 2 to 3 months before conception and during the first trimester of pregnancy. Taking the recommended 400 mcg of folic acid before conception and throughout the first trimester of pregnancy would reduce the risk of neural tube defect cases by 50% to 70% (Dalal et al., 2006).

Homocyteine: According to several studies, a deficiency of folate, vitamin B_{12}, or vitamin B_6 may increase serum homocysteine level, increasing risk for heart disease and stroke (Rimm et al., 1998; Refsum et al., 1998; Siri et al., 1998).

Hypertension: A higher folic acid intake from food and supplements appears to lower the risk of hypertension (Forman et al., 2005).

To overcome these risk factors, it is recommended that extreme diet plans be avoided. If moderation, variety, and balance of all foods from all food groups cannot be consumed to get the minimum amount of folate and other B vitamins needed, then taking 400 mcg to 800 mcg of folic acid daily is recommended.

OTHER NUTRITIONAL ANEMIAS

Copper-Deficiency Anemia

Copper and other heavy metals are essential for the proper formation of hemoglobin. Ceruloplasmin, a copper-containing protein, is required for normal mobilization of iron from its storage sites to the plasma. In a copper-deficient state, iron cannot be released, leading to low serum iron and hemoglobin levels, even in the presence of normal iron stores. Other consequences of copper deficiency suggest that copper proteins are needed for use of iron by the developing erythrocyte and for optimal functions of the erythrocyte membrane (see Chapter 3). The amounts of copper needed for normal hemoglobin synthesis are so minute that they are usually amply supplied by an adequate diet; however, copper deficiency may occur in infants who are fed cow's milk or a copper-deficient infant formula. It may also be seen in children or adults who have a malabsorption syndrome or who are receiving long-term total parenteral nutrition that does not supply copper.

Anemia of Protein-Energy Malnutrition

Protein is essential for the proper production of hemoglobin and red blood cells. Because of the reduction in cell mass and thus oxygen requirements in protein-energy malnutrition (PEM), fewer red blood cells are required to oxygenate the tissue. Because blood volume remains the same, this reduced number of red blood cells with a low hemoglobin level (**hypochromic,** normocytic anemia), which can mimic an iron deficiency anemia, is actually a physiologic (nonharmful) rather than harmful anemia. In acute PEM, the loss of active tissue mass may be greater than the reduction in the number of red blood cells, leading to polycythemia. The body responds to this red blood cell production, which is not a reflection of protein and amino acid deficiency but of an oversupply of red blood cells. Iron released from normal red blood cell destruction is not reused in red blood cell production but is stored, so that iron stores are often adequate. Iron deficiency anemia can reappear with rehabilitation when red blood cell mass expands rapidly.

The anemia of PEM may be complicated by deficiencies of iron and other nutrients and by associated infections, parasitic infestation, and malabsorption. A diet lacking in protein is usually deficient in iron, folic acid, and, less frequently, vitamin B_{12}. The nutrition counselor plays an important role in assessing recent and typical dietary intake of these nutrients.

Sideroblastic (Pyridoxine-Responsive) Anemia

Sideroblastic anemia has four primary characteristics: (1) microcytic and hypochromic red blood cells; (2) high serum and tissue iron levels (causing increased transferrin saturation); (3) the presence of an inherited defect in the formation of δ-aminolevulinic acid synthetase, an enzyme involved in heme synthesis (pyridoxal-5-phosphate is necessary in this reaction); and (4) a buildup of iron-containing immature red blood cells (sideroblasts, for which the anemia is named). The iron that cannot be used for heme synthesis is stored in the mitochondria of immature red blood cells. These iron-laden mitochondria do not function normally, and the development and production of red blood cells become ineffective. The symptoms are those of both anemia and iron overload. The neurologic and cutaneous manifestations of vitamin B_6 deficiency are not observed. The anemia responds to the administration of pharmacologic doses of pyridoxine and thus is referred to as vitamin B_6 (pyridoxine)–responsive anemia, to distinguish it from anemia caused by a dietary vitamin B_6 deficiency.

Treatment consists of a therapeutic trial dose of 50 to 200 mg daily of pyridoxine or pyridoxal phosphate, which is 25 to 100 times the RDA. If the anemia responds to one or the other, pyridoxine therapy is continued for life. However, the anemia is only partially corrected; a normal **hematocrit** value is never regained. Patients respond to this treatment to varying degrees, and some may achieve near-normal hemoglobin levels.

Unlike the familial sideroblastic anemia just mentioned, acquired sideroblastic anemias such as those attributable to drug therapy (isoniazid, chloramphenicol), copper deficiency, hypothermia, and alcoholism are not responsive to vitamin B_6 (pyridoxine administration).

Vitamin E–Responsive Anemia

Hemolytic anemia occurs when defects in red blood cell membranes lead to oxidative damage and eventually to cell lysis. Vitamin E, an antioxidant, is involved in protecting the membrane against oxidative damage, and one of the few signs noted in vitamin E deficiency is early hemolysis of red blood cells (see Chapter 3). Vitamin E–responsive hemolytic anemia in neonates is discussed in Chapter 43.

NONNUTRITIONAL ANEMIAS

Sports Anemia (Hypochromic Microcytic Transient Anemia)

Increased red blood cell destruction, along with decreased hemoglobin, serum iron, and ferritin concentrations, may occur at the initiation and early stages of a vigorous training program. Once called march hemoglobinuria, this anemia was believed to arise in soldiers as a result of mechanical trauma incurred by erythrocytes (red blood cells) during long marches. The red blood cells in the capillaries are compressed every time the foot lands until they burst, releasing hemoglobin. It was thought that a similar situation existed in runners, especially long-distance runners; however, it is now thought that it is a physiologic anemia (i.e., a transient problem of blood volume and dilution) (see Chapter 23 for further discussion).

Athletes who have hemoglobin concentrations below those needed for optimal oxygen delivery may benefit from consuming nutrient and iron-rich foods; ensuring that their diets contain adequate protein; and avoiding tea, coffee, antacids, H_2-blockers, and tetracycline, all of which inhibit iron absorption. No athlete should take iron supplements unless true iron deficiency is diagnosed based on a complete blood cell count with differential, serum ferritin level, se-

rum iron level, TIBC, and percent saturation of iron-binding capacity. Athletes who are female, vegetarian, involved in endurance sports, or entering a growth spurt are at risk for iron deficiency anemia and therefore should undergo periodic monitoring.

Anemia of Pregnancy

Another physiologic anemia is the anemia of pregnancy, which is related to increased blood volume and usually resolves with the end of the pregnancy; however, demands for iron during pregnancy are also increased so that inadequate iron intake may also play a role (see Chapter 5 for further discussion).

Anemia of Chronic Disease

Anemia of chronic disease from inflammation, infection, or malignancy occurs because there is decreased red blood cell production, possibly as a result of disordered iron metabolism. Why this happens is unclear, but it may be caused by the presence of inflammatory cytokines such as interleukin-1 and tumor necrosis factor, which decrease iron absorption and erythroblast activity (Spivak, 2002). Ferritin levels are normal or increased, but serum iron levels and TIBC are low (see Chapter 15 for further discussion). It is important that this form of anemia, which is mild and normocytic, not be mistaken for iron deficiency anemia and that iron supplements be given inappropriately. Recombinant erythropoietin therapy usually corrects this anemia.

Sickle Cell Anemia

Pathophysiology

Sickle cell anemia, a chronic hemolytic anemia also known as hemoglobin S disease, affects 1 of 600 blacks in the United States as a result of homozygous inheritance of hemoglobin S. This results in defective hemoglobin synthesis, which produces sickle-shaped red blood cells that get caught in capillaries and do not carry oxygen well. The disease is usually diagnosed toward the end of the first year of life.

Clinical Findings

In addition to the usual symptoms of anemia, sickle cell anemia is characterized by episodes of pain resulting from the occlusion of small blood vessels by the abnormally shaped erythrocytes. The occlusions frequently occur in the abdomen, causing acute, severe abdominal pain. The hemolytic anemia and vasoocclusive disease result in impaired liver function, jaundice, gallstones, and deteriorating renal function. The constant hemolysis of erythrocytes increases iron stores in the liver; however, iron deficiency anemia and sickle cell anemia can coexist. Iron overload is less common and is usually a problem only in those who have received multiple blood transfusions.

Typically serum homocysteine levels are elevated in these children, which may be due to low concentrations of vitamin B_6. Children with sickle cell anemia were found to have these lower vitamin B_6 levels despite B_6 intakes comparable to those of unaffected children (Segal et al., 2004).

Medical Management

No specific treatment exists for sickle cell anemia other than relieving pain during a crisis, keeping the body oxygenated, and possibly administering an exchange transfusion. It is important that sickle cell anemia not be mistaken for iron deficiency anemia, which can be treated with iron supplements, because iron stores in the patient with sickle cell anemia secondary to transfusions are frequently excessive.

Zinc can increase the oxygen affinity of both normal and sickle-shaped erythrocytes. Thus zinc supplements may be beneficial in managing sickle cell disease, especially because decreased plasma zinc is common in children with the SS genotype sickle cell disease and is associated with decreased linear and skeletal growth, muscle mass, and sexual maturation. Zinc supplementation (as little as 10 mg daily) may also prevent the deficit in growth that appears in these children (Zemel et al., 2002). Curiously this growth and development retardation is more apparent in males than in females (Modebe and Ifenu, 1993). Because zinc competes with copper for binding sites on proteins, the use of high doses of zinc may precipitate copper deficiency.

Medical Nutrition Therapy

Children with sickle cell anemia and their families should receive instruction about how they can develop a well-balanced food plan providing enough calories and protein for growth and development. Their dietary intake can be low because of the abdominal pain characteristic of the disease. They also have increased metabolic rates, by as much as 16% in adolescents, leading to a need for a higher caloric intake (Buchowski et al., 2002). This hypermetabolism is probably due to a constant inflammation and oxidative stress (Akohoue et al., 2007; Hibbert et al., 2005). Therefore their diets must be high enough in calories to meet these needs and must provide foods high in the vitamin folate (see Table 31-4) and the trace minerals zinc and copper (see Appendix 58 and Chapter 3 for sources of these minerals). In addition, they may be low in vitamins A, C, D, and E; and this needs to be addressed in food choices (Schall et al., 2004; Buison et al., 2004).

When assessing the nutrition status of patients with sickle cell anemia, the questions related to the use of vitamin and mineral supplements, the consumption of alcohol (which increases iron absorption), and sources of protein (animal sources being high in both zinc and iron) in the diet must be given special attention. A multivitamin/mineral supplement containing 50% to 150% of the RDA for folate, zinc, and copper (not iron) is recommended; 2 to 3 quarts of water daily is also important. Finally it is important to remember that patients with sickle cell disease may require higher than RDA amounts of protein.

If it is necessary for the diet to be low in absorbable iron, the diet should emphasize vegetable proteins. Iron-rich foods, such as liver, iron-fortified formula, iron-fortified cereals, and iron-fortified energy bars are excluded. Substances such as alcohol and ascorbic acid supplements, both of which enhance iron absorption should be avoided. However, it is important to remember that iron deficiency may be present in some patients with sickle cell anemia owing to repeated phlebotomies, excessive transfusions, or hematuria secondary to renal papillary necrosis. This should be assessed, and the diet adjusted appropriately. The diet should be high in folate (400 to 600 mcg daily) because the increased production of erythrocytes needed to replace the cells being continuously destroyed also increases folic acid requirements (see Table 31-4).

Thalassemias

Thalassemias (α and β) are severe inherited anemias characterized by microcytic, hypochromic, and short-lived red blood cells resulting from defective hemoglobin synthesis, which affects mostly persons in the Mediterranean region. The ineffective erythropoiesis leads to an increase in plasma volume, progressive splenomegaly, and bone marrow expansion with the result of facial deformities, osteomalacia, and bone changes. Ultimately there is increased iron absorption and progressive iron deposition in tissues, resulting in oxidative damage. The accumulation of iron causes dysfunction of the heart, liver, and endocrine glands. Because these patients require transfusions to stay alive, they must also have regular chelation therapy to prevent the damaging buildup of iron that can occur. Malnutrition is common and is an important factor in the stunted growth in these children (Fuchs et al., 1996).

⊙ FOCAL POINTS

- Anemia is a worldwide problem in persons of all ages; it is not a diagnosis but rather a sign or symptom of an underlying disorder.
- The goal of anemia management is to investigate and understand the different stages of anemia and its pathophysiologic mechanism so that proper treatment can begin.
- Thorough assessment is important. Determination of the underlying cause in nonnutritional anemias (such as anemia of inflammation) leads to appropriate medical treatment and eventual resolution.
- Identification of the etiology of a nutritional anemia as the result of inadequate intake, absorption, use, or increased requirement is essential to support the provision of targeted medical nutrition therapy.
- The registered dietitian is most effective with a complete understanding of the types of anemia and the ability to translate this understanding into practical advice for the patient.

Dedicated to the memory of Victor Herbert, MD, a pioneer in the area of macrocytic anemia and folic acid and vitamin B_{12} deficiencies.

✦ CLINICAL SCENARIO 1

Dana is a 30-year-old mother of a 2-year-old and is now planning to become pregnant with her second child. Struggling to lose the last 10 pounds from her first pregnancy, her diet of choice over this past year has been a version of the low-carbohydrate diet. Dana's food intake lacks variety and balance. She is low on fruits, vegetables, and grains. She complains of diarrhea, loss of appetite, weakness, and irritability. Her blood work reveals a normal hemoglobin level but a low serum folate level. She has scheduled an appointment to see you.

✳Nutrition Diagnosis: Inadequate B vitamin intake related to consumption of very low–carbohydrate diet as evidenced by low serum folate level

1. What are the risks of following a low-carbohydrate diet, especially before pregnancy?
2. What folate-containing, nutrient-dense foods could be included in her diet that would be beneficial to her pending pregnancy?
4. What supplements, if any, and in what amounts, would you recommend to Dana?
5. Which websites can you refer Dana to for her to learn more about the role of folate and neural tube defects?
6. What information do you need to gather before developing a plan for Dana? Of what would this plan consist?

✦ CLINICAL SCENARIO 2

Sarah is a 22-year-old recent college graduate who has joined the Peace Corp. On arrival in southern Africa, Sarah began feeling fatigued and weak. The site's nurse suggested that her symptoms were indicative of anemia and asked Sarah whether she was taking any multivitamin/mineral supplements. Sarah said she was taking a multivitamin (without iron) and also taking 1000 mg of vitamin C daily. The nurse gave Sarah a 15-mg iron supplement to be taken daily. Sarah's symptoms never subsided, and now, 10 months later, Sarah has begun experiencing abdominal pain, aching joints, and irregular menses. Sarah, now back in the United States, has made an appointment with you.

✳Nutrition Diagnosis: Inadequate iron intake related to iron supplementation less than appropriate as evidenced by progression of anemia

1. What questions are most relevant for you to ask during her initial evaluation?
2. What potential problems does Sarah face if her condition progresses?
3. What nutrition recommendations would you give to Sarah?
4. Do you think a vegetarian lifestyle would be more or less helpful? Why?
5. Discuss the genetic possibilities (i.e., hemochromatosis/thalassemia) as well as the environmental concerns you have regarding her case.
6. It is clear to you that Sarah needs to make an appointment with her physician. Write a letter to her physician discussing your thoughts and concerns. Also include your care plan and recommendations for laboratory tests that Sarah should have done.

USEFUL WEBSITES

Anemia Institute for Research and Education
www.anemiainstitute.org/

Anemia Lifeline
www.anemia.com/

Iron Disorders Institute
www.irondisorders.org/disorders/aio/

Iron Overload Disease Association
www.ironoverload.org/

National Institutes of Health
www.niddk.nih.gov/ health/hematol

Dietary Guidelines for Americans, 2005
www.health.gov/dietaryguidelines

low-density lipoproteins (LDLs) class of lipoproteins that are the predominant cholesterol carriers in the blood and considered atherogenic; main target for interventions because high levels are associated with increased risk of cardiovascular disease

metabolic syndrome constellation of risk factors—glucose intolerance, hypertension, abdominal obesity, low high-density–lipoprotein cholesterol, and hypercholesterolemia—that increases the risk of cardiovascular disease

myocardial infarction (MI) ischemia in one or more of the coronary arteries resulting in necrosis, tissue damage, and sometimes sudden death

nitric oxide key vasodilator produced by endothelial cells; also known as endothelium-derived relaxing factor or EDRF; prevents low-density lipoprotein oxidation

plaque early lesions seen in atherosclerosis; composed of cholesterol, calcium, and fibrin

risk factors characteristics found in healthy individuals that increase the likelihood of a person developing a disease; for coronary heart disease, major risk factors are hypercholesterolemia, hypertension, obesity, and cigarette smoking

stroke occlusion or hemorrhage of a cerebral artery resulting in impaired function, tissue damage, or death

thrombus a group of blood factors, primarily platelets and fibrin, which, if small, can contribute to the growth of plaque and, if large, can obstruct a blood vessel, resulting in angina, myocardial infarction, or sudden death

very low–density lipoproteins (VLDLs) primary triglyceride-carrying lipoproteins that transport endogenous lipid from the liver to the peripheral circulation

xanthoma cholesterol deposits (from low-density lipoproteins) seen on tendons and elbows

EPIDEMIOLOGY

Since 1900 cardiovascular disease (CVD) has been the leading cause of death in the United States for every year except 1918 (Thom et al., 2006). Of these deaths from CVD, 53% are from **coronary heart disease** (impaired blood flow in the coronary arteries that results in angina, myocardial infarction, and sudden death), and 17% are from stroke. The morbidity and mortality associated with CVD make it a major public health problem, with approximate costs in 2006 exceeding $403 billion.

Although most CVD deaths occur in persons older than 65 years of age, one third of deaths occur prematurely or before average life expectancy is reached. This observation has led to extensive research on prevention. Epidemiologic studies (observational studies such as cohort and cross-sectional studies) and experimental studies (clinical or community trials) have delineated the **risk factors** associated with CVD development, which has been a major breakthrough for prevention and treatment. One of the greatest public health successes in the twentieth century has been the decline in age-adjusted mortality rates from CVD (Thom et al., 2006).

Prevalence and Incidence

The United States ranks thirteenth and seventeenth among industrialized nations for the prevalence of CVD in women and men, respectively. More than 71 million Americans have at least one form of CVD (i.e., hypertension, coronary heart disease [CHD], stroke, rheumatic heart disease, or heart failure). Most CHD and strokes are the result of **ischemia,** or impaired blood flow. The distribution of CVD varies by race and ethnic group (Thom et al., 2006). In 2003 the prevalence of CVD was highest in non-Hispanic blacks (41% for men, 45% women), followed by non-Hispanic whites (34% men, 32% women) and Mexican-Americans (29% men, 29% women) (Thom et al., 2006). Non-Hispanic blacks are also more likely to have hypertension and stroke than non-Hispanic whites.

Native Hawaiians, Pacific Islanders, American Indians, or Alaskan natives are more likely to have CHD than the other groups. Hispanics, Latinos, and Asians have the lowest rates of all forms of CVD. With aging the prevalence of CVD increases, with a doubling of rates between middle (ages 35 to 44 years) and later ages (65 to 74 years of age). The incidence of CHD is high; 700,000 Americans had a new coronary attack and 500,000 had a recurrent attack in 2000. Men experience earlier incidence than women.

Mortality

Diseases of the heart and stroke cause most deaths in both sexes of all ethnic groups. CHD expressed as **myocardial infarction (MI)** or ischemia in one or more of the coronary arteries resulting in necrosis and tissue damage is the main form of heart disease responsible for these deaths. Mortality from all heart diseases increases with age in all races. Until the age of 65 years, black men have the highest rates of CHD deaths; thereafter white men have the highest rates. Black women have higher rates than white females at all ages. One in 30 women will die from breast cancer compared to 1 in 2.6 from CVD (Thom et al., 2006). Of all causes of death, stroke is the third leading cause of death, behind CHD and cancer. From 1993 to 2003 the number of deaths from stroke decreased by 19% (Thom et al., 2006). More blacks than whites die of strokes, especially blacks who live in the southeastern part of the United States, which is often called the "stroke belt." The age-adjusted death rates for CHD and stroke have been declining since the late 80s. Between the genders, CVD rates have fallen more in men than women.

PATHOPHYSIOLOGY

Atherosclerosis

Atherosclerosis is the most common cause of CHD and related mortality. The first observable event in the process of atherosclerosis is the accumulation of **plaque** (cholesterol from low-density lipoproteins [LDLs], calcium, and fibrin) in large and medium arteries. This plaque can grow and produce ischemia either by insufficient blood flow if there is a high oxygen demand or by rupturing, forming a thrombus and occluding the lumen (Rudd et al., 2005). Only high-risk or vulnerable plaque forms thrombi. Characteristics of vulnerable plaque are lesions with a thin fibrous cap, few smooth muscle cells, many macrophages (inflammatory cells), and a large lipid core (Figure 32-1) (Rudd et al., 2005).

The site of plaque formation or atherogenesis is the endothelium in the artery wall. Normally the endothelium promotes dilation of the blood vessel, less smooth muscle cell growth, and prevention of an antiinflammatory response (Davignon and Ganz, 2004). In atherosclerosis the endothelium becomes dysfunctional before an **atheroma** or plaque, a more serious lesion, develops. This **endothelial dysfunction** results in the production of less **nitric oxide,** a key vasodilator, and the blood vessel becomes more constricted. It also becomes more permeable and allows LDL cholesterol to be taken up by macrophages, which then accumulate and form foam cells and eventually an early lesion known as a **fatty streak** (Figure 32-2).

Endothelial dysfunction initiates atherosclerosis; fortunately the dysfunction is reversible (Viles-Gonzales et al., 2004). Some of the factors that cause endothelial dysfunction are **dyslipidemia** (abnormality in any of the lipoprotein fractions), especially elevated LDLs and decreased high-density lipoproteins (HDLs); hypertension; cigarette smoking; diabetes; obesity; hyperhomocysteinemia; and diets high in saturated fat and cholesterol. *Therefore endothelial dysfunction is an end point that can be modified by diet and other lifestyle changes.* With prevention the goal is to reduce inflammation, endothelial dysfunction, thrombosis, and vulnerable plaque (Naghavi et al., 2006).

Arterial changes begin in infancy and progress asymptomatically throughout adulthood if the person has risk factors, is susceptible to arterial thrombosis, or has a genetic susceptibility to getting atherosclerosis (Figure 32-3) (Naghavi et al., 2006). Consequently, atherosclerosis is called a silent disease because many individuals are asymptomatic until the first MI, which is often fatal.

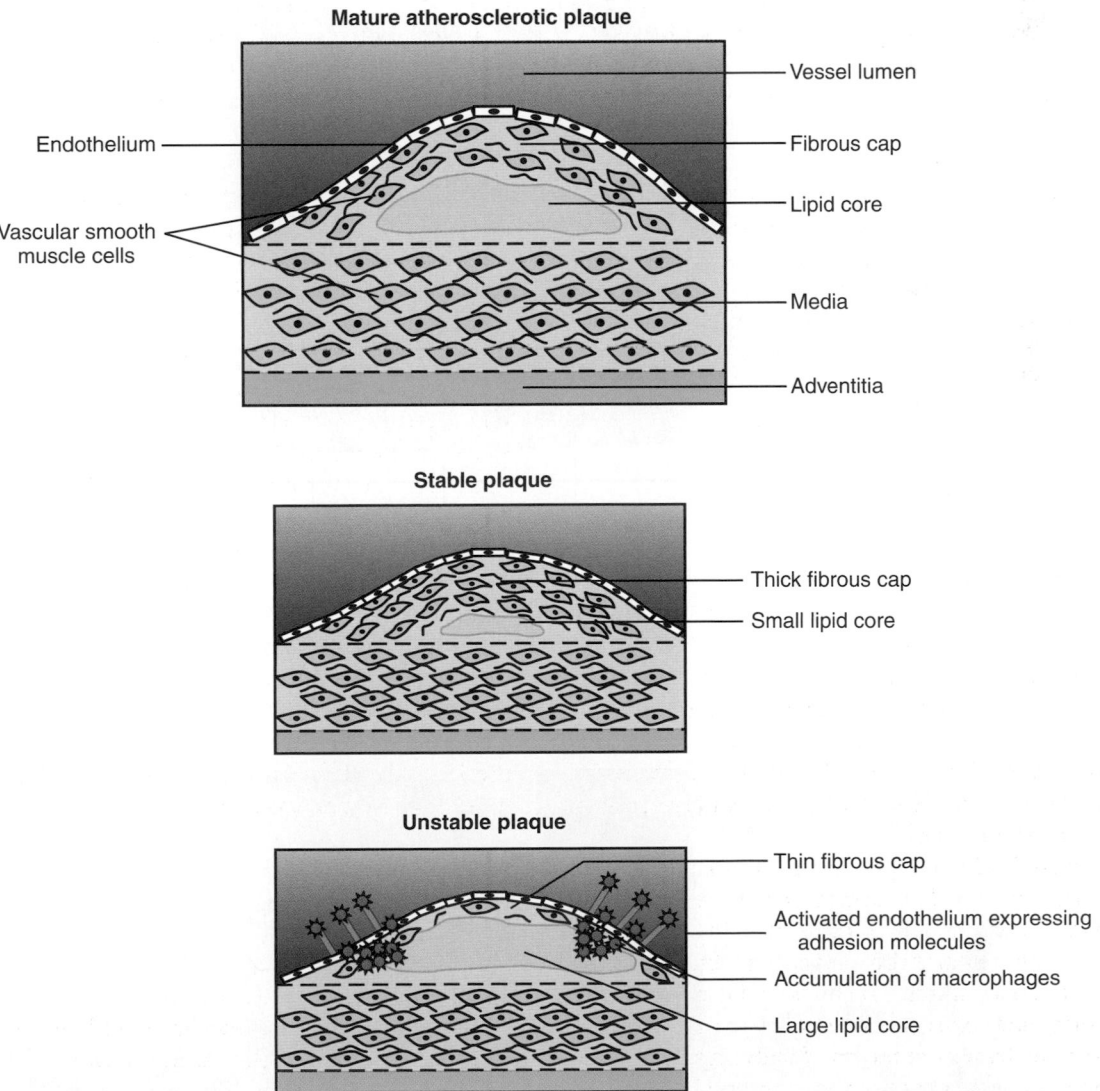

FIGURE 32-1 The structure of mature, stable, and unstable plaque. *(From Rudd JHF et al: Imaging of atherosclerosis—can we predict plaque rupture?* Trends Cardiovasc Med *15:17, 2005.)*

The clinical outcome of impaired arterial function arising from atherosclerosis depends on the location of the impairment. In the coronary arteries atherosclerosis causes angina, MI, and sudden death (Figure 32-4); in the cerebral arteries it causes **strokes** and transient ischemic attacks; and in the peripheral circulation it causes intermittent claudication, limb ischemia, and gangrene. Thus atherosclerosis is the underlying cause of many forms of CVD.

Many theories have been tested to explain how atherosclerosis develops. It is now known that atherogenesis, the process of development of **atherosclerosis,** is a chronic, lo-cal, inflammatory response to many risk factors, such as high levels of LDL-cholesterol, that are injurious to the arterial wall (Heinecke, 2006; Badimon et al., 2006). Hence lesion formation, progression, and eventual plaque rupture result from the release of inflammatory proteins known as cytokines (Paoletti et al., 2004; Esteve, 2005). Proinflammatory (e.g., tumor necrosis factor-alpha [TNF-α], interleukin-6 [IL-6], and C-reactive protein [CRP]) and antiinflammatory cytokines (e.g., IL-9, IL-10) are the key proteins that must be balanced to prevent plaque rupture and subsequent clinical events (Tedgui and Mallat, 2006).

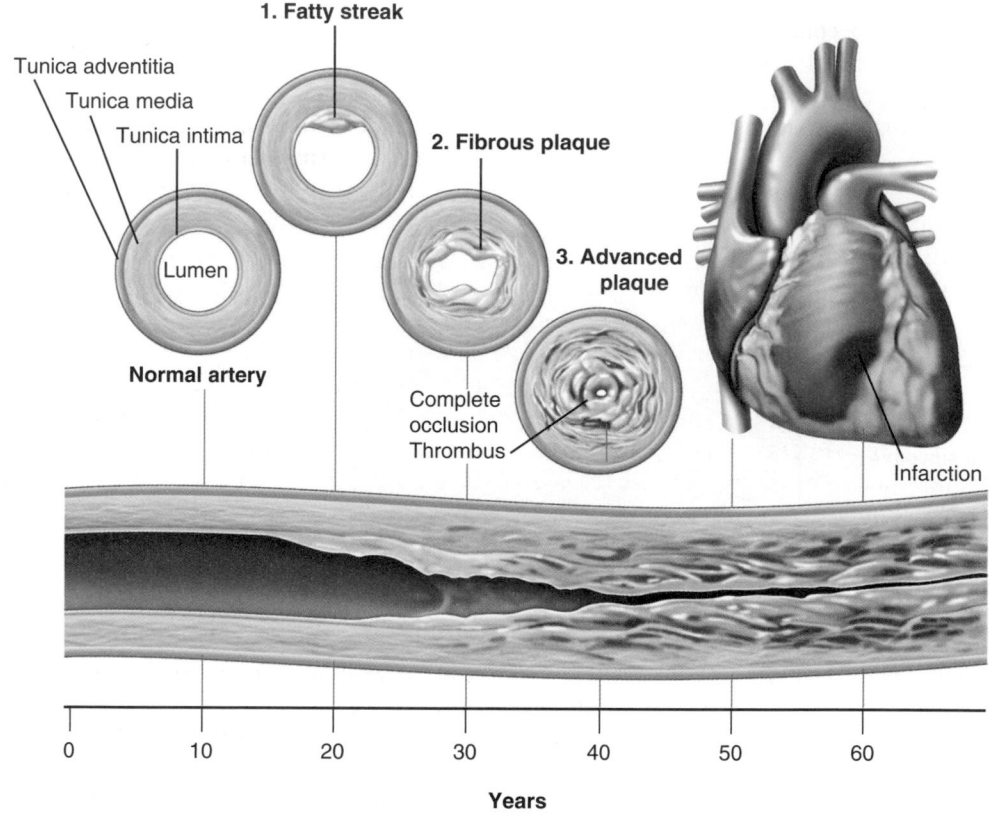

FIGURE 32-2 Natural progression of atherosclerosis. *(From Harkreader H: Fundamentals of nursing: caring and clinical judgment, Philadelphia, 2007, Saunders.)*

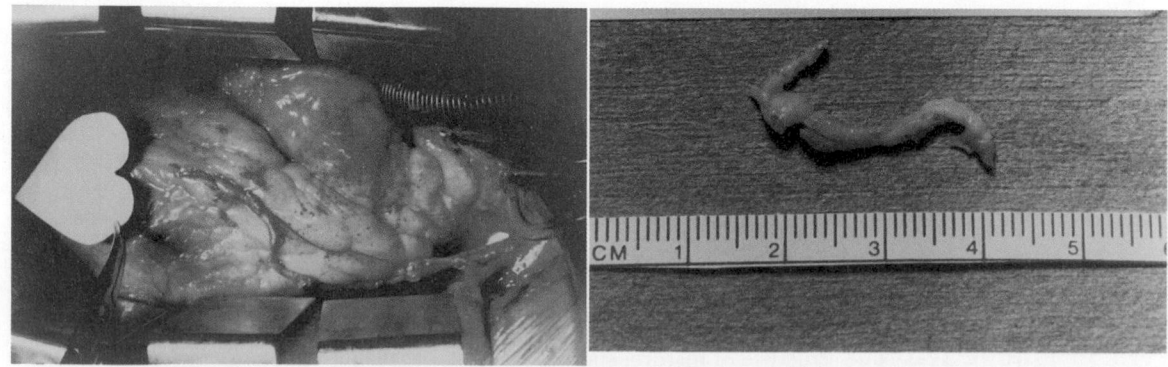

FIGURE 32-3 Plaque that can be surgically removed from the coronary artery. *(Photographs courtesy Ronald D. Gregory and John Riley, MD.)*

Clinical Evaluation

Noninvasive tests such as electrocardiograms, treadmill stress tests, thallium scans, and echocardiography are used initially to establish a diagnosis of CHD. A more definitive, invasive test is angiography (cardiac catheterization), in which a dye is injected into the arteries and radiographic images of the heart are obtained. Most narrowing and blockages from atherosclerosis are readily apparent on angiograms; however, smaller lesions are often not visible, nor are lesions that have undergone remodeling, a process where the blood vessel enlarges to accommodate the narrowing lumen.

Magnetic resonance imaging scans show smaller lesions and can be used to follow atherosclerosis progression or regression following treatments (Desai et al., 2005). The imaging method varies by arterial bed. In the carotid arteries an ultrasound measuring intimal thickness is the preferred noninvasive method, whereas in the coronary arteries intravascular ultrasound is preferred for invasive assessment of atherosclerosis (Sankatsing et al., 2005). Measuring the intimal thickness of the carotid artery has been found to be predictive of MI and stroke (Sankatsing et al., 2005). At present there is no method for detecting vulnerable plaque; however, new techniques, such as intracoronary thermography, are being refined to determine the presence of vulnerable plaque (Madjid et al., 2006). Lumen size, measured by flow-mediated dilation, is an estimate of endothelial dysfunction (Sankatsing et al., 2005). Finally, the calcium in atherosclerotic lesions can be assessed. A study of 4000 asymptomatic people using electron beam computed tomography that measures calcium in the coronary arteries, showed that persons with a positive scan were eight times more likely to have a future coronary event than those with a negative scan (Rich and McLaughlin, 2002). Despite these findings, atherosclerosis imaging in asymptomatic individuals is a controversial public health topic because of the costs associated with screening (O'Malley, 2006; Raggi, 2006).

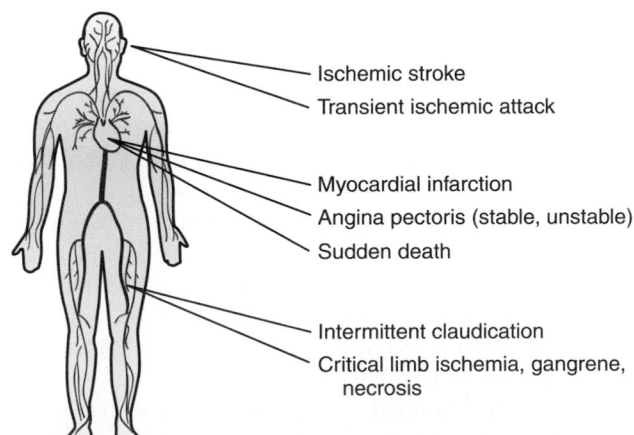

FIGURE 32-4 Major clinical manifestations of atherothrombotic disease. *(Viles-Gonzalez JF et al: Atherothrombosis: a widespread disease with unpredictable and life-threatening consequences,* Eur Heart J *25:1197, 2004.)*

End Points

Approximately two thirds of the cases of acute coronary syndromes (unstable angina and acute MI) happen in arteries that are minimally or mildly obstructed. This illustrates the importance of thrombosis in clinical events. In the ischemia of an infarction, the myocardium (or other tissue) is deprived of oxygen and nourishment. Whether the heart is able to continue beating depends on the extent of the musculature involved, the presence of collateral circulation, and the oxygen requirement.

LIPOPROTEINS

Blood Lipids and Lipoproteins

Blood lipids (cholesterol, triglycerides, and phospholipids) are transported in the blood bound to proteins. These complex particles, called **lipoproteins,** vary in composition, size, and density (Table 32-1). Lipoproteins measured in clinical practice (i.e., chylomicrons, very low–density lipoproteins [VLDLs], LDLs, and HDLs) consist of varying amounts of triglyceride, cholesterol, phospholipid, and protein. Each class of lipoproteins actually represents a continuum of particles.

The ratio of protein to fat determines the density; thus particles with higher levels of protein are the most dense (e.g., HDLs have more protein than LDLs). The physiologic role of lipoproteins includes transporting lipid to cells for energy, storage, or use as substrate for synthesis of other compounds such as prostaglandins, thromboxanes, and leukotrienes. Because of different metabolic roles, the lipoproteins also vary in atherogenicity.

Total Cholesterol

A total cholesterol measurement captures cholesterol contained in all lipoprotein fractions: 60% to 70% is carried on LDL, 20% to 30% on HDL, and 10% to 15% on VLDL. Cross-population, within-population, and clinical studies have consistently shown that a high serum cholesterol level and specifically a high LDL cholesterol is one of the key causes of CHD, stroke, and mortality. Furthermore, diet, serum cholesterol, and CHD are also positively related. Populations that consume diets high in saturated fatty acids (SFAs) have increased blood cholesterol levels **(hypercholesterolemia),** CHD incidence, and mortality. The most current report of the National Cholesterol Education Program (NCEP) (Third Report of the Expert Panel on Detection, Evaluation, and Treatment of High Blood Cholesterol in Adults—Adult Treatment Panel III [ATP-III]) reaffirms that "lowering total cholesterol and LDL cholesterol reduces CHD risk" (NCEP, 2002). A 10% reduction in total cholesterol would decrease CHD incidence by about 30% (NCEP, 2002). Whereas total cholesterol was previously recommended as a screening tool, ATP-III now recommends a complete lipoprotein profile for screening.

Numerous factors affect serum cholesterol levels, including age; diets high in fat, saturated fat, and cholesterol

TABLE 32-1

Characteristics and Functions of the Plasma Lipoproteins

Characteristics	Classes of Lipoproteins				
	Chylomicron	VLDL	IDL	LDL	HDL
Density, g/ml	<0.95	0.95-1.006	1.006-1.019	1.019-1.063	1.063-1.210
Electrophoretic mobility		Pre-β	Pre-β to β	β	α
Origin	Intestine	Liver and intestine	In circulation secondary to catabolism of other lipoproteins	Liver	Liver and intestine
Physiologic role	Transport of dietary triglyceride	Transport of endogenous triglyceride	LDL precursor	Major cholesterol transport lipoprotein	Reverse cholesterol transport
Relative atherogenicity	0	+	+++	++++	Negatively correlated with atherosclerosis
Composition (%)					
Triglyceride	90	60	40	10	5
Cholesterol	5	10	30	50	20
Phospholipid	3	18	20	15	25
Protein	2	10	10	25	50
Major apolipoproteins	A-1 A-IV B-48 C-I C-II C-III	B-100 C-I C-II C-III E	B-100 E	B-100	A-I A-II

From Kris-Etherton PM et al: The effect of diet on plasma lipids, lipoproteins, and coronary heart disease, *J Am Diet Assoc* 88:1373, 1988. Copyright the American Dietitic Association.

HDL, High-density lipoprotein; *IDL*, intermediate-density lipoprotein; *LDL*, low-density lipoprotein, *VLDL*, very low–density lipoprotein.

and other factors discussed later: genetics; endogenous sex hormones (absence in postmenopausal women or presence during menstrual cycle); exogenous hormones (anabolic steroids, oral contraceptive agents, hormone replacement therapy); drugs (β-blockers, thiazide diuretics); body weight; glucose tolerance; physical activity level; presence of other diseases (diabetes, obesity, anorexia nervosa, cancer, thyroid or liver disease); and season of the year. Since 1960 serum cholesterol levels in the U.S. population have been declining; in 2002 the average total cholesterol level was 203 mg/dl (5.34 mmol/L) (Carroll, 2005). The proportion of adults with high blood cholesterol (>240 mg/dl) fell to 17%, which is below the *Healthy People 2010* goal (*Healthy People 2010*, 2000). Because HDL cholesterol was not significantly different during this period, the decline in total cholesterol levels was due to decreased LDL cholesterol. Of note, the percentage of Americans on cholesterol-lowering drugs significantly increased from 3% in 1988-1994 to 9% in the 1999-2002 National Health and Nutrition Examination Survey (NHANES IV) (Carroll, 2005). CHD mortality rates have also been declining during this timeframe.

Total Triglyceride

The triglyceride-rich lipoproteins include chylomicrons, VLDLs, and any remnants or intermediary products formed in metabolism. Of these triglyceride-rich lipoproteins, chylomicrons and VLDL remnants are known to be atherogenic because they activate platelets and the coagulation cascade and lead to clot formation (Olufadi and Byrne, 2006). All contain the apo B lipoprotein. Fasting triglyceride levels are classified as normal (<150 mg/dl), borderline high (150 to 199 mg/dl), high (200 to 499 mg/dl), and very high (>500 mg/dl) (NCEP, 2002).

Patients with familial dyslipidemias have triglyceride levels in the borderline high or high range (**hypertriglyceridemia**). Triglycerides in the very high range place the patient at risk for pancreatitis. These patients usually have hyperchylomicronemia and require diets very low in fat (i.e., 10% to 15% of calories derived from fat). Similarly, patients lacking lipoprotein lipase (LPL), the enzyme that hydrolyzes triglycerides into fatty acids before entry into the cell, also have very high triglyceride levels and need a very low–fat diet. Drugs are often necessary to lower triglyceride levels in these patients. Triglyceride measurements are now considered in relationship to other risk factors such as glucose intolerance, hypertension, low HDL cholesterol, and high LDL cholesterol that can be part of the metabolic syndrome (see Chapters 9 and 30).

Lipoproteins and Metabolism

Chylomicrons

The largest particles, the **chylomicrons**, transport dietary fat and cholesterol from the small intestine to the liver and periphery (see Table 32-1). Once in the bloodstream, the triglycerides in the chylomicrons are hydrolyzed by LPL, located on the endothelial cell surface in muscle and adipose tissue. Apo C-II, one of the apolipoproteins in chylomicrons, is a cofactor for LPL. **Apolipoproteins** not only carry lipids in the blood but also control the metabolism of the lipoprotein molecule. When about 90% of the triglyceride is hydrolyzed, the particle is released back into the blood as a remnant. The liver metabolizes these chylomicron remnants, but some deliver cholesterol to the arterial wall and thus are considered atherogenic. Consumption of high-fat meals produces more chylomicrons and remnants. When fasting plasma studies are done, chylomicrons are normally absent.

Very Low–Density Lipoprotein

Very low–density lipoprotein (VLDL) particles are synthesized in the liver to transport endogenous triglyceride and cholesterol. Sixty percent of the VLDL particle is triglyceride. The large, buoyant VLDL particle is believed to be nonatherogenic. Vegetarian and low-fat diets increase the formation of large VLDL particles. Smaller VLDL particles (i.e., remnants) are formed from triglyceride hydrolysis by LPL. Normally these remnants, called *VLDL remnants* or **intermediate-density lipoproteins (IDLs)**, which are atherogenic, are taken up by receptors on the liver or are converted to LDLs. In metabolic syndrome the remnants are present and atherogenic (Olufadi et al., 2006). Some of the smaller LDL particles stay in the blood, are oxidized, and are then taken into the arterial wall. Clinically a total triglyceride level is a measurement of the triglycerides carried on VLDLs, remnants, and IDLs.

Low-Density Lipoprotein

Low-density lipoprotein (LDL) is the primary cholesterol carrier in blood and is formed by the breakdown of VLDL. After LDL formation, 60% is taken up by LDL receptors on the liver, adrenals, and other tissues. The remainder is metabolized via nonreceptor pathways. Both the number and activity of these LDL receptors are major determinants of LDL cholesterol levels in the blood. Ninety-five percent of the apolipoproteins in LDLs are apo B-100, known, as apo B. Apo B is also present in smaller amounts in VLDLs and IDLs of hepatic origin. Persons with a high triglyceride level usually have high apo B levels, giving these particles a longer time to deposit lipid in the arterial wall (Marcovina and Packard, 2006). Since lowering LDL cholesterol is the main focus for intervention, it is discussed in that section.

High-Density Lipoprotein

High-density lipoprotein (HDL) particles contain more protein than any of the other lipoproteins, which accounts for their metabolic role as a reservoir of the apolipoproteins that direct lipid metabolism. Apo A-I, the main apolipoprotein in HDL, is an antiinflammatory, antioxidant protein that also helps to remove cholesterol from the arterial wall to the liver (Choi et al., 2006; Barter and Rye, 2006). Numerous groups are recommending that apo A-I or the ratio of apo B to apo A-I be added to determine risk and tailor treatment (Marcovina and Packard, 2006; Walldius and Jungner, 2006; Barter and Rye, 2006). The lower the ratio, the lower the risk would be for getting CHD. Both apo C and apo E on HDL are transferred to chylomicrons. Apo E helps receptors metabolize chylomicron remnants and also inhibits appetite (Gotoh et al., 2006). Therefore high HDL levels are associated with low levels of chylomicrons; VLDL remnants; and small, dense LDLs and subsequently lower atherosclerotic risk. The exception is in patients with **familial hypercholesterolemia (FH)** who can have a triglyceride-enriched HDL_3 fraction that is proatherogenic (Ottestad et al., 2006).

GENETIC HYPERLIPIDEMIAS: CLASSIFICATION AND DIAGNOSIS

The study and identification of the genes responsible for the familial forms of hyperlipidemia have provided insight into the roles of enzymes, apolipoproteins, and receptors on cells involved in lipid metabolism. Several forms of hyperlipidemia have strong genetic components.

Familial Hypercholesterolemia

FH (type IIa hyperlipidemia) is a monogenetic disorder that is seen around the world, with an estimated 10,000,000 people being affected (Table 32-2). It is major risk factor for CHD; 85% of males and 50% of females with FH will have a coronary event before the age of 65 years unless the hypercholesterolemia is successfully treated (Civeira, 2004). Unfortunately few patients (<10%) are diagnosed, and less than 25% of patients are treated with LDL-lowering medication. Early detection is critical. Defects in the LDL receptor gene cause FH; 800 mutations have been identified, and screening is becoming possible (Civeira et al., 2005; Lombardi et al., 2006). Ultrasound of the Achilles tendon for **xanthomas** (cholesterol deposits from LDL) correctly identified 80% of FH patients (Junyent et al., 2005).

A person is heterozygous for FH if he or she carries one defective gene for the LDL receptor and homozygous if both genes are inherited. In these patients LDL levels range from 190 mg/dl to 400 mg/dl. Tendon xanthomas occur in 7% of patients with heterozygous FH at 20 to 30 years of age and in 38% of patients at 51 to 60 years of age and are highly related to risk factors and premature CHD, suggesting the need for aggressive treatment (Civeira et al, 2005). Recently it has been shown that patients with FH have a higher level of pro-inflammatory markers (TNF-α, IL-8) and HDL$_3$, which is high in triglyceride and considered proatherogenic (Ottestad et al, 2006). Antioxidant supplementation (vitamins C and E) in children with FH did not alter their lipid or inflammatory markers (Aldamiz-Echevarria, 2006).

Homozygotes have more severe hypercholesterolemia (as much as 1000 mg/dl) and atherosclerosis; thus many have an MI or die in the first or second decade of life (Steinberg, 2005). The standard treatment for homozygotes is apheresis, in which LDL is removed from the blood (Morelli et al., 2005). For all patients with FH, dietary modification is necessary because of putative benefits and because it enhances the effectiveness of medications (Civeira et al., 2005). Early detection with aggressive drug therapy and lifestyle change (no smoking, healthy diet, physical activity) can prevent or delay CHD. LDL goals are similar to the NCEP goals and are discussed in following paragraphs. However, a goal of 100 mg/dl may not be possible because of the limited efficacy of drugs, their cost, and side effects (Civeira, 2004). As with other diseases, education is imperative. A recent Swedish study showed a significant negative correlation between adherence and LDL cholesterol level; therefore patients who were more faithful to their diet and medication regimen had lower LDL cholesterol levels than those who did not (Hollman et al., 2006).

Polygenic Familial Hypercholesterolemia

Polygenic familial hypercholesterolemia is the result of multiple gene defects that have yet to be identified. The diagnosis is based on two or more family members having LDL cholesterol levels above the 90th percentile without any tendon xanthomas. Usually these patients have lower LDL cholesterol levels than patients with the nonpolygenic form, but they remain at high risk for premature disease. The apo E-4 allele is common in polygenic familial hypercholesterolemia. The treatment is similar to that for heterozygous familial hypercholesterolemia: therapeutic lifestyle changes (TLCs) in conjunction with cholesterol-lowering drugs.

Familial Combined Hyperlipidemia

Familial combined hyperlipidemia (FCHL) is a disorder in which two or more family members have serum LDL cholesterol or triglyceride levels above the 90th percentile. Several lipoprotein patterns may be seen in patients with FCHL. These patients can have (1) elevated LDL levels with normal triglyceride levels (type IIa), (2) elevated LDL levels with elevated triglyceride levels (type IIb), or (3) elevated VLDL levels (type IV). Often these patients have the small, dense LDL associated with CHD. Consequently all forms of FCHL cause premature disease; about 15% of patients who have an MI before the age of 60 have FCHL. The defect in FCHL is hepatic overproduction of apo B-100 (VLDL) or a defect in the gene that produces hepatic lipase, the liver enzyme involved in triglyceride removal from the bloodstream. Patients with FCHL usually have a constellation of other risk factors (i.e., obesity, hyperten-

---

TABLE 32-2

Selected Genetic Hyperlipidemias

Gene Defect	Lipoproteins Elevated	Diagnosis	Clinical Findings	U.S. Incidence	Treatment
Familial Hypercholesterolemia					
Heterozygous LDL-receptor	LDL	Serum cholesterol >300 mg/dl, normal TGs, affected first-degree relative	Tendon xanthomas, archus corneae, premature CHD	1/500	TLC, drug therapy
Homozygous LDL-receptor	LDL	Serum cholesterol from 500 mg/dl to 1000 mg/dl, skin biopsy with measure of LDL receptor activity	Xanthomatosis progresses rapidly, CHD in first decade of life	1/1,000,000	Plasmapheresis to remove LDL, liver transplant
Familial Defective apo B-100					
Apo B-100	LDL	Elevated serum cholesterol, normal TG	Tendon xanthomas, premature CHD	1/1000	TLC, drug therapy

Table created by Amy Plum MEd, RD, LD. Adapted from Kasper DL et al., editors: *Harrison's principles of internal medicine*, ed 16, New York, 2005, McGraw-Hill.

CHD, Coronary heart disease; *HDL*, high-density lipoprotein; *LDL*, low-density lipoprotein; *LP*, lipoprotein lipase; *PVD*, peripheral vascular disease; *TG*, trigyceride; *TLC*, therapeutic life change; *VLDL*, very low–density lipoprotein.

sion, diabetes, such as seen in metabolic syndrome). If lifestyle measures are ineffective, treatment includes TLC, weight reduction, diabetes control, increased physical activity, and medication Patients with elevated triglyceride levels also need to avoid alcohol.

Familial Dysbetalipoproteinemia

Familial dysbetalipoproteinemia (type III hyperlipoproteinemia) is relatively uncommon. Catabolism of VLDL and chylomicron remnants is delayed because apo E-2 replaces apo E-3 and apo E-4. For dysbetalipoprotein-

emia to be seen, other risk factors such as older age, hypothyroidism, obesity, or diabetes; or other dyslipidemias such as FCHL must be present. Total cholesterol levels range from 300 to 600 mg/dl, and triglyceride levels range from 400 to 800 mg/dl. This condition creates increased risk of premature CHD and peripheral vascular disease. Diagnosis is based on determining the isoforms of apo E. Treatment involves weight reduction, control of hyperglycemia and diabetes, and dietary restriction of saturated fat and cholesterol. If the dietary regimen is not effective, drug therapy is recommended.

TABLE 32-2

Selected Genetic Hyperlipidemias—cont'd

Gene Defect	Lipoproteins Elevated	Diagnosis	Clinical Findings	U.S. Incidence	Treatment
Polygenic Hypercholesterolemia (Nonfamilial Hypercholesterolemia)					
Unknown	LDL	Elevated LDL >95th percentile, absence of secondary causes of hypercholesterolemia, <10% of first-degree relatives affected	Absence of tendinous xanthomas	1/20 to 1/100	TLC, drug therapy
Familial Dysbetalipoproteinemia (Type III Hyperlipoproteinemia)					
Apo E	Chylomicrons, VLDL remnants	Lipoprotein electrophoresis or ratio of VLDL to total plasma TG	Palmar and tuberoeruptive xanthomas, CHD, PVD	1/10,000	Weight reduction, low-fat, low-cholesterol diet, minimize alcohol consumption, estrogen replacement in women, drug therapy
Familial Combined Hyperlipidemia					
Unknown	TGs, total cholesterol, HDL	Plasma TGs 200-800 mg/dl, cholesterol 220-400 mg/dl, HDL <40 mg/dl, family history of hyperlipidemia/ premature CHD, elevated plasma apo B	Often present: visceral adiposity, glucose intolerance, insulin resistance, hypertension, hyperuricemia, premature CHD	1/200	TLC, drug therapy, aggressive blood glucose control
Familial Hypertriglyceridemia					
Unknown	VLDL, sometimes chylomicrons	Elevated TGs, normal to mildly increased cholesterol, reduced plasma HDL Identification of first-degree relatives with high TGs Rule out other causes of high TGs	Possibility of pancreatitis and chylomicronemia	1/500	TLC, drug therapy if levels >400-600 mg/dl after TLC

RISK FACTORS AND PREVENTION

A landmark achievement of epidemiologic research has been the identification of risk factors for atherosclerosis, CHD, and stroke (Box 32-1). The primary prevention of these CVDs involves the assessment and management of the risk factors in the asymptomatic person. Persons with multiple risk factors are the target population for primary prevention (NCEP, 2002). Risk factor reduction has been shown to reduce CHD in persons of all ages. In a large study of men, 62% of coronary events could have been prevented if the men would have adopted a healthy lifestyle (eating a heart-healthy diet, exercising regularly, managing weight, and not using tobacco) and adhered to taking lipid and hypertension medications (Chiuve et al., 2006). Computer modeling studies have shown that approximately one quarter of the decline in CHD is attributable to improved treatment and 53% to 72% may be the result of positive changes in risk factors (Laatikainen et al., 2005). Over 200 risk factors have been identified. Only those that are the most prevalent, have strong evidence, or are related to diet are presented in this chapter.

Prevention of CHD and Stroke

In the medical model, primary prevention of CVD, in particular CHD and stroke, involves altering risk factors toward a healthy patient profile. CHD and stroke share most of the same risk factors. For ischemic stroke, atherosclerosis is the underlying disease. Therefore optimal lipid levels as determined by NCEP for hypercholesterolemia are also the target levels to prevent stroke. The latest NCEP report, ATP-III, focuses on LDL cholesterol as the target lipoprotein. The goal for LDL cholesterol depends on other risk factors and scores on risk assessment as described in the following paragraphs (Table 32-3).

Based on findings from recent clinical trials, an LDL cholesterol of less than 70 mg/dl is appropriate for some patients classified as very high risk. TLCs are the cornerstone of treatment for elevated LDL. The focus on LDL cholesterol supports the lipid hypothesis of atherosclerosis that high blood cholesterol levels cause atherosclerosis and CHD. As more is known about the disease, other risk factors will become more important. Future goals of prevention could include how to maintain endothelial function, stabilize plaque (versus reducing plaque), and prevent inflammation.

The American Heart Association (AHA) recommends that primary prevention of CHD begins in childhood (over the age of 2 years) (Gidding et al., 2006). Dietary recommendations are a bit more liberal than seen with adults (Box 32-2). Activity is emphasized in maintaining ideal body weight. Early screening for dyslipidemia is recommended for children with a family history of hypercholesterolemia or CHD (Fletcher et al., 2005). Goals for total cholesterol levels for 2- to 19-year-olds are shown in Table 32-4.

Assessing Risk

Several methods have been proposed to assess risk in asymptomatic persons. The first is from the Framingham

---

BOX 32-1

Modifiable Cardiovascular Risk Factors

Markers in Blood

Lipoprotein profile
  Low-density–lipoprotein cholesterol
  Total triglycerides
  High-density–lipoprotein cholesterol

Inflammatory Markers

Fibrinogen
C-Reactive protein

Lifestyle Risk Factors

Tobacco
Physical inactivity
Poor diet
Stress
Excessive alcohol consumption

Related Diseases/Syndrome

Hypertension
Diabetes
Obesity
Metabolic syndrome

BOX 32-2

Primary Prevention in Children and Youth

Dietary Modification

Limit foods with
  Saturated fats to <10% calories/day
  Cholesterol to <300 mg/day
  Trans-fatty acids to <1% calories/day

Physical Activity

Increase moderate to rigorous activities to ≥60 min/day
Limit sedentary activities ≤2 hr/day

Identification of Dyslipidemia

Selective screening
  Family history of CHD
  One parent with blood cholesterol ≥240 mg/dl
  No parental history, but CHD risk factors present
  One or more of the following risk factors present: high blood pressure; smoking; sedentary lifestyle; obesity; alcohol intake; use of drugs or diseases associated with dyslipidemia

From Fletcher B et al: Managing abnormal blood lipids: a collaborative approach, *Circulation* 112:3184, 2005.

CHD, Chronic heart disease.

TABLE 32-3

Revised ATP-III Goals for LDL-Cholesterol and Initiation of TLC and Drug Therapy

Risk Category	LDL-C Goal	Initiate TLC	Consider Drug Therapy**
High risk: CHD* or CHD risk equivalents† (10-year risk >20%)	<100 mg/dl (optional goal: <70 mg/dl)‖	≥100 mg/dl#	≥100 mg/dl†† (<100 mg/dl: consider drug options)**
Moderately high risk: 2+ risk factors‡ (10-year risk 10% 20%)§§	<130 mg/dl¶	≥130 mg/dl#	≥130 mg/dl (100-129 mg/dl; consider drug options)‡‡
Moderate risk: 2+ risk factors‡ (10-year risk <10%)§§	<130 mg/dl	≥130 mg/dl	≥160 mg/dl
Lower risk: 0-1 risk factor§	<160 mg/dl	≥160 mg/dl	≥190 mg/dl (160-189 mg/dl: LDL-lowering drug optional)

Modified from Grundy S et al: Implications of recent clinical trials for the NCEP-ATP III Guidelines, *Circulation* 110:227, 2004.

CHD, Coronary heart disease; *LDL,* low-density lipoprotein; *LDL-C,* low-density–lipoprotein cholesterol; *TLC,* therapeutic lifestyle changes.

*CHD includes history of myocardial infarction, unstable angina, stable angina, coronary artery procedures (angioplasty or bypass surgery), or evidence of clinically significant myocardial ischemia.

†CHD risk equivalents include clinical manifestations of noncoronary forms of atherosclerotic disease (peripheral arterial disease, abdominal aortic aneurysm, and carotid artery disease [transient ischemic attacks or stroke of carotid origin or >50% obstruction of a carotid artery]), diabetes, and 2+ risk factors with 10-year risk for hard CHD >20%.

‡Risk factors include cigarette smoking, hypertension (BP 140/90 mm Hg or on antihypertensive medication), low high-density–lipoprotein cholesterol (HDL-C) (<40 mg/dl), family history of premature CHD (CHD in male first-degree relative <55 years of age; CHD in female first-degree relative <65 years of age), and age (men ≥45 years; women ≥55 years).

§§Electronic 10-year risk calculators are available at www.nhlbi.nih.gov/guidelines/cholesterol.

§Almost all people with zero or 1 risk factor have a 10-year risk <10%, and 10-year risk assessment in people with zero or 1 risk factor is thus not necessary.

‖Very high risk favors the optional LDL-C goal of <70 mg/dl and in patients with high triglycerides, non-HDL-C <100 mg/dl.

¶Optional LDL cholesterol goal <100 mg/dl.

#Any person at high risk or moderately high risk who has lifestyle-related risk factors (e.g., obesity, physical inactivity, elevated triglycerides, low HDL-C, or metabolic syndrome) is a candidate for therapeutic lifestyle changes to modify these risk factors regardless of LDL-C level.

**When LDL-lowering drug therapy is used, it is advised that intensity of therapy be sufficient to achieve at least a 30% to 40% reduction in LDL-C levels.

††If baseline LDL cholesterol is <100 mg/dl, institution of an LDL-lowering drug is a therapeutic option on the basis of available clinical trial results. If a high-risk person has high triglycerides or low HDL cholesterol, combining a fibrate or nicotinic acid with an LDL-lowering drug can be considered.

‡‡ For moderately high-risk persons, when LDL-C level is 100 to 129 mg/dl, at baseline or on lifestyle therapy, initiation of an LDL-lowering drug to achieve an LDL-C level <100 mg/dl is a therapeutic option on the basis of available clinical trial results.

study (see *Focus On:* Framingham Heart Study). In this method risk factors are counted (Figures 32-5 and 32-6), and then an algorithm is used to determine 10-year risk (Figure 32-7). This system categorizes a patient into one of three categories: (1) very high risk (these individuals have a greater than a 30% chance of developing CHD or have a recurrent event within 10 years); (2) high risk (20% to 30% chance of new CHD within 10 years); (3) moderate risk (a 10% to 20% risk of new CHD within 10 years); or (4) low risk (less than a 10% risk). With each additional risk factor, the estimated 10-year risk for CHD or stroke increases markedly. Although the Framingham 10-year risk method is used widely, its accuracy in prediction varies between populations, and more validation has been recommended (Brindle et al., 2006).

The second risk assessment involves some of the imaging tools mentioned earlier (carotid intima media thickness [CIMT], ankle-brachial index, and the coronary artery calcium score [CACS]) (Naghavi et al., 2006). The National Screening for Heart Attack Prevention and Education (SHAPE) Program recommends screening in asymptomatic men 45 to 74 years of age and in women 55 to 75 years of age, excluding only those who are at low risk and then treating the subclinical atherosclerosis to prevent progression, symptoms, and events (Naghavi et al., 2006).

Markers in Blood

Lipoprotein Profile

A standard lipoprotein profile report includes measurement of total cholesterol, LDL cholesterol, HDL cholesterol, and total triglyceride levels, and thus should be measured after a person has fasted for 8 to 12 hours. Most clinical laboratories cannot quantify LDL cholesterol directly; therefore the Friedewald formula is used to estimate LDL cholesterol (NCEP, 2002). The Friedewald formula is:

$$\text{LDL-C} = (\text{TC}) - (\text{HDL-C}) - (\text{TG/5})$$

⊙ FOCUS ON

Framingham Heart Study

Since 1948 various leading investigators (Dr. Joseph Mountain, Dr. Thomas Dawber, Dr. William Kannel, and Dr. William Castelli) have been studying the population (28,000) of Framingham, Massachusetts, to determine the prevalence and incidence of cardiovascular disease and factors related to its development. This is the largest epidemiologic study of cardiovascular disease in the world. Initial study participants ($n = 5209$) were healthy adults between 30 and 62 years of age, and the study continues today looking at the offspring of the original cohort and now the grandchildren. Through this cohort study, the concept of risk factors and thus prevention was born. Modifiable risk factors not only predict disease in healthy adults but also contribute to the disease process in those who have atherosclerotic disease. The seven major risk factors identified by the Framingham study were age, sex, blood pressure, total and high-density–lipoprotein cholesterol, smoking, glucose intolerance, and left-ventricular hypertrophy (Opie et al., 2006).

Highlights of the Framingham Study: Most Significant Milestones

1960 Cigarette smoking found to increase the risk of heart disease

1961 Cholesterol level, blood pressure, and electrocardiogram abnormalities found to increase the risk of heart disease

1967 Physical activity found to reduce the risk of heart disease, and obesity found to increase the risk of heart disease

1970 High blood pressure found to increase the risk of stroke

1976 Menopause found to increase the risk of heart disease

1978 Psychosocial factors found to affect heart disease

1988 High levels of high-density–lipoprotein cholesterol found to reduce risk of death

1994 Enlarged left ventricle (one of two lower chambers of the heart) found to increase the risk of stroke

1996 Progression from hypertension to heart failure described

2006 Beginning of the Genetic Research Study to identify genes underlying cardiovascular and other chronic diseases in 9000 participants from three generations

In 1971 the offspring study was begun to measure the influence of heredity and environment on the offspring of the original cohort. The younger group appears to be more health conscious because they have lower rates of smoking, lower blood pressures, and lower cholesterol levels than their parents at the same age. The Generation III Cohort Study of the grandchildren is also presently underway.

From www.nhlbi.nih.gov/about/framingham/timeline.htm, accessed October 1, 2006.

TABLE 32-4

Cholesterol Levels for 2- to 19-Year-Olds

Levels	Total Cholesterol (mg/dl)	LDL-C (mg/dl)
Acceptable	<170	<110
Borderline	170-199	110-129
High	≥200	≥130

Modified from Fletcher B et al: Managing abnormal blood lipids: a collaborative approach, *Circulation* 112:3184, 2005.

---

where LDL-C is low-density–lipoprotein cholesterol, TC is total cholesterol, HDL-C is high-density–lipoprotein cholesterol, and TG is triglyceride. Calculating the LDL cholesterol level by difference can be done only when triglyceride levels are less than 400 mg/dl.

A desirable lipoprotein profile is a total cholesterol level of less than 200 mg/dl, LDL cholesterol less than 130 mg/dl, HDL cholesterol greater than 40 mg/dl, and triglyceride level less than 150 mg/dl (NCEP, 2002). An LDL cholesterol level less than 100 mg/dl is recommended for persons with two or more risk factors (high-risk patients). Based on new clinical findings, an LDL cholesterol less than 70 mg/dl is encouraged for very high–risk patients (Grundy et al., 2004).

Adults older than 20 years of age should have a fasting lipoprotein profile done every 5 years (NCEP, 2002). If nonfasting values are obtained, only total cholesterol and HDL cholesterol are usable. In this case, a total cholesterol of 200 mg/dl or higher or HDL cholesterol of less than 40 mg/dl necessitates a fasting analysis for appropriate LDL management. The ATP-III classification for prevention and treatment is shown in Table 32-3.

Low-Density–Lipoprotein Cholesterol. As discussed, LDL cholesterol has been the focus of much research since it is conclusively linked to atherosclerosis, CHD development, and acute clinical events, including MI and stroke. Consequently LDL cholesterol is the primary target for intervention efforts. A decrease of 1 mg/dl in LDL cholesterol results in about a 1% to 2% decrease in the relative risk for CHD. The mean LDL cholesterol levels for American children and adults are ≈100 mg/dl and 123 mg/dl, respectively (AHA, 2006). For persons who are without disease, LDL levels are classified as optimal (≤100 mg/dl), near optimal (≤129 mg/dl), borderline high risk (130 to 159 mg/dl), high risk (160 to 189 mg/dl), and very high risk (≥190 mg/dl).

Factors that increase LDL cholesterol include aging, genetics, diet, reduced estrogen levels (as occurs in postmenopausal women), progestins, diabetes, hypothyroidism, nephrotic syndrome, obstructive liver disease, obesity, and some steroid and antihypertensive drugs. Of these factors, an imprudent diet and obesity are the most prevalent. Diets high in saturated fat and cholesterol elevate LDL by down-regulating

Age	Points
20–34	−7
35–39	−3
40–44	0
45–49	3
50–54	6
55–59	8
60–64	10
65–69	12
70–74	14
75–79	16

HDL	Points
≥60	−1
50–59	0
40–49	1
<40	2

Total cholesterol	Points at age 20–39	Points at age 40–49	Points at age 50–59	Points at age 60–69	Points at age 70–79
<160	0	0	0	0	0
160–199	4	3	2	1	1
200–239	8	6	4	2	1
240–279	11	8	5	3	2
≥280	13	10	7	4	2

	Points at age 20–39	Points at age 40–49	Points at age 50–59	Points at age 60–69	Points at age 70–79
Nonsmoker	0	0	0	0	0
Smoker	9	7	4	2	1

Systolic BP	If untreated	If treated
<120	0	0
120–129	1	3
130–139	2	4
140–159	3	5
≥160	4	6

Point total	10-year risk (%)	Point total	10-year risk (%)
<9	<1	20	11
9	1	21	14
10	1	22	17
11	1	23	22
12	1	24	27
13	2	≥25	≥30
14	2		
15	3		
16	4		
17	5		
18	6		
19	8		

FIGURE 32-5 Estimate of 10-year coronary heart disease risk for women: Framingham point scores. (*National Heart, Lung, and Blood Institute:* Detection, evaluation, and treatment of high blood cholesterol in adults *[Adult Treatment Panel III]. Final report. U.S. Department of Health and Human Services, NIH Publication No. 02-5215, Bethesda, Md, September 2002.*)

the LDL receptors in the liver. With suppression of LDL receptor activity, less LDL is cleared from the plasma; thus levels rise. Obesity increases production of apo B–containing lipoproteins: VLDLs and consequently LDLs. Oxidation of LDLs in the vessel wall hastens the atherogenic process by recruiting macrophages, stimulating autoantibodies, increasing LDL uptake, and increasing vascular tone and coagulability. Lowering LDL cholesterol has been shown to shrink lesions; delay progression of atherogenesis; and reduce events, morbidity, and mortality in both primary and secondary pre-

vention trials. The target LDL cholesterol level for persons with disease is less than 70 mg/dl (see Table 32-3). Nutritional factors that affect LDL cholesterol are shown in Box 32-3.

Triglyceride Levels. In ATP-III elevated triglyceride levels are now recognized as an independent risk factor for CHD. Hypertriglyceridemia is most common in metabolic syndrome. Because of their roles in metabolism, triglyceride and HDL cholesterol levels are inversely related (i.e., when a patient has high triglyceride levels, the HDL cholesterol

Poor Diet

It is known that diet is the predominant environmental cause of coronary atherosclerosis and that diet modification unequivocally can reduce risk of CHD. Not surprisingly, caloric intake increased by ≈300 kcal between 1985 and 2000 (Thom et al., 2006). A major environmental, dietary contributor to obesity is the increase in portion sizes that has occurred over the last 20 years. Further evidence of a poor diet in this country is the low number of individuals who consume 9 to 12 fruits and vegetables a day; only 22% of adults consume five servings daily. The many dietary factors that affect the disease process are discussed in "Medical Nutrition Therapy," p. 852.

Stress

Type A personality (time-urgent, impatient, and compulsive) and perceived stress are associated with increased CVD risk. However, interventions for factors that may be amenable to intervention (i.e., stress) have not demonstrated a decrease in risk, and more research is needed.

Alcohol Consumption

Moderate alcohol consumption (i.e., one or two drinks a day) is associated with a significant reduction in CHD risk (Parks and Booyse, 2002), but the use of alcohol is not recommended as an intervention strategy. The limits on alcohol to no more than two drinks per day for men and one drink per day for women are made because alcohol also raises blood pressure (AHA, 2006a).

Alcohol raises both total triglyceride and HDL cholesterol levels. The effects of alcohol on triglyceride levels are dose dependent and are greater in persons with triglyceride levels exceeding 150 mg/dl. Wine contains resveratrol, an antifungal compound in grape skins that has been associated with an 11% to 16% increase in HDL cholesterol and 8% to 15% reduction in fibrinogen (Hansen et al., 2005) The French may experience lower rates of CVD, despite a high-fat diet, because of their consumption of red wine: "the French paradox" (Sun et al., 2002) (see Chapter 12).

Related Diseases and Syndromes

Hypertension

Hypertension is a risk factor for CHD, stroke, and heart failure. About 33% of all adult Americans have hypertension, defined as having an average blood pressure of higher than 140 mm Hg systolic pressure or 90 mm Hg diastolic pressure, using antihypertensive medication, or receiving a hypertension diagnosis (Thom et al., 2006). The prevalence increases with age, and it is seen more often in blacks than in non-Hispanic whites. Hypertension contributes to disease development by causing vascular injury and stress to the myocardium. About 69% of first MI patients, 77% of first stroke, and 74% who have heart failure (HF) have blood pressures higher than 140/90 mm Hg (Thom, 2006). Hypertension is frequently present with other risk factors such as hypercholesterolemia and obesity and is one of the risk factors used to determine the presence of metabolic syndrome. Treating hypertension decreases the incidence of stroke, CHD, and HF (see Chapter 33).

The left ventricle increases in size in response to high blood pressure and increased workload secondary to obesity. In the Framingham Study left ventricular hypertrophy (LVH) was found to be a strong risk factor for CVD, HF, and sudden death. LVH is a risk factor in all age, gender, and ethnic groups. Intervention trials are being conducted to determine whether regressing LVH will improve the clinical course. In the meantime, the presence of LVH necessitates more intensive risk factor management (see Chapter 34).

Diabetes

Diabetes, like hypertension, is both a disease and a risk factor. The prevalence of diabetes mirrors that of obesity in the United States. Since 1990, a 61% increase in the prevalence of diabetes has been observed, and it is becoming more prevalent in obese children (Thom et al., 2006). Any form of diabetes increases the risk for CHD, with occurrence at younger ages. Most people with diabetes die from CVD. Similarly, 75% of people with diabetes have more than two risk factors for CHD (McCollum et al., 2006). The age-adjusted prevalence of CVD in women with diabetes is twice that in women without diabetes or in men. Some of the increased risk for CHD seen in diabetic patients is attributable to the concurrent presence of other risk factors, such as dyslipidemia, hypertension, and obesity. Because of this, diabetes is now considered a CHD risk factor. Thus the LDL cholesterol treatment goal for persons with diabetes is 70 mg/dl (Pearson et al., 2003). Strict blood glucose control lessens microvascular complications in patients with type 1 and type 2 diabetes (see Chapter 30).

Obesity

Obesity is a disease and risk factor for CHD that has now reached epidemic levels in children and adults in many developed countries. BMI and CHD are positively related; as BMI goes up, the risk of CHD also increases. The prevalence of overweight and obesity is the highest that it has ever been in the United States; 65% of adults are overweight, and 31% are obese (Hedley et al., 2004). Obesity rates vary by race and ethnicity in women. Non-Hispanic black women have the highest prevalence, followed by Mexican-American women, American Indians and Alaskan natives, and non-Hispanic whites (Hedley et al., 2004). In men the rates of obesity vary from 25% to 28% of the population (Hedley et al., 2004). The epidemic of obesity and diabetes could reverse the downward trends in CHD mortality if it is not controlled in the near future, especially given the increasing rates seen in children and adolescents (Thompson et al., 2007) (see Chapter 21).

Carrying excess adipose tissue greatly impacts the heart through the many risk factors that are often present: hypertension, glucose intolerance, inflammatory markers (IL-6, TNF-α, CRP), obstructive sleep apnea, prothrombotic state, endothelial dysfunction, and dyslipidemia (small LDL, increased apo B, low HDL, high triglyceride levels) (Poirier et al., 2006). Many inflammatory proteins are now known to come from the adipocyte; this is an area of active research (Berg and Scherer, 2005) (see Chapter 21). These concurrent risk factors may help to explain the high morbidity and mortality rates observed in people who are obese.

Weight distribution (abdominal versus gynoid) is also predictive of CHD risk, glucose tolerance, and serum lipid levels. Central adiposity has also been strongly related to markers of inflammation; for example, CRP is 53% higher in individuals with central adiposity (Panagiotakos, 2005). Therefore a waist circumference of less than 35 inches for women and 40 inches for men is recommended (see Chapter 21). Small weight losses (10 to 20 lb) can improve risk factors such as LDL cholesterol, HDL cholesterol, triglycerides, high blood pressure, glucose tolerance, and CRP levels, even if an ideal BMI is not achieved. Weight loss has been correlated with lower fibrinogen and CRP levels (Tchernof et al., 2002). However, to restore vascular function, the amount of weight that must be lost, the time of weight maintenance, or the amount of improvement in endothelial function that lessens cardiovascular events is still unknown.

Metabolic Syndrome

Since the early findings of the Framingham study, it has been known that a clustering of risk factors markedly increases the risk of CVD. There has been a great debate about the clustering of "metabolic risk factors" and the identification of people with varying clusters (see *Clinical Insight:* The Metabolic Syndrome in Chapter 9). In general, this **metabolic syndrome** consists of some level of atherogenic dyslipidemia, elevated blood pressure, elevated plasma glucose, and a prothrombotic and proinflammatory state (Grundy, 2006). To date, at least four definitions of metabolic syndrome exist, and each varies in its predictability of CVD events (Saely et al., 2006; Athyros et al., 2006; Diamantopoulos et al., 2006). The most recent is that proposed by the AHA and the National Heart, Lung, and Blood Institute (Grundy et al., 2005) (Table 32-5).

However, informing patients that they have metabolic syndrome based on definitions that have not been agreed on is not wise (Reaven et al., 2006). Rather it is suggested to effectively treat the underlying cause of the individual risk factors. This thought is predicated on the observation that insulin-mediated glucose uptake is highly variable in healthy individuals; only one third of these would truly be insulin resistant and at risk for increased expression of other risk factors and CVD. Adiposity (especially abdominal) explains 25% of variability in insulin action, physical fitness explains 25%, and genetics explains the rest (Reaven et al., 2006). Therefore changing lifestyle as described under "Therapeutic Lifestyle Changes (TLC)" later in the chapter is critical to improving risk in individuals with any combination of the "metabolic risk factors" (Stone, 2006).

Nonmodifiable Factors

Menopausal Status

Endogenous estrogen confers protection against CVD in premenopausal women, probably by preventing vascular injury. Loss of estrogen following natural or surgical menopause is associated with increased CVD risk. Rates of CHD in premenopausal women are low except in women with multiple risk factors. During the menopausal period total cholesterol, LDL cholesterol, and triglyceride levels increase; and HDL cholesterol level decreases, especially in women who gain weight.

Age

Age is a nonmodifiable risk factor for CHD. With increasing age, higher mortality rates from CHD are seen in both genders. However, gender is a factor for the assessment of risk. The incidence of premature disease in men 35 to 44 years of age is three times as high as the incidence in women of the same age. Therefore being older than 45 years of age is considered a risk factor for men (NCEP, 2002). For women the increased risk comes after the age of 55 years,

---

TABLE 32-5

AHA/NHLBI Criteria for Diagnosis of the Metabolic Syndrome*

Risk Factor	Defining Level
Abdominal obesity	Waist circumference
Men	>102 cm (>40 in)
Women	>88 cm (>35 in)
Triglycerides	≥150 mg/dl or drug treatment for hypertriglyceridemia
HDL cholesterol	
Men	<40 mg/dl or drug treatment for low HDL cholesterol
Women	<50 mg/dl or drug treatment for low HDL cholesterol
Blood pressure	≥130 mm Hg systolic blood pressure or ≥85 mm Hg diastolic blood pressure or on antihypertensive drug treatment in patients with a history of hypertension
Fasting glucose	≥100 mg/dl or on drug treatment for elevated blood glucose level

From Grundy SM et al: Diagnosis and management of metabolic syndrome: an American Heart Association/National Heart, Lung, and Blood Institute Scientific Statement, *Circulation* 112:2735, 2005.

*Any three factors constitute a diagnosis.

which is after menopause for most women. Overall the increased risk for CHD parallels increase in age.

Family History

A family history of premature disease is a strong risk factor, even when other risk factors are considered. A family history is considered to be positive when MI or sudden death occurs before the age of 55 years in a male first-degree relative or the age of 65 in a female first-degree relative (parents, siblings, or children). The presence of a positive family history, although not modifiable, will influence the intensity of risk factor management.

MEDICAL NUTRITION THERAPY

Medical nutrition therapy, which includes physical activity, is the primary intervention for patients with elevated LDL cholesterol. Physicians are encouraged to refer patients to registered dietitians (RDs) to help patients meet goals for therapy (NCEP, 2002) based on LDL cholesterol levels as presented in Table 32-3. With diet, exercise, and weight reduction, patients can often reach serum lipid goals. The complexity of changes, number of changes, and motivation of the patient will dictate how many patient visits it will take for the adherent client to be successful. An initial visit of (45 to 90 minutes) followed by two to six visits of 30 to 60 minutes each with the RD is recommended (ADA Evidence Library, 2006). Consequently these interventions are tried before drug therapy and also continue during pharmacologic treatment to enhance effectiveness of the medication (see *Pathophysiology and Care Management Algorithm:* Atherosclerosis).

Therapeutic Lifestyle Changes

The ATP-III recommends the TLC dietary pattern for primary and secondary prevention of CHD (Table 32-6). In agreement, the AHA recommends diet and lifestyle changes to reduce CVD risk in all people over the age of 2 years (Box 32-6) (Lichtenstein et al., 2006).

SFA recommendations are lower at less than 7% of calories; total fat content has a range of 25% to 35% of calories. Consuming 30% to 35% of calories from fat while maintaining a low SFA and *trans*-fatty acid intake is the dietary pattern recommended for individuals with insulin resistance or metabolic syndrome. This higher fat intake, emphasizing polyunsaturated fatty acids (PUFAs) and monounsaturated fatty acids (MUFA), can be beneficial in lowering triglycerides and raising HDL cholesterol. Also, with a more liberal fat intake, LDL cholesterol can be lowered without exacerbating blood glucose levels.

The time course for medical nutrition therapy is a 3- to 6-month process (Figure 32-8). Lowering SFAs and cholesterol is the first level of behavior change. The TLC diet is followed for 6 weeks. At visit two, the LDL response is evaluated, and therapy is intensified as warranted. Adjuncts such as plant sterols and stanols, fiber, and soy are incorporated into education at the second visit (dietary

compliance must be monitored during this period). At visit three metabolic syndrome treatment begins if target LDL is not reached. Once the maximum LDL reduction has occurred, management of metabolic syndrome or the cluster of risk factors becomes the target for medical nutrition therapy.

Increasing physical activity and decreasing energy intake to facilitate weight loss are critical to normalizing multiple risk factors. Behavioral strategies for weight management to reduce cardiovascular risk have been provided by the AHA (Klein et al., 2004). Learning outcomes include planning meals that fit the TLC plan, reading food labels, modifying recipes, preparing or purchasing appropriate foods, and choosing healthier choices when dining out.

Along with the TLC dietary pattern, the Dietary Approaches to Stop Hypertension (DASH) pattern is also very appropriate for CVD prevention and treatment (see Table 32-7). Both of these dietary patterns emphasize grains, cereals, legumes, vegetables, fruits, lean meats, poultry, fish, and nonfat dairy products. Strategies to accomplish dietary goals are shown in Box 32-7. Because animal fats provide about two thirds of the SFAs in the American diet, these foods are limited. High-fat choices are omitted, but low-fat choices can be included. Meat is limited to 5 oz/day, and eggs to four or fewer per week. Lean meats are high in protein, zinc, and iron; thus, if patients wish to consume meat, a 5-oz portion or less can be fit into the dietary plan if other low SFA choices are made. Similarly with dairy products, nonfat choices are

---

BOX 32-6

American Heart Association 2006 Diet Recommendations for Cardiovascular Disease Risk Reduction

- Balance calorie intake and physical activity to achieve or maintain a healthy body weight.
- Consume a diet rich in vegetables and fruits.
- Choose whole grain, high-fiber foods.
- Consume fish, especially oily fish, at least twice a week.
- Limit intake of saturated fat to <7% of energy, *trans*-fat to <1% of energy, and cholesterol to <300 mg/day by:
  - Choosing lean meats and vegetable alternatives.
  - Selecting fat-free (skim), 1%-fat, and low-fat dairy products.
  - Minimizing intake of partially hydrogenated fats.
- Minimize your intake of beverages and foods with added sugars.
- Choose and prepare foods with little or no salt.
- When consuming alcohol, do so in moderation.
- When eating food that is prepared outside of the home, follow the American Heart Association Diet and Lifestyle Recommendations.

Modified from Lichtenstein AH et al: Diet and lifestyle recommendations revision 2006: a scientific statement from the American Heart Association Committee, *Circulation* 114:83, 2006.

PATHOPHYSIOLOGY AND CARE MANAGEMENT ALGORITHM

Atherosclerosis

ETIOLOGY

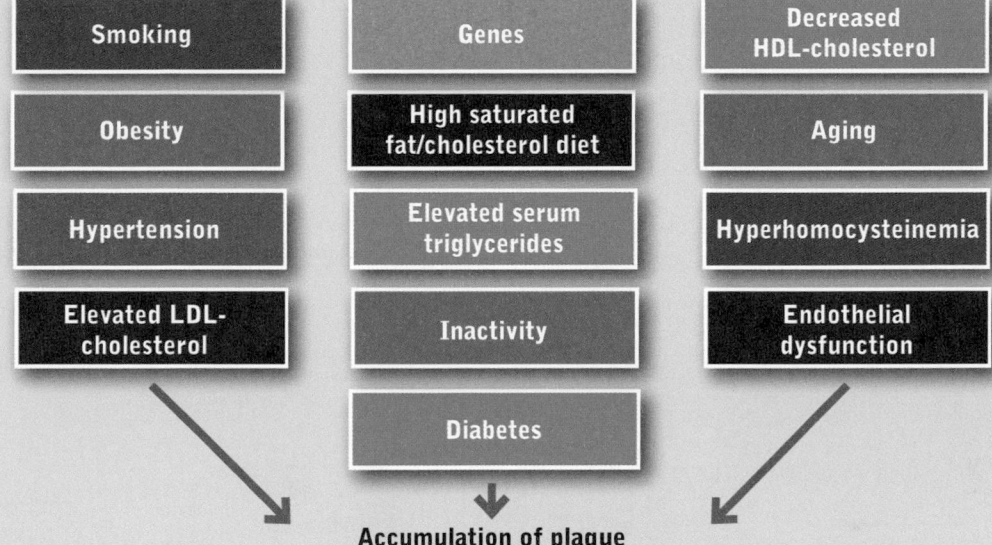

Smoking	Genes	Decreased HDL-cholesterol
Obesity	High saturated fat/cholesterol diet	Aging
Hypertension	Elevated serum triglycerides	Hyperhomocysteinemia
Elevated LDL-cholesterol	Inactivity	Endothelial dysfunction
	Diabetes	

Accumulation of plaque
Production of less nitric oxide
Oxidized LDL cholesterol taken up by macrophages
Formation of foam cells and fatty streaks

PATHOPHYSIOLOGY

Clinical Findings

- Elevated serum total cholesterol
- Elevated LDL cholesterol
- Elevated serum triglycerides
- Elevated C-reactive protein
- Low HDL-cholesterol

Nutrition Assessment

- BMI evaluation
- Waist circumference; waist to hip ratio (WHR)
- Dietary assessment for:
  SFA, *trans*-fatty acids, omega-3 fatty acids, fiber, sodium, alcohol, and refined carbohydrates

MANAGEMENT

Medical Management

- Bile acid sequestrants
- HMG CoA reductase inhibitors
- Nicotinic acid
- Triglyceride-lowering medication
- Blood pressure—lowering medication
- Medication for glucose management
- Percutaneous coronary intervention (PCI)
  - Balloon
  - Stent
- Coronary artery bypass graft (CABG)

Nutrition Management

- TLC dietary pattern—7% kcal from SFA
- AHA dietary pattern—7% kcal from SFA
- DASH dietary pattern
- Weight reduction if needed
- Increase dietary fiber to 25–30 g/day or more
- Add stanols and sterols (2–3 g/day) in multiple doses
- Add omega-3 fats
- Add soy protein
- Add fruits and vegatables for antioxidants
- Reduce dietary cholesterol—<200 mg/day

Developed by L. Kathleen Mahan, MS, RD, CDE, and Debra A. Krummel, PhD, RD, 2006.

TABLE 32-6

Nutrient Composition of the Therapeutic Lifestyle Change Dietary Pattern

Nutrient	Recommended Intake
Saturated fat*	Less than 7% of total calories
Polyunsaturated fat	Up to 10% of total calories
Monounsaturated fat	Up to 20% of total calories
Total fat	25%-35% of total calories
Carbohydrate†	50% to 60% of total calories
Fiber	25-30 g/day
Protein	Approximately 15% of total calories
Cholesterol	Less than 200 mg/day
Total calories (energy)‡	Balance energy intake and expenditure to maintain desirable body weight/prevent weight gain

From National Heart, Lung, and Blood Institute: *Detection, evaluation, and treatment of high blood cholesterol in adults* (adult treatment panel III), Final report, U.S. Department Of Health and Human Services, NIH Publication No. 02-5215, Bethesda, Md, September 2002.
*Trans-fatty acids are another low-density–lipoprotein raising fat that should be kept at a low intake.
†Carbohydrate should be derived predominantly from foods rich in complex carbohydrates, including grains, especially whole grains, fruits, and vegetables.
‡Daily energy expenditure should include at least moderate physical activity (contributing approximately 200 kcal/day).

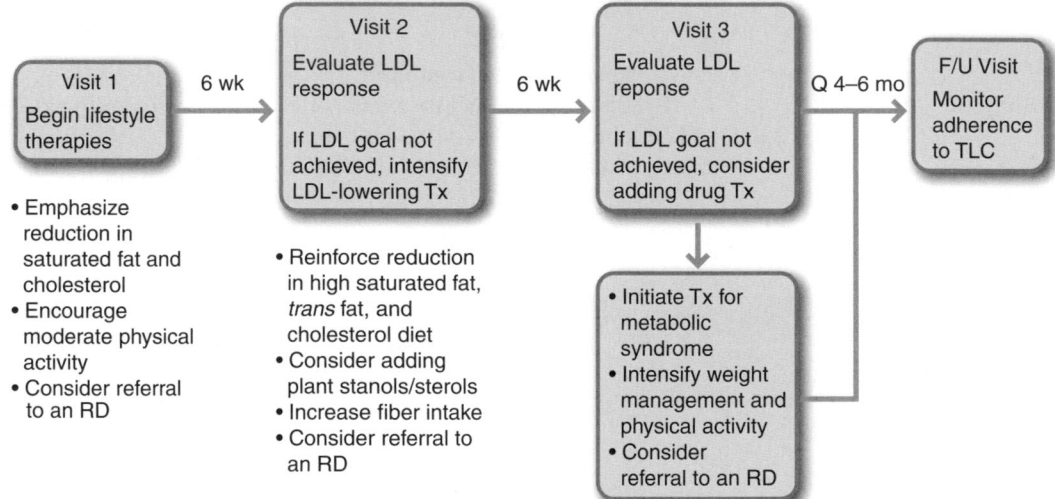

FIGURE 32-8 Steps in therapeutic lifestyle changes (TLC). *LDL*, Low-density lipoprotein; *RD*, registered dietitian; *Tx*, treatment; *F/U*, follow-up. (*From National Heart, Lung, and Blood Institute:* Detection, evaluation, and treatment of high blood cholesterol in adults *[Adult Treatment Panel III]. Final report. U.S. Department of Health and Human Services, NIH Publication No. 02-5215, Bethesda, Md, September 2002.*)

recommended. Neither food group has to be omitted; it is a matter of choice. Most people need to add the recommended two servings of fatty fish per week. Meeting sodium guidelines (1500 to 2300 mg daily) can be a challenge because lower-fat processed foods often contain salt to increase palatability. Patients may need to limit convenience and processed foods (see Chapter 33).

For highly motivated patients who want to avoid drug therapy, sometimes very low–fat diets are effective for reaching blood lipid goals. These diets can also be used as an adjunct to drug therapy for secondary prevention and possible regression of lesions. Such diets contain minimum amounts of animal products; thus SFA (<3%), cholesterol (<5 mg/day), and total fat (<10%) intakes are very low. The emphasis is on low-fat grains, legumes, fruits, vegetables, and nonfat

dairy foods. Because egg whites are allowed, the plan is a lacto-ovo-vegetarian regimen. To ensure nutritional adequacy, consulting with an RD is recommended (Box 32-8).

Dietary Factors

Fat

For more than 40 years epidemiologic studies, experimental studies, and clinical trials have shown that numerous dietary risk factors affect serum lipids, atherogenesis, and CHD. When studying the effects of fatty acids on serum lipids, two points of comparison are made. First, how do the fatty acids compare with the carbohydrate substitution, which is considered neutral? Second, how do they compare when they replace SFAs?

TABLE 32-7

DASH and TLC Dietary Patterns at 2000 kcal

Eating Pattern	DASH*	TLC†	Serving Sizes
Grains‡	6-8 serving/day	7 servings§/day	1 slice bread; 1 oz dry cereal¶; ½ c cooked rice, pasta, or cereal
Vegetables	4-5 servings/day	5 servings§/day	1 cup raw leafy vegetable, ½ c cut-up raw or cooked vegetable, ½ c vegetable juice
Fruits	4-5 servings/day	4 servings§/day	1 medium fruit; ¼ c dried fruit; ½ c fresh, frozen, or canned fruit; ½ c fruit juice
Fat-free or low-fat milk and milk products	2-3 servings/day	2 to 3 servings/day	1 c milk, 1 c yogurt, 1½ oz cheese
Lean meats,‖ poultry, and fish	<6 oz/day	≤5 oz/day	
Nuts, seeds and legumes	4-5 servings/week	Counted in vegetable servings	⅓ c (1½ oz), 2 Tbsp peanut butter, 2 Tbsp or ½ oz seeds, ½ c dry beans or peas
Fats and oils	2 to 3 servings#/day	Amount depends on daily calorie level	1 tsp soft margarine, 1 Tbsp mayonnaise, 2 Tbsp salad dressing, 1 tsp vegetable oil
Sweets and added sugars	5 or fewer servings per week	No recommendation	1 Tbsp sugar, 1 Tbsp jelly or jam, ½ c sorbet and ices, 1 c lemonade

From Lichtenstein AH et al: Diet and lifestyle recommendations revision 2006: a scientific statement from the American Heart Association Nutrition Committee, *Circulation* 114:82, 2006.

*Dietary Approaches to Stop Hypertension. For more information, please visit http://www.nhlbi.nih.gov/health/public/heart/hbp/dash.

†Therapeutic Lifestyle Changes. For more information, please visit http://www.nhlbi.nih.gov/cgi-bin/chd/step2intro.cgi. TLC includes two therapeutic diet options: Plan stanol/sterol (add 2 g/day) and soluble fiber (add 5 to 10 g/day).

‡Whole grain foods are recommended for most grain servings to meet fiber recommendations.

§This number can be less or more, depending on other food choices to meet 2000 calories.

¶Equals ½ to 1¼ cups, depending on cereal type. Check the product's Nutrition Facts Label.

‖Lean cuts include sirloin tip, round steak, and rump roast; extra lean hamburger; and cold cuts made with lean meat or soy protein. Lean cuts of pork are center-cut ham, loin chops, and pork tenderloin.

#Fat content changes serving counts for fats and oils: For example, 1 Tbsp of regular salad dressing equals 1 serving; 1 Tbsp of low-fat dressing equals ½ serving; 1 Tbsp of fat-free dressing equals 0 servings.

Saturated Fatty Acids. The predominant sources of SFAs in the American diet are animal foods (meat and dairy). SFAs are restricted because they have the most potent effect on LDL cholesterol, which rises in a dose-response fashion when increasing levels of SFAs are consumed. The most hypercholesterolemic-promoting or atherogenic SFAs in order of potency are myristic (C14:0), palmitic (C16:0), and lauric (C12:0) acids (see Chapter 3). Palmitic acid is the most prevalent hypercholesterolemic SFA in the American diet, constituting 60% of total SFA intake. Most dietary palmitate comes from animal foods. Myristic acid is found mostly in butterfat and coconut and palm kernel oils. It is less prevalent in the American diet than palmitic acid. Lauric acid, the only medium-chain SFA, is also found in palm kernel and coconut oils. Of all the added fats in the diet, the most hypercholesterolemic promoting are palm kernel, coconut, and palm oils; lard; and butter. In the NHANES IV the mean consumption of SFAs was 11% of kilocalories; less than 7% of energy is the population goal (Carroll et al., 2005; Lichtenstein et al., 2006).

SFAs raise serum LDL cholesterol by decreasing LDL receptor synthesis and activity. Regardless of form, all fatty acids lower fasting triglycerides if they replace carbohydrate in the diet. In secondary prevention trials replacement of SFAs with MUFAs, α-linolenic acid, and increased fruits and vegetables prevented fatal and nonfatal CVD events in persons with established disease (de Lorgeril, 1999). Thus fatty acids affect disease progression through lipids and other mechanisms and possibly through inflammation and thrombosis.

Monounsaturated Fatty Acids. The AHA does not have any recommendation for the *cis* form of MUFAs (Lichtenstein et al., 2006). Oleic acid (C18:1) is the most prevalent MUFA in the American diet. Substituting oleic acid for carbohydrate has almost no appreciable effect on blood lipids; however, replacing SFAs with MUFAs (as would happen when substituting olive oil for butter in a diet) lowers serum cholesterol levels, LDL cholesterol levels, and triglyceride levels to about the same extent as PUFAs. The effects of MUFAs on HDL

BOX 32-7

Practical Dietary Tips

Lifestyle

- Know your caloric needs to achieve and maintain a healthy weight.
- Know the calorie content of the foods and beverages you consume.
- Track your weight, physical activity, and calorie intake.
- Prepare and eat smaller portions.
- Track, and when possible, decrease screen time (e.g., watching television, surfing the Internet, playing computer games).
- Incorporate physical movement into habitual activities.
- Do not smoke or use tobacco products.
- If you consume alcohol, do so in moderation (equivalent of no more than one drink for women or two drinks for men per day).

Food Choices and Preparation

- Use the nutrition facts label and ingredients list when choosing foods to buy.
- Eat fresh, frozen, and canned vegetables and fruits without high-calorie sauces and added salt and sugars.
- Replace high-calorie foods with fruits and vegetables.
- Increase fiber intake by eating beans (legumes), whole-grain products, fruits, and vegetables.
- Use liquid vegetable oils in place of solid fats.
- Limit beverages and foods high in added sugars. Common forms of added sugars are sucrose, glucose, fructose, maltose, dextrose, corn syrups, concentrated fruit juice, and honey.

- Choose foods made with whole grains. Common forms of whole grains are whole wheat, oats/oatmeal, rye, barley, corn, popcorn, brown rice, wild rice, buckwheat, triticale, bulgur (cracked wheat), millet, quinoa, and sorghum.
- Cut back on pastries and high-calorie bakery products (e.g., muffins, doughnuts).
- Select milk and dairy products that are either fat free or low fat.
- Reduce salt intake by:
  - Comparing the sodium content of similar products (e.g., different brands of tomato sauce) and choosing products with less salt.
  - Choosing versions of processed foods, including cereals and baked goods, that are reduced in salt.
  - Limiting condiments (e.g., soy sauce, ketchup).
- Use lean cuts of meat and remove skin from poultry before eating.
- Limit processed meats that are high in saturated fat and sodium.
- Grill, bake, or broil fish, meat, and poultry.
- Incorporate vegetable-based meat substitutes into favorite recipes.
- Encourage the consumption of whole vegetables and fruits in place of juices.

From Lichtenstein AH et al: Diet and lifestyle recommendations revision 2006: a scientific statement from the American Heart Association Committee, *Circulation* 114: 86, 2006.

---

cholesterol depend on the total fat content of the diet. When intakes of both MUFA (>15% of total kilocalories) and total fat (>35% of kilocalories) are high, HDL cholesterol does not change or increases slightly compared with levels with a lower-fat diet. Oleic acid as part of the Mediterranean diet has been shown to have antiinflammatory effects.

In epidemiologic studies high-fat diets of people in Mediterranean countries have been associated with low blood cholesterol levels and CHD incidence (Trichopoulou et al., 2003). Among other factors, the main fat source is olive oil, which is high in MUFAs. This observation led to many studies on the benefits of high-fat and high-MUFA diets. More recently a Mediterranean-type step I diet was shown to reduce recurrent CVD by 50% to 70% (de Lorgeril et al., 1999). This diet emphasizes fruits, root vegetables (carrots, turnips, potatoes, onions, radishes), leafy green vegetables, breads and cereals, fish, foods high in α-linolenic acid (flax, canola oil), vegetable oil products (salad dressing and other products made with nonhydrogenated oils), and nuts and seeds (walnuts and flaxseed) (Kris-Etherton et al., 2001b) (see *Focus On:* The Mediterranean Diet: Is It Good For All of Us? and Figure 12-4 in Chapter 12).

Although higher-fat diets (low in SFAs with MUFAs as the predominant fat) can lower blood cholesterol, they should be used with caution because of the caloric density of high-fat diets and the results of clinical trials, which have shown new atherosclerotic lesions in men who consume higher-fat diets. The negative association between the Mediterranean diet and CHD could be the result of factors other than MUFA intake. For example, these populations consume more fruits and vegetables, bread, cereals, fish, and nuts, and less red meat than many populations. Olive oil is the primary source of fat, and eggs are consumed from zero to four times per week.

Trans-fatty acids (stereoisomers of the naturally occurring *cis*-linoleic acid) are produced in the hydrogenation process used in the food industry to increase shelf life of foods and to make margarines, made from oil, firmer. The AHA (Lichtenstein et al., 2006) recommends no more than 1% of calories (about 1-3 g/day) from *trans*-fatty acids. These fatty acids are limited mostly because they raise LDL cholesterol; effects on inflammation have been conflicting (Basu et al., 2006). Most *trans*-fatty acids intake comes from partially hydrogenated vegetable oils (Table 32-8).

BOX 32-8

Quick Tips for Aggressive Lipid-Lowering Diets

ABCs of the Reversal Eating Plan

A. Fat intake of 12-14 g/day
B. Vegetarian eating (i.e., no meat, poultry, fish)
C. No added fats (i.e., fat or oil is not added to any food)
D. Higher-fat foods are not used (e.g., nuts, seeds, avocado, olives)
E. No "fat-free" foods with fat in the ingredient list (e.g., whipped topping mix, dairy creamers)

Use These Foods Daily

A. Nonfat dairy foods
B. Nonfat egg substitutes and egg whites
C. Nonfat meat substitutes such as preformed fat-free soy burgers, textured soy nuggets, and wheat gluten
D. Fat-reduced tofu
E. Dried beans and peas
F. Breads, cereals, pasta, starches, rice, and grains
G. Vegetables and fruits

To Make Foods Taste Good: Use for Sauces, Gravies, and Seasonings

A. Nonfat vegetable broth
B. Fat-free, meat-based broth
C. Herbs and seasonings
D. Nonfat butter-flavored sprinkles and liquids
E. Also use, but sparingly: vegetable cooking spray

From Reversal Eating Plan, ©1996 Gerry Krag, MA, RD, Grosse Pte Park, Mich.

Polyunsaturated Fatty Acids. The essential fatty acid linoleic acid (LA) is the predominant PUFA consumed in the American diet. Population studies have demonstrated a negative correlation between LA intake and CHD rates (Wijendran and Hayes, 2004). Similarly, a metaanalysis of 60 controlled human trials found that replacing PUFAs for carbohydrate in the diet resulted in a decline in serum LDL cholesterol (Mensink et al., 2003). When SFAs are replaced with PUFAs in a low-fat diet, LDL and HDL cholesterol levels will be lowered. Overall, eliminating SFAs is twice as effective in lowering serum cholesterol levels as increasing PUFAs.

The lipid-lowering effects of LA depend on the total fatty acid profile of the diet (Wijendran and Hayes, 2004). When added to study diets, large amounts of LA diminished levels of HDL cholesterol serum levels, but studies of more moderate LA levels as in the NCEP Step 1 diet have demonstrated only modest HDL lowering effects (Karmally, 2005). Studies suggest that high intakes of n-6 PUFAs may exert adverse effects on the function of vascular endothelium or stimulate production of proinflammatory cytokines. A low ratio of omega-6:omega-3 PUFAs is recommended (Basu et al., 2006; Gebauer et al., 2006).

Omega-3 Fatty Acids. The main omega-3 fatty acids (i.e., eicosapentaenoic acid (EPA) and docosahexaenoic acid [DHA]) are high in fish oils, fish oil capsules, and ocean fish. Many studies have shown that eating fish is associated with a decreased CVD risk. The recommendation for the general population for fish consumption is to eat fish high in omega-3 fatty acids (salmon, tuna, mackerel, sardines) at least twice a week (Psota et al., 2006). For patients who have CVD, 1 g of EPA and DHA combined is recommended from fish if possible but, if not, then from supplements (Lichtenstein et al., 2006). Patients who have hypertriglyceridemia need 2 to 4 g of EPA and DHA per day for effective lowering (Lichtenstein et al., 2006). Omega-3 fatty acids lower triglyceride levels by inhibiting VLDL and apo B-100 synthesis and by decreasing postprandial lipemia.

α-Linolenic acid (ALA), an omega-3 fatty acid from vegetables, has antiinflammatory effects. CRP levels were reduced when male patients consumed 8 g of ALA daily; similar results have not been observed for fish oil supplementation (Basu et al., 2006). Omega-3 fatty acids also interfere with blood clotting by altering prostaglandin synthesis. Therefore high intakes prolong bleeding times, a condition that is common in Eskimo populations with high omega-3 fat dietary intakes and low incidence of CHD.

Amount of Dietary Fat. Total fat intakes are related to obesity, which affects many of the major risk factors for atherosclerosis. Also, high-fat diets increase postprandial lipemia and chylomicron remnants, both of which are associated with increased risk of CHD. When fat is reduced in the diet and carbohydrate is the replacement source of calories, triglycerides and HDL levels are affected. Low-fat diets (<25% of total kilocalories from fat) raise triglyceride levels and lower HDL cholesterol levels. Although these changes appear to be negative, they are not associated with CHD risk because (1) LDL cholesterol levels are low in persons consuming low-fat diets; and (2) the VLDLs that are produced are large, triglyceride-rich VLDLs, which are not associated with risk.

Dietary Cholesterol. Dietary cholesterol raises total cholesterol and LDL cholesterol but to a lesser extent than SFAs. The AHA and TLC dietary patterns contain no more than 200 mg of cholesterol each day. There is a threshold beyond which addition of cholesterol to the diet has minimal effects. When cholesterol intakes reach 500 mg/day, only small increments in blood cholesterol occur. Cholesterol responsiveness also varies widely among individuals. Some people are hyporesponders (i.e., their plasma cholesterol level does not increase after dietary cholesterol challenge), whereas others are hyperresponders (i.e., their plasma cholesterol level responds more strongly than expected to a cholesterol challenge). It has been suggested that hyperresponders may have the apo E-4 allele and poor rates of conversion of cholesterol to bile acids, which causes elevated LDL cholesterol. Feeding choles-

TABLE 32-8

Examples of Major Sources of *Trans*-Fatty Acids

Food	Serving Size	*Trans*-Fatty Acids (g/serving)
Cake, pound, cholesterol-free	2 oz	3.04
Cookie, (chocolate) with caramel and chocolate coating	2 oz	3.88
Cookie, (vanilla) with crème filling	3 cookies	2.13
Crackers, snack crackers, cheese flavored	14 crackers	1.04
Donut, cake or yeast	1 donut	1.72
French fries, made from frozen	10 fries	1.27
French fries, fast-food	30-40 fries	3.43
Hamburger, 25% fat patty, broiled	3 oz, cooked	1.14
Margarine, corn and soy, 80% fat, stick	1 Tbsp	2.76
Margarine, stick	1 Tbsp	2.72
Popcorn, microwave popped	3.5 c	2.11
Sandwich meat, bologna	1 oz	1.62
Shortening	1 Tbsp	2.44
Soy spread, 70% fat	1 Tbsp	2.69
Tortilla chips	1 oz	1.15

terol to animals enriches lipoproteins, which are atherogenic beyond just the rise in serum cholesterol.

In addition to the effects of dietary cholesterol alone on serum lipids, dietary SFAs and cholesterol have a synergistic effect on LDL cholesterol level. Together they decrease LDL receptor synthesis and activity, increase VLDLs enriched with apo E, increase all lipoproteins, and decrease chylomicron size (which is associated with CHD risk). The effect of dietary cholesterol on inflammatory factors has been inconsistent (Basu et al., 2006).

Fiber

With the AHA, TLC, and DASH dietary patterns' emphasis on fruits, vegetables, legumes, and whole grains, there would be adequate fiber to lower LDL cholesterol. In particular, the soluble fibers in pectins, gums, mucilages, algal polysaccharides, and some hemicelluloses lower LDL cholesterol. The quantity of fiber needed to produce the lipid-lowering effect varies by food source; higher quantities of legumes are needed than of pectin or gums. Proposed mechanisms for the hypocholesterolemic effect of soluble fiber include the following: (1) the fiber binds bile acids, which lowers serum cholesterol as it repletes the bile acid pool; and (2) bacteria in the colon ferment the fiber to produce acetate, propionate, and butyrate, which inhibit cholesterol synthesis. The

role of fiber, if any, on inflammatory pathways is not well established (Erkkila and Lichtenstein, 2006).

Insoluble fibers such as cellulose and lignin have no effect on serum cholesterol levels. Of the total recommended fiber intake (25 to 30 g daily for adults), approximately 6 to 10 g should be from soluble fiber. This level is easy to achieve with the recommended five or more servings of fruits or vegetables per day and six or more servings of grains (if whole grains and high-fiber cereals are chosen). The AHA does not recommend fiber supplements for prevention of CVD.

Antioxidants

Two dietary components that affect the oxidation potential of LDL cholesterol are the level of LA in the particle and the availability of antioxidants. Vitamins C, E, and β-carotene at physiologic levels have antioxidant roles in the body. Vitamin E is the most concentrated antioxidant carried on LDLs, the amount being 20 to 300 times greater than any other antioxidant. A major function of vitamin E is to prevent oxidation of PUFAs in the cell membrane. Epidemiologic studies suggest that vitamin E and carotenoids are inversely related to CVD, but randomized trials have not supported these observations (Lee et al., 2005; Lichtenstein et al., 2006). Because data have not shown vitamin E to be protective, the AHA does not recommend vitamin E supplementation for CVD prevention (Lichtenstein et al., 2006). However, RRR-α-tocopherol, the natural form of vitamin E, shows promise as an antiinflammatory agent (Basu et al., 2006).

Foods with concentrated amounts of the phytonutrients catechins, have been found to improve vascular reactivity. These foods are red grapes, red wine, tea (especially green tea), chocolate, and olive oil, and should be worked into any CVD preventive eating plan (Kay et al., 2006).

Soy Protein

Only very large intakes of soy protein (at least half of a person's daily protein intake) may decrease LDL cholesterol by a few percent when it replaces animal protein (Sacks et al., 2006). Using soy foods such as tofu, soy butter, or soy nuts may have benefits for cardiovascular health in that they contain other protective nutrients such as PUFAs and fiber. A 1-2 oz serving of soy daily is recommended (Table 32-9).

Stanols and Sterols

Since the early 1950s, plant stanols and sterols isolated from soybean oils or pine tree oil have been known to lower blood cholesterol (Lichtenstein et al., 2001). Recently they have been esterified and made into margarines. Consuming between 2 to 3 g/day lowers cholesterol by 9% to 20% (Lichtenstein et al., 2001). The mechanism for cholesterol lowering is by inhibiting absorption of dietary cholesterol. ATP-III includes stanols as part of dietary recommendations for lowering LDL cholesterol in adults. Because these esters can also affect the absorption of and cause lower β-carotene, α-tocopherol, and lycopene levels, further safety studies are needed for use in normocholesterolemic individuals, children, and pregnant women.

TABLE 32-9

Supplements and Functional Foods: Lipid Effects

Supplement/ Functional Foods	Mechanism	Lipid Lowering (Average % Change)	Usefulness for Lipid Management
Vitamin E	Antioxidant	No significant change in TC/LDL; lowers HDL$_2$	No clear benefit
Vitamin C, beta carotene	Antioxidant	No significant change in lipid profile	No clear benefit
n-3 Fatty acids (fish oils)	Inhibits VLDL synthesis	Lowers TG 15% to 40%; dose 1 to 3 g/day	Useful adjunct for hypertriglyceridemia; may be useful in diabetes
Garlic	Unknown	Lowers TC/LDL ≈5%	No major role
Soy protein	May have phytoestrogen effect	Lowers TC/LDL ≈5% to 10%, nonsignificant increase in HDL; dose 25 g/day	Modest role; best used in place of high saturated-fat foods
Plant sterols/ stanols	Decreases dietary and biliary cholesterol absorption	Lowers TC/LDL 9% to 20%, no change in HDL; dose 2-3 g/day	Moderate effect; may be useful adjunct
Fiber	Bile acid–binding action, decreases dietary cholesterol absorption	Lowers TC/LDL ≈5 to 15%; dose 25 to 30 g/day of dietary sources of fiber	Modest role; best used in place of high saturated fat foods

Modified from Fletcher B et al: Managing abnormal blood lipids: a collaborative approach, *Circulation* 112:3184, 2005.

HDL, High-density lipoprotein; *LDL*, low-density lipoprotein; *TC*, total cholesterol, *TG*, triglyceride.

Weight Loss

In a recent review, 11 out of 12 short studies (<6 months) showed that weight loss improves endothelial function measured using different methods (Brook, 2006). In a group of patients with extreme obesity (BMI = 52), flow-mediated dilation, which is an estimate of endothelial function, improved after the patients lost a mean of 23 kg (Williams et al., 2005). Overall it is not known how much weight has to be lost, how long the effect lasts, and whether the improvement in endothelial function reduces coronary events (Brook, 2006).

OTHER TREATMENT

Pharmacologic Management

Determination of drug therapy depends on risk category and attainment of the LDL cholesterol goal (see Table 32-3). Many drugs are available for LDL lowering (Table 32-10). Regardless of the drug used or category of risk, the TLCs underpin all treatment. A regimen combining diet and drugs enables more patients to achieve blood lipid goals than a drug-only regimen. A TLC dietary pattern with drugs can reduce serum cholesterol levels by up to 40% (Van Horn and Ernst, 2001). More restrictive diets with drugs have not been investigated.

The classes of drugs include the following: (1) **bile acid sequestrants** such as cholestyramine (adsorbs bile acids); (2) nicotinic acid; (3) **HMG CoA reductase inhibitors** (inhibit the rate-limiting enzyme in cholesterol synthesis) also known as statins (lovastatin, pravastatin); (4) fibric acid derivatives (clofibrate, gemfibrozil); and (5) probucol. Classes 1, 2, and 3 are the first choices for treatment (NCEP, 2001). In a review of pharmacologic therapy, 78% of patients were treated with a statin; treatment success rate was highest in diabetic patients with CVD (60%) and nondiabetics patients with CVD (52%), and lowest in diabetic patients without CVD (45%) (Yan et al., 2006).

Drugs used to lower CRP are lipid-lowering agents (statins, ezetimibe, fenofibrate, niacin), angiotensin-converting enzyme inhibitors (ramipril, captopril, fosinopril), angiotensin receptor blockers (valsartan, irbesartan, olmesartan, telmisartan), antidiabetic agents (rosiglitazone, pioglitazone), and platelet aggregation inhibitors (clopidogrel, abciximab) (Prasad, 2006).

Medical Intervention

Medical interventions such as percutaneous coronary intervention (PCI) are now being performed in patients with asymptomatic ischemia or angina (Smith et al., 2005). PCI, previously known as percutaneous transluminal coronary angioplasty (PTCA), is a procedure that uses a catheter with a balloon that once inflated, will break up plaque deposits in an occluded artery. Because the procedure is performed with the patient under local anesthesia in a cardiac catheterization laboratory, recovery is quicker than with bypass surgery. This procedure increased by 326% between 1987 and 2003; coronary stent (a wire mesh tube that holds an artery open and releases medication) insertion increased 147% between 1996 and 2000 (Thom et al., 2006). PCI is often possible because of earlier detection of

TABLE 32-10

Effects of Selected Cholesterol-Lowering Cardiovascular Disease Medications on Nutrition Status

Drug Class, Generic Name, and Dosage	Effects on Blood Lipids		Nutritional Considerations/Common Side Effects
HMG CoA reductase inhibitors—statins*	LDL	↓ 18%-55%	Take with meals; nausea, constipation, flatulence, dyspepsia, abdominal pain
	HDL	↑ 5%-15%	
	TG	↓ 7%-30%	
Fibric acid derivatives—Fibrates†	LDL	↓ 5%-20%	Take ½ hr before meals; dyspepsia, abdominal pain, nausea, gallstones, change in bowel function, flatulence
	HDL	↑ 10%-20%	
	TG	↓ 20%-50%	
Nicotinic acid‡	LDL	↓ 5%-25%	Gastrointestinal (GI) distress: nausea/vomiting, abdominal pain, change in bowel function, hyperglycemia; take with food to diminish GI distress; avoid with substantial alcohol consumption
	HDL	↑ 15%-35%	
	TG	↓ 20%-50%	
Omega-3 fatty acids§	LDL	↑ 3%-7%	Dyspepsia, fishy aftertaste
	TG	↓ 20%-30%	
Bile acid sequestrants¶	LDL	↓ 15%-30%	GI distress: nausea/vomiting, abdominal pain, belching, dyspepsia, constipation
	HDL	↑ 3%-5%	

Data from Szapary P, Rader DJ: Third Report of the National Cholesterol Education Program Expert Panel on Detection, Evaluation, and Treatment of High Blood Cholesterol in Adults, Bethesda, Md, 2001, National Heart, Lung, and Blood Institute; *Powers and Moore's Food medication interactions*, ed 13, NIH Publication No. 01-3670, Bethesda, Md; May, 2001-2004; Physicians Desk Reference, ed 57, Montvale, NJ, 2003, Thompson Healthcare.

*Lovastatin (20-80 mg), Pravastatin (20-80 mg), Simvastatin (20-80 mg), Fluvastatin (20-80 mg), Atorvastatin (10-80 mg).

†Gemfibrozil (600 mg bid), Fenofibrate (2000 mg), Clofibrate (1000 mg bid).

‡Immediate-release (crystalline) nicotinic acid (1.5-3g), extended-release nicotinic acid (Niaspan) (1-2 g), sustained-release nicotinic acid (1-2 g), sustained release nicotinic acid (1-2 g).

§Fish oil capsules (3-5 g).

¶Cholestyramine (4-16 g), Colestipol (5-20 g), Colesevelam (2.6-3.8 g).

GI, Gastrointestinal; *HDL*, high-density lipoprotein; *HMG CoA*, hydroxymethylglutaryl enzyme; *LDL*, low-density lipoprotein.

blockages. The most common problem with PCI is restenosis of the artery. A recent study of over 2200 patients, half of whom received intervention of medication and lifestyle changes such as quitting smoking, exercise and nutrition, and half of whom received this as well as angioplasty showed some interesting results. After 5 years it was observed that the number who had heart attacks or who were hospitalized or died because of their heart problems was virtually identical in both groups. There did not seem to be benefit from angioplasty over lifestyle changes combined with medication (Boden et al., 2007).

In coronary artery bypass graft (CABG) surgery, an artery from the chest is used to redirect blood flow around a diseased vessel. Candidates for CABG usually have more than two occluded arteries. CABG surgeries have decreased since 1995 because more PCI procedures are being done, but this may change. These surgeries improve survival time, relieve symptoms, and markedly improve the quality of life for patients with CHD. However, CABG does not cure atherosclerosis; the new grafts are also susceptible to atherogenesis. Consequently restenosis is common within 10 years of surgery. Risk factor modification, including at a minimum TLCs and probably more aggressive dietary changes, is needed to stop progression.

In the postoperative period CABG patients, like others undergoing major surgery, are in a catabolic state; therefore adequate nutritional intake via oral routes is essential. Patients with complications may be at risk for developing cardiac cachexia, which is often associated with heart failure (see Chapter 34). If oral intake is inadequate, tube feeding is indicated to meet increased energy, protein, and nutrient needs (see Chapter 20). In some facilities, after either cardiac surgery or an acute MI, the dietary regimen starts with a "cardiac liquid" diet (i.e., full liquids with no added salt, the omission of caffeine, and restriction of cholesterol). For example, eggnog, high-fat cream soups, caffeinated soda, coffee, and chocolate are excluded. Once the patient is stabilized and ready to progress to a more complex diet, he or she may choose selections from the appropriate menu. A weight-loss regimen may be recommended in addition to the cardiac restrictions. Patients are discharged on the TLC, AHA, or DASH dietary pattern.

- Lifestyle changes, with medical nutrition therapy at the cornerstone, are pivotal to maintaining cardiovascular health.
- In the past the focus has been on lipid lowering; however, more research is uncovering the role of diet in inflammation and endothelial dysfunction, which are involved in atherogenesis.

- LDL-C levels are the primary target for medical nutrition therapy.
- The AHA, TLC, and DASH dietary patterns are recommended in both the primary and secondary prevention of CVD.

✳ CLINICAL SCENARIO 1

Lenora is a 60-year-old black woman with dyslipidemia, hypertension, and obesity. She lives with her husband of 40 years and maintains a moderate amount of activity. Because their children are grown, many meals are consumed at restaurants. In the past she has been unsuccessful in maintaining any weight losses. Her family history for chronic heart disease (CHD) is positive. Her height is 5 ft 4 in, and her weight is 250 lb. Her medications are Diabinese, Diazide, Enalapril, and Premarin. At her last checkup, the laboratory tests revealed the following:

TG: 400 mg/dl
Total cholesterol: 253 mg/dl
HDL cholesterol: 37 mg/dl
LDL cholesterol: 185 mg/dl

Her diet history reveals intake of an average of 45% of kcal from fat and over 360 mg of cholesterol daily from high cholesterol foods.

✳**Nutrition Diagnosis:** Abnormal lab values related to high fat intake from foods (45% of kcal from fat), especially those consumed at restaurant meals as evidenced by TG level of 400 mg/dl, high LDL (185 mg/dl), and low HDL (37 mg/dl) cholesterol levels

1. What are Lenora's risk factors for CHD?
2. What type of diet would you recommend for Lenora? What additional information needs to be obtained before teaching her about a new eating plan?
3. What suggestions for restaurant eating will help Lenora adhere to the new eating plan?
4. What dietary factors could optimize Lenora's lipid profile?

✳ CLINICAL SCENARIO 2

Jeremiah is a single 30-year-old Hispanic male migrant worker with elevated serum cholesterol, serum homocysteine, and blood pressure. He recently emigrated from Mexico to the United States and has become a citizen. He has been referred to your ambulatory nutrition clinic for follow-up after a general medical evaluation. His diet history reveals that he skips meals frequently and cannot predict his income for planning meals. He does not drink milk, but he will eat fruits and vegetables when he can afford them. He seldom eats fish but is willing to eat lean poultry. When he does eat a meal, he uses mostly fast-food sandwiches and fried foods.

✳**Nutrition Diagnosis:** Undesirable food choices related to use of fast foods, skipping of meals, and omission of several food groups as evidenced by abnormal lab values and lack of access to a predictable income and food supply

1. What information do you need to provide further guidance for him?
2. What community resources may be available to assist him with obtaining food on a more regular basis?
3. What type of simple menus can you give Jeremiah that will include foods from the DASH diet plan that he may be willing to consume?

USEFUL WEBSITES

American Association of Cardiovascular and Pulmonary Rehabilitation
www.aacvpr.org/

American Dietetic Association, Evidence Analysis Library (Hyperlipidemia)
www.eatright.org

American Heart Association
www.americanheart.org/

NCEP Adult Treatment Panel Guidelines
www.nhlbi.nih.gov/guidelines/cholesterol/atp_iii.htm

References

Aldamiz-Echevarria L et al: A randomized single-blind trial of the effects of vitamin C and E in familial hypercholesterolemia, *An Peadiatr Barc* 65:101, 2006.

American Heart Association (AHA1): *Healthy lifestyle diet and nutrition*, from http://www.heart.org/presenter.jhtml?identifier=1200010, accessed September 10, 2006a.

American Heart Association (AHA2): *Primary prevention in the adult*, from http://www.americanheart.org/presenter.jhtml?identifier=4704, accessed September 10, 2006b.

American Dietetic Association (ADA): *Evidence analysis library on hyperlipidemia*, from www.eatright.org, accessed 2006.

Athyros VG et al: Prevalence of vascular disease in metabolic syndrome using three proposed definitions, *Int J Cardiol* 117: 204, 2006.

Aygun AD et al: Proinflammatory cytokines and leptin are increased in serum of prepubertal obese children, *Mediators Inflamm* 3:180, 2005.

Badimon L et al: Cell biology and lipoproteins in atherosclerosis, *Curr Mol Med* 6:439, 2006.

Barter PJ, Rye KA: The rationale for using apoA-I as a clinical marker of cardiovascular risk, *J Intern Med* 259:447, 2006.

Bartolucci AA, Howard G: Meta-analysis of data from the six primary prevention trials of cardiovascular events using aspirin, *Am J Cardiol* 98:746, 2006.

Basu A et al: Dietary factors that promote or retard inflammation, *Arterioscler Thromb Vasc Biol* 26:995, 2006.

Behavioral Risk Factor Surveillance System, Prevalence of heart disease—United States, 2005, CDC: *MMWR* 56(6):113, 2007.

Berg AH, Scherer PE: Adipose tissue, inflammation and cardiovascular disease, *Circ Res* 96:939, 2006.

Blum CA et al: Low-grade inflammation and estimates of insulin resistance during the menstrual cycle in lean and overweight women, *J Clin Endocrinol Metab* 90:3230, 2005.

Boden WE et al: Optimal medical therapy with or without PCI for stable coronary disease, *N Engl J Med* 356:1503, 2007.

Brindle P et al: Accuracy and impact of risk assessment in the primary prevention of cardiovascular disease: a systematic review, *Heart* 92:1752, 2006.

Brook RD: Obesity, weight loss, and vascular function, *Endocrine* 29:21, 2006.

Carroll MD et al: Trends in serum lipids and lipoproteins of adults, 1960-2002, *JAMA* 294:1773, 2005.

Chiuve SE et al: Healthy lifestyle factors in the primary prevention of coronary heart disease among men: benefits among users and nonusers of lipid-lowering and antihypertensive medications, *Circulation* 114:160, 2006.

Choi BH et al: The role of high-density lipoprotein cholesterol in atherothrombosis, *Mt Sinai J Med* 73:690, 2006.

Civeira F: Guidelines for the diagnosis and management of heterozygous familial hypercholesterolemia, *Atherosclerosis* 173:55, 2004.

Civeira F et al: Tendon xanthomas in familial hypercholesterolemia are associated with cardiovascular risk independently of the low-density lipoprotein receptor gene mutation, *Arterioscler Thromb Vasc Biol* 25:1960, 2005.

Davignon J, Ganz P: Role of endothelial dysfunction in atherosclerosis, *Circulation* 109(23 suppl 1):III27, 2004.

de Lorgeril M et al: Mediterranean diet, traditional risk factors, and the rate of cardiovascular complications after myocardial infarction, *Circulation* 99:779, 1999.

Desai MY et al: Atherosclerosis imaging using MR imaging: current and emerging applications. *Magn Reson Imaging Clin N Am* 13:171, 2005.

Diamantopoulos EJ et al: Metabolic syndrome and pre-diabetes identify overlapping but not identical populations, *Exp Clin Endocrinol Diabetes* 114:377, 2006.

Erkkila AT, Lichtenstein AH: Fiber and cardiovascular disease risk: how strong is the evidence? *J Cardiovasc Nurs* 21:3, 2006.

Esposito K, Giugliano D: Diet and inflammation: a link to metabolic and cardiovascular diseases, *Eur Heart J* 27:15, 2006.

Esteve E: Dyslipidemia and inflammation: an evolutionary conserved mechanism, *Clin Nutr* 24:16, 2005.

Fletcher B et al: Managing abnormal blood lipids: a collaborative approach, *Circulation* 112:3184, 2005.

Gao X et al: Plasma C-reactive protein and homocysteine concentrations are related to frequent fruit and vegetable intake in Hispanic and non-Hispanic white elders, *J Nutr* 134:913, 2004.

Gebauer SK et al: n-3 fatty acid dietary recommendations and food sources to achieve essentiality and cardiovascular benefits, *Am J Clin Nutr* 83(6 suppl):1526s, 2006.

Gidding SS et al: Dietary recommendations for children and adolescents: a guide for practitioners, *Pediatrics* 117:544, 2006.

Gotoh K et al: Apolipoprotein A-IV interacts synergistically with melanocortins to reduce food intake, *Am J Physiol Regul Integr Comp Physiol* 290:R202, 2006.

Grundy SM: Does a diagnosis of metabolic syndrome have value in clinical practice? *Am J Clin Nutr* 83:1248, 2006.

Grundy SM et al: Implications of recent clinical trials for the National Cholesterol Education Program Adult Treatment Panel III Guidelines, *Circulation* 110:227, 2004.

Grundy SM et al: Diagnosis and management of metabolic syndrome: an American Heart Association/National Heart, Lung, and Blood Institute Scientific Statement, *Circulation* 112:2735, 2005.

Hamer M, Steptoe A: Influence of specific nutrients on progression of atherosclerosis, vascular function, haemostasis and inflammation in coronary heart disease patients: a systematic review, *Br J Nutr* 95:849, 2006.

Hankey GJ: Is plasma homocysteine a modifiable risk factor for stroke? *Nat Clin Pract Neurol* 2:26, 2006.

Hansen AS et al: Effect of red wine and red grape extract on blood lipids, haemostatic factors, and other risk factors for cardiovascular disease, *Eur J Clin Nutr* 59:449, 2005.

Healthy People 2010: ed 2, Washington DC, 2000, U.S. Dept of Health and Human Services.

Hedley A et al: Prevalence of overweight and obesity among U.S. children, adolescents, and adults, 1999-2002, *JAMA* 292:2847, 2004.

Heinecke JW: Lipoprotein oxidation in cardiovascular disease: chief culprit or innocent bystanders? *J Exp Med* 203:813, 2006.

Hollman et al: Disease knowledge and adherence to treatment in patients with familial hypercholesterolemia, *J Cardiovasc Nurs* 21:103, 2006.

Junyent M et al: The use of Achilles tendon sonography to distinguish familial hypercholesterolemia from other genetic dyslipidemias, *Aterioscler Thromb Vasc Biol* 25:2203, 2005.

Karmally W: Balancing unsaturated fatty acids: what's the evidence for cholesterol lowering? *J Am Diet Assoc* 105:1068, 2005.

Kaul S et al: Homocysteine hypothesis for atherothrombotic cardiovascular disease: not validated, *J Am Coll Cardiol* 48:914, 2006.

Kay CD et al: Effects of antioxidant rich foods on vascular reactivity: review of the clinical evidence, *Curr Atheroscler Rep* 8:510, 2006.

Kelly AS et al: Inflammation, insulin, and endothelial function in overweight children and adolescents: the role of exercise, *J Pediatr* 145:731, 2004.

Klein S et al: Clinical implications of obesity with specific focus on cardiovascular disease: a statement for professionals from the American Heart Association Council on Nutrition, Physical Activity, and Metabolism: endorsed by the American College of Cardiology Foundation, *Circulation* 110; 2952, 2004.

Kris-Etherton PM et al: Lyon Diet Heart Study: benefits of a Mediterranean-style, National Cholesterol Education Program/American Heart Association Step I dietary pattern on cardiovascular disease, *Circulation* 103:1823, 2001b.

Laatikainen T et al: Explaining the decline in coronary heart disease mortality in Finland between 1982 and 1997, *Am J Epidemiol* 162:764, 2005.

Lee IM et al: Vitamin E in the primary prevention of cardiovascular disease and cancer: the Women's Health Study; a randomized controlled trial, *JAMA* 294:56, 2005.

Lichtenstein AH et al: Stanol/sterol ester-containing foods and blood cholesterol levels, *Circulation* 103:1177, 2001.

Lichtenstein AH et al: Diet and lifestyle recommendations revision 2006: a scientific statement from the American Heart Association Nutrition Committee, *Circulation* 114:82, 2006.

Lombardi MP et al: Molecular genetic testing for familial hypercholesterolemia in the Netherlands: a stepwise screening strategy enhances the mutation detection rate, *Genet Test* 10:77, 2006.

Madjid M et al: Intracoronary thermography for detection of high-risk vulnerable plaques, *J Am Coll Cardiol* 47:C80, 2006.

Marcovina S, Packard CJ: Measurement and meaning of apolipoprotein A-I and apolipoprotein B plasma levels, *J Intern Med* 259:437, 2006.

McCollum M et al: Prevalence of multiple cardiac risk factors in U.S. adults with diabetes, *Curr Med Res Opin* 22:1031, 2006.

Mensink RP et al: Effects of dietary fatty acids and carbohydrates on the ratio of serum total to HDL cholesterol and on serum lipids and apolipoproteins: a meta-analysis of 60 controlled trials, *Am J Clin Nutr* 77:1146, 2003.

Morelli F et al: Hypercholesterolemia and LDL apheresis, *Int J Artif Organs* 28:1025, 2005.

Naghavi M et al: From vulnerable plaque to vulnerable patient. Part III: Executive summary of the Screening for Heart Attack Prevention and Education (SHAPE) Task Force Report, *Am J Cardiol* 98(2A):2H, 2006.

National Cholesterol Education Program (NCEP): Expert Panel on Detection, Evaluation, and Treatment *of* High Blood Cholesterol in Adults (Adult Treatment Panel III) final report, *Circulation* 106:3143, 2002.

Olufadi R, Byrne CD: Effects of VLDL and remnant particles on platelets, *Pathophysiol Haemost Thromb* 35:281, 2006.

O'Malley PG: Atherosclerosis imaging of asymptomatic individuals, *Arch Intern Med* 166:1065, 2006.

Opie LH et al: Controversies in stable coronary artery disease, *Lancet* 367:69, 2006.

Ottestad IO et al: Triglyceride-rich HDL3 from patients with familial hypercholesterolemia are less able to inhibit cytokine release or to promote cholesterol efflux, *J Nutr* 136:877, 2006.

Panagiotakos DB: The implication of obesity and central fat on markers of chronic inflammation: the ATTICA study, *Atherosclerosis* 183:308, 2005.

Paoletti R et al: Inflammation in atherosclerosis and implications for therapy, *Circulation* 109:III-20, 2004.

Parks DA, Booyse FM: Cardiovascular protection by alcohol and polyphenols: role of nitric oxide, *Ann NY Acad Sci* 957:115, 2002.

Pearson T et al: Markers of inflammation and cardiovascular disease: application to clinical and public health practice: a statement for healthcare professionals from the Centers for Disease Control and Prevention and the American Heart Association, *Circulation* 107:499, 2003.

Plaisance EP, Grandjean PW: Physical activity and high-sensitivity C-reactive protein, *Sports Med* 36:443, 2006.

Poirier P et al: Obesity and cardiovascular disease: pathophysiology, evaluation, and effect of weight loss, *Circulation* 113:898, 2006.

Prasad K: C-reactive protein (CRP)-lowering agents, *Cardiovasc Drug Rev* 24:33, 2006.

Psota TL et al: Dietary omega-3 fatty acid intake and cardiovascular risk, *Am J Cardiol* 98:3, 2006.

Raggi P: Noninvasive imaging of atherosclerosis among asymptomatic individuals, *Arch Intern Med* 166:1068, 2006.

Rawson ES et al: Body mass index, but not physical activity, is associated with C-reactive protein, *Med Sci Sports Exerc* 35:1160, 2003.

Reaven GM et al: The metabolic syndrome: is this diagnosis necessary? *Am J Clin Nutr* 83:1237, 2006.

Rich S, McLaughlin VV: Detection of subclinical cardiovascular disease: the emerging role of electron beam computed tomography, *Prev Med* 34:1, 2002.

Rudd JHF et al: Imaging of atherosclerosis—can we predict plaque rupture? *Trends Cardiovasc Med* 15:17, 2005.

Sacks FM et al: Soy protein, isoflavones, and cardiovascular health: a summary of a statement for professionals from the American Heart Association Nutrition Committee, *Arterioscler Thromb Vasc Biol* 26:1689, 2006.

Saely CH et al: Adult Treatment Panel III 2001 but not International Diabetes Federation 2005 criteria of the metabolic syndrome predict clinical cardiovascular events in subjects who underwent coronary angiography, *Diabetes Care* 29:901, 2006.

nately effective screening and lifestyle modification approaches are available to achieve this objective.

Lowering blood pressure in patients with diabetes and hypertension is associated with a decrease in CVD events and renal failure (Sowers, 2003). The target blood pressure goal for antihypertensive therapy in individuals with diabetes is 130/80 mm Hg. In 2000 only 25% of individuals with diabetes receiving antihypertension therapy met this blood pressure goal (Hajjar and Kotchen, 2003). With the increased prevalence of diabetes in the United States, uncontrolled hypertension with diabetes is an important public health problem that warrants attention.

MORBIDITY AND MORTALITY

Although hypertensive patients are often asymptomatic, hypertension is not a benign disease. Cardiac, cerebrovascular, and renal systems are affected by chronically elevated blood pressure (Table 33-2). High blood pressure was the primary or a contributory cause in 261,000 of the 2.4 million U.S. deaths in 2002 (AHA, 2005). Between 1992 and 2002 the age-adjusted death rate from hypertension increased by 27%; overall deaths from hypertension increased by 57%. Death rates from hypertension are about 3.5 times higher in blacks than in whites (AHA, 2005). Hypertension is a major contributing factor to atherosclerosis, the underlying cause of much CVD (Kher and March, 2004). In adults with blood pressures ranging from 115/75 to 185/115 mm Hg, the risk of CVD doubles with a 20 mm Hg increase in SBP or a 10 mm Hg increase in DBP (Lewington et al., 2002). Stroke and myocardial infarction also are major contributors to morbidity; between 500,000 and a million people have nonfatal events each year. The factors associated with a poor prognosis in hypertension are shown in Box 33-1.

TABLE 33-2

Manifestations of Target Organ Disease from Hypertension

Organ System	Manifestations
Cardiac	Clinical, electrocardiographic, or radiologic evidence of coronary artery disease; left ventricular hypertrophy; left ventricular malfunction or cardiac failure
Cerebrovascular	Transient ischemic attack or stroke
Peripheral	Absence of one or more pulses in extremities (except for dorsalis pedis) with or without intermittent claudication; aneurysm
Renal	Serum creatinine >130 μmol/L (1.5 mg/dl), proteinuria (1+ or greater); microalbuminuria
Retinopathy	Hemorrhages or exudates, with or without papilledema

From the Joint National Committee on Prevention, Detection, Evaluation, and Treatment of High Blood Pressure: Fifth report (JNC V), *Arch Intern Med* 153:149, 1993.

BOX 33-1

Risk Factors and Adverse Prognosis in Hypertension

Risk Factors

Black race
Youth
Male gender
Persistent diastolic pressure >115 mm Hg
Smoking
Diabetes mellitus
Hypercholesterolemia
Obesity
Excessive alcohol intake
Evidence of end organ damage

Cardiac

Cardiac enlargement
Electrocardiographic signs of ischemia or left ventricular strain
Myocardial infarction
Congestive heart failure

Eyes

Retinal exudates and hemorrhages
Papilledema

Renal

Impaired renal function

Nervous system

Cerebrovascular accident

Fisher ND, Williams GH: Hypertensive vascular disease. In Kasper DL et al., editors: *Harrison's principles of internal medicine*, ed 16, New York, 2005, McGraw-Hill.

PATHOPHYSIOLOGY

Blood pressure is a function of cardiac output multiplied by peripheral resistance (the resistance in the blood vessels to the flow of blood). The diameter of the blood vessel markedly affects blood flow. When the diameter is decreased (as in atherosclerosis) resistance and blood pressure increase. Conversely, when the diameter is increased (as with vasodilator drug therapy), resistance decreases and blood pressure is lowered.

Many systems maintain homeostatic control of blood pressure. The major regulators are the sympathetic nervous system (for short-term control) and the kidney (for long-term control). In response to a fall in blood pressure, the sympathetic nervous system secretes norepinephrine, a vasoconstrictor, which acts on small arteries and arterioles to increase peripheral resistance and raise blood pressure. The kidney regulates blood pressure by controlling the extracellular fluid volume and secreting renin, which activates the renin-angiotensin system (Figure 33-2). When the regulatory mechanisms falter, hypertension develops.

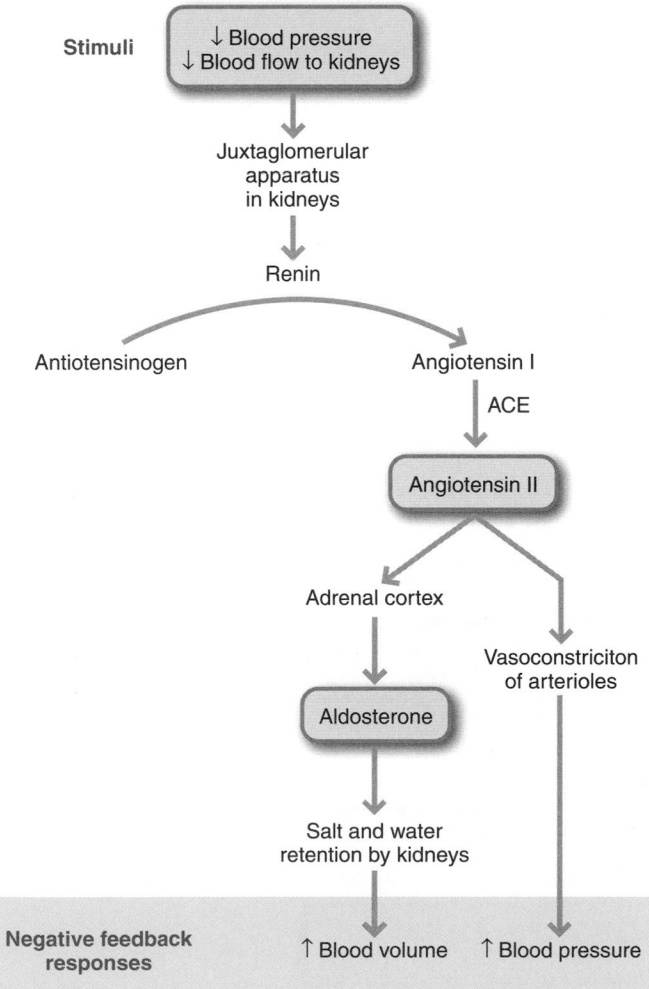

FIGURE 33-2 Renin-angiotensin cascade. *ACE,* Angiotensin-converting enzyme. *(Reprinted with permission from Fox SI: Human physiology, ed 6, New York, 1999, McGraw-Hill.)*

Plausible causes of hypertension are a hyperactive sympathetic nervous system, an over-stimulated renin-angiotensin system, a low-potassium diet, and use of the drug cyclosporine (Figure 33-3). All of these cause renal vasoconstriction, which results in ischemia or arterial changes. Chronic inflammation may be involved in the development of hypertension as well. Inflammatory markers, in particular C-reactive protein, have been shown to be elevated in patients with hypertension (Sesso et al, 2003). C-reactive protein inhibits formation of nitric oxide by endothelial cells, which in turn may promote vasoconstriction, leukocyte adherence, platelet activation, and thrombosis (Bautista et al., 2001).

The etiology of abnormal blood pressure is likely multifactorial. In most cases of hypertension, peripheral resistance increases. This resistance forces the left ventricle of the heart to increase its effort in pumping blood through the system. With time, left ventricular hypertrophy and eventually congestive heart failure can develop.

PRIMARY PREVENTION

The National High Blood Pressure Education Program (NHBPEP) is one of the most successful prevention programs in the twentieth century (Moser, 2002). Through educational efforts the detection, awareness, and treatment of hypertension have improved over the 35 years since its inception. These changes have contributed to the decline in cardiovascular mortality seen during the same time period.

Primary prevention of hypertension can improve quality of life and costs associated with medical management of hypertension and its complications. A strategy for the population would be to reduce blood pressure in those with prehypertension (above 120/80) but below the cut points for stage 1 hypertension. A downward shift of 3 mm Hg in SBP would decrease the mortality from stroke by 8% and from coronary heart disease by 5% (Appel, 2003). Persons at highest risk (Box 33-2) should be strongly encouraged to adopt healthier lifestyles.

Changing lifestyle factors has documented efficacy in the primary prevention and control of hypertension. These factors are presented in Table 33-3 and include losing weight if overweight; limiting alcohol intake; adopting a dietary pattern that emphasizes fruits, vegetables, and low-fat dairy products; reducing fat, especially saturated fat, and cholesterol; reducing intake of dietary sodium; increasing physical activity; and stopping smoking (NIH, 2004). In individuals with normal blood pressure, modification of these lifestyle factors has been shown to lower blood pressure and thereby has the potential to prevent hypertension and lower the risk of blood pressure–related complications. A substantial body of evidence strongly supports these lifestyle modifications as a means of significantly lowering blood pressure in individuals with hypertension.

Weight Reduction

There is a strong association between BMI and hypertension among men and women in all race or ethnic groups and in most age-groups. Based on the NHANES III survey, the prevalence of high blood pressure in persons with a BMI greater than 30 kg/m² is 42% for men and 38% for women, compared with 15% for men and women with a normal BMI (<25 kg/m²) (Brown, 2000). The risk of developing elevated blood pressure is two to six times higher in overweight than in normal-weight persons (NIH, 2004). Risk estimates from population studies suggest that 30% or more of cases of hypertension can be directly attributed to obesity (AHA, 2001). Weight gain during adult life is responsible for much of the rise in blood pressure seen with aging.

Some of the physiologic changes proposed to explain the relationship between excess body weight and blood pressure

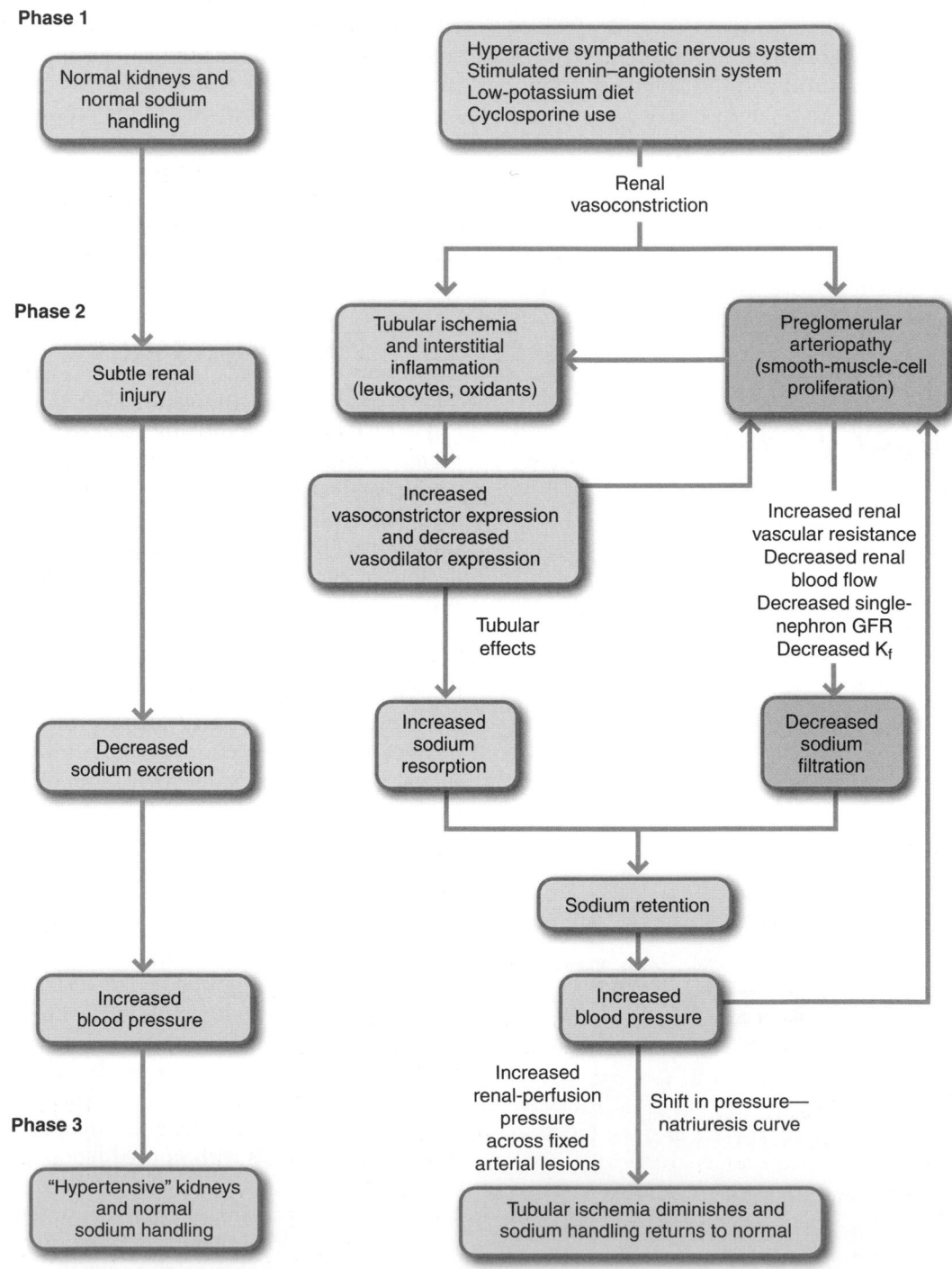

FIGURE 33-3 Physiology of the development of hypertension. *GFR,* Glomerular filtration rate. *(From Johnson R et al: Subtle acquired renal injury as a mechanism of salt-sensitive hypertension, N Engl J Med 346(12):913, 2002. Copyright 2002, Massachusetts Medical Society.)*

are overactivation of the sympathetic nervous and renin-angiotensin systems (Engeli and Sharma, 2001) and elevated levels of inflammatory pathways (Meerarani et al., 2006).

Virtually all clinical trials on weight reduction and blood pressure support the efficacy of weight loss on lowering blood pressure. In phase I of the Trial of Hypertension Prevention (He et al., 2000), normotensive individuals who lost an average of 3.5 kg in an 18-month intervention reduced their SBP and DBP by 5.8 mm Hg and 3.2 mm Hg, respectively. Seven years after treatment cessation, the incidence of hypertension was 18.9% in the weight-loss group and 40.5% in the control group. These findings suggest that improvements in blood pressure persist long after treatment cessation.

A metaanalysis of 25 randomized controlled trials, totaling nearly 5000 participants from different ethnic groups, showed a blood pressure reduction of 4.4/3.3 mm Hg for a 5-kg weight loss by means of energy restriction, increased physical activity, or both (Neter et al., 2003). Reductions in blood pressure occurred without attainment of desirable body weight in most participants. Larger blood pressure reductions were achieved in participants who lost more weight and who were also taking antihypertensive medications. This latter finding suggests a possible synergistic effect between weight loss and drug therapy.

Weight reduction and maintenance of a healthy body weight is a major effort for many persons, especially women. Interventions to prevent weight gain are ideal, particularly before an individual reaches midlife. BMI is recommended as a screening tool in adolescence for future health risk (Gardin et al., 2002). In adults a BMI above 30 is the cutoff for obesity, and referral to a registered dietitian (RD) is warranted. When a large percentage of the population is obese and hypertensive, better strategies are needed to prevent excess weight gain and improve compliance with treatment (NIH, 2004) (see Chapter 21).

Dietary Patterns

Several dietary patterns have been shown to lower blood pressure. Vegetarian dietary patterns have been associated

---

BOX 33-2

Cardiovascular Disease Risk Factors

Major Risk Factors

Hypertension*

Age (older than 55 years for men, 65 years for women)†

Diabetes mellitus*

Elevated LDL (or total) cholesterol, or low HDL cholesterol*

Estimated GFR <60 ml/min

Family history of premature CVD (men <55 years of age, or women <65 years of age)

Microalbuminuria

Obesity* (BMI >30 kg/m²)

Physical inactivity

Tobacco use, particularly cigarettes

Modified from National Institutes of Health, National Heart, Lung, and Blood Institute National High Blood Pressure Education Program: The Seventh Report of the Joint National Committee on Prevention, Detection, Evaluation, and Treatment of High Blood Pressure, NIH Publication No. 04-5230, August 2004.

BMI, Body mass index; *CVD*, cardiovascular disease; *GFR*, glomerular filtration rate; *HDL*, high-density lipoprotein; *LDL*, low-density lipoprotein.

*Components of the metabolic syndrome. Reduced HDL and elevated triglycerides are components of the metabolic syndrome. Abdominal obesity also is a component of metabolic syndrome.

†Increased risk begins at approximately 55 and 65 years of age for men and women, respectively. Adult Treatment Panel III used earlier age cut points to suggest the need for earlier action.

TABLE 33-3

Lifestyle Modifications to Prevent and Manage Hypertension*

Modification	Recommendation	Approximate SBP Reduction (Range)†
Weight reduction	Maintain normal body weight (body mass index 18.5-24.9 kg/m²).	5-20 mm Hg/10 kg
Adopt DASH eating plan	Consume a diet rich in fruits, vegetables, and low-fat dairy products with a reduced content of saturated and total fat.	8-14 mm Hg
Dietary sodium reduction	Reduce dietary sodium intake to no more than 100 mmol per day (2.4 g of sodium or 6 g of sodium chloride).	2-8 mm Hg
Physical activity	Engage in regular aerobic physical activity such as brisk walking (at least 30 min/day most days of the week).	4-9 mm Hg
Moderation of alcohol consumption	Limit consumption to no more than 2 drinks (e.g., 24 oz of beer, 10 oz of wine, or 3 oz of 80-proof whiskey) per day in most men and to no more than 1 drink per day in women and lighter weight persons.	2-4 mm Hg

From National Institutes of Health, National Heart, Lung, and Blood Institute National High Blood Pressure Education Program: The Seventh Report of the Joint National Committee on Prevention, Detection, Evaluation, and Treatment of High Blood Pressure, NIH Publication No. 04-5230, August 2004.

DASH, Dietary Approaches to Stop Hypertension; *SBP*, systolic blood pressure.

*For overall cardiovascular risk reduction, stop smoking.

†The effects of implementing these modifications are dose and time dependent and could be greater for some individuals.

with lower SBP in observational studies and clinical trials. Average SBP reductions of 5 to 6 mm Hg have been reported. Specifically, the **Dietary Approaches to Stop Hypertension (DASH) Diet** Study shows that this low-fat dietary pattern (including lean meats and nuts while emphasizing fruits, vegetables, and nonfat dairy products) decreased SBP an average of 6 to 11 mm Hg and DBP by 3 to 6 mm Hg (Appel et al., 1997). The DASH diet is found to be more effective than just adding fruits and vegetables to a low-fat dietary pattern (NIH, 2006).

The OmniHeart Trial examined the effects of three versions of the DASH diet on blood pressure and serum lipids. The diets studied included the original DASH diet, a high-protein version of the DASH diet (25% of energy from protein, about half from plant sources), and a high–unsaturated fat DASH diet (31% of calories from unsaturated fat, mostly monounsaturated). Although each diet lowered SBP, substituting some of the carbohydrate (approximately 10% of total calories) in the DASH diet with either protein or monounsaturated fat achieved the best reduction in blood pressure and blood cholesterol (Appel et al., 2005; Miller et al., 2006). This could be achieved by substituting some more nuts for some of the fruit, bread, or cereal servings.

Because many hypertensive patients are overweight, hypocaloric versions of the DASH diet have also been tested for efficacy in promoting weight loss and blood pressure reduction. The WELL diet study (Nowson et al., 2005) found that, for the same 5-kg weight loss, a hypocaloric DASH diet versus a low-calorie/low-fat diet produced a greater reduction in SBP and DBP.

Although the DASH diet is safe and currently being advocated by the JNC 7 (NIH, 2004) and the American Heart Association (AHA) (Appel et al., 2006) for preventing and treating prehypertension and hypertension, the diet is high in potassium, phosphorus, and protein, depending on how it is planned. For this reason the DASH diet would not be advisable for individuals with end-stage renal disease (Appel et al., 2006).

Excessive Consumption of Sodium Chloride

Evidence from a variety of sources (i.e., epidemiologic studies, intervention trials and metaanalyses) support lowering blood pressure by reducing dietary sodium. Large population studies have demonstrated a positive association between dietary sodium intake and blood pressure over a wide range of sodium intakes. Intervention studies such as the Phase 2 of the Trials of Hypertension Prevention (TOHP) have shown that sodium reduction with or without weight loss can reduce the incidence of hypertension by 20% (TOHP Collaborative Research Group, 1997).

Several metaanalyses (He and MacGregor, 2002, 2004) of randomized sodium reduction trials have confirmed positive effects of sodium reduction on blood pressure in both normotensive and hypertensive individuals. A high salt intake has also been implicated in hypertensive target organ disease, including cardiovascular and renal damage (Milan et al, 2002). Such data provide the basis for current dietary guidelines for all Americans to limit salt intake to 6 g/day or

sodium intake to 2.4 g/day, and for those with hypertension to limit sodium intake to 1.5 g/day (USDHHS, 2005) (see Chapter 12).

There is heterogeneity in individual responsiveness to sodium. Some persons with hypertension show a greater decrease in their blood pressures in response to reduced sodium intake than others. The term "**salt-sensitive hypertension**" has been used to identify these individuals. This versus "**salt-resistant hypertension**," which refers to individuals with hypertension whose blood pressures do not change significantly with lowered salt intakes. Current thinking on salt sensitivity is that the relationship between salt and blood pressure is "not binary" (Appel et al., 2006). Salt sensitivity has a continuous distribution within diverse populations with individuals having greater or lesser degrees of blood pressure reduction (Obarzanek et al., 2003). In general, individuals who are more sensitive to the effects of salt/sodium tend to be individuals who are black, obese, or middle-age and older, or those who have diabetes, chronic kidney disease, or hypertension (Johnson et al., 2002). Currently there are no practical methods for identifying the salt-sensitive individual from the salt-resistant individual.

Physical Activity

Less active persons are 30% to 50% more likely to develop hypertension than their active counterparts. Despite the benefits of activity and exercise in reducing disease, many Americans remain inactive. Hispanics (33% men, 40% women), blacks (27% men, 34% women), and whites (18% men, 22% women) all have a high prevalence of sedentary lifestyles (AHA, 2005).

Two metaanalyses have demonstrated the beneficial effects of exercise on blood pressure. The first analysis showed that walking reduced blood pressure in adults by an average of 2% (Kelley et al., 2001). Second, in 54 randomized clinical trials, aerobic exercise reduced blood pressure an average of 4 mm Hg for SBP and 2 mm Hg for DBP in patients with and without high blood pressure, irrespective of body weight change (Whelton et al., 2002). Thus increasing the amount of physical activity of low-to-moderate intensity to 30 to 45 minutes most days of the week is an important adjunct to other strategies for the primary prevention of hypertension.

Alcohol Consumption

Five to 7% of the hypertension in the population is the result of alcohol consumption (Appel et al., 2006). A three drink–per-day amount (a total of 3 oz of alcohol) is the threshold for raising blood pressure and is associated with a 3-mm Hg rise in SBP. For preventing high blood pressure, alcohol intake should be less than two drinks per day (24 oz of beer, 10 oz of wine, or 3 oz of 80-proof whiskey) in men. In women and lighter-weight men, no more than one drink a day is recommended (NIH, 2004).

Potassium

In observational studies dietary potassium and blood pressure are inversely related (i.e., higher potassium intakes are associated with lower blood pressures). Results from clinical trials on potassium and blood pressure have been less consistent. However, a metaanalysis of these trials found that high dietary potassium may help prevent and control hypertension (Whelton et al., 1997). On average a median dose of 2.4 g/day of supplemental potassium reduced SBP and DBP by 4.4 and 2.5 mm Hg in hypertensives, and 1.8 and 1 mm Hg in normotensives. The effects of potassium were greater in blacks than whites and in those with higher intakes of sodium.

Potassium intake has also been related to stroke mortality. In a large population-based cohort, a higher potassium intake was associated with a 38% lower risk of stroke (Ascherio et al., 1998). Data from the NHANES III survey suggests that low dietary potassium intake is associated with an increased risk of stroke (Bazzano et al., 2001). However, more statistically significant effects are found for improved diet, aerobic exercise, alcohol and sodium restriction, and fish oil supplements than for potassium supplements (Dickinson et al., 2006a).

The large number of fruits and vegetables recommended in the DASH diet makes it easy to meet dietary potassium recommendations of the JNC 7 and the AHA—approximately 4.7 g/day (NIH, 2004; Appel et al., 2006). In individuals with medical conditions that could impair potassium excretion (e.g., chronic renal failure, diabetes, and congestive heart failure), a potassium intake less than 4.7 g/day would be appropriate to prevent hyperkalemia.

Other Dietary Factors

Calcium

Higher dairy calcium versus nondairy calcium has been associated with a lower incidence of stroke among men and women (Ascherio et al, 1998). These findings suggest that the effects of calcium may differ, depending on the food source, or alternatively that other constituents of dairy may be responsible for the observed associations. Peptides derived from milk proteins, especially fermented milk products, have been shown to function as angiotensin-converting enzymes, thereby lowering blood pressure (Seppo et al, 2003). At present the JNC 7 report recommends a diet rich in fruits, vegetables, and low-fat dairy products over calcium supplementation for the prevention and management of elevated blood pressure (Chobanian et al., 2003). An intake of dietary calcium to meet the goal of 1000 to 2000 mg daily is recommended.

Magnesium

Magnesium is a potent inhibitor of vascular smooth-muscle contraction and may play a role in blood pressure regulation as a vasodilator. In observational studies dietary magnesium was inversely related to blood pressure (Ascherio et al., 1998). Less consistent findings have been reported from randomized clinical trials of magnesium supplementation for blood pressure control (Dickinson et al., 2006b). The DASH dietary pattern emphasizes foods rich in magnesium, including green leafy vegetables, nuts, and whole grain breads and cereals. Overall food sources of magnesium rather than supplemental doses of the nutrient are encouraged to prevent or control hypertension (Chobanian et al, 2003).

Lipids

Fewer vegans have hypertension than omnivores, even though their salt intake is not significantly different. The vegan diet tends to be higher in polyunsaturated fatty acids (PUFAs), among other nutrients, and lower in total fat, saturated fatty acids, and cholesterol. PUFAs are precursors of prostaglandins, whose actions affect renal sodium excretion and relax vascular musculature. Thus an effect on blood pressure is plausible.

Both the amount and type of fat have been studied with respect to blood pressure. In several large prospective observational studies and clinical trials, intake of total fat and specific fatty acids had little effect on blood pressure (Ascherio et al, 1998). More recently, studies have shown that supplementation with large doses of fish oil (median dose of 3.7 g/day) can give a modest reduction in SBP and DBP, especially in older hypertensive persons (Geleijnse et al., 2002). Side effects of supplementation with fish oils are frequent and include belching, gastrointestinal distress, and halitosis. For this reason and the high dose requirement, fish oils are not routinely recommended as a means of lowering blood pressure (Appel et al, 2006).

Factors other than dietary fat, such as increased potassium levels, appear to lower blood pressure in vegans. Although dietary lipids do not seem to affect blood pressure, they strongly affect CVD risk; thus the Therapeutic Lifestyle Change diet is recommended for preventing complications from hypertension and CVD (see Chapter 32). Although fatty acids may not directly affect blood pressure, an olive oil–enriched diet has been shown to result in a 48% reduction in need for antihypertensive medication (Ferrara et al., 2000). Soy protein is another factor that may contribute to the lowering of blood pressure (Hecker, 2001).

Combination of Risk Factors for Cardiovascular Disease

Hypertension often occurs with other risk factors for CVD. In the NHANES III survey (Must et al., 1999), 40% of persons with hypertension also had high blood cholesterol levels (>240 mg/dl). Fifty-five percent of overweight men have hypertension compared with 27% of normal-weight men. Researchers have long noted a larger than normal clustering of CVD risk factors, including abdominal obesity, high triglyceride levels, low high-density–lipoprotein cholesterol, high blood pressure, and high fasting glucose. The National Cholesterol Education Program (NCEP) recommendations for cholesterol management define the occurrence of three or more of these risk factors as the metabolic syndrome (NCEP, 2001).

Recent blood pressure treatment guidelines highlight the importance of evaluating patients for the presence of multiple CVD risk factors (see Box 33-2), and individualizing lifestyle modification and drug therapies to target coexisting abnormalities (NIH, 2004). Health problems related to the metabolic syndrome are expected to rise dramatically unless effective population-based health promotion strategies are promoted. Fortunately lifestyle modifications can prevent metabolic syndrome from developing (see Chapter 32, and *Clinical Insight:* The Metabolic Syndrome in Chapter 9).

Medications

A number of medications either raise blood pressure or interfere with the effectiveness of antihypertensive drugs. These include oral contraceptives, steroids, nonsteroidal antiinflammatory drugs, nasal decongestants and other cold remedies, appetite suppressants, cyclosporin tricyclic antidepressants, and monoamine-oxidase inhibitors (see Chapter 16 and Appendix 31).

MEDICAL MANAGEMENT

The goal of hypertension management is to reduce morbidity and mortality from stroke, hypertension-associated heart disease, and renal disease. According to the JNC 7 recommendations, three objectives for evaluating patients with hypertension are to (1) identify the possible causes; (2) assess the presence or absence of target organ disease and clinical CVD; and (3) identify other CVD risk factors that will help guide treatment (NIH, 2004). Weight history; leisure-time physical activity; and assessment of dietary sodium, alcohol, saturated fat, and other patterns (e.g., intake of fruits, vegetables, and dairy products) are essential components of the medical and diet history. The presence of risk factors and target organ damage determines treatment aggressiveness. As shown in Table 33-3, lifestyle changes are primary therapy in all patients with hypertension. However, pharmacologic therapy is necessary in many.

Pharmacologic Treatment

If blood pressure remains elevated after 6 to 12 months of lifestyle changes, antihypertensive medications are started. Most patients with hypertension more severe than stage 1 hypertension require drug treatment; however, lifestyle modifications are still a part of therapy even when drugs are used. The standard treatment for hypertension includes diuretics and β-blockers, although other drugs (β-angiotensin-converting enzyme inhibitors, α-receptor blockers, and calcium antagonists) are equally effective. All these drugs can affect nutrition status (see Chapter 16).

Diuretics lower blood pressure in some patients by promoting volume depletion and sodium loss; however, thiazide diuretics increase urinary potassium excretion, especially in the presence of a high salt intake, thus leading to potassium loss and possibly hypokalemia. Except in the case of a potassium-sparing diuretic such as spironolactone or triamterene, additional potassium is usually required.

NUTRITION MANAGEMENT

Lifestyle Modifications

Lifestyle modifications are definitive therapy for some and adjunctive therapy for all persons with hypertension. Several months of compliant lifestyle modifications should be tried before drug therapy is initiated. An algorithm for treatment of hypertension, established by the JNC 7 committee, is shown in Figure 33-4 (NIH, 2004). Even if lifestyle modifications cannot completely correct the blood pressure, they will help increase the efficacy of pharmacologic agents and improve other CVD risk factors. Management of hypertension requires a lifelong commitment.

Weight Reduction

Weight loss is an effective means of lowering blood pressure in hypertensive individuals. For each kilogram of weight lost, reductions in SBP and DBP of approximately 1 mm Hg are expected (Neter et al., 2003). Hypertensive patients who weigh more than 115% of ideal body weight should be placed on an individualized weight-reduction program that focuses on both hypocaloric dietary intake and exercise. Practical suggestions for assisting clients in increasing physical activity and reducing calories include reducing time spent watching television or being online, increasing time spent walking or in activities that raise the heart rate, reducing portion sizes for meals and snacks, reducing the size and frequency of calorie-containing drinks, and limiting fat intake.

In the Diet, Exercise, and Weight Loss Intervention study, the goal for energy intake to facilitate weight loss was 25 kcal/kg minus approximately 500 kcal daily to produce a 0.4-kg/week (about 1-lb) deficit that would reach a total weight loss of 4.5 kg (Miller et al., 2002). This modest caloric reduction was associated with a significant lowering of SBP and DBP, and low-density–lipoprotein cholesterol levels. For the same degree of weight loss, hypocaloric diets that include a low-sodium DASH dietary pattern have produced more significant blood pressure reductions than low-calorie diets emphasizing only low-fat foods (Nowson et al., 2005).

Another benefit of weight loss on blood pressure is the synergistic effect with drug therapy. In subjects who lost weight and were taking one antihypertensive drug, lowering of blood pressure was greater than in those taking the drug alone (Neter et al., 2003). Therefore weight loss should be an adjunct to drug therapy because it may decrease the dose or number of drugs necessary to control blood pressure.

Once weight is lost, maintenance is critical. Unfortunately relapse and weight gains are common following dieting to lose weight. Some factors associated with effective weight maintenance are exercise, positive self-statements related to weight-reduction efforts, self-monitoring activities (use of a food diary, goal setting, early attention to weight regain), and problem-solving skills in lieu of eating during stressful times (see Chapter 21).

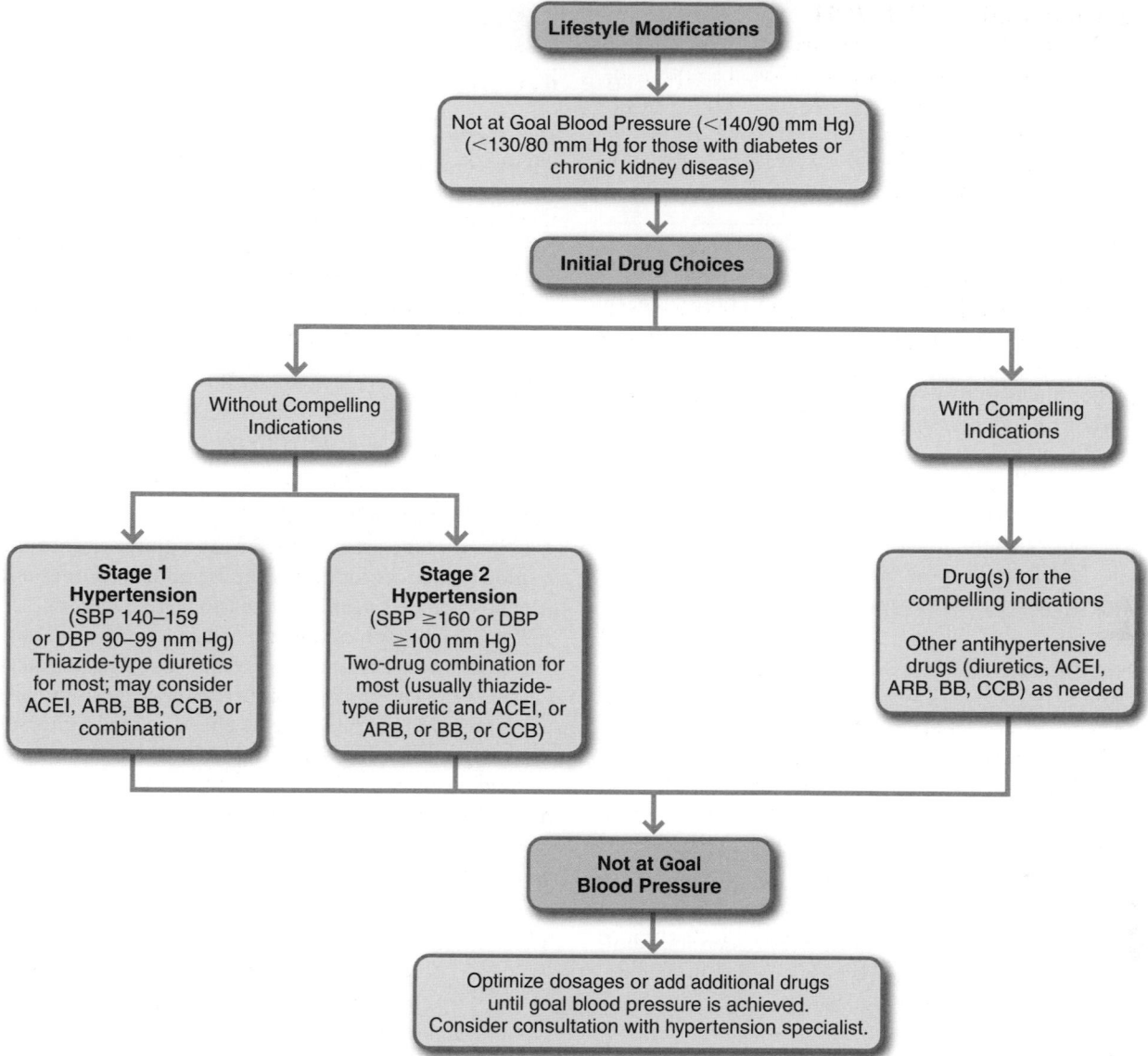

FIGURE 33-4 Algorithm for treatment of hypertension. *ACEI*, Angiotensin-converting enzyme inhibitor; *ARB*, angiotensin-receptor blocker; *BB*, β-blocker; *CCB*, calcium channel blocker; *DBP*, diastolic blood pressure; *SBP*, systolic blood pressure. *(National Institutes of Health, National Heart, Lung, and Blood Institute National High Blood Pressure Education Program: The Seventh Report of the Joint National Committee on Prevention, Detection, Evaluation, and Treatment of High Blood Pressure, NIH Publication No. 04-5230, August 2004.)*

Changing Dietary Patterns

The DASH diet is used for both preventing and controlling high blood pressure (see Appendix 33). Successful adoption of this diet requires many behavioral changes: eating twice the average number of daily servings of fruits, vegetables, and dairy products; limiting by one third the usual intake of beef, pork, and ham; eating half the typical amounts of fats, oils, and salad dressings; and eating one quarter the number of snacks and sweets (Blackburn, 2001). Lactose-intolerant persons may need to incorporate lactase enzyme or use other strategies to replace milk (see Chapter 27). Assessing patients' readiness to change and engaging patients in problem solving, decision making, and goal setting are behav-

ioral strategies that may improve adherence (Windhauser et al., 1999) (Box 33-3; see Chapter 19).

The high number of fruits and vegetables consumed on the DASH diet is a marked change from typical patterns of Americans. To achieve the 8 to 10 servings, two to three fruits and vegetables should be consumed at each meal (see Appendix 33). Importantly, because the DASH diet is high in fiber, gradual increases in fruit, vegetables, and whole grain foods should be made over time. Slow changes can reduce potential short-term gastrointestinal disturbances associated with a high-fiber diet such as bloating and diarrhea. The DASH pattern has been incorporated into the current AHA nutrition guidelines (Krauss et al., 2000).

BOX 33-3

Getting Started

It's easy to adopt the DASH eating plan. Here are some ways to get started:

Change Gradually

- If you now eat one or two vegetables a day, add a serving at lunch and another at dinner.
- If you don't eat fruit now or have juice only at breakfast, add a serving to your meals or have it as a snack.
- Gradually increase your use of fat-free and low-fat milk and milk products to three servings a day. For example, drink milk with lunch or dinner, instead of soda, sugar-sweetened tea, or alcohol. Choose fat-free (skim) or low-fat (1%) milk and milk products to reduce your intake of saturated fat, total fat, cholesterol, and calories and to increase your calcium.
- Read the Nutrition Facts label on margarines and salad dressings to choose those lowest in saturated fat and *trans*-fat.

Treat Meats as One Part of a Meal, Instead of the Focus

- Limit lean meats to 6 oz a day—all that's needed. Have only 3 oz at a meal, which is about the size of a deck of cards.
- If you now eat large portions of meats, cut them back gradually—by a half or a third at each meal.
- Include two or more vegetarian-style (meatless) meals each week.
- Increase servings of vegetables, brown rice, whole wheat pasta, and cooked dry beans in meals. Try casseroles, whole wheat pasta, and stir-fry dishes, which have less meat and more vegetables, grains, and dry beans.

Use Fruits or Other Foods Low in Saturated Fat, *Trans*-Fat, Cholesterol, Sodium, Sugar, and Calories as Desserts and Snacks

- Fruits and other lower-fat foods offer great taste and variety. Use fruits canned in their own juice or packed in water. Fresh fruits require little or no preparation. Dried fruits are a good choice to carry with you or to have ready in the car.
- Try these snacks ideas: unsalted rice cakes; nuts mixed with raisins; graham crackers; fat-free and low-fat yogurt and frozen yogurt; popcorn with no salt or butter added; raw vegetables.

Try These Other Tips

- Choose whole grain foods for most grain servings to get added nutrients such as minerals and fiber. For example, choose whole wheat bread or whole grain cereals.
- If you have trouble digesting milk and milk products, try taking lactase enzyme pills (available at drugstores and groceries) with milk products. Or buy lactose-free milk, which has the lactase enzyme already added to it.
- If you are allergic to nuts, use seeds or legumes (cooked dried beans or peas).
- Use fresh, frozen, or low-sodium canned vegetables and fruits.

From National Institutes of Health, National Heart, Lung, and Blood Institute: YOUR GUIDE TO Lowering Your Blood Pressure With DASH, U.S. Department of Health and Human Services, NIH Publication No. 06-4082, 2006.

Servings for different calorie levels are shown in Appendix 33. A quick assessment tool can help RDs and patients monitor progress (Table 33-4).

Salt Restriction

Moderate sodium restriction (2300 mg sodium daily or 6 g of salt) is recommended for treatment of hypertension (NIH, 2004). To achieve nutrient adequacy, an adequate intake (AI) level of sodium has been set at 1.5 g/day (Institute of Medicine, 2004). The DASH-Sodium trial showed that people consuming diets of 1.5g/day of sodium had greater blood pressure benefits than those with higher intakes (Appel et al., 1997). Lower-sodium diets were also shown to maintain low blood pressure over time and enhance the efficacy of certain blood pressure–lowering medications. Although it may be advisable for individuals with elevated blood pressure to restrict sodium to AI levels, adherence to diets containing less than 2 g/day of sodium is difficult to achieve.

Because most dietary salt comes from processed foods and eating out, changes in food preparation and processing can help patients reach the sodium goal. Sensory studies show that commercial processing could develop and revise recipes using lower sodium concentrations and reduce added sodium without affecting consumer acceptance. In addition to advice to select minimally processed foods, dietary counseling to lower sodium should include instruction on reading food labels for sodium content, avoidance of discretionary salt in cooking or meal preparation (1 tsp salt = 2400 mg sodium), and use of alternative flavorings to satisfy individual taste. Because the DASH eating plan is rich in fruits and vegetables, which are naturally lower in sodium that many other foods, adopting the DASH diet will enable individuals to consume less salt and sodium. *Focus On:* Sodium and the Food Industry discusses how difficult it is to follow a sodium-restricted diet in American society.

Other Dietary Modifications

Minerals

Consuming a diet rich in potassium has been shown to lower blood pressure and blunt the effects of salt on blood

TABLE 33-4

What's On Your Plate? How Much Are You Moving?

Date: **Number of Servings by DASH Food Group**

Food	Amount (serving size)	Sodium (mg)	Grains	Vegetables	Fruits	Fat-Free or Low-Fat Milk Products	Meats, Fish, and Poultry	Nuts, Seeds, and Legumes	Fats and Oils	Sweets and Added Sugars
Example: Whole wheat bread, with soft (tub) margarine	2 slices 2 tsp	299 52	2						2	
Breakfast										
Lunch										
Dinner										
Snacks										
Day's Totals										
Compare yours with the DASH eating plan at 2000 calories	2300 or 1500 mg/ day	6-8/ day	6-8/ day	4-5/ day	4-5/ day	2-3/ day	6 oz or less/day	4-5/ week	2-3/ day	5 or less/ week

Physical Activity Log

Record your minutes per day for each activity. Aim for at least 30 minutes of moderate-intensity physical activity on most days of the week.

From National Institutes of Health, National Heart, Lung, and Blood Institute: YOUR GUIDE TO Lowering Your Blood Pressure With DASH, U.S. Department of Health and Human Services, NIH Publication No. 06-4082, 2006.

⊙ FOCUS ON

Sodium and the Food Industry

Most foods sold in supermarkets and restaurants are too high in salt. The dramatic differences in sodium from brand to brand suggest that many companies could easily achieve significant reductions without sacrificing taste. According to the Center for Science in the Public Interest, processed foods and restaurant foods contribute about 80% of the sodium in Americans' diets; 10% comes from salt added during cooking at home or at the table; the remaining 10% is naturally occurring. Americans now consume about 4000 mg of sodium per day—about twice the recommended amount. The 2005 Dietary Guidelines for Americans recommend that young adults consume less than 2400 mg of sodium per day. People with hypertension, blacks, and middle-age and elderly people—almost half the population—are advised to consume no more than 1500 mg/day. Requesting that the food industry help with this change is worth the efforts in advocacy.

Data from Center for Science in the Public Interest: Food industry accused of "salt assault" on America, CSPI Newsroom, 2005, http://www.cspinet.org/new/200508171.html, accessed December 6, 2006.

pressure in some individuals (Appel et al., 2006). The recommended intake of potassium for adults is 4.7 g/day (Institute of Medicine, 2004). Potassium-rich fruits and vegetables include leafy green vegetables, fruits, and root vegetables. Examples of such foods include oranges, beet greens, white beans, spinach, bananas, and sweet potatoes. Although meat, milk, and cereal products contain potassium, the potassium from these sources is not as well-absorbed as that from fruits and vegetables (USDA, 2005).

Increased intakes of calcium and magnesium may have blood pressure benefits, although there is not enough data at present to support a specific recommendation for increasing levels of intake. Rather, recommendations suggest meeting the AI intake for calcium and the recommended dietary allowance for magnesium from food sources rather than supplements. The DASH diet plan encourages foods that would be good sources of both nutrients, including low-fat dairy products, dark green leafy vegetables, beans, and nuts.

Lipids

Current recommendations for lipid composition of the diet are those recommended by the NCEP (see Chapter 32) to help control weight and decrease the risk of CVD (NCEP, 2001).

Alcohol

The diet history should contain information about alcohol consumption. As discussed previously, alcohol intake should be limited to no more than 2 drinks daily in men, which is equivalent to 2 oz of 100-proof whiskey, 10 oz of wine, or 24 oz of beer. Women or lighter-weight men should consume half this amount.

Exercise

Moderate physical activity, defined as 30 to 45 minutes of brisk walking on most days of the week, is recommended as an adjunct therapy in hypertension. Overweight or obese hypertensive patients should strive for 300 to 500 kcal expended in exercise per day or 1000 to 2000 kcal/week to promote weight loss or weight control. Because exercise is strongly associated with success in weight-reduction and weight-maintenance programs, any increase in activity level should be encouraged. Sixty to 90 minutes of daily moderate-intensity physical activity is recommended for individuals trying to maintain a new lower weight after having lost weight (USDA, 2005).

Treatment of Blood Pressure in Children and Adolescents

The prevalence of primary hypertension among children in the United States is increasing in concert with rising obesity rates and increased intakes of high-calorie, high-salt foods (Mitsnefes, 2006; Munter et al., 2004). Hypertension tracks into adulthood and has been linked with carotid intimal-medial thickness (CIMT); left ventricular hypertrophy (LVH); and fibrotic plaque formation; all of which are determinants of adverse cardiovascular events in adults (Davis et al., 2001; Daniels, 1998). In addition, it has been noted that intrauterine growth retardation leads to hypertension in childhood (Shankaran, 2006). Secondary hypertension is more common in preadolescent children, mostly from renal disease; primary hypertension is more common in adolescents from obesity or a family history of hypertension (Luma and Spiotta, 2006).

High blood pressure in youth is based on a normative distribution of blood pressure in healthy children. Hypertension is defined as a SBP and/or DBP >95th percentile for age, sex, and height. New diagnostic recommendations have included a designation for prehypertension in children which is SBP and/or DBP >90th percentile (NIH, NHLBI and NHBPEP, 2005). Therapeutic lifestyle changes are recommended as an initial treatment strategy for children and adolescents with prehypertension or hypertension (Table 33-5). These lifestyle modifications include regular physical activity, avoiding excess weight gain, limiting sodium, and consuming a DASH-type diet. Of these, weight reduction is considered the primary therapy for obesity-related hypertension in children and adolescents.

Unfortunately sustained weight loss is difficult to achieve in this age-group. The Framingham Children's Study showed that children with higher intakes of fruits, vegetables (a combination of four or more servings per day) and dairy products (two or more servings per day) had lower SBP compared with those with lower intakes of these foods (Moore et al., 2005). Because adherence to dietary interventions may be particularly problematic among children, in-

TABLE 33-5

Classification, Monitoring, and Therapy Recommendations for Children and Adolescents with Hypertension

	SBP or DBP Percentile*	Frequency of BP Measurement	Therapeutic Lifestyle Changes	Pharmacologic Therapy
Normal	<90th	Recheck at next scheduled physical examination	Encourage healthy diet, sleep, and physical activity	—
Prehypertension	90th to <95th or if BP exceeds 120/80 mm Hg even if below 90th percentile up to <95th percentile†	Recheck in 6 months	Weight-management counseling if overweight; introduce physical activity and diet management‡	None, unless compelling indications such as CKD, diabetes mellitus, heart failure, or LVH exist
Stage 1 hypertension	95th percentile to the 99th percentile plus 5 mm Hg	Recheck in 12 weeks or sooner if the patient is symptomatic; if persistently elevated on two additional occasions, evaluate or refer to source of care within 1 month	Weight-management counseling if overweight; introduce physical activity and diet management‡	Initiate therapy based on indications
Stage 2 hypertension	>99th percentile plus 5 mm Hg	Evaluate or refer to source of care within 1 week or immediately if the patient is symptomatic	Weight-management counseling if overweight, introduce physical activity and diet management‡	Initiate therapy§

From National Institutes of Health, National Heart, Lung, and Blood Institute, National High Blood Pressure Education Program, The Fourth Report on the Diagnosis, Evaluation, and Treatment of High Blood Pressure in Children and Adolescents, NIH Publication No. 05-5267, originally printed September 1996 (96-3790), revised May 2005.

BP, Blood pressure; *CKD*, chronic kidney disease; *DBP*, diastolic blood pressure; *LVH*, left ventricular hypertrophy; *SBP*, systolic blood pressure.

*For sex, age, and height measured on at least three separate occasions; if systolic and diastolic categories are different, categorize by the higher value.

†This occurs typically at 12 years old for SBP and at 16 years old for DBP.

‡Parents and children trying to modify the eating plan to the Dietary Approaches to Stop Hypertension (DASH) eating plan could benefit from consultation with a registered dietitian.

§More than one drug may be required.

novative nutrition intervention approaches that address the unique needs and circumstances of this age-group are needed. Strategies for improving intake patterns among children and adolescents can be found in Chapters 7 and 8.

Treatment of Blood Pressure in Older Adults

More than half of the older population has hypertension; this is not a normal consequence of aging, but CVD risk in older adults is two to three times higher than in the middle-age population. The lifestyle modifications discussed previously are the first step in treatment of older adults, as with younger populations. The Trial of Nonpharmacologic Interventions in the Elderly (TONE) study found that losing weight (8 to 10 lb) and reducing sodium intake (to 1.8 g/day daily) can lessen or eliminate the need for drugs in obese, hypertensive older adults (60 to 80 years of age) (Whelton et al., 1998). At the end of the 30-month study, 31% of the sodium-reduction-alone group, 33% of the weight-reduction-alone group, and 53% of the combination group were off medications.

Although this study showed that losing weight and decreasing sodium in older adults were very effective in lowering blood pressure, knowing how to facilitate these changes and promote adherence remains an obstacle for health professionals. Only 38% in the TONE study were able to reach the sodium intake goals. Looking at dose-

PATHOPHYSIOLOGY AND CARE MANAGEMENT ALGORITHM

Treatment of Hypertension

ETIOLOGY

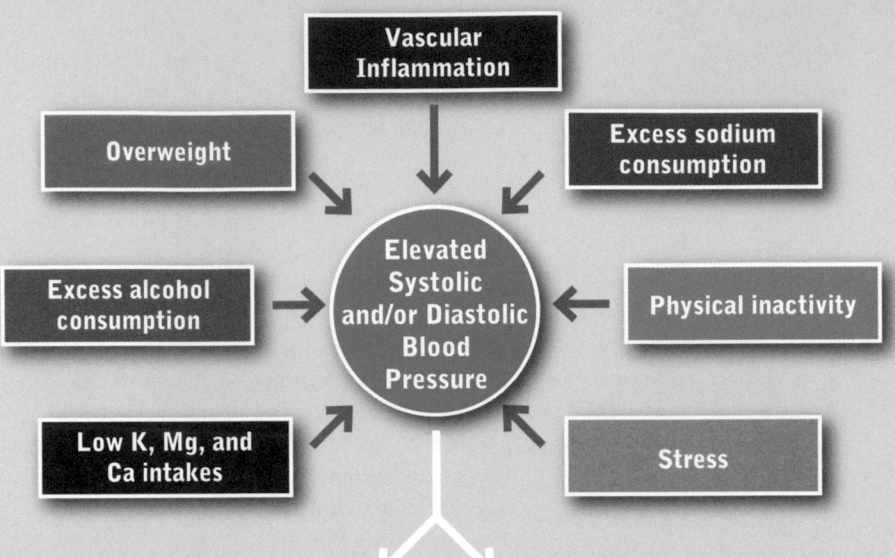

Vascular Inflammation

Overweight

Excess sodium consumption

Excess alcohol consumption

Elevated Systolic and/or Diastolic Blood Pressure

Physical inactivity

Low K, Mg, and Ca intakes

Stress

PATHOPHYSIOLOGY

Diagnosis of Hypertension

- Prehypertension
  - Systolic BP 120–139 mm Hg
  - Diastolic BP 80–89 mm Hg
- Systolic BP >139 mm Hg
- Diastolic BP >89 mm Hg

Target Organ Disease

- Cardiac
- Cerebrovascular
- Peripheral
- Renal
- Retinopathy

MANAGEMENT

Medical Management

Antihypertensive Drug Therapy
- Diuretics
- Beta blockers
- Vasodilators
- ACE inhibitors
- Calcium channel blockers
- α_1-Receptor blockers

Lifestyle Modification
- Exercise
- Stress reduction
- Lifestyle counseling

Nutrition Management

- Weight reduction
- Adopt a DASH eating plan
- Dietary sodium restriction to 2.4 g/day or less
- Moderation of alcohol consumption
- Nutrition education

Algorithm content developed by John J.B. Anderson, PhD, and Sanford C. Garner, PhD, 2002.

response analyses, those with greater sodium reduction had fewer occurrences of average SBP over 150 or DBP over 90 (Appel et al., 2001). Severe sodium restrictions are not adopted because these could lead to volume depletion in older patients with renal damage (NIH, 2004).

Drug treatment in the older adult is supported by very strong data. Based on these data, the JNC recommends that blood pressures be controlled regardless of age, initial blood pressure level, or duration of hypertension (NIH, 2004).

FOCAL POINTS

- Lifestyle changes can lower blood pressure and prevent or control hypertension (see *Pathophysiology and Care Management Algorithm:* Treatment of Hypertension).
- Weight control, physical activity, and a low-fat diet rich in fruits and vegetables with nonfat dairy foods and nuts incorporated have all been shown to lower blood pressure.
- The DASH diet and other nutritional therapies are useful for many individuals with hypertension.
- A major reason for inadequate control of high blood pressure is poor adherence to therapy.

- The *Healthy People 2000* objective was to increase to at least 90% the number of people with hypertension who were trying to normalize their blood pressure; this goal was not achieved since 31% of subjects in NHANES III with high blood pressure were not even aware they had hypertension. Barriers to adherence need to be investigated and remedied.

CLINICAL SCENARIO 1

Bob is a 56-year-old white man who works as a truck driver. He is on the road every week and recently saw his physician about headaches, dizziness, and insomnia. He was diagnosed as having hypertension, with three blood pressure tests of 160/90, 175/95, and 177/92. His physician gave him a diuretic, Lasix, and a β-blocker (Inderal). Bob was also given a diet sheet with a brief overview of a no-added-salt diet. Bob has contacted you for assistance in planning menus he can follow.

*Nutrition Diagnosis: Food- and nutrition-related knowledge deficit related to sodium content of foods as evidenced by patient requesting assistance with implementing a no-salt added diet

1. Write a week's set of menus that Bob can agree to follow, starting with a meal at home for breakfast, at a restaurant for lunch, and from a carryout deli late at night.
2. Bob generally consumes one or two beers before bedtime and is willing to give up that habit. What healthy snacks might Bob have in the evening?
3. Because Bob is on the road so much, food safety might be a problem. What tips would you suggest for meals and snacks that he can keep in his truck that would also fit with his eating plan?

CLINICAL SCENARIO 2

Nell is a 27-year-old white woman who follows traditional Judaism. In her meal planning she uses many foods that have been prepared in a kosher manner (added salt being part of this process). Nell's blood pressure has been identified as being high, with readings between 150/95 and 160/100. Nell works in an office and does not participate in any physical activity. She will drink milk, but does not commonly include milk in her daily diet. She buys her lunch at work, which consists of noodle soup, deli sandwich with large pickle, bottled club soda, and packaged cookies. Nell cooks her own breakfast, consisting typically of eggs, toast, and coffee with real cream. Her dinner is usually a roast such as brisket, with potatoes and vegetables, and a traditional dessert. She entertains guests frequently and loves to cook. Nell is 5 ft 2 in tall and weighs 170 lb.

Continued

⬡ CLINICAL SCENARIO 2—cont'd

✳**Nutrition Diagnosis:** Excessive sodium intake related to consumption of high sodium foods as evidenced by diet history revealing more than 4-g sodium consumed daily

1. What advice will you give Nell about her meal planning?
2. Write a second PES statement related to her BMI.

3. What resources are there to help her prepare meals that are higher in potassium, calcium, and magnesium? Would you suggest the DASH diet? How would you help her implement it?
4. What tips about activity will you share with Nell?
5. If Nell begins a weight-loss program, how much weight should she lose, and how quickly?

USEFUL WEBSITES

American Heart Association
http://www.americanheart.org

DASH Diet
www.nhlbi.nih.gov/health/public/heart/hbp/dash/

National High Blood Pressure Education Program
www.nhlbi.nih.gov

World Hypertension League
www.mco.edu/org/whl

References

American Heart Association: *2001 Heart and stroke statistical update*, Dallas, 2001, American Heart Association.

American Heart Association: *2005 Heart and stroke statistical update*, Dallas, 2005, American Heart Association.

Appel LJ: Lifestyle modification as a means to prevent and treat high blood pressure, *J Am Soc Nephrol* 14:S99, 2003.

Appel LJ et al: A clinical trial of the effects of dietary patterns on blood pressure, *N Engl J Med* 336:1117, 1997.

Appel LJ et al: Effects of reduced sodium intake on hypertension control in older individuals, *Arch Intern Med* 161:685, 2001.

Appel LF et al: Effects of protein, monounsaturated fat, and carbohydrate intake on blood pressure and serum lipids: results from the OmniHeart randomized trial, *JAMA* 294:2455, 2005.

Appel LJ et al: Dietary approaches to prevent and treat hypertension: a scientific statement from the American Heart Association, *Hypertension* 47: 296, 2006.

Ascherio A et al: Intake of potassium, magnesium, calcium, and fiber and risk of stroke among U.S. men, *Circulation* 98:1198, 1998.

Bautista LE et al: Is C-reactive protein an independent risk factor for essential hypertension? *J Hypertens* 19:857, 2001.

Bazzano LA et al: Dietary potassium intake and risk of stroke in U.S. men and women: National Health and Nutrition Examination Survey I epidemiologic follow-up study, *Stroke* 32:1473, 2001.

Blackburn GL: The public health implications of the dietary approaches to stop hypertension trial, *Am J Clin Nutr* 74:1, 2001.

Brown CD et al: Body mass index and the prevalence of hypertension and dyslipidemia, *Obes Res* 8:605, 2000.

Chobanian AV et al: The Seventh Report of the Joint National Committee on Prevention, Detection, Evaluation, and Treatment of High Blood Pressure: the JNC 7 Report, *JAMA* 289:2560, 2003.

Dickinson HO et al: Lifestyle interventions to reduce raised blood pressure: a systematic review of randomized controlled trials, *J Hypertens* 24:215, 2006a.

Dickinson HO et al: Magnesium supplementation for the management of essential hypertension in adults, *Cochrane Database Syst Rev* 3:CD004640, 2006b.

Engeli S, Sharma AM: The renin-angiotensin system and natriuretic peptides in obesity-associated hypertension, *J Mol Med* 79:21, 2001.

Ferrara LA et al: Olive oil and reduced need for antihypertensive medications, *Arch Intern Med* 160:837, 2000.

Fields LE et al: The burden of adult hypertension in the United States, 1999 to 2000: a rising tide, *Hypertension* 44:398, 2004.

Gardin JM et al: Demographics and correlates of five-year change in echocardiographic left ventricular mass in young black and white adult men and women: the Coronary Artery Risk Development in Young Adults (CARDIA) study, *J Am Coll Cardiol* 40:529, 2002.

Geleijnse JM et al: Blood pressure response to fish oil supplementation: meta-regression analysis of randomized trials, *J Hypertens* 20:1493, 2002.

Hajjar I, Kotchen TA: Trends in prevalence, awareness, treatment and control of hypertension in the United States, 1988-2000, *JAMA* 290:199, 2003.

He FJ, MacGregor GA: Effect of modest salt reduction on blood pressure: a meta-analysis of randomized trials: implications for public health, *J Hum Hypertens* 16:761, 2002.

He FJ, MacGregor GA: Effect of longer-term modest salt reduction on blood pressure, *Cochrane Database Syst Rev* 3: CD004937, 2004.

He J et al: Long-term effects of weight loss and dietary sodium reduction on incidence of hypertension, *Hypertension* 35:544, 2000.

Hecker KD: Effects of dietary animal and soy protein on cardiovascular disease risk factors, *Curr Atheroscler Rep* 3:471, 2001.

Hyman DJ, Pavlik VN: Characteristics of patients with uncontrolled hypertension in the United States, *N Engl J Med* 345:479, 2001.

Institute of Medicine: *Dietary reference intakes: water, potassium, sodium chloride and sulfate*, ed 1, Washington, DC, 2004, National Academies Press.

Jian-Jun L et al: Is hypertension an inflammatory disease? *Med Hypotheses* 64:236, 2005.

Johnson R et al: Subtle acquired renal injury as a mechanism of salt-sensitive hypertension, *N Engl J Med* 346:913, 2002.

Kelley GA et al: Walking and resting blood pressure in adults: a meta-analysis, *Prev Med* 33:120, 2001.

Kher N, March JD: Pathobiology of atherosclerosis—a brief review, *Semin Thromb Hemost* 30:665, 2004.

Krauss RM et al: Dietary guidelines revision 2000: a statement for healthcare professionals from the Nutrition Committee of the American Heart Association, *Circulation* 102:2284, 2000.

Lewington S et al: Age-specific relevance of usual blood pressure to vascular mortality: a meta-analysis of individual data for one million adults in 61 prospective studies: prospective studies collaboration, *Lancet* 360:1903, 2002.

Luma GB, Spiotta RT: Hypertension in children and adolescents, *Am Fam Physician* 73(9):1558, 2006.

Meerarani P et al: Metabolic syndrome and diabetic atherothrombosis: implications in vascular complications, *Curr Mol Med* 6a95a0:501, 2006.

Milan A et al: Salt intake and hypertension therapy, *J Nephrol* 15(1):1, 2002.

Miller ER III et al: Results of the Diet, Exercise and Weight Loss Intervention Trial (DEW-IT), *Hypertension* 40:612, 2002.

Miller ER III et al: The effects of macronutrients on blood pressure and lipids: an overview of the DASH and Omni Heart Trials, *Curr Atheroscler Rep* 8:460, 2006.

Mitsnefes MM: Hypertension in children and adolescents, *Pediatr Clin North Am* 53(3):493, 2006.

Moore LL et al: Intake of fruits, vegetables and dairy products in early childhood and subsequent blood pressure change, *Epidemiology* 16:4, 2005.

Moser M: Update on the management of hypertension: do recent clinical trial results indicate a change in national recommendations for therapy? *J Clin Hypertens* 4:(suppl 2)20, 2002.

Munter P et al: The impact of JNC-VI guidelines on treatment recommendations in the U.S. population, *Hypertension* 39:897, 2002.

Munter P et al: Trends in blood pressure among children and adolescents, *JAMA* 291:2107, 2004.

Must A et al: The disease burden associated with overweight and obesity, *JAMA* 282:1532, 1999.

National Cholesterol Education Program (NCEP): Summary of the Third Report of the National Cholesterol Education Program Expert Panel on Detection, Evaluation, and Treatment of High Blood Cholesterol in Adults (Adult Treatment Panel III), *JAMA* 285:2486, 2001.

National Institutes of Health, National Heart, Lung, and Blood Institute, National High Blood Pressure Education Program: The Seventh Report of the Joint National Committee on Prevention, Detection, Evaluation, and Treatment of High Blood Pressure, NIH Publication No. 04-5230, August 2004.

Neter JE et al: Influence of weight reduction on blood pressure: a meta-analysis of randomized controlled trials, *Hypertension* 42:878, 2003.

Nowson CA et al: Blood pressure change with weight loss is affected by diet type in men, *Am J Clin Nutr* 81:983, 2005.

Obarzanek E et al: Individual blood pressure responses to changes in salt intake: results from the DASH-Sodium trial, *Hypertension* 42:459, 2003.

Qureshi AI et al: Prevalence and trends of prehypertension and hypertension in United States: National Health and Nutrition Examination Surveys 1976 to 2000, *Med Sci Monit* 22:CR403, 2005.

Seppo L et al: A fermented milk high in bioactive peptides has a blood pressure–lowering effect in hypertensive subjects, *Am J Clin Nutr* 77:326, 2003.

Sesso HD et al: C-reactive protein and the risk of developing hypertension, *JAMA* 290:2945, 2003.

Shankaran S et al: Fetal origin of childhood disease: intrauterine growth restriction in term infants and risk for hypertension at 6 years of age, *Arch Pediatr Adolesc Med* 160(9):977, 2006.

Sowers JR: Recommendations for special populations: diabetes mellitus and the metabolic syndrome, *Am J Hypertens* 16:41S, 2003.

Trials of Hypertension Prevention Collaborative Research Group: Effects of weight loss and sodium reduction intervention on blood pressure and hypertension incidence in overweight people with high normal blood pressure: the Trials of Hypertension Prevention, phase II, *Arch Intern Med* 157:657, 1997.

United States Department of Health and Human Services, U.S. Department of Agriculture: Dietary Guidelines for Americans 2005, accessed on March 3, 2006, from www.healthierus.gov/dietaryguidelines.

Whelton PK et al: Effects of oral potassium on blood pressure: meta-analysis of randomized controlled clinical trials, *JAMA* 277:1624, 1997.

Whelton PK et al: Sodium reduction and weight loss in the treatment of hypertension in older persons: a randomized controlled trial of nonpharmacologic interventions in the elderly (TONE), *JAMA* 279:839, 1998.

Whelton PK et al: Effect of aerobic exercise on blood pressure: a meta-analysis of randomized controlled trials, *Ann Intern Med* 136:493, 2002.

Windhauser MM et al: Dietary adherence in the dietary approaches to stop hypertension trial, *J Am Diet Assoc* 99(supp):S76, 1999.

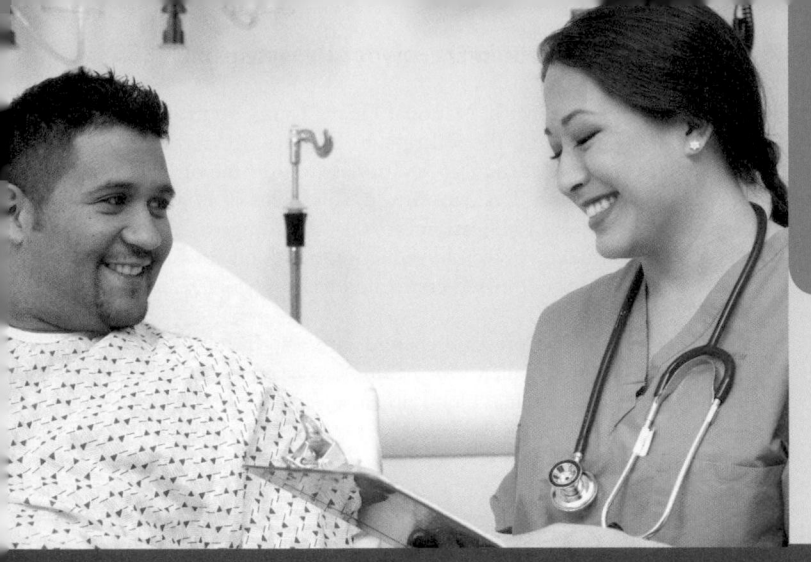

CHAPTER 34

Debra A. Krummel, PhD, RD

Medical Nutrition Therapy for Heart Failure and Transplant

KEY TERMS

cachectic heart a soft, flabby heart characterized by loss of myocardial mass as the result of extreme malnutrition

cardiac cachexia a serious complication of heart failure associated with high mortality rates and characterized by unintentional weight loss (body wasting) due to a loss of fat, muscle, and bone

dyslipidemia an abnormal pattern of blood lipoproteins that increases risk for heart disease

dyspnea perceived difficulty with breathing; shortness of breath (SOB), the hallmark of heart failure

edema abnormal accumulation of fluid in body tissues such as lungs, ankles, or feet

ejection fraction the percentage of blood pumped by the ventricles when the heart beats; is reduced in heart failure

heart failure a clinical syndrome characterized by progressive deterioration of cardiac function, inadequate tissue perfusion, fatigue, shortness of breath, and fluid retention

left ventricular hypertrophy enlargement of the left ventricle of the heart; a major risk factor for heart failure

myocardial infarction blockage in a coronary artery that can result in damage to the heart muscle; also known as a heart attack

orthopnea respiratory distress while in a recumbent position

syncope lack of oxygen to the brain causing a brief loss of consciousness

Some categories of heart disease such as heart failure and cardiac cachexia occur when the heart deteriorates and can no longer meet the body's need for blood flow. Nutritional care in these conditions is concerned primarily with the consequences of poor circulation throughout the body. In end-stage heart disease cardiac transplantation becomes necessary for survival.

HEART FAILURE

Normally the heart pumps adequate blood to perfuse tissues and meet metabolic needs (Figure 34-1). In **heart failure** (HF), the heart cannot provide adequate blood flow to the rest of the body, causing symptoms of fatigue, shortness of breath **(dyspnea),** and fluid retention (Hunt et al., 2005). Diseases of the heart (valves, muscle, blood vessels) and vasculature (hypertension) can lead to HF (see *Pathophysiol-*

ogy and Care Management Algorithm: Heart Failure). Once the heart is diseased, conditions such as **myocardial infarction** (MI), blockage in a coronary artery that can lead to heart damage or "heart attack," dietary sodium excess, medication noncompliance, arrhythmias, pulmonary embolism, infection, and anemia can precipitate HF. The prognosis for HF depends on the causative factors and the individual's response to treatment. Overall 80% of men and 70% of women under the age of 65 years who are diagnosed with HF will die within 8 years (Thom et al., 2006).

Prevalence and Incidence

HF is a major public health problem that affects over 5 million Americans. Unlike other cardiovascular diseases, the number of people being discharged with an HF diagnosis increased by 174% from 1979 to 2003 (Thom et al., 2006). The prevalence of HF increases with age and differs by race and ethnicity. Eighty percent of hospitalized patients with

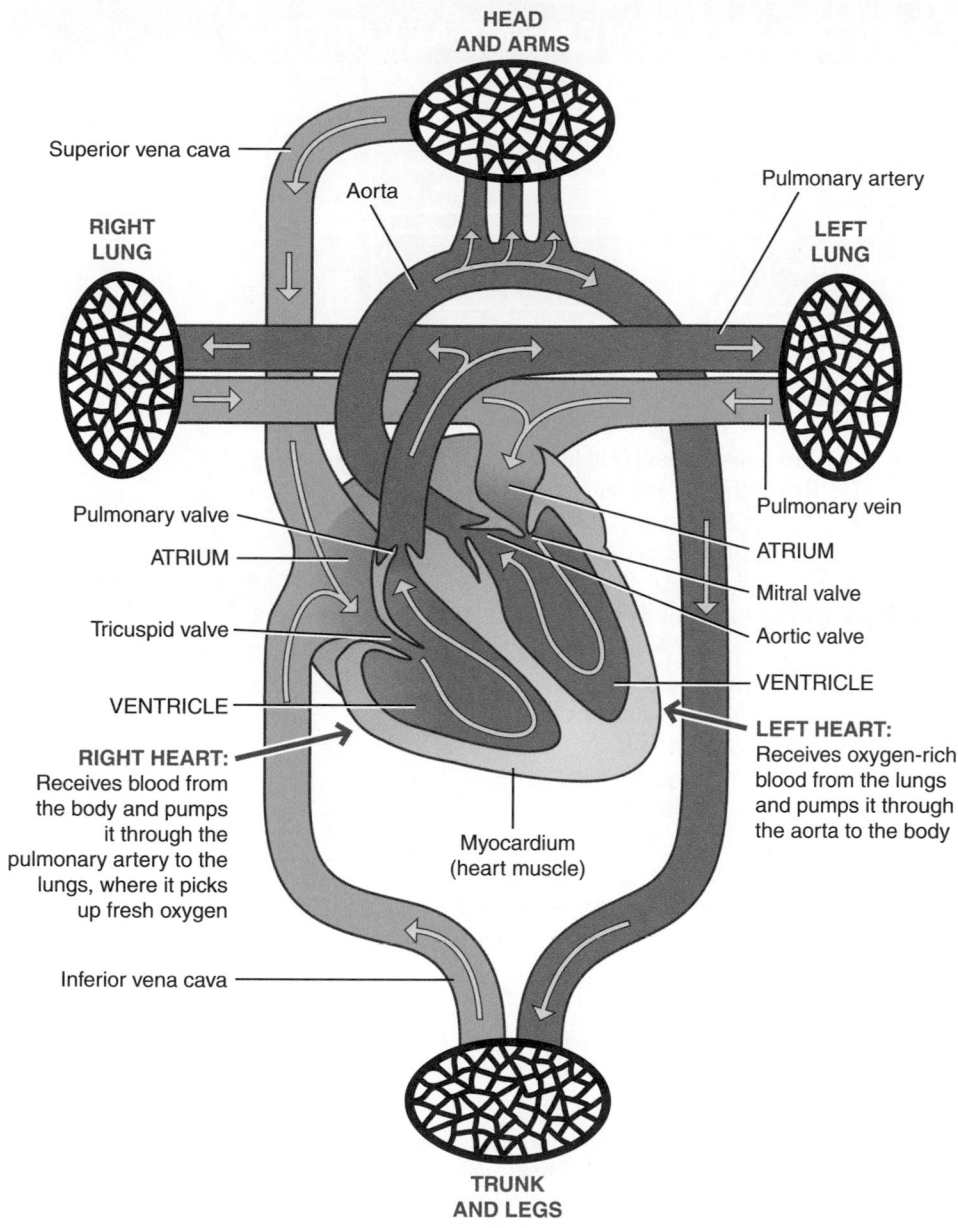

FIGURE 34-1 Structure of the heart pump

HF are over the age of 65 years (Hunt et al., 2005). Black women have the highest rates of HF, followed by black men, Mexican-American men, white men, white women, and Mexican-American women (Thom et al., 2006). The incidence (new cases) of HF has risen over the last 20 years because of an aging population, the increased number of people being saved from a MI, and the increase in obesity and associated hypertension (Rich, 2005).

Risk Factors

The Framingham Study is a 50-year epidemiologic study of the incidence, prevalence, and risk factors for cardiovascular diseases (see *Focus On:* Framingham Heart Study in Chapter 32). In the Framingham population the risk factors for HF are hypertension, diabetes, coronary heart disease, and **left ventricular hypertrophy** (enlargement of the left ventricle of the heart). Hypertension precedes HF in many men and women. Since the lifetime risk of developing hypertension is 75% and the prevalence of hypertension is high, control-

ling blood pressure is a major preventive strategy for HF (Vasan et al., 2002).

Individuals who have diabetes mellitus and ischemic heart disease more frequently develop HF compared with patients without diabetes (Rosano et al., 2006). Diabetes is an especially strong risk factor for HF in women. The prevalence of both hypertension and diabetes increases with age, making the elderly particularly vulnerable to HF. Even fasting blood glucose elevations (60 mg/dl increase) were predictive of new cases of HF in a sample of elderly people, mean age 72 years (Barzilay et al., 2004). Another large cohort study of older adults (70 to 79 years) showed that waist circumference and percentage of body fat were the strongest predictors of who would develop HF (Nicklas et al., 2006). Numerous changes in cardiovascular structure and function also place the elderly at high risk for developing HF (Box 34-1). Features of HF in the elderly differ from those seen in middle-age persons with HF (Table 34-1).

PATHOPHYSIOLOGY AND CARE MANAGEMENT ALGORITHM

Heart Failure

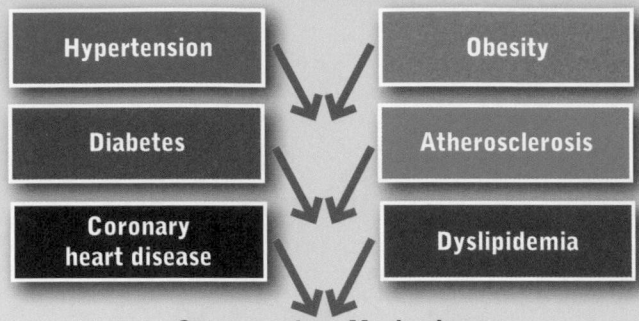

ETIOLOGY

Hypertension	Obesity
Diabetes	Atherosclerosis
Coronary heart disease	Dyslipidemia

Compensatory Mechanisms
Sympathetic nervous system
Renin-angiotensin system
Cytokine system

Left Ventricular Hypertrophy or Hemodynamic Stress on a Diseased Heart

Dietary sodium excess
Medication noncompliance
Arrhythmias
Pulmonary embolism
Infection
Anemia

Heart Failure

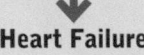

PATHOPHYSIOLOGY

Clinical Findings

- Shortness of breath
- Fatigue
- Fluid retention
- Peripheral vasoconstriciton
- B-natriuretic peptide
- Mental confusion
- Memory loss
- Anxiety
- Insomnia
- Syncope and headache
- Dry cough

Nutrition Assessment

- Anorexia
- Nausea, abdominal pain and feeling of fullness
- Constipation
- Malabsorption
- Malnutrition
- Cardiac cachexia
- Hypomagnesemia

MANAGEMENT

Medical Management

- ACE inhibitors
- Angiotensin receptor blockers
- Aldosterone blockers
- β-blockers
- Digoxin
- Vasodilators
- Implantable defibrillator
- Heart transplant

Nutrition Management

- Diet low in saturated fat, *trans* fat, cholesterol
- Restricted sodium diet—<2 gm/day
- Increased use of whole grains, fruits, vegetables
- Limit fluid to 2 L per day
- Lose to or maintain appropriate weight
- Magnesium supplementation
- Thiamin supplementation
- Increase physical activity as tolerated
- Avoid tobacco
- Avoid alcohol

Developed by L. Kathleen Mahan, MS, RD, CDE.

TABLE 34-1

Heart Failure in Middle Age vs. Heart Failure in Elderly

	Middle Age	Elderly
Prevalence	<1%	≈10%
Sex	Men > Women	Women > Men
Etiology	CAD	Hypertension
Clinical features	Typical	Atypical
LVEF	Reduced	Normal
Comorbidities	Few	Multiple
RCTs	Many	Few
Therapy	Evidence-based	Empiric
Physician treating HF	Cardiologist	Primary care

From Rich MW: Office management of heart failure in the elderly, *AM J Med* 118:342, 2005.

CAD, Coronary artery disease; *LVEF,* left ventricular ejection fraction; *RCT,* randomized clinical trial.

Prevention

Because long-term survival rates for persons with HF are low, prevention is critical. HF is categorized into four stages ranging from persons with risk factors (stage A—primary prevention) to persons with advanced HF (stage D—severe disease) (Figure 34-2). For stages A and B the aggressive treatment of underlying risk factors and diseases such as **dyslipidemia** (abnormal pattern of blood lipoproteins), hypertension, and diabetes is critical to prevent structural damage to the myocardium and the appearance of HF symptoms (see Chapters 30 and 32). Such prevention has been very effective. In seven studies of the elderly with these conditions, the use of antihypertensive therapy reduced the risk of HF by 22% to 68% (Rich, 2005). Even patients who had an MI can reduce the risk of HF by 81% with antihypertensive therapy (Kostis et al., 1997).

Along with pharmacologic therapy, lifestyle changes include adopting a heart-healthy diet that is low in saturated fatty acids, *trans*-fatty acids, cholesterol, and sodium, with increased use of whole grains, fruits, and vegetables; maintaining or losing body weight as needed; increasing physical activity as tolerated, and avoiding tobacco and alcohol. The use of nutrition supplements for the sole purpose of preventing structural heart disease is not recommended for patients at high risk for developing HF (Hunt et al., 2005).

For stages C and D, secondary prevention strategies to prevent further cardiac dysfunction are warranted. These strategies include the use of angiotensin-converting enzyme (ACE) inhibitors (first line of therapy), angiotensin receptor blockers, aldosterone blockers, β-blockers, and digoxin. Use of neurohormonal antagonists, ACE inhibitors, and β-blockers has been shown to reduce HF mortality (Prendergast, 2005). Early detection, correction of asymptomatic left ventricular dysfunction, and aggressive management of risk factors are needed to lower the incidence and mortality of HF.

Pathophysiology and Symptoms

The progression of HF is similar to that of atherosclerosis because there is an asymptomatic phase when damage is silently occurring (stages A and B). HF is initiated by damage or stress to the heart muscle either of acute MI or insidious (hemodynamic pressure or volume overloading) onset (Mann et al., 2002). This progressive insult alters the function and shape of the left ventricle such that it hypertrophies in an effort to sustain blood flow, a process known as cardiac remodeling. Symptoms do not usually arise until months or years after cardiac remodeling begins (Hunt et al., 2005).

Many compensatory mechanisms from the sympathetic nervous system, renin–angiotensin system, and cytokine system are activated to restore homeostatic function. Proinflammatory cytokines, such as tumor necrosis factor-α (TNF-α), interleukin (IL)-1, and IL-6 are increased in blood and the myocardium and have been found to regulate cardiac remodeling (Gullestad et al., 2005).

Another substance, B-natriuretic peptide (BNP), is secreted by the ventricles in response to pressure and is predictive of the severity of HF and mortality at any level of body mass index (BMI) (Horwich et al., 2006). Patients are asymptomatic during these first two stages. BNP is often highly elevated in patients with HF (greater than 100 pg/ml is abnormal, and some patients come in with levels over 3000 pg/ml). Nesiritide (recombinant human BNP) provides symptomatic and hemodynamic improvement in acute decompensated HF and is now standard procedure (Arora et al., 2006).

Eventually overuse of compensatory systems leads to further ventricle damage, remodeling, and appearance and then worsening of symptoms (stage C). HF patients have elevated levels of norepinephrine, angiotensin II, aldosterone, endothelin, and vasopressin, all of which are neurohormonal factors that increase the hemodynamic stress on the ventricle by causing sodium retention and peripheral vasoconstriction. These neurohormones and the proinflammatory cytokines contribute to disease progression; hence current therapies are being studied to inhibit these undesirable pathways and promote desirable ones (Gullestad et al., 2005).

Medical Management

Therapy recommendations correspond to the stage of HF (see Figure 34-2). For patients at high risk of developing HF (stage A), treatment of the underlying conditions (hypertension, dyslipidemia, thyroid disorders, arrhythmias), avoidance of high-risk behaviors (tobacco, alcohol, illicit drug use), and lifestyle changes (weight reduction, exercise, reduction of sodium intake, heart-healthy diet) are recommended. All these recommendations are carried through the other stages. In addition, an implantable defibrillator, which shocks the heart when it stops, can be placed in patients at risk of sudden death (Cesario and Dee, 2006). Pharmacologic treatment of HF is the hallmark of therapy with progressive stages. The last stage also includes surgically implanted ventricular assist devices, heart transplantation, and continual intravenous therapy.

The short-term goals for the treatment of HF are to relieve symptoms and improve the quality of life and reduce depression if it is present. The long-term goal of treatment is to prolong life by lessening, stopping, or reversing left ventricular dysfunction. Medical management is tailored to clinical and hemodynamic profiles (evidence of hypoperfusion and congestion) (Hunt et al., 2005). In some cases surgical procedures are needed to alleviate the HF caused by valvular disease. Medical management is relatively limited in these instances.

Initial management of HF includes a restricted sodium diet (less than 2000 mg daily) and regular activity, as symptoms permit (Hunt et al., 2005). Bed rest is no longer recommended except for those with acute failure. The heart becomes deconditioned with less exercise, whereas with regular exercise capacity can be increased. Standard fluid restrictions are to limit total fluid intake to 2 L (2000 ml) daily (Hunt, et al., 2005). When patients are severely decompensated, a more restrictive fluid intake (1000 to 1500 ml daily) may be warranted for adequate diuresis. A sodium-restricted diet should be maintained despite low-sodium blood levels because in this case the sodium has shifted from the blood to the tissues. Serum sodium appears low in a patient who is fluid overloaded due to dilution; diuresis improves the levels by decreasing the amount of water in the vascular space.

An ACE inhibitor is the first line of pharmacologic treatment for HF. As the stages progress, a β-blocker or angiotensin receptor blocker may be added. In Stages C and D selected patients may also take a diuretic, aldosterone antagonists, digitalis, and vasodilators (e.g., hydralazine) (Hunt et al., 2005). Basically these medications reduce excess fluid, dilate blood vessels, and increase the strength of the heart's contraction.

Several of these medications have neurohormonal benefits along with their primary mechanism of action. For example, ACE inhibitors (e.g., captopril, enalapril) not only inhibit the renin-angiotensin system (see Chapter 33) but also improve symptoms, quality of life, exercise tolerance, and survival. Similarly spironolactone has both diuretic and aldosterone-blocking functions that result in reduced morbidity and mortality in patients. Most of these medications can affect nutrition status (see Chapter 16 and Appendix 31).

Medical Nutrition Therapy

The registered dietitian (RD) as part of a multidisciplinary (physician, pharmacist, psychologist, nurse, and social worker) team provides medical nutrition therapy (MNT), which includes assessment, establishing a nutrition diagnosis, and interventions (education, counseling) for patients (Coats, 2005). Such a team with an RD positively impacts outcomes of readmission to the hospital (decreased by 42%), days in the hospital (decreased by 2 days), improved compliance with restricted sodium and fluid intakes, and improved quality of life scores in HF patients (Tangalos, 2002; Kuehneman et al., 2002).

Nutrition screening for HF in older adults can help prevent disease progression and improve disease management, overall health, and quality of life outcomes. The first step in screening is determination of body weight. Altered fluid balance complicates assessment of body weight in the patient with HF. Weights should be taken before eating and after voiding at the same time each day. A dry weight (weight without edema) should be determined on the scale at home (Rich, 2005). Patients should record daily weights and advise their care providers if weight gain exceeds more than 1 lb a day for patients with severe HF, more than 2 lb a day for patients with moderate HF, and more than 3 to 5 pounds with mild HF (Rich, 2005; Tangalos, 2002). Restricting sodium and fluids along with diuretic therapy may restore fluid balance and prevent full-blown HF.

In malnourished patients with HF, body weight can be either normal or increased as a result of fluid retention. Patients with cardiac cachexia may lose 10% to 15% of their body weight. Other markers of malnutrition (i.e., serum prealbumin and transferrin) may be disproportionately low because of the dilutional effect of excess extracellular fluid. Therefore to assess lean body mass anthropometrics must be used. Mid–upper arm circumference is an inexpensive method for assessing protein-energy malnutrition in HF patients (see Chapter 14).

Dietary assessment in free-living, stable, nonobese HF patients revealed that 54% had malnutrition: 16% with protein-calorie malnutrition and 39% with protein malnutrition and a normal body weight (Aquilani et al., 2003). Negative energy balance and negative nitrogen balances were observed in 70% and 60% of patients, respectively. These negative balances were noted despite comparable caloric and nitrogen intakes in controls without HF. A caloric intake of 31.8 kcal/kg and 1.37 g of protein per kilogram is recommended for malnourished HF patients and 28.1 kcal/kg and 1.12 g of protein per kilogram for HF patients with normal nutrition status (Aquilani, 2003).

In overweight patients caloric reduction must be carefully monitored to avoid excessive and rapid body protein catabolism. Numerous indices can be used to evaluate the effectiveness of MNT. Nutrition education to promote behavior change is a critical component of MNT. Since HF patients ranked diet as fifth out of seven educational topics that are important to learn for managing their disease, the benefits of MNT should be communicated to patients (Clark and Lan, 2004).

The total diet must be addressed in patients with HF (Silver, 2003). Because underlying risk factors are often present, dietary changes to modify these risk factors are an important component of MNT. Therefore for dyslipidemia or atherosclerosis, a heart-healthy diet low in saturated fatty acids, *trans*-fatty acids, and cholesterol, and high in fiber, whole grains, fruits, and vegetables would be recommended (see Chapter 32). For persons with hypertension the DASH-sodium diet is recommended (see Chapter 33). Both of these dietary patterns emphasize lower sodium foods as described in the following section. Also, both of the plans are high in potassium, which may be a problem for patients on large doses of certain diuretics. Even with high potassium intake, some patients require the use of potassium supplements. Since total energy expenditure is higher in HF patients because of the catabolic state, adequate protein and energy should be provided (Pasini et al., 2004).

Sodium

Edema in patients with decompensated HF results from impaired cardiac function. Inadequate blood flow to the kidneys leads to aldosterone and antidiuretic hormone secretion. Both these hormones act to conserve fluid, thus trying to restore blood flow. Aldosterone promotes sodium resorption, and antidiuretic hormone promotes water conservation in the distal tubules of the nephron. Sodium and fluid thus accumulate in the tissues. Even asymptomatic patients with mild HF and no edema can retain sodium and water if consuming a high-salt diet as most Americans do.

The degree to which sodium and possibly fluids are restricted depends on the individual. There is no consensus on the optimal level of sodium restriction. For the healthy elderly population (over 71 years), the adequate intake is 1200 mg (50 mmol)/day. Recommendations for HF patients vary between 1200 to 2400 mg/day. For patients taking large doses of lasix (80 mg/day), a sodium intake of less than 2 g/day is recommended to optimize the effects of the diuretic (Tangalos, 2002). Severe restrictions (500 mg/day) are unpalatable and nutritionally inadequate.

Adherence to sodium restrictions can be problematic for some patients, and individualized instruction is recommended (Rich, 2005). Of patients who reported that they were avoiding sodium, 94% reported consuming a high-sodium food on the previous day (Sneed and Paul, 2003).

Ethnic differences in sodium consumption must be considered. For blacks living in the southern part of the United States, eight high-sodium foods or preparation methods (salt in cooking, fast food, fried chicken, canned vegetables, corn bread, cheese, processed meats, and cold cereal) were consumed at least once a week (Kollipara et al., 2006). Poor adherence to low-sodium diets occurs as a result of lack of knowledge by the patient, the patient's perception that the diet interferes with social aspects of eating, and lack of food choices (Bentley et al., 2005). Following nutrition counseling sodium knowledge scores significantly increased, as did the number of patients who could read the nutrition label (Neily et al., 2002). Also

---

BOX 34-2

High-Sodium Foods

1. Smoked, processed, or cured meats and fish (e.g., ham, bacon, corned beef, cold cuts, hot dogs, sausage, salt pork, chipped beef, pickled herring, anchovies, tuna, and sardines)
2. Tomato juices and tomato sauce, unless labeled otherwise
3. Meat extracts, bouillon cubes, meat sauces, monosodium glutamate (MSG), and taco seasoning
4. Salted snacks (potato chips, tortilla chips, corn chips, pretzels, salted nuts, popcorn, and crackers)
5. Prepared salad dressings, condiments, relishes, ketchup, Worcestershire sauce, barbecue sauce, cocktail sauce, teriyaki sauce, soy sauce, commercial salad dressings, salsa, pickles, olives, and sauerkraut
6. Packaged mixes for sauces, gravies, casseroles, and noodle, rice, or potato dishes; macaroni and cheese; stuffing mix
7. Cheeses (processed and cheese spreads)
8. Frozen entrees and pot pies
9. Canned soup
10. Foods eaten away from home

This list is not comprehensive. NOTE: Reading labels is most important; some brands are lower in sodium than others.

---

positive outcomes (i.e., decreased urinary sodium excretion, less fatigue, less frequent edema) have been observed in HF patients receiving MNT (Ramirez et al., 2004).

The type of sodium restriction prescribed should be the least restrictive diet that will still achieve the desired results. The first step is to minimize or eliminate the use of table salt and high-sodium foods (Box 34-2). Table 34-4 lists serving sizes for some common high-sodium foods that should be used only sparingly in the sodium-restricted diet. Table 34-5 lists the sodium content of food groups and the number of servings from each group that can be included at each level of sodium restriction. See Appendix 37 for further explanation of the sodium restricted diet.

There are multiple websites for other helpful tips for consumers trying to reduce sodium intake, and many are noted at the end of this chapter.

Dietary Sources of Sodium

Dietary sources of sodium include (1) salt used at the table; (2) salt or sodium compounds added during preparation or processing of foods; (3) inherent sodium in foods; and (4) chemically softened water. The average American consumes approximately 4 to 6 g of sodium daily, much more than the minimum 250 mg (9 mEq) required by the human to maintain life. As much as 20% comes from salt added to food during preparation or at the table, and 80% comes from processed foods. With enactment of the Nutrition Labeling and Education Act of 1990, the Food and Drug Administration requires labeling of sodium content on foods and provides legal definitions for the terms low sodium, moderately low sodium, and reduced sodium (Table 34-6). The daily value for sodium used on the food label is set at 2400 mg. Patients can use the percent daily value to determine whether a certain food would fit into their dietary prescription.

LiteSalt (contains 20% to 50% less sodium) can be calculated into a mildly restricted diet. However, it is important to note that LiteSalt contains potassium, a problem when patients are also given potassium-sparing diuretics.

Spices, herbs, and other seasonings (horseradish, Tabasco sauce, lemon juice, and vinegar) can be used to improve the flavor of low-sodium foods. Herb or spice salts such as garlic salt should be avoided. In addition to the sodium in food and water, incidental amounts may be ingested in the form of medicines and toothpastes. Barbiturates, sulfonamides, antibiotics, and other drugs, as well as cough medications, stomach alkalizers, laxatives, and mouthwashes, may contain large amounts of sodium. For example, some antacids can add 1200 to 7000 mg of sodium daily when used as therapy for heartburn. Similarly aspirin used in large doses would need to be counted since it contains 50 mg of sodium per tablet. The label or product manufacturer could be used to determine the sodium content. Most other medicines contain less than 5 mg of sodium per dose and would not have to be counted in the total sodium allotment.

Animal protein foods such as milk, cheese, eggs, meat, poultry, and fish have relatively high sodium content because sodium chloride surrounds animal cells. Depending on food choices, these foods may have to be limited. Because kosher meats and poultry are soaked in salt water for 1 hour after slaughter to remove the blood, and even though the meat is washed thoroughly before cooking, the sodium content of such foods may still be increased as much as four times to a level of 90 to 115 mg/oz. Acceptable alternatives are to boil the meat and discard the broth before eating, or to use low-sodium kosher meats that are available.

Between 4% and 27% of dietary sodium comes from ingested water. The amount of sodium in drinking water is an issue if the sodium concentration in the water is greater than 40 ppm (40 mg or 2 mEq/L) and large quantities of water are consumed. Because of fluid restrictions, this should not be an issue for most patients with HF.

In summary, five behaviors aid in following a low sodium diet: (a) put away the salt shaker; (b) choose low-sodium versions of favorite foods; (c) choose foods that are naturally low in sodium; (d) read food labels carefully when purchasing foods; and (e) select foods carefully when dining out (see *Focus On:* Sodium and Salt Measurement Equivalents.

Alcohol and Caffeine

Alcohol contributes to fluid intake and raises blood pressure. Many cardiologists recommend avoiding alcohol. Chronic alcohol ingestion leads to cardiomyopathy and HF (Li and Ren, 2006). Although heavy drinking should be discouraged, moderate drinking may lower the risk of HF through beneficial effects of alcohol on coronary artery disease (Klatsky et al., 2005). If alcohol is consumed, intake should not exceed 1 drink per day for women and 2 drinks per day for men. A drink is equivalent to 1 ounce of alcohol (1 ounce of distilled liquor), 5 ounces of wine, or 12 ounces of beer.

Caffeine generally is not recommended in HF patients. If used, moderation is best (Houston, 2005).

Weight Maintenance

The energy needs of patients with HF depend on their current dry weight, activity restrictions, and the severity of the HF. Overweight patients with limited activity must achieve and maintain an appropriate weight that will not stress the

---

TABLE 34-4

Foods Containing About 400 mg of Sodium per Serving

Serving Sizes of Foods Containing 400 mg of Sodium (±50 mg)	Na (mg)
Meats and Cheeses	
3 small cocktail wieners	354
4 thin slices (1.3 oz) lunchmeat	450
2 slices bacon	370
2 oz pork sausage	425
2 oz. ham	443
1.25 oz corned beef	402
4.5 oz canned tuna	432
4.5 oz canned crab	426
2.5 oz canned salmon	393
½ c cottage cheese	425
2 oz cheese	352
Soups	
⅔ c beef broth	428
½ c tomato soup	371
½ c cream of mushroom	434
Condiments	
⅙ tsp salt	393
1¼ tsp soy sauce	380
6 tsp Worcestershire	394
2⅓ Tbsp catsup	391
2 Tbsp mustard	350
2 Tbsp chili sauce	457
2½ Tbsp barbeque sauce	390
4⅔ Tbsp tartar sauce	418
2 Tbsp French dressing	382
Miscellaneous	
8 medium olives	424
3 Tbsp sweet pickle relish	373
20 small pretzels	412
1½ slices thin crust cheese pizza (14-in diameter)	447
3 servings (½ c) each canned vegetables	407
¼ c sauerkraut	390
2 oz potato chips	366
¼ large dill pickle	433

From Krummel DA et al: Used University of Minnesota Nutrition Data System for Research (NDS-R 2005).

TABLE 34-5

Food Servings for Sodium-Controlled Diets

Food Group	Serving Size	Sodium Content		Suggested Number of Servings for Various Restricted Diets			
		mg Na⁺	mEq Na⁺	3 g	2 g	1 g	500 mg
Milk, low sodium	8 oz	7	—				1
Milk, regular	8 oz	120	5	2	2	2	1
Buttermilk, salted	8 oz	280	13	—	—	—	—
Cottage cheese, regular	¼ c	130	6	1	1	1	—
Cheese, regular	1 oz	200	9	1	—	—	—
Meat, fish, poultry, unsalted cheese, tofu (½ c)	1 oz	25	1	6	6	6	5
Fresh shellfish	1 oz	50	2	1	1	—	—
Peanut butter, regular	1 Tbsp	80	3	1	1	—	—
Egg	1	70	3	Not restricted		1	1
Vegetables, cooked, fresh, frozen	½ c	10	—		Not restricted		
Vegetables, naturally higher in sodium	½ c	40	2		Not restricted		1
Vegetable, canned, regular	½ c	230	10				
Vegetable juices, canned	½ c	200	9				
Fruits	½ c	2	—		Not restricted		
Bread, regular	1 slice	150	7	4	4	1	—
Bread, low sodium	1 slice	5	—		Not restricted		
Quick bread, muffin	1 serving	300	14	1	—	—	—
Cereal, ready-to-eat, salted	1 c	300	14	1	—	—	—
Cereal, unsalted	½ c	5	—		Not restricted		
Butter or margarine, salted	1 tsp	50	2	3	3	2	—
Butter or margarine, unsalted	1 tsp	1	—		Not restricted		
Mayonnaise, regular	1½ tsp	50	2	1	1	1	1
Salad dressing, regular	1 Tbsp	350	16	1	—	—	—
Soup, regular	1 c	900	42	—	—	—	—
Soup, low sodium	1 c	25	1		Not restricted		
Desserts, regular	1 serving	300	14	1	—	—	—
Desserts, low sodium	1 serving	15	—		Not restricted		
Salt	1 tsp	2300	10	½ tsp	¼ tsp	—	—

myocardium. For the obese patient, hypocaloric diets (1000 to 1200 kcal daily) reduce the stress on the heart and facilitate weight reduction. However, the nutrition status of the obese patient must be assessed to ensure that the patient is not malnourished.

In patients with severe HF, energy needs are increased by 30% to 50% above basal level as a result of the increased energy expenditure of the heart and lungs; 31 to 35 kcal/kg of body weight is often used as the starting point for determining caloric requirements. Patients with cardiac cachexia may require further increases in energy to 1.6 to 1.8 times the resting energy expenditure for nutritional repletion.

Calcium and Vitamin D

Patients with HF are at increased risk of developing osteoporosis because of low activity levels, impaired renal function, and prescription drugs that alter calcium metabolism (Zittermann et al., 2006). Cachectic HF patients have lower bone mineral density and lower calcium levels than HF patients without cachexia or normal subjects (Anker et al., 1997a, 1997b). Caution must be used with calcium supplements because they may aggravate cardiac arrhythmias. Before transplant most HF patients only have subtle changes in bone. However, patients with a polymorphism of the vitamin D receptor gene have higher rates of bone loss than HF patients without this genotype (Nishio et al., 2003).

Another positive role for vitamin D is improving inflammation in HF patients (Vieth and Kimball, 2006). In a double-blind, randomized, placebo-controlled trial, supplementation with vitamin D (50 mcg or 2000 international units of vitamin D₃ per day) for 9 months increased the antiinflammatory

Hunt SA et al: *ACC/AHA 2005 guideline* update for the diagnosis and management of chronic heart failure in the adult: a report of the American College of Cardiology/American Heart Association Task Force, *J Am Coll Cardiol* 46:e1, 2005.

Jankowska E et al: Autonomic imbalance and immune activation in chronic heart failure—pathophysiological links, *Cardiovasc Res* 70:434, 2006.

Kahn J et al: The impact of overweight on the development of diabetes after heart transplantation, *Clin Transplant* 20:62, 2006.

King DE et al: Dietary magnesium and C-reactive protein, *J Am Coll Nutr* 24:166, 2005.

Kistorp C et al: Plasma adiponectin, body mass index, and mortality in patients with chronic heart failure, *Circulation* 112:1756, 2005.

Klatsky AL et al: Alcohol drinking and risk of hospitalization for heart failure with and without associated coronary artery disease, *Am J Cardiol* 96:346, 2005.

Kollipara U et al: High-sodium food choices by southern, urban African-Americans with heart failure, *J Card Fail* 12:144, 2006.

Kostis J et al for the SHEP Cooperative Research Group: Prevention of heart failure by antihypertensive drug treatment in older persons with isolated systolic hypertension, *JAMA* 278:212, 1997.

Krack A et al: The importance of the gastrointestinal system in the pathogenesis of heart failure, *Eur Hear J* 26:2368, 2005.

Kuehneman T et al: Demonstrating the impact of nutrition intervention in a heart failure program, *J Am Diet Assoc* 102:1790, 2002.

Lainscah M et al: Body composition changes in patients with systolic heart failure treated with β-blockers: a pilot study, *Int J Cardiol* 106:319, 2006.

Levy HB, Kohlhaas HK: Considerations for supplementing with coenzyme Q during statin therapy, *Ann Pharmacother* 40:290, 2006.

Li Q, Ren J: Cardiac overexpression of metallothionein attenuates chronic alcohol intake-induced cardiomyocyte contractile dysfunction, *Cardiovasc Toxicol* 6:173, 2006.

Mann DL et al: New therapeutics for chronic heart failure, *Annu Rev Med* 53:59, 2002.

Mendoza C et al: Reversal of refractory congestive heart failure after thiamine supplementation: report of a case and review of the literature, *J Cardiovasc Pharmacol Ther* 8:313, 2003.

Miller LW, Missov ED: Epidemiology of heart failure, *Cardio Clin* 19:547, 2001.

Nagaya N, Kangawa K: Therapeutic potential of ghrelin in treatment of heart failure, *Drugs* 66:439, 2006.

Neily JB et al: Potential contributing factors to noncompliance with dietary sodium restriction in patients with heart failure, *Am Heart J* 143:29, 2002.

Nicklas B et al: Abdominal obesity is an independent risk factor for chronic heart failure in older people, *J Am Geriatr Soc* 54:413, 2006.

Nishio K et al: Congestive heart failure is associated with the rate of bone loss, *J Intern Med* 253:439, 2003.

Nohria A et al: Medical management of advanced heart failure, *JAMA* 287:628, 2002.

Pasini E et al: Inadequate nutritional intake for daily life activity of clinically stable patients with chronic heart failure, *Am J Cardiol* 93(suppl):41A, 2004.

Pirlich M et al: Prevalence of malnutrition in hospitalized medical patients: impact of underlying disease, *Dig Dis* 21:245, 2003.

Pisani B, Mullen G: Prevention of osteoporosis in cardiac transplant recipients, *Curr Opin Cardiol* 17:160, 2002.

Prendergast HM et al: Management of chronic heart failure: an old disease with a new face, *Emerg Med Aust* 17:143, 2005.

Ramirez R et al: Effects of a nutritional intervention on body composition, clinical status, and quality of life in patients with heart failure, *Nutrition* 20:890, 2004.

Rich MW: Office management of heart failure in the elderly, *Am J Med* 118:342, 2005.

Rosano GM et al: Metabolic therapy for patients with diabetes mellitus and coronary artery disease, *Am J Cardiol* 98(5A):14J, 2006.

Sanders S et al: The impact of coenzyme Q_{10} on systolic function in patients with chronic heart failure, *J Card Fail* 12(6):464, 2006.

Schleithoff SS et al: Vitamin D supplementation improves cytokine profiles in patients with congestive heart failure: a double-blind, randomized, placebo-controlled trial, *Am J Clin Nutr* 83:754, 2006.

Silver MA: Dietary research in heart failure, *J Am Coll Cardiol* 42:1224, 2003.

Sneed NV, Paul SC: Readiness for behavioral change in patients with heart failure, *Am J Crit Care* 12:444, 2003.

Springer J et al: Prognosis and therapy approaches of cardiac cachexia, *Curr Opin Cardiol* 3:229, 2006.

Strassburg S et al: Muscle wasting in cardiac cachexia, *Int J Biochem Cell Biol* 37:1938, 2005.

Tangalos EG: *Congestive heart failure: nutrition management for older adults*, Washington, DC, 2002, Nutrition Screening Initiative (NSI).

Taylor D et al: The registry of the international society for heart and lung transplantation: twenty-first official adult heart transplant report—2004, *J Heart Lung Transplant* 23:796, 2004.

Thom T et al: Heart disease and stroke statistics—2006 update from the American Heart Association Statistics Committee, *Circulation* 113:e85, 2006.

Vasan RS et al: Residual lifetime risk for developing hypertension in middle-aged women and men: the Framingham Heart Study, *JAMA* 287:1003, 2002.

Vieth R, Kimball S: Vitamin D in congestive heart failure, *Am J Clin Nutr* 83:731, 2006.

Vorlat A: Regular use of margarine-containing stanol/sterol esters reduces total and low-density lipoprotein (LDL) cholesterol and allows reduction of statin therapy after cardiac transplantation: preliminary observations, *J Heart Lung Transplant* 22(9):1059, 2003.

Wenke K: Management of hyperlipidaemia associated with heart transplantation, *Drugs* 64(10):1053, 2004.

Wenke K et al: Impact of simvastatin therapy after heart transplantation an 11-year prospective evaluation, *Herz* 30:431, 2005.

Witte KK et al: The effect of micronutrient supplementation on quality of life and left ventricular function in elderly patients with chronic heart failure, *Eur Heart J* 26:2238, 2005.

Zitterman A et al: Markers of bone metabolism in congestive heart failure, *Clin Chim Acta* 366:27, 2006.

CHAPTER 35

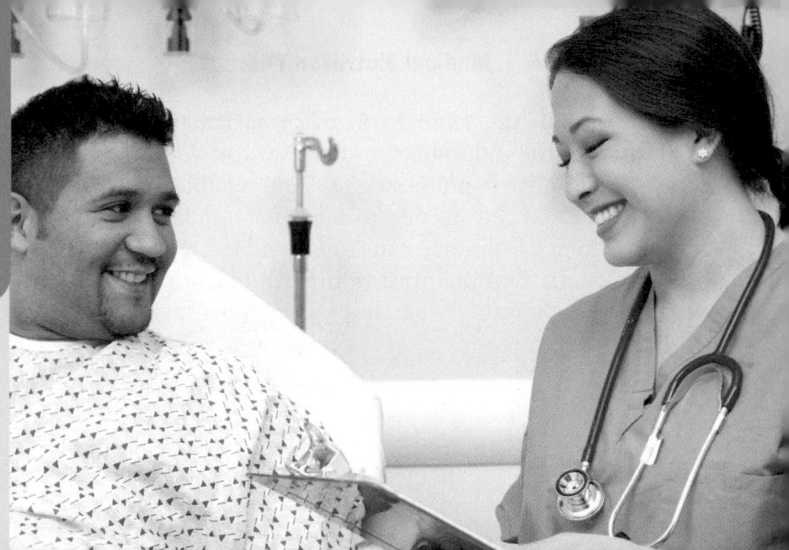

Donna H. Mueller, PhD, RD, FADA, LDN

Medical Nutrition Therapy for Pulmonary Disease

KEY TERMS

acute respiratory distress syndrome a life-threatening condition characterized by severe hypoxia, bilateral pulmonary fluid infiltration, and decreased lung compliance; usually occurring without prior lung disease but secondary to catastrophic illness

asthma a condition of hypersensitive airways from allergic and nonallergic causes generated by immunologic responses

bronchopulmonary dysplasia (BPD) a chronic lung disease of infancy that commonly arises following respiratory distress syndrome (RDS) and treatment with oxygen; characterized by broncheolar metaplasia and interstitial fibrosis; now referred to as chronic lung disease of prematurity

chronic bronchitis a chronic, productive cough with inflammation of one or more of the bronchi and secondary changes in lung tissue

chronic lung disease of prematurity (CLD) a diagnosis made at 36 weeks' postmenstrual age of an infant who has continued requirement for supplemental oxygen, an abnormal pulmonary physical examination, and an abnormal chest radiograph

chronic obstructive pulmonary disease (COPD) a process characterized by the presence of chronic bronchitis, emphysema, or both, leading to the development of airway obstruction

cor pulmonale a heart condition characterized by right ventricular enlargement and failure that results from resistance to the passage of blood through the lungs

cystic fibrosis (CF) an autosomal-recessive disorder characterized by dysfunction of the exocrine glands and production of abnormally thick secretions that obstruct airways and pancreatic and other ducts

distal intestinal obstruction syndrome (DIOS) recurrent distal intestinal impaction; formerly termed meconium ileus equivalent

dyspnea shortness of breath

elastase protein-digesting enzyme secreted by the pancreas and involved in hydrolysis of peptide bonds; presence in feces is marker of adequacy of pancreatic enzyme supplementation

emphysema a condition of the lung characterized by abnormal, permanent enlargement of alveoli, accompanied by destruction of their walls without obvious fibrosis

hypercapnia excessive carbon dioxide in the blood

pancreatic enzyme replacement therapy use of exogenous pancreatic enzymes to produce more normal digestion in persons with pancreatic insufficiency

pulmonary aspiration the drawing of foreign bodies such as food or liquid into the lungs during inspiration

pulmonary function tests a group of procedures designed to measure the ability of the respiratory system to exchange oxygen and carbon dioxide

respiratory quotient (RQ) the ratio of the volume of carbon dioxide expired to the volume of oxygen inspired (CO_2/O_2)

surfactant a substance composed of phospholipids (especially dipalmitophosphatidylcholine) and protein that is produced by type II cells of the alveolar epithelium; it lowers surface tension to permit gas exchange at the gas-liquid interface

sweat test a test performed using pilocarpine iontophoresis to determine levels of sodium and chloride in sweat; elevated levels are diagnostic of cystic fibrosis

tachypnea abnormal rapidity of respiration that, if prolonged, can lead to excess loss of CO_2 and respiratory alkalosis

tuberculosis (TB) a bacterial disease caused by mycobacteria, specifically *Mycobacterium tuberculosis*, *M. bovis*, or *M. africanum*; spread by inhalation of organisms dispersed as droplets from the sputum of infected persons (the bacteria-laden droplets can float in the air for several hours)

During fetal life, from birth to maturity and throughout adulthood, the pulmonary system is intertwined with nutrition. An optimal pulmonary system enables the body to obtain the oxygen needed to meet its cellular demands for bioenergetics from macronutrients and to remove metabolic by-products. Optimal nutrition permits the proper growth and development of the: respiratory anatomy; supporting structures of the skeleton and muscles; and related nervous, circulatory, and immunologic systems. Overall a person's nutritional well-being, as well as the proper metabolism of specific nutrients themselves, is essential for the formation, development, growth, maturity, and protection of healthy lungs and other associated body structures and processes throughout life (Andreoli et al., 2004).

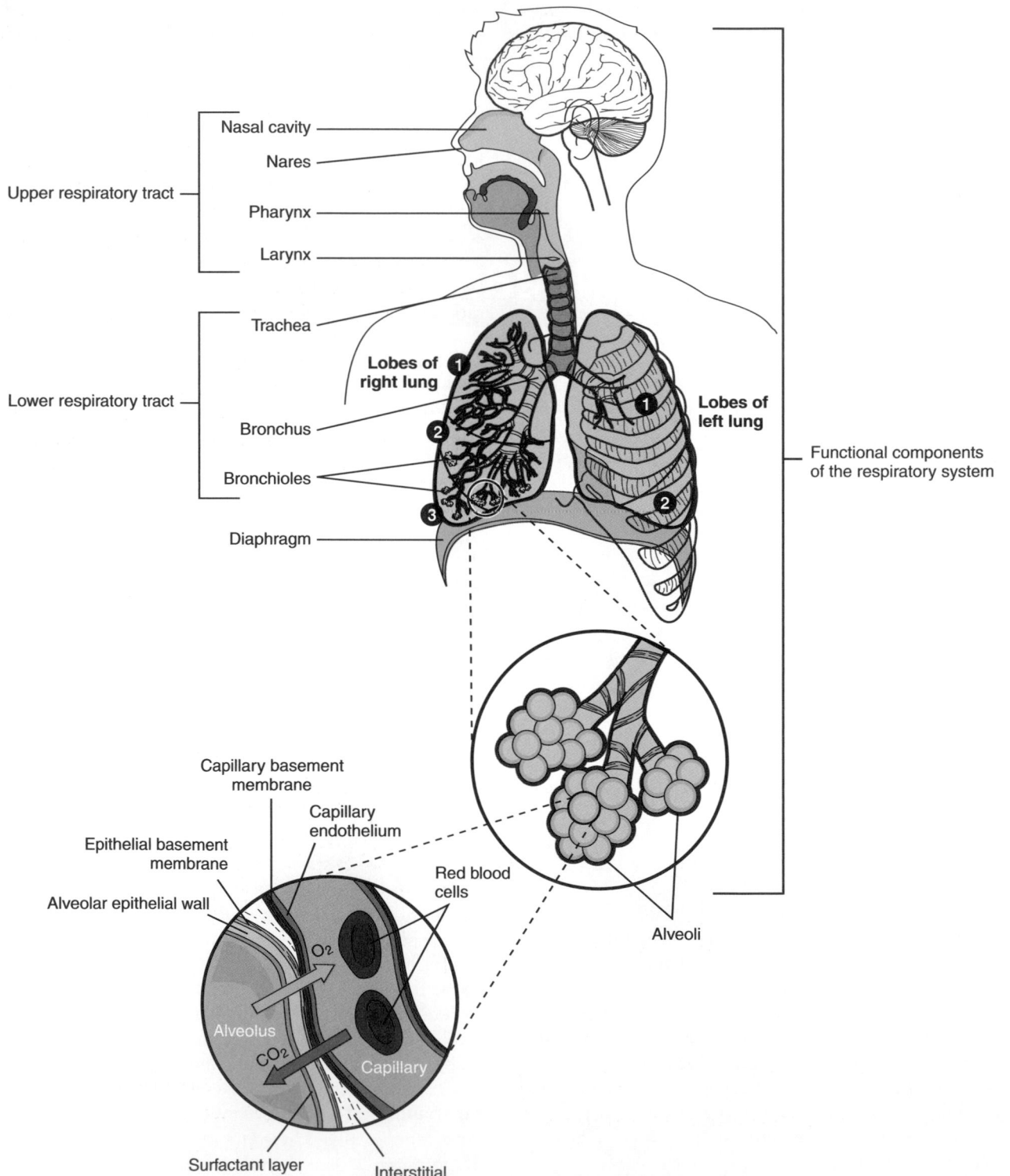

FIGURE 35-1 The anatomy of the pulmonary system is highly complex and interdependent.

Respiratory alterations can occur anytime throughout the life span: from the premature infant with insufficient surfactant production, to the emaciated teenager with anorexia nervosa, to the young adult with street-drug overdose, to the older adult with severe osteoporosis. Primary pulmonary system disorders include asthma, cystic fibrosis (CF), and emphysema. For best possible outcomes, medical nutrition therapy for all persons with pulmonary problems requires attention to the individual's nutrition status, nutritional intake, and other treatment procedures.

RELATIONSHIPS BETWEEN NUTRITION AND THE PULMONARY SYSTEM

Optimal Nutrition and the Pulmonary System

The respiratory structures include the nose, pharynx, larynx, trachea, bronchi, bronchioles, alveolar ducts, and alveoli. Supporting structures include the skeleton and the muscles (e.g., the intercostal, abdominal, and diaphragm muscles). Nerves, blood, and lymph supply all tissues (Figure 35-1). Within a month after conception pulmonary system structures are recognizable. The pulmonary system grows and matures during gestation and childhood. Aging results in diminished lung integrity.

Gas exchange is the major function of the pulmonary system (Figure 35-2). The lungs enable the body to obtain the oxygen needed to meet its cellular metabolic demands and to remove the carbon dioxide produced by these processes. The lungs also function to filter, warm, and humidify inspired air; synthesize surfactant; regulate body acid-base balance; synthesize arachidonic acid; and convert angiotensin I to angiotensin II.

The relationship between nutrition and lung immune defense mechanisms needs special highlight (Figure 35-3). First, inspired air is laden with particles and microorganisms. The mucus in the airways keeps the airways moist and traps the particles and microorganisms from inspired air. Most cells that line the trachea, bronchi, and bronchioles have cilia. These constantly beating cilia sweep the particles upward toward the pharynx. Each time a person swallows, the particle- and microorganism-containing mucus passes into the digestive tract. Second, the epithelial surface of the alveoli contains macrophages (Figure 35-4). By the process of phagocytosis, these alveolar macrophages engulf inhaled inert materials and microorganisms and digest them. Third, although the molecular mechanism of action is unknown, the antioxidant nutrients may protect lung tissues from oxidative injury.

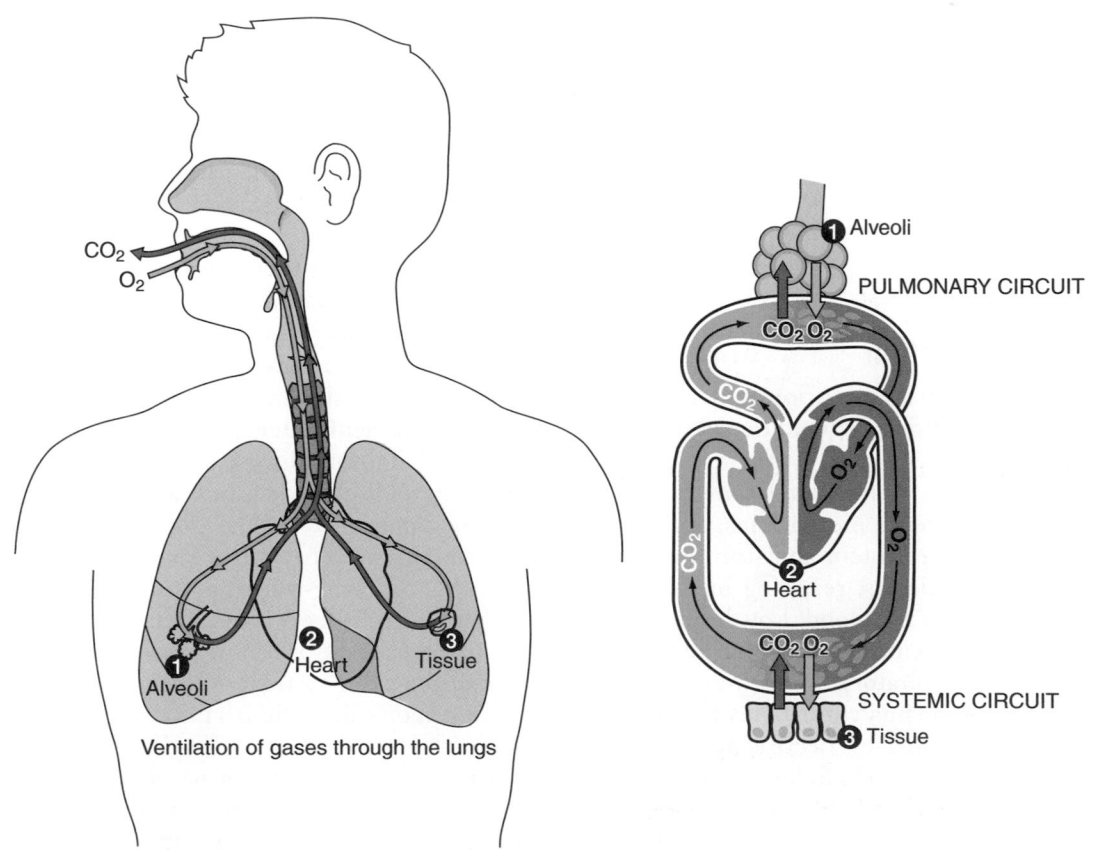

FIGURE 35-2 The major function of the respiratory tract is to provide the oxygen for cellular metabolism and to remove the carbon dioxide that is produced but not needed.

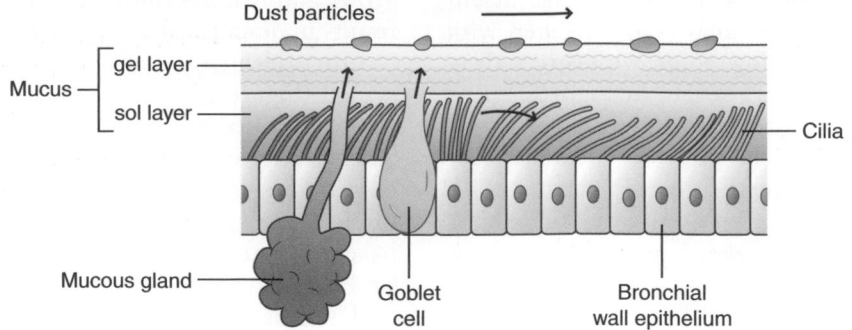

FIGURE 35-3 One of the roles of the respiratory tract is to function as a protective physical barrier against inhaled particles and microorganisms, preventing them from gaining entrance into the body. *(Modified from West JB:* Pulmonary pathophysiology: the essentials, *Baltimore, 1998, Williams & Wilkins.)*

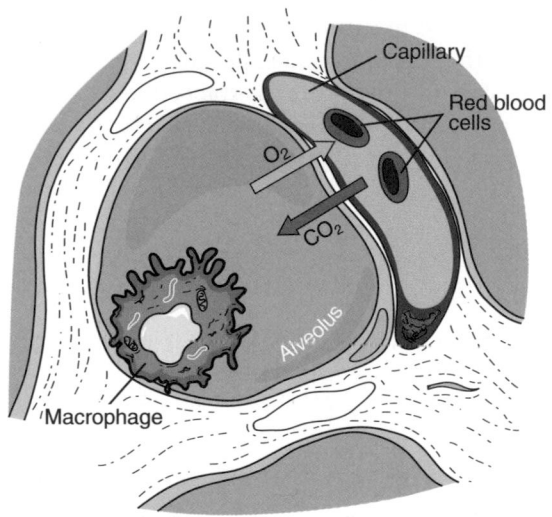

FIGURE 35-4 Alveolar macrophages are part of the body's systemic immune response. Macrophages are a main defense of the body against harmful cellular debris and microorganisms.

Impact of Malnutrition on the Pulmonary System

The relationship between malnutrition and respiratory disease has long been recognized (Gaultier et al., 1999). Malnutrition adversely affects lung structure, elasticity, and function; respiratory muscle mass, strength, and endurance; lung immune defense mechanisms; and control of breathing. For example, protein and iron deficiencies result in low hemoglobin levels, resulting in diminished oxygen-carrying capacity of the blood. Low levels of other minerals such as calcium, magnesium, phosphorus, and potassium compromise respiratory muscle function at the cellular level. Hypoproteinemia contributes to the development of pulmonary edema by decreasing colloid osmotic pressure, which allows body fluids to move into the interstitial space. Decreased levels of **surfactant,** a compound synthesized from proteins and phospholipids, contribute to the collapse of alveoli and thus increase the work of breathing. The supporting connective tissue of the lungs is composed of collagen, which requires vitamin C for its synthesis. Normal airway mucus is a substance consisting of water, glycoproteins, and electrolytes.

Weight loss from inadequate energy intake is significantly correlated with a poor prognosis in persons with pulmonary diseases. Malnutrition leading to impaired immunity places any patient at high risk for developing respiratory infections. Patients with pulmonary disease who are hospitalized and who are also malnourished are likely to have lengthy stays and are susceptible to increased morbidity and mortality.

Impact of Pulmonary System Disease on Nutrition Status

Pulmonary disease substantially increases energy requirements. This factor explains the rationale for including body composition and weight parameters in nearly all medical, surgical, pharmacologic, and nutrition research studies of people with respiratory diseases. The complications of pulmonary diseases or their treatments can make adequate intake and digestion difficult and absorption, circulation, cellular use, storage, and excretion of most nutrients problematic. Some adverse effects of lung disease on nutrition status are listed in Box 35-1.

Drug-nutrient interactions of medications commonly used in pulmonary disease, such as bronchodilators, antibiotics, steroids, and diuretics, are described in Chapter 16 and in Appendix 31. The nutritional implications of the medications need to be appreciated.

With the long-standing interest in natural remedies rather than reliance on manufactured pharmaceuticals, people use botanicals to treat respiratory ailments. For example, herbal remedies to treat symptomatically the cough from the common cold or flu fall into two groups: cough suppressants and expectorants. Cough suppressants include the volatile oils of eucalyptus or peppermint. These oils are added to lozenges to increase the production of saliva, thereby increasing the frequency of swallowing to suppress the cough reflex. Teas brewed from herbs are consumed for the mucilages they contain, which may form a protective

Cystic

ETIOLOGY

PATHOPHYSIOLOGY

MANAGEMENT

Obst

Secret
mucus

Med

• Ge
• Ora
• Ae
• Inh
• Ch

Algo
LDN

BOX 35-1

Adverse Effects of Lung Disease on Nutrition Status

Increased Energy Expenditure

Increased work of breathing
Chronic infection
Medical treatments (e.g., bronchodilators, chest physical therapy)

Reduced Intake

Fluid restriction
Shortness of breath
Decreased oxygen saturation when eating
Anorexia resulting from chronic disease
Gastrointestinal distress and vomiting

Additional Limitations

Difficulty preparing food because of fatigue
Lack of financial resources
Impaired feeding skills (for infants and children)
Altered metabolism

---

layer over the mucous membranes of the pharynx, larynx, and trachea. Expectorant herbs include anise, fennel, and thyme (see Chapter 18). This means that the clinician needs to ask about these therapies during the assessment of the patient (see Appendix 35).

OVERVIEW OF MEDICAL NUTRITION THERAPY IN PULMONARY DISEASE

Individualized nutrition assessment, nutrition diagnosis, and interventions such as nutrient delivery and counseling are integral components of care for each patient with pulmonary system disease. Pulmonary system disorders may be categorized as primary, such as tuberculosis (TB), bronchial asthma, and cancer of the lung, or secondary, such as those associated with cardiovascular disease, obesity, HIV infection, sickle cell disease, and scoliosis. Examples of acute conditions include aspiration of enteral feeding liquids, airway obstruction from foods like peanuts, and allergic anaphylaxis from consumption of shellfish. Examples of chronic conditions include CF and lung cancer. Table 35-1 categorizes some pulmonary conditions having nutritional implications.

To determine pulmonary status, the clinician uses the results of numerous diagnostic and monitoring tests such as imaging procedures, arterial blood gas determinations, sputum cultures, and biopsies. Also important are **pulmonary function tests,** a group of procedures designed to measure the ability of the respiratory system to exchange oxygen and carbon dioxide.

TABLE 35-1

Selected Pulmonary Conditions Having Nutritional Implications

Category	Examples
Neonatal	Bronchopulmonary dysplasia
	Chronic lung disease of prematurity
Obstructive	Cystic fibrosis
	Chronic obstructive pulmonary disease
	• Emphysema
	• Chronic bronchitis
	Asthma
	Aspiration (foreign body, food, fluid)
Tumor	Lung cancer
Infection	Pneumonia
	Tuberculosis
Respiratory failure	Acute respiratory failure
	Lung transplantation

Other System Abnormalities

Neuromuscular	Muscular dystrophy
Skeletal	Paralysis
	Osteoporosis
	Scoliosis
Cardiovascular	Pulmonary edema
Endocrine	Severe obesity
	Prader-Willi syndrome

Assessment of the cardiovascular, renal, neurologic, and hematologic systems also is important because diseases involving these systems often produce complications affecting pulmonary anatomy, physiology, and biochemistry.

Nutritionally relevant, common presenting signs and symptoms of pulmonary disease include cough, early satiety, anorexia, weight loss, **dyspnea** (shortness of breath) during preparing food and eating, and fatigue. As pulmonary disease progresses, other related conditions may interfere with food intake or overall nutrition status, especially abnormal production of sputum, vomiting, **tachypnea** (rapid breathing), hemoptysis, thoracic pain, nasal polyps, anemia, depression, and altered taste secondary to medications. Assessment of nutrition status is important and should precede any nutritional interventions or medical treatment unless the treatment is emergent (see Chapters 14-16).

ASPIRATION

Pulmonary aspiration, or the movement of food or fluid into the lungs, can result in pneumonia or even death. Proper body positioning when eating is essential for everyone. At increased risk are infants; toddlers; older adults; and persons with oral, upper gastrointestinal, neurologic, or muscular abnormalities. Besides liquids, foods that are most easily

sweat test, is perf
vated levels of so
lected sweat samp
diagnosis of CF ir
the presence of c
malabsorption, or
2006). Genotypir

CF can have a
(Constantine et a
have the diagno:
other causes. Abe
pancreatic insuff
quantity of dige:
into the small in
causes maldigest
Decreased bicar
tive enzyme activ
utes further to fa

The presence
nal tract may in
crovilli. Gastroi
smelling stools;
prolapse; and li
damage to the e
impaired glucos
diabetes mellitu

Medical Nut

Assessment

Individuals wit
digestion and
complications
creased nutrie:
intake and rete
and cough-ind
anorexia durir
sense of smell
and difficulty
common prob
demonstrate g
ally improves.
quate, growth
achieved (Ha
Management
As lung di
and weight fc
relationship
vival is not ki
long-term ba
factor to incr
Compreh
CF was first
1992 (Ramse
et al., 2002;
some compo
practice guic

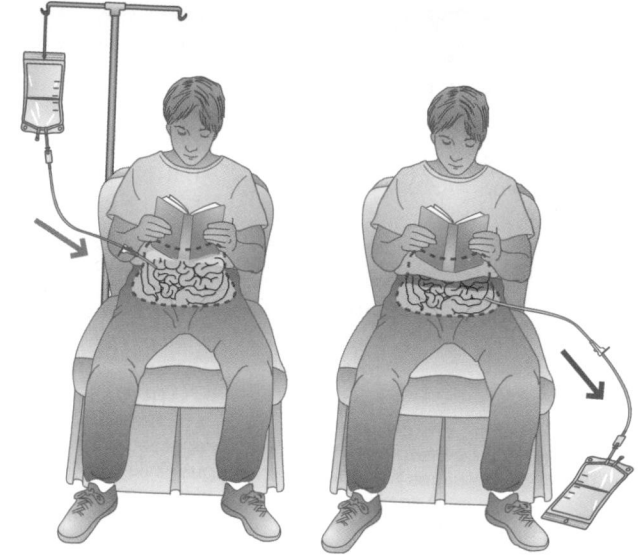

The peritoneal cavity is filled with dialysate, using gravity.

At the end of the exchange, the dialysate is drained into the bag, again using gravity.

FIGURE 36-6 Continuous ambulatory peritoneal dialysis; 20-minute exchanges are given four to five times daily every day.

availability of a hemodialysis helper to assist with therapy, type of water supply to the home, capability of the patient or involved family (including eyesight and ability to perform sterile technique), previous abdominal surgeries, membrane characteristics of the individual's peritoneal membrane, body size, cardiac status, presence of poor vascular access, desire to travel, and a host of other considerations.

Psychological Support

Patients with renal failure must deal not only with conflicting feelings about depending on artificial means of survival but also with changes in the quality of their lives and the necessity for adapting to a chronic, progressive illness. Control becomes a central issue because they must devote large quantities of time to dialysis, follow fairly strict dietary regimens, and take as many as 9 to 12 medications a day. Those who work with renal dialysis patients must be especially empathic to their feelings of depression, thirst, anorexia, and taste changes caused by uremia. Social workers are a part of the federally mandated dialysis team, and renal dietitians work closely with them.

Medical Nutrition Therapy

Goals of medical nutrition therapy in the management of ESRD are the following:

1. To prevent deficiency and maintain good nutrition status (and, in the case of children, growth) through adequate protein, energy, vitamin, and mineral intake
2. To control edema and electrolyte imbalance by controlling sodium, potassium, and fluid intake
3. To prevent or retard the development of renal osteodystrophy by controlling calcium, phosphorus, and vitamin D intake

4. To enable the patient to eat a palatable, attractive diet that fits his or her lifestyle as much as possible

Even with the development of dialysis methods and transplantation techniques, nutritional care remains essential to enhance dialysis, maintain optimal nutrition status, and prevent complications.

Because most treatment is outpatient or dialysis is done at home, almost all patients with ESRD assume responsibility for their diets. Most long-term patients know their diets very well (Figure 36-7), having been instructed many times by renal dietitians at their dialysis units. Patients who are relatively new to dialysis may require more intensive education. Regardless of length of time on dialysis, periodic professional counseling helps all patients who face long-term compliance with difficult diet regimens. Monitoring the patient's long-term nutrition status is an important role of the registered dietitian. Table 36-5 presents a guide for teaching patients about their blood values and control of their disease. The renal dietitian working in a dialysis unit is often responsible for coordinating the patient's nutritional care with RDs, nurses, and physicians working with the patient in acute-care facilities or skilled nursing facilities to ensure consistency of care.

Fluid and Sodium Balance

The kidney's ability to handle sodium and water in ESRD must be assessed frequently through measurement of blood pressure, presence of edema, amount of fluid weight gain, serum sodium level, and dietary intake. Sodium and fluid intake are then modified accordingly.

The vast majority of dialysis patients need to restrict intake of sodium, with a concomitant decrease in fluid intake (see Appendix 37). Excessive sodium intake is responsible for increased thirst, increased fluid gain, and resultant hypertension. Even those patients who do not experience these symptoms but put out minimum urine will benefit from a reduced sodium intake to limit their thirst and prevent large intradialytic fluid gains (Ahmad, 2004).

In the patient who is maintained on hemodialysis, sodium and fluid intake are regulated to allow for a weight gain of 4 to 5 lb (2 to 3 kg) from increased fluid in the vasculature between dialyses. This is about 2% to 5% of body weight. A sodium intake of 87 to 130 mEq (2 to 3 g) daily and a limit on fluid intake (usually about 1000 ml/day plus the amount equal to the urine output) is usually sufficient to meet these guidelines. Only fluids that are liquid at room temperature are included in this calculation. The fluid contained in solid foods is not included in the 1000-ml limit. Solid foods in the average diet contribute approximately 500 to 800 ml/day of fluid. This fluid in solid food is calculated to approximately replace the 500 ml/day net insensible water loss as shown in Table 36-1.

Fluid and sodium requirements can increase in the presence of perspiration, vomiting, or fever. Hypotension and the possibility of clotting at the shunt site from over restriction of fluid and sodium intake must be avoided, although this rarely occurs unless patients on CCPD are not eating at

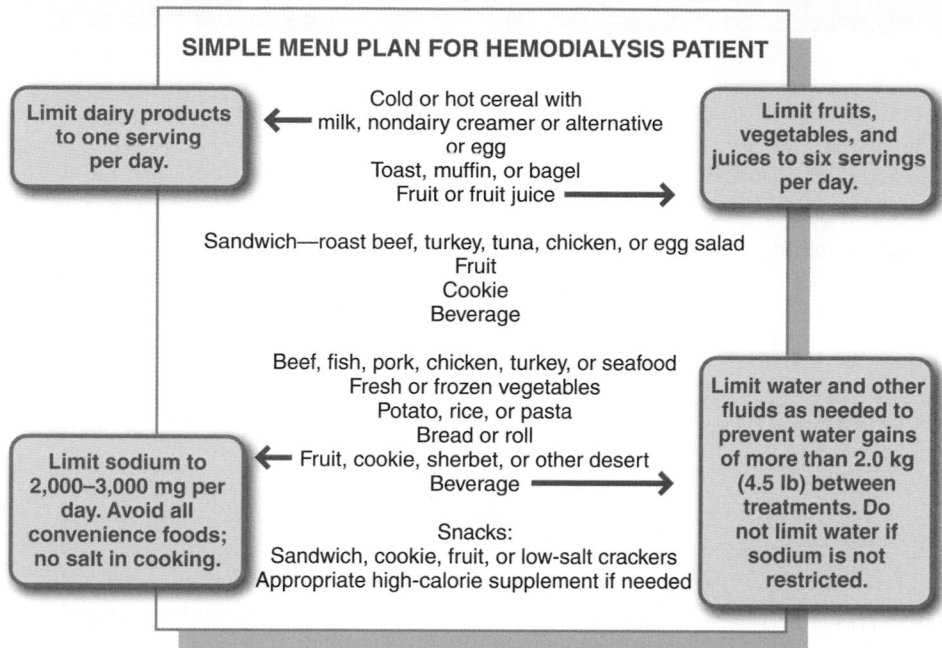

FIGURE 36-7 A simple menu plan for a patient on hemodialysis. The diet should allow for less than 4% fluid weight gain between dialyses.

all. Patients who have severe gastropathy or other fluid and electrolyte losses such as ileostomy or colostomy are much more at risk for these problems.

An 86- to 130-mEq (2 to 3 g) sodium diet allows for no salt in cooking; no salt at the table; no salted, smoked, or cured meat or fish; and no salted snack foods, canned soups, or high-sodium convenience foods. In today's increasing convenience food–oriented marketplace, it is estimated that 75% to 90% of patients' sodium intake is consumed in convenience foods, with only 10% to 25% added to foods in cooking or at the table. It is important to remember that the easiest way to reduce the renal patient's thirst and fluid intake is to decrease sodium intake (Rigby et al., 2000). Appendix 37 gives the details of a low-sodium meal plan.

Remembering that the underlying cause of thirst and high fluid gains is a high sodium intake, when educating about fluid balance, the health care provider must teach the patient how to deal with thirst without drinking. Sucking on a few ice chips, cold sliced fruit, or sour candies; using artificial saliva; or chewing "sports gum" that contains citric acid may help to alleviate the dryness. Patients must be taught to measure their fluid intake and urine output, examine their ankles for edema, weigh themselves regularly each morning, and record their weight. Occasionally (in about 15% to 20% of patients) hypertension is not alleviated even after meticulous attention to fluid and water balance. In these patients hypertension is usually perpetuated by a high level of renin secretion and requires medication for control.

Although most patients with ESRD retain sodium, a small number may lose it. Examples of conditions with a salt-losing tendency are polycystic disease of the kidney, medullary kidney disease, chronic obstructive uropathy, chronic pyelonephritis, and analgesic nephropathy. To prevent hypotension, hypovolemia, cramps, and further deterioration of renal function, extra sodium may be required. A diet for these types of patients may contain 130 mEq (3 g) or more of sodium per day, which is the amount in a normal diet without added salt. Adding salt or salty foods can satisfy the need for extra sodium. The number of patients who require this higher sodium intake is small, but these patients exemplify the need for individual consideration of the diet prescription and a thorough understanding of the patient's underlying disease and present diet.

Potassium

Potassium (K^+) usually requires restriction, depending on the individual's body size, the serum K^+ level, urine output, and the frequency of hemodialysis. The daily intake of potassium for most Americans is 75 to 100 mEq (3 to 4 g). This is usually reduced in ESRD to 60 to 80 mEq (2.3 to 3.1 g)/day and is reduced for the anuric patient on dialysis to 51 mEq (2 g)/day. Some patients (i.e., those on high-flux dialysis or with increased dialysis times or frequencies) will be able to tolerate higher intakes. Again, a close monitoring of the patient's laboratory values, K^+ content of the dialysate, and dietary intake is invaluable.

The potassium content of foods is listed in Box 4-1 in Chapter 4, and in Appendixes 36 and 56. When counseling hemodialysis patients on a low-potassium diet, one should take care to point out that some low-sodium foods contain potassium chloride (KCl) as a salt substitute rather than sodium chloride (NaCl). Salt substitutes, LiteSalt, and low-sodium herb mixtures must all be checked carefully to be sure they do not contain dangerous levels of potassium. Low-sodium soy sauces, sauerkraut, and other special dietary products may need particular review by a trained professional. Reviewing such practices not only with the patient but with other people who may be cooking for the patient such as a church group or neighbors who may use salt substitutes in the mistaken belief they are helping the patient avoid salt is also advisable.

Text continues p. 940.

TABLE 36-5

Guide to Blood Values

This guide is to help in understanding laboratory reports. In the following table, the normal values are for people with good kidney function. Acceptable values for dialysis patients are also given.

Many things affect blood values. Diet is only one of these. Underlying disease, adequacy of treatment, medications, and complications all may affect laboratory values.

Substance	Normal Values	Normal for People on Dialysis	Function	Diet Changes
Sodium	135-145 mEq/L	Same	Found in salt and many preserved foods. A diet high in sodium makes the patient thirsty. When patients drink too much fluid, it may actually dilute their sodium, and serum levels will be low. If patients eat too much sodium and do not drink water, sodium may be high. Too much sodium and water raise blood pressure and can cause fluid overload, pulmonary edema, and congestive heart failure.	High: Check fluid status. If high fluid gains, tell patient to eat fewer salty foods (give sodium brochure). If low fluid gains, make sure patient is gaining about 1.5 kg between runs (or <4% body weight) and are not dehydrated (this is rare). Low: If high fluid gains, tell patient to eat less salt and fluid. Check fluid status—patient is probably drinking too much fluid. Limit weight gains to under 4% of body weight between runs, and ask patient to eat fewer salty foods (give sodium brochure) and to limit fluid to 3 c plus urine output (give fluid brochure).
Potassium	3.5-5.5 mEq/L	3.5-5.5 mEq/L	Found in most high-protein foods, fruits, and vegetables. It affects muscle action, especially the heart. High levels can cause the heart to stop. Low levels can cause symptoms such as muscle weakness and atrial fibrillation.	High: Ascertain that no other causes, such as gastrointestinal bleeding, trauma, or medications are creating high potassium values. Tell patient to avoid foods with over 250 mg/serving and limit daily intake to 2000 mg. Consider lowering potassium in dialysate bath. Recheck blood level next treatment. Low: Add one high-potassium food/day, and recheck blood level (give potassium brochure). Consider raising potassium in dialysate bath if diet changes are not working.
Urea nitrogen (blood urea nitrogen [BUN])	7-23 mg/dl	50-100 mg/dl	Waste product of protein breakdown. Unlike creatinine, this is affected by the amount of protein in the diet. Dialysis removes urea nitrogen.	High: Patient is probably underdialyzed. Check eKT/V. Check nPNA. Low: Underdialysis is also a cause. BUN may decrease if patient is not eating because of uremic symptoms. May also decrease with loss of muscle.

Developed by Katy G. Wilkens, MS, RD, Northwest Kidney Centers, Seattle, Washington.
N/A, Not applicable.

TABLE 36-5

Guide to Blood Values—cont'd

Substance	Normal Values	Normal for People on Dialysis	Function	Diet Changes
Creatinine	0.6-1.5 mg/dl	Less than 15 mg/dl	A normal waste product of muscle breakdown. This value is controlled by dialysis. Patients have a higher amount because the patient is not dialyzing 24 hours a day, 7 days a week, like the normal kidney does.	Dialysis normally controls creatinine. Low creatinine may indicate good dialysis or low body muscle. Check the clearance of urea during dialysis (KT/V) to assess dialysis adequacy. If the patient is losing weight, he or she breaks down more muscle, so creatinine may be higher. The patient may need to eat more protein and calories to stop weight loss.
Urea reduction ratio (URR)	N/A	Above 65% (or 0.65)	A measure of reduction of urea that occurs during a dialysis treatment. Postdialysis BUN is subtracted and divided by predialysis BUN to give a percentage.	No diet changes, but catabolism or anabolism will affect values, as with KT/V and equilibrated clearance of urea during dialysis (eKT/V).
eKT/V	N/A	Above 1.2	A mathematic formula that attempts to quantify how well a patient is dialyzed. Represents the clearance of urea by the dialyzer, multiplied by the minutes of treatment, and divided by the volume of water the patient's body carries.	No diet changes. Low: Values below 1.2 are associated with increased morbidity and mortality. High: Higher values are associated with better outcomes.
KT/V		Above 1.4: hemodialysis Above 2: peritoneal dialysis	Not adjusted for urea quilibration	No diet changes.
Normalized protein-nitrogen appearance (nPNA)	N/A	0.8-1.4	A calculation used to look at the rate of protein turnover in the body. Assumes the patient is not catabolic because of infection, fever, surgery, or trauma. Can be a good indicator of stable patient's protein intake, when combined with dietary history and albumin. The term *normalized* means that values have been adjusted to the patient's "normal" or ideal weight.	High: Patient may need to decrease protein intake. Have patient consult with nutritionist. Patient may be catabolic. Patient may be eating large amounts of protein. Low: Patient may need to increase protein intake. If patient is putting out urine, a small urine volume can make a big difference in results. Have patient keep a 48-hour urine collection (give patient protein brochure).

Continued

TABLE 36-5

Guide to Blood Values—cont'd

Substance	Normal Values	Normal for People on Dialysis	Function	Diet Changes
Albumin	3.5-5 g/dl (bromcresol green)	Same	Albumin is a protein made in the liver. It is a good measure of health. Protein is lost with all dialysis. If albumin is below 2.9, fluid will "leak" from blood vessels into the tissue, thus causing edema. When fluid is in the tissue, it is more difficult to remove with dialysis.	Low: Increase intake of protein-rich foods; meat, fish, chicken, eggs (give patient protein brochure). A protein supplement may be needed. Intravenous albumin corrects short-term problems with oncotic pressure but does not change serum albumin levels.
	3-4.5 g/dl (bromcresol purple)	Above 3.4 g/dl	Low albumin is closely associated with increased risk of death in dialysis patients.	
Calcium	8.5-10.5 mg/dl	8.5-10.5 mg/dl	Found in dairy products and in some green vegetables. Dialysis patients' intakes are usually low. The body uses it to help muscle movement and build bones. Active vitamin D is needed for absorption. The calcium value multiplied by the phosphorus value should not exceed 59, or patient will get calcium deposits in soft tissue. Because it is bound to albumin, calcium can be falsely lower if albumin is low. Ionized calcium is a more accurate test in this case.	High: Check with doctor if patient is taking calcium supplement or active vitamin D (DHT, Rocaltrol, Hectorol, Calcijex, Zemplar). These should be temporarily stopped. Low: If albumin is low, suggest an ionized calcium be drawn. Patient may need a calcium supplement between meals and/or active vitamin D. Check with physician.
Phosphorus	2.5-4.8 mg/dl	3-6 mg/dl	Found in milk products, dried beans, nuts, and meats. It is used to build bones and helps the body produce energy. Acceptable levels depend on a variety of factors, including calcium, parathyroid hormone (PTH) levels, and the level of phosphorus in the diet. If calcium and PTH levels are normal, a slightly higher-than-normal level of phosphorus is acceptable.	High: Limit milk and milk products to 1 serving per day. Remind patient to take phosphate binders as ordered with meals and snacks. Noncompliance with binders is the most common cause of high phosphorus. Low: Add 1 serving milk product or other high-phosphorus food per day or decrease phosphate binders.

TABLE 36-5

Guide to Blood Values—cont'd

Substance	Normal Values	Normal for People on Dialysis	Function	Diet Changes
PTH intact (I—PTH)	10-65 pg/ml	200-300 pg/ml	A high level of PTH indicates that calcium is being pulled out of bone to maintain serum calcium levels. This syndrome is called secondary hyperparathyroidism and can lead to osteodystrophy. Pulsed doses of oral or intravenous (IV) vitamin D usually lowers PTH.	High: Check whether patient is taking oral or IV active vitamin D. Contact patient's physician regarding therapy. If patient has no symptoms (high phosphorus, bone pain, fractures), treat less aggressively. Low: No treatment available.
Aluminum	0-10 mcg/L	Less than 40 mcg/L	Patients taking aluminum hydroxide phosphate binders may develop aluminum toxicity, which can cause bone disease and dementia. Value should be checked every 6 months.	High: Discontinue aluminum hydroxide treatment. Some patients benefit from deferoxamine treatment, but this also has complications.
Magnesium	1.5-2.4 mg/dl	Same	Magnesium is normally excreted in the urine and can become toxic to dialysis patient. High levels may be caused by antacids or laxatives that contain magnesium such as Milk of Magnesia or Maalox.	No dietary changes, except to use nontoxic methods such as fiber to aid in constipation. Magnesium can also be used as a phosphate binder; if so, levels will need to be checked more often.
Ferritin	Male: 20-350 mcg/L Female: 6-350 mcg/L	>300-800 mcg/L with erythropoietin (EPO); 50 mcg/L without EPO	This is the way iron is stored in the liver. If iron stores are low, red blood cell production is decreased.	Low: Iron in food is not well absorbed. Most patients need an oral and/or IV iron supplement. Patients should not take iron at same time as phosphate binders.
CO_2 (carbon dioxide)		22-25 mEq/L	Dialysis patients are often acidotic because they do not excrete metabolic acids in their urine. Acidosis may increase the rate of muscle and bone catabolism.	Low: Review eKT/V, BUN, nPNA. Oral sodium bicarbonate may be given to raise CO_2, but it presents a significant sodium load to patient.
Glucose	65-114 mg/dl	Same for nondiabetic patients Less than 300 mg/dl (patients with diabetes)	This sugar in the blood is made from starches and sugar in the diet. The body uses glucose for energy. Because the kidney metabolizes insulin, low blood sugar levels caused by a longer half-life of insulin are possible. For patients with diabetes: a high blood sugar may increase thirst.	Most people need 6 to 11 servings of breads/starches or cereals per day and 2 to 4 servings of fruit per day to provide energy. Patients with diabetes should avoid concentrated sweets, unless blood sugar level is low.

When a thorough diet history does not reveal the source of an increased intake of potassium and a reason for elevated serum potassium, other nondietetic sources of potassium should be researched. Examples include poor dialysis adequacy or missed dialysis treatments, too high a concentration of potassium in the dialysate bath, very elevated blood sugar in patients with diabetes, acidosis, significant gastrointestinal bleeding, some medications, blood transfusions, major trauma, chemotherapy, or radiation therapy. Occasionally blood samples may have been handled improperly, resulting in a hemolyzed sample and elevated potassium; thus laboratory comments should be carefully reviewed.

Protein

Dialysis is a drain on body protein, and the daily intake should be increased to compensate for this. Protein losses of 20 to 30 g can occur during a 24-hour PD, with an average of 1 g/hr. Hourly losses in hemodialysis are similar. Patients who receive hemodialysis three times per week require a daily protein intake of 1.2 g/kg of body weight. Patients receiving PD need 1.2 to 1.5 g/kg of body weight. At least 50% should be HBV protein. Studies of patients on dialysis indicate that those with low albumin levels have a much higher mortality rate; consequently emphasis is placed on adequate protein intake (Jones et al., 2002). Protein requirements for patients on different types of dialysis are summarized in Table 36-4. Serum blood urea nitrogen and serum creatinine levels, uremic symptoms, and weight should be monitored; and the diet should be adjusted accordingly (see *Clinical Insight: When Protein Supplements Are Not Healthful*).

Serum albumin is a poor indicator of protein status; acute or chronic inflammation limits its specificity in renal failure. A decreased serum albumin level is predictive of poor survival in ESRD; however, the cause of hypoalbuminemia is multifactorial and related to poor nutrition, inflammation, and comorbid disease (Cooper et al., 2004; Jones et al., 2002). In addition, when interpreting albumin values, it is important to know the laboratory's methodology for measuring serum albumin (see Table 36-5).

Most patients find it challenging to consume adequate protein and still have a palatable diet. In addition, the uremia itself causes some taste aberrations, notably to red meats, sometimes making it difficult to achieve the HBV percentage.

Kinetic Modeling

A method for evaluating the efficacy of dialysis relies on measuring the removal of urea from the patient's blood over a given period of time. This method, often called **KT/V** (where *K* is the urea clearance of the dialyzer, *T* is the length of time of dialysis, and *V* is the patient's total body water volume), should ideally produce a result higher than 1.4 per dialysis, or 3.2 per week. These calculations are somewhat complex and are typically calculated using a computer program. A more accurate method for determining adequacy of dialysis is the eKT/V where *e* stands for *equilibrated* and takes into account the amount of time it takes for urea to

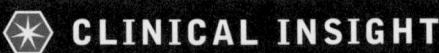

CLINICAL INSIGHT

When Protein Supplements Are Not Healthful

The use of protein supplements, especially amino acid supplements, commonly called "aminos," has become popular lately. They seem harmless because they "are naturally" from protein—and for most people they probably are. But for those with preend-stage or end-stage renal failure, these supplements can be toxic. Because the kidney metabolizes and excretes amino acids, the amino acid profile in renal failure is quite different from that of people who produce good-quality urine. Supplements such as glucosamine, arginase and arginine, lysine, creatine, glutamine, and others may act as toxins in the bodies of patients who cannot metabolize and excrete them. No studies have evaluated these products in patients on dialysis, and use of them should also be discouraged in patients with preend-stage or chronic kidney disease because they could be harmful.

equilibrate across cell membranes after dialysis has stopped. An acceptable eKT/V is 1.2 or greater.

Another method to determine effective dialysis treatment is the **urea reduction ratio,** which looks at the reduction in urea before and after dialysis. The patient is considered well dialyzed when a 65% or greater reduction in the serum urea occurs during dialysis. Unlike KT/V, this calculation can be done quickly at the patient's bedside by the practitioner.

The method for calculating the efficacy of PD is somewhat different, but a weekly KT/V of 2.0 is the goal. The KT/V can be altered by several patient- and dialysis-associated variables. The calculations for KT/V can also be used to determine the patient's protein-nitrogen appearance (PNA) rate, which is a simplified nitrogen balance test in the dialysis patient. The PNA values should be between 0.8 and 1.4.

Energy

Energy intake must be adequate to spare protein for tissue protein synthesis and to prevent its metabolism for energy (Byham-Gray, 2006). Depending on the patient's nutrition status and degree of stress, between 25 and 40 kcal/kg of body weight should be provided, with the lower amount for transplantation and PD patients and the higher level for the nutritionally depleted patient (Neyra et al., 2003). Tools have been developed to allow the renal dietitian to assess the quality of the patient's nutrition status using the Subjective Global Assessment. This technique has been modified because of the special circumstances surrounding basic physiologic and immunologic changes in ESRD (Kalantar-Zadeh et al., 1999).

Calcium, Phosphorus, and Vitamin D

A major complication of ESRD is metabolic bone disease, or **renal osteodystrophy.** The disease is essentially of three types: osteomalacia, or bone demineralization; osteitis fibrosa cystica, caused by hyperparathyroidism; and metastatic calcification of joints and soft tissues. A fourth type of bone disease, unique to renal failure patients treated with active vitamin D is **low turnover bone disease,** in which oversuppression of the parathyroid gland with too much active vitamin D causes decreased bone formation and fragile bones with very little matrix.

As the GFR decreases, phosphorus, the level of which is controlled by renal excretion, is retained in the plasma. The serum calcium level declines for several reasons. Decreased $1,25\text{-}(OH)_2D_3$, brought about by decreased ability of the kidney to convert the inactive form, appears to be most important. In addition, the calcium-phosphate product, which increases as phosphate increases, leads to extraosseous calcifications throughout the body at a calcium $\times$ phosphorus product greater than 55, and ultimately brings about a decreased calcium level.

The low calcium level triggers several mechanisms by which the healthy body increases calcium to normal. These include the release of PTH from the parathyroid glands as well as increased synthesis of the active form of vitamin D by the kidney. This in turn acts on the gut to increase absorption of both calcium and phosphate and, in concert with PTH, acts to increase bone resorption, thus liberating both calcium and phosphate. Because of the large molecular weight of the phosphate molecule, it is not easily removed by dialysis, and patients experience a net "gain" of about one half of the phosphate they consume daily (Pohlmeir and Vienken, 2001).

PTH, sometimes called parathormone, also acts on the kidney to increase secretion of phosphate while retaining extra calcium. With decreased ability to produce $1,25\text{-}(OH)_2D_3$, the patient with failing kidneys cannot increase gut absorption of calcium and therefore must rely on the effects of PTH to keep calcium levels up through bone resorption. Thus the dependence of calcium-phosphate control on increasing levels of PTH leads to a characteristic hyperplastic demineralized bone disease, **osteitis fibrosa cystica,** characterized by dull, aching bone pain.

Even though the serum calcium level is elevated in response to PTH, the serum phosphate concentration remains high as the GFR falls lower. If the product of the serum calcium level (mg/100 ml) multiplied by the serum phosphate level (mg/100 ml) is greater than 70, metastatic calcification is imminent. Clinical management aims to keep the product below 55 by preventing transient elevations in serum phosphate concentration (Block and Port, 2000; Block et al., 2004).

In essence, calcium and phosphorus intake must be controlled to as great a degree as possible to avoid aggravation of the delicate situation posed by hyperparathyroidism, phosphate retention, and hypocalcemia in renal failure. In practical terms calcium intake is kept high, and phosphorus intake is kept low. This is a problem as far as food is concerned because most high-calcium foods (milk and milk products) are also high in phosphorus (see Appendix 36). In addition, a high-protein diet, recommended because of protein losses during dialysis, is also of necessity high in phosphorus. Consequently patients must rely on medications in addition to dietary manipulation to reduce their phosphate levels.

Phosphate intake is lowered by restricting dietary sources to 1200 mg/day or less. A better way to estimate phosphorus restriction is to allow about 17 mg per kilogram of body weight per day. The difficulty in implementing the phosphorus restriction comes because of the necessity of a high-protein diet. All metabolically active tissue such as animal muscle contains high levels of phosphorus, found in the form of ATP; thus limiting phosphorus causes a limit in protein intake. At certain body weight and protein needs, the amount of phosphorous contributed by protein in the diet may exceed the phosphorus recommendation. The following regression equation exists for estimating phosphorus intake based on protein intake:

$$128 + 14 \text{ (grams of protein in the diet)} =$$
$$\text{milligrams of phosphorus per day in the diet}$$

In addition, the American diet, which contains more and more processed food has increased in type and amount of phosphorus that is available for absorption, thus making compliance even more difficult (Uribarri and Calvo, 2003).

Dietary restrictions alone are not adequate to control serum phosphorus, and nearly all patients who undergo dialysis require phosphate-binding medication. In the past aluminum hydroxide products such as Basaljel and Amphojel were used, but the resulting aluminum toxicity in many ESRD patients has caused this treatment largely to be abandoned. However, current medication treatment still relies on the use of agents to bind phosphorus in the gut. Calcium carbonate, acetate, lactate, or gluconate are routinely used with each meal or snack. Calcium citrate is avoided because of its ability to increase aluminum absorption.

A complication of use of these calcium-based binders with concomitant use of active vitamin D is hypercalcemia. Because of this some clinicians have returned to limited short-term use of aluminum binders in combination with calcium-based binders and sometimes even magnesium-based binders. Obviously serum levels of aluminum and magnesium need to be watched closely in these patients. A different type of binder, sevelamer hydrochloride (Renagel), a phosphate-binding resin, is able to reduce serum phosphorus without raising serum calcium because of its composition. However, this medication usually requires more doses of medication, and the pill burden to patients may interfere with compliance (Tomasello et al., 2004). Lanthanum carbonate, (Fosrenol), is another binder that is significantly less absorbable than aluminum. Gastrointestinal upset is one of the side effects of most phosphate binders and may also interfere with compliance (Shaw-Stewart and Stuart, 2000).

Side effects of taking large doses of all of these medications over long periods of time are common. Several types may cause gastrointestinal distress, diarrhea or gas (Table 36-6). Severe constipation, leading to intestinal impaction, is a potential risk of excessive consumption of some types of

TABLE 36-6

Common Medications for Patients with ESRD

1. Phosphate Binders
- Taken with meals and snacks to prevent dietary phosphorus absorption

Calcium carbonate	TUMS, Os-Cal, Calci-Chew, Calci-Mix
Calcium acetate	PhosLo
Mg/Ca^{++} carbonate	MagneBind
Sevelamer hydrochloride	Renagel
Lanthanum carbonate	Fosrenol
Aluminum hydroxide	AlternaGEL

2. Vitamins
- Increased need for water-soluble vitamins because of losses during dialysis
- Fat-soluble vitamins A, D, and K are not supplemented
- Vitamin E may be supplemented

Dialysis Recommendations:

Vitamin C	60 mg (not to exceed 200 mg daily)
Folic acid	1 mg
Thiamin	1.5 mg
Riboflavin	1.7 mg
Niacin	20 mg
Vitamin B$_6$	10 mg
Vitamin B$_{12}$	6 mcg
Pantothenic acid	10 mg
Biotin	0.3 mg

Brand names include Nephrocap, Neph-ron FA, Nephplex, Renal Caps, Tabron, and Dialtxy

3. Intradialytic Parenteral Nutrition (IDPN)
- Glucose, amino acid, and lipid solution infused during hemodialysis. Solution may include:

CHO	70% dextrose
Protein	15% amino acids
Lipid	20% lipid
Multivitamin	10 ml MVI-12 infusion

- Fluid volume is removed during the run
- Insulin often is given for hyperglycemia

4. Iron
- Iron needs are increased because of EPO therapy

IV iron	Iron dextran (Infed), Aron gluconate (Ferrlecit), iron sucrose (Venofer)

5. Erythropoietin
- Stimulates bone marrow to produce red blood cells

IV or IM	Epogen or EPO

6. Activated Vitamin D
- Used for the management of hyperparathyroidism

Oral	Calcitriol (Rocaltrol), doxercalciferol (Hectorol)
IV	Calcitriol (Calcijex), Paricalcitriol (Zemplar)

7. Biphosphonates
- Inhibit bone resorption by blocking osteoclasts

Oral	Alendronate (Fosamax)
IV	Pamidronate (Aredia)

8. Calcium Supplements
TUMS, Os-Cal, Calci-Chew

9. Phosphorus Supplements
Kphos, NutraPhos, NutraPhos K

10. Cinacalcet (Sensipar)
Calcimimetics
- Mimic calcium and binds to parathyroid gland

11. Heavy Metal Chelator
- Binds aluminum and iron and is dialyzed off

IV	Desferal (deferoxamine or DFO)

12. Cation Exchange Resin
- For the treatment of hyperkalemia

Oral or rectal	Sodium polystyrene sulfonate or SPS (Kayexalate)

Developed by Fiona Wolf, RD, and Thomas Montemayor, RPh, Northwest Kidney Centers, Seattle, Washington, 2006.
EPO, Epoetin; *ESRD,* end-stage renal disease; *IV,* intravenous.

phosphate binders. Occasionally this may lead to perforation of the intestine, resulting in peritonitis and death. Constipation is often the reason patients do not take prescribed phosphate binders. Suggestions for using bran or other high-fiber foods and regular light exercise may contribute to patient compliance. Bulking agents such as Citrucel and Metamucil are low in phosphorus and potassium and are often used; however, they require extra fluid mixed with them, which needs to be considered. Doss (Docusate sodium, Badrivishal Chemicals) or MiraLax (Braintree Laboratories) are also acceptable for use with ESRD patients, since their use does not require additional fluid.

As with calcium supplementation, the early initiation of phosphate reduction therapies is advantageous for delaying hyperparathyroidism and bone disease. Phosphate is elevated fairly early in renal failure, but often serum phosphate is not monitored. Unfortunately most patients are asymptomatic during the early phase of hyperparathyroidism and hyperphosphatemia and are not attentive about following a modified diet and taking calcium supplements and phosphate binders with meals. The active participation of a renal dietitian can be invaluable to the patient at this stage.

Because of potential hypermagnesemia, which can exacerbate the already existent bone disease, magnesium-containing antacids such as Maalox, Gelusil, Milk of Magnesia, or Mylanta should not be used. Often patients in skilled nursing facilities may be receiving these at their request; thus a review of PRN medications with the staff is appropriate.

The dual problems of hypocalcemia and hyperphosphatemia can be complex in renal failure. Added to this milieu is the fact that calcium is present in the dialysate bath. The amount can be adjusted to help stabilize low calcium values or to decrease serum calcium in patients who have developed hypercalcemia from active vitamin D administration. Patients who receive too large a calcium load may develop **calciphylaxis,** which occurs when calcium phosphate is deposited in soft tissues. The challenge becomes balancing the patient's need for phosphate binders without causing deposition in soft tissues.

Calcium intake is increased with calcium supplements in the form of calcium carbonate (e.g., Tums), calcium acetate (PhosLo), lactate, malate, or gluconate, along with the 300 to 500 mg calcium provided in the diet. These supplements are given between meals to increase calcium absorption. Starting calcium supplementation early is more likely to prevent hyperparathyroidism.

Many patients on dialysis suffer from hypocalcemia, despite calcium supplementation. Because of this the routine drug of choice is active vitamin D, 1,25-$(OH)_2D_3$ (Maung et al., 2001), which is available as calcitriol (Rocaltrol [Roche Labs] and Calcijex [Abbott Labs]). Analogs such as Hectorol and Zemplar are also all effective in lowering PTH and raising calcium levels with less enhancement of gut absorption of calcium than the 1,25 forms. Other mechanisms for controlling PTH include the medication Cinacalcet (Sensipar), a calcimimetic or calcium-imitating drug that binds to sites on the parathyroid gland and gives the gland a false impression that calcium levels are elevated (Block et al., 2004). The drug is very effective in suppressing PTH production and may also lower calcium levels dramatically, which can be a useful feature, but close monitoring is essential (Slatopolsky et al., 2000).

For effective phosphorus control patients must be responsible for following a low-phosphate diet; for taking calcium or some other binder with all food to bind phosphate in the meals; and for maintaining compliance with their dialysis regime, since about one half of daily phosphate consumption is removed by dialysis.

Iron

The hypoproliferative, normochromic, normocytic anemia of chronic renal failure usually stabilizes with dialysis; however, it manifests itself in complaints of fatigue. It is caused by both an inability of the kidney to produce EPO, a hormone that stimulates the bone marrow to produce red blood cells, and an increased destruction of red blood cells secondary to circulating uremic waste products.

A synthetic form of EPO, recombinant human EPO (rHuEPO), is used to treat the anemia of ESRD. Clinical trials have demonstrated a dramatic effect in correcting anemia and restoring a general sense of well-being. Initial use of EPO may occasionally cause a rise in serum K^+. Whether this is caused by increased blood viscosity impairing dialysis, increased breakdown of erythrocytes causing increased K^+, or an increase in the patient's appetite resulting from an increased sense of well-being is unclear. The patient who does not respond to rHuEPO therapy may be malnourished or in a state of stress or inflammation; this should be evaluated further (Locatelli et al., 2006).

Patients should be monitored closely while the EPO dose is adjusted, and they may need increased dialysis or a lower level of K^+ in the dialysate bath. Almost always accompanying the rise in hematocrit is an increased need for iron that requires supplementation intravenously. Oral iron alone is not effective in maintaining adequate iron stores in patients who take EPO. Unless a documented allergic reaction exists, almost all patients taking EPO require periodic IV or intramuscular iron. For patients who are allergic to IV iron, several much better–tolerated forms are now available. Iron dextran (Infed), iron gluconate (Ferrlecit), and iron sucrose (Venofer) are examples.

For a small minority of patients, oral iron is the only alternative and is usually given as 325 mg of $Feso_4$ in three divided doses. Because of its ability to bind with phosphate binders, oral iron should be taken between meals and not with calcium phosphate binders. Care should also be taken that large doses of vitamin C (over 500 mg/day) not be given to increase oral iron absorption, since intake above this level may cause kidney stone formation (Massey et al., 2005).

Blood transfusion is not recommended for most patients with ESRD because of (1) its depression of EPO in the bone marrow, (2) the possibility of overexpansion of the blood volume, (3) the risk of bloodborne pathogens, (4) the additional potassium load, and (5) the risk of hemochromatosis and hemosiderosis caused by increased iron stores (see Chapter 31).

Serum ferritin is an accurate indicator of iron status in renal failure. Patients who have received several transfusions and who are storing extra iron may have serum ferritin levels of 800 to 5000 ng/ml (a normal level is 68 ng/ml for women and 150 ng/ml for men; see Appendix 30). In patients who are receiving EPO, ferritin is kept above 300 ng/dl but below 800ng/dl. When ferritin values fall below 100 ng/ml, IV iron is usually given. The percent of transferrin saturation (% SAT) is another useful indicator of iron status in these patients and should be between 25% to 30%.

Vitamins

Water-soluble vitamins are lost during dialysis. In general, ascorbic acid and most B vitamins are lost through dialysate at about the same rate they would have been lost in the urine (depending on the type and duration of treatment), with the exception of folate, which is highly dialyzable. Patients who still produce urine may be at increased risk of loss of water-soluble vitamins. Folate is recommended to be supplemented at 1 mg/day based on extra losses. Because vitamin B_{12} is protein-bound, losses of this B vitamin during dialysis are minimal. Altered metabolism and excretory function, as well as drug administration, also may alter vitamin levels. Little is known about gastrointestinal absorption in uremia, but it may be significantly decreased. Uremic toxins may interfere with the activity of some vitamins (e.g., the phosphorylation of pyridoxine [vitamin B_6] and its analogs may be inhibited).

Another cause of decreased vitamin intake in uremia is the restriction of dietary phosphorus and potassium. Water-soluble vitamins are usually abundant in high-potassium foods such as citrus fruits and vegetables and high-phosphorus foods such as milk. Diets for patients on dialysis tend to be low in folate, niacin, riboflavin, and vitamin B_6. Ascorbic acid intake may be marginal. With frequent episodes of anorexia or illness, vitamin intake is decreased further.

Levels of fat-soluble vitamins do not usually change as much as levels of the water-soluble vitamins in renal disease. Circulating levels of retinol-binding protein are often high in patients with renal failure, a typical indicator of vitamin A toxicity. Whether this indicates toxicity in renal patients is unclear. They may actually have an increased capacity to tolerate vitamin A because of the extra carrying capacity. Because little is known about this, supplementation of vitamin A is not usually recommended.

Vitamin D should only be given in the active D_3 form $(1,25\text{-}[OH]_2D_3)$ by prescription because ESRD patients do not activate this vitamin in its normal dietary or usual supplemental form or that available from exposure to sunlight.

Little is known about vitamin E supplementation in chronic renal failure, although some evidence suggests that it does help protect against red blood cell fragility in the uremic patient. However, supplementation is not routinely recommended.

Vitamin K supplements are usually avoided because of the large number of these patients who take anticoagulants such as warfarin (Coumadin). Since many of these patients need to restrict dark-green leafy vegetables (good sources of vitamin K, but also high in potassium), excessive vitamin K is not usually a problem.

Several vitamin supplements that fit the needs of the uremic patient or the dialysis patient are now available by prescription: Nephrocaps (Fleming and Co.), Tabron (Parke-Davis), Neph-plex (Nephro-Tech Inc.), Dialya-Vit (Hillestad Pharmaceuticals) and Renal Caps (Cypress Pharmaceuticals Inc.). An over-the-counter supplement containing a vitamin B complex and vitamin C is often used and can be less expensive, but additional supplements of folic acid and pyridoxine may need to be given. Folic acid supplementation is recommended at 1 mg/day. This level is above that allowed in over-the-counter vitamin preparations and requires a prescription. For this reason, depending on the patient's financial needs and dietary intake, only 800 mg of folate may be recommended, particularly in light of recent supplementation of the U.S. food supply with folic acid. Occasionally megadoses of 3 to 6 mg/day of folic acid are given to patients with ESRD as a therapy to help

reduce homocysteine levels, which may affect cardiac function. Renax (5.5 mg) (Everett Laboratories) and Dialtx (5 mg) (Pam Laboratories) are both high–folic acid vitamins appropriate for these patients. Many dialysis patients routinely use some form of oral nutritional supplement, the majority of which contain complete vitamin supplementation to the level of the newly defined dietary reference intakes (DRIs) in three to four cans of formula. Patients may be getting a significant amount of their vitamin nutriture from these supplements and may not require oral vitamin preparations in addition to their diets. A thorough analysis of the patient's nutrient intake is needed before increasing their already large burden of capsules.

Lipid

Atherosclerotic cardiovascular disease is the most common cause of death among patients maintained on long-term dialysis (Bennett et al., 2006). This appears to be a function of both underlying disease (e.g., diabetes mellitus, hypertension, nephrotic syndrome) and a lipid abnormality common among patients with ESRD. The patient with ESRD typically has an elevated triglyceride level with or without an increase in cholesterol. The lipid abnormality likely represents both increased synthesis of very low–density lipoprotein and decreased clearance.

Treatment of hyperlipidemia with diet or pharmacologic agents remains controversial. Epidemiologic evidence demonstrating increased incidence of atherosclerotic coronary disease is balanced by studies that demonstrate that patients with clearly defined clinical evidence of atherosclerosis at the initiation of dialysis are at no increased risk for a cardiovascular event. Although routine treatment appears unwarranted, a good case can be made for dietary and pharmacologic treatment of patients with ESRD with underlying lipid disorders and evidence of accelerated atherosclerosis. Lipid-lowering drugs, including most statins, may have a significant impact on management (see Chapter 32).

Enteral Tube Feeding

Patients with ESRD who require enteral tube feeding often do quite well on standard formulas used for most tube-fed patients (see Chapter 20). Patients should receive standard formulas before they try a "specialty" formula because the former are usually less expensive and typically have lower osmolality than the specific renal products. If electrolyte or fluid concerns arise, patients can switch to one of the formulas now available that are specifically designed for renal patients: Nepro (Ross Labs), Magnacal Renal (Mead Johnson), Travasorb Renal (Travenol), Novasource Renal (Novartis), and ReNeph (Ross Labs), to name a few (see Appendix 32). If patients are receiving these "renal" products only, they may develop problems with a low phosphorus level if they are experiencing "refeeding syndrome" or if they are taking phosphate binders. The dosage of the phosphate binders may need to be adjusted or eliminated. In some cases patients may need a phosphorus supplement or the addition of milk to their feeding to maintain an acceptable serum phosphorus level.

Parenteral Nutrition

When a patient with ESRD becomes too ill to maintain an adequate oral intake and when tube feeding is not advisable because of gastrointestinal complications, parenteral nutrition should be considered. Parenteral nutrition in ESRD is similar to parenteral nutrition used for other malnourished patients. The use of essential amino acid solutions such as Nephramine formerly was recommended in cases of ARF or when a patient was not receiving dialysis treatment; but this practice has been largely discontinued because these patients seem to tolerate regular amino acid infusions well. Patients who receive dialysis therapy tolerate routine amino acid solutions such as FreAmine (McGaw), Travasol 8.5 (Clintec), and Aminosyn (Abbott Labs).

Vitamins and Minerals in Parenteral Feedings. Most researchers agree that vitamin needs for ESRD, during parenteral nutrition, are different from normal requirements but do not agree on recommendations for individual nutrients. It is generally accepted that folate, pyridoxine, and biotin should be supplemented and that vitamin A should not be provided parenterally unless retinol-binding protein is monitored because it is elevated in patients with renal failure. However, there is currently no parenteral vitamin that is specifically designed for patients with renal failure; thus in practice a standard vitamin preparation is usually administered. Table 36-7 presents vitamin supplementation guidelines.

Little information relating to trace mineral supplementation during parenteral nutrition in renal failure is available. Because most trace minerals, including zinc, chromium, and magnesium, are excreted in the urine, a close monitoring of these minerals in the serum seems to be appropriate.

Hypophosphatemia is a potential complication of parenteral nutrition in ESRD. When the patient is consuming some food and receiving phosphate binders, this may be of even greater concern. If adequate protein and calories are provided and the patient becomes anabolic, the phosphate-binder regimen may need to be altered to prevent hypophosphatemia and potential respiratory arrest. In some cases phosphorus may need to be supplemented.

Intradialytic Parenteral Nutrition. Malnourished patients with chronic renal failure who are on hemodialysis have easy access to parenteral nutrition because of the requirements of the dialysis therapy itself. Because direct access to the blood must be made at every treatment, intradialytic parenteral nutrition can be administered if necessary without additional invasive procedures or surgery. It is typically administered through a connection to the venous side of the extracorporeal circuit during dialysis (see Figure 36-3). Because of the high blood flow rate achieved through use of the surgically created fistula and the high blood pump speeds that are attained, hypertonic glucose and protein can be administered without danger of phlebitis. Lipids may also be administered (Tables 36-8 and 36-9). Reimbursement issues surrounding this therapy are complex since it is a supplemental feeding that requires the patient to have at least a functioning gastrointestinal tract and only supplies an

TABLE 36-7

Guidelines for Daily Parenteral Vitamin Supplementation in Total Parenteral Nutrition for Patients With Renal Failure*

Vitamin	Silberman	Kopple
A, as retinol (units)	3300	0
E, tocopherol (units)	10	10
K (mg)		7.5
Niacin (mg)	40	20
Thiamin HCl (mg)	3	2
Riboflavin (mg)	3.6	2
Pantothenic acid (mg)	15	10
Pyridoxine (mg)	5	10
Ascorbic acid (mg)	100	100
Biotin (mg)	60	200
Folic acid (mg)	1	2
B_{12} (mg)	5	3

From Kouba J: Vitamin and electrolytes in patients with renal failure requiring total parenteral nutrition. In *Dietitians in critical care*, Chicago, 1985, American Dietetic Association.
*These are general guidelines and may need more specific evaluation and adjustment in patients with severe stress or with gastrointestinal losses from diarrhea, ostomies, fistula drainage, etc.

average of 500 calories a day, or about 1000 calories every hemodialysis treatment.

Complications. Complications are similar to those encountered in usual TPN, with the exception of postdialysis hypoglycemia caused by the abrupt ending of the glucose supply. To avoid this problem, glucose administration typically is tapered up and down during the first and last half hour of the 3- to 5-hour treatment. Insulin is given often, usually in the bag of dextrose–amino acid solution, so that the patient does not become hypoglycemic if the infusion must be stopped. Blood sugar levels are typically monitored during the therapy. Some patients may benefit from a snack of complex carbohydrate toward the end of the treatment to avoid posttreatment rebound hypoglycemia.

Amino acid losses through the dialysate average about 10%. Vitamins and trace minerals are typically not administered with these solutions because patients are able to tolerate oral vitamin preparations and also have some oral dietary intake.

Another method of nutrition support in peritoneal dialysis patients is a peritoneal dialysate solution that contains amino acids instead of dextrose. Typically one bag of this solution is used per day. Some patients experience side effects from this treatment, and reimbursement issues are significant.

ESRD in Patients With Diabetes

Because renal failure is a complication of diabetes, approximately 40% to 50% of all new patients starting dialysis have diabetes (Zhang et al., 2005). Because of the need to control blood sugar, these patients require even more specialized diet therapy. The diet for diabetes management (see Chapter 30) can be modified for the patient on dialysis. In addition, the diabetic patient on dialysis often has other complications such as retinopathy, neuropathy, gastroparesis, and amputation, all of which can place this patient at high nutritional risk. The National Kidney Foundation (NKF) has established guidelines for managing diabetes in the presence of CKD (Nelson and Tuttle, 2007).

Increased osmolarity caused by high serum levels of glucose may cause water and potassium to be pulled out of cells, with resultant hyperkalemia. Interpretation of commonly used laboratory values change when a diabetic patient develops renal failure, since the hemoglobin A1C is affected by the half life of red blood cells (Joy et al., 2002; Rigalleau et al., 2006).

Education of Patients with ESRD

Now that biochemical parameters have been discussed, it is important to look at the long-range goals for educating the patient with ESRD about his or her nutritional needs. The average patient survives on dialysis an average of 7 to 10 years. Patients with a relatively benign diagnosis may look forward to life spans of 20 to 30 years, particularly if they receive kidney transplants as a part of their treatment. The challenge for the RD is educating a patient with a chronic disease who will be primarily responsible for implementing any nutritional recommendations for the rest of his or her life. In this respect, the nutrition therapy for ESRD and that for diabetes share many similarities.

It is incumbent on the RD to develop a long-standing rapport with the patient and family and to serve as an ally to help them make the best nutritional choices for the patient over an extended period of time. Understanding the burdens of a complex, challenging, and ever-changing diet and developing skills that allow the nutrition counselor to transfer the information to the renal patient in a workable, flexible, and easily understood manner are just as challenging, if not more so, than maintaining a patient's iron status or keeping the patient at a good body weight.

Exchange lists are not always used in educating the patient about a renal diet. Rather a booklet, *The National Renal Diet* (Schiro-Harvey, 2002), available from the American Dietetic Association (see Useful Websites), provides information about food sources of nutrients, adapting patients' usual intakes to meet requirements based on their laboratory values, and decreasing certain foods when values rise (Wiggins and Schiro-Harvey, 2002) (see Table 36-5). A renal diet for dialysis can be found in Appendix 36.

Chronic Kidney Disease in Children

Although chronic kidney disease (CKD) may occur in children at any age, from the newborn infant through the adolescent, it is a relatively uncommon diagnosis. Etiologies in children include congenital, anatomic defects (e.g., urologic malformations or dysplastic kidneys), inherited disease (e.g., autosomal-recessive polycystic kidney disease), metabolic disorders that eventually result in renal failure (e.g., cystinosis or methylmalonic aciduria), or acquired

---

TABLE 36-8

Regimen for Intermittent Parenteral Nutrition Administered During Hemodialysis Therapy

Infusion	Quantity	Calories (kcal)	Volume (ml)
70% dextrose	350 g dextrose	1190	500
15% amino acids	37.5 g protein	Protein should not be counted on to provide calories	250
20% lipid emulsion	50 g fat	450	250
TOTAL		1640	1000*

Monitor serum glucose, sodium, potassium, bicarbonate, phosphate, triglycerides

Developed by Katy G. Wilkens, MS, RD, Northwest Kidney Centers, Seattle, Wash.
*Additional volume may include insulin and vitamins.

TABLE 36-9

Regimen for Total Parenteral Nutrition by Subclavian Vein for Dialysis Patients

Infusion	Quantity	Calories (kcal)	Volume (ml)
70% glucose	700 g glucose	2380	1000
15% amino acids	75 g protein	Protein should not be counted on to provide calories.	500
20% lipid emulsion	100 g fat	900	500
TOTAL		3280	2000*

Monitor serum glucose, sodium, potassium, bicarbonate, phosphate, triglycerides.

Developed by Katy G. Wilkens, MS, RD, Northwest Kidney Centers, Seattle, Washington.
*Additional volume may include insulin and vitamins.

conditions or illnesses (e.g., untreated kidney infections, physical trauma to kidneys, exposure to nephrotoxic chemicals/medications, hemolytic anemia, often due to *E. coli* 0157 ingestion, or glomerular nephritis). As with all children, the major concern is to promote normal growth and development. Without aggressive monitoring and encouragement, the child with renal failure rarely meets his or her nutritional requirements. If the renal disease is present from birth, nutrition support needs to begin immediately to avoid losing the growth potential of the first few months of life (Ekim et al., 2003).

Growth in children with CKD is usually retarded. Although no specific therapy ensures normal growth, factors capable of responding to therapy include metabolic acidosis, electrolyte depletion, osteodystrophy, chronic infection, and protein-calorie malnutrition. Energy and protein needs for children with chronic renal disease are at least equivalent to the DRIs for normal children of the same height and age. If nutrition status is poor, energy needs may be even higher to promote weight gain and linear growth. Feeding by tube is required in the presence of poor intake, particularly in the critical growth period of the first 2 years of life. Gastros-

tomy tubes are almost always placed in these children to enhance nutritional intake and facilitate growth. TPN is rarely initiated unless the gastrointestinal tract is nonfunctional. Table 36-10 presents the nutritional requirements of children with renal failure.

Control of calcium and phosphorus balance is especially important for maintaining good growth. The goal is to restrict phosphorus intake while promoting calcium absorption with the aid of $1,25\text{-}(OH)_2D_3$. This helps prevent renal osteodystrophy, which can cause severe growth retardation during childhood. Use of calcium carbonate formulations to supplement the dietary intake enhances calcium intake while binding excess phosphorus. Aluminum-containing preparations are used only in patients with extreme hyperphosphatemia and only on a short-term basis. Aluminum binders should never be used routinely in children under the age of 10 years.

Persistent metabolic acidosis is often associated with growth failure in infancy. In chronic acidosis the titration of acid by the bone causes calcium loss and contributes to bone demineralization. Bicarbonate may be added to the infant formula to counteract this effect.

TABLE 36-10

Energy, Protein, Fluid, Sodium, Potassium, and Phosphorus Needs of Children With ESRD Based on Type of Therapy

Therapy	Energy	Protein	Fluid	Sodium	Potassium	Phosphorus
Conservative (children with CKD before end stage)	EER for age and size (adjust for comorbid conditions)	RDA for age	Maintenance/ unrestricted (increased if polyuria)	Limit to 1-3 mEq/kg if hypertension or edema; supplement if sodium wasting	Limit to 1-3 mEq/kg if high serum levels	600-800 mg/ day if serum levels elevated
Peritoneal dialysis	EER for age minus calories from dextrose absorption	RDA + 0.7 to 1g/kg/ day	Unrestricted, unless anuria; then insensible losses + urine output + fluid removed with dialysis	Same as above	Same as above	Same as above
Hemodialysis	EER for age and size (adjust for comorbid conditions)	RDA + 0.4 g/kg/day	Insensible losses + urine output + fluid removed with dialysis	Limit to 1-3 mEq/kg if hypertension/ edema	Limit to 1-3 mEq/kg if high serum levels	Same as above
Transplantation	EER for age and size	RDA × 1.75-2 (1st month) then RDA × 1.25	Increased to 1.5 to 3 L or more per day to keep kidney well perfused	Limit to 2-3 mEq/kg/day if edema/ hypertension	Limit to 1-3 mEq/kg if high levels (first month)	Increased needs; supplement if serum levels are low

Adapted by Lori S. Brizee MS, RD, CSP, from *Nutrition Management of Renal Diseases.* In *Pediatric Manual of Clinical Dietetics*, Chicago, American Dietetic Association, 2001, Tables 28-1 through 28-3, p 416.

CKD, Chronic kidney disease; *EER,* estimated energy requirements; *RDA,* recommended dietary allowance.

Restriction of protein in pediatric diets is controversial. The so-called "protective" effect on kidney function must be weighed against the clearly negative effect of possible protein malnutrition on growth. The recommended dietary allowance for protein for age is usually the minimum amount given.

Each child's diet should be adjusted to his or her food preferences, family eating patterns, and biochemical needs. This is often not an easy task. In addition, care must be taken not to place too much emphasis on the diet to avoid its becoming a manipulative tool and an attention-getting device. Special encouragement, creativity, and attention are required to help the child with CKD consume the necessary energy. When possible, CCPD, which is intermittent during the day and continuous at night, is a viable therapy of choice for children because it allows liberalization of the diet. The child is more likely to meet nutritional requirements with fewer dietary restrictions and therefore experience better growth.

Other treatments that help renal disease in children include the use of rHuEPO and rDNA-produced growth hormone (rHGH). These are usually started when the child's serum hemoglobin falls below 10 g/dl, with a goal of maintaining hemoglobin between 11 and 12 g/dl. Correction of anemia with the use of rHuEPO may increase appetite, intake, and feeling of well-being, but it has not been found to affect growth, even with seemingly adequate nutrition support.

The Team Approach

The position of the RD in the care of dialysis patients is unique, being a federally mandated position. So, too, is the RD's place on the mandated Health Care Team, which exists within each dialysis unit. The team approach in all health care is important, but nowhere is it more obviously applied than with the interdisciplinary team of the renal nurse, renal social worker, nephrologist, and renal dietitian. The care of these complex, long-term patients uses the skill and compassion of all members of the health care team working together to improve quality of life for patients with ESRD (Unruh et al., 2005).

NEPHROLITHIASIS (KIDNEY STONES)

Nephrolithiasis, or the presence of kidney stones, is an increasingly significant health problem in the population. In the almost 20 years between the two National Health and Nutrition Examination Surveys, NHANES II (1976-1980) and NHANES III (1988-1994), the prevalence of kidney stone disease in the United States increased from 3.8% to 5.2%. It is characterized by frequent occurrences between the ages of 30 and 50, predominance in males (three times more common) highest prevalence among whites compared with blacks and Mexican-Americans, and a high recurrence rate (Goldfarb et al., 2005). The

---

BOX 36-2

Urinary Risk Factors for Stone Development

Increased Risk	Decreased Risk
Low urine volume	High urine volume and flow
Oxalate	Citrate
Uric acid	Glycoproteins
Acid pH	Magnesium
Stasis	
Calcium	

---

risk doubles in those with a family history of kidney stones (Stamatelou et al., 2003).

Pathophysiology

Kidney stone formation is a complex process that consists of saturation, supersaturation; nucleation; crystal growth or aggregation; crystal retention; and stone formation in the presence of promoters, inhibitors, and complexors in urine. Calcium stones are the most common: calcium oxalate (60%), calcium oxalate and calcium phosphate (10%), calcium phosphate (10%), and uric acid (5% to 10%), struvite (5% to 10%), and cystine (1%). Low urine volume is the single most important risk factor for urolithiasis (Box 36-2).

Medical Management

Uric acid stones are the only type amenable to dissolution therapy. Shockwave lithotripsy and endourologic techniques have almost replaced the open surgical procedures of stone removal of 20 years ago. Management strategies are now aimed at kidney stone prevention and should include a patient evaluation and metabolic workup to identify causes (Meschi et al., 2004; Taylor and Curhan, 2004) (Table 36-11).

Medical Nutrition Therapy

After corrective treatment for medical disorders, patients should receive nutrition counseling for diet and fluid modification to reduce urinary risk factors for stone formation. Specific medical nutrition therapy based on comprehensive metabolic evaluation (Table 36-12), dietary counseling, and metabolic monitoring is more effective in reducing stone recurrence than nonspecific measures and limited screening. The effectiveness of any medical nutrition therapy should be monitored with evaluation of subsequent 24-hour urine collections. This will give the nutritionist and patient a measure of the impact of dietary changes (Taylor and Curhan, 2006).

Fluid and Urine Volume

A low urine volume is by far the most common abnormality noted on metabolic evaluation of stone formers, and its correction with a high fluid intake should be a focus of attention in the management of all types of kidney stones (Siener and Hesse, 2005). The objective is to maintain urinary solutes in the undersaturated zone to inhibit nucleation by

TABLE 36-11

Causes and Composition of Renal Stones

Pathogenetic Causes	Composition of Stone
Hypercalciuria	
Hyperoxaluria	
Hyperuricosuria	Calcium oxalate
Hypocitraturia	
Primary hyperparathyroidism	
Cystinuria	Cystine
Infection	Struvite
Acid urine pH	
Hyperuricosuria	Uric acid
Renal tubular acidosis	
Alkaline urine pH	Calcium phosphate

Modified from Martini LA, Wood RJ: Should dietary calcium and protein be restricted in patients with nephrolithiasis? *Nutr Rev* 58:111, 2000.

TABLE 36-12

Baseline Information and Metabolic Evaluation of Urolithiasis

Information	Description/Data
History of urolithiasis	History of onset, frequency
	Family history
	Spontaneous passage or removal
	Retrieval, analysis of stone
	Current status with radiologic examination
Medical history, investigation	Hyperparathyroidism
	Renal tubular acidosis
	Urinary tract infection
	Sarcoidosis
	Hypertension
	Osteoporosis
	Inflammatory bowel disease, malabsorption syndrome, intestinal bypass surgery for obesity
Blood tests	Serum—calcium, phosphorus, creatinine, uric acid, CO_2, albumin, parathyroid hormone
Urinalysis	Urine analysis with pH
	Urine culture
24-hr urine collection	Volume, calcium, oxalate, uric acid, sodium
	Citrate, magnesium, phosphorus
	Urea
	Creatinine
	Qualitative cystine
Medications and vitamins	Thiazide, allopurinol, vitamin C, vitamin B_6, vitamin D, cod liver oil, calcium carbonate, glucocorticoid therapy
Occupation history and strenuous exercise	Dermal losses, dehydration, low urine volume
	Type of job and activity level
Environment	Hard water area
Dietary evaluation	Intake of calcium, oxalate, animal protein, salt, purines, herbal products
	Volume of fluid intake
	Type of fluids

both an increase in urine volume and a reduction of solute load. High urine flow rate will tend to wash out any formed crystals, and a urine volume of 2 to 2.5 L/day has been shown to prevent stone recurrence (Meschi et al., 2004; Taylor et al., 2004; Curhan et al., 2004).

Achieving a urine volume of 2 to 2.5 L/day requires an intake of 250 ml of fluid at each meal, between meals, at bedtime, and when arising to void at night. Hydration during sleep hours is important to break the cycle of a "most-concentrated" morning urine. Half of this daily 2.5 L should be taken as water. Even higher fluid intake, perhaps as much as 3 L/day, may be necessary to compensate for gastrointestinal fluid loss, excessive sweating from strenuous exercise, or an excessively hot or an excessively dry environment (such as a commercial airplane cabin). Patients who form idiopathic calcium stones with low urine volume and who are unable to increase urine volume may have altered thirst sensitivity and vasopressin release, and this needs to be evaluated and treated.

In two large cohort studies consumption of tea, coffee, beer, and wine was associated with reduced risk of stone formation, but grapefruit juice was not (Taylor and Curhan, 2004). However, in a separate study, grapefruit juice ingestion caused no changes in lithogenicity, presumably because the increase in oxalate from the grapefruit juice was offset by the beneficial increase in citrate; therefore there was no net change in calculated supersaturation (Goldfarb and Asplin, 2001). Because these observations are still unexplained, it is still recommended to avoid grapefruit juice. Soft drinks and colas that contain phosphoric acid should also be avoided because of their urine acidifying effect. Carbonated beverages with caffeine are associated with excess calciuria (Heany and Rafferty, 2001).

Despite the high oxalate content of tea, when it is taken with milk it does not seem to increase stone formation. The recommendation for tea drinkers is to drink only a moderate amount of weak tea (about 2 c per day) with milk. Herbal teas have much lower oxalate content and are an acceptable alternative.

Cranberry juice acidifies urine and is useful in the treatment of urinary tract infections and struvite stones (Kessler et al., 2002). Black currant juice increases urinary citrate and oxalate and, because of its urine alkalizing effect, may prevent the occurrence of uric acid stones.

Calcium Stones

Calcium

Hypercalciuria is defined as a mean value of calcium in excess of 300 mg (7.5 mmol)/day in men or 250 mg (6.25 mmol)/day in women, or 4 mg (0.1 mmol)/kg/day for either in random urine collections of outpatients on unrestricted diets. Thirty to 40% of patients with calcium stones are hypercalciuric. Hypercalciuria is idiopathic when serum calcium is normal and the usual causes can be excluded. Idiopathic hypercalciuria can result from an exaggerated dietary calcium intake, increased intestinal absorption of calcium that may or may not be vitamin D–mediated, decreased renal tubular resorption of calcium, or prolonged bed rest. It can also result from low serum phosphorus levels caused by a renal phosphate leak that stimulates 1,25-dihydroxy vitamin D_3 production and consequent increase in intestinal calcium absorption (Morton et al., 2002). Calcium-loading studies show that urinary calcium rises with an increase in dietary calcium of up to 800 mg (20 mmol)/day. Beyond that point, animal protein may be responsible for the rise in urine calcium (Morton et al., 2002) (Box 36-3).

For decades low-calcium diets were recommended to reduce the high incidence of hypercalciuria in patients who form stones. However, chronic prolonged calcium restriction may damage the bones of calcium stone patients because of deficient calcium to meet requirements and increased losses of calcium from hypercalciuria. Vertebral mineral density is decreased in calcium stone formers with idiopathic hypercalciuria, and vertebral fracture risk is increased by nearly fourfold among urolithiasis patients in comparison with the expected incidence in the general population. Bone resorption may also be enhanced by a high protein intake of nondairy origin. An inadequate calcium and high protein intake also induces metabolic acidosis as a result of marked acid load, increased urinary ammonium and calcium excretion, and lower urine pH, and predisposes to mineral loss and fracture (Asplin et al., 2003, Caudarella et al., 2004). Patients with absorptive hypercalciuria type I have a double risk of nephrolithiasis and vast bone loss. A moderate calcium restriction, about 800 mg/day, in combination with thiazides and potassium citrate is recommended

to eliminate recurrent stone formation and increase bone density (Pak et al., 2003).

The relationship between dietary calcium and the incidence of symptomatic kidney stones was examined in two separate long-term prospective studies in men (Taylor et al., 2004) and women (Curhan et al., 2004). The higher the dietary calcium intake, the lower the risk of kidney stones. However, calcium supplements did not have the same protective effect as dietary calcium had and were associated with an increased risk because they may not have been taken with meals to reduce oxalate absorption. If taken as a supplement, it appears that the timing of calcium intake is important. Calcium supplements taken with meals increase urinary calcium and citrate and decrease urinary oxalate; thus the increase in citrate and decrease in oxalate counterbalance the effects of elevated urinary calcium. Therefore, if used, calcium supplements should be taken with meals to prevent hypercalciuria and to bind dietary oxalate and reduce its absorption (Stitchantrankul et al., 2004; Domrongkitchaiporn et al., 2004). It has been observed that a calcium intake of 1200 mg, coupled with restriction of both animal protein and salt intake, is more effective than calcium restriction (400 mg/day) and low oxalate intake in preventing recurrent calcium oxalate stones (Borghi et al., 2002).

Clearly calcium restriction does not prevent stone formation and may cause or worsen osteoporosis (Martini, 2002). Current DRIs recommend 1000 mg/day of calcium for men and women age 50 years or younger and 1200 mg/day of calcium for those older than 50 years, which aligns well with calcium recommendations for kidney stone formers (Martini and Wood, 2000).

Oxalate

Hyperoxaluria (>40 mg of oxalate in urine/day) plays an important role in calcium stone formation and is observed in 10% to 50% of recurrent stone formers. Normal healthy adults daily excrete 15 to 40 mg of oxalate in urine, and this can be increased by 50% by large intakes of oxalate-rich foods. The oxalate content of a typical diet is in the range of 44 to 350 mg/day, but it can be as high as 1980 mg/day in vegetarian diets (Holmes and Kennedy, 2000).

Dietary oxalate affects urinary oxalate because oxalate cannot be metabolized in the body and the renal route is the only mode of excretion. The dietary contribution to urinary oxalate varies from 24% to 40% at oxalate intakes of 10 mg/day to 180 to 250 mg/day (Holmes et al., 2001). Oxalate is found in all plant foods. A single food can vary twofold to fifteenfold in its oxalate content, depending on the variety, growth conditions, and season. Only limited data on food oxalate content are available because of inconsistent methodologies used for analysis. Further, only a few foods have been tested for oxalate bioavailability. High-oxalate foods should not be avoided based on their oxalate content alone when only a limited amount is bioavailable. Foods with a low oxalate content but higher bioavailability may be more of a problem in increasing urinary oxalate (Box 36-4).

Dietary counseling to reduce oxalate absorption is beneficial for stone-forming individuals who have large intakes

---

BOX 36-3

Dietary Factors Associated With Risk of Calcium Stones

Increased Risk	Decreased Risk
Animal protein	Calcium
Oxalate	Potassium
Sodium	Magnesium
Vitamin C	Fluid intake
	Fiber/phytate
	Vitamin B_6

of high oxalate foods and who excrete more than 30 mg (350 μmol) of oxalate per day. The amount of oxalate in the low-oxalate diet is about 200 mg/day, higher than the traditional low oxalate diet, which provided about 60 mg/day. To keep the diet plan simple, the patient is told to avoid those foods that are high in oxalate that have been in his or her diet. In addition, the patient is advised to consume a high-calcium food (150 mg of calcium to bind 100 mg of oxalate) at the same time to reduce oxalate absorption from the higher oxalate–containing foods in the meal (Meschi et al., 2004; Massey, 2003) (see EVOLVE website "Intervention Tools: Kidney Stones and Oxalate").

Because much less oxalate than calcium exists in urine (the ratio is 1:5), changes in oxalate concentration have a greater impact than changes in calcium concentration on the relative supersaturation of calcium-oxalate crystals. However, oxalate absorption, which is 3% to 8% of the amount in food, is affected by the amount of dietary calcium. On very low calcium intakes of ≈200 mg/day, oxalate absorption rose to 17%, whereas it fell to 2.6% when 1200 mg of calcium was ingested. Higher calcium doses did not result in further reduction (von Unruh et al., 2004).

Urinary oxalate also comes from endogenous synthesis, and this is proportional to lean body mass (Massey, 2003). Ascorbic acid accounts for 35% to 55%, and glyoxylic acid accounts for 50% to 70% of urinary oxalate. Several amino acids are precursors of oxalate via glyoxylate or glycolate. Because pyridoxine acts as a cofactor in the conversion of glyoxylate to glycine, its deficiency could increase endogenous oxalate production (Figure 36-8).

Patients with inflammatory bowel diseases or gastric bypass develop hyperoxaluria because of fat malabsorption. The bile acids produced during the digestive process normally are resorbed in the proximal gastrointestinal tract. When this fails to occur, bile salts and fatty acids increase colonic permeability to oxalate. The unabsorbed fatty acids also bind calcium to form soaps, thus making less calcium in soluble form available to bind oxalate and allowing for increased oxalate absorption from the gut (see Chapter 27). Urinary oxalate excretion increases up to five times normal in enteric hyperoxaluria after bypass surgery. It does not increase after small bowel surgery; but, among patients with colon surgery, low urine volume, low urine pH, and supersaturation with uric acid, the formation of stones is more common (Parks et al., 2003).

Primary hyperoxaluria is a feature of an autosomal-recessive genetic defect of a hepatic enzyme that results in overproduction of oxalate and a urinary oxalate concentration three to eight times the normal rate. Multiple stones occur in these children and cause renal failure and early death.

The health-promoting benefits of probiotics in the prevention of calcium oxalate stone disease using oxalate degrading bacteria, oxalobacter formigenes, is under study (Hoesl and Altwein, 2005).

Animal Protein

Epidemiologic studies find a correlation between improved standard of living, high animal protein intake, and a rising incidence of kidney stones. Excessive animal protein intake modulates several urinary risk factors such as hypercalciuria, hyperuricosuria, hyperoxaluria, low urine pH, and hypocitraturia, all of which increase the risk of kidney stones (Martini and Wood, 2000). Urinary urate acts as a promoter of heterogeneous nucleation of calcium oxalate, and approximately a third of calcium stone formers are sensitive to meat protein in terms of oxalate excretion. The mechanism does not seem to involve vitamin B_6 deficiency. Prevalence of stone formation in vegetarians is 1.2% as compared to 3.8% in the general population (Nguyen et al., 2001).

After 14 years of follow-up, the Male Health Professionals' Study (MHPS) demonstrated a 38% increased risk of kidney stones with a 77-g versus 50-g animal-protein diet if body mass index (BMI) was less than 25 (Taylor et al., 2004).

BOX 36-4

Foods That Raise Urinary Oxalate Excretion

Rhubarb
Spinach
Strawberries
Chocolate
Wheat bran and whole grain wheat products
Nuts (almonds, peanuts, or pecans)
Beets
Tea (green, black, iced, or instant)

Data from Siener R et al: Oxalate content of cereals and cereal products, *J Agric Food Chem* 54:3008, 2006; Brinkley LJ et al: A further study of oxalate bioavailability in foods, *J Urol* 144:94, 1990; French AM et al: Urine compositions in normal subjects after oral ingestion of oxalate-rich foods, *Clin Sci* 60:411, 1981; and Massey LK et al: Effect of dietary oxalate and calcium on urinary oxalate and risk of formulation of calcium oxalate kidney stones, *J Am Diet Assoc* 93:901, 1993.

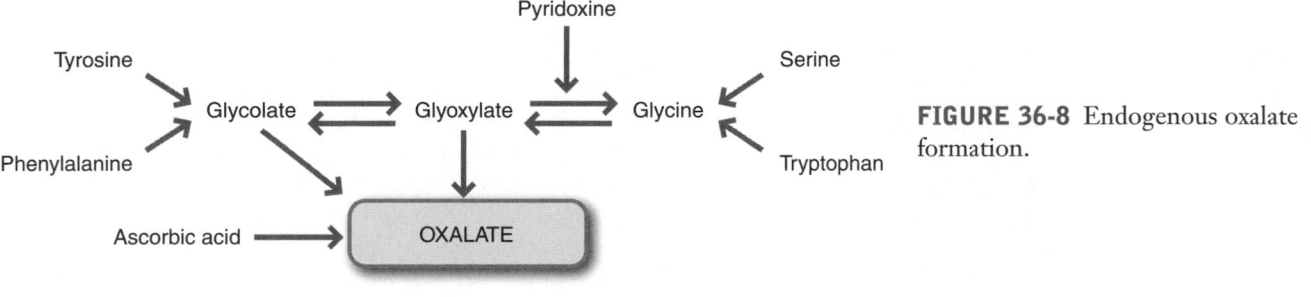

FIGURE 36-8 Endogenous oxalate formation.

A 5-year randomized trial of men on a diet of a normal level of calcium but low in salt and animal protein (52 g total with 21 g from meat or fish and 31 g from milk and derivatives) showed a 51% reduced stone incidence as a result of decreased urine calcium, oxalate, and calcium-oxalate saturation (Borghi et al., 2002). It is probably useful to recommend a lower protein diet (50-60 g/day) with at least half of the protein coming from other than meat sources.

Citrate

Citrate is a urinary stone inhibitor. It forms a complex with calcium in urine; thus less calcium is available to bind urinary oxalate, which helps prevent the formation of calcium oxalate or calcium phosphate stones. Distal RTA, acidosis accompanied by hypokalemia, malabsorption syndrome with enteric hyperoxaluria, and excessive meat intake (acid ash) are associated with decreased urinary citrate levels (Morton et al., 2002). In fact, one study showed 50% of recurrent calcium stone formers had hypocitraturia (urinary citrate of <300 mg/day), and it was predominately of dietary origin. They had lower fruit intakes and, as a consequence, also lower potassium intakes. Fruit intake should be particularly noted in the nutrition assessment of these recurrent stone formers

(Domrongkitchaiporn et al., 2006). Normal daily urinary citrate level should be more than 640 mg/day. Lemonade made with lemon juice (4 oz.) diluted to 2 L with water should be encouraged in patients with low urinary citrate (Seltzer et al., 1996). Fruit intake should also be encouraged (*Clinical Insight*: Acid Ash and Alkaline Ash Diets).

Magnesium

Magnesium is a low-molecular-weight–inhibitor that forms soluble complexes with oxalate. Like calcium, it inhibits oxalate absorption and may have a role to play in hyperoxaluric patients. Magnesium was associated with a 29% relative risk reduction in stone formers in the MPHS (Taylor et al., 2004). A combination of magnesium potassium citrate (21 mEq of magnesium) given over 3 years reduced recurrence risk of stone by 85% (Borghi et al., 2002).

Sodium

The daily amount of sodium chloride in modern diets reaches excessive levels of up to 10 g/day. The amount of sodium in the urine and hypercalciuria are directly correlated because sodium and calcium are resorbed at common sites in the renal tubule. A linear increase in urinary calcium

---

✦ CLINICAL INSIGHT

Acid Ash and Alkaline Ash Diets

Dietary intake can influence the acidity or alkalinity of the urine. The acid-forming potential is contributed by chloride, phosphorus, and sulfur (anions); and the base-forming potential by sodium, potassium, calcium, and magnesium (cations). Before the use of medication to acidify or alkalinize the urine, dietary changes were commonly used.

In general, fruits and vegetables contribute alkaline "ash" to the urine, except in the case of prunes, plums, and cranberries. These fruits contain benzoic and quinic acids that are excreted in the urine as hippuric acid.

High-protein foods (meat, fish, poultry, eggs, and cheese) and breads and cereals are the primary contributors of acid "ash." Milk contributes to both categories. However, because factors of digestion, absorption, use of salt or medications, hormonal status, and homeostatic mechanisms all affect renal excretion and urine production, urine pH cannot be predicted by calculation of intake. Such information can be obtained only by direct measurement of the urine.

The following food lists serve as a guide to influencing urine pH.

Potentially Acid or Acid Ash Foods

Meat: Meat, fish, fowl, shellfish, eggs, all types of cheese, peanut butter, peanuts
Fat: Bacon, nuts (Brazil nuts, filberts, walnuts)
Starch: All types of bread (especially whole wheat), cereal, crackers, macaroni, spaghetti, noodles, rice

Potentially Acid or Acid Ash Foods—cont'd

Vegetables: Corn, lentils
Fruits: Cranberries, plums, prunes
Desserts: Plain cakes, cookies

Potentially Basic or Alkaline Ash Foods

Milk: Milk and milk products, cream, buttermilk
Fat: Nuts (almonds, chestnuts, coconut)
Vegetables: All types (except corn and lentils), especially beets, beet greens, Swiss chard, dandelion greens, kale, mustard greens, spinach, turnip greens
Fruit: All types (except cranberries, plums, and prunes)
Sweets: Molasses

Neutral Foods

Fats: Butter, margarine, cooking fats, oils
Sweets: Plain candies, sugar, syrup, honey
Starches: Arrowroot, corn, tapioca
Beverages: Coffee, tea

Modified from Nelson JK et al: *Mayo Clinic diet manual*, ed 6, St. Louis, 1994, Mosby.

occurs as urinary sodium increases from 40 to 200 mmol (920 to 4600 mg)/day. For every 60-mmol (1380-mg) increase in urine sodium, the relative risk of hypercalciuria increases by 1.63 times. The risk for nephrolithiasis is significantly higher in hypertensive compared to normotensive individuals. Alterations in calcium homeostasis may act as a common cause of stone formation and hypertension. Sodium intake should be lowered in patients with hypercalciuria to less than 100 mmol (2300 mg)/day (Morton et al., 2002; Straub and Hautmann, 2005) (see Chapter 34, and Appendices 36 and 37).

Potassium

Stone formers often have a low-to-normal potassium intake and high sodium intake. Potassium intake is inversely related to urinary citraturia and the risk of kidney stones. Men who were in the highest quintile of potassium intake compared with those in the lowest showed a 46% reduction in the incidence of kidney stones (Taylor et al., 2004). The level of potassium used in a recent study that reduced stone incidence by 50% was 120 mmol (4680 mg)/day (Borghi et al., 2002). Estimation of fruit and vegetable intake should be included in the metabolic evaluation, and stone formers should be encouraged to increase the potassium in their diets by choosing low-oxalate fruit and vegetables many times throughout the day (see Appendix 56, and Box 36-4) (Domrongkitchaiporn et al., 2006).

Vitamins

Vitamin C. Use of vitamin C supplements has been controversial. Improper storage and processing of urine samples led to a conversion of ascorbic acid to oxalate and became the basis for recommendations against vitamin C supplementation (Gerster, 1997). The MHPS demonstrated no difference in relative risk of kidney stones between those with vitamin C intakes of less than 250 mg/day and those with intakes equal to or greater than 1500 mg/day, thus suggesting that routine restriction of vitamin C is not warranted (Curhan et al., 1999). But, in the same study after 14 years of follow-up, men who consumed 1000 mg or greater of vitamin C per day had a 41% higher risk of stones than those who consumed less than the recommended dietary allowance of 90 mg/day (Taylor et al., 2004) A randomized controlled cross-over design trial in a metabolic unit using 1000 mg twice a day of ascorbic acid found increased urine oxalate and Tiselius index for calcium oxalate kidney stones in 40% of participants, both stone formers and nonstone formers (Traxer et al., 2000). Up until now recommendations have stated an upper limit of 2000 mg/day of vitamin C with the avoidance of mega doses. However, since health benefits of more than 500 mg of ascorbic acid are not substantiated, individuals at risk for calcium oxalate stones would be wise to not exceed 500 mg/day until there is further research (Massey et al., 2005).

Vitamin B$_6$. Vitamin B$_6$ in the form of pyridoxal phosphate is a required co-factor in oxalate metabolism. The proposed mechanism is that deficiency of vitamin B$_6$ increases oxalate production and oxaluria because glyoxylate converts to oxalate instead of to glycine (see Figure 36-8). However, observational data fail to identify an association between vitamin B$_6$ consumption and risk of kidney stone formation in men (Taylor and Curhan, 2004; Taylor et al., 2004), but large doses of vitamin B$_6$ (40 mg/day) in women may reduce the risk (Curhan et al., 1999).

Studies using 2 or 10 mg/day of vitamin B$_6$ reduced urinary oxalate in some calcium oxalate stone formers. Marginal B$_6$ status may contribute to excessive oxalate excretion in some stone formers but is not likely to be a significant cause of increased oxalate in a healthy population (Kaelin et al., 2004; Massey, 2003).

Obesity

Obesity and weight gain are associated with an increased risk of nephrolithiasis, and the effect of obesity on stone risk seems to be greater in women. In prospective studies of three large cohorts (MHPS, NHSI and NHSII) after an adjustment for relevant variables, the relative risk with a BMI of 30 or greater versus 21 to 22.9 in men was 1.33, and in older and younger women 1.90 and 2.09, respectively. Waist circumference was positively associated with risk in all three cohorts (Taylor et al., 2004).

Obesity is associated with insulin resistance and hyperinsulinemia that may contribute to the development of calcium stones by increasing urinary calcium excretion (Maalouf et al., 2004).

Higher weight is also associated with a lower urine pH, and a defect in the ability to excrete acid. Urinary uric acid excretion is also higher in heavier patients. Men with a BMI of 30 or greater excreted 19% more uric acid per day than men with a BMI of less than 25 (Siener et al., 2004).

As body weight increases, the excretion of calcium, oxalate and uric acid also increases. In contrast, even a small drop in body weight in subjects with calcium stone disease is associated with considerable reduction of lithogenous salts in their urine (Meschi et al., 2004), an additional reason to encourage weight control. In stone formers a BMI of 18 to 25 kg/m² is recommended.

Fiber and Phytate

The large prospective observational study, NHSII, showed that in younger women dietary phytate is inversely associated with incident kidney stone formation (Curhan et al., 2004). Dietary phytate strongly influences urinary phytate and exhibits an inhibitory effect on the crystallization of calcium oxalate and calcium phosphate (Taylor and Curhan, 2004). Some calcium oxalate stone formers exhibit abnormally low urinary phytate levels. Phytate found in high-fiber foods may complex with calcium to decrease hypercalciuria, but it may also prevent oxalate absorption from the gut. The eating of oxalate-containing bran has not appeared to be a risk factor for hyperoxaluria. No change in urinary calcium or oxalate was observed when fiber intake was increased to 25 g/day from fruit, vegetables, and cereal sources (Rotily et al., 2000).

Omega-3 Fatty Acids

Dietary fatty acids can modulate the urinary excretion of calcium and oxalate. Fish oil supplementation lowers urinary calcium and oxalate in idiopathic calcium oxalate stone formers. The plasma and red blood cell membrane phospholipids of idiopathic calcium stone formers contain an increased amount of arachidonic acid (an omega-6 fatty acid), which results in increased production of prostaglandin E_2–induced hypercalciuria. The arachidonic acid content of red blood cell membranes directly correlates with red blood cell oxalate exchange. Fish oil (omega-3 fatty acids) supplementation reduces plasma arachidonic acid levels and normalizes red blood cell oxalate exchange (Baggio et al., 2000). However, fish protein contains high concentrations of purines, which could increase serum uric acid levels (see following paragraphs) and result in hyperuricosuria and hypercalciuria. If the intake of omega-3 fatty acids is to be increased, it should probably be with omega-3 fat supplements rather than with excessive amounts of fish.

Herbal Products

A study of the lithogenic properties of cranberry-concentrate pills in healthy volunteers demonstrated a 43% increase in urinary oxalate, sodium, and calcium (Terris et al., 2001). Patients at risk of nephrolithiasis should be educated to avoid ingestion of cranberry-concentrate pills. Long-term use of several products such as wild yam, flaxseed, zinc, copper, vitamin A, evening primrose oil, and goldenrod, which are promoted to reduce the risk of kidney stones, is not supported by scientific evidence.

Uric Acid Stones

Uric acid is an end product of purine metabolism. The sources of purine are food, de novo synthesis, and tissue catabolism. About half of the purine load is from endogenous sources and is constant. Exogenous dietary sources provide the other half and account for the variation in uric acid presence in the urine.

Solubility of uric acid depends on urine volume, the amount excreted, and urine pH (Table 36-13). Uric acid stones form when urine is supersaturated with undissociated uric acid, which occurs at urinary pH less than 5.5. Therefore conditions such as inflammatory bowel disease, which results in chronically acidic urine from dehydration, and gastrointestinal bicarbonate loss from diarrhea predispose patients to uric acid stones. Uric acid stones are also associ-

ated with lymphoproliferative and myeloproliferative disorders, with increased cellular breakdown that releases purines and thus increases uric acid load. Patients with recurrent uric acid stones are also found to be severely insulin resistant compared to healthy controls (Abate et al., 2004). In a population-based study of stone formers, those with uric acid stones had a greater percentage of diabetes compared to those with other types, 40% versus 9%. Diabetes, obesity, and hypertension appear to be associated with nephrolithiasis; and diabetes may be a factor in uric acid stone development (Lieske et al., 2006).

Besides diabetes management for patients with uric acid lithiasis and hyperuricosuric calcium oxalate stones, dietary purines should also be restricted. Animal flesh proteins (meat, fish, and poultry) are rich in purines and acid ash and should be used in moderation to meet protein requirements (see *Clinical Insight:* Acid Ash and Alkaline Ash Diets). Foods specifically high in purines should be avoided, including organ meats, anchovies, herrings, sardines, meat-based broth, and gravy (see Box 40-2 in Chapter 40). Noncompliance with dietary measures or persistence of hyperuricosuria warrants use of medication such as allopurinol. Uric acid stones are the only stones amenable to dissolution therapy by urine alkalinization to a pH of 6.0 to 6.5. Potassium citrate has been used as the therapy of choice. Sodium bicarbonate increases urinary monosodium urate and calcium and should not be used.

Cystine Stones

Cystine stones represent 1% to 2% of urinary calculi and are caused by homozygous cystinuria. Cystine stones affect about one in 15,000 persons in the United States. Whereas normal individuals daily excrete 20 mg or less of cystine in their urine, stone-forming cystinuric patients excrete more than 250 mg/day. Cystine solubility increases when urine pH exceeds 7.0; therefore an alkaline urine pH must be maintained 24 hours per day, even while the patient sleeps. This is almost always achieved with the use of medication; however, in the past dietary changes have been recommended to change urine pH (see *Clinical Insight:* Acid Ash and Alkaline Ash Diets). Fluid intake of more than 4 L daily is recommended to prevent cystine crystallization. Lower sodium intake may be useful in reducing cystine in the urine.

Methionine is the metabolic precursor of cystine. Severe protein restriction to avoid methionine is impractical, but avoiding excess may be beneficial. Restriction of methionine-containing foods such as milk, meat, and eggs results in a small decrease in total urine cystine excretion which may not be clinically significant or worth the effort involved. *d*-Pencillamine is commonly used as a cystine-binding agent to treat cystinuria because the cysteine-pencillamine product is 50 times more soluble than cystine itself.

Struvite Stones

Struvite stones are comprised of magnesium ammonium phosphate and carbonate apatite. They are also known as triple-phosphate or infection stones. Unlike most urinary

---

TABLE 36-13

Effect of Urine pH on Stone Formation

pH	State of Urate	Likely Stone Development
<5.5	Undissociated urate	Uric acid stones
5.5-7.5	Dissociated urate	Calcium oxalate stones
>7.5	Dissociated urate	Calcium phosphate stones

stones, they occur more commonly in women than in men, at a ratio of 2:1. They form only in the presence of bacteria such as *Pseudomonas*, *Klebsiella*, *Proteus mirabilis*, and *Urealyticum* that carry urease, a urea-splitting enzyme. Urea breakdown results in ammonia and CO_2 production, thus raising urine pH and the level of carbonate. Struvite stones grow rapidly to large staghorn calculi in the renal pelvic area. The mainstay of treatment is surgical removal or extracorporeal shockwave lithotripsy with adjunctive culture-specific antimicrobial therapy that uses urease inhibitors. The goal is to eliminate or prevent urinary tract infections by regularly screening and monitoring urine cultures.

Diet and fluid modification should be advocated as a first step for the prophylaxis of kidney stone disease to improve the urinary risk profile and reduce recurrence. These modifications, summarized in Table 36-14, are simple, economical, and without side effects.

The authors would like to thank Lori S. Brizee MS, RD, CSP, of Children's Hospital & Medical Center, Seattle, Wash, for her expertise in writing the section on renal failure in children; Alysun Deckert MS, RD, CD, and Elizabeth Mullins, RD, CD, of the University of Washington Medical Center, Seattle, Washington, for their expertise in writing the section on renal transplantation; and Fiona Wolf, RD, of Northwest Kidney Centers, Seattle, Washington, for her work in reviewing the chapter.

TABLE 36-14

Recommendations for Diet and 24-Hour Urine Monitoring

Diet Component	Intake Recommendation	24-Hour Urine
Protein	Normal intake: avoid excess	Monitor urinary urea
Calcium	Normal intake: 1000 mg; age ≤50 years 1200 mg; age >50 years	Urinary calcium <150 mg/L (<3.75 mmol/L)
Oxalate	Avoid moderate- to high-oxalate foods initially; further restrict if necessary	Urinary oxalate <20 mg/L (<220 µmol/L)
Fluid	2.5 L or more; assess type of fluids consumed; provide guidelines	Urine volume >2 L/day
Purines	Avoid excessive protein intake; avoid specific high-purine foods	Uric acid <2 mmol/L (<336 mg/L)
Vitamin C	≤ 500 mg/day	Monitor urinary oxalate
Vitamin D; cod liver oil	Supplements not recommended	
Vitamin B_6	40 mg or more/day reduces risk No recommendation made	
Sodium	<100 mmol/day	Monitor urinary sodium

⊛ FOCAL POINTS

- Renal diseases are very complex and often silent in origin. One in nine people in the United States have CKD and don't know it.
- 350,000 Americans are on dialysis, a life-saving therapy that costs billons of dollars every year.
- With an aging population and increasing incidence of type 2 diabetes and its association with CKD and ESRD, the number of people with this major organ failure will increase dramatically.
- Early detection of kidney disease and screening for renal risk factors should result in better and appropriate medical nutrition therapy, with increased life expectancy and decreased economic burden.

- There is new research indicating the effectiveness of dietary components, nutrients and fluid to influence urine pH and saturation in the prevention of nephrolithiasis and in its management once it has developed.
- Effective health care teams include RDs, who are familiar with the complex nature of therapy for renal disease and nephrolithiasis, and who play important roles in the management of these patients.
- With a "global" professional approach to renal nutrition, patients with CKD, ESRD, and nephrolithiasis all over the world will have a brighter future.

✱ CLINICAL SCENARIO 1

Mark is a 36-year-old man with a history of drug abuse and cocaine addiction. Recently he was admitted to the local hospital with acute renal failure and has been started on hemodialysis. He has no prior medical problems or hyperten-sion. His laboratory values include BUN, 90; creatinine, 7; potassium, 6.1; all other laboratory values are currently normal. He is 6 ft 2 in and weighs 190 lb.

✱**Nutrition Diagnosis:** Altered nutrition-related laboratory values as evidenced by hyperkalemia

1. What would you suggest for the dialysis nutrition prescription?
2. His physician suggests daily use of a multivitamin supplement containing B-complex vitamins but not fat-soluble vitamins. Why?

3. What level of protein would you suggest for Mark during dialysis? How much should Mark receive in the way of protein foods?
4. If he goes home without dialysis but has chronic renal failure, what might his doctor suggest for a protein level?
5. What foods will be monitored according to the National Renal Diet?

✱ CLINICAL SCENARIO 2

Kelsey is a 33-year-old woman with glomerulonephritis who has been on hemodialysis for 8 years. She takes the following medications: erythropoietin, Benadryl, folic acid, prednisone, Nephrocaps, Basaljel, and Tums. The patient dialyzes against the following dialysate fluid: 3 mEq of potassium, 3.5 mg of calcium, 35 mEq of bicarbonate, 200 g of dextrose. The patient is currently awaiting a cadaveric transplant. She asks you how her diet will change with the transplant. If the transplant does not happen soon, she is considering peritoneal dialysis to give her more freedom from the machine. Her current laboratory values are the following:

Na: 135	K: 5.9	CO_2: 16
Creat: 9	Ca: 8.7	PO_4: 6.9
Alb: 3.4	Ferritin: 82	Wt: 57.2 kg
Ht: 172	Fluid gains: 2.9-3.7 kg	BUN: 70
AMA: <50%	Anthropometrics are =	
AFA: >8%	Wt: 57.2 kg,	
	Ht: 172 cm	

Peritoneal dialysis will be started tomorrow.

✱**Nutrition Diagnosis:** Food- and nutrition-related knowledge deficit related to medical nutrition therapy for peritoneal dialysis as evidenced by patient statements

1. Explain why you would expect to see each of the laboratory value discrepancies and what could be done nutritionally to affect each value. Also assess the patient's weight and anthropometric values to determine appropriate nutrition therapy.
2. Comment on the appropriateness of each medication. For what is each used? Would you suggest any changes or additional medications?

✱ CLINICAL SCENARIO 3

Arnold is a 28-year-old man with a history of recurrent urolithiasis, two episodes of kidney stones, both passed spontaneously, requiring no surgical intervention, laser treatment, or lithotripsy. The stones were analyzed and found to be calcium oxalate. Review of laboratory data shows a normal creatinine, calcium, phosphorus and PTH. The serum electrolytes are within normal limits and do not suggest a medical diagnosis of complete RTA. There is no history of urinary tract infection. Arnold is not on any medications that would predis-pose him to urolithiasis, and there is no family history of urolithiasis. His height is 175 cm and he has a BMI of 31 kg/m². The 24-hour urine collection shows a volume of 1100 ml, urine calcium at 1.80 mmol, urine oxalate of 559 µmmol, urine uric acid at 4 mmol, and a urine urea of 300 mmol. Urine citrate is at 0.8 mmol. Urine cystine testing is negative. Diet history indicates a very high intake of animal protein (125% of needs); he supplements his diet with protein powder. He eats beets, nuts, and chocolate frequently and hates drinking plain water.

✱ CLINICAL SCENARIO 3—cont'd

✱Nutrition Diagnosis: Excessive protein intake related to very high animal protein intake and use of protein powders as evidenced by intake of protein at 125% of estimated requirements and recent kidney stones

1. List the risk factors for kidney stones that you identify from the analysis of the 24-hour urine collection.
2. What does a low urine calcium suggest?
3. Would you recommend additional dietary calcium, and if so, how would you suggest it be taken?

4. What strategies could you use to help him increase his urine volume?
5. Identify and educate to modify other risk factors from medical and diet history that could reduce his risk for kidney stones in the future.

USEFUL WEBSITES

American Dietetic Association and the National Renal Diet
www.eatright.org; www.Ikidney.com

Life Options
www.lifeoptions.org

National Institute of Diabetes and Digestive and Kidney Diseases (NIDDKD)
www.niddk.nih.gov/health/kidney/kidney.htm

National Kidney Foundation
www.kidney.org

Nationwide End-Stage Renal Network
www.esrdnetwork.org

Northwest Kidney Centers (source of "The Art of Good Eating," a free workbook for people on dialysis)
www.nwkidney.org

Renal Network
www.renalnet.org

United States Renal Data Systems
http://www.usrds.org/

References

Abate N et al: The metabolic syndrome and uric acid nephrolithiasis: novel features of renal manifestation of insulin resistance, *Kidney Int* 65(2):386, 2004.

Ahmad S: Dietary sodium restriction for hypertension in dialysis patients, *Semin Dial* 17:284, 2004

Appel GB: Improved outcomes in nephrotic syndrome, *Cleve Clin J Med* 73(2):161, 2006.

Asplin JR et al: Bone mineral density and urine calcium excretion among subjects with and without nephrolithiasis, *Kidney Int* 63(2):662, 2003.

Baggio B et al: Plasma phospholipid arachidonic acid content and calcium metabolism in idiopathic calcium nephrolithiasis, *Kidney Int* 58:1278, 2000.

Bennett SJ et al: Nutrition in chronic heart failure with coexisting chronic kidney disease, *J Cardiovasc Nurs* 21(1):56, 2006.

Beto J: Highlights of the consensus conference on prevention of progression in chronic renal disease: implications for dietetic practice, *J Ren Nutr* 4:122, 1994.

Block G, Port F: Re-evaluation of risks associated with hyperphosphatemia and hyperparathyroidism in dialysis patients: recommendations for a change in management, *Am J Kidney Dis* 35:1226, 2000.

Block G et al: Cinacalcet for secondary hyperparathyroidism in patients receiving hemodialysis, *New Engl J Med* 350:1516, 2004.

Borghi L et al: Comparison of two diets for the prevention of recurrent stones in idiopathic hypercalciuria, *N Engl J Med* 346:77, 2002.

Byham-Gray LD: Weighing the evidence: energy determinations across the spectrum of kidney disease, *J Ren Nutr* 16(1):17, 2006.

Caudarella et al: Osteoporosis and urolithiasis, *Urol Int* 72(suppl 1):17, 2004.

Cooper B et al: Protein malnutrition and hypoalbuminemia as predictors of vascular events and mortality in ESRD, *Am J Kidney Dis* 43:61, 2004.

Curhan GC et al: Intake of vitamins B_6 and C and the risk of kidney stones in women, *Urol Int* 10:840, 1999.

Curhan GC et al: Dietary factors and the risk of incident kidney stones in younger women. Nurses' Health Study II, *Arch Intern Med* 164:885, 2004.

Domrongkitchaiporn S et al: Schedule of taking calcium supplement and risk of nephrolithiasis, *Kidney Int* 65(5):1835, 2004.

Domrongkitchaiporn S et al: Hypocitraturia in recurrent calcium stone formers: focusing on urinary potassium excretion, *Am J Kidney Dis* 48:546, 2006.

Ekim M et al: Evaluation of nutritional status and factors related to malnutrition in children on CAPD, *Perit Dial Int* 23:557, 2003.

Gerster H: No contribution of ascorbic acid to renal calcium oxalate stones, *Ann Nutr Metabol* 41:269, 1997.

Giordano C: Early diet to slow the course of chronic renal failure. In Zurukzoglu W, Papadimetrious M, editors: *Eighth International Congress of Nephrology, June 1981*, Basel, 1981, S Karger.

Goldfarb DS, Asplin JR: Effect of grapefruit juice in urinary lithogenicity, *J Urol* 166:263, 2001.

Goldfarb DS et al: A twin study of genetic and dietary influences on nephrolithiasis: a report from the Vietnam Era Twin (VET) Registry, *Kidney Int* 67 (3):1053, 2005.

Heany RP, Rafferty K: Carbonated beverages and urinary calcium excretion, *Am J Clin Nutr* 74:343, 2001.

Hoesl CE, Altwein JE: The probiotic approach: an alternative treatment option in urology, *Eur Urol* 47(3):288, 2005.

Holmes RP et al: Contribution of dietary oxalate to urinary oxalate excretion, *Kidney Int* 59:270, 2001.

Holmes RP, Kennedy M: Estimation of oxalate content of foods and daily oxalate intake, *Kidney Int* 57:1662, 2000.

Howell A et al: Inhibition of the adherence of P-fimbriated *Escherichia coli* to uroepithelial-cell surface by proanthocyanidin extracts from cranberries [Letter], *N Engl J Med* 339:1085, 1998.

Jones CH et al: The relationship between serum albumin and hydration status in hemodialysis patients, *J Ren Nutr* 12:209, 2002.

Joy M et al: Long-term glycemic control measurements in diabetic patients receiving hemodialysis, *Am J Kidney Dis* 39:297, 2002

Kaelin A et al: Vitamin B_6 metabolites in idiopathic calcium stone formers: no evidence for a link to hyperoxaluria, *Urol Res* 32(1):61, 2004.

Kalantar-Zadeh K et al: A modified quantitative Subjective Global Assessment of nutrition for dialysis patients, *Nephrol Dial Transplant* 14:1732, 1999.

Kessler T et al: Effect of black currant, cranberry, and plum juice consumption on risk factors associated with kidney stone formation, *Eur J Clin Nutr* 56(10):1020, 2002.

Kontiokari T et al: Cranberry juice and bacterial colonization in children—a placebo-controlled randomized trial, *Clin Nutr* 24(6):1065, 2005.

Lieske JC et al: Diabetes mellitus and the risk of urinary tract stones: a population-based case controlled study, *Am J Kidney Dis* 48:897, 2006.

Locatelli F et al: Nutritional-inflammation status and resistance to erythropoietin therapy in haemodialysis patients, *Nephrol Dial Transplant* 21:991, 2006.

Maalouf NM et al: Association of urinary pH with body weight in nephrolithiasis, *Kidney Int* 65:1422, 2004.

Martini LA: Stop dietary calcium restriction in kidney stone–forming patients, *Nutr Rev* 60:212, 2002.

Martini LA, Wood RJ: Should dietary calcium and protein be restricted in patients with nephrolithiasis? *Nutr Rev* 58:111, 2000.

Massey LK: Dietary influences on urinary oxalate and risk of kidney stones, *Front Biosci* 8:S584, 2003.

Massey LK et al: Ascorbate increases human oxaluria and kidney stone risk, *J Nutr* 135:1673, 2005.

Maung H et al: Efficacy and side effects of intermittent intravenous and oral doxercalciferol in dialysis patients with secondary hyperparathyroidism: a sequential comparison, *Am J Kidney Dis* 37:532, 2001.

Meschi T et al: Body weight, diet and water intake in preventing stone disease, *Urol Int* 72(suppl 1):29, 2004.

Morton AR et al: Nephrology. 1. Investigation and treatment of recurrent kidney stones, *Can Med Assoc J* 166:213, 2002.

National Kidney Foundation (NKF): DOQI clinical practice guidelines for nutrition in chronic renal failure, *Am J Kidney Dis* 35(suppl 2):35, 2000.

Nelson RG, Tuttle KR: The new KDOQI clinical practice guidelines and clinical practice recommendations for diabetes and CKD, *Blood Purif* 25:112, 2007.

Neyra R et al: Increased resting energy expenditure in patients with end-stage renal disease, *JPEN J Parenter Enteral Nutr* 27:36, 2003.

Nguyen QY et al: Sensitivity to meat protein intake and hyperoxaluria in idiopathic calcium stone formers, *Kidney Int* 59:2273, 2001.

Pak CY et al: Prevention of stone formation and bone loss in absorptive hypercalciuria by combined dietary and pharmacological interventions, *J Urol* 169(2):465, 2003.

Parks JH et al: Urine stone risk factors in nephrolithiasis patients with and without bowel disease, *Kidney Int* 63:255, 2003.

Pennell JP: Optimizing medical management of patients with preend-stage renal disease, *Am J Med* 111:559, 2001.

Pohlmeir R, Vienken J: Phosphate removal and hemodialysis conditions, *Kidney Int* 59:S190, 2001.

Remuzzi G, Bertani T: Pathophysiology of progressive nephropathies, *N Engl J Med* 339:1448, 1998.

Rigalleau V et al: Cockcroft-Gault formula is biased by body weight in diabetic patients with renal impairment, *Metabolism* 55:108, 2006.

Rigby A et al: Sodium, not fluid, contributes to interdialytic weight gain, *Nephrol News Issues* 21:1, 2000.

Rotily M et al: Effects of protein or high-fibre diets on urine composition in calcium nephrolithiasis, *Kidney Int* 57:1115, 2000.

Schiro-Harvey K: *The national renal diet*, ed 2, Chicago, 2002, American Dietetic Association.

Seltzer MA et al: Dietary manipulation with lemonade to treat hypocitraturic calcium nephrolithiasis, *J Urol* 156:907, 1996.

Shaw-Stewart N, Stuart A: The effect of an educational patient compliance program on serum phosphate levels in patients receiving hemodialysis, *J Ren Nutr* 10:80, 2000.

Siener R, Hesse A: Recent advances in nutritional research on urolithiasis, *World J Urol* 23:304, 2005.

Siener R et al: The role of overweight and obesity in calcium oxalate stone formation, *Obes Res* 12(1):106, 2004.

Slatopolsky E et al: A novel mechanism for skeletal resistance in uremia, *Kidney Int* 58:753, 2000.

Stamatelou KK et al: Time trends in reported prevalence of kidney stones in the United States, 1976-1994, *Kidney Int* 63:1817, 2003.

Stitchantrakul W et al: Effects of calcium supplements on the risk of renal stone formation in a population with low oxalate intake, *Southeast Asian J Trop Med Public Health* 35(4):1028, 2004.

Straub M, Hautmann RE: Developments in stone prevention, *Curr Opin Urol* 15:119, 2005.

Strejc JM: Considerations in the nutritional management of patients with acute renal failure, *Hemodial Int* 9(2):135, 2005.

Taylor EN, Curhan GC: Role of nutrition in the formation of calcium containing kidney stones, *Nephron Physiol* 98:55, 2004.

Taylor EN, Curhan GC: Diet and fluid prescription in stone disease, *Kidney Int* 70:835, 2006.

Taylor EN et al: Dietary factors and the risk of incident kidney stones in men: new insights after 14 years of follow-up, *J Am Soc Nephrol* 15(12):3225, 2004.

Terris MK et al: Dietary supplementation with cranberry concentrate tablets may increase the risk of nephrolithiasis, *Urology* 57:26, 2001.

Tomasello S et al: Phosphate binders, KDOQI guidelines and compliance: the unfortunate reality, *Dial Transplant* 33:236, 2004.

Traxer O et al: Stone forming risk of ascorbic acid, *J Endourol* 14(suppl 1):A9, 2000.

Unruh ML et al: Choices for healthy outcomes in caring for end-stage renal disease (CHOICE) study, *Am J Kidney Dis* 46(6):1107, 2005.

Uribarri J Calvo M: Hidden sources of phosphorus in the typical American diet: does it matter in nephrology? *Semin Dial* 16:186, 2003.

von Unruh GE et al: Dependence of oxalate absorption on the daily calcium intake, *J Am Soc Nephrol* 15(6):1567, 2004.

Wiggins K: *Guidelines for nutritional care of renal patients*, ed 3, Chicago, 2002, American Dietetic Association.

Wiggins KL, Schiro-Harvey K: A review of guidelines for nutrition care of renal patients, *Ren Nutr* 12:190, 2002.

Zhang R et al: Kidney disease and the metabolic syndrome, *Am J Med Sci* 330:319, 2005.

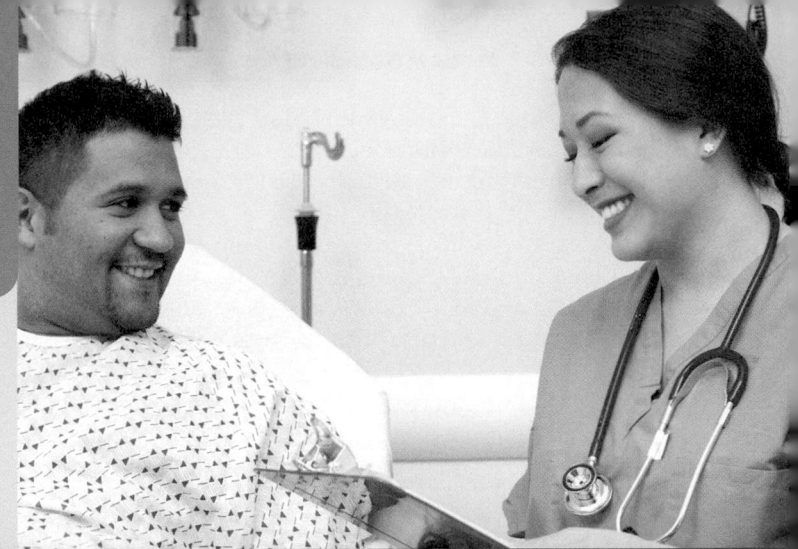

CHAPTER 37

Barbara Grant, MS, RD

Medical Nutrition Therapy for Cancer

KEY TERMS

ageusia loss or absence of the sense of taste

antioxidants molecules such as some vitamins that block action of activated oxygen molecules (free radicals) that can damage cells

cancer abnormal division and reproduction of cells that can spread throughout the body, crowding out normal cells and tissues

cancer cachexia weight loss and lessening of the body's fat and muscle stores that accompany advanced cancer, even with adequate nutrition; may be related to elevated levels of tumor necrosis factor

carcinogen an agent (physical, chemical, or viral) that induces cancer in humans and animals

case control studies studies in which the diets of individuals with cancer are compared with those of cancer-free controls matched for age, sex, and other key factors

chemotherapy the use of chemical agents (cytotoxics, immunologic preparations, hormonals) or medications to prevent the development, maturation, or spread of neoplastic cells

cohort studies studies in which diets of different groups of subjects are determined before cancer onset and the incidences of developing cancers in each group are compared

control to extend the length of life when a cure is not possible; to obscure microscopic metastases after tumors are surgically removed; to shrink tumors before surgery or radiation therapy

cross-sectional studies studies in which the diets of different groups of subjects are compared, using the same measures at a single point in time

cure to obtain a complete response to treatment of a specific cancer

cytokines protein mediators produced by inflammatory cells in response to exogenous stimuli

dysgeusia impaired taste

epidemiologic studies studies looking at cancer in populations, including who gets specific types and what factors play a part in the development of cancer

graft-versus-host disease (GVHD) a disease caused by the immune response of histoincompatible, immunocompetent donor cells against the tissues of an immunoincompetent host; an immunologic reaction of allogeneic donor cells (graft) reacting against the patient (host) tissues

hematopoietic stem cell transplantation (HSCT) the use of chemotherapy and radiation therapy to ablate bone marrow, followed by an intravenous infusion of autologous, allogenec, or syngeneic stem cells

hypogeusia decreased taste acuity

immunotherapy the use of biologic response modifiers that are made through cloning and genetic engineering, as cytotoxic agents or indirectly as stimulators of the individual's own natural defenses to kill tumor cells; examples are α-interferon and interleukin-2; also includes supportive care agents (hematopoietics) such as cytokines that stimulate the marrow to develop faster

initiation the initial stage of tumorigenesis, involving transformation of cellular deoxyribonucleic acid

malignant neoplasm a mass of cancer cells that invades surrounding tissues or spreads to distant areas of the body; if left untreated, it will likely worsen and become possibly fatal

metastasis growth of malignant tissue that spreads to surrounding tissues or organs

mucositis inflammation of a mucous membrane

myelosuppression suppression of bone marrow cell production

neoplasm a new and abnormal formation of tissue that serves no useful function

neutropenia a reduction in white blood cell count (neutrophils) that can be caused by chemotherapy or radiation therapy and that, in turn, results in increased susceptibility to potentially life-threatening infections

palliative care to provide support and comfort when cure or control is not possible; to improve quality of life; to reduce tumor burden and help relieve cancer-related symptoms

pancytopenia a reduction in all cellular elements of the blood

phytochemicals nonnutritive compounds in plants thought to influence the process of tumorigenesis

progression the phase in which tumor cells aggregate, grow autonomously, and form benign tumors that eventually lead to a malignant phenotype with the capacity for tissue invasion and metastasis

promotion the stage of tumorigenesis in which initiated cells are activated by a promoting agent to multiply and form a discrete tumor

radiation therapy use of high-energy rays (ionizing radiation) in multiple fractionated doses to cure, control, or palliate cancer

radiation-induced enteritis inflammation that can occur after radiation to the intestinal tract and that leads to diarrhea and malabsorption

sinusoidal obstructive syndrome (SOS) a symptomatic occlusion of the small hepatic venules caused by hepatotoxins and radiation therapy or chemotherapy; may resolve after removal of the offending agent or may progress to portal hypertension and liver failure

staging a classification system known as TNM that is used to identify the "extent" of the tumor: its size, the degree of growth and spread; T stands for the size of the tumor, N for the degree of spread to lymph nodes, and M for the presence of metastasis

tumor a solid cancer that causes a swelling or a lump; commonly defined as a malignant neoplasm

tumor markers different chemical substances that are found in the blood and body fluids and are used to identify and diagnose different types of cancer and monitor response to treatment

tumor necrosis factor (cachectin) a hormonelike protein that releases fat from fat stores, reduces the concentration of enzymes required for the production and storage of fat, and induces a state of anorexia

xerostomia dryness of the mouth

lular deoxyribonucleic acid. The transformation occurs rapidly, but the resultant cell remains dormant for a variable period until it is activated by a promoting agent.

During **promotion,** initiated cells multiply and escape the mechanisms set in place to protect the body from the growth and spread of such cells; a **neoplasm,** or new and abnormal tissue with no useful function, is established. From there **progression,** the phase in which tumor cells aggregate and grow, proceeds, leading eventually to a fully **malignant neoplasm** or a **tumor** with the capacity for tissue invasion that may eventually spread to distant tissues and organs, a process known as **metastasis** (see *Pathophysiology and Care Management Algorithm:* Cancer). The classification of tumors is based on their tissue of origin, their growth properties, and their invasion of other tissues. Tumors that are not malignant are typically described as benign.

Because cancer occurs in cells that are replicating, the patterns of cancer are quite different in children and adults. In early life the brain, nervous system, bones, muscles, and connective tissue are still growing. Thus in children these tissues are more commonly involved with cancerous lesions than they are in adults. Conversely, common adult tumors involve epithelial linings. Leukemias and lymphomas, which are cancers of the immune system, occur in both children and adults.

The American Cancer Society (ACS) predicts that the lifetime risk for developing cancer in the United States is slightly less than one in two for men and a little more than one in three for women (ACS, 2006). The leading types of new cancer cases annually diagnosed in the United States are prostate, lung and bronchus, colorectal, and urinary bladder cancers for men; and breast, lung and bronchus, colorectal, and uterine cancers for women. In 2006 the ACS estimated that almost 1,400,000 Americans would be diagnosed with cancer within the year, and that about a third of the almost 570,000 cancer deaths expected to occur will be related to nutrition, physical inactivity, and overweight and obesity. It is still anticipated that an additional 170,000 cancer deaths will be caused by tobacco use (ACS, 2006).

Currently the National Cancer Institute (NCI) estimates that there are 10.1 million Americans living with a history of cancer (e.g., cancer free, living with evidence of disease, or undergoing cancer treatment) (NCI, 2006b). As a result of improvements in early detection of cancer and the development of new anticancer therapies, the relative survival rate for all cancers diagnosed between 1995 and 2001 is now 65%, up from 50% in 1974 to 1976 (ACS, 2006).

Cancer, abnormal division and reproduction of cells that can spread throughout the body, is usually thought of as a single disease but consists of almost 100 disorders caused by nearly 300 different growths. Carcinogenesis, the origin or development of cancer, is thought to be a biologic, multistage process that proceeds on a continuum but is often described in three progressive phases: initiation, promotion, and tumor progression. **Initiation** involves a transformation of the cell produced by the interaction of chemicals, radiation, or viruses with cel-

CANCER DIAGNOSIS AND MEDICAL TREATMENT

Cancer diagnosis is determined by several methods. These diagnostic methods include medical history and physical examination; evaluation for **tumor markers** (e.g., AFP, BRCA, CA-125, CA 19-9, CEA, PSA or other substances in blood or body fluids that identify cancer); cytology stud-

PATHOPHYSIOLOGY AND CARE MANAGEMENT ALGORITHM

Cancer

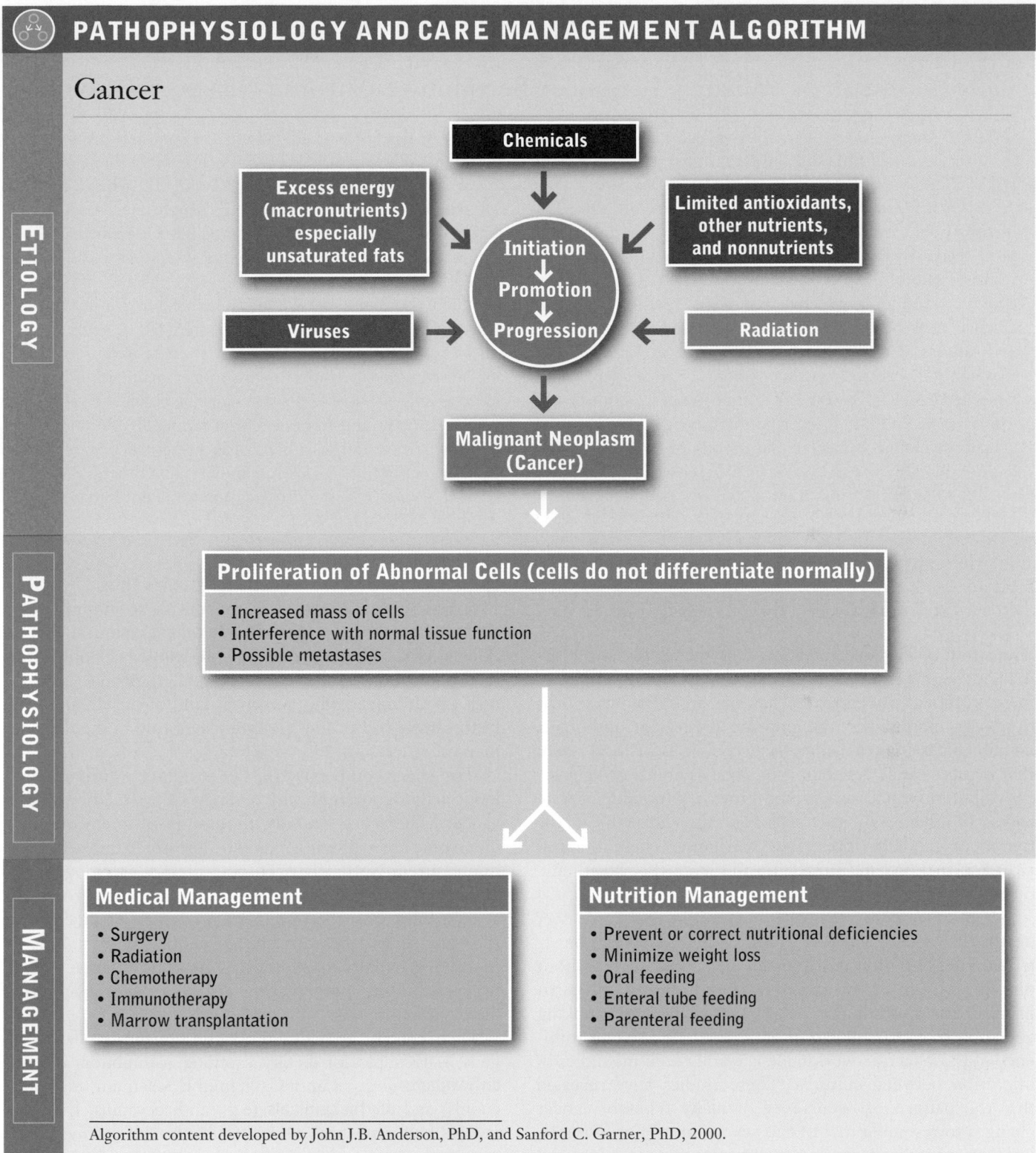

ETIOLOGY

Chemicals

Excess energy (macronutrients) especially unsaturated fats

Limited antioxidants, other nutrients, and nonnutrients

Initiation → Promotion → Progression

Viruses

Radiation

Malignant Neoplasm (Cancer)

PATHOPHYSIOLOGY

Proliferation of Abnormal Cells (cells do not differentiate normally)

- Increased mass of cells
- Interference with normal tissue function
- Possible metastases

MANAGEMENT

Medical Management

- Surgery
- Radiation
- Chemotherapy
- Immunotherapy
- Marrow transplantation

Nutrition Management

- Prevent or correct nutritional deficiencies
- Minimize weight loss
- Oral feeding
- Enteral tube feeding
- Parenteral feeding

Algorithm content developed by John J.B. Anderson, PhD, and Sanford C. Garner, PhD, 2000.

ies and tumor biopsy (e.g., fluid, sputum, tissue, urine); imaging studies (e.g., x-rays or computed tomography, magnetic resonance imaging, positron emission tomography scans), and **staging** (e.g., radiographic, pathologic, surgical, or staging for tumor size [T], nodes [N], metastasis [M]). The clinical intent of cancer treatment is to cure, control, or palliate (see *Clinical Insight*: Cure, Control, or Palliate—Is Cancer Becoming a Chronic Disease for

Some?). Response to treatment is defined as complete, partial, stable, or progressive.

Conventional modalities of cancer treatment include chemotherapy, immunotherapy, radiation therapy, and surgery used alone or in combination. In addition, solid tumors and hematologic malignant diseases such as leukemias, lymphomas, and multiple myelomas can be treated by hemopoietic cell transplantation.

✳ CLINICAL INSIGHT

Cure, Control, or Palliate—Is Cancer Becoming a Chronic Disease for Some?

Fewer Americans are dying from cancer, a trend that began over 15 years ago, and the rate of new cancers remains stable. The *Annual Report to the Nation on the Status of Cancer, 1975-2003, Featuring Cancer among U.S. Hispanic/Latino Populations* published in October 2006, states that death rates have decreased for common cancers in men and women as a result of reduced exposure to tobacco, earlier screening and detection, and more effective treatments. Among women incidence rates have decreased for colon and rectum cancers and cancers of the uterus, ovarian cancer, oral cancers, and stomach and cervical cancers. Among men incidence rates have decreased for colon and rectum cancers, stomach and oral cancers, and lung cancer but have increased for prostate cancer; myeloma; leukemia; and cancers of the liver, kidney, and esophagus. The full report may be viewed at www.interscience.wiley.com/cancer/report2006 (accessed 12/11/06).

Cure of cancer has been defined as a complete response to treatment. When treatments cannot cure, often they can control cancer. **Control** is defined as extending life when a cure is not possible by getting rid of microscopic metastases after tumors are surgically removed, shrinking tumors before surgery or radiation therapy, or reducing symptoms and side effects of cancer presence.

When a cure or control is not possible and death is likely, palliative care (comfort measures) is offered. The goals are to relieve pain and physical symptoms; alleviate isolation, anxiety and fear; and help those with cancer maintain independence as long as possible. Patients may be eligible for hospice care, either in an inpatient unit or at home. Hydration needs are usually met, and pain control is attempted. Patients are made as comfortable as possible in the dying process. Generally with palliative care, nutrition support is not initiated.

NUTRITION IN THE ETIOLOGY OF CANCER

The study of diet and nutrition as it relates to cancer addresses the causes and consequences of cancer and its treatment. Although the exact mechanisms are unknown, nutrition may modify the carcinogenic process at any stage, including **carcinogen** (a physical, chemical, or viral agent that induces cancer) metabolism, cellular and host defense, cell differentiation, and tumor growth. Nutrition is also adversely affected by several factors: the cancer itself, the treatment modality prescribed (including chemotherapy, radiation therapy, and surgery), and the current health and nutrition status of the individual.

Scientific evidence suggests that one third of the cancer deaths that occur each year in the United States can be attributed to nutrition and lifestyle behaviors such as poor diet, physical inactivity, overweight and obesity, and alcohol use, and another third is related to cigarette smoking and tobacco use (Mokdad et al., 2004). The strong influence of these factors worldwide is readily seen in studies of migration between cultures. These studies have revealed that the pattern of occurrence of many types of cancer changes to resemble that of the new country. For example, in Japan mortality from breast and colon cancer is low, and mortality from stomach cancer is high, whereas the reverse is true in Japanese living in the United States. After two or three generations, their cancer pattern becomes similar to that of the population in their new country (Wynder et al., 1991; NIH, 1996).

Studies of the role of diet in the etiology of cancer seek to identify relationships between the diets of population groups and categories of individuals and the incidence of specific cancers. Sets of individuals are compared in **case control, cohort,** or **cross-sectional studies** (Box 37-1). The strongest evidence comes from consistent findings from these different types of **epidemiologic studies** in diverse populations. In cancer research epidemiologists look at human populations and evaluate how many people are diagnosed with cancer, who gets what kind of cancer, and what factors such as diet and lifestyle play a role in the development of cancer.

The sheer complexity of diet presents a difficult challenge when contemplating a study of its relationship to cancer. There are literally thousands of chemicals in a diet; some are well known, and others are little known and unmeasured. Naturally occurring dietary carcinogens are natural pesticides produced by plants for protection against fungi, insects, or animal predators; or mycotoxins that are secondary metabolites produced by molds in foods (e.g., aflatoxins, fumosins or ochratoxin A). Food preparation and preservation are also major sources of dietary carcinogens.

Diets contain both inhibitors and enhancers of carcinogenesis. Examples of dietary carcinogen inhibitors include: **antioxidants** (e.g., vitamin C, vitamin E, selenium, and carotenoids) and **phytochemicals** (e.g., anthrocyanins, lycopene, indoles, sulforaphanes). Dietary enhancers of carcinogenesis may be the fat in red meat or the polycyclic aromatic hydrocarbons that form with the grilling of meat at high heat (see "Fat" on p. 963). Complicating the study of diet and cancer is the fact that, when one major component of the diet is altered, other changes take place simultaneously. For example, decreasing animal protein also decreases animal fat. This makes the interpretation of research findings difficult because the effects cannot be clearly associated with a single factor.

Many cancers have a long latency period, in which case the diet at the time of initiation or promotion—not at the time of diagnosis—may be important. Some prospective epidemiologic studies attempt to circumvent this difficulty by measuring diet at one point in time and following the same subjects for several years. Studies done with laboratory animals are used to test the effect of food and nutrition on cancer. Since the early part of the last century, laboratory scientists have shown that various nutritional manipulations influence the occurrence of tumors in animals. In concert with epidemiologic work, animal studies can be used to provide hypotheses to guide epidemiologic research and reveal modifiable pathways to cancer in humans.

Energy Intake, Body Weight, Obesity, and Physical Activity

In animal studies chronic restriction of food and or nutrition support (e.g., total parenteral nutrition [TPN]) inhibited the growth of most experimentally induced cancers and the occurrence of many spontaneous cancers. This effect was observed even when underfed animals ingested more fat than control animals ingested (Kritchevsky, 2001). Caloric restriction appears to extend life span and decrease molecular damage, at least in animals (Spindler, 2005) (see *New Directions:* Will Eating Less Make You Live Longer? in Chapter 2).

Currently 65% of all American adults are overweight or obese (body mass index [BMI] >25) (Hedley et al., 2004). Obesity increases the risk for developing and dying from cancer, heart disease, and diabetes (Eyre et al., 2004). The relationship between body weight, BMI, or relative body weight and site-specific cancer has been widely investigated, and in most epidemiologic studies a positive association has been seen with cancers of the breast, endometrium, kidney, colon, and prostate. In breast cancer a positive association with weight gain is seen in postmenopausal women (Abu-Abid et al., 2002; Biachini et al., 2002).

A study that followed 4.5 million male veterans for up to 27 years found that obesity was associated with significantly higher risks of cancers in men, specifically cancers of the lower esophagus, stomach, small intestine, colon, rectum, gallbladder, ampulla of Vater, breast, prostate, bladder, thyroid, connective tissue, melanoma, multiple myeloma, and two types of leukemia (Samanic et al., 2004). Results from the Cancer Prevention Study II showed that BMI was significantly associated with higher death rates from 11 types of cancer in men and 12 types of cancer in women (Calle et al., 2003). BMI in adolescence has implications for risk of cancer mortality in later life; measures of BMI throughout life are needed to determine the period of greatest risk from obesity (Okasha et al., 2002).

Being overweight or obese also appears to increase risk of cancer recurrence (Rock and Demark-Wahnfried, 2002) and cancer survival (Calle et al., 2003). A prospective study of Japanese women diagnosed with colon cancer found that study participants who were overweight and obese (BMI >25) had decreased overall and disease-free survival (Tamakoshi et al., 2004). Another study reported that significantly obese men (BMI ≥35) who had undergone radical prostatectomies for localized prostate cancer were at a higher risk for abnormal PSA measurements than normal or overweight participants (Freeland et al., 2004).

Physical inactivity, high energy intake, and large body mass are associated with an increased risk of developing colon cancer in men and women (Kushner, 2002). Conversely the benefit of regular physical activity in reducing the risk of breast and colon cancer has been demonstrated. Regular physical activity helps to control body weight; whereas excess body weight increases the amount of circulating estrogens, androgens, insulin, and insulin-like growth factors, all of which are associated with cell and tumor growth (NCHS, 2001). The ACS encourages all Americans to strive to maintain a BMI between 18.5 and 25 kg/m^2 and to engage in regular physical activity most days of the week.

Fat

Experimental and epidemiologic data show a link between some cancers and the amount of fat in the diet. Diets high in fat also tend to be high in calories and contribute to obesity, which in turn is associated with increased risk of cancers at several sites, including the colon and rectum, esophagus, gallbladder, breast among postmenopausal women, endometrium, pancreas, and kidney. Because dietary fat intake is correlated with intake of other nutrients and dietary components, it is difficult to distinguish between the effects of dietary fats and protein, total calories, and fiber. A complex interaction of fat with these or other factors may account for inconsistent results of epidemiologic and experimental investigations.

Several studies have shown that it is the type of fat such as that in red meats and dairy products that is associated with an increased risk of prostate, breast, and lung cancer (Augustsson et al., 2003; Kushi and Giovannuci, 2002). A prospective analysis of over 90,000 women participating in the Nurses' Health Study II found that the intake of animal fat from red meat and high-fat dairy during premenopausal years was associated with an increased risk of breast cancer (Cho et al., 2003). Goodstine and colleagues (2003) found that eating more omega-3 fat in relation to omega-6 fat may reduce risk of premenopausal breast cancer; other researchers have reported this same association for decreased breast cancer risk in postmenopausal women (Wirfalt et al., 2002). When choosing red meat, it is recommended to select leaner cuts and smaller portions; fish, poultry, or legumes are desirable alternatives to beef, pork, and lamb.

With respect to secondary cancer prevention and dietary fat intake, researchers from the Women's Interventional Nutrition Study of over 2400 women with a history of breast cancer have reported that breast cancer recurrence was reduced by eating a low-fat (less than 20% energy from fat) compared to a standard diet. Participants diagnosed with breast cancer reduced their risk of recurrence significantly by eating the low-fat diet.

Protein

Understanding the role of protein in cancer development is complicated by the fact that most diets high in protein are also high in meat and fat and low in fiber. The effect of protein on experimental carcinogenesis depends on the tissue of origin and the type of tumor as well as on the type of protein and the caloric adequacy of the diet. In general, tumor development is suppressed by diets that contain levels of protein below that required for optimal growth, whereas it is enhanced by protein levels two to three times the amount that is required. The effects may be attributable to specific amino acids, a general effect of protein, or, in the case of low-protein diets, depressed food intake. Epidemiologic data are limited and conflicting.

Increased red meat intake (e.g., beef, pork, lamb) has been found to be associated with an increased risk of colon cancer and prostate cancer. Recommendations for lowering cancer risk and improving overall health that are provided by the ACS American Institute for Cancer Research (AICR) encourage Americans to consume plant foods and limit the intake of animal sources of foods, including red meats, especially those high in saturated fat and processed foods (Byers et al., 2002). Numerous studies have shown that individuals consuming a plant-based diet (a diet composed of vegetables, fruits, whole grains, and legumes) rather than a diet comprised of foods from animal sources have the lowest risk of cancer (Leitzmann, 2005; Slattery et al., 2004).

Because animal studies demonstrate that certain amino acid deficiencies inhibit some tumors, the feeding of amino acid–deficient diets or amino acid antagonists has been proposed as an adjunct to cancer therapy. Although this hypothesis has theoretic appeal, currently there is no active clinical research in this area.

Soy and Phytoestrogens

Soy is a plant-based protein, and it contains phytoestrogens (e.g., weak plant-based estrogens and compounds such as isoflavones and lignans). A soy-containing diet may be protective against breast cancer (Dai et al., 2001; Yan and Spitznagel, 2004), especially if the soy diet is consumed before reaching adulthood (Shu et al., 2001; Wu et al., 2002). Researchers propose that it is the exposure to the weak estrogenic effects of isoflavones early in life that may reduce the risk of breast cancer (Cotroneo et al., 2002).

The use of soy remains controversial for individuals already diagnosed with cancer. There is concern that the phytoestrogens found in soy and soy-containing foods may be harmful if consumed by women diagnosed with estrogen-receptor–positive breast cancer. Commercially prepared soy supplement powders and foods made from soy protein isolates (e.g., energy bars, cereals, soy beverages, and phytoestrogen supplements) generally contain isoflavones at much higher concentrations than traditional whole soy foods such as edemame, tofu, and miso (USDA, 2006).

Animal studies have reported possible cancer-promoting effects of isoflavones (Bouker and Hilakivi-Clark, 2000). Investigators and clinicians in this area of study suggest that moderate use of traditional whole soy foods can be a part of a healthy plant-based diet and that commercially prepared soy supplements should be limited in women with breast cancer (Brown et al., 2003; Maskarinec, 2005).

Carbohydrates: Fiber, Sugars, and Glycemic Index

High-fiber foods such as whole grains comprise an important part of a healthy diet. Early studies focused much attention on the possible protective role of fiber in preventing cancer of the colon, rectum, breast, and ovaries. Most studies of the relationship between fiber and cancer have measured fiber-rich foods or total dietary crude fiber rather than fiber components. The intake of dietary fiber influences the intake of meat, fat, and refined carbohydrates, as well as a number of nutrients and nonnutrients with identified impact on cancer risk.

A number of observational and case-control studies indicate that fiber-rich diets are associated with a protective effect against the development of colon cancer; however, the role of genetics (e.g., family history of colorectal cancer) must also be considered. A study evaluating the dietary habits of over 61,000 women found that participants consuming 4.5 servings or more of whole grains daily had a 35% lower risk of colon cancer when compared to those eating less than 1.5 servings of whole grains each day (Larsson et al., 2005).

Two randomized intervention trials evaluating the effect of fiber intake on polyp and adenoma recurrence failed to show a significant reduction in recurrence between individuals consuming high fiber intakes compared to those who did not (Schatzkin et al., 2000; Alberts et al., 2000). Adenomas are small growths in the intestinal tract that are believed to be precursors to colorectal cancer. Therefore, although the association between fiber intake and cancer risk remains inconclusive (Martinez, 2005), consumption of high-fiber foods should still be recommended because of their overall health benefit (lowering heart disease risk) and because these foods contain other substances that contribute to cancer risk reduction.

A high consumption of simple sugars on a regular basis can increase blood glucose and triglyceride levels and raise levels of insulin and other hormones that may stimulate cancer cell growth (Augustin et al., 2001). High serum levels of insulin may increase the risk of dying from breast cancer, especially in women who are postmenopausal (Borugian et al., 2004). Numerous studies have shown an association between the consumption of high–glycemic index foods and increased risk of cancers, including ovary, endometrium, breast, colorectal, pancreas, and lung (Potischman et al., 2004; Augustin et al., 2003). It is prudent to limit processed and refined sugar intake and emphasize whole grains or complex carbohydrates as a part of a healthy diet for decreasing cancer risk (Slattery, 2004).

Fruits and Vegetables

A comprehensive review of epidemiologic studies examined the relationship between fruit and vegetable intake and the incidence of cancer and found a statistically significant protective effect in 128 of 156 dietary studies (Block et al., 1992). Increased consumption of fruits and vegetables has been shown to be associated with a lower risk of cancers of the mouth, pharynx, larynx, esophagus, lung, stomach, kidney, colon, rectum, ovary, and bladder (IARC, 2003).

A recent study evaluating the diets of over 280,000 women living in 12 European countries found no connection between eating fruits and vegetables and reduced breast cancer risk (van Gils et al., 2005). However, a closer analysis of the data reveals that women consuming about one serving of fruits and vegetables each day were compared to women consuming two to just over three servings of fruits a day. They all had low intakes of fruits and vegetables. Current recommendations of cancer prevention organizations recommend eating a minimum of five to nine servings of fruits and vegetables a day for decreasing cancer risk (NCI, 2006a).

Epidemiologic investigators report that consumption of the following groups and types of vegetables and fruits is comparatively low in those who subsequently develop cancer: raw and fresh vegetables, leafy green vegetables, cruciferous vegetables (i.e., broccoli and cabbage), lettuce, carrots, and raw and fresh fruit. Consumption of flavonoids, including soybeans, is thought to contribute to the low incidence of hormone-dependent cancers in Asian countries (Le Marchand, 2002).

Generally fruits and vegetables are low in energy and good sources of fiber, vitamins, minerals, and biologically active substances. Anticarcinogenic agents are found in fruits and vegetables, including antioxidants (vitamins C and E, selenium) and phytochemicals, nonnutritive compounds in plants thought to influence tumorigenesis. Phytochemicals include carotenoids, flavonoids, plant sterols, *Allium* compounds, indoles, phenols, and terpenes. At this time, it is unclear which specific substances of fruits and vegetables are protective against cancer (IARC, 2003). These substances have both complementary and overlapping mechanisms of action, including the induction of detoxification enzymes, inhibition of nitrosamine formation, provision of substrate for formation of chemotherapy agents, dilution and binding of carcinogens in the digestive tract, alteration of hormone metabolism, and antioxidant effects. It appears extremely unlikely that any one substance is responsible for all of the observed associations.

The national "5 A Day to Better Health" program seeks to encourage individuals to consume five to nine servings of vegetables and fruits each day (NCI, 2006a). Only 23% of Americans surveyed in 2003 consumed five or more servings a day (BRFS, 2004). Heber (2004) suggests that phytochemicals consumed from different vegetables and fruits each day have a synergistic and additive effect to inhibit cell growth via their antioxidant and anticancer properties (see Table 9-1). Adopting a color code system when selecting vegetables and fruits can help individuals change dietary patterns to ensure that a variety of phytochemicals are consumed (Table 37-1). To most effectively reduce cancer risk, the ACS suggests consuming these substances from food sources rather than supplements.

Nonnutritive Sweeteners

The Food and Drug Administration (FDA) has approved five nonnutritive sweeteners (ascesulfame-K, aspartame, neotame, saccharin, and sucralose) for use in the food supply and regulates them as food additives (ADA, 2004); they

---

TABLE 37-1

Color Code System of Vegetables and Fruits

Color	Phytochemical	Vegetables and Fruits
Red	Lycopene	Tomatoes and tomato products, pink grapefruit, watermelon
Red/purple	Anthocyanins, polyphenols	Berries, grapes, red wine, prunes
Orange	α-, β-carotene	Carrots, mangoes, pumpkin
Orange/yellow	β-cryptoxanthin, flavonoids	Cantaloupe, peaches, oranges, papaya, nectarines
Yellow/green	Lutein, zeaxanthin	Spinach, avocado, honeydew, collard and turnip greens
Green	Sulforaphanes, indoles	Cabbage, broccoli, Brussels sprouts, cauliflower
White/green	Allyl sulphides	Leeks, onion, garlic, chives

Data from Heber D: Vegetables, fruits and phytoestrogens in the prevention of diseases, *J Postgrad Med* 50:145, 2004.

appear to be safe when used in moderation. Described as "high-intensity" sweeteners, nonnutritive sweeteners provide little or no energy because they sweeten in minute amounts.

Nonnutritive sweeteners have been investigated primarily in relation to potential adverse health concerns, including long-term safety and carcinogenicity. Cyclamate was banned as a food additive by the FDA in 1969, and saccharin was banned in 1977 because their use was reported to cause bladder tumors in experimental laboratory animals fed a mixture of cyclamate and saccharin of doses up to 2500 mg/kg/day (Renwick, 1990). In 2000, after several intensive reviews were completed, the National Toxicology Program of the National Institutes of Health concluded that saccharin could be removed from the list of potential carcinogens. The Cancer Assessment Committee of the FDA has concluded that cyclamate does not cause cancer in humans or laboratory animals, and a petition to reapprove cyclamate is currently under review. After comprehensive review evaluating the safety of aspartame, including the possible incidence of brain tumors (Butchko et al., 2002), the Scientific Committee on Food (SCF) concluded that aspartame is not a carcinogen and is not associated with neurobehavioral disorders (SCF, 2002).

At this time five other nonnutritive sweeteners are under review for approval by the FDA. These nonnutritive sweeteners include alitame, a blend of nonnutritive sweeteners; cyclamates; neohesperidine, GRAS (Generally Regarded As Safe) approved for use as a flavor ingredient; thaumatin, GRAS approved for use as a flavor adjunct; and stevia, which can be sold in the United States as a dietary supplement, but not as a sweetener (ADA, 2004).

Alcohol

Epidemiologic studies indicate that alcohol consumption is associated with increased cancer risk, especially for cancers of the mouth, pharynx, larynx, esophagus, lung, colon, rectum, liver, and breast (USDHHS, 2000). Alcohol appears to have an increased effect on tissues directly exposed to it during its consumption. The malnutrition associated with alcoholism is also likely to be important in the increased risk for certain cancers in the alcoholic individual.

Alcohol has been associated with an increased risk for colorectal cancer in a number of studies. The association between increased colorectal cancer risk and alcohol use with low dietary intake of folate has also been investigated. The positive relationship between alcohol intake and breast cancer risk has been documented repeatedly. Horn-Ross and colleagues (2004) found that women having more than one to two alcoholic drinks per day were at increased risk of breast cancer, especially if there was also a history of regular alcohol use, benign breast disease, and estrogen or hormone replacement therapy. A study evaluating dietary intake and alcohol use in over 17,000 women found that the increased risk of breast cancer associated with regular alcohol use disappeared when women had dietary intakes of at least 400 mcg of folate (Baglietto et al., 2005).

The ACS recommends that, if alcoholic beverages are consumed, intake be limited to no more than two drinks per day for men and one drink per day for women and that folate intake be adequate (Byers et al., 2002).

Coffee and Tea

Coffee intake has been investigated in a variety of cancers. Investigators involved with two large prospective studies (the Nurse's Health Study [women] and the Health Professionals' Follow-Up Study [men]) explored the association between colorectal cancer incidence and consumption of coffee and tea (Michels et al., 2005). The investigators concluded that the regular consumption of caffeinated coffee or caffeinated tea or caffeine intake was not associated with the incidence of colon or rectal cancer in either cohort. Another study found that the regular drinking of green tea and other sources of polyphenols may reduce the risk of stomach cancer (Owuor and Kong, 2002). Some studies have shown that the consumption of very hot drinks has been associated with an increased risk of esophageal cancer (Sharp et al., 2001). At this time the regular consumption of coffee or tea has no significant relationship with the risk of cancer at any site.

Methods of Food Preparation and Preservation

Methods of food preparation and preservation are major sources of dietary carcinogens. Studies have shown a possible increased cancer risk posed by the formation of dietary carcinogens (e.g., polycyclic aromatic hydrocarbons and heterocyclic amines) when high-heat cooking methods such as grilling, broiling, barbecuing, and smoking of meats are used (Sugimura et al., 2004; Wu et al., 2001). These toxic substances are formed during combustion of carbon fuel and pyrolysis of protein. Some epidemiologic studies have also linked high consumption of processed meat to an increased risk of cancers of the colon, rectum, and stomach (Byers et al., 2002).

A study evaluating the diet and cooking methods of over 1500 Chinese women found that women who ate the most red meat and used deep frying to cook the meat to very well done appeared to have an increased risk of breast cancer (Dai et al., 2002). Participants with BMIs of 25 or more had the greatest risk for developing breast cancer.

Other dietary carcinogens include N-nitrosocompounds (NOCs) that are formed in smoked, salted, and pickled foods cured with nitrate or nitrite. Sodium and potassium nitrates are present in a variety of foods, and they give hot dogs and luncheon meats their pink color, but the main dietary sources are vegetables and drinking water. Nitrates can be readily reduced to nitrite, which in turn can interact with dietary substrates such as amines and amides to produce NOCs (e.g., N-nitroso compounds or nitrosamines and nitrosamides). This conversion, known as N-nitrosation, has been demonstrated to occur in saliva, as well as in the stomach, colon, and bladder. Nitrosamines are also present in tobacco and tobacco smoke. Diets with high amounts of fruits and vegetables that contain vitamin C and phytochemicals that can retard the conversion of nitrites to nitrosamines should be encouraged (Byers et al., 2002).

A group of Swedish scientists reported finding acrylamide, a carcinogen, in carbohydrate-rich foods such as potatoes and baked goods that had been cooked at high temperatures (Tareke et al., 2002). Acrylamide is a by-product that is formed during frying, roasting, and baking. At this time no studies in humans have demonstrated an association between consumption of foods containing acrylamide and increased cancer risk (Friedman, 2003; Pelucchi et al., 2005), although acrylamide remains under investigation. The ACS recommends eating fewer foods containing NOCs and healthier cooking alternatives for meats, including boiling, poaching, steaming, stewing, braising, baking, microwaving, and roasting (Byers et al., 2002).

Cancer Chemoprevention

Cancer chemoprevention involves pharmacologic intervention with specific nutrients or other chemicals to suppress or reverse carcinogenesis. Studies have been directed at reversing precancerous lesions, preventing disease in populations at high risk for recurrent or new disease, and reducing the incidence of specific tumors in the general population by using vitamin and mineral supplements as chemoprevention agents.

Several large-scale, randomized, intervention trials have examined the effects with mixed results. There was a high incidence of lung cancer in smokers associated with β-carotene supplementation, especially with heavy alcohol intake (ATBC Cancer Prevention Study Group, 1994; Omenn et al., 1996). The Physician's Health study found neither increased risk nor benefit from β-carotene supplementation after 12 years of follow-up study of patients with lung cancer; however, only 11% of the group studied were current smokers (Hennekens et al., 1996).

Overall findings from these β-carotene supplementation trials were unexpected, and other carotenoids have been studied as a result. Lower risks of lung cancer are observed for the highest versus the lowest quintiles of lycopene (28%), lutein and zeaxanthin (17%), α-cryptoxanthin (15%), total carotenoids (16%), β-carotene (19%), and serum retinol (27%), thus suggesting that high fruit and vegetable consumption, particularly a diet rich in carotenoids, tomatoes, and tomato-based products, may reduce the risk of lung cancer (Holick et al., 2002).

Two large studies were conducted in Linxian, China, to test the effects of vitamin and mineral supplements on cancer incidence in an area that has one of the highest esophageal and gastric cancer mortality rates in the world and a diet low in micronutrients. After 5 years the group that received two to three times the RDA for β-carotene, vitamin E, and selenium showed significant reduction in mortality due to cancer, especially stomach cancer. No significant effect on mortality was observed for other supplement regimens (Blot, 1994; Blot et al., 1993).

In the United States a number of randomized cancer prevention trials using vitamins, minerals, or chemical agents are ongoing or have been concluded (Thompson et al., 2005). The NCI began the Selenium and Vitamin E Cancer Prevention Trial (SELECT) to determine whether selenium and vitamin E can prevent prostate cancer (Klein, 2004). Examples of new studies under development include the following agents: epigallacatechin gallate (green tea) and curcumin, folic acid, as well as genistein (soy) and lycopene (tomatoes).

Chemoprevention is also an active area of clinical research that holds promise for patients with cancers commonly associated with recurrence such as head and neck cancers and for identified high-risk populations such as former smokers with bronchial metaplasia. The development of second primary tumors is a major cause of treatment failure in patients with head and neck cancers treated in an early stage. Early clinical trials with isotretinoin, a retinoid, decreased recurrence; however, significant side effects prevented many patients from completing the treatment (Hong et al., 1990). Doses with reduced toxicity side effects have shown mixed results in reducing recurrence of disease.

Trials with precursor lesions are more promising. Antioxidant compounds have been shown to be effective in reversing oral leukoplakia, precursor lesions with a high rate of transformation to malignant disease. Effort to decrease the risk of colorectal cancer has involved the use of calcium combined with vitamin D supplementation and is associated with a moderate reduction in the risk of recurrent colorectal adenomas (Grau et al., 2003).

Cancer Prevention Recommendations: Nutrition and Physical Activity

National health organizations, as well as the new Dietary Guidelines for Americans 2005, recommend healthful diet and lifestyle practices to reduce cancer risk (Eyre et al., 2004; USDHHS, 2006). Specifically the guidelines of the ACS are comprised of four recommendations: (1) eating a variety of healthful foods, with an emphasis on plant sources (eating five or more servings of a variety of vegetables and fruits, choosing whole grains, and limiting consumption of red meats); (2) adopting a physically active lifestyle; (3) achieving and maintaining a healthy body weight throughout life; and (4) limiting consumption of alcoholic beverages. In addition, the ACS presents one key recommendation—community action—which underscores the importance of community measures to support healthy behaviors by increasing access to healthful food choices and opportunities to be physically active.

Studies indicate that adults who strongly believe in a diet-cancer connection decrease the percentage of energy derived from fat and increase their fiber intake (Pierce et al., 2002; Patterson et al., 2003) and women with cancer prevention knowledge are more likely to make changes in their diet. The importance of diet and lifestyle change is evident in recommendations from the AICR as well. Box 37-2 summarizes guidelines for cancer prevention; Table 37-2 summarizes the benefit versus harm regarding nutrition and physical activity for cancer prevention.

Nutrition and Physical Activity Recommendations for Cancer Survivors

From the time of diagnosis through the balance of life, the ACS defines anyone living with a diagnosis of cancer as a cancer survivor (Brown et al., 2003). The ACS guidelines on nutrition and physical activity for cancer prevention, as well as the AICR recommendations (see Box 37-2) provide sound diet and nutrition advice for primary cancer prevention and health for all individuals, including cancer survivors. The ACS has produced a guide with a grading system to help cancer survivors and health professionals caring for them evaluate the strength of existing scientific evidence related to dietary factors and specific cancers (Table 37-3).

Cancer survivors represent one of the largest groups of people living with chronic illness. Many patients with cancer are able to return to full function and regain their quality of life. This trend is expected to continue because of recent awareness in cancer prevention, advances in cancer detection, development of more effective anticancer therapies, and advancements in determining the genetic causes of cancer (see *Clinical Insight*: Cure, Control, or Palliate—is Cancer Becoming a Chronic Disease for Some? on p. 962).

NUTRITIONAL IMPLICATIONS OF CANCER

The adverse nutritional effects of cancer can be severe and may be compounded by the effects of the treatment regimens and the psychological impact of cancer (Schattner and Shike, 2006). The result is often a profound depletion of nutrient stores. Anorexia, weight loss, and poor nutrition status are found in many individuals at the time of diagnosis, even in children (Goldman et al., 2006). Even small amounts of weight loss (less than 5% of body weight) before treatment are associated with a poor prognosis, thus reinforcing the importance of early nutrition assessment and intervention (Figure 37-1).

Cancer Cachexia

A common secondary diagnosis in patients with advanced cancer is a variant of protein-energy malnutrition. This syndrome is termed **cancer cachexia** and is characterized by progressive weight loss, anorexia, generalized wasting and weakness, immunosuppression, altered basal metabolic rate, and abnormalities in fluid and energy metabolism. The etiology of this complex metabolic derangement is not entirely understood and can manifest both in individuals with metastatic disease and in individuals with localized disease.

Cytokines, protein mediators produced by inflammatory cells through broad physiologic actions, produce metabolic changes and wasting in the tumor-bearing host that are similar but not identical to those seen in sepsis and inflammation (Tisdale, 2003). Cytokines that are thought to play a role in cancer cachexia include **tumor necrosis factor (TNF-α and TNF-β)** cachectin, interleukin-1, interleukin-6, and interferon-α (Argiles et al., 2003). These cytokines have overlapping physiologic activities, which makes it likely that no single substance is the sole cause of cancer cachexia. A pool of anticytokine antibodies or other cytokine inhibitors might be considered as a potential intervention for the treatment of cancer cachexia.

Energy Metabolism

In chronic starvation the resting energy expenditure (REE) is reduced as the body adapts to conserve energy and preserve body tissue. However, in comparison with control groups, hospitalized cancer patients were reported to be hypometabolic, normometabolic, or hypermetabolic (Knox et al., 1983). The difference in findings is most likely a result of the stages of illness and of nutrition status among the subjects, differing because of methods used in accurately measuring acutely ill individuals. Researchers have found that the site of cancer or tumor type does not predictably increase energy needs or REE (Jatoi et al., 2001).

Protein, Fat, and Carbohydrate Metabolism

Energy metabolism is intimately related to carbohydrate, protein, and lipid metabolism, all of which are altered by tumor growth. Tumors exert a consistent demand for glucose. Neoplastic cells exhibit a characteristically high rate of anaerobic metabolism and yield lactate as the end product. This expanded lactic acid pool requires an increased rate of host gluconeogenesis via Cori cycle activity, which is increased in some patients with cancer but not in others. Both protein breakdown and lipolysis take place at increasing rates to maintain high rates of glucose synthesis. A relative state of insulin resistance characterized by excess fatty acid oxidation and decreased uptake and use of glucose, especially in muscle, may develop. Alterations in protein metabolism appear to be directed toward providing adequate amino acids for tumor growth. Most notable is the loss of skeletal muscle protein.

TABLE 37-2

The American Cancer Society Workgroup Grading System for Benefit vs. Harm: Nutrition and Physical Activity for Cancer Prevention

To review the strength of the scientific evidence, a guidelines subcommittee used a method of summarizing the evidence similar to the methods used by other expert panels. For example, the U.S. Preventive Services Task Force judged the scientific evidence related to clinical preventive services with a system that considered both the source and strength of the evidence: from at least one controlled clinical trial, good uncontrolled trials, multiple good observation studies, expert opinion, and case reports. They then characterized those guidelines on a five-point grading scheme according to the strength of the guideline: "good for recommending, fair for recommending, insufficient to recommend for or against, fair for not recommending, good for not recommending. The AICR-World Cancer Research Fund project summarized the nature of the scientific evidence for nutritional factors in cancer prevention as being either "Convincing, Probable, Possible, or Insufficient." The American Cancer Society subcommittee used a method similar to that or both groups. For each issue, the committee judged the likelihood of benefit to the general public as follows:

A1 Convincing evidence for a benefit
A2 Probable benefit
A3 Possible benefit
B   Insufficient evidence to conclude benefit or risk
C   Evidence of lack of benefit
D   Evidence of harm

Nutritional Factor	Colorectal Cancer	Breast Cancer	Prostate Cancer	Lung Cancer	Oral, Esophageal Cancer	Stomach Cancer	Pancreatic Cancer	Bladder Cancer	Endometrial Cancer
Increasing vegetable and fruit intake	A2	A3	A3	A2	A2	A2	A3	A3	A3
Limiting intake of red meats	A2	B	A3	B	B	C	A3	C	B
Increasing physical activity	A1	A1	B	B	B	B	B	B	A2
Avoiding overweight	A1	A1	C	B	A2	C	A3	C	A1
Limiting alcohol intake	A3	A2	C	B	A1	C	A3	C	B
Consuming soy foods	B	B	B	B	B	B	B	B	B
Taking β-carotene supplements	B	B	C	D	B	B	B	B	B
Taking vitamin E supplements	B	B	A3	C	B	B	B	B	B
Taking vitamin C supplements	B	B	B	B	B	B	B	B	B
Taking folic acid supplements	A3	A3	B	B	B	B	B	B	B
Taking selenium supplements	A3	B	A3	A3	B	B	B	B	B

From Byers T et al: American Cancer Society's Guidelines on nutrition and physical activity for cancer prevention: reducing the risk of cancer with healthy food choices and physical activity, *Ca Cancer J Clin* 52:92, 2002.

TABLE 37-3

The American Cancer Society Workgroup Grading System for Benefit vs. Harm: Nutrition During and After Cancer Treatment

To summarize the strength of the scientific evidence, the ACS Workgroup used a method of summarizing the evidence similar to those used by other expert panels. For example, the U.S. Preventive Services Task Force judged the scientific evidence related to clinical preventive services using a system that considered both the source and strength of the evidence and categorized them as follows: from at least one controlled clinical trial, good uncontrolled trials, multiple good observation studies, expert opinion, and case reports. They then characterized those recommendations on a five-point grading scheme as to the strength of the recommendation: "Good for recommending, fair for recommending, insufficient to recommend for or against, fair for not recommending, or good for not recommending. The AICR-World Cancer Research Fund project summarized the nature of the scientific evidence for nutritional factors in cancer prevention as being either "Convincing, Probable, Possible, or Insufficient."

The ACS committee used a method of summarizing the evidence that was similar to those used by both groups. For each issue, the committee judged the likelihood of benefit to cancer survivors as follows:

A1   Proven benefit
A2   Probable benefit, but unproven
A3   Possible benefit, but unproven
B   Insufficient evidence to conclude benefit or risk
C   Evidence of possible harm as well as possible benefit
D   Evidence of lack of benefit
E   Evidence of harm

The following table presents a summary of ACS assessments regarding the benefit or harm of 25 dietary factors with respect to their impact on cancer survivors throughout the phases of survivorship.

Dietary Factor	Prostate Cancer	Breast Cancer	Gastrointestinal Cancer	Lung Cancer
Food safety	A1	A1	A1	A1
Intentional weight loss during treatment (if overweight)	E	E	E	E
Intentional weight loss after recovery (if overweight)	B	A2	A3	B
Decreased dietary fats	A3	A2	A3	B
Increased fruits and vegetables	B	A3	A2	A2
Increased physical activity	A3	A2	A2	B
Decreased alcohol	B	A3	A3	B
Fasting therapies	D	D	D	D
Juice therapies	B	A3	A3	A3
Macrobiotic therapies	C	C	C	C
Vegetarian diets	A3	A3	A2	A3
Vitamin and mineral supplements	A3	B	B	C
Flaxseed oil	B	B	B	B
Fish oils	B	B	A3	B
Ginger	B	B	B	B
Soy foods	C	C	B	B
Teas	B	B	B	B
Vitamin E supplements	A3	B	B	B
Vitamin C supplements	B	B	B	B
β-carotene supplements	C	C	C	E
Selenium	A3	B	A3	A3

From Brown J et al: Nutrition during and after cancer treatment: a guide for informed choices by cancer survivors, *CA Cancer J Clin* 51:153, 2001.

Note: Information contained in this table represents studies in progress and presents the best data available at this time. This table will be updated periodically.

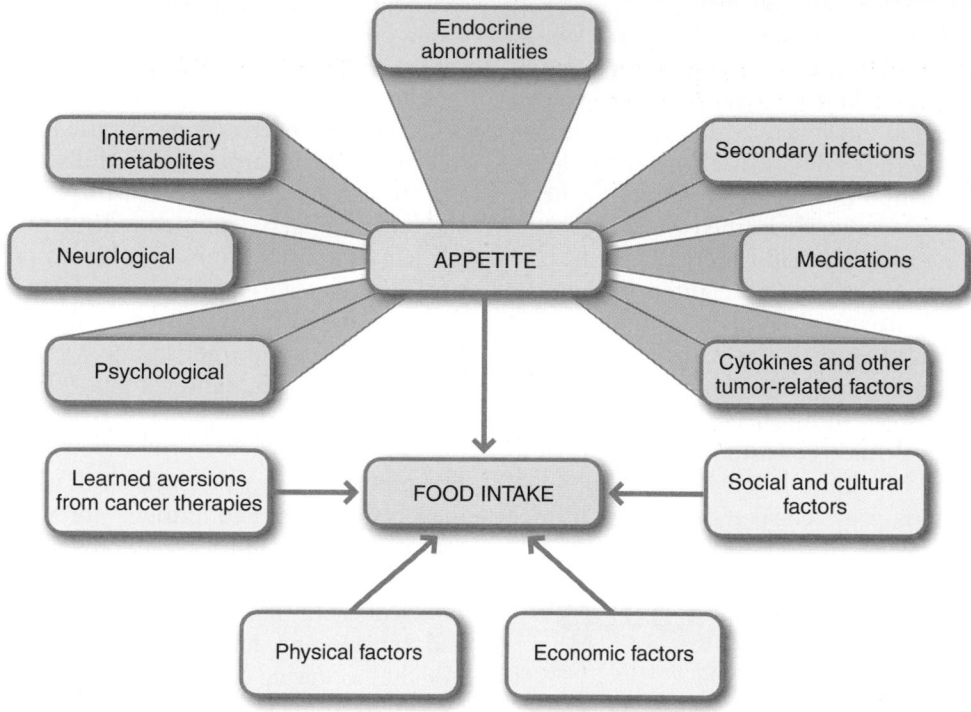

FIGURE 37-1 Factors that affect appetite, an especially important consideration in cancer patients.

Nutrition, Tumor Growth and Treatment Outcome

Nutrition or nutrition support (e.g., enteral or parenteral nutrition) when given to tumor-bearing animals may increase tumor mass and markers of tumor growth (Terosian and Daly, 1986). Although dietary intake and nutrition support show benefit in preserving lean body mass, minimizing toxicity to therapy, and improving quality of life, nutrition support also benefits the malignancy (Canada, 2002). In a prospective randomized trial of over 1000 patients with locally advanced head and neck cancer treated with radiation, patients receiving nutrition support before and during therapy had less weight loss and **mucositis** (inflammation of a mucous membrane) but also had increased incidence of recurrence and decreased overall survival (Rabinovitch et al., 2006). Although a commonly held belief among both health care professionals and cancer patients is that aggressive food or nutrition support "helps to fight cancer," further research is needed to clearly evaluate the effect of food and aggressive nutrition support in individuals diagnosed with cancer.

Other Metabolic Abnormalities

Hypercalcemia can occur in individuals with bone metastases and is caused by the osteolytic activity of tumor cells releasing calcium into the extracellular fluid. Hypercalcemia is a potentially fatal condition and is most commonly seen in metastatic breast cancer and multiple myeloma; symptoms include nausea, weakness, fatigue, lethargy, and confusion. Current medical management of hypercalcemia includes rehydration and use of biphosphonates and other antihypercalcemic agents (Percherstorfer et al., 2003) (see

Chapter 24). Health care professionals concur that restricting the intake of foods containing calcium is not indicated since the consumption of these foods has little effect in the overall management of hypercalcemia; common sense dictates that oral calcium supplements should be avoided.

Critical imbalances in fluid and electrolyte status can occur in individuals who have cancers that promote excessive diarrhea or vomiting. Profuse and often severe diarrhea can result from partial bowel obstructions; endocrine-secreting tumors such as those secreting serotonin (carcinoid syndrome), calcitonin, or gastrin (Zollinger-Ellison syndrome); and steatorrhea. The use of certain chemotherapy agents (e.g., antimetabolites, alkylating agents) and antibiotics is associated with the development of sometimes severe diarrhea (Grant, 2006). In some instances immunocompromised individuals may experience profuse diarrhea that is caused by *Clostridium difficile*.

Persistent vomiting is associated with intestinal obstruction, radiation therapy to the abdomen or whole brain, highly emetogenic chemotherapy agents, intracranial tumors, and terminal cancer (Grant, 2006). Careful assessment and evaluation of the etiology of the diarrhea or vomiting is critical for effective management.

The activities of several enzyme systems can be affected, as can certain endocrine functions. The nature of the alterations varies by tumor type. The individual's immunologic function can be impaired, apparently as the result of both the neoplasm and progressive malnutrition. In addition to the cancer-induced metabolic effects, the mass of the tumor may anatomically alter the normal physiology of specific organ systems.

Loss of Appetite and Sensory Changes

During the course of disease many individuals report a loss of appetite and a decreased voluntary food intake. Alterations in taste and smell are common, and they can contribute to the anorexia commonly seen in individuals with cancer. Taste alterations are associated with the disease itself, certain chemotherapy agents, and radiation therapy or surgery of the head and neck. Chemotherapy-induced, learned taste aversions have been reported in both adults and children.

Individuals may also experience a heightened sense of smell that results in sensitivity to food preparation odors and aversions to nonfood items such as soaps or perfumes. Dietary interventions that decrease the aroma of foods such as serving foods cold instead of hot may be helpful. These sensation abnormalities do not consistently correlate with the tumor site, extent of tumor involvement, tumor response to therapy, or food preferences and intake.

NUTRITION CARE OF ADULTS

Goals of Nutrition Care

Whether newly diagnosed, undergoing active therapy, recovering from treatment, or in remission and trying to prevent cancer recurrence, nutrition is an important component of cancer care and management. Best practice dictates that individuals diagnosed with cancer should be instructed to consume a nutritionally adequate diet. Ideally a diet that contains the recommended amounts of essential nutrients, including protein, carbohydrate, fat, vitamins and minerals, and water consumed through a variety of foods each day should be encouraged. The impact of cancer and its treatment increases nutritional needs, and individuals can benefit from individualized nutrition intervention to ensure adequate nutrition intake and weight maintenance (Schattner and Shike, 2006). The goals of nutrition intervention in cancer are to prevent or reverse nutrient deficiencies, to preserve lean body mass, to minimize nutrition-related side effects, and to maximize the quality of life (Eldridge et al., 2001).

Nutrition Screening and Risk Assessment

Early nutrition intervention is essential. Nutrition screening and assessment for risk of nutrition problems should be interdisciplinary and instituted at the time of diagnosis and reevaluated and monitored throughout treatment and recovery (McCallum, 2006). With the recent shift of care from the hospital setting to outpatient settings, nutrition screening and assessment throughout the continuum of cancer care are essential. Basic concepts of dietary and clinical assessment, as well as nutrition intervention and diet modification, are outlined in Chapters 14 and 17.

Nutrition status is evaluated by taking a careful review of the individual's appetite and oral intake, nutrition impact symptoms (e.g., nausea, vomiting, and diarrhea), weight loss, comorbidities, and laboratory studies. A nutrition-focused physical examination of the individual's body, including assessment of subcutaneous fat stores, muscle mass, and fluid status, provides vital information to fully evaluate the individual's nutrition status and degree of risk (Fuhrman, 2004).

The Patient-Generated Subjective Global Assessment (PG-SGA) has been adapted for use in cancer patients. This validated tool incorporates sections completed by the patient or caregiver on weight history, food intake, symptoms and functioning. Sections completed by a health care member (e.g., physician, nurse, registered dietitian (RD), social worker) evaluate weight loss, disease, metabolic stress, and a nutrition-focused physical examination (McCallum, 2006; nutritional risk and intervention are then determined by a scoring system (McMahon et al., 1998).

Body Weight

Best practice dictates that individuals who are able to maintain their body weight and nutrient stores may be better able to tolerate treatment impact symptoms and recover more quickly from therapy. Thus individuals should be advised to consume sufficient energy and protein to maintain their nutrition stores and achieve and maintain appropriate weight for height. Weight lost during cancer therapy is often more likely caused by the loss of muscle (lean body mass) rather than fat stores. Therefore, even if individuals are overweight, the maintenance of lean body mass should be encouraged throughout treatment and recovery (Brown et al., 2003). A widely used tool to estimate body weight for height is the BMI that is described in Chapter 14 and Appendix 23. Based on current available evidence, keeping a BMI between 18.5 and 25 throughout life is associated with best overall health.

Energy, Protein, Fluid, and Micronutrient Requirements

Energy

Methods used to estimate energy requirements for individuals diagnosed with cancer include standardized equations and indirect calorimetry using a metabolic cart. See Chapter 2 for validated methods for determining energy requirements such as the Mifflin-St. Jeor and Ireton-Jones equations. Which method is used is based on the individual's clinical status and the availability of assessment information and equipment (e.g., patient data, laboratory values, and access to a metabolic chart). To ensure that adequate energy (calories) is being provided, the health care professional needs to consider the individual's diagnosis, presence of other diseases, intent of treatment (e.g., curative, control, or palliation), anticancer therapies (e.g., surgery, chemotherapy, or radiation therapy), presence of fever or infection, and other metabolic complications.

The Harris-Benedict equations often overestimate needs in healthy individuals. Once the REE is calculated, activity and stress factors are added to estimate total energy requirements. Factors from 1.1 to 1.6 times greater than usual may be used, especially for the patients with a stem cell transplant, sepsis, or surgery (Charuhas, 2006; Hurst and Gallagher, 2006). Close monitoring and follow-up are essential to ensure adequate energy is being provided.

Protein

An individual's need for protein is increased during times of illness and stress. Additional protein is required by the body to repair and rebuild tissues affected by cancer therapy and to maintain a healthy immune system (Hurst and Gallagher, 2006). For the body to most effectively use the protein, adequate energy should be provided, or the body will use its lean body mass as a fuel source. When determining protein requirements, the health care professional needs to consider the degree of malnutrition, extent of disease, degree of stress, and ability to metabolize and use protein (Russell and Malone, 2004). Daily protein requirements are generally based on actual body weight, but in patients with body weight greater than 125% of ideal body weight, an adjusted body weight can be used. See Box 37-3 for protein requirements.

Fluid

The goals of fluid management are to ensure the maintenance of adequate hydration, tissue perfusion and electrolyte balance. Careful evaluation of an individual's hydration status is critical to identify possible causes for alterations in fluid balance such as fever, ascites, edema, profuse vomiting and diarrhea, multiple concurrent intravenous (IV) therapies, impaired renal function, or medications (diuretics). Calculations for estimating fluid requirements include:

Daily fluid requirements:
Body surface area: 1500 ml/m² or BSA × 1500 ml
Daily requirement method: 1 ml of fluid per 1 kcal of estimated needs
Holliday-Seger method: >20 kg of body weight = 1500ml + 20 ml/kg for each kg >20 kg
Age-based method:
<55 years of age: 30-40 ml/kg
55-65 years of age: 30 ml/kg
>65 years of age: 25 ml/kg (Russell and Malone, 2004; Hurst and Gallagher, 2006)

Micronutrients

Individuals diagnosed with cancer often take large amounts of vitamin and mineral supplements because they believe

---

BOX 37-3

Daily Protein Requirements for Patients With Cancer

RDA for adults: 0.8 g/kg
Normal maintenance: 0.8 to 1 g/kg
Nonstressed cancer patient: 1 to 1.2 g/kg
Hypercatabolic cancer patient: 1.2 to 1.6 g/kg
Severely stressed cancer patient: 1.5 to 2.5 g/kg
Hematopoietic stem cell transplant patient: 1.5 to 2 g/kg

Data from Charuhas PM et al: Medical nutrition therapy in bone marrow transplantation: energy, protein, micronutrient, and fluid requirement. In Elliott L et al, editors: *The clinical guide to oncology nutrition*, ed 2, Chicago, 2006, American Dietetic Association.

---

that these products can enhance their immune system. Many individuals may have existing nutritional deficiencies when they are diagnosed with cancer because of poor diet and lifestyle choices and the metabolic effects of the cancer itself (Kucuk and Ottery, 2002). Therefore, if individuals are experiencing difficulty with eating and treatment-related side effects, the use of a multivitamin and mineral supplement that provides no more than 100% of the dietary reference intakes (DRIs) is generally considered safe (Brown et al., 2003). Supplementation or restriction of specific micronutrients may be required above or below DRI levels, depending on medical diagnosis and laboratory analysis (e.g., iron supplementation for iron-deficiency anemia or vitamin K restriction if on therapeutic anticoagulation therapy).

Antioxidants During Anticancer Therapy

Controversy over whether the use of antioxidant supplements such as vitamins A, C, E, β-carotene, zinc, and selenium actually inhibits or enhances the antitumor effects of radiation therapy and chemotherapy continues (Conklin, 2000; Prasad et al., 2001). From a review of 19 randomized trials with control groups the authors report the lack of a negative impact of antioxidant supplemention on the effectiveness of chemotherapy (Block et al., 2007). Continued research is still necessary, so individuals should be cautioned about the concurrent use of antioxidant dietary supplements with chemotherapy or radiation therapies (D'Andrea, 2005; Kucuk and Ottery, 2002).

CANCER TREATMENT AND NUTRITIONAL IMPLICATIONS

Chemotherapy

Chemotherapy is the use of chemical agents or medications to treat cancer. Whereas surgery and radiation therapy are used to treat localized tumors, chemotherapy is a systemic therapy that affects the whole body. The target of action of chemotherapeutic agents is not limited to malignant tissue; it affects normal cells as well. Cells of the body with a rapid turnover such as bone marrow, hair follicles, and the mucosa of the alimentary tract are typically the most affected. Commonly experienced nutrition impact symptoms include **myelosuppression** (suppression of bone marrow production), anemia, fatigue, nausea and vomiting, loss of appetite, mucositis, changes in taste and smell, **xerostomia** (mouth dryness), dysphagia, and changes in bowel function (Table 37-4A). As a result, dietary intake and nutrition status can be adversely affected.

Classifications of chemotherapy agents include alkylating agents, nitrosoureas, antitumor antibiotics, hormones, hormone antagonists, antimetabolites, vinca alkaloids, taxanes, camptothecins, epipodophyllotoxins, and immunologics Routes of administration for chemotherapy include oral (capsule, pill or liquid), IV (delivery of medication via an injection or an indwelling catheter into a vein), intraperitoneal (delivery

TABLE 37-4A

Nutrition Impact of Chemotherapy and Immunotherapy

Chemotherapeutic Agents	Common Nutrition Impact Symptoms
Cytotoxic	
Alkylating agents (cisplatin, ifosfamide, cyclophosphamide, busulfan)	Myelosuppression, anorexia, nausea, vomiting, fatigue, renal toxicities
Antibiotics (doxorubicin, mitomycin, bleomycin)	Myelosuppression, anorexia, nausea, vomiting, fatigue, diarrhea, mucositis
Antimetabolites (5-Fluorouracil, methotrexate, fludarabine)	Myelosuppression, anorexia, nausea, vomiting, fatigue, diarrhea, mucositis
Antimitotic agents (vincristine, vinorelbine, paclitaxel, docetaxel)	Myelosuppression, anorexia, nausea, vomiting, diarrhea, mucositis, fatigue, peripheral neuropathy
Hormonal	
Glucocorticoids (prednisone, dexamethasone)	Sodium and fluid retention, gastrointestinal upset, glucose intolerance, potassium wasting, osteoporosis
Antiandrogens (flutamide)	Nausea, diarrhea, hot flashes
Antiestrogens (tamoxifen citrate)	Nausea, bone pain, fluid retention, hot flashes, hypercalcemia
Progestins (megestrol acetate)	Increased appetite, weight gain, fluid retention, hypercalcemia
Gonadotropin-releasing hormone analog (leuprolide)	Nausea, bone pain
Immunotherapy	
Immunologic—Biologic Response Modifers	
Interferon alfa	Myelosuppression, anorexia, nausea, vomiting, flulike symptoms
Interleukin	Myelosuppression, nausea, vomiting, hypotension, chills, fatigue, capillary leak syndrome
Monoclonal antibodies (rituximab, trastuzumab)	Myelosuppression, nausea, vomiting, fever, chills, rash
Immunologic—Hematopoietic	
Epoetin alpha (erythropoietin, EPO)	Fever; iron supplementation may be necessary
Filgrastim (granulocytic colony-stimulating factor, G-CSF)	Fever, bone pain, flulike symptoms
Sargramostim (granulocytic macrophage-stimulating factor, GM-CSF)	Fever, bone pain, flulike symptoms

Data in Table 37-4 from Eldridge B et al: Nutrition and the patient with cancer. In Coulston AM et al, editors: *Nutrition in the prevention and treatment of disease*, San Diego, 2001, Academic Press; Elliott L et al., editors: *The clinical guide to oncology nutrition*, ed 2, Chicago, 2006, American Dietetic Association; Cancer Therapy Evaluation Program, Common Terminology Criteria for Adverse Events, Version 3.0, DCTD, NCI, NIH, DHHS, March 31, 2003, http://ctep.cancer.gov, August 9, 2006.

of medication via a catheter directly into the abdominal cavity), intravesicular (delivery of medication via a Foley catheter directly into the bladder), or intrathecal (delivery of medication via an injection into the central nervous system using an Ommaya reservoir or a lumbar puncture).

The severity of the side effects depends on the specific agent(s) used, dosage, duration of treatment, number of treatment cycles, accompanying drugs, individual response, and current health status. The timely and appropriate use of supportive therapies such as antiemetics, antidiarrheals, hematopoietic agents, and antibiotics, as well as dietary changes, is important to the effective management of treatment-related side effects, especially those that have a nutrition impact. The reality is that, despite the supportive care, many patients still experience significant side effects, especially in "dose-intensive" multiple-agent chemotherapy regimens; **neutropenia** (reduced white blood cells or neutro-phils) and myelosuppression are the primary factors limiting chemotherapy administration.

Commonly experienced chemotherapy-induced toxicities for the gastrointestinal system include diarrhea, constipation, or adynamic ileus (inhibition of bowel motility). Chemotherapy-related taste abnormalities can lead to anorexia and oligophagy (eating few foods). Symptoms of gastrointestinal toxicity are usually not long lasting; however, some multiagent chemotherapy regimens have severe and prolonged gastrointestinal effects.

Some agents, especially corticosteroids, can cause tissue breakdown and promote excessive urinary loss of protein, potassium, and calcium. The intestinal mucosa and digestive processes are affected, thus altering digestion and absorption to some degree. Protein, energy, and vitamin metabolism may be impaired, although the consequences of this are not known. Total lymphocyte count is depressed and does not accurately reflect nutrition status after chemotherapy administration.

Health care professionals should be alert to possible drug-nutrient interactions since some chemotherapy agents can cause potentially severe adverse events. For example, individuals with certain types of lung cancer who are being treated with pemetrexed (Alimta) require vitamin B_{12} and folic acid supplementation to avoid significant anemia associated with this chemotherapy agent; or a severe hypertensive event is possible when tyramine-rich foods and beverages are consumed while taking procarbazine (Mutalane), a chemotherapy agent commonly used to treat brain cancer. Health care professionals can gain valuable insights regarding drug-nutrient interactions and contraindications by reviewing product medication inserts, pharmacy resource books, and medication databases or by consulting with pharmacy personnel (see Chapter 16 and Appendix 31).

Immunotherapy

Immunotherapy involves using biologic response modifiers that are natural products that are made in quantities through cloning and genetic engineering. Used directly as cytotoxic agents or indirectly as stimulators of the individual's own natural defenses, biologic agents can kill tumor cells. α-Interferon is used to treat hairy-cell leukemia. Interleukin-2 is used in the treatment of individuals with malignant melanoma and renal cell carcinoma.

Immunotherapy also includes supportive care agents (hematopoietics) such as colony-stimulating factors (i.e., cytokines that stimulate the marrow to develop faster) that are used to shorten periods of neutropenia and thrombocytopenia for individuals and to enrich the graft for myeloid precursors before harvest of marrow from donors (Isola et al., 1997). Individuals in whom these agents are used may experience fatigue, chills, fever, flulike symptoms, and decreased food intake (see Table 37-4A).

Radiation Therapy

Radiation therapy uses high-energy rays (ionizing radiation) in multiple fractionated doses to cure, control, or palliate cancer. Radiation therapy can be delivered externally into the body from a megavoltage machine (e.g., linear accelerator, cyclotron, or cobalt-60 unit) or with brachytherapy by placing a radioactive source (implant) in or near the treatment tumor volume to deliver a highly localized dose. Advances in technology to deliver radiation therapy with extreme accuracy include stereotactic radiosurgery (Gamma knife) and intensity-modulated radiation therapy. Whereas chemotherapy is a systemic therapy, radiation therapy affects only the tumor and the surrounding area. The side effects of radiation therapy are usually limited to the specific site being irradiated. Chemotherapy agents may also be given in combination with radiation therapy to produce a radiation-enhancing effect. Patients receiving multimodality therapy often experience more toxic side effects sooner.

The acute side effects of radiation therapy when used alone generally manifest around the second or third week of treatment and usually resolve within 2 to 4 weeks after the radiation therapy has been completed. Late effects of radiation therapy may occur several weeks, months, or even years after treatment. Regardless of the specific area being irradiated, commonly experienced nutrition impact symptoms include fatigue, loss of appetite, skin changes, and hair loss in the area being treated (Table 37-4B).

Radiation therapy to the head and neck can cause a variety of acute nutritional symptoms: sore mouth, altered taste and smell, dysphagia and odynophagia, mucositis, xerostomia, anorexia, fatigue, and weight loss. Current multimodality protocols for treatment of head and neck cancer that use chemotherapy and surgery, as well as radiation therapy, should not be used without aggressive enteral nutrition (Scolapio et al., 2001). Late effects of radiation therapy may include dental caries, permanent xerostomia, trismus (lockjaw), and osteoradionecrosis. Before beginning therapy, individuals should undergo a dental evaluation and thorough teeth cleaning and receive instruction in good oral hygiene and care, including daily brushing and rinsing (NOHIC, 2006). After therapy has been completed, individuals should continue to have close dental monitoring and follow-up. Individuals may also benefit from a referral to a speech pathologist for assessment and evaluation of swallowing function.

Nutrition impact symptoms of radiation therapy to the thorax can include heartburn and acute esophagitis characterized by dysphagia and odynophagia. Late effects include possible esophageal fibrosis and stenosis. When this occurs, individuals are generally only able to swallow liquids; esophageal dilations and nutrition support (enteral nutrition) may be necessary to meet nutritional needs.

Radiation therapy to the abdomen may produce acute gastritis or enteritis accompanied by nausea, vomiting, diarrhea, and anorexia. Late effects can include severe gastrointestinal damage that is manifested by malabsorption of disaccharides, fats, and electrolytes. **Radiation-induced enteritis** can develop into a chronic form of the condition, with symptoms of ulceration or obstruction intensifying the risk of malnutrition (Engelking, 2004).

Chronic radiation enteritis combined with massive bowel resection, which results in extensive bowel dysfunction, is called short bowel syndrome (see Chapter 27). The severity of this condition depends on the length and location of the nonfunctional or resected bowel; it is generally diagnosed when the individual has less than 150 cm of remaining small intestine. The sequelae include maldigestion, malabsorption, malnutrition, dehydration, and potentially lethal metabolic aberrations. Initially TPN is required, and frequent monitoring of fluids and electrolytes may be required for weeks or months. The diet may need to be restricted to defined formula tube feedings or to frequent small meals high in complex carbohydrate and protein, low in fat and oxalate, and lactose free. Medications such as antidiarrheals can be given to decrease intestinal motility. Multivitamin supplements that include vitamin B_{12}; folic acid; and vitamins A, E, and K should be given to prevent deficiencies. Serum concentrations of various minerals should be monitored and adjusted as needed.

Total-body irradiation (TBI) is a technique of radiation therapy that is used in hematopoietic stem cell transplantation

TABLE 37-4B

Nutrition Impact of Cancer Therapies: Radiation

Site of Radiation Therapy	Common Nutrition Impact Symptoms
Central nervous system (brain and spinal cord)	**Acute effects**: Nausea, vomiting Elevated blood glucose caused by steroid administration Fatigue Loss of appetite **Late effects (>90 days after treatment)**: Headache, lethargy
Head and neck area (tongue, larynx, pharynx, oropharynx, nasopharynx, tonsils, salivary glands)	**Acute effects**: Xerostomia Sore mouth and throat Dysphagia, odynophagia Mucositis Alterations in taste and smell Fatigue Loss of appetite **Late effects (>90 days after treatment)**: Mucosal—atrophy and dryness, ulceration Salivary glands—xerostomia, fibrosis Osteoradionecrosis Trismus Alterations in taste and smell
Thorax (esophagus, lung, breast)	**Acute effects**: Dysphagia, odynophagia Heartburn Fatigue Loss of appetite **Late effects (>90 days after treatment)**: Esophageal—fibrosis, stenosis, neurosis Cardiac—angina on effort, pericarditis, cardiac enlargement Pulmonary—dry cough, fibrosis, pneumonitis
Abdomen and pelvis	**Acute affects**: Nausea, vomiting Changes in bowel function—diarrhea, cramping, bloating, gas Changes in urinary function—increased frequency, burning sensation with urination Acute colitis or enteritis Lactose intolerance Fatigue Loss of appetite **Late effects (>90 days after treatment)**: Diarrhea, malabsorption, maldigestion Chronic colitis or enteritis Intestinal—stricture, ulceration, obstruction, perforation, fistula Urinary—hematuria, cystitis

to eradicate malignant cells, to ablate the bone marrow to make room for the engraftment of the infused hematopoietic cells, and to suppress the immune system of the recipient to decrease the risk of graft rejection in allogeneic transplants. Acute effects of TBI are often difficult to discern since it is given in conjunction with conditioning chemotherapy (Lawton, 2003). Commonly encountered side effects are fever, nausea, vomiting, headache, parotitis (inflammation of the parotid glands), xerostomia, diarrhea, and fatigue.

Surgery

The surgical resection or removal of any part of the alimentary tract, as well as the malignant disease process itself, can impair digestion and absorption significantly (Thomas,

2006). Surgery may be used as the only mode of cancer treatment, or it may be combined with preoperative or post-operative adjuvant chemotherapy or radiation therapy. After surgery individuals commonly experience fatigue, temporary changes in appetite and bowel function caused by anesthesia, and pain. They require additional energy and protein for wound healing and recovery. Most side effects are temporary and dissipate after a few days following surgery. However, some surgical interventions have long-lasting nutritional implications. See Table 37-4C for common nutrition impact symptoms associated with specific surgical interventions for the treatment of cancer (see Chapter 27).

Individuals with head and neck cancer often have impaired mastication and swallowing caused by the tumor mass or the specific surgical intervention required. These patients also present additional problems because of their frequent history of smoking, alcohol use, and poor dietary intake. They are at high risk for malnutrition and postoperative complications. Surgery often necessitates temporary or permanent reliance on enteral nutrition, including percutaneous endoscopic gastrostomy or nasogastric tube feedings (see Chapter 20). Individuals who resume oral intake often have prolonged dysphagia and require modifications of food consistency and extensive training in chewing and swallowing. Referrals to a speech therapist can yield dramatic positive results through evaluation and individualized instruction in swallowing and positioning techniques.

Surgical treatment of esophageal tumors may require partial or total removal of the esophagus. The stomach is commonly used for esophageal reconstruction. A feeding nasojejunostomy or jejunostomy tube can be placed at the time of surgery, permitting early postoperative tube feedings. Usually the individual is able to progress to oral intake with specific dietary recommendations to minimize nutrition impact symptoms, which include dumping syndrome, dysmotility, gastroparesis, early satiety, vomiting, and fluid and electrolyte imbalances. Postsurgical dietary recommendations include a low-fat diet with small, frequent feedings of nutrient-dense foods and avoidance of large amounts of fluids at any one time.

Surgery is the most common treatment for cancer of the stomach, although chemotherapy and radiation therapy can be used before or after surgery to improve survival and control disease (Layke and Lopez, 2004). Surgical interventions include partial or subtotal gastrectomy or total gastrectomy. Placement of a jejunostomy feeding tube at surgery is advisable, and enteral nutrition support is generally feasible within a few days after surgery (see Chapter 20).

Postgastrectomy syndrome encompasses a myriad of nutritional intolerances and deficiencies. Its symptoms include dumping syndrome, fat malabsorption, gastric stasis, lactose intolerance, anemias, and metabolic bone disease (e.g., osteoporosis, osteopenia, osteomalacia) (Schattner and Shike, 2006). Dumping syndrome is a common complication of gastric surgery, and it is manifested by the rapid transit of foods or liquids (especially those high in simple carbohydrate content) and the dilutional response of the small re-maining stomach to highly osmotic bolus feedings. Individuals may experience gastrointestinal and vasomotor symptoms such as abdominal cramps, diarrhea, nausea, vomiting, flushing, faintness, diaphoresis, and tachycardia (Radigan, 2004).

Malabsorption is another complication of gastric surgery; deficiency of iron, folate, and less commonly vitamin B_{12} can lead to anemia. Micronutrient deficiencies of calcium and fat-soluble vitamins are also common (Radigan, 2004). Individuals benefit from consumption of six to eight small meals per day, with fluids taken between meals. Fat intolerance may also be experienced, especially if the vagal nerve is severed. Administration of pancreatic enzymes with meals may be beneficial for patients for whom the mixing of food and pancreatic juices is inadequate.

Pancreatic cancer, with its attendant surgical resection, has significant nutritional consequences. The Whipple procedure and the pylorus-sparing pancreatic duodenectomy are the most commonly used pancreatic cancer surgeries. Postsurgical complications include delayed gastric emptying, early satiety, glucose intolerance, bile acid insufficiency, diarrhea, and fat malabsorption. Pancreatic enzyme replacement may be used to aid digestion and absorption, and a fat-restricted diet may be indicated. Individuals benefit from the use of small, more frequent feedings and, if indicated, avoidance of simple carbohydrates.

Partial or total resections of the intestinal tract may induce profound losses of fluid and electrolytes, the severity of which is related to the length and site of the resection. Resections of as little as 15 cm of the terminal ileum can result in bile salt losses that exceed the liver's capacity for resynthesis, and vitamin B_{12} absorption is affected. With depletion of the bile salt pool, steatorrhea develops. Nutrition support consists of a diet low in fat, osmolality, lactose, and oxalate (see Chapter 27, and Box 36-4 in Chapter 36).

Hematopoietic Stem Cell Transplantation

Hematopoietic stem cell transplantation (HSCT) is performed for the treatment of certain hematologic malignant diseases such as leukemia and lymphoma, malignant solid tumors, and autoimmune disorders. The stem cells used for HSCT arise from bone marrow, peripheral blood, or umbilical cord blood. The preparative regimen includes cytotoxic chemotherapy, with or without total-body irradiation, to suppress immunologic reactivity and eradicate malignant cells. This treatment regimen is followed by IV infusion of hematopoietic cells from the individual (autologous) or from a histocompatible related or unrelated donor (allogeneic) or from an identical twin (syngeneic) (NMDP, 2006) (see *Pathophysiology and Care Management Algorithm:* Hematopoietic Stem Cell Transplantation [HSCT]).

HSCT procedures can significantly affect nutrition status. There should be a thorough nutrition assessment of the patient before the initiation of therapy and reassessments and monitoring throughout the entire transplant course. The acute toxicities of immunosuppression that can last for 2 to 4 weeks after the transplant include nausea, vomiting, anorexia, dysgeusia, stomatitis, oral and esophageal mucositis,

TABLE 37-4C

Nutrition Impact of Cancer Therapies: Surgery

Anatomic Site	Common Nutrition Impact Symptoms	Anatomic Site	Common Nutrition Impact Symptoms
Oral cavity	Difficulty with chewing and/or swallowing Aspiration potential Sore mouth Xerostomia Alterations in taste and smell	Hepatocellular —cont'd	Hypertriglyceridemia Fluid and electrolyte imbalance Vitamin and mineral malabsorption (vitamins A, D, E, K, and B_{12}; folic acid, magnesium, zinc)
Larynx	Alterations in normal swallowing, dysphagia Aspiration potential	Pancreas	Gastroparesis Fluid and electrolyte imbalance Hyperglycemia Fat malabsorption Vitamin and mineral malabsorption (vitamins A, D, E, K, and B_{12}; calcium, zinc, iron)
Esophagus	Gastroparesis Indigestion and/or acid reflux Alterations in normal swallowing, decreased motility Anastomotic leak	Small bowel	Chyle leak Lactose intolerance Bile acid depletion Diarrhea Fluid and electrolyte imbalance Vitamin and mineral malabsorption (vitamins B_{12}, A, D, E, and K; calcium, iron, zinc)
Lung	Shortness of breath Early satiety		
Stomach	Dumping syndrome Dehydration Early satiety Gastroparesis Fat malabsorption Vitamin and mineral malabsorption (vitamins B_{12} and D; calcium, iron)	Colorectal	Increased transit time Diarrhea Dehydration Bloating, cramping, and/or gas Fluid and electrolyte imbalance Vitamin and mineral malabsorption (vitamin B_{12}, sodium, potassium, magnesium, calcium)
Gallbladder and bile duct	Gastroparesis Hyperglycemia Fluid and electrolyte Fat malabsorption Vitamin and mineral malabsorption (vitamins B_{12}, A, D, E, and K; magnesium, zinc, calcium, iron)	Gynecologic	Early satiety Bloating, cramping, and/or gas
Hepatocellular	Hyperglycemia	Brain	Nausea and vomiting If taking corticosteroids, possible hyperglycemia

fatigue and diarrhea. In addition, immunosuppressive medications can also adversely affect nutrition status (Charuhas, 2006).

Individuals typically have little or no oral intake during the first few weeks following transplant; therefore enteral or parenteral nutrition support is usually considered and has become a standardized component of care. Because the function of the gastrointestinal tract is compromised, TPN is often used. Gastrostomy tubes are useful for long-term nutrition support, and TPN should be reserved for individuals who are unable to tolerate oral or enteral feeding (Sheehan, 2005). However, the administration of optimal levels of TPN is complicated by the frequent need to interrupt it for the infusion of antibiotics, blood products, and medications. This in turn necessitates careful monitoring and the use of more concentrated nutrient solutions, increased flow rates, and double- or triple-lumen catheters.

Autologous HSCT involves the use of the individual's own stem cells to reestablish hematopoietic stem cell function after the administration of high-dose chemotherapy. In some cases the use of mobilized stem cell progenitors has replaced autologous bone marrow as the source of hematopoietic progenitors for transplantation. Their use has shortened the period of **pancytopenia** (reduction in the cellular components of the blood), when patients are at risk for bleeding and serious infections that may lead to sepsis. These advances, along with improved prophylactic antibiotic regimens that are relatively easy to administer, have allowed patients to receive autologous marrow transplantation in the outpatient setting. This change has substantially reduced the cost of transplantation and thus has made it available to an increased number of patients. However, because a majority of these patients receive much of their care outside the hospital, nutrition assessment and monitoring are of critical importance.

PATHOPHYSIOLOGY AND CARE MANAGEMENT ALGORITHM

Hematopoietic Stem Cell Transplantation (HSCT)

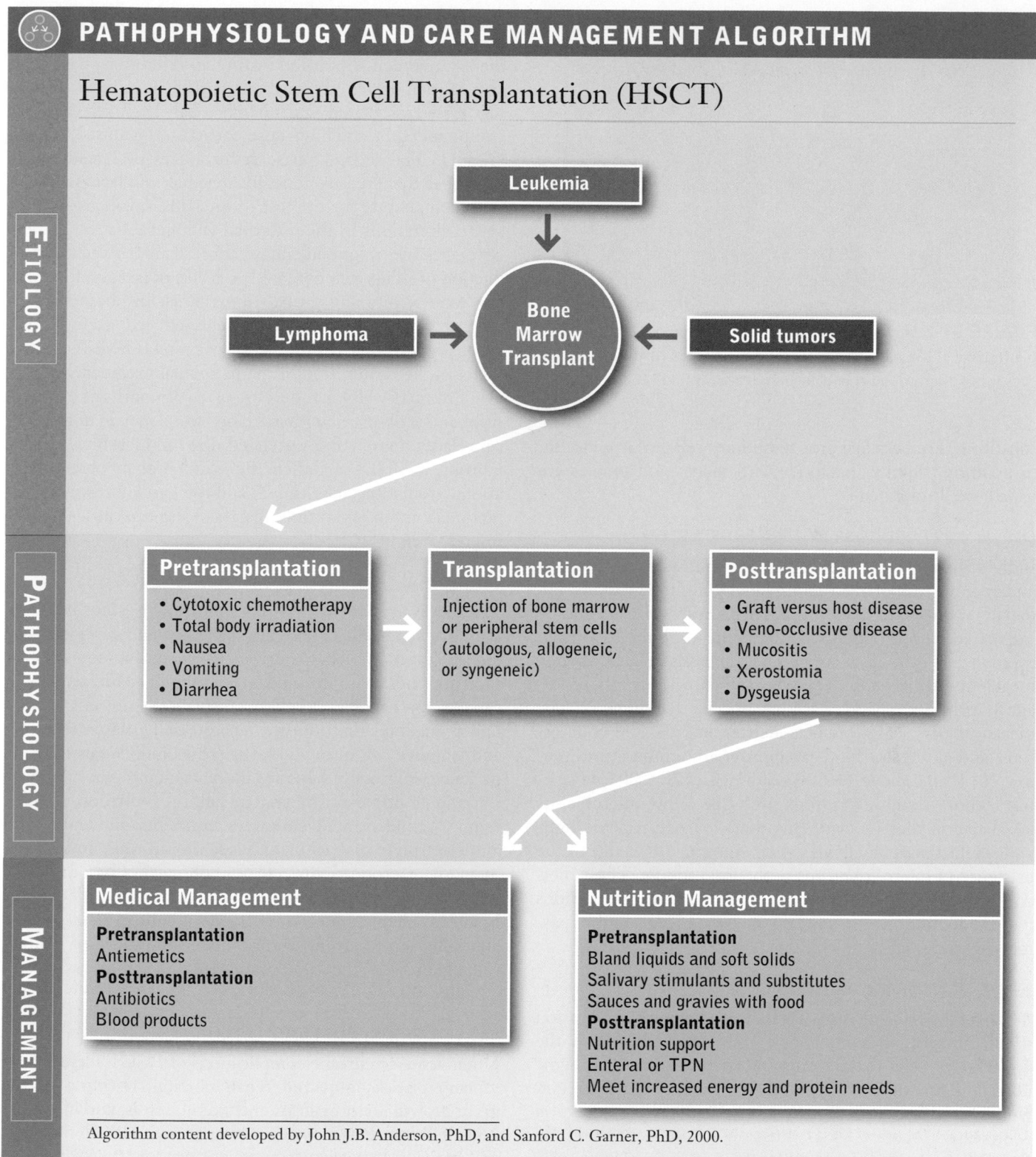

ETIOLOGY

Leukemia

Lymphoma → Bone Marrow Transplant ← Solid tumors

PATHOPHYSIOLOGY

Pretransplantation
- Cytotoxic chemotherapy
- Total body irradiation
- Nausea
- Vomiting
- Diarrhea

Transplantation
Injection of bone marrow or peripheral stem cells (autologous, allogeneic, or syngeneic)

Posttransplantation
- Graft versus host disease
- Veno-occlusive disease
- Mucositis
- Xerostomia
- Dysgeusia

MANAGEMENT

Medical Management

Pretransplantation
Antiemetics
Posttransplantation
Antibiotics
Blood products

Nutrition Management

Pretransplantation
Bland liquids and soft solids
Salivary stimulants and substitutes
Sauces and gravies with food
Posttransplantation
Nutrition support
Enteral or TPN
Meet increased energy and protein needs

Algorithm content developed by John J.B. Anderson, PhD, and Sanford C. Garner, PhD, 2000.

The HSCT procedure is associated with severe nutritional consequences and requires prompt, aggressive intervention. Nausea, vomiting, and diarrhea are caused by the cytotoxic conditioning regimen and may later accompany antibiotic administration. Antiemetics may be helpful. Complications of delayed onset include varying degrees of mucositis, xerostomia, and dysgeusia. Mucositis, which is often severe and extremely painful, develops in more than 75% of transplant patients (Figure 37-2).

Bland liquids and soft solids are usually better tolerated in individuals with treatment-related mucositis. Strong-flavored, acidic, or spicy foods should also be avoided. Herpes simplex virus and *Candida albicans* account for most oral infections (Eisen et al., 1997). Salivary stimulants and

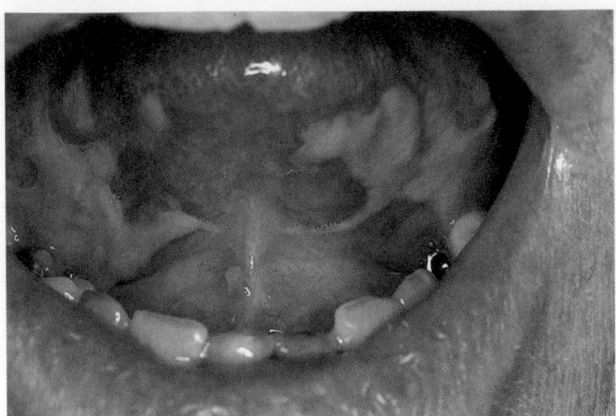

FIGURE 37-2 Severe oral mucositis after marrow transplantation. This patient also received a course of high-dose cyclophosphamide and whole-body radiation.

substitutes are beneficial for temporary relief of dry mouth; in addition, liquids and foods with sauces and gravies are usually well tolerated.

Dietary Precautions With Neutropenia

Individuals receiving HSCT become immunocompromised and require supportive therapy, including medications and dietary changes, to prevent infection. Individuals should be instructed on food safety practices, including the following: avoidance of foods that contain unsafe levels of bacteria (raw meats, spoiled or moldy foods, and unpasteurized beverages); thorough hand washing; special handling of raw meats, poultry, eggs, utensils, cutting boards, and countertops; and storage of foods at appropriate temperatures (below 40° F and above 140° F) (Eldridge et al., 2001; Charuhas, 2006). Many institutions prescribe a low-microbial or low-bacteria diet (neutropenic diet) for neutropenic individuals. Its use is chiefly based on empiric knowledge of the existence of microorganisms in the food supply. These diets consist primarily of cooked foods, and the major restrictions include avoiding fresh, raw, or uncooked foods and unpasteurized beverages.

Graft-Versus-Host Disease (GVHD)

Graft-versus-host disease (GVHD) is a major complication seen primarily after allogeneic transplants, in which the donor stem cells react against the tissues of the "foreign" host. The functions of several target organs (skin, liver, gut, lymphoid cells) are disrupted, and susceptibility to infection is increased. Acute GVHD is usually manifested within the first 100 days after the transplant and may be seen as early as 7 to 10 days posttransplant. It may resolve, or it may develop into a chronic form that requires long-term treatment and dietary management. Skin GVHD is characterized by a maculopapular rash. GVHD of the liver, evidenced by jaundice and abnormal liver function tests, often accompanies gastrointestinal GVHD and further complicates nutrition management.

The symptoms of acute gastrointestinal GVHD are severe, and individuals may experience gastroenteritis, including secretory diarrhea, abdominal pain, nausea, and vomiting. In addition to immunosuppressive medications, a phased dietary regimen should be instituted. The first phase consists of total bowel rest until the diarrhea is reduced. Nitrogen losses associated with diarrhea can be severe and are compounded by the high-dose corticosteroids used to treat GVHD. The second phase reintroduces oral feedings of beverages that are isosmotic, low residue, and lactose free so as to compensate for the loss of intestinal enzymes secondary to alterations in the intestinal villi and mucosa. If these beverages are tolerated, phase three includes the reintroduction of solids that contain low levels of lactose, fiber, fat, and total acidity and no gastric irritants. In phase four dietary restrictions are progressively reduced as foods are gradually introduced and tolerance is established. Phase five includes the resumption of the individual's regular diet.

Chronic GVHD can develop up to 3 months after transplant and is observed with increased frequency in nonidentical related donors and unrelated donors (Charuhas, 2006). Chronic GVHD can affect the skin, oral mucosa (ulcerations, stomatitis, xerostomia) and the gastrointestinal tract (anorexia, reflux symptoms, diarrhea) and can cause changes in body weight.

Sinusoidal Obstructive Syndrome

Another transplant-related complication is **sinusoidal obstructive syndrome (SOS)** (it is also known as venoocclusive disease), and it is characterized by chemotherapy- and or radiation therapy–induced damage to the hepatic venules. It can develop 1 to 3 weeks after transplant. Symptoms of right upper quadrant discomfort, hepatomegaly, fluid retention, and jaundice can occur; in severe cases individuals may experience progressive hepatic failure leading to encephalopathy and multiple-organ system failure. Nutrition support requires concentrated parenteral nutrients, judicious fluid and electrolyte management, close monitoring, and adjustment of macronutrients and micronutrients based on the tolerance and response of the individual patient. The use of branched-chain amino acid formulas is controversial. Serum ammonia level may not be a reliable indicator of protein tolerance or of the development of encephalopathy (see Chapter 28).

Other Complications of HSCT

Other acute or chronic complications of HSCT include pulmonary disease, impaired renal function, rejection of the graft, growth abnormalities in children, sepsis, and infection. Nutrition impact symptoms associated with HSCT may persist; individuals receiving outpatient marrow transplantation require frequent assessment and intervention by an RD.

MANAGEMENT OF NUTRITION IMPACT SYMPTOMS

Cancer and its treatment can impact nutritional needs significantly and affect digestion, absorption, and metabolism.

Symptoms with a nutrition impact include nausea and vomiting, changes in taste and smell, bowel changes, dysphagia, anorexia, pain, and fatigue (Schattner and Shike, 2006).

Determining Routes of Nutrition Therapy

Regardless of which routes of providing nutrition care and support are used, nutritional goals should be specific, achievable, and individualized in scope to encourage cooperation. Goals need to be directed toward a visible means of feedback such as body weight or some other meaningful index. Another goal is to minimize the effects of nutrition impact symptoms and to maximize the individual's nutritional parameters. Consultation with the individual, caregivers, or family members regarding expected problems and their possible solutions should be initiated early in the course of cancer therapy and should continue in conjunction with follow-up nutrition assessment and care.

Oral Nutrition Management Strategies

Ideally the preferred route of feeding is oral, although individuals who experience nutrition impact symptoms such as nausea, anorexia, early satiety, and dysphagia may resist it. Strategies for modifying nutrient intake depend on the specific feeding problem and the extent of depletion. Oral intake may be encouraged with modifications of food and its presentation. Liquid nutritional supplements may be considered for individuals unable to consume sufficient energy and protein to maintain their weight and optimal nutrition status (see Chapter 20).

Individuals with altered taste acuity (**dysgeusia, hypogeusia, ageusia**) may benefit from increased use of flavorings and seasonings during food preparation. Meat aversions may require the elimination of red meats, which tend to be strong in flavor, or the substitution of alternative protein sources. Dysphagia secondary to surgical interventions, radiation therapy–induced inflammation of the esophagus, or mucositis from chemotherapy involving the oral and esophageal tissues can be lessened with the intake of foods that are soft or liquefied and served at moderate or room temperature.

Artificial saliva preparations and saliva stimulants are often useful in cases of diminished salivation, as are foods with high moisture content and plenty of fluids throughout the day and with meals. Individuals with gastrointestinal symptoms may require dietary modifications of lactose, fat, and fiber content, as well as alterations in texture. Commercially prepared liquid nutritional supplements can be included in many dietary plans. Management of diarrhea and steatorrhea is discussed in Chapter 27.

The timing of food presentation also deserves consideration. Individuals with cancer often report a decreased ability to eat as the day progresses, which means that the morning is often the best time for eating. This phenomenon may be attributable to sluggish digestion and gastric emptying as a result of decreased production of digestive secretions, gastrointestinal mucosal atrophy, and gastric muscle atrophy. It may also be experienced as a result of treatment-related fatigue.

Fatigue is one of the most common symptoms reported by individuals with cancer and is often characterized as physical tiredness, mental slowness, and lack of emotional resilience. Individuals should be encouraged to consume more frequent, small feedings, with particular emphasis on morning feedings, and easy-to-eat foods that require less preparation and are easier to consume. Pain can also adversely affect individuals' appetite and ability to eat. Pain can be a result of the tumor itself or a consequence of treatment, or it can have a psychological component. Appropriate pain management medications such as topical anesthetics, anti-inflammatory agents, and opioid analgesics should be used (Wojtaszek et al., 2002).

The timing of meals or snacks relative to the gastrointestinal side effects of cancer treatment may have a bearing on subsequent learned food aversions. These aversions develop when specific foods are associated with unpleasant symptoms such as nausea and vomiting and psychological stimuli such as anxiety. The effect may not be limited to new food items but may also involve foods that were included in the individual's usual diet before treatment. Exposure of individuals to a "scapegoat" food or beverage just before chemotherapy or radiation therapy can markedly reduce the incidence of treatment-related aversions to foods in the usual diet (Puccio and Nathanson, 1997).

Management of Chemotherapy-Induced Nausea and Vomiting

Chemotherapy-induced nausea and vomiting are commonly classified as anticipatory, acute, or delayed, each of which is manifested by distinct pathophysiologic events and requires different therapeutic interventions (Bubalo et al., 2004). Currently the most effective agents for treatment-related (acute) nausea and vomiting are the 5-hydroxytryptamine 3 (5-HT) antagonists (i.e., ondansetron, granisetron, and dolasetron). Although costly, they are used in conjunction with highly and moderately emetogenic chemotherapeutic regimens. Although effective in managing acute nausea and vomiting, these agents are generally thought to be ineffective in the management of delayed nausea and vomiting (occurring 24 to 96 hours after treatment); other antiemetic agents, including neurokinin 1 (NK-1) antagonists (aprepitant), corticosteroids, and dopamine antagonists such as phenothiazines (prochlorperazine) and benzamides (metoclopramide) may be used (Ettinger et al., 2006; Von Roenn, 2006).

Other alternatives include cannabinoids (dronabinol) and benzodiazepines (lorazepam and diazepam). The anticipatory form of nausea and vomiting is a conditioned response that develops by the third or fourth cycle of treatment in about one third of individuals receiving chemotherapy. It is primarily a psychological issue and so responds best to behavioral interventions such as relaxation training, guided imagery, or systematic desensitization (Fessele, 1996).

Pharmaceutical Management of Anorexia-Cachexia Syndrome

A number of pharmacologic agents are under investigation in the management of the anorexia-cachexia syndrome and cancer-related weight loss, including appetite stimulants, metabolic agents and cytokine blockers, prokinetic agents, and anabolic agents (Von Roenn, 2006; Box 37-4).

Several trials have shown improved appetite and increased energy intake and body weight in cancer patients treated with megestrol acetate, a progestational agent. The benefits of megestrol acetate are dose dependent, with greater benefit at higher doses (Von Roenn, 2006). Prolonged use of corticosteroids is associated with negative side effects such as osteoporosis, fluid retention, adrenal suppression, glucose intolerance, electrolyte imbalance, or even arm and leg muscle wasting. Dronabinol, synthetically produced marijuana, stimulates appetite in patients with cancer-related anorexia. Oxandrolone, a synthetic anabolic steroid, combined with a resistance exercise program, has been found to increase total body weight and lean tissue weight (Von Roenn, 2006). Growth hormones have been studied in patients with wasting associated with human immunodeficiency virus, but few data are available regarding their use with cancer cachexia and anorexia.

In summary, the pharmacologic management of cachexia and anorexia requires careful evaluation based on the patient's treatment goals and prognosis and on close monitoring of symptoms and prescribed medications that may interfere with adequate intake. Ideally these agents are prescribed in combination with nutrition counseling and physical activity assessment, monitoring, and evaluation.

BOX 37-4

Pharmacologic Management of Anorexia-Cachexia Syndrome

Appetite Stimulants

- Megestrol acetate
- Dronabinol
- Corticosteroids

Metabolic Agents and Cytokine Blockers

- Melatonin
- Pentoxifylline
- Hydrazine sulfate
- Eicosapentaenoic acid (EPA)

Prokinetic Drugs

- Metoclopramide

Anabolic Agents

- Growth hormone
- Oxandrolone
- Nandrolone

Data from Von Roenn JH: Pharmacologic interventions for cancer-related weight loss, *Oncology Issues* 17(suppl):20, 2002; and Murphy S, Von Roenn JH: Pharmacological management of anorexia and cachexia. In McCallum PD, Polisena CG, editors: *The clinical guide to oncology nutrition*, Chicago, 2000, American Dietetic Association.

Enteral Nutrition

When individuals with cancer are unable to meet their nutritional needs because of malnutrition, prolonged anorexia, mechanical obstruction, or treatment-related toxicities (e.g., dysphagia, odynophagia, or mucositis), other more aggressive routes of nutrition support need to be considered. If the gut is functional, enteral nutrition is the preferred route of nutrition support. Enteral nutrition helps to preserve immune and gut barrier function. It is associated with fewer postoperative complications and shortened lengths of stay (Bozzetti et al., 2001). In patients with head and neck cancer receiving radiation therapy, the placement of a feeding tube and enteral nutrition support before the initiation of therapy has been shown to prevent weight loss and reduce treatment interruptions and hospitalizations for dehydration (Scolapio et al., 2001).

Nasogastric or nasojejunal feeding tubes are used most commonly for the short-term administration of enteral nutrition formulas. Gastrostomy or jejunostomy feeding tubes are used when longer-term enteral nutrition support (for greater than 3 to 4 weeks) is indicated (see Chapter 20).

The selection of the enteral nutrition formula for an individual with cancer is determined by several factors, including the functional capacity of the gut, the individual's nutrition status, considerations of cost and convenience, and the physical characteristics of the formula such as osmolality, presence of fructooligosaccharides (FOS), protein content, energy density, and nutrient content (Robinson, 2006). Appendix 32 describes available enteral preparations. General-purpose commercially prepared formulas serve most needs. However, individuals with preexisting medical conditions or treatment-related side effects (e.g., radiation enteritis, malabsorption) may benefit from elemental or peptide-based formulas (see Chapter 20).

Use of immune-enhancing enteral nutrition formulas that are supplemented with arginine, glutamine, and omega-3 fatty acids have been shown to reduce postsurgical complications and result in cost savings in individuals who are undergoing gastrointestinal surgery. Their use is generally indicated for 5 to 7 days (orally) before surgery and for a minimum of 5 days (orally or enterally) after surgery (Sax, 2001).

Of note, tumor development at the percutaneous feeding tube stoma site has been documented in over 20 individuals between 1989 and 2002 (Thakore et al., 2003). Researchers suspect that the metastases may be spread by a direct seeding of tumor cells at the feeding tube site after the tube has passed or been pulled through the area of primary disease in the digestive region during tube-feeding placement (Maccabee and Sheppard, 2003; Sinclair et al., 2001). The researchers suggest that methods of tube-feeding placement be used that avoid such contact.

Parenteral Nutrition

The use of parenteral nutrition support may be appropriate for some individuals with cancer for whom oral intake or enteral nutrition is not tolerated. Factors to consider include the individual's prognosis, prescribed therapy, degree of malnutrition, and gastrointestinal function (e.g., severe diarrhea or malabsorption necessitating bowel rest, radiation enteritis, intractable nausea and vomiting, GVHD, bowel obstruction or ileus, or severe pancreatitis). See Chapter 20 for an in-depth discussion of PN.

Parenteral nutrition has been shown to improve long-term survival in patients undergoing HSCT (Weisdorf et al., 1987) and reduce surgical complications in malnourished gastrointestinal cancer patients (Bozzetti et al., 2001). Ziegler and associates (1998) found that patients receiving parenteral nutrition supplemented with glutamine had improved clinical outcomes, as evidenced by fewer infections and shortened hospital stays. A retrospective study of over 50 patients with advanced-stage, incurable cancer and gastrointestinal failure showed that patients derived benefit from receiving home parenteral nutrition (Hoda et al., 2005).

The type of parenteral nutrition support is determined by the clinical and nutrition status of the patient and the type of IV access (DeChicco and Steiger, 2006). Individuals diagnosed with cancer often have central IV access to accommodate multiple IV therapies (i.e., chemotherapy, blood products, hydration, and IV medications). Parenteral nutrition support can be delivered via central IV access or peripheral catheter. Peripheral parenteral nutrition mixtures are administered via peripheral catheters, usually are lower in osmolarity, and are lipid-based formulas (see Chapter 20).

Potential complications associated with parenteral nutrition support include fluid overload in individuals who receive multiple IV therapies, hyperglycemia resulting from the high concentration of dextrose, insulin resistance associated with illness and stress, electrolyte imbalance, and infection (DeChicco and Steiger, 2006). Intense monitoring and specialized care are required. Successful outpatient use of parenteral nutrition can be achieved when the individual and family are cooperative and receive individualized instruction and follow-up.

Rehabilitation and Physical Activity

Rehabilitation is an important part of cancer care. The effect of cancer and cancer treatment on the individual's quality of life should be addressed throughout the treatment period and continue until the individual is able to successfully resume activities of daily living. Recovery from cancer treatment also requires physical activity to rebuild muscle and regain strength and energy (Brown et al., 2003).

Fatigue and impairment of physical performance and well-being are common and often severe problems for individuals diagnosed with cancer. Poor or inadequate nutritional intake contributes to fatigue; conversely, fatigue may hinder eating and nutrition support regimens. Appropriate physical activity and exercise may be helpful in managing primary fatigue. In addition, physical activity may improve immune function (Fairey et al., 2002), reduce anxiety and depression, improve mood and self-esteem, and reduce symptoms (Brown et al., 2003). Before participating in any type of physical activity and exercise program, individuals should be advised to undergo evaluation by qualified professionals, who can then design an individualized physical assessment and activity plan.

Individuals With Advanced Cancer Receiving Palliative Care

McCallum and Fornari (2006) define **palliative care** as the active total care of an individual when curative measures are no longer considered an option by either the medical team or the individual. The objectives of palliative care are to provide for optimal quality of life; relieve physical symptoms; alleviate isolation, anxiety, and fear associated with advanced disease; and to help patients maintain independence as long and as comfortably as possible (McCallum and Fornari, 2006). Hospice care focuses on relieving symptoms and supporting individuals with a life expectancy of months, not years (NHPCO, 2006).

Nutrition is an important component in the care and management of individuals with advanced cancer. The goals of nutrition intervention should focus on managing nutrition impact symptoms such as pain, weakness, loss of appetite, early satiety, constipation, weakness, dry mouth, and dyspnea (McCallum and Fornari, 2006). Another important goal is maintaining strength and energy to enhance quality of life, independence, and ability to perform activities of daily living.

Nutrition should be provided "as tolerated or as desired" along with emotional support and awareness of and respect for individual needs and wishes. Thus the pleasurable aspects of eating should be emphasized, without concern for quantity or nutrient and energy content. The use of nutrition support and hydration in individuals with advanced, incurable cancer is a difficult and often controversial issue and should be determined on a case-by-case basis (Stagno et al., 2000).

NUTRITION CARE
OF CHILDREN

Like adults diagnosed with cancer, children with cancer can experience malnutrition and nutrition impact symptoms as a result of their cancer and its treatment (Ringwald-Smith et al., 2006). The incidence of malnutrition ranges from 6% to 50% in the pediatric population, depending on the type, stage, and location of the cancer. It usually has greater severity in the presence of more aggressive cancers in the later stages of the disease (Andrassy and Chwals, 1998).

It is not uncommon for families and caregivers to express their fears of dying through an extreme preoccupation with eating and maintaining weight. Psychogenic food refusal in children requires interventions that address underlying psychological issues. Creative efforts are required to minimize the psychological effects of fear, unpleasant hospital routines, unfamiliar foods, learned food aversions, and pain. Nutrition intervention strategies that use oral intake should stress the maximum use of favorite, nutrient-dense foods during times when intake is likely to be best and food aversions are least likely to occur. Oral nutritional supplements can be useful, but their

Fairey AS et al: Physical exercise and immune system function in cancer survivors: a comprehensive review and future directions, *Cancer* 94:539, 2002.

Fessele KS: Managing the multiple causes of nausea and vomiting in the patient with cancer, *Oncol Nurs Forum* 23:1409, 1996.

Freeland SJ et al: Impact of obesity on biochemical control after radical prostatectomy for clinically localized prostate cancer: a report shared by the Shared Equal Access Regional Cancer Hospital Database Study Group, *J Clin Oncol* 22:446, 2004.

Friedman M: Chemistry, biochemistry, and safety of acrylamide: a review, *J Agric Food Chem* 51:4504, 2003.

Fuhrman MP: Nutrition-focused physical assessment. In Charney P, Malone A, editors: *Nutrition assessment*, Chicago, 2004, American Dietetic Association.

Goldman A et al: Symptoms in children/young people with progressive malignant disease: United Kingdom Children's Cancer Study Group/Paediatric Oncology Nurses Forum survey, *Pediatrics* 117(6):e1179, 2006.

Goodstine SL et al: Dietary (n-3)/(n-6) fatty acid ratio: possible relationship to premenopausal but not postmenopausal breast cancer risk in U.S. Women, *J Nutr* 133:1409, 2003.

Grant B, Byron J: Nutritional implications of chemotherapy. In Elliott L et al, editors: *The clinical guide to oncology nutrition*, ed 2, Chicago, 2006, American Dietetic Association.

Grau MV et al: Vitamin D, calcium supplementation, and colorectal adenomas: results of a randomized trial, *J Natl Cancer Inst* 95:1765, 2003.

Heber D: Vegetables, fruits and phytoestrogens in the prevention of diseases, *J Postgrad Med* 50:145, 2004.

Hedley A et al: Prevalence of overweight and obesity among U.S. children, adolescents and adults, 1999-2002, *JAMA* 291:2847, 2004.

Hennekens CH et al: Lack of effect of long-term supplementation with β-carotene on the incidence of malignant neoplasms and cardiovascular disease, *N Engl J Med* 334:1145, 1996.

Hoda D et al: Should patients with advanced, incurable cancers ever be sent home with total parenteral nutrition? A single institution's 20-year experience, *Cancer* 103:863, 2005.

Holick CN et al: Dietary carotenoids, serum β-carotene, and retinol and risk of lung cancer in the alpha-tocopherol, β-carotene cohort study, *Am J Epidemiol* 156:536, 2002.

Hong WK et al: Prevention of second primary tumors with isotretinoin in squamous-cell carcinoma of the head and neck, *N Engl J Med* 323:795, 1990.

Horn-Ross PL et al: Patterns of alcohol consumption and breast cancer risk in the California Teachers Study cohort, *Cancer Epidemiol Biomarkers Prev* 13:405, 2004.

Hurst JD, Gallagher AL: Energy, protein, micronutrient, and fluid requirement. In Elliott L et al, editors: *The clinical guide to oncology nutrition*, ed 2, Chicago, 2006, American Dietetic Association.

International Agency for Research on Cancer (IARC): *IARC handbooks of cancer prevention*, vol 8, *fruits and vegetables*, Lyon, France, 2003, IARC Press.

Ireton-Jones C et al: Clinical pathways in home nutrition support, *J Am Diet Assoc* 97:1003, 1997.

Isola LM et al: A pilot study of allogeneic bone marrow transplantation using related donors stimulated with G-CSF, *Bone Marrow Transplant* 20:1033, 1997.

Jatoi A et al: Do patients with nonmetastatic non-small cell lung cancer demonstrate altered resting energy expenditure? *Ann Thorac Surg* 72:348, 2001.

Kemper KJ et al: Herbs and other dietary supplements: healthcare professionals' knowledge, attitudes, and practices, *Altern Ther Health Med* 9:42, 2003.

Klein EA: Selenim and vitamin E cancer prevention trial, *Ann NY Acad Sci* 1031:234, 2004.

Knox LS et al: Energy expenditure in malnourished cancer patients, *Ann Surg* 197:152, 1983.

Kritchevsky D: Caloric restriction and cancer, *J Nutr Sci Vitaminol* 47:13, 2001.

Kucuk O, Ottery FD: Dietary supplements during cancer treatment, *Oncology Issues* 17(suppl):24, 2002.

Kushi LH et al: The macrobiotic diet in cancer, *J Nutr* 131(suppl):3056, 2001.

Kushi L, Giovannucci E: Dietary fat and cancer, *Am J Med* 113(suppl 9):63S, 2002.

Kushner RF: Medical management of obesity, *Semin Gastrointest Dis* 13:123, 2002.

Larsson SG et al: Whole grain consumption and risk of colorectal cancer: a population-based cohort of 60,000 women, *Br J Cancer* 92:1803, 2005.

Lawton C: Radiation therapy for bone marrow or stem cell transplantation. In Cox JD, Ang KK, editors: *Radiation oncology: rationale, technique, results*, ed 8, St Louis, 2003, Mosby.

Layke JC, Lopez PP: Gastric cancer: diagnosis and treatment options, *Am Fam Physician* 69:1133, 2004.

Le Marchand L: Cancer preventive effects of flavonoids: a review, *Biomed Pharmacother* 56:296, 2002.

Leitzmann C: Vegetarian diets: what are the advantages? *Forum Nutr* 57:147, 2005.

Luthringer S: Nutritional implications of radiation therapy. In Elliott L et al, editors: *The clinical guide to oncology nutrition*, 2nd ed. Chicago, 2006, American Dietetic Association.

Maccabee D, Sheppard BC: Prevention of percutaneous endoscopic gastrostomy stoma metastases in patients with active oropharyngeal malignancy, *Surg Endosc* 17:1678, 2003.

Martinez ME: Primary prevention of colorectal cancer: lifestyle, nutrition, exercise, *Recent Results Cancer Res* 166:177, 2005.

Maskarinec G: Soy foods for breast cancer survivors and women at high risk for breast cancer, *J Am Diet Assoc* 105:1524, 2005.

McCallum PD, Fornari A: Nutrition therapy in palliative care. In Elliott L et al, editors: *The clinical guide to oncology nutrition*, ed 2. Chicago, 2006, American Dietetic Association.

McCallum PD: Nutrition screening and assessment in oncology. In Elliott et al, editors: *The clinical guide to oncology nutrition*, ed 2. Chicago, 2006, American Dietetic Association.

McMahon K et al: Integrating proactive nutritional assessment in clinical practices to prevent complications and cost, *Semin Oncol* 25(2 suppl 6):20, 1998.

Michels KB et al: Coffee, tea, and caffeine consumption and incidence of colon and rectal cancer, *J Natl Cancer Inst* 16:282, 2005.

Mokdad AH et al: Actual causes of death in the U.S. 2000, *JAMA* 291:1238, 2004.

National Cancer Institute (NCI): *5 A day for better health program: Division of Cancer Control and Population Services*, from http://dccps.nci.nih.gov/5ad_2evi.html or www.5aday.com, accessed May 30, 2006a.

National Cancer Institute: *SEER stat fact sheets—cancer of all sites/2006*, from http://seer.cancer.gov/statfacts/html/all_print.html, accessed May 30, 2006b.

National Center for Complementary and Alternative Medicine (NCCAM) website: http://nccam.nih.gov/, accessed May 30, 2006.

National Center for Health Statistics (NCHS): *Health, United States 1998, with socioeconomic status and health chartbook,* Hyattsville, Md, 2001, National Center for Health Statistics.

National Hospice and Palliative Care Organization (NHPCO): *What is hospice?* from http://www.nhpco.org, accessed May 30, 2006.

National Institutes of Health (NIH): Racial/ethnic patterns for cancer in the United States, 1988-1992. In Miller BA, et al, editors: *SEER monograph,* NIH Publication No. 96-4104, Bethesda, Md, 1996, National Cancer Institute.

National Marrow Donor Program (NMPP): *Types of transplants,* from http://www.marrow.org, accessed May 30, 2006.

National Oral Health Information Clearinghouse (NOHIC): *Oncology reference guide to oral health: prevention and management of oral complication from head and neck therapy, chemotherapy, and blood and marrow transplant,* from http://www.nohic.nidcr.nih.gov, accessed May 23, 2006.

Okasha M et al: Body mass index in young adulthood and cancer mortality: a retrospective cohort study, *J Epidemiol Commun Health* 56:780, 2002.

Omenn GS et al: Effects of a combination of β-carotene and vitamin A on lung cancer and cardiovascular disease, *N Engl J Med* 334:1150, 1996.

Owuor ED, Kong AN: Antioxidants and oxidants regulated signal transduction pathways, *Biochem Pharmacol* 64:765, 2002.

Patterson RE et al: Changes in food sources of dietary fat in response to an intensive low-fat dietary intervention: early results from the women's health initiative, *J Am Diet Assoc* 103:454, 2003.

Pelucchi C et al: Dietary acrylamide and human cancer, *Int J Cancer* 118:467, 2006.

Percherstorfer M et al: Current management strategies for hypercalcemia, *Treat Endocrinol* 2:273, 2003.

Pierce JP et al: Women's Health and Living (WHEL) study group: a randomized trial of the effect of a plant-based dietary pattern on additional breast cancer events and survival: the Women's Health and Living (WHEL) study, *Control Clin Trials* 23:728, 2002.

Potischman N et al: Increased risk of early stage breast cancer related to consumption of sweet foods among women less than age 45 in the United States, *Cancer Causes Control* 13:937, 2002.

Prasad KN et al: Scientific rationale for using high-dose multiple micronutrients as an adjunct to standard and experimental cancer therapies, *J Am Coll Nutr* 20:450S, 2001.

Puccio M, Nathanson L: The cancer cachexia syndrome, *Semin Oncol* 24:277, 1997.

Rabinovitch R et al: Impact of nutrition support on treatment outcome in patients with locally advanced head and neck squamous cell cancer treated with definitive radiotherapy: a secondary analysis of RTOG trial 90-03, *Head Neck* 28:287, 2006.

Radigan AE: Post-gastrectomy: managing the nutrition fall-out, *Pract Gastroenterol* 18:63, 2004.

Renwick AG: Acceptable daily intake and the regulation of intense sweeteners, *Food Addit Contam* 7:463, 1990.

Richardson MA et al: Complementary/alternative medicine use in a comprehensive cancer center and the implications for oncology, *J Clin Oncol* 18:2505, 2000.

Ringwald-Smith K et al: Medical nutrition therapy in pediatric oncology. In Elliott L et al, editors: *The clinical guide to oncology nutrition,* ed 2, Chicago, 2006, American Dietetic Association.

Robinson CA: Enteral nutrition in adult oncology. In Elliott L et al, editors: *The clinical guide to oncology nutrition,* ed 2, Chicago, 2006, American Dietetic Association.

Rock CL, Demark-Wahnfried W: Nutrition and survival after the diagnosis of breast cancer: a review of the evidence, *J Clin Oncol* 20:3302, 2002.

Russell M, Malone A: Nutrient requirements. In Charney P, Malone A, editors: *Nutrition assessment,* Chicago, 2004, American Dietetic Association.

Samanic C et al: Obesity and cancer risk among white and black United States veterans, *Cancer Causes Control* 15:35, 2004.

Sax HC: Effect of immune enhancing formulas (IEF) in general surgery patients, *JPEN J Parenter Enteral Nutr* 25(2 suppl):S19, 2001.

Schattner M, Shike M: Nutrition support of the patient with cancer. In Shils ME et al, editors: *Modern nutrition in health and disease,* ed 10, Philadelphia, 2006, Lippincott, Williams & Wilkins.

Schatzkin A et al: Lack of effect of a low-fat, high-fat diet on the recurrence of colorectal adenomas, Polyp Prevention Trial Study Group, *N Engl J Med* 342:1149, 2000.

Scientific Committee on Food (SCF): Opinion of the Scientific Committee on Food: update on the safety of aspartame, Brussels, SCF/CS/ADD/EDUL/222 Final, 2002.

Scolapio JS et al: Prophylactic placement of gastrostomy feeding tubes before radiotherapy in patients with head and neck cancer: is it worthwhile? *J Clin Gastroenterol* 33:215, 2001.

Sharp L et al: Risk factors for squamous cell carcinoma of the oesophagus in women: a case-control study, *Br J Cancer* 85:1667, 2001.

Sheehan PM: Nutrition support of blood or marrow transplant recipients: how much do we really know? *Pract Gastroenterol* 26:84, 2005.

Shu XO et al: Soyfood intake during adolescence and subsequent risk of breast cancer among Chinese women, *Cancer Epidemiol Biomarkers Prev* 10:483, 2001.

Sinclair JJ et al: Metastasis of head and neck carcinoma to the site of percutaneous endoscopic gastrostomy: case report and literature review, *JPEN J Parenter Enteral Nutr* 25:282, 2001.

Slattery ML et al: Plant foods, fiber, and rectal cancer, *Am J Clin Nutr* 79:274, 2004.

Spindler SR: Rapid and reversible induction of the longevity, anticancer and genomic effects of caloric restriction, *Food Addit Contam* 126(9):960, 2005.

Stagno SJ, et al: Bioethics: communication and decision-making in advanced disease, *Semin Onocol* 27:94, 2000.

Sugimura T et al: Heterocyclic amines: mutagens/carcinogens produced during cooking of meat and fish, *Cancer Sci* 95:290, 2004.

Tamakoshi K et al: JACC Study Group: a prospective study of body size and colon cancer mortality in Japan: the JACC Study, *Int J Obes Relat Metab Disord* 28:551, 2004.

Tareke E et al: Analysis of acrylamide, a carcinogen formed in heated foodstuffs, *J Agric Food Chem* 50:4998, 2002.

Terosian MH, Daly JM: Nutritional support in the cancer-bearing host: effects on host and tumor, *Cancer* 58:1915, 1986.

Thakore JN et al: Percutaneous endoscopic gastrostomy associated with gastric metastasis, *J Clin Gastroenterol* 37:307, 2003.

Thomas S: Nutrition implications of surgical oncology. In Elliott L et al, editors: *The clinical guide to oncology nutrition,* ed 2, Chicago, 2006, American Dietetic Association.

Thompson IM et al: Phase III prostate cancer prevention trials: are the costs justified? *J Clin Oncol* 23:8161, 2005.

Tisdale MJ: Pathogenesis of cancer cachexia, *J Support Oncol* 1:159, 2003.

U.S. Department of Agriculture (USDA): *USDA-Iowa State University database on the isoflavone content of foods*, from http://www.nal.usda.gov/fnic/foodcomp/Data/isoflav/isoflav.html, accessed May 30, 2006.

USDHSS: *Dietary Guidelines for Americans*, ed 6, from http://www.healthierus.gov/dietaryguidelines, accessed May 30, 2006.

USDHSS: Ninth Report on Carcinogens, Research Triangle Park, NC, 2000, Public Health Service, National Toxicology Program.

van Gils CH et al: Consumption of vegetables and fruits and risk of breast cancer, *JAMA* 293:183, 2005.

Von Roenn JH: Pharmaceutical management of nutrition impact symptoms associated with cancer. In Elliott L et al, editors: *The clinical guide to oncology nutrition*, ed 2, Chicago, 2006, American Dietetic Association.

Weisdorf SA, et al: Positive effect of prophylactic total parenteral nutrition on long-term outcome of bone marrow transplantation, *Transplantation* 43:833, 1987.

Wirfalt E et al: Postmenopausal breast cancer is associated with high intakes of omega-6 fatty acids (Sweden), *Cancer Causes Control* 13:883, 2002.

Wojtaszek CA et al: Nutrition impact symptoms in the oncology patient, *Oncology Issues* 17(suppl):17, 2002.

Wu AH et al: Dietary heterocyclic amines and microsatellite instability in colon adenocarcinomas, *Carcinogenesis* 22:1681, 2001.

Wu AH et al: Adolescent and adult soy intake and risk of breast cancer in Asian-Americans, *Carcinogenesis* 23:1491, 2002.

Wynder EL et al: Comparative epidemiology of cancer between the United States and Japan: a second look, *Cancer* 67:746, 1991.

Yan L, Spitznagel E: A meta-analysis of soy foods and risk of breast cancer in women, *Int J Cancer* 1:281, 2004.

Yates JS et al: Prevalence of complementary and alternative medicine use in cancer patients during treatment, *Support Care Cancer* 13:806, 2005.

Ziegler TR et al: Effects of glutamine supplementation on circulating lymphocytes after bone marrow transplantation: a pilot study, *Am J Med Sci* 315:4, 1998.

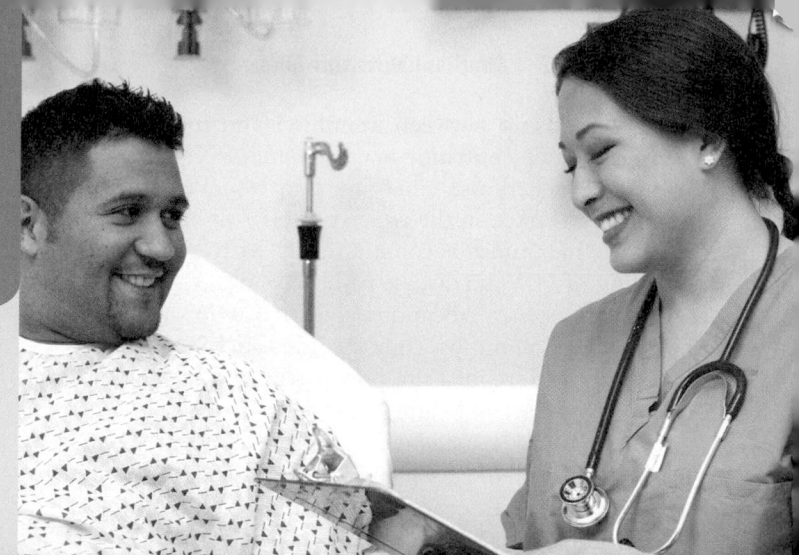

CHAPTER 38

Marcy Fenton, MS, RD
Ellyn C. Silverman, MPH, RD

Medical Nutrition Therapy for Human Immunodeficiency Virus (HIV) Disease

KEY TERMS

acquired immune deficiency syndrome (AIDS) HIV infection along with a CD4 cell count of 200 or less (or less than 14%), dementia, wasting syndrome, cancers such as Kaposi's sarcoma or non-Hodgkin's lymphoma, or one of 20 other opportunistic conditions

acute HIV infection the 4- to 7-week period of rapid viral replication immediately after exposure to the virus, characterized by fever, malaise, and other flulike symptoms

AIDS enteropathy changes in the small and large bowel thought to be attributable to direct HIV infection with no other identifiable pathogen; manifested as chronic diarrhea and possibly malabsorption

antiretroviral therapy (ART) combination of medications used to kill or suppress viral replication and progression of HIV disease; also called highly active antiretroviral therapy (HAART)

CD4+ cells T-helper lymphocyte cells

constitutional disease affecting the whole functioning make-up of the body, such as with HIV infection: persistent fever, night sweats, chronic or intermittent fatigue, malaise, or diarrhea of unknown etiology

cytomegalovirus (CMV) group of herpes viruses with special affinity for salivary glands; manifesting as mononucleosis-like symptoms

dysesthesia a painful and persistent sensation induced by gentle touch of the skin

HIV-associated nephropathy a syndrome of progressive renal failure with HIV infection

HIV encephalopathy (AIDS dementia) degenerative disease of the brain caused by HIV infection

HIV wasting syndrome catabolic condition with loss of weight and lean body and fat mass

human immunodeficiency virus (HIV) the retrovirus isolated and recognized as the etiologic agent of AIDS

Kaposi's sarcoma a malignant neoplastic vascular proliferation characterized by the development of bluish-red cutaneous nodules, usually on the surface of the skin or in the oral cavity

lipodystrophy a disturbance in the way the body produces, uses, and distributes fat

myalgia diffuse muscle pain, usually accompanied by vague feelings of discomfort or weakness

opportunistic infection infection by an organism that causes disease in someone with an impaired immune response

protease inhibitors antiviral drugs that inhibit the viral protease enzyme and prevent viral replication

retrovirus a virus such as HIV that replicates using an enzyme (reverse transcriptase) to copy RNA into DNA when RNA is its natural genetic state; most cells have DNA in their natural state and transcribe to RNA during replication

viral load testing measurement of the quantity of HIV RNA (free virus) in the blood, expressed as copies per milliliter of blood plasma, by polymerase chain reaction or bDNA tests; undetectable is optimal

The relationship between immunity and nutrition is well established. The nutrition management of HIV/AIDS draws from established and emerging nutritional science as it is applied and tested in the context of HIV disease. The nutrition provider must become familiar with evolving understanding of HIV: its disease pathophysiology, complications and treatments; medications and interactions; populations affected; and common comorbidities such as insulin resistance, lipid dysregulation, bone, liver and kidney diseases, substance abuse, and eating disorders.

The medical management of HIV disease is directed by robust research and frequently updated national guidelines available via the Internet. Although HIV nutrition does not have comparable research and guidelines, some resources are available. Further, it is "necessary for the patient to be entered into a continuum of medical care and services, including social, psychosocial, and nutritional services" (Panel on Clinical Practices for the Treatment of HIV, 2007). Prevention and treatment are different in economically disadvantaged countries.

PATHOPHYSIOLOGY, ETIOLOGY, AND CLASSIFICATION

The **acquired immune deficiency syndrome (AIDS)** was first described by the Centers for Disease Control and Prevention (CDC) in 1981 (Fee and Brown, 2006). Previously healthy young men were reported to have unusual **opportu-**nistic infections (OIs) associated with severe depression of cellular immunity: *Pneumocystis jirovecii* pneumonia, cytomegalovirus (CMV), candidiasis, or rare Kaposi's sarcoma. These cases presented a previously unknown disorder. In 1983 researchers isolated the etiologic **retrovirus** and named it **human immunodeficiency virus (HIV).** The oldest known case of HIV was confirmed using a 1959 blood sample of a man living in what was then called the Belgian Congo (Zhu et al., 1998). A 2006 report identified the origin of HIV in southeast Cameroon, where wild chimpanzees were found to have viruses most like the HIV found in humans globally (Keele et al., 2006).

Primary infection with HIV is the underlying cause of AIDS. HIV invades the genetic core of the **CD4+** cells, also called *T-helper lymphocyte cells*, which are the principal agents involved in protection against infection (Figure 38-1). The CD4+ cell count in blood is the common laboratory test used. The virus also resides in other distinct compartments, such as semen, vaginal secretions, the lymph system, and the central nervous system (CNS), and evolves independently. HIV infection causes a progressive depletion of CD4+ cells, which eventually leads to immunodeficiency, **constitutional disease** (persistent fever, night sweats, chronic fatigue, malaise, and diarrhea), neurologic complications, OIs, and neoplasms (Box 38-1).

While HIV viral load is a major determinant, HIV progression depends on complex interactions between viral and genetic host factors and differs among individuals. Better understanding of host responses is resulting in new therapeutic approaches for early treatment, immune modulation,

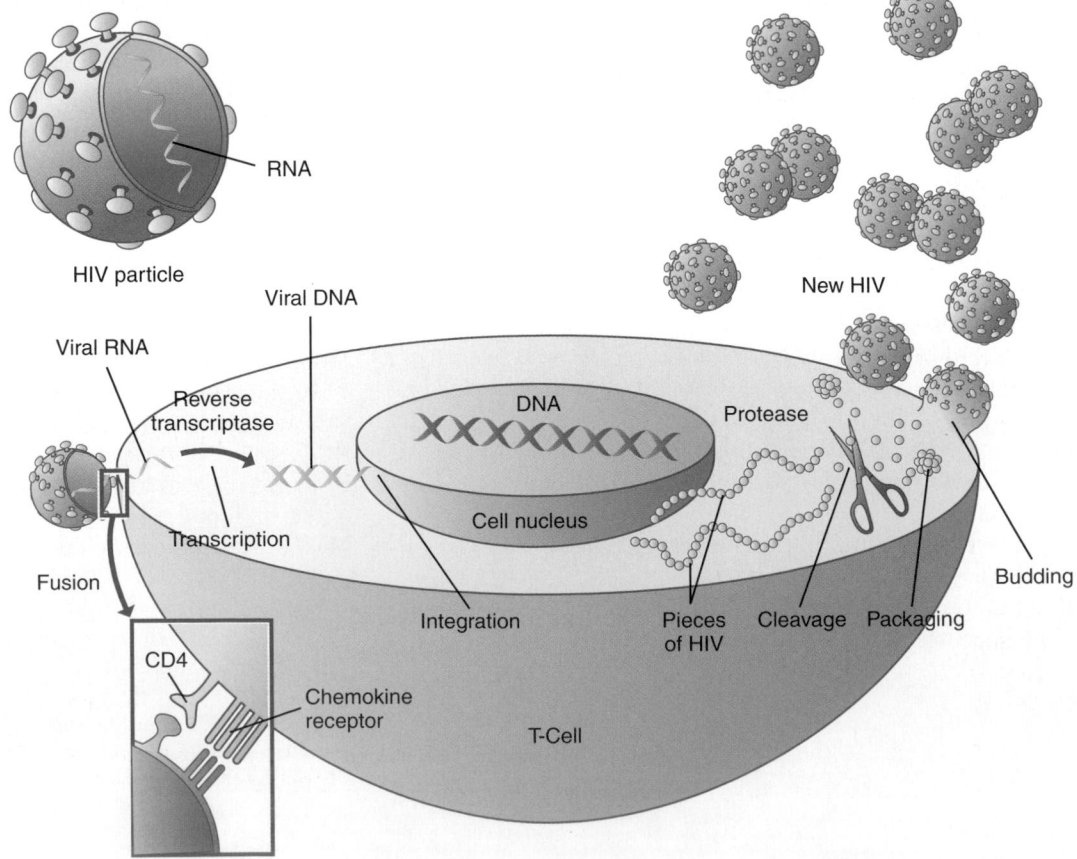

FIGURE 38-1 HIV life cycle. *(Copyright Community Research Initiative on AIDS, New York, 1998. Courtesy AIDS Community Research Initiative of America [ACRIA], New York.)*

BOX 38-1

Classification System for HIV Infection and Expanded AIDS Surveillance Case Definition for Adolescents and Adults

Clinical Categories

The clinical categories are defined as follows:

Category A—one or more of the conditions listed here occurring in an adolescent or adult with documented human immunodeficiency virus (HIV) infection. Conditions listed in categories B and C must not have occurred.

- Asymptomatic HIV infection
- Persistent generalized lymphadenopathy
- Acute (primary) HIV infection with accompanying illness or a history of acute HIV infection

Category B—symptomatic conditions occurring in an HIV-infected adolescent or adult that are not included among conditions listed in clinical category C and that meet at least one of the following criteria:

1. The conditions are attributed to HIV infection and/or indicate a defect in cell-mediated immunity.
2. The conditions are considered by physicians to have a clinical course or management that is complicated by HIV infection.

Examples of conditions in clinical category B include but are not limited to the following:

- Bacterial endocarditis, meningitis, pneumonia, or sepsis
- Candidiasis (vulvovaginal) that is persistent (1 month duration) or is poorly responsive to therapy
- Candidiasis, oropharyngeal (thrush)
- Cervical dysplasia, severe, or carcinoma
- Constitutional symptoms such as fever ($\geq$38.5° C) or diarrhea lasting >1 month
- Hairy leukoplakia, oral
- Herpes zoster (shingles), involving at least two distinct episodes or more than one dermatome
- Idiopathic thrombocytopenic purpura
- Listeriosis
- *Mycobacterium tuberculosis* infection, pulmonary
- Nocardiosis
- Pelvic inflammatory disease
- Peripheral neuropathy

Category C—any condition listed in 1987 surveillance case definitions for acquired immune deficiency syndrome (AIDS) and affecting an adolescent or adult. The conditions in clinical category C are strongly associated with severe immunodeficiency, occur frequently in HIV-infected individuals, and cause serious morbidity or mortality. Among the conditions listed in the 1993 AIDS surveillance case definition (assuming HIV positivity) are the following:

- Candidiasis of bronchi, trachea, or lungs
- Candidiasis, esophageal
- CD4 lymphocyte counts <200 or a CD4 percent of total lymphocytes <14 if the absolute count is not available
- Cervical cancer, invasive
- Coccidioidomycosis, disseminated or extrapulmonary (Valley fever)
- Cryptococcosis, extrapulmonary
- Cryptosporidiosis, chronic intestinal (>1 month duration)
- Cytomegalovirus disease (other than liver, spleen, or nodes)
- Cytomegalovirus retinitis (with loss of vision)
- HIV encephalopathy
- Herpes simplex: chronic ulcer(s) (>1 month duration) or bronchitis, pneumonitis, or esophagitis
- Histoplasmosis, disseminated or extrapulmonary
- Isosporiasis, chronic intestinal (>1 month duration)
- Kaposi's sarcoma
- Lymphoma, Burkitt's (or equivalent term)
- Lymphoma, immunoblastic (or equivalent term)
- Lymphoma, primary in brain
- *M. avium* complex or *M. kansasii*, disseminated or extrapulmonary
- *M. tuberculosis*, any site, pulmonary or extrapulmonary
- *Mycobacterium*, other species or unidentified species, disseminated or extrapulmonary
- *Pneumocystis jirovecii* pneumonia
- Pneumonia, recurrent
- Progressive multifocal leukoencephalopathy
- *Salmonella* septicemia, recurrent
- Toxoplasmosis of brain
- Wasting syndrome secondary to HIV

CD4+ T-Lymphocyte Categories	Asymptomatic, Acute (Primary) HIV	B Symptomatic, not (A) and not (C)	AIDS Indicator
Category 1: $\geq$500 cells/μl	A1	B1	C1
Category 2: 200-499 cells/μL	A2	B2	C2
Category 3: <200 cells/μL	A3	B3	C3

From Centers for Disease Control and Prevention: 1993 Revised classification system for HIV infection and expanded surveillance case definition for AIDS among adolescents and adults, *MMWR* 41:17, 1992, from www.cdc.gov/mmwr/preview/mmwrhtml/00018871.htm.

structured treatment interruptions, and new chemotherapeutic agents and vaccine development.

HIV can be transmitted via blood, semen, presemenal fluid, vaginal fluid, breast milk, and other body fluids that contain blood. Cerebrospinal fluid surrounding the brain and spinal cord, synovial fluid surrounding bone joints, and amniotic fluid surrounding a fetus are other fluids that can transmit HIV. Saliva, tears, and urine do not contain enough HIV for transmission. The most common way HIV is transmitted is via blood and semen during unprotected anal or vaginal intercourse with an HIV-infected person. Risk of transmission through oral sex is considered low but not risk-free (CDC, 2001c). Individuals with a sexually transmitted disease (STD) who are sexually exposed to HIV increase their chance of infection by two to five times. STD/HIV co-infected individuals are more likely to transmit HIV sexually than those without an STD.

Transmission can also occur by sharing contaminated needles and injecting contaminated blood products. Transferring HIV from an infected mother to her baby before or during birth or through breast-feeding is a major global concern. All persons working with body fluids should use universal precautions to protect both themselves and others. The virus is not transmitted by casual contact such as touching, hugging, or kissing or through using the same plates, silverware, or drinking glasses.

HIV-1 and HIV-2 are types of HIV and are transmitted the same way. Most people have HIV-1; unless specified, it is the type discussed. HIV-2, first isolated in West Africa, is less easily transmitted, and the time between infection and illness takes longer. HIV-1 mutates readily and has become

distributed unevenly throughout the world in different strains, subtypes, and groups.

EPIDEMIOLOGY AND TRENDS

The United States

The HIV/AIDS surveillance system of CDC works with state and local health departments, collects information to track the HIV epidemic, and directs funding for prevention. States and U.S. territories were federally mandated to implement confidential name-based reporting of AIDS cases to the CDC. However, AIDS data do not reflect the number of people living with HIV, nor do they reflect accurate trends of the infection.

Since 2000 confidential name-based HIV reporting was implemented in 35 areas (Figure 38-2). Even with more precise data collection, the picture is still limited (Figure 38-3). In October 2006 the record of HIV name-based cases became a determinant for federal HIV/AIDS funding allocated to states and cities, and areas without this system changed (CDC, 2006a; AVERT, 2006a). Health providers must seek information to stay aware of epidemiologic trends and ramifications by monitoring CDC, state, and local surveillance reports at websites listed in CDC Surveillance Reports.

HIV/AIDS is found in all sections of the United States population, which reached 300 million people in 2006. The CDC estimated that by the end of 2004 almost 1.2 million people in the United States were living with HIV/AIDS, of which one fourth were undiagnosed. Diagnosis of AIDS

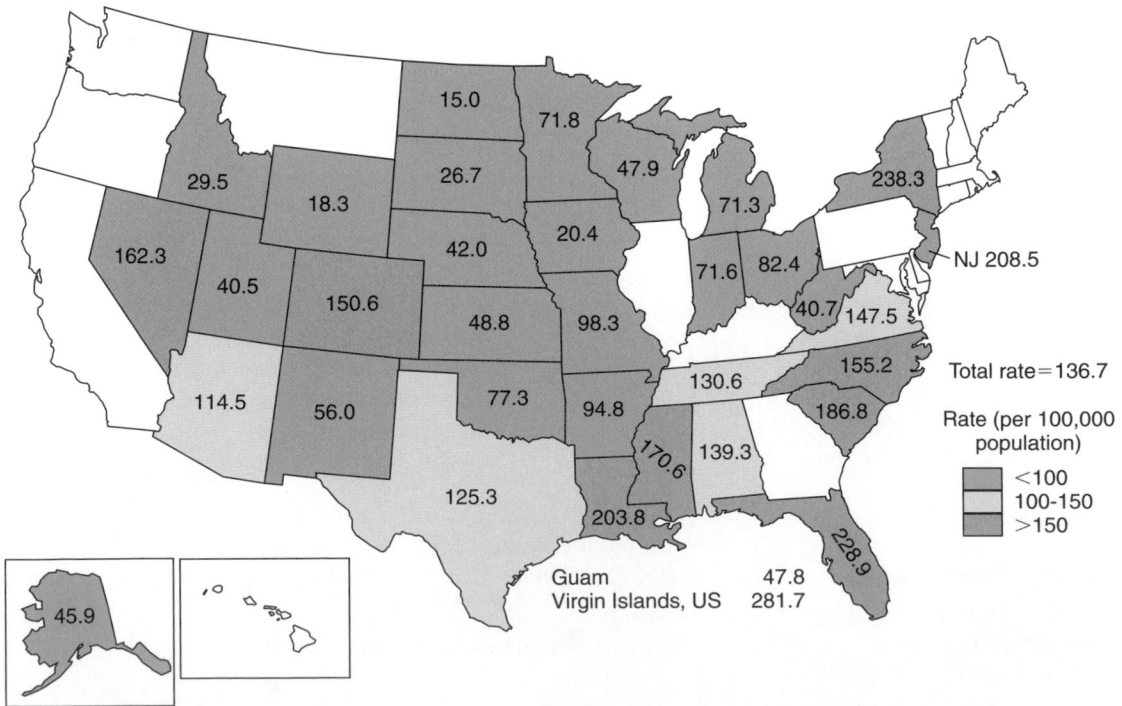

FIGURE 38-2 Estimated prevalence rates for adults and adolescents living with HIV infection (not AIDS), 2004—35 areas. *(From CDC: HIV/AIDS surveillance—general epidemiology [through 2004] http://www.cdc.gov/hiv/topics/surveillance/resources/slides/general/index.htm.)*

continues, with most cases in the age-group of 40 to 44 years. Compared to the U.S. population distribution, blacks and Latinos remain disproportionately affected (CDC, 2004; CDC, 2006b).

The largest of newly infected behavior risk groups in the United States are those with male-to-male sexual contact (42%), followed by those with heterosexual contact (31%), and injection drug use (22%) (CDC, 2006b). Half of all new HIV infections are in people ages 13 to 24 years. For women AIDS diagnosis increased to total 27% of all new AIDS cases. Blood-handling management has significantly decreased rates of HIV infection for hemophiliacs and other blood transfusion recipients.

The rate of AIDS diagnosis for black women is 25 times that of white women and four times that of Hispanic women (CDC, 2004). Women are still not diagnosed early and have limited access to quality health care and treatments. Numbers of people living with AIDS in the United States by region in 2004 were highest in the South, followed by the Northeast. The South also has the greatest proportion of AIDS cases in rural areas (CDC, 2006a). Mother-to-child transmission of HIV infections in the United States continues to decline; reductions can be attributed to prenatal HIV counseling and testing and use of perinatal antiretroviral drug therapy.

People 50 years and older now represent more than 10% of the total number of AIDS cases reported, becoming a larger percentage. Postmenopausal women, often uninformed about intravenous transmission, may have sexually active partners who use condoms less often or not at all. The physiology of older women increases the risk of transmis-

sion because the vaginal walls are thin, with easy access for the virus (CDC, 2006a; Gebo, 2004).

High-risk groups are marginalized by society. Users of crystal methamphetamine are three times more likely to get HIV than nonusers (San Francisco Department of Health, 2005). Men of all ethnicities may have male-to-male sexual contact, are not identified as homosexual or bisexual, and may also have male-to-female sexual contact. The male-to-female transgender group has an extremely high rate of HIV infection (Eliminating Disparities Working Group, 2004).

Homelessness and mental illness are growing problems, compounded with higher rates of HIV infection. State and federal correctional facilities also have high rates of confirmed AIDS (Kantor, 2003), especially among incarcerated women (De Groot, 2000).

Leading causes of death among people with HIV disease are infection, cancer, cardiac disease, trauma, and liver disease (Crum et al., 2006). Almost 16,000 deaths were reported in 2004. By 2006 cumulative deaths in the United States from AIDS exceeded 530,000, with 5515 of those being children. Black and American Indian/Alaska Native children have the fewest months of survival after an AIDS diagnosis (CDC, 2006). Deaths of adults and adolescents with AIDS in the United States have declined dramatically with increased use of antiretroviral therapy (ART) and treatment of OIs.

The largest source of public health funding for HIV/AIDS care in the United States is through Medicaid, followed by Medicare and then the Ryan White Comprehensive AIDS Resources Emergency (CARE) Act funding (Kaiser Family Foundation, 2006). HIV medical nutrition therapy services are now mandated through the Ryan White

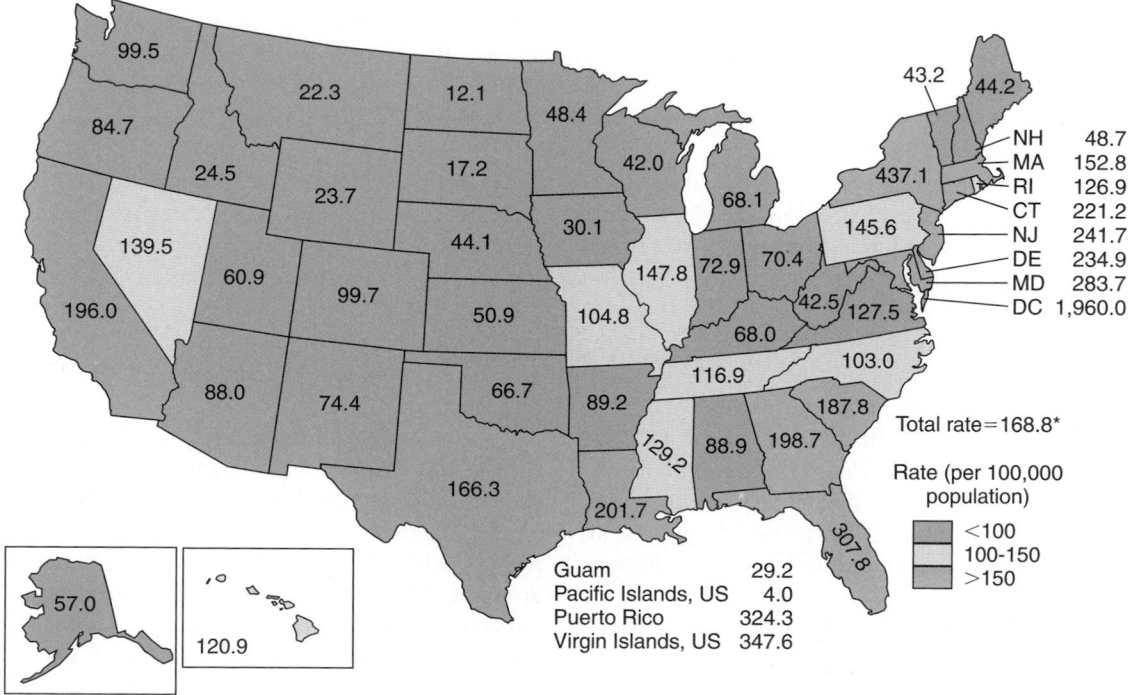

FIGURE 38-3 Estimated prevalence rates for adults and adolescents living with AIDS (per 100,000 population) 2004—United States. *(From CDC: AIDS surveillance—general epidemiology [through 2004] www.cdc.gov/hiv/topics/surveillance/resources/slides/epidemiology/index.htm.)*

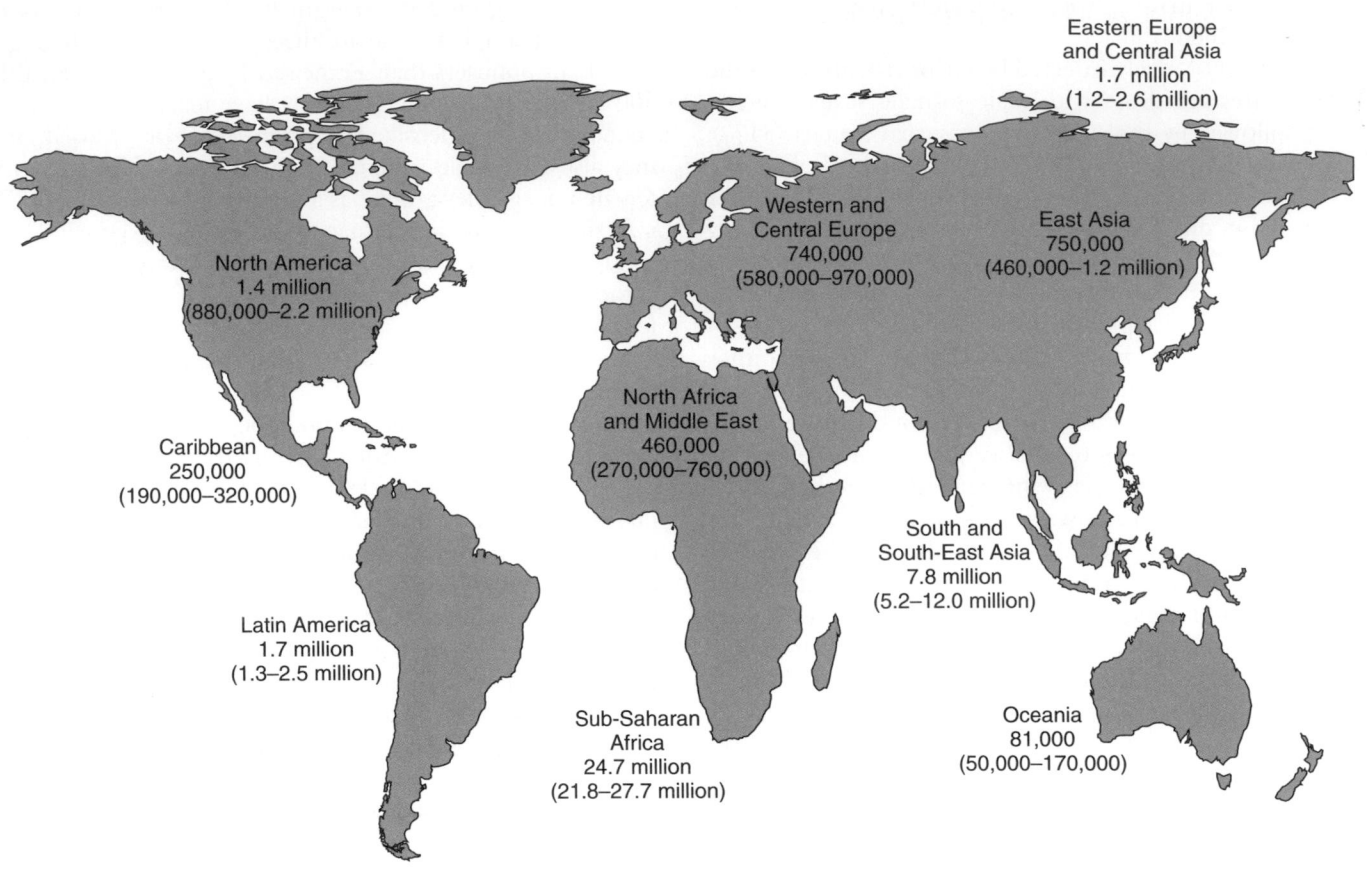

Adults and children estimated to be living with HIV in 2006

Eastern Europe
and Central Asia
1.7 million
(1.2–2.6 million)

Western and
Central Europe
740,000
(580,000–970,000)

East Asia
750,000
(460,000–1.2 million)

North America
1.4 million
(880,000–2.2 million)

North Africa
and Middle East
460,000
(270,000–760,000)

Caribbean
250,000
(190,000–320,000)

South and
South-East Asia
7.8 million
(5.2–12.0 million)

Latin America
1.7 million
(1.3–2.5 million)

Oceania
81,000
(50,000–170,000)

Sub-Saharan
Africa
24.7 million
(21.8–27.7 million)

Total: 39.5 million (34.1–47.1 million)

FIGURE 38-4 Worldwide presence of HIV: number of adults and children estimated to be living with HIV in 2006. *(From Joint United Nations Programme on HIV/AIDSAIDS Epidemic Update, Geneva, Switzerland, 2006, http://data.unaids.org/pub/EpiReport/2006/12-Maps_2006_EpiUpdate_eng.pdf. Reproduced with permission of UNAIDS, 2006.)*

Act. This mandate is encouraging because improving nutrition status is essential. Primary care programs through Title III CARE Act funding must provide nutrition services on site or at another facility, and the provider has to be a registered dietitian (RD) (HRSA, 2002).

Worldwide

The enormous disparity of HIV infection, access to health care, and AIDS-related deaths throughout the world became visible at the thirteenth World AIDS Conference in Durban, South Africa, in 2000. Ninety-five percent of the world's cases of HIV, including those caused by perinatal HIV transmission, are in the developing nations (see Figure 38-4) (AVERT, 2006b).

Over three million died from AIDS-related causes in 2005, and more than 25 million people have died of AIDS since 1981 (UNAIDS/WHO, 2005). High death rates in many countries cause decreased life expectancy, along with a reduction in the work force, a decrease in national incomes, slowed economic growth, and decreased economic potential. Globally the overall number of new HIV infections and the number of people living with HIV continues to increase. Steepest increases have occurred in Eastern Europe, Central Asia, and East Asia. Access to food, potable water, effective drugs, housing, and economic stability remains a concern.

STAGES OF HIV INFECTION

After exposure and transmission of HIV into the host, HIV spreads throughout the body, and blood CD4+ cell counts fall dramatically. An immune response can return CD4+ cells to almost normal, reduce virus in the blood, and establish equilibrium with HIV replication. Major reservoirs of infection are the CNS and the gastrointestinal tract. A period of apparent clinical latency follows for an average of 8 to 10 years until active HIV virus replication decreases CD4+ cells and increases risks of OIs (Table 38-1) and AIDS.

Untreated, HIV replicates billions of virion particles a day. The disease has four stages: (1) acute HIV infection; (2) asymptomatic chronic HIV infection; (3) symptomatic HIV infection; and (4) AIDS or advanced HIV (see *Pathophysiology*

TABLE 38-1

CD4 Cell Counts and Associated Conditions

CD4 Cell Count	Condition	Common Physical Problems and Symptoms
>550/mm³	Acute retroviral syndrome	May include fever, adenopathy, pharyngitis, rash, myalgias, diarrhea, headache, nausea and vomiting, hepatosplenomegaly, weight loss, thrush, neurologic symptoms
	Candidal vaginitis	Fungal infection causing itching and swelling of the vulva, thick white-yellow or cheesy discharge, and burning on urination
	Persistent generalized lymphadenopathy	Chronic, diffuse, noncancerous lymph node enlargement
	Guillain-Barré syndrome	The most common form of sudden generalized paralysis
	Myopathy	Progressive muscle weakness
	Aseptic meningitis	An inflammation of the meninges (membranes surrounding the brain or spinal cord), which may be caused by a bacterium, fungus, or virus
200-500/mm³	Oropharyngeal candidiasis (thrush)	Loss of appetite, white plaques, mouth discomfort, change in taste
	Kaposi's sarcoma	Slightly raised purplish lesions on the skin, mucous membranes, or lymph nodes; usually painless
	Pulmonary tuberculosis reactivation	Cough, blood-stained sputum (hemoptysis); fever; night sweats; weight loss; chest pain; prolonged fatigue; anorexia
	Herpes zoster (shingles) virus	Vesicular skin lesions along dermatomes, pain
	Cryptosporidiosis, self-limited	Watery diarrhea lasting 1 to 4 days or as long as 4 weeks
	Oral hairy leukoplakia	Whitish lesions that appear on the side of the tongue and cheeks with a "hairy" surface
	Pneumococcal and other bacterial pneumonia/bacterial sinusitis	Inflammation of the nasal cavity and sinuses, congestion, fever, pain, tearing of the eyes and sensitivity to light
	Herpes simplex (virus)	Weeping skin lesions (oral, perirectal), bleeding, rectal discharge, pain
	Cervical intraepithelial neoplasia	Dysplasia of the cervix epithelium, often premalignant, characterized by abnormal keratinization and condylomata
	Cervical cancer	Watery, blood-tinged vaginal discharge more often seen after sexual intercourse
	B-cell lymphoma	The type of lymphoma most commonly associated with HIV in which certain cells of the lymphatic system grow abnormally
	Anemia	A lower than normal number of red cells; fatigue
	Mononeuronal multiplex	A rare type of neuropathy that may be related to the cytomegalovirus
	Idiopathic thrombocytopenic purpura	A condition in which the body produces antibodies against the platelets in the blood
	Hodgkin's lymphoma	See B-cell lymphoma
	Lymphocytic interstitial pneumonitis	A type of pneumonia that affects 35%-40% of children with AIDS and causes a hardening of the lung membranes involved in absorbing oxygen
100-200/mm³	*Pneumocystis jirovecii* pneumonia (fungi)	Fever, chills, night sweats, cough with or without sputum production, shortness of breath, antibiotic side effects, weight loss, weakness
	Disseminated histoplasmosis and coccidioidomycosis	Fever, weight loss, skin lesions, difficulty breathing, anemia, lymphadenopathy, possibly pneumonia
	Miliary/extrapulmonary tuberculosis	Refers to the tiny discrete granulomatous lesions in lungs and other organs that result when bloodborne tubercle bacilli seeds many tissues
	Progressive multifocal leukoencephalopathy	Progressive weakness and dementia, speech problems, forgetfulness, perceptual problems, visual problems, incontinence
	Wasting	Loss of weight and body cell mass
	Peripheral neuropathy	Painful, burning feet or numbness in the feet and/or hands

Modified from Martin J et al: *AIDS home care and hospice manual*, ed 2, San Francisco, 1990, Visiting Nurses and Hospice of San Francisco; Phair JP, Murphy R: *Contemporary diagnosis and management of HIV/AIDS infections*, Newton, Pa, 1997, Health Care Co; Bartlett JG, Gallant JE: *Medical management of HIV infection*, 2001-2002 edition, Baltimore, Md, 2002, Johns Hopkins University, Division of Infectious Diseases.

Continued

TABLE 38-1		
CD4 Cell Counts and Associated Conditions—cont'd		
CD4 Cell Count	**Condition**	**Common Physical Problems and Symptoms**
100-200/mm³ —cont'd	HIV-associated dementia	Loss of coordination, mood swings, loss of inhibitions, widespread cognitive dysfunctions
	Cardiomyopathy	Disease of the myocardium associated with ventricular dysfunction
	Vascular myelopathy	Disease of the spinal cord
	Progressive polyradiculopathy	Radiating pain and paresthesias that cause mild sensory loss and lower extremity areflexia
	Non-Hodgkin's lymphoma	Depends on location, lumps, fatigue, and/or pain
50-100/mm³	Microsporidiosis	An intestinal infection from a parasite (microsporidia) that causes diarrhea and wasting in persons with HIV
	Candidal esophagitis	A *Candida* infection of the esophagus that can cause severe problems with swallowing
	Disseminated herpes simplex	A virus that causes cold sores on the mouth and around the eyes or can be transmitted to the genitals
	Cryptococcus (meningitis)	Headache and fevers, malaise, nausea, fatigue, loss of appetite
	Primary tuberculosis	Cough, blood-stained sputum (hemoptysis), fever, night sweats, weight loss, chest pain, prolonged fatigue, anorexia
	Cryptosporidiosis, chronic (protozoa)	Severe chronic, watery diarrhea (up to 15-20/day), severe weight loss, weakness, electrolyte imbalance, abdominal cramping, fever, nausea, vomiting, enlarged lymph nodes
	Toxoplasmosis (protozoa)	Fevers, swollen glands, headaches
0-50/mm³	Disseminated (cytomegalovirus)	Blindness or visual loss (retinitis), fever, fatigue and severe malaise, weight loss, facial edema (secondary to adrenalitis), enteritis, colitis
	Disseminated *Mycobacterium avium* complex	Fever, severe weight loss/cachexia, abdominal pain, diarrhea, malabsorption, antibiotic side effects
	Central nervous system lymphoma	A lymphoma limited to the cranial-spinal axis without systemic disease

and Care Management Algorithm: Human Immunodeficiency Virus Disease). Immunologic categories have been defined for adults (see Box 38-1) and children (Table 38-2).

Acute HIV infection occurs 2 to 4 weeks after infection and is a period of rapid viral replication. Forty percent to 90% of newly infected develop flulike symptoms: fever, maculopapular rash, oral ulcers, arthralgia, loss of appetite and weight loss, malaise, inflamed lymph nodes, pharyngitis, and **myalgia** (diffuse muscle pain). Lasting a few days to 4 weeks, diagnosis of HIV is often missed. The development of HIV antibodies is called *seroconversion* and may occur from 1 week to several months or more after the initial HIV infection. Once antibodies to HIV appear in the blood, individuals with and without symptoms will test positive for HIV. Viral load is extremely high, and individuals are extremely infectious at this time (see Box 38-1, Category A).

Asymptomatic HIV is the next stage in which few, if any, noticeable symptoms occur, lasting from a few months to as long as 10 years. However, subclinical changes may include a decrease in lean body mass without apparent total body weight change, vitamin B$_{12}$ deficiency, and increased susceptibility to foodborne and waterborne pathogens.

Symptomatic HIV occurs when symptoms appear (see Box 38-1, Category B). These non-AIDS defining symptoms may include fever, sweats, skin problems, or fatigue. A decline in nutrient status or body composition may also occur.

AIDS, or advanced HIV disease, is the diagnostic term reserved for persons with at least one well-defined, life-threatening clinical condition that is clearly linked to HIV-induced immunosuppression (see AIDS-defining conditions, Box 38-1, Category C).

A very small number of persons infected with HIV exhibit no signs of disease progression even after 12 or more years. Reasons for long-term nonprogression may include infection by a less virulent strain of the virus, protective genetic mutations, or particular protective characteristics of the host's immune system or genes. Study of long-term nonprogressors is ongoing in the hope of developing vaccines.

MEDICAL MANAGEMENT

Disease progression differs among individuals, and treatment decisions must be individualized. With the advent of **viral load testing** (measurement of the quantity of HIV deoxyribonu-

TABLE 38-2

Immunologic Categories for HIV-Infected Children Based on Age-Specific CD4+ T-Lymphocyte Counts and Percentage of Total Lymphocytes

Immunologic Category	Cell Counts (Cells/mcg [%]*) According to Age		
	<12 Months	1-5 Years	6-12 Years
No evidence of suppression	≥1500 (≥25)	≥1000 (≥25)	≥500 (≥25)
Evidence of moderate suppression	750-1499 (15-24)	500-999 (15-24)	200-499 (15-24)
Severe suppression	<750 (<15)	<500 (<15)	<200 (<15)

Modified from Centers for Disease Control and Prevention: 1997 USPHS/IDSA guidelines for the prevention of opportunistic infection in persons infected with human immunodeficiency virus, *MMWR* 46 (RR-12):27, 1997.

*Percentage of total lymphocytes.

TABLE 38-3

Indications for the Initiation of Antiretroviral Therapy in the Chronically HIV-1–Infected Patient

Clinical Category	CD4 + T Cell Count	Plasma HIV RNA	Recommendation
Symptomatic (AIDS, severe symptoms)	Any value	Any value	Treat
Asymptomatic, AIDS	CD + T cells <200 mm³	Any value	Treat
Asymptomatic	CD4 + T cells 201-350 mm³	Any value	Treatment should be offered
Asymptomatic	CD4 + T cells >350/mm³	>100,000 copies/ml	Some clinicians would recommend initiating therapy; most experienced clinicians defer therapy and monitor the CD4 + T cell count and level of plasma HIV RNA more frequently
Asymptomatic	CD4 + T cells >350/mm³	<100,000 copies/ml	Therapy should be deferred

Modified from Guidelines for the Use of Antiretroviral Agents in HIV-1-Infected Adults and Adolescents: *DHHS Panel on Antiretroviral Guidelines for Adults and Adolescents—a Working Group of the Office of AIDS Research Advisory Council (OARAC)*, October 10, 2006.

http://aidsinfo.nih.gov/ContentFiles/AdultandAdolescentGL.pdf, accessed April 9, 2007.

cleic acid [DNA] [free virus] in the blood, stated as copies per milliliter) and combination ART, clinical and therapeutic management of HIV disease in adults is based on numerous considerations (Table 38-3). Practitioners must use the latest evidence-based guidelines and research findings.

The overall goals of medical management of HIV are to reduce HIV-related morbidity and mortality, improve the quality of life, restore and preserve immunologic function, and maximize suppression of viral replication. To optimize and extend the usefulness of currently available therapies and minimize drug toxicity and manage side effects are important goals in both medical and nutritional management.

Antiretroviral therapy (ART) consists of a combination of at least two fully active antiretroviral agents known to kill the virus or suppress its replication. Antiretroviral medications are increasingly formulated with two single agents in one pill. The use of only one antiretroviral drug does not suppress viral activity and should not be used. Considerations in the choosing of ART and when to begin it include:

1. Viral load levels (HIV-ribonucleic acid [RNA]), which predict the risk of HIV disease progression
2. Current and lowest CD4+ cell counts for the extent of HIV-induced immune damage
3. Current and past clinical conditions and symptoms of HIV disease
4. Life stage: children, adolescents, and pregnant women warrant special considerations

PATHOPHYSIOLOGY AND CARE MANAGEMENT ALGORITHM

Human Immunodeficiency Virus Disease

ETIOLOGY

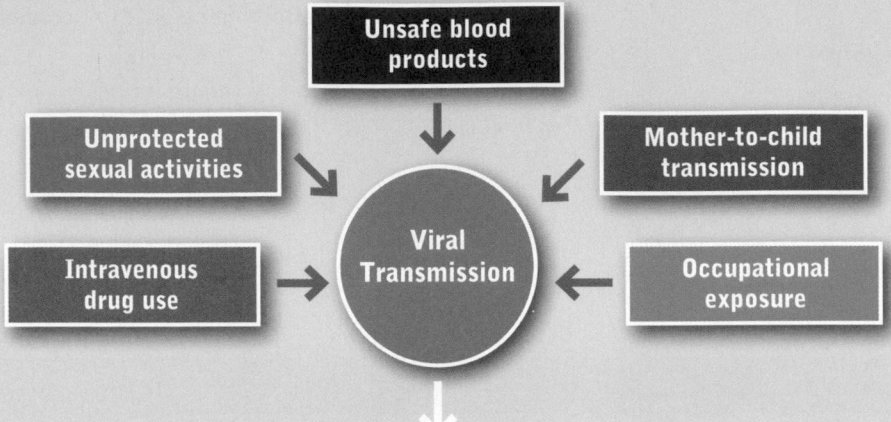

PATHOPHYSIOLOGY

Clinical Findings

Acute HIV infection (Acute retroviral syndrome) Fever, fatigue, rash, headache, generalized lympadenopathy, pharyngitis, myalgia, nausea/vomiting, diarrhea, night sweats, adenopathy, oral ulcers, genital ulcers, neurological symptoms, malaise, anorexia, weight loss, wasting syndrome

Seroconversion

HIV Positive Test HIV rapid tests; ELISA test, Western blot; PCR test

Asymptomatic HIV infection Abnormal metabolism, change of body composition (body cell mass loss with/without weight loss, lipoatrophy, lipohypertrophy), vitamin B_{12} deficiency, susceptibility to pathogens

Symptomatic HIV infection Weight loss, thrush, fever, loss of LBM with/without weight loss, diarrhea, oral hairy leukoplakia, herpes zoster, peripheral neuropathy, idiopathic thrombocytopenic purpura, pelvic inflammatory disease

Asymptomatic AIDS

Symptomatic AIDS (AIDS defined conditions) CD4 cell count <200/mm³, opportunistic infectious diseases (pneumocystitis jirovecii, pneumonia, others), Kaposi's sarcoma, lymphoma, HIV associated dementia, HIV associated wasting, vitamins/minerals deficiencies

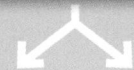

MANAGEMENT

Medical Management

Possible co-morbidities
Hyperglycemia, hyperlipidemia, hypertension, body composition changes, pancreatitis, kidney and liver diseases, hypothyroidism, hypogonadism, osteopenia, ↓ CD4 count, ↑ viral load, mental dysfunctions, others

Monitoring
Fasting blood lipid, fasting glucose/insulin level, protein status, blood pressure, TSH/testosterone level, CD4 cell count, and viral load

Medication
Antiretroviral therapy, lipid lowering agents, antidiabetic agents, antihypertensive agents, appetite stimulants, hormone replacement therapy, treatment for coinfectious diseases (i.e. hepatitis), prophylaxis and treatment for opportunistic infectious diseases

Nutrition Assessment (2-6+ times a year)

Anthropometric measurements: Height, weight, % of goal weight, IBW and UBW, BMI, fat, muscle and body cell mass, waist, hip, neck and thigh circumferences

Biochemical: Protein status (albumin, prealbumin), blood lipid profile, glucose/insulin status, blood pressure, hgb, hct, MCV, and liver function tests, electrolytes, bone mineral density

Clinical conditions: Oral/intestinal condition, nausea, vomiting, diarrhea, anorexia, appetite, functional capability, neuropathy

Dietary intake: Estimated intake and estimated need; food and nutrition security, dietary pattern/preferences, food intolerance/allergies

MANAGEMENT—CONT'D

Nutrition Management

- Emphasize importance of early/ongoing nutritional intervention
- Adequate intake of nutrients and fluids
- Emphasize importance of food and water safety and sanitation
- Regular exercise and physical activity
- Psycho-social economic barriers to food
- Additional food resources to meet needs
- Dietary multiple vitamin and mineral supplements
- Inform patient of possible side effects, symptoms and/or complications
- Monitor/manage metabolic abnormalities
- Small frequent, nutrient-dense meals; foods made should be mashed or ground
- Appetite stimulants if necessary
- Peripheral or total parental nutrition if necessary
- Anabolic therapies

Modified from Hayakawa M. and Fenton M., Los Angeles County Department of Public Health, Office of AIDS Programs and Policy, December 2006.

Management by the HIV primary care and nutrition care providers must consider factors such as viral resistance, medication adherence, medication tolerance, comorbidities, and costs of care. The largest decreases in the incidence of OIs have been seen in pneumonia, wasting syndrome, Kaposi's sarcoma, *Mycobacterium avium* complex, CMV retinitis, and cryptosporidiosis (Michaels et al., 1998). In the United States with the introduction of ART, the number of AIDS deaths has dropped dramatically. There are now 27 antiretroviral agents approved by the Food and Drug Administration (FDA).

Viral resistance impairs the activity of drugs. Without an adequate blood level of active drugs, HIV mutates rapidly, causing resistance to those drugs. High-level resistance to one medication can result in resistance to others of the same type. Increasingly people with new HIV infections have resistance to at least one class of medications (Kuritzkes et al., 2003).

At least 95% adherence to medication schedules is necessary for medications to work correctly (Carpenter et al., 2000), especially to minimize the amount of virus in the body and to minimize viral mutations. Late, missed, or harmful food-drug interactions increase suboptimal dosing, viral breakthrough, and the development of drug-resistant strains of HIV (Table 38-4). Barriers to medication adherence are: being busy, forgetting, being away from home, change in routines, depression, taking a "drug holiday," running out of medications, having too many medications to take, being worried about becoming immune to medications, side effects, not wanting others to notice (Gifford et al., 2000).

Not all patients tolerate antiretroviral drugs. Life-threatening reactions include hepatic necrosis, Stevens-Johnson syndrome, lactic acidosis, and hypersensitivity. Serious reactions include pancreatitis, Fanconi syndrome (nephrotoxicity), renal calculi, marrow suppression, and transaminasemia. Milder reactions include gastrointestinal intolerance, peripheral neuropathy, rash, insulin resistance, hyperlipidemia, and fat atrophy or hypertrophy (Bartlett, 2006).

Minor irritating adverse effects often diminish after the first few weeks of beginning medications. Common side effects are fever and night sweats, diarrhea, nausea, anorexia, **dysesthesia** (pain on skin being touched), severe headache, weight loss, vaginal symptoms, sinusitis, eye trouble, cough, shortness of breath, thrush, and oral pain.

Costs to treat HIV can be range from $14,000 to $34,000 annually per person, with sicker patients having the greater costs because of medications required to treat OIs and hospitalizations (Saag, 2002). Medications are not available to every patient; some state AIDS Drug Assistance Plans and private insurance policies do not cover all FDA-approved HIV-related medications. Many patients struggle to find financial resources.

OPPORTUNISTIC INFECTIONS, COMPLICATIONS, AND MALNUTRITION

OIs with bacteria, fungi, protozoa, or viruses that only cause disease in the immunocompromised are common in this population. They may cause diarrhea, malabsorption, fever, and weight loss, as well as many other symptoms. Common infections, their relationships to CD4+ counts, and their manifestations are summarized in Table 38-1.

Cancers

Kaposi's sarcoma (KS), non-Hodgkin's lymphomas, and cervical cancer are AIDS defining for someone with HIV (Box 38-1, category C). Although rates for these conditions have fallen with ART, rates for other malignancies have

Text continues on p. 1006.

TABLE 38-4

HIV Antiretroviral Medications and Nutritional Complications

Medication: Brand (generics and other names)	A	D	C	N	V	F	H	Food Effects and Recommendations	Other Considerations, Adverse Effects, and Notes (not all-inclusive)
Nucleoside Analogue Reverse Transcriptase Inhibitors (NRTIs)									
Combivir (lamivudine/zidovudine)	X			X		X	X	If possible, take on empty stomach; low-fat meal can reduce side effects;; avoid alcohol	See individual drugs (Retrovir and Epivir)
Emtriva (emtricitabine)		X		X		X	X	Take with or without food	Monitor patients with renal disease; may cause abnormal dreams, tingling in hands and feet, and lactic acidosis (www. emtriva.com)
Epivir (3TC, lamivudine)	X	X		X	X	X	X	Food may reduce gastrointestinal side effects; avoid alcohol	Malaise
Epzicom (abacavir sulfate and lamivudine)				X		X		Can be taken with or without food	See individual drugs (Ziagen and Epivir)
Hivid (ddC, zalcitabine)	X	X	X	X	X	X	X	Taken with food decreases complications by 14% (not clinically significant); avoid alcohol	Peripheral neuropathy, oral and esophageal ulcers, pancreatitis; avoid taking with antacids containing magnesium or aluminum
Retrovir (zidovudine, AZT, azidothymidine)		X		X	X	X	X	If possible, take on empty stomach; low-fat meal can reduce side effects; avoid alcohol	Dysphoria; bone marrow suppression (anemia, neutropenia); rash; peak plasma with food is decreased
Trizivir (fixed dose combination of Ziagen, Retrovir, and Epivir)				X	X	X	X	If possible, take on empty stomach; low-fat meal can reduce side effects; avoid alcohol	Rash (may be part of hypersensitivity reaction—*do not rechallenge*); see individual drugs (Ziagen, Retrovir, and Epivir)
Videx, Videx EC (didanosine, ddI, dideoxyinosine)	X	X	X	X	X	X	X	Take on empty stomach at least 30-60 min before or 2 hr after a meal; take with water; avoid alcohol	Peripheral neuropathy; pancreatitis; abnormal liver function tests; avoid antacids that contain magnesium or aluminum; chewable/dispersible, buffered tablets (or pediatric powder for oral formulation) thoroughly chewed, manually crushed, or dispersed in water (stable for 1 hour) before swallowing
Zerit (stavudine, d4T)	X	X	X	X	X	X	X	Food has little effect on absorption; avoid alcohol	Peripheral neuropathy; central nervous system (CNS) changes (agitation, dysphoria); pancreatitis

Drug	Possible complications	Nutritional considerations	Possible complication
Ziagen (abacavir)	X X X	Avoid alcohol; can be taken with or without food	Rash (may be part of hypersensitivity reaction—*do not rechallenge*)
Non-Nucleoside Analogue Reverse Transcriptase Inhibitors (NNRTIs)			
Rescriptor (delavirdine mesylate, DLV)	X X X X	Can be taken without regard to food; avoid alcohol; avoid taking with antacids; do not take St. John's wort	Rash; antacids that contain aluminum and magnesium and ddI reduce absorption and should be taken at least 1 hr after DLV
Sustiva (efavirenz)	X X	Low-fat meals improve tolerability; avoid high-fat meal (increases bioavailability and CNS effects); do not take if pregnant; do not take St. John's wort; alcohol may increase CNS side effects	Rash; CNS changes (vivid dreams, dizziness, euphoria, dysphoria, hallucinations); take in the evening to minimize CNS effects
Viramune (nevirapine)	X	Can be taken without regard to food; avoid alcohol; do not take St. John's wort	Rash
Nucleotide Analogue Reverse Transcriptase Inhibitors (NtRTIs)			In general: lactic acidosis and severe hepatomegaly with steatosis, including fatal cases, have been reported with the use of nucleoside analogues alone or in combination with other antiretrovirals
Viread (tenofovir disoproxil fumarate)	X X	Should be taken with special meal of 700-1000 kcal and 40%-50% fat to enhance drug bioavailability	Asthenia, abdominal pain, flatulence, and—for a few—anorexia; contains lactose; drug is not a substrate of the CYP450 enzymes
Fusion Inhibitor			
Fuzeon (enfuvirtide, T-20, ENF)	X X X		May cause pain at injection sites, dizziness, numbness in feet and hands, insomnia, pancreas problems
Protease Inhibitors (PIs)			PIs in general: lipodystrophy syndrome: fat maldistribution (increased fat in waist, neck, breasts; decrease in extremities, buttocks, face); elevated cholesterol and/or triglycerides; insulin resistance (or frank diabetes mellitus); abnormal liver function tests (increased enzymes: SGOT [AST] and SGPT [ALT], alkaline phosphatase, bilirubin, GGT); bone density, hair and nail changes; substrates of the CYP450 enzymes in varying degrees

Modified from Fenton M: *HIV antiretroviral medications and nutritional complications*, Los Angeles, 2001, AIDS Project Los Angeles. For more information on these and new medications, refer to most current version of Panel on Clinical Practices for the Treatment of HIV: guidelines for the use of antiretroviral agents in HIV-infected adults and adolescents, *MMWR* 1998 47(RR-5), updated July 2003, www.aidsinfo.nih.gov.

X, Possible complication; A, appetite loss; D, diarrhea; C, constipation; N, nausea; V, vomiting; F, fatigue; H, headache; AUC, area under the curve.

Continued

TABLE 38-4

HIV Antiretroviral Medications and Nutritional Complications—cont'd

Medication: Brand (generics and other names)	A	D	C	N	V	F	H	Food Effects and Recommendations	Other Considerations, Adverse Effects, and Notes (not all-inclusive)
Protease Inhibitors (PIs)—cont'd									
Agenerase (amprenavir)	X			X	X	X	X	Take with or without food; if taken with food, no more than 67 g of fat, which decreases absorption; do not take St. John's wort	Rash; tingling around the mouth (paresthesia); avoid extra vitamin E above a general multiple vitamin; each 150-mg capsule contains 109 units vitamin E; each milliliter of solution contains 46 units; high doses of vitamin E may exacerbate blood coagulation defects of vitamin K deficiency caused by anticoagulation therapy or malabsorption; grapefruit juice may be a concern; increase fluid intake; do not take antacids within 1 hr of taking medication; oral solution contains a propylene glycol excipient and is contraindicated in infants and children under 4 yr, pregnant women, patients with hepatic or renal failure, and patients receiving disulfiram or metronidazole
Aptivus (tipranavir TPV)				X	X	X	X	Must be used with low dose Norvir; take with food	Stomach pain; associated with hepatitis and liver damage; pregnancy category C drug
Crixivan (indinqvir sulfate)	X	X		X	X	X	X	Take on empty stomach at least 1 hr before or 2 hr after a meal; wait 2 hr after last meal/snack; take drug and wait 1 hr to eat again; may take with light meals that total no more than 2 g of fat, 5.6 g of protein, 65 g of carbohydrates, and fewer than 300 calories; must drink approximately 48 oz extra water daily; avoid grapefruit juice; do not take St. John's wort	Must be taken every 8 hr and requires careful meal/snack coordination; in combination with Ritonavir, it significantly increases blood levels of Indinavir, eliminating the need to fast; kidney stones; abdominal, back or flank pain; elevated serum bilirubin (jaundice); dizziness; dry skin; rash; take 1 hr before or after ddI (buffer in ddI impairs absorption)
Fortovase (saquinavir mesylate, no longer marketed)	X			X	X	X	X	Take with or up to 2 hr after a full (high-fat) meal to increase AUC 670%; avoid alcohol; do not take St. John's wort	Store capsules in the refrigerator

Drug	Possible complications	Take with food	Comments
Invirase (saquinavir mesylate)	X X	Take within 5 min or up to 2 hr after a full (high-fat) meal to increase absorption; grapefruit juice increases absorption; avoid alcohol; do not take St. John's wort	Another formulation is under development to be taken with Ritonavir
Kaletra (lopinavir/ritonavir)		Take with food to increase absorption; do not take St. John's wort	Store capsules in the refrigerator
Lexiva (Fosamprenavir Calcium, FPV)	X X X	Take with or without food; do not take St. John's Wort, garlic pills, or milk thistle	Less side effects than Agenerase; usually boosted by taking with Norvir
Norvir (ritonavir-ABT-538)	X X	Take with food to increase absorption; do not take St. John's wort	Oral and peripheral paresthesia; hyperesthesia; vasodilation; store capsules in the refrigerator; mix oral solution with chocolate milk or supplements or intensely flavored food to mask taste
Prezista (darunavir, DRV)	X	Must be boosted by taking with low-dose Norvir; should be taken with a meal or a snack	Sulfa containing drug; many drug interactions
Reyataz (atazanavir sulfate E)	X	Take with food and 1 hr away from antacids; do not take St. John's wort	Can cause high levels of bilirubin and jaundice, which dissipate after stopping medication; can cause tingling in hands and feet, abdominal pain, and depression (www.reyataz.com)
Viracept (nelfinavir mesylate, NFV)	X X	Food increases absorption 2 to 3 times more than fasted state and reduces gastrointestinal side effects; bioavailability was better with test meal of 500 kcal, 11.3 g of fat, 20.5 g of protein, 99.2 g of carbohydrates, than test meal of 125 kcal, 3.1 g of fat, 10 g of protein, 14.6 g of carbohydrates (Peterson et al., 2003); lactase enzyme or lactose-free dairy products may reduce diarrhea; avoid acidic food or liquid; do not take St. John's wort	Rash, flatulence, abdominal pain, asthenia
Multi-Class Combination			
Atripla (efavirenz, emtricitabine, and tenofovir disoproxil fumarate)	X	Taken once a day without food, preferably at bedtime	See individual drugs (Sustiva, Viread, and Emtriva)

X, Possible complication; A, appetite loss; D, diarrhea; C, constipation; N, nausea; V, vomiting; F, fatigue; H, headache; AUC, area under the curve.

risen among those who are older, who have had HIV longer, and who have a history of an OI.

Kaposi's sarcoma, associated with human herpesvirus 8 (HHV-8), affects people with AIDS 20,000 times more frequently than the general population and 300 times more than those with other immune disorders. KS manifests as purple nodules on the skin, mucous membranes, or lymph nodes or throughout the gastrointestinal tract. KS lesions in the oral cavity or esophagus may cause pain and difficulty with chewing and swallowing, and lesions in the intestinal tract have been implicated in diarrhea and intestinal obstruction. Antibacterial mouthwashes are used to prevent fungal infections. Localized KS lesions can be treated with surgery or radiation therapy, and chemotherapy is used for disseminated KS.

Lymphomas may involve the small bowel and can cause malabsorption, diarrhea, or intestinal obstruction. Primary lymphomas in the brain can cause alterations in personality and motor and cognitive abilities. Persons with HIV are at increased risk of developing Hodgkin's disease, and persons with AIDS have a risk 100 times greater than that in the general population to develop AIDS-related lymphoma.

Neuromuscular Diseases

Immediately following infection, HIV enters the brain and may result in **HIV encephalopathy (AIDS dementia),** myelopathy, peripheral neuropathy, and myopathy. Secondary neurologic complications may result from *Toxoplasma* encephalitis, progressive multifocal leukoencephalopathy, CMV encephalitis, radiculomyelitis, cryptococcal meningitis, primary CNS lymphoma, and neurosyphilis.

Symptoms of AIDS dementia may include deterioration in cognition (concentration, recall, new memory development, language), motor function (coordination, gait, bladder control), and behavior (psychosis, depression, withdrawal). The abnormal presence of one or more of these factors may be necessary for AIDS dementia to be identified: cytokines, calcium-mediated toxicity, excitatory amino acids (glutamate, quinolinic acid), arachidonic acid, oxidative mechanisms, platelet-activating factor, or apoptosis (programmed cell death). Viral load in the brain and the level of neurologic decline are not strongly correlated.

Myelopathy (disease of the spinal cord) may occur in as many as 25% of those with advanced HIV disease and can result in partial paralysis of the lower extremities (paraparesis). Myelopathy affects motor and sensory functions and is manifested by spasticity and, in some, weakness in the legs and bladder. Approximately 20% of patients with AIDS experience peripheral neuropathy with sensory loss, pain, weakness, and wasting of muscle in the hands or legs and feet. Peripheral neuropathy may be caused by the virus or by drugs (zalcitabine, didanosine, and stavudine).

HIV-Liver Disease

Hepatitis C (HVC) is now considered an HIV opportunistic infection, and liver disease is the predominant cause of death for people with HIV/AIDS. Those with both HIV and HVC have a faster progression to AIDS and death. Liver function may be compromised through the use of HIV ART and by infection with **cytomegalovirus (CMV),** herpes viruses with an affinity for salivary glands; cryptosporidium; hepatitis B; hepatic malignant diseases, such as KS or lymphoma. Dosing of drugs must be adjusted for those with liver failure. The FDA has approved α-interferon with ribavirin for treatment. When ribavirin is not tolerated, α-interferon alone is also FDA approved and used.

Tuberculosis and Lung Diseases

There has been a drop in deaths caused by tuberculosis (TB). Although most cases of TB caused by *M. tuberculosis* affect the lungs, the disease may also occur, especially in HIV-infected persons, in extrapulmonary sites such as in the larynx, lymph nodes, brain, kidneys, or bones. Medical conditions that increase the risk of TB infection include HIV infection; a body weight that is 10% or more below ideal weight; immunosuppressive therapy; and hematologic disorders such as leukemia and lymphomas.

M. tuberculosis and HIV co-infection may cause immune activation and a rapid increase in the rate of HIV replication. Early and aggressive treatment of TB and HIV is critical to controlling the progression of both diseases. Dietary recommendations include liberal amounts of protein and calories; sufficient, but not excessive, calcium and vitamin D; iron; supplemental vitamin B_6 and vitamin A since carotene is poorly converted; adequate fluids unless contraindicated; and adjustments of TB medications because of nutrient-drug interactions (see Appendix 31 and Chapter 35).

HIV-Associated Nephropathy

A syndrome of progressive renal failure, or **HIV-associated nephropathy,** may occur. Proteinuria may also result from repeated infections, volume depletion, or nephrotoxic drugs. Deaths from kidney disease have increased, and the number of dialysis centers serving HIV-infected patients has also increased. Dosing of drugs and nutrition therapy must be adjusted for those with renal failure (see Chapter 36).

Gastrointestinal and Pancreatic Issues

The gastrointestinal tract and the pancreas may also be affected. *M. avium* complex, greatly decreased in incidence since the use of powerful HIV medications, can be seen in the lymph nodes, liver, bone marrow, blood, and urine of patients with AIDS. Chronic diarrhea may persist in the absence of identifiable enteric pathogens as a result of what is known as **AIDS enteropathy.** Persons with HIV enteropathy may have villous atrophy and abnormal results on tests of small bowel function. Because of the vulnerability of persons with immune suppression to foodborne and waterborne pathogens, food and water safety is a concern (see *Focus On:* Reducing Infections).

Other Effects

CMV can affect the eye, causing retinitis; and if left untreated it may progress to blindness (Drew et al., 2003).

Reducing Infections

The CDC has emphasized the need to consider blood and other body fluids from all persons to be potentially infective (CDC, 2001a). In the hospital setting, nursing and nutrition service employees should follow their institution's appropriate universal precaution policies and procedures to prevent the transmission of HIV. Hospital personnel need not wear gowns, masks, or gloves while performing general patient care unless respiratory or strict isolation is indicated.

Persons with HIV and their caregivers should be instructed in food and water safety practices at home and for eating out or traveling abroad. Tips from the Centers for Disease Control to reduce the risk of cryptosporidiosis include careful hand washing; avoiding sex that involves contact with stool; avoiding touching of farm animals or the stool from pets; carefully washing and cooking of foods; exercising caution when swimming in pools, hot tubs, or lakes; drinking only safe water; and exercising caution with food and water while traveling.

WOMEN AND HIV

Prenatal Considerations

Risk of mother-to-child transmission of HIV infection is 15% to 25% when not breast-feeding. Perinatal use of ART sharply reduces HIV transmission from mother to baby. Zidovudine therapy can reduce perinatal HIV transmission by half. One dose of nevirapine given during labor and to the neonate within the first 72 hours also decreases transmission of HIV by almost half; this treatment is now widely used. Current guidelines call for standard ART to be offered to HIV-infected pregnant women. Guidelines also recommend counseling before conception for optimal nutrition status because malnutrition increases the risk of postcesarean complications and postpartum morbidity, which are especially prevalent in HIV-infected women (Public Health Service Task Force, 2006).

Poor nutrition status increases the risk of perinatal HIV transmission. A randomized, placebo-controlled study found that multiple vitamins (B, C, and E) without vitamin A reduced transmission of HIV at birth, whereas added vitamin A or vitamin A alone increased the risk of transmission (Dreyfuss and Fawzi, 2002; French et al., 2002). Nutrient deficiencies can result from the increased nutritional demands for fetal growth and development. HIV further increases these demands, especially in developing countries where deficiencies of vitamin A, folate, iron, and zinc are common.

Breast-Feeding

Breast-feeding increases the risk of mother-to-child transmission to 20% to 45%, yet exclusive breast-feeding is attributed to saving six million lives a year (O'Brien, 2005). Breast-feeding recommendations for developed and "resource-poor" settings are different. In the United States HIV-positive mothers are recommended to not breast-feed their infants (Public Health Services Task Force, 2006). Heating milk or using Pretoria Pasteurization or flash heating may be options for some mothers.

Among the challenges to resource-poor settings are unclean water, clinical and subclinical mastitis, and inadequate access to formula (Papathakis, 2006). Breast-feeding may be the better option for these women. As many as 1.45 million lives are lost as a result of suboptimal breast-feeding in developing countries; World Health Organization recommendations are to provide daily sulfonamide prophylaxis for HIV-infected pregnant or breast-feeding women (Lauer et al., 2006; Forna et al., 2006).

Other Considerations

Women should be counseled on real-life strategies and referrals to improve their health and nutrition status, living situation, access to food and income, and practical solutions. Some women access an RD through the Women, Infant, and Children (WIC) Program. When HIV status is not disclosed, the opportunity to receive appropriate HIV medical nutrition therapy is lost. Other barriers for HIV-positive women that prevent access to care include low socioeconomic situations, multiple children for whom they care and whose needs are placed before their own, lack of child care or transportation, isolation, and fear of disclosure. Moreover, women may have been or are currently at subsistence level and may eat a less than nutritionally adequate diet. Women may seek ways to lose weight quickly such as starvation or fad dieting to decrease weight and fat mass and may have no regular exercise regimen.

Women have lower viral loads than men but lose CD4+ cells and develop AIDS just as quickly (Sterling et al., 2001). Drug metabolism and excretion are different in women than in men; women experience more drug-related gastrointestinal symptoms and more weight gain.

PEDIATRIC CONSIDERATIONS

Children born to mothers with HIV are often born with weight and height below the 50th percentile, and HIV-infected children do not catch up. An earlier and more pronounced deficit in height for age is noted, especially by

15 months of age (Saavedra et al., 1995). Growth failure and neurodevelopmental deterioration may be manifestations of pediatric HIV disease.

Pediatric guidelines recognize that monitoring growth and development is essential and nutrition support is an intervention that affects immune function, quality of life, and bioactivity of antiretroviral drugs. Growth failure, a persistent decline in weight-gain velocity despite adequate nutrition support and without other explanation, is a reason to consider changing ART. Change in CD4+ percentage, not number, may be a better marker of identifying disease progression in children (Guidelines for the Use of Antiretroviral Agents in Pediatric HIV Infection, 2005). Every child with infection should be assessed within 3 months of diagnosis and every 1 to 6 months thereafter relative to age, problems, and nutrition status (Heller, 2000).

Current guidelines acknowledge that management of the complex and diverse needs of HIV-infected infants, children, adolescents, and their families requires a multidisciplinary team of physicians, nurses, social workers, psychologists, registered dietitians, outreach workers, and pharmacists. The health care professional's role may be direct or may involve referral to an appropriate agency or individual. When working with the HIV-infected child, one must consider the total family unit, including social and financial issues, cultural issues, and caregiver support. Adherence to medication schedules may involve setting meal and medication times or including particular foods in specific sequences.

Clinical trials of antiretroviral drugs often have not included children; as a result, 11 of the 15 antiretroviral drugs approved for adults and adolescents are used for children, although they are not labeled for this population. Current pediatric guidelines detail drug dosing for neonatal, pediatric, and adolescent patients and detail toxicities, interactions, and special instructions, including food and nutrition concerns. Some drugs are in liquid form for dosing according to weight and for easier administration. Tube feeding, more prevalent in this population, is sometimes initiated to administer crucial medications.

RELATIONSHIP BETWEEN MALNUTRITION AND AIDS

Weight Loss, Wasting, and Metabolic Disorders

Malnutrition is an important and complicated consequence of HIV infection. Problems leading to malnutrition may involve ingestion, absorption, digestion, metabolism, and use of nutrients. Without successful ART, protein-energy malnutrition (PEM) is a frequent complication of advanced HIV disease.

HIV wasting syndrome, a constitutional disease, is an AIDS-defining condition. The CDC definition is profound involuntary weight loss of greater than 10% of baseline body weight plus either chronic diarrhea or weakness and

documented fever longer than 30 days in the absence of a concurrent illness (CDC, 1992). Before widespread use of potent ART, HIV wasting syndrome was common. CDC no longer reports the incidence of wasting. However, wasting still occurs. Involuntary weight loss of 10% to 15% in AIDS is common, and as little as a 5% weight loss has been associated with a significantly increased risk of opportunistic infections and death (Wheeler et al., 1998). Weight loss, lean body mass depletion, decreased skin-fold thickness and midarm circumference, decreased iron-binding capacity, decreased serum potassium and intracellular water, and hypoalbuminemia are still reported.

Weight is the easiest measurement to obtain, and the provider must measure weight accurately and routinely, keep a weight chart in the medical record, and monitor changes to identify the following wasting and weight concerns: weight less than 90% ideal body weight or body mass index less than 18.5; weight loss more than 10% from weight before illness; or weight loss more than 5% in the previous 6 months.

Weight loss and wasting are multifactorial, related to lack of adequate intake, malabsorption, metabolic irregularities, uncontrolled opportunistic infection, or lack of physical activity. Decreased oral intake is very common and can result from anorexia secondary to medications; depression; infection; symptoms such as nausea, vomiting, diarrhea, dyspnea, or fatigue; or neurologic disease. Analysis of intake of participants in the Nutrition for Healthy Living Study found attitudinal, economic, and lifestyle factors played a large part, including lack of compensation; increased dietary requirements as illness progressed; food insecurity and hunger; absence of a caregiver; and drug use (Mangili et al., 2006).

Low oral intake can also be attributable to disorders of the mouth and esophagus, such as candidiasis (thrush), oral herpes, aphthous ulcers, or CMV. Malabsorption—often suspected in the event of loose stools, diarrhea, or vomiting—can be caused by medications; HIV infection; opportunistic infections such as CMV or cryptosporidiosis; or a developed intolerance to lactose, fat, or even gluten. At the same time, fevers and infection may increase energy and protein needs.

HIV-induced metabolic changes and host responses are poorly understood. Reports from the NHLS found a 1.9 kg lower weight for each 100-cell/mm³ decrease in CD4 cell count and that each log10 increase in HIV RNA viral load is associated with a 0.92-kg decrease in weight (Mangili et al., 2006). Women have been found to lose more body fat than lean body mass during both the early and advanced stages of wasting, whereas men lose greater amounts of lean body mass while sparing body fat.

The malnutrition associated with HIV infection and AIDS has characteristics similar to other infectious processes and some that are unique to HIV. Nutrition status is a major factor in survival, and, in the absence of disease, starvation usually leads to death when the victim reaches two thirds of ideal body weight for height. Persons with AIDS, men more than women, tend to lose body cell mass with less loss of fat, in contrast to uncomplicated starvation in which fat stores are depleted. As with HIV wasting syndrome, host resistance to infection causes changes in metabolism, as mediated by cytokines. The search for host mediators of metabolic disturbances initially resulted in the cachectin hypothesis, related to tumor necrosis factor (see Chapter 37). Other theories have also been evaluated.

Immune changes associated with AIDS are similar to those seen in PEM. Both conditions are marked by multiple opportunistic infections of viral, bacterial, parasitic, and fungal origin. KS and B-cell lymphomas have been reported in individuals in Central and East Africa, where PEM is common. Malnutrition may contribute to the frequency and severity of infection seen in AIDS by compromising immune function. Deficiencies of protein; calories; copper; zinc; selenium; iron; essential fatty acids; pyridoxine; folate; and vitamins A, C, and E all interfere with immune function. Severe weight loss can also result in organ damage, which may increase the risk of death from infections.

Direct and indirect mechanisms are responsible for the impact of nutrition on HIV. Directly, nutritional factors are required for specific immune-cell triggering, interaction, and expression. Clinical trials with supplementation of specific nutrients at different stages of HIV disease are needed. Indirectly, nutritional factors are essential for DNA and protein synthesis and for the physiologic integrity of cell tissues and organ systems, including lymphoid tissues.

Simply, maintaining and restoring weight and lean body mass requires (1) eliminating or mitigating the deleterious effects of the infectious agent; (2) providing ample caloric and nutrient intake; and (3) having sufficient exercise. Nutrition counseling is a necessary component in the treatment of HIV-associated wasting (Fisher 2001; New York State Department of Health AIDS Institute, 2001). Adequate resistance exercise is important to ensure gain in lean body mass (Roubenoff and Wilson, 2001).

Decreases in testosterone levels have been associated with lower libido and loss of bone density. Testosterone exists in serum both free and bound to albumin and to sex hormone–binding globulin. HIV-infected men and women should be routinely monitored for serum levels of both free and total testosterone and treated for testosterone deficiency. Testosterone is obtainable in injected, patch, gel, and oral synthetic forms.

Megestrol acetate (Megace), dronabinol (Marinol), and—experimentally—medical marijuana are appetite stimulants considered to combat HIV anorexia. Megestrol acetate, the more powerful appetite stimulant, reduces testosterone levels and increases body fat. Dronabinol, a derivative of marijuana, produces undesired CNS side effects. Weight gains from these agents are primarily but not entirely in the fat compartment (Mulligan et al., 2001). Although exercise is necessary to increase lean body mass, clinicians seek better appetite stimulants.

Prescriptive drug treatments used to prevent and help restore weight and body cell mass loss have become available. Other drug treatments that may be considered for use in wasting and preservation of lean body mass are anabolic agents to promote positive nitrogen balance and cytokine inhibitors to slow protein breakdown. Anabolic agents include nandrolone, oxandrolone, stanozolol, oxymetholone, nandrolone decanoate, and recombinant human growth hormone. Cytokine inhibitors include thalidomide, cyproheptadine, ketotifen, pentoxifylline, fish oil, and N-acetylcysteine.

Use of anabolic steroids is still controversial because of the increased risk for hepatotoxicity. Also, they require adequate caloric intake and progressive resistance exercise to maintain and maximize increases in lean body mass. One study found progressive resistance training with nutrition intervention (counseling and nutrition supplementation) more cost effective than oxandrolone (Shevitz et al., 2005).

Recombinant human growth hormone, a lipolytic agent, promotes lean body mass at the expense of fat stores, and adequate energy intake is necessary. Side effects vary and include mood changes, skin problems, hair growth, menstrual irregularities, changes in libido and potency, fluid retention, abnormal liver enzymes, altered blood glucose, and even diabetes.

Lipodystrophy and Metabolic Abnormalities

The use of HIV medications often results in a generalized **lipodystrophy** (abnormalities in fat metabolism with body shape changes and glucose dysregulation and dyslipidemia), bone disorders, mitochondrial toxicity, and lactatemia. Morphologic changes include lipoatrophy (loss of subcutaneous adipose tissue), resulting in thinning of the arms and legs, buttocks, and face (maxillary, nasolabial, and temporal areas).

The nucleoside reverse transcriptases inhibitors stavudine and zidovudine have been implicated in the cause of lipoatrophy, and patients have been delayed from starting or switched from ART containing those drugs. Other morphologic changes include accumulation of visceral adipose tissue (Figure 38-5), mammary adipose tissue, and adipose tissue in axillary regions; lipomas; and enlargement of the dorsocervical fat pad (buffalo hump). Prominent veins from loss of subcutaneous fat and ingrown toenails have also been reported. Peripheral and central lipoatrophy occur more in HIV-positive than in HIV-negative persons and can be detected by magnetic resonance imaging (MRI) but not noticed by the individual for some time (Bacchetti et al., 2005).

Metabolic alterations include low serum testosterone concentrations in both women and men and elevations in serum triglyceride, insulin, glucose, and blood pressure (Kotler, 2005). Resting energy expenditure (REE) may be increased with lipodystrophy and insulin resistance (Kosmiski et al., 2001). Insulin resistance has become a major problem (see Chapters 9, 30, and 32). Antiretrovirals, some more than others, have had a direct effect on insulin resistance (i.e., raising cholesterol, LDL, and triglyceride levels and lowering HDL level) (see Chapter 32).

ART treatment increases cardiovascular disease and diabetes. Use of fish oil alone or taken with fenofibrate sharply decreases triglyceride levels (Mascolini, 2006). Diet, exercise, and weight reduction if needed are fundamental to treatment of lipid and glucose dysregulation (see Chapter 30).

Factors for changes in bone metabolism may include low body mass, wasting, poor nutrition, previous corticosteroid use, or hormonal deficiencies. Potent ART seems to further

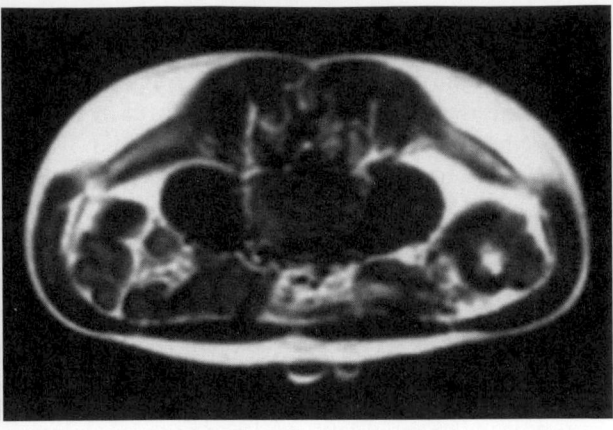

FIGURE 38-5 A, Abdominal magnetic resonance image (MRI) of an HIV-infected man with visceral adiposity syndrome. **B,** Abdominal MRI of a non–HIV-infected man similar in race, age, height, weight, and total adiposity. *(From Engelson et al: Fat distribution in HIV-infected patients reporting truncal enlargement quantified by whole-body magnetic resonance imaging,* Am J Clin Nutr *69(6):1162, 1999. Reproduced with permission by the American Journal of Clinical Nutrition. Copyright American Journal of Clinical Nutrition, Society for Clinical Nutrition.)*

increase new bone formation and bone destruction, with greater bone turnover and loss of bone mineral density. Early studies suggest that HIV-positive subjects who take **protease inhibitors** for a while and those with lipodystrophy syndrome may develop bone loss, osteopenia, and osteoporosis (Duran et al., 2001; Moyle, 2001). Suggestions include improved diet, use of calcium and vitamin D dietary supplements, exercise, and use of biphosphonates such as alendronate or risedronate (Mondy and Tebas, 2003) (see Chapter 24).

Avascular necrosis (asceptic necrosis or osteonecrosis) occurs at greater rates in the HIV-infected than in the non-infected person. Whether HIV is an independent risk factor is unknown. A suggested reason for the increased rate is the occurrence of the following risk factors in this population: hyperlipidemia, alcohol abuse, pancreatitis, corticosteroid use, and hypercoaguability (Scribner et al., 2000).

MEDICAL NUTRITION THERAPY

Nutrient deficiencies play important roles in the pathogenesis of HIV disease. Medical nutrition therapy with individualized counseling is critical in overall treatment. The goals of nutrition intervention are as follows:

1. Maintain and expand nutrition knowledge and sense of empowerment.
2. Maintain or restore healthy body weight and normal morphology.
3. Preserve or restore optimal somatic and visceral protein status.
4. Prevent nutrient deficiencies or excesses known to compromise immune function.
5. Treat or minimize HIV or medication-related complications that interfere with either intake or absorption of nutrients.

6. Correct metabolic abnormalities.
7. Support adherence to medications to achieve optimal therapeutic drug levels.
8. Prolong and optimize quality of life.

When adequately provided, timely HIV nutrition therapy should decrease health care costs. In the context of the unique HIV disease complications, the RD or nutrition practitioner should apply basic nutrition fundamentals in assessment and interventions.

Screening

All persons with HIV infection should be screened for nutrition-related problems by their primary care provider at the time of their first contact and on an ongoing basis. The presence of nutrition-related symptoms should trigger a referral for medical nutrition therapy by an RD. Figure 38-6 lists nutrition screening criteria for adults; Box 38-2 provides nutrition referral criteria specific to children.

Assessment

A comprehensive nutrition assessment should be performed. Factors include HIV infection–associated symptoms, dietary patterns, use of nontraditional therapies, and the impact of these treatments on the person (see Chapter 14). The diet should be evaluated for nutrient adequacy, especially for nutrients involved with immune function, and for a possible history of erratic and inadequate intakes. Individuals who follow nontraditional diet therapies should be made aware of any potentially harmful effects. Psychosocial conditions (fear, anxiety, depression, and social isolation) all affect appetite and nutrient intake. Illness or ostracism often leads to a lack of employment and subsequent loss of social contacts, as well as income and medical insurance.

Weight, percent of usual weight, percent of goal body weight, and percent of ideal body weight are helpful markers. Monitoring changes in anthropometric measurements over time is feasible because patients have multiple clinic visits. Useful measurements in addition to height and weight include waist, hip and neck circumferences, and measurements of either lean body mass (using triceps skin-fold and midarm muscle circumference) or body cell mass (using bioelectric impedance analysis or other techniques). These calculations can be compared with each other and with published reference data (see Chapter 14).

Laboratory values are useful when compared over time (see Chapter 15). Total lymphocyte count and delayed hypersensitivity skin testing should not be used since these immune values are impaired in this population. Values to monitor include fasting lipids, fasting blood sugar and insulin, serum albumin and C-reactive protein, serum alkaline phosphatase, and liver function tests. Evaluation of drug therapy is essential since many side effects complicate nutrition status (see Table 38-4 and Appendix 31).

Nutrition Diagnosis

The RD should carefully select the **p**roblem, its **e**tiology, and signs and **s**ymptoms (PES statement). The specific etiology determines the interventions that will lead to the desired outcome. In this population knowledge deficit is a common nutrition diagnosis, as is inadequate food and beverage intake.

Interventions

All persons with HIV infection and AIDS need early, ongoing medical nutrition therapy. It is essential to educate individuals about the importance of consuming a well-balanced diet, to provide adequate food and nutrients for maintenance or improvement in nutrition status, and to prevent protein-energy malnutrition and vitamin and mineral deficiencies. Counseling should be individualized, considering barriers to adequate intake, and supported with practical written materials. Mapping out one's meal and medication schedule is part of medical nutrition therapy and is an important component for supporting adherence to the drug regimen.

Energy and Protein

Energy and protein needs vary depending on the health status of the individual at the time of HIV infection, the progression of the disease, and the development of complications that impair nutrient intake and use. Hypermetabolism occurs. Energy requirements increase by 13% (Grunfeld and Feingold, 1992) and protein requirements by 10% for every degree Celsius of temperature elevation above normal. Improvements and reversal of HIV wasting are noted when using 500 kcal above estimated energy requirements (use 40 to 50 kcal/kg of current weight) and 1.6 to 1.8 g of protein per kilogram of current weight (McDermott et al., 2003). NHLS also found participants had a 90-kJ/day (21.5 kcal) increase in REE per 1–log10 copy/ml increase in HIV RNA and a 339-kJ/day (81 kcal) higher REE if they were receiving ART. These observations should be factored into estimates of energy needs using the Mifflin-St. Jeor equations with specific activity factors (see Chapter 2).

High-protein diets might safely promote positive nitrogen balance and lean body mass repletion, but studies to clarify the ability of a high-protein diet to reverse HIV-malnutrition and body composition changes are still needed. Protein requirements may be estimated at 1 to 1.4 g/kg for maintenance and 1.5 to 2 g/kg for repletion. Because of the increased protein requirements, protein restriction is indicated only in persons with severe hepatic or renal disease (see Chapters 28 and 36).

Fat

Fat tolerance varies from person to person. In individuals with malabsorption or diarrhea, use of a low-fat diet may aid in management. Use of the more readily absorbed medium-chain triglyceride (MCT) oil is considered better than long-chain triglyceride–based supplements for decreasing stool fat and stool nitrogen content and in reducing the number of bowel movements and abdominal symptoms.

Fish oil (omega-3 fatty acids), when given with MCT oil, may improve immune function because this combination is less inflammatory than the usual omega-6 fatty acids. If triglyceride and cholesterol levels are increased, following the guidelines of the National Cholesterol Education Program is recommended (see Chapter 32).

Fluids and Electrolytes

Fluid needs in HIV-infected individuals are similar to those of well individuals and are calculated to be 30 to 35 ml/kg (8 to 12 c for adults) per day, with additional amounts to compensate for losses from diarrhea, nausea and vomiting, night sweats, and prolonged fever. Replacement of electrolyte losses (sodium, potassium, and chloride) in the presence of vomiting and diarrhea is also recommended.

Vitamins and Minerals

Blood or serum micronutrient levels may not reflect actual status and measurements of the dietary intake; recorded intake from supplements may be more helpful in determining the nutritional condition (Kupka and Fawzi, 2002). The need for increased intake of micronutrients has been suggested, and it is commonly recommended that patients take a daily multivitamin and mineral supplement that provides 100% of the recommended dietary allowances (RDAs) and a basic B-complex supplement, and that they receive nutrition counseling (Woods et al., 2002).

Special Concerns in Pediatric Patients

In addition to supporting optimal function of the immune system, nutrition is especially critical for normal growth and development in children. Children should be growing consistently, and weight gain and linear growth must be monitored carefully from baseline and at least every 3 months (see Box 38-2). In some studies failure to thrive and growth stunting have been identified. Changes in adipose and muscle stores may occur as a result of metabolic changes. The goal is to preserve lean body mass.

Each infected child should undergo a baseline nutrition assessment with follow-up every 4 to 6 months, depending on

I. Nutrition Screen and Referral Criteria for Adults with HIV/AIDS

Today's Date_____

Name _____ Phone _____ Messages: ☐ Yes ☐ No ☐ Discreet

Gender _____ Language _____ DOB ___/___/___ Age _____ File # _____

Medicaid Waiver Client? ☐ Yes ☐ No   Insurance _____ Case Managed By _____

Referred By _____ Date _____ Phone_____

Screen every six months and/or per status change. Automatically refer to a registered dietitian for any of the following:
(Check and circle all that apply)

A. Medical Diagnosis and Nutrition Assessment
1. ☐ Newly diagnosed HIV infection
2. ☐ Newly diagnosed with AIDS
3. ☐ Any change in disease, diet or nutritional status
4. ☐ No nutrition assessment by a registered dietitian or not seen by a registered dietitian in six months

B. Physical Changes and Weight Concerns
1. ☐ ≥3% unintentional weight loss from usual body weight in the last 6 months or since last visit
   (% wt. loss formula: usual body weight − current body wt/usual body wt × 100)
2. ☐ Visible wasting, <90% ideal body weight, BMI <20 kg/m^2, or decrease in body cell mass (BCM)
3. ☐ Uses anabolic steroids or growth hormone for weight, muscle gain or metabolic complications
4. ☐ Lipodystrophy: lipoatrophy, central fat adiposity and/or fat accumulation on the neck, upper back, breasts or other areas
5. ☐ Abdominal obesity: Waist circumference >102 cm or 40 inches (men) and >88 cm or 35 inches (women)
6. ☐ Client or MD initiated weight management, or obesity: BMI >30 kg/m^2

C. Oral/GI Symptoms
1. ☐ Uses an appetite stimulant or suppressant
2. ☐ Loss of appetite, desire to eat or poor oral intake of food or fluid for >3 days
3. ☐ Missing teeth, severe dental caries, difficulty chewing and/or swallowing
4. ☐ Mouth sores, thrush, or mouth, tooth or gum pain
5. ☐ Persistant diarrhea, constipation or change in stools (color, consistency, frequency, smell)
6. ☐ Persistant nausea or vomiting
7. ☐ Persistant gas, bloating or heartburn
8. ☐ Changes in perception of taste or smell
9. ☐ Food allergies or food intolerances (fat, lactose, wheat, etc.)
10. ☐ Medication involving food or meal modification
11. ☐ Receives or needs evaluation for oral supplement or enteral or parental nutrition

D. Metabolic Complications and Other Medical Conditions
1. ☐ Diabetes mellitus, impaired glucose tolerance, impaired fasting glucose, insulin resistance, or
   history of hypoglycemia or hyperglycemia
2. ☐ Hyperlipidemia: cholesterol >200 mg/dL, triglycerides ≥150 mg/dL, LDL >100 g/dL, and/or
   HDL <40 mg/dL (men), <50 mg/dL (women)
3. ☐ Hypertension: two BP readings 120-139/80-90 mm Hg or diagnosed with HTN
4. ☐ Hepatic disease: Hepatitis C, Hepatitis B, cirrhosis, steatotosis, or other:_____
5. ☐ Osteopenia/osteoporosis risk, e.g., elevated alkaline phosphatase, DEXA of the hip and spine low T-scores
6. ☐ Other conditions: renal disease, anemia, heart disease, pregnancy, cancer or other:_____
7. ☐ Albumin <3.5 mg/dL, prealbumin <19 mg/dL, or cholesterol <120 mg/dL
8. ☐ Scheduled chemotherapy or radiation therapy

E. Barriers to Nutrition, Living Environment, Functional Status
Usually or always needs assistance with: Patient is:
1. ☐ Eating   4. ☐ Homebound   7. ☐ Has limited or no cooking skills
2. ☐ Preparing food   5. ☐ Homeless   8. ☐ Income at or below Federal Poverty Guidelines
3. ☐ Shopping for food and necessities   6. ☐ Unable to secure food   9. ☐ Has no stove or refrigerator

F. Behavioral Concerns or Unusual Eating Behaviors
1. ☐ Disordered eating, e.g., binges, purges, purposely skips meals, avoids eating when hungry, pica
2. ☐ Alcoholic consumption: >2/day (men), >1/day (women), or with contraindicated condition
3. ☐ Substance abuse, e.g., alcohol, tobacco, drugs
4. ☐ Vegetarianism
5. ☐ Client initiated vitamin and/or mineral supplementation, or complimentary or alternative diet or related therapies

FIGURE 38-6 Nutrition screen and referral criteria for adults with HIV/AIDS. *(From ADA MNT Evidence Based Guides for Practice ©2005, American Dietetic Association, March 2005. For interim revisions see www.hivaidsdpg.org.)*

the child's age, nutrition status, and nutritional symptoms (see Boxes 38-2 and 38-3). As in adults, nutrition changes in children with HIV/AIDS are not always apparent, and poor intake is usually the major reason for weight loss. General nutrition recommendations for children include high-energy, high-protein, nutrient-dense foods because protein and energy needs are significantly increased. Nutrient and caloric intake must be assessed. Children with severe encephalopathy may be bedridden and require fewer calories.

Weight loss may be attributable to poor energy intake, malabsorption, and opportunistic infections. Stunting and failure to thrive have been identified in nearly all HIV-infected children. Skin-fold measurements should be taken for comparison. The goal is simply to preserve lean body mass.

A multivitamin supplement is needed to provide at least 100% of the RDAs. Poor absorption may be a problem for vitamins A, C, B_6, B_{12}, and folate; iron; selenium; and zinc. Tube feeding via gastrostomy tube may improve the weight and fat mass of children with HIV.

Treatment for children with HIV includes the use of potent antiretroviral medications. When these medications are used in children, they are associated with adverse side effects and difficulty in maintaining a rigid dosage schedule. Children and their caregivers need assistance from RDs in identifying creative ways of adhering to medication schedules and reducing the flavor and smells of medications. Medications can be mixed into foods or beverages such as shakes, ice cream, cranberry or apple sauces, so that they are consumed in sufficient quantities to be effective. Table 38-4 presents HIV medications, along with their dietary considerations and side effects.

Mild-to-severe developmental delays may occur. A child's oral-motor and self-feeding skills, especially during the first 3 years of life, should be monitored closely. Oral and esophageal manifestations such as *Candida* or herpes simplex infections can make it painful for the child to eat. In such cases the family may benefit from guidelines and suggestions as to soft, cold, and nonacidic foods and beverages that can help support the child's nutrition status. Resolving barriers to adequate nutrition intake, ensuring regular access to food, eliminating stress in the environment, and increasing financial resources can help to improve the child's nutrition.

COMPLICATIONS WITH A NUTRITION IMPACT

If the disease progresses, signs and symptoms of HIV infection and AIDS will be manifested along with increased nutrition complications. Common nutrition-related complications are anorexia, fatigue, fever, dehydration, nausea, and fat and metabolic abnormalities. Successful lowering of the viral load, especially through the use of combination antiretroviral therapies, helps to maintain nutrition status.

BOX 38-2

Nutrition Referral Criteria for Children and Adolescents (Less than 18 Years) With HIV/AIDS

Refer to a registered dietitian (RD) when any one of the following conditions exist:
1. Not seen by a registered dietitian in 3 months
2. Weight for age <10th percentile (National Center for Health Statistics [NCHS])
3. Height for age <10th percentile if weight for age is also <10th percentile for age (NCHS)
4. Weight for height <95% of standard or weight for height <25th percentile
5. Downward crossing of one major "weight for age" percentile measurement
6. Visible wasting, <95% ideal body weight, body mass index <25th percentile for age and gender, or any decrease in body cell mass
7. Poor appetite, food or fluid refusals
8. Prolonged bottle-feeding or severe dental caries
9. Change in stool (color, consistency, frequency, smell)
10. For children 0-12 months: Low birth weight
11. For children 0-12 months: No weight gain for 1 month
12. For children 0-12 months: Diarrhea or vomiting for 2 days
13. For children 0-12 months: Poor suck
14. For children 1-3 years: No weight gain for several consecutive months
15. For children 1-3 years: Diarrhea or vomiting for 3 days
16. For children 4-16 years: No weight gain for 3 consecutive months
17. For children 4-18 years: Diarrhea or vomiting for 4 days
18. Poor feeding skills
19. Food allergies or intolerances (e.g., formula, fat, lactose, wheat)
20. Inborn error of metabolism
21. Prealbumin: 9-22 mg/dl (0-6 months), 11-29 mg/dl (6 months-6 years), 15-37 mg/dl (6-16 years)
22. Cholesterol <65 mg/dl or <175 mg/dl
23. Triglycerides <40 mg/dl and <160 mg/dl

Modified from Fenton M et al: Nutrition referral criteria for pediatrics (<18 years) with HIV/AIDS. In *Guidelines for implementing HIV medical nutrition therapy*, Los Angeles, 1999, Los Angeles County Commission on HIV Health Services.

BOX 38-3

Practical Eating Suggestions for Symptom Management

Nausea

Small, frequent meals
Avoidance of high-fat, greasy foods
Cool or room-temperature foods
Avoidance of lying down flat after eating
Take medications after meal

Sore Mouth or Throat

Soft, moist food
Avoidance of spicy or acidic foods
Experimentation with temperature of foods (avoidance of very hot or very cold foods; cool or room-temperature foods are best)
Use of nutrient- and energy-dense foods to maximize oral intake

Xerostomia (Dry Mouth)

Use of foods that are moist or served with a sauce or gravy
Consumption of liquids at mealtimes and extra fluids between meals
Emphasis on good oral hygiene: flossing, brushing, and rinsing; regular dental care
Use of fluoride gels or mouthwashes
Consideration of prophylactic antifungal therapy
Chewing of sugarless gum or sucking of mints

Difficulty With Breathing

Use of easy-to-eat foods
Use of nutrient- and energy-dense foods

Diarrhea

Fluid and electrolyte replacement
Low-insoluble and high-soluble–fiber diet
Possible benefits from low-lactose diet
Low-fat diet (may be indicated)
Avoidance of gas-causing foods and beverages
Avoidance of caffeine
Take medications after meal

Constipation

Increased fluid intake
Increased dietary fiber intake

Inadequate Oral Intake

Use of nutrient- and energy-dense foods, including nutritional supplements
Use of small, frequent meals and snacks
Consideration of alternative nutrition support or appetite stimulant such as Megace or Marinol

Fatigue

Adequate sleep, relaxation, exercise
Adequate diet, especially foods rich in vitamins B_{12}, A, C, folate, and carotene or zinc; inadequate amounts may cause fatigue
Avoidance of caffeine, alcohol, cigarette smoking, and recreational drug use
Avoidance of stress and treatment of anxiety or depression
Identification and management of possible causes for anemia:
Medications: AZT, Bactrim, dapsone, ganciclovir, interferon, pyrimethamine
Other causes: alcohol abuse, bleeding, *Mycobacterium avium* complex, tuberculosis, fungal infections, cytomegalovirus
Check lactic acid levels for indications of mitochondrial toxicity

Body Cell Mass Loss

Diet: 500 calories above daily energy requirement (40-50 kcal/kg current body weight and 1.6-1.8 g protein/kg current weight per day)
Mitigate associated symptoms: identify exacerbating and helpful foods
Resistance exercise
Correct for testosterone deficiency
Consider anabolic agents (Rx from MD)

Diarrhea and Malabsorption

Persons with the greatest risk of developing diarrhea are those with a CD4+ cell count of less than 200 to 250 cells/mm³. Causes of diarrhea can be multifactorial; etiology must be pursued. Pathogens and other factors that cause diarrhea are listed in Table 38-5.

Diarrhea and malabsorption are the major nutrition problems for this population, and they are often the most difficult problems to resolve. Abnormal *d*-xylose absorption and steatorrhea are common. Malabsorption of fat, monosaccharides, disaccharides, nitrogen, vitamin B_{12}, folate, minerals, and trace elements occurs in patients with intestinal infections of the small bowel. When the large bowel is infected, malabsorption of fluids and electrolytes is seen.

Regardless of whether the cause of diarrhea is identified, intervention and treatment must be pursued. Treatment often uses a combination of antidiarrheal agents, including cholestyramine and fiber supplements; antimotility agents such as codeine phosphate, Lomotil, Imodium, morphine, and paregoric; and hormones such as octreotide and Sandostatin. Table 38-6 provides information on the nutrition management of diarrhea.

Disorders of the Oral Cavity and Esophagus

Oral lesions are common and usually are neoplastic, bacterial, viral, or fungal in origin. They often are the first sign of HIV infection that leads to diagnosis and can mark immunodeficiency and disease progression. Symptoms of oral candidiasis (thrush) include soreness of the mouth and tongue, often described as a "burnt" feeling, and pain or difficulty in swallowing (Figure 38-7).

Dysgeusia may also be present secondary to medication, zinc and other nutrient deficiencies, candidiasis, xerostomia, or excessive mucus production. Necrotizing ulcerative periodontitis is often seen. Frequent dental care and routine hygiene are essential.

KS or herpes in the oropharyngeal or esophageal area can also inhibit normal chewing and swallowing, thus limiting nutritional intake. Patients with extensive or chronic lesions may require alternative nutrition support such as enteral or parenteral nutrition.

Use of specially designed formulas may slow the progressive decline toward malnutrition. Box 38-3 lists suggestions for improving the dietary intake of the patient who has a painful mouth. For painful mouth sores the patient can swish and spit "magic mouthwash," consisting of equal parts 2% viscous lidocaine, Benadryl, and Maalox, which can be prescribed by the physician and formulated by the pharmacist.

Neurologic Disorders

CNS manifestations of AIDS, ranging from psychomotor impairment to severe dementia, can significantly affect the ability of an infected individual to maintain adequate nutrition. Moreover, decreased sensory perception when chewing and swallowing can increase the risk of aspiration. Working closely with occupational and physical therapists, speech pathologists, the nursing staff, and others involved in overall patient care is important in helping the patient maintain adequate nutritional intake.

Alterations in Metabolism and Body Shape

Distinguishing body composition changes that indicate wasting, lipodystrophy, or obesity from a healthy and non-threatening weight loss is essential. Monitoring body composition provides a picture of body shape changes over time. Measuring waist, hip and waist-hip ratio, midarm, breast, and neck circumferences, in addition to weight should be done every 3 to 6 months.

Bioelectrical impedance analysis (BIA) (see Figure 14-17 in Chapter 14) is an inexpensive and easy tool for measuring body cell mass, loss of which may indicate wasting. BIA does not indicate regional differences in fat and therefore is not useful in identifying fat redistribution. Expensive tools such as dual-energy x-ray absorptiometry, computed tomography scans, and MRI are mostly used for research and provide the most accurate assessment of these body composition changes.

The use of potent anti-HIV therapies, especially protease inhibitors, has increased the incidence of insulin resistance, type 2 diabetes, hypercholesterolemia, pancreatitis, and hypertriglyceridemia in the HIV/AIDS population. Principles developed for diabetes or from the National Cholesterol Education Program are used in an effort to control these conditions (see Chapters 30 and 32). Oral hypoglycemics and insulin are being used, as are lipid-lowering drugs.

TABLE 38-5

Possible Causes of HIV-Related Diarrhea

Category	Specific Agents/Conditions
Bacteria	*Campylobacter* species
	Clostridium difficile
	Enteroadherent *Escherichia coli*
	Mycobacterium avium complex/ *M. tuberculosis*
	Salmonella species
	Shigella
	Vibrio
Parasites	*Cryptosporidium*
	Cyclospora
	Giardia
	Isospora
	Microsporidia
	Entamoeba histolytica
Fungi	*Histoplasma capsulatum*
Viruses	Adenovirus
	Cytomegalovirus
	Herpes simplex
	HIV (possibly)
Nutritional causes	Fat malabsorption
	High-fiber diet
	Hypoalbuminemia
	Lactose intolerance
	Kaposi's sarcoma
	Malnutrition
	Caffeine
	Sorbitol
Drugs/antacids/ antiretrovirals	Mg^{++}-containing
	Didanosine (Videx, ddl)
	Nelfinavir (Viracept)
	Ritonavir (Norvir)
	Saquinavir (Fortovase)
Antimicrobials	Amphotericin
	Macrolide antibiotics
	Azithromycin
	Clorithromycin
	Pentamidine
Vitamins (high dose)	Vitamin C

Modified from Dieterich DT: *Diarrhea in the HIV/AIDS patient*, 1997, Golden Colo., Medical Education Collaborative and Oestreicher Medical Communications, Inc.

Supplements often promoted for these conditions include omega-3 fatty acids, α-lipoic acid, and *l*-carnitine.

Treatment for body shape changes has been both difficult and confusing. The stigma and psychological discomfort associated with the condition can be devastating. Discontinuing ART is not a favorable option, and less offending regimens are under active study. Those who can afford them are using cosmetic surgery such as liposuction or implants,

TABLE 38-6

Nutrition Intervention for Diarrhea

Type of Diarrhea	Intervention
Treatable diarrhea	Maintain adequate nutritional intake for bowel regeneration
	Enhance absorption by using elemental diets
	Control infection and symptoms with antibiotics and antidiarrheals
	Provide fiber-containing supplements; follow general guidelines
Diarrhea resistant to treatment	Promote patient comfort
	Maintain adequate hydration; intravenous hydration may be indicated
	Control symptoms by using antidiarrheals or antispasmodics
	Total parenteral nutrition may be indicated
	Calcium carbonate (500 mg bid)
Diarrhea resulting from AIDS enteropathy	Incorporate small frequent meals into daily plan
	Avoid lactose-containing foods and medications or use lactase enzyme
	Reduce high fructose–containing foods (apple and pear juices, grapes, honey, dates, nuts, figs, soft drinks)
	Limit sorbitol, hexitols, and mannitol in "sugar-free" products
	Limit carbonated beverages
	Limit fat if steatorrhea is present; try medium-chain triglyceride oil
	Consider a lactobacillus replacement or probiotics if patient is receiving long-term antibiotic therapy
	Consider prescriptive pancreatic enzymes
	Consider l-glutamine (0.4 g/kg up to 30 g/day for 5-14 days, followed by 5-10 g/day)
	Recommend a multivitamin/mineral supplement
	Gradually reintroduce suspect foods, one at a time, and check for tolerance
General guidelines for diarrhea	Consume foods at room temperature
	Limit insoluble and bran-type, high-fiber foods
	Avoid foods that cause gas

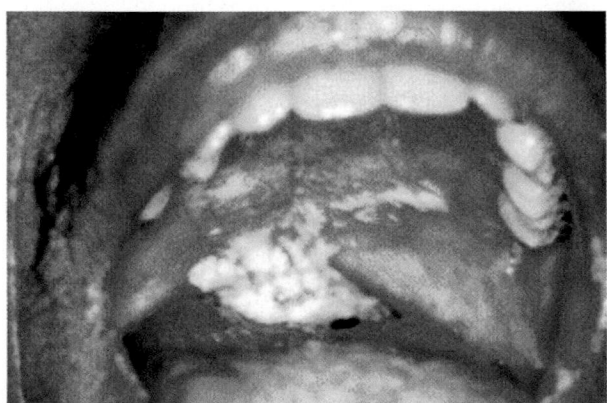

FIGURE 38-7 Fluconazole-resistant pseudomembranous candidiasis. *(Copyright 1996, 2000 David Reznik, DDS. All rights reserved. Used with permission by HIVdent and Dr. Reznik.)*

anabolic therapy, or a combination of these options. Aerobic exercise may have a role in reducing truncal adiposity, along with a moderate-fat, moderate-carbohydrate, and high-fiber diet (Roubenoff et al., 2002).

Growth hormone, approved for AIDS wasting or cachexia, may have a role in reducing HIV-associated fat accumulation. Transient worsening of both insulin sensitivity and glucose tolerance of most individuals and increased insulin-like growth factor I levels can occur. An oral glucose tolerance test has been recommended to identify those at risk for growth hormone–induced hyperglycemia (Lo et al., 2001).

A pilot study that used low-dose metformin resulted in reductions of insulin resistance and visceral adipose tissue; however, subcutaneous adipose tissue was also reduced, which was undesirable for some (Hadigan et al., 2000). Metformin has been associated with lactic acidosis and must be used cautiously in this population. The use of metformin and other insulin-sensitizing agents are being studied actively. Implementing changes in diet and exercise, core components in treating insulin resistance, are prudent while awaiting formal studies in this population (Grinspoon, 2001).

COMPLEMENTARY AND ALTERNATIVE THERAPIES

People with HIV disease often become frustrated with the lack of definitive medical therapies, and some turn to unconventional nutrition therapies. Among the major questions to consider in assessing these therapies are the following:

- Is the product or treatment harmful?
- Are there harmful drug-drug interactions with prescription or over-the-counter medications?
- Are unproven treatments being used while effective treatments are being delayed?
- Does the therapy work?
- Is the financial expense worth the benefit?

One must be wary of products or services when their promotion uses sensationalism, testimonials, or claims that they are based on a secret formula or when promotional literature accuses the government or traditional Western medicine of neglect.

Many herbs that might have been dismissed casually as safe are contraindicated when used with antiretroviral medications. St John's wort, an inducer of the cytochrome P450 pathway, decreases plasma concentrations of indinavir, which is metabolized in the cytochrome P450 pathway. Drug resistance and treatment failure could occur because of this pharmacokinetic interaction. Researchers and the FDA have cautioned that other protease inhibitors, nonnucleoside reverse transcriptase inhibitors, and other drugs using the same pathway would be negatively affected as well (Lumpkin and Alpert, 2000; Piscitelli et al., 2000). Garlic supplements reduced blood concentrations of saquinavir by about 50% (Piscitelli et al., 2001).

Concern has been raised about silymarin, the flavonoid extract from Silybum marianum (milk thistle). Although silymarin is promoted and used to protect the liver, one study showed that it reduced the activity of CYP3A4 enzyme in human hepatocyte cultures, which could lessen metabolism of coadministered medications and increase toxicity (Venkataramanan et al., 2000).

Specific dietary supplements often used by this population include Echinacea, St John's wort, cat's claw, protein supplements, creatine, anabolic steroids, and Chinese herbs.

Reiki, massage, yoga, and acupuncture are also used often (see Chapter 18). One study found that 56% of patients had informed their physicians about using alternative therapies, but the information was found in the medical charts of only 13% of the patients (Southwell et al., 2001).

Addressing alternative therapies should be a customary part of both the medical and nutrition assessment and intervention. Therapies that people living with HIV may try include dietary supplements, herbal medications, megavitamins, counseling, and prayer therapy. Nutrition supplements formulated and marketed for this population have yet to be substantiated.

✳ FOCAL POINTS

- HIV disease involves multiple systems and has complex psychological, social, and economic ramifications.
- Until recently, research, medical care, and education about HIV have been less than ideal throughout the world.
- Nutrition intervention has a role in improving the quality of life of those living with HIV infection and may even prolong life.
- Multiple factors must be considered to find the best ways to provide appropriate HIV medical nutrition therapy.
- Reimbursement for medical nutrition therapy in HIV patients through the Ryan White Act is a major breakthrough for this population.
- Advocacy for improving inequities will undoubtedly improve outcomes for people with HIV in the United States and in the rest of the world.

✳ CLINICAL SCENARIO 1

Gary is a 41-year-old male HIV-positive patient who also is diagnosed with hepatitis C and recently had shingles. His current HIV antiretroviral regimen is Viracept, Zerit, and Videx. His last viral load was 250,000; his CD4+ cell count was 14; and his serum triglycerides were 890 mg/dl. He lives alone and gets one meal per day from a community meal provider. He has chronic diarrhea, with four to five loose stools per day. He has recurrent heartburn and bloating after meals. He is on disability and has no extra money to join a gym. Gary smokes 1 pack of cigarettes per day and is in an outpatient alcohol recovery program. He is 5 ft 10 in and weighs 150 lb; his dietary intake as shown from a recent 24-hour recall is 1650 kcal with 40 g protein.

✳Nutrition Diagnosis: Inadequate protein-energy intake related to heartburn and bloating after meals as evidenced by 24-hour recall of 1650 kcal and 40 g of protein

1. What energy and protein recommendations would you make? How does this compare with the recommended amount for his age, sex, and size?
2. What recommendations would you make to his meal provider?
3. Would you recommend any other laboratory tests? If so, which ones?
4. What exercise recommendations would you make given his limited funds?

☸ CLINICAL SCENARIO 2

Miguel is a 34-year-old man infected with HIV for over 10 years. His current viral load is undetectable at below 50 copies, and his CD4+ count is 563. He is 6 ft 0 in and weighs 202 lb. He has been on antiretroviral therapy for 8 years and currently takes Kaletra, Epivir, and Rescriptor. Miguel drinks two alcoholic drinks per week and works out at the gym twice a week, where he walks on a treadmill for 30 minutes and weight trains for 1 hour. Over the last year he has noticed that his body composition has changed with an increasing abdominal girth. His last fasting lipid profile was abnormal with a total cholesterol of 280 mg/dl, triglycerides 455 mg/dl, HDL 29 mg/dl, and LDL 148 mg/dl. He has a positive family history for both cardiovascular disease and diabetes. He states that he has never been educated about NCEP guidelines.

✳Nutrition Diagnosis: Abnormal nutrition-related laboratory values related to knowledge deficit about lipodystrophy and current cholesterol management guidelines, as evidenced by elevated lipid panel and lack of prior education on that topic.

1. What do you think are the reasons for Miguel's expanding waist?
2. Calculate Miguel's daily energy and protein needs.
3. What risk factors does he have for developing diabetes or heart disease?
4. What are your dietary, exercise, and lifestyle recommendations?

USEFUL WEBSITES

AIDS organization
http://www.aids.org/

HIV at Medscape
www.medscape.com/hiv

Panel on Clinical Practices for the Treatment of HIV
www.aidsinfo.nih.gov

Research developments
www.clinicalcareoptions.com/HIV

United Nations AIDS Organization
http://www.unaids.org/en/

References

AVERT: United States HIV & AIDS Statistics Summary, from http://www.avert.org/statsum.htm, accessed March 25, 2006a.

AVERT: Worldwide HIV & AIDS epidemic statistics 2006b, www.avert.org/worlstatinfo.htm, accessed March 25, 2006.

Bartlett J: *Pocket guide adult HIV/AIDS treatment: Johns Hopkins University, 2006,* from http://hopkins-aids.edu/publications/pocketguide/pocketgd0106.pdf, accessed February 26, 2006.

Bacchetti P et al: Fat distribution in men with HIV infection, *J Acquir Immune Defic Syndr* 40(2):121, 2005.

Carpenter CCJ et al: Antiretroviral therapy in adults: updated recommendations of the International AIDS Society—USA Panel, *JAMA* 293:381, 2000.

Centers for Disease Control and Prevention: AIDS surveillance—General Epidemiology (through 2004), 2006a, from www.cdc.gov/hiv/topics/surveillance/resources/slides/epidemiology/index.htm, accessed March 26, 2006.

Centers for Disease Control and Prevention: *Basic statistics,* 2006b, from http://www.cdc.gov/hiv/basic.htm, accessed March 24, 2006.

Centers for Disease Control and Prevention: CDC report of the NIH Panel to define principles of therapy of HIV infection and guidelines for the use of antiretroviral agents in HIV-infected adults and adolescents, *MMWR* 47(RR-5):1, 1998.

Centers for Disease Control and Prevention: Characteristics of persons living with AIDS and HIV 2001, *HIV/AIDS Surveillance Suppl Rep* 9(2):1, 2003, www.cdc.gov/hiv/Topics/surveillance/basic.htm hasrsupp92/commentary.htm, accessed June 3, 2007.

Centers for Disease Control and Prevention: *HIV/AIDS among women,* updated December, 2004, from www.cdc.gov/hiv/pubs/facts/women.htm#2, accessed April 1, 2006.

Centers for Disease Control and Prevention: *HIV/AIDS surveillance report 2004,* vol 16, Atlanta, 2001b, U.S. Department of Health and Human Services, CDC, www.cdc.gov/hiv/topics/surveillance/resources/reports/2004report/default.htm (update 9/24/2001b resources), accessed June 3, 2007.

Centers for Disease Control and Prevention: HIV/AIDS surveillance report, 2006c, www.cec.gov/HIV/topics/surveillance, accessed March 26, 2006.

Centers for Disease Control and Prevention: 1993 Revised classification system for HIV infection and expanded surveillance case definition for AIDS among adolescents and adults, *MMWR* 41:17, 1992, www.cdc.gov/mmwr/.

Centers for Disease Control and Prevention: 1997 USPHS/IDSA guidelines for the prevention of opportunistic infection in persons infected with human immunodeficiency virus, *MMWR* 46(RR-12):27, 1997, website: www.cdc.gov/search, accessed June 3, 2007.

Centers for Disease Control and Prevention: Primary HIV infection associated with oral transmission, updated 2/2001c, www.cdc.gov/hiv/pubs/facts/oralsexqa.htm, accessed January 2, 2007.

Centers for Disease Control and Prevention: *Questions and answers: the science behind the new initiative,* from www.cdc.gov/hiv/topics/prev_prog/AHP/resources/qa/AdvancingFS.pdf, accessed March 5, 2006.

Crum NF et al: Comparisons of causes of death and mortality rates among HIV-infected persons: analysis of the pre-, early-, and late HAART (highly active antiretroviral therapy) eras, *J Acquir Immune Defic Syndr* 41(2):194, 2006.

De Groot AS: HIV infection among incarcerated women: epidemic behind bars, AIDS Reader 10(5):287, 2000.

Drew WL et al: New perspectives on CMV and other viruses in the immunocompromised patient, *Medscape Today,* March 2003, University of Minnesota, www.medscape.com/viewprogram/2255, accessed June 3, 2007.

Dreyfuss ML, Fawzi WW: Micronutrients and vertical transmission of HIV-1, *Am J Clin Nutr* 75:959, 2002.

Duran A et al: Bone loss associated with lipodystrophy syndrome [Abstract]. Conference on HIV Pathogenesis and Treatment, First IAS Conference in Buenos Aires, July, 2001, www.aids2001ias.org, accessed June 3, 2007.

Eliminating Disparities Working Group: An overview of US trans health priorities, August 2004, Washington, DC, National Coalition for LGBT Health, www.nctequality.org/HealthPriorities.pdf, accessed June 3, 2007.

Fee E, Brown TM: Michael S Gottlieb and the identification of AIDS, *Am J Public Health* 96(6):982, 2006.

Fisher K: Wasting and lipodystrophy in patients infected with HIV: a practical approach in clinical practice, *The AIDS Reader* 11(3):132, 2001.

Forna F et al: Systematic review of the safety of trimethoprim-sulfamethoxazole for prophylaxis in HIV-infected pregnant women: implications for resource-limited settings, *AIDS Rev* 8(1):24, 2006.

French AL et al: Vitamin A deficiency and genital viral burden in women infected with HIV-1, *Lancet* 359:1210, 2002.

Gebo KA: HIV in patients over 50: an increasing problem. The Hopkins HIV Report, November 2004, website: http://hopkins-aids.edu/publications/report/nov04_2.html.

Gifford AL et al: Predictors of self-reported adherence and plasma HIV concentrations in patients on multidrug antiretroviral regimens, *J Acquir Immune Defic Syndr* 23:386, 2000.

Grinspoon S: *Insulin resistance in HIV disease,* New York, June 2001, Physicians Research Network.

Grunfeld C, Feingold KR: Metabolic disturbances and wasting in the acquired immunodeficiency syndrome, *N Engl J Med* 327:329, 1992.

Guidelines for the use of antiretroviral agents in pediatric HIV infection, October 26, 2006 1-126 from *http://* www.aidsinfo.nih.gov/ContentFiles/PediatricGuidelines.pdf, accessed. June 3, 2007

Hadigan C et al: Metformin in the treatment of HIV lipodystrophy syndrome: a randomized controlled trial, *JAMA* 284:472, 2000.

Health Resources and Services Administration (HRSA): Health care and HIV: nutritional guide for providers and clients, June 2002, HRSA, HIV/AIDS Bureau, Rockville, Md, http://careacttarget.org/librarysearch2.asp, accessed June 3, 2007.

Heller L: Nutrition support for children with HIV/AIDS, *AIDS Reader* 10(2):109, 2000.

Kaiser Family Foundation: U.S. federal funding for HIV/AIDS: the FY 2007 budget request, February 2006, from www.kff.org/hivaids/upload/7029-03.pdf, accessed April 1, 2006.

Kantor E: *HIV transmission and preventions in prisons, HIV InSite Knowledge Base,* February 2003, http://hivinsite.ucsf.edu/InSite?page=KB, accessed March 25, 2006.

Keele BF et al: Chimpanzee reservoirs of pandemic and nonpandemic HIV-1, *Science* 313(5786):523, 2006.

Kosmiski LA et al: Fat distribution and metabolic changes are strongly correlated and energy expenditure is increased in the HIV lipodystrophy syndrome, *AIDS* 15:1193, 2001.

Kotler DP: HIV and insulin resistance in context, *AIDS Read* 15:220, 2005.

Kupka R, Fawzi W: Zinc nutrition and HIV infection, *Nutr Rev* 60(3):69, 2002.

Kuritzkes DR et al: Current management challenges in HIV: antiretroviral resistance, *AIDS Read,* 13:133, 2003.

Lauer JA et al. Deaths and years of life lost due to suboptimal breast-feeding among children in the developing world: a global ecological risk assessment, *Public Health Nutr* 9(6):673, 2006.

Lo JC et al: The effects of recombinant human growth hormone on body composition and glucose metabolism in HIV-infected patients with fat accumulation, *J Clin Endocrinol Metabol* 86(8):3480, 2001.

Lumpkin MM, Alpert A: Risk of drug interactions with St John's wort and indinavir and other drugs, FDA Public Health Advisory, February 2000, from http://www.fds.gov/cder/drug/advisory/stjwort.htm, accessed March 26, 2006.

Mangili A et al: Nutrition and HIV infection: Review of weight loss and wasting in the era of highly active antiretroviral therapy from the Nutrition for Healthy Living Cohort, *Clin Infect Dis* 42:836, 2006.

Mascolini M: Fish oil lowers triglycerides in randomized study of HIV-infected patients, *Clin Care Options,* February 14, 2006, website http://clinicalcareoptions.com/HIV/.aspx, accessd June 3, 2007.

McDermott AY et al: Nutrition treatment for HIV wasting: a prescription for food as medicine, *Nutr Clin Pract* 18:86, 2003.

Michaels S et al: Differences in the incidence rates of opportunistic processes before and after the availability of protease inhibitors, Fifth Conference on Retrovirus and Opportunistic Infections, Chicago, February 1-5, 1998.

Mondy K, Tebas P: Emerging problems of bone in HIV disease, *Clin Infect Dis* 36:1015, 2003.

Moyle G: Adverse events with antiretrovirals, Highlights from the First International AIDS Society (IAS) Conference on HIV Pathogenesis and Treatment, July 8-11, 2001, Buenos Aires, Argentina 2001.

Mulligan K et al: Body composition changes in HIV-infected men consuming self-selecting diets during a placebo-controlled inpatient study of cannabinoids, Eighth Conference on Retroviruses and Opportunistic Infections, [Abstract No. 647], 2001.

New York State Department of Health AIDS Institute: General nutrition, weight loss and wasting syndrome, Adult HIV Guidelines, March 2001, www.hivguidelines.org/public_html/CENTER/clinicalguidelines/adult_hiv_guidelines/ADULTS.htm, accessed March 26, 2006.

O'Brien J: Six million babies now saved every year through exclusive breastfeeding, UNICEF, Nov, 2005, www.unicef.org/nutrition/index_30006.html, accessed March 26, 2006.

O'Neill JF: *Guidelines for the Use of Antiretroviral Agents in HIV-Infected Adults and Adolescents,* from http://aidsinfo.nih.gov/Guidelines/GuidelineDetail.aspx?MenuItem=Guidelines&Search=Off&GuidelineID=7&ClassID=1, accessed April 9, 2007.

Panel on Clinical Practices for the Treatment of HIV: Guidelines for the use of antiretroviral agents in HIV-infected adults and adolescents, from http://aidsinfo.nih.gov/contentfiles/AdultandAdolescent.pdf, accessed March 24, 2007.

Papathakis P: Personal communication, April, 2006.

Peterson C et al: Pharmacokinetics of nelfinavir (Virecept 250-mg tablet): effect of food intake on single-dose PK parameters, Abstracts of the Tenth Conference on Retroviruses and Opportunistic Infections, Chicago, February 2003.

Piscitelli SC et al: Indinavir concentrations and St John's wort, *Lancet* 355:547, 2000.

Piscitelli SC et al: The effect of garlic supplements on the pharmacokinetics of saquinavir, *Clin Infect Dis* electronic edition, 12/3/2001.

Public Health Service Task Force: Safety and toxicity of individual antiretroviral agents in pregnancy, *MMWR* 47 (RR-2), 1998, updated December 5, 2001a, from http://aidsinfo.nih.gov, accessed June 3, 2007.

Public Health Service Task Force: Recommendations for use of antiretroviral drugs in pregnant HIV-1 infected women for maternal health and interventions to reduce perinatal HIV-1 transmission in the United States, www.aidsinfo.nih.gov, accessed April 9, 2007.

Public Health Service Task Force: Safety and Toxicity of Individual Antiretroviral Agents in Pregnancy: *MMWR* 47 (RR-2), 1998, updated as a Living Document on December 5, 2001b, www.aidsinfo.nih.gov, accessed April 9, 2007.

Roubenoff R, Wilson IB: Effect of resistance training on self-reported physical functioning in HIV infection, *Med Sci Sports Exerc* 33:1811, 2001.

Roubenoff R et al: Reduction of abdominal obesity in lipodystrophy associated with human immunodeficiency virus by means of diet and exercise: case report and proof of principle, *Clin Infect Dis* 34:390, 2002.

Saag M: Current controversies in antiretroviral therapy, XIV international AIDS conference, Barcelona, 7/10/2002.

Saavedra J et al: Longitudinal assessment of growth in children born to mothers with human immunodeficiency virus infection, *Arch Pediatr Adolesc Med* 149:497, 1995.

San Francisco Department of Health: Crystal meth use triples the number of new HIV infections, August 15, 2005, www.dph.sf.ca.us/press/2005PR/pr08152005B.shtml, accessed March 26, 2006.

Scribner AN et al: Osteonecrosis in HIV: a case-control study, *J Acquir Immune Defic Syndr* 25:19, 2000.

Shevitz AH et al: A comparison of the clinical and cost-effectiveness of 3 intervention strategies for AIDS wasting, *J Acquir Immune Defic Syndr* 38:399, 2005.

Southwell H et al: Use of alternative therapy among HIV-infected patients at an urban tertiary center, [Abstract No. 497], Eighth Conference on Retroviruses and Opportunistic Infections, 2001.

Sterling T et al: Initial plasma HIV-1 RNA levels and progression to AIDS in women and men, *N Engl J Med* 344:720, 2001.

United Nations Programme on HIV/AIDS (UNAIDS) and World Health Organization (WHO): *AIDS epidemic update*, 2005, www.unaids.org/epi/2005/doc/EPIupdate2005_pdf_en/epi-update2005_en.pdf, www.unaids.org/worldaidsday/2001/Epiupdate2001/EPIupdate2001_en.doc, accessed March 26, 2006.

Venkataramanan R et al: Milk thistle, an herbal supplement, decreases the activity of CYI and uridine diphosphglucuronosyl transferase in human hepatocyte cultures, *Drug Metab Dispos* 28(11):1270, 2000.

Wheeler D et al: Weight loss as a predictor of survival and disease progression in HIV infection, *J AIDS Hum Retroviral* 18:80, 1998.

Woods MN et al: Nutrient intake and body weight in a large HIV cohort that includes women and minorities, *J Am Diet Assoc* 102:203, 2002.

Zhu T et al: An African HIV-1 sequence from 1959 and implications for the origin of the epidemic, *Nature* 391:594, 1998.

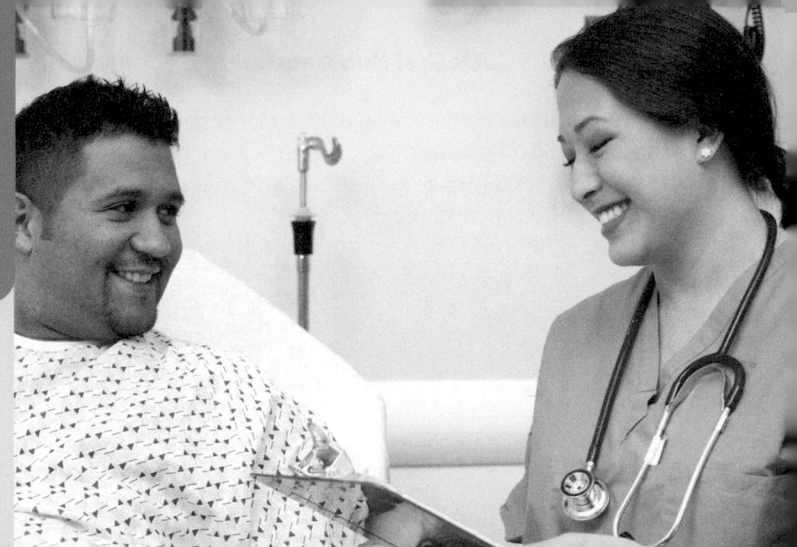

CHAPTER 39

Marion F. Winkler, MS, RD, LDN, CNSD
Ainsley M. Malone, MS, RD, CNSD

Medical Nutrition Therapy for Metabolic Stress: Sepsis, Trauma, Burns, and Surgery

KEY TERMS

acute-phase proteins secretory proteins in the liver that are altered in response to injury or infection; positive acute-phase proteins, C-reactive protein, α_1-antitrypsin, and fibronectin are increased; negative acute-phase proteins, immunoglobulin G and M, complement, transthyretin, transferrin, ceruloplasmin, and albumin are decreased

adrenocorticotropic hormone a hormone secreted by the anterior pituitary gland that acts primarily on the adrenal cortex, thus stimulating its growth and secretion of corticosteroids

bacterial translocation morphologic changes from acute insult to the gastrointestinal tract that may allow entry of bacteria from the gut lumen into the body; associated with a systemic inflammatory response that may contribute to multiple organ dysfunction syndrome

catecholamines hormones (epinephrine and norepinephrine) released by the adrenal medulla in response to shock and a higher glucagon/insulin ratio; stimulate hepatic glycogenolysis, fat mobilization, and gluconeogenesis

cortisol a glucocorticoid released by the adrenal cortex

cytokines proinflammatory proteins released by macrophages that act as mediators of shock, multiple organ dysfunction syndrome, and sepsis; examples include tumor necrosis factor, interleukin-1, and interleukin-6

ebb phase initial response to bodily insult characterized by lower blood pressure, cardiac output, body temperature, and oxygen consumption; associated with hypovolemia, hypoperfusion, and lactic acidosis

flow phase a neuroendocrine response to physiologic stress that follows the ebb phase; characterized by hypermetabolism and hypercatabolism

Glasgow Coma Scale (GCS) system for determining the degree of neurologic insult and a patient's level of consciousness by assessing responses to eye opening and motor and verbal response

glutamine an amino acid that is the preferential fuel for enterocytes in the gut mucosa, especially during stress; it enhances cell mass and the height of the mucosal villi

growth hormone (GH) an anabolic agent mediated by insulin-like growth factor 1 (IGF-1); thought to accelerate growth in children and improve protein synthesis in injured patients

gut-associated lymphoid tissue a component of the gut intestinal mucosal barrier that may protect against multiple organ dysfunction syndrome; contains 40% of the immune effector cells in the body

hemodynamic relating to physiologic processes involving blood flow in circulation; blood pressure and cardiac output are key components in hemodynamic stability

ileus loss of intestinal peristalsis or lack of effective coordinated peristalsis

interleukin-1 a cytokine mediator induced by tumor necrosis factor and produced by endothelial cells and monocytes; induces fever by stimulating prostaglandin production

multiple organ dysfunction syndrome (MODS) organ dysfunction that results from direct injury, trauma, or disease or as a response to inflammation; the response usually is in an organ remote from the original site of infection or injury

sepsis the systemic response to an identifiable infectious agent

shock sudden disturbance of mental equilibrium; profound hemodynamic and metabolic disturbance characterized by failure of the circulatory system to maintain adequate perfusion of vital organs

structured lipid fat composed of rearranged triglycerides that contain both medium- and long-chain fatty acids; may improve hepatic protein synthesis and reduce protein catabolism and energy expenditure

systemic inflammatory response syndrome (SIRS) sepsis that occurs without evidence of invasive bacterial or fungal infection; can result in multiple organ dysfunction syndrome

tumor necrosis factor a cytokine produced by activated cells, Kupffer cells in the liver, and macrophages that is stimulated by endotoxin or by bacterial, viral, and fungal infection; initiates an inflammatory response and stimulates skeletal muscle catabolism

Trauma from motor vehicle accidents, gunshots, stab wounds, falls, and burns is a major cause of death and disability. Unintentional injuries and motor vehicle accidents are ranked as the fifth leading cause of death—after heart disease, malignant neoplasm, cerebrovascular disease, and chronic respiratory diseases. Injury results in profound metabolic alterations beginning at the time of injury and persisting until wound healing and recovery are complete. Whether the event is **sepsis** (infection), trauma (including burns), or surgery, once the systemic response is activated, the physiologic and metabolic changes that follow are similar and may lead to shock and other negative outcomes (Figure 39-1). Variable responses relate in part to the patient's age, previous state of health, preexisting disease, type of infection, and presence of multiple organ dysfunction syndrome (MODS).

METABOLIC RESPONSE TO STRESS

The metabolic response to critical illness, traumatic injury, sepsis, burns, or major surgery is complex and involves most metabolic pathways. This state is characterized by an accelerated catabolism of lean body or skeletal mass that clinically results in negative nitrogen balance and muscle wasting. The response to critical illness, injury, and sepsis characteristically involves both ebb and flow phases (Table 39-1). The **ebb phase**, occurring immediately following injury, is associated with hypovolemia, shock, and tissue hypoxia. Typically decreased cardiac output, oxygen consumption, and body temperature characterize this phase. Insulin levels fall in direct response to the increase in glucagon, most likely as a signal to increase hepatic glucose production (Souba and Wilmore, 1994).

Increased cardiac output, oxygen consumption, body temperature, energy expenditure, and total body protein catabolism characterize the **flow phase** which follows fluid resuscitation and restoration of oxygen transport. Physiologically a marked increase occurs in glucose production, free fatty acid release, circulating levels of insulin, **catecholamines** (epineph-

rine and norepinephrine released by the adrenal medulla), glucagon, and cortisol. The magnitude of hormonal response appears to be associated with the severity of injury.

Hormonal and Cell-Mediated Response

Metabolic stress is associated with an altered hormonal state that results in an increased flow of substrate but poor use of carbohydrate, protein, fat, and oxygen Counter-regulatory hormones, which are elevated after injury and sepsis, play a role in the accelerated proteolysis that characteristically is seen. Glucagon promotes gluconeogenesis, amino acid uptake, ureagenesis, and protein catabolism. **Cortisol,** which is released from the adrenal cortex in response to stimulation by **adrenocorticotropic hormone** secreted by the anterior pituitary gland, enhances skeletal muscle catabolism and promotes hepatic use of amino acids for gluconeogenesis, glycogenolysis, and acute-phase protein synthesis (Table 39-2).

After injury or sepsis, energy production becomes increasingly protein-dependent. Branched-chain amino acids (leucine, isoleucine, and valine) are oxidized from skeletal muscle as a source of nitrogen, energy for the muscle, and carbon skeletons for the glucose-alanine cycle and muscle glutamine synthesis. The fate of amino acid generation from muscle catabolism is shown in Figure 39-2.

The mobilization of **acute-phase proteins,** those secretory proteins in the liver that are altered in response to injury or infection, results in rapid loss of lean body mass and an increased negative nitrogen balance, which continues until the cause of the stress is relieved. Breakdown of protein tissue also causes increased urinary losses of potassium, phosphorus, and magnesium. Protein-C plays a role in host defense against infection along with a role in hemostasis; depleted levels of protein-C may be an indicator of morbidity and mortality in septic patients (Shorr et al., 2006).

Lipid metabolism is also altered in stress and sepsis. Increased circulation of free fatty acids is thought to result from increased lipolysis caused by elevated catecholamines and cortisol, as well as a marked elevation in the ratio of glucagon to insulin. The free fatty acids can be oxidized and used to form ketones, which provide energy to nonglucose-dependent tissues, or to resynthesize triglycerides.

Most notable is the hyperglycemia observed during stress. This initially results from a marked increase in glucose production and uptake secondary to gluconeogenesis and elevated levels of hormones, including epinephrine, that diminish insulin release. Stress also initiates the release of aldosterone, a corticosteroid that causes renal sodium retention, and vasopressin (antidiuretic hormone), which stimulates renal tubular water resorption. The action of these hormones results in conservation of water and salt and support of the circulating blood volume (see Table 39-2).

The response to injury is also regulated by metabolically active **cytokines** (proinflammatory proteins) such as **interleukin-1,** interleukin-6, and **tumor necrosis factor,** which are released by phagocytic cells in response to tissue damage, infection, inflammation, and some drugs and chemicals. Cytokines are thought to stimulate hepatic amino acid uptake and protein synthesis, accelerate muscle breakdown,

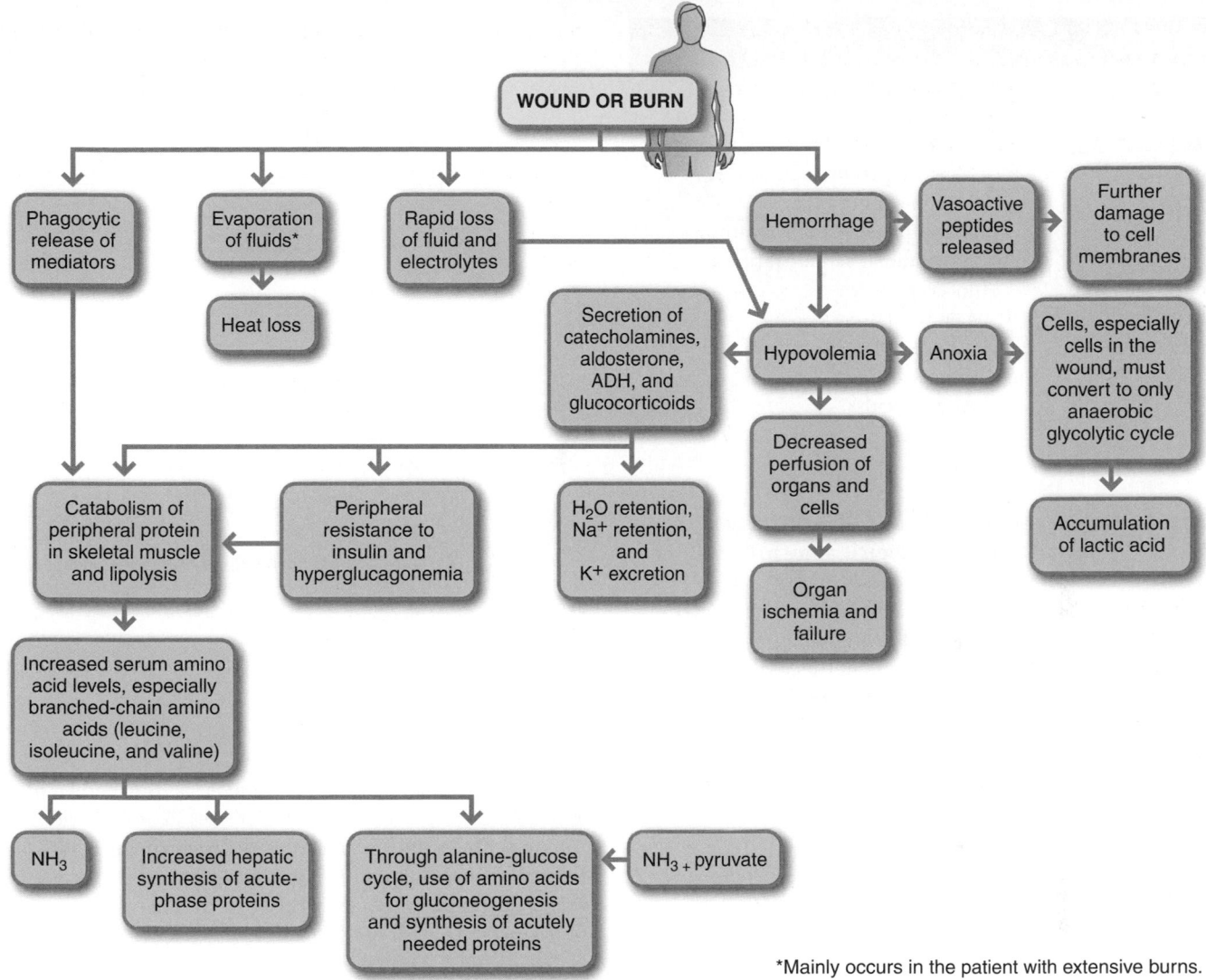

FIGURE 39-1 Physiologic and metabolic changes immediately after an injury or burn. The extent of these changes depends on the severity of the trauma. *ADH*, Antidiuretic hormone (or vasopressin); *NH₃*, ammonia.

TABLE 39-1

Characteristic of Metabolic Phases Occurring After Severe Injury

| EBB-Phase Response | Flow Phase | |
	Acute Response	Adaptive Response
Hypovolemic Shock	**Catabolism Predominates**	**Anabolism Predominates**
↓ Tissue perfusion	↑ Glucocorticoids	Hormonal response gradually diminishes
↓ Metabolic rate	↑ Glucagon	↓ Hypermetabolic rate
↓ Oxygen consumption	↑ Catecholamines	Associated with recovery
↓ Blood pressure	Release of cytokines, lipid mediators	Potential for restoration of body protein
↓ Body temperature	Production of acute-phase proteins	Wound healing depends in part on nutrient intake
	↑ Excretion of nitrogen	
	↑ Metabolic rate	
	↑ Oxygen consumption	
	Impaired use of fuels	

From *Enteral nutrition support in critical care*, Columbus, Oh, 1994, Ross Products Division, Abbott Labs.

TABLE 39-2

Metabolic Responses During Sepsis

Organ	Response
Liver	↑ Glucose production
	↑ Amino acid uptake
	↑ Acute-phase protein synthesis
	↑ Trace metal sequestration
Central nervous system	Anorexia
	Fever
Circulation	↑ Glucose
	↑ Triglycerides
	↑ Amino acids
	↑ Urea
	↓ Iron
	↓ Zinc
Skeletal muscle	↑ Amino acid efflux (especially glutamine), leading to loss of muscle mass
Intestine	↓ Amino acid uptake from both luminal and circulating sources, leading to gut mucosal atrophy
Endocrine	↑ Adrenocorticotropic hormone
	↑ Cortisol
	↑ Growth hormone
	↑ Epinephrine
	↑ Norepinephrine
	↑ Glucagons
	↑ Insulin (usually)

From Michie HR: Metabolism of sepsis and multiple organ failure, *World J Surg* 20:461, 1996.

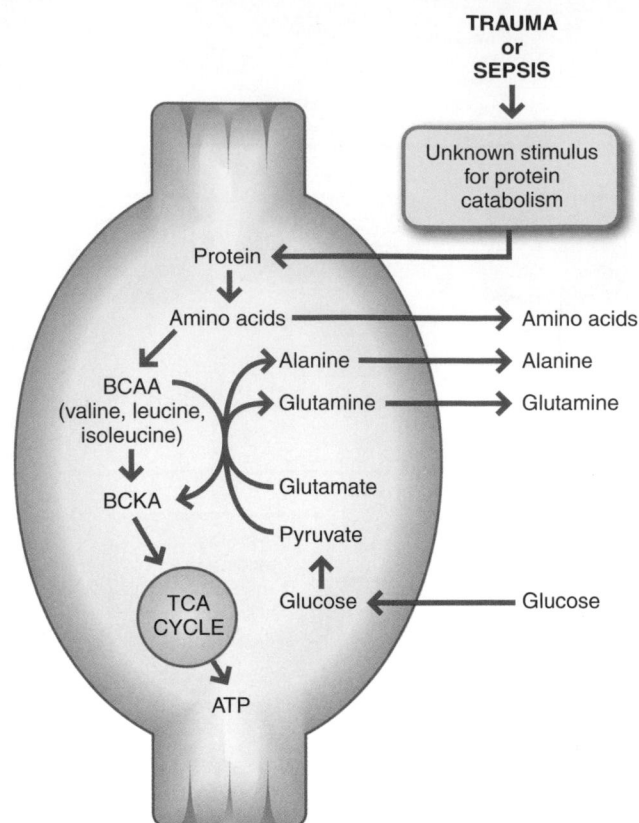

FIGURE 39-2 Skeletal muscle proteolysis. Breakdown of skeletal muscle protein leads to increases in amino acid levels. Amino acids are transaminated with glutamate or pyruvate to form alanine and glutamine. The muscle preferentially uses branched-chain amino acids (BCAAs) for energy through transamination with the formation of branched-chain ketoacids (BCKAs), which can enter the tricyclic acid (TCA) cycle for energy production. *(From Simmons RL, Steed DL: Basic science review for surgeons, Philadelphia, 1992, Saunders.)*

and induce gluconeogenesis. IL-1 appears to have a major role in stimulating the acute-phase response. The vagus nerve helps to regulate cytokine production through a "cholinergic antiinflammatory pathway," with release of nicotinic acetylcholine receptor alpha 7 (nAChR alpha7), which is being studied for treatment of diseases affected by excessive cytokine activity (Galloswitsch-Puerta and Tracey, 2005).

As part of the acute-phase response, serum iron and zinc levels also decrease, and levels of ceruloplasmin increase, primarily because of sequestration and, in the case of zinc, increased urinary zinc excretion. The net effect of the hormonally and cell-mediated response is an increase in oxygen supply and a greater availability of substrates for metabolically active tissues.

STARVATION VERSUS STRESS

The metabolic response to critical illness is very different from simple or uncomplicated starvation, in which loss of muscle is much slower in an adaptive response to preserve lean body mass. Stored glycogen, the primary fuel source in early starvation, is depleted in about 24 hours. After the depletion of glycogen, glucose is available from the break-

down of protein to amino acids, depicted in Figure 39-3. The depressed glucose levels lead to decreased insulin secretion and increased glucagon. During the adaptive state of starvation, protein catabolism is reduced, and hepatic gluconeogenesis decreases. Lipolytic activity is also different in starvation and in stress. After 1 week of fasting or food deprivation, a state of ketosis—in which ketones supply the bulk of energy needs, thus reducing the need for gluconeogenesis and conserving body protein to the greatest possible extent—develops. In late starvation, as in stress, ketone body production is increased, and fatty acids serve as a major energy source for all tissues except the glucose-obligated brain, nervous system, and red blood cells.

Starvation is characterized by decreased energy expenditure, diminished gluconeogenesis, increased ketone body production, and decreased ureagenesis. Conversely, energy expenditure in stress is markedly increased, as are gluconeogenesis, proteolysis, and ureagenesis. As discussed, the stress response is activated by hormonal and cell mediators—counter-regulatory hormones such as catecholamines, cortisol, and growth hormone. This media-

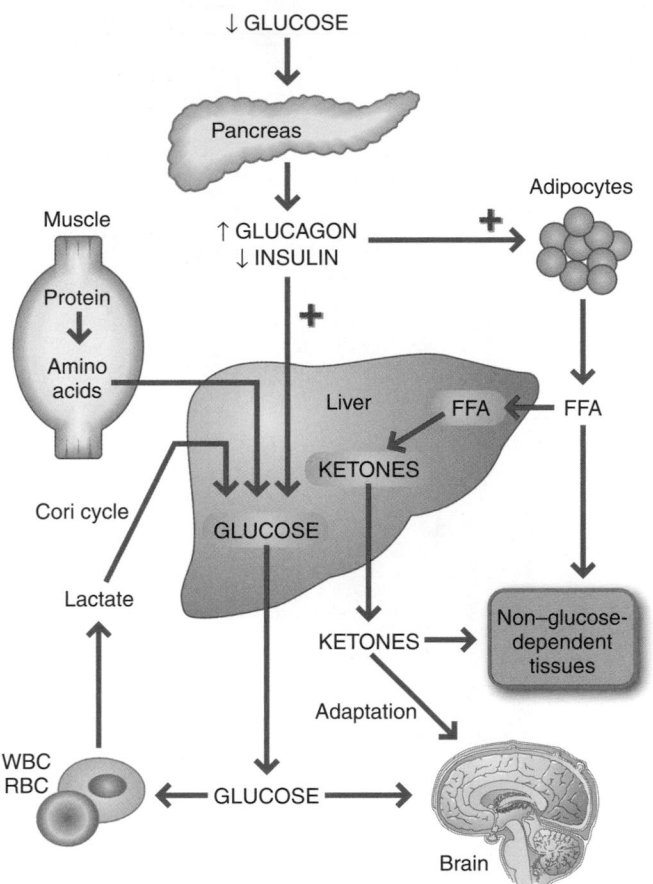

FIGURE 39-3 Metabolic changes in starvation. *FFAs,* Free fatty acids; *RBCs,* red blood cells; *WBCs,* white blood cells. *(From Simmons RL, Steed DL: Basic science review for surgeons, Philadelphia, 1992, Saunders.)*

TABLE 39-3

Comparison of Starvation and Stress Hypermetabolism*

	Starvation	Stress Hypermetabolism
Resting energy expenditure	Decreased	Increased
Respiratory quotient	(0.6-0.7)	(0.8-0.9)
Mediator activation	—	+++
Primary fuels	Fat	Mixed
Proteolysis	+	+++
Branched-chain oxidation	+	+++
Hepatic protein synthesis	+	+++
Ureagenesis	+	+++
Urinary nitrogen loss	+	+++
Gluconeogenesis	+	+++
Ketone body production	+ + + +	+

From Barton RG: Nutrition support in critical illness, *Nutr Clin Pract* 9:127, 1994. Modified from the American Society for Parenteral and Enteral Nutrition (ASPEN).

*Patients fall in a continuum between the extremes of starvation and stress hypermetabolism.

tor activation does not occur in starvation. Table 39-3 highlights the physiologic differences between starvation and stress.

SYSTEMIC INFLAMMATORY RESPONSE SYNDROME AND MULTIPLE ORGAN DYSFUNCTION SYNDROME

Pathophysiology

Sepsis and the systemic inflammatory response syndrome often complicate the course of a critically ill patient. The term *sepsis* is used when a patient has a documented infection and an identifiable organism. Bacteria and their toxins lead to a stronger inflammatory response. Other microorganisms that lead to an inflammatory response include viruses, fungi, and parasites.

Systemic inflammatory response syndrome (SIRS) is the preferred terminology to describe the widespread inflammation that can occur in infection, pancreatitis, ischemia, burns, multiple trauma, hemorrhagic shock, and immunologically mediated organ injury. The inflammation is usually present in areas remote from the primary site of injury and affects otherwise healthy tissue. Each condition leads to release of cytokines, proteolytic enzymes, or toxic oxygen species (free radicals) and activation of the complement cascade. SIRS is diagnosed according to criteria shown in Box 39-1.

A common complication of SIRS is the development of **multiple organ dysfunction syndrome (MODS).** The syndrome generally begins with lung failure and is followed by failure, in no particular order, of the liver, intestines, and kidney. Hematologic and myocardial failures usually manifest later; however, central nervous system changes can occur at any time (Deitch, 1992). MODS can be primary and the direct result of injury to an organ from trauma. Examples of primary MODS include pulmonary contusion, renal failure caused by rhabdomyolysis, or coagulopathy from multiple blood transfusions (Bone, 1992). Secondary MODS occurs in the presence of inflammation or infection in organs remote from the initial injury.

Patients with SIRS and MODS are clinically hypermetabolic and exhibit high cardiac output, low oxygen consumption, high venous oxygen saturation, and lactic acidemia. Patients generally have a strong positive fluid balance associated with massive edema and a decrease in plasma protein concentrations.

Multiple hypotheses have been proposed to explain the development of SIRS or MODS. In some animal models and clinical studies, SIRS leading to MODS appears to be

---

BOX 39-1

Diagnosis for Systemic Inflammatory Response Syndrome (SIRS)

Site of infection established and at least two of the following are present:

- Body temperature above 38° C or less than 36° C
- Heart rate more than 90 beats/min
- Respiratory rate greater than 20 breaths/min (tachypnea)
- $Paco_2$ of less than 32 mm Hg (hyperventilation)
- White blood cell count above 12,000/mm³ or less than 4000/mm³
- Bandemia—the presence of more than 10% bands (immature neutrophils) in the absence of chemotherapy-induced neutropenia and leukopenia

Data from Bone et al: ACCP/SCCM Consensus Conference: Definitions for sepsis and organ failure and guidelines for the use of innovative therapies in sepsis, *Chest* 101:1664, 1992.

---

mediated by excessive production of proinflammatory cytokines and other mediators of inflammation. The gut hypothesis suggests that the trigger is injury or disruption of the gut barrier function, with corresponding translocation of enteric bacteria into the mesentery lymph nodes, liver, and other organs (Figure 39-4). Unique gut-derived factors carried in the intestinal lymph but not the portal vein lead to acute injury- and shock-induced SIRS and MODS (Deitch et al., 2006).

Shock and resulting gut hypoperfusion are inciting events; the reperfused gut is a source of proinflammatory mediators; early gut hypoperfusion causes an **ileus** or lack of peristalsis in both the stomach and small bowel, and late infections cause further worsening of this gut dysfunction (Hassoun et al., 2001). Enteral feeding is thought to restore gut function and influence this clinical course. Alterations in intestinal gut barrier function associated with malnutrition are thought to occur through weight loss and villous atrophy. Because enteral feeding promotes the maintenance of villous height and brush border enzymes, feedings may be better tolerated when initiated promptly while this absorptive area remains intact (see Chapter 20).

Aspects of gut barrier function related to immunity and the route and type of nutrition support are active areas of research. Experimental and clinical data demonstrate that cells processed within the **gut-associated lymphoid tissue** can migrate outside of the intestine to the respiratory tract and other mucosal surfaces and induce immunity (Kudsk, 2002). Lack of enteric stimulation is associated with mucosal atrophy and decreased intestinal absorption; this is thought to negatively affect the host defense against bacterial and toxin products in the intestine in septic patients. This **bacterial translocation** from the intestinal lumen to the mesenteric lymph nodes is well documented in animals, especially rats, but does not occur to the same extent in humans (Alpers, 2002).

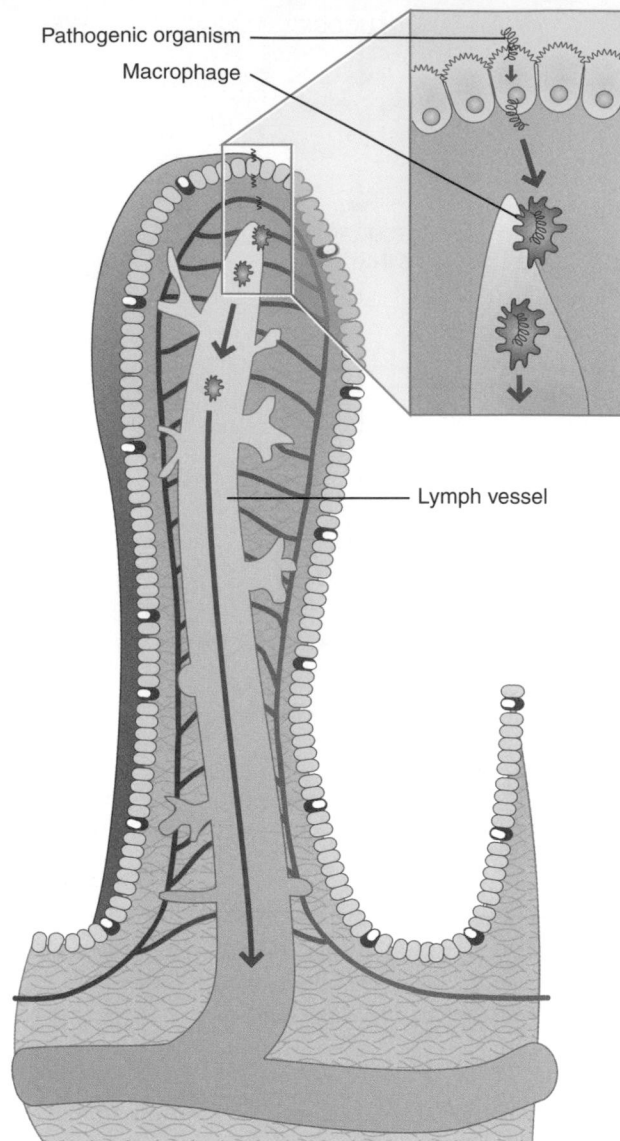

FIGURE 39-4 Bacterial translocation across microvilli and spread into the bloodstream.

Medical Nutrition Therapy

Nutritional Assessment

The critically ill patient typically enters an intensive care unit (ICU) because of a cardiopulmonary diagnosis, intraoperative or postoperative complication, multiple trauma, burn injury, or sepsis. Patients often have numerous catheters for intravenous (IV) fluids and invasive **hemodynamic** (related to cardiac output and blood flow) monitoring, as well as tubes for drainage of body fluids.

Traditional methods of assessing nutritional status are often of limited value in the critical care setting. The severely injured patient is usually unable to provide a dietary history. Values for weight may be erroneous after fluid resuscitation, and anthropometric measurements are not easily attainable nor are they sensitive to acute changes. Abnormal serum albumin may result both from the effects of

BOX 39-2

Factors to Consider in Screening an ICU Patient

Factors to Consider With ICU Medical Admission

Preadmission nutrition status
Organ function
Use of pharmacologic agents, vasopressors, and other paralytic agents
Ability to predict clinical course (i.e., length of intubation or ventilator dependence)
Need for enteral or parenteral nutrition

Factors to Consider With Postoperative ICU Admission

Intraoperative complications
Preoperative nutrition status
Cardiopulmonary event
Diagnosis
Sepsis or systemic inflammatory response syndrome
Gastrointestinal function
Ability to predict return of gastrointestinal function
Nutrition support access options

Factors to Consider With Burn or Trauma ICU Admission

Preinjury nutrition status
Type of trauma
Extent of injury
Surgical findings
Gastrointestinal function
Enteral access options

undernutrition and the severity of illness or underlying disease. Other plasma proteins such as transthyretin and transferrin often drop precipitously, related not to nutrition status but to an inflammatory-induced decrease in hepatic synthesis and changes caused by compartmental shifts in body fluid. This is part of the acute-phase response in which secretory and circulating proteins are altered in response to inflammation or injury. Because of the difficulties in conducting a nutrition assessment in a critically ill patient, clinical judgment must play a major role in deciding when to offer nutrition support.

In general, assessment focuses on the preadmission, preoperative, or preinjury nutrition status; presence of any organ system dysfunction; the need for early nutrition support; and options that exist for enteral or parenteral access. Care planning should consider the factors in Box 39-2. When monitoring critically ill patients, one must focus on laboratory data, not to define or determine nutrition status but to design the nutrition prescription (see Chapter 20).

Practitioners should review indices of organ system function, blood glucose, and laboratory abnormalities, specifically electrolytes and acid-base balance, which may impact enteral and parenteral formulations or the diet order. Urine urea nitrogen (UUN) excretion in grams per day has been used to evaluate the degree of hypermetabolism. A UUN value of 0 to 5 corresponds to no stress, 5 to 10 to mild hypermetabolism or level 1 stress, 10 to 15 to moderate hypermetabolism or level 2 stress, and greater than 15 to a severe hypermetabolic state or level 3 stress (Blackburn et al., 1977).

Goals of Nutrition Support

The goals of nutrition support during sepsis and after injury include minimization of starvation, prevention or correction of specific nutrient deficiencies, provision of adequate calories to meet energy needs while minimizing associated metabolic complications, and fluid and electrolyte management to maintain adequate urine output and normal homeostasis (see *Pathophysiology and Care Management Algorithm:* Hypermetabolic Response). The first emphasis of care is fluid resuscitation and the removal of the inflicting stress through wound repair, abscess drainage, burn wound debridement and grafting, or treatment of infection. Nutrition support should begin as soon as the patient is hemodynamically stable (stabilized vital functions, fluid and electrolyte and acid-base balance, and adequate tissue perfusion to allow transport of oxygen and fuel).

Trauma, sepsis, and surgery are associated with hypercatabolism and a negative nitrogen balance (Teng Chung and Hinds, 2006). The provision of nutrition support alone cannot abolish the hypermetabolic response (Wolfe and Martini, 2000). Critically ill patients who are injured, septic, or bedridden cannot be expected to gain weight, lean body mass, or strength until the source of hypermetabolism is treated or corrected and physical therapy or exercise is begun. This is the point at which the patient transitions into the anabolic phase of his or her disease course. The ASPEN practice guidelines for critical care at this stage are outlined in Box 39-3.

Nutritional Requirements

Energy. Critically ill patients should receive feedings at rates of 25 to 30 kcal/kg (ASPEN Board of Directors, 2002). Although adequate energy is essential to metabolically stressed patients, excess calories can result in complications such as hyperglycemia, hepatic steatosis, and excess carbon dioxide production, which can exacerbate respiratory insufficiency or prolong weaning from mechanical ventilation (see Chapter 35).

Persistent hyperglycemia can lead to hyperosmolar nonketotic coma and glucose-obligated diuresis, which may complicate fluid and electrolyte management. Hyperglycemia associated with insulin resistance in critically ill patients may also lead to complications and increased susceptibility to severe infection. A landmark study demonstrated that intensive insulin therapy maintaining blood glucose at or below 110 mg/dl is associated with reduced morbidity and mortality in cardiothoracic surgical ICU patients (Van Den Berghe et al., 2001). Research has confirmed that strict glycemic control can result in decreased wound infections, decreased subsequent organ failure, and

PATHOPHYSIOLOGY AND CARE MANAGEMENT ALGORITHM

Hypermetabolic Response

ETIOLOGY

Sepsis → Hypermetabolic Response

Trauma → Hypermetabolic Response

Fractures → Hypermetabolic Response

Burns → Hypermetabolic Response

Stress → Hypermetabolic Response

Major surgery → Hypermetabolic Response

PATHOPHYSIOLOGY

EBB Phase

Hypovolemia
Shock
Tissue hypoxia
Decreased:
• Cardiac output
• O_2 consumption
• Body temperature

Flow Phase

Acute-phase proteins
Hormonal responses
Immune responses (cell-mediated and antibody)
Increased:
• Cardiac output
• O_2 consumption
• Body temperature
• Energy expenditure
• Protein catabolism

MANAGEMENT

Medical Management

• Treat cause of hypermetabolism
• Physical therapy
• Exercise

Nutrition Management

• Minimize catabolism
• Meet energy requirements, but do not overfeed
  • Non-obese: 25-30 kcal/kg/day
  • Obese: 18-20 kcal/kg/day
• Meet protein, vitamin, and mineral needs
• Establish and maintain fluid and electrolyte balance
• Plan nutrition therapy (oral, enteral, and/or parental nutrition)

Algorithm content developed by John J.B. Anderson, PhD, and Sanford C. Garner, PhD, 2000. Updated by Marlon F. Winkler, MS, RD, LDN, CNSD, and Ainsley Malone, MS, RD, CNSD, 2002.

decreased mortality in both medical and surgical ICU patients (Butler et al., 2005; Bochicchio et al., 2005; Finney et al., 2003).

Energy requirements can be estimated with the new dietary reference intake (DRI) equations (see Chapter 2). Avoidance of overfeeding the critically ill, stressed patient is important. Some clinicians favor the use of specific predictive equations for energy expenditure that include physiologically based variables such as minute ventilation and core temperature (Penn State Equation, Swinamer Equation [Swinamer et al., 1990]) rather than the static variables of height and weight. Minute ventilation and core temperature better reflect the physiologic effects of disease state and clinical status than do height and weight, which are fixed. More research is needed to validate this practice (Frankenfield et al., 2004).

BOX 39-3

ASPEN Practice Guidelines for Critical Care

- Patients with critical illnesses are at nutritional risk and should undergo nutrition screening to identify those who require formal nutrition assessment with development of a nutrition care plan.
- Specialized nutrition support should be initiated when it is anticipated that critically ill patients will be unable to meet their nutrient needs orally for a period of 5 to 10 days.
- Enteral nutrition is the preferred route of feeding in critically ill patients who require specialized nutrition support.
- Parenteral nutrition should be reserved for patients who require specialized nutrition support and in whom enteral nutrition is not possible.

Data from ASPEN Board of Directors: Guidelines for the use of parenteral and enteral nutrition in adult and pediatric patients, *JPEN J Parenter Enteral Nutr* 26(suppl):1S, 2002.

Once the patient is hemodynamically stable and ambulating or undergoing rehabilitation, caloric delivery can be in a higher anabolic range, and energy requirements may be estimated at >30 kcal/kg. However, it is important not to overestimate the caloric requirements of mechanically ventilated and sedated patients; neuromuscular paralysis may decrease energy requirements, even in septic patients, by as much as 30%.

The amount of energy to provide critically ill obese patients is a topic of current interest. Recent research has demonstrated improved glycemic control and positive clinical outcomes in obese patients who were provided with 22 kcal/kg of ideal weight in conjunction with increased protein intakes (Choban and Dickerson, 2005). Energy requirements are difficult to predict in critically ill obese patients because of the metabolic response to critical illness and degree of stress. Indirect calorimetry (see Chapter 2) provides a good estimate of energy expenditure; however, its predictive value is more variable when body mass index exceeds 50 (Glynn et al., 1999).

There is some debate in practice as to what value should be used for weight in predictive equations. Breen and Ireton-Jones conclude that actual body weight is a better predictor of energy expenditure than ideal body weight in obese individuals (Breen and Ireton-Jones, 2004). A thorough evaluation of the literature suggests that the Mifflin-St. Jeor equation is the most effective of several predictive equations (Frankenfield et al., 2005).

Research suggests that hypocaloric, high-protein nutrition support or "permissive underfeeding" in critically ill obese patients results in achievement of net protein anabolism and minimizes complications resulting from overfeeding. Dickerson (2005) recently summarized this research in a review of studies using hypocaloric specialized nutrition support in obese ICU patients. Although there is no agreement as to what constitutes hypocaloric feeding, studies suggest that this approximates 18 to 20 kcal/kg/day.

Indirect calorimetry is the preferred method for measurement of oxygen consumption in severely injured patients (Epstein et al., 2000). Oxygen consumption is an essential component in the determination of energy expenditure. Many investigators have examined the alterations in energy expenditure associated with critical illness and have documented substantial increases, particularly in septic and trauma patients (Moriyama et al., 1999; Uehara et al., 1999). Indirect calorimetry can be performed serially as a patient's clinical status changes (Compher et al., 2006); this allows a more accurate assessment of energy requirements over a patient's course in the ICU (see Chapter 2).

Indirect calorimetry is not appropriate for all patients, however, and should be performed and interpreted by experienced clinicians (Compher et al., 2006). High oxygen requirements, the presence of a chest tube, acidosis, and the use of supplemental oxygen are several factors that produce invalid results. In these situations measurement of energy expenditure by indirect calorimetry is not recommended (Malone, 2002).

Glucose is the primary caloric substrate in a parenteral nutrition formulation. The maximum rate of glucose oxidation is approximately 5 to 7 mg/kg/min or 7.2 g/kg/day (Wolfe et al., 1979). Part of this glucose load is provided endogenously via gluconeogenesis. Carbohydrate should constitute approximately 60% to 70% of goal energy intake. Parenteral nutrition should be initiated with a low dextrose infusion rate, and blood glucose should be closely monitored in patients with diabetes, preexisting hyperglycemia, or risk of glucose intolerance. Insulin should be administered to maintain blood glucose levels at desirable levels. In some cases continuous insulin infusion may be useful. The exact desirable blood glucose level varies for each patient, and iatrogenic hypoglycemia must also be avoided (Turina et al., 2006).

Fat should be 15% to 40% of energy intake. Fat is used not only to prevent essential fatty acid deficiency but also to meet elevated energy requirements, particularly in the presence of glucose intolerance. The use of IV fat emulsion in stressed, and trauma patients should be monitored carefully because fatty acids modulate the immune response (Fritsche, 2006).

Protein. Amino acids are supplied to critically ill patients as part of the total nutrition regimen to support the synthesis of proteins required for defense and recovery, to spare lean body mass, and to reduce the amount of endogenous protein catabolism for gluconeogenesis. For the unstressed adult patient with adequate organ function requiring nutrition support, 0.8 g/kg/day may be adequate, but requirements may rise with metabolic demands to levels of about 2 g/kg/day (ASPEN Board of Directors, 2002). Providing exogenous amino acids does not alter the catabolic state, but it does decrease the characteristic negative nitrogen balance by supplying the liver with substrates for protein synthesis and subsequently reducing the need for endogenous proteins from peripheral tissue.

Vitamins, Minerals, and Trace Elements. No specific guidelines exist for the provision of vitamins, minerals, and trace elements in metabolically stressed individuals. Micronutrient needs are elevated during acute illness because of increased urinary and cutaneous losses and diminished gastrointestinal absorption, altered distribution, and altered carrier protein concentrations (Prelack and Sheridan, 2001). With increased caloric intake there may be an increased need for B vitamins, particularly thiamin and niacin. Catabolism and loss of lean body tissue increase the loss of potassium, magnesium, phosphorus, and zinc. Gastrointestinal and urinary losses, organ dysfunction, and acid-base imbalance necessitate that mineral and electrolyte requirements be determined and adjusted individually. Fluid and electrolytes should be provided to maintain adequate urine output and normal serum electrolytes.

Feeding Strategies. The preferred route for nutrient delivery is an oral diet. However, critically ill patients are often unable to eat because of endotracheal intubation and ventilator dependence. Furthermore, oral feeding may be delayed by impairment of chewing, swallowing, or anorexia induced by pain-relieving medications or posttraumatic shock and depression. Patients who are able to eat may not be able to meet the increased energy and nutrient requirements associated with metabolic stress and recovery and often require combinations of oral nutritional supplements, enteral tube nutrition, and parenteral nutrition. When enteral nutrition fails to meet nutritional requirements or when gastrointestinal feeding is contraindicated, parenteral nutrition support should be initiated (Figure 39-5).

Timing and Route of Feeding. Enteral is the preferred method for nutrition support because it is more physiological and leads to fewer infectious complications (DiSario, 2006). Successful enteral nutrition for surgical or stressed patients may require access to the small bowel. Critically ill patients are presumed to be at a higher risk of aspiration because of conditions such as respiratory insufficiency, gastric dysmotility, or neuromuscular paralysis. Although transpyloric feeding may be useful for those with regurgitation and aspiration of gastric feeds, the rate of aspiration when patients are fed into the stomach versus the small bowel is not significantly different (Kattelmann et al., 2006; Malik and Zaloga, 2003).

Gastric motility is usually impaired for 12 to 24 hours after laparotomy, whereas a colonic ileus may last up to 5 days. Generally small bowel motility returns within 4 to 6 hours after surgery. An enteric feeding tube may be placed if the patient is expected to be unable to consume food by mouth for an extended period. Tubes can be placed under x-ray guidance, endoscopically, or intraoperatively into the stomach or small bowel (see Chapter 20).

Initially patients with multiple intestinal injuries, small bowel ileus, high-output intestinal fistulas, or other severe intestinal insults may require total parenteral nutrition (TPN). However, because of the demonstrated benefits of early enteral nutrition, tube feedings can often be administered simultaneously with TPN at low rates to maintain gut integrity. This allows adequate nutrient delivery while helping to preserve the intestinal mucosa.

Although early enteral feeding has proven benefits, waiting until the patient is hemodynamically stable before beginning remains important. Anaerobic metabolism during shock and after resuscitation differs, and the aggressive delivery of enteral nutrients when the intestines are in a state of hypoperfusion may result in increased intestinal ischemia and necrosis (Tappenden et al., 1998).

Formula Selection. Choosing an enteral product should be based on fluid, energy, and nutrient requirements, as well as gastrointestinal function. Most standard polymeric enteral formulas can be used to feed the critically ill patient. Some critically ill patients demonstrate intolerance to standard diets because of the fat content of the formula and temporarily require a lower-fat diet or a product containing a higher ratio of medium-chain triglycerides. Several commercially available products are marketed specifically for patients with trauma and metabolic stress. These products typically have higher protein content and a higher ratio of BCAAs or additional glutamine or arginine (see Appendix 32).

Specialized enteral formulas designed to enhance the immune system have been investigated for their role in improving patient outcomes. Complex pharmaconutrient formulas that contain arginine, glutamine, and omega-3 fatty acids have been proven to shorten hospital stay, decrease the incidence of infection, and reduce hospital costs in selected groups of patients (Alexander, 2002). The effects are greatest in patients with severe trauma, including burn injury; and major surgical procedures, especially when malnourished. However, in the septic population there is concern that the use of specialized enteral formulas may have a detrimental effect (Consensus Recommendations, 2001).

Figure 39-6 depicts **glutamine** metabolism and demonstrates its uptake by the kidney and the intestine as a preferential fuel for enterocytes. Glutamine can attenuate gut permeability following critical illness and injury, and it attenuates the systemic inflammatory response driven by the gut (Wischmeyer, 2006). Specialty supplemented enteral formulas administered to critically ill or injured patients and surgical patients have been documented to be beneficial in a number of randomized prospective studies (Kudsk, 2006). However, routine use of immune-enhancing formulas in the critically ill patient is not recommended (American Dietetic Association, 2006). Parenteral nutrition formulations have not traditionally contained glutamine because of instability in the solution, and, as a result, TPN has been thought to contribute to this deficiency.

Dietary fiber is known to maintain colonic integrity. The colonic fermentation of fiber and other nondigestible carbohydrates produces the short-chain fatty acids (SCFAs) propionate, acetate, and butyrate. These substances are readily

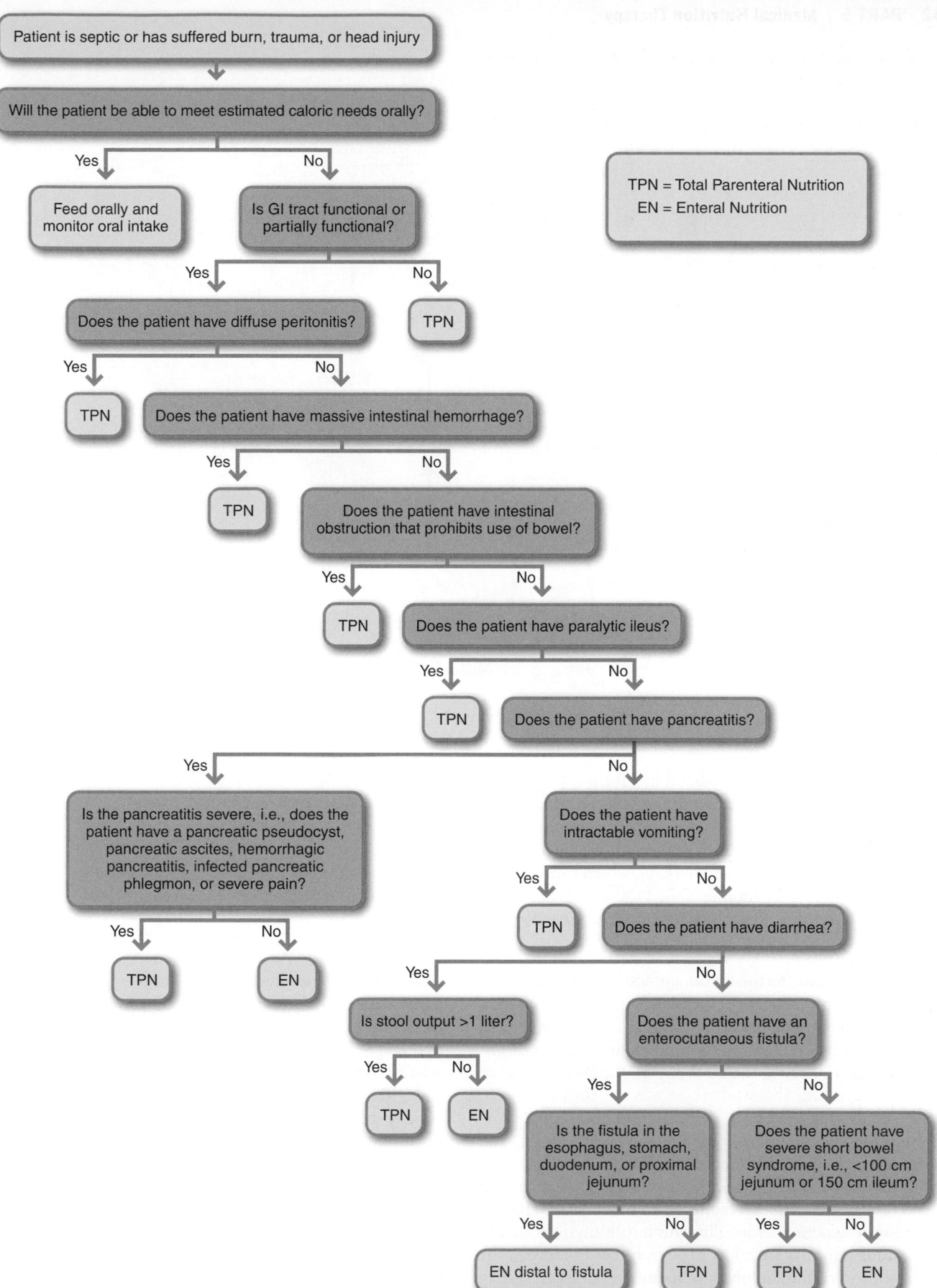

FIGURE 39-5 Determining the route of nutrition support in the critically ill patient. *GI*, Gastrointestinal. (*ASPEN Nutrition Support Practice Manual*: Determining the route of nutrition support in the critically ill, *Silver Spring, Md, 1998, ASPEN. [ASPEN does not endorse the use of this material in any form other than in its entirety.]*)

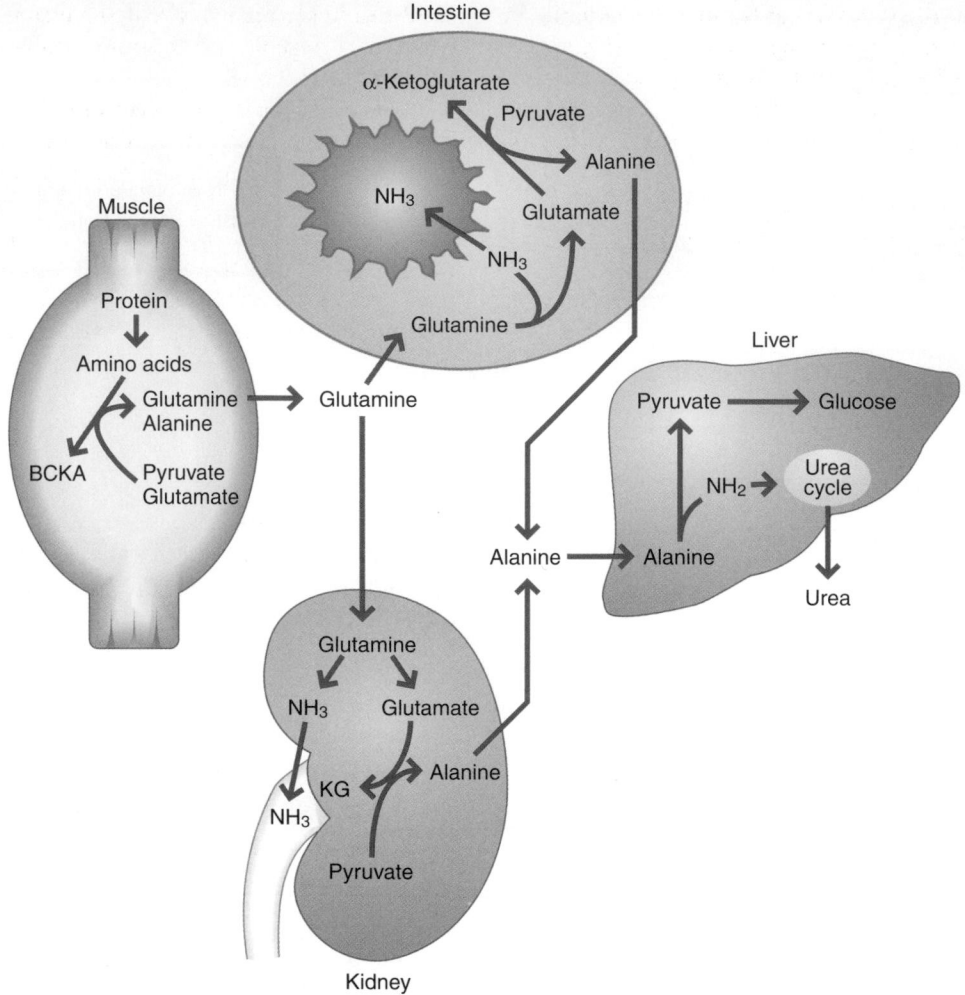

FIGURE 39-6 Glutamine metabolism. Glutamine is generated by skeletal muscle from glutamate by transamination. Glutamine is taken up by the intestine and kidney, where deamination and ammonia elimination occur. The glutamate formed is transaminated with pyruvate to form alanine, which goes to the liver for gluconeogenesis, and α-ketoglutarate (KG), which can be used for energy production by the muscle or kidney. *NH₂*, Amine; *NH₃*, ammonia. (*From Simmons RL, Steed DL: Basic science review for surgeons, Philadelphia, 1992, Saunders.*)

absorbed, are trophic to the colonocyte, stimulate water and sodium absorption, and may provide a significant source of energy. Research continues on additional roles of SCFAs in reducing risk of developing gastrointestinal disorders, cancer, and cardiovascular disease (Wong et al., 2006).

Anabolic Hormones

Combinations of anabolic hormones, growth factors, and specific nutrients have been used to enhance nutrition support and modify the metabolic response to trauma and critical illness. **Growth hormone (GH)** stimulates growth, antagonizes the action of insulin, and has lipolytic activity.

In trauma patients with low growth hormone levels, the administration of human growth hormone has been shown to improve protein and fat metabolism (Jeevanandam et al., 1992, 1995). The administration of growth hormone to pediatric burn patients has shown positive results, especially in lean body mass and growth (Przkora et al., 2006).

In addition, many small clinical studies indicate that treatment with recombinant human (rh) GH is a safe and effective means of limiting the catabolic response; however, two large prospective randomized controlled trials demonstrated that administration of rhGH to long-stay critically ill adults increases morbidity and mortality (Teng Chung and Hinds, 2006). Caution in the use of growth hormone therapy in critically ill patients.

HEAD INJURY

Pathophysiology

Patients with traumatic brain injury (TBI) are severely hypermetabolic and catabolic. The more severe the head injury, the greater is the release of catecholamines (norepinephrine and epinephrine) and cortisol and the hypermetabolic response. Although most brain-injured patients are well nourished before injury, without aggressive nutrition support, rapid loss in lean body mass and immunosuppression can occur. With evidence that neurons are capable of regenerating, it becomes crucial to provide an environment conducive for repair. The **Glasgow Coma Scale (GCS)** is a commonly used tool for quantifying a patient's state of consciousness. A score of 14 to 15 indicates minor head injury; 9 to 13 corresponds to moderate injury; and a less than 8 reflects severe injury (Hester, 1993) (see Chapter 41).

Medical Nutrition Therapy

Energy Requirements

Energy metabolism of the brain is highly aerobic, with little capacity for anaerobic glycolysis and limited tissue stores of glucose; a steady supply of oxygen and glucose is essential. Mitochondrial respiratory oxidative phosphorylation and calcium transport are compromised by TBI. Energy expenditure in TBI is often as much as 40% greater than normal. Patients with a GCS of 4 to 5 often have the highest energy expenditure. On the other hand, brain-dead patients or those who receive sedatives, barbiturates, or musculoskeletal blocking agents often have lower-than-predicted energy expenditure, averaging about 14% less (Hester, 1993). The use of indirect calorimetry is helpful in determining the caloric requirements of these patients because overfeeding or underfeeding can be harmful (see Chapter 2).

Protein Requirements

Because achieving early nitrogen equilibrium is very difficult, minimizing catabolism is paramount. Protein requirements are generally estimated at 1.5 to 2.2 g/kg of body weight. An adequate amount of nonprotein calories is essential for protein sparing; thus including 30% to 40% of kcal from fat and especially omega-3 fatty acids is important (Twyman, 1997).

Vitamins, Minerals, and Fluid

Although the requirements for vitamins and minerals are not well established for brain-injured individuals, studies have shown decreased plasma levels of many B vitamins and vitamin C. Urinary zinc excretion increases significantly during stress, and serum zinc levels are often low. Because salt wasting occasionally occurs in the brain-injured patient, treatment may consist of restricting fluids, providing additional sodium, or both. In addition, osmotic dehydration may be performed to control cerebral swelling.

Methods of Nutrition Support

Some brain-injured individuals are unable to take oral nutrition, and many experience dysphagia. Impairment can be physiologic or cognitive. These individuals may have a delayed or absent swallowing reflex, reduced lingual control, prolonged oral transit time, reduced pharyngeal peristalsis, or laryngeal incompetence (see Chapter 41). Patients may be easily distracted, which greatly prolongs mealtime and

results in inadequate intake. Conversely some brain-injured patients eat rapidly and consume excessive amounts of food, even nonfood items.

Early nutrition support is essential and may help decrease intestinal permeability to toxins. Furthermore, prompt use of the gut should maintain the intestinal absorptive area. Patients commonly experience impaired gastric emptying, which hinders the ability to feed via a nasogastric or gastrostomy tube. Access to the small bowel has allowed for successful enteral feeding in many instances, and parenteral and enteral nutrition support often is combined.

MAJOR BURNS

Pathophysiology

Major burns result in severe trauma. Energy requirements can increase as much as 100% above resting energy expenditure (REE), depending on the extent and depth of the injury (Figure 39-7). Exaggerated protein catabolism and increased urinary nitrogen excretion accompany this hypermetabolism. Protein is also lost through the burn wound exudate. Burn patients are particularly susceptible to infection, and this markedly increases requirements for both energy and protein. Because patients with major burns may develop an ileus and are anorexic, nutrition support can be a real challenge.

Medical Management

Fluid and Electrolyte Repletion

The first 24 to 48 hours of treatment for thermally injured patients are devoted to fluid and electrolyte replacement. A variety of formulas have been developed to calculate the volume of resuscitation fluid needed. Most providers agree that half of the calculated volume for the first 24 hours should be given during the first 8 hours because this is the period of greatest intravascular loss.

The volume of fluid needed is based on the age and weight of the patient and the extent of the burn. Variations of a standard known as the Lund and Browder chart (Lund and Browder, 1944) can be used to determine the percentage of total body surface area (TBSA) burned. Once resuscitation is complete, ample fluids must be given to cover both maintenance requirements and evaporative losses that continue through open wounds. Evaporative water loss can be estimated at 2 to 3.1 ml/kg of body weight per 24 hours per percent of TBSA burn. Serum sodium, osmolar concentrations, and body weight are used to monitor fluid status. Providing adequate fluids and electrolytes as early as possible after injury is paramount for maintaining circulatory volume and preventing ischemia.

Wound Management

Wound management depends on the depth and extent of the burn. Current surgical management promotes early debridement, excision, and grafting. Energy expenditure may

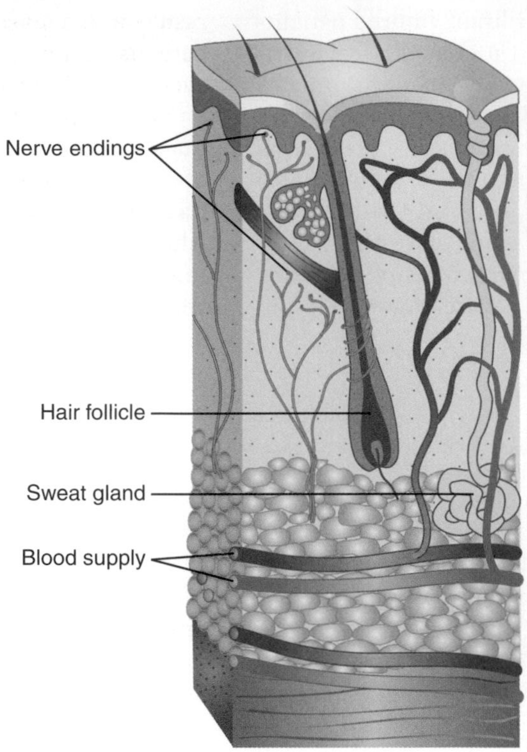

FIGURE 39-7 Interpretation of burn classification based on damage to the integument.

TISSUE LAYER	SKIN THICKNESS (inches)	DEPTH OF BURN
Epidermis	0.010	1
Dermis	0.020	2
Subcutaneous tissue	0.035	3
Muscle	0.040	4

be reduced slightly by the practice of covering wounds as early as possible to reduce evaporative heat and nitrogen losses and prevent infection.

Ancillary Measures

Physical therapy helps prevent muscle wasting and atrophy. A warm environment minimizes heat loss and the expenditure of energy to maintain body temperature. Thermal blankets, heat lamps, and individual heat shields are often used to maintain environmental temperature near 30° C (86° F). Minimizing fear and pain with reassurance from the staff and adequate pain medication can also reduce catecholamine stimulation and help to avoid increases in energy expenditure. Finally, antacids are given to patients with major burns to prevent formation of stress-related Curling's ulcers in the gastric or duodenal mucosa.

Medical Nutrition Therapy

Along with early wound coverage and infection control, nutrition support is recognized as one of the most significant aspects of care for the burned patient. Weight loss is a common complication in the burn unit (Lee et al., 2005). Wound healing can occur only in an anabolic state. Feeding should be initiated soon after resuscitation is complete. In fact, very early enteral feeding (within 4 to 12 hours of hospitalization) has been shown to be successful in decreasing the hypercatabolic response, thus decreasing the release of catecholamines, decreasing glucagon, reducing weight loss, and shortening the length of hospital stay (McClave et al., 2002).

Achievement of enteral access and provision of a sufficient volume of enteral nutrients early in the hospital course of a critically ill burned patient affords an opportunity to improve the outcome of that patient. Enteral feeding provides a conduit for the delivery of immune stimulants and serves as effective prophylaxis against stress-induced gastropathy and gastrointestinal hemorrhage. Tube placement beyond the stomach into the small bowel in hypermetabolic, severely ill patients prone to ileus and disordered gut motility may aid delivery of enteral nutrients while reducing risk of aspiration. Placement of enteral tubes during surgery has been practiced at some burn centers in an effort to minimize the length of time a burn patient is without nutrition support. See Box 39-4 for the nutritional care goals for the burned person.

Energy Requirements

The increased energy needs of the burned patient vary according to the size of the burn. Various formulas have been developed for estimating energy needs. The Curreri formula (1979) is as follows:

$$\text{Energy} = 24 \text{ kcal} \times \text{usual body wt (kg)} + 40 \text{ kcal} \times \%\text{TBSA burned}$$

The measurement of metabolic rate by indirect calorimetry has confirmed that the Curreri formula exceeds actual energy expenditure (Saffle et al., 1990). The Curreri formula may overestimate energy expenditure because of overall improvements in burn care and management since the formula was developed (Gottschlich and Ireton-Jones, 2001).

Once a burn exceeds 50% to 60% TBSA, minimum increases in energy expenditure occur. Some formulas do not establish an upper limit to the number of calories required. When these formulas are used, it should be noted that the maximum caloric load that the body can handle is approximately 100% above resting metabolic expenditure (2 × REE).

BOX 39-4

Nutrition Care Goals for Burned Patients

1. Minimize metabolic response by:
   - Controlling environmental temperature
   - Maintaining fluid and electrolyte balance
   - Controlling pain and anxiety
   - Covering wounds early
2. Meet nutritional needs by:
   - Providing adequate calories to prevent weight loss of greater than 10% of usual body weight
   - Providing adequate protein for positive nitrogen balance and maintenance or repletion of circulating proteins
   - Providing vitamin and mineral supplementation as indicated
3. Prevent Curling's ulcer by:
   - Providing antacids or continuous enteral feedings

Measuring energy expenditure via indirect calorimetry is the most reliable method for assessing energy expenditure in burned patients. Increasing energy expenditure by 20% to 30% is necessary to account for energy expenditure associated with wound care and physical therapy. An alternate equation for assessing energy expenditure in the burned patient has been developed that accounts for burn injury and ventilatory status. The Ireton-Jones equation, which follows, has been repeatedly validated since its initial development (Gagliardi et al., 1995; Ireton-Jones et al., 1992; Ireton-Jones and Jones, 1997, 2002; Wall et al., 1995).

$$EEE = 1784 - 11(A) + 5(W) + 244(G) + 239(T) + 804(B)$$

EEE = Estimated Energy Expenditure
  A = Age
  W = Weight (kg)
  G = Gender (male = 1, female = 0)
  T = Diagnosis of trauma (absent = 0, present = 1)
  B = Diagnosis of burn (absent = 0, present = 1)

Additional calories may be required to meet the needs because of fever, sepsis, multiple traumas, or the stress of surgery. Although weight gain may be desirable for the severely underweight patient, this is generally not feasible until after the acute illness. Weight maintenance should be the goal for overweight patients until the healing process is complete. Obese individuals may be at higher risk of wound infection and graft disruption. The energy requirement for the obese burned person is probably more than that calculated when ideal body weight is used but less than that calculated when actual body weight is used. Indirect calorimetry is the most accurate method of determining the energy needs of the obese person who is burned.

An accurate formula for calculating the nutritional needs of the pediatric burn patient remains to be developed. Be-cause basic requirements depend on the stage of growth and development and gender, providing a formula to cover all age-groups is difficult. The commonly used Galveston formula estimates the caloric requirements as 1800 kcal/m² + 2200 kcal/m² TBSA burned (Hildreth et al., 1989). However, it has also been documented that burned boys have higher REEs than do burned girls; thus this needs to be taken into account in determining their energy requirements (Mlcak et al., 2006). Mayes and Gottschlich (2003) estimate caloric need for children younger than 3 years of age as 108 + (68 × kg weight) + 3.9 × % TBSA.

Energy Sources

Carbohydrates are excellent for protein sparing. However, although carbohydrate is recommended as the chief energy source in burn patients, there appears to be a maximum glucose load of 7 mg/kg/min, above which glucose is not oxidized but rather is converted to fat (Wolfe et al., 1979). This state of lipogenesis causes increased oxygen consumption and carbon dioxide production (see Chapter 35). Excessive carbohydrate can aggravate hyperglycemia and cause osmotic diuresis, dehydration, and respiratory difficulty.

Although lipids are a concentrated source of calories, high levels of lipids may cause deleterious immunologic responses and increased susceptibility to infections. The composition of the lipid is important because diets high in omega-3 fatty acids may result in improved immune response and tube-feeding tolerance (Alexander and Gottschlich, 1990). The omega-3 fatty acids inhibit the production of prostaglandin E_2 and leukotrienes, which have immunosuppressive properties. However, omega-3 fatty acids are not usually added during the early stages because of their antiinflammatory effect.

The administration, both enterally and parenterally, of a low-fat formula results in less pneumonia, improved respiratory function, faster recovery of nutrition status, and a shorter length of care (Garrel et al., 1995). A reasonable approach is to begin by limiting lipids to 12% to 15% of the nonprotein calories, giving attention to indicators of immune function, feeding tolerance, and serum triglycerides before higher amounts are used (Mayes and Gottschlich, 2003).

Both medium-chain triglycerides and **structured lipids**, composed of both medium- and long-chain fatty acids, are currently under investigation. Medium-chain triglycerides are theoretically preferentially oxidized, thus leaving little tendency for deposition in adipose tissue or clogging of the reticuloendothelial system of the mitochondria (Tredget and Yu, 1992). Structured lipids may improve hepatic protein synthesis and reduce protein catabolism and energy expenditure.

Protein

The protein needs of burned patients are elevated because of losses through urine and wounds, increased use in gluconeogenesis, and wound healing. Recent evidence promotes the feeding of high amounts of protein. Providing 20% to 25% of total calories as protein of high biologic value is also recommended (Mayes and Gottschlich, 2003). Protein need in thermally injured children is generally agreed to be higher than the recommended RDA. Feeding 2.5 to 3 g/kg of protein has been suggested (Cunningham et al., 1990). The ability of pediatric burn patients to tolerate protein depends on their renal function and fluid balance.

The BCAAs seem to have no beneficial effect in burn patients. However, the conditionally essential amino acid, arginine, may improve cell-mediated immunity and wound healing (Mayes and Gottschlich, 2003; Tredget and Yu, 1992). Arginine may also affect anabolic hormone production. Glutamine enhances the ability of neutrophils to kill certain bacteria (Ogle et al., 1994). For all patients who receive high-protein diets, blood urea nitrogen, serum creatinine, and hydration must be monitored.

Assessment of Energy and Protein Adequacy

The adequacy of protein and energy intake is best evaluated by monitoring wound healing, graft take, and basic nutrition assessment parameters. Wound healing or graft take may be delayed if weight loss exceeds 10% of the usual weight. An exact evaluation of weight loss may be difficult to obtain because of fluid shifts or edema or because of differences in the weights of dressings or splints. The coordination of weight measurement with dressing changes or hydrotherapy may allow recording of a weight without dressings and splints (Mayes and Gottschlich, 2003). Generally the fluid gained during the resuscitation period is lost within 2 weeks. Weight-change trends can then be identified.

Nitrogen balance often is used to evaluate the efficacy of a nutritional regimen, but it cannot be considered accurate without accounting for wound losses. The following formulas are used to estimate wound nitrogen losses (Mayes and Gottschlich, 2003):

$$<10\% \text{ open wound} = 0.02 \text{ g nitrogen/kg/day}$$

$$11\% \text{ to } 30\% \text{ open wound} = 0.05 \text{ g nitrogen/kg/day}$$

$$>31\% \text{ open wound} = 0.12 \text{ g nitrogen/kg/day}$$

Nitrogen excretion should begin to decrease as wounds heal or are grafted or covered; however, serum albumin levels usually remain depressed until major burns are healed. Proteins with shorter half-lives such as serum transthyretin, retinol-binding protein, and transferrin help to assess the protein status of burn patients (see Chapter 15).

Vitamins and Minerals. Vitamin needs generally increase for burn patients, but exact requirements have not been established. Supplements may be needed for patients who are eating food; however, most patients who receive tube feeding or TPN receive amounts of vitamins in excess of the DRIs because of the high calorie intake. Vitamin C is involved in collagen synthesis and immune function and may be required in increased amounts for wound healing. Doses of 500 mg twice daily are the routine protocol at some burn centers (Mayes and Gottschlich, 2003). Vitamin A is also an important nutrient for immune function and epithelialization. Provision of 5000 units of vitamin A per 1000 calories of enteral nutrition is often recommended (Mayes and Gottschlich, 2003).

Electrolyte imbalances that involve serum sodium or potassium are usually corrected by adjusting fluid therapy. Hyponatremia may be seen in patients whose evaporative losses are reduced drastically by the application of dressings or grafts; who have had changes in maintenance fluids; or who have been treated with silver nitrate soaks, which tend to draw sodium from the wound. Restricting the oral consumption of free water and sodium-free fluids may help correct hyponatremia. Hypokalemia often occurs after the initial fluid resuscitation and during protein synthesis. Slightly elevated serum potassium may indicate inadequate hydration.

Depression of serum calcium levels may be seen in patients with burns that involve more than 30% TBSA. Hypocalcemia often accompanies hypoalbuminemia. Calcium losses may be exaggerated if the patient is immobile or being treated with silver nitrate soaks. Early ambulation and exercise should help minimize these losses. Administration of calcium supplements may be necessary to treat symptomatic hypocalcemia.

Hypophosphatemia has also been identified in patients with major burns. This occurs most commonly in patients who receive large volumes of resuscitation fluid along with parenteral infusion of glucose solutions and large amounts of antacids for stress ulcer prophylaxis. Serum levels need to be monitored, and appropriate phosphate supplementation provided. Magnesium levels may also require attention because a significant amount of magnesium can be lost from the burn wound. Supplemental phosphorus and magnesium are often given parenterally to prevent gastrointestinal irritation.

A depressed serum zinc level has been reported in burn patients, but whether this is representative of total body zinc nutriture or is an artifact of hypoalbuminemia is unclear, because zinc is bound to serum albumin. Zinc is a cofactor in energy metabolism and protein synthesis. Supplementation with 220 mg of zinc sulfate is appropriate (Mayes and Gottschlich, 2003). The anemia initially seen following a burn is usually unrelated to iron deficiency and is treated with packed red blood cells.

Methods of Nutrition Support. Methods of nutrition support need to be implemented on an individual basis. Most patients with burns of less than 20% TBSA are able to meet their needs with a regular high-calorie, high-protein diet (see *Focus On*: Maximizing Oral Nutrient Intake). Often the use of concealed nutrients such as adding protein to puddings, milks, and gelatins is helpful because consuming large volumes of foods can be overwhelming to the patient and can lead to overeating after the burns are healed.

Patients with major burns, extraordinarily high energy expenditure, or poor appetites usually require tube feeding or TPN. Enteral feeding is the preferred method of nutrition support for burn patients, but parenteral nutrition may be necessary with early excision and grafting to avoid the frequent interruptions in enteral nutrition support required for anesthesia. Because ileus is often present only in the stomach, severely burned patients can be successfully fed by tube into the small bowel. This is a routine practice in many burn cen-

⊙ FOCUS ON

Maximizing Oral Nutrient Intake

A 58-year-old woman suffered third-degree burns over her lower extremities that resulted in a 15% total body surface burn. Because of her small overall burn size, the registered dietitian recommended providing optimal nutrition via the oral route. The patient's energy and protein requirements were determined to be approximately 2100 kcal/day (measured via indirect calorimetry) and 155 g protein/day. A high-calorie, high-protein diet was provided via three meals and two snacks daily. *Nutrition diagnosis:* Increased energy requirements related to 15% TBSA burn as evidenced by indirect calorimetry results indicating 2100 kcal/day. *Intervention:* calorically enhanced meals and snack items as follows:

Breakfast

Orange juice with added Polycose
Cereal with fortified whole milk*
Scrambled eggs
Toast with butter and jelly

Lunch

Cream-of-potato soup
Ham and cheese sandwich with mayonnaise
Whole milk yogurt with fruit
Chocolate pudding with added protein supplement

Afternoon Snack

Milkshake made with a vitamin/mineral fortified protein
  powder supplement

Dinner

Tossed salad with Parmesan cheese and Italian dressing
Spaghetti with meat sauce
Cheesecake
Fortified whole milk

Evening Snack

Fruit slush with protein supplement
This meal plan offers approximately 2700 kcal/day and
  175 g protein.

*Milk supplemented with protein (nonfat dry milk powder or general protein supplement).

Note: Enteral nutrition manufacturers offer a wide variety of fortified foods for maximizing oral nutrient intake; please refer to individual manufacturers for specific items (see Appendix 32).

ters. Insulin-like growth factor 1 and human growth hormone in conjunction with nutrition support have been shown to blunt the stress response and improve nitrogen balance in burn patients (Losada et al., 2002; Goodwin, 1993).

TPN may be needed for patients with persistent ileus who do not tolerate tube feedings or who have a high risk of aspiration. With careful monitoring, central lines for TPN can be maintained through burn wounds.

SURGERY

Although surgical morbidity correlates best with the extent of the primary disease and the nature of the operation performed, malnutrition may compound the severity of complications (Eneroth et al., 2006). A well-nourished patient usually tolerates major surgery better than a severely malnourished patient. Malnutrition is associated with a high incidence of operative complications, morbidity, and death (Hasse, 2006).

Preoperative nutrition support is beneficial, especially for moderately or severely malnourished patients such as those individuals with gastrointestinal cancers (Wu et al., 2006). The National Veterans Affairs Surgical Risk Study evaluated 87,000 noncardiac surgeries in 44 Veterans' Administration medical centers and found preoperative serum albumin to be the strongest predictor of postoperative mortality (Khuri et al., 1997).

Medical Nutrition Therapy

Preoperative Nutrition Care

A chemically defined or elemental liquid diet with minimum residue can be used before surgery for patients at nutritional risk. Preoperative TPN should be limited to patients who exhibit signs of severe malnutrition, unless other specific indications exist. Except for patients who are unable to take food enterally or who are malnourished, no conclusive evidence suggests that perioperative nutrition support (other than in the form of oral intake) is effective in reducing operative complications and death. Preoperative nutrition support should be administered for 7 to 14 days to moderately or severely malnourished patients who are undergoing major gastrointestinal surgery if the operation can be safely postponed (ASPEN Board of Directors, 2002).

It is important that the stomach be empty of food at the time of the operation to avoid the danger of vomitus aspiration during the induction of anesthesia or on awakening. In elective cases no food is allowed by mouth for at least 6 hours before surgery. In emergency cases gastric lavage is advisable to remove stomach contents before anesthesia is started.

Before abdominal surgery, the colon should be free of residue to prevent postoperative infection. Colonic bacteria are reduced when less food residue is present. Low-fiber foods or a liquid diet is commonly given for 1 to 2 days before surgery, and the patient receives an enema a few hours before going to the operating room. Enteral products that are low in residue can be used for colon preparation before surgery (see Appendix 32).

Postoperative Nutrition Care

In a prolonged postoperative period nutrition support is used to reduce nutritional deficits that ordinarily develop in untreated patients during the period of nothing by mouth (NPO) after surgery. The length of time a patient can tolerate remaining NPO after surgery without complications is unknown, but it is definitely influenced by the patient's preexisting nutrition status, the severity of the operative stress, and the nature and severity of the illness. Postoperative nutrition support should be administered to patients when it is anticipated that they will be unable to meet their nutrient needs orally for a period of 7 to 10 days (ASPEN Board of Directors, 2002). The addition of omega-3 fatty acids, especially to support immune modulation after liver, tumor, or abdominal surgery is recommended (Heller et al., 2006; Senkal et al., 2005).

The introduction of solid food depends on the condition of the gastrointestinal tract. Oral feeding is often delayed for the first 24 to 48 hours after surgery to await the return of bowel sounds or passage of flatus. A general practice has been to progress over a period of several meals from clear liquids to full liquids and finally to solid foods. However, no physiologic reason exists for solid foods not to be introduced as soon as the gastrointestinal tract is functioning and a few liquids are being tolerated. Multiple studies have now demonstrated that after surgery patients can be fed a regular solid-food diet rather than a clear liquid diet (Pearl et al., 2002; Martindale, 1998).

If oral feeding is not possible or an extended NPO period is anticipated, an access device for enteral feeding should be inserted at the time of surgery. Combined gastrostomy-jejunostomy tubes offer significant advantages over standard gastrostomies because they allow for simultaneous gastric drainage from the gastrostomy tube and enteral feeding via the jejunal tube.

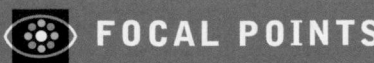

FOCAL POINTS

- The combined impact of metabolic alterations that occur in stress and bed rest can lead to rapid and severe depletion of lean body mass.
- Nutrition support cannot fully prevent or reverse the metabolic alterations and disruptions in body composition associated with critical illness; however, nutrition support likely ameliorates the rate of net protein catabolism.
- Initial assessment of the critically ill patient should include an evaluation of the patient's preexisting nutrition status.
- Clinical judgment is paramount in making decisions about the need to initiate nutrition support.
- For patients who will require enteral or parenteral nutrition, it should begin as soon as hemodynamic stability is achieved.
- Critically ill patients who are injured, septic, or bedridden cannot be expected to gain weight, lean body mass, or strength until the hypermetabolism resolves and physical therapy, exercise, and rehabilitation begin.

CLINICAL SCENARIO 1

Michael, a 22-year-old man, was involved in a motor vehicle accident as an unbelted rear-seat passenger and sustained a skull fracture, left subdural hematoma, and right pneumothorax that requires a chest tube. Glasgow Coma Scale was 10. Michael's weight on admission to the surgical intensive care unit was 162 lb, and his height is 6 ft 4 in. He had no previous significant medical or nutrition history. Michael was stabilized and given slightly less than his maintenance fluid requirements and a diuretic to prevent brain swelling. He was maintained on a respirator. A nasogastric tube was placed for drainage.

On hospital day 4, TPN was initiated because of bilious nasogastric drainage and radiologically confirmed ileus. Michael began running high fevers. The diuretic was discontinued, and the fluid restriction was liberalized because he was becoming too dehydrated. Using the Harris-Benedict equation with an injury factor of 1.4, the registered dietitian calculated his energy requirements at 2681 kcal/day. Indirect calorimetry indicated that Michael's measured energy expenditure was 2990 kcal/day. The nutritional goal was to feed the patient his actual measured energy needs. Protein requirements were calculated to provide approximately 1.5 g/kg, or 110 g of protein per day. The serum albumin level of 4.3 g/dl on admission dropped to 2.9 g/dl after rehydration.

A concentrated, intact nutrient formula was started at 20 ml/hr via the nasogastric tube on hospital day 8 following resolution of his ileus. Feeding advancements were impaired by frequent elevated gastric residual volumes (>300 ml); and by hospital day 11 the tube-feeding infusion remained at 40 ml/hr. On hospital day 12, a nasojejunal tube replaced the nasogastric tube secondary to poor gastric emptying and the inability to advance feedings. Feedings were successfully advanced to the goal rate of 85 ml/hr by day 14. This provided 3060 calories and 124 g of protein per day. Total parenteral nutrition was discontinued as Michael continued to tolerate enteral nutrition. Rapid turnover proteins were low; retinol-binding protein was 1.3 mg/dl (normal 3 to 6 mg/dl); and prealbumin was 4.8 mg/dl (normal 10 to 40 mg/dl). Zinc was normal at 83 (63 to 147 mg/dl). Total urinary nitrogen excretion was 27 g/day.

Michael continued to run a fever and was often treated with a cooling blanket. Because of anticipated continued ventilator dependence and neurologic impairment, gastrostomy (G-tube) and jejunostomy (J-tube) tubes were surgically placed. Since the initiation of nutrition support, Michael has received 90% or more of his measured nutritional requirements. His weight is now 132 lb. Diarrhea and copious airway secretions began during hospital week 3. An infectious cause of diarrhea was ruled out. A less concentrated tube-feeding formula is provided for hydration and to perhaps lessen stooling.

✸ CLINICAL SCENARIO 1—cont'd

✳**Nutrition Diagnosis 1:** Hypermetabolism as evidenced by recent trauma and surgery

✳**Nutrition Diagnosis 2:** Altered GI function related to inability to advance enteral feedings as evidenced by poor gastric emptying

✳**Nutrition Diagnosis 3:** Altered GI function related to intolerance of formula as evidenced by diarrhea

1. What indications of hypermetabolism are evident in this patient's history?
2. Compare Michael's measured energy expenditure with that calculated by the Harris-Benedict equation. What are the differences? Also compare it in kcal/kg body weight.
3. What nutritional recommendations would you make for the remainder of his hospital stay?

✸ CLINICAL SCENARIO 2

Thomas, a 61-year-old man, was admitted with gastric outlet obstruction secondary to gastric carcinoma. Surgical intervention was planned, but because of his history of a 30-lb weight loss over 2 months, preoperative parenteral nutrition was initiated, with surgery scheduled for his fifth day of hospitalization. His weight on admission was 135 lb, and his height was 5 ft 10 in. Thomas' usual body weight is 165 lb, which he also reported weighing 3 months ago. According to Thomas, he was easily able to consume liquids when his symptoms initially began, but within the past 2 weeks he has had difficulty consuming liquids without emesis. He has not been able to consume solid foods during the past 3 months. His initial laboratory work included a BUN of 2 mg/dl, an albumin of 3.5 g/dl, and serum triglycerides of 65 mg/dl. Indirect calorimetry testing revealed a resting energy expenditure of 1460 kcal/day. His respiratory quotient (RQ) was 0.72. His past medical history was significant for type I diabetes mellitus and chronic bronchitis.

Thomas underwent a total gastrectomy with jejunostomy tube placement on his fifth hospital day. He experienced blood pressure instability in the initial postoperative period and required multiple fluid boluses and large amounts of pharmacologic agents to maintain adequate blood pressure. On postoperative day 1, Thomas' abdomen was firm and distended, and bowel sounds were absent. His laboratory work after surgery included a blood glucose level of 275 mg/dl, a serum albumin of 1.9 g/dl, and a prealbumin of 5.7 mg/dl. Repeated indirect calorimetry revealed an energy expenditure of 1925 kcal/day and an RQ of 0.85. Urinary urea nitrogen excretion was 21 g/day.

On postoperative day 3, Thomas' abdomen was soft and nondistended, and bowel sounds were hypoactive. An intact nutrient formula with added arginine, omega-3 fatty acids, and nucleotides was initiated at 20 ml/hr via the jejunostomy tube. Thomas tolerated this initial enteral regimen but demonstrated abdominal distention and pain when attempts were made to advance his feeding rate. Consequently his TPN continued at the goal rate. On postoperative day 7, the tube-feeding rate was increased to 30 ml/hr with subsequent tolerance. Feeding advancement continued and reached the goal rate of 55 ml/hr. TPN infusion remained at the goal rate. On postoperative day 8 Thomas' serum glucose level was 310 mg/dl, and his arterial Pco_2 was 52 mg/dl. His TPN was slowly discontinued over 2 hours, and on postoperative day 9 his glucose is now 205 mg/dl, and his arterial Pco_2 has decreased to 38 mg/dl. Insulin has been administered.

✳**Nutrition Diagnosis 1:** Involuntary weight loss related to inability to consume solid foods as evidenced by loss of 30 lb over 2 months

✳**Nutrition Diagnosis 2:** Altered GI function as evidenced by lack of bowel sounds and distended abdomen

✳**Nutrition Diagnosis 3:** Altered lab values related to type 1 diabetes and recent surgery as evidenced by blood glucose of 275 mg/dl on postop day 1

1. Describe Thomas' nutrition status. What assessment parameters are used for evaluation? Was preoperative TPN indicated?
2. What are the differences in metabolic response between Thomas' initial presentation and his postoperative status?
3. Why may an immune-enhancing enteral formula be beneficial for Thomas?
4. What may have been the explanation for Thomas' increased glucose and Pco_2 levels during his combined TPN and tube feeding therapies?

USEFUL WEBSITES

American College of Surgeons
www.facs.org

American Society for Clinical Nutrition (ASCN)
www.faseb.org/ASCN

American Society for Parenteral and Enteral Nutrition (ASPEN)
www.clinnutr.org

Burn Nutrition
http://www.burnsurgery.org/Modules/burnmetabolism/pt2/index_nutrition.htm

Burn Survivor Resource Center
www.burnsurvivor.com/nutrition.html

National Guidelines for Nutrition Support of the Trauma Patient
http://www.guideline.gov/summary/summary.aspx?ss = 15&doc_id = 2961&nbr = 2187#s23

References

Alexander JW: Nutritional pharmacology in surgical patients, *Am J Surg* 183:349, 2002.

Alexander JW, Gottschlich MM: Nutritional immunomodulation in burn patients, *Crit Care Med* 18:S149, 1990.

Alpers DH: Enteral feeding and gut atrophy, *Curr Opin Clin Nutr Metabol Care* 5:679, 2002.

American Dietetic Association: Evidence-analysis library, www.eatright.org, accessed December 1, 2006.

ASPEN Board of Directors: Guidelines for the use of parenteral and enteral nutrition in adult and pediatric patients, *JPEN J Parenter Enteral Nutr* 26:1S, 2002.

Blackburn GL et al: Nutritional and metabolic assessment of the hospitalized patient, *JPEN J Parenter Enteral Nutr* 1:11, 1977.

Bochicchio GV et al: Persistent hyperglycemia is predictive of outcome in critically ill trauma patients, *J Trauma* 58:921, 2005.

Bone RC: Toward an epidemiology and natural history of SIRS (systemic inflammatory response syndrome), *JAMA* 268:3452, 1992.

Breen H, Ireton-Jones C: Predicting energy needs in obese patients, *Nutr Clin Pract* 19:284, 2004.

Butler SO et al: Relationship between hyperglycemia and infection in critically ill patients, *Pharmacotherapy* 25:963, 2005.

Choban PS, Dickerson RN: Morbid obesity and nutrition support: is bigger different? *Nutr Clin Pract* 20:480, 2005.

Compher C et al: Best practice methods to apply to measurement of resting metabolic rate in adults: a systematic review, *J Am Diet Assoc* 106:881, 2006.

Consensus recommendations from the U.S. summit on immune-enhancing enteral therapy, *JPEN J Parenter Enteral Nutr* 25:S61, 2001.

Cunningham J et al: Calorie and protein provision for recovery from severe burns in infants and young children, *Am J Clin Nutr* 51:553, 1990.

Curreri PW: Nutritional replacement modalities, *J Trauma* 19:904, 1979.

Deitch EA: Multiple organ failure, *Ann Surg* 216:117, 1992.

Deitch EA et al: Role of the gut in the development of injury- and shock-induced SIRS and MODS: the gut-lymph hypothesis, a review, *Front Biosci* 11:520, 2006.

Dickerson RN: Hypocaloric feeding of obese patients in the intensive care unit, *Curr Opin Clin Nutr Metabol Care* 8:189, 2005.

DiSario JA: Endoscopic approaches to enteral nutrition support, *Best Pract Res Clin Gastroenterol* 20:605, 2006.

Eneroth M et al: Nutritional supplementation decreases hip fracture–related complications, *Clin Orthop Relat Res* 451:212, 2006.

Epstein CD et al: Comparison of methods of measurements of oxygen consumption in mechanically ventilated patients with multiple trauma: the Fick method versus indirect calorimetry, *Crit Care Med* 28:1363, 2000.

Finney SJ et al: Glucose control and mortality in critically ill patients, *JAMA* 290:2041, 2003.

Frankenfield D et al: Validation of 2 approaches to predicting resting metabolic rate in critically ill patients, *JPEN J Parenter Enteral Nutr* 28:259, 2004.

Frankenfield D et al: Comparison of predictive equations for resting metabolic rate in healthy nonobese and obese adults: a systematic review, *J Am Diet Assoc* 105:775, 2005.

Fritsche K: Fatty acids as modulators of the immune response, *Annu Rev Nutr 2006*, 26:45, 2006.

Gagliardi E et al: Predicting energy expenditure in trauma patients: validation of the Ireton-Jones equations, *JPEN J Parenter Enteral Nutr* 19(suppl):22S, 1995 [abstract].

Galloswitsch-Puerta M, Tracey KJ: Immunologic role of the cholinergic anti-inflammatory pathway and the nicotinic acetylcholine alpha 7 receptor, *Ann NY Acad Sci* 1062:209, 2005.

Garrel DR et al: Improved clinical status and length of care with low-fat nutrition support in burn patients, *JPEN J Parenter Enteral Nutr* 19:482, 1995.

Glynn CC et al: Predictive versus measured energy expenditure using limits-or-agreement analysis in hospitalized, obese patients, *JPEN J Parenter Enteral Nutr* 23:147, 1999.

Goodwin CW: Parenteral nutrition in thermal injuries. In Rombeau J, Caldwell MD, editors: *Clinical nutrition: parenteral nutrition*, ed 2, Philadelphia, 1993, Saunders.

Gottschlich MM, Ireton-Jones CS: The Curreri formula: a landmark process for estimating caloric needs of burn patients, *Nutr Clin Pract* 16:172, 2001.

Hasse J: Examining the role of tube feeding after liver transplantation, *Nutr Clin Pract* 21:299, 2006.

Hassoun HT et al: Post-injury multiple organ failure: the role of the gut, *Shock* 15:1, 2001.

Heller AR et al: Omega-3 fatty acids improve the diagnosis-related clinical outcome, *Crit Care Med* 34:972, 2006.

Hester DD: Neurologic impairment. In Gottschlich MM et al, editors: *Nutrition support dietetics core curriculum*, ed 2, Silver Spring, Md, 1993, American Society for Parenteral and Enteral Nutrition, from http://adaevidencelibrary.com/topic.cfm?cat=1034, accessed November 23, 2005.

Hildreth MA et al: Caloric needs of adolescent patients with burns, *J Burn Care Rehabil* 10:523, 1989.

Ireton-Jones CS, Jones JD: Why use predictive equations for energy expenditure assessment? *J Am Diet Assoc* 97(suppl):A-44, 1997 [abstract].

Ireton-Jones C, Jones JD: Improved equations for predicting energy expenditure in patients: the Ireton-Jones equations, *Nutr Clin Pract* 17:29, 2002.

Ireton-Jones CS et al: Equations for the estimation of energy expenditures in patients with burns with special reference to ventilatory status, *J Burn Care Rehabil* 13:330, 1992.

Jeevanandam M et al: Decreased growth hormone levels in the catabolic phase of severe injury, *Surgery* 111:495, 1992.

Jeevanandam M et al: Adjuvant recombinant human growth hormone normalizes plasma amino acids in parenterally fed trauma patients, *JPEN J Parenter Enteral Nutr* 19:137, 1995.

Kattelmann KK et al: Preliminary evidence for a medical nutrition therapy protocol: enteral feedings for critically ill patients, *J Am Diet Assoc* 106:1226, 2006.

Khuri SF et al: Risk adjustment of the postoperative mortality rate for the comparative assessment of the quality of surgical care: results of the National Veterans Affairs Surgical Risk Study, *J Am Coll Surg* 185:315, 1997.

Kudsk KA: Current aspects of mucosal immunology and its influence by nutrition, *Am J Surg* 183:390, 2002.

Kudsk KA: Immunonutrition in surgery and critical care, *Annu Rev Nutr* 26:463, 2006.

Lee JO et al: Nutrition support strategies for severely burned patients, *Nutr Clin Pract* 20:325, 2005.

Losada F et al: Effects of human recombinant growth hormone on donor-site healing in burned adults, *World J Surg* 26(1):2, 2002.

Lund CL, Browder NC: The estimation of areas of burns, *Surg Gynecol Obstet* 79:352, 1944.

Malik PE, Zaloga GP: Gastric versus post-pyloric feeding: a systematic review, *Crit Care* 7(3):46, 2003.

Malone AM: Methods of assessing energy expenditure in the intensive care unit, *Nutr Clin Pract* 17:21, 2002.

Martindale R: Clear liquid diets: tradition or intuition? *Nutr Clin Pract* 13:186, 1998.

Mayes T, Gottschlich MM: Burns and wound healing. In Matarase LE, Gottschlich MM, editors: *Contemporary nutrition support practice: a clinical guide*, ed 2, Philadelphia, 2003, Saunders.

McClave SA et al: Enteral access for nutrition support: rationale for utilization, *J Clin Gastroenterol* 35:209, 2002.

Mlcak RP et al: The influence of age and gender on resting energy expenditure in severely burned children, *Ann Surg* 244:121, 2006.

Moriyama S et al: Evaluation of oxygen consumption and resting energy expenditure in critically ill patients with systemic inflammatory response syndrome, *Crit Care Med* 27:2133, 1999.

Ogle CK et al: Effect of glutamine on phagocytosis and bacterial killing by normal and pediatric burn patient neutrophils, *JPEN J Parenter Enteral Nutr* 18:128, 1994.

Pearl ML et al: A randomized controlled trial of a regular diet as the first meal in gynecologic oncology patients undergoing intraabdominal surgery, *Obstet Gynecol* 100:230, 2002.

Prelack K, Sheridan RL: Micronutrient supplementation in the critically ill patient: strategies for clinical practice, *J Trauma* 51:601, 2001.

Przkora R et al: Beneficial effects of extended growth hormone treatment after hospital discharge in pediatric burn patients, *Ann Surg* 243:796, 2006.

Saffle JR et al: A randomized trial of indirect calorimetry-based feedings in thermal injury, *J Trauma* 30:776, 1990.

Senkal M et al: Preoperative oral supplementation with long-chain omega-3 fatty acids beneficially alters phospholipid fatty acid patterns in liver, gut mucosa, and tumor tissue. *JPEN J Parenter Enteral Nutr* 29:236, 2005.

Shorr AF et al: Protein C concentrations in severe sepsis: an early directional change in plasma levels predicts outcome, *Crit Care* 10(3):1292, 2006.

Souba W, Wilmore D: Diet and nutrition in the case of the patient with surgery, trauma and sepsis. In Shils ME et al, editors: *Modern nutrition in health and disease*, vol 2, ed 8, Philadelphia, 1994, Lea & Febiger.

Swinamer DL et al: Predictive equation for assessing energy expenditure in mechanically ventilated critically ill patients, *Crit Care Med* 18:657, 1990.

Tappenden KA et al: Early enteral nutrition may have detrimental effects in patients with gastrointestinal hypoperfusion [abstract]. Presented at the Twenty-second Clinical Congress, American Society for Parenteral and Enteral Nutrition, January 1998.

Teng Chung T, Hinds CJ: Treatment with GH and IGF-1 in critical illness, *Crit Care Clin* 22:29, 2006.

Tredget EE, Yu YM: The metabolic effects of thermal injury, *World J Surg* 16:68, 1992.

Turina M et al: Diabetes and hyperglycemia: strict glycemic control, *Crit Care Med* 34:S291, 2006.

Twyman D: Nutritional management of the critically ill neurologic patient, *Crit Care Clin* 13:39, 1997.

Uehara M et al: Components of energy expenditure in patients with severe sepsis and major trauma: a basis for clinical care, *Crit Care Med* 27:1295, 1999.

Van Den Berghe G et al: Intensive insulin therapy in critically ill patients, *N Engl J Med* 345:1359, 2001.

Wall J et al: A validation of equations for predicting the energy expenditures of hospitalized patients, *J Am Diet Assoc* 9524S, 1995 [abstract].

Wischmeyer PE: Glutamine: role in gut protection in critical illness, *Curr Opin Nutr Metab Care* 9:607, 2006.

Wolfe RR, Martini WZ: Changes in intermediary metabolism in severe surgical illness, *World J Surg* 24:639, 2000.

Wolfe R et al: Glucose metabolism in man: responses to intravenous glucose infusion, *Metabolism* 28:210, 1979.

Wong JM et al: Colonic health: fermentation and short-chain fatty acids, *J Clin Gastroenterol* 40:235, 2006.

Wu GH et al: Perioperative artificial nutrition in malnourished gastrointestinal cancer patients, *World J Gastroenterol* 12:2441, 2006.

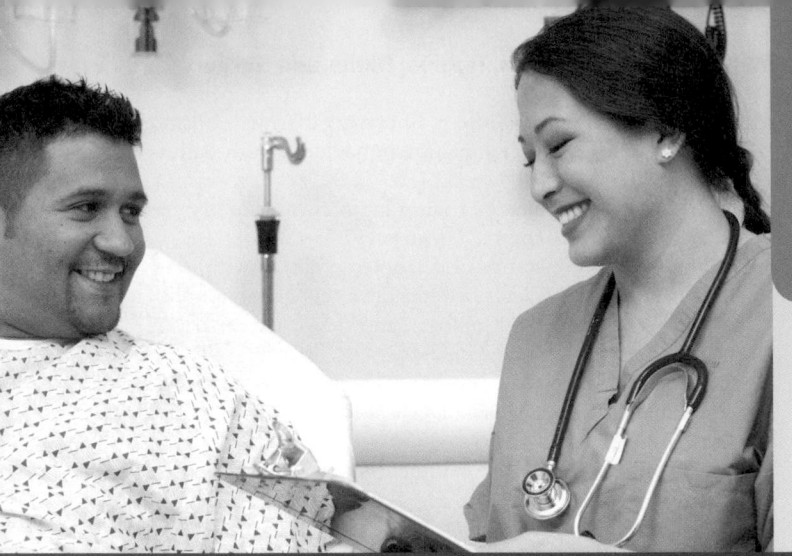

CHAPTER 40

Kristine Duncan, MS, RD, CDE

Medical Nutrition Therapy for Rheumatic Disease

KEY TERMS

activities of daily living (ADLs) includes walking, bathing, dressing, use of the toilet and performing household chores; the ability to perform these activities can be used to evaluate the severity of rheumatic disease for an individual

arachidonic acid a polyunsaturated fatty acid with four double bonds on the 5, 8, 11, and 14 carbon positions; a precursor for eicosanoid production

chronic fatigue syndrome (CFS) a disorder characterized by extreme fatigue that doesn't improve with rest and may worsen with physical or mental activity; may also present with weakness; headaches; difficulty concentrating; and painful joints, muscles, and lymph nodes

cytokines small proteins, including lymphokines and monokines, that are produced by immunocytes, macrophages, and fibroblasts and that mediate or increase an inflammatory response

fibromyalgia a chronic disorder characterized by widespread muscle pain, fatigue, and multiple tender points, especially in the neck, spine, shoulder, and hip

gout a type of inflammatory arthritis resulting from deposits of needlelike crystals of uric acid in connective tissue, the joints, or both

juvenile rheumatoid arthritis an inflammatory autoimmune disease of the synovium (lining of the joint), resulting in pain, stiffness, swelling, and joint damage and loss of function; most common form of arthritis in childhood; may also be associated with rash or fever; often presents symmetrically

osteoarthritis (OA) a nonsystemic joint disease characterized by degeneration of the joint cartilage, resulting in pain, stiffness, and loss of motion most commonly affecting the spine, knee, and hip; may also result in bone spurs (osteophytes) in and around the joint; also called degenerative joint disease

prostaglandins (PGs) a group of components derived from unsaturated 20-carbon fatty acids that are extremely potent mediators of a diverse group of physiologic processes; the series is designated with a subscript 1, 2, or 3, depending on the number of double bonds in the hydrocarbon skeleton and the fatty acid from which it was synthesized

purines the nitrogenous bases adenine and guanine, which are constituents of nucleoproteins, the metabolic end product of which is uric acid

Raynaud's syndrome ischemia or coldness in the small extremities such as the fingers

rheumatic disease (RD) manifestations of inflammation and loss of function of connecting and supporting body structures, including joints, tendons, ligaments, bones, muscles, and even internal organs; includes spondyloarthropathies, polymyalgia rheumatica, bursitis, tendonitis, and psoriatic, infectious or reactive arthritis

rheumatoid arthritis (RA) inflammatory autoimmune disease of the synovium (lining of the joint), resulting in pain, stiffness, swelling, joint damage, and loss of function of the joint; often presents symmetrically

rheumatoid factor abnormal circulating proteins found in the serum of individuals with rheumatoid arthritis; a group of immunoglobulins that have been classified as antibodies

scleroderma umbrella term for a group of diseases involving abnormal growth of connective tissue that supports the skin and internal organs; literally means "hard skin"; can also affect blood vessels and joints; also called systemic sclerosis

Sjögren's syndrome autoimmune disease targeting moisture-producing glands most commonly resulting in diminished production of both saliva and tears

Sections of this chapter were written by Lisa Dorfman, MS, RD, LMHC for the previous edition of this text.

synovial fluid transparent, alkaline fluid secreted by the synovial membrane and located in joints

systemic lupus erythematosus (SLE) an autoimmune disease that involves inflammation resulting in extreme fatigue, arthritis, unexplained fever, skin rashes, and kidney problems

temporomandibular disorders (TMDs) collection of medical and dental conditions affecting the temporomandibular joint and the muscles of mastication, as well as contiguous tissue components

Rheumatic disease (RD) and related conditions include more than 100 different manifestations of inflammation and loss of function of connecting and supporting body structures, including joints, tendons, ligaments, bones, muscles, and sometimes internal organs. RD is thought to have an autoimmune component. Because no identifiable cause or cure is known, pharmacotherapy, physical and occupational treatment, and medical nutrition therapy (MNT) play important roles in managing the symptoms (Table 40-1).

RD affects all population groups. Osteoarthritis (OA) affects 21 million Americans, gout affects 5.1 million (Kramer and Curhan, 2002); fibromyalgia affects 3.7 million; rheumatoid arthritis (RA), 3 million; and systemic lupus erythematosus (SLE), about 240,000. According to the National Institute of Arthritis and Musculoskeletal and Skin Diseases (NIAMS),

conditions such as Sjögren's syndrome (affecting 1 to 4 million) and scleroderma also have a great impact on the American population (NIAMS, 2001). Estimates for the number of people in the United States with systemic sclerosis range from 40,000 to 165,000 (NIAMS, 2006b).

Arthritis is a generic term that comes from the Greek word *arthro*, which means joint, and the suffix *-itis*, which means inflammation of. There are two distinct categories of disease: systemic, autoimmune RD and nonsystemic OA. The autoimmune arthritis group, the more debilitating group, includes RA, **juvenile rheumatoid arthritis,** gout, Sjögren's syndrome, fibromyalgia, lupus, and scleroderma. The OA group includes OA, bursitis, and tendonitis. Other RDs include spondyloarthropathies, polymyalgia rheumatica, and polymyositis.

Body changes associated with aging—including decreased body protein, body fluid, and bone density and increased proportion of total body fat—may contribute to the onset and progression of arthritis. The aging body mass causes changes in neuroendocrine regulators, immune regulators, and metabolism, which affect the inflammation process.

Therefore recent increases in the frequency of these conditions may be the result of aging of the U.S. population. By 2030 about 20% of Americans (about 72 million people) will have passed their 65th birthday and subsequently will be at high risk for OA and rheumatic disease (NIAMS, 2006a).

Arthritis and other RDs are among the most prevalent chronic disease conditions in the United States and are as-

TABLE 40-1

Overview of Medical Nutrition Therapy for Rheumatic Diseases

Disease	Medical Nutrition Therapy	Complementary Therapy	Supplements or Herbs That Can Be Safely Considered	Therapies Without Adequate Evidence
Rheumatoid arthritis	Monitored fast 7-10 days; vegetarian or vegan diet; appropriate calories for maintenance of normal body weight; RDA for protein unless malnutrition present; moderate-fat diet with emphasis on omega-3 fats; modifications as needed for jaw pain, anorexia, etc.; low-mercury fish 1-2 ×/week	Exercise, meditation, tai chi, spirituality, relaxation techniques	Supplement diet as needed to meet DRI for antioxidants, calcium, folate, vitamins B_6, B_{12}, D; GLA; fish oils	China root, willow bark, valerian, feverfew, boswellia, curcumin, ginger, copper or copper salts, devil's claw, thunder god vine
Osteoarthritis	Weight management; diet adequate antioxidants, calcium, folate, vitamins B_6, B_{12}, D	Exercise, acupuncture	Supplement diet as needed to meet DRI for antioxidants, calcium, folate, vitamins B_6, B_{12}, D; glucosamine and chondroitin	Shark cartilage, SAM-e

DRI, Dietary reference intake; *GLA,* Gamma-linolenic acid; *RDA,* recommended dietary allowance; *SAM-e,* S-adenosyl-L-methionine.

Continued

TABLE 40-1

Overview of Medical Nutrition Therapy for Rheumatic Diseases—cont'd

Disease	Medical Nutrition Therapy	Complementary Therapy	Supplements or Herbs That Can Be Safely Considered	Therapies Without Adequate Evidence
Gout	Weight management; purine-controlled diet; adequate fluid consumption; 40% complex carbs, 30% fat (mostly unsaturated), 30% protein with moderate calorie restriction; restrict or eliminate alcohol	Exercise; alkaline-ash foods		
Lupus	Tailor diet to individual needs; calories to promote IBW; restriction of protein, fluid, and sodium if renal involvement; possible gluten intolerance		Supplement diet as needed to meet DRI for antioxidants	
Scleroderma	Adequate fluid; high-energy protein supplements as needed; moist foods; modifications for GERD if needed			
Fibromyalgia/chronic fatigue	Increase in sodium and fluid if hypotension present; vegan diet	Exercise, massage, stress management		Biofeedback, relaxation, chlorella, homeopathy, guaifenesin, magnesium, SAM-e DHEA
Sjögren's syndrome	Balanced diet with adequate B_{12}, folate; limit or avoid sugary foods; modifications as needed for dysphagia			
TMD	Mechanically soft foods in small pieces			

DHEA, Dehydroepiandrosterone; *GERD*, gastroesophageal reflux disease. *IBW*, ideal body weight; *TMD*, temporomandibular disorder.

sociated with total direct and indirect costs to the U.S. economy of $86 billion per year in medical care and lost wages (CDC, 2004).

ETIOLOGY

The etiology of most rheumatic conditions remains unknown. In addition, some forms of rheumatic conditions can affect other organs such as the skin or blood vessels. Rheumatic conditions have no known cure and are usually chronic but may present as acute episodes with short or intermittent duration. Chronic arthritic conditions are associated with alternating periods of remission, without symptoms, and flares with worsening symptoms that occur without any identifiable etiology. Risk factors that appear to increase the likelihood of developing an RD include repetitive joint injury, inherited cartilage weakness, genetic susceptibility, family history, gender, and environmental triggers.

PATHOPHYSIOLOGY OF INFLAMMATION IN RHEUMATIC DISEASE

Inflammation, the predominant cause of pain, is the most debilitating component of all forms of arthritis. Pain reflects a neuroendocrine process associated with levels of corticotrophin-releasing hormone, methyl-D-aspartate, inflammatory mediators, unmyelinated C fibers sensitized to noradrenaline, and biologically active peptides. The inflammatory process normally occurs to protect and repair tissue damaged by infections, injuries, toxicity, or wounds via accumulation of fluid and cells. Once the cause is resolved, the inflammation usually subsides. Whether inflammation is attributable to stress on the joints (OA) or is an autoimmune response (RA), in most forms of arthritis the inflammatory reaction continues out of control, thus causing more damage than repair.

The complex inflammatory process is initiated by the production of histamine, prostaglandins (PGs), plasma proteases, and plasma-activating factors. Many specific PGs and other mediators (i.e., PGE_1 and PGE_2, thromboxanes and leukotrienes) potentiate the effects of inflammatory mediators such as histamine. **Arachidonic acid,** a polyunsaturated fatty acid that is a precursor for eicosanoid production, when released from cell membranes, is oxygenated to several classes of eicosanoids, including PGs, thromboxanes, leukotrienes, and prostacyclins (PGI_2s), all of which are proinflammatory.

Thromboxanes activate platelet aggregation to initiate clotting and release growth factors and proteases. Leukotrienes stimulate the attraction of neutrophils, macrophages, and fibroblasts into the circulating joint fluid. PGI_2 has the opposite effect of PGE_1 and PGE_2; it relaxes the smooth muscle and inhibits platelet aggregation.

Prostaglandins (PGs), the group of components derived from arachidonic and other unsaturated, long-chain fatty acids, are potent mediators of a diverse group of physiologic processes, including inflammation. They are produced by neutrophils, macrophages, and synovial fibroblasts in large quantities in synovial tissue as a response to specific **cytokines** (activating protein hormones such as tumor necrosis factors [TNF-αs], interferons, and interleukins [ILs]) acting on oxygenated arachidonic acid. PGs play a major role in the depletion of bone in RA, and TNF-α has assumed particular importance.

LABORATORY TESTS FOR RHEUMATIC DISEASE

A thorough history of symptoms and detailed physical examination are the cornerstones of an accurate diagnosis of RD. However, laboratory testing can help to further refine the diagnosis and identify appropriate treatment.

Acute-phase proteins are defined as proteins with plasma concentrations that change by 25% during inflammatory states. Two acute-phase proteins traditionally used to screen for and monitor RD are erythrocyte sedimentation rate (ESR) and C-reactive protein (CRP), as both values increase during an acute phase inflammatory response. However, both proteins are non-specific and may also indicate an infection or even a recent cardiac event. The American College of Rheumatology recommends periodic measurements of CRP and ESR in addition to a detailed assessment of symptoms and functional status, and radiographic examination to determine the current level of disease activity in RD patients.

Antinuclear antibodies appear to be present in many autoimmune diseases and can assist with proper diagnosis, when used correctly, while antineutrophil cytoplasmic antibodies and myositis-specific antibodies can provide information about the presence of RD as well. Measurements of rheumatoid factor, a group of antibodies found in the serum of those with RA, and anticyclic citrullinated peptide antibodies may provide unique data in the management of RA (Colgazier and Sutej, 2005). Routine blood testing for RD may include complement, complete blood count, creatinine,

hematocrit, and white blood cell count, in addition to analysis of urine or **synovial fluid** secreted by the synovial membrane in the joints (NIAMS, 2002).

PHARMACOTHERAPY FOR RHEUMATIC DISEASE

Many of the drugs used in treating rheumatic diseases provide relief from pain and inflammation, with hopes of controlling symptoms rather than providing a cure. Analgesics such as acetaminophen (Tylenol), are effective pain relievers. Drugs commonly used to reduce inflammation affect the synthesis of prostaglandins, usually by diminishing their production.

Glucocorticoid therapy decreases the release of arachidonic acid from cell membrane phospholipids by binding to the receptor in the cell cytoplasm. This forms a complex that moves into the nucleus as a transcription factor and interferes with expression for the enzyme phospholipase.

Nonsteroidal antiinflammatory drugs (NSAIDs), which include ibuprofen (Advil or Motrin) and naproxen (Aleve) slow down the body's production of PGs by inhibiting cyclooxygenase (COX-1). They are considered useful tools in the management of most rheumatic disorders. Long-term use of NSAIDs may cause gastrointestinal problems such as irritation, ulcers, abdominal burning, pain, cramping, nausea, GI bleeding, or even renal failure (Table 40-2) (see Chapter 16 and Appendix 31).

Disease-modifying antirheumatic drugs (DMARDs) may be prescribed because of their unique ability to slow or prevent further joint damage caused by arthritis. These include methotrexate (MTX), sulfasalazine (Azulfidine), hydroxychloroquine (Plaquenil), azathioprine (Imuran), and leflunomide (Arava). In fact, the American College of Rheumatology (ACR) recommends that the majority of patients with newly diagnosed RA be prescribed a DMARD within 3 months of diagnosis. Depending on which drug is selected, side effects can include myelosuppression or macular or liver damage (ACR, 2002).

An adverse effect of the DMARD MTX treatment is folate antagonism. Treatment with MTX induces a significant rise in serum-homocysteine, which is corrected by folic acid supplementation (Slot, 2001). For many patients a properly balanced diet is sufficient to avoid folate deficiency; however, folic acid supplementation is advised to offset the toxicity of this drug, for protection against gastrointestinal disturbances, and for maintenance of red blood cell production (van Ede et al., 2001). Fortunately folic acid supplementation does not decrease the efficacy of MTX therapy. Long-term supplementation in patients on MTX is important to prevent neutropenia and to avoid discontinuation of treatment because of mouth ulcers, nausea, and vomiting (see Appendix 31 and Chapter 31).

Additional DMARDs include gold salt therapy, antimalarials, and d-penicillamine and may lead to a remission in RA symptoms. Proteinuria may occur with administration of

TABLE 40-2

Nutritional Side Effects of Arthritis Medications

Side Effects	NSAIDs — Traditional NSAIDs	NSAIDs — COX-2s	NSAIDs — Salicylates	Biologic Response Modifiers	Analgesics	Corticosteroids	DMARDs
GI ulceration/bleeding	X*	X†	X			X	
Dyspepsia	X	X	X				X
Nausea/vomiting	X	X	X		X		X
Oral ulcers							X
Diarrhea	X	X	X				X
Polyuria						X	
Polydipsia						X	
Constipation					X		
Dry mouth					X		
Loss of appetite					X		X
Abdominal/stomach cramps	X	X	X	X			X
Metallic taste in mouth							X
Irritation and soreness of tongue							X
Irritated or bleeding gums							X
Folate antagonism							X
Increased excretion or decreased absorption of vitamin C	X		X				
Iron loss	X						
Potassium loss						X	
Vitamin B$_6$ loss						X	X
Increased potassium level	X						
Magnesium loss						X	
Edema	X	X	X			X	
Liver disease							X
Gallbladder disease							X
Renal disease							X
Proteinuria							X
Change in blood pressure				X		X	X
Hyperglycemia						X	
Osteoporosis						X	
Weight gain						X	
Urinary retention					X		
Thrombotic cardiovascular events		X					

Data from ACR: Guidelines for the management of rheumatoid arthritis, *Arthritis Rheum* 46:2, 2002; Arthritis Foundation: *Arthritis today, 2005 drug guide*; Boullata JI, Armenti VT, editors: *Handbook of drug-nutrient interactions*, Totowa, NJ, 2004, Humana Press.

*Less with diclofenac sodium with misoprostol, but increased risk of abdominal pain and diarrhea.

† Less than traditional NSAIDs.

DMARD, Disease-modifying antirheumatic drug; *GI*, gastrointestinal; *NSAID*, nonsteroidal antiinflammatory drug.

gold and *d*-penicillamine; therefore toxicity from these drugs must be monitored continually. Minocycline (Minocin) is an antibiotic often used to treat mild RA (Cannon, 2005).

Biologic response modifiers, another class of drugs, are given by injection and include adalimumab (Humira), anakinra (Kineret), etanercept (Enbrel), and infliximab (Remicade). These drugs block the reaction of TNF-α and cytokine IL-1, and thus help reduce inflammation and protect the joints. However, the cost of biologic agents can be a barrier for their use. The costs range from $13,000 to $30,000 annually (ACR, 2006). Patients taking these drugs should be monitored for chronic infections (ACR, 2002).

Corticosteroids (cortisone [Cortone], prednisone [Deltasone], methylprednisolone [Medrol], and hydrocortisone [Cortef]) suppress the immune system and decrease inflammation, making them desirable treatment for many of the RDs. Possible side effects of corticosteroids include hypertension, hyperglycemia, weight gain, and osteoporosis (ACR, 2002). Low-dose steroids control most of the inflammatory features of early polyarticular RA (Conn, 2001).

As the most potent of the antiinflammatory drugs used to treat RA, steroids have extensive catabolic impact that can result in negative nitrogen balance. Hypercalciuria and reduced calcium absorption can increase the risk of osteoporosis (see Chapters 16 and 24). Concomitant calcium (1 g/day) and vitamin D (at least 500 International units/day) and monitoring of bone status can minimize osteopenia (Conn, 2001). Care must be taken to avoid serum calcium levels greater than 11 mg/dl and 25-OH vitamin D levels less than 35 ng/ml. Edema often occurs and may require diet modification, including a sodium- and fluid-restricted diet. Other side effects of steroid use include cushingoid syndrome, and gastrointestinal bleeding.

COX-2 inhibitors (COX-2 selective NSAIDs) such as celecoxib (Celebrex), valdecoxib (Bextra), and rofecoxib (Vioxx) have been shown to provide relief comparable to other NSAIDs with potentially less gastrointestinal toxicity. However, research has identified an increased risk of thrombotic cardiovascular events, including nonfatal myocardial infarction and nonfatal strokes associated with their use, especially at higher doses. As a result, the manufacturers of valdecoxib and rofecoxib voluntarily removed these drugs from the market. In early 2005 the Food and Drug Administration (FDA) determined that naproxen and celecoxib appeared to be safer than other NSAIDs and offered a reasonable risk-benefit profile. Further research is needed to better determine the cardiovascular risks of both types of NSAIDs, but labeling changes have been proposed to highlight these concerns in the interim (FDA, 2005).

Salicylates are commonly used to treat RA. However, chronic aspirin ingestion is associated with gastric mucosal injury and bleeding, increased bleeding time, and increased urinary excretion of vitamin C. Taking aspirin with milk, food, or an antacid often alleviates the gastrointestinal symptoms. Vitamin C supplementation is prescribed when serum and platelet levels of ascorbic acid are abnormally low.

Gout is treated with drugs that inhibit or eliminate uric acid synthesis. Probenecid (Benemid) and sulfinpyrazone decrease the blood uric acid level by increasing elimination through the kidneys. Allopurinol inhibits uric acid production. Both probenecid and sulfinpyrazone are often used in conjunction with colchicine, a drug that has no effect on uric acid metabolism but has been shown to relieve the joint pain of gouty arthritis. Colchicine is most valuable during the acute stage but may be needed during symptom-free periods as a preventive measure. Other antiinflammatory agents such as indomethacin or phenylbutazone are sometimes used in the acute stage of gout.

Plaquenil, an antimalarial drug, appears to be effective in clearing up skin lesions for some individuals with lupus but has side effects that include nausea, abdominal cramping, and diarrhea. Immunosuppressives such as cyclophosphamide may be used with renal involvement, but gastrointestinal and fertility problems may occur.

Tricyclic antidepressants and selective serotonin reuptake inhibitors (SSRIs) are commonly used with chronic fatigue syndrome (CFS) patients. They may be helpful in treating depression and sleep disturbances common with this syndrome (Craig and Kakaumanu, 2002). Side effects may include agitation, dry mouth, drowsiness, and weight gain. There are other pharmaceutic options such as tramadol (Ultram) for treating patients with fibromyalgia.

Medications for Sjögren's syndrome address the issues of dry eyes and dry mouth. These include artificial tears and immunosuppressant drops such as cevimeline (Evoxac) and pilocarpine (Salagen), respectively (Arthritis Foundation [AF], 2005a).

OSTEOARTHRITIS

Pathophysiology

Osteoarthritis (OA), formally known as degenerative arthritis or degenerative joint disease, is the most prevalent form of arthritis. Obesity, aging, female gender, white ethnicity, greater bone density, and repetitive-use injury associated with athletics have been identified as risk factors (see *Pathophysiology and Care Management Algorithm:* Osteoarthritis).

OA is a chronic joint disease that involves the loss of habitually weight-bearing articular (joint) cartilage. This cartilage normally allows bones to glide smoothly over one another. The loss can result in pain, swelling, loss of motion, and changes in joint shape, in addition to abnormal bone growth, which can result in osteophytes (bone spurs) (Radin, 2004) (Figure 40-1).

The major difference between OA and RA is that OA is not systemic or autoimmune in origin but involves cartilage destruction with asymmetric inflammation. It is caused by joint overuse, whereas RA is a systemic autoimmune disorder that results in symmetric joint inflammation.

The joints most often affected in OA are the distal interphalangeal joints; the thumb joint; and, in particular, the joints of the knees, hips, ankles, and spine, which bear the bulk of the body's weight (Figure 40-2). The elbows, wrists, and ankles are less often affected. OA generally presents as pain that worsens with weight bearing and activity and improves with rest, and patients often report morning stiffness and "gelling" of the affected joint after periods of inactivity. Diseases of the joints influenced by congenital and mechanical derangements may contribute to OA as well. Inflammation occurs at times but is generally mild and localized.

Medical Management

According to ACR Guidelines, the patient's medical history and level of pain should determine the most appropriate treatment. This should include nonpharmacologic modalities (patient education, physical and occupational therapy),

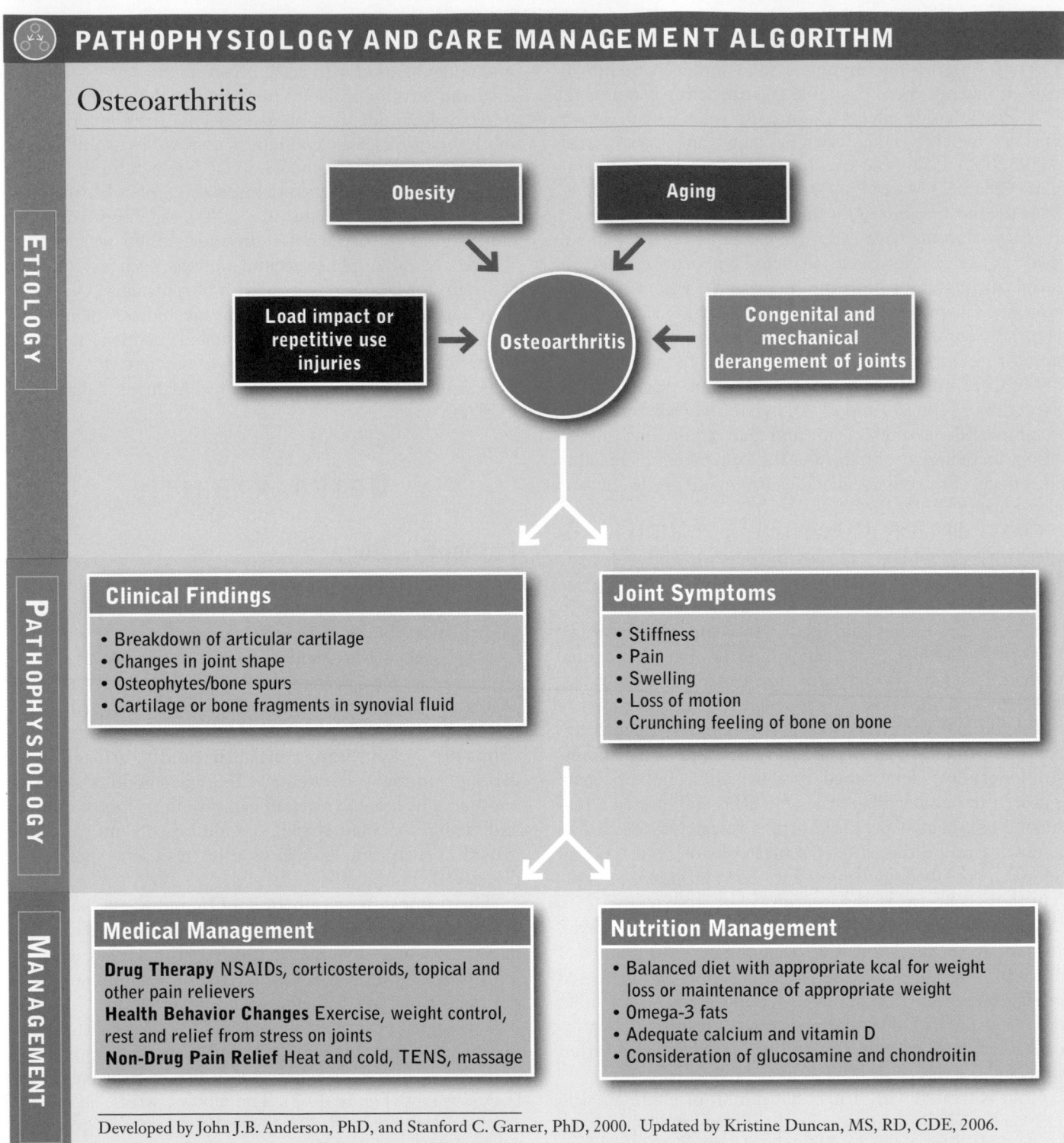

PATHOPHYSIOLOGY AND CARE MANAGEMENT ALGORITHM

Osteoarthritis

ETIOLOGY

Obesity

Aging

Load impact or repetitive use injuries

Osteoarthritis

Congenital and mechanical derangement of joints

PATHOPHYSIOLOGY

Clinical Findings

- Breakdown of articular cartilage
- Changes in joint shape
- Osteophytes/bone spurs
- Cartilage or bone fragments in synovial fluid

Joint Symptoms

- Stiffness
- Pain
- Swelling
- Loss of motion
- Crunching feeling of bone on bone

MANAGEMENT

Medical Management

Drug Therapy NSAIDs, corticosteroids, topical and other pain relievers
Health Behavior Changes Exercise, weight control, rest and relief from stress on joints
Non-Drug Pain Relief Heat and cold, TENS, massage

Nutrition Management

- Balanced diet with appropriate kcal for weight loss or maintenance of appropriate weight
- Omega-3 fats
- Adequate calcium and vitamin D
- Consideration of glucosamine and chondroitin

Developed by John J.B. Anderson, PhD, and Stanford C. Garner, PhD, 2000. Updated by Kristine Duncan, MS, RD, CDE, 2006.

pharmacologic agents, and surgical procedures with the goals of pain control, improved function and health-related quality of life, and avoidance of toxic effects from treatment (ACR, 2000; Barnes and Edwards, 2005).

Surgery

According to the ACR, patients with severe symptomatic OA pain that has not responded adequately to medical treatment and who have been progressively limited in their **activities of daily living (ADLs)** such as walking, bathing, dressing and

toileting, should be evaluated by an orthopedic surgeon. Surgical options include arthroscopic debridement (with or without arthroplasty), total joint arthroplasty, and osteotomy. Surgical reconstruction has been quite successful but should not be viewed as a replacement for overall good nutrition, maintenance of healthy body weight, and exercise.

Exercise

OA limits the ability to increase energy expenditure through exercise. It is critical that the exercise to be done in correct

A Healthy Joint

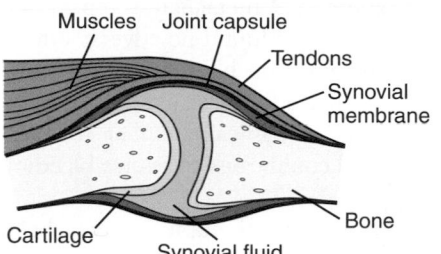

A Joint with Osteoarthritis

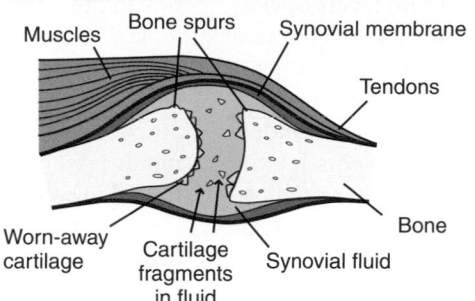

FIGURE 40-1 A healthy joint and a joint with severe osteoarthritis. *(From National Institute of Arthritis and Musculoskeletal and Skin Diseases:* Handout on health: osteoarthritis, *National Institutes of Health, Department of Health and Human Services, NIH Publication Number 06-4617, July 2002, revised May 2006.)*

form so as not to cause damage or exacerbate an existing problem. Physical and occupational therapists can provide unique expertise for OA patients by making individualized assessments and recommending appropriate exercise programs and assistive devices, in addition to offering guidance regarding joint protection and energy conservation. Nonloading aerobic (swimming), range-of-motion, and weight-bearing exercises have all been shown to reduce symptoms, increase mobility, and lessen continuing damage from OA. Nonweight-bearing exercise may also serve as an adjunct to NSAID use (Nicolakis et al., 2002).

The Fitness Arthritis and Seniors Trial concluded that exercise should be prescribed as part of the treatment for OA (Ettinger et al., 1997). Sports or strenuous activities that subject joints to repetitive high impact and loading increase the risk of joint cartilage degeneration. Therefore increased muscle tone and strength, correct form, general flexibility, and conditioning will help protect these joints in the habitual exerciser. A walking program and lower extremity strength training are beneficial for individuals with knee OA (Mikesky et al., 2006).

Medical Nutrition Therapy

Excess weight puts an added burden on the weight-bearing joints. Epidemiologic studies have shown that obesity and injury are the two greatest risk factors for OA. The risk for knee OA increases as the body mass index increases (Coggon et al., 2001). Controlling obesity can reduce the burden of ostearthritis through both disease prevention and improvement in symptoms (Messier et al., 2005).

A well-balanced diet that is consistent with established dietary guidelines and promotes attainment and maintenance of a desirable body weight is an important part of MNT for OA. When combined with moderate exercise, diet-induced weight loss has been shown to be an effective intervention for knee OA (Messier et al., 2004). There may be an antiinflammatory effect from weight loss in OA management because the reduced fat mass results in the presence of less inflammatory mediators from adipose tissue (see Chapter 24).

Vitamins and Minerals

Cumulative damage to tissues mediated by reactive oxygen species has been implicated as a pathway that leads to many of the degenerative changes seen with aging. Large doses of

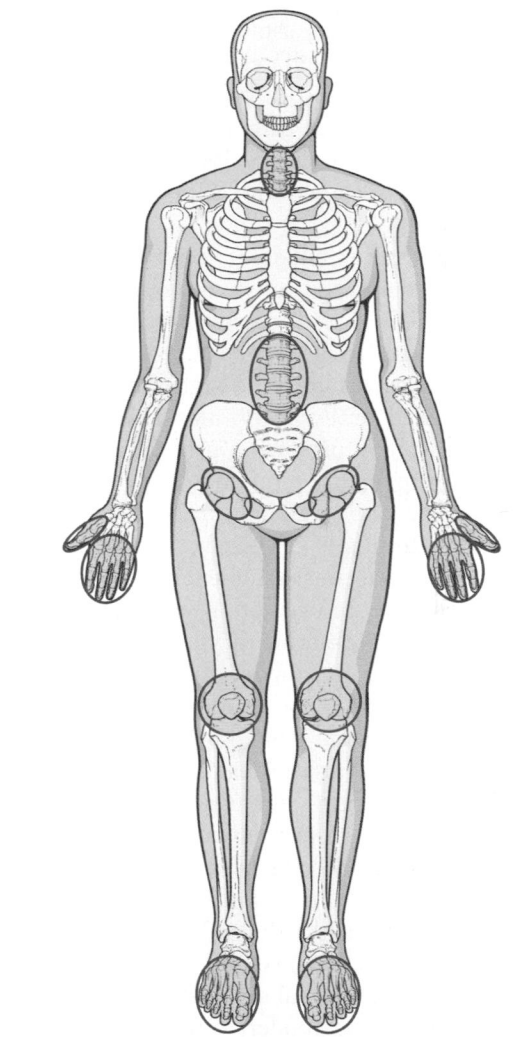

FIGURE 40-2 Joints commonly affected by osteoarthritis.

dietary antioxidants, including vitamin C, the tocopherols (vitamin E), β-carotene, and selenium, may be beneficial in OA management (Darlington and Stone, 2001). However, several studies showed no benefit for the management of symptomatic OA with a daily vitamin E supplement (Wluka et al., 2002; Brand et al., 2001). Preliminary research has suggested that antioxidants with antiinflammatory properties may protect against cartilage damage when injected intraarticularly (McAlindon and Biggee, 2005). Further studies are needed before routine supplementation of antioxidants can be recommended.

Many patients with OA consume deficient levels of dairy products, calcium, and vitamin D. Low serum levels of vitamin D are being studied for a role in OA progression (McAlindon and Biggee, 2005). Improving intake to at least dietary reference intakes (DRIs) is important. Comprehensive nutrition interviewing and counseling should include a determination of acceptable sources of all nutrients for the OA patient, as well as supplementation of the diet to achieve the recommended levels (with special attention given to vitamin B_6, vitamin D, and folate).

Alternative Therapies

Some alternative "therapies" that are being used to help lessen the need for NSAIDs, aspirin, and acetaminophen are glucosamine, chondroitin sulfate, oils, and herbs. Advocates of these alternative modalities cite reports of progressive and gradual decline of joint pain and tenderness, improved mobility, sustained improvement after drug withdrawal, and a lack of toxicity associated with short-term use of these agents (AF, 2005b).

Sodium chondroitin sulfate (chondroitin sulfate) and glucosamine hydrochloride (glucosamine) are both molecules that are involved in cartilage production, but their mechanism for eliminating pain has not been identified. In an analysis of studies, limited data suggest that glucosamine sulfate administered orally, intravenously, intramuscularly, or intraarticularly may produce a gradual and progressive reduction in joint pain and tenderness, as well as improved range of motion and walking speed (DaCamara and Dowless, 1998). Results of trials have also shown that glucosamine has produced consistent benefits, including greater than 50% improvement in symptom scores in patients with OA. In some cases glucosamine may be equal or superior to ibuprofen (McAlindon and Biggee, 2005). Together glucosamine and chondroitin rank third among all top-selling nutritional products in the United States.

The National Institutes of Health (NIH) undertook the Glucosamine/Chondroitin Arthritis Intervention Trial (GAIT), the first, large-scale, multicenter clinical trial in the United States to test the effects of these supplements on knee OA. A dose of 1500 mg of glucosamine (given as 500 mg, three times daily) with 1200 mg of chondroitin (given as 400 mg, three times daily) resulted in statistically significant pain relief for a small subset of study participants who were classified as having moderate-to-severe pain but not for those in the mild pain subset. Compared to 54% of those taking placebo, 79% of those taking glucosamine/chondroitin reported a 20% or greater reduction in pain. Because of the small sample size of this subset of patients, the researchers suggest that these findings be considered preliminary pending further studies (NIH, 2006).

Although it is not effective for all afflicted individuals, the AF suggests a safe dose of glucosamine and chondroitin sulfate to be 1500 mg/day and 1200 mg/day in divided doses, respectively (AF, 2005b). There is some concern about the potential for glucosamine to negatively affect insulin regulation in individuals with insulin resistance or diabetes (McAlindon and Biggee, 2005), although GAIT found no change in glucose

tolerance (NIH, 2006). Possibly chondroitin can elicit a reaction in those with shellfish allergies. A metaanalysis report that looked at over 3000 human subjects found no adverse effects of oral glucosamine administration on blood, urine, or fecal parameters and no serious or fatal side effects (Anderson et al., 2005). However, chondroitin is chemically similar to commonly used blood thinners and could cause excessive bleeding if used in combination.

A variety of complementary therapies have been proposed as a solution to managing pain in OA, including topical aids, manipulative therapies, and acupuncture. Capsaicinoids, derived from chili peppers, have a fatty acid receptor that stimulates, then blocks, small-diameter pain fibers by depleting them of the neurotransmitter substance P, thought to be the principal chemomediator of pain impulses from the periphery (Robbins, 2000). Capsaicin, applied with glyceryl trinitrate to reduce on-site burning, can reduce pain in OA patients (McCleane, 2000).

Certain pulsed electromagnetic fields can also affect the growth of bone and cartilage with potential use in OA, and use of static magnets may provide temporary pain relief under certain circumstances (Trock, 2000).

According to the AF, S-adenosyl-L-methionine (SAM-e) has also shown promise for reducing pain and improving mobility in people with OA at doses of 600 to 1200 mg/day but should not be taken without a doctor's supervision (AF, 2007). Two recent randomized controlled trials found a benefit for OA patients treated with acupuncture (Berman et al., 2004; Witt et al., 2005).

RHEUMATOID ARTHRITIS

Rheumatoid arthritis (RA) is a debilitating and frequently crippling autoimmune disease with overwhelming personal, social, and economic effects. Although less common than OA, RA is usually more severe. RA affects the interstitial tissues, blood vessels, cartilage, bone, tendons, and ligaments, as well as the synovial membranes that line joint surfaces. RA occurs more frequently in women than in men. Although the peak onset commonly occurs between 20 and 45 years of age, it often strikes individuals in their twenties or thirties. Numerous remissions and exacerbations generally follow its onset, although for some people it lasts just a few months or years and then goes away completely.

The exact cause of RA is still unknown, but there are some clues. Certain genes have been discovered that play a role in the development of RA, but it appears that something must occur to trigger the disease in those who are susceptible. Like other autoimmune diseases, the most likely trigger is a viral or bacterial infection. It's also possible that changing hormone levels in women related to pregnancy, breast-feeding, or contraceptive use may also be a factor (NIAMS, 2004).

Pathophysiology

RA is a chronic, autoimmune, systemic disorder. The inflammatory process, which involves cytokines, seems to play a role. RA has articular manifestations that involve chronic inflammation that begins in the synovial membrane and progresses to subsequent damage in the joint cartilage (see *Pathophysiology and Care Management Algorithm:* Rheumatoid Arthritis).

Although any joint may be affected by RA, involvement of the small joints of the extremities—typically the proximal interphalangeal joints of the hands and feet—is most common (Figure 40-3).

Pain, stiffness, swelling, and loss of function are frequent complaints. The swelling or puffiness is caused by the accumulation of synovial fluid in the membrane lining the joints and inflammation of the surrounding tissues (Figure 40-4). The appearance of **rheumatoid factor,** an abnormal circulating protein that is an immunoglobulin-classified antibody, may precede symptoms of RA (Kelly et al., 1997). Anemia may also be present.

Medical Management

Pharmacologic therapy to control pain and inflammation is the mainstay of treatment for RA. Salicylates and NSAIDs are often the first line of treatment, and MTX is commonly

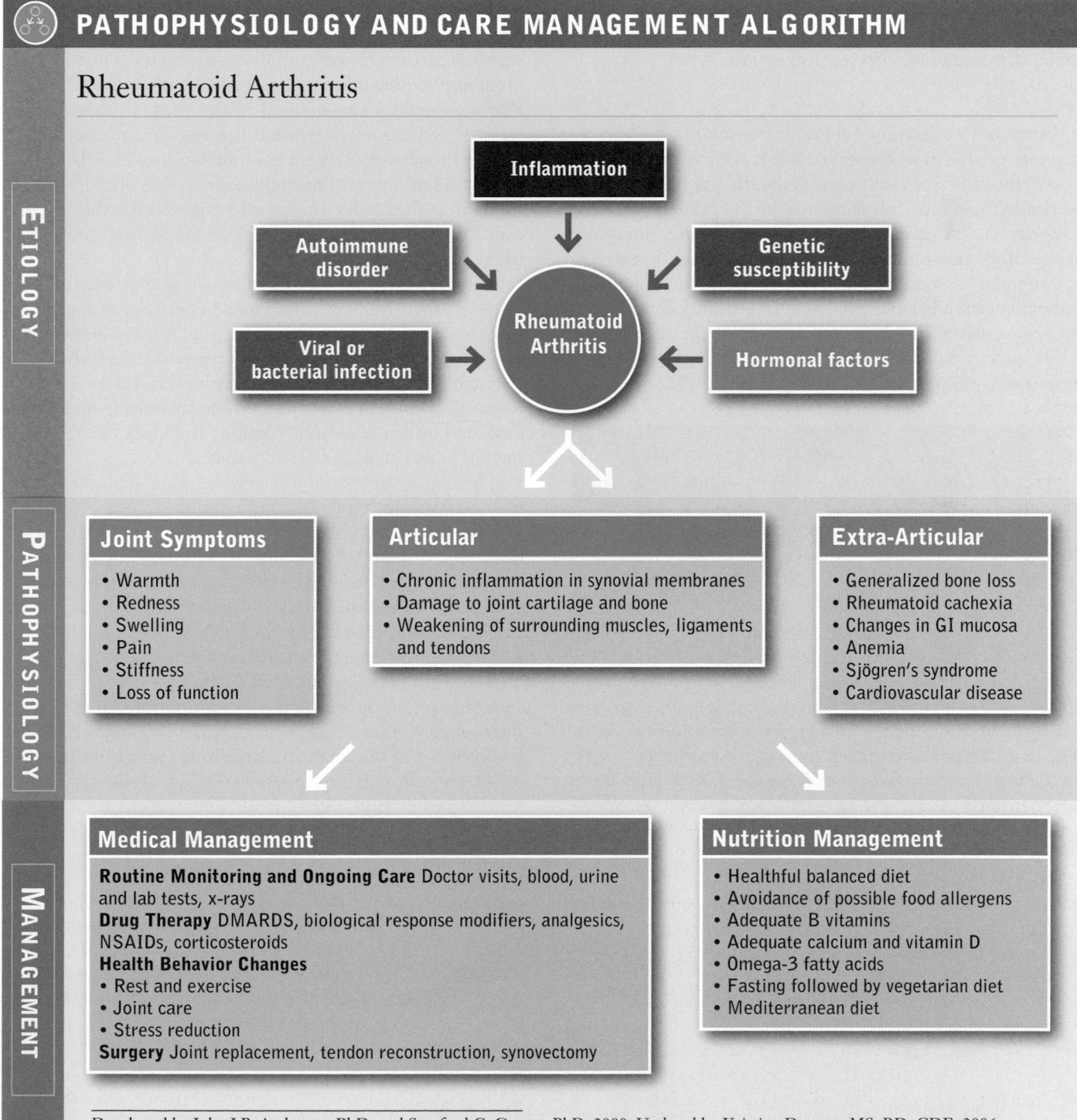

PATHOPHYSIOLOGY AND CARE MANAGEMENT ALGORITHM

Rheumatoid Arthritis

ETIOLOGY

Inflammation

Autoimmune disorder

Genetic susceptibility

Viral or bacterial infection

Rheumatoid Arthritis

Hormonal factors

PATHOPHYSIOLOGY

Joint Symptoms
- Warmth
- Redness
- Swelling
- Pain
- Stiffness
- Loss of function

Articular
- Chronic inflammation in synovial membranes
- Damage to joint cartilage and bone
- Weakening of surrounding muscles, ligaments and tendons

Extra-Articular
- Generalized bone loss
- Rheumatoid cachexia
- Changes in GI mucosa
- Anemia
- Sjögren's syndrome
- Cardiovascular disease

MANAGEMENT

Medical Management

Routine Monitoring and Ongoing Care Doctor visits, blood, urine and lab tests, x-rays
Drug Therapy DMARDS, biological response modifiers, analgesics, NSAIDs, corticosteroids
Health Behavior Changes
- Rest and exercise
- Joint care
- Stress reduction
Surgery Joint replacement, tendon reconstruction, synovectomy

Nutrition Management
- Healthful balanced diet
- Avoidance of possible food allergens
- Adequate B vitamins
- Adequate calcium and vitamin D
- Omega-3 fatty acids
- Fasting followed by vegetarian diet
- Mediterranean diet

Developed by John J.B. Anderson, PhD, and Stanford C. Garner, PhD, 2000. Updated by Kristine Duncan, MS, RD, CDE, 2006.

prescribed as well, but these drugs may cause significant side effects for some individuals. The choice of drug class and type is based on patient response to the medication, incidence and severity of adverse reactions, and patient compliance. Drug-nutrient side effects can occur with any of the drugs. Side effects of drug use may influence ingestion, digestion, and absorption, and hence nutrition status.

Surgery

Surgical treatment for RA may be considered if pharmacologic and nonpharmacologic treatment cannot adequately control the pain or maintain acceptable levels of functioning. Common surgical options include synovectomy, joint replacement, and tendon reconstruction.

Exercise

Physical and occupational therapy are often part of the initial therapy for newly diagnosed RA but may also be integrated into the treatment plan as the disease progresses and ADLs are affected. To maintain joint function, recommendations may be given for energy conservation, along with range-of-motion and strengthening exercises. Although the patient may be reluctant at first, research has shown that individuals with RA can participate in conditioning exercise programs without increasing fatigue or joint symptoms while improving joint mobility, muscle strength, aerobic fitness, and psychological well-being (ACR, 2002).

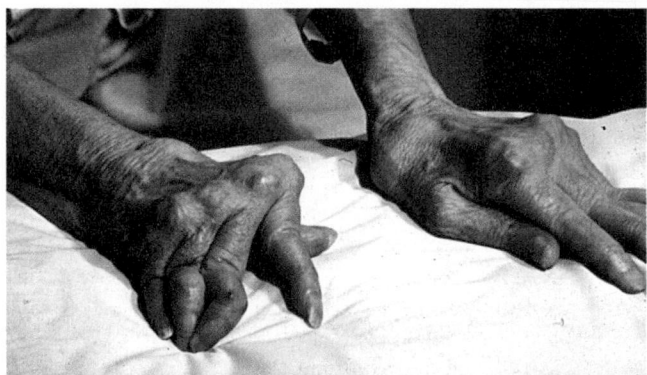

FIGURE 40-3 A patient with advanced rheumatoid arthritis. The twisted hands and the puffiness of the metacarpal joints are typical of the disease. *(From Damjanov I:* Pathology for the health-related professions, *ed 3, Philadelphia, 2006, Saunders.)*

A loss of body cell mass that accompanies RA, called *rheumatoid cachexia,* involves the skeletal muscle, viscera, and immune system. This can lead to muscle weakness and loss of function, which may hasten morbidity and mortality in RA. Physical activity, including both aerobic exercise and strength training, seems to be the most important tool to combat rheumatoid cachexia. Any exercise program for an RA patient must take into account the individual's disease status (Walsmith and Roubenoff, 2002).

Medical Nutrition Therapy

The American Dietetic Association's Nutrition Care Process and Model serves as a guide for implementing MNT with RA patients (Lacey and Pritchett, 2003). The first step, a comprehensive nutrition assessment of individuals with RA, is essential. The medical history should include a review of systems to determine the systemic impact of the disease process. A physical examination provides diagnostic signs and symptoms of nutrient deficits. Use of a "likelihood of malnutrition index" has been suggested for this population (Alarcon and Morgan, 1997), considering the number of medications often used.

Current weight and history of weight change over time are the least expensive, least invasive, and most reliable assessment tools to use with this population. Studies demonstrate that weight change is an important measure in RA severity. The characteristic progression of malnutrition in RA is attributed to excessive protein catabolism evoked by inflammatory cytokines and by disuse atrophy resulting from functional impairment (Fukuda et al., 2005; Morgan et al., 1997).

The diet history should review the usual diet, the impact of the handicap; types of food consumed; and changes in food tolerance secondary to oral, esophageal, and intestinal disorders. Impact of the disease on food shopping and preparation, self-feeding ability, appetite, and intake also need to be assessed. The use of elimination or other diets purported to treat or cure arthritis should be evaluated. The information gathered from the nutrition assessment can be used to formulate the nutrition diagnosis.

Articular and extraarticular manifestations of RA affect the nutrition status of individuals in several ways. Articular involvement of the small and large joints may limit the ability to perform nutrition-related ADLs, including shopping for, preparing, and eating food. Involvement of the tem-

Normal Joint

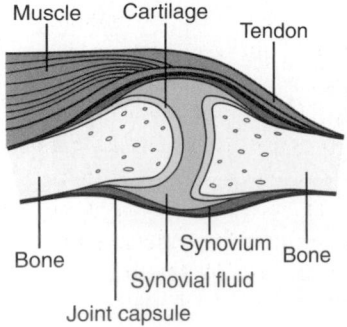

Joint Affected by Rheumatoid Arthritis

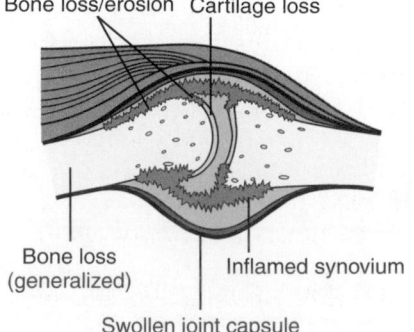

FIGURE 40-4 Comparison of a normal joint and one affected by rheumatoid arthritis, which has swelling of the synovium. *(From National Institute of Arthritis and Musculoskeletal and Skin Diseases:* Handout on health: rheumatoid arthritis, *NIH Publication Number 04-4179, January 1998, Revised May 2004.) National Institutes of Health, Department of Health and Human Services.*

poromandibular joint can impact the ability to chew and swallow and may necessitate changes in diet consistency. Extraarticular manifestations include increased metabolic rate secondary to the inflammatory process, Sjögren's syndrome, and changes in the gastrointestinal mucosa.

The increase in metabolic rate secondary to the inflammatory process leads to increased nutrient needs, often in the face of a diminishing nutrient intake. Taste alterations secondary to xerostomia and dryness of the nasal mucosa; dysphagia secondary to pharyngeal and esophageal dryness; and anorexia secondary to medications, fatigue, and pain may reduce dietary intake. Changes in the gastrointestinal mucosa affect intake, digestion, and absorption. The impact of RA and the medications used may be evident throughout the gastrointestinal tract, from the oral cavity to the small and large intestines. Based on the patient's unique profile, a registered dietitian can determine the most appropriate nutrition intervention, followed by appropriate monitoring and evaluation.

The association of foods with disease flares should be discussed because of the possibility of undetected food allergies (see Chapter 29). Whether food intake can modify the course of RA is an issue of continued scientific debate and interest. Dietary manipulation by either modifying food composition or reducing body weight may give some clinical benefit in improving RA symptoms. Some benefits may be related to a reduction in immunoreactivity to food antigens eliminated by a change in diet (Karatay et al., 2005) (see *Clinical Insight*: Fasting and Vegetarian Diets in Rheumatoid Arthritis).

A recent prospective cohort was inconclusive with regard to identifying consumption of particular dietary components as risk factors for RA but suggested that, if food does play a role, it most likely does so a few years before clinical diagnosis (Pedersen et al., 2005). Red meat has been identified as having proinflammatory properties as a source of arachidonic acid; no link has been identified between RA and coffee or tea (Choi, 2005).

Energy

Objective measures of actual energy needs for this population have not been determined. It is important to remember that the actual impact of the inflammatory response on the metabolic rate is unknown and may vary from individual to individual. In addition, activity levels vary greatly.

Although traditional measures to assess energy requirements can be used, weight should be monitored, and energy intake modified as needed to achieve desirable or usual body weight. Methods to determine energy requirements are noted in Chapter 2. For patients who are totally sedentary, calculations should be estimated at the resting energy expenditure and adjusted for weight changes that occur over time. When intakes are poor, enteral or parenteral supplementation may be required, and home nutrition support is beneficial for chronic cases.

Protein

Well-nourished individuals require protein at levels comparable to the DRIs for age and sex. Patients with RA have increased whole-body protein breakdown (regardless of age), which correlates with growth hormone factor, glucagon, and TNF-α production (Rall et al., 1996b). Rall and associates also concluded that strength training for patients receiving MTX yielded normal rates of protein catabolism (Rall et al., 1996a). Protein may be given as 1.5 to 2 g/kg/day.

Lipids

The generation of reactive oxygen species is an important factor in the development and maintenance of RA (Darlington and Stone, 2001). Low-fat diets (including use of low-fat substitutes) lead to low serum levels of vitamins A and E and actually stimulate lipid peroxidation and eicosanoid production, thus aggravating RA (Adam et al., 1995). Therefore the typical emphasis on low-fat or fat-free dieting that has been the cornerstone of healthy eating in the United

✷ CLINICAL INSIGHT

Fasting and Vegetarian Diets in Rheumatoid Arthritis

Scientific literature suggests fasting for control of joint inflammation. Fasting followed by a vegetarian diet may produce a sustained positive response and that has been measured clinically and by laboratory variables of inflammation (Muller et al., 2001). Researchers pooled the results of four controlled studies lasting three months or more from 31 studies and showed a statistically and clinically significant long-term effect of fasting followed by a vegetarian diet (Muller et al., 2001).

A vegan, gluten-free diet causes improvement in some patients, possibly because of the reduction of immunoreactivity to food antigens. Similarly, a very low-fat vegan diet can improve symptoms in patients with moderate-to-severe RA (McDougall et al., 2002). Uncooked, lactobacilli- and

antioxidant-rich, vegan diets have also been suggested to have a positive outcome (Hanninen et al., 2000). Large amounts of living lactobacilli and chlorophyll-rich drinks and increased fiber intake seem to have positive effects on objective measures of RA and decrease the need for medications (Nenonen et al., 1998). It does not appear that the improvement comes from the body weight reducing effect of these diets (Sköldstam et al., 2005). Plant-based diets have long been regarded as appropriate interventions for prevention or treatment of cardiovascular disease, hypertension, cancer, renal disease, and diabetes and may serve as a reasonable template for a lifelong diet for reducing the risk of more than just rheumatic disease (ADA and DC, 2003; Leitzmann, 2005).

BOX 40-1

Production of Eicosanoids from Omega-3 and Omega-6 Fatty Acids

Omega-3: Linolenic Acid 18:3, Eicosapentaenoic Acid 20:5

Thromboxane A_3: Weak vasoconstrictor and weak platelet aggregator

Prostacyclin PGI_{3+}: Vasodilator and platelet antiaggregator

Leukotriene B_5: Weak inflammation inducer and weak chemotactic agent

Omega-6: Linoleic Acid 18:2 and Arachidonic Acid 20:4

Thromboxane A_2: Vasoconstrictor and potent platelet aggregator

Prostaglandin E_2: Vasodilator and platelet antiaggregator

Leukotriene B_4: Inflammation inducer and potent leukocyte chemotaxis and adherence inducer

From Simopoulos AP: Omega-3 fatty acids in inflammation and autoimmune diseases, *J Am Coll Nutr* 21:6, 2002.

States may actually be counterproductive for patients susceptible to or afflicted by RA.

RA patients are at increased risk for cardiovascular disease, explained by a systemic inflammatory response for both conditions (Snow and Mikuls, 2005). This is especially significant considering the new findings regarding COX-2 selective NSAIDs. In fact, many of the drugs used to treat RA can result in hyperhomocysteinemia, hypertension, and hyperglycemia, which have all been identified as risk factors for cardiovascular disease. Conveniently, treatment aimed at reducing inflammation may benefit both diseases (Snow and Mikuls, 2005).

Rather than eliminating fat, changing the type of fat in the diet is useful and would likely offer advantages for both the arthritis and cardiovascular systems. Omega-3 fatty acids, either in tablet form or as they occur in oils, have increased in popularity in the management of RA because of their role in inflammatory pathways (Box 40-1; *Focus On:* Omega-3 Fatty Acids and the Inflammatory Process). A shift from a traditional Western diet to a Mediterranean diet (higher in omega-3 fatty acids) has been shown to cause a reduction in inflammatory activity,

◎ FOCUS ON

Omega-3 Fatty Acids and the Inflammatory Process

Two classes of polyunsaturated fatty acids—omega-6 and omega-3—are metabolized competitively, including conversion of their 20-carbon chain by oxygenase enzymes to form eicosanoids (*eicosa* means 20 in Greek). Prostaglandins, thromboxanes, leukotrienes, and prostacyclins are eicosanoids. Eicosapentaenoic acid (EPA) has a 20-carbon chain, and docosahexaenoic acid (DHA) has a 22-carbon chain; these are the omega-3 polyunsaturated fatty acids that are abundant in fish such as salmon, mackerel, herring, tuna, and some other fish oils. α-Linolenic acid (ALA) has an 18-carbon chain with an omega-3 bond and is found in abundance in flaxseed, walnuts, and soy and canola (rapeseed) oils.

EPA, DHA, and ALA have all been shown to reduce the synthesis of aggressive inflammatory response cytokines by interfering with the conversion of arachidonic acid in various pathways, thus suppressing activation of cytokines in the cell membrane. Cytokines are produced by antagonistic omega-6 polyunsaturated acids that are mostly formed from linoleic acid found in safflower and other oils (Grimble and Tappia, 1998).

Arachidonic acid comes exclusively from animal foods. The type of inflammatory mediator that is produced is determined by the composition of cellular membrane lipids, which in turn is influenced by the nature of the fatty acids in the diet. By increasing the amount of omega-3 fatty acids in the diet, the production of mediators with antiinflammatory effects is increased. Similarly, reducing the amount of arachidonic acid appears to minimize inflammation in rheumatoid arthritis independently and can enhance the benefits of fish oil supplementation (Adam et al., 2003).

Studies over the past two decades have clearly shown beneficial changes in cytokine and eicosanoid metabolism with fish oil supplementation in patients with rheumatoid arthritis (James et al., 2000; Tidow-Kebritchi and Mobahan, 2001). Although fish oil seems to exert an antiinflammatory effect in short-term studies, these effects may vanish during long-term treatment because of decreased numbers of autoreactive T cells via apoptosis. In already existing disease increased consumption might not be beneficial over a long period (Ergas et al., 2002).

Although most studies (Ariza-Ariza et al., 1998; Hansen et al., 1998) have demonstrated improvement in arthritic conditions and modulation of the inflammatory response with the administration of omega-3, lowered intake of omega-6 fatty acids and increased intake of omega-3 oils should not replace conventional drug therapies. These oils should be used in conjunction with improved eating habits. A diet that includes baked or broiled fish one to two times/week, and/or an omega-3 supplement (approximate daily dose: EPA: 50 mg/kg/day, DHA: 30 mg/kg/day) can be recommended for rheumatoid arthritis patients. However, the Food and Drug Administration has identified shark, swordfish, king mackerel, and tilefish as high-mercury fish that should be avoided. It's possible that additional benefits may come from a combination of fish oils and olive oil (Berbert et al., 2005) (see Box 40-2). Counselors should advise their patients that, although the quality of fish oil supplements is steadily improving, these supplements are not without their own side effects, such as increased bleeding time, gastrointestinal distress, fishy taste or odor, and possible mercury contamination (if not obtained from a reputable manufacturer).

increase in physical function, and improved vitality for RA patients (Sköldstam et al., 2003).

Some other oils of marine origin and a range of vegetable oils (olive and evening primrose oil) have indirect antiinflammatory actions probably mediated via PGE_1 (Belch and Hill, 2000; Darlington and Stone, 2001). Flaxseed oil contains the 18-carbon, omega-3 fatty acid α-linolenic acid, which can be converted to eicosapentaenoic acid after ingestion; it can be just as effective as fish oil in inhibiting arachidonic acid conversion to eicosanoids (James et al., 2000).

Minerals, Vitamins, and Antioxidants

Animal studies have shown that vitamin E—in addition to omega-3 and omega-6 fatty acids—may also affect cytokine and eicosanoid production by decreasing proinflammatory cytokines and lipid mediators (Tidow-Kebritchi and Mobahan, 2001). In one human study several antioxidant enzymes were efficient suppressors of oxygen radical overproduction in RA patients (Ostrakhovitch and Afanas'ev, 2001). Selenium, used in some trials, does not show specific clinical benefits (Peretz et al., 2001). Synovial fluid and plasma trace element concentrations, excluding Zn, change in inflammatory RA, but not in OA; altered trace element concentrations in inflammatory RA might be a result of the changes of the immunoregulatory cytokines (Yazar et al., 2005).

Earlier studies have shown that juvenile arthritis patients have reduced serum concentrations of antioxidants in comparison to healthy controls and may benefit from dietary supplements when the dietary intake does not reach desired levels (Helgeland et al., 2000). Clinical trials have shown significant pain reduction in RA patients treated with vitamin E and other antioxidants (Ostrakhovitch and Afanas'ev, 2001; Tidow-Kebritchi and Mobahan, 2001).

Degradation of collagen and eicosanoid stimulation are associated with oxidative damage; therefore increased intakes of supplemental antioxidants have been linked with beneficial effects in terms of both prevention and therapy for RA (Aaseth et al., 1998; Hansen et al., 1998); however,

---

BOX 40-2

Olive Oil as Medicine

The benefits of olive oil as a component of a healthy diet are well established (Wahle et al., 2004), but preliminary research suggests that it may be used as an alternative to medication. A component of olive oil has been shown to inhibit cyclooxygenase enzymes in the synthesis of prostaglandins just as ibuprofen can. This action has been attributed to oleocanthal, a compound in newly pressed extra virgin olive oil that has natural antiinflammatory activity (Beauchamp et al., 2005). More studies are needed to determine an effective dose and identify any limits to its use for patients with rheumatic disease. The addition of an antioxidant would be required to improve the oxidative stability of olive oil (Lee et al., 2006).

---

there are not significant data to support routine supplementation with vitamin C, vitamin A, or β-carotene.

RA patients often have nutritional intakes below the dietary recommended intakes (DRI) for calcium, folic acid, vitamin E, zinc, vitamin B, and selenium (Stone et al., 1997; Morgan et al., 1993). Calcium and vitamin D malabsorption and bone demineralization are characteristic of advanced stages of the disease, leading to osteoporosis or osteomalacia. Prolonged use of glucocorticoids can also lead to osteoporosis (ACR, 2002). Supplementation with calcium and vitamin D has been shown to help prevent and reduce the severity of these detrimental conditions (Oelzner and Hein, 1997).

Results from animal studies have shown that the role of vitamin D as a selective immunosuppressant is illustrated by its ability to either prevent or markedly suppress animal models of RA and SLE, although the action of vitamin D depends on the animal's maintenance of a normal or high-calcium diet in almost every case. Greater intake of vitamin D may be associated with a lower risk of RA in older women, although this finding is yet to be confirmed with more studies (Merlino et al., 2004).

Use of MTX in rheumatoid RA may be associated with elevated homocysteine levels caused by low folate levels. Thus in patients with RA, paying special attention to adequate intakes of folate and vitamins B_6 and B_{12} makes sense (Morgan et al., 1998; Roubenoff et al., 1997).

Elevated levels of copper and ceruloplasmin in serum and joint fluid are seen in RA. Plasma copper levels correlate with the degree of joint inflammation, decreasing as the inflammation is diminished. Elevated plasma levels of ceruloplasmin, the carrier protein for copper, may have a protective role because of its antioxidant activity.

Variations in serum ferritin levels are less common in elderly persons than in young adults; this is true in RA as well (Lammi-Keefe et al., 1996). Plasma transferrin receptor levels are reliable for assessing iron status in this population. No special requirement for iron supplementation appears to exist in cases of RA.

Independent of drug-induced alterations in specific vitamin or mineral levels, mounting evidence supports supplementation beyond the minimum levels for some nutrients. Vitamin therapy may complement conventional drug therapy, especially in the case of vitamin E (Tidow-Kebritchi and Mobahan, 2001), folic acid (Dervieux et al., 2006), and vitamin D (Deluca and Cantorna, 2001).

Herbs and Complementary Therapy

The increasing popularity of the use of complementary and alternative treatments appears to be particularly evident with people afflicted with chronic diseases. One therapy that has been identified to have a potential benefit in the treatment of RA is herbal therapy (Little and Parsons, 2001; Tao et al., 2001); however, concerns of toxicity must also be addressed because the FDA provides relatively little regulation of herbal therapies.

Gamma-linolenic acid (GLA) is an omega-6 fatty acid found in the oils of black currant, borage, and evening primrose that can be converted into the antiinflammatory

PGE_1 or into arachidonic acid (AA), a precursor of the inflammatory PGE_2. Because of competition between omega-3 and omega-6 fatty acids for the same enzymes, the relative dietary contribution of these fats appears to affect which pathways are favored. The enzyme delta-5 desaturase converts GLA into AA, but a diet high in omega-3 fats will pull more of this enzyme to the omega-3 pathway, allowing the body to use GLA to produce PGE_1. This antiinflammatory PG may relieve pain, morning stiffness, and joint tenderness with no serious side effects. Further studies are required to establish optimum dosage and duration (Little and Parsons, 2001), but the AF suggests 2 to 3 g daily from oil or capsules.

Thunder god vine (*Tripterygium wilfordii*) has been used in China to treat patients with a number of autoimmune diseases. It has been shown to inhibit mitogen-stimulated lymphoproliferation and inhibit production of proinflammatory cytokines by monocytes, lymphocytes, and PGE_2 production via the COX-2 pathway (Lipsky and Tao, 1997). Doses greater than 360 mg/day are associated with a clinical benefit in patients with RA (Tao et al., 2001; Tao et al., 2002). However, currently there are no consistent, high-quality thunder god vine preparations being manufactured in the United States. High doses and long-term use of thunder god vine may suppress the immune system and/or reduce bone density (NCCAM, 2005).

SJÖGREN'S SYNDROME

Sjögren's syndrome, a chronic autoimmune disorder, is characterized by polyglandular tissue destruction leading to keratoconjunctivitis, diminished production of tears and saliva, xerostomia, and xerophthalmia (Tabbara and Vera-Cristo, 2000). Half of the patients with Sjögren's syndrome also have RA. Patients may also suffer from disorders of the skin, lung, kidney, nerve, connective tissue, and digestive system because of more extensive glandular damage.

The goal of dietary management in individuals with Sjögren's syndrome is relief of symptoms and eating discomfort, which can result in lack of appetite, weight loss, fatigue, difficulty chewing and swallowing, mouth infections such as candidiasis, and anemia. Management of xerostomia should also include strategies for reducing the risk of dental decay (see Chapter 25), including frequent rinsing with water, toothbrushing, using topical fluorides, or chewing sugar-free gum. It's also a good idea to limit or avoid sugary foods altogether to minimize cavities. If sugary foods or beverages are consumed, the teeth should be brushed immediately. Changes in the sense of smell are also a possible result of xerostomia.

Because swallowing is a problem, ready-to-eat foods may be useful. Foods should all be moist, and extremes in temperature should be avoided. The tartness of artificially sweetened lemon drops may help stimulate salivary flow. Artificial saliva or products such as lemon glycerin may also be recommended by dental professionals or dietetic professionals.

It has been suggested that nutrient intake may play a role in the development or progression of Sjögren's syndrome. One study found a higher energy-adjusted intake of supplemental calcium and a lower energy-adjusted intake of non-supplemental vitamin C, polyunsaturated fat, linoleic acid, and omega-3 fatty acid in Sjögren's patients compared to controls (Cermak et al., 2003). Malnutrition does not seem to be more common in this population (Hay et al., 2001); however, iron and vitamin deficiencies such as low vitamin B_{12} and folate are possible and should be treated with a well-balanced diet (Lundstrom and Lindstrom, 2001).

Dehydroepiandrosterone (DHEA), a hormone made by the adrenal glands, the production of which declines with aging, has benefited some patients and has been suggested as an adjunct treatment to corticosteroids (Straub et al., 2000). However, a clinical trial of 200 mg of oral DHEA failed to show efficacy (Pillemer et al., 2004).

TEMPOROMANDIBULAR DISORDERS

Temporomandibular disorders (TMDs) affect the temporomandibular joint, which connects the lower jaw (mandible) to the temporal bone. TMDs can be classified as myofascial pain, internal derangement of the joint, or degenerative joint disease. One or more of these conditions may be present at the same time, causing pain or discomfort in the muscles or joint that control jaw function. Besides experiencing a severe jaw injury, there is little scientific evidence to suggest a cause for TMD, but it is generally agreed that physical or mental stress may aggravate TMD.

The goal of dietary management is to alter food consistency to reduce chewing pain. According to the National Institute of Dental and Craniofascial Research (NIDCR), diet should be mechanically soft in consistency, all foods should be cut into bite-size pieces to minimize the individual's need to chew or open the jaw widely, and gum-chewing should be avoided (NIDCR, 2005). Nutrient intake of TMD patients appears to be the same as the general population with regard to total calories, protein, fat, carbohydrates and dietary fiber, calcium, and iron, but during times of acute pain their intake of fiber appears to be reduced (Raphael et al., 2002).

GOUT

Pathophysiology

Gout, one of the oldest diseases in recorded medical history, is a disorder of **purine** metabolism in which abnormally high levels of uric acid accumulate in the blood (hyperuricemia). As a consequence, sodium urates are formed and deposited as tophi in the small joints and surrounding tissues. Renal disease is common, and uric acid nephrolithiasis can occur. In chronic gout a classic site is the helix of the ear (Figure

40-5); a more common site is the large toe or the elbow (Figure 40-6).

The prevalence of gout is increasing (Choi and Curhan, 2005). The disease usually occurs after the age of 35 years and predominantly affects men. However, it becomes equally distributed in both sexes in the older years (Saag and Choi, 2006).

Gout is characterized by the sudden and acute onset of localized arthritic pain that usually begins in the big toe and continues up the leg. In one retrospective study those with familial gout had an onset 7.5 years earlier than environmentally afflicted subjects and had lower serum triglyceride and cholesterol levels and less hypertension than nonfamilial gout sufferers (Chen et al., 2001). These urate deposits can destroy joint tissues, leading to chronic symptoms of arthritis (Figure 40-7).

One comorbidity of gout is obesity (World Health Organization, 2000). Increased visceral adipose tissue seems to aggravate the risk of insulin resistance in gout and may leave these patients at an increased risk for atherosclerotic disease (Takahashi et al., 2001). Although weight loss appears to be protective (Choi et al., 2005a; Dessein et al., 2000), ketosis associated with fasting or a low-carbohydrate diet can also precipitate an attack. Occasionally the disturbance follows surgery. As the disease advances, symptoms occur more frequently and are more prolonged. Trivial injury or unaccustomed exertion may precipitate the episodes, and attacks have been related to environmental lead exposure, and excessive eating, drinking, and exercise. Hypertension and use of diuretics appear to be risk factors for gout as well (Choi et al., 2005b). Epidemiologic studies suggest an association between gout and dyslipidemia, diabetes mellitus, and insulin resistance syndrome (Fam, 2005).

Medical Management

The goals of treatment are to reduce the pain associated with acute attacks, to prevent future attacks, and to avoid the formation of tophi and nephrolithiasis. The primary treatment for gout involves pharmacologic therapy, but the patient can take an active role by adhering to the nutrition guidelines for the management of gout as well.

Medical Nutrition Therapy

Uric acid, derived from the metabolism of purines, constitutes a part of nucleoproteins. Although gout has traditionally been treated with a low-purine diet, drugs have largely replaced the need for rigid restriction of the diet. It appears that about two thirds of the daily purine load results from endogenous cell turnover, with just one third supplied by the diet (Fam, 2005).

Low-fat dairy products, ascorbic acid, and wine consumption appear to be protective (Lee et al., 2006), possibly because of the alkaline ash effect of these foods (see *Clinical Insight*: Acid Ash and Alkaline Ash Diets, in Chapter 36). Otherwise specific dietary changes are not clear. It is prudent to advise patients to consume meat, seafood, and alcoholic beverages in moderation; control food portion size; and reduce noncomplex carbohydrate intake to achieve weight loss and improve insulin sensitivity (Lee et al., 2006).

Results from the Third National Health and Nutrition Examination Survey (NHANES) found that higher levels of meat and seafood consumption were associated with increased serum uric acid levels in adults, but total protein intake was not (Choi et al., 2005a). A moderate intake of purine-rich vegetables is not associated with an increased risk of gout (Choi et al., 2004).

Even though limiting dietary purines is unlikely to decrease the uric acid pool significantly, individuals with gout can be encouraged to limit or avoid foods high in purines to avoid metabolic stress (ketosis from excessive dieting). If purine is restricted, as in severe gout, it should be restricted to 100 to 150 mg/day; the groupings in Box 40-3

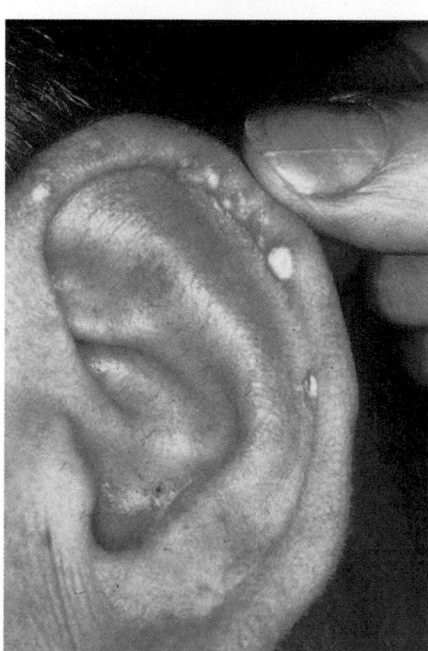

FIGURE 40-5 Tophi on the ear of a patient who has had gout for many years. (*Courtesy American College of Rheumatology, Atlanta.*)

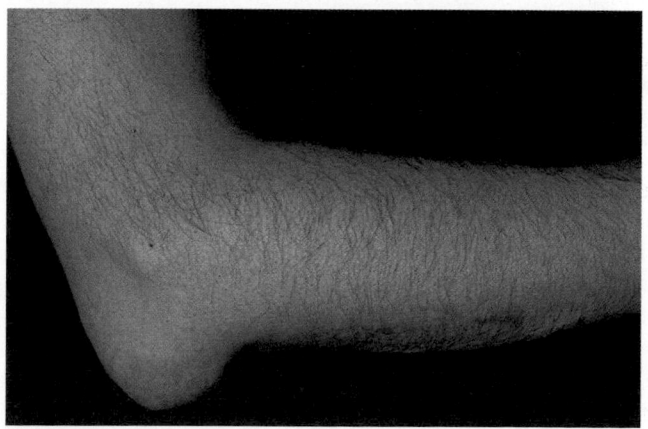

FIGURE 40-6 Gout. This markedly enlarged olecranon bursa is caused by gout. (*From the Clinical Slide Collection on the Rheumatic Diseases, copyright 1991, 1995, 1997. Used by permission of the American College of Rheumatology, Atlanta.*)

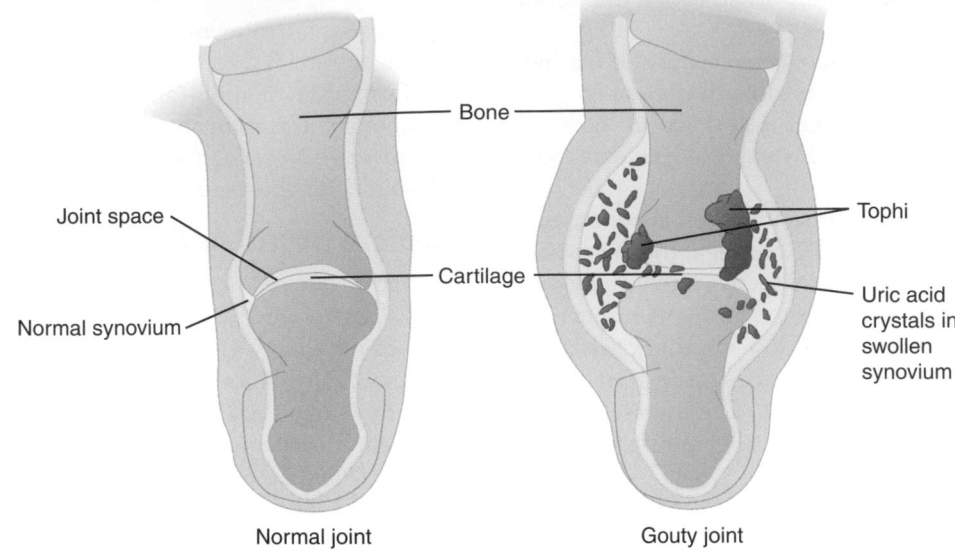

FIGURE 40-7 Comparison of a gouty joint and a normal joint in the toe. *(From Black JM et al: Medical surgical nursing, ed 7, Philadelphia, 2005, Saunders.)*

BOX 40-3

Foods Grouped According to Purine Content

Group 1: High Purine Content (100 to 1000 mg of Purine Nitrogen per 100 g of Food)

Anchovies	Meat extracts
Bouillon	Mincemeat
Brains	Mussels
Broth	Partridge
Consommé	Roe
Goose	Sardines
Gravy	Scallops
Heart	Sweetbreads
Herring	Yeast (baker's and brewer's),
Kidney	taken as supplement
Mackerel	

Foods in this list should be omitted from the diet of patients who have gout (acute and remission stages).

Group 2: Moderate Purine Content (9 to 100 mg of Purine Nitrogen per 100 g of Food) (except those listed in group 1)

Meat and Fish	**Vegetables**
Fish	Asparagus
Poultry	Beans, dried
Meat	Lentils
Shellfish	Mushrooms
	Peas, dried
	Spinach

One serving (2 to 3 oz) of meat, fish, or fowl or 1 serving (½ c) of vegetables from this group is allowed daily.

Group 3: Negligible Purine Content

Bread, white, and crackers	Fruit
Butter or margarine	Gelatin desserts
(in moderation)*	Herbs
Cake and cookies	Ice cream
Carbonated beverages	Milk
Cereal beverage (e.g., Postum)	Macaroni products
Cereals and cereal products	Noodles
Cheese	Nuts
Chocolate	Oil
Coffee	Olives
Condiments	Pickles
Cornbread	Popcorn
Cream (in moderation)*	Puddings
Custard	Relishes
Eggs	Rennet desserts
Fats (in moderation)*	Rice
Vegetables (except those	Salt
in group 2)	Sugar and sweets
	Tea
	Vinegar
	White sauce

Foods included in this group may be used daily.

*Recommended in moderation because of fat content.

can be used, allowing for considerable individualization among patients.

Intake of fluids (3 L/day) should be encouraged to assist with the excretion of uric acid and to minimize the possibility of renal calculi formation. A calorie-restricted diet (1600 kcal), consisting of 40% carbohydrate (primarily complex), 30% protein, and 30% fat (primarily monounsaturated and polyunsaturated), reduces frequency of attacks, serum uric acid levels, total cholesterol, and low-density lipoprotein–cholesterol and high-density lipoprotein–cholesterol in adult men with gout (Dessein et al., 2000).

A suspected association between gout and alcohol consumption is long-standing. Recent studies suggest that the type of alcoholic beverage may make a difference. Beer intake appears to increase uric acid levels and subsequently the risk of gout, whereas moderate wine consumption appears to do neither (Choi and Curhan, 2005).

SCLERODERMA

Pathophysiology

Scleroderma is a progressive, systemic sclerosis characterized by deposition of fibrous connective tissue in the skin and visceral organs, including the gastrointestinal tract (Escott-Stump, 2007). It is considered an autoimmune disease with a genetic component. Free-radical, oxidative damage from cytokines, where fibroblast proteins are modified, is involved (Kurien et al., 2006). Women tend to be afflicted four times more often than men.

One manifestation of scleroderma is **Raynaud's syndrome** with ischemia or coldness in the small extremities, which causes difficulty in preparation and consumption of meals. Sjögren's syndrome is often also present. Gastrointestinal symptoms include gastroesophageal reflux, nausea and vomiting, dysphagia, diarrhea, constipation, fecal incontinence, small bowel bacterial overgrowth and chronic intestinal pseudoobstruction (Attar, 2002). Joint stiffness and pain, renal dysfunction, hypertension, pulmonary fibrosis, and pulmonary arterial hypertension are common (Scleroderma Research Foundation, 2005). Treatments for the pulmonary hypertension and renal crises have shown the best results overall (Charles et al., 2006). The 5-year survival rate after diagnosis is 80% to 85%.

Medical Management

The disease is progressive, and no current treatment corrects the overproduction of collagen; therefore treatment is aimed at relieving symptoms and limiting damage. Pharmacologic therapy is often involved. Some studies have been undertaken with the use of anti-TNF therapies with some promising results (Alexis and Strober, 2005).

Medical Nutrition Therapy

Dysphagia may be one symptom that requires nutrition intervention (see Appendix 35). Malabsorption of lactose, vitamins, fatty acids, and minerals can cause further nutri-

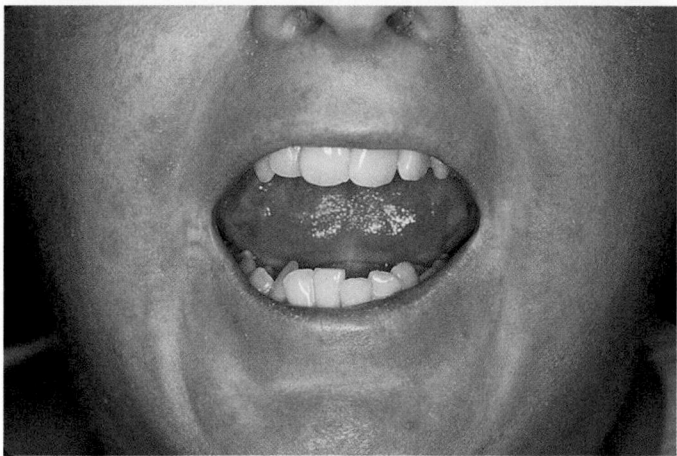

FIGURE 40-8 Facial scleroderma. Taut smooth skin over the face and reduced oral aperture of a woman with long-standing disease. *(From Wigley FM, Hummers LK: Clinical features of systemic sclerosis. In Hochberg MC et al., editors:* Practical rheumatology, *ed 3, Toronto, 2004, Mosby.)*

tion problems; supplementation may be required. A high-energy, high-protein supplement or enteral feeding may be effective in correcting or preventing weight loss, which is a common manifestation. Home enteral or parenteral nutrition support is often required when problems such as chronic diarrhea persist (see Chapter 20).

Dry mouth with resultant tooth decay, loose teeth, and tightening facial skin can make eating difficult (Figure 40-8). Consuming adequate fluids, choosing moist foods, chewing sugarless gum, and using saliva substitutes may offer some relief and help moisten the mouth. If gastroesophageal reflux is a concern, small, frequent meals are recommended along with avoidance of late-night eating, alcohol, caffeine, and spicy or fatty foods (see Chapter 26).

SYSTEMIC LUPUS ERYTHEMATOSUS

Pathophysiology

Systemic lupus erythematosus (SLE) has an etiology related to genetic predisposition and overproduction of type 1 interferon and other cytotoxic cells (Banchereau and Pascual, 2006). The condition is most prevalent in women of childbearing age and is more common in blacks and women of Hispanic, Asian, and Native American descent than in whites. Common symptoms include extreme fatigue, painful or swollen joints, unexplained fever, skin rashes, mouth ulcers, and kidney problems (NIAMS, 2003).

Medical Management

SLE is considered to be an autoimmune disease that affects all organ systems. Renal function is deranged, thus causing excessive excretion of protein and often renal failure.

The disease itself, as well as the medications (corticosteroids, NSAIDs, immunosuppressants, antimalarials) that are commonly used to treat SLE affect nutrient metabolism, needs, and excretion. Recent therapies include B cell depletion with rituximab. B cell depletion helps promote remission while maintaining normal levels of IgG and IgM levels (Smith et al., 2006).

Medical Nutrition Therapy

At this time no specific dietary guidelines for managing SLE exist. Rather, the diet needs to be tailored to the individual needs of the patient. Priorities include addressing the sequelae of the disease and the pharmacologic effects on organ function and nutrient metabolism (see Table 40-1). Protein requirements are altered as a result of disordered renal function caused by the disease and steroid-induced side effects. Sodium and fluid intakes are typically restricted for the same reasons.

The effect of dietary modifications has been extensively studied in lupus animal models. Energy needs should be tailored to the individual's dry weight. The goal in determining caloric requirements should be to attain and maintain the usual body weight. Calorie, protein, and especially fat restriction may cause a significant reduction in immune-complex deposition in the kidney and proteinuria and may prolong the life span (Leiba et al., 2001). Adding polyunsaturated fatty acids (30 g of ground flaxseed daily for 1 year) in a small group of subjects protected the kidneys; large-scale studies are recommended (Clark et al., 2001). Nutrition support may be required in chronic cases.

Antioxidant status may provide insight into this disease. SLE patients have been found to have lower plasma antioxidant levels and dietary antioxidant intake than control subjects (Bae et al., 2002). Similarly, a 4-year prospective study of women with SLE found that vitamin C intake was inversely associated with the risk of active disease (Minami et al., 2003). Anemia is also common, regardless of iron intake (Shah et al., 2004).

It has been suggested that gluten sensitivity could be the true culprit in patients mistakenly diagnosed with lupus (Hadjivassiliou et al., 2004). Because there appears to be significant crossover of symptoms among several autoimmune diseases, specific MNT guidelines prove to be a challenge.

CHRONIC FATIGUE SYNDROME AND FIBROMYALGIA

Disorders such as **chronic fatigue syndrome (CFS)** and **fibromyalgia** have rheumatic symptoms but unknown pathophysiology and no proven cure. Some experts believe that CFS and fibromyalgia are variations on the same pain and fatigue syndrome. In fact, 50% to 70% of people with a diagnosis of fibromyalgia also meet the criteria for CFS and vice versa (Davis, 2005). Women are affected two to four times more often than men (Mayo Clinic Staff, 2005).

In CFS chronic fatigue is the major symptom. It lasts 6 months or longer and is accompanied by hypotension, sore throat, multiple joint pains, headaches, postexertion lethargy, muscle pain, and impaired concentration. CFS mimics autoimmune disorders such as SLE or hypothyroidism. Viral pathogens, immune dysregulation, central nervous system dysfunction, clinical depression, musculoskeletal disorders, and allergies have been suggested in the etiology of the syndrome (Craig and Kakaumanu, 2002).

In fibromyalgia nonarticular aches and fatigue cause disabling symptoms that are similar to those of RA. Muscle tenderness, sleep disturbances, fatigue, morning stiffness, numbness and tingling, chronic headaches, irritable bowel, and irritable bladder have all been reported to be associated with the "fibromyalgia syndrome." Several hypotheses have been proposed, including central pain derangement, central nervous system dysfunction, nutrient deficiencies of magnesium, malic acid, manganese, or thiamin, and other systemic abnormalities.

Medical Management

A treatment program for CFS should be multidisciplinary and include exercise, MNT, appropriate sleep hygiene, low-dose tricyclic antidepressants or SSRIs, and cognitive behavior therapy (Lucas, 2006; Craig and Kakaumanu, 2002).

Exercise has been shown to be effective with fibromyalgia patients. In one study three 30-minute classes for 23 weeks appeared to be successful in improving mood and physical function (Gowans et al., 2001). Similarly a multidisciplinary rehabilitation program consisting of supervised exercise therapy, group pain and stress management lectures, massage therapy sessions, and a dietary lecture resulted in improved self-perceived health status and average pain intensity (Lemstra and Olszynski, 2005). Management of concomitant disorders, including irritable bowel syndrome, depression, and migraine headaches, can improve quality of life for these patients.

Medical Nutrition Therapy

Data regarding MNT for CFS are extremely limited. Since symptoms of CFS can mimic those present with a nutrient deficiency, inadequate nutrition has been theorized as a possible cause. When hypotension is identified medically in CFS patients, increases in sodium and fluid intakes have been suggested.

A vegan diet may have beneficial effects on fibromyalgia patients, at least for the short term (Donaldson et al., 2001; Kaartinen et al., 2000). A low-salt, uncooked-vegetable, lactobacteria-rich diet may yield improvements in pain, joint stiffness, and sleep quality. In another study a vegan "living food" diet of berries, fruits, vegetables and roots, nuts, germinated seeds, and sprouts rich in carotenoids and vitamins C and E resulted in a decrease in joint stiffness (Hanninen et al., 2000). Longer studies are needed to confirm these findings.

Regular meal spacing is recommended. The intake of omega-3 fatty acids should be high since they can decrease the inflammatory effects of CFS and depression (Maes et al., 2005). Finally, the natural antiinflammatory flavonoids in quercetin show promise (Lucas et al., 2006).

Complementary Therapy

The treatment options for fibromyalgia appear to be limited and generally unsatisfactory. Patients often seek complementary and alternative medicine (CAM) treatments for relief from symptoms. A survey of fibromyalgia patients found that 98% had used some type of CAM in the previous 6 months, including massage therapy, chiropractic therapy, and vitamin or mineral supplements (Wahner-Roedler et al., 2005). A review of CAM studies for fibromyalgia found that acupuncture, massage therapy, and supplements of magnesium and SAM-e offer the most hope and empiric evidence for effectiveness (Holdcraft et al., 2003).

CONTROVERSIES AND LIMITATIONS OF UNCONVENTIONAL THERAPIES FOR RHEUMATIC DISEASE

Because modern medicine cannot promise a cure or even permanent relief of symptoms, many persons with RDs understandably turn to alternative and complementary medical approaches for help. With growing access to the Internet, RD patients have a greater exposure to remedies and controversial treatments that have little scientific evidence to support their effects or claims of benefits.

Favorable effects of self-help treatments are often reported anecdotally, but as a rule no cause-and-effect relationships are documented. Any amelioration can usually be attributed to the placebo effect or to characteristic cycles of worsening followed by periods of improvement. The American College of Rheumatology "supports the integration of those therapies scientifically proven safe and effective and advises caution for those not studied scientifically" (ACR, 2004).

Some seemingly "natural" remedies have their roots in medicine, as in the case of willow bark and copper bracelets. Salicylates, as in aspirin and derived from willow bark, have been around as a medicinal remedy for pain and inflammation since 1763; some have even traced their use back to ancient Egypt (Vane, 2000). Willow bark and ginger may relieve pain since their chemical composition is similar to NSAIDs, but excessive blood thinning is a concern (Marcus, 2005). Although the folk remedy of wearing a copper bracelet to relieve arthritis pain has been suggested as a means of promoting copper absorption through the skin, no clinical studies have substantiated this claim.

Additional research is needed on valerian, feverfew, boswellia, and curcumin before recommendations can be made for their usefulness in treating RA (NCCAM, 2005). The AF recommends against the use of copper or copper salts, devil's claw, echinacea, guaifenesin, alfalfa, wild yam, and MSM. Feedback, relaxation, chlorella supplements, magnet therapies, homeopathy, botanical oils and dietary modifications need further study before general recommendations for fibromyalgia patients can be made (Holdcraft et al., 2003).

Shark cartilage is a popular remedy because it is a cheap source of chondroitin sulfate, but there are no studies of the effect of shark cartilage on joint disease. Even with positive-effect evidence for cow trachea chondroitin sulfate and other promising "natural" remedies, some difficulties persist, including the following: (1) lack of regulation of such supplements in terms of dosage, purity, or claims; (2) the fact that using these nonregulated remedies is, in effect, self-medication without monitoring; and (3) lack of understanding of interactions with drugs or long-term safety. Although much of the dietary experimentation is harmless, except for the costs, some self-treatment modalities can be harmful. Both comfrey and alfalfa are herbs that have been promoted as potential cures for arthritis, yet both have been deemed toxic by the scientific community.

Clinical trials have shown positive effects of mind-body therapies in the treatment of RA, including meditation, tai chi, relaxation techniques, and spirituality (NCCAM, 2005). There is preliminary evidence that thermotherapy and transcutaneous electrical nerve stimulations may offer pain reduction for OA patients, but not electrotherapy, homeopathy, static magnets or manual therapy (Sarzi-Puttini et al., 2005; NCCAM, 2005). Finally the use of pulsed electromagnetic fields has been shown to affect the growth of bone and cartilage in vitro with potential application as an arthritis treatment, but data are limited (NCCAM, 2005).

Registered dietitians can serve as a valuable resource for RD patients regarding the safety and effectiveness of new, alternative, and complementary treatments for their disease, specifically in responding to questions about dietary strategies and nutrition supplements. Registered dietitians can use their unique skills in providing care for this population, including making referrals when appropriate and encouraging patients to share their use of these treatments with their primary care physician and the entire health care team.

⊙ FOCAL POINTS

- No known cure for rheumatic disorders exists, but MNT plays a key role in their treatment and holds promise for patients for the span of their lifetimes.
- Pharmacotherapy, physical therapy, occupational therapy, and MNT can help to manage the symptoms associated with rheumatic disorders.
- Alternative diet therapies, supplements, and programs currently under investigation promise to reduce the need for high doses of toxic medications, to alleviate some of the symptoms, and to manage pain.
- Since rheumatic disease is likely linked to other chronic diseases such as diabetes, cardiovascular disease, and obesity, which have a nutritional component, MNT should provide the optimal balance of immediate relief from rheumatic symptoms and preservation of short-term health.
- A diet rich in omega-3 fatty acids, fruits and vegetables, and whole grains can be safely recommended for all patients with rheumatic disease.

CLINICAL SCENARIO 1

Maryanne is a 63-year-old woman who has been diagnosed with early stage osteoarthritis in her right knee and both thumbs. Until diagnosis she enjoyed walking with her neighbor on the weekends, chasing after her two grandchildren, cooking for her family, and knitting. She's afraid the arthritis will limit her ability to keep up with these activities. Her weight has been slowly increasing over the years, and she is currently at 160 lbs. with a height of 5 ft 5 in. Her physician has prescribed a nonsteroidal antiinflammatory drug (NSAID) for pain and suggested that she speak with a registered dietitian about a weight-loss program to decrease her symptoms and the progression of the disease. She comes to see you and presents a list of supplements and herbs that her friends have suggested she take to control her osteoarthritis naturally because the NSAID seems to affect her stomach.

*** Nutrition Diagnosis 1:** Food and nutrition knowledge deficit related to appropriate diet for weight loss as evidenced by weight gain

*** Nutrition Diagnosis 2:** Food and nutrition knowledge deficit related to use of herbs and supplements as evidenced by questions regarding use for arthritis treatment

*** Nutrition Diagnosis 3:** Food medication interaction related to NSAID use as evidenced by gastric pain following medication

1. How would you approach Maryanne's diet, considering her current situation?
2. What type of complementary therapy might you recommend as a possibility to help improve her weight and manage the pain?
3. What are the benefits and risks of NSAID use that you could discuss with her?
4. What advice would you give her regarding the use of herbs and supplements? What type of information is available (e.g., research; websites; organizations that may be able to provide information on the efficacy, safety, and hazards of consuming specific vitamin/mineral supplements and herbs)?

CLINICAL SCENARIO 2

Mike is a 43-year-old man who lives alone in a large city. He is 5 ft 10 in and weighs 250 lb. He has hypertension and a family history of diabetes and has recently been diagnosed with gout. He is a long-haul truck driver; thus he is often away from home for extended periods and relies on restaurants for most of his meals. He limits his alcohol intake when he's on the road but likes to indulge on the weekends with his favorite beer and wine. His physician has referred him to a registered dietitian to help improve his eating habits and his long-term health.

*** Nutrition Diagnosis:** Food and nutrition knowledge deficit related to medical nutrition therapy for gout as evidenced by patient report

1. What type of diet or meal plan would you recommend for Mike to manage his gout?
2. How will his hypertension and risk of diabetes impact this plan?
3. Are there specific foods you would encourage him to choose less often or more often? What about fluid?
4. How would exercise benefit his current situation?
5. Mike does not mention his overweight. How would you bring up the subject, and what steps would you recommend for him?

USEFUL WEBSITES

American College of Rheumatology
www.rheumatology.org

Arthritis Foundation
www.arthritis.org
www.arthritis.org/conditions/supplementguide

Lupus Foundation of America
www.lupus.org

National Center for Complementary and Alternative Medicine
http://nccam.nih.gov/

National Fibromyalgia Association
www.fmaware.org

National Institute of Arthritis and Musculoskeletal and Skin Diseases
www.nih.gov/niams

Scleroderma Foundation
www.scleroderma.org

Scleroderma Research Foundation
www.srfcure.org

Sjögrens Syndrome Foundation
www.sjogrens.org

References

Aaseth J et al: Rheumatoid arthritis and metal compounds: perspectives on the role of oxygen radical detoxification, *Analyst* 123:3, 1998.

Adam O et al: Low-fat diet decreases alpha-tocopherol levels and stimulates LDL oxidation and eicosanoid biosynthesis in man, *Eur J Med Res* 1:65, 1995.

Adam O et al: Anti-inflammatory effects of a low arachidonic acid diet and fish oil in patients with rheumatoid arthritis, *Rheumatol Int* 23:1, 2003.

Alarcon GS, Morgan SL: Guidelines for folate supplementation in rheumatoid arthritis patients treated with methotrexate: comment on the guidelines for monitoring drug therapy, *Arthritis Rheum* 40:391, 1997.

Alexis AF, Strober BE: Off-label dermatologic uses of anti-TNF-α therapies, *J Cutan Med Surg* 9(6):296, 2005.

American College of Rheumatology: Recommendations for the medical management of osteoarthritis of the hip and knee, *Arthritis Rheum* 43:9, 2000.

American College of Rheumatology: Guidelines for the management of rheumatoid arthritis, 2002 update, *Arthritis Rheum* 46:2, 2002.

American College of Rheumatology: *Biologic agents for rheumatic disease*, 2006, http://www.rheumatology.org/publications/position/biologics.asp, accessed April 9, 2007.

American College of Rheumatology: *Position statement: complementary and alternative therapies for rheumatic diseases*, 2004, www.rheumatology.org, accessed April 1, 2007.

American Dietetic Association, Dietitians of Canada: Position of the American Dietetic Associations and Dietitians of Canada: vegetarian diets, *J Am Diet Assoc* 103:6, 2003.

Anderson JW et al: Glucosamine effects in humans: a review of effects on glucose metabolism, side effects, safety considerations and efficacy, *Food Chem Toxicol* 43(2):187, 2005.

Ariza-Ariza R et al: Omega-3 fatty acids in rheumatoid arthritis: an overview, *Semin Arthritis Rheum* 27:366, 1998.

Arthritis Foundation: *Arthritis today, 2007 drug guide*, 2007, www.arthritis.org/conditions/drugguide/, accessed April 9, 2007.

Arthritis Foundation: *Herbs and supplements and their uses*, 2005a, www.arthritis.org, accessed April 9, 2007.

Arthritis Foundation: *Arthritis today, supplements and vitamins*, 2005b. www.arthritis.org, accessed April 9, 2007.

Attar A: Digestive manifestations in systemic sclerosis, *Ann Med Interne* (Paris) 153:4, 2002.

Bae SC et al: Impaired antioxidant status and decreased dietary intake of antioxidants in patients with systemic lupus erythematosus, *Rheumatol Int* 22:6, 2002.

Bancherau J, Pascual V: Type I interferon in systemic lupus erythematosus and other autoimmune diseases, *Immunity* 25(3):383, 2006.

Barnes EV, Edwards NL: Treatment of osteoarthritis, *South Med J* 98:5, 2005.

Beauchamp GK et al: Phytochemistry: ibuprofen-like activity in extra-virgin olive oil, *Nature* 437:7055, 2005.

Belch JJ, Hill A: Evening primrose oil and borage oil in rheumatologic conditions, *Am J Clin Nutr* 71: 352S, 2000.

Berbert AA et al: Supplementation of fish oil and olive oil in patients with rheumatoid arthritis, *Nutrition* 21:2, 2005.

Berman BM et al: Effectiveness of acupuncture as adjunctive therapy in osteoarthritis of the knee: a randomized, controlled trial, *Ann Intern Med* 141:12, 2004.

Brand C et al: Vitamin E is ineffective for symptomatic relief of knee osteoarthritis: a six-month double blind, randomized, placebo-controlled study, *Ann Rheum Dis* 60:946, 2001.

Cannon M: *Minocycline*, www.rheumatology.org, accessed April 2005.

Centers for Disease Control and Prevention: Update: direct and indirect costs of arthritis and other rheumatic conditions—United States, 1997, *MMWR* 53:18, 2004.

Centers for Disease Control and Prevention: Racial/ethnic differences in the prevalence and impact of doctor-diagnosed arthritis—United States, 2002, *MMWR* 54:5, 2005.

Cermak JM et al: Nutrient intake in women with primary and secondary Sjögren's syndrome, *Eur J Clin Nutr* 57:2, 2003.

Charles C et al: Systemic sclerosis: hypothesis-driven treatment strategies, *Lancet* 367(9523):1683, 2006.

Chen SY et al: Clinical features of familial gout and effects of probable genetic association between gout and its related disorders, *Metabolism* 50:1203, 2001.

Choi HK: Dietary risk factors for rheumatic diseases, *Curr Opin Rheumatol* 17:2, 2005.

Choi HK et al: Purine-rich foods, dairy and protein intake, and the risk of gout in men, *N Engl J Med* 350:11, 2004.

Choi HK et al: Intake of purine-rich foods, protein, and dairy products and relationship to serum levels of uric acid: the Third National Health and Nutrition Examination Survey, *Arthritis Rheum* 52:1, 2005a.

Choi HK et al: Obesity, weight change, hypertension, diuretic use, and risk of gout in men: the health professionals' follow-up study, *Arch Intern Med* 165:7, 2005b.

Choi HK, Curhan G: Gout: epidemiology and lifestyle choices, *Curr Opin Rheumatol* 17:3, 2005.

Clark WF et al: Flaxseed in lupus nephritis: a two-year nonplacebo-controlled crossover study, *J Am Coll Nutr* 20:143S, 2001.

Coggon D et al: Knee osteoarthritis and obesity, *Int J Obes Relat Metab Disord* 25: 622, 2001.

Colgazier CL, Sutej PG: Laboratory testing in the rheumatic diseases: a practical review, *South Med J* 98:2, 2005.

Conn DL: Resolved: low-dose prednisone is indicated as a standard treatment in patients with rheumatoid arthritis, *Arthritis Rheum* 45: 462, 2001.

Craig T, Kakaumanu S: Chronic fatigue syndromes: evaluation and treatment, *Am Fam Physician* 65:6, 2002.

DaCamara CC, Dowless GV: Glucosamine for osteoarthritis, *Ann Pharmacother* 32:58, 1998.

Darlington LG, Stone TW: Antioxidants and fatty acids in the amelioration of rheumatoid arthritis and related disorders, *Br J Nutr* 85:251, 2001.

Davis C: *What's in a name: fibro vs. CFS*, Arthritis Foundation, www.arthritis.org, accessed July 24, 2005.

Deluca HF, Cantorna MT: Vitamin D: its role and uses in immunology, *FASEB J* 15:2579, 2001.

Dervieux T et al: Pharmacogenomic and metabolic biomarkers in the folate pathway and their association with methotrexate effects during dosage escalation in rheumatoid arthritis, *Arthritis Rheum* 54:3095, 2006.

Dessein PH et al: Beneficial effects of weight loss associated with moderate calorie/carbohydrate restriction and increased proportional intake of protein and unsaturated fat on serum urate and lipoprotein levels in gout: a pilot study, *Ann Rheum Dis* 59:7, 2000.

Donaldson MS et al: Fibromyalgia syndrome improved using a mostly raw vegetarian diet: an observational study, *BMC Complement Altern Med* 1:1, 2001.

Ergas D et al: N-3 fatty acids and the immune system in autoimmunity, *Isr Med Assoc* J 4:34, 2002.

Escott-Stump S: *Nutrition and diagnosis-related care*, ed 6, Baltimore, 2007, Lippincott Williams & Wilkins.

Ettinger WH Jr et al: A randomized trial comparing aerobic exercise and resistance exercise with a health education program in older adults with knee osteoarthritis: the Fitness Arthritis and Seniors Trial (FAST), *JAMA* 277:1, 1997.

Fam AG: Gout: excess calories, purines and alcohol intake and beyond: response to a urate-lowering diet, *J Rheumatol* 32:5, 2005.

Food and Drug Administration: *FDA announces important changes and additional warnings for COX-2 selective and nonselective nonsteroidal anti-inflammatory drugs (NSAIDs)*, from www.fda.gov, accessed April 7, 2005.

Fukuda W et al: Malnutrition and disease progression in patients with rheumatoid arthritis, *Mod Rheumatol* 15:2, 2005.

Gowans SE et al: Exercise can improve mood and physical function, *Arthritis Rheum* 45:519, 2001.

Grimble RF, Tappia PS: Modulation of pro-inflammatory cytokine biology by unsaturated fatty acids, *Z Ernahrungswiss* 37:57, 1998.

Hadjivassiliou M et al: Gluten sensitivity masquerading as systemic lupus erythematosus, *Ann Rheum Dis* 63:11, 2004.

Hanninen O et al: Antioxidants in vegan diet and rheumatic disorders, *Toxicology* 155:45, 2000.

Hansen G et al: Nutritional status of Danish patients with rheumatoid arthritis and effects of a diet adjusted in energy intake, fish content and antioxidants, *Ugeskr Laeger* 160:3074, 1998.

Hay KD et al: Quality of life and nutritional studies in Sjögren's syndrome patients with xerostomia, *NZ Dent J* 97:430, 2001.

Helgeland M et al: Dietary intake and serum concentrations of antioxidants in children with juvenile arthritis, *Clin Exp Rheumatol* 18:637, 2000.

Holdcraft LC: Complementary and alternative medicine in fibromyalgia and related syndromes, *Best Pract Res Clin Rheumatol* 17:4, 2003.

James MJ et al: Dietary polyunsaturated fatty acids and inflammatory mediator production, *Am J Clin Nutr* 71:343S, 2000.

Kaartinen K et al: Vegan diet alleviates fibromyalgia symptoms, *Scand J Rheumatol* 29:308, 2000.

Karatay S et al: General or personal diet: the individualized model for diet challenges in patients with rheumatoid arthritis, *Rheumatol Int* 26:556, 2005.

Kelly WN et al: *Textbook of rheumatology*, vol 2, Philadelphia, 1997, Saunders.

Kramer HM, Curhan G: The association between gout and nephrolithiasis: the National Health and Nutrition Examination Survey III, 1988-1994, *Am J Kidney Dis* 40:1, 2002.

Kurien BT et al: Oxidatively modified autoantigens in autoimmune diseases, *Free Radic Biol Med* 41(4):549, 2006.

Lacey K, Pritchett E: Nutrition care process and model: ADA adopts road map to quality care and outcomes management, *J Am Diet Assoc* 103:1062, 2003.

Lammi-Keefe C et al: Day-to-day variation in iron status indexes is similar for most measures in elderly women with and without rheumatoid arthritis, *J Am Diet Assoc* 96:247, 1996.

Lee SJ et al: Recent developments in diet and gout, *Curr Opin Rheumatol* 18(2):193, 2006.

Lee JH et al: Antioxidant evaluation and oxidative stability of structured lipids from extra virgin olive oil and conjugated linoleic acid, *J Agric Food Chem* 54:5416, 2006.

Leiba A et al: Diet and lupus, *Lupus* 10:246, 2001.

Leitzmann C: Vegetarian diets: what are the advantages? *Forum Nutr* 57:147, 2005.

Lemstra M, Olszynski WP: The effectiveness of multidisciplinary rehabilitation in the treatment of fibromyalgia: a randomized controlled trial, *Clin J Pain* 21:2, 2005.

Lipsky PE, Tao XL: A potential new treatment for rheumatoid arthritis: thunder god vine, *Semin Arthritis Rheum* 26:713, 1997.

Little C, Parsons T: Herbal therapy for treating rheumatoid arthritis, *Cochrane Database Syst Rev* (1):CD002928, 2001.

Lucas HJ: Fibromyalgia—new concepts of pathogenesis and treatment, *Int J Immunopathol Pharmacol* 19(1):5, 2006.

Lundstrom IM, Lindstrom FD: Iron and vitamin deficiencies, endocrine and immune status in patients with primary Sjögren's syndrome, *Oral Dis* 7:144, 2001.

Maes M et al: In chronic fatigue syndrome, the decreased levels of omega-3 poly-unsaturated fatty acids are related to lowered serum zinc and defects in T cell activation, *Neuro Endocrinol Lett* 26:745, 2005.

Marcus D: *Herbal and Natural Remedies*, from www.rheumatology.org, accessed 2005.

Mayo Clinic Staff: Chronic fatigue syndrome, overview, from www.mayoclinic.com, accessed June 23, 2005.

McAlindon TE, Biggee BA: Nutritional factors and osteoarthritis: recent developments, *Curr Opin Rheumatol* 17:5, 2005.

McCleane G: The analgesic efficacy of topical capsaicin is enhanced by glyceryl trinitrate in painful osteoarthritis: a randomized, double-blind, placebo-controlled study, *Eur J Pain* 4:355, 2000.

McDougall J et al: Effects of a very low–fat, vegan diet in subjects with rheumatoid arthritis, *J Altern Complement Med* 8:1, 2002.

Merlino LA et al: Vitamin D intake is inversely associated with rheumatoid arthritis: results from the Iowa Women's Health Study, *Arthritis Rheum* 50:1, 2004.

Messier SP et al: Exercise and dietary weight loss in overweight and obese older adults with knee osteoarthritis: the Arthritis, Diet and Activity Promotion Trial, *Arthritis Rheum* 50:5, 2004.

Messier SP et al: Weight loss reduces knee-joint loads in overweight and obese older adults with knee osteoarthritis, *Arthritis Rheum* 52:7, 2005.

Mikesky AE et al: Effects of strength training on the incidence and progression of knee osteoarthritis, *Arthritis Rheum* 55(5):690, 2006.

Minami Y et al: Diet and systemic lupus erythematosus: a 4-year prospective study of Japanese patients, *J Rheumatol* 30:4, 2003.

Morgan SL et al: Dietary intake and circulating vitamin levels of rheumatoid arthritis patients treated with methotrexate, *Arthritis Care Res* 6:4, 1993.

Morgan S et al: Nutrient intake patterns, body mass index, and vitamin levels in patients with rheumatoid arthritis, *Arthritis Care Res* 10:9, 1997.

Morgan S et al: Folic acid supplementation prevents deficient blood folate levels and hyperhomocysteinemia during long-term, low-dose methotrexate therapy for rheumatoid arthritis: implications for cardiovascular disease prevention, *J Rheumatol* 25:441, 1998.

Muller H et al: Fasting followed by a vegetarian diet in patients with rheumatoid arthritis: a systemic review, *Scand J Rheumatol* 30:1, 2001.

National Center for Complementary and Alternative Medicine: *Rheumatoid arthritis and complementary and alternative medicine*, from http://nccam.nih.gov/, accessed December 1, 2005.

National Institute of Arthritis and Musculoskeletal and Skin Diseases: *Questions and answers about Sjögren's syndrome*, from www.niams.nih.gov, accessed 2001.

National Institute of Arthritis and Musculoskeletal and Skin Diseases: *Questions and answers about arthritis and rheumatic disease*, from www.niams.nih.gov, accessed 2002.

National Institute of Arthritis and Musculoskeletal and Skin Diseases: *Systemic lupus erythematosus, handout on health*, from www.niams.nih.gov, accessed 2003.

National Institute of Arthritis and Musculoskeletal and Skin Diseases: *Rheumatoid arthritis, handout on health*, from www.niams.nih.gov, accessed 2004.

National Institute of Arthritis and Musculoskeletal and Skin Diseases: *Osteoarthritis, handout on health*, 2006a, from www.niams.nih.gov, accessed 2006.

National Institute of Arthritis and Musculoskeletal and Skin Diseases: *Scleroderma, handout on health*, 2006b, from www.niams.nih.gov, accessed 2006.

National Institute of Dental and Craniofacial Research: TMD: temporomandibular disorders, from www.nidcr.nih.gov, accessed May, 2005.

National Institutes of Health: *Questions and answers: NIH glucosamine/chondroitin arthritis intervention trial (GAIT)*, from www.nccam.nih.gov, accessed February 2006.

Nenonen T et al: Uncooked, lactobacilli-rich, vegan food and rheumatoid arthritis, *Br J Rheumatol* 37:274, 1998.

Nicolakis P et al: Long-term outcome after treatment of temporomandibular joint osteoarthritis with exercise and manual therapy, *Cranio* 20:23, 2002.

Oelzner P, Hein G: Inflammation and bone metabolism in rheumatoid arthritis: pathogenetic viewpoints and therapeutic possibilities, *Med Klin* 92:607, 1997.

Ostrakhovitch EA, Afanas'ev IB: Oxidative stress in rheumatoid arthritis leukocytes: suppression by rutin and other antioxidants and chelators, *Biochem Pharmacol* 62:743, 2001.

Pederson M et al: Diet and risk of rheumatoid arthritis in a prospective cohort, *J Rheumatol* 32:7, 2005.

Peretz A et al: Selenium supplementation in rheumatoid arthritis investigated in a double blind, placebo-controlled trial, *Scand J Rheumatol* 30:208, 2001.

Pillemer SR et al: Pilot clinical trial of dehydroepiandrosterone (DHEA) versus placebo for Sjögren's syndrome, *Arhritis Rheum* 51:4, 2004.

Radin EL: Who gets osteoarthritis and why? *J Rheumatol* 31:S 70, 2004.

Rall LC et al: Effects of progressive resistance training on immune response in aging and chronic inflammation, *Med Sci Sports Exerc* 28:1356, 1996a.

Rall LC et al: Protein metabolism in rheumatoid arthritis and aging: effects of muscle strength training and tumor necrosis factor cc, *Arthritis Rheum* 39:1115, 1996b.

Raphael KG et al: Dietary fiber intake in patients with myofascial face pain, *J Orofac Pain* 16:1, 2002.

Robbins W: Clinical applications of capsaicinoids, *Clin J Pain* 16:86S2, 2000.

Roubenoff R et al: Abnormal homocysteine metabolism in rheumatoid arthritis, *Arthritis Rheum* 40:718, 1997.

Saag KG, Choi H: Epidemiology, risk factors, and lifestyle modifications for gout, *Arthritis Res Ther* 8:S2, 2006.

Sarzi-Puttini P et al: Osteoarthritis: an overview of the disease and its treatment strategies, *Semin Arthritis Rheum* 35(suppl 1):1, 2005.

Scleroderma Research Foundation: *Treatment information*, from www.srfcure.org, accessed October 9, 2005.

Shah M et al: Nutrient intake and diet quality in patients with systemic lupus erythematosus on a culturally sensitive cholesterol lowering dietary program, *J Rheumatol* 31:71, 2004.

Sköldstam L et al: An experimental study of a Mediterranean diet intervention for patients with rheumatoid arthritis, *Ann Rheum Dis* 62:3, 2003.

Sköldstam L et al: Weight reduction is not a major reason for improvement in rheumatoid arthritis from lacto-vegetarian, vegan or Mediterranean diets, *Nutrition J* 4:15, 2005.

Slot O: Changes in plasma homocysteine in arthritis patients starting treatment with low-dose methotrexate subsequently supplemented with folic acid, *Scand J Rheumatol* 30:305, 2001.

Smith KG et al: Long-term comparison of rituximab treatment for refractory systemic lupus erythematosus and vasculitis: remission, relapse, and re-treatment, *Arthritis Rheum* 54:2970, 2006.

Snow MH, Mikuls TR: Rheumatoid arthritis and cardiovascular disease: the role of systemic inflammation and evolving strategies for prevention, *Curr Opin Rheumatol* 17:3, 2005.

Stone J et al: Inadequate calcium, folic acid, vitamin E, zinc, and selenium intake in rheumatoid arthritis patients: results of a dietary survey, *Semin Arthritis Rheum* 27:180, 1997.

Straub RH et al: Replacement therapy with DHEA plus corticosteroids in patients with chronic inflammatory diseases—substitutes of adrenal and sex hormones, *Z Rheumatol* 59,108S2, 2000.

Tabbara KF, Vera-Cristo CL: Sjögren syndrome, *Curr Opin Opthalmol* 11:449, 2000.

Takahashi S et al: Increased visceral fat accumulation further aggravates the risks of insulin resistance in gout, *Metabolism* 50: 393, 2001.

Tao X et al: A phase I study of ethyl acetate extract of the Chinese antirheumatic herb *Tripterygium wilfordii* hook F in rheumatoid arthritis, *J Rheumatol* 28:2160, 2001.

Tao X et al: Benefit of an extract of *Tripterygium wilfordii* hook F in patients with rheumatoid arthritis: a double-blind, placebo-controlled study, *Arthritis Rheum* 46:7, 2002.

Tidow-Kebritchi S, Mobahan S: Effects of diets containing fish oil and vitamin E on rheumatoid arthritis, *Nutr Rev* 59:335, 2001.

Trock DH: Electromagnetic fields and magnets. Investigational treatment for musculoskeletal disorders, *Rheum Dis Clin N Am* 26:57, 2000.

Van Ede AE et al: Effect of folic or folinic acid supplementation on the toxicity and efficacy of methotrexate in rheumatoid arthritis: a forty-eight week, multicenter, randomized, double-blind, placebo-controlled study, *Arthritis Rheum* 44:1515, 2001.

Vane JR: The fight against rheumatism: from willow bark to COX-1 sparing drugs, *J Physiol Pharmacol* 51:573, 2000.

Wahle KW et al: Olive oil and modulation of cell signaling in disease prevention, *Lipids* 39:12, 2004.

Wahner-Roedler DL et al: Use of complementary and alternative medical therapies by patients referred to a fibromyalgia treatment program at a tertiary care center, *Mayo Clin Proc* 80:6, 2005.

Walsmith J, Roubenoff R: Cachexia in rheumatoid arthritis, *Int J Cardiol* 85:1, 2002.

Witt C et al: Acupuncture in patients with osteoarthritis of the knee: a randomized trial, *Lancet* 366:9480, 2005.

Wluka AE, et al: Supplementary vitamin E does not affect the loss of cartilage volume in knee osteoarthritis: a 2-year double-blind randomized placebo-controlled study, *J Rheumatol* 29:12, 2002.

World Health Organization: Obesity: preventing and managing the global epidemic: report of a WHO consultation, *World Health Organ Tech Rep Ser* 894:i, 1, 2000.

Yazar M et al: Synovial fluid and plasma selenium, copper, zinc and iron concentrations in patients with rheumatoid arthritis and osteoarthritis, *Biol Trace Elem Res* 106:2, 2005.

CHAPTER 41

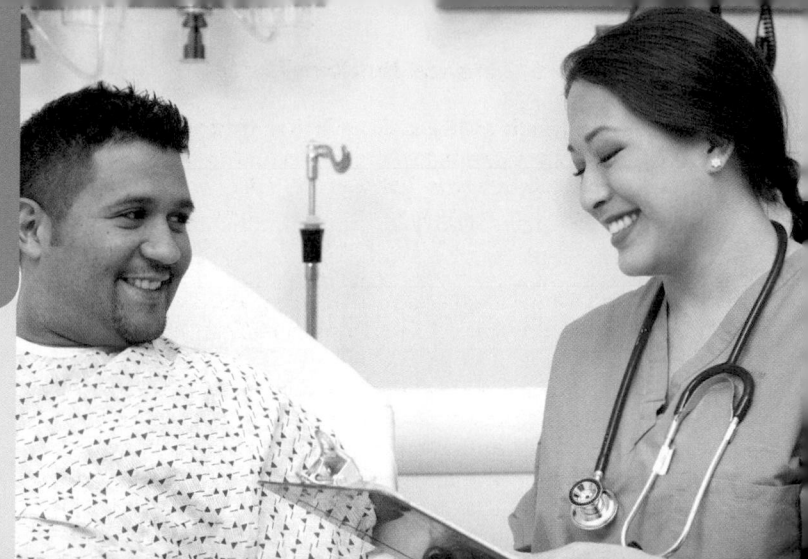

Valentina M. Remig, PhD, RD, LD, FADA

Medical Nutrition Therapy for Neurologic Disorders

KEY TERMS

absence seizure formerly known as petit mal seizure; generalized in nature in which the patient may appear to be daydreaming during an episode, but recovers consciousness within a few seconds and has no postictal fatigue or disorientation

adrenomyeloleukodystrophy (ALD) a rare congenital enzyme deficiency that affects the metabolism of very long–chain fatty acids (vlcfas) in young men; characterized by the accumulation of vlcfas in the brain and adrenal glands and the development of myelopathy, peripheral neuropathy, and cerebral demyelination

agnosia, agnosis loss of recognition that occurs as a manifestation of Alzheimer's disease; may affect any of the senses

Alzheimer's disease (AD) a complex neurodegenerative disease characterized by the presence in the brain of abnormal clumps of β-amyloid and neurofibrillary tangles composed of misplaced proteins; begins gradually, advances, and eventually leads to confusion, personality and behavior changes, and impaired judgment

amyotrophic lateral sclerosis (ALS) a progressive neurodegenerative disease of the motor neurons characterized by weakness and atrophy of muscles

anomia inability to remember names of objects; a common manifestation of Alzheimer's disease

anosmia absence of smell

aphasia loss of speech or expression

apraxia inability to perform purposeful movements although no sensory or motor impairment exists

ataxia impaired muscular movement, especially voluntary movement

corpus callosum the bridge between the two hemispheres of the brain, consisting of white matter

cortical blindness blindness resulting from a lesion of visual area of cerebral cortex

deglutitory dysfunction swallowing irregularity

diffuse axonal injury injury of axons throughout the brain, usually in the brainstem

dysarthria impairment of the tongue or other muscles essential to speech, which makes speaking difficult

dysgeusia impaired taste

dysomia distortion of normal smell

dysphagia difficulty swallowing

echolalia repeating spoken words by others; manifestation of Alzheimer's disease and psychotic disorders

embolic stroke occlusion of an artery by cholesterol plaque, depriving part of the oxygen supply of the brain

epidural hematoma usually from trauma; bleeding between the skull and the dura mater

Guillain-Barré syndrome (GBS) acute onset, inflammatory, demyelinating polyneuropathy that affects proximal motor nerves, including the cranial nerves and the diaphragm

hemiparesis weakness affecting only one side of the body

hemianopsia blindness for half of the visual field or vision in one eye

hemotympanum fluid or blood behind the eardrum or leaking from the ear, suggesting a skull base fracture

hydrocephalus accumulation of cerebrospinal fluid within ventricles of the brain

hyperosmia increased sensitivity of smell

migraine syndrome an episodic intense, throbbing head pain that lasts from 4 to 72 hours; usually on one side of the head and becomes worse with exertion; may be accompanied by nausea, a prodrome of visual disturbances or unusual olfactory and gustatory perception, and transient visual aura, including flashing lights

Sections of this chapter were written by Cecilia Romero, MD for the previous edition of this text.

multiple sclerosis (MS) a progressive disease characterized by disseminated demyelination of nerve fibers of the brain and spinal cord

myasthenia gravis (MG) an autoimmune disorder of the neuromuscular junction in which the body's immune system raises a response to acetylcholine receptors

myelopathy any pathologic condition of the spinal cord

nystagmus constant, involuntary movement of the eyeball

otorrhea clear fluid running from the ear, suggesting a skull base fracture

paresthesia numbness sensation, heightened sensitivity, experienced in central and peripheral nerve lesions and locomotor ataxia

Parkinson's disease (PD) a progressive, disabling, neurodegenerative disease characterized by slow and decreased movement, muscular rigidity, resting tremor, postural instability, and decreased dopamine transmission to the basal ganglia

peripheral neuropathy functional disturbance or pathologic changes in the peripheral nervous system; noninflammatory lesions in the peripheral nervous system

rhinorrhea salty fluid dripping from the nose or down the pharynx

subarachnoid hemorrhage (SAH) bleeding into subarachnoid space, often caused by a ruptured aneurysm in the arteries at the base of the brain

subdural hematoma blood collection between the dura mater and arachnoid membrane

thromboembolic event obstruction of a blood vessel by a thrombus that has become detached from its site of formation

thrombotic stroke the rupturing of a cholesterol plaque in an artery, with subsequent platelet aggregation to clot an already narrowed artery

tonic-clonic seizure "grand mal" seizure characterized by generalized involuntary muscular contraction and cessation of respiration; may occur singly or in close succession with a sensory warning or aura preceding each seizure; followed by deep sleep, headache, confusion, and muscle soreness

transient ischemic attack a brief attack lasting from a few minutes to hours of cerebral dysfunction of vascular origin with no persistent neurologic defect

Wernicke-Korsakoff syndrome (WKS) a disease of the cerebellum and brainstem that results from chronic thiamin deficiency with continued carbohydrate ingestion

Diseases of the nervous system pose serious health problems of worldwide magnitude despite knowledge and understanding of the nutrients required to prevent neurologic diseases. For example, between 1991 and 1994, when sudden economic and political changes occurred in Cuba, the Cuban Ministry of Public Health reported over 50,000 cases of optic and peripheral neuropathy among its population of 10.8 million. The pathogenesis was associated with an acute nutritional deficiency combined with the toxic effects of tobacco. A significant number of patients improved after treatment with parenteral administration of vitamin B–complex vitamins (high doses of thiamin, riboflavin, B_6, and B_{12}); oral supplements of vitamins A, E, and folic acid; and consumption of a high-protein diet for 10 days. Prophylactic vitamin supplements were subsequently distributed to the entire population, and after only 2 months the incidence of disease had plummeted (Ordunez-Garcia et al., 1996). Fortunately in this situation, nutrition was assessed, and inexpensive vitamin B therapy prevented a major catastrophe.

NEUROLOGIC DISEASE CLASSIFICATION

The medical or health history is often the most important part of the neurologic evaluation. Numerous symptoms and malnutrition may accompany the various types of neurologic disease. Complaints of even minor symptoms such as headaches, dizziness, insomnia, weakness, pain, and discomfort must be skillfully evaluated for the presence of a nutrition component in their cause and treatment.

Primary prevention is the cornerstone of management for neurologic diseases that arise from nutritional deficiencies as described in the previous section or from nutritional excesses. Although not all neurologic diseases have a nutrition etiology, nutritional considerations are integral to effective medical and clinical management (Table 41-1). Some neurologic dysfunctions such as **peripheral neuropathy,** occur secondary to a deficiency of a single or several vitamins, whereas other diseases of the nervous system may be attributed to dietary excess (Table 41-2).

In those neurologic diseases with a nonnutrition etiology, nutrition therapies are adjuncts to medical management. Many elements of nutrition care for neurologic disease are similar, regardless of the origin of the disease process.

NERVOUS SYSTEM WIRING AND LESIONS

The central nervous system (CNS) in mammals is differentiated functionally into three dimensions. This implies that lesions of the nervous system can leave a unique "calling card" of localized dysfunction. Localizing the defect (lesion) to muscle, nerve, spinal cord, or brain is part of the diagnosis. This chapter provides an emphasis on conditions with nutritionally significant dysfunction.

Nerve tracts coming to and from the brain cross to opposite sides in the CNS (Figure 41-1). Therefore a lesion in the brain that affects the right arm would be found on the left side of the brain. Signs of weakness are the most quantifiable clinical signs of nervous system disease.

The neurons in the motor strip (upper motor neurons) receive input from all parts of the brain and project their

TABLE 41-1

Nutritional Considerations for Neurologic Conditions

Medical Condition	Relevant Nutrition Therapy
Adrenoleukodystrophy	Dietary avoidance of very-long-chain fatty acids (VLCFAs) has not been proven
	Lorenzo's oil lowers VLCFA levels
Alzheimer's disease	Assess nutrition status of patient
	Minimize distractions at mealtime
	Initiate smell or touch of food
	Hand guide to initiate eating
	Provide nutrient-dense foods and omega-3 fatty acids
Amyotrophic lateral sclerosis	Intervene to prevent malnutrition and dehydration
	Monitor dysphagia
Epilepsy	Ketogenic diet
Guillain-Barré	Attain positive energy balance with high-energy, high-protein tube feedings
	Assess dysphagia
Migraine headache	Follow general recommendations about food avoidance
	Maintain adequate dietary and fluid intake
	Keep extensive records of symptoms and foods
Myasthenia gravis	Provide nutritionally dense foods at beginning of meal
	Small, frequent meals are recommended
	Limit physical activity before meals
	Place temporary feeding tube
Multiple sclerosis	Antioxidant supplements
	Possibly linoleic acid supplement
	Evaluate health and especially vitamin D status of patient
	Nutrition support may be needed in advanced stages
	Distribute fluids throughout waking hours; limit before bed
Neurotrauma	Enteral or parenteral nutrition support needed
Parkinson's disease	Focus on drug-nutrient interactions
	Minimize dietary protein at breakfast and lunch
	Ensure nutritionally complete diet
Pernicious anemia	Administer vitamin B_{12} injections
	Provide diet liberal in high biological value (HBV) protein
	Provide diet supplemented with Fe^+, vitamin C, and B complex vitamins
Spinal trauma	Provide enteral/parenteral nutrition support
	Provide high-fiber, adequate hydration to minimize constipation
	Provide dietary intake to maintain nutrition health and adequate weight
Stroke	Dietary alterations for primary prevention
	Maintain good nutrition status
	Assess possible dysphagia
	Enteral or parenteral nutrition support may be needed
Wernicke-Korsakoff syndrome	Thiamin supplementation
	Provide adequate hydration
	Provide diet liberal in high-thiamin foods
	Eliminate alcohol
	Dietary protein may need to be restricted

axons all the way to their destinations in the spinal cord. Here they connect to the spinal cord motor neurons (lower motor neurons). These neurons extend from the spinal cord to muscles without interruption. The location of a lesion in the nervous system can often be deduced clinically by observing stereotypical abnormalities of either upper or lower motor neurons (Table 41-3).

Localizing Signs of Mass Lesions

The frontal lobes in the brain are the source of our most complex activities and therefore commonly offer the most complex presentations. Psychiatric manifestations such as depression, mania, or personality change may herald a tumor or other frontal lobe mass, either right or left (see Chapter 42 for additional information on psychiatric

TABLE 41-2

Neurologic Syndromes Attributes to Nutritional Deficiency or Excess

Nutritional Deficiency

Site of Major Syndrome	Name
Encephalon	Hypocalcemia and tetany seizures from lack of vitamin D
	Mental retardation (protein-calorie deprivation)
	Cretinism (lack of iodine)
	Wernicke-Korsakoff syndrome (thiamin)
Corpus callosum	Marchiafava-Bignami disease
Optic nerve	Nutritional deficiency optic neuropathy ("tobacco-alcohol amblyopia")
Brainstem	Central pontine myelinolysis
Cerebellum	Alcoholic cerebellar degeneration
	Vitamin E deficiency in bowel disease
Spinal cord	Combined system disease (B_{12} deficiency)
	Tropical spastic paraparesis
Peripheral nerves	Beriberi (thiamin), pellagra (nicotinic acid)
	Hypophosphatemia
	Tetany (vitamin D deficiency)
Muscle	Myopathy of osteomalacia

Nutritional Excess

Syndrome	Condition	Agent
Increased intracranial pressure	Self-medication	Vitamin A
Encephalopathy	Phenylketonuria	Phenylalanine
	Water intoxication	Water
	Hepatic encephalopathy	Protein (and NH_3)
	Ketotic or nonketotic coma in diabetes	Glucose
Stroke	Hyperlipidemia	Lipid
Peripheral neuropathy	Hypochondriasis	Pyridoxine
	Insomnia, anxiety	Tryptophan
Myopathy	Anorexia nervosa, bulimia	Emetine, ipecac
Myoglobinuria	Constipation	Licorice

TABLE 41-3

Clinical Differences Between Upper and Lower Motor Neuron Lesions

Upper Motor Neuron Findings	Lower Motor Neuron Findings
Weakness	Weakness
Stiff limbs	Floppy limbs
Sensory loss less common	Sensory loss more common
Increased reflexes	Decreased reflexes

conditions). If the tumor is near the base of the skull, one may lose the sense of smell or have visual changes because the olfactory and optic nerves track along the bottom of the frontal lobes.

Chemosensory losses of smell have been described in stages: **anosmia** (absence of smell), **hyperosmia** (increased sensitivity of smell), and **dysomia** (distortion of normal smell). Compensation for taste and smell losses with flavor-enhanced food has been found to improve palatability and intake, increase salivary flow and immunity, reduce chemosensory complaints in both healthy and sick elderly, and lessen the need for table salt.

Lesions in the central portion of the frontal lobes may present as a motor **apraxia**. With apraxia the patient cannot properly execute a complex activity, although he or she is strong and understands a request to perform the activity. The frontal lobes are larger than normal, and the posterior portions of the frontal lobes are where the motor strips are located. Lesions here exhibit upper motor neuron signs in the part of the body governed by this cortex. Temporal lobes control memory and speech functions; thus lesions here may affect these abilities.

Although any lesion of cerebral gray matter may produce seizures, the temporal lobes are particularly prone to seizures. Masses in the right parietal lobe may cause the patient to exhibit chronic inability to focus attention, thus completely ignoring the left side of the body. The speech centers are located near the junction of the left temporal, parietal, and frontal lobes. Pathology in this region may

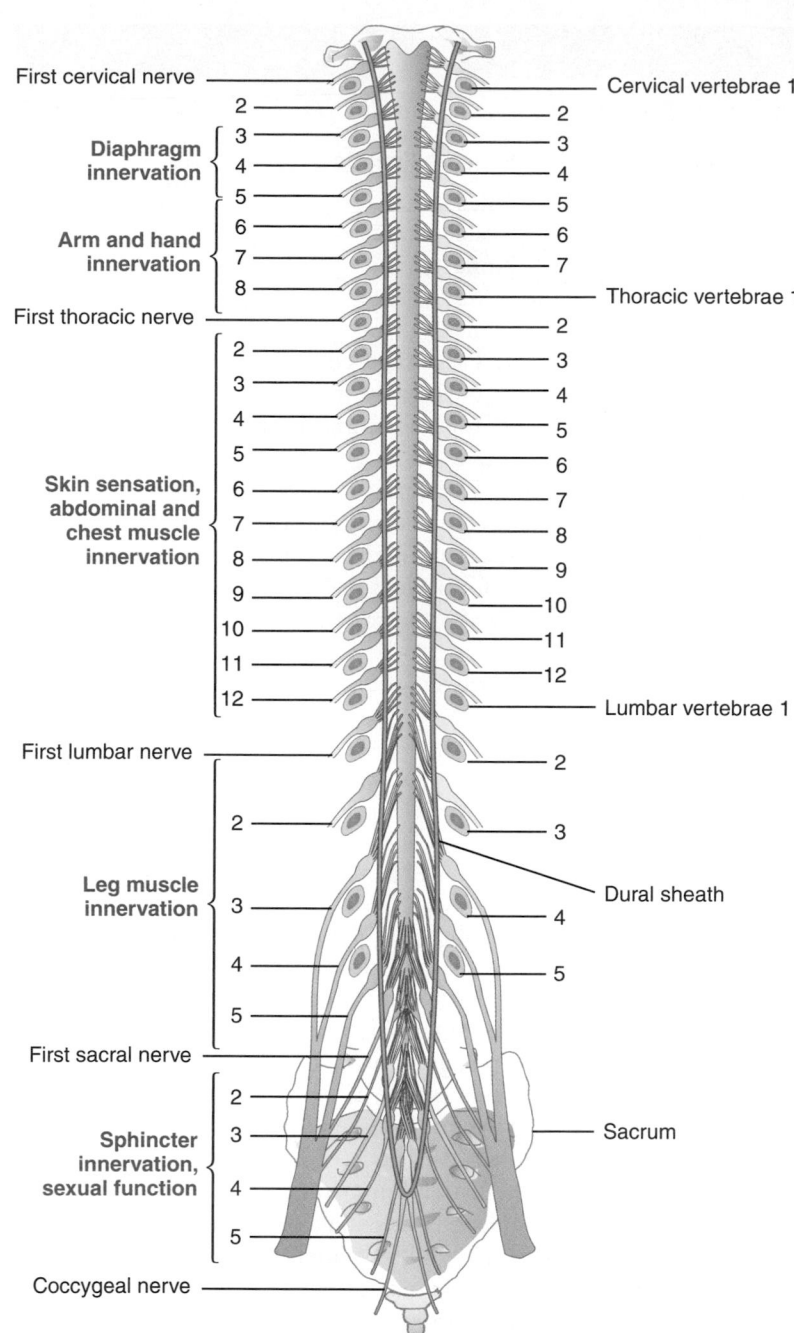

First cervical nerve
2
Diaphragm innervation { 3 4 5
Arm and hand innervation { 6 7 8
First thoracic nerve
2
3
4
5
Skin sensation, abdominal and chest muscle innervation { 6 7 8 9 10 11 12
First lumbar nerve
2
Leg muscle innervation { 3 4 5
First sacral nerve
2
3
Sphincter innervation, sexual function { 4 5
Coccygeal nerve

Cervical vertebrae 1
2
3
4
5
6
7
Thoracic vertebrae 1
2
3
4
5
6
7
8
9
10
11
12
Lumbar vertebrae 1
2
3
Dural sheath
4
5
Sacrum

FIGURE 41-1 Spinal cord lying within the vertebral canal. Spinal nerves are numbered on the left side; vertebrae are numbered on the right side; body areas supplied by various levels are in blue.

cause speech problems. The occipital lobes are reserved for vision, and dysfunction here may bring about **cortical blindness** of varying degrees. In this condition the patient is unaware that he or she cannot see. Lesions at other points along the visual pathway can cause several different types of visual field deficits.

Lesions of the cerebellum and brainstem may obstruct the ventricular system where it is the narrowest. This obstruction may precipitate life-threatening **hydrocephalus,** a condition of increased intracranial pressure (ICP) that may quickly result in death. Other signs of hydrocephalus include trouble with balance, walking and coordination abnormalities, and marked sleepiness. The person may complain of a headache that is worse on awakening. Lesions in the brainstem may infiltrate any of the cranial nerves (Table 41-4) that enervate

structures of the face and head, including the eyes, ears, jaw, tongue, pharynx, and facial muscles. These lesions have consequences for nutrition because the patient is often unable to eat without risking aspiration of food or liquids into the lung. Tumors or other lesions in the medulla may infiltrate respiratory and cardiac centers, and dysregulation of these centers has grim consequences. Providing nutrition through other means is often necessary.

Lesions in the spinal cord are much less common than brain tumors and ordinarily cause lower motor neuron signs at the level of the lesion and upper motor signs in segments below the level of the lesion (NIH, 2006). Spinal cord injury (SCI) is the most common cause of pathology in this region. Other examples of spinal cord abnormalities are multiple sclerosis (MS), amyotrophic lateral sclerosis (ALS), tumor,

TABLE 41-4

Basic Functions of Cranial Nerves

Number	Cranial Nerve Motor Function	Sensory Function
Olfactory (I)	None	Smell
Optic (II)	None	Vision
Oculomotor (III)	1. Eye movement 2. Pupil constriction	None
Trochlear (IV)	Eye movement	None
Trigeminal (V)	Mastication	1. Facial heat, cold, and touch 2. Noxious odors 3. Input for corneal reflex
Abducens (VI)	Eye movement	None
Facial (VII)	1. All muscles of facial expression 2. Corneal reflex	1. Facial pain 2. Taste on anterior two thirds of tongue
Vestibulocochlear (VIII)	None	Hearing and head acceleration and input for oculocephalic reflex
Glossopharyngeal (IX)	1. Swallowing 2. Gag reflex	Palatal, glossal, and oral sensation
Vagus (X)	1. Heart rate, gastrointestinal activity, sexual function 2. Cough reflex	Taste on posterior third of tongue
Spinal accessory (XI)	1. Trapezius 2. Sternocleidomastoid	None
Hypoglossal (XII)	Tongue movement	None

syrinx (fluid-filled neurologic cavity), chronic meningitis, vascular insufficiency, and mass lesions of the epidural space.

Lesions of the pituitary gland and hypothalamus are often heralded by systemic manifestations that may include electrolyte and metabolic abnormalities secondary to adrenocortical, thyroid, and antidiuretic hormone dysregulation. Because of the proximity to the visual pathways, visual field, acuity, and binocular deficits are also often present. The syndrome of inappropriate secretion of antidiuretic hormone is often a complication, and consideration of volume status is important here; hyponatremia is essential to the diagnosis. Because the hypothalamus is the regulatory center for hunger and satiety, lesions here may present as anorexia or overeating.

Finally, disorders of peripheral nerves and the neuromuscular junction can certainly affect one's ability to maintain proper nutrition. Disorders such as Guillain-Barré syndrome (the most commonly acquired demyelinating neuropathy) or myasthenia gravis may aggravate the patient's natural efforts to maintain metabolic balance. To eat and drink effectively, many parts of the nervous system are required; thus a problem at any step along the way can result in an inability to meet metabolic demands.

MEDICAL NUTRITION THERAPY

The nutritional management of patients with neurologic disease is complex. Severe neurologic impairments often compromise the mechanisms and cognitive abilities needed for adequate nourishment. Not only do many of these patients have dysphagia (difficulty swallowing), but the ability to obtain, prepare, and present food to the mouth is compromised. As a result, all neurologic patients are at risk for malnutrition. Early recognition of signs and symptoms, implementation of an appropriate care plan to meet the nutritional requirements of the individual, and counseling for the patient and family members on dietary choices are first steps. Regular evaluation of the patient's nutrition status in relation to the disease management is essential, with the ultimate goal of improving outcomes and the patient's quality of life.

Nutrition assessment is the first step in managing the patient (see Chapters 14 and 15, and Appendix 30). It should include a detailed diet history, as well as a history of weight loss or gain. The diet history is helpful to assess patterns of normal chewing, swallowing, and rate of ingestion. Weight loss history establishes a baseline weight, and a weight loss of 10% or more is indicative of nutritional risk. Anemias should be noted because the synthesis of the neurotransmitters dopamine and serotonin require adequate iron.

PROBLEMS WITH ACCESS TO FOOD

With chronic neurologic diseases, a decline in function may hinder the ability for self-care. Fulfilling nutritional needs and malnutrition are concerns. Access to food and satisfying basic needs may depend on the involvement of family, friends,

TABLE 41-5

Common Disorders of Neurologic Diseases

Site in the Brain	Impairment	Results
Cortical lesions of the parietal lobe (perception of sensory stimuli)	Sensory deficits	Fine regulation of muscle activities impossible if the patient is unable to perceive joint position and motion and tension of contracting muscles
Lesions of the nondominant hemisphere	Hemiinattention syndrome (neglect)	Patient neglects that side of the body
Optic tract lesions (usually of the middle cerebral artery or the artery near the internal capsule)	Visual field cuts	Patient reads one half of a page, eats from only half of the plate, etc. (see Figure 43-2).
Loss of subcortically stored pattern of motor skills	Apraxia	Inability to perform a previously learned task (e.g., walking, rising from a chair), but paralysis, sensory loss, spasticity, and incoordination are not present
No identification with a particular brain disorder or a specifically located lesion	Language apraxia	Inability to produce meaningful speech, even though oral muscle function is intact and language production has not been affected
Lesion of Broca's area	Nonfluent aphasia	Thought and language formulation are intact, but the patient is unable to connect them into fluent speech production
Lesion of Wernicke's area	Fluent aphasia	Flow of speech and articulation seem normal, but language output makes little or no sense
Extensive brain damage	Global aphasia	Both expression and speech perception are severely impaired
Brainstem lesions, bilateral hemispheric lesions, cerebellar disorders	Dysarthria	Inability to produce intelligible words with proper articulation

From Steinberg FU: Rehabilitating the older stroke patient: what's possible? *Geriatrics* 41:85, 1986.

or professionals. With acute neurologic situations such as trauma, stroke, or Guillain-Barré syndrome, the entire process of eating can be interrupted abruptly, and the patient may require enteral nutrition support for a period of time until overall function improves and eating can be resumed.

Meal Preparation

Confusion, dementia, impaired vision, or poor ambulation also may contribute to difficulty with meal preparation, thus hindering even the enjoyment of eating. An increased reliance on comfort or convenience foods such as prepackaged single servings can be encouraged as a way to maintain nourishment obtained independently.

Feeding Issues: Presentation of Food to the Mouth

The patient with neurologic disease may be unable to feed himself or herself because of limb weakness, poor body positioning, hemianopsia, apraxia, confusion, or neglect. Tremors as in Parkinson's disease; spastic movements; or involuntary motor manifestations as occur with cerebral palsy, Huntington's disease, or tardive dyskinesia may further restrict dietary intake. The affected region of the CNS determines the resulting disability (Table 41-5).

If limb weakness or paralysis occurs on the dominant side of the body, poor coordination resulting from a new reliance on the nondominant side may make eating difficult and unpleasant. The patient may have to adjust to eating with one hand and also to using the nondominant hand. Small, frequent feedings can help if fatigue or early satiety is a problem. An occupational therapist may help recommend specific adaptive eating utensils.

Hemiparesis is weakness on one side of the body that causes the body to slump toward the affected side; it may increase a patient's risk of aspiration. It is important to have the patient sit as upright (at a 90-degree angle) as possible. If the patient must be in bed during mealtime, pillows can be used to bank and support the paretic side.

Hemianopsia is blindness for one half of the field of vision. The patient must learn to recognize that he or she no longer has a normal field of vision and must compensate by turning the head. Neglect is inattention to a weakened or paralyzed side of the body; this occurs when the nondominant (right) parietal side of the brain is affected. The patient ignores the affected body part, and his or her perception of the body's midline is shifted. Hemianopsia and neglect can occur together and severely impair the patient's function. A patient may eat only half of the contents of a meal because he or she recognizes only half of it; assistance or supervision may be needed (Figure 41-2).

Another potential interference with self-feeding is apraxia because the person is unable to carry out an action and

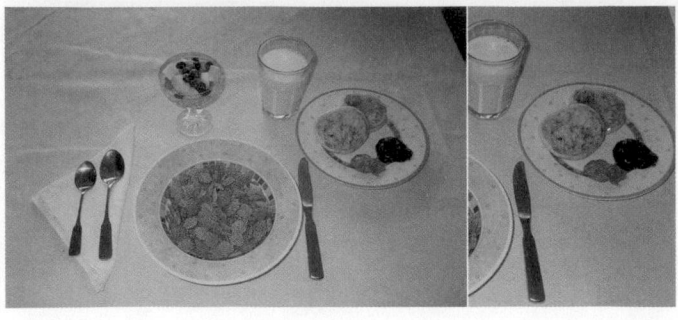

FIGURE 41-2 A, Normal vision. **B,** Vision with hemianopsia.

follow directions. Demonstration may make it possible to do the action; however, judgment may be affected as well and can result in the performance of dangerous tasks. This makes leaving the patient alone unsafe.

Eating: The Oral Process

Dysphagia (difficulty swallowing) often accompanies neurologic disease. Symptoms include drooling, choking, or coughing during or following meals; inability to suck from a straw; a gurgly voice quality; holding pockets of food in the buccal recesses (of which the patient may be unaware); absent gag reflex; and chronic upper respiratory infections.

Dysphagia often leads to malnutrition because of inadequate intake. A swallowing evaluation by a speech pathologist is important. The speech pathologist specializes in assessing and treating swallowing disorders and is often consulted for individuals following traumatic brain injury, stroke, cancers of the head and neck and those at risk of aspiration or with other conditions that result in a lack of coordination in swallowing. Many registered dietitians (RDs) have acquired additional training in swallowing therapies to help coordinate this evaluative process. Patients with intermediate or late-stage Parkinson's disease, MS, ALS, dementia, or stroke are likely to have dysphagia.

Weight loss and anorexia are key concerns. Environmental distractions and conversations during mealtime increase the risk for aspiration and should be curtailed. Reports of coughing and unusually long mealtimes are associated with tongue, facial, and masticator muscle weakness. Observation during meals allows the nurse or RD to screen informally for signs of dysphagia problems and bring them to the attention of the health care team. Changing the consistency of foods served may be beneficial. See Appendix 35 for the different stages of the National Dysphagia Diet.

Swallowing

Proper position for effective swallowing should be encouraged (i.e., sitting bolt upright with the head in a chin-down position). Concentrating on the swallowing process can also help reduce choking. Initiation of the swallow begins voluntarily but is completed reflexively. Normal swallowing allows for safe and easy passage of food from the oral cavity through the pharynx and esophagus into the stomach by propulsive muscular force, with some benefit from gravity.

The process of swallowing can be organized into three phases as shown in Figure 41-3.

Oral Phase

During the preparatory and oral phases of swallowing, food is placed in the mouth, where it is combined with saliva, chewed if necessary, and formed into a bolus by the tongue. The tongue pushes the food to the rear of the oral cavity by gradually squeezing it backward against the hard and soft palate (see Figure 41-3). Increased ICP or intracranial nerve damage may result in weakened or poorly coordinated tongue movements and lead to problems in completing the oral phase of swallowing. Weakened lip muscles result in the inability to completely seal the lips, form a seal around a cup, or suck through a straw. Patients are embarrassed by drooling and may not want to eat in front of others. The patient may have difficulty forming a cohesive bolus and moving it through the oral cavity. Food can become pocketed in the buccal recesses, especially if sensation in the cheek is lost or facial weakness exists.

Pharyngeal Phase

The pharyngeal phase is initiated when the bolus is propelled past the faucial arches. Four events must occur in rapid succession during this phase. The soft palate elevates to close off the nasopharynx and prevent oropharyngeal regurgitation. The hyoid and larynx elevate, and the vocal cords adduct to protect the airway. The pharynx sequentially contracts while the cricopharyngeal sphincter relaxes, allowing the food to pass into the esophagus. Breathing resumes at the end of the pharyngeal phase. Symptoms of poor coordination during this phase include gagging, choking, and nasopharyngeal regurgitation.

Esophageal Phase

The final or esophageal phase, during which the bolus continues through the esophagus into the stomach, is completely involuntary. Difficulties that occur during this phase are generally the result of a mechanical obstruction, but neurologic disease cannot be ruled out. For example, impaired peristalsis can arise from a brainstem infarct.

Liquids

Swallowing liquids of thin consistency such as juice or water requires the most coordination and control. Liquids are easily aspirated into the lungs and may pose a life-threatening event because aspiration pneumonia may ensue, even from sterile water in the lungs. Sterile water is no longer sterile once it is introduced to the bacterial load of the oral cavity.

If a patient has difficulty consuming thin liquids, fluid requirements may be met by thickening liquids. Liquids of all types can be thickened with nonfat dry milk powder, cornstarch, modular carbohydrate supplements, or commercial thickeners that contain a modified cornstarch thickener. Thick liquids that contain a high percentage of water are needed to maintain fluid balance. Fatigue and malaise are often associated with a "mild chronic dehydration" that results from decreased fluid intake. Popsicles, ice, and fresh

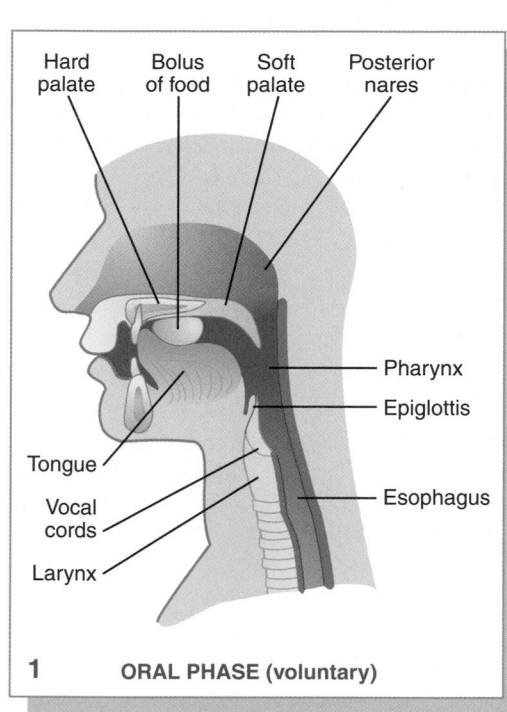

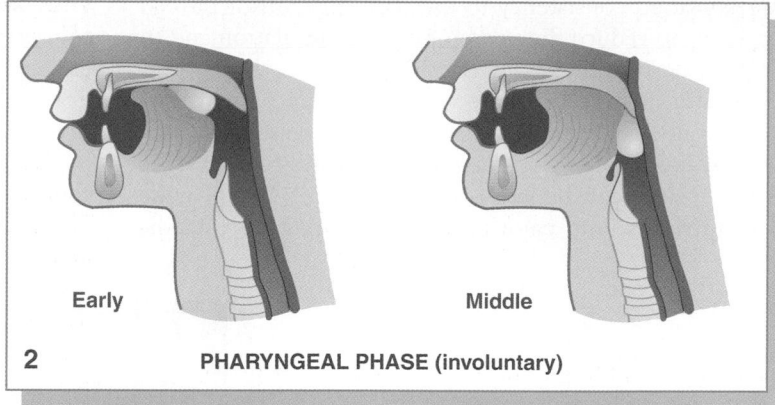

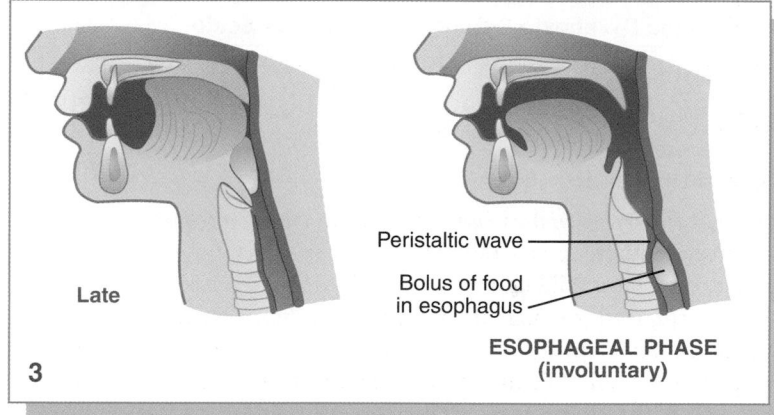

FIGURE 41-3 Swallowing occurs in three phases: *(1) Voluntary or oral phase:* Tongue presses food against the hard palate, forcing it toward the pharynx. *(2) Involuntary, pharyngeal phase:* Early: wave of peristalsis forces a bolus between the tonsillar pillars. Middle: soft palate draws upward to close posterior nares, and respirations cease momentarily. Late: vocal cords approximate, and the larynx pulls upward, covering the airway and stretching the esophagus open. *(3) Involuntary, esophageal phase:* Relaxation of the upper esophageal (hypopharyngeal) sphincter allows the peristaltic wave to move the bolus down the esophagus.

fruit are additional sources of free water. Use of noncaffeinated beverages should be encouraged because caffeine has a diuretic effect that contributes to dehydration, fatigue, and thickened saliva.

Milk is considered a liquid with unique properties. Some people associate consumption of milk with symptoms of excess mucus production; however, no statistically significant data have proven a link between milk or dairy products and symptoms of mucus production. However, the dysphagic patient often reports increased phlegm after milk consumption, which may actually be a consequence of poor swallowing ability rather than mucus production. Patients are encouraged to "chase" the milk products with appropriately thickened liquids to help flush the throat rather than eliminate dairy products.

Liquid intake is a concern in those with neurogenic bladder (the main feature is urinary retention), which is a common sign and management issue in patients with a **myelopathy,** a pathologic condition of the spinal cord, or SCI. This predisposes the individual to urinary tract infections (UTIs) and miscalculation of fluid balance. Alternately myelopathy and SCI may result in urinary urgency, frequency, and in-

continence. To minimize these problems, distributing fluids evenly throughout the waking hours and limiting them before bedtime is helpful. Some patients limit fluid intake severely to decrease urgency or frequent urination. This practice increases the risk of UTI and is not recommended. One nontraumatic cause of myelopathy and neurogenic bladder is MS, an unpredictable severe, progressive disease of the CNS. Individuals with MS (women are affected more often than men) have a higher incidence of UTIs. Increased intake of cranberry juice may reduce the frequency of UTIs (see Chapter 36).

Textures

As chronic disease progresses, cranial nerves become damaged, thus leading to neurologic deficits manifested by dysphagia and possible elimination of entire food groups. Nutrition intervention should be individualized according to the type and extent of dysfunction. Vitamin and mineral supplementation may be necessary. If chewable supplements are not handled safely, liquid forms may be added to acceptable foods. The health professional can ensure that the diet remains palatable and nutritionally adequate by recommending changes in food consistency to mechanically soft or pureed consistency to reduce the need for oral manipulation and to conserve energy while eating (Box 41-1).

Presented with small, frequent meals, the patient may be encouraged to eat more. Swallowing can also be improved by emphasizing the taste, texture, and temperature of foods. Juices can be substituted for water and provide flavor, nutrients, and calories. A cool temperature facili-

tates swallowing; therefore, cold food items may be better tolerated. Carbonation may also be better tolerated because there is the beneficial effect of texture. Sauces and gravies lubricate foods for ease in swallowing and can help prevent fragmentation of foods in the oral cavity. Moist pastas, casseroles, and egg dishes are well tolerated. Avoid foods that crumble easily in the mouth, as they can increase the risk of choking.

BOX 41-1

Guidelines for Feeding the Dysphagic Patient

Part One: The Dysphagia Outcome and Severity Scale

Full PO: Normal Diet

Level 7: Normal in All Situations
- Normal diet
- No strategies or extra time needed

Level 6: Within Functional Limits/Modified Independence
- Normal diet; functional swallow
- Patient may have mild oral or pharyngeal delay, retention, or trace epiglottal undercoating but independently and spontaneously compensates and clears
- May need extra time for meal
- No aspiration with different consistencies

Full PO: Modified Diet and Independence

Level 5: Mild Dysphagia: Distant Supervision; May Need One Diet Consistency Restricted
May exhibit one or more of the following:
- Aspiration of thin liquids only but with strong reflexive cough to clear completely
- Airway penetration midway to cords or to cords with one consistency but clears spontaneously
- Retention in pharynx that is cleared spontaneously
- Mild oral dysphagia with reduced mastication or oral retention that is cleared spontaneously

Level 4: Mild-Moderate Dysphagia: Intermittent Supervision/Cueing; One to Two Diet Consistencies Restricted
May exhibit one or more of the following:
- Retention in pharynx that is cleared with cue
- Retention in oral cavity that is cleared with cue
- Aspiration with one consistency; airway penetration to the level of the vocal cords with cough with two consistencies, or airway penetration to the level of the vocal cords without cough with one consistency

Level 3: Moderate Dysphagia: Total Assist, Supervision, or Strategies; Two or More Diet Consistencies Restricted
May exhibit one or more of the following:
- Moderate retention in pharynx that is cleared with cue
- Moderate retention in oral cavity that is cleared with cue
- Airway penetration to the level of the vocal cords without cough with two or more consistencies or aspiration with two consistencies

Nonoral Nutrition Necessary

Level 2: Moderately Severe Dysphagia: Maximum Assistance or Maximum Use of Strategies With Partial PO Only
May exhibit one or more of the following:
- Severe retention in pharynx; unable to clear or needs multiple cues
- Severe oral stage bolus loss or retention; unable to clear or needs multiple cues
- Aspiration with two or more consistencies, no reflexive cough and weak volitional cough; or aspiration with one or more consistencies, no cough, and airway penetration to cords with one or more consistencies no cough

Level 1: Severe Dysphagia: NPO: Unable To Tolerate Any PO Safely
May exhibit one or more of the following:
- Severe retention in pharynx; unable to clear
- Severe oral stage bolus loss or retention; unable to clear
- Silent aspiration with two or more consistencies; nonfunctional volitional cough or unable to achieve swallow

Part Two: Techniques for Improving Acceptance

Feeding individuals with dysphagia requires extra care and consideration. Food is enjoyed with all of the senses. Pureed meals need to look good, smell good, and taste good. Here are some ideas to improve the sensory experience for those with dysphagia. Start simple and build a puree program to be creative; serve attractive meals.

Aroma
- Good-smelling food and a pleasant atmosphere may increase appetite and improve consumption.
- Serve foods seasoned with aromatic ingredients such as garlic, pepper, onions, and cinnamon.

Seasoning
- Individuals with dysphagia often have a dulled sense of taste.
- Taste all foods and adjust seasoning as needed.
- Serve foods that have stronger flavors such as chili, spaghetti, and apple pie.

Modified from the American Dietetic Association: *National dysphagia diet: standardization for optimal care*, Chicago, 2003, ADA.

BOX 41-1

Guidelines for Feeding the Dysphagic Patient—cont'd

Part Two: Techniques for Improving Acceptance—cont'd

Layering/Swirling

- Swirling vegetables together is simple and makes a great plate presentation; peas and carrots are striking together and taste great.
- Use standardized recipes to make attractive layered casseroles such as shepherd's pie, lasagna, or chicken á la king.

Piping

- Place pureed food into a pastry bag and pipe for a lovely plate presentation.
- Keep it simple and have fun with pureed pasta.

Molding

- To mold, use a thickener or a shaping or enhancing product.
- For hot foods: prepare per recipe, freeze and heat to temperature before serving.
- For cold foods: prepare per recipe, freeze, set on plate, and serve (will thaw quickly).

Slurries

- Prepare slurry with thickener and juice or milk.
- Prepare slurry with a liquid that goes well with the food being prepared.
- Slurry shortcake with juice and serve with pureed strawberries.
- Slurry sugar cookies with milk.
- Slurries work well with biscuits, cakes, graham crackers, muffins, and brownies.

Garnishing

- Garnishing is often overlooked but makes a big visual impact.
- Only garnish with foods appropriate for the diet consistency.
- Use sauces, gravies, and syrups and try putting in squeeze bottles and decorating plates.
- Pipe garnishes around edges such as piping lettuce around the edge of a pureed sandwich.
- Cut shapes out of cranberry sauce and serve with turkey.

These are a few simple ideas to keep in mind when serving modified-consistency foods. Beautiful plate presentations and good-tasting foods will help maintain good consumption and ultimately positive nutrition status. Resident and patient dignity is very important. Good-looking and good-tasting food can help people feel more dignified.

Nutrition Support

Patients with acute and chronic neurologic diseases may benefit from nutrition support. In acute disease it may be required initially until a degree of function is regained, whereas in chronic neurologic disease it may be required in the late stages to meet changing metabolic demands. Well-managed nutrition support helps to prevent pneumonia and sepsis, which can complicate these diseases.

Enteral tube feedings may be necessary if the risk of aspiration from oral intake is high or if the patient cannot eat enough to meet his or her nutritional needs. In the latter case nocturnal tube feedings can bridge the gap between oral intake and actual nutritional requirements. This should allow the normal sensation of hunger to be generated and provide freedom from tube feeding during the day.

In most instances the gastrointestinal tract function remains intact, and enteral nutrition is the preferred method of administering nutrition support. One noted exception occurs after SCI. In this instance ileus is common for 7 to 10 days after the insult, and parenteral nutrition may be necessary.

Although a nasogastric tube can be a short-term option, a percutaneous endoscopic gastrostomy (PEG) or gastrostomy-jejunostomy (PEG/J) tube, placed with the patient under local anesthesia, is preferred for long-term management. These should be considered for patients whose swallowing function is inadequate to ensure their nutritional health (see Chapter 20). Malnutrition itself can produce neuromuscular weakness that affects quality of life; it is a prognostic factor for poor survival.

In the acutely ill but previously well-nourished individual who is unable to resume oral alimentation within 7 days, nutrition support is used to prevent decline in nutritional health and aid in recovery until oral nourishment can be resumed. Conversely in the chronically ill, nutrition support is an issue that each patient must eventually address because it may result in prolonged therapy. However, adequate nutriture can prolong health of the individual, and may be a welcome relief to an overburdened patient.

Some patients may decline early placement of a feeding tube because of the emotional, economic, or physical impact of this choice. In advanced stages of disease the patient may refuse tube feedings, choosing not to prolong life. Nutrition support should enhance the quality of life and the health care team plays an important role in alleviating patient and family concerns and fostering informed decisions (Mitsumoto and Del Bene, 2000). The patient needs to be fully informed about the impact of tube feeding on daily life. Discussion of both the advantages and disadvantages of nutrition support should be initiated with the patient and family well ahead of need; options should include a description of feeding schedules, tube placement procedures, and appropriate training (see Chapter 20).

NEUROLOGIC DISEASES ARISING FROM NUTRITIONAL DEFICIENCIES OR EXCESSES

Beriberi and Pellagra

The major manifestations of thiamin deficiency in humans involve the cardiovascular (wet beriberi) and nervous (dry beriberi, neuropathy, or Wernicke-Korsakoff syndrome) systems. Pellagra (niacin deficiency) also affects the nervous system: it is less common in the United States today than decades ago because of the variety of foods consumed (see Chapter 3).

Pernicious Anemia

Historically pernicious anemia and vitamin B_{12} (cobalamin) deficiencies have been the more common neurologic syndromes caused by lack of a single nutrient. The classic triad of anemia, neurologic deficits, and epithelial atrophy of the tongue was well recognized at the turn of the century. Until 1926 when replacement therapy was introduced, the term *pernicious* appropriately described the fatal outcome. Consumption of liver was prescribed empirically, and only in 1948 was vitamin B_{12} recognized as the healing agent. Sufficient intrinsic factor, a protein that helps the body absorb vitamin B_{12}, is also needed.

Given the technology for measuring vitamin B_{12} levels in the blood, early detection during the preclinical phase of disease is the rule. As a result, pernicious anemia is rarely seen in medical centers in developed countries. Among those who develop pernicious anemia, most are over 60. The effectiveness of diagnosis and treatment has been remarkable in that over 90% of symptomatic patients after treatment with vitamin B_{12} regain independence in conducting activities of daily living (ADLs) (see Chapter 31).

Pathophysiology

Nerve and blood cells require vitamin B_{12} to function properly; deficiency can cause a wide variety of symptoms, including fatigue, shortness of breath, tingling sensations, difficulty walking, and diarrhea.

In the nervous system lesions occur initially in the myelin sheaths of optic nerves, cerebral white matter, and peripheral nerves.

Medical Treatment

Early diagnosis of pernicious anemia can be somewhat complicated because hematologic and neurologic signs do not always correlate. A significant component of primary prevention is the determination of serum vitamin B_{12} because it is the best, most readily available test for evaluating vitamin B_{12} status. Serum levels less than 150 mg/ml are considered to represent deficiency (see Chapters 15 and 31, and Figure 31-3).

Most neurologic manifestations of vitamin B_{12} deficiency are associated with the typical macrocytic anemia of pernicious anemia. General weakness and especially **paresthesia** (numbness sensation and heightened sensitivity in the nerve lesions) constitute the earliest and most common symptoms, with tingling or the feeling of "pins and needles" in hands or feet. This tends to be constant and steadily progressive. If left untreated, the following signs may ensue: **dysgeusia** (impaired taste); impaired gait, spasticity, contracture; mental signs of irritability, apathy, somnolence, emotional instability, marked confusion, and depression; and visual impairment. Fortunately for the majority of patients today, the disease can be detected before neurologic symptoms or signs develop.

The duration of symptoms before treatment is the factor most likely to influence treatment response; neurologic manifestations that occur in less than 3 months are rapidly and completely reversible. Amelioration of symptoms occurring between 6 and 12 months is variable, and in extreme cases, arrest of disease progression is the most that can be accomplished. Prompt initiation of therapy is imperative. A monthly maintenance injection of B_{12} is administered for life if lack of intrinsic factor is apparent (see Chapter 31).

Medical Nutrition Therapy

For the majority of individuals with pernicious anemia, inadequate dietary intake of vitamin B_{12} is unrelated to this disease; most have inadequate absorption. It is recommended that, in addition to the injections of vitamin, the diet be liberal in use of high-biologic value proteins and supplemented with iron, vitamin C, and other B vitamins, including folic acid. Oral immediate-release B_{12} is increasingly used, but effectiveness in reversing neurologic abnormalities has yet to be established (Solomon, 2006).

Wernicke-Korsakoff Syndrome

Wernicke-Korsakoff syndrome (WKS) is a disease of the cerebellum and brainstem that results from chronic thiamin deficiency with continued carbohydrate ingestion. WKS is actually two separate diseases (Wernicke's encephalopathy and Korsakoff's psychosis); their common association has led to inclusion into one syndrome with characteristic memory defects.

WKS is one of the gravest consequences of alcoholism. The incidence of WKS may be underreported because it is often undiagnosed. Alcoholism is more prevalent in the homeless in which access to medical care is limited. Because clinical findings are subtle, diagnosis of WKS is often made at autopsy. In North America and Europe this nutritional disorder is the most commonly encountered manifestation acquired from thiamin deficiency; it develops after severe or repeated attacks of postalcoholic delirium tremens. It has also been seen in patients who are nutritionally depleted from anorexia nervosa, gastrointestinal disease, or HIV infection. It also may follow ischemic stroke or subarachnoid or thalamic hemorrhage.

Pathophysiology

Thiamin deficiency is the accepted primary cause of WKS. Depletion of body stores of thiamin can happen rapidly, within 7 to 8 weeks, especially in alcoholics. The pathology in this acute and severe nutritional deficiency is restricted to the CNS. The exact relationship between the lesions induced by thiamin deficiency and their effect on the brain remains unclear. However, one certain thing is the effect of treatment on outcome. Wernicke's encephalopathy is responsive to thiamin, whereas Korsakoff's psychosis is not; the mental derangements precipitated by Korsakoff's psychosis are irreversible.

Wernicke's disease is characterized by the triad of disturbances in mentation (encephalopathy), vision (**nystagmus** or involuntary movement of the eyeball), and gait (**ataxia** or impaired movement); but they are not always present simultaneously, and clinical diagnosis is often deferred until autopsy. Korsakoff's psychosis presents as an amnesia, a confabulatory mental disorder in which retentive memory is significantly impaired in comparison to other cognitive functions. Memory is diminished; the patient is unable to learn new things; conceptual or perceptual functions decline; and, as the disease progresses, confabulation is less apparent.

Medical Treatment

Treatment with thiamin should be started immediately, and adequate hydration should be provided if WKS is suspected. Thiamin is administered prophylactically to alcoholics to prevent disease progression and even to reverse the brain abnormalities that are not yet permanent changes. From 50 to 100 mg of parenteral thiamin should be administered for several days because of the possibility of coexisting gastrointestinal malabsorption. Glucose must never be given before thiamin because sudden increases in brain glucose levels may precipitate symptoms of WKS in patients with marginal thiamin reserves. Infusion of glucose and metabolic stress also increase requirements for thiamin.

The response to therapy depends on the conversion of thiamin to its active form in the liver. With concomitant liver disease response may be delayed. Ophthalmologic symptoms generally respond rapidly to thiamin, whereas ataxia and encephalopathy respond more slowly. Mental deficits of Korsakoff's psychosis do not improve. A decrease in erythrocyte transketolase activity also correlates well with improvement in the clinical picture since a normal value is a sensitive measure of adequate thiamin nutriture.

Medical Nutrition Therapy

First and foremost, the nutritional deficiency should be corrected if possible. With thiamin deficiency, not only should therapeutic supplementation be administered, but nutrient-dense foods containing thiamin such as whole grain or enriched breads and cereals should also be incorporated into the patient's diet. Alcohol must be eliminated. Because no singular food item contains large amounts of thiamin, one serving of a nutrient-dense food item contributes about 10% of an individual's daily need. A diet consisting of a variety of food items is required to ensure that the recommended dietary allowance for thiamin is met (see Chapter 3). In the presence of concomitant encephalopathy, repletion of dietary protein may be limited or restricted; refer to Chapter 28.

Stroke

Stroke is the most rampant clinical entity of cerebrovascular disease in developed countries. It is defined as an acute onset of focal or global neurologic deficit lasting more than 24 hours and is attributable to diseases of the intracranial or extracranial neurovasculature. Severe strokes are often preceded by **transient ischemic attacks,** brief attacks lasting from a few minutes to hours of cerebral dysfunction of vascular origin with no persistent neurologic defect.

Stroke is the third most common cause of death in the United States and the most common cause of disability in the United States (NIH, 2006). Old age is the most significant risk factor. Among modifiable risk factors, hypertension and smoking contribute most to the risk of stroke. Other factors include obesity, coronary heart disease, diabetes, physical inactivity, and genetics (Goldstein et al., 2006) (see Chapter 32). Stroke is a disease of the twentieth century that in large part has resulted from tobacco use and obesity. Although the incidence of stroke has declined over the past 30 years, it appears now to have leveled off. High costs are attributed in part to the large degree of disability imparted by cerebrovascular events.

Pathophysiology

Embolic stroke occurs when a cholesterol plaque is dislodged from a proximal vessel, travels to the brain, and blocks an artery, most commonly the middle cerebral artery (MCA). In patients with dysfunctional cardiac atria, clots may be dislodged from there and embolize. In **thrombotic stroke** a cholesterol plaque within an artery ruptures, and platelets subsequently aggregate to clog an already narrowed artery. Most strokes are incited by a **thromboembolic event,** which may be aggravated by atherosclerosis, hypertension, diabetes, and gout (see *Pathophysiology and Care Management Algorithm*: Stroke).

Intracranial hemorrhage is less common (15% of strokes) but more often fatal immediately. Both varieties of intracranial hemorrhage occur more commonly in individuals with hypertension. The first is intraparenchymal hemorrhage, when a vessel inside the brain ruptures. A variation of intraparenchymal hemorrhage is a lacunar (deep pool) infarct.

These smaller infarcts occur in the deep structures of the brain such as the internal capsule, basal ganglia, pons, thalamus, and cerebellum. Even a small lacunar infarct can produce significant disability because the brain tissue in the deep structures is so densely functional. The second type of intracranial hemorrhage is **subarachnoid hemorrhage (SAH).** This occurs most commonly as a result of head trauma but more often as a result of a ruptured aneurysm of a vessel in the subarachnoid space.

Medical Treatment

The medical history can give some evidence about the mechanism of a new infarct. Hemorrhage is suspected when the patient presents with headache, decreased level of consciousness, and vomiting, all of which evolve over minutes to hours. A thromboembolic stroke is more likely to occur when the patient is fully conscious, but onset of motor or sensory changes occurs suddenly. As with all neurologic disease, the clinical presentation depends on the location of

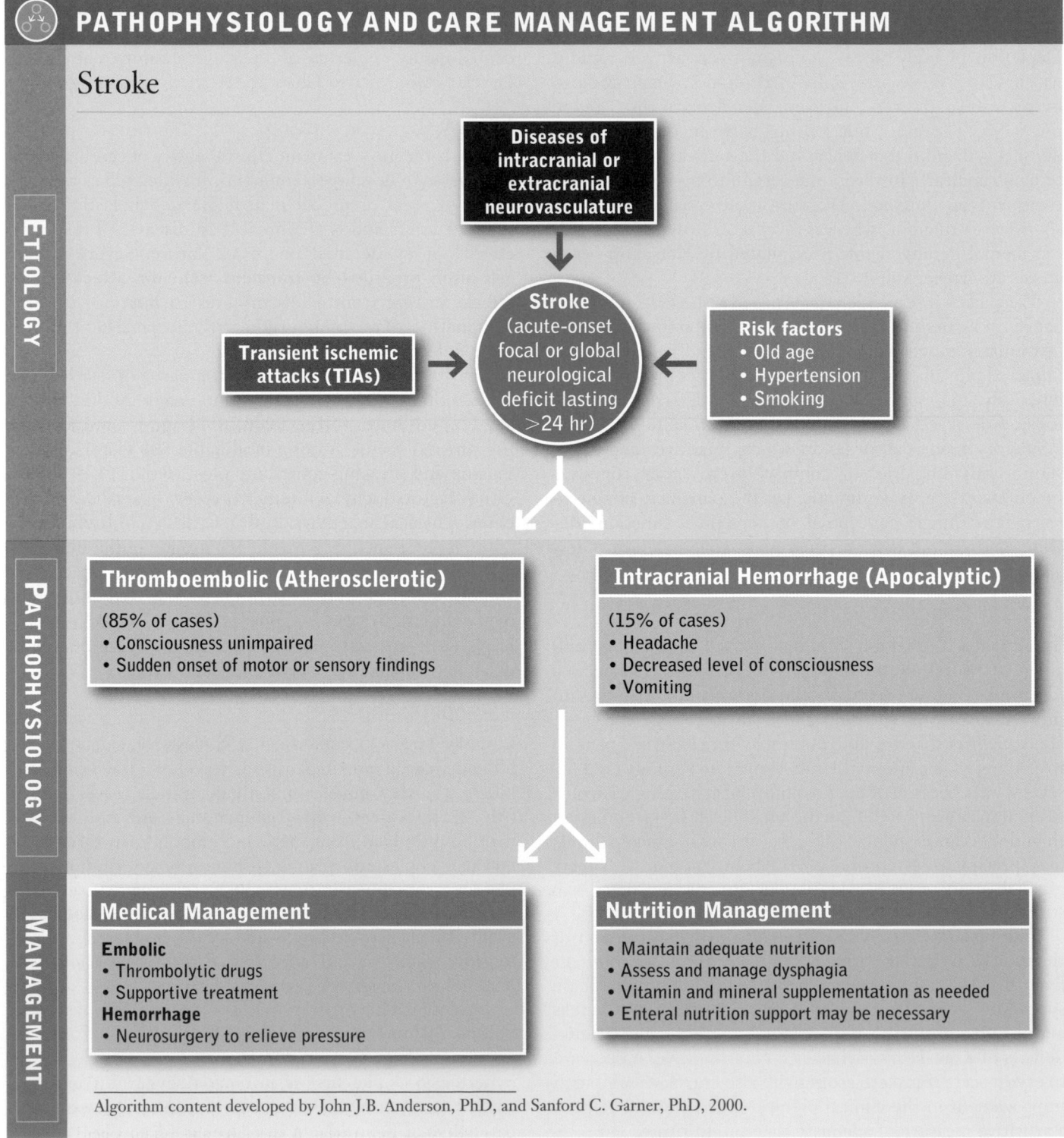

PATHOPHYSIOLOGY AND CARE MANAGEMENT ALGORITHM

Stroke

ETIOLOGY

Diseases of intracranial or extracranial neurovasculature

↓

Transient ischemic attacks (TIAs) → Stroke (acute-onset focal or global neurological deficit lasting >24 hr) ← Risk factors
• Old age
• Hypertension
• Smoking

PATHOPHYSIOLOGY

Thromboembolic (Atherosclerotic)

(85% of cases)
• Consciousness unimpaired
• Sudden onset of motor or sensory findings

Intracranial Hemorrhage (Apocalyptic)

(15% of cases)
• Headache
• Decreased level of consciousness
• Vomiting

MANAGEMENT

Medical Management

Embolic
• Thrombolytic drugs
• Supportive treatment
Hemorrhage
• Neurosurgery to relieve pressure

Nutrition Management

• Maintain adequate nutrition
• Assess and manage dysphagia
• Vitamin and mineral supplementation as needed
• Enteral nutrition support may be necessary

Algorithm content developed by John J.B. Anderson, PhD, and Sanford C. Garner, PhD, 2000.

the abnormality. An infarction of a particular cerebrovascular territory can be suspected by seeking out various constellations of neurologic deficits. An MCA occlusion produces paresis, with sensory deficits of limbs on the opposite side of the body because this artery supplies the motor and sensory strips. If the left MCA is occluded, **aphasia,** or loss of speech or expression may also be present.

In the past, treatment for embolic stroke was supportive; it focused on prevention of further brain infarction and rehabilitation. Recently use of thrombolytic or "clot-busting" drugs has allowed reversal of brain ischemia by lysing thromboembolic clots in selected patients. Evaluation and initiation of therapy needs to occur within 6 hours of the onset of symptoms. Use of aspirin may be of some value in preventing further cerebrovascular events, but its effectiveness has not yet been demonstrated definitively.

Controlling ICP while maintaining sufficient perfusion of the brain is the treatment for intracranial hemorrhage. This may include surgical evacuation of large volumes of intracranial blood, ventricular drainage, or other neurosurgical interventions. Rehabilitation is a key component of therapy. Hemorrhage, particularly SAH, commonly has more severe functional consequences and therefore has a longer period of convalescence than ischemic stroke.

Medical Nutrition Therapy

Primary prevention is the cornerstone for managing stroke. This can be accomplished in part by dietary means as well as by other lifestyle behaviors (Goldstein et al., 2006). These nutrition-related factors have shown a salutary effect on reducing the incidence of stroke and have been compiled from various large population–based prospective studies in (Box 41-2).

Given the prevalence of stroke and its associated burden of disease, treatment for those afflicted with this disease cannot be ignored. In 2003 stroke cost the United States an estimated $51 billion in lost productivity and health, including $12 billion in nursing home costs (CDC, 2006). Once stroke does occur, dietary reduction of cholesterol, fat, and salt are of questionable benefit. Efforts should be directed toward maintaining the overall health of the patient.

Malnutrition predicts a poor outcome. Under ideal circumstances nutrition status would be maintained; however, even in the presence of adequate intake, good nutriture is a challenge. Feeding difficulties are determined by the extent of the stroke and the area of the brain affected. Dysphagia, an independent predictor of mortality, commonly accompanies stroke and contributes to complications and poor outcome from malnutrition, pulmonary infections, disability, increased length of hospital stay, and institutional care. In some instances nutrition support is required to maintain nutritional health until oral alimentation can be resumed. As motor functions improve, eating and other ADLs are fundamental to the patient's rehabilitation process and necessary for resuming independence.

NEUROLOGIC DISEASES WITH NONNUTRITIONAL ETIOLOGIES

Adrenomyeloleukodystrophy

Pathophysiology

Adrenomyeloleukodystrophy (ALD) is a rare congenital enzyme deficiency that affects the metabolism of very long–chain fatty acids (VLCFAs) in young men. This leads to accumulation of VLCFAs, particularly hexacosanoic acid ($C_{26:0}$) and tetracosanoic acid ($C_{24:0}$) in the brain and adrenal glands (Deon et al., 2006). The mental and physical deterioration progresses to dementia, aphasia, apraxia, dysarthria, and blindness. The incidence is 1/21,000 male births and 1/14,000 female (Moser, 2006). It is an X-linked recessive disorder characterized by myelopathy, peripheral neuropathy, and cerebral demyelination.

Medical Treatment

First clinical manifestations usually occur before age 7 and may manifest as adrenal insufficiency or cerebral decompensation. **Dysarthria** (impairment of the tongue or other muscles needed for speech) or dysphagia may interfere with oral alimentation. Bronzing of the skin is a late clinical sign. In the face of adrenal insufficiency, physiologic replacement of steroids is indicated, which may improve neurologic symptoms and prolong life. Numerous therapies have been directed at the root of the disorder but have been disappointing. The selective use of bone marrow transplant is one current therapy; gene therapy holds promise for the future.

Medical Nutrition Therapy

Nutritional therapy by dietary avoidance of VLCFAs has not been proven. It does not lead to biochemical change because of endogenous synthesis. A specialty altered fatty acid product,

---

BOX 41-2

Nutrition-Related Factors and Stroke Risk

Risk Factors for Stroke

BMI >27 kg/m2 in women
Weight gain >11 kg over 16 years in women
Waist-to-hip ratio >0.92 in men
Diabetes
Hypertension
Cholesterol in hemorrhagic stroke

Protective Factors for Stroke

High intake of total dietary fat
Daily consumption of fresh fruit
Flavonoid consumption >4.7 cups green tea/daily
Fish consumption in white and black women and black men
Cholesterol in ischemic stroke

BMI, Body mass index.

Lorenzo's oil (C18:1 oleic acid and C22:1 erucic acid), lowers the VLCFA level; however, the clinical course is not significantly improved (Suzuki et al., 2001). Slower decline in function may be the more important result.

Alzheimer's Disease

Alzheimer's disease (AD) is the most common form of dementia with "patterns and rates of cognitive decline that are far from uniform" (Soto et al., 2005). It is named after Alois Alzheimer, who first described the clinical features and pathologic changes of this complex degenerative brain disease in 1907. AD begins gradually; advances; and eventually leads to confusion, personality and behavior changes, and impaired judgment. A loss of independence, disordered eating behavior, and weight loss may accompany other symptoms.

Manifestations of AD result in a progressive dementia, with increasing loss of memory, intellectual function, and disturbances in speech. Persons with poor physical function have been shown to be at greater risk for developing dementia and AD (from a prospective cohort study of 2288 persons ages 65+); delayed onset of symptoms was reported in that same study for those with higher physical function (Wang, 2006).

Initially day-to-day events are forgotten—possessions are misplaced, and appointments are forgotten—while memories are retained. Cerebral function declines, but this decline only becomes evident after the loss in memory is pronounced. Speech becomes impaired; names of objects are not remembered **(anomia)**, words spoken by others are repeated **(echolalia)**, and comprehension is lost **(agnosia)**. Over time motor skills deteriorate, as evidenced by changes in reflexes and a shuffling gate. Clinical findings are consistent when disease progression reaches the terminal stage. Bowel and bladder control is lost; limb weakness and contractures occur; and intellectual activity ceases. The patient becomes completely incapacitated in a vegetative state as death approaches.

The incidence rate of new cases of AD is similar for both sexes and throughout the world, increasing exponentially after age 40. The higher prevalence rate seen in women (three times higher than in men) is because women tend to live longer than men. Given its prevalence, the personal, familial, financial, and clinical impact of AD is staggering.

Pathophysiology

Alzheimer's disease (AD) is a progressive, neurodegenerative disease characterized in the brain by abnormal clumps of β-amyloid and neurofibrillary tangles composed of misplaced proteins (NIH, 2006). Age is the most important risk factor for AD; the number of people with the disease doubles every 5 years beyond age 65. Symptoms of AD include memory loss, language deterioration, impaired ability to mentally manipulate visual information, poor judgment, confusion, restlessness, and mood swings. Eventually AD destroys cognition, personality, and the ability to function. The early symptoms of AD, which include forgetfulness and loss of concentration, are often missed because they resemble natural signs of aging (see *Pathophysiology and Care Management Algorithm*: Alzheimer's Disease).

Three genes have been discovered that cause early-onset, familial AD. Other genetic mutations that cause excessive accumulation of amyloid protein are associated with age-related (sporadic) AD. Several genes have been identified as increasing the susceptibility for developing AD. Apolipoprotein-E4 (Apo-E4) has nutritional implications. Apo-E4 is a protein located on chromosome 19; it binds β-amyloid and is involved in the transport of cholesterol. Damage to key mitochondrial components (Kidd, 2005), impaired insulin signaling, and the factors related to heart disease and stroke (elevated homocysteine, low folate, high serum cholesterol) may also be part of the etiology.

Medical Treatment

There currently is no cure for AD. It is diagnosed by histopathology. Clinically, the diagnosis is presumptive and one of exclusion. As a result, studies may be subjected to criticism because of the absence of a confirmatory diagnosis. Treatment directed at the impairment of brain metabolism may improve neuropsychological function. No definitive treatment currently exists; cerebral vasodilators; stimulants; levodopa (L-dopa); and megadoses of vitamins B, C, and E remain unproven therapies.

Drug treatment remains experimental, and nonsteroidal antiinflammatory drugs (NSAIDs) in combination with nutrition supplements (e.g., acetylcholine, vitamin E, other antioxidants, and omega-3 fatty acids) are currently believed to be most effective. Tacrine, the first cholinesterase inhibitor approved by the Food and Drug Administration (FDA) for use in the treatment of AD, gives only modest improvement in both function and cognition. Some other medications are used to suppress aberrant behavior, disturbed sleep, anxiety, or agitation.

Primary care management is the most effective treatment. Collaborative interdisciplinary care has been shown to improve behavioral and psychological symptoms of dementia (Callahan et al., 2006). Empathic support and caregiver awareness are important, especially since the disease is progressive with a decline over 5 to 20 years.

Medical Nutrition Therapy

Determination of the nutrition status of the patient is essential because this population is often malnourished. Although a gluttonous appetite may develop in some individuals with AD with accompanying weight increase, generally the presentation is weight loss. Whether increased resting metabolic rate or increased energy expenditure causes weight loss is unclear. The latter is probably true because energy output associated with constant pacing may be increased. For others, eating is neglected, and weight loss is caused by an inadequate food intake resulting from decreased independence and impaired self-feeding. In still other cases weight loss may be secondary to higher basal energy expenditure from infections. Weight loss in turn increases the risk of infections, skin ulcers, and consequently a decreased quality of life.

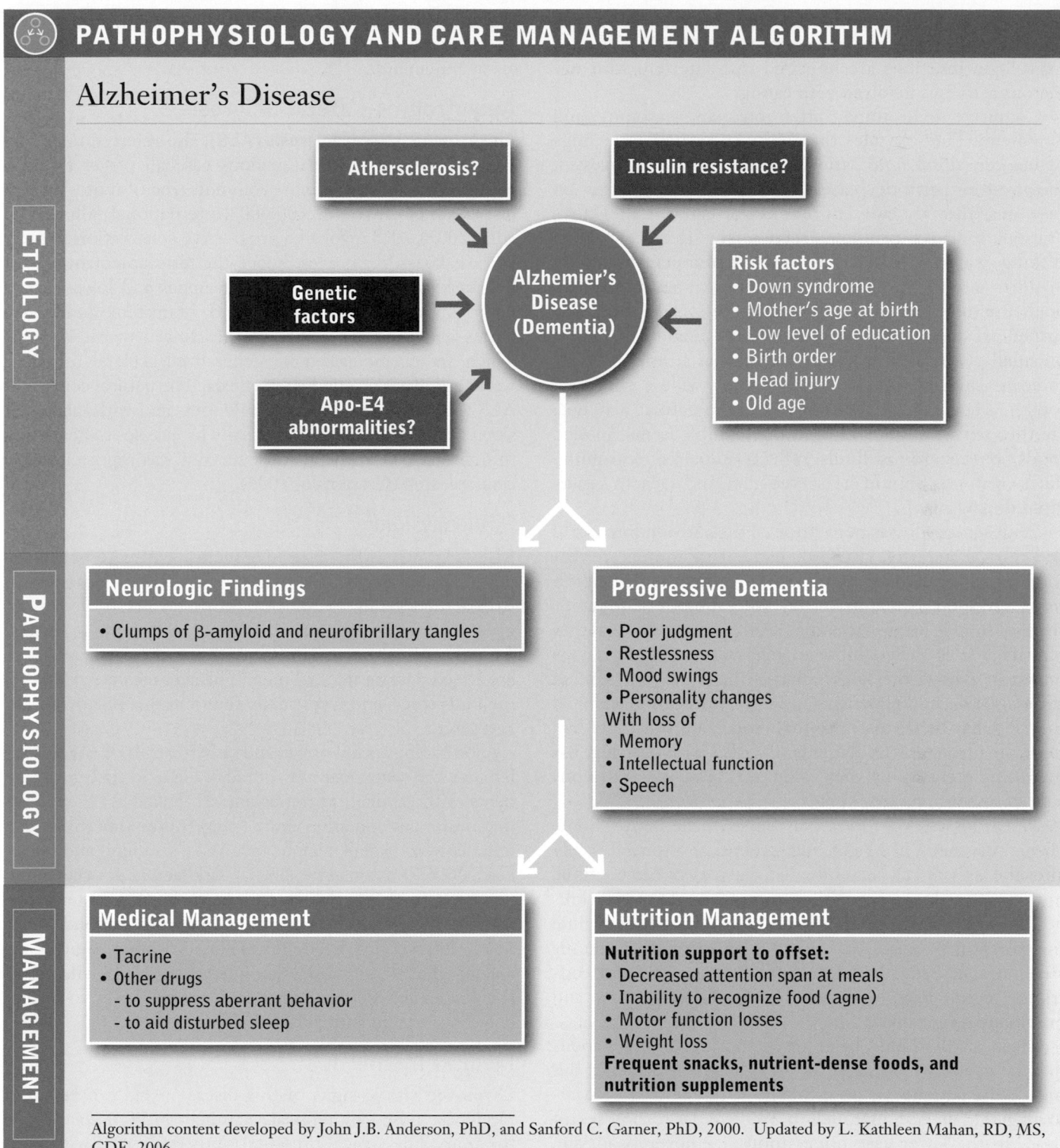

PATHOPHYSIOLOGY AND CARE MANAGEMENT ALGORITHM

Alzheimer's Disease

ETIOLOGY

Atherosclerosis?

Insulin resistance?

Genetic factors

Alzhemier's Disease (Dementia)

Apo-E4 abnormalities?

Risk factors
- Down syndrome
- Mother's age at birth
- Low level of education
- Birth order
- Head injury
- Old age

PATHOPHYSIOLOGY

Neurologic Findings
- Clumps of β-amyloid and neurofibrillary tangles

Progressive Dementia
- Poor judgment
- Restlessness
- Mood swings
- Personality changes
With loss of
- Memory
- Intellectual function
- Speech

MANAGEMENT

Medical Management
- Tacrine
- Other drugs
  - to suppress aberrant behavior
  - to aid disturbed sleep

Nutrition Management
Nutrition support to offset:
- Decreased attention span at meals
- Inability to recognize food (agne)
- Motor function losses
- Weight loss
Frequent snacks, nutrient-dense foods, and nutrition supplements

Algorithm content developed by John J.B. Anderson, PhD, and Sanford C. Garner, PhD, 2000. Updated by L. Kathleen Mahan, RD, MS, CDE, 2006.

Proper inclusion of antioxidants and specific nutrients may protect the AD patient from further decline (Meydani, 2001). Garlic and its constituents have been proposed as neuroprotective for AD, but work with mice models remains inconclusive, and extrapolation to humans is still needed (Chauhan, 2005). Resveratrol is also being studied; its antioxidant properties may help to prevent neuronal decline with aging (Anekonda, 2006). Some studies suggest that high intake of vitamins C, E, B$_6$, B$_{12}$, and folate; un-

saturated fatty acids; and fish is related to a low risk of AD; but reports are inconsistent, and an overall dietary regimen for AD is not yet defined (Luchsinger and Mayeux, 2004).

Problems with Self-Feeding and Nutritional Intake

Alzheimer's disease is a disease of cortical neurons. The frontal lobe controls behavior, reasoning, emotion, and cognition; the temporal lobe controls hearing, memory, smell, and language; and the parietal lobe controls sensory perception, hearing, and body image. As a result, a wide range of neurologic functions are impaired that interfere with numerous activities involved with eating.

Cognitive losses impair attention span, reasoning, and judgment. This includes the ability to recognize feelings of hunger, thirst, and satiety. As the disease progresses, the attention span decreases, and meals may be forgotten as soon as they are eaten or may not be eaten at all. Dehydration is also a problem; recognizing thirst and then seeking water is often neglected. Attempts should be made to minimize distractions at mealtimes. Noise can be distracting; therefore the radio or television should be turned off during mealtime. Food may need to be placed on small plates or bowls and given one at a time so as not to stress the individual by offering too wide a choice of foods. As social inhibitions decrease, the patient may take another person's food. Consuming inedible items, spoiled foods, or hazardous fluids reflects impaired reasoning. These patients should be served first and closely supervised during meals.

With sensory losses perception of the surrounding world and related auditory, visual, or tactile recognition are distorted; this is called agnosia. Visual agnosia, the inability to recognize food, is manifested by not eating. The touch or smell of food is needed to initiate eating responses. Another sensory loss is the inability to recognize food when it is served in a bowl the same color as the food item. Use of colored bowls and plates that are in contrast to the color of the food may be necessary so that food can be distinguished from the place setting. Patients may also have difficulty using eating utensils, but they can model behaviors if demonstrated by staff or caregivers.

Motor losses occur over the course of the illness. Some clients may need hand guidance to initiate eating. Usually after the activity has been initiated, the patient can continue the activity as long as verbal cues continue. As motor skills decline, use of eating utensils becomes limited; over time the patient may be able to use only a spoon. Eating utensils should not be removed prematurely because this may contribute to agitation, excessive disability, lack of eating, and eventually weight loss.

Motor skills should be assessed routinely. Finger foods may be useful when use of utensils becomes difficult, but only if the patient has no difficulty with chewing or swallowing and is not inclined to swallow large boluses of food. In the latter case finger foods are not appropriate. Although adaptive equipment is useful in certain situations, it may be unfamiliar to the patient with AD and not as helpful. As end-stage disease approaches, swallowing often becomes impossible; dysphagia should be assessed to prevent aspiration.

Frequent snacks, nutrient-dense foods, and nutrition supplements need to be provided to combat weight loss. Behavior modification, along with altered food items, improve the quality of life of the individual for as long as possible. Evaluation of nutrition status is needed throughout the stages of AD to ensure that objectives of nutrition

therapy continue to be met. Table 41-6 lists additional interventions for eating-related behavioral problems in individuals with dementia.

Amyotrophic Lateral Sclerosis

Amyotrophic lateral sclerosis (ALS), also referred to as Lou Gehrig's disease after the famous baseball player afflicted with the disease, is the most common type of motor system disease. Incidence is 2/100,000 (International Alliance of ALS, 2007). ALS involves a progressive denervation atrophy and weakness of muscles; hence the term amyotrophy, the hallmark sign and symptom. Both upper and lower motor neurons are lost in the spinal cord, brainstem, and motor cortex and thus contribute to the clinical manifestations, which are characterized by generalized skeletal muscular weakness, atrophy, and hyperreflexia. The natural course for ALS is unpleasant. Decline is relentless and without remissions, relapses, or plateaus; it finally progresses to death in 2 to 6 years, 3.45 years' average survival was reported in recent research (Czaplinski, 2006).

Pathophysiology

ALS is known as the neurodegenerative disease of the aging nervous system. The pathologic basis of weakness in ALS is the selective death of motor neurons in the ventral gray matter of the spinal cord and in the motor cortex. The prevalence is constant throughout the world, and men are affected more than women. The average age of onset is the mid-fifties, and it is usually found in the 40- to 70-year age-group.

The etiology is unknown, and only 5% to 10% of cases are familial; the remainder are sporadic. Genetic analysis of patients with familial, chromosome 21–linked ALS suggests that misfolding mutations in the copper-zinc superoxide dismutase (SOD1) gene may be involved (Nordlund and Oliveberg, 2006; Jonsson et al., 2002). Risk factors of occupation, trauma, diet, or socioeconomic status are not consistent. The possible role of antioxidant status in prevention and therapeutic intervention needs further investigation. Studies involving the use of polyunsaturated fatty acids, vitamin E (Veldink et al., 2006) and vitamin C are underway to further define the role of antioxidant therapy in ALS.

Medical Treatment

Given the classic signs of this disease, ALS can be accurately diagnosed by clinical examination 90% to 95% of the time. The typical presentation is evidenced with both lower motor neuron (weakness, wasting, fasciculation) and upper motor neuron deficits (hyperactive tendon reflexes, Hoffman signs, Babinski signs, or clonus). Muscle weakness begins in the legs and hands and progresses to the proximal arms and oropharynx. As these motor nerves deteriorate, almost all of the voluntary skeletal muscles are at risk for atrophy and complete loss of function. The loss of spinal motor neurons causes the denervation of voluntary skeletal muscles of the neck, trunk, and limbs, resulting in muscle wasting, flaccid weakness, and fasciculations leading to loss of mobility.

The progressive loss of function in cortical motor neurons can lead to spasticity of jaw muscles, resulting in slurred speech and dysphagia. The onset of dysphagia is usually insidious. Swallowing difficulties usually follow speech difficulties. Although some weight loss is inevitable given the muscle atrophy, consistent or dramatic loss may be an indicator of chewing difficulties or dysphagia (Bulat and Orlando, 2005).

Eye movement and eye blink are spared, as are the sphincter muscles of the bowel and bladder; thus incontinence is rare. Sensation remains intact, and except in rare cases mental acuity is maintained. No effective therapy can cure or even slow the disease progression. Research has shown no benefit from immunosuppression, immunoenhancement, plasmapheresis, lymph node irradiation, glutamate antagonists, nerve growth factors, or antiviral agents.

The Amyotrophic Lateral Sclerosis Severity Scale (ALSSS) is used to assess the functional level of swallowing, speech, and upper and lower extremities. Once the severity of deficits has been identified, the appropriate interventions can be implemented (Box 41-3). Although mechanical ventilation can extend the life of patients, most decline this option because the quality of life is poor in advanced ALS. Therefore only supportive measures are used.

TABLE 41-6

Practical Interventions for Eating-Related Behavioral Problems Common in Individuals With Dementia

Behavioral Problem	Intervention	Behavioral Problem	Intervention
Attention/or concentration deficit	Verbally direct client through each step of eating process Place utensils in hand Make food and fluids available and visible	Forgetful or disoriented	Follow simple routines Provide constant environment Provide assigned seating Minimize distractions Limit choices
Combative, throws food	Identify provocative agent, remove Feeder stands or sits on nondominant side Provide nonbreakable dishes with suction holder Give one food at a time Reward appropriate mealtime behavior	Forgets to swallow	Tell client to swallow Feel for swallow before offering next bite Stroke upward on larynx
		Inappropriate emotional expression	Engage in conversation Ignore emotional display Provide quiet environment
Chews constantly	Tell client to stop chewing after each bite Serve soft foods to reduce the need to chew Offer small bites	Paces	Sit beside client at table Change dining location Provide aerobic exercise before meals Offer finger foods Use cups with covers or spouts
Eats nonedible things	Remove nonedibles from reach Provide finger foods Provide edible centerpiece or table decorations	Plays in food	Serve one food at a time Fill glass or plate half full at refill Offer finger foods Use cups with covers or spouts
Eats too quickly	Set utensils down between bites Offer food items separately Offer bulky foods that require chewing Use a smaller spoon or cup	Shows paranoia	Provide structured routine Present food in consistent manner Serve foods in closed containers Do not put medicine in food
Eats too slowly	Monitor eating place and provide verbal cues: "chew," "take a bite" Serve first to allow more time Use insulated dishes to maintain proper temperatures	Spits	Evaluate chewing and swallowing ability Tell client not to spit Place away from others who would be offended Provide mealtime supervision
		Will not go into dining room	Ask why Change dining location Provide a single dining partner versus a group Serve meals in room

Modified from the Nutrition Screening Initiative, a project of the American Academy of Family Physicians, The American Dietetic Association, and the National Council on the Aging, Inc., and funded in part by a grant from Ross Products Division, a division of Abbott Labs.

Amyotrophic Lateral Sclerosis Severity Scale

Swallowing Scale Rating

Normal Eating Habits

10 Normal Swallowing: Person denies any difficulty chewing or swallowing. Examination demonstrates no abnormality.

9 Nominal Abnormality: Only the individual with amyotrophic lateral sclerosis (ALS) notices slight indicators, such as food lodging in the recesses of the mouth or sticking in the throat.

Early Eating Problems

8 Minor Swallowing Problems: Complains of some swallowing difficulties. Maintains essentially a regular diet. Isolated choking episodes.

7 Prolonged Eating Time or Small Bite Size: Mealtime has significantly increased, and smaller bite sizes are necessary. Must concentrate on swallowing liquids.

Dietary Consistency Changes

6 Soft Diet: Diet is limited primarily to soft foods. Requires some special meal preparation.

5 Liquefied Diet: Oral intake adequate. Nutrition limited primarily to liquefied diet. Thin liquid intake usually a problem. May force self to eat.

Needs Tube Feeding

4 Supplemental Tube Feedings: Oral intake alone is no longer adequate. Person uses or needs a tube to supplement intake. Person continues to take significant nutrition (greater than 50%) by mouth.

3 Tube Feeding With Occasional Oral Nutrition: Primary nutrition and hydration accomplished by tube. Receives less than 59% of nutrition by mouth.

Nothing by Mouth

2 Secretions Managed With Aspirator/Medication: Cannot safely manage any oral intake. Secretions managed by aspirator and/or medications. Swallows reflexively.

1 Aspiration of Secretions: Secretions cannot be managed noninvasively. Rarely swallows.

Speech Scale Rating

Normal Speech Processes

10 Normal Speech: Individual denies any difficulty speaking. Examination demonstrates no abnormality.

9 Nominal Speech Abnormality: Only the individual with ALS or spouse notices that speech has changed. Maintains normal rate and volume.

Detectable Speech Disturbance

8 Perceived Speech Changes: Speech changes are noted by others, especially during fatigue or stress. Rate of speech remains essentially normal.

7 Obvious Speech Abnormalities: Speech is consistently impaired. Affected are rate, articulation, and resonance. Remains easily understood.

Behavioral Modifications

6 Repeats Messages on Occasion: Rate is much slower. Repeats specific words in adverse listening situations. Does not limit complexity or length of message.

5 Frequent Repeating Required: Speech is slow and labored. Extensive repetition or a "translator" is commonly needed. Person probably limits the complexity or length of message.

Use of Augmentative Communication

4 Speech Plus Augmentative Communication: Speech is used in response to questions. Intelligibility problems need to be resolved by writing or a spokesperson.

3 Limits Speech to One-Word Response: Vocalizes one-word response beyond yes/no; otherwise writes or uses a spokesperson. Initiates communication nonvocally.

Loss of Useful Speech

2 Vocalizes for Emotional Expression: Uses vocal inflection to express emotion, affirmation, and negation.

1 Nonvocal: Vocalization is difficult, limited in duration, and rarely attempted. May vocalize for crying or pain.

X Tracheostomy

Upper Extremities Scale Rating

Normal Function

10 Normal Function: Person denies any weakness or unusual fatigue of upper extremities. Examination demonstrates no abnormality.

9 Suspected Fatigue: Person suspects fatigue in upper extremities during exertion. Cannot sustain work for as long as normal. Atrophy not evident on examination.

Independent and Complete Self-Care

8 Slow Self-Care Performance: Dressing and hygiene performed more slowly than usual.

7 Laborious Self-Care Performance: Requires significantly more time (usually double or more) and effort to accomplish self-care. Weakness is apparent on examination.

Intermittent Assistance

6 Mostly Independent: Handles most aspects of dressing and hygiene alone. Adapts by resting, modifying (electric razor), or avoiding some tasks (e.g., buttons, tie).

5 Partial Independence: Handles some aspects of dressing and hygiene alone. However, routinely requires assistance for many tasks such as makeup, combing, and shaving.

Needs Attendant for Self-Care

4 Attendant Assists Person: Attendant must be present for dressing and hygiene. Person performs the majority of each task with the assistance of the attendant.

3 Person Assists Attendant: The attendant assists the person with ALS for most tasks. The person moves in a purposeful manner to assist the attendant. Does not initiate self-care tasks.

From Hillel AD et al: ALS Severity Scale, *J Neuroepidemiol* 8:142, 1989. Reproduced with permission of J. Karger AG, Basel, Switzerland.

BOX 41-3

Amyotrophic Lateral Sclerosis Severity Scale—cont'd

Upper Extremities Scale Rating—cont'd

Total Dependence

2 Minimum Movement: Minimum movement of one or both arms. Cannot reposition arms.

1 Paralysis: Flaccid paralysis. Unable to move upper extremities.

Lower Extremities Scale Rating

Normal

10 Normal Ambulation: Person denies any weakness or fatigue. Examination detects no abnormality.

9 Fatigue Suspected: Person suspects weakness or fatigue in lower extremities during exertion.

Early Ambulation Problem

8 Difficulty With Uneven Terrain: Difficulty and fatigue when walking long distances, climbing stairs, and walking over uneven ground (even thick carpet).

7 Observed Changes in Gait: Noticeable change in gait. Pulls on railing when climbing stairs. May use leg brace.

Walks With Assistance

6 Walks With Mechanical Device: Needs or uses canes, walker, or assistant to walk. Probably uses wheelchair away from home.

5 Walks With Mechanical Device and Attendant: Does not attempt to walk without an attendant. Ambulation limited to less than 50 feet. Avoids stairs.

Functional Movement Only

4 Able to Support Weight: At best can shuffle a few steps with the help of an attendant for transfers.

3 Purposeful Leg Movements: Unable to take steps but can position legs to assist an attendant in transfers. Moves legs purposefully to maintain mobility in bed.

No Purposeful Leg Movement

2 Minimum Movement: Minimum movement of one or both legs. Cannot reposition legs independently.

1 Paralysis: Flaccid paralysis. Cannot move lower extremities.

Medical Nutrition Therapy

Although not all of the nutritional changes during the different stages of ALS have been well documented, those presented in Table 41-7 can have a major impact. There are decreases in body fat, lean body mass, muscle power, and nitrogen balance and an increase in resting energy expenditure as death approaches. A hypermetabolic status as evidenced by increased resting energy expenditure measurements has been confirmed (Desport et al., 2001).

The relationship between dysphagia and respiratory status in disease progression is important. As ALS progresses, a progressive loss of function in bulbar and respiratory muscles contributes to oral and pharyngeal dysphagia. In late stages the respiratory status is impaired such that the patient is not a good candidate for PEG placement; and alternative placements may be required (Chio et al., 2004). Although a PEG is placed under local anesthesia, the patient may not be able to lie prone for tube placement without respiratory decompensation. This reinforces the need for early versus late education about dysphagia management and discussion about whether to place a feeding tube.

The clinician should become familiar with common clinical findings throughout the natural history of the disease to prevent secondary complications of malnutrition and dehydration. The functional status of each patient should be monitored closely so that timely intervention with the appropriate management techniques can be started. In particular, dysphagia should be monitored closely. Oropharyngeal weakness affects survival in ALS by placing the patient at continuous risk of aspiration, pneumonia, and sepsis and by curtailing the adequate intake of energy and protein. These problems can compound the deteriorating effects of the disease (see *Focus On:* Dysphagia Intervention for ALS).

Epilepsy

Epilepsy is an intermittent derangement of the nervous system presumably caused by a sudden, excessive, disorderly discharge of cerebral neurons. It is estimated that 2.3 million individuals in the United States have epilepsy (200,000 new cases each year); 45,000 children under the age of 15 develop epilepsy each year according to the Epilepsy Foundation in 2006. Direct medical costs for persons with continued seizure activity are reported to be 55% higher than the average costs for all persons with epilepsy (Mandel et al., 2002).

Pathophysiology

Most seizures begin in early life, but a resurgence of epileptic events occurs after age 60. The first occurrence of a seizure in adults should prompt investigation into a cause. A clinical workup usually reveals no anatomic abnormalities, and the cause of the seizure may remain unknown (idiopathic). Seizures before age 2 are usually caused by developmental defects, birth injuries, or a metabolic disease (see Chapters 44 and 45). The medical history is the key component for suggesting further avenues of diagnostic investigation and potential treatments, especially in children. An electroencephalogram can help to delineate seizure activity. It is most helpful in localizing partial complex seizures.

Medical Treatment

The dramatic **tonic-clonic (grand mal) seizure** is the most common image of a seizure (lasting 1 to 2 minutes), yet

TABLE 41-7

Nutritional and Metabolic Changes During the Progression of Amyotrophic Lateral Sclerosis

	Early Phase	Late Phase
Pathophysiology	Cycles of muscle denervation, muscle catabolism and atrophy, reinnervation, and protein synthesis	Net muscle catabolism and atrophy
Functional status	Mild functional restriction of physical activity	Progressive limitation of physical activity
	Mild impairment of respiration	Increased work of ventilation
Nutritional and metabolic changes	Positive nitrogen balance	Negative nitrogen balance
	Normal resting energy expenditure	Increased resting energy expenditure
	Probable neutral energy balance	Decrease in body fat

From Kasarskis EJ et al: Nutritional status of patients with amyotrophic lateral sclerosis: relation to the proximity of death, *Am J Clin Nutr* 63:130, 1996. Printed in USA. Copyright 1996 *Am J Clin Nutr*, American Society for Clinical Nutrition.

numerous classifications of seizures, each with a different and often less dramatic clinical presentation, exist. A generalized seizure is one that involves or appears to involve the entire brain cortex from its beginning phases. The tonic-clonic seizure comes under this heading. After such a seizure the patient wakes up slowly after a time; he or she will be groggy and disoriented for minutes to hours after the event. This is termed the *postictal phase* and is characterized by deep sleep, headache, confusion, and muscle soreness.

The **absence seizure (petit mal)** is also generalized in nature. A patient with absence seizures may appear to be daydreaming during an episode, but he or she recovers consciousness within a few seconds and has no postictal fatigue or disorientation. Partial seizures occur when there is a discrete focus of epileptogenic brain tissue. A simple partial seizure involves no loss of consciousness, whereas a complex partial seizure is characterized by a change in consciousness. Failure of partial seizure control may prompt consideration of seizure surgery. A localized focus resected from nonessential brain renders a patient seizure free in 75% of cases.

Determining the seizure type is key to implementing effective therapy. Generalized seizures are ordinarily managed with valproate or phenytoin. Phenytoin metabolism has unusual kinetics; thus toxic levels may be attained with very small dosage adjustments. These drugs interact with other drugs metabolized in the liver and may cause liver damage. Liver enzymes and serum drug levels must be monitored periodically. Gabapentin has been introduced recently, and it is rapidly gaining popularity because of its safety and ease of use. Carbamazepine or phenytoin can usually control partial seizures.

Medications used in anticonvulsant therapy may alter the nutrition status of the patient. Phenobarbital has been associated with decreased intelligence quotient (IQ) when used in children. It is occasionally considered for use after failure of other antiepileptic drugs. Phenobarbital, phenytoin, and primidone interfere with intestinal absorption of calcium by increasing vitamin D metabolism in the liver. Long-term therapy with these drugs may lead to osteomalacia in adults or rickets in children. Vitamin D supplementation is recommended. Folic acid supplementation interferes with phenytoin metabolism; thus it contributes to

difficulties in achieving therapeutic levels. For this reason sporadic folic acid supplementation should be avoided.

Phenytoin and phenobarbital are bound primarily to albumin in the bloodstream. Decreased serum albumin levels in malnutrition or with reduced albumin synthesis secondary to advanced cirrhosis limit the amount of drug that can be bound. This results in an increased free drug concentration and possible drug toxicity with a standard dose.

New treatment guidelines for medication use and for preventing photic- and pattern-induced seizures have been released by the Epilepsy Foundation. These guidelines emphasize the public health nature of seizure management and the special needs of women and older Americans in optimizing strategies. Use of just one antiseizure medication is recommended initially, resorting to combination therapies only when needed.

Continuous enteral feeding slows the absorption of phenytoin, thus necessitating an increase in the dose to achieve a therapeutic level. Decreased serum phenytoin concentrations associated with enteral feeding may increase the risk of seizures; a patient-specific care plan that includes consideration of the enteral feeding formulation and method of administration, as well as the phenytoin dosage form, schedule of administration, and monitoring, is needed (Au Yeung and Ensom, 2000). Recommendations to separate phenytoin suspension from tube-feeding formulas are common. Stopping the tube feeding before and after the phenytoin dose is generally suggested. The most common recommendation is a 2-hour feeding-free interval before and after the dose of phenytoin is administered (Au Yeung and Ensom, 2000). Whenever tube feedings are stopped, the dose of phenytoin needs to be adjusted to avoid toxicity. Absorption of phenobarbital is delayed by the consumption of food; therefore administration of the drug must be staggered around mealtimes if it is used.

Medical Nutrition Therapy

A *ketogenic diet* has been used for treatment of all types of seizures in children in whom drug therapies have failed. This diet is also used in the management of several inborn errors of metabolism (Roman, 2006). The ketogenic diet is financially beneficial, particularly in comparison to total costs for care (Mandel et al., 2002). A report that evaluated medical

Dysphagia Intervention for Amyotrophic Lateral Sclerosis

Strand and colleagues (1996) outlined the timing of dysphagia intervention on a continuum of five stages that correlate to the amyotrophic lateral sclerosis (ALS) severity scale. They include:

1. *Normal Eating Habits (ALS Severity Scale Rating 10-9).* Early assessment and intervention are critical for maintaining nutritional health in ALS. This is the appropriate time to begin educating the patient, before the development of speech or swallowing symptoms. Hydration and maintenance of nutritional health are critical at this stage. Fluid intake of at least 2 q/day from noncaffeinated sources is important because caffeine has a diuretic effect that contributes to dehydration. Dehydration contributes to fatigue and thickens saliva. For patients with spinal ALS, emphasis on fluids is important because they may intentionally limit fluid intake because of difficulties with toileting. The diet history is helpful to assess patterns of normal chewing, swallowing, and the rate of ingestion; weight loss history establishes a baseline weight. A weight loss of 10% or more is indicative of nutritional risk.

2. *Early Eating Problems (Severity Scale Rating 8-7).* At this point patients begin to report difficulties eating; reports of coughing and unusually long mealtimes are associated with tongue, facial, and masticator muscle weakness. Dietary intervention begins to focus on modification of consistency, avoidance of thin liquids, and use of foods that are easier to chew and swallow.

3. *Dietary Consistency Changes (Severity Scale Rating 6-5).* As symptoms progress, the oral transport of food becomes difficult as dry, crumbly foods tend to break apart and cause choking. Foods that require more chewing (e.g., raw vegetables or steak) are typically avoided. As dysphagia progresses, ingestion of thin liquids, especially water, may become more problematic. Often the patient has fatigue and malaise, which may be associated with a mild chronic dehydration resulting from a decreased fluid intake. Dietary intervention should change food consistency to mechanically soft or pureed (see Appendix 35) to reduce the need for oral manipulation and to conserve energy. Small, frequent meals may also increase intake. Thick liquids that contain a high percentage of water, as well as attempts to increase fluid intake, need to be emphasized to maintain fluid balance. Popsicles, gelatin, ice, and fresh fruit are additional sources of free water. Liquids can be thickened with a modified cornstarch thickener. Swallowing can be improved by emphasizing taste, texture, and temperature. Juices can be substituted for water to provide taste, nutrients, and calories. A cool temperature facilitates the swallowing mechanism; therefore cold food items may be better tolerated; heat does not provide the same advantage. Carbonation may also be better tolerated because of the beneficial effect of texture. Instructions for preventing aspiration should be addressed: safe swallowing includes sitting bolt upright with the head in a chin-down position. Concentrating on the swallowing process can also help reduce choking. Avoid environmental distractions and conversation during mealtime; however, families should be encouraged to maintain a normal mealtime routine. As dysphagia progresses, the limitation of food consistencies may result in the exclusion of entire food groups. Vitamin and mineral supplementation may be necessary. If chewable supplements are not handled safely, liquid forms may be added to acceptable foods. Fiber may also need to be added along with fluids for constipation problems.

4. *Tube Feeding (Severity Scale Rating 4-3).* Dehydration will occur acutely before malnutrition, a more chronic state, is exhibited. This may be an early indication of the need for nutrition support. Weight loss from muscle wasting and dysphagia will eventually lead to placement of a percutaneous endoscopic gastrostomy (PEG) tube for nutrition and protection against aspiration caused by dysphagia. Enteral nutrition support is preferred because the gastrointestinal tract should be functioning properly. Given the progressive nature of ALS, placing feeding tubes with signs of dysphagia and dehydration is better than initiating this therapy later, after the patient has become overtly malnourished or when respiratory status is marginal. The decision of whether to place a feeding tube for nutrition support is part of the decision-making process each patient must face. Adequate nutriture can maintain health of the individual longer and may be a welcome relief for the patient. The purpose of nutrition support should be to enhance the quality of life. Long-term access should be considered via a PEG or percutaneous endoscope jejunostomy tube (see Chapter 20).

5. *Nothing by Mouth NPO (Severity Scale Rating 2-1).* The final level of dysphagia is reached when the patient can neither eat orally nor manage his or her own oral secretions. Although saliva production is not increased, it tends to pool in the front of the mouth as a result of a declining swallow response. Once the swallowing mechanism is absent, mechanical ventilation is required to manage saliva flow. Tube feeding is permanent at this stage.

Data from Strand EA et al: Management of oral-pharyngeal dysphagia symptoms in amyotrophic lateral sclerosis, *Dysphagia* 11:129, 1996.

costs for children (2 to 28 years of age) with drug refractory epilepsies demonstrated cost advantage, reduction in seizures, and a reduced need for drugs with the use of a ketogenic diet (Mandel et al., 2002).

The ketogenic diet has minimum side effects. However, data on the long-term impact on growth or cardiovascular risk are lacking. One recent report on growth change in children did find that subjects on the ketogenic diet showed a growth delay; additional research is needed (Peterson et al., 2005). Although the diet is initially demanding, it completely controls epilepsy in one third of the children whose seizures are otherwise uncontrollable. Practice guidelines released by the American Academy of Neurology and the American Epilepsy Society can be retrieved from the Epilepsy Foundation website (Epilepsy Foundation, 2006).

The diet is designed to create and maintain a state of ketosis (Bough and Rho, 2007). Although its mechanism of action is not clearly understood, the beneficial effect in epilepsy may be caused by a change in neuronal metabolism, whereby a ketone body behaves as an inhibitory neurotransmitter, thus producing an anticonvulsant effect on the body. Two forms of the ketogenic diet are in use: the "traditional" approach, developed in the 1920s, and the medium-chain triglyceride (MCT)-based approach (Liu et al., 2003). With either approach the child fasts in the hospital for 24 to 72 hours until a 4+ ketonuria is produced. For the majority of patients, if the diet is going to work, it usually works during the initial fasting period. It should also be noted that antiepileptic drugs need to be stopped when administering the ketogenic diet.

In the traditional approach, once ketosis is established, caloric intake is resumed in a ratio of 4:1 for fat kcal:protein/carbohydrate kcal in the diet. For a child the diet is calculated so that 75% of the kilocalories are from fat. Protein is calculated to provide appropriate intake for growth (about 1 g/kg/day). Carbohydrates are added to make up the remaining portion of protein and carbohydrate calories, which is usually a minimum to negligible amount. The Exchange Lists (see Appendix 34) can be used to adjust the carbohydrate amount. A multiple vitamin/mineral and extra calcium supplement is recommended to ensure that the diet is nutritionally complete; this should be provided in a sugar-free form. Mild dehydration is used to prevent dilution of the level of ketones circulating at any time (Berryman, 1997). Fluids are carefully controlled—not to exceed 2 L/day (Kinsman et al., 1992).

The MCT-based ketogenic diet replaces the long-chain fats of the traditional diet with MCT. MCT oil is an odorless, colorless, tasteless oil and was originally used as a means of improving the palatability of the diet. A greater amount of nonketogenic foods such as fruits and vegetables and small amounts of bread and other starches can be allowed because ketosis from MCT can be more readily achieved (Table 41-8). Fluids are not limited in the MCT ketogenic diet.

Inititiating the ketogenic diet is intense. Further, the diet may seem unpalatable as well as complex, thus making compliance difficult to achieve. To be successful, children may benefit from behavioral techniques, whereas parents most often require substantial psychosocial support. Attention

required during the follow-up phase varies and is affected by the patient's health status, growth, and development and the caregiver's level of anticipation. For the child whose epilepsy is controlled on the diet, complying with the diet is much easier than dealing with devastating seizures and associated injuries. Fortunately the duration of the diet is limited; it can often be discontinued after 2 to 3 years.

Guillain-Barré Syndrome

Guillain-Barré syndrome (GBS) is an acute-onset, inflammatory, demyelinating polyneuropathy that has a predilection for proximal motor nerves, including the cranial nerves and the diaphragm. The incidence is approximately 2/100,000, and the cause is most likely mediated by the immune system. GBS is the most common paralytic illness of children and adolescents in countries with established immunization programs (Joseph and Tsao, 2002).

Pathophysiology

In 60% of cases the disorder follows an infection, surgery, or an immunization. Some of the more common organisms are *Campylobacter jejuni* and *Mycoplasma*. Several pathologic varieties exist, and the nature of the distinction is related to the segment of the immune system that is inflicting nerve damage. The clinical course of GBS is similar regardless of subtype, although GBS after a *Campylobacter* infection tends to be more severe. Relatively symmetric weakness with paresthesia usually begins in the legs and progresses to the arms.

The loss of function in affected nerves occurs because of demyelination. Myelin is the specialized fatty insulation that envelops the conducting part of the nerve, the axon. In GBS the immune system recognizes myelin and mounts an attack against it. Presumably myelin shares a common characteristic with the pathogen from the antecedent infection; thus the immune system cannot differentiate what is foreign (the pathogen) from what is native (myelin). When the nerve is demyelinated, its ability to conduct signals is severely impaired, and this results in neuropathy.

Medical Treatment

The most common sequence of symptoms is areflexia (absence of reflexes), followed by proximal limb weakness, and followed finally by cranial nerve weakness and respiratory insufficiency. These symptoms may progress for up to 1 month but normally peak by 2 weeks. Diagnosis is ordinarily made on clinical grounds, but nerve conduction studies are revealing. Before the clinical course is apparent, myelopathic disorders need to be considered. GBS reveals itself in a matter of days.

Because of the potentially precipitous progression of GBS, hospitalization is in order, if only for observation. Vital capacity and swallowing function may rapidly deteriorate such that intensive care is sometimes necessary. Intubation and respiratory support should be instituted early in the face of respiratory decline to avoid the need for resuscitation. Plasmapheresis, the exchange of the patient's plasma for albumin, is often helpful. This reduces the load of circu-

TABLE 41-8

Typical Ketogenic Diet Menu Using MCT Oil

Food Item	Amount (g)	Carbohydrates (g)	Protein (g)	Fat (g)	Energy (kcal)
Breakfast					
White bread	5	2.8	0.4	0.2	13
Egg, scrambled	48		6.1	5.5	74
Cream, heavy whipping	10	0.3	0.3	3.8	36
Margarine or butter	5			5.0	45
MCT oil	12			12.0	108
Fat	11			11.0	99
Drink sweetened with nonnutritive sweetener	240				
TOTAL		2.8	6.8	37.5	375
Lunch					
American cheese	12	2.2	2.8	3.6	52
Ham	23	0.7	3.7	3.9	53
MCT oil mayonnaise	11			11.0	99
Fat	19			19.0	171
Drink sweetened with nonnutritive sweetener	240				
TOTAL		2.9	6.5	37.5	375
Dinner					
Turkey	19		6.3	0.7	32
Tomato	10	0.5	0.1	0.0	3
Green beans	10	0.6	0.2	0.0	3
Potatoes	12	1.4	0.2	0.0	8
Margarine	15			15.0	135
MCT oil mayonnaise	11			11.0	99
Fat	10			10.0	90
Drink sweetened with nonnutritive sweetener	240				
TOTAL		2.8	6.8	36.7	370
DAILY TOTAL		8.5	20.1	111.7	1120

MCT, Medium-chain triglyceride.

lating antibodies. Also intravenous immunoglobulin has been shown to be of benefit. Steroids may also be used.

Medical Nutrition Therapy

Guillain-Barré syndrome evolves quickly, and during this acute stage the metabolic response of GBS is similar to the stress response that occurs in neurotrauma. Researchers studied 21 patients with GBS admitted to an intensive care unit and found that energy needs assessed by indirect calorimetry were 40 to 45 nonprotein kcal/kg and protein needs were 2 to 2.5 g/kg. Supportive care by immediate attainment of positive energy balance provided by high-energy and protein tube feedings may help to reestablish a positive nitrogen balance and attenuate muscle wasting (Roubenoff et al., 1992).

For a small percentage of patients, oropharyngeal muscles may be affected, leading to dysphagia and dysarthria. In this situation a visit by the RD at mealtime can be an invaluable way to observe any difficulties the patient may have with chewing or swallowing. Such difficulties warrant evalu-

ation by a swallowing specialist. The speech therapist can evaluate the degree of dysphagia and make appropriate dietary recommendations pertaining to texture. As the patient recovers, it is important to discuss safe food handling and future prevention of *C. jejuni* infection.

Migraine Headache

The **migraine syndrome** is defined clinically as an episodic intense, throbbing head pain that lasts from 4 to 72 hours. It is usually on one side of the head and becomes worse with exertion. It may be accompanied by nausea and classically is associated with a prodrome of visual disturbances or unusual olfactory and gustatory perception. Most persons report an associated transient visual aura, including flashing lights. Migraines are more common between the ages 15 and 55 and affect women more often than men.

Pathophysiology

Although the cause is unknown, migraine headache is thought to be vascular in origin and follows a family history of migraines or of visual prodromata. The leading theory proposes that dural blood vessels become dilated and the pulsatile blood flow through these vessels distends and irritates the highly pain-sensitive dura mater. This would explain the throbbing quality of the headache. An inflammatory component to migraine headache has also been proposed.

Medical Treatment

Treatment depends on the frequency of attacks and the presence of comorbid illness. A thorough history is the key to diagnosis. To qualify for a diagnosis of migraine headache, the headache must be throbbing, episodic, and supremely intense. The excruciating headache must not be prematurely considered a migraine. A history of intercurrent nausea, vomiting, photophobia, and visual or olfactory auras should be present.

Numerous medicines are used to prevent or abort migraine, indicating a less than crystal clear understanding of its pathophysiology. NSAIDs are often the first line, followed by sympathomimetics and serotonin agonists such as sumatriptan. Prophylaxis can include calcium channel antagonists, α-adrenergic blockers, and serotonin antagonists.

Medical Nutrition Therapy

Migraine attacks are triggered by a variety of factors, including food, drugs, odors, changes in sleep habits; they respond to a variety of treatments (Dowson et al., 2006). Since foods implicated in one individual may not trigger attacks in another and food intolerance thresholds vary over time, generalized recommendations about food avoidance are ill advised. There has been attention to biogenic amines such as tyramine or phenylethylamine in foods as causes of migraine headaches, but subsequent research does not appear to validate this, and their avoidance cannot be generally recommended (D'Andrea et al., 2004; Janssen et al., 2003).

In some patients dehydration may be the instigator of a migraine headache; one simple measure is to drink more water to rehydrate (Blau 2005; Spigt et al, 2005). An obstacle to dietary management occurs when restriction of the offending foods contributes to inadequate nutritional intake. Because suspect food items can only be correctly identified if eliminated and then reintroduced into the diet, the RD should offer alternative food suggestions so that optimal nutrition status can be maintained. See Chapter 29 for a Food and Symptom Diary Form to record intake and timing of symptoms, and in consultation with a health practitioner, to determine which foods may be a problem.

Many patients will try herbs or botanical products or nutritional supplementation to manage their headaches. Feverfew is used by many migraine sufferers, even though a Cochrane Database Review did not show that feverfew was any more effective than placebo in reducing frequency or severity of migraine (Pittler and Ernst, 2004).

Because of their roles in energy metabolism, two nutrients, riboflavin and CoQ_{10}, have been studied for migraine prophylaxis (Hershey et al., 2007; Woolhouse, 2005). Magnesium has also been studied in children. When given daily over a period of 16 weeks, magnesium oxide reduced the severity but not the frequency of headaches (Wang et al., 2003). However, the studies have limitations, and conclusions on effectiveness must be drawn with caution (Damen et al., 2006).

Myasthenia Gravis

Myasthenia gravis (MG) is not only the most well known disorder of the neuromuscular junction, but it is also one of the most well-characterized autoimmune diseases, a class of disorders in which the body's immune system raises a response to acetylcholine receptors (AChRs). The incidence of MG is low, about 14 in 100,000 people.

Pathophysiology

The neuromuscular junction is the site on the striated muscle membrane where a spinal motor neuron connects. Here the signal from the nerve is carried to the muscle via a submicron-size gap, a synapse. The molecule that carries the signal from the nerve ending to the muscle membrane is acetylcholine (ACh), and acetylcholine receptors (AChRs) populate the muscle membrane. These receptors translate the chemical signal of ACh into an electrical signal that is required for contraction of muscle fibers.

In MG the body unwittingly makes antibodies to AChR. These antibodies are the same that fight off colds and give immunity. The AChR antibodies bind to AChR and make them unresponsive to ACh. There is no disorder of nerve conduction and no intrinsic disorder of muscle. The characteristic weakness in MG occurs because the signal of the nervous system to the muscle is garbled at the neuromuscular junction. Patients with MG commonly have an overactive thymus gland. This gland resides in the anterior thorax and plays a role in the maturation of B lymphocytes, the cells that are charged with synthesizing antibodies.

Medical Treatment

Relapsing and remitting weakness and fatigability, the period which varies from minutes to days, characterize MG. The most common presentation is diplopia (double vision) caused by extraocular muscle weakness, followed by dysarthria, facial muscle weakness, and dysphagia. Swallowing disorders resulting from fatigue following mastication or dysphagia may cause malnutrition. Less commonly proximal limb weakness (i.e., in hips and shoulders) may be present. In some patients severe diaphragmatic weakness can result in respiratory difficulty. No involvement of sensory nerves occurs.

Anticholinesterases are medicines that inhibit acetylcholinesterase. They serve to increase the amount of ACh in the neuromuscular junction. Removal of the thymus results in symptomatic improvement in most patients. Corticosteroids are immunosuppressive.

Medical Nutrition Therapy

Chewing and swallowing are often compromised in MG. Because this occurs with fatigue, it is important to provide nutritionally dense foods at the beginning of meals before the patient tires. Small, frequent meals that are easy to chew and swallow are helpful. Difficulties holding a bolus on the tongue have also been observed, suggesting that foods that do not fall apart easily may be better tolerated. For patients treated with anticholinesterase drugs, it is crucial to time medication with feeding to facilitate optimal swallowing.

Physical activity should be limited before mealtime to ensure maximum strength to eat a meal. It is also important not to encourage food consumption once the patient begins to tire because this may contribute to aspiration. If and when respiratory crisis occurs, it is usually temporary. Nutrition support via nasogastric tube may be implemented in the interim to assist in maintaining vital functions of the patient until the crisis subsides. Once extubated, a swallow evaluation using cinefluoroscopy is appropriate to assess the degree of **deglutitory dysfunction** (swallowing irregularity) or risk of aspiration associated with an oral diet.

Multiple Sclerosis

Multiple sclerosis (MS) is a chronic disease that affects the CNS and is characterized by destruction of the myelin sheath, the function of which is transmission of electrical nerve impulses. MS is called *multiple* because multiple areas of optic nerves, spinal cord, and brain undergo "sclerosis," whereby myelin is replaced with sclera or scar tissue. As with other complex conditions and diseases, no single test can ascertain whether a patient has MS; however, diagnostic criteria (known as the McDonald criteria) were developed for use by practicing clinicians (McDonald et al., 2001). Following use of those criteria, evidence-based revisions helped to establish the latest guidelines (Polman et al., 2005).

The signs and symptoms of MS are easily distinguished features, despite remitting to a varying extent, and they recur over the natural history of this disease. In the worst scenario MS can render a person unable to write, speak, or walk; fortunately the majority of patients are only mildly affected.

The prevalence is lower in equatorial areas, southern United States, and southern Europe; it is higher in Canada, northern Europe, and the northern United States. MS is the most common demyelinating disorder of the CNS, affecting 2.5 million people worldwide (Freedman, 2006).

Pathophysiology

The precise cause of MS remains undetermined. A number of well-established findings have been incorporated into a hypothesis to explain the etiology of MS. Although a familial predisposition to MS has been noted in a minority of cases, familial tendency is not well established; no consistent pattern of mendelian inheritance has emerged (Victor and Ropper, 2005). Thus environmental factors compete for this distinction, and two of these are geographic latitude and diet. Epidemiologic studies have linked the incidence of MS to geographic location rather than to a particular ethnic group.

The increased incidence from the equator northward has been explained by sun exposure. Exogenous 1,25-dihydroxyvitamin D_3 (hormonal form of vitamin D_3) has been associated with preventing experimental autoimmune encephalomyelitis in mice, thus focusing attention on the relationship of MS to vitamin D. Researchers hypothesize that the degree of sunlight exposure catalyzing the production of vitamin D_3 in skin is an environmental factor and that the hormonal form of vitamin D_3 is a selective immune system regulator inhibiting this autoimmune disease (Mark and Carson, 2006). Low sunlight exposure yields insufficient vitamin D_3, which limits 1,25-dihydroxyvitamin D_3 and increases the risk for MS. Further, in cross-sectional evaluations of MS and vitamin D, an increased prevalence of clinical vitamin D deficiency was associated with decreased bone density (Mark and Carson, 2006).

Data from two large cohorts (the Nurses Health Study with 92,422 individuals and the Nurses Health Study II with 95,389) have been analyzed for associations between intakes of total and specific types of fat and the risk of MS (Zhang et al., 2000). Most investigators report that dietary fats are unrelated or inconclusive for risk of MS (Payne, 2001; Zhang et al., 2000).

Medical Treatment

Fluctuating symptoms and spontaneous remissions make treatments difficult to evaluate. Currently no proven treatment for changing the course of MS, preventing future attacks, or preventing deterioration exists. Initially recovery from relapses is nearly complete, but over time, neurologic deficits remain (Figure 41-4). Therefore measures to maximize recovery from initial attacks or exacerbations, prevent fatigue and infection, and use all of the available rehabilitative measures to postpone the bedridden stage of disease are imperative. Physical and occupational therapies are standard for weakness, spasticity, tremor, incoordination, and other symptoms.

Drugs for spasticity can be initiated at a low dose and cautiously increased until the patient responds. Physical therapy for gait training and range-of-motion exercises helps. Steroid therapy is used in treating exacerbations; adrenocorticotropic hormone (ACTH) and prednisolone are the drugs of choice. However, treatment is not consistently effective and tends to be more useful in cases of less than 5 years' duration. Side effects of short-term steroid treatment include increased appetite, weight gain, fluid retention, nervousness, and insomnia. Reduced cerebrospinal fluid and serum levels of vitamin B_{12} and folate have been noted in MS patients who receive high-dose steroids. Methotrexate may also be

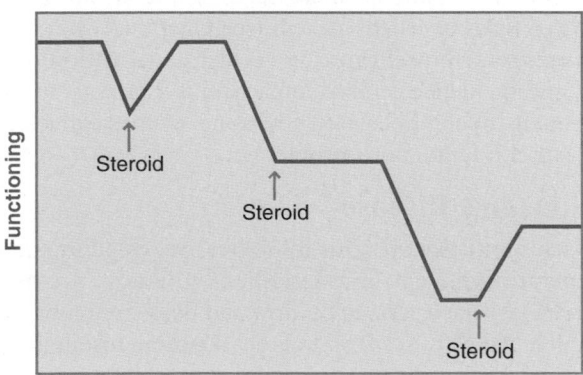

FIGURE 41-4 The progression of multiple sclerosis.

used with ACTH, causing anorexia and nausea. Drug therapies may be a challenge (see Chapter 16 and Appendix 31).

Medical Nutrition Therapy

With respect to nutritional research, environmental factors such as nutrition have dominated over therapeutic trials aimed at treating the disease once it has occurred. Several dietary regimens for managing MS have been studied, all of which have yielded equivocal results. Past trials of various diets such as allergen-free, gluten-free, pectin-free, and fructose-restricted diets; the raw food diet; the MacDougal diet (no gluten, low sugar and no refined sugar, low-fat diet high in polyunsaturated fatty acids, and megadoses of vitamins/minerals); the Cambridge liquid diet (330 kcal/day with 22 g of protein); and vitamin and mineral therapies (zinc phosphates, calcium, other combinations) have been ruled ineffective (Wozniak-Wowk, 1993).

Although no valid clinical trials have supported the efficacy of nutrition in delaying the progression of MS, the registered dietitian's careful evaluation of the patient to maximize nutritional intake is imperative. Vitamin D supplementation may be warranted, but total intake should be monitored from multivitamin and mineral supplements and fortified foods (Brown, 2006).

As the disease progresses, neurologic deficits and dysphasia may occur as the result of damaged cranial nerves. Thus diet consistency may need to be modified from solids to mechanically soft or pureed items, even progressing to thick liquids to prevent aspiration. Additional problems include impaired vision, dysarthria, and poor ambulation, making eating less enjoyable by turning meal preparation into a difficult task. In this situation reliance on comfort foods or prepackaged, single-serving, or convenience foods often permits independent preparation of meals. Given the chronic nature of this debilitating disease, patients may require enteral nutrition support.

Neurogenic bladder is common, causing urinary incontinence, urgency, and frequency. To minimize these problems, distributing fluids evenly throughout the waking hours and limiting them before bed is helpful. Some patients limit fluid intake severely to decrease frequency of urination but thereby increase the risk of UTIs. UTIs are common in patients with MS, and some patients increase their intake of cranberry juice as a form of self-treatment (see Chapter 36).

Neurogenic bowel can cause either constipation or diarrhea, and incidence of fecal impaction is increased in MS. A diet that is high in fiber with additional prunes and adequate fluid can moderate both problems.

Parkinson's Disease

Parkinson's disease (PD) is a progressive, disabling, neurodegenerative disease, first described by James Parkinson in 1817. PD is characterized by slow and decreased movement, muscular rigidity, resting tremor, postural instability, and decreased dopamine (a neurotransmitter) transmission to the basal ganglia. Although the natural history of this disease can be remarkably benign in some cases, approximately 66% of patients are disabled within 5 years, and 80% are disabled after 10 years (Victor and Ropper, 2005).

PD is one of the most common neurologic diseases in North America; it affects approximately 1% of the population over 65 years of age. The incidence is similar across socioeconomic groups, although PD is less common in blacks and Asians in comparison to whites. It most commonly occurs between the ages of 40 and 70.

Pathophysiology

Although the cause of PD remains unclear, it is presumably multifactorial, and the pathogenesis is well described. It involves an interaction of inheritance with environmental factors. There is a marked loss of dopaminergic neurons (pigmented cells) in the substantia nigra, as well as tyrosine hydroxylase, the rate-limiting enzyme for dopamine. Three theories are postulated for the etiology of PD: (1) altered dopamine metabolism from neural injury; (2) exposure to environmental neurotoxins; and (3) predisposition (Standaert and Stern, 1993).

In studying the brains of people with PD after they die, accumulations of protein called *Lewy bodies* (named after the doctor who first found them) are found. There is new interest in a protein called α-synuclein (found in large amounts in the Lewy bodies). Over 10 genes causing familial PD have been identified, but Ueki and Otsuka (2004) report that no genetic polymorphism has been confirmed for a majority of patients with sporadic PD. Genetic testing for PD is not warranted at this time, but the clinical impact of continued investigations holds promise.

The role of endogenous toxins from cellular oxidative reactions has emerged because aging has been associated with a loss of neurons containing dopamine and an increase in monoamine oxidase. When metabolized (enzymatic oxidation and autooxidation), dopamine produces endogenous toxins (hydrogen peroxide and free radicals), causing peroxidation of membrane lipids and cell death. In the presence of an inherited or acquired predisposition, severe oxidative injury can lead to substantial loss of dopaminergic neurons similar to that observed in PD.

Several other environmental factors have also been implicated in the etiology of PD, and this theory of etiology has been strengthened considerably by the observation of intravenous drug users who self-administered an opiate substance, 1-methyl-4-phenyl-1,2,3,6-tetrahydropyridine. This neurotoxin produces a rapidly progressive Parkinsonian syndrome that selectively destroys dopamine cells in the substantia nigra (Gelinas and Martinoli, 2002). The connection between smoking and a lowered risk for PD has also been evaluated, but results are inconsistent among younger and older persons with PD (Zhang et al., 2006). In older patients drug-induced PD may occur as a side effect of neuroleptics or metoclopramide (see Chapter 16 and Appendix 31).

Nutrient-related findings are biologically plausible and support the hypothesis that oxidative stress may contribute to the pathogenesis of PD. The interrelationships of folate, plasma homocysteine levels, lack of fiber, and caloric deficits as contributors to PD are being evaluated. Vitamin B_6 intake may decrease the risk of PD, but the exact mechanism is not yet known (De Lau et al., 2006). Vitamin E has also been studied, and results are inconclusive until larger trials are completed.

The final environmental factor associated with the incidence of PD is geography. There is a greater incidence of PD in industrialized countries and agrarian areas where toxins are more commonly used. No one chemical toxin or heavy metal has been shown to definitely cause PD (Victor and Ropper, 2005). An overload of dietary iron and manganese may be related (Powers et al., 2003), but more research is needed.

Medical Treatment

The "classic triad" of signs—tremor at rest, rigidity, and bradykinesia—first described by James Parkinson, remain the accepted clinical criterion for diagnosis. However, it was well over a century before an effective therapy, L-dopa (a precursor to dopamine and the current cornerstone of treatment), was introduced for controlling symptoms.

A cholinesterase inhibitor, Exelon, available for treatment of mild-to-moderate PD dementia was approved by the FDA in 2006. The use of monoamine oxidase inhibitors has also been tested and found to be somewhat helpful in Parkinson's disease patients (Henchcliffe et al., 2005). Pharmacotherapy agents, surgical interventions, and physical therapy are the best adjunctive therapies for treating PD. Current symptomatic treatment strategies have time limitations and ultimately undesirable side effects.

Medical Nutrition Therapy

The primary nutrition intervention in counseling patients with PD, especially patients having refractory fluctuations of dyskinesias, should be to focus on drug-nutrient interactions, especially between dietary protein and L-dopa. Interactions between pyridoxine and aspartame should be considered as well. Fiber and fluid adequacy lessen constipation, a common concern for persons with PD.

For some patients dyskinesia may be reduced by limiting dietary protein at breakfast and lunch and adding it to the evening meal. Table 41-9 presents a sample menu for this diet. Recent research suggests that a ketogenic diet may be more beneficial (Vanitallie et al., 2005) (see previous paragraphs).

Pyridoxine has been studied for a possible interaction with L-dopa. Decarboxylase, the enzyme required to convert L-dopa to dopamine, is dependent on pyridoxine. If excessive amounts of the vitamin are present, L-dopa may be metabolized in the periphery and not in the CNS where its therapeutic activity occurs. Therefore vitamin preparations containing pyridoxine should not be taken with doses of L-dopa. In addition, manganese in supplements should be carefully monitored to avoid excesses above DRI levels.

Side effects of medications for PD include anorexia, nausea, reduced sense of smell, constipation, and dry mouth. To diminish the gastrointestinal side effects of L-dopa, it should be taken with meals. Avoid foods that contain natural L-dopa such as broad beans (fava beans).

As the disease progresses, rigidity of the extremities can interfere with the patient's ability to care for self, including self-feeding. Rigidity also interferes with the ability to control the position of the head and trunk, necessary for eating. Eating is slowed; mealtimes can take up to 1 hour. Simultaneous movements such as those required to handle both a knife and fork become difficult. Tremor in the arms and hands may make self-feeding of liquids impossible without spilling. Perception and spatial organization can become impaired.

Dysphagia is a late complication. A large number of patients may be silent aspirators, which affects nutrition status. One study identified a fourfold increase in weight loss

TABLE 41-9	
Protein Redistribution in L-Dopa Therapy	
	Amount of Protein (g)
Breakfast	
½ c oatmeal	2
1 orange	0.5
1 c Rice Dream beverage	0.5
Egg Replacer (unlimited)	0
Low-protein bread toast	0
Margarine or butter (unlimited)	0
Jelly or jam (unlimited)	0
Sugar or sugar substitute (unlimited)	0
Coffee or tea (unlimited)	0
Lunch	
½ c vegetable soup	2
1 c tossed salad	1
Salad dressing (unlimited)	0
1 banana	1
Low-protein pasta (unlimited)	0
Margarine or butter (unlimited)	0
Low-protein cookies (unlimited)	0
Soda pop, coffee, tea, or water	0
Afternoon Snack	
Gum drops or hard candy (unlimited)	0
Apple or cranberry juice (unlimited)	0
TOTAL	7
Dinner	
4 oz (at least) beef, pork, veal, chicken	28 or more
1 c stuffing	4
Gravy	0
½ c peas	2
1 c pudding	8
1 c milk	8
Evening Snack	
1 oz cheese	7
4 crackers	2
Soda pop	0
DAILY TOTAL	66 or more

greater than 10 lb in patients with PD than matched control patients (Beyer et al., 1995). Experimental treatment procedures are being tested and reported with increasing frequency (e.g., progress with deep brain penetration, other surgical interventions), and efforts with stem cell research continue in hopes that the "cure" is not far off.

Neurotrauma

Head trauma refers to any of the following, alone or in combination: brain injury, skull fractures, extraparenchymal hemorrhage—epidural, subdural, subarachnoid—or hemorrhage into the brain tissue itself, including intraparenchymal or intraventricular hemorrhage. In the United States trauma is the leading cause of death in persons up to 44 years of age, and more than one half of these deaths are the result of head injuries (Victor and Ropper, 2005). The annual incidence is estimated to be 200/100,000 people, with a peak frequency between 15 and 24 years of age.

Even though relatively much is known about different types of head injuries, it is difficult to accurately predict neurologic recovery. Headache is one of the most common complaints. Morbidity is high. Motor vehicle collisions are the major source of injury. Despite intensive intervention, long-term disability occurs in a large portion of the survivors of severe head injury.

Pathophysiology

Brain injury can be subdivided into three types: concussion, contusion, and diffuse axonal injury. A concussion is described as a brief loss of consciousness (<6 hours) with no evidence of damage found on computed tomography (CT) or magnetic resonance imaging (MRI) scans. Microscopic studies have failed to find any evidence of structural damage in areas of known concussion, although evidence of change in cellular metabolism exists.

Contusion is similar to a bruise on the skin. It is characterized by damaged capillaries and swelling, followed by resolution of the damage. Note that large contusions may dramatically increase ICP and may lead to ischemia or herniation. Contusions can be detected by CT or MRI scans.

Diffuse axonal injury results from the shearing of axons by a rotational acceleration of the brain inside the skull. Damaged areas are often found in the **corpus callosum** (the bridge between the two hemispheres) and the upper outer portion of the brainstem.

Skull fractures of the calvarium and the base are described in the same manner as other fractures. Comminution refers to splintering of bone into many fragments. Displacement refers to a condition in which bones are displaced from their original apposition to one another. *Open* or *closed* describes whether a fracture is exposed to air. Open fractures dramatically increase the risk of infection (osteomyelitis), and open skull fractures in particular carry an increased risk for meningitis because the dura mater is often violated.

Epidural and subdural hematomas are often corrected by surgical intervention. The volume of these lesions often displaces the brain tissue and may cause diffuse axonal injury and swelling. When the lesion becomes large enough, it may cause herniation of brain contents through various openings of the skull base. Consequent compression and ischemia of vital brain structures may rapidly lead to death.

Medical Treatment

The body's response to stressors such as that seen in neurotrauma results in the production of cytokines such as interleukin 1, interleukin 6, interleukin 8, and tumor necrosis factor. These are elevated in the body after head injury and associated with the hormonal milieu that negatively affects metabolism and organ function. Some of the metabolic events include fever, neutrophilia, muscle breakdown, altered amino acid metabolism, production of hepatic acute-phase reactants, increased endothelial permeability, and expression of endothelial adhesion molecules (see Chapter 39). It has also been proposed that specific cytokines cause organ demise. Specific tissue damage has been observed in the gut, liver, lung, and brain.

The molecular basis of functional recovery is poorly understood. Several metabolites are implicated in neuronal degeneration; levels of intracellular adenosine triphosphate (energy source) and pH are decreased, whereas levels of extracellular glutamate; intracellular calcium ions; and oxidative damage to ribonucleic acid and deoxyribonucleic acid, protein, and lipid are increased (Liu et al., 2002).

Clinical findings of brain injury often include a transient decrease in level of consciousness. Headache and dizziness are relatively common and not worrisome unless they become more intense or are accompanied by vomiting. Focal neurologic deficits, progressively decreasing level of consciousness, and penetrating brain injury demand prompt neurosurgical evaluation.

Skull fractures are suspected underneath lacerations, can often be felt as a "drop off" or discontinuity on the surface of the skull, and are readily identifiable by CT scan. Basilar skull fractures are manifested by **otorrhea**, **hemotympanum** (fluid or blood behind the eardrum or leaking from the ear), and **rhinorrhea** (salty fluid dripping from the nose or down the pharynx). Other signs include raccoon eyes and Battle's sign—blood behind the mastoid process. Basilar skull fractures may precipitate injuries to cranial nerves, which are essential for chewing, swallowing, taste, and smell.

Hematomas are neurosurgical emergencies because they may rapidly progress to herniation of brain contents through the skull base and to subsequent death. These lesions may present similarly, with decreased level of consciousness, contralateral hemiparesis, and pupillary dilation. Classically the **epidural hematoma** presents with progressively decreasing consciousness after an interval of several hours in which the patient has been awake following a brief loss of consciousness. The **subdural hematoma** usually features progressively decreasing consciousness from the time of injury. These lesions damage brain tissue by gross displacement and traction.

Sequelae most often include epilepsy and the postconcussive syndrome, a constellation of headache, vertigo, fatigue, and memory difficulties. Treatment approaches for these patients can become highly complex, but the two goals of any therapeutic intervention are to maintain cerebral perfusion and to regulate ICP. Of the possible interventions, perfusion and pressure control have implications for nutrition therapy in the patient with a head injury.

Medical Nutrition Therapy

The goal of nutritional management is to oppose the hypercatabolism and hypermetabolism associated with the inflammation. Hypercatabolism is manifested by protein degradation evidenced by profound urinary urea nitrogen excretion. Data in non–head-injured patients show that a 30% weight loss increases mortality rate; further, starved head-injured patients lose sufficient nitrogen to reduce weight by 15% per week (Brain Trauma Foundation, 2000).

Nitrogen catabolism in a fasting normal human is only 3 to 5 g of nitrogen per day, whereas nitrogen excretion is 14 to 25 g of nitrogen per day in the fasting patient with severe head injury. In the absence of nutritional intake, this degree of nitrogen loss can result in a 10% decrease in lean mass within 7 days. If sequelae were to continue unabated, a weight loss of 30% could lead to death (Brain Trauma Foundation, 2000).

Hypermetabolism contributes to increased energy expenditure. Correlations between the severity of brain injury as measured by the Glasgow Coma Scale and energy requirements have been shown. One hundred percent to 140% replacement of resting metabolism expenditure with 15% to 20% nitrogen calories reduces nitrogen loss (Brain Trauma Foundation, 2000). In patients medicated with barbiturates, metabolic expenditure may be decreased to 100% to 120% of basal metabolic rate. This decreased metabolic rate in pharmacologically paralyzed patients suggests that maintaining muscle tone is an important part of metabolic expenditure.

Nutriture of the neurologically critically ill patient is accomplished by administering either enteral or parenteral nutrition support. Nutrition support is usually begun within 72 hours after injury and is necessary to achieve nutritional replacement by 7 days after injury (Brain Trauma Foundation, 2000). Both modes of therapy must be initiated at levels below actual requirements and increased gradually to meet nutritional requirements. For more guidelines, refer to Chapter 39.

Spine Trauma

Spine trauma encompasses many types of injuries, ranging from stable fractures of the spinal column to catastrophic transsection of the spinal cord. Of nutritional significance is neurologic injury. A complete SCI is defined as a lesion in which there is no preservation of motor or sensory function more than three segments below the level of the injury. With an incomplete injury there is some degree of residual function, motor or sensory, more than three segments below the lesion. SCI is somewhat less common than head injury. Like head injury, SCI is most often seen in the young. Motor vehicle collisions account for one third to one half of SCIs; the balance is caused by athletic injuries and domestic and industrial accidents.

Pathophysiology

The spinal cord responds to insult in a manner similar to the brain. Bleeding, contusion, and shorn axons appear first, followed by a several-year remodeling process consisting of gliosis and fibrosis. Liquefactive necrosis may predispose to the formation of a *syrinx*, a fluid collection in the center of the spinal cord, the mass effect of which may manifest as a slowly progressive neurologic deficit. Although SCI may strike at a single location, the significance of the injury lies more in the disruption of descending axons at that level than in injury to the segment itself.

Traumatic extraparenchymal hematomas in the spine are unusual; however, SCIs are almost invariably associated with spinal column fractures and ligament instability. Such processes may be amenable to either surgical or nonsurgical reduction and stabilization.

Medical Treatment

Spinal cord injuries have numerous clinical manifestations, depending on the level of the injury. Complete transsection results in complete loss of function below the level of the lesion, including the bladder and sphincters. Numerous incomplete cord syndromes have been identified.

After the patient is stabilized hemodynamically, the doctor evaluates the degree of neurologic deficit. Patients with suspected SCI are usually immobilized promptly in the field. Complete radiographic evaluation of the spinal column is obligatory in multitrauma and unconscious patients. In the awake patient clinical evidence of spine compromise is usually sufficient to determine the need for further workup. CT and MRI are used to more accurately delineate bony damage and spinal cord compromise. A dismal 3% of patients with complete spinal cord insults recover some function after 24 hours. Failure to regain function after 24 hours predicts a 0% chance of reestablishment of function in the future. Incomplete spinal cord syndromes may have somewhat improved outcomes.

Medical Nutrition Therapy

Morbidity and mortality rates associated with SCI have improved dramatically, particularly in the last two decades. Advances in acute-phase care have reduced early mortality and prevented complications frequently associated with early death such as respiratory failure and pulmonary emboli. Fewer than 10% of patients with SCI die from the acute injury. Technologic advances in enteral and parenteral feeding techniques and formulas have also played a role in maintaining nutrition status of these patients. Although the metabolic response to neurotrauma has been studied extensively, the acute metabolic response to SCI has not; but it is similar to that seen in neurotrauma during the acute phase. Initially paralytic ileus may occur but may resolve within 72 hours after injury (see "Medical Nutrition Therapy for Neurotrauma" earlier in the chapter).

For those who survive the injury but are disabled for life, there are significant alterations in lifestyle as well as the possibility of secondary complications. In general the number and frequency of complications, constipation, pressure ulcers, obesity, and pain vary but are interrelated to nutrition.

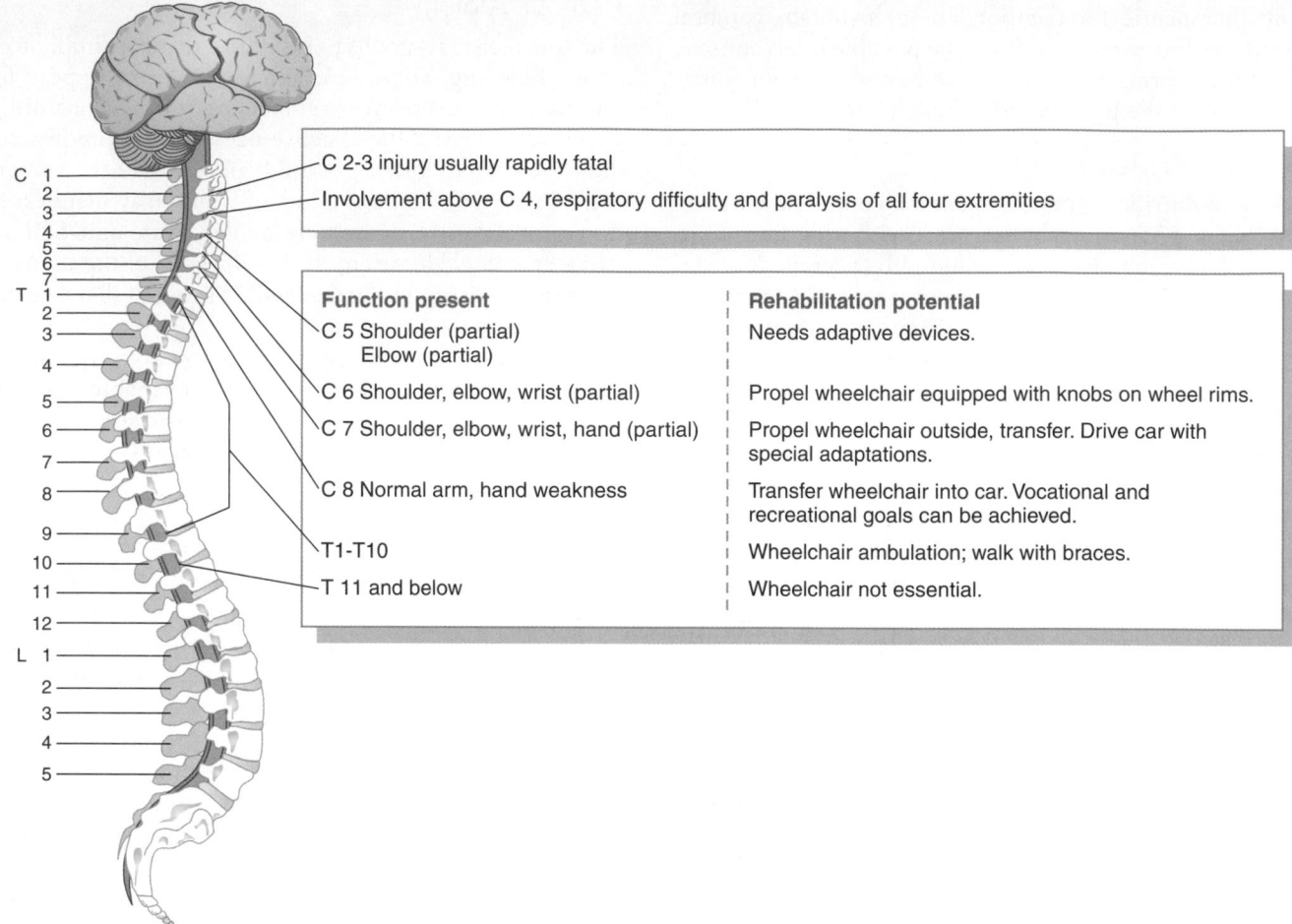

C 2-3 injury usually rapidly fatal

Involvement above C 4, respiratory difficulty and paralysis of all four extremities

Function present	Rehabilitation potential
C 5 Shoulder (partial) Elbow (partial)	Needs adaptive devices.
C 6 Shoulder, elbow, wrist (partial)	Propel wheelchair equipped with knobs on wheel rims.
C 7 Shoulder, elbow, wrist, hand (partial)	Propel wheelchair outside, transfer. Drive car with special adaptations.
C 8 Normal arm, hand weakness	Transfer wheelchair into car. Vocational and recreational goals can be achieved.
T1-T10	Wheelchair ambulation; walk with braces.
T 11 and below	Wheelchair not essential.

FIGURE 41-5 Sequelae of spinal cord injury and rehabilitation changes.

Figure 41-5 describes the rehabilitation potential based on the level of injury.

Constipation is a problem that can adversely affect appetite. Therapeutic diets of high fiber and adequate water intake alone do not suffice for treatment of constipation. More than likely a routine bowel preparation program is required. The individual with SCI is at risk for developing pressure ulcers, which, if left uncared for, can contribute to morbidity. Maintenance of nutritional health is one factor in preventing the development of pressure ulcers because poor nutrition is an underlying risk factor for infection. Sufficient intake of calories, protein, and micronutrients (vitamins C, A, B-complex, and zinc) is critically important.

Loss of muscle tone caused by skeletal muscle paralysis below the level of injury contributes to decreased metabolic activity, initial weight loss, and predisposition to osteoporosis. Acutely the patient experiences some weight loss. Guidelines for accepted weights adjusted for paraplegia and quadriplegia are as follows: the paraplegic should weigh 10 to 15 lb less than the ideal body mass index (BMI) would indicate; the quadriplegic should weigh 15 to 20 lb less than ideal weight dictated by the BMI. The higher the injury, the lower the metabolic rate, and the lower the kcaloric requirement. Quadriplegic patients have lower metabolic rates than paraplegic patients, proportional to the amount of denervated muscle, which is caused in part by the loss of residual motor function.

In the rehabilitation phase, quadraplegics may require approximately 25% to 50% fewer calories than conventional equations would predict. Thus these patients have the potential to become overweight. It has been proposed that obesity may actually influence the eventual rehabilitation process by limiting functional outcome. As a consequence of bone loss resulting from the loss of mineralization caused by immobilization, SCI is associated with osteopenia and osteoporosis, and the prevalence of long-bone fractures is increased.

FOCAL POINTS

- Although not all neurologic conditions originate with nutritional deficits, diet directly impacts quality of life.
- Widely diverse physical and psychosocial issues such as ability to swallow, anemia, respiratory paralysis, pneumonia, ileus, pressure ulcers, hemorrhage, neurogenic bowel and bladder, depression, and social support affect the nutrition status of patients with neurologic condition(s).
- Nutritional intake is a critical component of managing neurologic conditions; nutrients such as vitamin D may play a role in the treatment of epilepsy and the etiology of MS, and excesses of iron or manganese may contribute to PD.

- The RD plays a key role in acute- and long-term care as patients adjust to life with differing levels of self-management, mobility, functionality, and independence.
- Targeted interventions relate to methods, types, and frequency of feedings; exercise; maintaining optimal health; and attaining nutritional intakes which promote recovery and positive outcomes.

CLINICAL SCENARIO

Clarence A., a hospitalized patient receiving enteral nutrition support, is having mild seizure activity. Tube feedings have been infused via a PEG over 12 hours. Therapeutic serum level for phenytoin has not been achieved, despite receiving a normal prescribed dose of phenytoin. The physicians would like input regarding the drug-nutrient interaction to achieve therapeutic serum phenytoin levels for control of the seizures.

*Nutrition Diagnosis: Food-medication interaction related to enteral feedings and phenytoin as evidenced by subtherapeutic phenytoin levels

1. As the clinician managing the nutrition care of this patient, what would be the most appropriate action based on the current enteral support regimen?
   a. Hold the feedings 2 hours before and after administering the phenytoin.
   b. Change the tube-feeding regimen to gravity drip infusions of 480 ml four times per day.
   c. Change the tube-feed formula to a blenderized formula.

   d. Suggest dosing phenytoin once per day via sustained-release capsule so that the tube feeding formula will not bind with the medication.
   e. Continue present enteral support regimen because answers a and c will not result in therapeutic phenytoin levels without increasing the dose of phenytoin.
2. Clarence's wife has suggested adding bolus feedings so the patient can walk with her more often. How would you design the feeding frequency and how will this affect the phenytoin administration?

USEFUL WEBSITES

Alzheimer's Disease Education and Referral Center
http://www.nia.nih.gov/alzheimers/

American Stroke Association
http://www.strokeassociation.org/

Epilepsy Foundation
http://www.epilepsyfoundation.org/

Migraine Awareness Group
http://www.migraines.org/

Myasthenia Gravis
http://www.myasthenia.org/

National Headache Foundation
http://www.headaches.org/

National Human Genome Research Institute
http://www.genome.gov

National Institute of Neurological Disorders and Stroke
http://www.ninds.nih.gov/

NIH—Swallowing Disorders
http://www.ninds.nih.gov/disorders/swallowing_disorders/swallowing_disorders.htm

NINDS Stroke Page
http://www.ninds.nih.gov/disorders/stroke/stroke.htm

References

Anekonda TS: Resveratrol—a boon for treating Alzheimer's disease? *Brain Res Brain Res Rev* 52:316, 2006.

Au Yeung SC, Ensom MH: Phenytoin and enteral feedings: does evidence support an interaction? *Ann Pharmacother* 34: 896, 2000.

Berryman MS: The ketogenic diet revisited, *J Am Diet Assoc* 97: S192, 1997.

Beyer PL et al: Weight change and body composition in patients with Parkinson's disease, *J Am Diet Assoc* 95:979, 1995.

Blau JN: Water deprivation: a new migraine precipitant? *Headache* 45:757, 2005.

Bough KJ, Rho JM: Anticonvulsant mechanisms of the ketogenic diet, *Epilepsia* 48:43, 2007.

Brain Trauma Foundation, The American Association of Neurological Surgeons, The Joint Section on Neurotrauma and Critical Care: Nutrition, *J Neurotrauma* 17:539, 2000.

Brown SJ: The role of vitamin D in multiple sclerosis, *Ann Pharmacother* 40:1158, 2006.

Bulat RD, Orlando RC: Oropharyngeal dysphagia, *Curr Treat Options Gastroenterol* 8:269, 2005.

Callahan CM et al: Effectiveness of collaborative care for older adults with Alzheimer disease in primary care, *JAMA* 295:2148, 2006.

Centers for Disease Control and Prevention: *Heart disease and stroke*, from http://www.cdc.gov/nccdphp/scientific.htm, accessed June 30, 2006.

Chauhan NB: Multiplicity of garlic health effects and Alzheimer's disease, *J Nutr Health Aging* 9:421, 2005.

Chio A et al: Percutaneous radiological gastrostomy: a safe and effective method of nutritional tube placement in advanced ALS, *J Neurol Neurosurg Psychiatry* 75:645, 2004.

Czaplinski A et al: Amyotrophic lateral sclerosis: early predictors of prolonged survival, *J Neurol* 13 June:2226(on-line), 2006.

Damen L et al: Prophylactic treatment of migraine in children. Part 1. A systematic review of non-pharmacological trials, *Cephalalgia* 26:373, 2006.

D'Andrea G et al: Elevated levels of circulating trace amines in primary headaches, *Neurol* 62:1701, 2004.

De Lau LM et al: Dietary folate, vitamin B_{12}, and vitamin B_6 and the risk of Parkinson disease, *Neurology* 67:315, 2006.

Deon M et al: The effect of Lorenzo's oil on oxidative stress in X-linked adrenoleukodystrophy, from *J Neurol Sci* www.sciencedirect.com/science? accessed June 28, 2006.

Desport JC et al: Factors correlated with hypermetabolism in patients with amyotrophic lateral sclerosis, *Am J Clin Nutr* 74:328, 2001.

Dowson AJ et al: Review of clinical trials using acute intervention with oral triptans for migraine management, *Int J Clin Pract* 60:698, 2006.

Epilepsy Foundation: Statistics, website http://www.epilepsyfoundation.org/answerplace/statistics.cfm, accessed June 30, 2006.

Freedman MS: Disease-modifying drugs for multiple sclerosis: current and future aspects, *Expert Opin Pharmacother* 7:S1, 2006.

Gelinas S, Martinoli MG: Neuroprotective effect of estradiol and phytoestrogens on MPP+-induced cytotoxicity in neuronal PC12 cells, *J Neurosci Res* 70:90, 2002.

Goldstein LB et al: Primary prevention of ischemic stroke: a guideline from the American Heart Association/American Stroke Association Stroke Council: cosponsored by the Atherosclerotic Peripheral Vascular Disease Interdisciplinary Working Group; Cardiovascular Nursing Council; Clinical Cardiology Council; Nutrition, Physical Activity and Metabolism Council; and the Quality of Care and Outcomes Research Interdisciplinary Working Group, *Stroke* 37:1583, 2006.

Henchcliffe C et al: Recent advances in Parkinson's disease therapy: use of monoamine oxidase inhibitors, *Expert Rev Neurother* 5:811, 2005.

Hershey AD et al: Coenzyme Q10 deficiency and response to supplementation in pediatrics and adolescent migraine, *Headache* 47:73, 2007.

International Alliance of ALS: *What is ALS/MND?* from www.alsmndalliance.org/whatis.html, accessed March 26, 2007.

Janssen SC et al: Intolerance to dietary biogenic amines: a review, *Ann Allergy Asthma Immunol* 91:233, 2003.

Jonsson P et al: CuZn-superoxide dismutase in D90A heterozygotes from recessive and dominant ALS pedigrees, *Neurobiol Dis* 10:327, 2002.

Joseph SA, Tsao CY: Guillain-Barré syndrome, *Adolesc Med* 13:487, 2002.

Kidd PM: Neurodegeneration from mitochondrial insufficiency: nutrients, stem cells, growth factors, and prospects for brain rebuilding using integrative management, *Altern Med Rev* 10:268, 2005.

Kinsman SL et al: Efficacy of the ketogenic diet for intractable seizure disorders: review of 58 cases, *Epilepsia* 33:1132, 1992.

Liu PK et al: The association between neuronal nitric oxide synthase and neuronal sensitivity in the brain after brain injury, *Ann NY Acad Sci* 962:226, 2002.

Liu YC et al: A prospective study: growth and nutritional status of children treated with the ketogenic diet, *J Am Diet Assoc* 103:707, 2003.

Luchsinger JA, Mayeux R: Dietary factors and Alzheimer's disease, *Lancet Neurol* 3:579, 2004.

Mandel A et al: Medical costs are reduced when children with intractable epilepsy are successfully treated with the ketogenic diet, *J Am Diet Assoc* 102:396, 2002.

Mark BL, Carson JA: Vitamin D and autoimmune disease—implications for practice from the multiple sclerosis literature, *J Am Diet Assoc* 106:418, 2006.

McDonald WI et al: Recommended diagnostic criteria for multiple sclerosis: guidelines from the international panel on the diagnosis of multiple sclerosis, *Ann Neurol* 50:121, 2001.

Meydani M: Antioxidants and cognitive function, *Annu Rev Nutr* 59:75S, 2001.

Mitsumoto H, Del Bene M: Improving the quality of life for people with ALS: the challenge ahead, *Amytroph Lateral Scler Other Motor Neuron Disord* 1:329, 2000.

Moser HW: Therapy of X-linked adrenoleukodystrophy, *NeuroRx* 3:246, 2006.

National Institutes of Health: Stroke, website http://www.ninds.nih.gov/, accessed December 2, 2006.

Nordlund A, Oliveberg M: Folding of Cu/Zn superoxide dismutase suggests structural hotspots for gain of neurotoxic function in ALS: parallels to precursors in amyloid disease, *Proc Natl Acad Sci USA* 103:10218, 2006.

Ordunez-Garcia et al: Cuban epidemic neuropathy, 1991 to 1994: history repeats itself a century after the "amblyopia of the blockade," *Am J Public Health* 86:738, 1996.

Payne A: Nutrition and diet in the clinical management of multiple sclerosis, *J Hum Nutr Diet* 14:349, 2001.

Peterson SJ et al: Changes in growth and seizure reduction in children on the ketogenic diet as a treatment for intractable epilepsy, *J Am Diet Assoc* 105:718, 2005.

Pittler MH, Ernst E: Feverfew for preventing migraine, *Cochrane Database Syst Rev* (1):CD002286, 2004.

Polman CH et al: Diagnostic criteria for multiple sclerosis: 2005 revisions to the "McDonald" criteria, *Ann Neurol* 58:840, 2005.

Powers KM et al: Parkinson's disease risks associated with dietary iron, manganese, and other nutrient intakes, *Neurology* 60:1761, 2003.

Roman GC: Nutritional disorders of the nervous system. In Shils ME et al, editors: *Modern nutrition in health and disease*, ed 10, Baltimore, 2006, Lippincott Williams & Wilkins.

Roubenoff RA et al: Hypermetabolism and hypercatabolism in Guillain-Barré syndrome, *JPEN J Parenter Enteral Nutr* 16:464, 1992.

Solomon LR: Disorders of cobalamin (vitamin B$_{12}$) metabolism: emerging concepts in pathphysiology, diagnosis, and treatment, *Blood Rev* 21:113, 2007.

Soto ME et al: Rapid cognitive decline: Searching for a definition and predictive factors among elderly with Alzheimer's disease, *J Nutr Health Aging* 9:158, 2005.

Spigt MG et al: Increasing the daily water intake for the prophylactic treatment of headache: a pilot trial, *Europ J Neurol* 12:715, 2005.

Standaert DG, Stern MB: Update on the management of Parkinson's disease, *Med Clin North Am* 77(1):169, 1993.

Strand EA et al: Management of oral-pharyngeal dysphagia symptoms in amyotrophic lateral sclerosis, *Dysphagia* 11:129, 1996.

Suzuki Y et al: The clinical course of childhood and adolescent adrenoleukodystrophy before and after Lorenzo's oil, *Brain Dev* 23:30, 2001.

Ueki A, Otsuka M: Life style risks of Parkinsons's disease: association between decreased water intake and constipation, *J Neurol* 251(suppl 7):1706, 2004.

Vanitallie TB et al: Treatment of Parkinson disease with diet-induced hyperketonemia: a feasibility study, *Neurology* 64:728, 2005.

Veldink JH et al: Intake of polyunsaturated fatty acids and vitamin E reduces the risk of developing amyotrophic lateral sclerosis, accessed April 2006 from *J Neurol Neurosurg Psychiatry* www.jnnp.com.

Victor M, Ropper AH: *Adams and Victor's principles of neurology*, ed 8, New York, 2005, McGraw-Hill, Health Professions Division.

Wang F et al: Oral magnesium oxide prophylaxis of frequent migrainous headache in children: a randomized, double-blind, placebo-controlled trial, *Headache* 43:601, 2003.

Wang L et al: Performance-based physical function and future dementia in older people, *Arch Intern Med* 166:1115, 2006.

Woolhouse M: Migraine and tension headache—a complementary and alternative medicine approach, *Aust Fam Physician* 34:647, 2005.

Wozniak-Wowk CS: Nutrition intervention in the management of multiple sclerosis, *Nutr Today* 28(6):12, 1993.

Zhang S et al: Dietary fat in relation to risk of multiple sclerosis among two large cohorts of women, *Am J Epidemiol* 152:1056, 2000.

Zhang ML et al: Dietary factors and smoking as risk factors for PD in a rural population in China: a nested case-control study, *Acta Neurol Scand* 113:278, 2006.

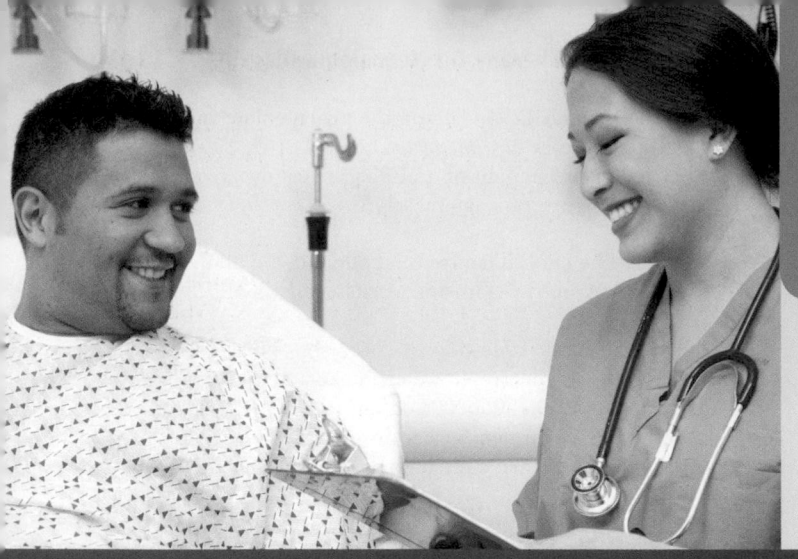

CHAPTER 42

Monika M. Woolsey, MS, RD

Medical Nutrition Therapy for Psychiatric Conditions

KEY TERMS

α-linolenic acid (ALA) precursor for the *n*-3 fatty acids eicosapentaenoic acid and docosahexaenoic acid

axis I disorders disorders that are primarily biologic in origin, resulting from alterations in brain structure (either inherited or generated as a result of stress, trauma, nutrition status, or illness), biochemistry, or exposure to other environmental factors

axis II disorders personality disorders, not biologic

docosahexaenoic acid (DHA) omega-3 fatty acid (22:6 *n*-3) primarily found in fish; important for infant nutrition

eicosapentaenoic acid (EPA) omega-3 fatty acid (20:5 *n*-3) primarily found in fish; shows some promise as a therapeutic agent in the treatment of schizophrenia and possibly other psychiatric disorders

Minnesota Multiphasic Personality Inventory valid psychological examination used to assess psychiatric disorders

---

Discussion of mental health has been included in this textbook because research is rapidly accumulating information that nutrition has a significant role in the development, prevention, and management of mental health disorders. Nutrition professionals with an interest in mental health have a special opportunity to help some of humanity's best, brightest, and most creative individuals minimize the devastation these diseases can impose and maximize their contributions to society (see *Focus On*: Who Has Suffered from Mental Illness?).

MENTAL ILLNESS: AXIS I AND AXIS II DISORDERS

Mental illness is an alteration in brain or nervous system function that results in altered perception and response to the environment. The American Psychiatric Association classifies mental illness into two different categories, *Axis I* and *Axis II disorders* (APA, 1994).

Axis I disorders often do not improve without medication. In fact, left unchecked, they can be degenerative and permanently destructive to brain and nervous system tissue. The primary Axis I disorders include depression, anxiety disorder, obsessive-compulsive disorder, bipolar disorder, attention deficit/hyperactivity disorder, schizophrenia, and posttraumatic stress disorder (PTSD) (APA, 1994).

The eating disorders (anorexia nervosa, bulimia nervosa, and binge eating disorder) are also classified as Axis I disorders. Because of this classification, it is important to note that eating disorders are not merely behavioral issues. They require medical, nutritional, and often pharmacologic treatment *in addition to psychotherapy* to correct underlying pathologies (see Chapter 22). These interventions can be the foundation for successful response to psychotherapy. It is quickly becoming clear that nutrition is crucial for the rehabilitation of *every* mental health issue, not just the eating disorders.

Despite their strong physiologic component, Axis I disorders are diagnosed primarily through behavioral criteria and psychological testing (e.g., **Minnesota Multiphasic**

◎ FOCUS ON

Who Has Suffered from Mental Illness?

April 20, 1999, Littleton, Colorado: 13 students and one teacher were killed, 23 students and one teacher wounded in a shootout at Columbine High School.

August 24, 2005, Peoria, Arizona: Two Walmart employees were randomly shot and killed in the parking lot of the store where they worked.

December 7, 2005, Miami, Florida: A 44-year-old man was shot and killed by air marshals as he ran from a plane claiming he was carrying a bomb.

What do these news items have in common? Each of these tragedies involved a person with a mental illness. In addition, in each of the news stories cited, for various reasons, the individual was not using medications to help his condition at the time he was involved in the tragic event. Unfortunately, when mental health issues appear in the news, they are often related to tragedies such as these. What is often overlooked is that some of history's most illustrious and creative individuals accomplished their greatest achievements while also managing the mental chaos, disruption in logical thinking, and hypersensitivity to stress that mental diagnoses can impose on the brain and nervous system. It is to the credit of all of these individuals and to the benefit of all of us who enjoy the fruits of their labor that they persisted and created in spite of their struggles and emotional turmoil. Famous living and historical figures who had mental illness include Isaac Newton, Ernest Hemingway, Charles Dickens, Michelangelo, Tennessee Williams, Ludwig van Beethoven, Terry Bradshaw, Brooke Shields, Abraham Lincoln, Winston Churchill, and Vincent van Gogh (NAMI, 2006).

Personality Inventory). Because there currently is no definitive diagnostic testing (e.g., blood tests, brain scans) for these disorders, it can be difficult to convince a person with such a diagnosis that he or she has a medical issue requiring treatment. It can also be difficult for the friend, family member, or colleague to understand that challenging behaviors affecting relationships and productivity are medical and biochemical in origin. For both parties, frustration, shame, and destructive behavior can result from attempting to willfully change behaviors that will not respond to anything less than intensive biologic intervention.

A person's food behaviors are often the first indication that an Axis I disorder exists. For example, a person with obsessive-compulsive disorder may struggle in grocery stores and restaurants, where a multitude of choices exist. They may seek help from a registered dietitian (RD) for specific direction (e.g., "just tell me what to eat") to lessen the stress that these daily activities can induce. A person with bipolar disorder may alternate between periods of mania, during which consumption of sugar, caffeine, and large quantities of food are extreme, to depression so severe that food is not eaten at all. These mood fluctuations often manifest as weight fluctuations and can even be misidentified as hypoglycemia. Often the medical comorbidity, not the core mental health diagnosis, brings an individual in for an initial nutrition consultation.

A nutritionist's job is not to diagnose or treat mental health disorders. However, it is important to recognize behaviors indicative of their existence so that appropriate recommendations for treatment can be made. In general, when an individual seems to be genuinely trying to follow nutrition treatment recommendations or to change behavior yet seems to be driven to behaviors that counter those intentions, the existence of an Axis I disorder should always be considered, and the individual should be evaluated.

Axis II disorders are also called personality disorders (APA, 1994). The personality disorders listed in the American Psychological Association, Diagnostic and Statistical Manual—Version IV (DSM- IV) include antisocial, narcissistic, histrionic, schizoid, avoidant, dependent, and borderline behavior. These disorders are primarily learned behaviors and do not respond to medication. Psychotherapy is required to achieve symptom relief. One exception to this rule is borderline personality disorder; evidence suggests that fish oil supplementation may help to reduce the rapid mood swings and impulsive behaviors of this disorder.

Axis I and Axis II disorders are often comorbid conditions. When an Axis I diagnosis impairs an individual's ability to interact with his or her environment, an Axis II disorder may develop as a coping mechanism. For example, a person with PTSD is likely to be easily overstimulated and fluctuate between periods of intense anxiety and depression. Borderline personality disorder is a common condition occurring comorbidly with PTSD. This person with this personality type often engages in extreme behaviors (e.g., hypersexuality, emotional volatility, poor impulse control, manipulative behavior, and suicide attempts) to (1) provide an emotional diversion from the physical wear and tear that the PTSD inflicts, and (2) maintain relationships with loved ones the individual perceives might otherwise abandon them.

Axis II disorders differ from Axis I disorders because, to the individual who has an Axis II disorder, it serves an important purpose. A person with low self-esteem or who knows from experience that he or she struggles with interpersonal relationships may develop an Axis II disorder to prevent abandonment. For a person who does not have alternative communication, conflict resolution, or coping skills, the perceived potential loss of that connection to others can be traumatizing. Whereas treating an Axis I disorder can provide great relief and improved well-being, treating an Axis II disorder may actually temporarily *increase* distress and behavioral acting out as treatment progresses.

◎ FOCUS ON

Addiction and Substance Abuse

Substance-abuse disorders include a variety of behavioral or psychological anomalies resulting from ingestion of or exposure to a drug of abuse, medication, or toxin. Addiction is a chronic brain disorder that involves compulsive and relapsing behavior. Three predisposing factors exist: biochemical, psychological, and social vulnerability. The personality type is often perfectionistic and prone to depression. The master "pleasure" molecule of addiction is dopamine; it is triggered by heroin, amphetamines, marijuana, alcohol, nicotine, and caffeine. Abnormalities in the metabolism of dopamine, serotonin, and norepinephrine may contribute to substance dependency. In some cases use of antidepressant medications alleviates the dependency. Changes in appetite, either decreases or increases, occur with substance abuse and with medications. Eating disorders and substance abuse have similarities, and many clients have both. The nutrition counselor must be aware of the various types of malnutrition and counseling techniques appropriate for this population.

Data from Escott-Stump S: *Nutrition and diagnosis-related care*, ed 6, Baltimore, 2007, Lippincott-Williams & Wilkins.

The primary responsibility of an RD working with individuals with mental health diagnoses is to impart information and support for eating choices that minimize the negative impact of these illnesses on both the client and their affected loved ones. Therapy for behavioral issues is primarily the responsibility of the psychotherapy team. However, it is important to consider that "change" as the goal of nutrition counseling, especially in individuals with an Axis II disorder, is a goal that they do not always embrace.

The long-term outcome of healthy food and lifestyle changes is most certainly positive. However, the process of incorporating *any* change, in food choices, relationships, or any life situation, for a person with a mental illness, regardless of intelligence, can be overwhelming or even frightening (see Chapter 19). This stress from the need for change extends to individuals with addictions and substance abuse also (see *Focus On*: Addiction and Substance Abuse).

When working with the mentally ill, the RD needs to understand the differing Axis I and Axis II responses to stress and change in order to support these individuals through what may be the very first change in their life that is associated with a positive outcome. A positive experience with an RD can build a foundation and motivation to attempt other positive changes long after nutrition counseling is finished.

NUTRITIONAL ASPECTS OF BRAIN AND NERVOUS SYSTEM STRUCTURE AND FUNCTION

One of the most important contributions of nutrition to mental health is the maintenance of the structure and function of the neurons and brain centers coordinating communication within the body and between the body and the environment. Sixty percent of the brain's dry weight is fat, and under optimal conditions 25% of this fat is **docosahexaenoic acid (DHA),** an omega-3 fatty acid (see Chapter 3). Omega-3 (*n*-3) fatty acids appear to be the type of fat preferred by the brain and nervous system. Each of the three *n*-3 fatty acids have been studied with regard to mental health, and each has been found to have unique, important, and noninterchangeable contributions to overall brain and nervous system functioning (see *Pathophysiology and Care Management Algorithm:* Psychiatric Disorders).

α-Linolenic Acid

α-linolenic acid (ALA) is also known to chemists as 18:3 *n*-3, with a chain length 18 carbons long and three bonds that are unsaturated. ALA is found in flax and flaxseed oil, canola oil, soybeans, and perilla (Kurowska et al., 2003), as well as in several varieties of nuts and their oils (Maguire et al., 2004).

Pure ALA has been found to have many health benefits, especially in the inhibition of inflammatory processes associated with cardiovascular disease, autoimmune disease, diabetes, and bowel disease (Simopoulos, 2002a). Its secondary benefit is that it can function as a precursor for the *n*-3 fatty acids eicosapentaenoic acid and docosahexaenoic acid (DHA). However, this conversion is low even in the most optimum nutritional conditions, and a diet lacking a variety of vitamins and minerals (common in persons with mental health diagnoses) further limits this conversion. Most experts in the area of nutrition and mental health do not recommend a reliance on ALA as a source of DHA or EPA. Table 42-1 provides a summary of "good sources" of ALA; this information is provided to illustrate that some sources of this *n*-3 fatty acid are efficient to consume, whereas others can be rather impractical.

Eicosapentaenoic Acid and Docosahexaenoic Acid

Eicosapentaenoic acid (EPA) (20:5 *n*-3) is primarily found in fish. In addition, under conditions of tissue DHA (22:6 *n*-3) saturation, DHA can "retroconvert" into EPA (Stark and Holub, 2004.) This process is so named because under normal conditions, conversion from EPA into DHA is the

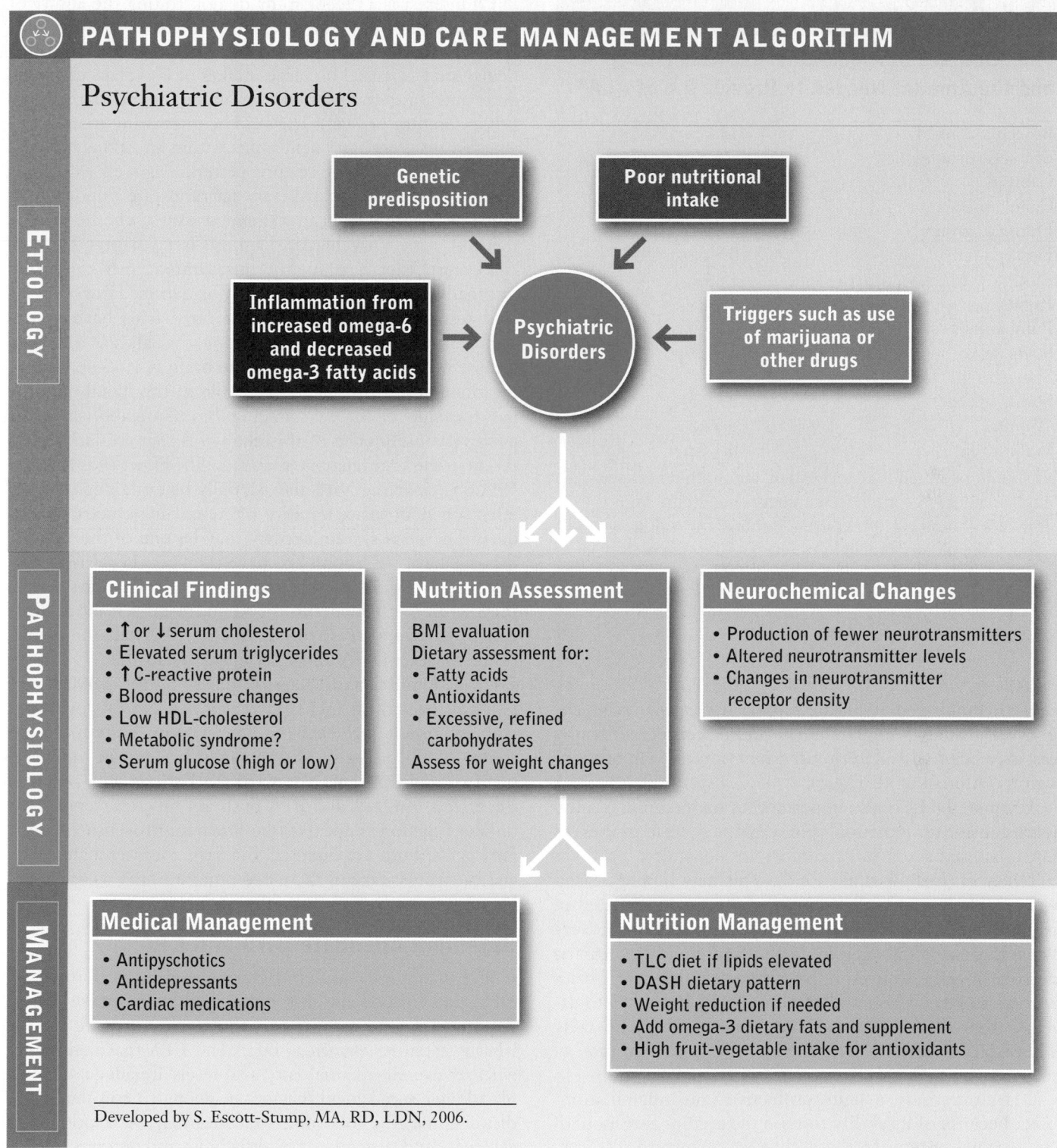

PATHOPHYSIOLOGY AND CARE MANAGEMENT ALGORITHM

Psychiatric Disorders

ETIOLOGY

Genetic predisposition

Poor nutritional intake

Inflammation from increased omega-6 and decreased omega-3 fatty acids → Psychiatric Disorders ← Triggers such as use of marijuana or other drugs

PATHOPHYSIOLOGY

Clinical Findings

- ↑ or ↓ serum cholesterol
- Elevated serum triglycerides
- ↑ C-reactive protein
- Blood pressure changes
- Low HDL-cholesterol
- Metabolic syndrome?
- Serum glucose (high or low)

Nutrition Assessment

BMI evaluation
Dietary assessment for:
- Fatty acids
- Antioxidants
- Excessive, refined carbohydrates
Assess for weight changes

Neurochemical Changes

- Production of fewer neurotransmitters
- Altered neurotransmitter levels
- Changes in neurotransmitter receptor density

MANAGEMENT

Medical Management

- Antipyschotics
- Antidepressants
- Cardiac medications

Nutrition Management

- TLC diet if lipids elevated
- DASH dietary pattern
- Weight reduction if needed
- Add omega-3 dietary fats and supplement
- High fruit-vegetable intake for antioxidants

Developed by S. Escott-Stump, MA, RD, LDN, 2006.

more common biochemical process. As with ALA, EPA has been found to have many benefits in the possible delay and prevention of inflammatory diseases.

DHA is also primarily found in fish. Fish do not synthesize DHA; they obtain DHA in their diets by eating marine algae (Innis, 2003). Humans benefit from the fact that this DHA is stored in the muscle tissue of the fish that they consume. It is also possible to purchase supplements of DHA obtained from marine algae.

OMEGA-3 FATTY ACIDS AND BRAIN FUNCTION

DHA is the brain's building block. When provided with a choice of different fatty acids, the brain appears to prefer DHA (Williard et al., 2002). This fatty acid provides structure to neurons and is an anchor point for neurotransmitter receptors. In rats fed a DHA-deficient diet, neuron atrophy was observed in the parietal cortex

TABLE 42-1

Food Sources of Alpha-Linolenic Acid (ALA) and the Amount Needed to Provide 2 g of ALA*

Broccoli, cooked	122 c
Brussels sprouts	7.6 c
Cabbage	12 c
Canola oil	1.7 tbsp
Flaxseed, ground	1 tbsp
Flaxseed oil	0.3 oz
Kale	15.4 c
Parsley	400 c
Pumpkin seeds	42.5 oz
Soybean oil	2.4 tbsp
Spinach	50 c
Spring greens	21.7 c
Walnuts	0.9 oz
Walnut oil	0.3 tsp

It should be noted that soybean oil and walnut oil have higher omega-6 content than omega-3 content. Their intake will improve total omega-3 intake but will not reduce the dietary omega-6 to omega-3 ratio, which is an important dietary strategy for management of mental health disorders.

*Daily intake as recommended by the ISSFAL.

(logical thinking center), the hippocampus (memory center), and the hypothalamus (hormone center). Atrophy was associated with deteriorated function in each of these regions (Ahmad et al., 2002).

Adequate DHA is also important for maintaining healthy neurotransmitter function. For example, the densities of dopamine and serotonin receptors are dependent on brain DHA levels (Delion et al., 1996). This may be one reason why, in the patient with anorexia who is often depleted in fat, antidepressants are not effective for promoting recovery (when there is minimal fat in the diet and tissues) but can be effective in relapse prevention (when the diet and tissues have more fat) (Walsh and Devlin, 1992). For neurotransmitters to work as they should, an adequate receptor density is necessary to interact with the increased concentration of neurotransmitters.

DHA may have a neuroprotective (antiinflammatory) effect because of its ability to raise the seizure threshold of the nervous system. In the early days of seizure research, very high–fat diets were found to be therapeutic for reducing seizure frequency and intensity (see Chapter 41). As this research progressed, it was found that the fats with the most therapeutic value for seizure management were the fish oils (Voskuyl et al., 1998). As new uses of seizure medications are evolving, this finding may be pertinent for several psychiatric diagnoses. Fish oil may have the potential to either reduce or eliminate the dose of many medications with potential for metabolic side effects such as weight gain.

Of interest is a recent study demonstrating the ability of the Atkins diet to reduce seizure activity in persons with epilepsy (Kossoff et al., 2003) (see Chapter 41). This particular study focused on large intakes of fat versus carbohydrate and was not designed to evaluate the fat source (e.g., fish vs. poultry or beef). It would be interesting to consider whether different fatty acid ratios within an Atkins high-fat diet produce different seizure patterns, as well as weight changes. It may be that dietary fat ratios are important in individuals with weight management issues, whether or not they also have a psychiatric diagnosis (see Chapter 21).

Because they are highly unsaturated, fish oils were originally thought of as agents of oxidation. However, recent research suggests that these fatty acids have a very important antioxidant effect (Erdogan et al., 2004). Since the preferred energy source of the brain is glucose, reducing the amount of glucose available in the metabolic mix has the side effect of reducing brain metabolism. The positive consequence of this change is that oxidative processes in the brain may be reduced. The effect of DHA and EPA on seizure activity may partially be explained by their effect on neuron excitability or neural hyperactivity. Reducing nervous system activity may be one of the reasons fish oils have been found to have therapeutic value in diseases that tend to worsen under stress. In laymen's terms, they "chill out" the nervous system, making it more difficult to engage a stress response. Box 42-1 lists the conditions in which DHA and EPA may play a role.

To date most of the research regarding the nervous system has focused on DHA. However, EPA has its own specific important influence on the nervous system. It has shown special promise as a therapeutic agent in the treatment of schizophrenia (Peet, 2003). Experts who research the effects of DHA and EPA on brain function report that unique functions appear to be attributed to each of these fatty acids. Both are essential, they are not interchangeable, and the daily intake of these two omega-3 fatty acids should be roughly equivalent (Peet, 2003).

Obtaining Adequate DHA and EPA

Unlike many essential nutrients, obtaining and retaining DHA and EPA depend not only on adequate intake but on important lifestyle and "macro" nutritional choices. It is often what is eaten *in addition to* DHA and EPA that determines whether overall essential fatty acid levels are adequate. Simply taking a supplement may not be enough. Over the course of a lifetime, the following strategies may be important to achieving and sustaining a healthy brain and nervous system.

During Pregnancy and Lactation

Unfortunately fetal nervous system growth may be suffering from warnings from government experts about eating fish during pregnancy. It is true that certain fishes (shark, tilefish, mackerel, and swordfish) may contain toxic levels of mercury that can be harmful to fetal development if consumed in large amounts (FDA, 2005). However, foods such as fish-oil–supplemented margarine and omega-3 eggs can provide essential fatty acids without the heavy metal risk.

BOX 42-1

Conditions for Which Fish Oils Are Beneficial

Anxiety disorder (Song et al., 2003)

Attention deficit-hyperactivity disorder (Young et al., 2004)

Autism (Vancassel et al., 2001)

Borderline personality disorder (Zanarini and Frankenburg, 2003)

Eating disorders (Ayton et al., 2004)

Epilepsy and bipolar disorder (Appleton et al., 2006; Lee et al., 2006; Stoll et al., 1999)

Postpartum depression (Marangell et al., 2003)

Schizophrenia (Emsley et al., 2003)

And many fish such as wild caught salmon, sardines, herring, halibut, and tuna are safe oil sources.

For pregnant women who are concerned that heavy metals may be present in fish oil supplements, a good general guideline is to only use products with the U.S. Pharmacopeia (USP) symbol on the label because this symbol identifies companies with manufacturing processes and product quality and purity that have been inspected and approved and have received endorsement by an independent third party (USP Verified, 2005).

Omega-3–supplemented foods have started to appear on the market; these products can be another alternative to fish and fish oils. When evaluating such foods, it is important to confirm that the omega-3 source is DHA and/or EPA. Many foods labeled as containing omega-3 fat are supplemented with flax, a beneficial food, but not high enough in DHA and EPA to be a realistic source of these essential fatty acids. Currently DHA and EPA are appearing in foods in four different forms: (1) as menhaden oil; (2) as microencapsulated fish oil powder; (3) as DHA produced by another animal; and (4) as marine algae.

Menhaden. Menhaden is a pelagic, surface feeding fish that is not typically consumed by humans because its bony structure does not render much edible flesh. However, in 1997 the oil of this fish was designated by the Food and Drug Administration to be on the Generally Regarded As Safe (GRAS) list, provided that maximum intake of this product did not exceed 3 g/person/day (Food Navigator, 2005). Since then food manufacturers have been working to create food products containing this additive. The first of these, a margarine, appeared on grocery store shelves in 2004. Future menhaden-supplemented products may include soup bases, creamy sauces, salad dressings, and mayonnaise (Menhaden Resource Council, 2005).

Microencapsulated Fish Oil Powder. Microencapsulated fish oil powder is produced by forcing fish oil through a sieve and creating small flakes that can be incorporated into food products such as bread (Wallace et al., 2000; Yep et al., 2002).

In 2005 a new heat-stable powder product was introduced in the United States, providing an alternative to fish and fish oils for individuals who do not consume fish or cannot tolerate the capsules (Omega-3 Brain Booster, 2005).

DHA and EPA Produced by Other Livestock. Humans do not efficiently convert ALA into EPA and DHA, but this is not the case with other animals. For example, when they are fed a sufficient amount of flaxseed, chickens produce eggs with an elevated amount of DHA in the yolks (Lewis et al., 2000). Cows that feed on grasses high in omega-3 fatty acids (as opposed to traditional feed) produce milk with a higher-than-average EPA and DHA content. Likewise, wild deer, elk, and other animals that feed primarily on grasses have a higher tissue content of omega-3 fatty acids in their meat than livestock raised on traditional feed. Currently animal scientists are also researching cost-effective methods for increasing the overall supply of omega-3 fatty acids by altering the composition of livestock feed by supplementing traditional feed with fish oil (Bourre, 2005).

Marine Algae. The DHA and EPA that humans obtain when they eat fish originate in marine algae that are eaten by small fish. It then moves up the food chain, as the smaller fish are consumed. Food scientists have developed marine algae products that can be incorporated into supplements or food. Baby formulas were the first product to contain marine algae as a DHA source. In 2006 the first marine algae–supplemented cereals began to appear in grocery stores.

It is important to note that of all of these sources of DHA and EPA, eggs and marine algae–based products contain DHA *only*.

One particularly high-risk group for essential fatty acid deficiency (and mental health–related medical problems) may be women with a history of eating disorders or restrictive or vegetarian eating who become pregnant. Previous dietary choices may have depleted tissue DHA stores. As fetal growth accelerates during the third trimester, body image issues may arise that trigger food restriction. A tendency to be fearful about food may provoke a woman to overgeneralize about the dangers of fish, resulting in no seafood intake at all. Practitioners working with women in the perinatal period may have one of the most important intervention opportunities in the health care field. At a time when the nutritional need for DHA is at its highest and intake of this fatty acid is likely to be at its nadir, it is important for women to have accurate and positive guidance through choices that maximize mental health status in both mother and baby (see Chapters 5 and 6).

During Infancy

One of the most important sources of DHA and EPA is mother's milk. In recent times duration of the nursing experience has either shortened significantly or disappeared completely. Whereas babies were often nursed for up to 2 years of age in times past, economic and social changes have reduced the time that many women spend with their

---

BOX 42-2

Questionnaire: Early Feeding History and Fatty Acid Intake

Were you born at term?

If you were born early, how early?

Did your premature birth affect how and what you were fed?

Did your mother have prolonged postpartum depression after you were born? If yes, did this influence your feeding? How?

Were you nursed or bottle fed? For how long? In what country? With what formula?

How many children did your mother have/nurse and for how long each time? (include miscarriages and stillbirths.)

Where do you rank in the overall lineup of your siblings? (Essential fatty acid availability may decrease with successive pregnancies.)

How many children have you nursed? For how long? Did your lactation cease after weaning or did it seem to continue longer than it should have?

---

babies. This change has reduced the availability of omega-3 fatty acids to babies. Until 2002 omega-3 fatty acids were not added to baby formula in the United States (Broughton et al., 2004). Now a number of formulas have been introduced that contain DHA. In baby formulas the ingredient source is marine algae. Although this is a definite improvement over other formulas, it is important to note that supplemented formulas contain only DHA. They have not been used long enough to determine if the absence of EPA is a beneficial, detrimental, or neutral factor. Box 42-2 lists questions about fatty acids and a person's early feeding history that may be useful in a nutrition assessment.

During Adulthood

Depression affects many adults. Long-chain fatty acid (LCFA) supplements will often improve depression and its related pathology. They should be used with vitamin E supplementation to make sure that they are not oxidized and are thus effective (Appleton et al., 2006; Osher et al., 2006). Patients with bipolar disorder, postpartum depression, schizophrenia, dementia, alcoholism, tardive dyskinesia and other psychiatric conditions may also improve with LCFA supplementation (Lee et al., 2006; Lim et al., 2006).

NUTRITION RECOMMENDATIONS

Goal 1: Consumption of Dietary DHA and EPA

The amount of these omega-3 fatty acids needed daily to sustain healthy brain and nervous system function remains under debate. The International Society for the Study of

Fatty Acids and Lipids (ISSFAL) recommends a daily minimum of 220 mg each of both DHA and EPA (Simopoulos et al., 2005). However, needs may be much higher (Simopoulos, 2002b). ISSFAL does not clarify whether its recommendations are specifically for an apparently healthy population with a significant fish intake (e.g. Japan, Norway), or if this is what is needed in a population such as in the United States with less fish intake and a pandemic deficiency of omega-3 fatty acids. As more information about the importance of DHA and EPA for adequate mental health is elucidated, it is likely that these recommendations will be increased.

One of the biggest misperceptions about fish is that only the "fatty fishes"—salmon, tuna, and trout—are significant sources of beneficial oils. In reality, *all* seafood is beneficial with regard to omega-3 content. Because these foods may help to reduce the need for medications used to manage mental health disorders, an investment in seafood may also create a financial savings in the long run. However, psychotropic medications should never be discontinued without consulting the prescribing physician.

Goal 2: Maintenance of a Diet With a Low Total Daily Omega-6 to Omega-3 Ratio

The natural consequence of the public "war on saturated fat" in years past has been a significant increase in the intake of omega-6 (n-6) fatty acids. With this shift in fat intake, researchers have gained a better understanding of n-3 fatty acid function. A high n-6:n-3 ratio (>10) appears to promote inflammation and oxidation. Originally the focus of this research was in the cardiovascular and endocrine systems; however, mental health research is suggesting that one consequence inflammation may have for the brain and nervous system is an increase in mental illnesses. Experts estimate that the average American may consume a diet with an n-6:n-3 ratio as high as 17:1. A beneficial ratio is probably close to 2:1 (Davis and Kris-Etherton, 2003).

When considering a recommendation of fish or fish oil supplements, consider that the inclusion of fish in a meal improves the overall balance of fat, saturated fat, and polyunsaturated fat in addition to increasing the n-3 intake. It is the n-6:n-3 *ratio*, not the total amount of n-3 that is important. More total DHA and EPA will be needed to achieve this ratio if the strategy is simply to add supplements to an n-6–rich diet. The most efficient choice, requiring less supplementation, would be to regularly consume fish and seafood as a protein of choice.

Even very low–fat diets can have high n-6:n-3 ratios. Ironically some of the highest ratios can be found in vegan vegetarian diets. Unless a vegetarian is diligent about including n-3 fatty acids in the diet, this ratio can very easily escalate. In fact, vegan vegetarians have been found to have lower tissue DHA concentrations than nonvegetarians (Salem et al., 2001). Vegetarians who have been diagnosed with mental illness may benefit from using a marine algae–based omega-3 supplement. These supplements do not contain EPA, but once tissues are saturated with DHA,

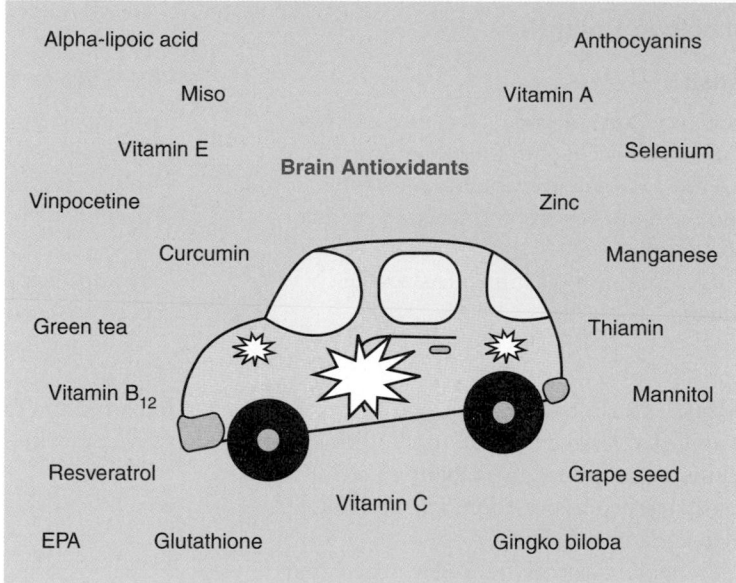

FIGURE 42-1 The brain can be thought of as a car that is damaged by oxidation, but can be protected by several vitamins, minerals and phytochemicals that function as antioxidants. (©2006 After the Diet Network.)

retroconversion can promote EPA synthesis (Stark and Holub, 2004). This strategy may require more time to be effective than if fish oils were used, but for the staunch, uncompromising vegetarian, it may very well be the only nutrition solution for chronic diseases and mental health issues related to inflammation.

Goal 3: Avoidance of Restrictive Diets That Encourage Rapid Weight Loss

Unfortunately dietary manipulation and restriction cannot specify which type of fat is lost during periods of calorie restriction. Dieting may create a "double whammy," in that n-3 fatty acids are being liberated and oxidized through calorie restriction at an accelerated pace at the same time that dietary choices may be restricting the foods that might help to replace n-3 fatty acids that are lost. In fact, supplementation with the omega-3 ALA during a weight loss diet has been found not to preserve n-3 stores in tissues (Arivazhagan and Panneerselvam, 2000). Two or more generations of restrictive eating specifically creating a DHA deficiency has been shown to affect brain function, specifically spatial learning and olfactory-cued reversal learning tasks (Arivazhagan et al., 2002; Farr et al., 2003). These deficiencies were present, even though hippocampal mass did not appear to be deficient.

Goal 4: Increased Antioxidant Intake

The two major goals for the maintenance of healthy fatty acid levels are to increase the levels through dietary choices and to prevent their oxidation through dietary food choices. Although DHA is an antioxidant, antioxidants in other foods may have importance in preserving these fats as well. A diet rich in fruits and vegetables is an important strategy. These foods contain many vitamins, minerals, and antioxi-

---

BOX 42-3

Compounds With Known Antioxidant Activity in the Brain and Nervous System

α-Lipoic acid	Miso
Anthocyanins	Quercetin
Curcumin	Resveratrol
Eicosapentaenoic acid	Selenium
Gingko biloba	Thiamin
Glutathione	Vitamin A
Grapeseed	Vitamin B$_{12}$
Green tea	Vitamin C
Manganese	Vitamin E
Mannitol	Zinc

Data from Arivazhagan P, Panneerselvam C: Effect of DL-alpha-lipoic acid on neural antioxidants in aged rats, *Pharmacol Res* 42:219, 2000; Arivazhagan P et al: Effect of DL-α-lipoic acid on the status of lipid peroxidation and protein oxidation in various brain regions of aged rats, *J Nutr Biochem* 13:619, 2002; and Farr SA et al: The antioxidants alpha-lipoic acid and *N*-acetylcysteine reverse memory impairment and brain oxidative stress in aged SAMP8 mice, *J Neurochem* 84:1173, 2003.

---

dants that can help protect and preserve the brain and nervous system. In addition, when prepared with vinaigrettes and marinades, they can be important carriers for the omega-3 fatty acids that are the foundation for brain and nervous system health. Omega–3 supplements, or any LCFA supplements should also contain the fat-soluble antioxidant vitamin E or be taken with vitamin E. A summary of antioxidants identified to be important for brain and nervous system integrity is found in Box 42-3 and Figure 42-1. Table 42-2 gives more specific guidance about nutrition in other psychiatric conditions.

TABLE 42-2

Nutrition for Specific Psychiatric Conditions

Mental Disorder	Explanation	Relevance to Nutrition
Acute stress disorder or posttraumatic stress disorder	Development of anxiety and dissociative and other symptoms within 1 month following exposure to an extremely traumatic event; the symptoms include reexperiencing the event, avoidance of trauma-related stimuli.	May impact appetite, with increase or decrease accordingly. Overall nutrition status may decline, or obesity may result.
Adjustment disorder	Maladaptive reaction to identifiable stressful life events.	May impact appetite, with increase or decrease accordingly. Overall nutrition status may decline, or obesity may result.
Amnestic disorder	Mental disorder characterized by acquired impairment in the ability to learn and recall new information, sometimes accompanied by inability to recall previously learned information, and not coupled with dementia or delirium.	Impaired ability to retain new information from nutrition counseling.
Anxiety disorders	A group of mental disorders in which anxiety and avoidance behavior predominate, including panic disorders, agoraphobia, specific phobias, social phobia, obsessive-compulsive disorder, posttraumatic stress disorder, acute stress disorder, generalized anxiety disorder, and substance-abuse anxiety disorder.	May impact appetite, with increase or decrease accordingly. Overall nutrition status may decline, or obesity may result. May respond to increased intake of omega-3 fats to 1-3 g/day.
Attention deficit disorder	Mental disorder characterized by inattention (such as distractibility, forgetfulness, not finishing tasks, and not appearing to listen), hyperactivity and impulsivity (such as fidgeting and squirming, difficulty in remaining seated, excessive running or climbing, feelings of restlessness, difficulty awaiting one's turn, interrupting others, and excessive talking) or both types of behavior (see Chapter 7).	Impaired ability to retain and use new information after nutrition counseling. May respond to increased intake of omega-3 fats, especially DHA, to 1-3 g/day
Autistic disorder	Severe pervasive developmental disorder with onset usually before three years of age and a biologic basis related to neurologic or neurophysiologic factors. Characterized by qualitative impairment in reciprocal social interaction (e.g., lack of awareness of the existence of feelings of others, failure to seek comfort at times of distress, lack of imitation), verbal and nonverbal communication, and capacity for symbolic play and by restricted and unusual repertoire of activities and interests.	May impact appetite, with increased needs common. Overall nutrition status may decline. May respond to increased intake of omega-3 fats, especially DHA, to 1-3 g/day. Gluten-free, casein-free diet may be useful (see Chapters 7 and 27).
Binge eating disorder	An eating disorder characterized by repeated episodes of binge eating, as in bulimia nervosa, but not followed by inappropriate compensatory behavior such as purging, fasting, or excessive exercise.	May impact nutrition status; health may decline, or obesity may result (see Chapter 22).
Bipolar disorders	Mood disorders characterized by a history of manic, mixed, or hypomanic episodes, usually with concurrent or previous history of one or more major depressive episodes.	May impact appetite, with increase or decrease accordingly. Overall nutrition status may decline, or obesity may result. May respond to increased intake of omega-3 fats to 1-3 g/day.
Body dysmorphic disorder	A mental disorder in which a normal-appearing person is either preoccupied with some imagined defect in appearance or is overly concerned about some very slight physical anomaly.	Likely to cause altered eating habits with potential for decline in intake. May lead to eating disorder (see Chapter 22). May be prone to food fads or use of herbs or steroids.

Data from *Merck manual of medical information*, http://www.mercksource.com/pp/us/cns/cns_home.jsp, accessed July 23, 2006.

TABLE 42-2

Nutrition for Specific Psychiatric Conditions—cont'd

Mental Disorder	Explanation	Relevance to Nutrition
Catatonic disorder	Immobilization caused by the physiologic effects of a general medical condition.	May impact appetite, with decrease accordingly. Overall nutrition status may decline.
Childhood disintegrative disorder	Pervasive developmental disorder characterized by marked regression in a variety of skills, including language, social skills or adaptive behavior, play, bowel or bladder control, and motor skills after at least 2, but less than 10 years of apparently normal development.	May impact appetite, with increase or decrease accordingly. Overall nutrition status may decline, or obesity may result (see Chapter 45).
Conduct disorder	A type of disruptive behavior disorder of childhood and adolescence characterized by a persistent pattern of conduct in which rights of others or age-appropriate societal norms or rules are violated.	No specific nutritional challenges except that mealtimes may be disrupted.
Conversion disorder	Mental disorder characterized by conversion symptoms (loss or alteration of voluntary motor or sensory functioning suggesting physical illness, such as seizures, paralysis, dyskinesia, anesthesia, blindness, or aphonia) having no demonstrable physiologic basis.	May impact appetite, with increase or decrease accordingly. Overall nutritional status may decline or obesity may result.
Delusional disorder	Mental disorder marked by well-organized, logically consistent delusions, but lacking other psychotic symptoms. Most functioning is not markedly impaired, the criteria for schizophrenia are not met; symptoms of a major mood disorder are present only briefly, if at all.	May impact appetite, with increase or decrease accordingly. Overall nutrition status may decline, or obesity may result.
Depersonalization disorder	Dissociative disorder characterized by one or more severe episodes of depersonalization (feelings of unreality and strangeness in one's perception of self or one's body image) not caused by another mental disorder such as schizophrenia. The perception of reality remains intact; patients are aware of their incapacitation. Episodes are usually accompanied by dizziness, anxiety, of fears of going insane.	May impact appetite, with increase or decrease accordingly. An eating disorder or obesity can result; overall nutrition status may decline.
Depressive disorders	Mood disorders in which depression is unaccompanied by manic or hypomanic episodes.	May impact appetite, with increase or decrease accordingly. Nutrition status may decline. May respond to increased intake of omega-3 fats to 1-3 g/day.
Dissociative disorders	Mental disorders characterized by sudden, temporary alterations in identity, memory, or consciousness, segregating normally integrated memories or parts of the personality from the dominant identity of the individual.	May impact appetite, with increase or decrease accordingly. Overall nutrition status may decline, or obesity may result.
Dissociative identity disorder	A disorder characterized by the existence in an individual of two or more distinct personalities, each having unique memories, characteristic behavior, and social relationships. Multiple personality disorder.	May impact appetite, with increase or decrease accordingly. Overall nutrition status may decline, or obesity may result.
Dysthymic disorder	Mood disorder characterized by depressed feeling (sad, blue, low), loss of interest or pleasure in one's usual activities, and by at least some of the following: altered appetite, disturbed sleep patterns, lack of energy, low self-esteem, poor concentration or decision-making skills, and feelings of hopelessness. Symptoms have persisted >2 years but are not severe enough to meet the criteria for major depressive disorder.	May impact appetite, with increase or decrease accordingly. Overall nutrition status may decline, or obesity may result. May coexist with an eating disorder. May respond to increased intake of omega-3 fats to 1-3 g/day.

Continued

TABLE 42-2

Nutrition for Specific Psychiatric Conditions—cont'd

Mental Disorder	Explanation	Relevance to Nutrition
Eating disorders	Any of several disorders in which abnormal feeding habits are associated with psychological factors; in DSM-IV these include anorexia nervosa, bulimia nervosa, pica and rumination disorder.	May impact appetite, with increase or decrease accordingly. Overall nutrition status may decline, or obesity may result, depending on the specific condition. May respond to increased intake of omega-3 fats to 1-3 g/day (see Chapter 22).
Generalized anxiety disorder	Disorder characterized by the presence of excessive, uncontrollable anxiety and worry about two or more life circumstances for 6 months or longer, accompanied by some combination of restlessness, fatigue, muscle tension, irritability, disturbed concentration or sleep, and somatic symptoms.	May impact appetite, with increase or decrease accordingly. Overall nutrition status may decline, or obesity may result. May coexist with an eating disorder. May benefit from increased intake of omega-3 fats, especially DHA, 1-3 g/day.
Impulse control disorders	Group of mental disorders characterized by repeated failure to resist an impulse to perform some act harmful to oneself or others.	May impact appetite, with increase or decrease accordingly. Overall nutrition status may decline, but more likely obesity may result.
Motor skills disorder	Any disorder characterized by inadequate development of motor coordination severe enough to limit locomotion or restrict the ability to perform tasks, schoolwork, or other activities.	No specific nutritional changes, but may have difficulty preparing food (see Chapter 45).
Obsessive-compulsive disorder	Anxiety disorder characterized by recurrent obsessions or compulsions that are severe enough to interfere significantly with personal or social functioning. Performing compulsive rituals may release tension temporarily, and resisting them causes increased tension.	May impact appetite, with increase or decrease accordingly. May avoid specific foods or food groups. Overall nutrition status may decline, or obesity may result.
Oppositional defiant disorder	A type of disruptive behavior disorder characterized by a recurrent pattern of defiant, hostile, disobedient, and negativistic behavior directed toward those in authority, including such actions as defying the requests or rules of adults, deliberately annoying others, arguing, spitefulness, and vindictiveness that occur much more frequently than would be expected on the basis of age and developmental stage.	May impact appetite, with increase or decrease accordingly. Overall nutrition status may decline, or obesity may result. Mealtimes and thus quality of nutritional intake may be disrupted.
Pain disorder	A somatoform disorder characterized by a chief complaint of severe chronic pain that causes substantial distress or impairment in functioning; the pain is neither feigned nor intentionally produced, and psychological factors appear to play a major role in its onset, severity, exacerbation, or maintenance.	May impact appetite, with increase or decrease accordingly. Overall nutrition status may decline, or obesity may result. May benefit from increased intake of omega-3 fats, especially EPA, for their inflammatory effect, 1-3 g/day.
Panic disorder	Anxiety disorder characterized by recurrent panic (anxiety) attacks, episodes of intense apprehension; fear; or terror associated with somatic symptoms such as dyspnea, palpitations, dizziness, vertigo, faintness, or shakiness, and with psychological symptoms such as feelings of unreality or fears of dying, going crazy, or losing control. There is usually chronic nervousness and tension between attacks; almost always associated with agoraphobia.	May impact appetite, with increase or decrease accordingly. May turn to food to soothe. Overall nutrition status may decline, or obesity may result.

TABLE 42-2

Nutrition for Specific Psychiatric Conditions—cont'd

Mental Disorder	Explanation	Relevance to Nutrition
Personality disorders	Mental disorders characterized by enduring, inflexible, and maladaptive personality traits that deviate markedly from cultural expectations; are self-perpetuating; pervade a broad range of situations, and either generate subjective distress or result in significant impairments in social, occupational, or other functioning. Onset in adolescence or early adulthood.	May impact appetite, with increase or decrease accordingly. Overall nutrition status may decline, or obesity may result. May respond to increased intake of omega-3 fats to 1-3 g/day.
Pervasive developmental disorders	Group of disorders characterized by impairment of development in multiple areas, including the acquisition of reciprocal social interaction, verbal and nonverbal communication skills, and imaginative activity and by stereotyped interests and behaviors; included are autism, Rett syndrome, childhood disintegrative disorder and Asperger's syndrome.	May not be able to comprehend information shared during nutrition counseling. Autism and Asperger's syndrome may benefit from dietary and nutrition changes (see Chapters 7 and 45).
Premenstrual dysphoric disorder	Premenstrual syndrome viewed as a psychiatric disorder.	May impact appetite, with increase or decrease accordingly. Overall nutrition status may decline, or obesity may result. May benefit from increasing intake of omega-3 fats to 1-3 g/day. Gamma-linoleic acid from evening primrose oil may be effective.
Rumination disorder	Eating disorder seen in infants under 1 year of age; after a period of normal eating habits, the child begins excessive regurgitation and rechewing of food, which is then ejected from the mouth or reswallowed.	If untreated, death from malnutrition may occur. May require enteral or parenteral nutrition.
Schizoaffective disorder	A mental disorder in which a major depressive episode, manic episode, or mixed episode occurs along with prominent psychotic symptoms characteristic of schizophrenia. Symptoms of the mood disorder are present for a substantial portion of the illness, and the disturbance is not the result of the effects of a psychoactive substance.	May impact appetite, with increase or decrease accordingly. Overall nutrition status may decline, or obesity may result. May respond to increased intake of omega-3 fats to 1-3 g/day.
Seasonal affective disorder	A cyclic mood disorder characterized by depression, extreme lethargy, increased need for sleep, hyperphagia, and carbohydrate craving. It intensifies most commonly in winter months and is hypothesized to be related to melatonin levels. In DSM-IV terminology called "mood disorder with seasonal pattern."	May impact appetite, with increase or decrease accordingly. Overall nutrition status may decline, or obesity may result. May respond to increasing omega-3 fat intake to 1-3 g/day. May benefit from increasing protein intake to balance blood sugar levels.
Sleep disorder	Chronic disorders involving sleep. Primary sleep disorders comprise dyssomnias and parasomnias. Causes of secondary sleep disorders may include a general medical condition, mental disorder, or psychoactive substance.	May impact appetite, with increased intake common; night eating syndrome may present. Obesity may result.

⊛ FOCAL POINTS

- For humans, the first exposure to DHA and EPA occurs in utero. Omega-3 fatty acids in the mother cross the placenta and are provided to the developing fetus, where they are used as building blocks for the brain and nervous system.
- Fatty acid transfer accelerates in the third trimester, when the brain and nervous system are most rapidly developing.
- Brain development in general depends on DHA; but learning, memory, hormone, and visual centers appear to be especially dependent on DHA for proper growth, development, and function.

- Promotion of appropriate dietary inclusion of omega-3 fatty acids, antioxidants, and the phytochemicals in fruits and vegetables is important in the prevention and management of psychiatric disorders.
- Regular inclusion of foods that contain targeted nutrients is essential for lifelong mental wellness.
- Dietitians play a major role in helping with management and recovery of psychiatric and substance-abuse patients, and improving nutrition status is a priority for a return to wellness.

⊛ CLINICAL SCENARIO 1

Nels is a 20-year-old white male who was recently admitted to the adult psychiatric unit of your hospital. He has exhibited signs of psychosis, and his medical record indicates a family history of schizophrenia, diabetes, and bipolar disorder. He has been prescribed aripiprazole and bupropion; he is becoming more alert. His fasting blood glucose is normal at 100 mg/dl, but his serum LDL cholesterol is low at 70 mg/dl. His diet has been poor lately, and he has been consuming mostly snack foods and sweetened carbonated beverages. He seldom eats fish and eats fewer than three fruits and vegetables weekly.

> *Nutrition Diagnosis 1:** Inadequate intake of food fats (i.e., omega-3 fatty acids) related to poor diet as evidenced by low serum cholesterol

*Nutrition Diagnosis 2:** Inadequate bioactive substance intake related to antioxidants and phytochemicals as evidenced by intake of fewer than three fruits and vegetables weekly

1. What information will you need to assess his nutritional history more thoroughly?
2. What dietary components will you suggest?
3. What are the nutritional side effects of the medications he is taking?
4. What long-term nutrition care will he need?

⊛ CLINICAL SCENARIO 2

Marylin is a 57-year-old Asian female with a family history of diabetes and depression. She has been admitted to your inpatient psychiatric unit for a 2-week stay. She has been exhibiting signs of severe depression and has been placed on two antidepressants, Prozac and Tofranil. Her appetite has been poor, and she has lost 25 lb over the past 3 months. She is 5 ft 0 in and currently weighs 90 lb. From her food history and intake records, you have noted that she is eating about 50% of her meals but will drink beverages between meals. Her food preferences include seafood and fish, rice and pasta, and salads and vegetables. She dislikes fruit and desserts of all kinds.

*Nutrition Diagnosis:** Unintentional weight loss related to depression and poor intake as evidenced by 25-lb weight loss in 3 months and BMI of 18

1. What kinds of foods and snacks might you recommend for Marylin?
2. Since medications such as antidepressants take several weeks to work effectively, what types of monitoring and evaluation will you do for Marylin?
3. How might you adapt the meals served to Marylin to enhance calories and energy intake?

USEFUL WEBSITES

American Association on Mental Retardation
http://www.AAMR.org

**American Academy of Child
and Adolescent Psychiatry**
http://www.aacap.org/

American Psychiatric Association
http://www.psych.org/

**National Depressive & Manic-Depressive
Association**
http://www.ndmda.org/

Internet Mental Health
www.mentalhealth.com

National Alliance for the Mentally Ill
http://www.nami.org/

References

Ahmad A et al: Decrease in neuron size in docosahexaenoic acid-deficient brain, *Pediatr Neurol* 26:210, 2002.

American Psychiatric Association (APA): *Diagnostic and statistical manual of mental disorders DSM-IV,* ed 4, Arlington, Vir, 1994, The Association.

Appleton KM et al: Effects of *n*-3 long-chain polyunsaturated fatty acids on depressed mood: systematic review of published trials, *Am J Clin Nutr* 84:1308, 2006.

Arivazhagan P, Panneerselvam C: Effect of DL-alpha-lipoic acid on neural antioxidants in aged rats, *Pharmacol Res* 42:219, 2000.

Arivazhagan P et al: Effect of DL-alpha-lipoic acid on the status of lipid peroxidation and protein oxidation in various brain regions of aged rats, *J Nutr Biochem* 13:619, 2002.

Ayton AK et al: A pilot open case series of ethyl-EPA supplementation in the treatment of anorexia nervosa, *Prostaglandins Leukot Essent Fatty Acids* 71:205, 2004.

Bourre JM: Where to find omega-3 fatty acids and how feeding animals with diet enriched in omega-3 fatty acids to increase nutritional value of derived products for human: what is actually useful? *J Nutr Health Aging* 9:232, 2005.

Broughton KS: Diet and Ovulation, Presentation at Polycystic Ovary Syndrome: the Perfect Endocrine Storm, Tucson, Az, April 24, 2004.

Davis BC, Kris-Etherton PM: Achieving optimal essential fatty acid status in vegetarians: current knowledge and practical implications, *Am J Clin Nutr* 78:640S, 2003.

Delion S et al: Alpha-linolenic acid dietary deficiency alters age-related changes of dopaminergic and serotoninergic neurotransmission in the rat frontal cortex, *J Neurochem* 66:1582, 1996.

Emsley R et al: Clinical potential of omega-3 fatty acids in the treatment of schizophrenia, *CNS Drugs* 17:1081, 2003.

Erdogan H et al: Effect of fish oil supplementation on plasma oxidant/antioxidant status in rats, *Prostaglandins Leukot Essent Fatty Acids* 71:149, 2004.

Farr SA et al: The antioxidants alpha-lipoic acid and N-acetylcysteine reverse memory impairment and brain oxidative stress in aged SAMP8 mice, *J Neurochem* 84:1173, 2003.

FDA: *Backgrounder for the 2004 FDA/EPA Consumer Advisory: What you need to know about mercury in fish and shellfish,* from http://www.epa.gov/waterscience/fishadvice/factsheet.html, accessed December 15, 2005.

Food Navigator: *FDA amends fish oil GRAS. Food Navigator USA, 01/24/04,* from http://www.foodnavigator-usa.com/news/ng.asp?n=49276-fda-amends-fish, accessed December 15, 2005.

Innis SM: Perinatal biochemistry and physiology of long-chain polyunsaturated fatty acids, *J Pediatr* 143:1S, 2003.

Kossoff EH et al: Efficacy of the Atkins diet as therapy for intractable epilepsy, *Neurology* 61:1789, 2003.

Kurowska EM et al: Bioavailability of omega-3 essential fatty acids from Perilla seed oil, *Prostaglandins Leukot Essent Fatty Acids* 68:207, 2003.

Lee S et al: Current applications of omega-6 and omega-3 fatty acids, *Nutr Clin Pract* 21:323, 2006.

Lewis NM et al: Enriched eggs as a source of *n*-3 polyunsaturated fatty acids for humans, *Poult Sci* 79:971, 2000.

Lim WS et al: Omega 3 fatty acids for the prevention of dementia, *Cochrane Database Syst Rev* (1):CD005379, Jan 25, 2006.

Maguire LS et al: Fatty acid profile, tocopherol, squalene, and phytosterol content of walnuts, almonds, peanuts, hazelnuts, and the macadamia nut, *Int J Food Sci Nutr* 55: 171, 2004.

Marangell LB et al: Omega-3 fatty acids for the prevention of postpartum depression: negative data from a preliminary, open-label, pilot study, *Depress Anxiety* 19(1):20, 2003.

Menhaden Resource Council: from www.menhaden.org, accessed December 15, 2005.

National Association for Mental Illness (NAMI): from http://www.NAMI.org/Content/Microsites88/NAMI_Olmsted_County/Home84/Links6/Famous_People/famous_people_with_mental_illness.doc, accessed January 11, 2006.

Omega-3 Brain Booster: *Omega-3 frequently asked questions,* from www.omega3brainbooster.com, accessed December 15, 2005.

Osher Y et al: Clinical trials of PUFAs in depression: state of the art, *World J Biol Psychiatry* 7:323, 2006.

Peet M: Eicosapentaenoic acid in the treatment of schizophrenia and depression: rationale and preliminary double-blind clinical trials, *Prostaglandins Leukotr Essent Fatty Acids* 69:477, 2003.

Salem N Jr et al: Alterations in brain function after loss of docosahexaenoate due to dietary restriction of *n*-3 fatty acids, *J Mol Neurosci* 16:299, 2001.

Simopoulos AP: Omega-3 fatty acids in inflammation and autoimmune diseases, *J Am Coll Nutr* 21:495, 2002a.

Simopoulos AP: The importance of the ratio of omega 6/omega 3 fatty acids, *Biomed Pharmacother* 56:365, 2002b.

Simopoulos AP et al: *Workshop on the essentiality and recommended dietary intakes for omega-6 and omega-3 fatty acids,* from http://www.issfal.org.uk/adequateintakes.htm, accessed December 16, 2005.

Song C et al : Effects of dietary *n*-3 or *n*-6 fatty acids on interleukin-1 beta-induced anxiety, stress, and inflammatory responses in rats, *J Lipid Res* 44:1984, 2003.

Stark KD, Holub BJ: Differential eicosapentaenoic acid elevations and altered cardiovascular disease risk factor responses after supplementation with docosahexaenoic acid in postmenopausal women receiving and not receiving hormone replacement therapy, *Am J Clin Nutr* 79:765, 2004.

Stoll AL: *The omega-3 connection: the groundbreaking anti-depression and brain program*, New York, 2001, The Free Press.

Stoll AL et al: Omega-3 fatty acids in bipolar disorder: a preliminary, double-blind, placebo-controlled trial, *Arch Gen Psychiatry* 56:407, 1999.

United States Department of Agriculture: Food Composition Tables, from http://www.nal.usda.gov/fnic/foodcomp/Data/, accessed December 22, 2005.

United States Pharmacopeia: USP Verified: Supplements, from http://www.usp.org/USPVerified/, accessed December 15, 2005.

Vancassel S et al: Plasma fatty acid levels in autistic children, *Prostaglandins Leukot Essent Fatty Acids* 65(1): 1, 2001.

Voskuyl RA et al: Anticonvulsant effect of polyunsaturated fatty acids in rats, using the cortical stimulation model, *Eur J Pharmacol* 341:145, 1998.

Wallace JM et al: Bioavailability of *n*-3 polyunsaturated fatty acids (PUFA) in foods enriched with microencapsulated fish oil, *Ann Nutr Metab* 44:157, 2000.

Walsh BT, Devlin MJ: The pharmacologic treatment of eating disorders, *Psychiatr Clin North Am* 15(1):149, 1992.

Williard DE et al: Comparison of 20-, 22-, and 24-carbon *n*-3 and *n*-6 polyunsaturated fatty acid utilization in differentiated rat brain astrocytes, *Prostaglandins Leukot Essent Fatty Acids* 67:99, 2002.

Yep YL et al: Bread enriched with microencapsulated tuna oil increases docosahexaenoic acid and total omega-3 fatty acids in humans, *Asia Pac J Clin Nutr* 11:285, 2002.

Young GS et al: Blood phospholipid fatty acid analysis of adults with/without attention deficit/hyperactivity disorder, *Lipids* 39:117, 2004.

Zanarini MC, Frankenburg FR: Omega-3 fatty acid treatment of women with borderline personality disorder: a double-blind, placebo-controlled study, *Am J Psychiatry* 160:167, 2003.

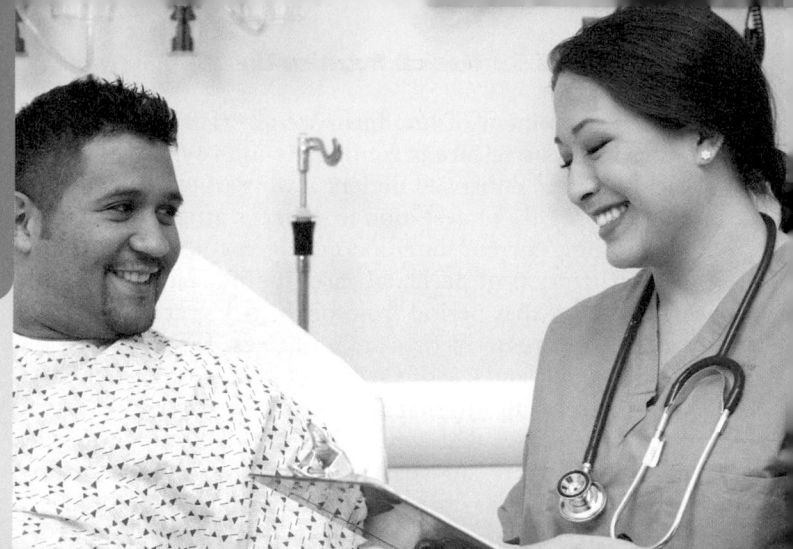

CHAPTER 43

Diane M. Anderson, PhD, RD, CSP, FADA

Medical Nutrition Therapy for Low-Birth-Weight Infants

KEY TERMS

appropriate for gestational age (AGA) describes the size of an infant whose birth weight is between the 10th and 90th percentiles for gestational age on an intrauterine growth grid

extremely low birth weight (ELBW) a birth weight of less than 1000 g (2¼ lb)

gastric gavage a feeding method that involves inserting a soft feeding tube through the mouth or nose into the stomach

gestational age the age of an infant at birth as determined by the length of the pregnancy (the number of weeks since the last menstrual period) or a clinical assessment

glucose load the amount of glucose received intravenously

hemolytic anemia anemia caused by oxidative destruction of mature red blood cells; sometimes caused by vitamin E deficiency

human milk fortifiers supplements of protein, carbohydrate, fat, minerals, and vitamins added to human milk to meet the increased nutrient needs of premature infants

infancy birth to 1 year of age

infant mortality rate the number of infant deaths in the first year of life per 1000 live births

intrauterine growth restriction (IUGR) decreased fetal growth rate as determined by the obstetrician during pregnancy

large for gestational age (LGA) refers to the size of an infant whose birth weight is above the 90th percentile of the standard weight for gestational age according to the intrauterine growth chart

low birth weight (LBW) a birth weight of less than 2500 g (5½ lb)

necrotizing enterocolitis inflammation or death of the gastrointestinal tract

neonatal period the first 28 days of life

neutral thermal environment the environmental temperature at which an infant expends the least amount of energy to maintain body temperature

osteopenia of prematurity reduced bone mass in a premature infant resulting from a decreased bone synthesis rate; often attributable to inadequate calcium and phosphorus intake

perinatal period from 28 weeks of gestation to 4 weeks after birth

premature (preterm) infant an infant born before 37 weeks' gestation

respiratory distress syndrome lung disease caused by a surfactant deficiency; develops shortly after birth and is common in preterm infants

small for gestational age (SGA) referring to the size of an infant whose birth weight is lower than the 10th percentile of the standard weight for gestational age

surfactant a mixture of lipoproteins secreted by alveolar cells into the alveoli and respiratory air passages that contributes to the elastic properties of pulmonary tissue

term infant an infant born between 37 and 42 weeks of gestation

very low birth weight (VLBW) a birth weight of less than 1500 g (3⅓ lb)

The management of low-birth-weight (LBW) infants requiring intensive care is continually improving. With new technologies, enhanced understanding of **perinatal period** (from 28 weeks of gestation to 4 weeks after birth) pathophysiology, current nutrition management principles, and regionalization of perinatal care, the mortality rates during **infancy,** that period from birth to 1 year of age, continue to decrease in the United States. In particular, the development and use of **surfactant**—a mixture of lipoproteins secreted by alveolar cells into the alveoli and respiratory air passages that contributes to the elastic properties of pulmonary tissue—has increased the survival of preterm infants, as has the use of antepartum corticosteroids. Most LBW infants have the potential for long and productive lives (Wilson-Costello and Hack, 2006).

Nutrition can be provided to LBW infants in many ways, each of which has certain benefits and limitations. The infant's size, age, and clinical condition dictate the nutrition requirements and the way they can be provided. Because of the complexities involved in the neonatal intensive care setting, a team that includes a registered dietitian trained in neonatal nutrition should make the decisions necessary to facilitate optimal nutrition. In regionalized perinatal care systems, the neonatal nutritionist may also consult with health care providers in community hospitals and public health settings.

PHYSIOLOGIC DEVELOPMENT

Gestational Age and Size

At birth an infant who weighs less than 2500 g (5½ lb) is classified as having a **low birth weight (LBW);** an infant weighing less than 1500 g (3⅓ lb) has a **very low birth weight (VLBW);** and an infant weighing less than 1000 g (2¼ lb) has an **extremely low birth weight (ELBW).** LBW may be attributable to a shortened period of gestation, prematurity, or a retarded intrauterine growth rate, which makes the infant small for gestational age.

The **term infant** is born between the 37th and 42nd weeks of gestation. A **premature (preterm) infant** is born before 37 weeks of gestation, whereas a postterm infant is born after 42 weeks of gestation.

Antenatally an estimate of the infant's **gestational age** is based on the date of the mother's last menstrual period, clinical parameters of uterine fundal height, the presence of quickening (the first movements of the fetus that can be felt by the mother), fetal heart tones, or ultrasound evaluations. After birth, gestational age is determined by clinical assessment. Clinical parameters fall into two groups: (1) a series of neurologic signs, which depend primarily on postures and tone; and (2) a series of external characteristics that reflect the physical maturity of the infant. The New Ballard Score (Ballard et al., 1991) examination is a frequently used clinical assessment tool. An accurate assessment of gestational age is important for establishing nutritional goals for individual infants and differentiating the premature infant from the term SGA infant.

An infant who is **small for gestational age (SGA)** has a birth weight that is lower than the 10th percentile of the standard weight for that gestational age. An SGA infant whose intrauterine weight gain is poor but whose linear and head growth are between the 10th and 90th percentiles on the intrauterine growth grid has experienced asymmetric **intrauterine growth restriction (IUGR).** An SGA infant whose length and occipital frontal circumference are also below the 10th percentile of the standards has symmetric IUGR. Symmetric IUGR, which usually reflects early and prolonged intrauterine deficit, is apparently more detrimental to later growth and development. Some infants can be SGA because they are genetically small, and these infants should do well.

An infant whose size is **appropriate for gestational age (AGA)** has a birth weight between the 10th and 90th percentiles on the intrauterine growth chart. The obstetrician diagnoses IUGR when the fetal growth rate decreases. Serial ultrasound measurements document this reduction in fetal anthropometric measurements, which may be caused by maternal, placental, or fetal abnormalities. The future growth and development of infants who have had IUGR is diverse, depending on the specific cause of the IUGR and treatment. Some infants who suffered from IUGR are SGA, but many may plot as AGA infants at birth. Decreased fetal growth does not always result in an infant who is SGA.

An infant whose birth weight is above the 90th percentile on the intrauterine growth chart is **large for gestational age (LGA).** Box 43-1 summarizes the weight classifications. Figure 43-1 shows the classification of neonates based on maturity and intrauterine growth.

Infant Mortality and Statistics

In 2002 the **infant mortality rate** in the United States rose to 7 deaths per 1000 live births. This is the first time that the infant mortality rate increased since 1958 (MacDorman et al., 2005). At the same time the number of premature and LBW infants increased. Infant mortality and morbidity are higher for the premature infant than the infant born at term.

BOX 43-1

Classification of Birth Weight and Intrauterine Growth

Low birth weight <2500 g
Very low birth weight <1500 g
Extremely low birth weight <1000 g
Small for gestational age = Birth weight <10th percentile of standard for gestational age
Appropriate for gestational age = Birth weight between the 10th and 90th percentile of standard for gestational age
Large for gestational age = Birth weight >90th percentile of standard for gestational age

An inverse relationship exists between birth weight and infant mortality rate. The risk for infant death for those who weigh 1500 to 2499 g is six times higher than for infants who weigh more than 2500 g; for infants who weigh less than 1500 g, the risk is 100 times higher (Hoyert et al., 2006). Maternal factors associated with infant mortality include teenage pregnancy, age 40 years or older, unmarried status, high school not completed, late prenatal care, and smoking during pregnancy (Hoyert et al., 2006). Teenage pregnancy is at its lowest rate in the last 60 years, and the incidence of smoking during pregnancy has decreased. Paternal smoking also has a negative effect on fetal growth (Nakamura et al., 2004).

Multiple births contribute to the high infant mortality rate. Greater than 50% of twins and 90% of triplets are premature or LBW. In 2003 the older mother of 45 to 54 years had an increased rate of multiple births with more than 1 in 5 births as compared to 1 in 50 in 1990. This growth in the number of multiple births is related to women delaying childbirth, because multiple gestations are associated with mothers of older ages. In addition, fertility-enhancing therapies are frequently used (Hoyert et al., 2006) (see Chapter 5).

The United States' infant mortality rate remains higher than many Western countries (Hoyert et al., 2006). This discrepancy may be attributable to the inconsistent collection of mortality data among nations, which may falsely lower mortality rates in other countries. However the high incidence of LBW infants born in the United States contributes to this high infant mortality rate.

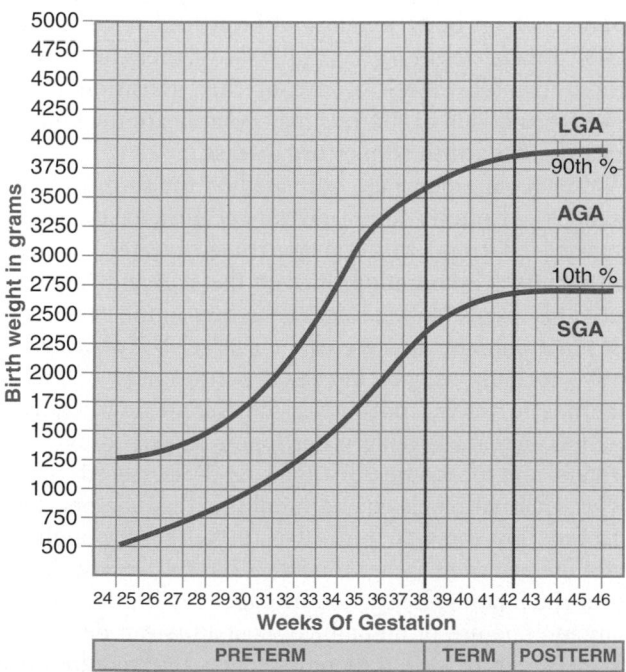

FIGURE 43-1 Classification of neonates based on maturity and intrauterine growth (small for gestational age [SGA], appropriate for gestational age [AGA], or large for gestational age [LGA]). *(From Battaglia FC, Lubchenco LO: A practical classification of newborn infants by weight and gestational age,* J Pediatr *71:159, 1967).*

Characteristics of Immaturity

The premature or LBW infant has not had the chance to develop fully in utero and is physiologically different from the term infant (Figure 43-2). Because of this, LBW infants have various clinical problems in the early **neonatal period,** depending on their intrauterine environment, degree of prematurity, birth-related trauma, and function of immature or stressed organ systems. Certain problems occur with such frequency that they are considered typical of prematurity (Table 43-1). Premature infants are at high risk for poor nutrition status because of poor nutrient stores, physiologic immaturity, illness (which may interfere with nutritional management and needs), and the nutrient demands required for growth.

Most fetal nutrient stores are deposited during the last 3 months of gestation; therefore the premature infant begins life in a compromised nutritional state. Because metabolic (i.e., energy) stores are limited, nutrition support in the form of parenteral nutrition (PN), enteral nutrition, or both should be initiated as soon as possible. In the preterm infant weighing 1000 g, fat constitutes only 1% of total body weight; by contrast the term infant (3500 g) has a fat percentage of about 16%. For example, a 1000-g AGA premature infant has a glycogen and fat reserve equivalent to about 110 kcal/kg of body weight. With basal metabolic needs of approximately 50 kcal/kg/day, it is obvious that this infant will rapidly run out of fat and carbohydrate fuel unless adequate nutrition support is established. The depletion time is even shorter for preterm infants weighing less than 1000 g at birth. Nutrient reserves are depleted most quickly by tiny infants who have IUGR as a result of their increased basal metabolic rate.

However, it is often difficult to provide adequate nutrition during the first several days of life because of immature organ systems and severe medical problems. When an adequate dietary intake cannot be established and fat and glycogen reserves have been exhausted, the infant begins to catabolize vital body protein tissue for energy. Theoretic

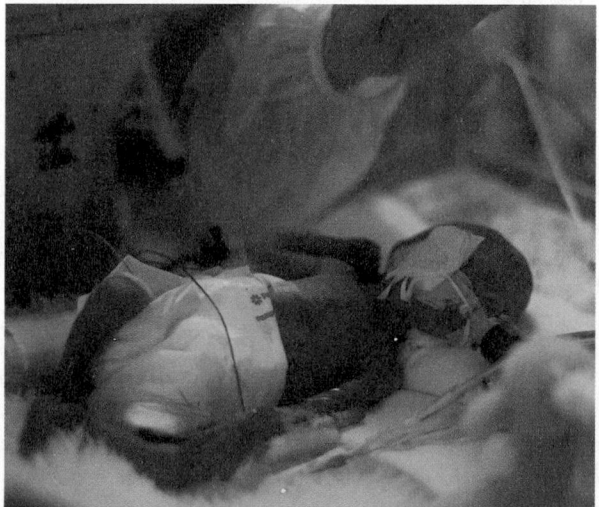

FIGURE 43-2 A.R., born at 27 weeks of gestation; birth weight of 870 g (1 lb, 14 oz).

TABLE 43-1

Common Problems Among Premature Infants

System	Problem
Respiratory	Respiratory distress syndrome, chronic lung disease (bronchopulmonary dysplasia)
Cardiovascular	Patent ductus arteriosus
Renal	Fluid and electrolyte imbalance
Neurologic	Intraventricular hemorrhage, periventricular leukomalacia (cerebral necrosis)
Metabolic	Hypoglycemia, hyperglycemia, hypocalcemia, metabolic acidosis
Gastrointestinal	Hyperbilirubinemia, feeding intolerance, necrotizing enterocolitis
Hematologic	Anemia
Immunologic	Sepsis, pneumonia, meningitis
Other	Apnea, bradycardia, cyanosis, osteopenia

Modified from Zerzan J, O'Leary MJ: Nutrition for preterm and low-birth-weight infants. In Trahms CM, Pipes PL, editors: *Nutrition in infancy and childhood*, ed 6, New York, 1997, WBC/McGraw-Hill.

TABLE 43-2

Expected Survival Time of Starved (H_2O Only) and Semistarved ($D_{10}W$) Infants

Birth Weight (g)	Estimated Survival Time (Days)	
	H_2O	$D_{10}W$
1000	4	11
2000	12	30
3500	32	80

Data from Heird WC et al: Intravenous alimentation in pediatric patients, *J Pediatr* 80:351, 1972.

estimates of survival time of starved and semistarved infants are shown in Table 43-2. These estimates assume depletion of all glycogen and fat and about one third of body protein tissue at a rate of 50 kcal/kg/day. The effects of fluids such as intravenously provided water (which has no exogenous calories) and 10% dextrose solution ($D_{10}W$) are shown. Even with protein tissue catabolism, the projected survival times are alarmingly short.

The small premature infant is particularly vulnerable to undernutrition. Malnutrition in premature infants may increase the risk of infection, prolong chronic illness, and adversely affect brain growth and function. In fact, Lucas and colleagues (1998) reported that the type of milk used for the neonatal diet may be directly linked to neurodevelopment at 18 months of age. Human milk or premature infant formula fed the first month of life resulted in improved development.

NUTRITION REQUIREMENTS: PARENTERAL FEEDING

Many critically ill preterm infants have difficulty progressing to full enteral feedings in the first several days or even weeks of life. The infant's small stomach capacity, immature gastrointestinal tract, and illness make the progression of enteral feedings difficult (see *Pathophysiology and Care Management Algorithm:* Nutrition Support of Premature Infants). PN becomes essential for nutrition support, either as a supplement to enteral feedings or as the total source of nutrition. Chapter 20 offers a complete discussion of PN; only aspects related to feeding of the preterm infant are presented here.

Fluid

Because fluid needs vary widely for preterm infants, fluid balance must be monitored. Inadequate intake can lead to dehydration, electrolyte imbalances, and hypotension; excessive intake can lead to edema, congestive heart failure, and possible opening of the ductus arteriosus. Additional neonatal clinical complications reported with high fluid intakes include necrotizing enterocolitis, and bronchopulmonary dysplasia (BPD) (see Chapter 35).

The premature infant has a greater percentage of body water (especially extracellular water) than the term infant (see Figure 4-1 in Chapter 4). The amount of extracellular water should decrease in all infants during the first few days of life. This reduction is accompanied by a normal loss of 10% to 15% of body weight and improved renal function. ELBW infants often lose up to 20% of their birth weight without complications. Failure of this transition in fluid dynamics and lack of diuresis may complicate the course of preterm infants with respiratory disease.

Water requirements are estimated by the sum of the predicted losses from the lungs and skin, urine, and stool and the water needed for growth. A major route of water loss in preterm infants is evaporation through the skin and respiratory tract. This insensible water loss is highest in the smallest and least mature infants because of their larger body surface area relative to body weight, increased permeability of the skin epidermis to water, and greater skin blood flow relative to metabolic rate. Insensible water loss is increased by radiant warmers and phototherapy lights and decreased by heat shields, thermal blankets, and humidified incubators. Insensible water loss can vary from 50 to 100 ml/kg/day on the first day of life and increase up to 120 to 200 ml/kg/day, depending on the infant's size, gestational age, day of life, and environment. The use of humidified incubators can decrease insensible water losses and thereby reduce fluid requirements.

Excretion of urine, the other major route of water loss, varies from 40 to 85 ml/kg/day. This loss depends on the fluid volume and solute load presented to the kidneys. The infant's ability to concentrate urine increases with maturity. Stool water loss is generally 5 to 10 ml/kg/day, and 10 to 15 ml/kg/day is suggested as optimal for growth (Dell and Davis, 2006).

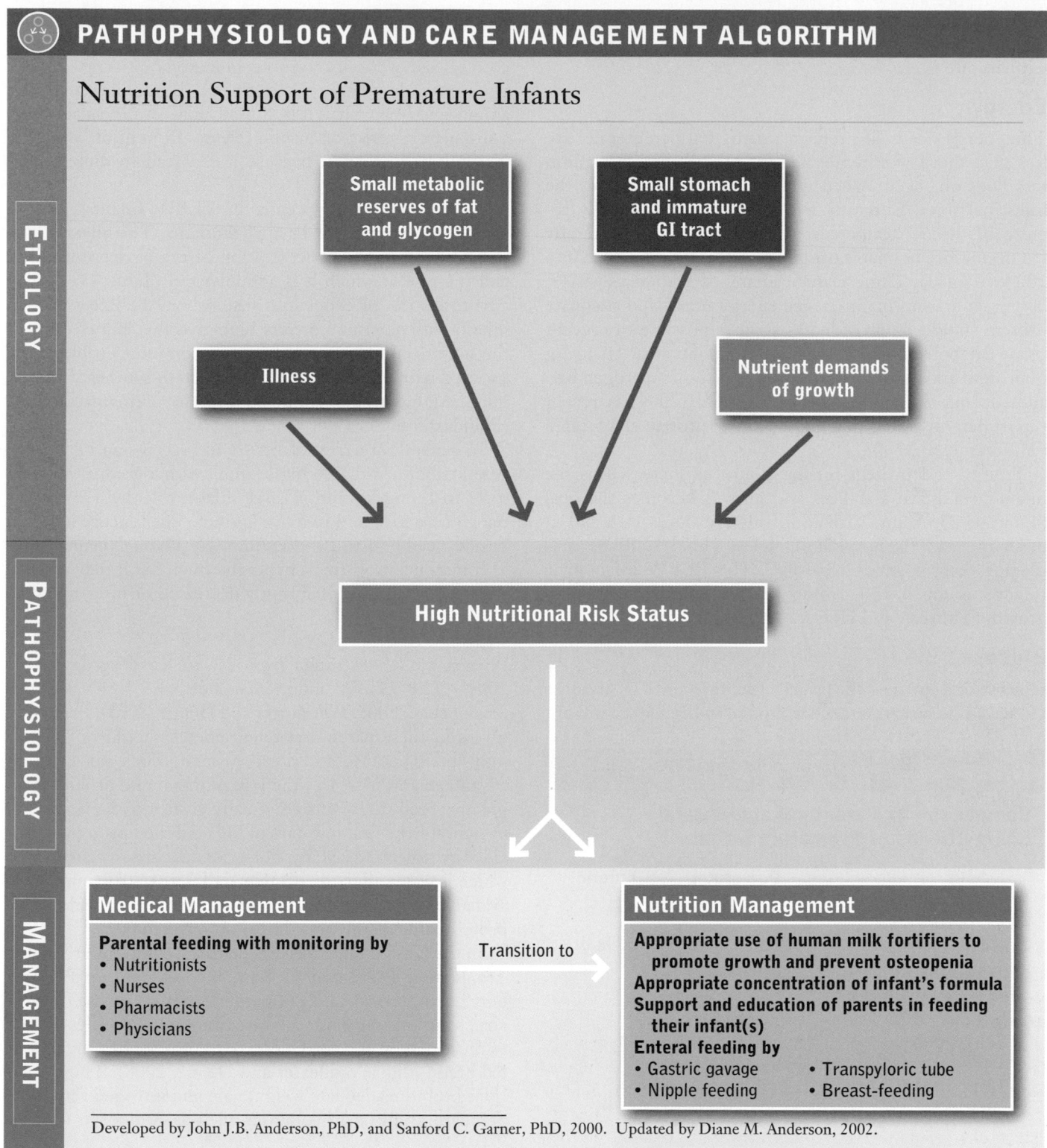

PATHOPHYSIOLOGY AND CARE MANAGEMENT ALGORITHM

Nutrition Support of Premature Infants

ETIOLOGY

Small metabolic reserves of fat and glycogen

Small stomach and immature GI tract

Illness

Nutrient demands of growth

PATHOPHYSIOLOGY

High Nutritional Risk Status

MANAGEMENT

Medical Management

Parental feeding with monitoring by
- Nutritionists
- Nurses
- Pharmacists
- Physicians

Transition to

Nutrition Management

Appropriate use of human milk fortifiers to promote growth and prevent osteopenia
Appropriate concentration of infant's formula
Support and education of parents in feeding their infant(s)
Enteral feeding by
- Gastric gavage
- Nipple feeding
- Transpyloric tube
- Breast-feeding

Developed by John J.B. Anderson, PhD, and Sanford C. Garner, PhD, 2000. Updated by Diane M. Anderson, 2002.

Because of the many variables affecting neonatal fluid losses, fluid needs must be determined on an individual basis. Usually fluid is administered at a rate of 80 to 105 ml/kg/day the first day of life to meet insensible losses and urine output. Fluid needs are then evaluated by assessing fluid intake and comparing it with the clinical parameters of urine volume output; specific gravity or osmolality; and serum electrolyte, creatinine, and urea nitrogen levels. Assess-

ments of weight, blood pressure, peripheral perfusion, skin turgor, and mucous membrane moisture are performed daily. Daily fluid administration generally increases by 10 to 20 ml/kg/day. By the end of the second week of life, preterm infants may receive fluids at a rate of 140 to 160 ml/kg/day. Fluid restriction may be necessary in preterm infants with patent ductus arteriosus, congestive heart failure, renal failure, or cerebral edema. However, more fluids are needed by preterm infants who are placed under phototherapy lights or a radiant warmer or when the environmental or body temperature is elevated.

Energy

The energy needs of preterm infants fed parenterally are less than those of enterally fed infants because absorption loss does not occur when nutritional intake bypasses the intestinal tract. Enterally fed preterm infants usually require 105 to 130 kcal/kg/day to grow, whereas parenterally fed premature neonates can grow well if they receive 90 to 100 kcal/kg/day (American Academy of Pediatrics [AAP], 2004). Minimum maintenance energy needs and adequate protein should be provided as soon as possible to prevent tissue catabolism. Providing VLBW infants with 1.5 to 2 g of protein and 30 to 50 kcal/kg/day promotes nitrogen balance during the first 3 days of life (AAP, 2004). A recent report demonstrated that 3 g/kg/day of protein is tolerated (Thureen et al., 2003).

Energy and protein intake should be increased as the infant's condition stabilizes and growth becomes the goal (Table 43-3). Many VLBW infants are born AGA but at discharge from the hospital weigh less than the 10th percentile for their postmenstrual age. The ELBW infant may require as much 130 to 150 kcal/kg/day to catch up in growth (Thureen and Heird, 2005; Tsang et al., 2005).

Glucose

Glucose or dextrose is the principal energy source (3.4 kcal/g). However, glucose tolerance is limited in premature infants,

especially in VLBW infants, because of inadequate insulin production, insulin resistance, and continued hepatic glucose release while intravenous glucose is infusing. Hyperglycemia is less likely when glucose is administered with amino acids than when it is infused alone. Amino acids exert a stimulatory effect on insulin release. Prevention of hyperglycemia is important because it can lead to diuresis and dehydration.

To prevent hyperglycemia in VLBW infants, glucose should be administered in small amounts. The **glucose load** is a function of the concentration of the dextrose infusion and the rate at which it is administered (Table 43-4). The administration of exogenous insulin may be necessary for infants with persistent or very high glycemia, but changes in the infant's blood glucose level are common problems associated with its use. In addition, protein synthesis may be inhibited by insulin administration in premature infants (Poindexter et al., 1998).

In general, preterm infants should receive an initial glucose load of less than 6 mg/kg/min, with a gradual increase to 11 to 12 mg/kg/min. ELBW infants tolerate a lower initial glucose load of 4 to 6 mg/kg/min. The glucose load can be advanced by 1 to 2 mg/kg/min/day. Hypoglycemia is not as common a problem as hyperglycemia, but it may occur if the glucose infusion is abruptly decreased or interrupted.

Amino Acids

Protein guidelines range from 2.7 to 3.5 g/kg/day (AAP, 2004). The ELBW infant may need 3.5 to 4 g/kg/day (Tsang et al., 2005, Poindexter and Denne, 2005). Protein in excess of these parenteral requirements should not be administered because additional protein offers no apparent advantage and increases the risk of metabolic problems. In practice preterm infants are usually given 1 to 2 g/kg/day of protein for the first few days of life, and then protein is provided as tolerated. Many nurseries will stock starter PN, which is water, glucose, protein, and perhaps calcium and is available 24 hours a day. Infants can then be provided with protein immediately on admission to the nursery.

In the United States several pediatric solutions are in use: Trophamine (B. Braun/McGaw, Inc.), Aminosyn PF (Abbott Laboratories), and Premasol (Baxter). The use of pediatric solutions results in plasma amino acid profiles similar to those of fetal and cord blood or to those of healthy infants fed breast milk (Poindexter and Denne, 2005). These solutions promote adequate weight gain and nitrogen retention. Standard amino acid solutions such as Aminosyn (Abbott

TABLE 43-3

Comparison of Parenteral and Enteral Energy Needs of Premature Infants

	Parenteral	Enteral
Maintenance		
Gradually increase intake to meet energy needs by the end of the first week	30-50 cal/kg/day	50 kcal/kg/day
Growth		
Meet energy needs as soon as the infant's condition is stable	90-100 cal/kg/day	105-130 kcal/kg/day

TABLE 43-4

Guidelines for Glucose Load in Premature Infants

Birth Weight (g)	Initial Load (mg/kg/min)*	Daily Increments (mg/kg/min)	Maximum Load (mg/kg/min)
<1000	4-6	1-2	11-12
1001-2000	<6	1-2	11-12

*Use the following formula to calculate glucose load: (% Glucose × ml/kg/day) × (1000 mg/g glucose) ÷ (1440 min/day). For example: (0.10 ×150 ml/kg/day) × (1000 mg/g glucose) ÷ (1440 min/day) = 10.4 mg/kg/min.

Laboratories), FreAmine (B. Braun/McGaw, Inc.), and Travasol (Baxter) were not designed to meet the particular needs of immature infants and may provoke imbalances in plasma amino acid levels. For example, cysteine, tyrosine, and taurine levels in these solutions are low relative to the needs of the preterm infant; but the methionine and glycine levels are relatively high. Because premature infants do not effectively synthesize cysteine from methionine because of decreased concentrations of the hepatic enzyme cystathionase, a cysteine supplement has been suggested. Cysteine is insoluble and unstable in solution; thus it is added as cysteine hydrochloride when the PN solution is prepared. In one study nitrogen retention was increased with cysteine supplementation, although this finding has not consistently been reported (Poindexter and Denne, 2005; Rivera et al., 1993). Metabolic acidosis can also occur with the use of cysteine hydrochloride, but it can be corrected by decreasing the dose of the supplement or by adding additional acetate to the solution.

In addition to plasma amino acid imbalances, other metabolic problems associated with amino acid infusions in preterm infants include metabolic acidosis, hyperammonemia, and azotemia. These problems can be minimized by using the crystalline amino acid products that are available and by keeping the protein load within the recommended guidelines (Table 43-5).

Lipids

Intravenous fat emulsions are used for two reasons: (1) to meet essential fatty acid (EFA) requirement; and (2) to provide a concentrated source of energy. EFA needs can be met by providing 0.5 to 1 g/kg/day of lipids. Biochemical evidence of EFA deficiency has been noted during the first week of life in VLBW infants fed parenterally without fat. The clinical consequences of EFA deficiency may include coagulation abnormalities, abnormal pulmonary surfactant, and adverse effects on lung metabolism.

Lipids should be introduced slowly in preterm infants, with periodic monitoring of plasma triglyceride levels, which ideally remain less than 150 mg/dl. Elevated plasma triglyceride levels may develop in infants with a decreased ability to hydrolyze triglycerides. This problem is most commonly associated with lower gestational age, SGA status, infection, surgical stress, and malnutrition. Under these conditions, close monitoring of serum triglyceride levels is indicated, and less than 3 g/kg/day of fat may be required. Once the infant is medically stable and additional energy is needed for growth, lipid loads can slowly be increased. Intralipids can be given to the infant with hyperbilirubinemia. At the present recommendation of 3g/kg/day, given over 24 hours, the displacement of bilirubin from albumin-binding sites does not occur (AAP, 2004).

Lipids should be administered over 24 hours at a maximum rate of 0.15 g/kg/hr to prevent a rise in triglycerides and free fatty acids. A daily increment of 0.5 to 1 g/kg/day is added until a rate of 3 g/kg/day is being provided (Table 43-6). The total lipid load is usually less than 30% to 40% of nonprotein calories, but it should not exceed 60% of nonprotein calories. (The lipid emulsions currently in use are described in Chapter 20.) In preterm infants 20% solutions providing 2 kcal/ml are recommended because plasma triglyceride, cholesterol, and phospholipid levels are generally lower with these than with the 10% emulsions. The lower plasma fat levels may be attributable to a decreased phospholipid load per gram of fat in the 20% emulsion.

Carnitine is frequently added to PN solutions provided to premature infants. Carnitine facilitates the mechanism by which fatty acids are transported across the mitochondrial membrane, allowing their oxidation to provide energy. Enhanced lipid use has been documented with carnitine supplementation in LBW infants receiving PN for longer than 1 month (Pande et al., 2005). Other short-term investigations have failed to show an improvement in fatty acid oxidation. When high doses of carnitine are provided, protein oxidation increases and the rate of weight gain decreases. Carnitine supplementation may be helpful for preterm infants who are receiving only PN at 2 to 4 weeks of age.

TABLE 43-5

Guidelines for Administration of Parenteral Amino Acids for Premature Infants

Initial Rate (g/kg/day)*	Increments (g/kg/day)	Maximum Rate (g/kg/day)
1.5-2	Advance to meet needs	3.5-4†

From Tsang RC et al: Summary of reasonable nutrient intakes. In Tsang RC: *Nutrition of the preterm infant*, ed 2, Cincinnati, Oh, 2005, Digital Educational Publishing, Inc.

*Use the following formula to calculate protein load:
% Protein × ml/kg/day = Protein g/kg/day.
For example: 2% amino acid parenteral solution provided at 150 ml/kg/day = 0.02 ×150 ml/kg/day = 3 g/kg/day.

†4 g/kg/day is recommended for infants weighing less than 1000 g.

TABLE 43-6

Guidelines for Administration of Parenteral Lipids for Premature Infants

Initial Rate (g/kg/day)*	Increments (g/kg/day)	Maximum Rate (g/kg/day)
0.5-1	0.5-1	3-4†

Tsang and colleagues (2005) recommend up to 4 g/kg/day of lipids.
From Tsang RC et al: Summary of reasonable nutrient intakes. In Tsang RC, editor: *Nutrition of the preterm infant*, ed 2, Cincinnati, Oh, 2005, Digital Educational Publishing, Inc.

*Use the following formula to calculate lipid load:
% Lipid × ml/kg/day = Lipid g/kg/day.
For example: 0.20 × 15 ml/kg = 3 g/kg/day.

†AAP (2004) recommends 3 g/kg/day. (American Academy of Pediatrics, Committee on Nutrition: Nutritional needs of preterm infants. In Kleinman RE, editor: *Pediatric nutrition handbook*, ed 5, Elk Grove, Ill, 2004, AAP.)

Electrolytes

After the first few days of life, sodium, potassium, and chloride are added to parenteral solutions to compensate for the loss of extracellular fluid. To prevent hyperkalemia and cardiac arrhythmia, potassium should be withheld until renal flow is demonstrated. In general, the preterm infant has the same electrolyte requirements as the term infant, but actual requirements vary, depending on factors such as renal function, state of hydration, and the use of diuretics (Table 43-7). Very immature infants may have a limited ability to conserve sodium and thus may require increased amounts of sodium to maintain a normal serum sodium concentration. Serum electrolyte levels should be monitored periodically. Urine electrolytes should be quantified when serum levels are abnormal to detect inappropriate electrolyte excretion.

Minerals

Calcium and phosphorus are important components of the PN solution. Premature infants who receive PN with low calcium and phosphorus concentrations are at risk for developing osteopenia of prematurity. This poor bone mineralization is most likely to develop in VLBW infants who receive PN for prolonged periods. Calcium and phosphorus status should be monitored using serum calcium, phosphorus, and alkaline phosphatase levels and radiographic bone studies.

Preterm infants have higher calcium and phosphorus needs than term infants. However, it is difficult to add enough calcium and phosphorus to parenteral solutions to meet these higher requirements without causing precipitation of the minerals. Calcium and phosphorus should be provided simultaneously in PN solutions. Alternate-day infusions are not recommended because abnormal serum mineral levels and decreased mineral retention develop.

Current recommendations for parenteral administration of additional calcium, phosphorus, and magnesium are presented in Table 43-8. The intakes are expressed per liter of solution, at a rate of 120 to 150 ml/kg/day, with 2.5 g of amino acids or protein. Lower fluid volumes or lower protein concentrations may cause the minerals to precipitate out of solution. The addition of cysteine hydrochloride increases the acidity of the fluid, which inhibits precipitation of calcium and phosphorus.

Trace Elements

Zinc should be given to all preterm infants receiving PN. If enteral feedings cannot be started by 2 weeks of age, additional trace elements should be added. However, the amounts of copper and manganese should be reduced for infants with obstructive jaundice; and the amounts of selenium, chromium, and molybdenum should be reduced in infants with renal dysfunction. Parenteral iron is not routinely provided because treated infants often receive blood transfusions soon after birth, and enteral feedings, which provide a source of iron, can often be initiated. The dosage for parenteral iron is approximately 10% of the enteral dosage; guidelines range from 0.1 to 0.2 mg/kg/day (Rao and Georgieff, 2005). Recommended guidelines have not yet been established for parenteral administration of fluoride to preterm infants (Table 43-9).

Vitamins

Shortly after birth all newborn infants receive an intramuscular injection of 0.5 to 1 mg of vitamin K to prevent hemorrhagic disease of the newborn from vitamin K deficiency. Stores of vitamin K are low in newborn infants, and little intestinal bacterial production of vitamin K occurs until bacterial colonization takes place. Because initial di-

---

TABLE 43-7

Guidelines for Administration of Parenteral Electrolytes for Premature Infants

Electrolyte	Amount (mEq/kg/day)
Sodium	2-4
Chloride	2-4
Potassium	1.5-2

TABLE 43-8

Guidelines for Administration of Parenteral Minerals for Premature Infants

Minerals	Amount (mg/kg/day)*
Calcium	80-100
Phosphorus	43-62
Magnesium	6-10

From American Academy of Pediatrics, Committee on Nutrition: Nutritional needs of preterm infants. In Kleinman RE, editor: *Pediatric nutrition handbook*, ed 5, Elk Grove, Ill, 2004, American Academy of Pediatrics.

*These recommendations assume an average fluid intake of 120 to 150 ml/kg/day with 2.5 g of amino acids per 100 ml. The amino acid concentration prevents the precipitation of these minerals.

TABLE 43-9

Guidelines for Administration of Parenteral Trace Elements for Premature Infants

Trace Elements	Amount (mcg/kg/day)
Zinc	400
Copper	20*
Manganese	1*
Selenium	2†
Chromium	0.2†
Molybdenum	0.25†
Iodine	1

From American Academy of Pediatrics, Committee on Nutrition: Nutritional needs of preterm infants. In Kleinman RE, editor: *Pediatric nutrition handbook*, ed 5, Elk Grove, Ill, 2004, AAP.

*Reduced or not provided for infants with obstructive jaundice.

†Reduced or not provided for infants with renal dysfunction.

etary intake of vitamin K may be limited, neonates would be at nutritional risk if they did not receive this intramuscular supplement.

Only intravenous multivitamin preparations currently approved and designed for use in infants should be given to provide the appropriate vitamin intake and prevent toxicity from additives used in adult multivitamin injections. The AAP (2004) recommends using the American Society of Clinical Nutrition's guideline of 40% of the MVI-Pediatric 5-ml vial per kilogram of weight. The maximum dose of 5 ml would be given to an infant with a weight of 2.5 kg (Greene et al., 1988) (Table 43-10).

Respiratory distress syndrome (RDS) is a disease that occurs in premature infants shortly after birth because these infants are deficient in the lung substance surfactant. Surfactant is responsible for keeping the lung elastic with breathing; thus surfactant supplements are given to the infant to prevent RDS or to lessen the illness. Lipids and proteins are components of surfactant, and phospholipids are the major lipid. Choline is required for phospholipid synthesis, but choline supplementation does not increase the production of phospholipids (van Aerde and Narvey, 2006). Choline is a conditionally essential nutrient because the infant can synthesize choline (see Chapter 5 for a discussion of requirement for choline in pregnancy). Choline is added to premature infant formulas at the level contained in human milk. The upper level is extrapolated from the adult safe level of intake (Klein, 2002).

Large supplemental doses of vitamin A have been suggested for the prevention of BPD because of the role of the vitamin in facilitating tissue repair and because of reports of preterm infants having low vitamin A stores. Several reports suggest that providing premature infants with intramuscular injections of vitamin A at 5000 units/day three times per week during the first month of life decreases the incidence of BPD (Tyson et al., 1999). However, more research is needed regarding dose toxicity (Darlow and Graham, 2002).

TABLE 43-10

Guidelines for Administration of Parenteral Vitamins for Premature Infants

	Preterm*
Percentage of one 5-ml vial of MVI-Pediatric†	40%/kg

*Data from American Academy of Pediatrics, Committee on Nutrition: Nutritional needs of preterm infants. In Kleinman RE, editor: *Pediatric nutrition handbook*, ed 5, Elk Grove, Ill, 2004, American Academy of Pediatrics.

Maximum volume intake is 5 ml/day, which is achieved at 2.5 kg body weight.

†MVI-Pediatric (5 ml) contains the following vitamins: 80 mg of ascorbic acid, 2300 USP units of vitamin A, 400 USP units of vitamin D, 1.2 mg of thiamin, 1.4 mg of riboflavin, 1 mg of vitamin B_6, 17 mg of niacin, 5 mg of pantothenic acid, 7 USP units of vitamin E, 20 mcg of biotin, 140 mcg of folic acid, 1 mcg of vitamin B_{12}, and 200 mcg of vitamin K.

TRANSITION FROM PARENTERAL TO ENTERAL FEEDING

It is beneficial to begin enteral feedings for preterm infants as early as possible because the feedings stimulate gastrointestinal enzymatic development and activity, promote bile flow, increase villous growth in the small intestine, and promote mature gastrointestinal motility. These initial enteral feedings can also decrease the incidence of cholestatic jaundice and the duration of physiologic jaundice and can improve subsequent feeding tolerance in preterm infants. At times small, initial feedings are used only to prime the gut and are not intended to optimize enteral nutrient intake until the infant demonstrates feeding tolerance or is clinically stable.

When making the transition from parenteral to enteral feeding, it is important to maintain parenteral feeding until enteral feeding is well established to maintain adequate net intake of fluid and nutrients. In VLBW infants it may take 7 to 14 days to provide a full enteral feeding, and it may take longer for infants with feeding intolerances or illness. The smallest, sickest infants usually receive increments of only 10 ml/kg/day. Larger, more stable preterm infants may tolerate increments of 20 to 30 ml/kg/day (see Chapter 20 for a more detailed discussion of transitional feeding).

NUTRITION REQUIREMENTS: ENTERAL FEEDING

Enteral alimentation is preferred for preterm infants because it is more physiologic than parenteral alimentation and is nutritionally superior. Initiating a tiny amount of an appropriate milk feeding whenever possible is beneficial. However, determining when and how to provide enteral feedings is often difficult and involves consideration of the degree of prematurity, history of perinatal insults, current medical condition, function of the gastrointestinal tract and respiratory status, and several other individual concerns (Table 43-11).

Preterm infants should be fed enough to promote growth similar to that of a fetus at the same gestational age but not so much that nutrient toxicity develops. Although the exact nutrient requirements are unknown for preterm infants, several useful guidelines exist. In general the requirements of premature infants are higher than those of term infants because the preterm infant has smaller nutrient stores, decreased digestion and absorption capabilities, and a rapid growth rate. Stress, illness, and certain therapies for illness may further influence nutrient requirements. It is also important to remember that, in general, enteral nutrient requirements are different from parenteral requirements.

Energy

The energy requirements of premature infants vary with individual biologic and environmental factors. It is estimated that an intake of 50 kcal/kg/day is required to meet

TABLE 43-11

Factors to Consider Before Initiating or Increasing the Volume of Enteral Feedings

Category	Factors
Perinatal	Birth asphyxia
Respiratory	Stability of ventilation, blood gases, apnea, bradycardia, cyanosis
Medical	Vital signs (heart rate, respiratory rate, blood pressure, temperature)
Gastrointestinal	Anomalies (gastroschisis, omphalocele), patency, gastrointestinal tract function (bowel sounds present, passage of stool), risk of necrotizing enterocolitis
Procedure	Pending intubation or extubation

Modified from Zerzan J, O'Leary MJ: Nutrition for preterm and low-birth-weight infants. In Trahms CM, Pipes PL, editors: *Nutrition in infancy and childhood*, ed 6, New York, 1997, WCB/McGraw-Hill.

maintenance energy needs, compared with 105 to 130 kcal/kg/day for growth (Table 43-12). However, energy needs may be increased by stress, illness, and rapid growth. Likewise, energy needs may be decreased if the infant is placed in a **neutral thermal environment** (the environmental temperature at which an infant expends the least amount of energy to maintain body temperature). It is important to consider the infant's rate of growth in relation to average energy intakes. Some premature infants may need at least 130 to 150 kcal/kg/day to sustain an appropriate rate of growth; ELBW infants or those with BPD often require such increased amounts. To provide such a large number of calories to infants with a limited ability to tolerate large fluid volumes, it may be necessary to concentrate the feedings to a level of more than 24 kcal/oz.

Protein

The amount and quality of protein must be considered when establishing protein requirements for the preterm infant. Amino acids must be provided at a level that meets demands without inducing amino acid or protein toxicity.

Amount

A reference fetus model has been used to determine the amount of protein that needs to be ingested to match the quantity of protein deposited into newly formed fetal tissue (Ziegler et al., 2002). To achieve these fetal accretion rates, additional protein must be supplied to compensate for intestinal losses and obligatory losses in the urine and skin.

Based on this method for determining protein needs, the advisable protein intake is 3.5 to 4 g/kg/day. This amount of protein is apparently well tolerated by stable infants who are growing rapidly. However, it may increase stress for sick infants who are not growing.

Type

The quality or type of protein is an important consideration because premature infants have different amino acid needs than term infants because of immature hepatic enzyme pathways. The amino acid composition of whey protein, which differs from that of casein (see Chapter 6), is more

TABLE 43-12

Estimation of the Energy Requirement of the Low-Birth-Weight Infant

Activity	Average Estimation (kcal/kg/day)
Energy expended	40-60
Resting metabolic rate	40-50*
Activity	0-5*
Thermoregulation	0-5*
Synthesis	15†
Energy stored	20-30†
Energy excreted	15
Energy intake	90-120

Modified from American Academy of Pediatrics, Committee on Nutrition: Nutritional needs of preterm infants. In Kleinman RE, editor: *Pediatric nutrition handbook*, ed 5, Elk Grove, Ill, 2004, AAP; Committee on Nutrition of the Preterm Infant, European Society of Paediatric Gastroenterology and Nutrition (ESPGAN): *Nutrition and feeding of preterm infants*, Oxford, 1987, Blackwell Scientific.

*Energy for maintenance.

†Energy cost of growth.

appropriate for premature infants. The essential amino acid cysteine is more highly concentrated in whey protein, and premature infants do not synthesize cysteine well. In addition, the amino acids phenylalanine and tyrosine are lower, and the preterm infant has difficulty oxidizing them. Furthermore, metabolic acidosis decreases with consumption of whey-predominant formulas. Because of the advantages of whey protein for premature infants, breast milk or formulas containing predominate whey proteins should be chosen whenever possible.

Taurine is a sulfonic amino acid that may be important for preterm infants. Human milk is a rich source of taurine, and taurine is added to most infant formulas. Term and preterm infants develop low plasma and urine concentrations of taurine without a dietary supply, but the clinical significance of this requires additional study.

Energy must be provided at sufficient levels to allow protein to be used for growth and not merely for energy expenditure. A range of 10.2% to 12.4% of calories from protein has been suggested. Inadequate protein intake is growth limiting, whereas excessive intake causes elevated plasma amino acid levels, azotemia, and acidosis.

Lipids

Amount

The growing preterm infant needs an adequate intake of well-absorbed dietary fat to help meet the high energy needs of growth, provide essential fatty acids, and facilitate absorption of other important nutrients such as the fat soluble vitamins and calcium. However, neonates in general, and premature and SGA infants in particular, digest and absorb lipids inefficiently.

The percentage of total calories as fat relative to carbohydrate and protein is another important consideration. Fat should constitute 40% to 50% of total calories. Furthermore, a diet that is high in fat and low in protein may yield more fat deposition than is desirable for the growing preterm infant. To meet essential fatty acid needs, linoleic acid should comprise 3% of the total calories, and α-linolenic acid should be added in small amounts (AAP, 2004). Additional longer-chain fatty acids—arachidonic acid (ARA) and docosahexaenoic acid (DHA)—are present in human milk and have recently been added to infant formulas for term and premature infants meeting the Food and Drug Administration's guidelines for amounts and sources. The premature infant has a greater need than the term infant for ARA and DHA supplementation. These fatty acids accumulate in fatty tissue and the brain during the last 3 months of gestation; thus the premature infant will have decreased fatty acid stores. Premature infants fed formulas supplemented with ARA and DHA from birth to 92 weeks' postmenstrual age (12 months after term) demonstrate greater gain in weight and length and higher psychomotor development scores than premature infants not receiving the fatty acid supplementation (Clandinin et al., 2005).

Type

Preterm infants have low levels of pancreatic lipase and bile salts, and this decreases their ability to digest and absorb fat. Lipases are needed for triglyceride breakdown, and bile salts solubilize fat for ease of digestion and absorption. Because medium-chain triglycerides (MCTs) do not require pancreatic lipase and bile acids for digestion and absorption, they have been added to the fat mixture in premature infant formulas.

Human milk and vegetable oils contain the EFA linoleic acid, but MCT oil does not. Premature infant formulas must contain vegetable oil and MCT oil to provide the essential long-chain fatty acids.

The composition of dietary fat also plays a role in the digestion and absorption of lipid. In general, infants absorb vegetable oils more efficiently than saturated animal fats, although one exception is the saturated fat in human milk.

Infants digest and absorb human milk fat better than the saturated fat in cow's milk or the vegetable oil in standard infant formulas. Human milk contains two lipases that facilitate fat digestion and has a special fatty acid composition that aids absorption.

Carbohydrates

Carbohydrates are an important source of energy, and the enzymes for endogenous production of glucose from carbohydrate and protein are present in preterm infants.

Amount

Approximately 40% of the total calories in human milk and standard infant formulas are derived from carbohydrates. Too little carbohydrate may lead to hypoglycemia, whereas too much may provoke osmotic diuresis or loose stools. The recommended range for carbohydrate intake is 40% to 50% of total calories.

Type

Lactose, a disaccharide composed of glucose and galactose, is the predominant carbohydrate in almost all mammalian milks and may be important to the neonate for glucose homeostasis, perhaps because galactose can be used for either glucose production or glycogen storage. Generally galactose is used for glycogen formation first, and then it becomes available for glucose production as blood glucose levels decrease. Because infants born before 28 to 34 weeks of gestation have low lactase activity, the premature infant's ability to digest lactose may be marginal. In practice, malabsorption is not a clinical problem because lactose is hydrolyzed in the intestine or fermented in the colon and absorbed. Sucrose is another disaccharide that is commonly found in commercial infant formula products. Because sucrase activity early in the third trimester is at 70% of newborn levels, sucrose is well tolerated by most premature infants. Sucrase and lactase are sensitive to changes in the intestinal milieu. Infants who have diarrhea, are undergoing antibiotic therapy, or are undernourished may develop temporary intolerances to lactose and sucrose.

Glucose polymers are common carbohydrates in the preterm infant's diet. These polymers, consisting mainly of chains of five to nine glucose units linked together, are used to achieve the isoosmolality of certain specialized formulas. Glucosidase enzymes for digesting glucose polymers are active in small preterm infants.

Minerals and Vitamins

Premature infants require the same vitamins and minerals as term infants, but poor body stores, physiologic immaturity, illness, and rapid growth increase their needs. Formulas and **human milk fortifiers** that are developed especially for preterm infants contain higher vitamin and mineral concentrations to meet the needs of the infant, obviating the need for additional supplementation in most cases (Table 43-13). The major exception is infants receiving human milk with a fortifier that does not contain iron. An iron supplement of 2 mg/kg/day should be sufficient to meet their needs (AAP, 2004).

TABLE 43-13

Recommendations for Enteral Administration of Vitamins for the Premature Infant

Vitamin	Amount (kg/day)
Vitamin A	700-1500 IU
Vitamin D	150-400 IU*
Vitamin E	6-12 IU
Vitamin K	8-10 mcg
Ascorbic acid	18-24 mg
Thiamin	180-240 mcg
Riboflavin	250-360 mcg
Pyridoxine	150-210 mcg
Niacin	3.6-4.8 mg
Pantothenate	1.2-1.7 mcg
Biotin	3.6-6 mcg
Folate	25-50 mcg
Vitamin B_{12}	0.3 mcg

From Tsang RC et al: Summary of reasonable nutrient intakes, In Tsang RC, editor: *Nutrition of the preterm infant,* ed 2, Cincinnati, Oh, 2005, Digital Educational Publishing, Inc.

*Maximum of 400 IU/day.

Calcium and Phosphorus

Calcium and phosphorus are just two of many nutrients that growing premature infants require for optimal bone mineralization. Intake guidelines have been established at levels that promote the bone mineralization rate that would occur in the fetus. An intake of 175 mg/100 kcal/day of calcium and 91.5 mg/100 kcal/day of phosphorus is recommended. Two thirds of the calcium and phosphorus body content of the term neonate is accumulated through active transport mechanisms during the last trimester of pregnancy. Infants who are born prematurely are deprived of this important intrauterine mineral deposition. With poor mineral stores and low dietary intake, preterm infants can develop **osteopenia of prematurity,** a disease characterized by demineralization of growing bones and documented by radiologic evidence of "washed-out" or thin bones. Very immature babies are particularly susceptible to osteopenia and may develop bone fractures or florid rickets with a prolonged dietary deficiency. Osteopenia of prematurity is most likely to develop in preterm infants who are (1) fed infant formula that is not specifically formulated for preterm infants; (2) fed human milk that is not supplemented with calcium and phosphorus; or (3) receiving long-term PN without enteral feedings.

Vitamin D

Human milk with human milk fortifier or infant formula for preterm infants provides adequate vitamin D when infants consume the entire calorie intake suggested. It was once common practice to provide 400 to 1000 IU/day of vitamin D as a supplement to prevent osteopenia of prematurity, but this was later shown to be ineffective. In fact, the current recommendations for intake range from 150 to 400 IU/day for preterm infants.

Vitamin E

Preterm infants require more vitamin E than term infants because of their limited tissue stores, decreased absorption of fat-soluble vitamins, and rapid growth. Vitamin E protects biologic membranes against oxidative lipid breakdown. Because iron is a biologic oxidant, a diet high in either iron or polyunsaturated fatty acids (PUFAs) increases the risk of vitamin E deficiency. The PUFAs are incorporated into the red blood cell membranes and are more susceptible to oxidative damage than when saturated fatty acids comprise the membranes.

A premature infant with vitamin E deficiency may experience **hemolytic anemia** (oxidative destruction of red blood cells). However, this anemia is uncommon today because of changes that have been made in infant formula composition. The fat blends in human milk and premature infant formulas now contain appropriate vitamin E/PUFA ratios for preventing hemolytic anemia. Preterm infants do not generally receive additional iron unless they are receiving recombinant erythropoietin therapy, and these infants should receive vitamin E supplementation of 15 to 25 IU/day (Ohls et al., 2001).

Because the dietary requirement for vitamin E depends on the PUFA content of the diet, the recommended intake of vitamin E is commonly expressed as a ratio of vitamin E to PUFA. The recommendation for vitamin E is 0.7 IU (0.5 mg of d-α-tocopherol) per 100 kcal, and at least 1 IU of vitamin E per gram of linoleic acid.

Pharmacologic dosing of vitamin E (50 to 100 mg/kg/day) has not proven to be helpful in preventing BPD or retinopathy of prematurity by reducing the toxic effects of oxygen. Furthermore, high doses of vitamin E have been associated with intraventricular hemorrhage, sepsis, necrotizing enterocolitis, liver and renal failure, and death.

Iron

Preterm infants are at risk for iron deficiency anemia because of the reduced iron stores associated with early birth. At birth most of the available iron is in the circulating hemoglobin. Thus frequent blood sampling further depletes the amount of iron available for erythropoiesis. Transfusions of red blood cells are often needed to treat the early physiologic anemia of prematurity. Recombinant erythropoietin therapy has been used to prevent anemia. Iron supplementation is indicated to facilitate red blood cell production, and a dosage of 6 mg/kg/day of enteral iron has been used (AAP, 2004). This therapy has not consistently prevented anemia and the need for blood transfusions (Ohls et al., 2001).

In general the recommendation for iron intake is 2 to 3 mg/kg/day. Infants fed human milk should be given ferrous sulfate drops beginning at 1 month of age. Formulas fortified with iron usually contain sufficient iron for preterm infants (AAP, 2004).

Folic Acid

Premature infants seem to have higher folic acid needs than infants born at term. Although serum folate levels are high at birth, they decrease dramatically, probably as a result of high folic acid use by the premature infant for deoxyribonucleic acid and tissue synthesis needed for rapid growth.

A mild form of folic acid deficiency causing low serum folate concentrations and hypersegmentation of neutrophils is not unusual in premature infants. Megaloblastic anemia is much less common. A daily folic acid intake of 25 to 50 mcg effectively maintains normal serum folate concentrations. Fortified human milk and formulas for premature infants meet these guidelines when full enteral feedings are established.

Sodium

Preterm infants, especially those with VLBW, are susceptible to hyponatremia during the neonatal period. These infants may have excessive urinary sodium losses because of renal immaturity and an inability to conserve adequate sodium. Furthermore, their sodium needs are high because of their rapid growth rate.

Daily sodium intakes of 4 to 8 mEq/kg or more may be required by some infants to prevent hyponatremia. Routine sodium supplementation of fortified human milk and infant formulas is not necessary. However, it is important to consider the possibility of hyponatremia and monitor infants by assessing serum or urinary sodium concentrations. Milk can be supplemented with sodium if repletion is necessary.

FEEDING METHODS

Decisions about breast-feeding, bottle-feeding, or tube-feeding depend on the gestational age and the clinical condition of the preterm infant. The goal is to feed the infant via the most physiologic method possible and supply nutrients for growth without creating clinical complications.

Gastric Gavage

Gastric gavage by the oral route is often chosen for infants who are unable to suck because of immaturity or problems with the central nervous system. Infants less than 32 to 34 weeks of gestational age, regardless of birth weight, may be expected to have poorly coordinated sucking and swallowing abilities because of their developmental immaturity. Consequently they have difficulty with nipple-feeding.

With the oral **gastric gavage** method, a soft feeding tube is inserted through the infant's mouth and into the stomach. The major risks of this technique include aspiration and gastric distention. Because of weak or absent cough reflexes and poorly developed respiratory muscles, the tiny infant may not be able to dislodge milk from the upper airway, which can cause reflex bradycardia or airway obstruction. However, electronic monitoring of vital functions and proper positioning of the infant during feeding minimize the risk of aspiration from regurgitation of stomach con-

tents. Gastric distention and vagal nerve stimulation with resultant bradycardia are potential problems when oral gastric gavage feedings are delivered on an intermittent bolus schedule. Occasionally elimination of the distention and vagal bradycardia requires the use of an indwelling tube for continuous gastric gavage feedings rather than intermittent administration of boluses. Continuous drip feedings are sometimes preferred for tiny, immature infants whose small gastric capacity and slow intestinal motility may impede the tolerance of large-volume bolus feeds. However, a randomized control trial was conducted with premature infants of 26 to 30 weeks of gestation to compare continuous and bolus feedings. Bolus feedings resulted in better weight gain and feeding tolerance than continuous infusion of feedings (Schanler et al., 1999b).

Nasal gastric gavage is sometimes better tolerated than oral tube feeding. However, because neonates must breathe through the nose, this technique may compromise the nasal airway in preterm infants and cause an associated deterioration in respiratory function. This method is helpful for infants who are learning to nipple-feed. An infant with a nasal gastric tube can still form a tight seal on the bottle nipple, but it can be difficult if an oral feeding tube is in place during feedings (see Chapter 20).

Transpyloric Feeding

Transpyloric tube-feeding is indicated for infants who are at risk for aspirating formula into the lungs or who have slow gastric emptying. The goal of this method is to circumvent the often slow gastric emptying of the immature infant by passing the feeding tube through the stomach and pylorus and placing its tip within the duodenum or jejunum. Infants with severe gastrointestinal reflux do well with this method, which prevents aspiration of feedings into the lungs. This method is also used for infants whose respiratory function is compromised and who are at risk for formula aspiration. The possible disadvantages of transpyloric feedings include decreased fat absorption, diarrhea, dumping syndrome, alterations of the intestinal microflora, intestinal perforation, and bilious fluid in the stomach. In addition, the placement of transpyloric tubes also requires considerable expertise and radiographic confirmation of the catheter tip location. Although associated with many possible complications, transpyloric feedings are used when gastric feeding is not successful (see Chapter 20).

Nipple-Feeding

Nipple-feeding may be attempted with infants whose gestational age is greater than 32 weeks and whose ability to feed from a nipple is indicated by evidence of an established sucking reflex and sucking motion. Before this time they are unable to coordinate sucking, swallowing, and breathing. Because sucking requires effort by the infant, any stress from other causes such as hypothermia or hypoxemia diminishes the sucking ability. Therefore nipple-feeding should be initiated only when the infant is under minimum stress and is sufficiently mature and strong to sustain the sucking effort. Initial oral feedings may be limited to one to three times per day to prevent undue fatigue or too much energy expenditure, either of which can slow the infant's rate of weight gain.

Before oral feedings begin, a standardized oral stimulation program can help infants successfully nipple-feed more quickly (Fucile et al., 2002). Healthy premature infants who are younger than 32 weeks of gestation may tolerate the introduction of one nipple-feeding per day (Simpson et al., 2002). This daily feeding can help infants learn and improve their oral feeding skills.

Breast-Feeding

When the mother of a premature infant chooses to breast-feed, nursing at the breast should begin as soon as the infant is ready. Before this time the mother must express her milk so that it can be tube-fed to her infant. These mothers need emotional and educational support for successful lactation. One study reports that premature breast-fed infants have better sucking, swallowing, and breathing coordination and fewer breathing disruptions than bottle-fed infants (Meier, 2001). Kangaroo baby care—allowing the mother to maintain skin-to-skin contact while holding her infant—facilitates her lactation. In addition, this type of contact promotes continuation of breast-feeding and enhances the mother's confidence in caring for her high-risk infant. The latter benefit may also apply to fathers who engage in kangaroo care with their infants (Meier, 2001).

Feeding infants with cups instead of bottles to supplement breast-feeding has been suggested for preterm infants based on the rationale that it may prevent infant "nipple confusion" (i.e., confusion between nursing at the breast and from a bottle). However, further study showed that it did not affect breast-feeding in the hospital, but there was an increase in the likelihood that these infants would be fully breast-fed at discharge and at home (Collins et al., 2004). Complications such as milk aspiration and low volume intakes need to be monitored.

Tolerance of Feedings

All preterm babies receiving enteral nutrition should be monitored for signs of feeding intolerance. Vomiting of feedings usually signals the infant's inability to retain the provided amount of milk. When not associated with other signs of a systemic illness, vomiting may indicate that feeding volumes were increased too quickly or are excessive for the infant's size and maturity. Simply reducing the feeding volume may resolve the problem. If it does not or if the infant has signs of a systemic illness, feedings may need to be interrupted until the infant's condition has stabilized. Bile-stained emesis may indicate that the infant has an intestinal blockage and needs additional evaluation or that the feeding tube has slipped into the intestine.

Abdominal distention may be caused by excessive feeding, organic obstruction, excessive swallowing of air, resuscitation, or sepsis (i.e., systemic infection). Observing infants for abdominal distention should be a routine practice for nurses. Abdominal distention often indicates the need to interrupt feeding until its cause is determined and the abdomen becomes soft and is not distended.

Gastric residuals, measured by aspiration of the stomach contents, should be determined routinely before each bolus gavage feeding and intermittently in all continuous drip feedings. Whether a residual amount is significant depends partly on its volume in relation to the total volume of the feeding. For example, a residual volume of more than 50% of a bolus feeding or equal to the continuous infusion rate might be a sign of feeding intolerance. However, when interpreting the significance of a gastric residual measurement, it is important to consider other concurrent signs of feeding intolerance and the previous pattern of residual volumes established for a particular infant. Bloody or bilious gastric residuals are more alarming than those that seem to be undigested milk.

The frequency and consistency of bowel movements should be constantly monitored when feeding preterm infants. Simple inspections can detect the presence of gross blood. However, occult blood is not always visible; a specific assay to detect small amounts of blood in the stool can be performed.

All feeding methods for preterm infants have associated complications. Unless close attention is paid to symptoms that indicate poor feeding tolerance, serious complications may ensue. Certain diseases can be recognized by recognizing signs of feeding intolerance. For example, **necrotizing enterocolitis** is a serious and potentially fatal disease associated with specific symptoms such as abdominal distention and tenderness, abnormal gastric residuals, and grossly bloody stools.

SELECTION OF ENTERAL FEEDING

During the initial feeding period premature infants may often require additional time to adjust to enteral nutrition feedings and may experience concurrent stress, weight loss, and diuresis. The primary goal of enteral feeding during this initial period is to establish tolerance to the milk being provided. When aggressive nutrition support is provided and expected to be tolerated from the onset of enteral feeding, the effort often fails. Infants seem to need a period of adjustment to be able to assimilate a large volume and concentration of nutrients. Thus enteral feedings often require supplementation with parenteral fluids until infants can tolerate adequate amounts of feedings by mouth.

After the initial period of adjustment, the goal of enteral feeding changes from establishing milk tolerance to providing complete nutrition support for growth and rapid organ development. All essential nutrients should be provided in quantities that support sustained growth. The following feeding choices are appropriate: (1) human milk supplemented with human milk fortifier and iron if the low-iron fortifier is used; (2) iron-fortified premature infant formula for infants who weigh less than 2 kg; or (3) iron-fortified standard infant formula for infants who weigh more than 2 kg.

Premature infants who are discharged from the hospital and going home can be given a transitional formula. Additional vitamins and iron supplements are not indicated with the use of this enriched formula. Breast-fed infants may be provided with two to three bottles of transitional formula daily to meet needs. The breast-fed premature infant should also receive 2 mg /kg/day of iron and a multiple vitamin for the first year of life (AAP, 2004). Premature infants discharged home on standard formula should receive a multivitamin until the infant reaches 3 kg in weight (AAP, 2004).

Human Milk

Human milk is the ideal food for healthy term infants and premature infants. Although human milk requires nutrient supplementation to meet the needs of premature infants, its benefits for the infant are numerous. During the first month of lactation, the composition of milk from mothers who have given birth to premature infants differs from that of mothers who have given birth to term infants; the protein and sodium concentrations of breast milk are higher in mothers with preterm infants (Klein, 2002). When premature infants are fed their own mother's milk, they grow more rapidly than infants fed banked, or mature, breast milk (Schanler et al., 2005).

In addition to its nutrient concentration, human milk offers nutritional benefits because of its unique mix of amino acids and long-chain fatty acids. The zinc and iron in human milk are more readily absorbed, and fat is more easily digested because of the presence of lipases. Moreover, human milk contains factors that are not present in formulas. These components include (1) live cells, macrophages, and T and B lymphocytes; (2) antimicrobial factors-secretory immunoglobulin A, lactoferrin, and others; (3) hormones; (4) enzymes; and (5) growth factors. The significance of many of these factors is currently being investigated. It has also been reported that human milk as compared to premature infant formula fed to preterm infants reduces the incidence of necrotizing enterocolitis and sepsis, improves neurodevelopment, facilitates a more rapid advancement of enteral feedings, and leads to an earlier discharge (Lucas et al., 1998; Schanler et al., 1999a).

However, one well-documented problem is associated with feeding human milk to preterm infants. Whether it is preterm, term, or mature, human milk does not meet the calcium and phosphorus needs for normal bone mineralization in premature infants. Therefore calcium and phosphorus supplements are recommended for rapidly growing preterm infants who are fed predominantly human milk. Currently three human milk fortifiers are available: Similac Natural Care (Ross Laboratories), which is available in liquid form, and Similac and Enfamil Human Milk Fortifiers (Ross Laboratories, Mead Johnson Nutritionals), which are available in powdered form. These contain calcium and phosphorus, as well as protein, carbohydrates, fat, vitamins, and minerals, and are designed to be added to expressed breast milk fed to premature infants (Table 43-14).

Providing human milk to a premature infant can be a very positive experience for the mother, one that promotes involvement and interaction. Because many preterm infants are neither strong enough nor mature enough to nurse at their mother's breast in the early neonatal period, their mothers usually express their milk for several days (and occasionally for several weeks) before nursing can be established. The proper technique of expression, storage, and transport of milk should be reviewed with the mother (see Chapter 5). Many summaries of the special considerations for nursing a preterm infant have been published (AAP and the American College of Obstetricians and Gynecologists [ACOG], 2006; Lawrence and Lawrence, 2005).

Premature Infant Formulas

Formula preparations have been developed to meet the unique nutritional and physiologic needs of growing preterm infants. The quantity and quality of nutrients in these products promote growth at intrauterine rates. These formulas, which have caloric densities of 20, 24, and 30 kcal/oz, are available only in a ready-to-feed form. These premature formulas differ in many respects from standard cow's milk–based formulas (see Table 43-14). The types of carbohydrate, protein, and fat differ to facilitate digestion and absorption of nutrients. These formulas also have higher concentrations of protein, minerals, and vitamins.

Transitional Infant Formulas

Formulas containing 22 kcal/oz have been designed as transition formulas for the premature infant. Their nutrient content is less than that of the nutrient-dense premature infant formulas and more than that of the standard infant formula (see Table 43-14). These formulas can be introduced when the infant reaches a weight of 1800 g or more, and they can be used throughout the first year of life. Not all premature infants need these formulas to grow appropriately. Infants who weigh less than 1250 g (2 lb, 11 oz) at birth and do not consume enough nutrients while hospitalized or cannot consume adequate amounts of standard formula to grow, may benefit from these formulas when discharged (Carver et al., 2001; Worrell et al., 2002). Transitional formulas are available in powder form for home use and in ready-to-feed form for use in hospitals.

Formula Adjustments

Occasionally it may be necessary to increase the energy content of the formulas fed to small infants. This may be appropriate when the infant is not growing quickly enough and is already consuming as much as possible during feedings.

Concentration

One approach to providing hypercaloric formula is to prepare the formula with less water, thus concentrating all its nutrients, including energy. Concentrated infant formulas with energy contents of 24 kcal/oz are available to hospitals as ready-to-feed nursettes. However, when using these concentrated formulas, it is important to consider the infant's fluid intake and losses in relation to the renal solute load of the concentrated feeding to ensure that a positive water balance is maintained. This method of increasing formula density is often preferred because the nutrient balance remains the same; infants who need more energy also need additional nutrients. As mentioned, the transitional formulas are available in ready-to-feed and powder form and can be concentrated from 24 to 30 kcal/oz. However, this formula is still inadequate for infants who need additional calcium (e.g., infants with osteopenia).

Recently a ready-to-feed 30 kcal/oz premature infant formula, Similac Special Care (Ross Laboratories), has become available. It meets the nutritional needs for premature infants who must be fluid restricted because of illness. This 30 kcal/oz formula can be diluted with Similac Special Care 24 to make 26, 27, or 28 kcal/oz milks. These milks are sterile and are the preferred source of providing concentrated milks to premature infants in the neonatal intensive care unit (NICU). Infant formula powder is not sterile and is not to be used with high-risk infants when a nutritionally adequate liquid, sterile product is available (Robbins and Beker, 2004).

Caloric Supplements

Another approach to increasing the energy content of a formula involves the use of caloric supplements such as corn oil, MCT oil (Mead Johnson Nutritionals), and glucose polymers such as Polycose (Ross Laboratories). These supplements increase the caloric density of the formula without markedly altering solute load or osmolality. However, they do alter the relative distribution of total calories derived from protein, carbohydrate, and fat. Because even small amounts of oil or carbohydrate dilute the percentage of calories derived from protein, adding these supplements to human milk or standard (20 kcal/oz) formulas is not advised. Caloric supplements should be used only when a formula already meets all nutrient requirements other than energy or when the renal solute load is a concern.

When a high-energy formula is needed, MCT oil and Polycose can be added to a base that has a concentration of 24 kcal/oz or greater (either full-strength premature formula or a concentrated standard formula), with a maximum of 50% of total calories from fat and a minimum of 9% of total calories from protein. For the infant who can tolerate long-chain fatty acids, an emulsified fatty acid product (Microlipid, Sherwood Medical) may be appropriate because it stays in solution better than the MCT oil or the corn oil, both of

---

TABLE 43-14

Comparison of the Nutritional Content of Human Milk and Formulas

	Human Milk	Fortified Human Milk*	Standard Formula†	Transitional Formula‡	Premature Formula§
Caloric density (kcal/oz)	20	24	20	22	20, 24, 30
Protein whey/casein ratio	70:30	Whey predominate	60:40, 48:52; 100:0	60:40, 50:50	60:40
Protein(g/L)	9	19-20	14-15	21	20, 24, 30
Carbohydrate	Lactose	Lactose, glucose polymers	Lactose or lactose and glucose polymers	Lactose, glucose polymers	Lactose, glucose polymers
Carbohydrate (g/L)	70	74-88	72-75	76-77	70, 84, 88
Fat	Human fat	Human fat, MCT oil	Vegetable oil	Vegetable oil, MCT oil	Vegetable oil, MCT oil
Fat (g/L)	35	39-45	34-36	39-41	37, 44, 67
Calcium (mg/L)	250	1150-1420	429-523	788-888	1105, 1440, 1830
Phosphorus (mg/L)	140	640-810	241-288	465-488	556, 800, 1010
Vitamin D (units/L)	13.2	1213-1513	402	525-592	1005, 1920, 1520
Vitamin E (units/L)	8	40-54	10-13.4	27-30	26.8, 50, 41
Folic acid (mcg/L)	140	370-390	101-107	188-192	248, 320, 375
Sodium (mEq/L)	11	18	7-8	11	13, 20, 19

Data from American Academy of Pediatrics and the American College of Obstetricians and Gynecologists: Breastfeeding infants with special needs. In Schanler RD et al., editors: *Breastfeeding handbook for physicians*, Evanston, Ill, 2006, AAP/ACOG; Nestle Infant Nutrition Nutrient Comparison Chart, 2004; Ross Laboratories Product Handbook (Internet) cited February 10, 2006, from http://www.ross.com/productHandbook/pedNut.asp; and Mead Johnson Product Handbook (Internet) cited February 10, 2006, from http://www.meadjohnson.com/professional/handbook.html.

*Based on the composition of term human milk fortified with either Enfamil or Similac Human Milk Fortifiers at four packets per 100 ml.

†Based on the composition of Enfamil, Lipil, Similac Special Care Advance, and Good Start Supreme formulas.

‡Based on the composition of Similac, NeoSure, Advance, Enfamil and EnfaCare formulas.

§Based on the composition of Enfamil, Premature Lipil, and Similac Special Care Advance formulas.

MCT, Medium-chain triglycerides.

which cling to the sides of the container. Adding fat at each feeding rather than mixing it with the daily supply of formula may prevent the oil from adhering to the storage container and thus not being taken in by the infant.

NUTRITION ASSESSMENT AND GROWTH

Dietary Intake

Dietary intake needs to be evaluated to ensure that the nutrition provided meets the infant's needs. Parenteral fluids and milk feedings are advanced as tolerated, and the nutrient intakes must be reviewed to ensure that they are within the guidelines for premature infants and that the infant is thriving on the nutrition provided. Appropriate growth and growth charts are reviewed in the following paragraphs.

Growth Rates and Growth Charts

All neonates typically lose some weight after birth. Preterm infants are born with more extracellular water than term infants and thus tend to lose more weight than term infants. However, the postnatal weight loss should not be excessive. Preterm infants who lose more than 15% to 20% of their birth weight may become dehydrated from the inadequate fluid intake or experience tissue wasting from poor energy intake. An infant's birth weight should be regained by the

second or third week of life. The smallest and sickest infants take the longest time to regain their birth weights.

During the first 98 days of life the Ehrenkranz growth chart is commonly used to assess weight progress (Ehrenkranz et al., 1999). This chart (Figure 43-3) longitudinally depicts daily weight changes and actual growth curves for 1660 infants who were born with a weight of 501 to 1500 g (1$\frac{1}{10}$ to 3$\frac{1}{3}$ lb). These infants received care in 12 different NICUs for various neonatal medical problems. Charts are also available for length, head circumference, and midarm circumference (Ehrenkranz et al., 1999) (see Useful Websites for a source to create a growth curve for an individual infant).

Intrauterine growth curves have also been developed using birth weight data of infants born at several successive weeks of gestation. However, these curves do not depict the initial period of postnatal weight loss and probably set unrealistic goals for preterm infants in the neonatal period. After an infant's condition stabilizes and the infant begins consuming all needed nutrients, the infant may be able to grow at a rate that parallels these curves. An intrauterine weight gain of 15 g/kg/day can be achieved before 38 weeks of gestation.

Although weight is an important anthropometric parameter, measurements of length and head circumference can also be helpful. A growth curve can be used to evaluate the adequacy of growth in all three areas (Figure 43-4). This chart has a built-in correction factor for prematurity, and the infant's growth can be followed from 22 to 50 weeks of

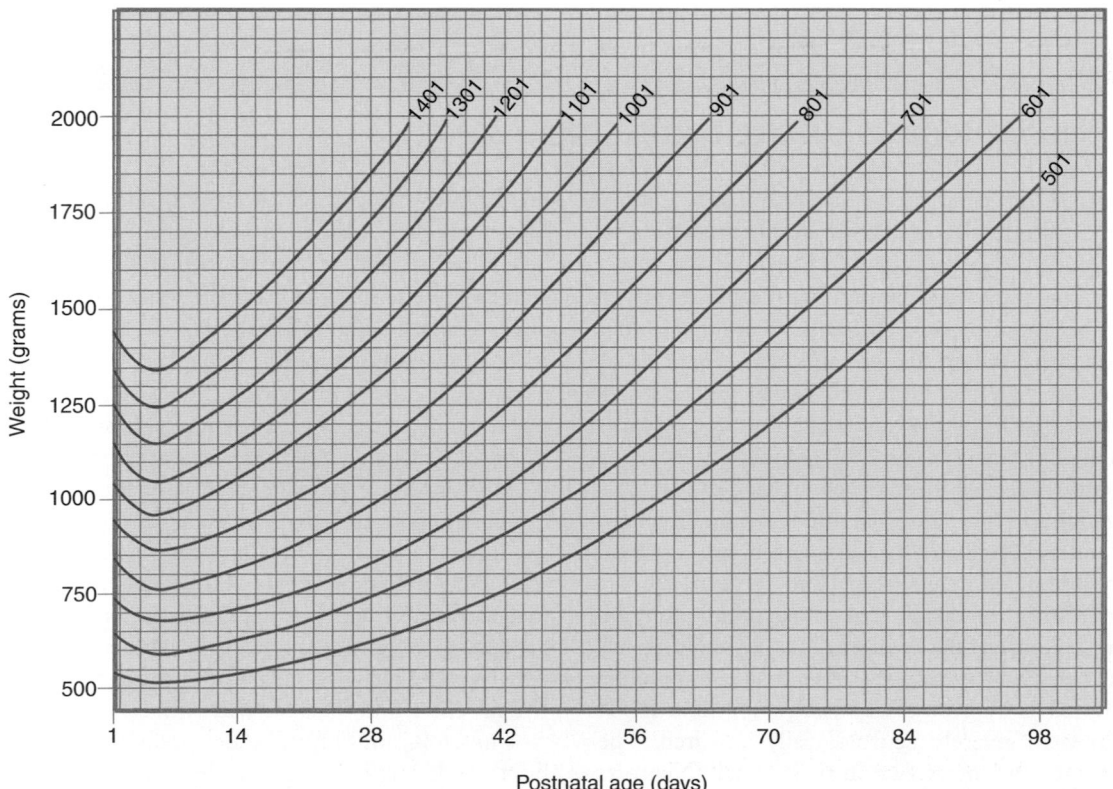

FIGURE 43-3 Weight chart for premature infants based on actual growth data. *(From Ehrenkranz RA et al: Longitudinal growth of hospitalized very–low-birth-weight infants, Pediatrics 104:283, 1999.)*

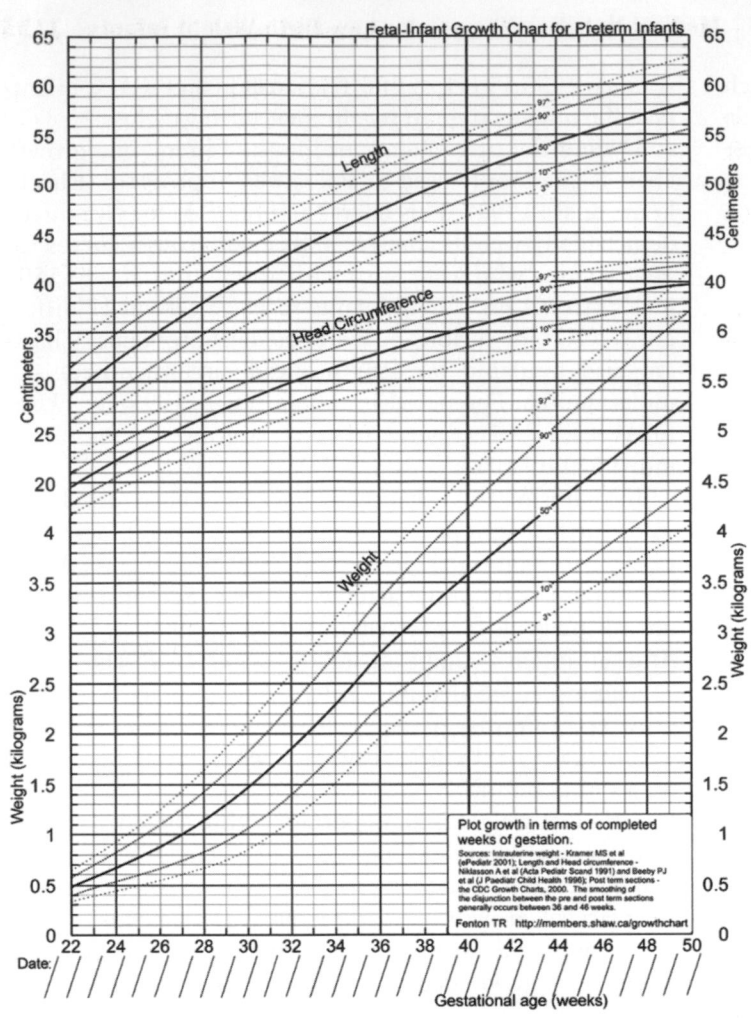

FIGURE 43-4 Example of a growth record of weight, length, and head circumference for infants from 22 to 50 weeks of gestation. This chart has a built-in correction factor for prematurity. *(From Fenton TR: A new growth chart for preterm babies: Babson and Benda's chart updated with recent data and a new format, BMC Pediatr 3:13, 2003.)*

◎ FOCUS ON

Long-Term Outcome for Premature Infants

As the survival of premature infants continues to improve, their physical growth, mental development, health, and quality of life are being investigated. Previously it was believed that, if premature infants experienced catch-up growth, it would only occur during the first few years of life. However, catch-up growth for weight, length, and head circumference can continue throughout childhood. Hack and colleagues (2003) reported that VLBW women catch up by 20 years of age but that VLBW men remain shorter and lighter.

Only recently have tools been developed and validated that assess how children report their health status and quality of life. Saigal and colleagues (2002) compared two groups of adolescents who ranged in age from 12 to 16 years. The first group included 150 children who were born prematurely with ELBW. The second group consisted of 122 children who were born at term and were not LBW infants. All children were interviewed in the same way except for nine ELBW children who were severely neurologically impaired. Their parents completed the interviews on their behalf. Neurosensory impairments were present in 24% of the children who were born prematurely and in 1.6% of the children born at term. The impairments included cerebral palsy, hydrocepha-

lus, cognitive impairments, autism, blindness, and deafness. Of the children who were preterm infants, 34% rated their health as "perfect" compared with 58% of the children who were born at term. Quality of life was also rated lower by the children who had been born prematurely. However, when the parents' scores for the nine adolescents with neurologic impairments were not included in the calculations, no difference was found between the two groups' assessments of their quality of life. Although children who were born prematurely may be more likely to have neurosensory impairments, they are optimistic about their quality of life. In addition, no difference was found between assessments of self-esteem by children who were born prematurely and children who were born at term (Saigal et al., 2002). Further evaluation showed that the two groups of children did not differ in their self-perception of behavior or social problems. Both groups reported to be active in school and social activities (Saigal et al., 2003).

Therefore not only are more premature infants surviving, but they also are growing into children who are enjoying their lives. The medical and nutrition care in the hospital nursery continues to progress, which improves outcome in the nursery and sets the stage for later development.

gestation. This chart represents cross-sectional data constructed from the anthropometric measurements taken at birth of infants born in Canada, Sweden, and Australia (Fenton, 2003).

The Centers for Disease Control and Prevention (CDC) 2000 Growth Charts from birth to 3 years of age can also be used for preterm infants after 40 weeks of gestation, as long as the age is adjusted (see *Focus On:* Long-Term Outcome for Premature Infants). For example, an infant born at 28 weeks of gestation is 12 weeks premature (40 weeks of term gestation minus 28 weeks of birth gestational age). Four months after birth, the growth parameters of a premature infant born at 28 weeks of gestation can be compared with those of a 1-month-old infant born at term (Box 43-2). When using growth grids, age should be adjusted for prematurity until at least 2½ to 3 years of corrected age. In Figure 43-5 A.R.'s pattern of growth is shown through 18 years of age. These charts are based on infants born with a birth weight greater than 1500 g (3⅓ lb). By using this chart, the infant's growth can be compared to the term infant to assess catch-up growth.

BOX 43-2

Steps for Adjusting Age for Prematurity on Growth Charts

Calculate the number of weeks the infant was premature:
- 40 weeks (term) − birth gestational age = number of weeks premature.
- The resulting number of weeks is the correction factor.

Calculate the adjusted age for prematurity:
- Chronologic age − Correction factor = Adjusted age for prematurity

For example:
40 weeks − 28 weeks of gestation = 12 weeks premature
Therefore 12 weeks (3 months) is the correction factor.
4 months (chronologic age) − 3 months (correction factor) = 1 month adjusted age

---

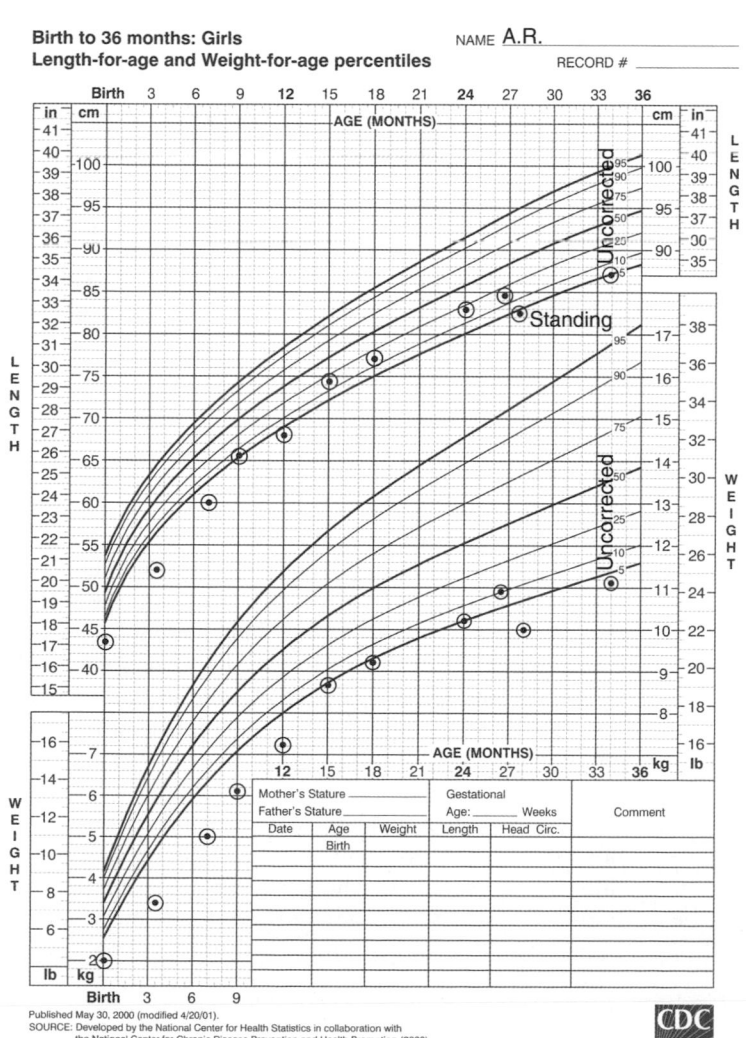

Birth to 36 months: Girls
Length-for-age and Weight-for-age percentiles
NAME A.R.
RECORD #

Published May 30, 2000 (modified 4/20/01).
SOURCE: Developed by the National Center for Health Statistics in collaboration with the National Center for Chronic Disease Prevention and Health Promotion (2000).
http://www.cdc.gov/growthcharts

FIGURE 43-5 A, Graphs showing how A.R. (from Figure 43-2), who was born at 27 weeks of gestation, grew after leaving the neonatal unit 1 day before her due date at a weight of 4½ lb. Heights and weights until age of 28 months are plotted on the grid at "corrected age" points and thereafter at "uncorrected age" points. A.R. experienced catch-up growth during the first 15 months. *Continued*

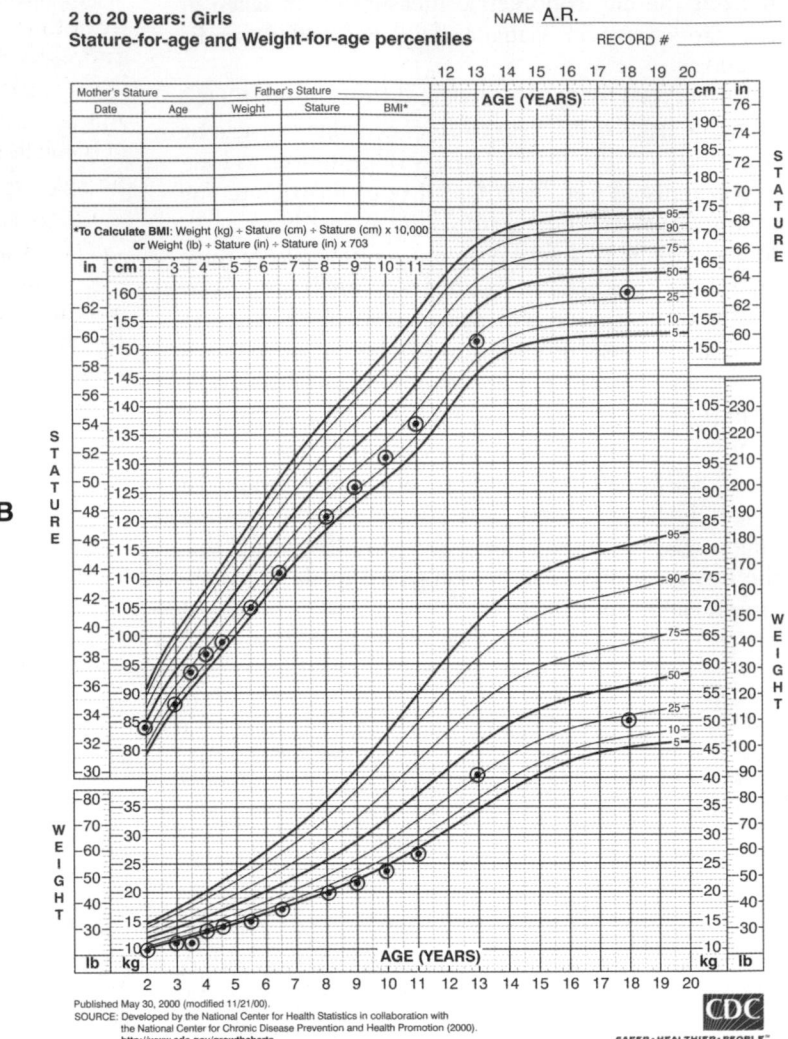

FIGURE 43-5, cont'd B, A.R.'s growth pattern from the age of 2 to 18 years. During the first 10 years she grew at the 5th percentile for weight and the 10th percentile for height. She followed her channel of growth but did not experience catch-up growth. However, between the ages of 10 and 13 she began to change growth channels and moved to the 25th percentile for weight and the 25th percentile for height (catch-up growth). At 18 years she crossed the 25th percentile for height and fell slightly below the 25th percentile for weight.

Laboratory Indices

Laboratory assessments usually involve measuring the following parameters: (1) fluid and electrolyte balance; (2) PN or EN tolerance; (3) bone mineralization status; and (4) hematologic status. In addition, serum protein, prealbumin, and retinol-binding protein levels may reflect recent changes in nutritional intake. However, these levels are also influenced by the infant's gestational age, illness, level of stress, and vitamin A and zinc status.

DISCHARGE CARE

Establishment of successful feeding is the pivotal factor determining whether a preterm infant can be discharged from the hospital nursery and go home. Preterm infants must be able to (1) tolerate their feedings and usually obtain all of their feedings from the breast or bottle; (2) grow adequately on a modified-demand feeding schedule (usually every 3 to 4 hours during the day for bottle-fed infants or every 2 to 3

hours for breast-fed infants); and (3) maintain their body temperature without the help of an incubator. In addition, it is important that any ongoing chronic illnesses, including nutrition problems, be manageable at home. Most important, the parents must be ready to care for their infant. In hospitals that allow parents to visit their infants in the nursery 24 hours a day, staff can help parents develop their caregiving skills and learn to care for their infant at home. Often, parents are permitted to "room in" with their infant (i.e., stay with the infant all day and night) before discharge, which helps build confidence in their ability to care for a high-risk infant (Figure 43-6).

Many preterm infants who are discharged from the hospital weigh less than 5½ lb. Although these infants must meet certain discharge criteria before they can go home, the stress of a new environment may lead to setbacks. Small preterm infants should be followed very closely during the first month after discharge, and parents should be given as much information and support as possible. Within the first week of discharge, a home visit by a

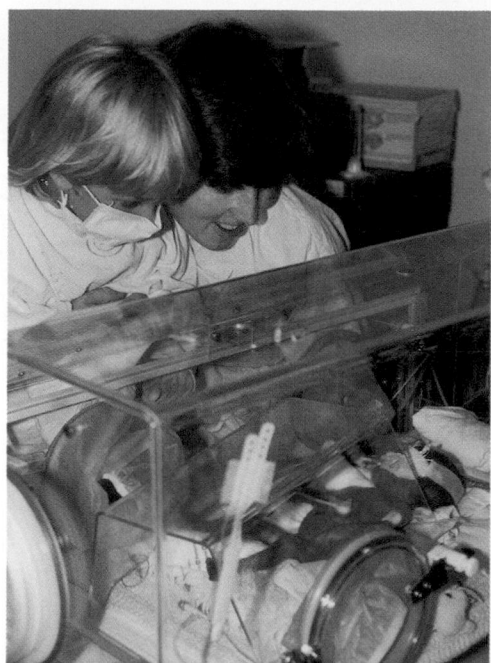

FIGURE 43-6 Family in the nursery with their premature infant.

nurse, nutritionist, or both and a visit to the pediatrician can be extremely helpful educationally; and they can provide early intervention for developing problems.

Factors that affect the feeding skills and behavior of preterm infants are particularly important after the infants have been discharged. Physical factors such as a variable heart rate, a rapid respiratory rate, and tremulousness are examples of physiologic events that interfere with feeding. In addition, infants weighing less than 5½ lb have poor muscle tone. Although muscle tone gradually improves as an infant becomes larger and more mature, it can deteriorate quickly in infants who are tired or weak. Feeding is often difficult for infants who have limited muscle flexion and strength and poor head and neck control, which are needed to maintain a good feeding posture. Positioning these infants in a manner that supports normal body flexion and ensures proper alignment of the head and neck during feedings may be helpful. Premature infants may also need their chin and cheeks supported while bottle-feeding.

Small infants tend to sleep more than larger and term infants. It is much easier for preterm infants to feed effectively if they are fully awake. To awaken a preterm infant, the caregiver should provide one type of gentle stimulation for a few minutes and then change to a different type, repeating this pattern until the infant is fully awake. Lightly swaddling of the infant and then placing him or her in a semi-upright position may also help.

The feeding environment should be as quiet as possible. Preterm infants are easily distracted and have difficulty focusing on feeding when noises or movements interrupt their attention. They also tire quickly and are easily overstimulated. When they are overstimulated, they may show only subtle signs of distress. It is important to teach parents of premature infants to recognize the subtle cues that indicate the need for rest or comfort and to respond to them appropriately.

After discharge, most preterm infants need approximately 180 ml/kg/day (2¾ oz/lb/day) of breast milk or standard infant formula containing 20 kcal/oz. This amount of milk provides 120 kcal/kg/day (55 kcal/lb/day). Alternatively transitional formula with a concentration of 22 kcal/oz can be provided at a rate of 160 ml/kg/day (or 2½ oz/lb/day). The best way to determine whether these amounts are adequate for individual infants is to compare their intake with their growth progress over time. Some infants may need a formula that provides 24 kcal/oz. As mentioned previously, powdered transitional formula can be readily altered to a concentration of 24 kcal/oz because ready-to-feed premature formulas providing 24 kcal/oz are higher in calcium and phosphorus than the concentrated formulas.

It is important to evaluate needs based on the three growth parameters: weight, length, and head circumference. Patterns of growth should be assessed to determine whether (1) individual curves at least parallel reference curves; (2) growth curves are shifting inappropriately across growth percentiles; (3) weight is appropriate for length; and (4) growth is proportionate in all three areas.

NEURODEVELOPMENTAL OUTCOME

It is possible to meet the metabolic and nutritional needs of premature infants sufficiently to sustain life and promote growth and development. In fact, more tiny premature infants are surviving than ever before because of adequate nutrition support and the recent advances in neonatal intensive care technology. There is concern that the ELBW infant is often smaller at discharge than the infant of the same postmenstrual age who was not born prematurely. Research in ongoing to see if nutrition interventions can promote catch-up growth without causing harm (Thureen and Heird, 2005).

The increased survival rate of VLBW infants has increased concerns about their short- and long-term neurodevelopmental outcomes. Many questions have been raised about the quality of life awaiting infants who receive neonatal intensive care. As a rule, VLBW infants should be referred to a follow-up clinic to evaluate their development and growth and begin early interventions (Wilson-Costello and Hack, 2006). The survival of ELBW infants has increased, with an increase in the number of children with neurodevelopmental disabilities, but also with an increase in the number of children who are developmentally normal (Wilson-Costello et al., 2006). Many of these premature infants reach childhood with no evidence of any disability (Figure 43-7).

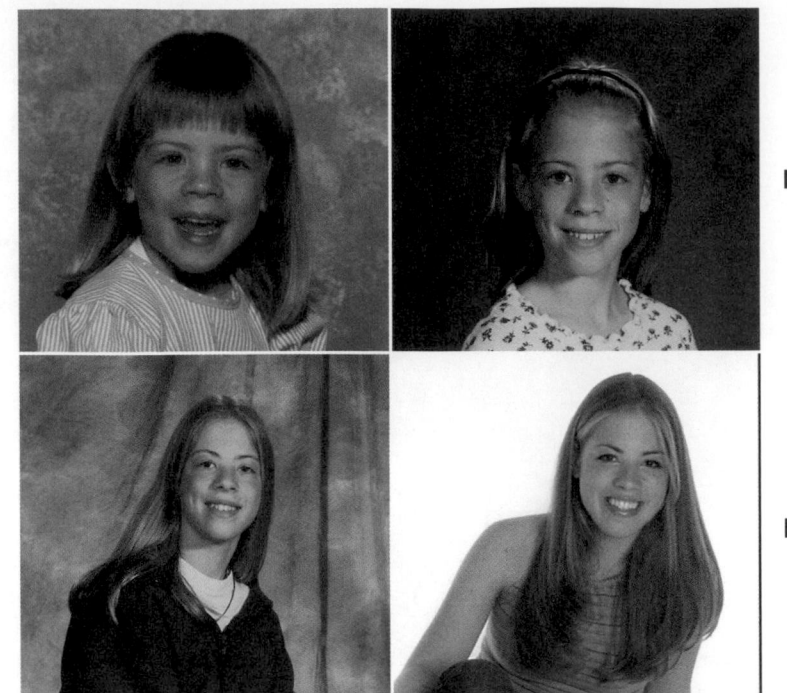

FIGURE 43-7 The premature infant A.R. (see Figures 43-2 and 43-6) as she grows up. **A,** 3½ years. **B,** 10 years. **C,** 14 years. **D,** 18 years. (*D Courtesy Yuen Lui Studio, Seattle, Wash.*)

◉ FOCAL POINTS

- Nutritional management of the LBW or premature infant is a dynamic process, as the nutritional needs change based on the rapid growth of the infant.
- Parenteral and enteral nutrition guidelines are used to feed these high-risk infants.
- Nutrition fortifiers for human milk and infant formulas, specially designed for the premature infant, help tremendously in meeting the large nutritional needs of these infants.

- Assessments and concerns for the neurodevelopmental outcome of premature infants reveal that the nutritional efforts provided help them reach adulthood in good health.

✱ CLINICAL SCENARIO 1

Sara, an infant born at 26 weeks of gestation, was admitted to the NICU. Her birth weight was 850 g (AGA). Sara had respiratory distress syndrome and had to receive a tube for mechanical ventilation. During the first few hours of her life, she was given surfactant, and her ventilator settings were lowered. She was also placed in a humidified incubator and given 100 ml/kg/day of starter PN ($D_{10}W$ with amino acids) intravenously. On the second day after her birth, she had gained 20 g, and her serum sodium concentration and urine volume output were low. She was diagnosed with a PDA and was given indomethacin to close the ductus arteriosus. On the fourth day after birth, her body weight had decreased 50 g—6% of her birth weight—and her serum electrolyte levels were normal. The protein concentration of her parenteral fluids was increased, as was the volume of intravenous fat being provided. By the sixth day, Sara was clinically stable. She began receiving feedings of milk from her mother—0.7 ml every 2 hours (10 ml/kg of her birth weight)—via bolus oral gastric tube. The feedings were tolerated well. She then began receiving 10 ml/kg/day of her mother's breast milk and less parenteral fluids. Full enteral feedings were established, and following extubation Sara was successfully breathing on her own.

✱ **Nutrition Diagnosis, Day 2:** Excessive fluid intake related to IV fluids as evidenced by gain of 20 g

✲ CLINICAL SCENARIO 1—cont'd

✲**Nutrition Diagnosis, Day 6+:** In adequate intake of protein and minerals related to need for HMF as evidenced by feeding only expressed breast milk.

1. On the second day after birth, should Sara's intravenous fluid volume have been (1) increased because she needed more calories; (2) decreased because she was overhydrated; or (3) changed to enteral feedings because she was clinically stable?

2. How should the intravenous fat that was given to Sara have been administered?
3. The breast milk from Sara's mother may have inadequate amounts of which nutrients? What do you recommend to resolve this?

✲ CLINICAL SCENARIO 2

Baby Jones was born at 29 weeks of gestation, and his birth-weight was 1400 g. He is now 1 week old or 30 weeks' postmenstrual age and weighs 1375 g. He is receiving parenteral nutrition at 130 ml/kg/day that contains 12.5% dextrose and 3.5% amino acids and a 20% intravenous fat emulsion at 15 ml/kg per day. The registered dietitian assesses the nutrient intake, and calculations are given below. The patient's intakes are compared to the parenteral guidelines of the AAP (2004) for premature infants.

Nutrient	Nutrient (kg/day)	Guidelines (kg/day)
Kilocalories kcal/ kg/day	103	90-100
Glucose mg/kg/min	11.3	4-12
Protein g/kg	4.6	1.5-4
Fat g/kg	3	0.5-4

✲**Nutrition Diagnosis:** Excessive protein intake (NI-52.2) related to protein intake 4.6 g/kg/day as evidenced by intake greater than recommendation of 3.5 g of protein per kilogram established by the AAP in 2004

1. The registered dietitian chooses the nutrition diagnosis and writes the PES statement (above). Interventions include decreasing the amino acid concentration to 2.7%, which will provide 3.5 g of protein per kilogram per day.
2. Monitor and evaluate infant's nutrition status in how many days?
3. What guidance is needed for the staff to evaluate for signs of dehydration?

USEFUL WEBSITES

American Academy of Pediatrics
www.aap.org

Fenton Growth Chart
http://members.shaw.ca/growthchart/

National Center for Education in Maternal and Child Health
www.ncemch.org

National Institute of Child Health and Human Development (NICHD), Neonatal Research Network

Growth Charts
http://neonatal.rti.orgs

References

American Academy of Pediatrics and the American College of Obstetricians and Gynecologists: Breastfeeding infants with special needs. In Schanler RD et al., editors: *Breastfeeding handbook for physicians*, Evanston, Ill, 2006, American Academy of Pediatrics.

American Academy of Pediatrics, Committee on Nutrition: Nutritional needs of preterm infants. In Kleinman RE, editor: *Pediatric nutrition handbook*, ed 5, Elk Grove, Ill, 2004, American Academy of Pediatrics.

Ballard JL et al: New Ballard score, expanded to include extremely premature infants, *J Pediatr* 119:417, 1991.

Carver JD et al: Growth of preterm infants fed nutrient-enriched or term formula after hospital discharge, *Pediatrics* 107:683, 2001.

Clandinin MT et al: Growth and development of preterm infants fed infant formulas containing docosahexaenoic acid and arachidonic acid, *J Pediatr* 146:461, 2005.

Collins CT et al: Effect of bottles, cups, and dummies on breast feeding in preterm infants: a randomized controlled trial, *Br Med J* 329: 193, 2004.

Darlow BA, Graham PJ: Vitamin A supplementation for preventing morbidity and mortality in very low birthweight infants, 2002, www.nichd.nih.gov/cochraneneonatal/, accessed August 1, 2006.

Dell KM, Davis ID: Fluid, electrolyte, and acid-base homeostasis. In Martin RJ et al, editors: *Neonatal-perinatal medicine diseases of the fetus and infant*, ed 8, Philadelphia, 2006, Mosby.

Ehrenkranz RA et al: Longitudinal growth of hospitalized very low birth weight infants, *Pediatrics* 104:280, 1999.

Fenton TR: A new growth chart for preterm babies: Babson and Benda's chart updated with recent data and a new format, *BMC Pediatrics* 3:13, 2003.

Fucile S et al: Oral stimulation accelerates the transition from tube to oral feeding in preterm infants, *J Pediatr* 141:230, 2002.

Greene HL et al: Guidelines for the use of vitamins, trace elements, calcium, magnesium, and phosphorus in infants and children receiving total parenteral nutrition: report of the Subcommittee on Pediatric Parenteral Nutrient Requirements from the Committee on Clinical Practice Issues of the American Society for Clinical Nutrition, *Am J Clin Nutr* 48(5):1324, 1988.

Hack M et al: Growth of very low birth weight infants to age 20 years, *Pediatrics* 112:e30, 2003.

Hoyert DL et al: Annual summary of vital statistics: 2004, Pediatrics 117:168, 2006.

Klein CJ, editor: Nutrient requirements for preterm infant formula, *J Nutr* 132:1395S, 2002.

Lawrence RA, Lawrence RM: Breastfeeding the premature infant. In *Breastfeeding: a guide for the medical profession*, ed 6, Philadelphia, 2005, Mosby.

Lucas A et al: Randomised trial of early diet in preterm babies and later intelligence quotients, *Br Med J* 317:1481, 1998.

MacDorman MF et al: Explaining the 2001-2002 infant mortality increase in the United States: data from the linked birth/infant death data set, *Int J Health Ser* 35:415, 2005.

Meier PP: Breastfeeding in the special care nursery: prematures and infants with medical problems, *Pediatr Clin North Am* 48:425, 2001.

Nakamura MU et al: Obstetric and perinatal effects of active and/ or passive smoking during pregnancy, *Sao Paulo Med J* 122:94, 2004.

Ohls RK et al: Effects of early erythropoietin therapy on the transfusion requirements of preterm infants below 1250 grams birth weight: a multicenter, randomized, controlled trial, *Pediatrics* 108:934, 2001.

Pande S et al: Lack of effect of L-carnitine supplementation on weight gain in very preterm infants, *J Perinatol* 25:470, 2005.

Poindexter BB, Denne SC: Parenteral nutrition. In Martin RJ et al, editors: *Neonatal-perinatal medicine diseases of the fetus and infant*, ed 8, Philadelphia, 2006, Mosby.

Poindexter BB et al: Exogenous insulin reduces proteolysis and protein synthesis in extremely low birth weight infants, *J Pediatr* 132:948, 1998.

Rao R, Georgieff M: Microminerals. In Tsang RC et al, editors: *Nutrition of the preterm infant*, ed 2, Cincinnati, Oh, 2005, Digital Educational Publishing, Inc.

Rivera A et al: Effects of intravenous amino acids on protein metabolism of preterm infants during the first three days of life, *Pediatr Res* 33:106, 1993.

Robbins ST, Beker LT, editors: *Infant feedings: guidelines for preparation of formula and breastmilk in health care facilities*, Chicago, 2004, American Dietetic Association.

Saigal S et al: Self-esteem of adolescents who were born prematurely, *Pediatrics* 109:429, 2002.

Saigal S et al: Psychopathology and social competencies of adolescents who were extremely low birth weight, *Pediatrics* 111:969, 2003.

Schanler RJ et al: Feeding strategies for premature infants: randomized trial of gastrointestinal priming and tube-feeding method, *Pediatrics* 103:434, 1999a.

Schanler RJ et al: Feeding strategies for premature infants: beneficial outcomes of feeding fortified human milk versus preterm formula, *Pediatrics* 103:1150, 1999b.

Schanler RJ et al: Randomized trial of donor human milk versus preterm formula as substitutes for mothers' own milk in feeding of extremely premature infants, *Pediatrics* 116:400, 2005.

Simpson C et al: Early introduction of oral feeding in preterm infants, *Pediatrics* 110:517, 2002.

Thureen PJ, Heird WC: Protein and energy requirements of the preterm/low birthweight (LBW) infant, *Pediatr Res* 57:95R, 2005.

Thureen PJ et al: Effect of low versus high intravenous amino acid intake on very low birth weight infants in the early neonatal period, *Pediatr Res* 53:24, 2003.

Tsang RC et al: Summary of reasonable nutrient intakes. In Tsang RC, editor: *Nutrition of the preterm infant*, ed 2, Cincinnati, Oh, 2005, Digital Educational Publishing, Inc.

Tyson JE et al: Vitamin A supplementation for extremely-low-birth-weight infants, *N Eng J Med* 340:1962, 1999.

van Aerde JE, Narvey M: Acute respiratory failure. In Thureen PJ, Hay WW, editors: *Neonatal nutrition and metabolism*, ed 2, Cambridge, 2006, Cambridge University Press.

Wilson-Costello DE, Hack M: Follow-up for high-risk neonates. In Fanaroff AA, Martin RJ, editors: *Neonatal-perinatal medicine diseases of the fetus and infant*, vol 2, ed 8, Philadelphia, 2006, Mosby.

Wilson-Costello DE et al: Improved survival rates with increased neurodevelopmental disability for extremely low birth weight infants in the 1990s, *Pediatrics* 115:997, 2006.

Worrell LA et al: The effects of the introduction of a high-nutrient transitional formula on growth and development of very-low-birth-weight infant, *J Perinatol* 22:112, 2002.

Ziegler EE et al: Aggressive nutrition of the very low birth weight infant, *Clin Perinatol* 29:225, 2002.

CHAPTER 44

Cristine M. Trahms, MS, RD, CD, FADA
Beth N. Ogata, MS, RD, CD

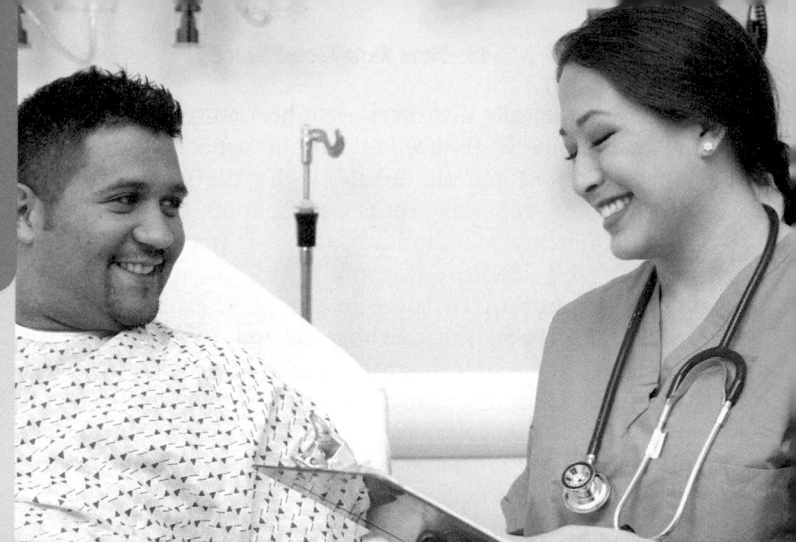

Medical Nutrition Therapy for Genetic Metabolic Disorders

KEY TERMS

argininosuccinic aciduria (ASA) the presence of argininosuccinic acid in the blood and urine as a result of argininosuccinate lyase deficiency

autosomal-recessive a trait (or genetic condition) that appears only when an individual has received two copies of a gene that is not on a sex chromosome

carbamyl-phosphate synthetase (CPS) deficiency a defect in urea cycle metabolism that causes hyperammonemia and elevated plasma glycine

L-carnitine a substance that functions as a carrier of fatty acids across the mitochondrial membranes; also competes with organic acids for excretion via the kidney

citrullinemia elevated citrulline in the blood and urine secondary to a deficiency of argininosuccinic acid synthetase in the metabolism of citrulline to argininosuccinic acid

galactosemia a disturbance in the conversion of galactose to glucose because of the absence of the enzyme galactokinase or galactose-1-phosphate uridyl transferase

genetic metabolic disorders inborn errors of metabolism

gluconeogenesis the formation of glucose from noncarbohydrate molecules, such as glycerol, and the carbon skeletons of amino acids

glycogen storage diseases a group of inherited disorders of glycogen metabolism, such as glycogenolysis, in which an enzyme deficiency causes glycogen to accumulate in abnormally large amounts in various parts of the body, especially the liver

glycogenolysis the breakdown of glycogen to glucose

ketone utilization disorder possibly mitochondrial 2-methylacetoacetyl-CoA thiolase deficiency; a disorder of isoleucine and ketone body metabolism

long-chain 3-hydroxyacyl-CoA dehydrogenase deficiency (LCHAD) a disorder of long-chain fatty acid oxidation

maple syrup urine disease (MSUD) or **branched-chain ketoaciduria** an autosomal-recessive metabolic defect in decarboxylation that affects the metabolism of branched-chain amino acids

medium-chain acyl-CoA dehydrogenase deficiency (MCAD) a disorder of medium-chain fatty acid oxidation

methylmalonic acidemia an excess of methylmalonic acid in the blood and urine because of a defect of methylmalonyl-CoA mutase or other similar enzyme

ornithine transcarbamylase (OTC) deficiency an X-linked recessive disorder in the conversion of ornithine and carbamyl-phosphate to citrulline; usually lethal in males

phenylketonuria (PKU) hyperphenylalaninemia in which phenylalanine is not metabolized to tyrosine because of a deficiency of phenylalanine hydroxylase

propionic acidemia an excess of propionic acid in the blood secondary to defective propionyl-CoA reductase

Genetic metabolic disorders are inherited traits that result in the absence or reduced activity of a specific enzyme or cofactor. Most genetic metabolic disorders are inherited as **autosomal-recessive** traits (see Chapter 13). The treatment for many metabolic disorders is medical nutrition therapy and medications specific to the disorder (e.g., phenylketonuria). In some instances when treatment is initiated early in the newborn period and meticulously continued for a lifetime, the affected individual usually is cognitively and physically normal. In other instances, for example galactosemia, treatment when meticulously applied early and continued does not always prevent cognitive and physical damage.

It is important to remember that biochemical disorders vary from normal variations in enzyme activity that are benign and do not require intervention to severe manifestations that are incompatible with life. For many of the metabolic disorders, significant questions related to diagnosis and treatment still need to be answered.

niques and treatment modalities, have improved the outcome for many of these infants.

Infants suspected of having a metabolic disorder should be afforded access to care offered by centers with expertise in treating these disorders. Infants who are afebrile for no apparent reason, lethargic, vomiting, in respiratory distress, or having seizures should be evaluated for an undiagnosed metabolic disorder. The initial assessment should include blood gas measurements, electrolyte values, glucose and ammonia tests, and a urine test for ketones.

Advances in newborn screening technology have offered opportunities for earlier diagnosis, prevention of neurologic crisis, and improved intellectual and physical outcomes. When tandem mass spectrometry techniques are used in newborn screening laboratories, infants with a broader range of metabolic disorders can be identified, and the disorder can be identified earlier (see *New Directions*: Newborn Screening).

NEWBORN SCREENING

Most inherited metabolic disorders are associated with severe clinical illness that often appears soon after birth. Mental retardation and severe neurologic involvement may be quickly apparent. Diagnosis of a specific disorder may be difficult, and appropriate treatment measures may be uncertain. Prenatal diagnosis is available for many metabolic disorders, but it usually requires the identification of a family at risk, which can be done only after the birth of an affected child. However, effective newborn screening programs, as well as advanced diagnostic techniques and treatment modalities, have improved the out-

GENERAL GOALS OF MEDICAL NUTRITION THERAPY

The goals of medical nutrition therapy for metabolic disorders are to maintain biochemical equilibrium for the affected pathway, provide adequate nutrients to support typical growth and development, and support social and emotional development. Nutrition interventions are designed to circumvent the missing or inactive enzyme by (1) restricting the amount of substrate available; (2) supplementing the amount of product; (3) supplementing the enzymatic cofactor; or (4) combining any or all of these approaches (Table 44-1).

⇄ NEW DIRECTIONS

Newborn Screening

Since the 1960s states across the United States have adopted mandatory newborn screening (NBS) as law (Waisbren, 2006). These programs were developed as a result of the efficacy of the Guthrie bacterial inhibition assay, in which dried blood spots were assayed. This simple, sensitive, and inexpensive screening test became the basis for population-based screening systems for newborns. Hemoglobinopathies, endocrine disorders, metabolic disorders, and some infectious disorders can be effectively identified in this way (Albers et al., 2001). In the 1990s tandem mass spectrometry (MS/MS) began to be used in NBS across the United States and as of 2004 was used by 35 states (Schoen, 2002). This technology makes it possible to identify multiple disorders from dried blood spots.

The number of disorders screened for varies widely by state, and expanded screening is also offered by private, for-

profit companies. Follow-up programs also vary; some states have a centralized program, whereas follow-up in other states is less coordinated. Successful early NBS programs include screening for congenital hypothyroidism, phenylketonuria, congenital adrenal hyperplasia, galactosemia, sickle cell disease, and maple syrup urine disease (Brosco et al., 2006). The Maternal and Child Health Bureau (MCHB) of the U.S. Health Resources and Services Administration commissioned a report from the American College of Medical Genetics. This expert panel identified 29 conditions for which newborn screening should be mandated and 25 secondary conditions that may be detected incidentally (MCHB, 2007). Other groups, including the World Health Organization, March of Dimes, and Massachusetts Newborn Screening Advisory Committee, have also issued recommendations.

Newborn Screening—cont'd

Providers who may be involved in the care and follow-up of families identified by NBS should have a good understanding of their state's system, as well as the factors that may affect results. Communication among families, primary health care providers, and tertiary clinics is critical to timely identification and treatment. Follow-up, including referral to the appropriate specialists, is important for any family who receives NBS test results. NBS fact sheets have been revised by the Committee on Genetics of the American Academy of Pediatrics regarding (1) newborn testing; (2) follow-up of abnormal screening results to facilitate timely diagnostic testing and management; (3) diagnostic testing; (4) disease management, which requires coordination with the medical home and genetic counseling; and (5) continuous evaluation and improvement of the NBS system (Kaye et al., 2006).

Further Thought

What are the disorders identified by newborn screening in your state?

What are the differences between screening and diagnostic tests?

What is the system for follow-up of presumptive positive results in your state?

DISORDERS OF AMINO ACID METABOLISM

Nutrition therapy for amino acid disorders most commonly consists of substrate restriction, which involves limiting one or more essential amino acids to the minimum requirement while providing adequate energy and nutrients to promote typical growth and development (e.g., restricting phenylalanine in phenylketonuria). An inadequate intake of an essential amino acid is often as detrimental as excess. Supplementation of the product of the specific enzymatic reaction is usually required in nutrition therapy for amino acid disorders; for example, tyrosine is supplemented in formulas for treatment of phenylketonuria.

Requirements for individual amino acids are difficult to determine because typical growth and development can be achieved over a wide range of intake. The data of Holt and Snyderman (1967) are often used as the basis for prescribing amino acid intakes (Table 44-2). Careful and frequent monitoring is required to ensure the adequacy of the nutritional prescription (Acosta and Yannicelli, 1994). Although nitrogen studies would be the most precise, weight gain in infants is a sensitive and easily monitored index of well-being and nutrition adequacy.

Phenylketonuria

Of the amino acid disorders, phenylketonuria provides a reasonable model for detailed discussion because it (1) occurs relatively frequently and most neonates are screened for it; (2) has a predictable course, with the greatest available documentation of "natural" and "intervention" history (see *Focus On*: Time Line of Events in the Diagnosis and Treatment of Phenylketonuria); and (3) has a successful medical nutrition therapy.

Phenylketonuria (PKU) is the most common of the hyperphenylalaninemias. In this disorder phenylalanine (Phe) is not metabolized to tyrosine (Tyr) because of a deficiency or inactivity of phenylalanine hydroxylase, as shown in Figure 44-1. Nutritional treatment involves restricting the substrate (Phe) and supplementing the product (Tyr) (see *Pathophysiology and Care Management Algorithm*: Phenylketonuria on p. 1150). Most affected infants exhibit phenylalanine hydroxylase deficiency; the remainder (less than 3%) have defects in associated pathways. Low-Phe nutrition therapy does not prevent the neurologic deterioration present in the disorders of associated pathways.

Diagnostic Criteria and Outcome

All states have newborn screening programs for PKU and other metabolic disorders. Diagnostic criteria for PKU include blood concentrations of Phe that consistently exceed 6 to 10 mg/dl (360 to 600 μmol/L) and Tyr concentrations of less than 3 mg/dl (165 μmol/L). The diagnostic process should also include evaluation for hyperphenylalaninemia that results from the deficiency of enzymes other than phenylalanine hydroxylase.

Outcome, measured in terms of intelligence quotient (IQ) attainment or intellectual function, depends on the age of the infant at diagnosis and start of nutrition therapy, as well as the individual's biochemical control over time. Because infants with PKU (i.e., phenylalanine hydroxylase deficiency) do not manifest any clinical signs of abnormality in the immediate postnatal period, the age of the infant at diagnosis and start of nutrition therapy depend on the effectiveness of the screening program and an organized follow-up program.

The advantage of rigorous nutrition therapy has been demonstrated by measurements of intellectual function. Individuals who do not receive diet therapy are severely mentally retarded (mean IQ of about 40), whereas individuals who are on therapy from the early neonatal period have IQs in the normal range of intellectual function (NIH, 2001).

Tetrahydrobiopterin (BH$_4$) has been studied to evaluate its effectiveness as an alternative treatment to severe dietary

Text continues on p. 1148

TABLE 44-1

Selected Genetic Metabolic Disorders That Respond to Dietary Treatment

Disorder	Affected Enzyme	Prevalence	Clinical/Biochemical Features	Medical Nutrition Therapy Diet Therapy	Medical Nutrition Therapy Adjunct Treatment
Urea Cycle Disorders					
Carbamyl-phosphate synthetase deficiency	Carbamyl-phosphate synthetase	1:30,000 (all UCDs)	Vomiting; seizures; sometimes, coma → death. Survivors usually have MR. ↑ Plasma ammonia, glutamine	Food: low protein Formula: without nonessential amino acids	L-carnitine, phenylbutyrate,* L-citrulline, L-arginine Hemodialysis or peritoneal dialysis during acute episodes
Ornithine transcarbamylase deficiency	Ornithine transcarbamylase (x-linked)	1:30,000 (all UCDs)	Vomiting; seizures; coma → death as a newborn. ↑ Plasma ammonia, glutamine, glutamic acid, alanine	Food: low protein Formula: without nonessential amino acids	L-carnitine, phenylbutyrate,* L-citrulline, L-arginine
Citrullinemia	Argininosuccinate synthetase	1:30,000 (all UCDs)	*Neonatal:* vomiting; seizures; coma → death. *Infantile:* vomiting; seizures; progressive developmental delay. ↑ Plasma citrulline, ammonia, alanine	Food: low protein Formula: without nonessential amino acids	L-carnitine, phenylbutyrate,* L-arginine
Argininosuccinic aciduria	Argininosuccinate lyase	1:30,000 (all UCDs)	*Neonatal:* hypotonia; seizures *Subacute:* vomiting; FTT; progressive developmental delay. ↑ Plasma argininosuccinic acid, citrulline, ammonia levels	Food: low protein Formula: lower protein SF (without nonessential amino acids)	L-carnitine, phenylbutyrate,*
Argininemia	Arginase	1:30,000 (all UCDs)	Periodic vomiting; seizures; coma. Progressive spastic diplegia, developmental delay. ↑ Arginine, ammonia with protein intake	Food: low protein Formula: lower protein SF (without nonessential amino acids)	L-carnitine, phenylbutyrate,*
Organic Acidemias					
Methylmalonic acidemia	Methylmalonyl-CoA mutase or similar	1:80,000	Metabolic acidosis; vomiting; seizures; coma; often death. ↑ Organic acid, ammonia levels	Food: low protein Formula: lower protein SF (without isoleucine, methionine, threonine, valine)	L-carnitine, vitamin B₁₂ IV fluids, bicarbonate during acute episodes

Disorder	Enzyme	Incidence	Clinical Features	Diet	Supplements
Propionic acidemia	Propionyl-CoA carboxylase or similar	1:80,000	Metabolic acidosis; ↑Ammonia, propionic acid; ↑Methylcitric acid in urine	Food: low protein; Formula: lower protein SF (without isoleucine, methionine, threonine, valine)	L-carnitine, biotin IV fluids, bicarbonate during acute episodes
Isovaleric acidemia	Isovaleryl-CoA dehydrogenase	1:80,000	Poor feeding; lethargy; seizures; metabolic ketoacidosis; hyperammonemia	Food: low protein; Formula: SF (without leucine)	L-carnitine, L-glycine
Ketone utilization disorder	2-methylacetoacetyl-CoA-thiolase or similar	Unknown	Vomiting; dehydration; metabolic ketoacidosis	Food: low protein; Formula: SF (without isoleucine); Avoid fasting, diet high in complex carbohydrates	L-carnitine, bicitra
Biotinidase deficiency	Biotinidase or similar	1:60,000	In infancy, seizures, hypotonia, rash, stridor, apnea; in older children, also see alopecia, ataxia, developmental delay, hearing loss		Supplemental oral biotin
Carbohydrate Disorders					
Galactosemia	Galactose-1-phosphate uridyl transferase	1:50,000	Vomiting; hepatomegaly; FTT; cataracts; MR; often, early sepsis; ↑urine/blood galactose	Eliminate lactose, low galactose, use soy protein isolate formula	
Hereditary fructose intolerance	Fructose-1-phosphate aldolase	?1:20,000	Vomiting; hepatomegaly; hypoglycemia, FTT, renal tubular defects after fructose introduction; ↑blood/urine fructose after fructose feeding	No sucrose; no fructose	
Fructose 1,6-diphosphatase deficiency	Fructose 1,6-diphosphatase	Unknown	Hypoglycemia; hepatomegaly; hypotonia; metabolic acidosis with fructose introduction; No ↑blood/urine fructose		

* Phenylbutyrate is a chemical administered to enhance waste ammonia excretion; other compounds producing the same effect are also used.

CoA, Coenzyme A; *FTT*, failure to thrive; *SF*, specialized formulas are available for medical nutrition therapy for this disorder; *MR*, mental retardation; *Phe*, phenylalanine; *UCD*, urea cycle disorder; *IV*, intravenous.

Continued

TABLE 44-1

Selected Genetic Metabolic Disorders That Respond to Dietary Treatment—cont'd

Disorder	Affected Enzyme	Prevalence	Clinical/Biochemical Features	Diet Therapy	Adjunct Treatment
Carbohydrate Disorders—cont'd					
Glycogen storage disease, type Ia	Glucose 6-phosphatase	1:60,000	Profound hypoglycemia; hepatomegaly	Low lactose, fructose, sucrose; low fat; high complex carbohydrate; avoid fasting	Raw cornstarch, iron supplements
Amino Acid Disorders					
Hyperphenylalaninemias					
Phenylketonuria	Phenylalanine hydroxylase	1:15,000	↑↑ Blood Phe ↑ Phenylketones in urine Progressive, severe MR, which can be prevented by early treatment	Food: low protein Formula: SF (without Phe, supplement tyrosine)	
Mild phenylketonuria	Phenylalanine hydroxylase	1:24,000	↑ Blood Phe	Food: low protein Formula: SF (without Phe, supplement tyrosine)	
Dihydropteridine reductase deficiency	Dihydropteridine reductase	Rare	↑ Blood Phe Irritability; developmental delay; seizures	Food: low protein Formula: SF (without Phe, supplement tyrosine)	Biopterin, 5- hydroxytryptophan, L-dopa, folinic acid
Biopterin synthase defect	Biopterin synthase	Rare	Mild ↑ blood Phe Irritability; developmental delay; seizures	None	L-dopa, tetrahydrobiopterin, 5-hydroxytryptophan
Tyrosinemia, type I	Fumaryl-acetoacetate hydrolase	<1:120,000	Vomiting; acidosis; diarrhea; FTT; hepatomegaly rickets ↑ Blood/urine tyrosine, methionine ↑ Urine parahydroxy derivatives of tyrosine Liver cancer	Food: low protein Formula: SF (without tyrosine, Phe, methionine)	Nitisinone*
Maple Syrup Urine Disease (MSUD)					
MSUD	Branched-chain ketoacid decarboxylase complex (<2% activity)	1:200,000	Seizures; acidosis Plasma leucine, isoleucine, valine 10 × normal	Food: low protein Formula: SF (without leucine, isoleucine, valine)	?Thiamin

Disorder	Enzyme	Incidence	Clinical features	Diet	Supplements
Intermittent MSUD	Branched-chain ketoacid decarboxylase complex (<20% activity between episodes)	Rare	Intermittent symptoms; Plasma leucine, isoleucine, valine 10 × normal during illness	Food: low protein; Formula: SF (without leucine, isoleucine, valine)	
Homocystinuria	Cystathionine synthase or similar	1:200,000	Detached retinas; thromboembolic and cardiac disease; mild to moderate MR; bony abnormalities; fair hair and skin; ↑ methionine; ↑ homocysteine	Food: low protein; Formula: SF (without methionine, supplement L-cystine)	Betaine, folate, ?vitamin B$_6$ if folate levels are normal
Fatty Acid Oxidation Disorders					
Long-chain acyl-CoA dehydrogenase (LCAD) deficiency	Long-chain acyl-CoA dehydrogenase	Rare	Vomiting, lethargy, hypoglycemia	Low fat, low long-chain fatty acids; avoid fasting	MCT oil, ?L-carnitine
Long-chain 3-hydroxy-acyl-CoA dehydrogenase deficiency (LCHAD)	Long-chain 3-hydroxy-acyl-CoA dehydrogenase	Rare	Vomiting, lethargy hypoglycemia	Low fat, low long-chain fatty acids; avoid fasting	MCT oil, ?L-carnitine
Medium chain acyl-CoA dehydrogenase (MCAD) deficiency	Medium-chain acyl-CoA dehydrogenase	1:20,000	Vomiting, lethargy, hypoglycemia	Low fat, low medium-chain fatty acids, avoid fasting	L-carnitine
Short-chain acyl-CoA dehydrogenase (SCAD) deficiency	Short-chain acyl-CoA dehydrogenase	Rare	Vomiting, lethargy, hypoglycemia	Low fat, low short-chain fatty acids, avoid fasting	L-carnitine
Very long-chain acyl-CoA dehydrogenase (VLCAD) deficiency	Very long-chain acyl-CoA dehydrogenase	Rare	Vomiting, lethargy, hypoglycemia	Low fat, low long-chain fatty acids, avoid fasting	?L-carnitine, MCT oil

*Nitisinone, Formerly NTBC, 2-(2-nitro-4-trifluoro-methyl-benzoyl-1,3-cyclohexanedione, commercially available as Orfadin; ? indicates patient may or may not respond to the compound.

TABLE 44-2

Approximate Daily Requirements for Selected Dietary Components and Amino Acids in Infancy and Childhood

Dietary Component/Amino Acid	Age/Requirement	
	Birth to 12 mo (mg/kg)	**1 to 10 yr (mg/day)**
Phenylalanine	1-5 mo: 47-90 6-12 mo: 25-47	200-500*
Histidine	16-34	
Tyrosine†	1-5 mo: 60-80 6-12 mo: 40-60	25-85 (mg/kg)
Leucine	76-150	1000
Isoleucine	1-5 mo: 79-110 6-12 mo: 50-75	1000
Valine	1-5 mo: 65-105 6-12 mo: 50-80	400-600
Methionine‡	20-45	400-800
Cyst(e)ine§	15-50	400-800
Lysine	90-120	1200-1600
Threonine	45-87	800-1000
Tryptophan	13-22	60-120
Energy	1-5 mo: 108 kcal/kg 6-12 mo: 98 kcal/kg	70-102 kcal/kg
Water	100 ml/kg	1000 ml
Carbohydrate	kcal × 0.5 ÷ 4 = g/day	kcal × 0.5 ÷ 4 = g/day
Total protein	1-5 mo: 2.2 g/kg 6-12 mo: 1.6 g/kg	16-18
Fat	kcal × 0.35 ÷ 9 = g/day	kcal × 0.35 ÷ 9 = g/day

Modified from Committee on Nutrition, American Academy of Pediatrics: Special diets for infants with inborn errors of metabolism, *Pediatrics* 57:783, 1976.

Compiled from amino acid data of Holt and Snyderman. Information on amino acid requirements of infants and children at different ages is limited; the figures given here are in excess of minimum requirements. Consequently, this table should be used only as a guide and should not be regarded as an authoritative statement to which individual patients must conform.

*More phenylalanine (>800 mg) is required in the absence of tyrosine.

†Total phenylalanine plus tyrosine should be considered in the prescription since most phenylalanine is converted to tyrosine.

‡More methionine is required in the absence of cyst(e)ine.

§More cyst(e)ine is required in presence of a blocked *trans*-sulfuration outflow pathway for methionine metabolism.

Phe restriction in PKU. Although BH₄ holds promise as an alternative therapy for some milder mutations, observations on long-term outcome are for less than 5 years so far (Perez-Duenas et al., 2004; Lambruschini et al., 2005).

Medical Nutrition Therapy for Infants and Children

Formula. For PKU dietary therapy is planned around the use of a formula/medical food with Phe removed from the protein. The formulas or medical foods described in Table 44-3 provide a major portion of the daily protein and energy needs for affected infants, children, and adults. In general, the protein source in the formula or medical food is L-amino acids, with the critical amino acid (i.e., Phe) omitted. Carbohydrate sources are corn syrup solids, modified tapioca starch, sucrose, and hydrolyzed cornstarch. Fat is provided by a variety of oils.

Some formulas and medical foods contain no fat or carbohydrate; therefore these components must be provided from other sources. If prescribing formulas without fat, sources of essential fatty acids must be provided; essential fatty acid deficiencies have been noted among individuals consuming fat-free formulas (Cleary et al., 2006; Rose, et al., 2005). Most formulas/medical foods contain calcium, iron, and all other necessary vitamins and minerals and are a reliable source of these nutrients; others are devoid of these nutrients and require supplementation to ensure nutritional adequacy.

Phe-free formula is supplemented with regular infant formula or breast milk during infancy and cow's milk in early childhood to provide high–biologic value protein, nonessential amino acids, and sufficient Phe to meet the individualized requirements of the growing child. The optimal amount of protein substitute depends on the individual's age (and thus requirements for growth) and enzyme activity and must be individually prescribed.

Time Line of Events in the Diagnosis and Treatment of Phenylketonuria

1934: A. Folling identifies phenylpyruvic acid in the urine of mentally retarded siblings.

Early 1950s: G. Jervis demonstrates a deficiency of phenylalanine oxidation in the liver tissue of an affected patient. H. Bickel demonstrates that dietary phenylalanine restrictions lower the blood concentration of phenylalanine.

Early 1960s: R. Guthrie develops a bacterial inhibition assay for measuring blood phenylalanine levels.

Mid-1960s: Semisynthetic formulas restricted in phenylalanine content become commercially available.

1965-1970: States adopt newborn screening programs to detect phenylketonuria (PKU).

1967-1980: Collaborative Study of Children Treated for Phenylketonuria is conducted. Data from this study form the basis for treatment protocols for PKU clinics in the United States.

Late-1970s: Detrimental effects of maternal PKU are recognized as a significant public health problem.

1980s: Lifelong restriction of phenylalanine intake becomes the standard of care for PKU clinics in the United States.

1983: The Maternal PKU Collaborative Study begins to study the effects of treatment on the pregnancy outcome of women with phenylketonuria.

1987: Techniques for carrier detection and prenatal diagnosis of PKU are developed.

Late-1980s: The gene for phenylalanine hydroxylase deficiency (MIM No. 261600) is located on chromosome 12q22-q24.1. Deoxyribonucleic acid mutation analysis can be accomplished with peripheral leukocytes.

1990s: Phenylalanine level of 1-6 mg/dl (60-360 μmol/L), lower than the previous level of less than 10 mg/dl (600 μmol/L), becomes the new standard of care for treatment of PKU.

1999: Tetrahydrobiopterin (BH₄)-responsive forms of PKU have been recognized, especially those with mild mutations.

Data from Maternal Child Health Bureau: Newborn screening: toward a uniform screening panel and system, *Genet Med* 8(Suppl1):1S, 2006; and Saugstad LF: From genetics to epigenetics, *Nutr Health*, 18:285, 2006.

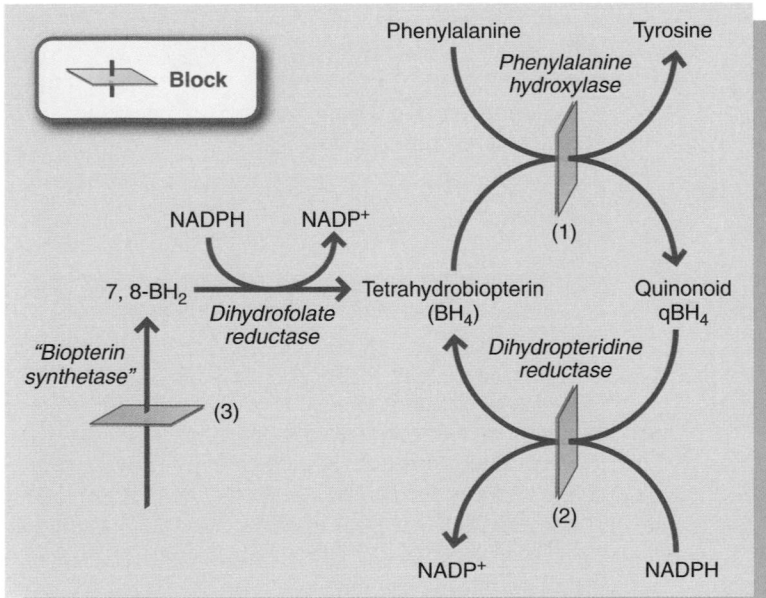

FIGURE 44-1 Hyperphenylalaninemias. *1*, Phenylalanine hydroxylase deficiency; *2*, Dihydropteridine reductase deficiency; *3*, Biopterin synthetase deficiency. *NADPH*, Nicotinamide-adenine dinucleotide phosphate (reduced form); *NADP+*, nicotinamide-adenine dinucleotide phosphate (oxidized form).

The Phe-free formula and milk mixture should provide about 90% of the protein and 80% of the energy needed by infants and toddlers. A method for calculating the appropriate quantities of a Phe-free formula is shown in Table 44-4. It must be stressed that calculations should provide adequate but not excessive energy for the infant, as well as appropriate fluid to maintain hydration. To support metabolic control effectively, formulas and medical foods must be consumed in three or four nearly equal portions throughout the day.

Low-Phenylalanine Foods. Foods of moderate- or low-Phe content are used as a supplement to the formula/medical food mixture. These foods are offered at the appropriate ages to support developmental readiness and to meet energy needs. Puréed foods from a spoon might be introduced at 5 to 6 months of age, finger foods at 7 to 8 months, and the cup at 8 to 9 months, using the same timing and progression of texture recommended for typical children. Table 44-5 suggests typical low-Phe food patterns for young children.

PATHOPHYSIOLOGY AND CARE MANAGEMENT ALGORITHM

Phenylketonuria

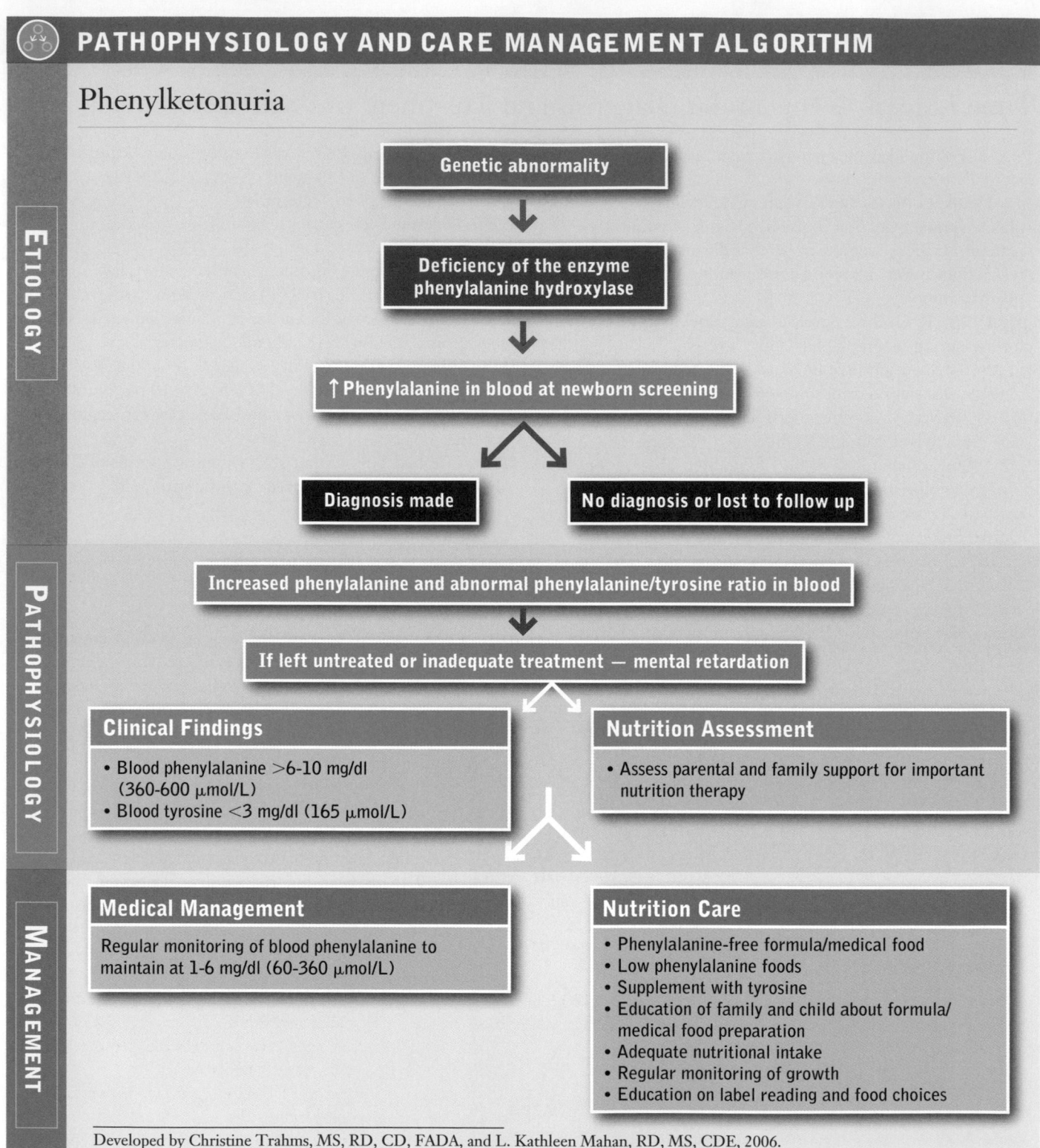

Developed by Christine Trahms, MS, RD, CD, FADA, and L. Kathleen Mahan, RD, MS, CDE, 2006.

Low-protein pastas, breads, and baked goods made from wheat starch add variety to the food pattern and allow children to eat some foods "to appetite." Table 44-6 compares low-protein and regular food items. Sources for low-protein products are given in *Clinical Insight*: Sources of Low-Protein Foods on p. 1154.

In many cases parents create recipes or adapt family favorites to meet the needs of their children. These recipes offer the children a variety of textures and food choices, al-lowing them to participate in family meals. Families are also able to meet the energy and Phe needs of their children without resorting to excessive intakes of sugars and concentrated sweets. Use of aspartame (NutraSweet), an artificial sweetener that contains Phe, has made food choices more difficult because it may be an ingredient in otherwise low-Phe foods (e.g., sugarless chewing gum).

A formula/medical food that is free of Phe and has a more appropriate amino acid, vitamin, and mineral compo-

TABLE 44-3

Formulas/Medical Foods for the Management of Selected Genetic Metabolic Disorders

Disorder	Formulas	Composition
Phenylketonuria	Phenex-1, Phenex-2, Phenex-2 Vanilla,* Phenyl-Free 2, Phenyl-Free HP,† XPhe Analog, Periflex‡	Protein: L-amino acids (each product has amino acids limited for a specific disorder), carbohydrate, fat, vitamins, and minerals. There are two versions of many of these products: (1) infant; and (2) child-adult, with age-appropriate protein, energy, fat, and vitamin/mineral modifications.
Maple syrup urine disease	Ketonex-1, Ketonex-2,* BCAD 1, BCAD 2,† MSUD Analog, Acerflex‡	
Isovaleric acidemia	I-Valex-1, I-Valex-2,* LMD,† XLeu Analog‡	
Glutaric aciduria, type 1	Glutarex-1, Glutarex-2,* GA,† XLys, XTrp Analog‡	
Homocystinuria	Hominex-1, Hominex-2,* HCY 1, HCY 2,† XMet Analog‡	
Propionic acidemia and methylmalonic acidemia	Propimex-1, Propimex-2,* OA 1, OA 2,† XMTVI Analog‡	
Tyrosinemia	Tyrex-1, Tyrex-2,* TYROS 1, TYROS 2,† XPhe, XTyr Analog,‡ XPTM Analog	
Urea cycle disorders	Cyclinex-1, Cyclinex-2,*	
Phenylketonuria	XPhe Maxamaid, XPhe Maxamum‡	Protein: L-amino acids (each product has amino acids limited for a specific disorder), carbohydrate, no fat, vitamins and minerals. (Maxamaid is designed for children, Maxamum for adults.)
Isovaleric acidemia	XLeu Maxamaid, XLeu Maxamum†	
Glutaric acidemia, type 1	XLys, XTrp Maxamaid; XLys, XTrp Maxamum‡	
Maple syrup urine disease	MSUD Maxamaid, MSUD Maxamum‡	
Homocystinuria	XMet Maxamaid, XMet Maxamum‡	
Propionic acidemia and methylmalonic acidemia	XMTVI Maxamaid, XMTVI Maxamum‡	
Tyrosinemia	XPhe, XTyr Maxamaid‡	
Phenylketonuria	Lophlex, Phlexy-10 System‡	L-amino acids only; may or may not have vitamins and minerals
Other products	Pro-Phree*; PFD 1, PFD 2†	Protein-free, carbohydrate, fat, vitamins, and minerals
	ProViMin*	Carbohydrate- and fat-free, protein, vitamins, and minerals
	RCF*	Carbohydrate-free, protein, fat, vitamins, and minerals
	Super soluble Duocal‡	Protein-free, carbohydrate and fat, not vitamins and minerals

*Ross, Abbott Laboratories, Abbott Park, Il, www.ros.com

†Mead Johnson Nutritionals, Evansville, In, www.meadjohnson.com

‡SHS North America, Gaithersburg, Md www.shsna.com

TABLE 44-4

Guidelines for Low-Phenylalanine Food Pattern Calculations

Case Study
Molly is a 6-month-old infant with phenylketonuria.

Baseline Data

Age	6 mo
Weight (kg)	7.7
Weight percentile	50th
Height (cm)	67.8
Length percentile	50th
Head circumference (cm)	43.3
General health	Good
Activity	Very active

Step 1 Calculate the child's requirement for phenylalanine, protein, and energy (kcal) by using the information in Table 44-2.
  A. Phenylalanine
     7.7 kg body weight × 60* mg phenylalanine/kg/day = 462 mg phenylalanine/day
  B. Protein
     7.7 kg body weight × 3.3† g protein/kg/day = 25.4 g protein/day
  C. Energy
     7.7 kg body weight × 115† kcal/kg/day = 885 kcal/day

Step 2 Determine the amount of phenylalanine-free formula required per day. This information is determined from the infant's protein requirement.
     For example: 25.4 g of protein per day × 90% of protein from phenylalanine-free formula powder (Phenex-1) = 23 g of protein = 145 g of formula powder per day.

Step 3 Determine the amount of standard infant formula to be included in the formula.

Step 4 Determine the amounts of phenylalanine, protein, and energy in the phenylalanine-free and infant formulas as shown in the following examples.

Step 5 Determine the amount of water to mix with the phenylalanine-free formula. The consistency of the formula will vary according to the infant's age and fluid requirements.
     For example: To prepare formula for the infant described in the case study, mix 145 g of Phenex-1 and 120 g of Enfamil powder with 4 oz of water to prevent lumps from forming. Then add water to make a total of 32 oz of formula. This provides 4 bottles of 8 oz each.

Formula	Phenylalanine (mg)	Protein (g)	Energy (kcal)
Phenex-1 powder (145 g)		23.0	695
Enfamil powder (120 g)	410	4.8	120
TOTAL	410	27.8	815

Step 6 Determine the amount of phenylalanine, protein, and energy to be obtained from foods other than the formula mixture.

Total phenylalanine	462 mg/day
Phenylalanine in formula	410 mg/day
Phenylalanine from other foods	52 mg/day
Total protein	25.4 g/day
Protein in formula	27.8 g/day
Protein from other foods	1-2 g/day
Total energy	885 kcal/day
Energy in formula	815 kcal/day
Energy from other foods	70 kcal/day

*A phenylalanine intake of 60 mg/kg/day is chosen as a moderate intake level. The prescription for phenylalanine must be adapted to individual needs as judged by growth and blood levels.

†Although these intakes are higher than the RDA, they are the intakes found by the Collaborative Study to promote normal growth with consumption of protein hydrolysate-based formula.

‡Total energy intake must be adjusted to meet individual needs, and an excess must be avoided.

TABLE 44-4

Guidelines for Low-Phenylalanine Food Pattern Calculations—cont'd

Step 7 Determine the amount of foods other than formula to be included in the dietary plan‡

	Phenylalanine (mg)	Protein (g)	kcal
Baby rice cereal, 1 Tbsp	9	0.2	9
Green beans, strained, 1 Tbsp	9	0.2	4
Banana, mashed, 50 g	22	0.6	44
Carrots, strained, 3 Tbsp	9	0.3	12
TOTAL	49	1.3	69

Step 8 Determine the actual amounts of phenylalanine, protein, and energy per kilogram of body weight by dividing the total available nutrients by the body weight (in kg).
Phenylalanine (mg)
460 mg of phenylalanine ÷ 7.7 kg body weight = 60 mg of phenylalanine per kilogram per day
Protein
29.1 g of protein ÷ 7.7 kg body weight = 3.8 g protein per kilogram per day
Energy
885 kcal ÷ 7.7 kg of body weight = 115 kcal per kilogram per day

TABLE 44-5

Typical Menus for a 3-Year-Old With Phenylketonuria

Tolerance: 300 mg of phenylalanine/day
Formula/medical food for 24 hours: 100 g of Phenyl-Free-2, 125 g of 2% milk, water to 34 oz
This formula mixture provides 25.8 g of protein, 670 kcal of energy, 200 mg of phenylalanine.

Tolerance: 400 mg of phenylalanine per day
Formula/medical food for 24 hours: 100 g of Phenyl-Free-2, 125 g of 2% milk, water to 34 oz
This formula mixture provides 25.8 g of protein, 670 kcal of energy, 200 mg of phenylalanine.

Menu for 100 mg of Phenylalanine From Food	Amount of Phenylalanine	Menu for 200 mg of Phenylalanine From Food	Amount of Phenylalanine
Breakfast		**Breakfast**	
Formula mixture, 10 oz		Formula mixture, 10 oz	
Kix cereal, 4 g (3 Tbsp)	15 mg	Rice Krispies, 20 g (¼ c)	22 mg
Peaches, canned, 60 g (¼ c)	9 mg	Nondairy creamer, ¼ c	19 mg
Lunch		**Lunch**	
Formula mixture, 8 oz		Formula mixture, 8 oz	
Low protein bread, ½ slice	7 mg	Vegetable soup (¼ c soup plus ¼ c water)	52 mg
Jelly, 1 tsp	0	Grapes, 50 g (10)	9 mg
Carrots, cooked, 40 g (¼ c)	13 mg	Low-protein crackers, 5	3 mg
Apricots, canned, 25 g (½ c)	6 mg	Low-protein cookie, 2	2 mg
Snack		**Snack**	
Apple slice, peeled, 4	4 mg	Rice cakes, 6 g (2 mini)	18 mg
Goldfish crackers, 10	18 mg	Jelly 1 tsp	0
Formula mixture, 8 oz		Formula mixture, 8 oz	
Dinner		**Dinner**	
Formula mixture, 8 oz		Formula mixture, 8 oz	
Low-protein pasta, ½ c, cooked	5 mg	Potato, diced, 50 g (5 Tbsp)	50 mg
Tomato sauce, 2 Tbsp	16 mg	Dairy-free margarine, 1 tsp	0 mg
Green beans, cooked, 17 g (2 Tbsp)	9 mg	Zucchini, sauteed, ¼ c (45 g)	18 mg
TOTAL PHENYLALANINE FROM FOOD	102 mg	TOTAL PHENYLALANINE FROM FOOD	193 mg

sition for an older child is generally introduced in the toddler or preschool period. The criteria for introduction of the "next step" formulas are that the child accept the food pattern and formula well and reliably consume a wide variety of foods from the low-Phe food list. Successful management with consistently low blood Phe levels is based on habit (i.e., the formula or medical food is offered and consumed without negotiation or threat). Children respond favorably to the regularity of the time of ingestion of the formula/medical food and the familiarity of its taste and presentation. Table 44-7 compares a restricted Phe food pattern with a typical food pattern for a child of the same age.

✳ CLINICAL INSIGHT

Sources of Low-Protein Foods

Low-protein products add energy, texture, and variety to restricted–amino acid and low-protein food patterns. A variety of low-protein pastas, rice, breads, rusks, crackers, cookies, egg replacers, and gelled dessert mixes are available. Wheat starch and a variety of low-protein baking mixes for breads, cakes, and cookies are also available.

These selected companies provide low-protein baking ingredients, breads, pastas, cereals, cookies, recipes, and low-protein cookbooks.

Company	Telephone	Web Address
Dietary Specialties Whippany, NJ 07951	(888) 640-2800	www.dietspec.com
Med-Diet Inc. Plymouth, MN 55447	(800) 633-3438	www.med-diet.com
Ener-G Foods Seattle, WA 98124-5787	(800) 331-5222	www.ener-g.com
Scientific Hospital Supplies Gaithersburg, MD 20884	(877) 482-7845	www.shsna.com
Cambrooke Foods Framingham, MA 01701	(866) 456-9776	www.cambrookfoods.com

TABLE 44-6

Comparison of Protein and Energy Content of Foods Used in Low-Protein Diets

Food Item	Energy (kcal)	Protein (g)
Pasta, ½ c, cooked		
Low-protein	107	0.15
Regular	72	2.4
Bread, 1 slice		
Low-protein	135	0.2
Regular	74	2.4
Cereal, ½ c, cooked		
Low-protein	45	0.0
Regular	80	1.0
Egg, 1		
Low-protein egg replacer	30	0.0
Regular	67	5.6

Blood Phenylalanine Control. The blood Phe concentration must be checked regularly, depending on the age and health status of the child, to be sure it remains within the range of 2 to 6 mg/dl or 120 to 360 μmol/L (NIH, 2001). Phe-containing foods are offered as tolerated as long as the blood concentration of Phe remains in the range of good biochemical control. The child's rate of growth and mental development must be carefully monitored.

Effective management requires a cohesive team in which the child, parents, registered dietitian, pediatrician, psychologist, social worker, and nurse work together to achieve and maintain biochemical control and provide an atmosphere for normal mental and emotional development. An essential management tool for parents, children, and clinicians is the food diary, an example of which is shown in Figure 44-2. Daily record-keeping supports compliance with treatment and builds self-management skills. An accurate record of food and formula intake for at least the 3 days before a laboratory specimen is obtained is mandatory for accurate interpretation of the results and subsequent adjustment of the Phe prescription.

Elevations in blood Phe concentration are generally caused by either excessive Phe intake or tissue catabolism. Intake of Phe in excess of the amount required for growth accumulates in the blood. Deficient energy intake or the trauma of illness or infection can result in protein breakdown and the release of amino acids, including Phe, into the blood. In general, the anorexia of illness limits energy intake. Preventing tissue catabolism by maintaining intake of formula/medical food as much as possible is essential. Although it may occasionally be necessary to offer only clear liquids during an illness, the Phe-free formula/medical food should be reintroduced as soon as it is feasible.

The necessity of continuing the restricted-Phe dietary therapy beyond adolescence is a consideration in the management of children with PKU. Progressively decreasing IQs, learning difficulties, poor attention span, and behavioral difficulties have been reported in children who have discontinued the dietary regimen. Children enrolled in the National Collaborative Study who maintained well-controlled blood Phe levels demonstrated comparatively higher intellectual achievement than those who did not (Azen et al., 1996). Good dietary control of blood Phe concentrations is

TABLE 44-7

Comparison of Menus Appropriate for Children With and Without Phenylketonuria (PKU)

Meal	Menu for PKU	Phenylalanine (mg)	Regular menu	Phenylalanine (mg)
Breakfast	Phenylalanine-free formula	0	Milk	450
	Rice Krispies		Rice Krispies	
	Orange juice		Orange juice	
Lunch	Jelly sandwich with low-protein bread	18	Jelly sandwich with white bread	260
	Banana		Banana	
	Carrot and celery sticks		Carrot and celery sticks	
	Low-protein chocolate chip cookies	4	Chocolate chip cookies	60
	Juice		Juice	
Snack	Phenylalanine-free formula	0	Milk	450
	Orange		Orange	
	Potato chips (small bag)		Potato chips	
Dinner	Phenylalanine-free formula	0	Milk	450
	Salad		Salad	
	Low-protein spaghetti with tomato sauce	8	Spaghetti	240
			Spaghetti with tomato sauce and meatballs	600
	Baskin-Robbins fruit ice	10	Ice cream	120
ESTIMATED INTAKE		40		2630

the best predictor of IQ, whereas "off-diet" blood Phe concentrations of greater than 20 mg/dl (1200 μmol/L) are the best predictors of IQ loss. Subtle deficits in higher-level cognitive function may persist even at blood Phe levels of 6 to 10 mg/dl (360 to 600 μmol/L); thus most clinics recommend treatment blood levels of 1 to 6 mg/dl (60 to 360 μmol/L). Restricted-Phe therapy should be continued for life to maintain normal cognitive function (NIH, 2001).

Education about Therapy Management. The energy needs and amino acid requirements of children with PKU do not differ appreciably from those of children in general. With proper management, typical growth can be expected (Figure 44-3). However, parents may tend to offer excessive energy as sweets because they feel the child is being deprived of food experiences. Health care providers and parents need to understand that children with PKU are well children who must make careful food choices for themselves, not chronically ill children who require food indulgences.

Appropriate clinical interaction with family members provides them with the information and skills to differentiate between food behaviors that are typical for the age and developmental level of the child and those related specifically to PKU (Ievers-Landis et al., 2005; Keickhefer and Trahms, 2000; Trahms, 1986). To avoid power struggles and conflicts over food, it is advisable to involve the child in choosing appropriate foods at an early age. Two-

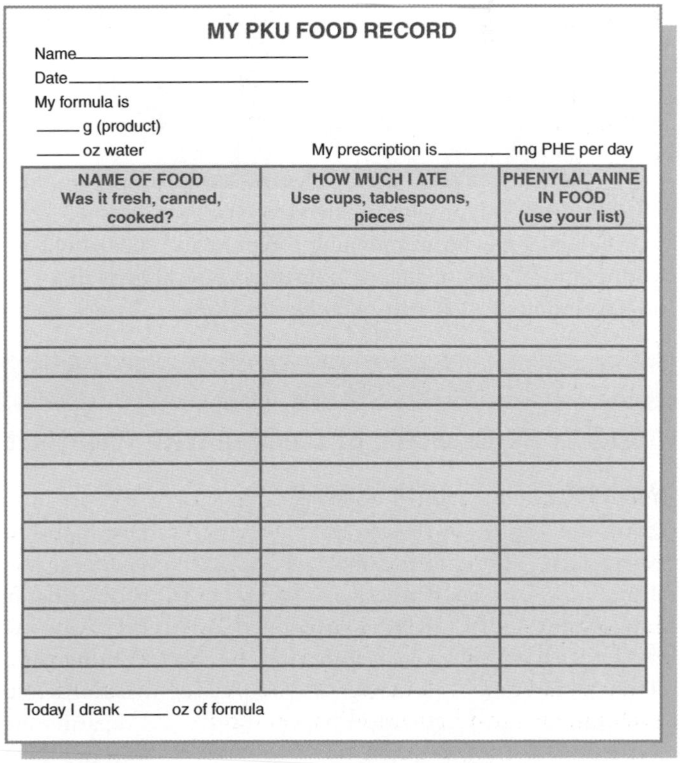

MY PKU FOOD RECORD

Name_____

Date_____

My formula is

_____ g (product)

_____ oz water   My prescription is_____ mg PHE per day

NAME OF FOOD Was it fresh, canned, cooked?	HOW MUCH I ATE Use cups, tablespoons, pieces	PHENYLALANINE IN FOOD (use your list)

Today I drank _____ oz of formula

FIGURE 44-2 Sample phenylketonuria (PKU) food record. *PHE*, Phenylalanine.

and 3-year-old children can master the concept of appropriate choices when foods are categorized as "yes foods" and "no foods."

The concept of an appropriate quantity of a food can be introduced to a 3- or 4-year-old child in terms of "how many" by counting crackers or raisins and then in terms of "how much" by weighing or measuring foods such as cereal or fruit. The child then moves to more complex tasks (e.g., formula and food preparation) and planning of meals (e.g., breakfast or a packed lunch). Responsibility for planning a full day's menu by calculating the quantity of Phe in portions of food and compiling the daily total is the ultimate goal. These age-related tasks are shown in Table 44-8.

Psychosocial Development. The necessity of carefully controlling food intake may prompt parents to overprotect their children and perhaps to restrict their social activities.

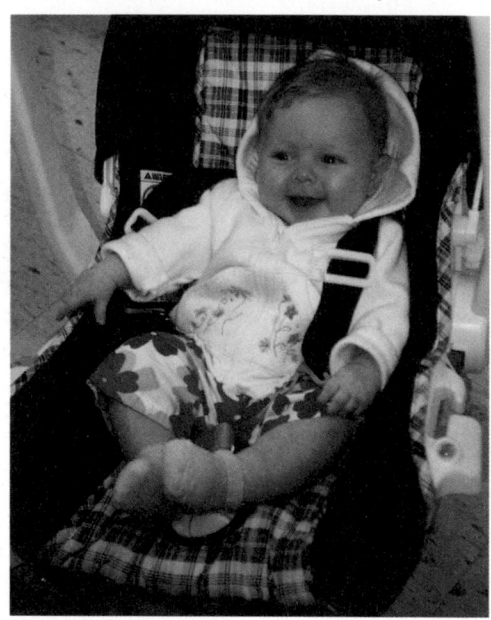

FIGURE 44-3 Infant with phenylketonuria, who was identified by a newborn screening program and started on treatment by 7 days of age, demonstrates typical growth and development. *(Courtesy Cristine M. Trahms, Seattle).*

The children, in turn, may react negatively to their parents and to their nutrition therapy. The ability of the family to respond to the stresses of PKU, as reflected by adaptability and cohesion scores, is demonstrated by improved blood Phe concentrations and the positive coping behaviors of older children with PKU (Kazak et al., 1988; Trahms et al., 1987). Thus continuing nutrition therapy beyond early childhood requires that children become knowledgeable about and responsible for managing their own food choices (Figure 44-4). The health care team becomes responsible for working with families and children to provide strategies that enable children and adolescents to participate in social and school activities, interact with peers, and progress through the typical developmental stages with self-confidence and self-esteem (Keickhefer and Trahms, 2000; Sullivan, 2001; Ievers-Landis et al., 2005).

Children require parental and professional support as they assume responsibility for their food management. Self-management of food choices avoids the risk of the child using dietary noncompliance as a wedge against parental restrictions. Normal intellectual development is a laudable goal of management of PKU, but to be entirely successful children with PKU concomitantly need to develop self-assurance and a strong self-image. This can be achieved in part by fostering self-management, problem-solving skills, independence, and a typical lifestyle.

Nutrition Care in Maternal PKU

A pregnant woman with elevated blood Phe concentrations endangers her fetus because of the amplified transport of amino acids across the placenta. The fetus is exposed to about twice the Phe level contained in normal maternal blood. Babies whose mothers have elevated blood Phe concentrations have an increased occurrence of cardiac defects, retarded growth, microcephaly, and mental retardation, as presented in Table 44-9.

The fetus appears to be at risk of damage even with minor elevations in maternal blood Phe levels, and the higher the level, the more severe the effect (Levy et al., 2001). Strict control of maternal Phe levels before conception and throughout pregnancy offers the best oppor-

TABLE 44-8

Tasks To Be Expected of Children With Phenylketonuria by Age Level

Age (yr)	School Level	Task
2-3	Preschool	Distinguishing between yes and no foods
3-4	Preschool	Counting: how many?
4-5	Preschool	Measuring: how much?
5-6	Kindergarten	Preparing own formula; using scale
6-7	Grade 1-2	Writing basic notes in food diary
7-8	Grade 2	Making some decisions on after-school snack
8-9	Grade 3	Preparing breakfast
9-10	Grade 4	Packing lunches
10-14	Middle school	Managing food choices with increasing independence
14-18	High school	Independently managing phenylketonuria

tunity for normal fetal development (AAP, 2001; Waisbren and Azen, 2003).

The management of nutrition therapy during pregnancy for women with hyperphenylalaninemia is complex. The changing physiology of pregnancy and changing nutritional needs are difficult to monitor with the precision required to maintain appropriately low blood-Phe concentrations. Even with meticulous attention to Phe intake, blood concentrations, and the nutritional requirements of pregnancy, a woman cannot be assured of a normal infant (Lee et al., 2005). The risks of abnormal development of the fetus, even with therapeutic dietary management and maintenance of blood Phe concentrations at 1 to 5 mg/dL (60 to 300 µmol/L), are an important consideration for young women with PKU considering pregnancy (Waisbren and Azen, 2003).

Nutritional management during pregnancy is difficult, even for women who have consistently followed a low-Phe dietary regimen since infancy. Women who have discontinued treatment find that reinstituting medical food consumption and limitation of food choices is difficult, if not overwhelming. Inadequate maternal nourishment (i.e., inadequate

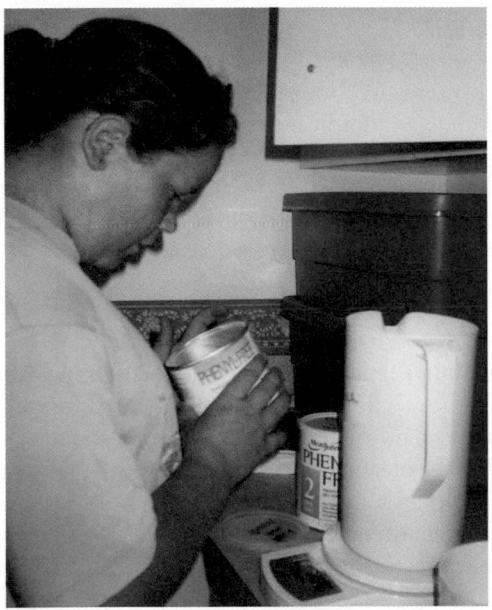

FIGURE 44-4 A preadolescent girl demonstrates her self-care skills by preparing her own formula/medical food. (*Courtesy Cristine M. Trahms, Seattle*).

intakes of total protein, fat, and energy) may also contribute to poor fetal development (Acosta et al., 2001). Adherence to nutrition therapy during pregnancy for even the well-motivated woman requires family and professional support, as well as frequent monitoring of biochemical and nutritional aspects of both pregnancy and PKU.

Medical Nutrition Therapy for Adults With Phenylketonuria

Many adults with PKU have had the benefits of early diagnosis and treatment and are less likely to be affected by neurologic damage. However, among those who have had some degree of mental retardation, hyperactivity and self-abuse are often major concerns. Not all patients have responded to the late institution of treatment with improved behavioral or intellectual function. For the difficult-to-manage older patient, a trial of a low-Phe food pattern is recommended. If successful, continued Phe restriction therapy may facilitate behavioral management.

Reinstituting a Phe-restricted food pattern is difficult after the eating pattern has been liberalized (Finkelson et al., 2001). However, the current recommendation of most clinics is effective management of blood Phe concentration throughout a lifetime. This recommendation is based on reports of declining intellectual capabilities and changes in the brain after prolonged, significant elevation of Phe concentrations (Waisbren and Azen, 2003). The efficacy of continued treatment throughout adulthood has been documented by reports of improved current intellectual performance, especially in terms of response time (Krause et al., 1985) and improved problem-solving abilities (Ris et al., 1994) when blood Phe levels are kept low.

Dietary management of PKU throughout the life span is similar to that of other chronic disorders but unlike many other chronic disorders, MNT results in a normal quality of life (Bosch et al., 2006).

Maple Syrup Urine Disease

Maple syrup urine disease (MSUD), or **branched-chain keto-aciduria,** results from a defect in enzymatic activity, specifically the branched chain α-ketoacid dehydrogenase complex. This decarboxylation defect prevents metabolism of the branched-chain amino acids (BCAAs) leucine, isoleucine, and valine (Figure 44-5).

TABLE 44-9

Frequency of Abnormalities in Children Born to Mothers With Phenylketonuria

Complication (% of Offspring)	Maternal Phenylalanine Levels (mg/dl)				
	20	16-19	11-15	3-10	Non-PKU Mother
Mental retardation	92	73	22	21	5.0
Microcephaly	73	68	35	24	4.8
Congenital heart disease	12	15	6	0	0.8
Low birth weight	40	52	56	13	9.6

Modified from Lenke RR, Levy HL: Maternal phenylketonuria and hyper-phenylalaninemia: an international survey of the outcome of untreated and treated pregnancies, *N Engl J Med* 303:1202, 1980.

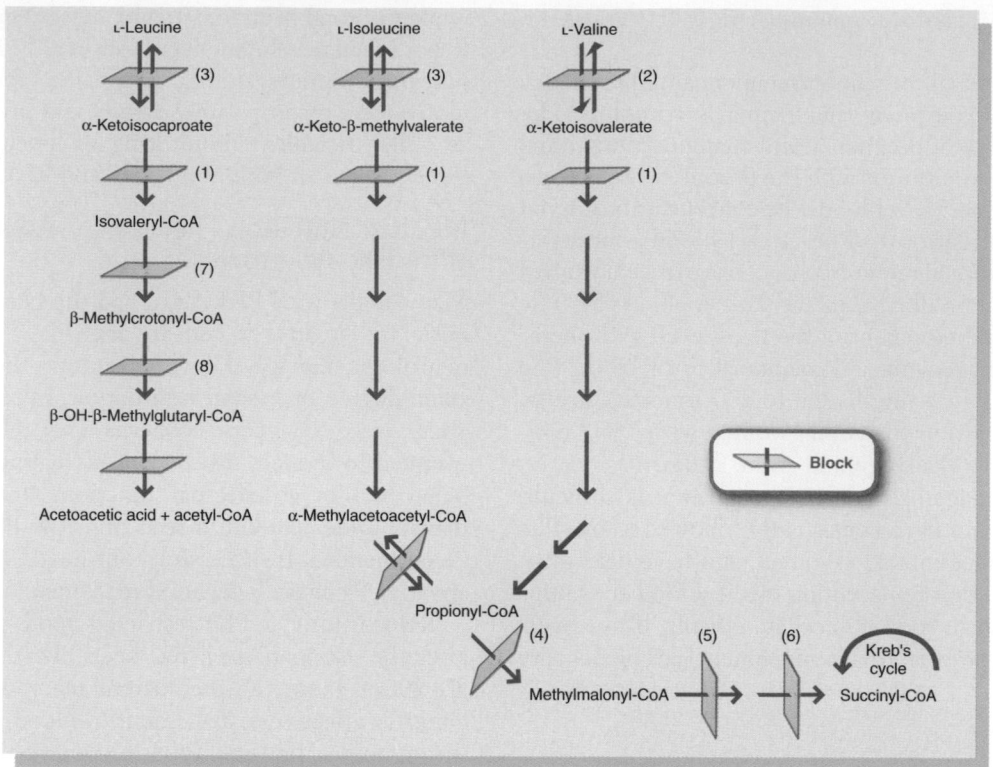

FIGURE 44-5 Organic acidemias and maple syrup urine disease (MSUD). *1*, Branched-chain ketoacid decarboxylase (MSUD); *2*, Valine aminotransferase; *3*, Leucine-isoleucine aminotransferase; *4*, Propionyl-CoA carboxylase (propionic acidemia); *5*, Methylmalonyl-CoA racemase (methylmalonic aciduria); *6*, Methylmalonyl-CoA mutase (methylmalonic aciduria); *7*, Isovaleryl-CoA dehydrogenase (isovaleric acidemia). *8*, β-methylcrotonyl-CoA carboxylase (biotin-responsive multiple carboxylase deficiency). *CoA*, Coenzyme A.

MSUD is an autosomal-recessive disorder. Infants appear normal at birth, but by 4 or 5 days of age they demonstrate poor feeding, vomiting, lethargy, and periodic hypertonia. A characteristic sweet, malty odor from the urine and perspiration can be noted toward the end of the first week of life. Failure to treat this condition leads to acidosis, neurologic deterioration, seizures, and coma, proceeding eventually to death. Management of acute disease often requires peritoneal dialysis and hydration (see Chapter 36).

BCAAs are introduced gradually into the diet when plasma leucine concentrations are sufficiently decreased (Chuang and Shih, 2001). The precise mechanism for the complete decarboxylase reaction and the resultant neurologic damage is not known. Neither is the reason why leucine metabolism is significantly more abnormal than that of the other two BCAAs understood. Clinical relapse is most often related to the degree of elevation of leucine concentrations, and these relapses often are related to infection. Acute infections represent life-threatening medical emergencies in this group of children. If the plasma leucine concentration increases rapidly during illness, BCAAs should be removed from the diet immediately, and intravenous therapy started.

Depending on the severity of the enzyme defect, early intervention and meticulous biochemical control can provide a more hopeful prognosis for infants and children with MSUD. Reasonable growth and intellectual development in the normal-to-low-normal range have been described. Diagnosis before 7 days of age and long-term metabolic control are critical factors in long-term normalization of intellectual development. Maintenance of plasma leucine concentrations in infants and preschool children should be as close to physiologically normal as possible (Hoffman, 2006). Concentrations above 10 mg/dl (760 μmol/L) are often associated with α-ketoacidemia and neurologic symptoms.

Nutrition therapy requires very careful monitoring of blood concentrations of leucine, isoleucine, and valine; growth and general nutritional adequacy. Several formulas specifically designed for the treatment of this disorder are now available to provide a reasonable amino acid and vitamin mixture (see Table 44-3). These are generally supplemented with a small quantity of standard infant formula or cow's milk to provide the BCAAs needed to support growth and development. Some infants and children may require additional supplementation with L-valine or L-isoleucine to maintain biochemical balance. Typical leucine-modified menus for young children are presented in Table 44-10.

Because the liver is the central site of metabolic control for amino acids and other compounds that cause acute degeneration of the brain during illness, therapeutic liver

TABLE 44-10

Typical Menus for a 2 Year Old With Maple Syrup Urine Disease (MSUD)

Tolerance: 450 mg of leucine per day
Formula/medical food for 24 hours: 100 g of Ketone-2,
    38 g of Isomil powder, water to 24 ounces
This formula mixture provides 34.8 g of protein, 608 kcal
    of energy, 388 mg of leucine

Tolerance: 550 mg of leucine per day
Formula/medical food for 24 hours: 100 g of Ketone-2,
    38 g of Isomil powder, water to 24 ounces
This formula mixture provides 34.8 g of protein, 608 kcal
    of energy, 388 mg of leucine

Menu for 50 mg of Leucine From Food	Amount of Leucine	Menu for 150 mg of Leucine From Food	Amount of Leucine
Breakfast		**Breakfast**	
Formula mixture, 6 oz		Formula mixture, 6 oz	
Kix cereal, 1 g (1 Tbsp)	5 mg	Rice Krispies, 6 g (¼ c)	35 mg
Peaches, canned, 60 g (¼ c)	9 mg	Nondairy creamer, 2 Tbsp	7 mg
Lunch		**Lunch**	
Formula mixture, 6 oz		Formula mixture, 6 oz	
Low protein bread, 1 slice	4 mg	Vegetable soup (2 Tbsp soup plus ¼ c water)	30 mg
Jelly, 1 tsp	0	Grapes, 50 g (10)	7 mg
Carrots, cooked, 20 g (2 Tbsp)	9 mg	Low-protein crackers, 5	3 mg
Apricots, canned, 25 g (½)	9 mg	Low-protein cookie, 3	3 mg
Snack		**Snack**	
Apple slices, peeled, 4	4 mg	Rice cakes, 1 g (1 mini)	7 mg
Low-protein crackers, 5	3 mg	Jelly, 1 tsp	0
Formula mixture, 6 oz		Formula mixture, 6 oz	
Dinner		**Dinner**	
Formula mixture, 6 oz		Formula mixture, 6 oz	
Low protein pasta, ½ c cooked	5 mg	Potato, diced, 30 g (3 Tbsp)	33 mg
Dairy-free margarine	0	Dairy-free margarine, 1 tsp	0
Green beans, cooked, 9 g (1 Tbsp)	7 mg	Zucchini, sautéed, 45 g (¼ c)	24 mg
TOTAL FROM FOOD	55 mg	**TOTAL FROM FOOD**	149 mg

transplantation has been proposed as an option for eliminating this risk in MSUD. Studies are underway to assess the long-term effects of this procedure on stabilization of biochemical and neurologic status (Kaller et al., 2005).

DISORDERS OF ORGANIC ACID METABOLISM

Pathophysiology

The organic acid disorders are a group of disorders characterized by the accumulation in the blood of nonamino acid organic acids. Most of the organic acids are efficiently excreted in the urine. Diagnosis is based on excretion of compounds not normally present or the presence of abnormally high amounts of other compounds in the urine.

Propionic acidemia is a defect of propionyl–coenzyme A (CoA) carboxylase in the pathway of propionyl-CoA to methylmalonyl-CoA, as illustrated in Figure 44-5. The clinical course can vary but is generally marked by vomiting,

lethargy, hypotonia, dehydration, seizures, and coma. Survivors often have permanent neurologic damage. Metabolic acidosis with a marked anion gap and hyperammonemia is characteristic. Long-chain ketonuria may also be present. Some patients with propionic acidemia may respond to pharmacologic doses of biotin (Fenton et al., 2001). Long-term outcome in propionic acidemia is variable; hypotonia and cognitive delay may result even in children who are diagnosed early and who receive rigorous treatment (North et al., 1995). Liver damage and cardiomyopathy are possible sequelae. Liver transplantation may limit mental retardation and cardiac changes (Barshes et al., 2006).

At least five separate enzyme deficiencies have been identified that result in **methylmalonic acidemia** or aciduria. The defect of methylmalonyl-CoA mutase apoenzyme is the most frequently identified (see Figure 44-5). The clinical features are similar to those of propionic acidemia. Acidosis is common, and diagnosis is confirmed by the presence of large amounts of methylmalonic acid in blood and urine. Other findings include hypoglycemia, ketonuria, and elevation of plasma ammonia and lactate levels. Some patients may respond to pharmacologic doses of vitamin B_{12};

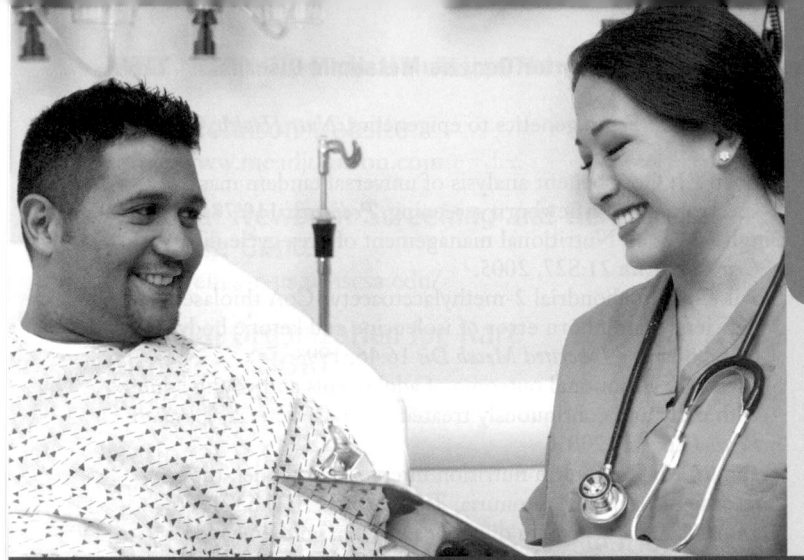

CHAPTER 45

Harriet Cloud, MS, RD, FADA

Medical Nutrition Therapy for Developmental Disabilities

KEY TERMS

Arnold Chiari malformation of the brain a structural disorder affecting the cerebellum frequently found in spina bifida that can affect swallowing and gagging

Asperger syndrome used to describe children with the problems of ASD but who have normal-to-high cognitive level

attention-deficit hyperactivity disorder (ADHD) a neurobehavioral problem associated with learning disorders, inappropriate degrees of impulsiveness, excessive inability to pay attention; diagnostic criteria are for three types: (1) combined type of hyperactivity and attention deficit; (2) predominately inattentive type; and (3) predominately hyperactive-impulse type

autism spectrum disorders (ASDs) a group of disorders diagnosed by the presence of qualitatively impaired reciprocal social interaction; impaired communication skills; and restricted, repetitive, stereotypical interests and behaviors; many children with autism also have mental retardation

cerebral palsy a disorder of motor control or coordination resulting from injury to the brain during its early development

cleft lip and cleft palate (CL/CP) incomplete merging and fusion of embryonic processes during formation of the face; cleft lip is a condition that creates an opening in the upper lip that can range from a slight notch to complete separation in one or both sides of the lips and extending upward; cleft palate occurs when the roof of the mouth has not joined completely; it can be either unilateral or bilateral and can range from just an opening at the back of the soft palate or separation of the roof of the mouth with both soft and hard palate involved

congenital anomaly a malformation present at birth that can affect various organs or structures of the body (e.g., cleft lip or palate)

developmental disability a condition caused by fetal abnormalities, birth defects, metabolic disorders, or chromosomal disorders

Down syndrome a chromosomal aberration of chromosome 21 (trisomy 21) that causes the physical and developmental features of short stature, congenital heart disease, mental retardation, decreased muscle tone, hyperflexibility of joints, speckling of the iris, upward slant of the eyes, epicanthal folds, small oral cavity, short broad hands with the single palmar crease, and wide gap between the first and second toes

hypotonia low tone of the muscles frequently found in Down syndrome, Prader-Willi syndrome, and other conditions such as prematurity

individualized education plan (IEP) individualized education plan mandated for children in special education

individualized family plan comprehensive care for children in early intervention programs

mental retardation significantly below average intellectual functioning along with related limitation in two or more of the following areas: communication, self-care, functional academics, and home-living and community use, self-direction, health and safety, leisure, work and social skills

midfacial hypoplasia a type of craniofacial deformity, common in cleft palate

mosaicism different cells within an individual who has developed from a single fertilized egg have a different chromosomal makeup; most common kind found at prenatal diagnosis involves Down syndrome

Prader-Willi syndrome (PWS) a chromosomal aberration characterized by developmental delays, poor muscle tone, short stature, small hands and feet, incomplete sexual development, unique facial features, and insatiable appetite leading to obesity

spastic quadriplegia a term used to describe an individual with spastic paralysis of the arms and legs

spina bifida a neurologic tube defect or derangement of spinal cord formation, which presents as either meningocele, myelomeningocele, or spina bifida occulta; myelomeningocele is most common; lesion may occur in the thoracic, lumbar, or sacral area and will influence the amount of paralysis; manifestations range from weakness in the lower extremities to complete paralysis and loss of sensation and incontinence and hydrocephalus; can be prevented with prenatal folic acid supplementation

syndrome a term used to identify a developmental disability with a cluster of distinctive features such as Down syndrome

Individuals with developmental disabilities were generally housed in institutions for the mentally retarded for the first half of the 20th century. Little attention was paid to their education, medical or nutritional care. In 1963 the Developmental Disabilities Assistance and Bill of Rights Act was passed. Through this Act federal funds supported the development and operation of state councils, protection and advocacy systems, university centers, and projects of national significance. This Act provided the structure to assist people with developmental disabilities to pursue meaningful and productive lives (Developmental Disabilities Act, 2000).

The institutions that housed these individuals were gradually closed or reduced in size. By 1975 this population of individuals, which comprises approximately 5% of the population, were cared for in the community—at home, in schools, and some in small residential facilities. In 1975 P.L. 94-142 was passed, opening up public schools to children with developmental disabilities. In 1985 P.L. 99-487 (102-119 in 1992), the Early Intervention Act, was passed, bringing services to children from birth to school age. Much has been learned about the role of nutrition in both the prevention of disabilities and intervention when a nutrition problem exists. Medical nutrition therapy (MNT) is an important component of both prevention and intervention. The role of the registered dietitian (RD) is changing in the provision of medical nutrition therapy for this population because of the abundance of information that parents and caretakers use from support groups and websites that may be untested scientifically. RDs will be required to provide counseling related to the information parents and caretakers are learning on their own.

DEFINING DEVELOPMENTAL DISABILITIES

A **developmental disability** is defined legislatively in the Developmental Disabilities Assistance and Bill of Rights Act (Public Law, 99-101-496 and revised in 2000 to PL 106-402) as a severe chronic disability of a person that is attributable to a mental or physical impairment or combination of mental and physical impairments. It is manifested before the person attains age 22; is likely to continue indefinitely; results in substantial functional limitations in three or more areas of major life activity (self-care, receptive and expressive language, learning, mobility, self-direction, capacity for independent living, and economic self-sufficiency); and reflects the person's need for a combination of special interdisciplinary or generic care, treatments, or other services that are lifelong or of extended duration and individually planned and coordinated.

It is important to recognize that developmental disabilities affect individuals of all ages and are not a disease state. It is a condition that is caused by fetal abnormalities, birth defects, and metabolic and chromosomal disorders. For this reason medical nutrition therapy will vary, depending on the individual and the physical or mental problem he or she may have. Throughout this chapter, many of the conditions associated with developmental disabilities and the applicable medical nutrition therapy will be addressed.

ETIOLOGY AND INCIDENCE

The etiology of developmental disabilities has been traced to many causes: chromosomal aberrations, **congenital anomalies,** specific syndromes, neuromuscular dysfunction, neurologic disorders, prematurity, cerebral palsy, untreated inborn errors of metabolism, toxins in the environment, and nutrient deficiencies.

The Centers for Disease Control and Prevention (CDC) reports that 17% of children under 18 years of age have some type of developmental disability (CDC, 2003). Other surveys have reported that there are 3 to 4 million Americans with developmental disabilities and another 3 million who have milder forms of cognitive disabilities or mental retardation (American Dietetic Association, 2004).

Mental retardation is the most common developmental disability and is characterized by significantly below-average intellectual functioning along with related limitations in two or more of the following areas: communication, self-care, functional academics, home-living, self-direction, health and safety, leisure, or work and social skills (Luckasson et al., 2002).

PRINCIPLES OF NUTRITION CARE

In a 2004 position paper the American Dietetic Association (ADA) stated, "It is the position of the American Dietetic Association that nutrition services are essential components of comprehensive care for infants, children and adults with developmental disabilities and special health care needs." The ADA also stated that nutrition services should be provided throughout the life cycle of health care and educational and vocational programs should provide MNT in a manner that is interdisciplinary, family centered, community based and culturally competent (ADA, 2004).

Numerous nutrition problems have been identified in the individual with developmental disability, including growth retardation, obesity, failure to thrive, feeding problems, metabolic disorders, medication-nutrient interactions, constipation, and renal problems. Other health problems exist, depending on the disorder. Table 45-1 lists the most common developmental disabilities and their associated nutrition problems.

In designing the medical nutrition therapy plan, four areas are considered: nutrition assessment (anthropometrics, biochemical assessment when available, dietary intake, feeding issues such as oral-motor problems, positioning problems and feeding skills), nutrition diagnosis (problem identification), intervention, and monitoring and evaluation.

Nutrition Assessment

Assessment for both children and adults with a developmental disability follows that of a normal individual, except in certain syndromes in which additional measures may be required (see Chapters 14 and 15).

Anthropometrics

Anthropometric measures are altered when an individual is unable to stand, suffers from contractions, or has other gross motor problems. Measuring body weight may require special equipment such as chair scales or bucket scales. Wheelchair scales are used in some clinics but require that the wheelchair weight be known. Obtaining height for the nonambulatory individual requires either a recumbent board that can be purchased or constructed. Other measures of height include arm span, knee-to-ankle height (Chumlea et al., 1994), or sitting height (Figure 45-1 and Appendix 20). An excellent depiction of these methods is included in the CDC website on obtaining measures to use with the CDC growth curves for infants, children, and adults to age 20 (www.cdc.gov, 2003). Examples of obtaining height measures are in Appendixes 19 and 20.

Standards for the comparison of height and weight were developed in 2000 by the CDC for children in two age-groups, 0 to 36 months and 2 to 20 years. Growth charts for children with various syndromes do exist; however, most clinicians recommend using the CDC charts (Appendixes 9 to 16) since the information in the charts for specialized populations is based on small numbers,

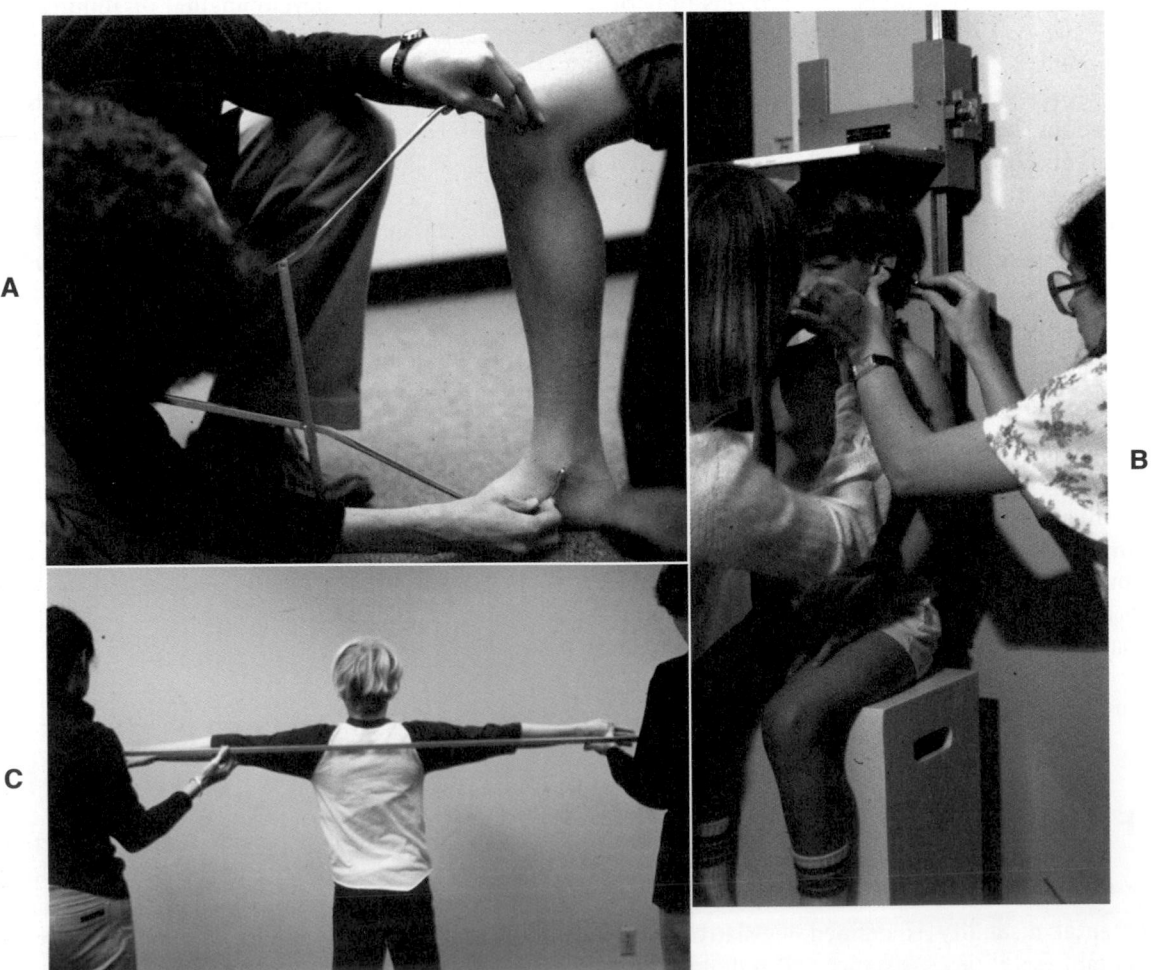

FIGURE 45-1 A, Knee height measure. **B,** Sitting height measure. **C,** Arm span measure. (©*Cristine M. Trahms, 2002.*)

TABLE 45-1

Selected Syndromes and Developmental Disabilities: Frequently Reported Nutrition Problems and Factors Contributing to Nutritional Risk

Syndrome/Disability	Altered Growth Underweight Obesity	Altered Energy Need	Constipation/Diarrhea	Feeding Problems	Others
Cerebral Palsy					
A disorder of muscle control or coordination resulting from injury to the brain during its early (fetal, perinatal, and early childhood) development; there may be associated problems with intellectual, visual, or other functions	Growth problems	Failure to thrive	Constipation	Oral/motor problems	Central nervous system involvement; Orthopedic problems; Medication/nutrient interaction related to seizure disorder
Down Syndrome (A Genetic Disorder)					
Results from an extra chromosome 21, causing development problems such as congenital heart disease, mental retardation, small stature, and decreased muscle tone	Risk for obesity	Related to short stature and limited activity	Constipation	Poor suck in infancy	Gum disease; Increased risk of heart disease; Osteoporosis; Alzheimer's disease
Prader-Willi Syndrome (A Genetic Disorder)					
A disorder characterized by uncontrollable eating habits, inability to distinguish hunger from appetite, severe obesity, poorly developed genitalia, and moderate-to-severe mental retardation	Risk for obesity	Failure to thrive in infancy	N/A	Weak suck in infancy; Abnormal food-related problems	Risk of diabetes mellitus
Autism					
Classified as a type of pervasive developmental disorder; diagnostic criteria include communication problems, ritualistic behaviors, and inappropriate social interaction	N/A	N/A	N/A	Limited food selection; Strong food dislikes	Pica; Medication/nutrient interaction
Spina Bifida (Myelomeningocele)					
Results from a midline defect of the skin, spinal column, and spinal cord; characterized by hydrocephalus, mental retardation, and lack of muscular control	Risk for obesity	Altered energy needs based on short stature and limited mobility	Constipation	Swallowing problems caused by Arnold Chiari malformation of the brain	Urinary tract infections

From American Dietetic Association: Position of the American Dietetic Association: providing nutrition services for infants, children, and adults with developmental disabilities and special health care needs, *J Am Diet Assoc* 104:97, 2004.

mixed populations, and data that are out of date. Other measures that can be used to further explore weight include arm circumference, triceps skin fold measures, and body mass index (BMI). BMI is a part of the CDC growth charts and can also be found in Appendixes 12, 16, and 23. Using the BMI for age can be helpful for the child with a developmental disability; however, there has been controversy related to its usefulness in identifying overweight in children who are overly fat because of decreased muscle mass and short stature.

Biochemical Assessment

Laboratory assessment for the child and adult with developmental disabilities is generally the same as that listed in Chapter 15 and Appendix 30 for any individual without developmental disabilities. Additional tests may be indicated for the individual with epilepsy or seizures who is receiving an anticonvulsant medication such as phenytoin (Dilantin), divalproex sodium (Depakote), topiramate (Topamax), or carbamazepine (Tegretol). Use of these medications can lead to low blood levels of folic acid, carnitine, ascorbic acid, calcium, vitamin D, alkaline phosphatase, phosphorus, and pyridoxine. Assessment of thyroid status is part of the protocol for children with Down syndrome (DS), and a glucose tolerance test is recommended for Prader-Willi syndrome (PWS) (www.medlineplus, 2005).

Dietary Intake

Dietary information should be obtained for the child with a developmental disability through a diet history such as would be used with any child. There are difficulties in obtaining an accurate recall when the parents work outside the home and the child is in a day-care center. Written diaries are also difficult to obtain when the child has multiple caretakers and when he or she is in school. When working with an adult with developmental disabilities, it is often difficult to obtain accurate information unless the individual has supervision such as in special residential housing. Use of pictures and food models can often assist the RD in obtaining a picture of the individual's intake.

Feeding Issues

Many children and adults with developmental disabilities display feeding problems that seriously decrease their ability to eat an adequate diet. Feeding problems have been defined as the inability or refusal to eat certain foods because of neuromotor dysfunction, obstructive lesions such as strictures, and psychosocial factors (Cloud et al., 2005). Other causes of feeding problems in this population include oral-motor difficulties, positioning problems, conflict in parent-child relationships, sensory issues, and tactile resistance post intubation (Tobin et al., 2005).

The nutritional consequences of feeding problems include inadequate weight gain, poor growth in length, poor immunity, anemia, vitamin and mineral deficiencies, dental caries, and psychosocial problems. Feeding problems should be assessed with an understanding of the normal

development of feeding and the physical makeup of the mouth and pharynx (Cloud et al., 2005) (see Figure 41-3 in Chapter 41).

Feeding problems are classified usually as oral motor, positioning, behavioral, and self-feeding. Oral-motor problems include suckling, sucking, swallowing, and chewing. They also include sensory motor integration and problems with self-feeding. Children with developmental disabilities such as DS, cerebral palsy, or cleft lip and palate often have oral-motor feeding problems that may be related to the cleft, muscle tone, and inability to accept texture changes. The oral-motor problem may also be related to the developmental level, which may be delayed. The oral-motor problem is described as an exaggeration of normal neuromotor mechanisms that disrupts the rhythm and organization of oral-motor function and interferes with the feeding process (see *Clinical Insight*: Oral-Motor Problems).

Positioning the child for feeding is very much related to his or her motor development, head control, trunk stability, and ability to have hips and legs at a right angle (Figures 45-2 and 45-3). This is frequently a problem for individuals with cerebral palsy, spina bifida, and DS, as will be discussed later. However, without proper positioning oral-motor problems are difficult to correct. The ability to self-feed may be delayed in the child with developmental disabilities and may require training by a feeding specialist and special equipment for feeding such as spoons, dishes, and cups.

A complete feeding evaluation is best completed with actual observation by a team composed of a speech thera-

---

✹ CLINICAL INSIGHT

Oral-Motor Problems

Problem	Description
Tonic bite reflex	Strong jaw closure when teeth and gums are stimulated
Tongue thrust	Forceful and often repetitive protrusion of an often bunched or thick tongue in response to oral stimulation
Jaw thrust	Forceful opening of the jaw to the maximum extent during eating, drinking, attempts to speak, or general excitement
Tongue retraction	Pulling back the tongue within the oral cavity at the presentation of food, spoon, or cup
Lip retraction	Pulling back the lips in a very tight smilelike pattern at the approach of the spoon or cup toward the face
Sensory defensiveness	A strong adverse reaction to sensory input (touch, sound, light)

Modified from Lane S, Cloud H: Feeding problems and intervention: an interdisciplinary approach, *Top Clin Nutr* 3:23, 1988.

pist, a dentist, a physical therapist, an occupational therapist, and a registered dietitian. An excellent interdisciplinary feeding evaluation form is called the Developmental Feeding Tool shown in Figure 45-4.

Behavioral issues may result from oral-motor or sensory problems, medical problems or medications, and the amount of emphasis placed on feeding. Issues such as control of the feeding process along with lack of autonomy for the child may create negative behavior. Environmental factors also influence the eating behavior of the child. Examples include where the child is fed, distractibility, serving sizes, delayed weaning, and frequency of feeding. Estimates are that feeding problems are found in 40% to 70% of children with special health care needs and 80% of children with developmental delays. See Table 45-1 for the potential feeding- and nutrition-related problems associated with specific conditions.

Nutrition Diagnosis: Problem Identification

Once the nutrition assessment has been completed, problems should be identified related to growth, including weight; dietary adequacy or inadequacy; fluid intake; and clinical problems such as constipation, diarrhea, allergies, reactions to medications, and feeding issues. The problems in addressing them should be listed so that priorities can be set. When possible, this information is shared with the parent or caregiver and the adult client before the intervention process begins.

Interventions

Before intervention or medical nutrition therapy can begin, consideration must be given to the motivational level of the parent or client, his or her cultural background, and how the therapy can be community based and family centered. This means that consideration must be given to where the client will be served so that it becomes a part of the **individualized education plan (IEP)** or the **individualized family plan**.

Intervention should include all aspects of an individual's treatment program to avoid issuing an isolated set of instructions relevant to only one treatment goal when there

are many involved in the care (Cloud, 2001). In some cases medical nutrition therapy may not be the family's first priority in the care of the child or adult, making it important for the RD to recognize the importance of waiting for the family's cues (see Chapter 19). Even when the family is ready for intervention, such as weight management for a child with spina bifida, many factors still require consideration (e.g., the parent or caregiver's educational level and income, potential language barriers, and how the family implements coping strategies).

Monitoring and Evaluation

Once some type of medical nutrition therapy has been initiated, the need for follow-up evaluation and monitoring either by the RD or another health care professional is important. Giving information in writing, followed by a phone call helps to repeat some of the discussion and answer questions that the parent may not have asked during the clinic session. This also provides an opportunity for a follow-up visit. A case manager who communicates with the adult with a developmental disability may be involved. The RD may also need to find appropriate resources to pay for supplemental nutrition products, tube feedings, and special food products as a part of the follow-up process. Community and agency resources will be discussed later in this chapter.

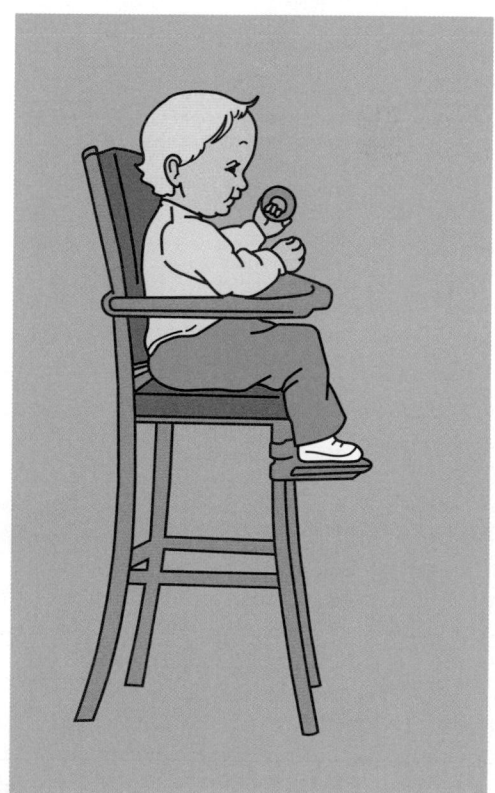

FIGURE 45-3 Good feeding position for a child ages 6 to 24 months, showing hip flexion, trunk in midline, and head in midline. Good foot support with a stool should continue throughout childhood. *(From Cloud H: Team approach to pediatric feeding problems, Chicago, 1987, American Dietetic Association. Used with permission.)*

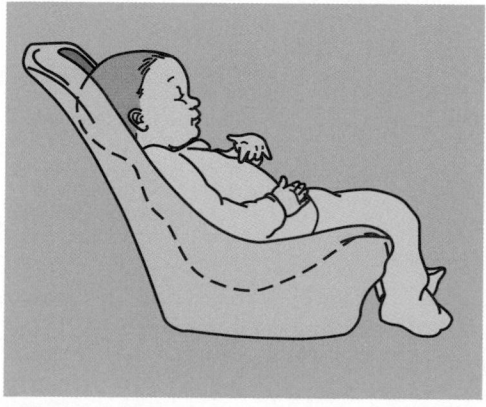

FIGURE 45-2 Proper feeding position for the infant. *(From Cloud H: Team approach to pediatric feeding problems, Chicago, 1987, American Dietetic Association. Used with permission.)*

Developmental Feeding Tool (DFT)

Parent/Guardian_____   Date_____

Address_____   Staff member_____

City_____ State_____ Zip _____   Child's name_____

County_____ Telephone_____   Birth date_____ Age_____ Sex_____ Race_____

Referrer_____   Head circumference (cm)____ (%ile NCHS)____ Hand dominance _____

Height (cm)_____ (%ile NCHS)_____ Weight (kg)_____ (%ile NCHS)_____

Weight for height (%ile NCHS)_____ Hematocrit_____ Urine screen_____

		PHYSICAL			NEUROMOTOR/ MUSCULAR			ORAL/MOTOR
Yes	No	Size	Yes	No	Tonicity	Yes	No	Facial Expression

PHYSICAL

Size

1. Weight (avg. %ile NCHS)
2. Underweight
3. Overweight
4. Stature (avg. %ile NCHS)
5. Short (below 5th %ile for ht. NCHS)
6. Tall (above 95th %ile for ht. NCHS)
7. Abnormal body proportions*
8. Head circumference (avg. %ile NCHS)
9. Microcephalic
10. Macrocephalic

Laboratory

11. Hematocrit (normal)
12. Urine screen (normal)*

Health Status

13. Bowel problems*
14. Diabetes
15. Vomiting
16. Dental caries
17. Anemia
18. Food allergies/ intolerance*
19. Medications*
20. Vitamin/mineral supplements*
21. Ingests non-food items
22. Therapeutic diet*
23. General appearance (normal)*
24. Head (normal)*
25. Eyes (normal)*
26. Ears (normal)*
27. Nose (normal)*
28. Teeth/gums (normal)*
29. Palate (normal)*
30. Skin (normal)*
31. Muscles (normal)*
32. Arms/hands (normal)*
33. Legs/feet (normal)*

NEUROMOTOR/ MUSCULAR

Tonicity

34. Body tone (normal)*

Head and Trunk Control

35. Head control (normal)*
36. Lifts head in prone
37. Head lags when pulled to sitting
38. Head drops forward
39. Head drops backward
40. Trunk control (normal)*

Upper Extremity Control

41. Range of motion (normal)*
42. Approach to object (normal)*
43. Grasp of object (normal)*
44. Release of object (normal)*
45. Brings hand to mouth
46. Dominance established

Reflexes

47. Grossly normal
48. Asymmetrical tonic neck reflex*
49. Symmetical tonic neck reflex*
50. Moro reflex*
51. Grasp reflex*

Body Alignment

52. Scoliosis
53. Kyphosis
54. Lordosis
55. Hip subluxation or dislocation, suspected

Position in Feeding

56. Mother's lap
57. Infant seat
58. High chair
59. Table and chair
60. Wheelchair
61. Other adaptive chair*

ORAL/MOTOR

Facial Expression

62. Symmetrical structure/ function*
63. Muscle tone lips/cheeks (normal)
64. Hypertonic muscle tone of lips
65. Hypotonic muscle tone of lips

Oral Reflexes

66. Gag (normal)*
67. Bite (normal)*
68. Rooting (normal)*
69. Suck/swallow (normal)*

Respiration

70. Mouth
71. Nose
72. Thoracic
73. Abdominal
74. Regular rhythm*

Oral Sensitivity

75. Inside mouth (normal)*
76. Outside mouth (normal)*
77. Hypersensitivity*
78. Hyposensitivity*
79. Intolerance to brushing teeth

FEEDING PATTERNS

Yes No Bottle-feeding

80. Suckling tongue movements
81. Sucking tongue movements
82. Firm lip seal*
83. Coordinated suck- swallow-breathing
84. Difficulty swallowing*

Cup-drinking

85. Adequate lip closure*
86. Loses less than 1/2 total amount*

Yes No

87. Wide up-and-down jaw movements
88. Stabilizes jaw by biting edge of cup
89. Stabilizes jaw through muscle control
90. Drinks through a straw

Feeding Patterns—Spoon-feeding

Yes No

91. Suckles as food approaches
92. Cleans food off lower lip
93. Cleans food off spoon with upper lip
94. Munching pattern

Lateralizes Tongue:

95. When food placed between molars

Yes No

96. When food placed in center of tongue
97. To move food from side to side
98. Vertical jaw movements
99. Rotary jaw movements

Feeding Patterns—Chewing

100. Lip closure during chewing*

FIGURE 45-4 Developmental feeding tool. (*Smith MAH et al:* Feeding management for a child with a handicap: a guide for professionals, *Memphis, 1982, University of Tennessee: The Boling Child Development Center, University of Tennessee Center for Health Sciences.*)

Developmental Feeding Tool (Cont'd)

Yes	No	Isolated, Voluntary Tongue Movements
____	____	101. Protrudes/retracts tongue
____	____	102. Elevates tongue outside mouth
____	____	103. Elevates tongue inside mouth
____	____	104. Depresses tongue outside mouth
____	____	105. Depresses tongue inside mouth
____	____	106. Lateralizes tongue outside mouth
____	____	107. Lateralizes tongue inside mouth
		Special Oral Problems
____	____	108. Drools*
____	____	109. Thrusts tongue when utensil placed in mouth*
____	____	110. Thrusts tongue during chewing/swallowing*
____	____	111. Other oral-motor problem*
		NUTRITION HISTORY
Yes	No	Past Status
____	____	112. Feeding problems birth—1 year*
____	____	113. Breast fed
____	____	114. Bottle fed
____	____	115. Weaned
		Current Status
____	____	116. Eats blended food
____	____	117. Eats limited texture
____	____	118. Eats chopped table foods
____	____	119. Eats table foods
____	____	120. Feeds unassisted
____	____	121. Feeds with partial guidance
____	____	122. Feeds with complete guidance
____	____	123. Drinks from a cup unassisted
____	____	124. Drinks from a cup assisted
____	____	125. Finger-feeds
____	____	126. Uses a spoon
____	____	127. Uses a fork
____	____	128. Uses a knife

Yes	No	
____	____	129. Average rate of eating
____	____	130. Fast rate of eating
____	____	131. Slow rate of eating
		Diet Review
____	____	132. Appetite normal
____	____	133. Eats 3 meals/day
____	____	134. Snacks daily
		Dietary Intake, Current
____	____	135. Milk/dairy products, 3-4/day
____	____	136. Vegetables, 2-3/day
____	____	137. Fruit, 2-3/day
____	____	138. Meat/meat substitute, 2-3/day
____	____	139. Bread/cereal, 3-4/day
____	____	140. Sweets/snacks, 1-2/day
____	____	141. Liquids, 2 cups/day
		SOCIAL/BEHAVIORAL
Yes	No	Child-Caregiver Relationship
____	____	142. Child responds to caregiver
____	____	143. Caregiver affectionate to child
		Social Skills
____	____	144. Eye contact
____	____	145. Smiles
____	____	146. Gestures, i.e. waves byebye
____	____	147. Clings to caregiver
____	____	148. Interacts with examiner
____	____	149. Responds to simple directions
____	____	150. Seeks approval
____	____	151. Toilet trained
____	____	152. Knows own sex
		Behavior Problems
____	____	153. Self abusive
____	____	154. Hyperactive
____	____	155. Aggressive
____	____	156. Withdrawn
____	____	157. Other*
		Play
____	____	158. Plays infant games, i.e., pat-a-cake
____	____	159. Solitary play
____	____	160. Parallel play
____	____	161. Cooperative play
____	____	162. Additional comments*

Number COMMENTS

FIGURE 45-4, cont'd Developmental feeding tool.

CHROMOSOMAL ABERRATIONS

Down Syndrome

Down syndrome (DS) is a chromosomal aberration of chromosome 21 (trisomy 21). It has an incidence of one in 700 live births and results from the presence of an extra chromosome in each cell of the body. This anomaly causes the physical and developmental features of short stature, congenital heart disease, mental retardation, decreased muscle tone, hyperflexibility of joints, speckling of the iris (Brushfield spots), upward slant of the eyes, epicanthal folds, small oral cavity, short broad hands with the single palmar crease, and wide gap between the first and second toes (Capone et al., 2005).

Normally every cell of the human body except for the gametes (spermo or ova) contains 46 chromosomes, which are arranged in pairs (see Chapter 13). With DS there is one extra (47) chromosome. There are three processes by which this anomaly can occur: nondysjunction, translocation, and mosaicism. In nondysjunction chromosome 21 fails to separate before conception and the abnormal gamete joins with a normal gamete at conception to form a fertilized egg with three of chromosome 21. This may also occur during the first cell division after conception. This type of DS is usually sporadic and has a recurrence rate of 0.5% to 1%. In translocation the extra chromosome is attached to another chromosome (usually 14, 15, or 22). About half the time, this type of DS is inherited from a parent who is a carrier; it has a much higher risk of recurrence. In **mosaicism** the abnormal separation of chromosome 21 occurs sometime after

conception. All future divisions of the affected cell result in cells with an extra chromosome. Therefore the child has some cells with the normal number of chromosomes and other cells with an extra chromosome. Frequently the child with this type of DS lacks some of the more distinctive features of the syndrome (Capone et al., 2005) (see *Pathophysiology and Care Management Algorithm*: Down Syndrome).

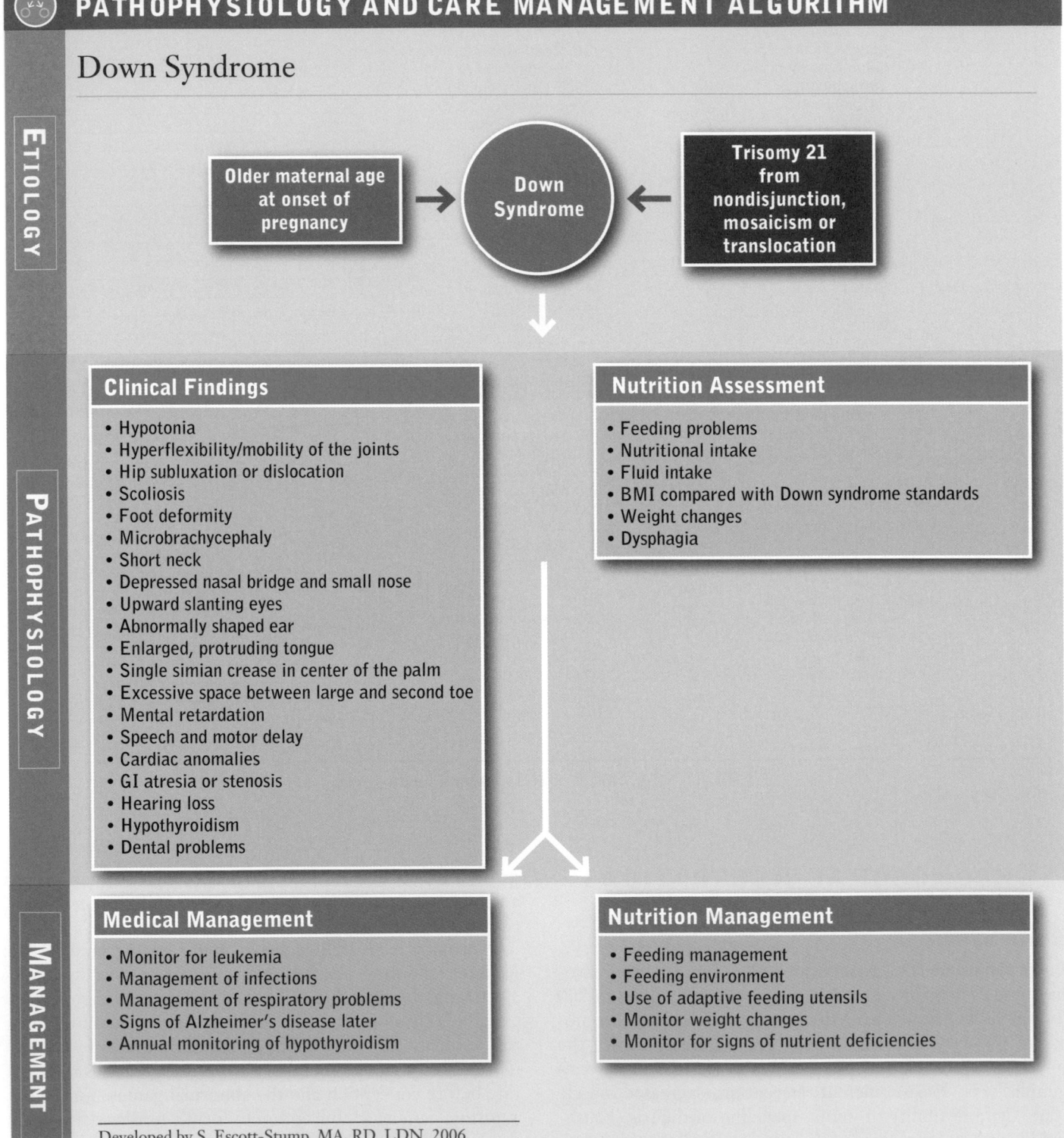

PATHOPHYSIOLOGY AND CARE MANAGEMENT ALGORITHM

Down Syndrome

ETIOLOGY

Older maternal age at onset of pregnancy → **Down Syndrome** ← Trisomy 21 from nondisjunction, mosaicism or translocation

PATHOPHYSIOLOGY

Clinical Findings

- Hypotonia
- Hyperflexibility/mobility of the joints
- Hip subluxation or dislocation
- Scoliosis
- Foot deformity
- Microbrachycephaly
- Short neck
- Depressed nasal bridge and small nose
- Upward slanting eyes
- Abnormally shaped ear
- Enlarged, protruding tongue
- Single simian crease in center of the palm
- Excessive space between large and second toe
- Mental retardation
- Speech and motor delay
- Cardiac anomalies
- GI atresia or stenosis
- Hearing loss
- Hypothyroidism
- Dental problems

Nutrition Assessment

- Feeding problems
- Nutritional intake
- Fluid intake
- BMI compared with Down syndrome standards
- Weight changes
- Dysphagia

MANAGEMENT

Medical Management

- Monitor for leukemia
- Management of infections
- Management of respiratory problems
- Signs of Alzheimer's disease later
- Annual monitoring of hypothyroidism

Nutrition Management

- Feeding management
- Feeding environment
- Use of adaptive feeding utensils
- Monitor weight changes
- Monitor for signs of nutrient deficiencies

Developed by S. Escott-Stump, MA, RD, LDN, 2006.

Health Concerns

The National Down Syndrome Congress has published a listing of the health concerns for individuals with DS; many have nutrition implications Table 45-2).

Nutrition Assessment

Anthropometric Measures. Height, weight, head circumference, triceps skin fold, and arm circumference are obtained for the child with DS with the usual measurements. BMI can be taken but may be higher than normal because of short stature. Growth measures are an important part of the assessment and ongoing nutrition therapy since these individuals tend to be short. Muscle tone is low, and gross motor ability is often delayed, leading to the possibility of the individual becoming overweight. Monitoring should be frequent, and growth plotted on the CDC charts (see Appendixes 9-16).

Biochemical Measures. There have been numerous studies showing biochemical and metabolic abnormalities in individuals with DS; however, many have involved small samples and were difficult to interpret (Capone et al, 2005). Although serum concentrations of albumin have been found to be low, the guidelines from the Down Syndrome Medical Congress do not list serum albumin assessment as routine. Increased glucose levels have been reported, with one study reporting an increased incidence of diabetes mellitus (Van Goor et al., 1997).

A number of studies have looked at zinc, copper, and selenium status, with some reporting that zinc and selenium levels are reduced, but the results for plasma levels of copper are conflicting (Ani et al., 2000). These studies, along with multiple studies involving vitamin A, carotene, and vitamin D

have concluded that these deficiencies do not exist. Studies involving vitamin E report decreased concentrations in DS (Shah and Johnson, 1989). It is suggested that trisomy 21 predisposes to increased oxidative stress and the increased use of antioxidants to protect against the stress; thus the low levels of vitamin E, an antioxidant. This theory of oxidative stress because of trisomy 21 has led parents of individuals with DS to purchase many vitamin supplements with the expected outcome of improved cognitive ability and growth. At this point there is no conclusive evidence that supplementation is effective.

Dietary Intake. During infancy the food intake of the infant with DS may differ from that of the normal infant. Although human breast milk is recommended, many infants with DS are formula fed. One recent study (Piscane et al., 2003) found that out of 560 children with DS, 57% were formula fed. The main reasons reported by the mothers were infants' illness and admission to the neonatal unit, frustration or depression, perceived milk insufficiency, and difficulty in suckling by the infant.

Progression to solid food has been found to be delayed in children with DS, mostly as a result of delays in feeding and motor development. Introduction of solid food may not be offered at 6 months if the infant has poor head control or is not yet sitting. Low tone and sucking problems also delay weaning from the breast or bottle to the cup. IEPs include feeding and feeding progression instruction and practice.

An important part of evaluating the dietary intake is determining energy and fluid needs since children with DS have a high prevalence of obesity. Studies have indicated that the resting energy expenditure (REE) of the child with DS is lower than for controls without DS (Luke et al., 1994)

TABLE 45-2

Health Concerns for Children With Down Syndrome

Health Concern	Implications	Treatment
Congenital heart disease	40%-50% of population	Medication or surgical repair
Hypotonia	Reduced muscle tone, increased range of joints	
Motor function problem	Early intervention for physical therapy, occupational therapy	
Delayed growth	Short stature	In some cases growth hormone
Developmental delays		Early intervention
Hearing concerns	Small ear canals, otitis media, conductive impairment	
Dental problems	Decreased saliva, reflux, and vomiting	Low sucrose intake
Ocular problems	Refractive errors, strabismus, cataracts	Corrective glasses
Cervical spine abnormality		None
Thyroid disease	Hypothyroidism	Thyroid supplement, tests repeated annually
Overweight	Excessive weight gain, inactivity	Decreased energy; increased activity
Seizure disorders		Medications
Emotional disorders	May occur late in childhood	Medication

Data from Saenz RB: Primary care of infants and young children with Down syndrome, *Am Fam Phys* 59:381, 1999.

and may be as much as 10% lower than the dietary reference intake for energy. For the child over the age of 5, calculations for energy requirements may need to be based on height rather than weight (Table 45-3) (see Chapter 2).

Feeding Skills. Feeding skills are delayed in the infant and child with DS. Some parents have found difficulty in initiating oral motor skills such as suckling and sucking. The infant with DS often has difficulty in coordinating sucking, swallowing, and breathing, which are the foundations for early feeding. When the infant has a congenital heart defect, which occurs in 40% to 60% of the DS infants, sucking is weakened, and fatigue interferes with the feeding process. Gastrointestinal anomalies are found in 8% to 12% of infants with DS, and these infants often require nasogastric or gastrostomy feedings.

Other physical factors that make feeding difficult in the first years of life include a **midfacial hypoplasia** (a craniofacial deformity common in cleft palate), a small oral cavity, a small mandible, delayed or abnormal dentition, malocclusion, nasal congestion, small hands, and short fingers. Weaning and self-feeding are usually late when compared to the normal infant and frequently do not emerge until 15 to 18 months of age. The DS infant strives for independence and autonomy about 6 months later than the child without DS.

Intervention Strategies

Overweight. The most effective intervention for the overweight child with DS is to design a calorie-controlled eating plan based on kilocalories per centimeter of height (see Table 45-3). Dietary management includes assessing the feeding developmental level of the child, working with a physical therapist related to gross motor skills to determine possible activity levels, and making environmental changes. Environmental changes should include following a regular eating schedule that includes three meals at regular times with the child sitting either in a high chair or at the table. Planned snacks should be low in fat and sugar. Soft drinks should be drastically limited if not eliminated, and milk should be low fat (after age 2). Physical activity should be encouraged. Counseling in which the parent helps determine a realistic plan should focus on serving sizes and food preparation and decreasing the number of times meals are purchased in fast-food restaurants. If the child or adolescent is school age, a prescription for a special meal at school can be obtained by using the school food service prescription (to be discussed later in the chapter).

Feeding Skills. Often parents wrongly expect different feeding development for the child with DS. Behavioral problems related to feeding usually develop based on what happens between the parent and child at mealtime. An example of this is the unnecessary delay of weaning to a cup or avoiding progression of food textures because of inadequate effort or education needed to enable this in the DS child. During intervention programs the feeding team can guide the parent in positioning the child and working toward attainable feeding skills related to the developmental level of the child. Close attention should be paid to feeding and the development of self-feeding skills.

Constipation. This is a frequent problem for the child with DS because of overall low tone followed by lack of fiber and fluid in the diet. Treatment should involve increasing fiber and fluid, with water consumption emphasized. Fiber content of the diet for children after age 3 is 5 to 6 g per year of age per day. For adults the recommendation is for 25 to 30 g of dietary fiber daily.

TABLE 45-3

Estimated Caloric Needs for Special Conditions

Condition	kcal/cm	Comments
Normal child	16	
Prader-Willi	Maintain growth: 10-11	For all children and adolescents
	Slow weight loss: 8.5	
Cerebral palsy		
Mild	14	Reliable for ages 5-11 yr
Severe, limited mobility	11	Reliable for ages 5-11 yr
Down syndrome	Girls: 14.3	Reliable for ages 5-11 yr
	Boys: 16.1	
Motor dysfunction		
Nonambulatory	7-11	Reliable for ages 5-12 yr
Ambulatory	14	Reliable for ages 5-12 yr
Spina bifida	Maintain weight: 9-11	For all children over 8 years of age and minimally
	Promote weight loss: 7	active

Modified from Rokusek C, Heindicles E: *Nutrition and feeding for persons with special needs*, with permission of the South Dakota University Affiliated Program, Interdisciplinary Center for Disabilities, 1992.

Prader-Willi Syndrome

Prader-Willi syndrome (PWS) was first described in 1956 by Drs. Prader, Willi, and Lambert. It is a genetic condition caused by the absence of chromosomal material from chromosome 15. PWS occurs with a frequency of 1/10,000 to 1/25,000 live births. Characteristics of the syndrome include developmental delays, poor muscle tone, short stature, small hands and feet, incomplete sexual development, and unique facial features. Insatiable appetite leading to obesity is the classic feature of PWS; however, in infancy the problem of **hypotonia** (low muscle tone) interferes with feeding and leads to failure to thrive (McCune and Driscoll, 2005). Developmental delays (affecting 50% of the population), learning disabilities, and mental retardation (affecting 10%) are associated with PWS.

The genetic basis of PWS is complex. Individuals with PWS have a portion of genetic material deleted from chromosome 15 received from the father. Of the cases of PWS, 70% are caused from the paternal deletion, occurring in a specific region on the q arm of the chromosome. PWS can also develop if a child receives both chromosome 15s from the mother. This is seen in approximately 25% of the cases of PWS and is called maternal uniparental disomy. Early detection of PWS is now possible because of the use of deoxyribonucleic acid methylation analysis, which correctly diagnoses 99% of the cases (McCune and Driscoll, 2005). This is an important development in the early identification and subsequent treatment of these children to prevent obesity and growth retardation and is used to identify the infant born with features and characteristics described above (McCune, Driscoll, 2005).

Health Concerns

Metabolic Abnormalities. Short stature in the individual with PWS has been attributed to growth hormone deficiency. In addition to decreased growth hormone release, children have low serum insulin-like growth factor-1 (IGR-1), low IGF binding protein-1, and low insulin compared to normal obese children. Growth hormone therapy was approved by the Food and Drug Administration (FDA) in 2000, and in one 5-year study in Japan 37 patients from age 3 to 21 years experienced significant increase in height gain velocity when given growth hormone (Obata et al., 2003).

In addition to the growth hormone deficiency, individuals have a deficiency in the hypothalamic-pituitary-gonadal axis, causing delayed and incomplete sexual development. Finally there is a decreased insulin response to a glucose load in children with PWS compared to age-matched non-PWS obese children (Schuster et al., 1996).

Appetite and Obesity. Appetite control and obesity are common problems with individuals with PWS. After the initial period of failure to thrive, children begin to gain excessively between the ages of 1 and 4, and appetite is excessive. This uncontrollable appetite, a classic feature of PWS, when combined with overeating, a low basal metabolic rate, and decreased activity, leads to the characteristic obesity. The cause of the uncontrollable appetite involves the hypo-

thalamus and the parvocellular oxytocin neurons, which are decreased in PWS brains (Swaab et al., 1995). Other hormones and peptides related to appetite control in animals were not found to be increased in the hypothalamus of individuals with PWS (Goldstone et al., 2002). Body composition is an important consideration in the evaluation of individuals with PWS. They have abnormal body composition, decreased lean body mass, and increased body fat, even in infancy. In a study of 16 infants (Bekx et al., 2003), the percent of body fat was significantly increased and the percent of fat free mass significantly decreased with reduced energy expenditure. Body fat is generally deposited in the thighs, buttocks, and abdominal area. The lowered energy expenditure is found in young children, adolescents, and adults with PWS, with one study showing adolescents with PWS having a total energy expenditure (TEE) 53% of that of normal obese adolescents (McCune and Driscoll, 2005). The low muscle tone contributes greatly to the lack of interest in physical activity.

Nutrition Assessment

Anthropometrics. As stated earlier, height measurements tend to be lower in PWS infants and young children, with the rate of height gain tapering off between the ages of 1 and 4. The usual measurements of length or height, weight, and head circumference should be taken and plotted on the CDC growth curves. Other measures of interest include arm circumference and triceps skin fold measures. BMI may be distorted for the individual with PWS because of the short stature; however, plotting the BMI over time is useful in determining unusual changes (see the tables found in Appendices 12 and 16). It is important that anthropometric measures be taken frequently and reported to the parents or caregiver.

Biochemical Measures. Biochemical studies are generally the same for the PWS individual, with the exception of either fasting blood glucose tests or glucose tolerance tests. These are added because of the risk for diabetes mellitus, possibly related to the obesity that usually accompanies PWS.

Dietary Intake. Dietary information varies for individuals with PWS, depending on their age. In infancy the dietary information should be obtained with a careful dietary history and analyzed for energy and nutrient intake. Infants are commonly difficult to feed because of their hypotonia, poor suck, and delayed motor skills. Generally their feeding development is slower than in the normal infant, and transitioning to food at 4 to 6 months of age may be difficult. Many of these infants have gastroesophageal reflux requiring medication or thickening of their formula.

During the toddler years weight gain may increase rapidly as dietary intake increases. This requires careful assessment of portion sizes, frequency of feeding, and types of foods served. Although some parents may report that the child with PWS does not eat more than other children in the family, they need to be informed that the energy needs are lower because of the reduced lean muscle mass and slow development of motor skills and activity. As the children get older, their interest in food increases; and, starting around ages 5 through 12, they may be hungry all the time and display difficult behaviors such as tantrums, stubbornness, and food stealing. Many parents have found it necessary to lock cabinets, refrigerators, and the kitchen door to control food intake (Dimitropoulas et al., 2001). Information gathered during the dietary interview should include asking about environmental control techniques.

Determination of energy needs for the infant with PWS is the same as for a normal infant. However, as the child enters the toddler years, he or she will need fewer calories to maintain weight gain along the growth curve. This will apply in adulthood when fewer calories are needed to maintain weight. Energy needs have been calculated according to centimeters of height from 2 years on. It has been recommended that the macronutrient intake of the diet be 25% protein, 50% carbohydrate, and 25% fat (see Table 45-3).

Feeding Skills. The infant with PWS often presents with weak oral skills and poor sucking skills in the first year of life. As the child matures, feeding skills are not a problem, but they may be delayed. Chewing and swallowing problems are not usually seen, although they may be associated with the low muscle tone. Behavioral feeding issues are associated with an insatiable appetite and not being provided with food. As stated earlier, this can bring about tantrums.

Intervention Strategies

Intervention for PWS should be at each developmental stage: infancy, toddler, preschool age, school age and adult.

Infancy. Providing adequate nutrition as established by the American Academy of Pediatrics (AAP) related to breast-feeding or formula feeding is recommended (see Chapters 5 and 6). Since feeding may be difficult related to sucking, concentrating the formula or breast milk may be necessary to promote adequate weight gain. Feeding intervention will assist in improving the sucking problems caused by hypotonia. As the infant matures, a concentrated formula is not necessary, and foods can be added when head control and trunk stability are achieved, usually around ages 4 to 6 months.

Toddler and Preschool Age. Most children begin to gain excessive weight between 1 and 4 years of age. Beginning a structured dietary protocol for the child and the family is important so that the toddler learns that meals are provided at specified times so that a pattern of grazing doesn't develop. Parents should be taught to provide small servings of meats, vegetables, grains, and fruits and limited amounts of sweets. Early intervention for these children in the preschool years is very important in working with feeding issues and intake control as they grow older. Weight, height, and nutrient intake should be monitored monthly, and energy needs adjusted if weight gain becomes excessive. Concurrently physical activity must be encouraged as a part of IEP, and physical therapy services made available if necessary.

School Age. For the school-age child, collaboration with the school food service program becomes important. Energy needs should be calculated per centimeter of height (see Table 45-3) and are generally 50% to 75% of the energy needs of unaffected children. This may require using the prescription for special meals through the school food service program.

At home environmental controls may be required, with cupboards and refrigerators being locked, since the child and adolescent have limited satiety and search for food away from mealtime. Some parents say that growth hormone therapy for their child helps, but it doesn't seem to change the child's lack of satiety. Appetite-suppressing medications have been used but are largely unsuccessful.

Adulthood. Prevention of obesity is truly the key for successful treatment of PWS; however, many adults who were not identified early became very obese. Weight management programs providing a very low 6 to 8 kcal per centimeter of height may be required. Nutrient values should be calculated, and vitamin-mineral supplements added, as well as essential fatty acids if indicated. Many dietary treatments have been tried such as the ketogenic diet and the protein-sparing modified-fast diets. However, with any approach strict supervision is usually required, and great emphasis must be placed on physical activity. A behavior management approach has also been recommended to implement both the dietary management and physical activity plans. In many states there are group homes for adults with PWS where supervised independent living is possible and meals can be very structured and exercise programs implemented.

Medical nutrition therapy of children and adults with PWS requires follow-up through many health care providers and schools. Fortunately parents of the individual with PWS now have access to a number of support groups and organizations dedicated to education, research, and establishing treatment programs.

NEUROLOGIC DISORDERS

Spina Bifida

Spina bifida is a neurologic tube defect that presents in a number of ways: meningocele, myelomeningocele (MM), and spina bifida occulta. Myelomeningocele is the most common derangement in the formation of the spinal cord and generally occurs between 26 to 30 days of gestation, with the date of occurrence affecting the location of the lesion. The lesion may occur in the thoracic, lumbar, or sacral area and will influence the amount of paralysis. The higher the lesion, the greater is the paralysis. Manifestations range from weakness in the lower extremities to complete paralysis and loss of sensation. Other manifestations include incontinence and hydrocephalus. The incidence of spina bifida is 1 per 600 births, whereas the incidence of myelomeningocele is 5 per 10,000 in the United States (Ekvall and Cerniglia, 2005).

The spinal lesion may be open and can be surgically repaired shortly after birth, usually within 24 hours to prevent infection. Although the spinal opening can be surgically repaired, the nerve damage is permanent, resulting in the varying degrees of paralysis of the lower limbs. In addition to physical and mobility issues, most individuals have some form of learning disability.

Prevention of spina bifida is now possible (Stevenson, 2000). In 1983 Smithells and colleagues published results of a multilevel study involving the preconception supplementation of mothers with folic acid plus multivitamins. This reduced the risk of a second pregnancy with spina bifida as an outcome. As a result of numerous studies showing folic acid supplementation before conception to be effective, the national recommendation is 400 mcg per day for all women of childbearing age. In addition, folic acid has been added to many flours and other cereal and grain products in the food supply (USDHHS FDA, 1996). These public health measures have resulted in increased folic acid blood levels in U.S. women of childbearing age and a decrease of 20% in the national rate of spina bifida (Robbins et al, 2006) (see Chapters 5 and 11).

Health Concerns

The spinal lesion affects many systems of the body and can result in weakness in the lower extremities, paralysis, and nonambulation; poor skin condition caused by pressure sores; loss of sensation and bladder incontinence; hydrocephalus; urinary tract infections; constipation; and obesity. Seizures also occur in approximately 20% of children with myelomeningocele and require medication. Chronic medication is required for prevention and treatment of urinary tract infections and for bladder control. The resultant nutrition problems include obesity, feeding problems, constipation, and drug-nutrient interaction problems. Children with spina bifida have been allergic to latex brought about by multiple surgeries. It has been recommended that they avoid certain foods: bananas, kiwi, and avocados. Mild reactions can occur from apples, carrots, celery, tomatoes, papaya, and melons (Cloud et al., 2005) (see Chapter 29).

Nutrition Assessment

Anthropometrics. Infants and children with neural tube defects are usually shorter because of reduced length and atrophy of the lower extremities, although other problems such as hydrocephalus, scoliosis, renal disease, and malnutrition may contribute to it. The level of the lesions can also affect the length and height of the individual.

Obtaining accurate length and height measures can be difficult, especially as the child grows older. An alternate measure for determining height, the arm span to height ratio, is used and modified, depending on leg muscle mass. Arm span can be used directly as a height measure (arm span × 1) if there is no leg muscle mass loss, as in a sacral

lesion. Arm span × 0.95 can be used to determine height if there is partial leg muscle loss, and arm span × 0.90 is used for a height measurement when there is complete leg muscle loss such as with a thoracic spinal lesion (Ekvall and Cerniglia, 2005).

Weight measures can be obtained for the child unable to stand by using chair scales, bucket scales, and wheelchair scales. To monitor the weight accurately, it should be obtained in a consistent manner, with the person in light clothing or undressed. Triceps skin fold measures can also be used, along with subscapular measures and abdominal and thorax measures, to determine the amount of body fat.

Head circumference should be measured in infants and toddlers up to age 3. A high percentage of children with spina bifida have head shunts as a result of their hydrocephalus. Unusual changes in the size of the head may indicate a problem with the shunt.

Biochemical Measures. Most protocols in the treatment of spina bifida include iron status tests, measurements of vitamin C and zinc levels, and other tests related to the nutritional consequences of medications needed for seizures and urinary tract infection control (see Chapter 16 and Appendix 31).

Dietary Intake. Many children with spina bifida eat a limited variety of foods, and they are frequently described as a "picky eaters" by the parents. When doing a dietary history, it is important to ask about the variety of foods, particularly of high-fiber foods. The school-age child may be prone to skipping breakfast since early morning preparations for school require more time than for the nonaffected child.

Energy needs are lower for the child with spina bifida (see Table 45-3), and calorie requirements must be determined carefully to prevent the obesity to which many are prone. Ekvall (2005) has found that for myelomeningocele children 8 years or older, the caloric need is 7 cal/cm of height for weight loss and 9 to 11 cal/cm of height to maintain weight. It is important to evaluate how the mother or caretaker perceives food for the child since it represents sympathy and love for many parents.

Fluid intake is very important to evaluate since so many children have urinary tract infections and may be drinking inadequate amounts of water and excessive amounts of soft drinks or tea. Physical activity must also be evaluated and may be found to be very limited, particularly when the child is nonambulatory. Ambulatory individuals with a shunt may be restricted from contact sports but can be involved in walking and running.

Feeding skills need evaluating, along with oral motor function in particular. Many children with spina bifida are born with **Arnold Chiari malformation of the brain,** which affects the brainstem and swallowing. Difficulty in swallowing may contribute to the child avoiding certain foods later in life. Because of this there may be delays in weaning from the breast or bottle to the cup, but there should be no delays in gaining self-feeding skills.

Clinical Evaluation. Evaluation should include looking for pressure sores and signs of dehydration, along with asking the amount and type of fluids consumed. Constipation may be caused by the neurogenic bowel combined with a diet low in fiber and fluids. The evaluation should include a review of food intake, fiber content, and fluids.

Intervention Strategies

From a nutritional standpoint many children with spina bifida have obesity as the number one problem because of the impact of other physical problems. It usually occurs when ambulation is a problem and there is a lack of awareness of energy needs coupled with a lack of exercise. Other problems include inadequate fluids and fiber and refusal to accept a wide variety of foods. Feeding frequently is both a oral-motor and a behavioral problem. Early intervention and counseling about introducing foods around age 6 months, limiting the intake of high-sucrose infant jar foods, and training the child in accepting a wide variety of flavors and textures are important.

Obesity prevention should include addressing the problems of limited physical activity and lack of fluids and fiber and should begin with a calculation of the appropriate amount of calories and fluid. Once the child is in school, the food service manager should be provided with a prescription for a low-calorie breakfast and lunch, and weight management should be listed as a part of the individualized education plan (IEP). Enrollment in a group weight management program has been used successfully with modification of the accompanying physical exercise. The ideal program uses a team approach with involvement of the RD, nurse, occupational therapist, physical therapist, educator, and psychologist.

In many clinics the child or adult with spina bifida is seen on a semiannual or annual basis. This frequent follow-up is necessary and should include monitoring of growth, particularly weight; food and fluid intake; and medication use. School programs and IEPs are excellent follow-up sites; however, the school often lacks appropriate scales for weighing a nonambulatory student. In this situation the parent should be encouraged to bring the child to the clinic for weight checks or, if distance is a problem, find a long-term care facility that will permit using its scales. Follow-up by phone contact or e-mail can be done for evaluating dietary intake and fluid management.

Cerebral Palsy

Cerebral palsy (CP) is a disorder of motor control or coordination resulting from injury to the brain during its early development. Among the causative agents of CP are prematurity; blood type incompatibility; placental insufficiency; maternal infection that includes German measles; other viral diseases; neonatal jaundice; anoxia at birth; and other bacterial infections of the mother, fetus, or infant that affect the central nervous system.

The problem in CP lies in the inability of the brain to control the muscles, even though the muscles themselves and the nerves connecting them to the spinal cord are normal. The extent and location of the brain injury determine the type and distribution of CP. The incidence of CP varies with different studies, but the most commonly used rate is 2 to 3 per thousand live births. The prevalence of premature births has contributed to maintenance of this figure despite electro-fetal monitoring.

There are various types of CP, which are classified according to the neurologic signs involving muscle tone and abnormal motor patterns and postures. The diagnosis of CP is generally made between 9 to 12 months of age and as late as 2 years with some types (Box 45-1).

Health Concerns

Poor nutrition status and growth failure, often related to feeding problems, are common in children with CP. Meeting energy and nutrient needs is particularly difficult in children and adults with more severe forms of CP such as spastic quadriplegia and athetoid CP. For example, bone mineral density of children and adolescents with moderate-to-severe CP was reduced in those with gross motor function and feeding difficulties (Henderson et al., 2005).

Other health problems include constipation, usually caused by inactivity and lack of fiber and fluids, often connected to feeding problems. Dental problems occur and are often related to malocclusion, dental irregularities, and fractured teeth. Lengthy and prolonged bottle-feedings of milk and juice promote the decay of the primary upper front teeth and molars (see Chapter 25). Hearing problems and especially visual impairments, mental retardation, respiratory problems, and seizures impact nutrition status. Seizures are controlled with anticonvulsants, and a number of drug-nutrient interaction problems occur (see Chapter 16 and Appendix 31).

BOX 45-1

Different Types of Cerebral Palsy

Spastic CP—increased muscle tone, persistent infant reflexes, increased deep tendon reflexes in one of three patterns: hemiplegia (arm and leg on one side of the body), diplegia (involving the lower extremities), and quadriplegia (all four extremities and may include the trunk, head, and neck)

Dyskinetic CP—abnormalities in muscle tone that affect the entire body; includes athetoid CP, which includes uncontrolled and continuous involuntary movements

Mixed CP—a condition in which both athetosis and spasticity are present

Ataxic CP—abnormalities of voluntary movement and balance such as unsteady gait

Athetoid dyskinetic CP—normal intelligence but difficulty walking, sitting, speaking clearly

Data from *4Mychild: what type of cerebral palsy does my child have?* from www.cerebralpalsy.org/types-of-cerebral-palsy/, accessed June 18, 2007.

CP, Cerebral palsy.

Nutrition Assessment

Anthropometrics. This is an important area of assessment because of the growth failure of the more severely involved child or adult with CP. Children with CP are often shorter, and, depending on the level of severity, some children with CP may need to be measured for length using recumbent length boards or standing boards even as they grow older. However, some of the measuring devices are inappropriate for the child with contractures and inability to be stretched out full length. Arm span can be used when the individual's arms are stretchable, as well as upper arm and lower leg length. Hogan (1999) and Stevenson (2005) have recommended lower leg length or knee height as a possible measure for determining height for both children and adults with lower-leg CP. Krick and colleagues (1996) developed growth charts for children with CP using weight and length data on 360 children. However, the CDC training module on use of the growth curves for children from birth to 20 years of age recommends using the CDC curves designed for nonaffected children and plotting sequentially for indications of malnutrition rather than using the disease-specific curves.

Weight measures should be collected over time. Scales may require modifications, with positioning devices for the individual with CP who has developed scoliosis, contractures, and spasticity. Working with a physical therapist to find a positioning device that can be placed in a chair scale or using a bucket scale often works well. Mid-upper arm circumference and triceps skin fold measures are recommended by Samson-Fang and Stevenson (2000) as the reliable way to screen for fat stores in children with CP. Head circumference should be measured regularly from birth to 36 months and plotted on the CDC growth curves.

Biochemical Measures. Although there are no specific laboratory values indicated for the child with CP, a complete blood count, including hemoglobin and hematocrit, should be done when food intake is limited and malnutrition is a possibility. Because bone fractures are a significant problem for many children and adults with spastic quadriplegia, bone mineral density may need evaluating. Medications for seizures may be given; many have nutrition interaction problems (see Appendix 31). Evaluation of vitamin D, calcium, carnitine, and vitamin K levels may be indicated (King et al., 2003).

Dietary Intake. Feeding may be an important problem limiting the intake of food and fluid, and caretakers may not provide sufficient food to meet nutritional needs. The energy needs of the individual with CP vary according to the type of CP. Studies show that the REE and TEE are lower in those with spastic quadriplegic CP than in normal controls (Bandini et al., 1991; Stallings et al., 1996). Estimated energy needs for the child with CP are shown in Table 45-3.

Intervention Strategies

A high percentage of children with CP have feeding problems that are largely the result of oral-motor, positioning, and behavioral factors. As infants they have difficulty swallowing and coordinating swallowing and chewing, so that the normal progression to solid foods is later than usual. All this may lead to inadequate intake and growth limitations. For those infants and children in IEPs, the team of dietitian, speech therapist, occupational therapist, and physical therapist should evaluate the problem and work together in planning therapy.

Gastroesophageal reflux also is frequently seen in these infants and toddlers and a tube feeding may be required if a modified barium swallow reveals aspiration. This then requires that the formula prescribed be evaluated for caloric and nutritional value and volume required and directions be given for inclusion of solid foods in addition to the formula.

The most usual problems identified in the evaluation will be altered growth, inadequate energy provided, inadequate fluid intake, drug-nutrient interaction problems, constipation, and feeding problems. Working out an intervention plan is most successful when it involves the parent as part of the team, addresses cultural issues, and recognizes the importance of the feeding problem.

Children with CP have complex problems that will require continuing follow-up with the family and in the community and will take time to correct. There are agencies within the state that provide tube-feeding formulas and special wheelchairs and equipment to assist with feeding problems These agencies vary from state to state and are addressed in the section on resources.

Autism

Autism is one of five disorders under the category Pervasive Developmental Disorder (PDD). PDD was first used in the 1980s to describe a class of disorders as shown in Table 45-4. All types of PDD are neurologic disorders that are usually evident by age 3. In general children who have a type of PDD have difficulty in talking, playing with other children, and relating to others, including their families.

Autism spectrum disorders (ASDs) affect 3.4 per 1000 (Yeargin-Allsopp et al., 2003) and are diagnosed by the presence of qualitatively impaired reciprocal social interaction; impaired communication skills; and restricted, repetitive, stereotypical interests and behaviors. Many children with autism also have mental retardation. ASD is four times more common in boys than in girls. The term **Asperger syndrome** is most often used to describe children with the problems of ASD but who have normal-to-high cognitive levels (Edelson and Rimland, 2003).

ASDs may occur with other developmental or physical disabilities. They have been associated with tuberous sclerosis, maternal rubella, and mental retardation. Macrocephaly has been a common finding in large surveys of individuals with autism and also among their relatives. Overall growth is usually normal, and medical problems nonexistent. It is possible that, with the limited variety of foods usually eaten by these children, vitamin and mineral intake could be inadequate.

Efforts to find the cause of ASD have led to many studies looking at a possible toxic environment, toxic food, a nutritionally deficient diet, immune system problems, oxidative stress, and emotional stress as important factors. Other studies have studied neurotransmitters such as elevated

---

TABLE 45-4

Pervasive Developmental Disorders

Disorder	Characteristics
1. Autistic disorder	Impairment in social interaction
	Poor communication skills
	Repetitive and stereotypical behavior
2. Rett syndrome	Normal until 6-18 months
	Loss of abilities in motor skills
	Loss of social interaction
	Deceleration of head growth between 5 and 48 mo
3. Childhood Disintegrative disorder	Before age 10
	Loss of expressive language, social skills, bowel or bladder control, play motor skills
4. Asperger's syndrome	Impairment in social interaction
	Restricted repetitive or stereotypical behavior
	Normal language development
	Normal cognitive development
5. Pervasive developmental disorder not otherwise specified	Deficits in social behavior
	Impairment in understanding speech and in speech development
	Does not meet the criteria for the other four disorders

serotonin levels and disturbances in gamma-amino butyric receptors, glutamate transmitters, and cholinergic activity.

Much research is needed to find a major link between heredity and neuropathology and autism. Some treatment and research programs are using genomic panels to identify specific intervention protocols. The genomic panel identifies single nucleotide polymorphisms, which are identified from blood samples or cell cultures (see Chapter 13). This work has revealed that the child with autism may need additional essential fatty acids; nutrients with antioxidant qualities such as vitamins A, C, E, and selenium; mineral supplementation with zinc, calcium, and magnesium; a mercury-free diet; or an allergy elimination diet (see Chapter 29).

Interest in a neurochemical cause of ASD was started in 1979 when Jaak Panksepp proposed that ASD simulated brain opioid dysfunction. Earlier studies discovered a unique urinary peptide pattern in adults with ASD and hypothesized that brain opioids came from an exogenous source. Gluten and casein were the suspected sources, and in the 1980s researchers found these urinary peptides in the urine and cerebrospinal fluid of autistic individuals. The condition of the intestine has played a role in this theory, with constipation and diarrhea common in the individual with ASD. Intestinal inflammation has been reported in children with ASD and has improved with dietary restriction of gluten and casein (Reichelt and Knivsberg, 2007).

Nutrition Assessment

Anthropometrics. Height and weight are determined for the child and adult with ASD using the equipment and growth charts for nonaffected individuals. Head circumference should be taken and has been found to be larger than that of the non-ASD individual.

Biochemical Measures. These tests vary, depending on the clinic where the child is followed. There is no standard pattern of tests that should be given other than the regular blood work for health monitoring. However, amino acid screening shortly after birth is indicated along with thyroid testing. For some children allergy testing may be indicated (see Chapter 29).

Dietary Intake. Evaluations are sometimes difficult to complete for the child with a very limited intake. An effective measure may be having the parents and caregivers keep a food diary for several days to determine the macronutrient intake in addition to the vitamin and mineral intake. Obtaining information related to when food is presented and the amount eaten is important along with fluid consumption. Often excessive fluids are provided to compensate for limited food consumption.

Evaluations should include an observation of the child during mealtime. Some children are slow in arriving at developmental milestones for self-feeding and require feeding. Others finger feed or insist on self-feeding. The texture of the food presented should be recorded since sensory integration is difficult for children with ASD, and they may be very resistant to texture progression or variety. This is reflected in their fixation on one food (e.g., crackers, dry cereal, or chips). Fugassi and colleagues (2003) found that 70% of 87 children with autism had food jags and picky eating. The feeding evaluation should also include a description of the feeding environment, whether there is a high chair or age-appropriate toddler chair, the timing of meals, and the location for meals.

Intervention Strategies

No one therapy or method will work for all individuals with ASD. Many professionals and families use a range of treatments simultaneously, including behavior modification, structured educational approaches, medication, speech therapy, occupational therapy, and counseling. Popular nutrition interventions include mineral and vitamin therapy and elimination diets such as a gluten-free–casein-free diet; allergy diet; essential fatty acids, megavitamins; specific carbohydrate diets; and the Body Ecology Diet (Box 45-2). Very little has been published to demonstrate the value of the diets, although there are anecdotal reports of success. The exclusion diets are now used in some treatment centers and are publicized on various websites (http://www.autismndi.com). See Table 45-5, which compares three exclusion diets. It is important for the RD to understand these various forms of therapy in order to counsel the parent effectively. Because of the increasing prevalence of ASD, research on potential medical nutrition therapy should be promoted.

BOX 45-2

Autism Spectrum Disorder

Gluten-Free and Casein-Free Diet

These diets are based on a number of theories, but the basic premise of the diet is the exclusion of gluten, a part of wheat, oats, barley, and rye, and casein, the primary protein in milk and dairy products.

Specific Carbohydrate Diet

This diet is based on the premise that limiting the diet to simple sugars, usually at least for a year, will starve out toxic organisms in the gastrointestinal tract and restore gut integrity and immune function. It eliminates starches and sugars and consists mainly of meat, poultry, eggs, fish, vegetables, fruits, nuts, and seeds. There has been concern about the high protein content of the diet and its effect on the kidneys.

Body Ecology Diet

This diet proposes to restore and maintain the inner ecology of the body by eliminating food products that could have disturbed the immune system. The premise of the diet is to add cultured foods to the diet, change the quality of fats and oils consumed, and drastically reduce the intake of carbohydrates and sugars. The diet was originally created to reverse fungal infections, including candidiasis, and establish an inner ecosystem within the intestinal tract.

One of the problems with the gluten-free and casein-free diet is cost, since special foods needed to provide sufficient food choices are expensive and sometimes difficult to find. See Chapter 27 for the gluten-free and casein-free diet. When medical nutrition therapy is used, taking a team approach and working with the occupational therapist, speech therapist, and other members of the team is important for success. Parents also should be members of the team and counseled that changes will take time.

Follow-up is an important component of all therapy. From a nutritional standpoint, routine measures of height and weight should be scheduled, and there should be regular evaluation of eating and feeding behavior related to increasing ability to self-feed and accept new and different foods.

Attention-Deficit Hyperactivity Disorder

Attention-deficit hyperactivity disorder (ADHD) is a neurobehavioral problem seen in children with increasing frequency. It has been associated with learning disorders, inappropriate degrees of impulsiveness, hyperactivity, and attention deficit. Diagnostic criteria were developed by the American Psychiatric Association and have designated three types: (1) combined type of hyperactivity and attention deficit; (2) predominately inattentive type; and (3) predominately hyperactive-impulse type. ADHD affects the child at home, in school, and in social situations.

Nutrition Assessment

Many factors should be considered, along with the usual anthropometric measures, particularly when the individual is on medication.

Anthropometric Measures. Measurements of height and weight should be taken and recorded on a regular basis since the medications used in treatment may cause anorexia if given at inappropriate times, resulting in inadequate energy intake and potential slowing of growth.

Biochemical Measures. These measurements should include a complete blood count and blood and tissue levels of vitamin and minerals if megavitamin therapy is used.

Dietary Intake. A detailed dietary history would include infant feeding history, food likes and dislikes, behavior at mealtimes, snacking behavior, food allergies or food intolerances, or use of special diets. If the individual is on medications, the time of administration in relation to mealtime is important. Information should be obtained regarding any specific diet for the child or individual and how closely it is being followed.

Feeding evaluations should include observing the individual at mealtime. Generally the problems around feeding will be behavioral and will not include oral-motor or positioning peculiarities. Evaluating the environment around mealtime is important since distractions can be problematic.

Intervention Strategies

Current treatment may include psychotropic medications and the use of consistent behavioral management techniques. The timing and type of medication must be adjusted so that there is minimum influence on the child's dietary intake.

Specific diets have been used for many years, but they are not based on scientific research. For example, parents have been advised to use the Feingold diet (Wolraich, 1998), which states that foods containing synthetic food colors and naturally occurring salicylates be removed from the diet because of their neurologic effect. Other recommendations have included the elimination of sugar, the elimination of caffeine, or the addition of large doses of vitamins (megavitamin therapy). A series of well-designed studies to evaluate the effectiveness of these recommendations have generally had negative results, and successful outcomes are largely anecdotal (see Chapter 7).

For the child or adult who is up and down throughout the meal, behavior modification may be indicated, and it should be a part of the overall behavioral management program. Distractions should be eliminated.

The most effective treatment for the individual with ADHD is a diet based on wholesome foods as outlined in the Dietary Guidelines or MyPyramid and in Chapter 12. The food should be served at regular times, with small servings followed by refills. This is an important concept because of the tendency of the child or individual to eat very small amounts and leave the table, planning to return or graze throughout the day. Some programs recommend

TABLE 45-5

Comparison of Foods Allowed in the Gluten-Free and Casein-Free Diet, Specific Carbohydrate Diet, and Body Ecology Diet

Food	GF/CF	SCD	BED
Gluten-containing grains (wheat, rye, barley, spelt, kamut, possibly oats) and any products from those grains	Not allowed	Not allowed	Not recommended
Rice	Unlimited	Not allowed	Not recommended
Corn	Unlimited	Not allowed	Some OK if tolerated
Millet, quinoa, amaranth, buckwheat	Unlimited	Not allowed	Unlimited (80/20 rule), presoaked
Eggs and meat (beef, fish, lamb, chicken, turkey)	Unlimited	Allowed; processed not permitted	Recommended organic free range/ wild caught preferred, use 80/20 rule
Vegetables	Unlimited	Fresh or frozen allowed; no canned; no potatoes and yams	Unlimited; fermented vegetables highly recommended
Fruits	Unlimited	Allowed, cooked in initial phase; no canned	Not recommended except lemon, lime, cranberry or black currants; no tomatoes
Milk products	Not allowed	Not initially; then 24 hr goat yogurt, dry curd cottage cheese, specific cheeses and butter	Raw butter and cream initially; kefir in 1 month
Sweeteners	Unlimited	Honey and saccharin	Stevia only
Vinegar	Unlimited	White or apple cider	Raw apple cider only
Juice	Unlimited	Those with no added sugar	Only those from fruits above
Oils	Unlimited	Unlimited	Olive, coconut, pumpkin seed
Condiments	Unlimited	No added sugars, spices	Wheat-free tamari, herbs and spices, Celtic sea salt
Nuts and seeds	Unlimited	Most nuts, no seeds for 3 months	Unlimited raw and soaked
Seaweed	Unlimited	Not allowed	Highly recommended
Beans	Unlimited	After 3 months and soaked 12 hr	Not recommended
Coffee and tea	Unlimited	Allowed weak	Only herb tea or green tea
Coconut products	Unlimited	Fresh only	All recommended
Gelatin	Unlimited	Allowed	Not recommended. Use agar-agar instead

Developed by G. A. Houston-Ludlam. Reprinted with permission from *The ANDI News*, Autism Network for Dietary Intervention, ©2005.

removing the food and returning it only once after explaining why this is being done. The intervention requires that the child or individual sit at the table in the high chair away from television or other distractions. These suggestions are most applicable to children in preschool settings and in the school cafeteria or classroom.

It has been suggested that a lack of essential fatty acids (EFAs) is a possible cause of hyperactivity in children. It is more likely the result of varying biochemical influences. These children have a deficiency of EFAs because they cannot metabolize linoleic acid normally, they cannot absorb EFA effectively from the intestine, or their EFA requirements are higher than normal. Older studies showed lower levels of docosahexaenoic acid (DHA) and arachidonic acid (ARA) in children with hyperactivity, and this has been replicated in more recent studies (Burgess et al., 2000).

Cleft Lip and Palate

Cleft lip and cleft palate (CL/CP) are the most commonly occurring craniofacial birth defects (Merritt, 2005). Cleft lip is a condition that creates an opening of the upper lip. It can range from a slight notch to complete separation in one or both sides of the lips, and extending upward. If it occurs on one side of the lip, it is called a *unilateral cleft lip;* if it occurs on both sides, it is called a *bilateral cleft lip.* The cleft palate occurs when the roof of the mouth has not joined completely; it can be either unilateral or bilateral. Cleft palate can range from just an opening at the back of the soft palate or separation of the roof of the mouth with both soft and hard palate involved. CL/CP result from incomplete merging and fusion of embryonic processes during formation of the face. There is also a condition called submucous cleft palate in which there is incomplete fusion of the muscular layers of the soft palate with fusion of the overlying mucosa (Figures 45-5 and 45-6).

Lip and palate development occur between 5 and 12 weeks of gestation. Lip development begins first, usually at 5 weeks of gestation, followed by the development of the maxilla prominences and the primary palate. Fusion of the hard palate is completed by 10 weeks of gestation and the soft palate by 12 weeks.

The incidence of CL/CP varies but is generally 1 in 700 live births. Cleft palate and cleft lip/palate have multiple etiologies and are often associated with underlying syndromes such as Pierre Robin sequence. The Pierre Robin syndrome or complex is a birth condition that involves the lower jaw being either small in size (micrognathia) or set back from the upper jaw (retrognathia) (Cleft Palate Foundation, 2006). As a result, the tongue tends to be displaced back toward the throat, where it can fall back and obstruct the airway. Most infants will have a cleft palate, but none will have a cleft lip. The incidence of Pierre Robin ranges from 1 in 2000 to 30,000 births, based on how strictly the diagnosis is made (Cohen, 1999). The basic cause appears to be the failure of the lower jaw to develop normally before birth.

Approximately 50% of children with cleft palate have an underlying syndrome or multiple anomalies. Wide ranges of studies in developmental biology have shown that both genetics and environmental factors are involved in the etiology of oral clefts. Some of the risk factors from the environment include maternal folic acid deficiency, smoking, alcohol use, anticonvulsant use, and some maternal illnesses. Genetic counseling can now identify high risk families.

Nutrition Assessment

Nutrition assessment for CL/CP includes the usual anthropometric measures for all infants and children. Biochemical measures are also those used with nonaffected children, and dietary intake information depends on the feeding problems that exist. Other problems include dental abnormalities and missing teeth, speech difficulties, and increased incidence of middle ear infections. The feeding evaluation is a major part of the assessment and is best accomplished with a team approach, making sure that the parent is part of the team.

Because the major problem in CL/CP is feeding and providing adequate intake, growth can be jeopardized and needs to be assessed regularly.

Intervention Strategies

Surgical repair of the cleft lip is generally done at 2 to 3 months of age, and cleft palate repair at 9 months. Other operations may involve minor improvements to the lip or nose and are usually completed before the child starts school.

Breast-feeding is difficult for these infants because of problems with sucking, although those infants with just the cleft lip may be successful. It is generally recommended that the mother who wishes to breast-feed express her milk and give it to her baby from a specialized bottle and nipple. Par-

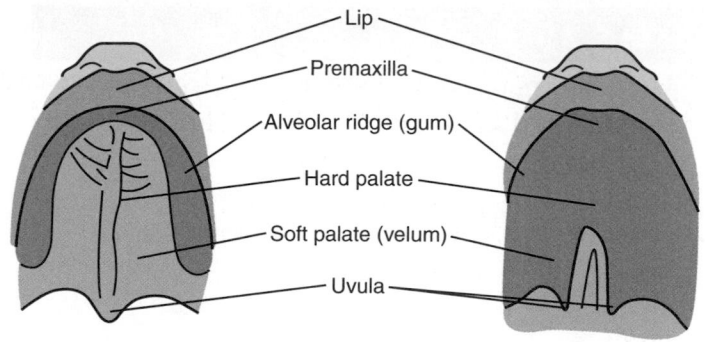

FIGURE 45-5 Cleft palate. *(From the Cleft Palate Foundation, www.cleftline.org, accessed December 28, 2006.)*

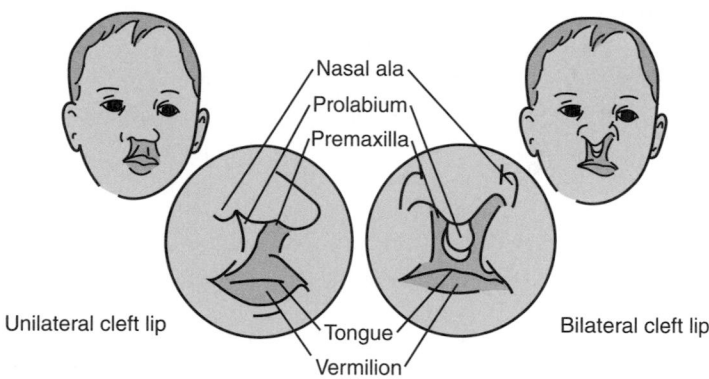

FIGURE 45-6 Cleft lip. *(From the Cleft Palate Foundation, www.cleftline.org, accessed December 28, 2006.)*

ents and caregivers need to be educated in the positioning of the child for feeding, nipple selection, bottle selection, and monitoring of intake.

Energy needs are generally the same as for a nonaffected infant or child, but, if the feeding process is too difficult, the energy needs may not be met. Strategies for solving that problem vary, with some professionals advising tube feeding, whereas others recommend continuing with appropriate bottles and nipples but using more concentrated formula or breast milk (Table 45-6).

Effective feeding requires that the infant be able to form a vacuum inside the mouth and form a seal around the nipple with the lips. This is achieved through the proper bottle, nipple, and position for feeding. Some of the acceptable nipples and bottles include a regular newborn nipple with enlarged holes, a lamb's nipple, a Ross cleft palate assembly, obturator nipples, and the orthodontic vented nipple. Bottles can vary from a very soft bottle with a cross-cut nipple to a Haberman feeder, squeeze bottles, and Asepto feeders.

Individuals with CL/CP are different; thus it is extremely important that the feeding team evaluate various types of equipment and carefully educate the parent in their use. Palate obturators have been used to cover the cleft palate until the child can have surgery to close it; their use results in improved intake, better feeding skills, increased weight

TABLE 45-6

Increasing Calories Through Concentration of Formulas and Addition of Oils and Carbohydrates

Caloric Density Required Per Ounce	Measures of Powder	Water Added
20 calories	1 scoop	2 oz
22 calories	2 scoops	3.5 fl oz
24 calories	3 scoops	5 fl oz
27 calories	3 scoops	4.25 fl oz
Using 22 Calorie Formulas		
22 cal	1 scoop	2 fl oz
24 cal	3 scoops	5.5 fl oz
27 cal	5 scoops	8 fl oz
Adding Oil or Carbohydrates		

Product	kcal	Source
Corn oil or safflower oil	9/g or 8.3/ml	Corn or safflower oil
Microlipid	4.5/ml	Safflower oil
MCT oil	8.3/g 7.6/ml	Fractionated coconut oil
Karo syrup	1 Tbsp = 58 kcal	Polysaccharides
Polycose liquid	2/ml or 60/fl oz	Glucose polymers
Polycose powder	3.8/g; 8/tsp; 23/Tbsp	Glucose polymers
Modulcal powder	30/Tbsp	Glucose polymers

gain, and growth of the dental arches. Disadvantages include cost and the inconvenience of refabricating the devices as the infant grows to maintain effectiveness. One recent study (Prahl et al., 2005) measured growth and the length of feeding between two groups, one using the obturator and one without, and found no significant difference in growth, leading the researchers to conclude that the obturator could be abandoned. Positioning in an upright position, choosing the appropriate nipple, and directing the liquid flow to the side or back of the mouth seem to be just as effective in promoting optimal feeding and are recommended. The baby should be given ample opportunities for frequent burping in an upright position.

Introduction of solid foods for the CL/CP infant can follow the usual protocol at 4 to 6 months of age. By this time the cleft lip should have been repaired, and the child has achieved good head control and trunk stability. Care needs to be taken that the food is presented slowly, allowing the infant to control each bite while gradually learning how to direct the food around the cleft until it is repaired. Following the repair and healing of the cleft palate, feeding along the developmental pathway should progress slowly but normally.

CONTROVERSIAL NUTRITION THERAPY

An important factor in providing medical nutrition therapy for children and adults with developmental disabilities is realizing that counseling may have been inadequate in helping the parent accept the limitations of the disorder. These limitations may include growth, feeding, and cognitive ability. As a result, many parents look for unusual medical or nutrition therapies. Major sources of information are often the Internet and parent support groups. Recent media coverage has promoted the use of antioxidant vitamins (A, C, and E) and minerals (zinc, copper, manganese, and selenium) along with the amino acids glucosamine, tyrosine, and tryptophan. The expected outcomes are improved growth; increased cognition, alertness, and attention span; and changed facial features.

There is little scientific information to back up these therapies. Research studies have addressed the vitamin needs of children with DS, spina bifida, fragile X syndrome, and autism, and findings do not indicate that the vitamin and mineral needs of these children with developmental disabilities are higher than normal (Ani, 2000). Numerous historical studies (Bennett et al., 1983) have searched for nutritional deficiencies as causative factors in DS. Traditionally the studies have included looking at numerous vitamins, minerals, fatty acids, digestive enzymes, lipotropic nutrients, and numerous drugs with no definitive results.

The key concept in the proposed nutrition interventions for DS is metabolic correction of genetic overexpression. It is postulated that presence of the third chromosome 21 causes overproduction of superoxide dismutase and cystathionine β-synthase, which disrupts active methylation pathways. Vitamin supplements of folic acid and antioxidants counteract this and are considered key to the treatment. However, these are just theories, and at this point nutrition supplements are considered an expensive, questionable approach.

Parents of children with ADHD report that omitting sugar from the children's diets decreases hyperactivity, but there is no scientific evidence to support this. However, it probably is a good idea to eliminate or at least reduce the sugar intake in any child's diet to promote better nutritional intake. Blue-green algae has been promoted for children with DS and other developmental disabilities, purportedly to increase attention span and concentration. It is of concern that little monitoring is part of the initiation of these treatments. High-dose supplementation of vitamin B_6 and magnesium has been proposed for autism to diminish tantrums and self-stimulation activities and improve attention and speech. Another proposed treatment is dimethyl glycine. Limited research is available to substantiate anything other than anecdotal reports that the child is helped (Cornish, 2002).

Name of student for whom special meals at school are requested:

_____

Disability or medical condition that requires the student to have a special diet. Include a brief description of the major life activity affected by the student's condition.

_____

_____

Foods omitted and substitutions (Please check food groups to be omitted. List specific foods to be omitted and suggest substitutions using the back of this form or attach information.)

- Meat and meat alternatives
- Milk and milk products
- Bread and cereal products
- Fruits and vegetables

Textures allowed: Please check the allowed texture
☐ Regular   ☐ Chopped   ☐ Ground   ☐ Pureed

Other information regarding diet or feeding:

I certify that the above named student needs special school meals prepared as described above because of the student's disability or chronic medical condition.

_____   _____
Physician/Recognized Medical Authority Signature   Office Phone Number/Date

FIGURE 45-7 Diet prescription for meals at school. *(Reprinted with permission from CARE: Special nutrition for kids, Birmingham, AL, 1999, Alabama Department of Education.)*

COMMUNITY RESOURCES

For many types of nutrition problems and medical nutrition therapy, the school system is an excellent resource through the school lunch and school breakfast programs (Cloud, 2001). Children and adolescents may receive modified meals at school. Child and Adult Care Food Programs must provide meals at no extra cost for children and adolescents with special needs and developmental disabilities. School food service is required to offer special meals at no additional cost to children whose disabilities restrict their diets as defined in U.S. Department of Agriculture's nondiscrimination regulations. The term "child with a disability" under Part B of the Individuals with Disabilities Education Act (IDEA) refers to a child evaluated in accordance with IDEA as having one of the 13 recognized disability categories: (1) autism; (2) deaf-blindness; (3) deafness; (4) mental retardation; (5) orthopedic impairments; (6) other health impairments caused by chronic or acute health problems such as asthma, nephritis, diabetes, sickle cell anemia, a heart condition, epilepsy, rheumatic fever, hemophilia, leukemia, lead poisoning, or tuberculosis; (7) emotional disturbances; (8) specific learning disabilities; (9) speech or language impairment; (10) traumatic brain injury; (11) visual impairment; (12) multiple disabilities; and (13) developmental delays. Attention deficit disorder may fall under one of the 13 categories.

When a referral is made to the school system for a special meal related to a developmental disability, it must be accompanied by a medical statement for a child with special dietary needs (Figure 45-7). The request requires an identification of the medical or other special dietary condition, the food or foods to be omitted, and the food or choice of foods to be substituted. The statement requires the signature of the physician or recognized medical authority. The school food service may make food substitutions for individual children who do not have a disability but who are medically certified as having a special medical or dietary need. An example would be the child with severe allergies or an inborn error of metabolism. The availability of school food service for children with developmental disabilities is an important resource in the long-term implementation of medical nutrition therapy.

⊙ FOCAL POINTS

- The nutritional needs of individuals with developmental disabilities are unique as a result of differences in body composition, metabolic functions, physical activity, medications, and behavioral issues. It is important to understand this so that medical nutrition therapy can be effective in the clinical setting, home, school, and community.
- The availability of school food service for children with developmental disabilities is an important

- resource in the long-term implementation of medical nutrition therapy.
- The key concept in prevention is potential correction of genetic overexpression from an adequate maternal diet during pregnancy.
- Medical nutrition therapy for the child with a developmental disability is most effective with an interdisciplinary team approach.

⬡ CLINICAL SCENARIO 1

Mitchell is a 2-month-old male with Down syndrome. He was born prematurely (30 weeks of gestation) and was started on gastrostomy tube feeding at 10 days of age because of his poor weight gain and severe gastroesophageal reflux. The poor weight gain was caused by a poor suck, although swallowing was not a problem. He was first seen by a nutritionist in an early intervention program at 4 months of age when he was 22.5 in tall and weighed 10 lb 7 oz.

By 21 months his height was 28 inches, and his weight 18.5 lb. He was at the fifth percentile for length and weight using the CDC growth curves but at the 25th percentile when the Down syndrome curves were used. He had been taking oral feeds since 7 months of age, but his total oral consumption was one jar of baby food a day. At 16 months he started eating table foods, and his tube-feeding formula was Pediasure. At 21 months of age he was crawling but not yet walking, and he had very limited self-feeding skills. Now at age 21 months his mother's highest priority is to stop the tube feeding and have Mitchell continue to grow well; she is concerned about his rate of weight gain. She is also concerned that constipation has become a problem requiring medication.

✳**Nutrition Diagnosis:** Self-feeding difficulty related to developmental delays as evidenced by inability to feed self most foods offered

1. What would be your approach in working with this mother and the other team members?
2. What do you think would be his nutritional needs, starting with energy?
3. How many ounces of a 30 cal/oz tube-feeding formula would you recommend for Mitchell to promote weight gain?
4. What steps should be taken to increase his oral intake and decrease the tube feeding?
5. What would you recommend for management of his constipation?

⬡ CLINICAL SCENARIO 2

Luke is a 2-year-old male with Prader-Willi syndrome. He was born weighing 7 lb and was 18 in long. A test done in the nursery determined that he had Prader-Willi syndrome. Typical of Prader-Willi syndrome, Luke was a very hypotonic infant with a very poor suck. Mom wanted to breast-feed, but Luke was unable to latch on at the breast, so she pumped her milk. Also it was recommended that human milk fortifier (HMF) be added to the breast milk. She was very concerned about adding the HMF since she had read about potential obesity as Luke grew older. After discharge from the hospital Luke entered an early intervention program with nutrition services. Eventually the mother changed Luke to an infant formula, but Luke continued to have a weak suck, and feeding services were needed.

✳**Nutrition Diagnosis:** Inability to feed self related to weak suck and hypotonia as evidenced by need for feeding services

1. What would be a good plan for continuing nutrition care for Luke?
2. What kind of information should the nutritionist provide to the mother related to her fear of eventual obesity for Luke?
3. As Luke grows older, what would be a good way to determine the number of calories he should receive to prevent obesity?

USEFUL WEBSITES

CDC Birth Defects Research
http://www.cdc.gov/ncbddd/bd/research.htm

March of Dimes
http://www.modimes.org/

National Center for Education in Maternal and Child Health
http://www.ncemch.org/

National Dissemination Center for Children With Disabilities
http://www.nichcy.org/

National Folic Acid Campaign
http://www.cdc.gov/folicacid/promote.htm

References

American Dietetic Association: Position of the American Dietetic Association: providing nutrition services for infants, children, and adults with developmental disabilities and special health care needs, *J Am Diet Assoc* 104:97, 2004.

Ani C et al: Nutritional supplementation of Down syndrome: theoretical considerations and current status, *Dev Med Child Neurol* 42:207, 2000.

Bandini LG et al: Body composition and energy expenditure in adolescents with cerebral palsy or myelodysplasia, *Pediatr Res* 29:70, 1991.

Bekx MR et al: Decreased energy expenditure is caused by abnormal body composition in infants with Prader-Willi syndrome, *J Pediatr* 143:372, 2003.

Bennett FC et al: Vitamin and mineral supplementation in Down's syndrome, *Pediatrics* 72:707, 1983.

Burgess JR et al: Long-chain polyunsaturated fatty acids in children with attention-deficit hyperactivity disorder, *Am J Clin Nutr* 71(suppl):327, 2000.

Capone G et al: Down syndrome. In Ekvall SW, Ekvall VK, editors: *Pediatric nutrition in chronic disease and developmental disorders*, New York, 2005, Oxford University Press.

Centers for Disease Control and Prevention: *Developmental disabilities*, Atlanta, Ga, from http://www.cdc.gov/ncbdddb/dd/default.htm, accessed June 18, 2007.

Chumlea WC et al: Prediction of stature from knee height for black and white adults and children with application to mobility—impaired or handicapped persons, *J Am Diet Assoc* 94(12):1385, 1994.

Cleft Palate Foundation: Information about Pierre Robin sequence/complex, 2006, http://www.Cleftline.Org/publications/pierre_robin, accessed April 14, 2007.

Cloud HH: Recent trends in care of children with special needs: nutrition services for children with developmental disabilities and special health care needs, *Topics Clin Nutr* 16(4):28, 2001.

Cloud HH et al: Feeding problems of the child with special health care needs. In Ekvall SV, Ekvall VK, editors: *Pediatric nutrition in chronic disease and developmental disorders*, ed 2, New York, 2005, Oxford University Press.

Cohen MM Jr: Robin sequence and complexes, *Am J Med Genetics* 84:311, 1999.

Cornish E: Gluten and casein free diets in autism: a study of the effects on food choice and nutrition, *J Hum Nutr Diet* 15:261, 2002.

Demitropoulas A et al: Emergence of compulsive behavior and tantrums in children with Prader-Willi syndrome, *Am J Ment Retard* 106:3:208, 2001.

Edelson SM, Rimland B: *Recovering autistic children*, San Diego, CA, 2003, Autism Research Institute.

Ekvall SW, Cerniglia F: Myelomeningocele. In Ekvall SW, Ekvall VK, editors: *Pediatric nutrition in developmental disabilities and chronic disorders*, ed 2, New York, 2005, Oxford University Press.

Fugassi P et al: The characteristics of autism and nutrition in children, *Am J Coll Nutr* 22:481, 2003.

Goldstone AP et al: Hypothalamic NPY and agouti-related protein are increased in human illness but not in Prader-Willi syndrome and other obese subjects, *J Clin Endocrinol Metab* 87:927, 2002.

Henderson RC et al: Longitudinal changes in bone density in children and adolescents with moderate to severe cerebral palsy, *J Pediatr* 146:769, 2005.

Hogan SE: Knee height as a predictor of recumbent length for individuals with mobility-impaired cerebral palsy, *J Am Coll Nutr* 18(2):201, 1999.

King W et al: Prevalence of reduced bone mass in children with spastic quadriplegia, *Dev Med Child Neurol* 45:12, 2003.

Krick J et al: Pattern of growth in children with cerebral palsy, *J Am Diet Assoc* 97:680, 1996.

Luckasson R et al: *Mental retardation: definition, classification, and systems of supports*, ed 10, Washington, DC, 2002, American Association on Mental Retardation.

Luke DA et al: Energy expenditure in children with Down syndrome: correcting metabolic rate of movement, *J Pediatr* 125(5 Pt 1):829, 1994.

McCune H, Driscoll D: Prader-Willi syndrome. In Ekvall SW, Ekvall, VK, editors: *Pediatric nutrition in chronic disease and developmental disorders*, ed 2, New York, 2005, Oxford University Press.

Merritt L: Physical assessment of the infant with cleft lip and/or palate, *Adv Neonatal Care* 5(3):125, 2005.

Obata K et al: Effects of 5 years' growth hormone treatment in patients with Prader-Willi syndrome, *J Pediatr Endocrinol Metab* 16(2):155, 2003.

Piscane A et al: Down syndrome and breastfeeding, *Acta Pediatr* 92:1479, 2003.

Prahl C et al: Infant orthopedics in UCLP: effect on feeding, weight, and length: a randomized clinical trial (Dutch cleft), *Cleft Palate Craniofac J* 42:171, 2005.

Reichelt K, Knivsberg AM: *Why use the gluten-free and casein-free diet? What the results have shown so far*, Autism Research Institute, 2003, www.autismwebsite.com/ARI/dan/reichelt.htm, accessed April 14, 2007.

Robbins JM et al: Hospitalizations of newborns with folate-sensitive birth defects before and after fortification of foods with folic acid, *Pediatrics* 118:906, 2006.

Samson-Fang LJ, Stevenson RD: Identification of malnutrition in children with cerebral palsy: poor performance of weight for height percentiles, *Dev Med Child Neurol* 43(3):162, 2000.

Schuster DP et al: Characterizations of alterations in glucose and insulin metabolism in Prader-Willi subject, *Metabolism* 45:1514, 1996.

Shah S, Johnson R: Antioxidant vitamin A and E status in children with Down syndrome subjects, *Nutr Res* 9:709, 1989.

Smithells RN et al: Further experience of vitamin supplementation for prevention of neural tube defect recurrences, *Lancet* 1:1027, 1983.

Stallings VA et al: Energy expenditure of children and adolescents with severe disabilities: a cerebral palsy model, *Am J Clin Nutr* 64:627, 1996.

Stevenson RD: Use of segmental measures to estimate stature in children with cerebral palsy, *Arch Paediatr Adolesc Med* 149:658, 2005.

Stevenson RE et al: Decline in prevalence of neural tube defects in a high-risk region of the United States, *Pediatrics* 106:825, 2000.

Swaab DF et al: Alterations in the hypothalamic paraventricular nucleus and its oxytocin neurons (putative satiety cells) in Prader Willi syndrome—a study of five cases, *J Clin Endocrinol Metab* 80:573, 1995.

Tobin SP et al: The role of an interdisciplinary feeding team in the assessment and treatment of feeding problems: building blocks for life: Pediatric Nutrition Practice Group, *J Am Diet Assoc* 28:3, 2005.

U.S. Department of Health and Human Services, Food and Drug Administration: Food standards: amendment of the standards of identity for enriched grain products to require addition of folic acid, *Fed Reg* 61:8781, 1996.

Van Goor JC et al: Increased incidence and prevalence of diabetes mellitus in Down syndrome, *Arch Dis Child* 77:183, 1997.

Wolraich M: Attention deficit hyperactivity disorder, *Prof Care Mother Child* 8:35, 1998.

Yeargin-Allsopp M et al: Prevalence of autism in a U.S. metropolitan area, *JAMA* 289:49, 2003.

Appendixes

Nutritional Facts* (Appendixes 38-58) unless otherwise noted created from the North Carolina Dietetic Association: *Nutrition care manual*, 2005, Raleigh, North Carolina; Agricultural Research Service (ARS) Nutrient Database for Standard Reference, Release 17, ARS single nutrient reports, 2002 revision of USDA Home and Garden Bulletin No. 72, *Nutritive value of foods*, accessed April 10, 2007, from http://www.health.gov/dietaryguidelines/dga2005/document/html/appendixB.htm; Institute of Medicine, Food and Nutrition Board: *Dietary reference intakes*, Washington, DC, 1997-2005, The National Academies Press. Compiled by Maria Montesano, East Carolina University Dietetic Intern, 2007.

APPENDIX 1   General Abbreviations

ABGs	arterial blood gases	FX	fracture
ACTH	adrenocorticotropic hormone	GB	gallbladder
AD	Alzheimer's disease	GFR	glomerular filtration rate
ADH	antidiuretic hormone	GI	gastrointestinal
ADI	acceptable daily intake	GIP	gastric inhibitory polypeptide
ADL	activities of daily living	GTF	glucose tolerance factor
AI	adequate intake	GTT	glucose tolerance test
AIDS	acquired immunodeficiency syndrome	GVHD	graft-versus-host disease
ALA	α-linolenic acid	HA	hyperalimentation
ALS	amyotrophic lateral sclerosis	HAV	hepatitis A virus
AP	angina pectoris	Hgb	hemoglobin
ARF	acute renal failure	HBV	hepatitis B virus
ASHD	atherosclerotic heart disease	HCT	hematocrit
ATP	adenosine triphosphate	HDL	high-density lipoprotein
BCAA	branched-chain amino acid	HE	hepatic encephalopathy
BEE	basal energy expenditure	Hgb	hemoglobin
BHA	butylated hydroxyanisole	HIV	human immunodeficiency virus
BHT	butylated hydroxytoluene	HPN	home parenteral nutrition
BMI	body mass index	HSL	hormone-sensitive lipase
BMR	basal metabolic rate	HTN	hypertension
BMT	bone marrow transplantation	HX	history
BPD	bronchopulmonary dysplasia	IBD	inflammatory bowel disease
BSA	body surface area	IBS	irritable bowel syndrome
BV	biologic value	IBW	ideal body weight
CA	cancer	ICU	intensive care unit
CAD	coronary artery disease	IF	intrinsic factor
CAPD	continuous ambulatory peritoneal dialysis	IgE	immunoglobulin E
CAVH	continuous arteriovenous hemofiltration	IGT	impaired glucose tolerance
CC	cardiac cachexia	IL-2	interleukin-2
CCK	cholecystokinin	IM	intramuscular
CCU	coronary care unit	INH	isonicotinic acid hydrazide
CDC	Centers for Disease Control and Prevention	INR	International normalized ratio
CHD	coronary heart disease	IV	intravenous
CHF	congestive heart failure	IVH	intravenous hyperalimentation
CHI	closed head injury	J	joule
CKD	chronic kidney disease	kcal (Cal)	kilocalorie
CNS	central nervous system	kJ	kilojoule
COPD	chronic obstructive pulmonary disease	KS	Kaposi's sarcoma
CPN	central parenteral nutrition	KUB	kidney, ureter, bladder
CSII	continuous subcutaneous insulin infusion	LBM	lean body mass
CSF	cerebrospinal fluid	LCT	long-chain triglyceride
CVA	cerebrovascular accident	LDL	low-density lipoprotein
DCCT	Diabetes Control and Complications Trial	LES	lower esophageal sphincter
DHA	docosahexaenoic acid	LFT	liver function test
DHHS	Department of Health and Human Services	LPL	lipoprotein lipase
DJD	degenerative joint disease	MAOI	monoamine oxidase inhibitor
DKA	diabetic ketoacidosis	MCH	mean corpuscular hemoglobin
DM	diabetes mellitus	MCT	medium-chain triglyceride
DNA	deoxyribonucleic acid	MCV	mean corpuscular volume
DRI	dietary reference intake	MET	metabolic equivalent
ECG/EKG	electrocardiogram	MFOS	mixed-function oxidase system
EDTA	ethylenediaminetetraacetate	MI	myocardial infarction
EFA	essential fatty acid	MOM	Milk of Magnesia
EPA	eicosapentaenoic acid	MSG	monosodium glutamate
EPO	erythropoietin	MSUD	maple syrup urine disease
ERT	estrogen replacement therapy	NANB	non-A, non-B hepatitis virus
ESR	erythrocyte sedimentation rate	NCEP	National Cholesterol Education Program
ESRD	end-stage renal disease	NCJ	needle catheter jejunostomy
FAD	flavin adenine dinucleotide	NG	nasogastric
FBG	fasting blood glucose	NPO	nothing by mouth
FBS	fasting blood sugar	NPU	net protein utilization
FFA	free fatty acid	NSAID	nonsteroidal antiinflammatory drug
FIGLU	formimino glutamic acid	NSP	nonstarch polysaccharide
FMN	flavin mononucleotide	N&V	nausea and vomiting
FPG	fasting plasma glucose	OCA	oral contraceptive agent
FTT	failure to thrive	OGTT	oral glucose tolerance test

Continued

APPENDIX 1 General Abbreviations—cont'd

OHA	oral hypoglycemic agent		SCA	sickle cell anemia
PBI	protein-bound iodine		SCT	short-chain triglycerides
PCM	protein-calorie malnutrition		SFA	saturated fatty acid
PEG	percutaneous endoscopic gastrostomy		SLE	systemic lupus erythematosus
PEM	protein-energy malnutrition		SMBG	self-monitoring of blood glucose
PER	protein efficiency ratio		SOB	shortness of breath
PG	prostaglandin		TBSA	total body surface area
PHE	phenylalanine		TC	total cholesterol
PKU	phenylketonuria		TEE	total energy expenditure
PLP	pyridoxal phosphate		TEF	thermic effect of food
PPN	peripheral parenteral nutrition		TG	triglyceride or triacylglycerol
PT	prothrombin time		THF	tetrahydrofolate
PTA	prior to admission		TIA	transient ischemic attack
PU	peptic ulcer		TIBC	total iron-binding capacity
PUFA	polyunsaturated fatty acid		TNF	tumor necrosis factor
RAST	radioallergosorbent test		TPN	total parenteral nutrition
RBC	red blood cell		TS	transferrin saturation
RDA	recommended dietary allowance		UL	upper intake level
RDS	respiratory distress syndrome		URI	upper respiratory infection
REE	resting energy expenditure		UTI	urinary tract infection
RMR	resting metabolic rate		VLCD	very low–calorie diet
RNA	ribonucleic acid		VLDL	very low–density lipoprotein
R/O	rule out		VOD	venous occlusive disease
ROS	review of systems		VS	vital signs
RQ	respiratory quotient		WNL	within normal limits
RTA	renal tubular acidosis			

APPENDIX 2 Unit Abbreviations

Along with the specialized vocabulary that is used in the medical, dietetic, and nursing fields, there are acceptable forms of abbreviations. The following is a list of abbreviations commonly used.

aa: Gr. *ana*; of each

ac: L. *ante cibum*; before meals

ad, add: L. *adde, addatus,* or *addantur*; add or added

ad lib: L. *ad libitum*; at pleasure, as desired

aq: L. *aqua*; water

aq dest: L. *aqua destillata*; distilled water

bid, bis in d: L. *bis in die*; twice a day

c̄: L. *cum*; with

c: cup

cc: cubic centimeter

Cent; cent; C: centigrade, Celsius

cm: centimeter

dilut: L. *dilutus*; dilute

div: L. *divide*; divide

fac: make

g: gram

gr: L. *granum*; grain

gtt: L. *guttae*; drops

hs: L. *hora somni*; at hour of sleep

IU: international unit

kcal: kilocalorie

kg: kilogram

kJ: kilojoule

lb: pound

mcg: microgram

mEq: milliequivalent

mg: milligram

mil or ml: milliliter

mM: millimole

μmol: micromol

mOsm: milliosmole

oz: ounce

prn: L. *pro re nata*; may be repeated according to instructions

pt: pint

pulv: L. *pulvis*; powder

qd: L. *quaque die*; every day

QID, qid: L. *quater in die*; four times daily

q3h: every 3 hours

qs: L. *quantum satis*; a sufficient quantity

qt: quart

RE: retinal equivalent

s̄: L. *sine*; without

sol: solution

ss: L. *semis*; half

stat: L. *statim*; immediately

t, tsp: teaspoon

T, Tbsp: tablespoon

tid: L. *ter in die*: three times a day

APPENDIX 3 Milliequivalents and Milligrams of Electrolytes

To Convert Milligrams to Milliequivalents

Divide milligrams by atomic weight and then multiply by the valence

$$\frac{\text{Milligrams}}{\text{Atomic weight}} \times \text{Valence} = \text{Milliequivalents}$$

Mineral Element	Chemical Symbol	Atomic Weight (mg)	Valence
Calcium	Ca	40	2
Chlorine	Cl	35	1
Magnesium	Mg	24	2
Phosphorus	P	31	2
Potassium	K	39	1
Sodium	Na	23	1
Sulfate	SO_4	96	2
Sulfur	S	32	

To Convert Specific Weight of Sodium to Sodium Chloride

Multiply by 2.54

Example:
1000 mg Sodium = 1000 × 2.54 = 2540 mg Sodium chloride (2.5 g)

To Convert Specific Weight of Sodium Chloride to Sodium

Multiply by 0.393

Example:
2.5 g Sodium chloride = 2.5 × 0.393 = 1000 mg Sodium

Milligrams	Sodium Values (Milliequivalents)	Grams of Sodium Chloride
500	21.8	1.3
1000	43.5	2.5
1500	75.3	3.8
2000	87.0	5.0

Modified from Nelson JK et al: *Mayo Clinic diet manual*, ed 7, St Louis, 1994, Mosby.

APPENDIX 4 Equivalents, Conversions,* and Portion (Scoop) Sizes

Liquid Measure—Volume Equivalents

1 tsp = ⅓ Tbsp = 5 ml or cc
1 Tbsp = 3 tsp = 15 ml or cc
2 Tbsp = 1 fluid oz = ⅛ cup = 30 ml or cc
2 Tbsp + 2 tsp = ⅙ cup = 40 ml or cc
4 Tbsp = ¼ cup = 2 fluid oz = 60 ml or cc
5 Tbsp + 1 tsp = ⅓ cup = 80 ml or cc
6 Tbsp = 3 fluid oz = ⅜ cup = 90 ml or cc
8 Tbsp = ½ cup = 120 ml or cc
10 Tbsp + 2 tsp = ⅔ cup = 160 ml or cc
12 Tbsp = ¾ cup = 180 ml or cc
48 tsp = 16 Tbsp = 1 cup (8 fluid ounces) = ½ pint = 240 ml or cc
2 cups = 1 pint (16 fluid oz) = 0.4732 L
4 cups = 2 pints = 1 quart (32 fluid oz) = 0.9462 L
1.06 quarts = 34 fluid oz = 1000 ml or cc
4 quarts = 1 gallon = 3785 ml or cc

Dry Measure

1 quart = 2 pints = 1.101 L
Dry measure and quarts are about ⅙ larger than liquid measure pints and quarts.

Weights

Avoirdupois	Metric
1 oz*	Approx 30 g
1 lb (16 oz)	454 g
2.2 lb	1 kg

Scoop Sizes

It is important to use the proper scoop size when portioning out foods to serve to patients. The dietitian will be expected to know this and provide staff guidance accordingly.

Number	Approximate Liquid Volume
6	⅔ cup (5 fluid oz)
8	½ cup (4 fluid oz)
10	⅜ cup (3¼ fluid ozs)
12	⅓ cup (2⅔ fluid oz)
16	¼ cup (2 fluid oz)
20	3⅕ Tbsp (1⅗ fluid oz)
24	2⅔ Tbsp (1⅓ fluid oz)
30	2⅕ Tbsp (1 fluid oz)
40	1⅗ Tbsp (0.8 fluid oz)
60	1 Tbsp (0.5 fluid oz)

Metric Conversion Factors

Multiply	By	To Get
Fluid ounces	29.57	Grams
Ounces (dry)	28.35	Grams
Grams	0.0353	Ounces
Grams	0.0022	Pounds
Kilograms	2.21	Pounds
Pounds	453.6	Grams
Pounds	0.4536	Kilograms
Quarts	0.946	Liters
Quarts (dry)	67.2	Cubic inches
Quarts (liquid)	57.7	Cubic inches
Liters	1.0567	Quarts
Gallons	3,785	Cubic centimeters
Gallons	3.785	Liters

From North Carolina Dietetic Association: *Nutrition care manual*, 2005, Raleigh, NC, The Association.

*In the United States' measuring systems the same word may have two meanings. For example, an ounce may mean 1/16 of a pound and 1/16 of a pint; but the former is strictly a weight measure, and the latter is a volume measure. Except in the case of water, milk, or other liquids of the same density, a fluid ounce and an ounce of weight are two completely different quantities. These measures are not to be used interchangeably.

APPENDIX 5 Focus on Nutrition Care Process: Nutrition Assessment

Step 1. Nutrition Assessment

Nutrition assessment is designed to identify nutrition-related problems and their etiology. A nutrition assessment matrix links nutrition assessment parameters with nutrition diagnoses.

Nutrition assessment data are organized into five categories.

Anthropometric Measurements	Biochemical Data, Medical Tests, and Procedures	Client History	Diet: Food/ Nutrition History	Examination Findings
Height, weight, body mass index, growth rate, and rate of weight change	Laboratory data (e.g., electrolytes, glucose, lipid panel) and tests (e.g., gastric emptying time, resting metabolic rate)	Medication and supplement use, medical/health history, and social, personal/family history	Food and nutrient intake, nutrition-related knowledge and practices, physical activity, and food availability	Oral health, physical appearance, muscle and subcutaneous fat, wasting, and mental status

Critical Thinking

- Determine appropriate data to collect and select valid and reliable tools.
- Distinguish relevant versus irrelevant data.
- Select appropriate norms and standards for comparing the data. This may include NHANES data, dietary reference intakes, and other standards of care.
- Organize, categorize, and synthesize the data about the individual, group, or population.

Text Chapters Involved

Chapter 13 aligns nutrition assessment with nutrigenomics.
Chapter 14 describes the basics of nutrition assessment.
Chapter 15 describes the role of laboratory data and biochemical parameters in assessment.
Chapter 16 provides details about potential food-drug interactions.
Chapter 17 provides a thorough review of the nutrition care process.

APPENDIX 6 Focus on Nutrition Care Process: Nutrition Diagnosis

Step 2. Nutrition Diagnosis

Nutrition diagnosis is designed to identify and describe a specific nutrition problem that can be resolved or improved through intervention by a registered dietitian (RD). Unlike a medical diagnosis, a nutrition diagnosis often can be resolved.

Steps to make a nutrition diagnosis: RDs use the data collected in the nutrition assessment to identify the patient/client's nutrition diagnosis using standard terminology. Each nutrition diagnosis follows a prescribed reference sheet. The specific definition, possible etiology, and common signs or symptoms are identified in this care process step.

Nutrition diagnoses are organized into three categories.

Intake	Clinical	Behavioral-Environmental
Too much or too little of a food or nutrient compared to actual or estimated needs	Nutrition problems that relate to medical or physical conditions	Knowledge, attitudes, beliefs, physical environment, access to food, or food safety

Format

The nutrition diagnosis is written as a PES statement to describe the problem, its root cause, and the signs and symptoms (assessment data) that provide evidence for that nutrition diagnosis. The PES statement is "Nutrition problem label related to _____ as evidenced by _____".

(P) Problem or Nutrition Diagnosis Label	(E) Etiology: Cause/Contributing Risk Factors	(S) Signs/Symptoms
Describes alterations in the patient/client's nutrition status	Linked to the nutrition diagnosis label by the words "related to"	Data used to determine that the patient or client has the nutrition diagnosis specified; linked to the etiology by the words "as evidenced by"

Critical Thinking

- Can the RD resolve or improve the problem stated in the nutrition diagnosis?
- Can the RD envision an intervention that would address the etiology and thus resolve or improve the problem?
  If not, is the intervention targeted to reducing or eliminating the signs and symptoms of the problem?
- How do nutrition assessment data support the selected nutrition diagnosis, its etiology, and its signs and symptoms?
- Is the etiology listed as the "root cause" that the RD can address through nutrition intervention?
- Will measuring the signs and symptoms indicate if the problem is resolved or improved?
- Signs and symptoms need to be specific enough to measure/evaluate changes at the next visit to document resolution or improvement.
- When all things are equal and there is a choice between two nutrition diagnosis labels in different categories, use the nutrition diagnosis from the Intake category.

Text Chapters Involved

Chapter 17 provides a thorough review of the nutrition care process, including nutrition diagnosis. All of the medical nutrition therapy chapters include case scenarios that highlight examples of nutrition diagnostic language.

APPENDIX 7 Focus on Nutrition Care Process: Nutrition Intervention

Step 3. Nutrition Intervention

Nutrition interventions are designed for the registered dietitian and team members to resolve or improve the identified nutrition diagnosis by planning and implementing appropriately tailored actions. Selection of a nutrition intervention is related to the **etiology** of the nutrition problem. Intervention strategies are purposefully selected to change nutritional intake, nutrition-related knowledge or behavior, risk factors, environmental conditions, or access to supportive care and services. Intervention goals provide the basis for monitoring progress and measuring outcomes.

Interventions are organized into four categories.

Food and/or Nutrient Delivery	Nutrition Education	Nutrition Counseling	Coordination of Nutrition Care
An individualized approach for food/nutrient provision, including meals and snacks, enteral and parenteral feeding, and supplements	A formal process to instruct or train a patient/client in a skill or to impart knowledge to help patients/clients voluntarily manage or modify food choices and eating behavior to maintain or improve health	A supportive process, characterized by a collaborative counselor-patient relationship, to set priorities, establish goals, and create individualized action plans that acknowledge and foster responsibility for self-care to treat an existing condition and promote health	Consultation with, referral to, or coordination of nutrition care with other health care providers, institutions, or agencies that can assist in treating or managing nutrition-related problems

The Two Distinct and Interrelated Processes of Intervention

Planning:
a. Prioritizing nutrition diagnoses
b. Consulting ADA's medical nutrition therapy evidence-based guides for practice and other practice guides
c. Determining patient-focused expected outcomes for each nutrition diagnosis
d. Conferring with patient/client/caregivers
e. Defining an intervention plan and strategies
f. Defining time and frequency of care
g. Identifying resources needed

Implementation:
a. Communicating the nutrition care plan
b. Carrying out the plan
c. Collecting data, documenting, and modifying the plan based on goals and progress

Critical Thinking

- Set goals and prioritize them.
- Define the nutrition prescription or clarify the basic plan.
- Make interdisciplinary connections.
- Initiate behavioral and other interventions.
- Match intervention strategies with client needs, values, and nutrition diagnoses.
- Choose from among alternatives to determine a course of action.
- Specify the time and frequency of care.

Text Chapters Involved

Chapter 17 provides a thorough review of the nutrition care process.
Chapter 18 reviews the use of supplementation as an intervention.
Chapter 19 summarizes counseling as an intervention.
Chapter 20 explains enteral and parenteral support as an intervention.
Chapters 21 to 25 contain content related to various prevention and wellness interventions.
Chapters 26 to 45 contain medical nutrition therapy interventions.

APPENDIX 8 Focus on Nutrition Care Process: Nutrition Monitoring and Evaluation

Step 4. Nutrition Monitoring and Evaluation

Nutrition monitoring and evaluation is designed to determine the amount of progress made and whether goals are being met. Nutrition monitoring and evaluation tracks patient/client outcomes relevant to the nutrition diagnosis and intervention plans and goals. Nutrition care outcomes—the desired results of nutrition care—have been defined, and specific indicators that can be measured and compared to reference standards or norms have been identified. The aim is to promote uniformity in assessing the effectiveness of nutrition intervention.

What To Measure

Selection of the appropriate nutrition care indicators is determined by the nutrition diagnosis, its etiology and signs or symptoms, and the nutrition intervention used. The medical diagnosis and health care outcome goals and quality management goals for nutrition also influence which nutrition care outcome indicators are chosen. Other factors such as practice setting, patient/client population, and disease state and/or severity also impact the indicator selection.

Outcomes for nutrition monitoring and evaluation are organized into four categories.

Nutrition-Related Behavioral and Environmental Outcomes	Food and Nutrient Intake Outcomes	Nutrition-Related Physical Signs and Symptoms Outcomes	Nutrition-Related Patient/ Client-Centered Outcomes
Patient/client's nutrition-related knowledge, behavior, access, and ability that impact food and nutrient intake	Patient/client's food and/or nutrient intake	Patient/client's anthropometric, biochemical, and physical examination parameters	Patient/client's perception of his or her nutrition intervention and its impact on life

Nutrition Monitoring and Evaluation = Monitor, Measure, and Evaluate

Monitor the patient/client progress: determine whether the nutrition intervention is being implemented and provide evidence that the nutrition intervention is or is not changing the patient/client behavior or status.

Measure the outcomes by selecting the appropriate nutrition care outcome indicator(s).

Evaluate and compare the patient's current findings or indicator with previous status, nutrition intervention goals, and/or reference standards (i.e., criteria).

Critical Thinking

- Select appropriate indicators/measures.
- Use appropriate reference standards for comparison.
- Define where patient/client is in terms of expected outcomes.
- Explain a variance from expected outcomes.
- Determine factors that help or hinder progress.
- Decide between discharge and continuation of nutrition care.

Text Chapters Involved

Chapter 17 provides a thorough review of the nutrition care process.

Chapters 26 to 45 contain medical nutrition therapy interventions.

© Copyright American Dietetic Association. Adapted with permission. Adapted from Snapshots designed by members of The Nutrition Care Process–Standardized Language Committee, 2002-2007; Chicago: The American Dietetic Association, March 19, 2007. The most current information on this topic is available in current publications from the American Dietetic Association.

APPENDIX 9 Birth to 36 Months: Boys Length-for-Age and Weight-for-Age Percentiles

NAME _____

RECORD # _____

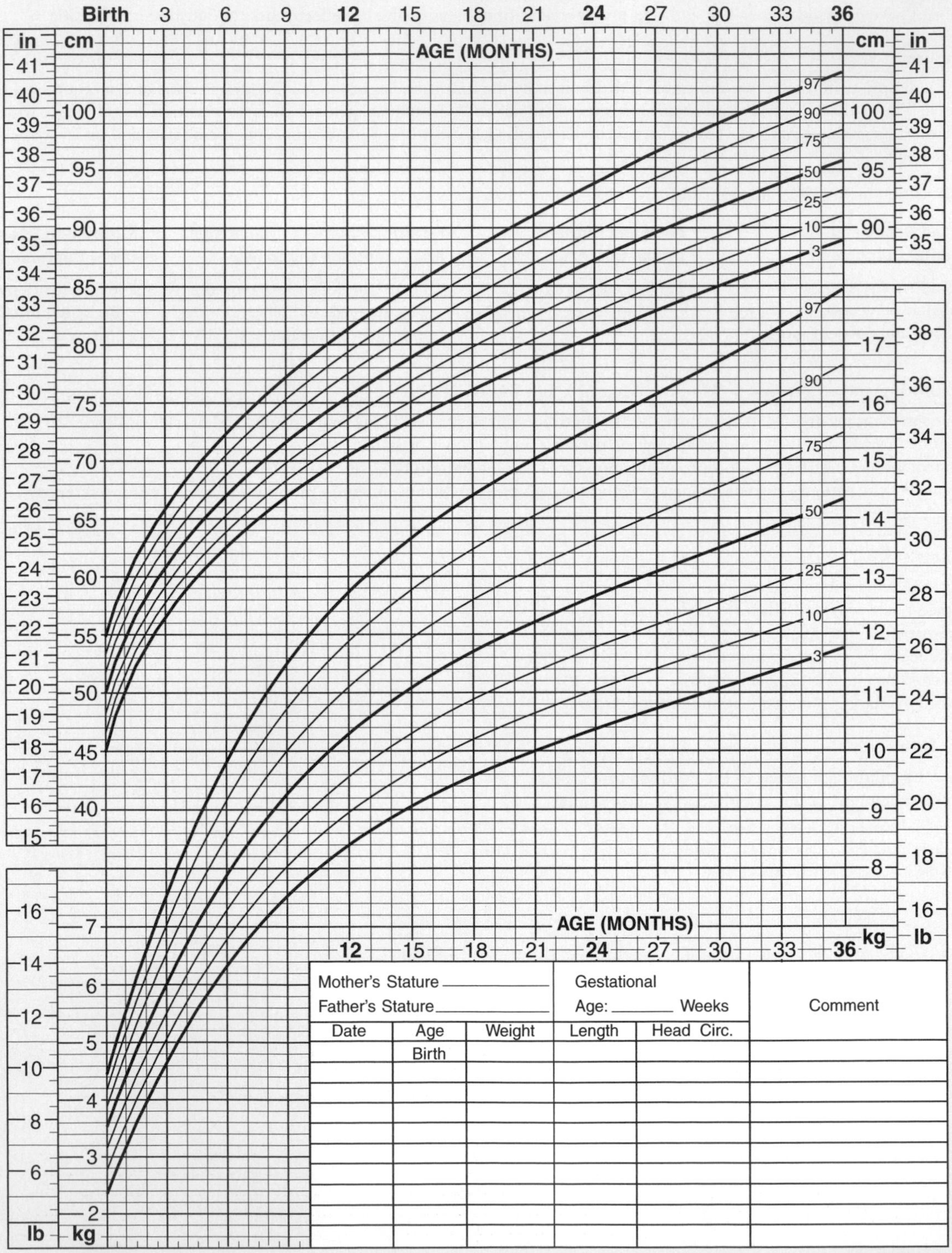

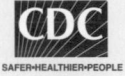

AGE (MONTHS)

LENGTH

WEIGHT

Mother's Stature _____
Father's Stature _____

Gestational Age: _____ Weeks

Comment

Date	Age	Weight	Length	Head Circ.
	Birth			

Published May 30, 2000 (modified 4/20/01).
SOURCE: Developed by the National Center for Health Statistics in collaboration with the National Center for Chronic Disease Prevention and Health Promotion (2000).
http://www .cdc.gov/growthcharts

APPENDIX 10 Birth to 36 Months: Boys Head Circumference-for-Age and Weight-for-Length Percentiles

NAME _____

RECORD # _____

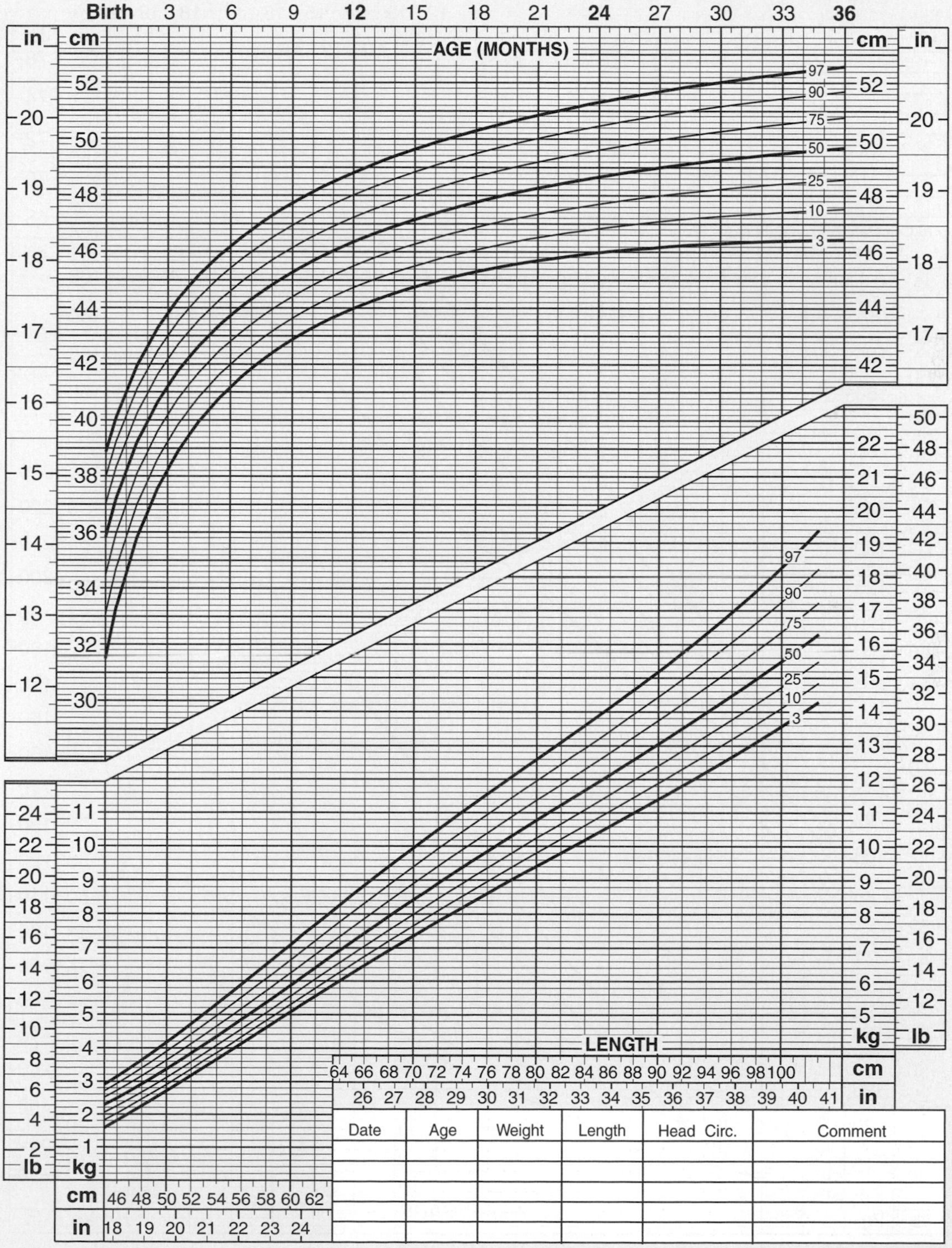

AGE (MONTHS)

Birth 3 6 9 12 15 18 21 24 27 30 33 36

HEAD CIRCUMFERENCE

97
90
75
50
25
10
3

LENGTH

97
90
75
50
25
10
3

WEIGHT

LENGTH
cm 64 66 68 70 72 74 76 78 80 82 84 86 88 90 92 94 96 98 100
in 26 27 28 29 30 31 32 33 34 35 36 37 38 39 40 41

Date	Age	Weight	Length	Head Circ.	Comment

cm 46 48 50 52 54 56 58 60 62
in 18 19 20 21 22 23 24

Published May 30, 2000 (modified 10/16/00).
SOURCE: Developed by the National Center for Health Statistics in collaboration with
the National Center for Chronic Disease Prevention and Health Promotion (2000).
http://www.cdc.gov/growthcharts

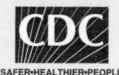
SAFER•HEALTHIER•PEOPLE

APPENDIX 11 2 to 20 Years: Boys Stature-for-Age and Weight-for-Age Percentiles

NAME _____

RECORD # _____

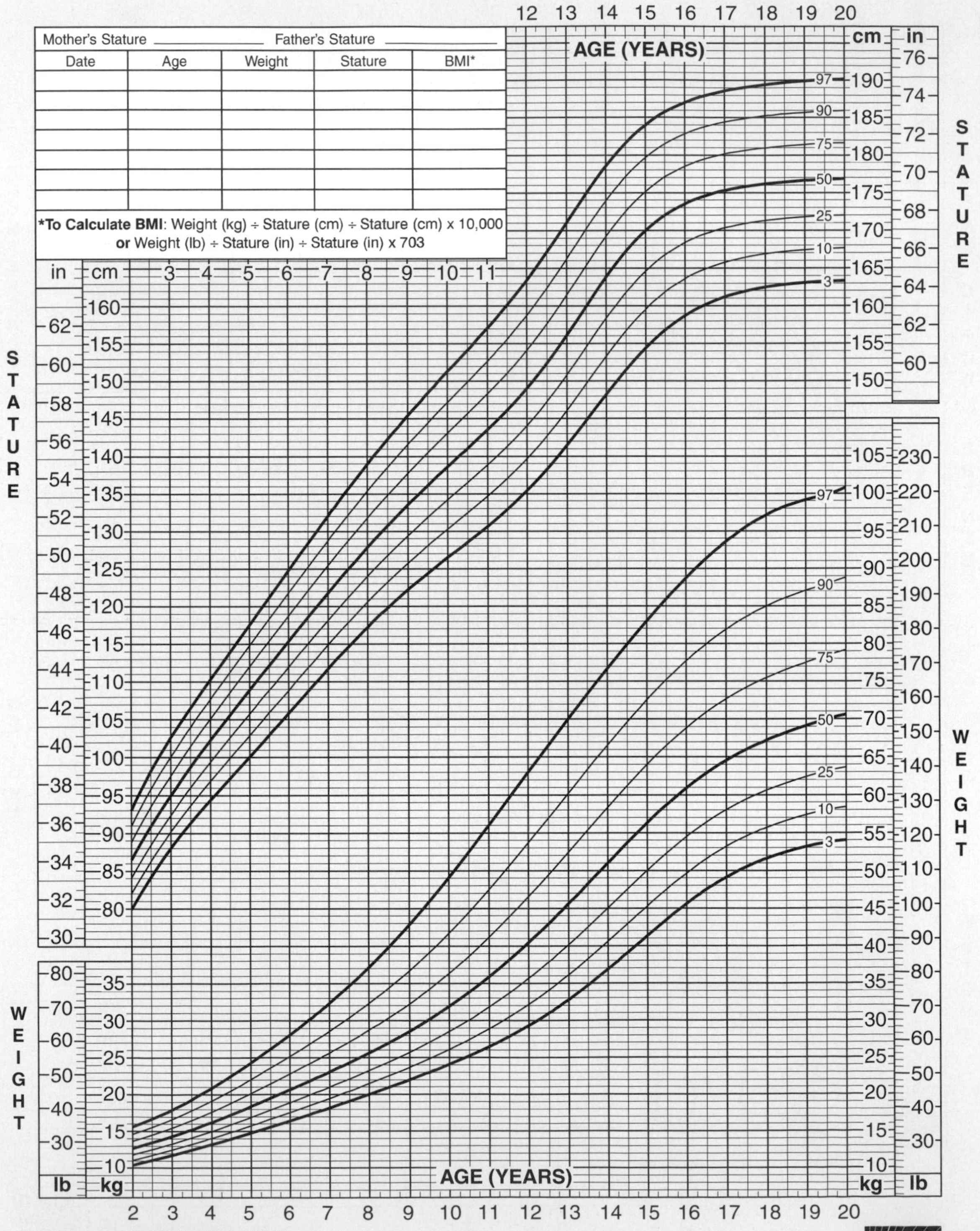

Mother's Stature _____		Father's Stature _____		
Date	Age	Weight	Stature	BMI*

*To Calculate BMI: Weight (kg) ÷ Stature (cm) ÷ Stature (cm) x 10,000
or Weight (lb) ÷ Stature (in) ÷ Stature (in) x 703

AGE (YEARS)

12 13 14 15 16 17 18 19 20

STATURE

STATURE

WEIGHT

WEIGHT

AGE (YEARS)

Published May 30, 2000 (modified 11/21/00).
SOURCE: Developed by the National Center for Health Statistics in collaboration with
the National Center for Chronic Disease Prevention and Health Promotion (2000).
http://www.cdc.gov/growthcharts

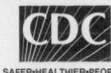
SAFER•HEALTHIER•PEOPLE

APPENDIX 12 Body Mass Index-for-Age Percentiles: Boys, 2 to 20 Years

NAME _____

RECORD # _____

Date	Age	Weight	Stature	BMI*	Comments

*To Calculate BMI: Weight (kg) ÷ Stature (cm) ÷ Stature (cm) x 10,000
or Weight (lb) ÷ Stature (in) ÷ Stature (in) x 703

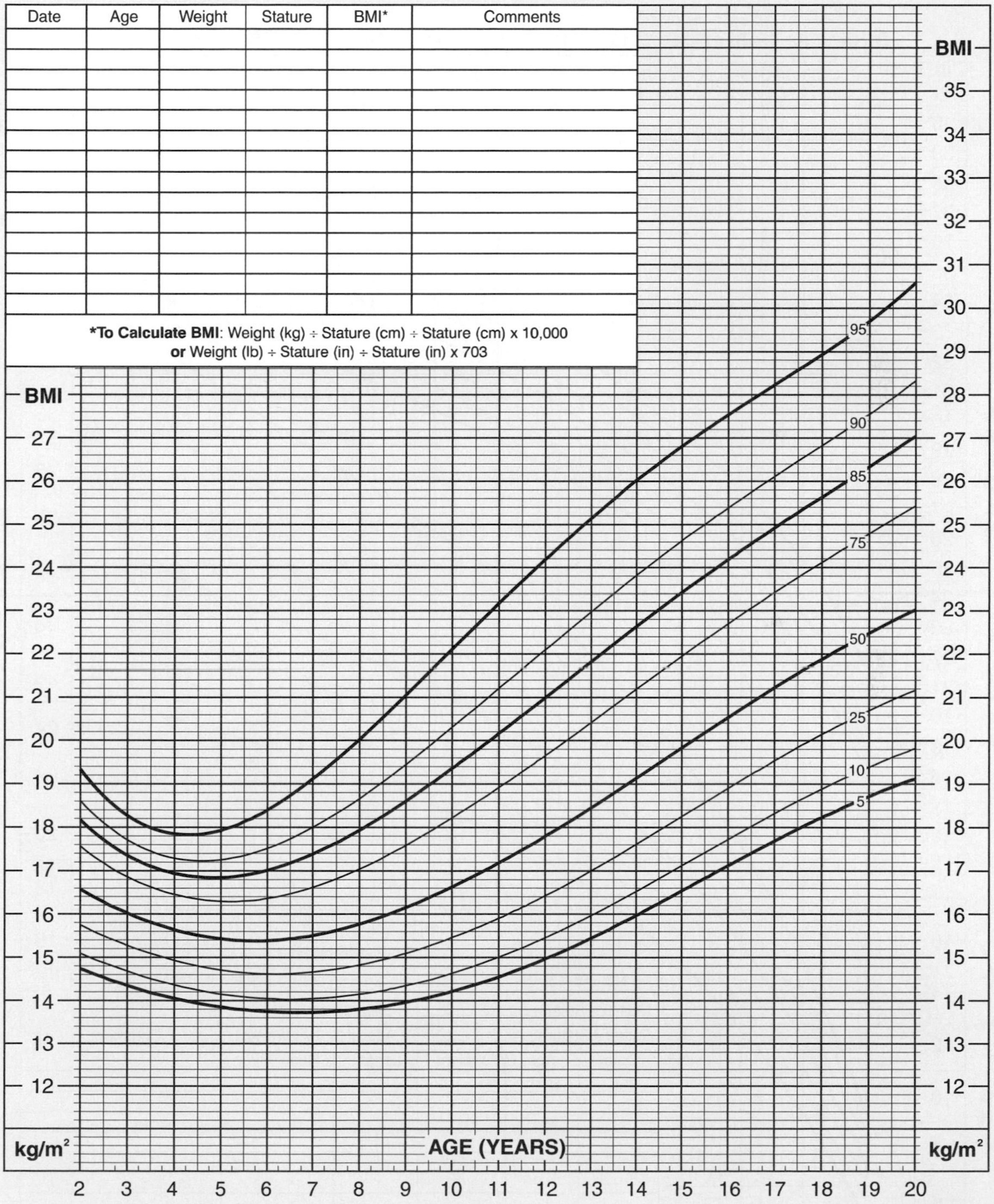

BMI

35
34
33
32
31
30
29
28
27
26
25
24
23
22
21
20
19
18
17
16
15
14
13
12

95
90
85
75
50
25
10
5

kg/m²

AGE (YEARS)

kg/m²

2 3 4 5 6 7 8 9 10 11 12 13 14 15 16 17 18 19 20

Published May 30, 2000 (modified 10/16/00).
SOURCE: Developed by the National Center for Health Statistics in collaboration with
the National Center for Chronic Disease Prevention and Health Promotion (2000).
http://www.cdc.gov/growthcharts

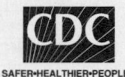

CDC
SAFER·HEALTHIER·PEOPLE

APPENDIX 13 Birth to 36 Months: Girls Length-for-Age and Weight-for-Age Percentiles

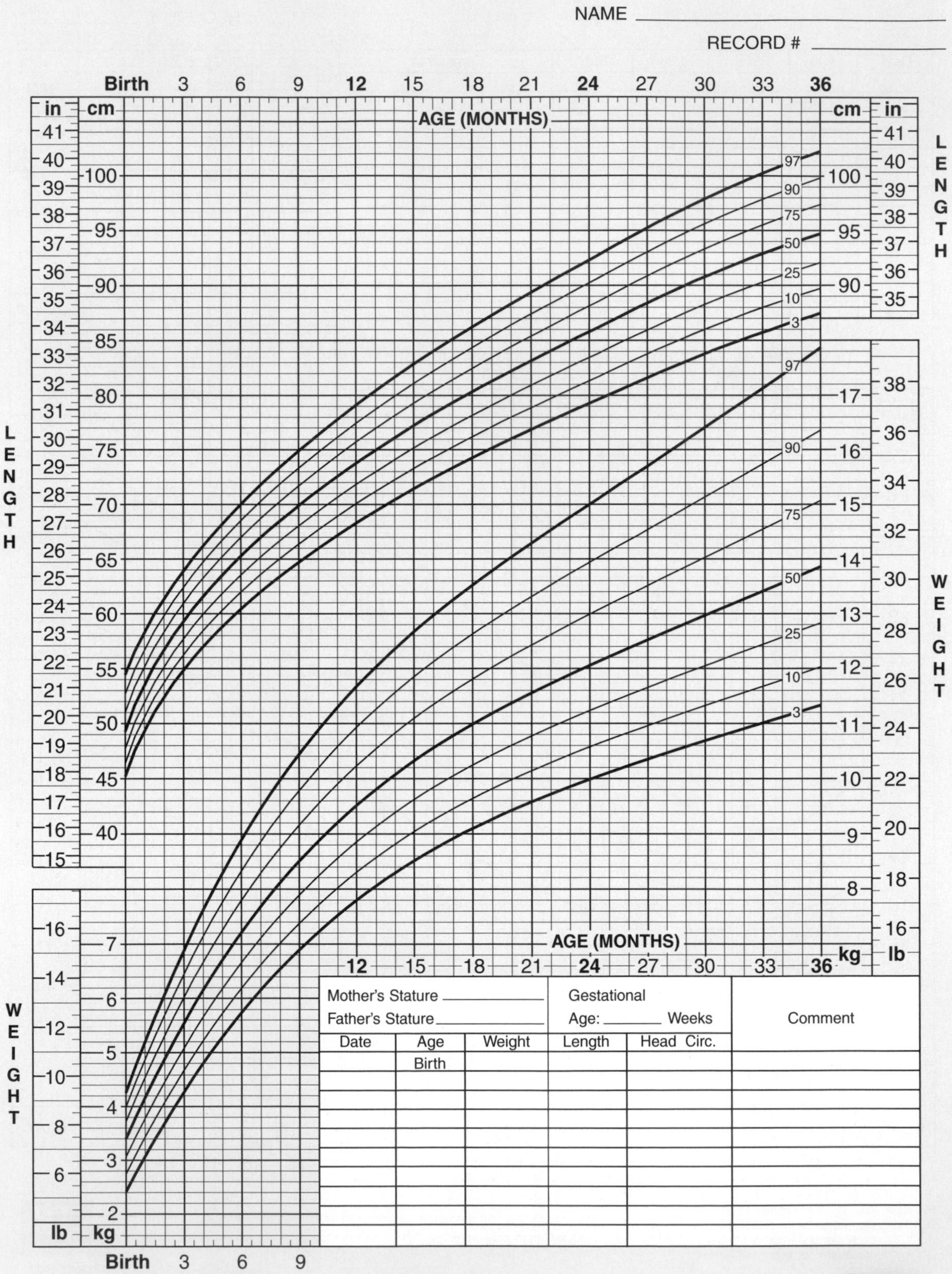
NAME
RECORD #
Birth 3 6 9 12 15 18 21 24 27 30 33 36
AGE (MONTHS)
in cm
LENGTH
WEIGHT
97 90 75 50 25 10 3
lb kg
Mother's Stature
Father's Stature
Gestational Age: Weeks
Comment
Date Age Weight Length Head Circ.
Birth

Published May 30, 2000 (modified 4/20/01).
SOURCE: Developed by the National Center for Health Statistics in collaboration with the National Center for Chronic Disease Prevention and Health Promotion (2000).
http://www.cdc.gov/growthcharts

CDC SAFER•HEALTHIER•PEOPLE

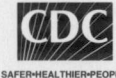

APPENDIX 14 Birth to 36 Months: Girls Head Circumference-for-Age and Weight-for-Length Percentiles

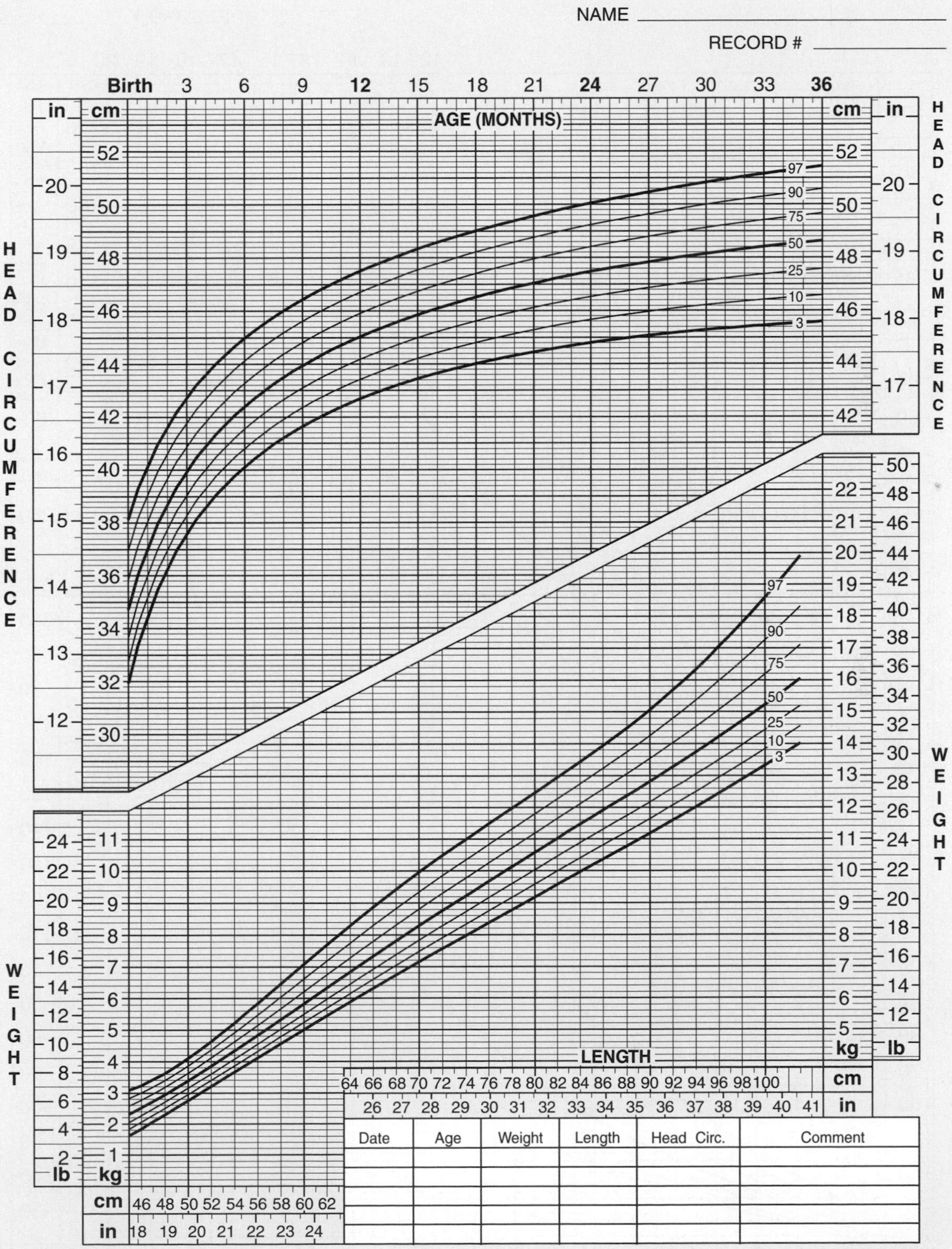

NAME _____

RECORD # _____

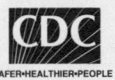

Published May 30, 2000 (modified 10/16/00).
SOURCE: Developed by the National Center for Health Statistics in collaboration with
the National Center for Chronic Disease Prevention and Health Promotion (2000).
http://www.cdc.gov/growthcharts

APPENDIX 15 2 to 20 Years: Girls Stature-for-Age and Weight-for-Age Percentiles

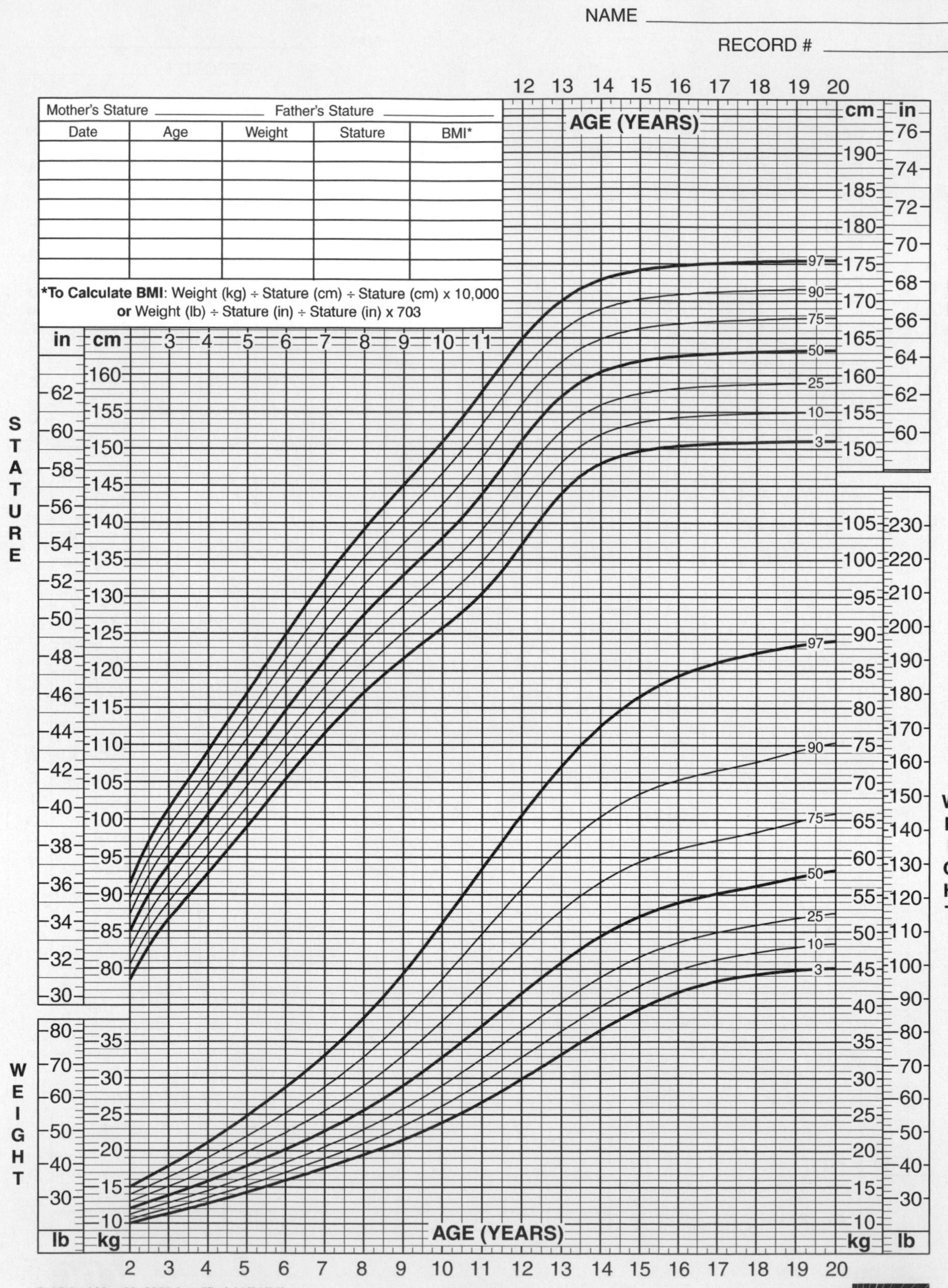

NAME _____

RECORD # _____

Mother's Stature _____ Father's Stature _____

Date	Age	Weight	Stature	BMI*

*To Calculate BMI: Weight (kg) ÷ Stature (cm) ÷ Stature (cm) x 10,000
or Weight (lb) ÷ Stature (in) ÷ Stature (in) x 703

AGE (YEARS)

STATURE

WEIGHT

AGE (YEARS)

Published May 30, 2000 (modified 11/21/00).
SOURCE: Developed by the National Center for Health Statistics in collaboration with
the National Center for Chronic Disease Prevention and Health Promotion (2000).
http://www.cdc.gov/growthcharts

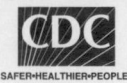
SAFER·HEALTHIER·PEOPLE

APPENDIX 16 Body Mass Index-for-Age Percentiles: Girls, 2 to 20 Years

NAME _____

RECORD # _____

Date	Age	Weight	Stature	BMI*	Comments

*To Calculate BMI: Weight (kg) ÷ Stature (cm) ÷ Stature (cm) x 10,000
or Weight (lb) ÷ Stature (in) ÷ Stature (in) x 703

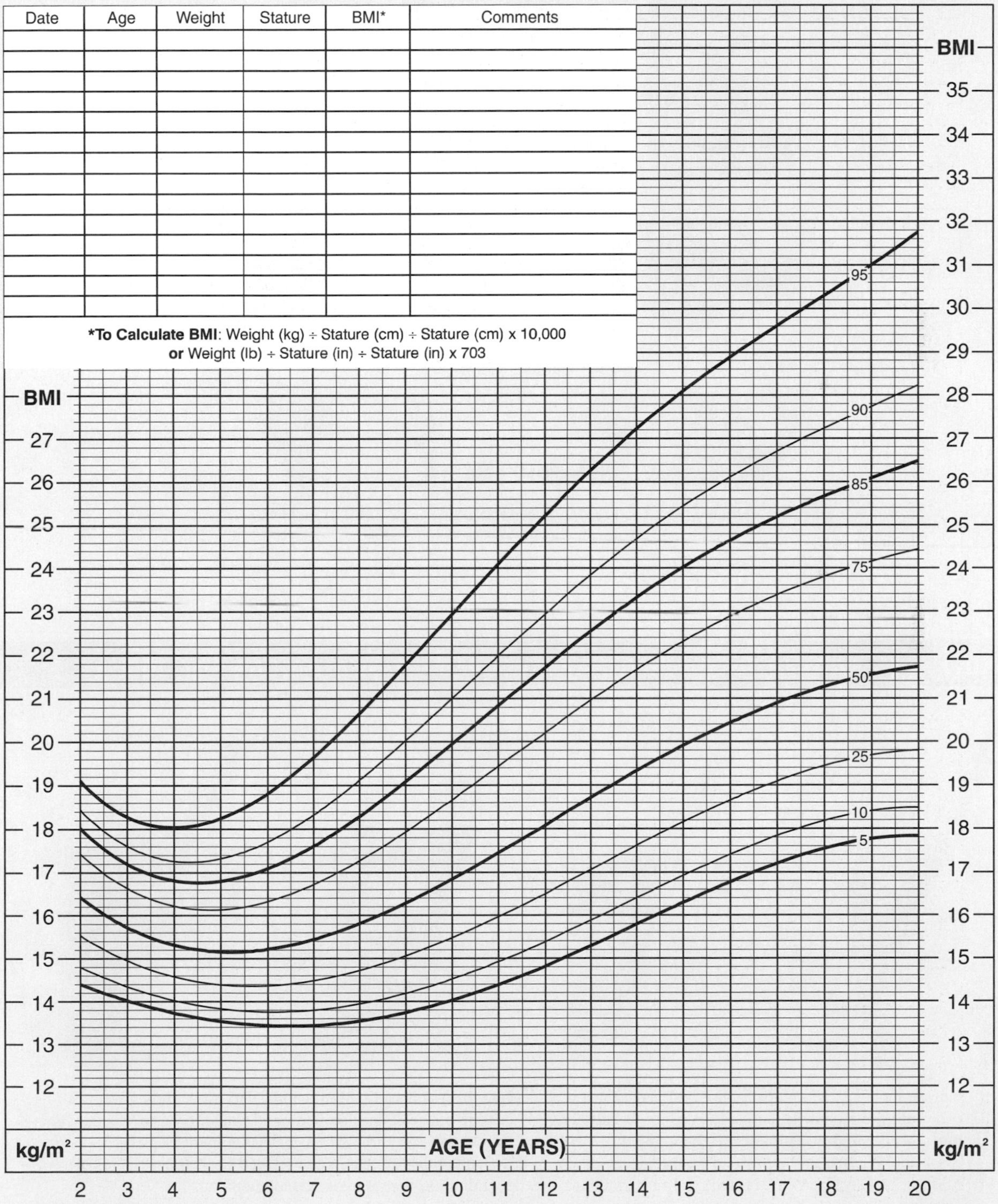

BMI

35
34
33
32
31
30
29
28
27
26
25
24
23
22
21
20
19
18
17
16
15
14
13
12

95
90
85
75
50
25
10
5

BMI

27
26
25
24
23
22
21
20
19
18
17
16
15
14
13
12

kg/m²

AGE (YEARS)

kg/m²

2 3 4 5 6 7 8 9 10 11 12 13 14 15 16 17 18 19 20

Published May 30, 2000 (modified 10/16/00).
SOURCE: Developed by the National Center for Health Statistics in collaboration with
the National Center for Chronic Disease Prevention and Health Promotion (2000).
http://www.cdc.gov/growthcharts

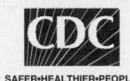

SAFER•HEALTHIER•PEOPLE

APPENDIX 17 Tanner Stages of Adolescent Development for Females

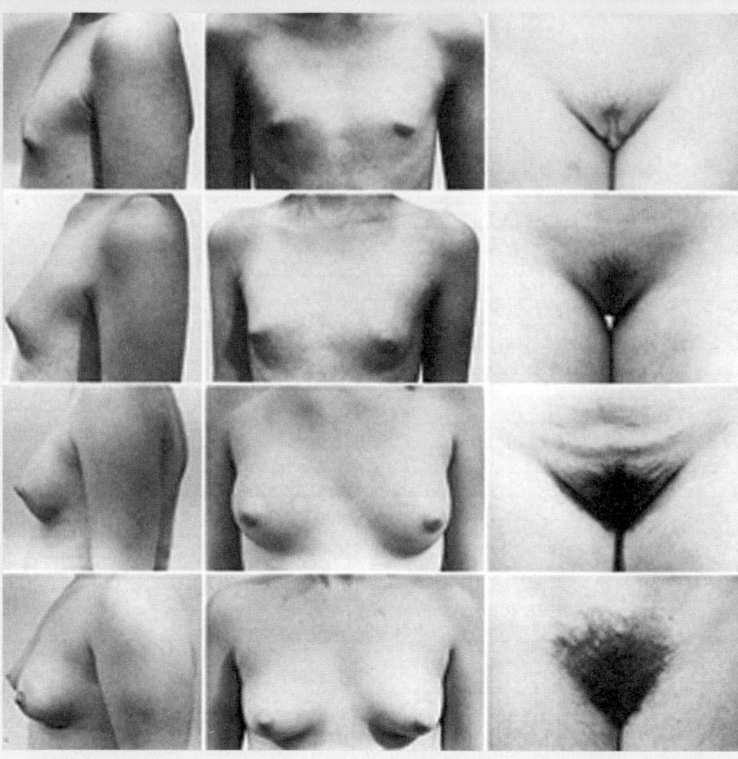

From Mahan LK, Rees JM: *Nutrition in adolescence*, St. Louis, 1984, Mosby.

APPENDIX 18 Tanner Stages of Adolescent Development for Males

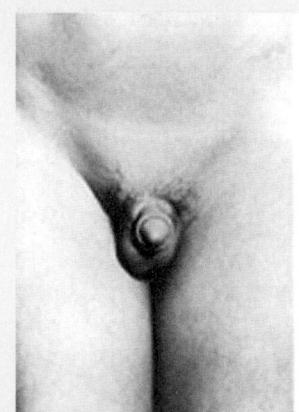 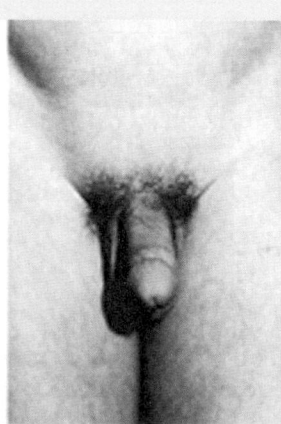 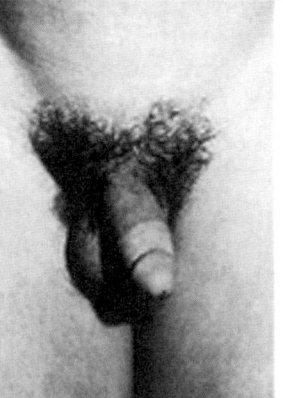 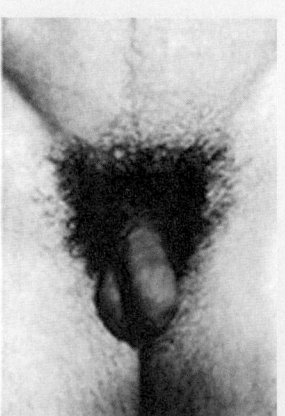

Chronologic age is not always the best way to assess adolescent growth because of individual variations in beginning and completing the growth sequence. A more useful way of describing pubertal development, and thus the varying needs for nutrients throughout adolescence, is to divide growth into stages of breast and pubic hair development in girls (Appendix 17) and pubic hair and penis and testicle development in boys (Appendix 18). These are termed the Tanner Stages of Adolescent Development. Nutritional requirements vary, depending on the stage of development.

From Mahan LK, Rees JM: *Nutrition in adolescence*, St. Louis, 1984, Mosby.

APPENDIX 19 Direct Methods for Measuring Height and Weight

Height

1. Height should be measured without shoes.
2. The individual's feet should be together, with the heels against the wall or measuring board.
3. The individual should stand erect, neither slumped nor stretching, looking straight ahead, without tipping the head up or down. The top of the ear and outer corner of the eye should be in a line parallel to the floor (the "Frankfort plane").
4. A horizontal bar, a rectangular block of wood, or the top of the statiometer should be lowered to rest flat on the top of the head.
5. Height should be read to the nearest ¼ inch or 0.5 cm.

Weight

1. Use a beam balance scale, not a spring scale, whenever possible.
2. Periodically calibrate the scale for accuracy, using known weights.
3. Weigh the subject in light clothing without shoes.
4. Record weight to the nearest ½ lb or 0.2 kg for adults and ¼ lb or 0.1 kg for infants. Measurements above the 90th percentile or below the 10th percentile warrant further evaluation.

APPENDIX 20 Indirect Methods for Measuring Height

Measuring Arm Span

Steps:
1. The arms are extended straight out to the sides at a 90-degree angle from the body.
2. The distance from the longest fingertip of one hand to the longest finger of the other hand is measured. See Figure 45-1, *C*.

Adult Recumbent

Steps:
1. Stand on right side of the body.
2. Align body so that the lower extremities, trunk, shoulders, and head are straight.
3. Place a mark at the top of the sheet in line with the crown of the head and one at the bottom of the sheet in line with the base of the heels.
4. Measure length between marks with measuring tape.

Knee Height*

Knee height measurement is highly correlated with upright height. It is useful in those who cannot stand and in those who may have curvatures of the spine.

Steps:
1. Use the left leg for measurements.
2. Bend the left knee and the left ankle to 90-degree angles. A triangle may be used if available. See Figure 45-1, *A*.
3. Using knee height calipers, open the caliper and place the fixed part under the heel. Place the sliding blade down against the thigh (approximately 2 inches behind the patella).
4. Measure from the heel to the anterior surface of the thigh, using a cloth measuring tape.
5. Obtain the measurement and convert it to centimeters by multiplying by 2.54.
6. Formulas to use to calculate estimated height from knee height:

$$\text{Men (height in centimeters)} = 64.19 - (0.04 \times \text{Age}) + (2.02 \times \text{Knee height in centimeters})$$

$$\text{Women (height in centimeters)} = 84.8 - (0.24 \times \text{Age}) + (1.83 \times \text{Knee height in centimeters})$$

*Data from Chumlea WC et al: *Nutritional assessment of the elderly through anthropometry*, Columbus, Ohio, 1984, Ross Laboratories.

Predicting Stature From Knee Height

Recommended equations for predicting stature from knee height in adults (18 to 60 years of age) and children (6 to 18 years of age)

Group	Equations
White men	Stature = 71.85 + (1.88 knee height)
	$R^2 = 0.65$; RMSE = 3.97; SEI = 3.97 cm; CV = 2.28
Black men	Stature = 73.42 + (1.79 knee height)
	$R^2 = 0.69$; RMSE = 3.60; SEI = 3.60 cm; CV = 2.08
White women	Stature = 70.25 + (1.87 knee height) − (0.06 age)
	$R^2 = 0.66$; RMSE = 3.60; SEI = 3.60 cm; CV = 2.23
Black women	Stature = 68.10 + (1.86 knee height) − (0.06 age)
	$R^2 = 0.69$; RMSE = 3.80; SEI = 3.80 cm; CV = 2.36
White boys	Stature = 40.54 + (2.22 knee height)
	$R^2 = 0.96$; RMSE = 4.16; SEI = 4.21 cm; CV = 2.79
Black boys	Stature = 39.60 + (2.18 knee height)
	R^2 50.95; RMSE = 4.44; SEI = 4.58 cm; CV = 2.99
White girls	Stature = 43.21 + (2.15 knee height)
	$R^2 = 0.95$; RMSE = 3.84; SEI = 3.90 cm; CV = 2.63
Black girls	Stature = 46.59 + (2.02 knee height)
	$R^2 = 0.94$; RMSE = 4.25; SEI = 4.39 cm; CV = 2.91

RMSE, Root mean square error; *SEI*, standard error for an individual; *CV*, coefficient of variation.

APPENDIX 21 Determination of Frame Size

Method 1*

Height is recorded without shoes.

Wrist circumference is measured just distal to the styloid process at the wrist crease on the right arm, using a tape measure. The following formula is used:

$$r = \frac{\text{Height (cm)}}{\text{Wrist circumference (centimeters)}}$$

Frame size can be determined as follows:

Males	Females
r >10.4 small	r >11.0 small
r = 9.6-10.4 medium	r = 10.1-11.0 medium
r <9.6 large	r <10.1 large

Method 2†

The patient's right arm is extended forward perpendicular to the body, with the arm bent so the angle at the elbow forms 90 degrees with the fingers pointing up and the palm turned away from the body. The greatest breadth across the elbow joint is measured with a sliding caliper along the axis of the upper arm on the two prominent bones on either side of the elbow. This is recorded as the elbow breadth. The following tables give the elbow breadth measurements for medium-framed men and women of various heights. Measurements lower than those listed indicate a small frame size; higher measurements indicate a large frame size.

Men		Women	
Height in 1″ Heels	**Elbow Breadth (inches)**	**Height in 1″ Heels**	**Elbow Breadth (inches)**
5′2″-5′3″	2½-2⅞	4′10″-4′11″	2¼-2½
5′4″-5′7″	2⅝-2⅞	5′0″-5′3″	2¼-2½
5′8″-5′11″	2¾-3	5′4″-5′7″	2⅜-2⅝
6′0″-6′3″	2¾-3⅛	5′8″-5′11″	2⅜-2⅝
6′4″	2⅞-3¼	6′0″	

*From Grant JP: *Handbook of total parenteral nutrition*, Philadelphia, 1980, Saunders.

†From Metropolitan Life Insurance Co., 1983.

APPENDIX 22 Adjustment of Desirable Body Weight for Amputees

The percentages listed below are estimates because body proportions vary in individuals. Use of these percentages provides an approximation of desirable body weight, which is more accurate than a comparison with the standards for normal adults.

Ideal body weight (IBW) must be adjusted downward to compensate for missing limbs or paralysis. It is estimated that 5% to 10% should be subtracted from IBW for a paraplegic and from 10% to 15% subtracted for a quadriplegic.

Adjustment of Ideal Body Weight for Amputees*

Body Segment	Average % of Total Weight
Lower arm and hand	2.3
Trunk without extremities	50
Entire arm	5.0
Hand	0.7
Entire lower leg	16.0
Below knee including foot	5.9
Foot	1.5

$$\text{Estimated IBW} = \frac{100 - \% \text{ amputation}}{100} \times \text{IBW for original height}$$

To use this information, you must know the patient's approximate height before the amputation. Span measurement is a rough estimate of height at maturity and is calculated as follows: with the upper extremities, including the hands, fully extended and parallel to the ground, measure the distance between the tip of one middle finger and the tip of the other middle finger. See Figure 45-1, *C*.

Use this height or actual measurement to calculate the desirable body weight for the normal body size; then adjust the figures according to the type of amputation performed.

Example: To determine the desirable body weight for a 5′10″ male with a below-the-knee amputation:

1. Calculate desirable body weight for a 5′10″ male: 166 lb
2. Subtract weight of amputated limb (6%) = 166 × 0.06: − 9.96 (approx. 10 lb)
3. Desirable weight of a 5′10″ male with a below-knee amputation: 156 lb

From North Carolina Dietetic Association: *Nutrition care manual*, 2005, Raleigh, NC, The Association.

*Data from Brunnstrom S: *Clinical kinesiology*, Philadelphia, 1972, FA Davis.

APPENDIX 23 Body Mass Index (BMI) Table

BMI	Normal Weight						Overweight					Obesity					
	19	**20**	**21**	**22**	**23**	**24**	**25**	**26**	**27**	**28**	**29**	**30**	**31**	**32**	**33**	**34**	**35**
Height	Weight (in pounds)																
4′10″ (58″)	91	96	100	105	110	115	119	124	129	134	138	143	148	153	158	162	167
4′11″ (59″)	94	99	104	109	114	119	124	128	133	138	143	148	153	158	163	168	173
5′ (60″)	97	102	107	112	118	123	128	133	138	143	148	153	158	163	168	174	179
5′1″ (61″)	100	106	111	116	122	127	132	137	143	148	153	158	164	169	174	180	185
5′2″ (62″)	104	109	115	120	126	131	136	142	147	153	158	164	169	175	180	186	191
5′3″ (63″)	107	113	118	124	130	135	141	146	152	158	163	169	175	180	186	191	197
5′4″ (64″)	110	116	122	128	134	140	145	151	157	163	169	174	180	186	192	197	204
5′5″ (65″)	114	120	126	132	138	144	150	156	162	168	174	180	186	192	198	204	210
5′6″ (66″)	118	124	130	136	142	148	155	161	167	173	179	186	192	198	204	210	216
5′7″ (67″)	121	127	134	140	146	153	159	166	172	178	185	191	198	204	211	217	223
5′8″ (68″)	125	131	138	144	151	158	164	171	177	184	190	197	203	210	216	223	230
5′9″ (69″)	128	135	142	149	155	162	169	176	182	189	196	203	209	216	223	230	236
5′10″ (70″)	132	139	146	153	160	167	174	181	188	195	202	209	216	222	229	236	243
5′11″ (71″)	136	143	150	157	165	172	179	186	193	200	208	215	222	229	236	243	250
6′ (72″)	140	147	154	162	169	177	184	191	199	206	213	221	228	235	242	250	258
6′1″ (73″)	144	151	159	166	174	182	189	197	204	212	219	227	235	242	250	257	265
6′2″ (74″)	148	155	163	171	179	186	194	202	210	218	225	233	241	249	256	264	272
6′3″ (75″)	152	160	168	176	184	192	200	208	216	224	232	240	248	256	264	272	279

Data from NIH/National Heart, Lung, and Blood Institute (NHLBI): *Evidence report of clinical guidelines on the identification, evaluation, and treatment of overweight and obesity in adults*, Bethesda, Md, 1998, NIH/NHLBI. For a BMI of greater than 30, please go to http://www.nhlbi.nih.gov/guidelines/obesity/bmi_tbl.pdf.

APPENDIX 24 Percentage of Body Fat Based on Four Skinfold Measurements*

Sum of Skinfolds (mm)	Males (Age in Years)				Females (Age in Years)			
	17-29	**30-39**	**40-49**	**50+**	**16-29**	**30-39**	**40-49**	**50+**
15	4.8	—	—	—	10.5	—	—	—
20	8.1	12.2	12.2	12.6	14.1	17.0	19.8	21.4
25	10.5	14.2	15.0	15.6	16.8	19.4	22.2	24.0
30	12.9	16.2	17.7	18.6	19.5	21.8	24.5	26.6
35	14.7	17.7	19.6	20.8	21.5	23.7	26.4	28.5
40	16.4	19.2	21.4	22.9	23.4	25.5	28.2	30.3
45	17.7	20.4	23.0	24.7	25.0	26.9	29.6	31.9
50	19.0	21.5	24.6	26.5	26.5	28.2	31.0	33.4
55	20.1	22.5	25.9	27.9	27.8	29.4	32.1	34.6
60	21.2	23.5	27.1	29.2	29.1	30.6	33.2	35.7
65	22.2	24.3	28.2	30.4	30.2	31.6	34.1	36.7
70	23.1	25.1	29.3	31.6	31.2	32.5	35.0	37.7
75	24.0	25.9	30.3	32.7	32.2	33.4	35.9	38.7
80	24.8	26.6	31.2	33.8	33.1	34.3	36.7	39.6
85	25.5	27.2	32.1	34.8	34.0	35.1	37.5	40.4
90	26.2	27.8	33.0	35.8	34.8	35.8	38.3	41.2
95	26.9	28.4	33.7	36.6	35.6	36.5	39.0	41.9
100	27.6	29.0	34.4	37.4	36.4	37.2	39.7	42.6
105	28.2	29.6	35.1	38.2	37.1	37.9	40.4	43.3
110	28.8	30.1	35.8	39.0	37.8	38.6	41.0	43.9
115	29.4	30.6	36.4	39.7	38.4	39.1	41.5	44.5
120	30.0	31.1	37.0	40.4	39.0	39.6	42.0	45.1
125	30.5	31.5	37.6	41.1	39.6	40.1	42.5	45.7
130	31.0	31.9	38.2	41.8	40.2	40.6	43.0	46.2
135	31.5	32.3	38.7	42.4	40.8	41.1	43.5	46.7
140	32.0	32.7	39.2	43.0	41.3	41.6	44.0	47.2
145	32.5	33.1	39.7	43.6	41.8	42.1	44.5	47.7
150	32.9	33.5	40.2	44.1	42.3	42.6	45.0	48.2
155	33.3	33.9	40.7	44.6	42.8	43.1	45.4	48.7
160	33.7	34.3	41.2	45.1	43.3	43.6	45.8	49.2
165	34.1	34.6	41.6	45.6	43.7	44.0	46.2	49.6
170	34.5	34.8	42.0	46.1	44.1	44.4	46.6	50.0
175	34.9	—	—	—	—	44.8	47.0	50.4
180	35.3	—	—	—	—	45.2	47.4	50.8
185	35.6	—	—	—	—	45.6	47.8	51.2
190	35.9	—	—	—	—	45.9	48.2	51.6
195	—	—	—	—	—	46.2	48.5	52.0
200	—	—	—	—	—	46.5	48.8	52.4
205	—	—	—	—	—	—	49.1	52.7
210	—	—	—	—	—	—	49.4	53.0

From Durnin JVGA, Wormersley J: Body fat assessed from total body density and its estimation from skinfold thickness: measurements on 481 men and women ages 16-72 years, *Br J Nutr* 32:77, 1974.

*Measurements made on the right side of the body, using biceps, triceps, subscapular, and suprailiac skinfolds.

APPENDIX 25 Arm Anthropometry for Children

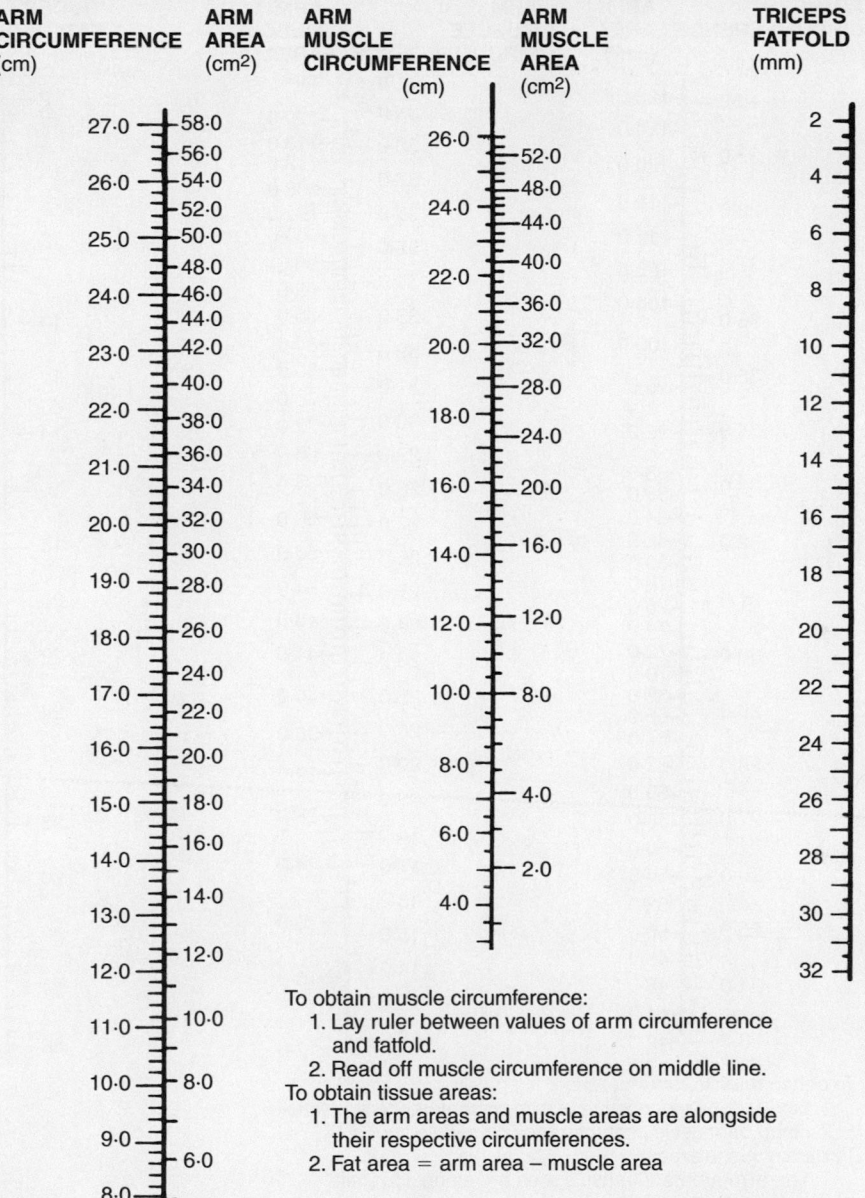

To obtain muscle circumference:
1. Lay ruler between values of arm circumference and fatfold.
2. Read off muscle circumference on middle line.

To obtain tissue areas:
1. The arm areas and muscle areas are alongside their respective circumferences.
2. Fat area = arm area – muscle area

From Gurney JM, Jelliffe DB: Arm anthropometry in nutritional assessment: nomogram for rapid calculation of muscle circumference and cross-sectional muscle fat areas, *Am J Clin Nutr* 26:913, 1973.

APPENDIX 26 Arm Anthropometry for Adults

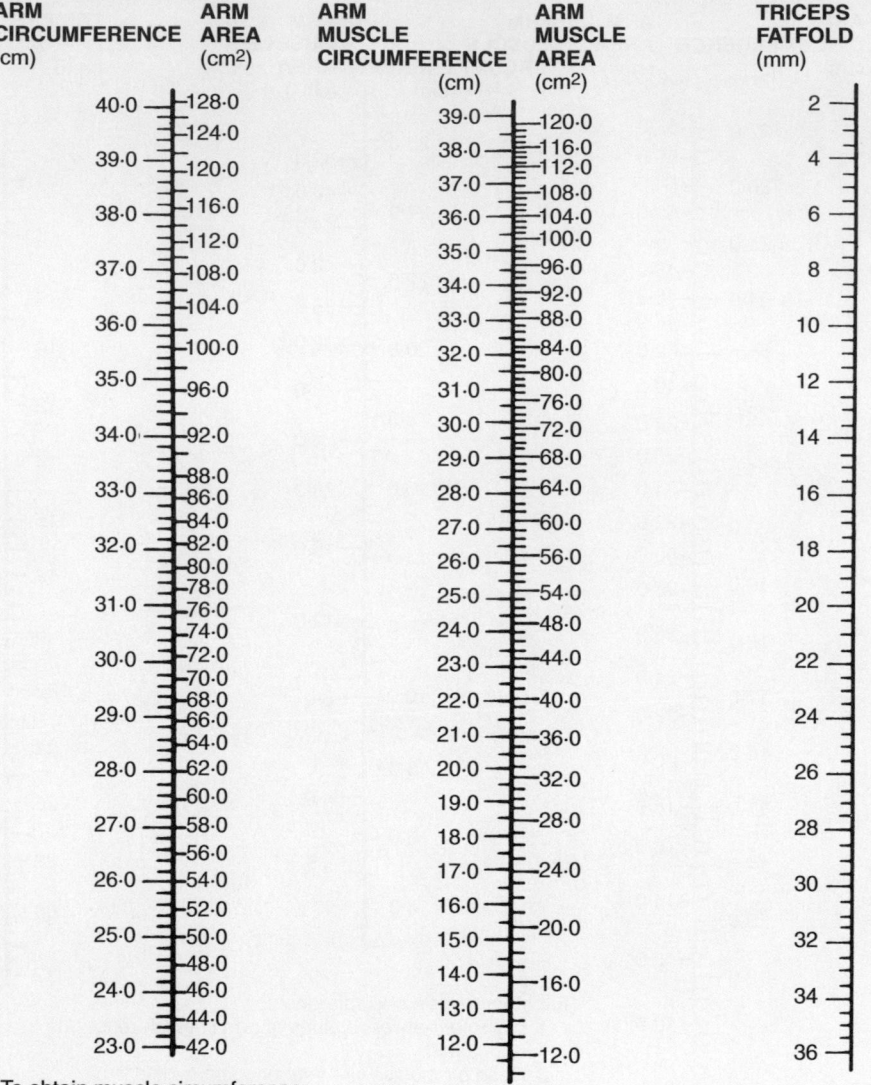

To obtain muscle circumference:
  1. Lay ruler between value of arm circumference and fatfold.
  2. Read off muscle circumference on middle line.
To obtain tissue areas:
  1. The arm area and muscle area are alongside their respective circumferences.
  2. Fat area = arm area − muscle area

From Gurney JM, Jelliffe DB: Arm anthropometry in nutritional assessment: nomogram for rapid calculation of muscle circumference and cross-sectional muscle fat areas, *Am J Clin Nutr* 26:913, 1973.

APPENDIX 27 Recommendations for Clinical Application of Bioelectrical Impedance Analysis (BIA)

Instruments/Material	Definition/Comments	Recommendations
Statiometer	Calibrated to 0.5 cm	Use tape measure for subjects who are unable to stand and for knee height or arm span
Scale	Calibrated to 0.1 kg	Regular cross-calibration with other scales
Subjects		
Height/weight	Measure height (0.5 cm) and weight (0.1 kg) at time of BIA measurement	Self-reported height and weight not valid

APPENDIX 27 Recommendations for Clinical Application of Bioelectrical Impedance Analysis—cont'd

Subjects—cont'd	Definition/Comments	Recommendations
Food, drink, alcohol	Fasting/no alcohol for >8 h recommended	Shorter periods of fasting may be acceptable for clinical practice (vs. research)
Bladder voided		Subject has voided before measurement
Physical exercise		No exercise for >8 h
Timing	Note time of measurement	For longitudinal follow-up, perform measurement at the same time of day; note menstrual cycle
Skin condition	Temperature	Ambient temperature
	Integrity	No skin lesions at sight of electrodes; change site of electrodes
	Cleaning	Clean with alcohol
Electrode position	Note body site of measurement; distance between electrodes	Always measure same body side
		Minimum of 5 cm between electrodes; if needed, move proximal electrode
Limb position	Abduction of limbs	Arms separated from trunk by about 30 degrees; legs separated by about 45 degrees
Body position	Supine, except for "scale" type BIA instruments	Ambulatory subjects supine for 5 to 10 min; for research protocol, standardize time that subjects are supine before measurement; note if subject is confined to bed (patients)
Environment	Electrical interference	No contact with metal frame of bed; neutral environment (no strong electrical or magnetic fields)
Body shape	Note body abnormalities	Note measurement validity (e.g., R or Xc outside of expected range for subject)
		Consider validity of measurement when interpreting results (e.g., abnormally low R suggests edema)
	Amputation	Measure nonaffected limb; not valid for research but permits determination of body compartment because measurement error is consistent
		Measure nonaffected side
	Atrophy/hemiplegia	Note abnormal condition
	Abnormal limb or trunk (e.g., scoliosis dystrophy (e.g., HIV, Cushing syndrome)	Limited validity in conditions of abnormal body compartment distribution
	Obesity	Use electricity-isolating material (e.g., towel) between arm and trunk and between thighs
Ethnic group		Note race; use race-specific BIA equation, if applicable
Disease Conditions		
Cardiac insufficiency	Edema interferes with measurement	Measure patient in stable condition
Liver failure	Ascites/edema interferes with measurement accuracy	Consider segmental BIA measurement
Kidney failure	Edema/altered ion balance interferes with measurement	
Abnormal serum electrolyte concentrations	Electrolyte concentration affects BIA measurement	Perform BIA when serum electrolytes are within normal range
		Compare BIA results when serum electrolyte concentrations are similar
Hypothyroid	Pachyderma	May invalidate measurement because of high skin resistance
Treatments		
Intravenous/electrolyte infusions	Peripheral edema interferes with measurement	Measurements are invalid if patient is abnormally hydrated
Drugs that affect water balance	Steroids, growth hormone, diuretics	If patient is in stable condition, measurement should be taken at same time after medication administration
Dialysis	Hemo-1 peritoneal dialysis	Use special protocols, standardize measurement procedure (i.e., measurement should be performed 20 to 30 minutes after dialysis)
Ascites puncture		Use special protocols; standardize measurement procedure
Orthopedic prosthesis/implants (metal)	Hip prosthesis, for example	Measure nonaffected body side; note prosthesis/implants
Pacemakers, defibrillators	Implanted cardiac defibrillator	No interference with pacemakers or defibrillators is anticipated; although there are no known incidents reported as a result of BIA measurement, the possibility cannot be eliminated that the induced field of current during the measurement could alter the pacemaker or defibrillator activity; therefore the patient should be monitored for cardiac activity

Reprinted from Kyle UG, Bosaeus I, et al. Bioelectrical impedance analysis—Part II: Utilization in clinical practice, *Clin Nutr* 23:1430, 2004.

BIA, Bioelectrical impedance analysis; *HIV,* human immunodeficiency virus; *PhA,* phase angle; *R,* resistance; *Xc,* reactance.

APPENDIX 28 Physical Activity and Calories Expended per Hour

Activity	Type	Body Weight							
		(110 lb)	(130 lb)	(150 lb)	(170 lb)	(190 lb)	(210 lb)	(230 lb)	(250 lb)
Aerobics class	Water	210	248	286	325	364	401	439	477
Aerobics class	Low impact	263	310	358	406	455	501	549	596
Aerobics class	High impact	368	434	501	568	637	702	768	835
Aerobics class	Step with 6- to 8-inch step	446	527	609	690	774	852	933	1014
Aerobics class	Step with 10- to 12-inch step	525	621	716	812	910	1003	1097	1193
Backpack	General	368	434	501	568	637	702	768	835
Badminton	Singles and doubles	236	279	322	365	410	451	494	537
Badminton	Competitive	368	434	501	568	637	702	768	835
Baseball	Throw/catch	131	155	179	203	228	251	274	298
Baseball	Fast or slow pitch	263	310	358	406	455	501	549	596
Basketball	Shooting baskets	236	279	322	365	410	451	494	537
Basketball	Wheelchair	341	403	465	528	592	652	713	775
Basketball	Game	420	496	573	649	728	802	878	954
Bike	10-11.9 mph, slow	315	372	430	487	546	602	658	716
Bike	12-13.9 mph, moderate	420	496	573	649	728	802	878	954
Bike	14-15.9 mph, fast	525	621	716	812	910	1003	1097	1193
Bike	16-19.9 mph, very fast	630	745	859	974	1092	1203	1317	1431
Bike	>20 mph, racing	840	993	1146	1299	1457	1604	1756	1908
Bike	50 watts, stationary, very light	158	133	215	243	273	301	329	358
Bike	100 watts, stationary, light	289	341	394	446	501	552	603	656
Bike	150 watts, stationary, moderate	368	434	501	568	637	702	768	835
Bike	200 watts, stationary, vigorous	551	652	752	852	956	1053	1152	1252
Bike	250 watts, stationary, very vigorous	656	776	895	1015	1138	1253	1372	1491
Bike	BMX or mountain	446	527	609	690	774	852	933	1014
Boxing	Punching bag	315	372	430	487	546	602	658	716
Boxing	Sparring	473	558	644	730	819	902	988	1074
Calisthenics	Back exercises	184	217	251	284	319	351	384	417
Calisthenics	Pull-ups, jumping jacks	420	496	573	649	728	802	878	954
Calisthenics	Push-ups or sit-ups	420	496	573	649	728	802	878	954
Circuit training	General	420	496	573	649	728	802	878	954
Football	Flag or touch	420	496	573	649	728	802	878	954
Football	Competitive	473	558	644	730	819	902	988	1074
Frisbee	General	158	133	215	243	273	301	329	358
Frisbee	Ultimate	420	496	573	649	728	802	878	954
Golf	Power cart	184	217	251	284	319	351	384	417
Golf	Pull clubs	226	267	308	349	391	431	472	513
Golf	Carry clubs	236	279	322	365	410	451	494	537
Handball	General	630	745	859	974	1092	1203	1317	1431
Hike	General	315	372	460	487	546	602	658	716
Hockey	Ice, field hockey	420	496	573	649	728	802	878	954
Jog	General	368	434	501	568	637	702	768	835
Jog	Jog/walk combination	315	372	430	487	546	602	658	716
Jump rope	Slow	420	496	573	649	728	802	878	954
Jump rope	Moderate	525	621	716	812	910	1003	1097	1193
Jump rope	Fast	630	745	859	974	1092	1203	1317	1431
Kayak	General	263	310	358	406	455	501	549	596
Martial arts	General	525	621	716	812	910	1003	1097	1193
Racquetball	Casual	368	434	501	568	637	702	768	835
Racquetball	Competition	525	621	716	812	910	1003	1097	1193
Rafting	Whitewater	263	310	358	406	455	501	549	596
Rock climb	General	420	496	573	649	728	802	878	954
Rugby	General	525	621	716	812	910	1003	1097	1193
Run	5 mph, 12 min/mile	420	496	573	649	728	802	878	954
Run	5.2 mph, 11.5 min/mile	473	558	644	730	819	902	988	1074

APPENDIX 28 Physical Activity and Calories Expended per Hour—cont'd

Activity	Type	Body Weight							
		(110 lb)	(130 lb)	(150 lb)	(170 lb)	(190 lb)	(210 lb)	(230 lb)	(250 lb)
Run	6 mph, 10 min/mile	525	621	716	812	910	1003	1097	1193
Run	6.7 mph, 9 min/mile	578	683	788	893	1001	1103	1207	1312
Run	7 mph, 8.5 min/mile	604	714	824	933	1047	1153	1262	1372
Run	7.5 mph, 8 min/mile	656	776	895	1015	1138	1253	1372	1491
Run	8 mph, 7.5 min/mile	709	838	967	1096	1229	1354	1481	1610
Run	8.6 mph, 7 min/mile	735	869	1003	1136	1274	1404	1536	1670
Run	9 mph, 6.5 min/mile	788	931	1074	1217	1366	1504	1646	1789
Run	10 mph, 6 min/mile	840	993	1146	1299	1457	1604	1756	1908
Run	10.9 mph, 5.5 min/mile	945	1117	1289	1461	1639	1805	1975	2147
Run	Cross country	473	558	644	730	819	902	988	1074
Skate, ice	General	368	434	501	568	637	702	768	835
Skate, inline	Inline/general	656	776	895	1015	1138	1253	1372	1491
Skateboard	General	263	310	358	406	455	501	549	596
Ski, downhill	Light	263	310	358	406	455	501	549	596
Ski, downhill	Moderate	315	372	430	487	546	602	658	716
Ski, downhill	Vigorous/race	420	496	573	649	728	802	878	954
Ski machine	General	368	434	501	568	637	702	768	835
Ski, cross-country	2.5 mph, slow	368	434	501	568	637	702	768	835
Ski, cross-country	4-4.9 mph, moderate	420	496	573	649	728	802	878	954
Ski, cross-country	5-7.9 mph, brisk	473	558	644	730	819	902	988	1074
Snowboard	General	394	465	537	609	683	752	823	895
Snowshoe	General	420	496	573	649	728	802	878	954
Soccer	Casual	368	434	501	568	637	702	768	835
Soccer	Competitive	525	621	716	812	910	1003	1097	1193
Softball	General	263	310	358	406	455	501	549	596
Stair stepper	General	473	558	644	730	819	902	988	1074
Stationary rower	50 watts, light	184	217	251	284	319	351	384	417
Stationary rower	100 watts, moderate	368	434	501	568	637	702	768	835
Stationary rower	150 watts, vigorous	446	527	609	690	774	852	933	1014
Stationary rower	200 watts, very vigorous	630	745	859	974	1092	1203	1317	1431
Stretch/yoga	General, Hatha	131	155	179	203	228	251	274	298
Swim	Lake, ocean, or river	315	372	430	487	546	602	658	716
Swim	Laps freestyle, slow/moderate	368	434	501	568	637	702	768	835
Swim	Laps freestyle, fast	525	621	716	812	910	1003	1097	1193
Swim	Backstroke	368	434	501	568	637	702	768	835
Swim	Sidestroke	420	496	573	649	728	802	878	954
Swim	Breaststroke	525	621	716	812	910	1003	1097	1193
Swim	Butterfly	578	683	788	893	1001	1103	1207	1312
Tennis	Doubles	315	372	430	487	546	602	658	716
Tennis	Singles	420	496	573	649	728	802	878	954
Treadmill, run	6 mph, 10 min/mile, 0% incline	525	621	716	812	910	1003	1097	1193
Treadmill, run	6 mph, 10 min/mile, 2% incline	578	683	788	893	1001	1103	1207	1312
Treadmill, run	6 mph, 10 min/mile, 4% incline	620	732	845	958	1074	1183	1295	1408
Treadmill, run	6 mph, 10 min/mile, 6% incline	667	788	909	1031	1156	1273	1394	1515
Treadmill, run	7 mph, 8.5 min/mile, 0% incline	604	714	824	933	1047	1153	1262	1372
Treadmill, run	7 mph, 8.5 min/mile, 2% incline	667	788	909	1031	1156	1273	1394	1515

Continued

APPENDIX 28 Physical Activity and Calories Expended per Hour—cont'd

Activity	Type	Body Weight							
		(110 lb)	**(130 lb)**	**(150 lb)**	**(170 lb)**	**(190 lb)**	**(210 lb)**	**(230 lb)**	**(250 lb)**
Treadmill, run	7 mph, 8.5 min/mile, 4% incline	719	850	981	1112	1247	1374	1503	1634
Treadmill, run	7 mph, 8.5 min/mile, 6% incline	767	906	1046	1185	1329	1464	1602	1741
Treadmill, run	8 mph, 7.5 min/mile, 0% incline	709	838	967	1096	1229	1354	1481	1610
Treadmill, run	8 mph, 7.5 min/mile, 2% incline	756	894	1031	1169	1311	1444	1580	1718
Treadmill, run	8 mph, 7.5 min/mile, 4% incline	814	962	1110	1258	1411	1554	1701	1849
Treadmill, run	8 mph, 7.5 min/mile, 6% incline	872	1030	1189	1347	1511	1665	1821	1980
Treadmill, run	3 mph, 20 min/mile, 0% incline	173	205	236	268	300	331	362	394
Treadmill, run	3 mph, 20 min/mile, 2% incline	194	230	265	300	337	371	406	441
Treadmill, run	3 mph, 20 min/mile, 4% incline	215	254	293	333	373	411	450	489
Treadmill, run	3 mph, 20 min/mile, 6% incline	236	279	322	365	410	451	494	537
Treadmill, run	4 mph, 15 min/mile, 0% incline	263	310	358	406	455	501	549	596
Treadmill, run	4 mph, 15 min/mile, 2% incline	294	348	401	455	510	562	614	668
Treadmill, run	4 mph, 15 min/mile, 4% incline	326	385	444	503	564	622	680	740
Treadmill, run	4 mph, 15 min/mile, 6% incline	352	416	480	544	610	672	735	799
Tread water	Moderate	210	248	286	325	364	401	439	477
Tread water	Vigorous	525	621	716	812	910	1003	1097	1193
Volleyball	Noncompetitive	158	133	215	243	273	301	329	358
Volleyball	Competitive	420	496	573	649	728	802	878	954
Walk	<2 mph	105	124	143	162	182	201	219	239
Walk	2 mph, 30 min/mile	131	155	179	203	228	251	274	298
Walk	2.5 mph, 24 min/mile	158	133	215	243	273	301	329	358
Walk	3 mph, 20 min/mile	173	205	236	268	300	331	362	394
Walk	3.5 mph, 17 min/mile	200	236	272	308	346	381	417	453
Walk	4 mph, 15 min/mile	263	310	358	406	455	501	549	596
Walk	4.5 mph, 13 min/mile	331	391	451	511	574	632	691	751
Walk	Race walking	341	403	465	528	592	652	713	775
Water polo	General	525	621	716	812	910	1003	1097	1193
Weight training	Free, nautilus, light/moderate	158	133	215	243	273	301	329	358
Weight training	Free, nautilus, vigorous	315	372	430	487	546	602	658	716
Wind surf	Casual	158	133	215	243	273	301	329	358

APPENDIX 29 Nutrition-Focused Physical Assessment

System	Normal Findings	Abnormal Findings	Possible Nutrition/Metabolic Associations	Nonnutritional Examples
General survey	Weight for height appropriate, well-nourished, alert, and cooperative	Loss of weight, muscle mass and fat stores, growth retardation	Protein-calorie deficiency	Endocrine disorders, osteogenic disorders, menopausal disorders secondary to estrogen depletion
Skin	Pink, soft, moist turgor with instant recoil, smooth appearance	Excess fat stores	Excess calorie intake	Diabetes, steroids
		Fatigue, anemia	Iron deficiency	
		Poor wound healing, ulcers	Protein, vitamin C, or zinc deficiency	Environmental or hygiene factors
		Dry with fine lines and shedding, scaly (xerosis)	Essential fat or vitamin A deficiency	
		Spinelike plaques around hair follicles on buttocks, thighs, or knees (follicular hyperkeratosis)	Vitamin A or essential fat deficiency	
		Pellagrous dermatitis (hyperpigmentation of skin exposed to sunlight)	Niacin or tryptophan deficiency	Thermal, sun, or chemical burns; Addison's disease
		Pallor	Iron or folic acid deficiency	Skin pigmentation disorders, hemorrhage
		Yellow pigmentation	Carotene excess	Jaundice
		Poor skin turgor	Fluid loss	
		Petechiae, ecchymoses	Vitamin K or C deficiency	Aspirin overdose, liver disease, or trauma
Nails	Smooth, translucent, slightly curved nail surface and firmly attached to nail bed; nail beds with brisk capillary refill	Spoon-shaped (koilonychia)	Iron deficiency	Chronic obstructive pulmonary disease (COPD), heart disease, aortic stenosis
		Dull, lackluster	Protein or iron deficiency	Chemical effects
		Pale, mottled	Vitamin A or C deficiency	Infection, chemical effects
Scalp	Pink, no lesions, tenderness; fontanels without softening, bulging	Softening or craniotabes	Vitamin D deficiency	
		Open anterior fontanel (usually closes by ≈18 months of age)	Vitamin D deficiency	Hydrocephalus
Hair	Natural shine, consistency in color and quantity, fine-to-coarse texture	Lack of shine and luster, thin, sparse	Protein, zinc, or linoleic acid deficiency	Hypothyroidism, chemotherapy, psoriasis, color treatment
		Easily pluckable	Protein deficiency	Hypothyroidism, chemotherapy, psoriasis, color treatment
		Alternating bands of light and dark hair in young children (flag sign)	Protein deficiency	Chemically processed or bleached hair
Face	Skin warm, smooth, dry, soft, moist with instant recoil	Diffuse depigmentation, swollen	Protein deficiency	Steroids and other medications
		Pallor	Iron, folate, or B$_{12}$ deficiency	Low-perfusion, low-volume states
		Moon face	Protein, calorie	Cushing's disease
		Bilateral temporal wasting	Protein, calorie	Neuromuscular disorders

From Hammond K: Physical assessment: a nutritional perspective, *Nurs Clin North Am* 32(4):779, 1997.

NOTE: This chart is not intended to be a comprehensive list for all nutritional or metabolic deficiencies or nonnutrition examples.

Continued

APPENDIX 29 Nutrition-Focused Physical Assessment —cont'd

System	Normal Findings	Abnormal Findings	Possible Nutrition/Metabolic Associations	Nonnutritional Examples
Eyes	Evenly distributed brows, lids, lashes; conjunctiva pink without discharge sclerae, without spots; cornea clear; skin without cracks or lesions	Pale conjunctiva	Iron, folate, or B₁₂ deficiency	
		Night blindness	Vitamin A deficiency	
		Dry, grayish, yellow or white foamy spots on whites of eyes (Bitot's spots)	Vitamin A deficiency	Pterygium, Gaucher's disease
		Dull, milky, or opaque cornea (corneal xerosis)	Vitamin A deficiency	
		Dull, dry, rough appearance to whites of eyes and inner lids (conjunctival xerosis)	Vitamin A deficiency	Chemical, environmental
		Softening of cornea (keratomalacia)	Vitamin A deficiency	
		Cracked and reddened corners of eyes (angular palpebritis)	Riboflavin, niacin deficiency	Infection, foreign objects
Nose	Uniform shape, septum slightly to left of midline, nares patent bilaterally, mucosa pink and moist, able to identify smells	Scaly, greasy, with gray or yellowish material around nares (nasolabial seborrhea)	Riboflavin, niacin, pyridoxine deficiency	
		Inflammation, redness of sinus tract, discharge, obstruction or polyps	Irritation of skin membranes	Need to reconsider if placing feeding tube; evaluate for nonfood allergies
Oral Cavity				
Lips/mouth	Pink, symmetric, smooth intact	Bilateral cracks, redness of lips (angular stomatitis)	Riboflavin, niacin, pyridoxine deficiency	Poor-fitting dentures, herpes, syphilis
		Vertical cracks of lips (cheilosis)	Riboflavin, niacin deficiency	Acquired immune deficiency syndrome (Kaposi's sarcoma), environmental exposure
Tongue	Pink, moist, midline, symmetric with rough texture	Magenta	Riboflavin deficiency	
		Smooth, slick, loss of papillae (atrophic filiform papillae)	Folate, niacin, riboflavin, iron, or B₁₂ deficiency	
		Beefy red color, atrophied taste buds, mucosa red and swollen	Niacin, folate, riboflavin, iron, B₁₂ or pyridoxine deficiency	Crohn's disease, infection
		Decreased taste (hypogeusia)	Zinc deficiency	Cancer therapy
Gums	Pink, moist without sponginess	Spongy, bleeding, receding	Vitamin C deficiency	Dilantin and other medication, poor hygiene, lymphoma, polycythemia, thrombocytopenia
Teeth	Repaired, no loose teeth; color may be various shades of white	Missing, poor repair, caries, loose	Excess sugar	Trauma, syphilis, aging, poor dental hygiene
		White or brownish patches (mottled)	Excess flouride	Enamel hypoplasia, erosion
Cranial nerves	Intact	Abnormal	Influences feeding route	
Gag reflex	Intact	Absent	Affects route of feeding	
Jaw	Proper alignment, movement from side to side	Improper alignment and movement	May influence intake by ability to chew properly	
Parotid gland	Located anterior to earlobe, no enlargement	Bilateral enlargement	Protein deficiency	Bulimia, cysts, tumors, hyperparathyroidism
Neck nodules	Trachea midline, freely movable without enlargement or nodules	Enlarged thyroid	Iodine deficiency	Cancer, allergy, cold infection

Cardiopulmonary

	Normal findings	Abnormal findings	Possible deficiency/cause	Possible other cause
Chest/lungs	Anterior and posterior thorax; adequate muscle and fat stores, respirations even and unlabored, symmetric rise and fall of chest during inspiration and expiration, lung sounds clear	Somatic muscle- and fat-wasting; labored respirations; breath sounds such as crackles, rhonchi, and wheezing; evaluate for fluid status vs. tenacious secretions that may labor breathing and increase energy expenditure; also consider increased rate and depth, decreased rate and depth	Protein-calorie deficiency / Metabolic acidosis / Metabolic alkalosis	Respiratory disease (e.g., copd)
Heart	Rhythm regular and rate within normal range; S_1 and S_2 heart sounds	Irregular rhythm	Potassium deficiency or excess / calcium deficiency / Magnesium deficiency or excess / phosphorus deficiency	Cardiopulmonary disease states
		Pounding pulse / Small, weak pulse / Palpitations / Tachycardia / Enlarged heart	Fluid overload (hypervolemia) / Fluid deficiency (hypovolemia) / Hypoglycemia / Thiamin deficiency / Thiamin deficiency associated with anemia and beriberi	Cardiopulmonary disease
Vascular access devices intact	No swelling, redness, drainage	Purulent drainage, swelling, excessive redness	Influences nutrition if device has to be removed	
Abdomen	Soft, nondistended, symmetric, bilateral without masses, umbilicus in midline, no ascites, bowel sounds present and normoactive; tympanic on percussion; feeding device intact without redness, swelling	Generalized symmetric distention	Obesity	Enlarged organs, fluid, or gas
		Protruding, everted umbilicus; tight glistening appearance (ascites) / Scaphoid appearance / Increased bowel sounds	Influences protein, fluid, sodium concerns of feeding / Protein-calorie deficiency / Influences nutrition in gastroenteritis (normal if hunger pains)	
		High-pitched tinkling	Influences nutrition if intestinal fluid and air present, indicating early obstruction	
		Decreased bowel sounds	Influences nutrition if peritonitis or paralytic ileus present	
Kidney, ureter, bladder	Urine golden yellow (ranges from pale yellow to deep gold), clear without cloudiness, adequate output	Decreased output, extremely dark, concentrated	Dehydration	

Continued

APPENDIX 29 Nutrition-Focused Physical Assessment—cont'd

System	Normal Findings	Abnormal Findings	Possible Nutrition/Metabolic Associations	Nonnutritional Examples
Musculoskeletal	Full range of motion without joint swelling or pain, adequate muscle strength	Inability to flex, extend, and rotate neck adequately	Influences nutrition by interfering with ability to feed or make hand-to-mouth contact	
		Decreased range of motion, swelling, impaired joint mobility of upper extremities; muscle wasting on arms, legs; skin folding on buttocks	Protein-calorie deficiency	
		Swollen, painful joints	Vitamin C deficiency	Connective tissue disease
		Enlargement of epiphyses at wrist, ankle, or knees	Vitamins D or C deficiency	Trauma, deformity, or congenital cause
		Bowed legs	Vitamin D deficiency, calcium deficiency	Renal rickets, malabsorption
		Beading of ribs	Vitamin D deficiency, calcium deficiency	
		Pain in calves, thighs	Thiamin deficiency	Deep vein thrombosis, other neuropathy
Neurologic	Alert, oriented, hand-to-mouth coordination; no weakness or tremors	Decreased or absent mental alertness; inadequate or absent hand-to-mouth coordination	Influences nutrition by the ability to feed or make hand-to-mouth contact	
	Cranial nerves intact: primary nutritionally focused ones include trigeminal, facial, glossopharyngeal, vagus, and hypoglossal	Psychomotor changes, confusion, peripheral neuropathy	Protein deficiency; thiamin, pyridoxine, vitamin B_{12} deficiency	Trauma, neurologic disease
	Reflexes (biceps, brachioradialis patella, and Achilles common in examination), functioning within normal range of 2^{++}	Tetany	Calcium, magnesium deficiency	
	Hypoactive reflexes	Hyperactive reflexes	Hypocalcemia	Tetany, upper motor neuron disease
		Hypokalemia	Associated with metabolic diseases such as diabetes mellitus and hypothyroidism	
		Hypoactive achilles, patellar reflex	Thiamin, vitamin B_{12}	Neurologic disorder

APPENDIX 30 Laboratory Values for Nutritional Assessment and Monitoring

I. Principles of Nutritional Laboratory Testing

A. Purpose

Laboratory-based nutritional testing, used to estimate nutrient availability in biologic fluids and tissues, is critical for assessment of both clinical and subclinical nutrient deficiencies. Laboratory data are the only objective data used in nutrition assessment that are "controlled"—that is, the validity of the method of its measurement is checked each time a specimen is assayed by also assaying a sample with a known value. The known sample is called a control, and if the value obtained for the sample is outside the range of normal analytic variability, both the specimen and control are measured again.

The nutrition professional can use laboratory data to support subjective data and clinical assessment findings. Furthermore, because numeric values do not themselves connote personal judgment, this kind of data can often be passed on to a patient or client without implicit or perceived blame.

B. Specimen Types

Ideally the specimen to be tested reflects the total body content of the nutrient to be assessed. However, often the best specimen is not readily available. The most common specimens for analysis are the following:

Whole blood—Must be collected with an anticoagulant if entire content of the blood is to be evaluated. The two common anticoagulants for whole blood analyses are ethylenediaminetetraacetic acid (EDTA), a calcium chelator used in hematologic analyses, and heparin (maintains the blood in its most natural state).*

Blood cells—Separated from anticoagulated whole blood for measurement of cellular analyte content.

Plasma—The uncoagulated fluid that bathes the formed elements (blood cells).

Serum—The fluid that remains after whole blood or plasma has coagulated. Coagulation proteins and related substances are missing or significantly reduced.

Urine—Contains a concentrate of excreted metabolites.

Feces—Important in nutritional analyses when nutrients are not absorbed and therefore are present in fecal material.

Hair—An easy-to-collect tissue; usually a poor indicator of actual body levels.

Other tissues—Buccal cells and solid organ biopsy specimens are rarely used in nutrition laboratory assessment.

C. Interpretation of Laboratory Data

As with all data, nutrition data may be quantitative (e.g., how much, how often, how fast), semiquantitative (e.g., many, most, few, a lot, usually, majority, several), or qualitative (e.g., color, shape, species). The advantage of quantitative data is that they are less ambiguous or more objective than other types of observations. Although objective laboratory data are extremely important resources in nutrition assessment, one should be extremely cautious about using a single isolated laboratory test value to make an assessment. One value is often misleading, especially when taken out of the context of an individual's habits, clinical status, and dietary and medical histories. The best data are obtained from analysis of changes in laboratory values.

When monitoring patients for changes in nutrition test values, one must consider how much change is necessary to give confidence that a difference is significant. The change required for statistical significance has been called the *critical difference*. It is calculated from measurement of the variances calculated from repeated measurements of an analyte: (1) specimens that have been obtained, at several different times, from each of several healthy persons (intrasubject variation); and (2) separate samples from a large specimen pool (analytic variation).

The critical differences for some plasma proteins of nutritional significance are the following:†

Protein	Critical Difference
Albumin	8%
Prealbumin/transthyrectin	32%

The statistical probability that two consecutive albumin measurements are statistically different requires that the concentration change by 8% or more. Therefore an albumin increase, for example, from 30 g/L to 32.4 g/L indicates that a statistically significant change has occurred. For prealbumin, an increase from 30 mg/dl to 39.6 mg/dl would be significant. There are two reasons for the large discrepancy in the critical differences for these three proteins. The major reason is that the albumin level is very stable in healthy persons, whereas prealbumin concentrations vary considerably. Also contributing to these differences is the fact that the currently available methods measure albumin more precisely than prealbumin.

In practice, assessments are not based on the measurement of a single analyte at one point in time. Changes in laboratory tests may have biologic significance (e.g., patient's condition is improving) long before statistical significance is achieved. The changes in laboratory data may precede changes in other nutritional indices, but generally, although not always, the data available should point to the same conclusion.

Appendix updated by Mary Demarest Litchford, PhD, RD, LDN, from original by Timothy Carlson, PhD, RD.

*Samples obtained for blood coagulation tests are diluted with solutions containing sodium citrate (a calcium chelator). Because of the dilutional effect of the anticoagulant solutions, citrated samples are not suitable for measurement of the concentrations of analytes.

†Clark GH, Fraser CG: Biological variation of acute phase proteins, *Ann Clin Biochem* 30:373, 1993.

‡Monsen ER: The *Journal* adopts SI units for clinical laboratory values, *J Am Diet Assoc* 37:356, 1987.

Continued

D. Reference Ranges

To determine whether a particular laboratory value is abnormal, particularly when serial data are not available, the value is generally compared to a reference range. The reference range is constructed from a large number of test values (20 to >1000). The average value and the standard deviation for these data are determined, and the reference range is calculated from the mean ± 2 standard deviations.

If the sample group is representative of the reference population, the reference range will include values that reflect those found in approximately 95% of the reference population. About 2.5% of this normal population will have values greater than the upper end of the reference range, and 2.5% will have values less than the lower end. This means that one normal individual in 20 would have a value below or above the reference range.

Reference ranges can be made for different populations. For example, reference ranges based on gender, age, race, and so forth, can be developed. In practice, the differences between populations are often ignored because the importance of small differences in a nutrient analyte is not usually significant. However, in the event of borderline values, the possible influence differences between the population of which the patient is a member and the reference population may need to be taken into account. Reference ranges often are determined by obtaining blood from personnel working in or near the clinical laboratory. This population is often skewed toward younger persons, has few minorities, and is overrepresented by women.

E. Units

Many types of units are used in reporting nutrient-dependent laboratory values. Two basic systems of units are in common use: the conventional system and the Système Internationale d'Unités (SI) system.‡ The conventional system sometimes lacks convention; thus different laboratories adopt different units to report the same analyte. For example, the conventional report of an ionized calcium value could be 2.3 mEq/L, 46 mg/L or 4.6 mg/dl. However, in the SI system only 1.15 mmol/L is allowed.

F. Nature of Nutritional Testing and Types of Tests

Typically laboratory tests are static assays (i.e., the concentration of an analyte is measured in a biologic fluid [e.g., a fasting blood specimen] at a point in time). Assessment of nutrient status made by this approach is often inaccurate or distorted as explained in Chapter 15.

Some nutrients can be assessed by tests that are based on measurements that reflect the endogenous availability of a nutrient to a measurable biologic function (e.g., biochemical, tissue, or organ). Most often, functional assessment of nutrient status may be done by measurement of a biochemical marker (i.e., a normal or abnormal metabolite) of function. The results of this type of testing can be reliably considered to reflect the adequacy of a nutrient pool (see Chapter 15).

APPENDIX 30 Laboratory Values for Nutritional Assessment and Monitoring—cont'd

II. A. Tests of Protein-Energy Status

Test	Principle and Requirements	Interpretation	Reference Range	Limitations
Urea urinary N (UUN)	The protein pool (visceral and somatic) N is catabolized to urea; urine urea represents ~80% of N catabolized; requires accurate estimate of protein intake; thus usually used only for total parenteral nutrition (TPN) or tube-feeding patients.	UUN is compared with the actual N intake. $$N \text{ balance} = \frac{\text{Protein (g)}}{6.25^*} - \text{UUN} + 4$$ *Factor = 5.95 for TPN; reflects severity of metabolic stress.	− = Catabolism 0 = Catabolism + = Anabolism (3-6 g/24 hr = optimal use range)	Urine collection must be quantitative (complete); UUN not appropriate in renal insufficiency; does not account for wound leakage, cell losses, or diarrhea; inaccurate in metabolically stressed patients.
Total urinary N (TUN)	Some N is excreted as nonurea N (e.g., ammonia and creatinine); 24-hour TUN reflects total protein catabolism, accounting for all sources of urinary N; as for UUN, requires accurate protein intake.	TUN is compared with the actual N intake; $$N \text{ balance} = \frac{\text{Protein (g)}}{6.25^*} - \text{TUN} + 2$$ *Factor = 5.95 for TPN; reflects severity of metabolic stress; TUN gives the most accurate estimation of total protein catabolism.	− = Catabolism 0 = Catabolism + = Anabolism (3-6 g/24 hr = optimal use range)	Urine collection must be quantitative (complete); TUN not appropriate in renal insufficiency; not done in many institutions; does not account for wound leakage, cell losses, or diarrhea.
Urea kinetics	Formulas used to estimate protein catabolic rate (PCR) from changes in blood urea nitrogen (BUN) concentration in patients with impaired renal function.	Urinary urea (residual renal urea clearance—KrU) and BUN levels (urea generation rate—GU) are used to determine PCR; 1- to 3-day diet intake compared with PCR.	In protein balance, PRC = protein intake	Urea lost in dialysis must be accounted for in calculating urea nitrogen appearance. Dietary protein intake hard to estimate.
Visceral Proteins				
Total protein (TP)	Protein concentration in serum is easily measured colorimetrically; largely reflects albumin (50%-60% of TP)	TP levels parallel clinical signs of malnutrition; plasma TP is 0.4 g/dl greater than serum TP.	6.4-8.3 g/dl (64-83 g/L)	Does not reflect status during inflammatory (acute-phase) response; conditions that affect individual protein affect TP. Not useful to assess protein status.
Albumin	Easily and quickly measured colometrically; large body pool (3-5 g/kg body weight); ~60% is outside the plasma in the extravascular pool); long half-life of 3 weeks.	Decreased levels can occur following short-term protein and energy deficiency; often associated with other deficiencies (i.e., zinc, iron, and vitamin A).	3.5-5 g/L) (35-50 g/L)	Significance confounded by acute stress reaction, liver disease, protein-losing enteropathy, nephrotic syndrome, pregnancy, oral contraceptive use, strenuous exercise, and hemodilution.
Transferrin	Iron transport protein, smaller extravascular pool than albumin; measured by immunoassay or calculated from total iron-binding capacity (TIBC) (see p. 1237); half-life ~ 9 days.	Levels increased during iron deficiency and decreased by protein-energy deficiency. Calculated values give inexact estimates of serum concentration.	F: 250-380 mg/dl (2.50-3.80 g/L) M: 215-365 mg/dl (2.15-3.65 g/L)	Significance confounded by acute stress reaction, liver disease, protein-losing enteropathy, nephrotic syndrome, pregnancy or estrogen administration, and hemodilution.

Continued

APPENDIX 30 Laboratory Values for Nutritional Assessment and Monitoring—cont'd

II. A. Tests of Protein-Energy Status—cont'd

Visceral Proteins—cont'd

Test	Principle and Requirements	Interpretation	Reference Range		Limitations
Prealbumin/transthyrectin	Transports thyroxin and acts as a carrier for retinol-binding protein; also called thyroxin-binding protein; half-life ≈2 days.	More sensitive protein-energy balance indicator than albumin or transferrin; responds rapidly to nutrition intervention; reportedly more sensitive to energy intake than to protein intake.	15-36 mg/dl		Very sensitive to stress response, also ↓ in liver disease, protein-losing enteropathy, nephrotic syndrome, hemodilution, and acute stress reaction.
Retinol-binding protein (RBP)	Transport retinol; because of low molecular weight, RBP is filtered by glomerulus and catabolized by the kidney tubule; half-life ≈0.5 days.	More sensitive protein-energy balance indicator than albumin or prealbumin; responds rapidly to nutritional intervention; reportedly more sensitive to protein intake than to energy intake.	2.6-7.6 mg/dl (1.43-2.86 μmol/L)		Very sensitive to stress response; also ↓ in liver disease, protein-losing enteropathy, nephrotic syndrome, vitamin A and zinc deficiencies, and hemodilution; ↑ in chronic renal disease.
Insulin-like growth factor-1 (IGF-1) (somatomedin C)	The peptide mediator of growth hormone activity produced by the liver; half-life of a few hours; much less sensitive to stress response than other proteins.	Low in chronic undernutrition; increases rapidly during nutrition support when albumin, transferrin, prealbumin, and RBP are not affected	F: 24-253 ng/ml M: 43-178 ng/ml		Reduced levels seen in hypopituitarism, hypothyroidism, and liver disease and with estrogen use.

Metabolic Indicators

Test	Principle and Requirements	Interpretation	Reference Range		Limitations
Urea/creatinine ratio	Urinary area/creatinine ratio (U:Cr) in fasting, first-void urine used to compare amino acid catabolism (BUN) with muscle mass (creatinine).	$$U:Cr = \frac{\text{Urine area (mg/dl)}}{\text{Urine creatinine (mg/dl)}}$$ Can be used in uncomplicated protein-energy deficiency to approximate status.	*Risk* Low Medium High	*Ratio* >12.0 6.0-12.0 <6.0	Affected by recent protein taken, therefore not useful for estimating long-term status; ratio not used for accurate assessment or monitoring.

II. B. Immunologic Tests

Test	Principle and Requirements	Interpretation	Reference Range	Limitations
Total lymphocyte count (TLC)	Calculated from the percentage of lymphocytes reported in the hemogram and the WBC count. Units = cells/μl or cells/mm³	Decreased in protein-energy malnutrition and immunocompromised state.	Normal: >2700 Moderate depletion: 900-1800 Severe depletion: <900	Decreased by viral infection, chemotherapy, radiation, and drugs (e.g., steroids, penicillin, sulfonamides, Lasix, phenylbutazone); increased by tissue necrosis and other types of infection.
Delayed cutaneous hypersensitivity	Anergy for antigens, such as mumps and *Candida*; occurs in malnutrition; antigens injected intradermally; redness (erythema) and hardness (induration) read 1, 2, or 3 days later.	Response affected by protein-energy status and vitamin A, iron, zinc, and vitamin B_6 deficiencies.	*Induration* 1+: <5 mm 2+: 6-10 mm 3+: 11-20 mm 4+: >20 mm Erythema Present or absent	Usefulness in acute care limited by drugs, effect of aging and disease (metabolic, malignant, and infectious diseases); difficult to administer and interpret results; semiquantitative.

II. C. Prognostic Indices

Test	Principle and Requirements	Interpretation	Reference Range	Limitations
Albumin	↓ Levels associated with increased incidence of medical or nutritional complications (morbidity), length of hospital stay, and mortality.	Levels <3.5 g/dl indicate need for further patient evaluation; <3 g/dl can be associated with edema; <2.5 g/dl implies extreme medical and nutritional risk.	See interpretation	Albumin responds slowly to treatment because of long t½; markedly decreased during the metabolic response to injury.

Continued

Test	Principle and Requirements	Interpretation	Reference Range	Limitations
Cholesterol	Low levels (<80 mg/dl) are associated with increased incidence of medical or nutritional complications and death.	Levels <150 indicate increased risk; concentration correlates with ↓ albumin, prealbumin, iron, zinc, and vitamins A and E.	See interpretation	Decreasing levels of total cholesterol may be more significant than absolute values.

III. Tests of Carbohydrate Absorption

Test	Principle and Requirements	Interpretation	Reference Range	Limitations
Lactose Intolerance				
Breath hydrogen	Lactose loading (2 g/kg) in lactase deficiency allows bacterial metabolism of lactose with production of H_2 gas. Breath analyzed for H_2 by gas chromatography.	Breath H_2 measured fasting and 0.5 and 2 hours after dosing with lactose; a significant increase is associated with malabsorption.	Normal increase: <50 parts/ million (i.e., <50 ppm)	Bacterial overgrowth can cause false-positive results; consumption of soluble fiber or legumes and smoking are associated with H_2 production; false-negative results caused by antibiotics.
Lactose tolerance test	Lactose loading (50 g) followed by blood sampling at 5, 10, 30, 60, 90, and 120 min after dose; glucose produced from lactose is assayed.	Lactase deficiency associated with <20 mg/dl increase in glucose.	Normal glucose increase ≥20 mg/dl	Test is not specific (many false positives) or sensitive (many false negatives).

IV. Tests of Lipid Status

Test	Principle and Requirements	Interpretation	Reference Range	Limitations
Fat Malabsorption				
Fecal fat screening	Microscopic inspection of fat-stained (Sudan stain) specimens for the presence of lipid droplets.	Trained observers are able to identify excessive fat in ~80% of persons with fat malabsorption.	Qualitative results	Patient must be consuming sufficient fat for analysis to reveal malabsorption. Semiquantitative.
Prothrombin time (PT)	Absorption of fat-soluble vitamins, including vitamin K, decrease in fat malabsorption; vitamin K impairs coagulation, causing an ↑ in PT	A prolonged PT is a relatively sensitive but nonspecific indicator of fat malabsorption.	10-15 sec	Oral anticoagulant and other drugs, ↓ plateler count, acquired and hereditary bleeding diseases, and liver disease ↑PT.
Serum carotene (total serum carotenoids)	Carotenoids, fat-soluble pigments in plant foods, are poorly absorbed in fat malabsorption; extracted by organic solvents for quantification.	A serum carotene level of less than 50 mg/dl is seen in ~85% of patients with fat malabsorption.	50-200 mcg/dl (0.74-3.72 µmol/L)	Decreased serum carotenoid levels are also seen in those with low vegetable/fruit diets (e.g., in TPN or tube feeding), liver failure, celiac disease, cystic fibrosis, human immunodeficiency virus, and some lipoprotein disorders.
Quantitative fecal fat determination	Patient must consume 100 g fat/ day (4 × 8 oz whole milk/day, and 2 Tbsp vegetable oil/meal) during and for 2 days before collection	Quantitative 72-hour stool collection required for accurate assessment; average daily discharge used for interpretation.	Normal: <5 g fat/24 hr Malabsorption: ≥10 g/24 hr	Failure to adhere to the diet invalidates the results.

APPENDIX 30 Laboratory Values for Nutritional Assessment and Monitoring—cont'd

IV. Tests of Lipid Status—cont'd

Test	Principle and Requirements	Interpretation	Reference Range	Limitations
Essential Fatty Acid Deficiency				
Fatty acid analysis	Levels of eicosapentaenoic acid (C20:3n9) and linoleic acid (C18:2n6) reflect essential fatty acid status; fatty acids in plasma or blood cell fractions assayed by gas chromatography.	Endogenous synthesis of C20:3n9 greatly increases during linoleic acid deficiency; plasma phospholipid C20:3n9/C18:2n6 ratio used to assess status.	C20:3n9/C18:2n6 ratio >0.2 confirms deficiency	Test available only from laboratories specializing in nutrition or lipid analyses.
Nonesterified Fatty Acids				
Serum-free fatty acids (FFAs or NEFA)	Measured by a simple colorimetric procedure.	↑ When medium-chain fatty acids are administered.	8-25 mg/dl (0.28-0.89 mmol/L)	Many conditions ↑ FFAs, including hyperthyroidism, alcoholism, diabetes, acute myocardial infarct; also ↑ in fasting and strenuous exercise.

V. Tests for Nutrition-Influenced Risk Factors for Atherosclerotic Diseases

Test	Principle and Requirements	Interpretation	Reference Range	Limitation
High-sensitivity C-reactive protein (hs-CRP)	CRP is an acute-phase protein used to assess inflammatory status; measured by a variety of immunoassay techniques.	When slightly increased, CRP has been shown to be associated with increased risk for coronary heart disease and other cardiovascular disease.	Low risk: <0.07 mg/dl Moderate risk: 0.07-0.38 mg/L High risk: >0.39 mg/L	Is not specific for risk of atherosclerotic disease; relatively minor injuries and other causes of inflammation also increase CRP levels.
Total serum or plasma cholesterol	Cholesterol is enzymatically released from cholesterol esters. Free cholesterol measured in automated enzyme assays.	Total cholesterol correlated with risk for cardiovascular diseases but not as good an indicator as high-density lipoprotein (HDL)-c and low-density lipoprotein (LDL)-c. See National Cholesterol Education Program (NCEP) guidelines.	Desirable: <200 mg/dl (<5.2 µmol/L) Borderline: 200-239 mg/dl (5.2-6.2 µmol/L) High risk: ≥240 mg/dl (≥6.2 µmol/L)	Cholesterol measurements have considerable within-subject variability. May partly result from variability in specimen collection or handling.
HDL cholesterol (HDL-c)	LDL-c (and VLDL-c) are precipitated from the serum before measurement of residual HDL-c; direct measurement of HDL-c is now done in some laboratories.	HDL-c is called "good cholesterol" to indicate that it is a negative risk factor.	Desirable: >40 mg/dl (>1 mmol/L) in men >50 mg/dl (>1.25 mmol/L) in women	Some precipitation methods cause underestimation of HDL. HDL can be divided into classes: HDL_1, HDL_2, and HDL_3; HDL_3 best correlates with risk of coronary heart disease (CHD).
LDL cholesterol (HDL-c)	LDL-c is estimated by the Friedewald formula, LDL-c = total cholesterol − HDL-c − TG/5, or by new direct assays.	LDL-c is called "bad cholesterol" to indicate that it is a positive risk factor. See NCEP guidelines.	Desirable: <100 mg/dl (<2.59 µmol/L) Borderline: 130-159 mg/dl (3.4-4.1 µmol/L) High risk: ≥160 mg/dl (≥4.1 µmol/L) F: 40-160 mg/dl (0.45-1.81 mmol/L) M: 35-135 mg/dl (0.40-1.55 mmol/L)	Calculation only valid when TG concentration is <400 mg/dl, so cannot be determined in nonfasting serum or plasma. Direct assay methods preferred.

Test	Principle and Requirements	Interpretation	Reference Range	Limitations
Triglycerides (TGs)	Lipases release glycerol and fatty acids from TGs; glycerol measured in automated enzyme assays.	The association of TGs and CHD has been shown.		Fasting specimen is essential; alcohol ingestion can increase; some anticoagulants affect.
Lipoprotein (a) (Lp[a]) LDL subclass pattern and size	Measured by a variety of immunoassay techniques. LDL particles of different sizes (densities) can be assessed by electrophoresis or other techniques.	Positive association exists between CHD risk and serum Lp(a). Pattern B (small, dense LDL) is associated with ↑ risk of CHD and is responsive to diet. Pattern A (larger, buoyant LDL) is not associated with risk.	F: 2.1-57.3 mg/dl M: 2.2-49.4 mg/dl	Results of different assay methods may not be comparable. Ultracentrifuge methods available in some laboratories.
Homocysteine (Hcy)	Total Hcy (oxidized + reduced forms) is measured by chromatography or by more rapid immunoassays that have recently become available.	Hcy level is an independent risk factor for CHD, venous thrombotic disease, and other diseases; folic acid and vitamins B_{12} and B_6 reduce plasma Hcy levels.	4-14 μmol/L	↑ Hcy and ↑ LDL cholesterol risk is increased even at slightly elevated levels.

VI. Tests of Micronutrient Status

Test	Principle and Requirements	Interpretation	Reference Range	Limitations
A. Vitamins				
Thiamin (B_1)[1]	Thiamin status is usually assessed by measuring the amount of thiamin pyrophosphate (TPP) needed to fully activate the red blood cell (RBC) enzyme transketolase.	The TPP needed to fully activate transketolase is inversely related to B_1 status; percent stimulation by TTP.	% Stimulation >20% (index >1.2) indicates deficiency	Amount (and activity) of enzyme affected by drugs, iron, folate, or vitamin B_{12} status, malignant or gastrointestinal diseases, and diabetes.
Riboflavin (B_2)	Riboflavin status is assessed by measuring the amount of flavin adenine dinucleotide (FAD) needed to fully activate RBC enzyme glutathione reductase (GR)	The FAD needed to fully activate GR is inversely related to B_2 status; percent stimulation.	% Stimulation >40% (index >1.4) indicates deficiency	Amount and/or activity of enzyme may change with age, iron status, liver disease, and glucose-6-phosphate dehydrogenase deficiency.
Niacin (B_3)[2] Pyridoxal phosphate (PLP) compounds (B_6)[3]	1. RBC enzymes, ALT (GPT) or AST (GOT), are assayed for the presence of PLP as the enzymes' cofactor.[4] 2. Plasma PLP can be directly measured by chromatography. 3. Tryptophan (Trp) load test, measures excretion of the PLP-dependent metabolite xanthurenic acid (XA).	1. Difference between enzyme activities before and after addition of PLP is inversely related to B_6 status. 2. PLP is major transport form of B_6; therefore serum levels reflect body stores. 3. In this functional test the levels of urinary XA should ↑ significantly when 2-5 g of Trp is ingested.	1. % ALT stimulation of >25% or AST activity of >50% in deficiency 2. Normal: 0.50-3.0 mcg/dl (20-120 nmol/L) 3. Marginal status: >50 mg/24 hr	1. Disease and drugs that affect the liver and heart and pregnancy confound interpretation. 2. Deficiency may be seen clinically before plasma PLP levels ↓. 3. Steroid drugs and estrogen ↑ enzyme activity; some drugs cause analytic errors.

[1] Red blood cells are separated from plasma by centrifugation and washed with saline; after hemolyzing the cells, the intracellular material is analyzed for vitamin availability.

[2] No biochemical tests have been developed to assess B_3 status; the fraction of whole blood niacin as NAD is a potentially useful test (see Powers HJ: Current knowledge concerning optimum nutritional status of riboflavin, niacin, and pyridoxine, *Proc Nutr Soc* 58:435, 1999).

[3] Several tests in addition to the ones described here have been used to assess B_6 status—for example, urinary B_6/creatinine ratios, urinary 4-pyridoxic acid excretion, and the kynurenine load test are tests for B_6, but these are not usually available for clinical use.

[4] Alanine aminotransferase (ALT) and glutamic-pyruvate transaminase (GPT) are the same enzyme; aspartate aminotransferase (AST) and glutamic-oxalacetic transaminase (GOT) are the same enzyme.

Continued

APPENDIX 30 Laboratory Values for Nutritional Assessment and Monitoring—cont'd

VI. Tests of Micronutrient Status—cont'd

Test	Principle and Requirements	Interpretation	Reference Range	Limitations
A. Vitamins—cont'd				
Folate[5]	1. Because of ↓ DNA synthesis, large RBCs are produced.	1. Deficiency leads to increase in mean cell volume (MCV)	1. Normal: MCV <100	1. Not sensitive or specific for folate.
	2. Shape of neutrophil nucleus affected by folate deficiency.	2. ↑Neutrophil lobe count seen in folate deficiency.	2. Normal: ≤4 lobes per neutrophil	2. Lobe count sensitive but not specific.
	3. Folate levels can be directly measured by radioimmunoassay.	3. Both RBC and serum folate are indicators of body stores.	3. 2-10 mcg/L serum; 140-960 ng/L RBC (3.2-22 nmol/L)	3. Plasma from nonfasted subjects may reflect recent intake; RBC folate is not measured accurately.
	4. Functional folate status assayed by formimino-glutamic acid (FIGLU) in 24-hour urine or after oral histidine loading.	4. After 2-15 g loading dose, 10-50 mg of FIGLU should be excreted in 8 hours.	4. Normal: <7.4 mg/24 hr (<42.6 μmol/24 hr) without loading	4. FIGLU affected by vitamin B$_{12}$, drugs, liver disease, cancer, tuberculosis, and pregnancy.
Cobalamin (B$_{12}$)	1. Because of ↓ DNA synthesis, large RBCs are produced.	1. Deficiency leads to increase in MCV (mean cell volume)	1. Normal: MCV <100	1. Not sensitive or specific for B$_{12}$.
	2. Shape of neutrophil nucleus is affected by B$_{12}$ deficiency.	2. ↑Neutrophil lobe count in B$_{12}$ deficiency.	2. Normal: ≤4 lobes per neutrophil	2. Lobe count sensitive but not specific.
	3. B$_{12}$ can be directly measured by radioimmunoassay.	3. Levels <150 ng/L indicate deficiency (age affects level).	3. 160-950 pg/ml (118-701 pmol/L)	3. Marginal deficiency not collated with level.
	4. Methylmalonic acid excretion reflects B$_{12}$ available for branched-chain amino acid (BCAA) metabolism.	4. Methylmalonic acid excretion >300 mg/24 hr in B$_{12}$ deficiency.	4. Normal excretion: ≤5 mg/24 hr (≤42 μmol/24 hr) Serum mmA 17-76 ng/ml (0.08-0.56 μmol/L)	4. Specific for B$_{12}$ but requires normal BCAA levels; done only in specialized laboratories.
	5. Schilling test for intrinsic factor and B$_{12}$ absorption assesses radiolabeled B$_{12}$ absorption as reflected by urinary excretion.	5. Abnormal B$_{12}$ absorption indicated by excretion <3% of B$_{12}$ radioactivity per 24 hours.	5. Normal excretion: ~8% of radioactivity per 24 hours	5. Test must be repeated with oral administration of intrinsic factor (IF) to differentiate IF deficiency and malabsorption.
Ascorbic acid (C)	Plasma or leukocyte C measured by (1) chromatography; (2) by ascorbate oxidase; (3) spectrophotometrically by reaction with 2,4-dinitrophenylhydrazine.	Leukocyte C is less affected by recent intake, but well-fasted plasma levels parallel leukocyte levels; plasma preferred for acutely ill patients because leukocyte level is affected by infection, some drugs, and hyperglycemia; <0.2 mg/dl (<10 mcg/10^8 WBC)	Plasma: 0.5-1.4 mg/dl (30-80 μmol/L) Leukocyte deficiency: 20-50 mcg/10^8 white blood cells (WBCs) (1.1-3 fmol/cell)	Blood samples must be carefully prepared for assay to prevent C breakdown. Oxalate, glucose, and proteins interfere with some assays; recent intake can mask deficiency.

Retinols (A)	Serum retinol and retinol esters extracted by organic solvents and measured by chromatography; functional tests (e.g., dark adaptation) only detect severe deficiency.	Retinol levels <100 g/L indicate severe deficiency; retinol ester >5% of total retinols indicates hypervitaminosis A.	30-80 mcg/dl (1-2.8 μmol/L)	Exposure of serum to bright light or oxygen destroys vitamin A; low RBP level associated with low vitamin A (see protein-energy section).
Tocopherols (E)	Serum tocopherols measured by chromatography; α- and β-tocopherols serve different antioxidant functions.	Lower values found in infants; level associated with deficiency not determined.	0.5-1.8 mg/dl (12-42 μmol/L)	Plasma level dependent on recent intake and level of lipids, especially TGs, in blood.
Cholecalciferol (D_3) calcidiol calcitriol Calciferol (D_2) ercalcidiol/ ercalcitriol	1. Alkaline phosphatase activity reflects level of bone activity and indirectly D status.	1. Serum levels >190 units/L D deficiency; 30% is the form from bone.	1. Adult: 25-100 U/L 1-12 yr <350 U/L	1. Not specific, but a sensitive indicator; serum Ca and PO_4 should also be ↑.
	2. Calcidiol and ercalcidiol (25-OH-D) are assayed together by chromatography or radioimmunoassay.	2. <3 ng/ml (7.4 nmol/L) indicates deficiency; >200 ng/ml (500 nmol/L) indicates hypervitaminosis D.	2. 15-80 mcg/L summer (37-200 nmol/L) 14-42 mcg/L winter (35-105 nmol/L)	2. Best indicator of status (liver stores), but hard to interpret.
	3. Calcitriol [1,25-(OH)2-D_3] is assayed by chromatographic or immunoassay procedures.	3. Used to show that vitamin D metabolism is occurring normally.	3. 2.5-4.5 ng/dl (60-108 pmol/L) (little seasonal change)	3. Poor indicator of status because of tight control of synthesis independent of body stores.
25-hydroxyvitamin D (25OHD)	Vitamin D malabsorption can lead to secondary malabsorption of calcium.	Vitamin D insufficiency is defined as the lowest threshold value for plasma 25OHD that prevents secondary hyperparathyroidism, ↑ bone turnover, bone mineral loss, or seasonal variations in plasma PTH.	>35 ng/ml	Not available in all laboratories.
Phylloquinone (K_1) and menadione (K_2)	Normal coagulation factor synthesis requires K; prothrombin (PT) assesses coagulation status.	In K deficiency, PT increases with increasing production of abnormal coagulation factors.[6]	10.4-12.8 slc (varies significantly with method)	The level of vitamin K available for vitamin K–dependent bone proteins may not be reflected by the PT.

[5]Microbiologic growth assays, the deoxyuridine suppression test, and recently developed research tests for folate and vitamin B_{12} are not generally offered in the contemporary clinical laboratory.

[6]More sensitive procedures for measurement of vitamin K include serum chromatography and determination of the serum level of vitamin K–dependent bone protein called osteocalcin. Deficiency significantly increases the amount of abnormal forms of this protein. These tests are not yet widely available.

Continued

APPENDIX 30 Laboratory Values for Nutritional Assessment and Monitoring—cont'd

VI. Tests of Micronutrient Status—cont'd

Test	Principle and Requirements	Interpretation	Reference Range	Limitations
B. Minerals				
Electrolytes Sodium (Na+)[7,8] Potassium (K+) Chloride (Cl−) Bicarbonate or total CO_2	Serum electrolytes, including bicarbonate, are usually measured together by ion-specific electrodes in autoanalyzers; sometimes Na and K are measured by flame emission spectrophotometry.	↑ Serum Na seen in water loss; ↓ Na occurs in many conditions. ↓ Serum K seen in renal diseases and ↓ Na; ↓ K usually indicates ↓ intake or ↑ cellular uptake. Chloride levels change with cation and osmotic changes in the body. Bicarbonate levels reflect acid-base balance.	135-145 mEq/L (135-145 mmol/L) 3.5-5 mEq/L (3.5-5 mmol/L) 100-110 mEq/L (100-110 mmol/L) 21-30 mEq/L (21-30 mmol/L)	Electrolytes change rapidly in response to changes in physiology (e.g., hormonal stimulus, renal and other organ dysfunction, acid-base balance changes, and drug action); serum electrolytes are minimally affected by diet.
Major minerals Calcium (Ca^{2+})	1. Total serum Ca^{2+} measured as chromogenic or fluorescent complexes or by atomic absorption. 2. Ionized (free) Ca^{2+} measured by ion-specific electrodes.	Usually slightly more than half of the serum Ca^{2+} is bound to albumin or complexed with other molecules; the remaining Ca^{2+} is called ionized Ca (ICA); ICA is available physiologically.	1. 8.6-10 mg/dl (2.15-2.5 mmol/L) 2. 4.64-5.28 mg/dl (1.16-1.32 mmol/L)	Calcium status is related to many factors, including vitamin D, phosphate, parathyroid function and malignancy, and renal function.
Phosphate (H_2PO_4, PO_4^{2-}, and PO_4^{3-}) (Phosphorus)	Usually measured spectrophotometrically after reaction with ammonium phosphomolybdate.	Abnormal P level is most closely associated with disturbed intake, distribution, or renal function.	2.7-4.5 mg/dl (0.87-1.45 mmol/L) (higher in children)	Reported as phosphorus (P), not phosphate; hemolyzed blood cannot be used because of high RBC phosphate levels.
Magnesium (Mg^{2+})	1. Total serum Mg^{2+} measured after reaction to form chromogenic or fluorescent complexes or by atomic absorption. 2. Ionized (free) Mg^{2+} measured by ion-specific electrodes.	Neuromuscular function (hyperirritability, tetany, convulsion, and electrocardiographic changes) affected when levels of total serum $Mg2+$ fall to <1 mEq/L.	1. 1.3-2.5 mEq/L (0.65-1.25 mmol/L) 2. 0.7-1.2 mEq/L (0.35-0.60 mmol/L)	Usually about 45% of the serum Mg^{2+} is complexed with other molecules; the remaining Mg^{2+} is called ionized magnesium; serum levels remain constant until body stores are nearly depleted.
Trace minerals Iron Complete blood count[9] (CBC) and RBC indices	1. Hematocrit (HCT) = % RBC in whole blood 2. Hemoglobin (Hb) = blood hemoglobin concentration 3. Mean corpuscular volume (MCV) = mean red blood cell volume	A CBC with RBC indices is one of the first set of tests that a patient receives; although CBC data are not specific for nutrition status, their universal and repeated presence in the patient's record make them very important.	1. F: 35-47% (0.35-0.47)[10] M: 42-52% (0.42-0.52) 2. F: 12-15g/dl (7.45-9.31 mmol/L) M: 14-17g/dl (8.44-10.6 mmol/L) 3. 82-99 μm³ (82-99 fL)	These tests are affected only when iron stores are essentially depleted; and HCT and Hb are sensitive to hydration status; low MCV also occurs in thalassemias and lead poisoning.

Substance	Method	Clinical significance	Reference values	Comments
Serum iron (Fe)	Serum Fe^{3+} reduced to Fe^{2+} and then complexed with chromogen.	Slightly higher in males than in premenopausal females; reflects recent Fe intake.	F: 40-150 mcg/dll (7.2-26.9 μmol/L) M: 50-160 mg/dll (8.9-28.7 mmol/L)	Very insensitive index of total Fe stores; extremely variable (day-to-day and diurnal).
Total iron binding capacity (TIBC)	TIBC determined by saturating serum transferrin with Fe and then remeasuring serum Fe.	Reflects transferrin concentration.	250-400 mcg/dll (45-71 μmol/L)	TIBC does not increase until Fe stores are essentially completely depleted.
Transferrin saturation (Tf-sat)	Tf-sat = serum Fe/TIBC × 100	Used like TIBC in assessment of Fe deficiency; useful in diagnosis of iron toxicity or excess storage (hemochromatosis).	M: 20%-50% F: 15%-50%	↓ When Fe stores essentially depleted; ↑ in ↓ vitamin B_6 aplastic anemia.
RBC distribution width (RDW)	Measurement of variation in RBC diameter (anisocytosis); reported to be helpful in distinguishing Fe deficiency and anemia associated with chronic inflammation.	Very sensitive indicator of Fe status; normal RDW reportedly rules out anemia caused by chronic inflammatory diseases.[11]	Normal value 13.4%-14.6% Microscopic electronic interpretation required.	Specificity of RDW for Fe deficiency is relatively low; interpretation confounded by red cell transfusion; measurement usually not reported.
Ferritin	Intracellular Fe-storage protein; serum levels parallel iron stores; measured by immunoassays.	Best biochemical index of uncomplicated iron deficiency or overload (iron toxicity) and excess storage.	M: 15-200 ng/ml (15-200 mcg/L) F: 12-263 ng/ml (12-263 mcg/L)	Increases during metabolic response to injury, even when Fe stores are adequate; not useful in anemia of chronic and inflammations diseases.
Zinc (Zn)[12]	Serum levels measured by atomic absorption spectrophotometry.	Serum levels affected by diet and the inflammatory response. Zinc deficiency associated with many diseases and trauma.	0.7-1.2 mg/L (11-18 μmol/L)	Serum levels detect frank—but not marginal—deficiency; blood must be collected in zinc-free tubes.
Copper (Cu)	1. Serum levels measured by flame emission atomic absorption spectrophotometry. 2. Ceruloplasmin is the major Cu-containing plasma protein; measured by immunoassay (e.g., nephelometry).	1. Cu deficiency is associated with neutropenia, anemia, and scurvylike bone disease and megadoses of zinc. 2. Ceruloplasmin is required for conversion of Fe^{2+} to Fe^{3+} during cellular Fe uptake; anemia can result from ↑ ceruloplasmin.	M: 70-140 mcg/dl (11-22 mmol/L) F: 80-155 mcg/dl (13-24 μmol/L) (2) 150-600 mg/L	1. Serum levels detect frank but not marginal deficiency; use of oral contraceptives ↑ serum Cu. 2. Ceruloplasmin not a useful marker of Cu status but can be used to assess changes in status after supplementation.
Selenium (Se)	1. Serum levels measured by atomic absorption spectrophotometry. 2. Whole blood levels (measured by same methods) better reflect long-term status.	Margin between deficiency and toxicity is narrower for Se than any other trace element; important component of the antioxidant enzyme glutathione peroxidase.	(1) 80-320 mcg/L (1-4 μmol/L) (2) 60-340 mcg/L (0.75-4.3 μmol/L)	Cutoff points for deficiency or toxicity are not well established.

[7] These substances are measured by similar techniques when the concentration in urine or other body fluids is determined.

[8] These tests are combined with serum glucose, creatinine, and BUN on a test battery or panel. This set of tests is among the first and most frequently administered laboratory tests.

[9] The CBC includes the red cell count, the red cell indices, Hb concentration, HCT, MCV, mean cell hemoglobin (MCH), mean cell hemoglobin concentration (MCHC), and white cell and platelet counts. Only HCT, Hb, and MCV are discussed here (see Savage RA: The red cell indices: yesterday, today, and tomorrow, *Clin Lab Med* 13:773-785, 1993).

[10] Ranges are for adult men and premenopausal women. Pregnant women, infants, and children have different reference ranges.

[11] See van Zeben D et al: Evaluation of microcytosis using serum ferritin and red cell distribution width, *Eur J Haematol* 44:106-109, 1990.

[12] Taste acuity tests can be used to supplement laboratory methods (see, e.g., Gibson RS et al: A growth limiting mild zinc deficiency syndrome in some Southern Ontario boys with low growth percentiles, *Am J Clin Nutr* 49:1266,1989).

Continued

APPENDIX 30 Laboratory Values for Nutritional Assessment and Monitoring—cont'd

Test	Principle and Requirements	Interpretation	Reference Range	Limitations
Iodine (I)	Urinary excretion is best indicator of I status, either mcg/24 hr or mcg/g creatinine; thyroid hormone level related to I status.	Excretion should be ≥ DRT for 24-hour urine or >50 mcg/g creatinine; thyroid hormone = T_3 or T_4.	No urinary I reference range T4 reference range: 5-12 mcg/dl (65-155 nmol/L)	Thyroid hormone levels are affected by many factors besides iodine status.
Ultra-Trace Minerals				
Chromium (Cr)	Urinary excretion usually tested by atomic absorption spectrophotometry.	Excretion should be ≥DRI; deficiency reported in patients on long-term TPN; ↓ levels in diabetes mellitus.	10-200 ng/dl (1.9-38 nmol/L)	Test not available in most clinical laboratories; special handling required to prevent specimen contamination during collection.

VII. Blood Gases and Water Status

Test	Principle and Requirements	Interpretation	Reference Range	Limitations
pH	pH = $-\log$ [H^+]; H^+ depends mainly on the CO_2 from respiration: CO_2 +. H_2O ⇔ H_2CO_3 ⇔ HCO_3^- + H^+. Measured by ion-selective electrodes (like those found in common pH meters)	In: Acidosis pH <7.35 Alkalosis pH >7.45 pH compatible with life 6.80-7.80.	Whole blood: Arterial: 7.35-7.45 Venous: 7.32-7.42	Blood must not be exposed to air before or during measurement.
pO₂ or Po₂ and O₂ saturation	Whole blood O_2 measured by oxygen electrode; Po_2 = "pressure" contributed by O_2 to the total "pressure" of all the gases dissolved in blood. Saturation = $\dfrac{\text{Content}}{\text{Capacity}}$ ($\times$ 100).	Affected by alveolar gas exchange, ventilation/perfusion inequalities, and generalized alveolar hypoventilation.	Arterial blood: pO₂: 83-108 mm Hg <40 mm Hg = critical value (gravely dangerous) O₂ saturation: 0.95-0.98 (95%-98%)	Blood must not be exposed to air before or during measurement.
pCO₂ or Pco₂	Measured by ion-selective electrode; "pressure" contributed by CO_2 to the total "pressure" of all the gases dissolved in blood.	↑ In respiratory acidosis (↑ CO_2 in inspired air or ↓ in alveolar ventilation) and ↓ in respiratory alkalosis (e.g., in hyperventilation from anxiety, mechanical ventilator, or closed head injury [damaged respiratory center]).	Whole blood: Arterial M: 35-48 mm Hg F: 32-45 mm Hg Venous 6-7 mm Hg higher	Blood must not be exposed to air before or during measurement.
Bicarbonate (HCO_3^-) and total CO_2 (tCO_2)	For whole blood [HCO_3^-] is calculated from the equation given in pH section.	↑ In compensated respiratory acidosis and in metabolic acidosis; ↓ in metabolic acidosis and in compensated respiratory alkalosis.	Whole blood: Arterial 18-23 mEq/L (18-23 mmol/L)	Blood must not be exposed to air before or during measurement.
Osmolality (Osmol)	Osmol is dependent on amount of particles (solutes) dissolved in a solution; measurement based on relationship between solute concentration and freezing point; serum osmol assesses hydration status and solute load.	Osmol increases in dehydration, diabetic coma, diabetic ketoacidosis; also estimated from the formula: mOsmol/L = 1.86 a(Na^+) + (Glucose)/18 + (BUN)/2.8	282-300 mOsmol/kg (1 Osmol = 1 mol of solute particles; 1 kg serum ≈ L)	Freezing point depression gives a more accurate estimate of osmol than the calculated value (e.g., in ketoacidosis).

Continued

VIII. Tests of Antioxidant Status/Oxidative Stress

Test	Principle and Requirements	Interpretation	Reference Range	Limitations
Water-soluble compounds	See Vitamin C.			
Lipid-soluble compounds: see Vitamin E Carotenoids Coenzyme Q_{10}	The carotenoids: lutein, xanthine zeaxanthin, α- and β-carotene, and lycopene; carotenoids and coenzyme Q_{10} (ubiquinone-10) are measured chromatographically.	Reference ranges for these compounds vary greatly, depending on the method used for their assay.	See reference for carotenoid range under fat malabsorption	Tests for carotenoids and coenzyme Q are not yet available for routine clinical use.
Total antioxidant capacity: (e.g., ORAC TEAC FRAP)	ORAC: Oxygen radical absorbance capacity TEAC: Trolox-equivalent antioxidant capacity FRAP: Ferric-reducing ability of plasma	These assays reflect the presence of all of plasma or serum antioxidants, including vitamins C and E, carotenoids, coenzyme $Q_{1}0$, glutathione, uric acid, bilirubin, superoxide dismutase, catalase, glutathione peroxidase, and albumin.		These assays are now commercially available but are currently performed only in specialized laboratories.
Oxidative stress markers: (e.g., o-tyrosine, nitro-tyrosine, 8-isoprostane, 4-hydroxynonenal, malondialdehyde)	Free radical oxidation products of lipids (e.g., malondialdehyde, 8-isoprostane), proteins (e.g., o-tyrosine and nitro-tyrosine), or secondary oxidation products (e.g., 4-hydroxynonenal) can be measured chromatographically or by immunoassay.	8-Isoprostane (also called 8-epiprostaglandin F_{2a}) increases in plasma or urine of patients with lung disease, hypercholesterolemia, or diabetes mellitus.		8-Isoprostane assays are now commercially available. Markers of oxidative stress are currently assayed only in specialized laboratories.

IX. Tests for Monitoring Nutrition Support

Test	Principle and Requirements	Interpretation	Reference Range	Limitations
CRP	CRP is an acute-phase protein used to assess inflammatory status. Measured by a variety of immunoassay techniques.	Large increases in CRP are associated with development of a catabolic state during the stress response; CRP levels begin to fall when the anabolic phase is entered.	<10 mg/L	Serial values rather than a single value must be used to specify the stage of the stress response.
Chemistry panel with phosphate and Mg^{2+}	Panel includes electrolytes, glucose, creatinine, BUN, and total CO_2 (bicarbonate); see earlier discussion for additional test information.	Used to monitor carbohydrate tolerance, hydration status, and major organ system function.	See earlier discussion	Very frequently ordered test panel.
Osmolality (see earlier discussion)	Can be measured or calculated from chemistry panel data.	Used to assess hydration status.	See earlier discussion	Measured value accounts for substances in blood not accounted for by calculation.
Protein-Energy Balance				
Serum proteins (see earlier discussion) Nitrogen balance: UUN, TUN (see earlier discussion)	Prealbumin, RBP, Tf, albumin most often available.	These visceral proteins aid in assessing protein and energy balance.	See earlier discussion Nitrogen balance in hospitalized patients ranges from −20g to +6 g/day	Stress reaction can markedly affect these and confound their interpretation as protein-energy indicators. UUN may greatly underestimate nitrogen excretion.

DRI, Dietary reference intake.

APPENDIX 30 Laboratory Values for Nutritional Assessment and Monitoring—cont'd

Test	Principle and Requirements	Interpretation	Reference Range	Limitations
Minerals: Zn, Cu, Se, Cr (see earlier discussion)			See earlier discussion	Most trace minerals are measured only in long-term nutrition support patients.
Vitamins C and A (see earlier discussion)	Because vitamins C and A are important in immune function and wound healing, they should be assessed regularly.	Vitamin C levels can ↓ sharply in response to stress.	See earlier discussion	Systematic, regular monitoring protocol should be followed.
Liver Function tests				
Bilirubin	Total serum bilirubin represents both the conjugated or direct and unconjugated or indirect bilirubin. Elevated levels suggest medical problem.	Conjugated bilirubin elevated levels with cancer of pancreas or liver and bile duct obstruction; unconjugated bilirubin level elevated with hepatitis, jaundice anemias	Total bilirubin: 0.3-1 mg/dl; 5.1-17 μmol/L Indirect bilirubin: 0.2-0.8 mg/dl; 3.4-12 μmol/L Direct bilirubin: 0.1-0.3 mg/dl; 1.7-5.1 μmol/L	Many medications are associated with elevated bilirubin levels.
Alanine amino transferase (ALT)	Enzyme found primarily in the liver.	Injury to the liver results in elevated levels of ALT. Depressed in malnutrition.	4-36 U/L	Many medications are associated with elevated ALT levels. ALT levels are often compared with AST for differential diagnosis.
Gamma glutamyl transferase (GGT)	Biliary excretory enzyme involved in transfer of amino acids across cell membranes.	Used to evaluate progression of liver disease and screening for alcoholism	F: 4-25 UL M: 12-38 UL	Many medications are associated with elevated GGT levels.
Alkaline phosphatase (ALP)	Enzyme found primarily in the bone, liver, and biliary tract; increased in an alkaline environment.	Elevated levels noted in liver and bone disorders.	30-120 U/L; 0.5-2 μKat/L	Nonspecific test; other tests need to confirm diagnosis. Many medications are associated with elevated ALP levels.
Aspartate aminotransferase (AST)	Enzyme primarily found in the heart, liver, and skeletal muscle cells.	Diagnostic tool when coronary occlusive heart disease or hepatocellular disease is suspected.	0-35 U/L; 0-0.58 μKat/L	Many medications are associated with elevated AST levels. AST levels are often compared with ALT for differential diagnosis.
Triglycerides (TG) (see earlier discussion)	Sepsis and stress can alter ability to metabolize fat, therefore TG should be regularly measured.	↑ TG indicates fat overload syndrome; measure TG before and after initial lipid infusion and postinfusion, weekly thereafter.	See earlier discussion	Measurement only after lipid infusion may make interpretation impossible.
Vitamin K status (TPN only) (see earlier discussion)	Contribution of the gut flora to vitamin K status is absent during TPN, and basic TPN formulas are devoid of it.	PTT is used to assess status.	See earlier discussion	PTT is affected by many other factors besides vitamin K status.
Thyroid Function Tests				
Thyroxine T4	Measures the total amount of T4 in the blood; free T4 active form	↑ Hyperthyroidism; ↓ hypothyroidism and malnutrition	F: 5-12 mcg/dl; 64-154 nmol/L M: 4-12 mcg/dl, 51-154 nmol/L	Tests are ordered to distinguish between euthyroidism, or hyperthyroidism and hypothyroidism
Triiodothyronine T3	Measures the total amount of T3 in the blood; free T3 active form	↑ Hyperthyroidism; ↓ hypothyroidism	20-50 yrs: 70-205 ng/dl; 1.2-3.4 nmol/L >50 yrs: 40-180 ng/dl; 0.6-2.8 nmol/L	Tests are ordered to distinguish between euthyroidism, or hyperthyroidism and hypothyroidism
Thyroid-stimulating hormone	Used to monitor exogenous thyroid replacement or thyroid suppression	↓ Hyperthyroidism; ↑ hypothyroidism	2-10 μU/ml	Tests are ordered to distinguish between euthyroidism, or hyperthyroidism and hypothyroidism.

X. Tests for Metabolic Disease

Test	Principle and Requirements	Interpretation	Reference Range	Limitations
Amino acidurias	Dietary treatment is the major therapy for many of these genetic diseases: phenylketonuria, cystinuria, maple syrup urine disease, tyrosinemia, homocystinuria, Hartnup disease.	Monitoring amino acid level in urine or serum is necessary to assess adequacy of treatment.	Examples: Phe 1-16 g/L (35-90 µmol/L) Cys 2-22 g/L (10-90 µmol/L) Val 17-37 g/L (145-315 µmol/L) Tyr 4-16 g/L (20-90 µmol/L)	There are several methods used to measure (e.g., phenylalanine); these usually do not have exactly equivalent reference ranges.
Diabetes Mellitus (See Chapter 30)				
Diabetes diagnosis	1. Serum or whole blood glucose: after fasting 8-16 hours or on a casual blood sample.	1. ≥2 fasting levels >126 mg/dl are diagnostic; casual level ≥200 followed by fasting level >126 are diagnostic. Fasting levels of 110 to 126 indicate impaired glucose tolerance (IGT).		1. Elevated glucose levels are normal in physiologic stress; whole blood gives slightly lower values.
	2. Glucose tolerance test (GGT); 75 g glucose (100 g during pregnancy) given after fasting; serum glucose measured by before and five times during the next 3 hours after oral dosing. Glucose measured by automated chemistry procedure.	2. Serum levels >200 at 2-hour point is diagnostic; 2-hour level <140 and all 0- to 2-hour levels <200 are normal; 140-199 at 2 hours indicates IGT. Gestational diabetes: fasting >105; 1-hour GGT >190; 2 hour GGT >165; and 3-hour GGT >145.		2. Often used for confirmation; ambulatory patient only; bed rest or stress impairs GGT; inadequate carbohydrate consumption before test invalidates results.
Diabetes monitoring	1. Blood glucose—monitoring requires that *the patient* monitor blood glucose level.	1. Tight diabetes control requires frequent monitoring of glucose levels.	1. 70-99 mg/dl (3.9-5.5 mmol/L)	A combination of glucose monitoring (by patient) and laboratory measurement of glycated proteins are needed to effectively monitor glucose control; fructosamine must be interpreted in light of plasma protein half-lives, and HbA$_{1c}$ must be interpreted in light of RBC half-life.
	2. Serum fructosamine—assesses medium-term glucose control by measured glycated serum proteins; currently only tested in the laboratory.	2. Allows assessment of average glucose levels for previous 2-3 weeks.	2. Normal levels: 1%-2% of total protein Ranges vary according to method used	
	3. Serum glycated hemoglobin or HbA$_{1c}$—assesses longer-term glucose control; currently only tested in the laboratory.	3. Allows assessment of average glucose levels for previous 2-3 months and verification of patient's serum glucose log.	3. Normal levels: Non-diabetic 2.2-4.8% Good diabetic control 2.5%-5.9% Fair diabetic control >6% <8% Poor diabetic control >8%	

Appendix created by Mary Demarest Litchford, PhD, RD, LDN.

APPENDIX 31 Nutritional Implications of Selected Drugs

Drug	Category	Drug Effect	Nutritional Implications/Cautions
Antiinfective Agents			
Penicillin	Antibacterial agents	Long-term use may lead to oral candidiasis, diarrhea, epigastric distress. Some products contain high amounts of potassium and/or sodium. May cause *Clostridium difficile* pseudomembranous colitis.	Caution with low-sodium diet or potassium supplements. Take most oral forms 1 hour before or 2 hours after food to improve absorption. Take amoxicillin/potassium clavulanate with food to decrease gastrointestinal (GI) distress. Focus on fluid and electrolyte replacement for diarrhea.
Selected Macrolides			
Azithromycin (Zithromax) Clarithromycin (Biaxin) Elythromycin (Ery-Tab)	Macrolide antibacterial agent Macrolide antibacterial agent Macrolide antibacterial agent	May cause GI distress, anorexia, stomatitis, bad taste in the mouth, or diarrhea. May increase sedative effect of alcohol. May cause *Clostridium difficile* pseudomembranous colitis.	Take with food to decrease GI distress. Eat frequent, small, appealing meals to counteract anorexia. Use mouth rinses, sugarless gum, or lemon water for abnormal taste in mouth. Focus on fluid and electrolyte replacement for diarrhea. Avoid alcohol.
Sulfamethoxazole/trimethoprim (Bactrim, Bactrim DS)	Sulfonamide combination antibacterial agent	May interfere with folate metabolism, especially with long-term use. May cause stomatitis, anorexia, nausea/vomiting, severe allergic reactions. May cause *Clostridium difficile* pseudomembranous colitis.	Take with food and 8 ounces of fluid to lessen nausea, vomiting, and anorexia. Folate supplement may be necessary. Discontinue drug and consult physician at first sign of allergic reaction. Focus on fluid and electrolyte replacement for diarrhea.
Selected Cephalosporins			
Cephalexin (Keflex) Cefprozil (Cefzil)	Cephalosporin antibacterial agent Cephalosporin antibacterial agent	May cause stomatitis, sore mouth and tongue and interfere with eating. May cause diarrhea. May cause *Clostridium difficile* pseudomembranous colitis.	Focus on fluid and electrolyte replacement for diarrhea. Eat moist, soft, low-salt foods as well as cold foods such as ice chips, sherbet, and yogurt for stomatitis and sore mouth.
Cefuroxime axetil (Ceftin)	Cephalosporin antibacterial agent	Food increases bioavailability of tablets and suspension. Antacids, calcium, and magnesium supplements may decrease bioavailability.	Take with a meal for optimal bioavailability. Take separately from antacids, calcium, or magnesium supplements
Selected Fluoroquinolones			
Ciprofloxacin (Cipro) Levofloxacin (Levaquin) Gatifloxacin (Tequin) Moxifloxacin (Avelox)	Fluoroquinolone antibacterial agents	Drug may rarely precipitate in renal tubules. Drug will bind to magnesium, calcium, zinc, and iron, forming an insoluble, unabsorbable complex. Ciprofloxacin inhibits the metabolism of caffeine, causing increased central nervous system stimulation. May cause *Clostridium difficile* pseudomembranous colitis.	Take drug with 8 ounces of fluid; maintain adequate fluid intake. Limit caffeine intake. Take drug at least 2 hours before or 6 hours after antacids, magnesium, calcium, iron, or zinc supplements or multivitamin with minerals. Focus on fluid and electrolyte replacement for diarrhea.
Linezolid (Zyvox)	Oxazolidinone antibacterial agent	Drug exhibits mild monoamine oxidase inhibition. May cause taste change, oral candidiasis, and pseudomembranous colitis.	Avoid significant amounts (>100 mg) of high tyramine/pressor foods. See chart in 14th edition of *Food Medication Interactions*. Eat multiple small meals of appealing foods if taste changes become a problem. Focus on fluid and electrolyte replacement for diarrhea.
Tetracycline (Sumycin)	Antibacterial agent	Drug may cause anorexia. Drug will bind to Mg^+, Ca^{++}, Zn^{++}, and Fe^{++}, forming an insoluble unabsorbable complex. May decrease bacterial production of vitamin K in intestinal tract. May cause vitamin B deficiency with long-term use. Drug combined with vitamin A may increase the risk of benign intracranial hypertension. May cause *Clostridium difficile* pseudomembranous colitis.	Take supplements separately by 3 hours. Eat frequent, small appealing meals to decrease anorexia. Avoid excessive vitamin A while taking drug. Vitamins K and B supplements may be necessary with long-term use. Focus on fluid and electrolyte replacement for diarrhea.

Drug	Type	Effect	Recommendation
Metronidazole (Flagyl)	Antibacterial agent/antiprotozoal agent	May cause anorexia, GI distress, stomatitis, and metallic taste in mouth. May cause disulfiram-like reaction when ingested with alcohol.	Take with food to avoid GI distress. Eat frequent, small, appealing meals to decrease anorexia. Avoid all alcohol during use and for 3 days after discontinuation.
Nitrofurantoin (Macrobid)	Nitrofuran Antibacterial agent	Drug may cause peripheral neuropathy, muscle weakness, and muscle wasting, especially in individuals with preexisting anemia, vitamin B deficiency, and electrolyte abnormalities. May cause *Clostridium difficile* pseudomembranous colitis.	Drug should be taken with adequate calories, protein, and vitamin B complex. Avoid in G-6-PD deficiency because of increased risk of hemolytic anemia. Focus on fluid and electrolyte replacement for diarrhea.
Gentamicin (Garamycin)	Aminoglycoside Antibacterial agent	Drug may be ototoxic and nephrotoxic. Dehydration increases risk of toxicity.	Adequate fluid intake/hydration necessary to lower risk of toxicity.
Amikacin (Amikin)	Aminoglycoside Antibacterial agent		
Isoniazid (Nydrazid)	Antitubercular agent	Drug may cause pyridoxine (vitamin B$_6$) and niacin (vitamin B$_3$) deficiency resulting in peripheral neuropathy and pellagra. Drug may affect vitamin D metabolism and decrease calcium and phosphate absorption. Drug possesses monoamine oxidase (MAO) inhibitor–like activity.	Avoid use in malnourished individuals and others at increased risk for peripheral neuropathy. Supplement with 25 to 50 mg of pyridoxine and possibly B-complex if skin changes occur. Avoid foods high in tyramine (e.g., aged cheeses). Maintain adequate calcium and vitamin D intake.
Rifampin (Rifadin)	Antitubercular agent	Drug may increase metabolism of vitamin D. Rare cases of osteomalacia have been reported.	May need vitamin D supplement with long-term use.
Ethambutol (Myambutol)	Antitubercular agent	Drug may decrease body copper and zinc. Drug may decrease the excretion of uric acid, leading to hyperuricemia and gout.	Increase intake of foods high in copper and zinc; take daily multivitamin with minerals when drug is used long term. Maintain adequate hydration and purine-restricted diet.
Pyrazinamide	Antitubercular agent	Drug may decrease the excretion of uric acid, leading hyperuricemia and gout.	Maintain adequate hydration and purine-restricted diet.
Amphotericin B (Fungizone)	Antifungal agent	Drug may cause anorexia and weight loss. Drug causes loss of potassium, magnesium, and calcium.	Eat frequent, small, appealing meals high in magnesium, potassium, calcium. Ensure adequate hydration.
Ketoconazole (Nizoral)	Antifungal agent	Drug does not dissolve at pH >5.0.	Take with food to increase absorption. Take with acidic liquid (e.g., cola), especially individuals with achlorhydria.
Amprenavir (Agenerase)	Antiretroviral agent	Drug provides 1744 IU of vitamin E with daily adult dose.	Avoid vitamin E supplements.
Hematologic Agents			
Warfarin (Coumadin)	Anticoagulant	Prevents the conversion of oxidized vitamin K to the active form. Produces a state of systemic anticoagulation. May inhibit mineralization of newly formed bone.	Consistent intake of dietary supplements (i.e., in vitamins) must be consistent to achieve desired state of anticoagulation. Monitor bone mineral density in individuals on long-term therapy.
Aspirin (Bayer Ecotrin)	Salicylate platelet inhibitor	Drug may cause GI irritation and bleeding. Drug may decrease uptake of vitamin C by leukocytes and increase systemic levels of iron, folic acid, sodium, and potassium, especially with high dose, long-term use.	Incorporate foods high in vitamin C and folic acid into diet. Monitor electrolytes, hemoglobin to determine need for potassium or iron supplements. Avoid alcohol consumption.

Continued

Appendix created by Sr. Jeanne P. Crowe, PharmD., RPh. Adapted from Pronsky, ZM: *Food medication interactions*, ed 14, 2006. Copyright retained by Waza, Inc. T/A Food Medication Interactions, Birchrunville, Pa. Permission granted for publication in Krause's *Food, nutrition, and diet therapy*, ed 12. May not be copied or reprinted for any reason without permission from Waza, Inc.

APPENDIX 31 Nutritional Implications of Selected Drugs—cont'd

Drug	Category	Drug Effect	Nutritional Implications/Cautions
Hormonal/Metabolic Agents			
Metformin (Glucophage)	Biguanide	Drug may decrease absorption of vitamin B_{12}, folic acid. May cause lactic acidosis.	Maintain prescribed diabetic diet. Increase foods high in vitamin B_{12} and folic acid or supplement if necessary. Avoid alcohol to decrease risk of lactic acidosis.
Prednisone (Deltasone) Methylprednisolone (Medrol)	Corticosteroid Corticosteroid	Drug induces protein catabolism, resulting in muscle wasting, atrophy of bone protein matrix, delayed wound healing. Drug decreases intestinal absorption of calcium; promotes urinary loss of calcium, potassium, zinc, vitamin C, nitrogen; causes sodium retention.	Maintain diet high in calcium, vitamin D, protein, potassium, zinc, and vitamin C, and low in sodium. Calcium and vitamin D supplements recommended for prevention of osteoporosis with long-term use of drug.
Alendronate (Fosamax) Risedronate (Actonel) Ibandronate (Boniva)	Biphosphonates	Drug may induce mild decrease in serum calcium.	Diet high in calcium or calcium and vitamin D supplement. Drug must be taken 30 minutes (alendronate and risedronate) or 1 hour (ibandronate) before first food or medication of the day on completely empty stomach with plain water only.
Estrogen (Premarin) Oral contraceptives	Sex hormones	Drug may decrease absorption and tissue uptake of vitamin C. Drug may increase absorption of vitamin A. May inhibit folate conjugate and decrease serum folic acid levels. Drug may decrease serum levels vitamin B_6, B_{12}, riboflavin, magnesium, zinc.	Maintain diet with adequate magnesium, folic acid, vitamin B_6 and B_{12}, riboflavin, and zinc. Calcium and vitamin D supplements may be recommended with estrogen as hormone replacement for postmenopausal women.
Cardiovascular Agents			
Digoxin (Lanoxin)	Cardiac glycoside	Drug may increase urinary loss of magnesium and decrease serum levels of potassium.	Hypokalemia, hypomagnesemia, and hypercalcemia increase drug toxicity. Maintain diet high in potassium and magnesium. Caution with calcium supplements and antacids.
Propranolol (Inderal) Metoprolol (Lopressor, Toprol XL) Atenolol (Tenormin)	β-Adrenergic antagonist β-Adrenergic antagonist β-Adrenergic antagonist	Drug may mask sympathetic signs of hypoglycemia. Drug may prolong hypoglycemia. Drug may decrease insulin release in response to hyperglycemia.	Maintain prescribed diabetic diet. Monitor blood glucose for hyperglycemia. Monitor for nonsympathetic signs of hypoglycemia.
Benazepril (Lotensin) Enalapril (Vasotec) Fosinopril (Monopril) Lisinopril (Zestril, Prinivil)	Ace inhibitor Ace inhibitor Ace inhibitor Ace inhibitor	Drug may increase serum potassium levels.	Caution with high potassium diet or potassium supplements. Avoid salt substitutes. Ensure adequate fluid intake/hydration. Check recommendation for each agent as regards ingestion with food. See monograph in 14th edition of *Food Medication Interactions.*
Candesartan (Atacand) Eprosartan (Teveten) Irbesartan (Avapro) Losartan (Cozaar) Olmesartan (Benecar) Telmisartan (Micardis) Valsartan (Diovan)	Angiotenson II receptor antagonist Angiotenson II receptor antagonist Angiotenson II receptor antagonist Angiotenson II receptor antagonist Angiotenson II receptor antagonist Angiotenson II receptor antagonist Angiotenson II receptor antagonist	Drug may increase serum potassium levels.	Caution with high potassium diet or potassium supplements. Avoid salt substitutes. Ensure adequate fluid intake/hydration. Avoid natural licorice. Avoid grapefruit/related citrus with Losartan.

Drug	Classification	Effect	Recommendation
Clonidine (Catapres)	Alpha-adrenergic agonist	Drug commonly causes dizziness, drowsiness, sedation.	Avoid alcohol/alcohol products. Drug increases sensitivity to alcohol, which may increase sedation caused by drug alone.
Hydralazine (Apresoline)	Peripheral vasodilator	Drug interferes with pyridoxine (vitamin B_6) metabolism. May result in pyridoxine deficiency.	Maintain a diet high in pyridoxine. Supplementation may be necessary.
Quinidine (Quinaglute)	Antiarrhythmic agent	Cardiac toxicity of drug is increased in the presence of hypokalemia, hypomagnesemia, and/or hypocalcemia.	Diet adequate in potassium, magnesium, calcium to maintain normal serum levels. Supplementation may be necessary.
Antihyperlipidemic Agents			
Atorvastatin (Lipitor)	HMG Co-A reductase inhibitor	Drug may cause significant reduction in coenzyme Q_{10}. Drug lowers low-density lipoprotein cholesterol; raises high-density lipoprotein cholesterol.	Supplementation with Coenzyme Q_{10} is controversial. Drug is adjunct to diet therapy. Maintain low-fat, low-cholesterol diet for optimal drug effect. Avoid grapefruit/related citrus with atorvastatin, lovastatin, or simvastatin.
Fluvastatin (Lescol)	HMG Co-A reductase inhibitor		
Lovastatin (Mevacor)	HMG Co-A reductase inhibitor		
Pravastatin (Pravachol)	HMG Co-A reductase inhibitor		
Rosuvastatin (Crestor)	HMG Co-A reductase inhibitor		
Simvastatin (Zocor)	HMG Co-A reductase inhibitor		
Gemfibrozil (Lopid)	Fibric acid derivative	Drug decreases serum triglycerides.	Maintain low-fat, low-sucrose diet; avoid alcohol for optimal therapeutic effect.
Fenofibrate (Tricor)	Fibric acid derivative		
Cholestyramine (Questran)	Bile acid sequestrant	Drug binds fat-soluble vitamins (A,E,D,K), β-carotene, calcium, magnesium, iron, zinc, and folic acid.	Take fat-soluble vitamins in water-miscible form or take vitamin supplement at least 1 hour before first dose of drug daily. Maintain diet high in folic acid, magnesium, calcium, iron, zinc, or supplements when necessary. Monitor serum nutrient levels with long-term use of drug.
Niacin (Niaspan)	Nicotinic acid	High dose may elevate blood glucose and uric acid.	Maintain diabetic, low-purine diet if necessary.
Diuretics			
Furosemide (Lasix)	Loop diuretic	Drug increases urinary excretion of sodium, potassium, magnesium, calcium.	Maintain diet high in potassium, magnesium, and calcium. Avoid natural licorice, which may counteract the diuretic effect of the drug. Monitor electrolytes; supplementation may be necessary.
Bumetanide (Bumex)	Loop diuretic		
Hydrochlorothiazide (Hydrodiuril)	Thiazide diuretic	Drug increases urinary excretion of sodium, potassium, magnesium. Drug increases renal resorption of calcium.	Maintain diet high in potassium and magnesium. Avoid natural licorice, which may counteract the diuretic effect of the drug. Monitor electrolytes; supplementation may be necessary. Caution with calcium supplements.
Triamterene (Dyrenium)	Potassium-sparing diuretic	Drug increases renal resorption of potassium.	Avoid salt substitutes. Caution with potassium supplements. Avoid excessive potassium intake in diet.
Spironolactone (Aldactone)	Potassium-sparing diuretic		
Analgesics			
Acetaminophen (Tylenol)		Drug may cause hepatotoxicity at high dose. Chronic alcohol ingestion increases the risk of hepatotoxicity.	Maximum safe adult dose is <4 g/day. Avoid alcohol or limit to <2 drinks/day.
Nonsteroidal antiinflammatory drugs (ibuprofen, naproxen, nabumetone)		Drug may cause GI irritation and bleeding; both acute and occult.	Take drug with food or milk to decrease risk of GI toxicity.

Continued

APPENDIX 31 Nutritional Implications of Selected Drugs—cont'd

Drug	Category	Drug Effect	Nutritional Implications/Cautions
Antidepressants			
Fluoxetine (Prozac)	Selective serotonin reuptake inhibitor	Fluoxetine may cause anorexia and weight loss. Fluoxetine may decrease the absorption of leucine.	Monitor weight and caloric intake if necessary. Avoid tryptophan, St. John's wort. Additive effects may produce adverse effects/serotonin syndrome.
Paroxetine (Paxil)	Selective serotonin reuptake inhibitor	Some herbal/natural products may increase toxicity.	
Sertraline (Zoloft)	Selective serotonin reuptake inhibitor		
Trazodone (Desyrel)	Unclassified antidepressant	Some herbal/natural products may increase toxicity.	Avoid tryptophan, St. John's wort. Additive effects may produce adverse effects/serotonin syndrome.
Venlafaxine (Effexor XR)	Unclassified antidepressant		
Mirtazapine (Remeron)	Unclassified antidepressant	Mirtazapine may cause significant increase in appetite and weight gain.	
Amitriptyline (Elavil)	Tricyclic antidepressant	Drug may cause increased appetite (especially for carbohydrates and sweets) and weight gain. High fiber may decrease drug absorption.	Monitor caloric intake. Maintain consistent amount of fiber in diet.
Phenelzine (Nardil)	MAO inhibitor	Drug may cause increased appetite (especially for carbohydrates and sweets) and weight gain. Risk for severe reaction with dietary tyramine.	Avoid foods high in tyramine during drug use and for 2 weeks after discontinuation to prevent hypertensive crisis. Monitor caloric intake to avoid weight gain.
Lithium carbonate (Lithobid)	Antimanic/antidepressant	Sodium intake affects drug levels. Low-sodium diet, dehydration, increased drug toxicity. Drug may cause GI irritation.	Drink 2 to 3 L of fluid daily to avoid dehydration. Maintain consistent dietary sodium intake. Take with food to decrease GI irritation.
Antipsychotic Agents			
Clozapine (Clozaril)	Second generation antipsychotic	Drug may cause increased appetite and weight gain. Drug may cause life-threatening toxic agranulocytosis.	Monitor for weight gain/calorie count. Individual must be enrolled in and adhere to requirements of Clozaril program, including a weekly white blood cell count.
Olanzapine (Zyprexa)	Second generation antipsychotic	Drug may cause increased appetite and weight gain.	Monitor weight and food intake.
Risperidone (Risperdal)	Second generation antipsychotic		
Chlorpromazine (Thorazine)	First generation antipsychotic, low potency	Drug may impair glucose tolerance and insulin release. May cause increased appetite and weight gain. Risk for tardive dyskinesia.	Closer monitoring of blood glucose in the diagnosed diabetic individual. Periodic check of blood glucose in the "at-risk" nondiabetic individual. Monitor weight/calorie count. Tardive dyskinesia may interfere with biting, chewing, swallowing.
Haloperidol (Haldol)	First generation antipsychotic, high potency	May cause increased appetite and weight gain. Risk for tardive dyskinesia.	Monitor weight/calorie count. Tardive dyskinesia may interfere with biting, chewing, swallowing.
Antianxiety and Hypnotic Agents			
Lorazepam (Ativan)	Benzodiazepine	Drugs may cause significant sedation.	Avoid concurrent ingestion of alcohol, which will produce CNS depression. Limit or avoid caffeine, which may decrease the therapeutic effect of the drug. Caution with herbal/natural products that cause CNS stimulation or sedation.
Diazepam (Valium)	Benzodiazepine		
Alprazolam (Xanax)	Benzodiazepine		
Clonazepam (Klonopin)	Benzodiazepine		
Temazepam (Restoril)	Benzodiazepine hypnotic		
Zolpidem (Ambien)	Nonbenzodiazepine hypnotic		
Anticonvulsant Agents			
Carbamazepine (Tegretol)		Drug may decrease biotin, folic acid, and vitamin D levels.	Maintain diet high in folic acid and vitamin D. Calcium and vitamin D supplementation may be necessary for long-term therapy to prevent loss of bone mineral density.
Phenytoin (Dilantin)	Hydantoin	Drug may decrease serum levels of folic acid, calcium, vitamin D, biotin, and thiamin.	Folic acid, calcium, and vitamin D supplement may be recommended with long-term use.

Drug	Classification	Effect	Nursing Considerations
Phenobarbital	Barbiturate	Drug may induce rapid metabolism of vitamin D and produce deficiency of vitamin D and calcium. Drug may increase the metabolism of vitamin K, decrease serum folic acid and vitamin B_{12} levels.	Increase dietary intake of calcium, vitamin D, and folic acid. May need calcium, vitamin D, folic acid, and vitamin B_{12} supplementation with long-term use of drug.
Anti-Alzheimer's Agents			
Donepezil (Aricept)	Cholinesterase inhibitor	Drug is highly cholinergic; may cause anorexia, nausea and vomiting, diarrhea, increased gastric acid secretion, GI bleeding.	Take drug with food to prevent GI irritation. Monitor food intake and weight.
Rivastigmine (Exelon)	Cholinesterase inhibitor		
Galantamine (Reminyl)	Cholinesterase inhibitor		
Memantine (Namenda)	NMDA receptor antagonist	Drug is cleared from the body almost exclusively by renal excretion. Urine pH >8 decreases renal excretion by 80%.	Avoid diet that alkalinizes the urine to avoid drug toxicity.
Gastrointestinal Agents			
Famotidine (Pepcid)	H_2 receptor antagonist	Drug may reduce the absorption of vitamin B_{12} and iron.	Monitor iron studies, vitamin B_{12} level while on long-term therapy. Supplement if necessary.
Nizatidine (Axid)	H_2 receptor antagonist		
Ranitidine (Zantac)	H_2 receptor antagonist		
Omeprazole (Prilosec)	Proton pump inhibitor	Inhibition of acid secretion may inhibit the absorption of iron and vitamin B_{12}.	Monitor iron studies and vitamin B_{12} levels with long-term use of drug. Supplement if necessary.
Lansoprazole (Prevacid)	Proton pump inhibitor		
Pantoprazole (Protonix)	Proton pump inhibitor		
Rabeprazole (Aciphex)	Proton pump inhibitor		
Metoclopramide (Reglan)	Prokinetic agent	Drug increases gastric emptying; may change insulin requirements in persons with diabetes; may increase CNS depressant effects of alcohol. Drug may cause tardive dyskinesia with extended use.	Monitor blood glucose in persons with diabetes carefully when drug is initiated. Avoid alcohol. Tardive dyskinesia may interfere with biting, chewing, swallowing.
Antineoplastic Agents			
Methotrexate	Folate antagonist	Drug inhibits dihydrofolate reductase; decreased formation of active folate. Drug may cause GI irritation or injury.	Maintain diet high in folic acid and vitamin B_{12}. Daily folic acid supplement recommended with antirheumatic doses. Leucovorin rescue may be necessary with antineoplastic doses.
Cyclophosphamide (Cytoxan)	Alkylating agent	Drug metabolite causes bladder irritation, acute hemorrhagic cystitis.	Maintain high fluid intake (2-3 L daily) to induce frequent voiding.
All antineoplastic agents		All agents are cytotoxic; potential to damage intestinal mucosal.	Extensive effects discussed in Chapter 16.
Anti-Parkinson Agents			
Carbidopa/levodopa (Sinemet)	Dopamine precursor	Carbidopa protects levodopa against pyridoxine-enhanced peripheral decarboxylation to dopamine.	Pyridoxine supplements in excess of 10-25 mg daily may increase carbidopa requirements and increase adverse effects of levodopa.
Bromocriptine (Parlodel)	Dopamine agonist	Drug may cause GI irritation, nausea, vomiting, and GI bleeding	Take drug with food to prevent GI irritation. Take drug at bedtime to decrease nausea.
Selegiline (Eldepyl)	MAO-B inhibitor	Drug selectively inhibits MAO-B at 10 mg or less per day. Drug loses selectivity at higher doses.	Avoid high-tyramine foods at doses greater than 10 mg/day. May precipitate hypertension.
Entacapone (Comtan)	COMT inhibitor	Drug chelates iron; may decrease serum iron levels.	Take iron supplement separately from drug.
CNS Stimulants			
Methylphenidate (Ritalin, Concerta)	CNS stimulant	Drug may cause anorexia, weight loss, and decreased growth.	Ensure adequate calorie intake. Limit ingestion of caffeine; avoid alcohol and herbal products. Monitor children's weight and growth.
Amphetamine (Adderall, Dexedrine)	CNS stimulant	Drug may cause anorexia, decreased weight loss, and decreased growth.	Ensure adequate calorie intake. Limit ingestion of caffeine; avoid alcohol and herbal products. High-dose vitamin C may decrease drug absorption, increase drug excretion, and decrease half-life of drug. Monitor children's weight and growth.

APPENDIX 32 System ABCD Enteral Formulary
Nutrition Information for Enteral Formulas and Oral Supplements

Enteral Formula	kcal/ml	Protein (g/L)	CHO (g/L)	Fat (g/L)	Total kcal:N ratio	mOsm	Na mg/L (mEq/L)	K (mg/L) (mEq/L)	PO_4 (mg/L) (mEq/L)	Mg (mg/L) (mEq/L)	Ca (mg/L) (mEq/L)	Vol to meet 100% RDI (ml)	Fiber (g/L)	Free H_2O (ml/L)	Formula Cost
Nutren 1.0	1	40	127	38	133:1	315	876(38)	1248(32)	668(22)	268(13)	668(33)	1500	0	850	$
Nutren 1.5	1.5	60	169	68	131:1	430	1168(51)	1872(48)	1000(33)	400(20)	1000(50)	1000	0	775	$
Nutren 2.0	2	80	196	104	131:1	745	1300(57)	1920(49)	1340(44)	536(27)	1340(67)	750	0	700	$
Probalance	1.2	54	156	41	114:1	350	764(33)	1560(40)	1000(33)	400(20)	1250(63)	1000	10	810	$
Nutren Replete	1	62	113	34	75:1	300	876(38)	1500(38)	1000(33)	400(20)	1000(50)	1000	0	845	$
Nutren Renal	2	70	204	104	151:1	650	740(32)	1256(32)	700(23)	200(10)	1400(70)	750	0	704	$$
Nutren Glytrol	1	45	100	48	114:1	280	740(32)	1400(36)	720(23)	286(14)	740(37)	1400	15	840	$$
Peptamen 1.5	1.5	68	188	56	116:1	550	1020(44)	1860(48)	1000(33)	400(20)	1000(50)	1000	0	771	$$
Crucial	1.5	94	134	68	67:1	490	1168(51)	1872(48)	1000(33)	400(20)	1000(50)	1000	0	772	$$$
Nutren Jr	1	30	110	50	183:1	350	460(20)	1320(34)	800(26)	200(10)	1000(50)	1000	0	852	$
Nutren Jr w/fiber	1	30	110	50	183:1	350	460(20)	1320(34)	800(26)	200(10)	1000(50)	1000	6	851	$

Oral Supplement	kcal/ml	Protein (g/svg)	CHO (g/svg)	Fat (g/svg)	Total Kcal:N ratio	mOsm	Na (mg/svg) (mEq/svg)	K (mg/svg) (mEq/svg)	PO4 (mg/svg) (mEq/svg)	Mg (mg/svg) (mEq/svg)	Ca (mg/svg) (mEq/svg)	Vol to meet 100% RDI (ml)	Fiber (g/L)	Free H_2O (ml/L)	Formula Cost
Boost	1	10	41	4	128:1	610-670	130(5.7)	400(10.2)	310(10)	105(5)	330(17)	1180	0	204	$
Boost Plus	1.5	14	45	14	139:1	630-670	170(7.4)	380(9.7)	310(10)	105(5)	330(17)	946	0	187	$
Boost Diabetic	1.06	14	20	12	89:1	400	260(11.3)	260(6.7)	220(7)	80(4)	276(14)	1180	3.5	203	$$
Boost Breeze	0.7	8	31	0	102:1	900-930	50(2.2)	230(6)	350(11)	40(2)	150(8)	—	0	214	$

Modular	kcal	Protein	CHO	Fat
Beneprotein	25/pkt	6 g/pkt	0	0
Microlipid	4.5/ml	0	0	7.5 g/15 ml
Polycose	60/ounce	0	15 g/ounce	0

Enteral Formula	Carbohydrate Source	Protein Source	Fat Source
Nutren 1.0	Maltodextrin, corn syrup solids	Calcium, potassium caseinate	Canola oil, MCT, corn oil
Nutren 1.5	Maltodextrin	Calcium, potassium caseinate	MCT, canola oil, corn oil
Nutren 2.0	Corn syrup solids, maltodextrin, sucrose	Calcium, potassium caseinate	MCT, canola oil, corn oil
Probalance	Maltodextrin, corn syrup solids, gum arabic	Calcium, potassium caseinate	MCT, corn oil
Nutren Replete	Maltodextrin	Calcium, potassium caseinate	Canola oil, MCT
Nutren Renal	Maltodextrin	Calcium, potassium caseinate	MCT, canola oil, corn oil
Nutren Glytrol	Maltodextrin, modified cornstarch, pea fiber, gum arabic	Calcium, potassium caseinate	Canola oil, high oleic sunflower oil, MCT
Peptamen 1.5	Maltodextrin, cornstarch	Hydrolyzed whey protein	MCT, soybean oil
Crucial	Maltodextrin, cornstarch	Hydrolyzed casein, L-arginine	MCT, fish oil, soybean oil
Nutren Jr	Maltodextrin, sucrose	Milk protein concentrate, whey protein concentrate	Canola oil, MCT
Nutren Jr w/fiber	Maltodextrin, sucrose, pea fiber, oligofructose	Milk protein concentrate, whey protein concentrate	Soybean oil, canola oil, MCT
Oral Supplement			
Boost	Corn syrup solids, sugar	Milk protein concentrate	Canola oil, high oleic sunflower oil, corn oil
Boost Plus	Corn syrup solids, sugar	Milk protein concentrate, calcium and sodium caseinates	Canola oil, high oleic sunflower oil, corn oil
Boost Diabetic	Tapioca dextrin, fructose, corn syrup solids	Calcium and sodium caseinates, L-arginine	Canola oil
Boost Breeze	Fructose, juice concentrate, sugar	Whey protein isolate	
Modular			
Beneprotein	—	Whey protein isolate	—
Microlipid	—	—	Safflower oil
Polycose	Cornstarch	—	—

Appendix created by Ainsley M. Malone, MS, RD, CNSD.

APPENDIX 33 DASH Diet

The DASH diet is an eating pattern that reduces high blood pressure. It is not the traditional low-salt diet. DASH uses foods high in the minerals calcium, potassium, and magnesium, which when combined helps lower blood pressure. It is also low in fat and high in fiber, an eating style recommended for everyone.

The Healthy Eating Pattern is the template for the DASH eating pattern, with inclusion of ½ to 1 serving of nuts, seeds, and legumes daily, limited fats and oils, and use of nonfat or low-fat milk. The eating pattern is reduced in saturated fat, total fat, cholesterol, and sweet and sugar-containing beverages and provides abundant servings of fruits and vegetables.

Although the DASH eating plan is naturally lower in salt because of the emphasis on fruits and vegetables, all adults should still make an effort to reduce packaged and processed foods and high-sodium snacks (such as salted chips, pretzels, and crackers) and use less or no salt at the table.

DASH can be an excellent way to lose weight. Because weight loss can help lower blood pressure, it is often suggested. In addition to following DASH, try adding in daily physical activity such as walking or other exercise. You may want to check with your doctor first.

Current recommendations include:

The DASH Diet

Food Group	1600 kcal Servings/Day	2000 kcal Servings/Day	2600 kcal Servings/Day	3100 kcal Servings/Day
Grains (whole grains)	6	7-8	10-11	12-13
Vegetables	3-4	4-5	5-6	6
Fruits and juices	4	4-5	5-6	6
Milk, nonfat or low-fat	2-3	2-3	3	3-4
Meats, poultry, and fish	1-2	2 or less	6	2-3
Nuts, seeds, and legumes	3/week	½-1	1	1
Fats and oils	2	2-3	3	4
Sweets	0	5/week	Less than 2	2

Dietary Guidelines

Food Group	Servings/Day	Serving Sizes	Examples	Significance of Each Food Group
Grains	6-13	1 slice bread ½ cup (1 oz) dry cereal* ½ cup cooked rice, pasta, or cereal and fiber	Whole-wheat bread, English muffin, pita bread, bagel, cereals, grits, oatmeal, crackers, unsalted pretzels, and popcorn	Major sources of energy
Vegetables	3-6	1 cup raw, leafy veg. ½ cup cooked veg. 6 oz veg. juice	Tomatoes, potatoes, carrots, peas, kale, squash, broccoli, turnip greens, collards, spinach, artichokes, beans, sweet potatoes	Rich sources of potassium, magnesium, antioxidants, and fiber
Fruits	4-6	6 oz fruit juice 1 medium fruit ¼ cup dried fruit ½ cup fresh, frozen, or canned fruit	Apricots, bananas, dates, grapes, oranges and juice, tangerines, strawberries, mangoes, melons, peaches, pineapples, prunes, raisins, grapefruit and juice	Important sources energy, potassium, magnesium, and fiber
Low-fat dairy	2-4	8 oz milk, 1 cup yogurt, or 1.5 oz cheese	Fat-free or 1% milk, fat-free or low-fat buttermilk, yogurt, or cheese	Major sources of calcium, vitamin D, and protein
Meat, poultry, fish	1-3	3 oz cooked meats, poultry, or fish 1 egg white†	Select only lean meats; trim away visible fats, broil, roast, boil, instead of frying; remove skin from poultry	Rich sources of protein, zinc, and magnesium
Nuts, seeds, legumes	3/wk– 1/day	1.5 oz (½ cup) nuts, ½ oz or 2 tbsp seeds, ½ cup cooked legumes	Almonds, filberts, mixed nuts, walnuts, sunflower seeds, kidney beans, lentils	Rich sources of energy, magnesium, protein, monounsaturated fats, and fiber
Fat	2-4	1 tsp soft margarine, veg. oil, 1 Tbsp low-fat mayo or salad dressing, or 2 Tbsp light salad dressing‡	Soft margarine, low fat mayo, veg. oil, light salad dressing	The DASH study had 27% of calories as fat, including fat in or added to foods Sweets should be low in fat

National Institutes of Health, National Heart, Lung, and Blood Institute: YOUR GUIDE TO Lowering Your Blood Pressure With DASH, U.S. Department of Health and Human Services, NIH Publication No. 06-4082, 2006.

*Serving sizes vary between ½ cup and 1¼ cup, depending on cereal type. Check the product's Nutrition Facts label.

†Since eggs are high in cholesterol, limit egg yolk intake to no more than four per week; two egg whites have the same protein content as 1 oz of meat.

‡Fat content changes serving amount for fats and oils. For example, 1 Tbsp of regular salad dressing equals one serving; 1 Tbsp of a low-fat dressing equals one-half serving; 1 Tbsp of a fat-free dressing equals zero servings.

Sample Menu

Breakfast	Lunch	Dinner
1 cup calcium-fortified orange juice	3-oz boneless skinless chicken breast	1 cup spaghetti with vegetarian/low-sodium tomato sauce
¾ cup Raisin Bran	2 slices reduced-fat cheese	3 Tbsp Parmesan cheese
1 cup skim milk	2 large leaves lettuce	½ cup green beans
Mini-whole wheat bagel	2 slices tomato	1 cup spinach, raw
1½ tsp soft margarine	1 Tbsp light mayonnaise	¼ cup mushrooms, raw
1 cup coffee	2 slices whole wheat bread	2 Tbsp croutons
2 tsp sugar	1 medium apple	2 Tbsp low-fat Italian dressing
	½ cup raw carrot sticks	1 slice Italian bread
	1 cup iced tea	½ cup frozen yogurt

Midmorning Snack	Midafternoon Snack	
1 cup apple juice	1 large banana	
2 oz walnuts		

Nutritional Analysis:

Kilocalories: 1980	Sodium: 2377 mg
Protein: 78 g	Potassium: 4129 mg
Fat: 56 g	Fiber: 32 g
Saturated fat: 13 g	Magnesium: 517 g
Carbohydrates: 314 g	

APPENDIX **34** Exchange Lists for Meal Planning

MENU PLAN

Meal Plan for: _____ Date: _____

Dietitian: _____ Phone: _____

	Grams	Percent
Carbohydrate	_____	_____
Protein	_____	_____
Fat	_____	_____
Calories	_____	_____

Time	Number of Exchanges/Choices	Menu Ideas	Menu Ideas
	_____ Carbohydrate group _____ Starch _____ Fruit _____ Milk _____ _____ Meat group _____ _____ Fat group _____		
	_____ _____ _____ _____ _____ _____ _____ Carbohydrate group _____ Starch _____ Fruit _____ Milk _____ _____ Vegetables _____ Meat group _____ Fat group		
	_____ _____ _____ _____ _____ _____ _____ Carbohydrate group _____ Starch _____ Fruit _____ Milk _____ _____ Vegetables _____ Meat group _____ Fat group		

The Exchange Lists are the basis of a meal planning system designed by a committee of the American Diabetes Association and the American Dietetic Association. Although designed primarily for people with diabetes and others who must follow special diets, the Exchange Lists are based on principles of good nutrition that apply to everyone. ©2003 American Diabetes Association, Inc., The American Dietetic Association. Used with permission.

Continued

APPENDIX 34 Exchange Lists for Meal Planning—cont'd

STARCH LIST

Cereals, grains, pasta, breads, crackers, snacks, starchy vegetables, and cooked beans, peas, and lentils are starches. In general, one starch is
- ½ cup cooked cereal, grain, or starchy vegetable
- 1 oz bread product, such as 1 slice of bread
- ¾ to 1 ounce of most snack foods (Some snack foods may also have added fat.)
- ⅓ cup cooked rice or pasta

Nutrition Tips

1. Most starch choices are good sources of B vitamins.
2. Foods made from whole grains are good sources of fiber.
3. Dried beans and peas are a good source of protein and fiber.

Selection Tips

1. Choose starches made with little fat as often as you can.
2. Starchy vegetables prepared with fat count as one starch and one fat.
3. Bagel or muffins can be 2, 3, or 4 oz in size and therefore can count as 2, 3, or 4 starch choices. Check the size you eat.
4. Beans, peas, and lentils are also found on the Meat and Meat Substitutes list.
5. A waffle or pancake is about the size of a compact disc (CD) and about ¼-inch thick.
6. Because starches often swell in cooking, a small amount of uncooked starch becomes a much larger amount of cooked food.
7. Most of the serving sizes are measured or weighed after cooking.
8. Always check Nutrition Facts on the food label.

ONE STARCH EXCHANGE EQUALS 15 g CARBOHYDRATE, 3 g PROTEIN, 0-1 g FAT, AND 80 CALORIES

Bread

Bagel, 4 oz	¼ (1 oz)
Bread, reduced-calorie	2 slices (1½ oz)
Bread, white, whole-wheat, pumpernickel, rye	1 slice (1 oz)
Bread sticks, crisp, 4 in long × ½ in	4 (⅔ oz)
English muffin	½
Hot dog or hamburger bun	½ (1 oz)
Naan, 8 × 2″	¼
Pita, 6 in. across	½
Pancake, 4 in across, ¼ in thick	1
Roll, plain, small	1 (1 oz)
Raisin bread, unfrosted	1 slice (1 oz)
Tortilla, corn, 6 in across	1
Tortilla, flour, 6 in across	1
Tortilla, flour, 10 in across	⅓
Waffle, 4½ in square, reduced-fat	1

Cereals and Grains

Bran cereals	½ cup
Bulgur	½ cup
Cereals, cooked	½ cup
Cereals, unsweetened, ready-to-eat	¾ cup
Cornmeal (dry)	3 tbsp
Couscous	⅓ cup
Flour (dry)	3 tbsp
Granola, low-fat	¼ cup
Grape-Nuts	¼ cup
Grits	½ cup
Kashi	½ cup
Millet	⅓ cup
Muesli	¼ cup
Oats	½ cup
Pasta	½ cup
Puffed cereal	1½ cups
Rice, white or brown	⅓ cup
Shredded Wheat	½ cup
Sugar-frosted cereal	½ cup
Wheat germ	3 Tbsp

Starchy Vegetables

Baked beans	⅓ cup
Corn	½ cup
Corn on cob, large	½ cob (5 oz)

Starchy Vegetables—cont'd

Mixed vegetables with corn, peas, or pasta	1 cup
Peas, green	½ cup
Plantain	½ cup
Potato, baked with skin	¼ large (3 oz)
Potato, boiled	½ cup or ½ medium (3 oz)
Potato, mashed	½ cup
Squash, winter (acorn, butternut, pumpkin)	1 cup
Yam, sweet potato, plain	½ cup

Crackers and Snacks

Animal crackers	8
Graham crackers, 2½ in square	3
Matzoh	¾ oz
Melba toast	4 slices
Oyster crackers	24
Popcorn (popped, no fat added or low-fat microwave)	3 cups
Pretzels	¾ oz
Rice cakes, 4 in across	2
Saltine-type crackers	6
Snack chips, fat-free (tortilla, potato)	15-20 (¾ oz)
Whole-wheat crackers, no fat added	2-5 (¾ oz)

Beans, Peas, and Lentils

(Count as 1 starch exchange, plus 1 very lean meat exchange)

Beans and peas (garbanzo, pinto, kidney, white, split, black-eyed)	½ cup
Lima beans	⅔ cup
Lentils	½ cup
Miso*	3 Tbsp

Starchy Foods Prepared With Fat

(Count as 1 starch exchange, plus 1 fat exchange)

Biscuit, 2½ in across	1
Chow mein noodles	½ cup
Corn bread, 2 in cube	1 (oz)
Crackers, round butter type	6
Croutons	1 cup
French-fried potatoes, oven-baked	1 cup (12 oz)
Granola	¼ cup
Hummus	⅓ cup
Muffin, 5 oz	1 (1½ oz)

*400 mg or more sodium per exchange serving.

APPENDIX 34 Exchange Lists for Meal Planning—cont'd

STARCH LIST—cont'd
ONE STARCH EXCHANGE EQUALS 15 g CARBOHYDRATE, 3 g PROTEIN, 0-1 g FAT, AND 80 CALORIES

Starchy Foods Prepared With Fat—cont'd

Popcorn, microwave .... 3 cups
Sandwich crackers, cheese or peanut butter filling 3
Snack chips (potato, tortilla)................9-13 (¾ oz)
Stuffing, bread (prepared)............................ ⅓ cup
Taco shell, 6 in across 2
Waffle, 4½ in square 11
Whole-wheat crackers, fat added .... 4-6 (1 oz)

Some uncooked food will weigh less after you cook it. Starches often swell in cooking, so a small amount of uncooked starch will become a much larger amount of cooked food. The following table shows some of the changes.

Food (Starch Group)	Uncooked	Cooked
Oatmeal	3 Tbsp	½ cup
Cream of Wheat	2 Tbsp	½ cup
Grits	3 Tbsp	½ cup
Rice	2 Tbsp	⅓ cup
Spaghetti	¼ cup	½ cup
Noodles	⅓ cup	½ cup
Macaroni	¼ cup	½ cup
Dried beans	¼ cup	½ cup
Dried peas	¼ cup	½ cup
Lentils	3 Tbsp	½ cup

Common Measurements

3 tsp = 1 Tbsp	4 oz = ½ cup
4 Tbsp = ¼ cup	8 oz = 1 cup
5½ Tbsp = ⅓ cup	1 cup = ½ pint

FRUIT LIST

Fresh, frozen, canned, and dried fruits and fruit juices are on this list. In general, one fruit exchange is
- 1 small (4 oz) fresh fruit
- ½ cup of canned or fresh fruit or unsweetened fruit juice
- ¼ cup of dried fruit

Nutrition Tips

1. Fresh, frozen, and dried fruits have about 2 g of fiber per choice. Fruit juices contain very little fiber.

Selection Tips

1. Count ½ cup cranberries or rhubarb sweetened with sugar substitutes as free foods.

2. Read the Nutrition Facts on the food label. If one serving has more than 15 grams of carbohydrate, you will need to adjust the size of the serving you eat or drink.
3. Portion sizes for canned fruits are for the fruit and a small amount of juice.
4. Whole fruit is more filling than fruit juice and may be a better choice.
5. Food labels for fruits may contain the words "no sugar added" or "unsweetened." This means that no sucrose (table sugar) has been added.
6. Generally, fruit canned in extra light syrup has the same amount of carbohydrate per serving as the "no sugar added" or the juice pack. All canned fruits on the fruit list are based on one of these three types of packs.

ONE FRUIT EXCHANGE EQUALS 15 g CARBOHYDRATE AND 60 CALORIES
THE WEIGHT INCLUDES SKIN, CORE, SEEDS, AND RIND

Fruit

Apple, unpeeled, small............................. 1 (4 oz)
Applesauce, unsweetened ....½ cup
Apples, dried .... 4 rings
Apricots, fresh .... 4 whole (5½ oz)
Apricots, dried.................................... 8 halves
Apricots, canned ....½ cup
Banana, small................................... 1 (4 oz)
Blackberries ....¾ cup
Blueberries...¾ cup
Cantaloupe, small ....⅓ melon (11 oz) or 1 cup cubes
Cherries, sweet, fresh .... 12 (3 oz)
Cherries, sweet, canned...............................½ cup
Dates 3
Figs, fresh..................... 1½ large or 2 medium (3½ oz)
Figs, dried 1½
Fruit cocktail ....½ cup
Grapefruit, large ....½ (11 oz)
Grapefruit sections, canned ....¾ cup
Grapes, small .... 17 (3 oz)
Honeydew melon ....1 slice (10 oz) or 1 cup cubes
Kiwi ....1 (3½ oz)
Mandarin oranges, canned ....¾ cup
Mango, small................... ½ fruit (5½ oz) or ½ cup
Nectarine, small.................................. 1 (5 oz)
Orange, small................................1 (6½ oz)

Papaya .... ½ fruit (8 oz) or 1 cup cubes
Peach, medium, fresh .... 1 (6 oz)
Peaches, canned.....................................½ cup
Pear, large, fresh ....½ (4 oz)
Pears, canned ....½ cup
Pineapple, fresh ....¾ cup
Pineapple, canned ....½ cup
Plums, small.. 2 (5 oz)
Plums, canned ....½ cup
Prunes, dried 3
Raisins ....2 Tbsp
Raspberries... 1 cup
Strawberries........................1¼ cup whole berries
Tangerines, small................................. 2 (8 oz)
Watermelon..............1 slice (13½ oz) or 1¼ cup cubes

Fruit juice

Apple juice/cider ....½ cup
Cranberry juice cocktail ....⅓ cup
Cranberry juice cocktail, reduced-calorie.................. 1 cup
Fruit juice blends, 100% juice ....⅓ cup
Grape juice...⅓ cup
Grapefruit juice.....................................½ cup
Orange juice..½ cup
Pineapple juice......................................½ cup
Prune juice...⅓ cup

Continued

APPENDIX 34 Exchange Lists for Meal Planning—cont'd

MILK LIST

Different types of milk and milk products are on this list. Cheeses are on the Meat list, and cream and other diary fats are on the Fat list. Based on the amount of fat they contain, milks are divided into fat-free/low-fat milk, and whole milk. One choice of these includes:

	Carbohydrate (g)	Protein (g)	Fat (g)	Calories
Fat-free/low-fat (½% or 1%)	12	8	0-3	90
Reduced fat 2%	12	8	8	150
Whole	12	8	8	150

Nutrition Tips

1. Milk and yogurt are good sources of calcium and protein. Check the Nutrition Facts on the food label.

2. The higher the fat content of milk and yogurt, the greater the amount of saturated fat and cholesterol. Choose lower-fat varieties.
3. For those who are lactose intolerant, look for lactose-reduced or lactose-free varieties of milk. Check the food label for total amount of carbohydrate per serving.

Selection Tips

1. One cup equals 8 fluid ounces or ½ pint.
2. Look for chocolate milk, frozen yogurt, and ice cream on the other Carbohydrates list.
3. Nondairy creamers are on the Free Foods list.

ONE MILK EXCHANGE EQUALS 12 G CARBOHYDRATE, 8 g PROTEIN, 0-8 g FAT, AND 90-150 kcal

Fat-Free and Low-Fat Milk 90 kcal (0–3 g fat per serving)

Fat-free milk	1 cup
½% milk	1 cup
1% milk	1 cup
Buttermilk, low-fat or fat-free	1 cup
Evaporated fat-free milk	½ cup
Fat free dry milk	⅓ cup dry
Yogurt, plain nonfat	¾ cup
Yogurt, fat-free, flavored, sweetened with nonnutritive sweetener and fructose	1 cup
Soy milk, low-fat or fat-free	1 cup

Reduced-Fat 120 kcal (5 g fat per serving)

2% milk	1 cup
Yogurt, plain lowfat	¾ cup
Sweet acidophilus milk	1 cup
Soy milk	1 cup

Whole Milk 150 kcal (8 g fat per serving)

Whole milk	1 cup
Evaporated whole milk	½ cup
Goat's milk	1 cup
Kefir	1 cup
Yogurt, plain (made from whole milk)	¾ cup

SWEETS, DESSERTS, AND OTHER CARBOHYDRATES LIST

You can substitute food choices from this list for a starch, fruit, or milk choice on your meal plan. Some choices will also count as one or more fat choices.

Nutrition Tips

1. These foods can be substituted in your meal plan, even though they contain added sugars or fat. However, they do not contain as many important vitamins and minerals as the choices on the Starch, Fruit, or Milk lists.
2. When planning to include these foods in your meal, include foods from the other lists to eat a balanced meal.

Selection Tips

1. Because many of these foods are concentrated sources of carbohydrate, fat, saturated fat, and *trans*-fat, the portion sizes are often very small.
2. Look for the words "hydrogenated" or "partially hydrogenated" on the label. The lower down the list these words appear, the fewer *trans*-fats there are.
3. Always check Nutrition Facts on the food label. It will be your most accurate source of information.
4. Many fat-free or reduced-fat products made with fat replacers contain carbohydrate. When eaten in large amounts, they may need to be counted. Talk with your dietitian to determine how to count these in your meal plan.
5. Look for fat-free salad dressings in smaller amounts on the Free Foods list.

ONE OTHER CARBOHYDRATE EXCHANGE EQUALS 15 g CARBOHYDRATE, OR 1 STARCH, OR 1 FRUIT, OR 1 MILK

Food	Serving Size	Exchanges per Serving
Angel food cake, unfrosted	1/12 cake (about 2 oz)	2 carbohydrates
Brownie, small, unfrosted	2 in. square (about 1 oz)	1 carbohydrate, 1 fat
Cake, unfrosted	2 in. square (about 1 oz)	1 carbohydrate, 1 fat
Cake, frosted	2 in. square (about 2 oz)	2 carbohydrates, 1 fat
Cookie, sugar-free	3 small or 1 large (⅔ oz)	1 carbohydrate, 1-2 fats
Cookie or sandwich cookie with cream filling	2 small or 1 large (⅔ oz)	1 carbohydrate, 1 fat
Cranberry sauce, jellied	¼ cup	1½ carbohydrates
Cupcake, frosted	1 small	2 carbohydrates, 1 fat
Doughnut, plain cake	1 medium (1½ oz)	1½ carbohydrates, 2 fats

APPENDIX 34 Exchange Lists for Meal Planning—cont'd

ONE OTHER CARBOHYDRATE EXCHANGE EQUALS 15 g CARBOHYDRATE, OR 1 STARCH, OR 1 FRUIT, OR 1 MILK—cont'd

Food	Serving Size	Exchanges per Serving
Doughnut, glazed	3¾ in across (2 oz)	2 carbohydrates, 2 fats
Energy, sport, or breakfast bar	2 oz	2 carbohydrates, 1 fat
Fruit juice bars, frozen, 100% juice	1 bar (3 oz)	1 carbohydrate
Fruit snacks, chewy (pureed fruit concentrate)	1 roll (¾ oz)	1 carbohydrate
Fruit spreads, 100% fruit	1½ Tbsp	1 carbohydrate
Gelatin, regular	½ cup	1 carbohydrate
Gingersnaps	3	1 carbohydrate
Granola bar or snack bar, regular or low-fat	1 bar	1½ carbohydrates
Honey	1 Tbsp	1 carbohydrate
Ice cream, light	½ cup	1 carbohydrate, 1 fat
Ice cream, fat-free, no sugar added	½ cup	1 carbohydrate
Jam or jelly, regular	1 Tbsp	1 carbohydrate
Milk, chocolate, whole	1 cup	2 carbohydrates, 1 fat
Pie, fruit, 2 crusts	⅙ of 8 in pie	3 carbohydrates, 2 fats
Pie, pumpkin or custard	⅛ of 8 in pie	2 carbohydrates, 2 fats
Pudding, regular (made with reduced fat milk)	½ cup	2 carbohydrates
Pudding, sugar-free (made with fat-free milk)	½ cup	1 carbohydrate
Reduced calorie meal replacement (shake)	1 can (10-11 oz)	1½ carbohydrates, 0-1 fat
Rice milk, low-fat, flavored	1 cup	1½ carbohydrates
Salad dressing, fat-free	¼ cup	1 carbohydrate
Sherbet, sorbet	½ cup	2 carbohydrates
Spaghetti or pasta sauce, canned*	½ cup	1 carbohydrate, 1 fat
Sport drink	1 cup (8 oz)	1 carbohydrate
Sugar	1 Tbsp	1 carbohydrate
Sweet roll or Danish	1 (2½ oz)	2½ carbohydrates, 2 fats
Syrup, light	2 Tbsp	1 carbohydrate
Syrup, regular	1 Tbsp	1 carbohydrate
Syrup, regular	¼ cup	4 carbohydrates
Vanilla wafers	5	1 carbohydrate, 1 fat
Yogurt, frozen	½ cup	1 carbohydrate, 0-1 fat
Yogurt, frozen, fat-free	⅓ cup	1 carbohydrate
Yogurt, low-fat with fruit	1 cup	3 carbohydrates, 0-1 fat

NONSTARCHY VEGETABLE LIST

Vegetables that contain small amounts of carbohydrates and calories are on this list. Vegetables contain important nutrients. Try to eat at least two or three vegetable choices each day. In general, one vegetable exchange is:

• ½ cup of cooked vegetables or vegetable juice
• 1 cup of raw vegetables

If you eat one to two vegetable choices at a meal or snack, you do not have to count the calories or carbohydrates because they contain small amounts of these nutrients.

Nutrition Tips

1. Fresh and frozen vegetables have less added salt than canned vegetables. Drain and rinse canned vegetables if you want to remove some salt.
2. Choose more dark green and dark yellow vegetables such as spinach, broccoli, romaine, carrots, chilies, and peppers.

3. Broccoli, Brussels sprouts, cauliflower, greens, peppers, spinach, and tomatoes are good sources of vitamin C.
4. Vegetables contain 1 to 4 g of fiber per serving.

Selection Tips

1. A 1-cup portion of broccoli is a portion about the size of a light bulb.
2. Tomato sauce is different from spaghetti sauce, which is on the Other Carbohydrates list.
3. Canned vegetables and juices are available without added salt.
4. Starchy vegetables such as corn, peas, winter squash, and potatoes that contain larger amounts of calories and carbohydrates are on the Starch list.

ONE NONSTARCHY VEGETABLE EXCHANGE EQUALS 5 g CARBOHYDRATE, 2 g PROTEIN, 0 g FAT, AND 25 CALORIES

Artichoke	Broccoli
Artichoke hearts	Brussels sprouts
Asparagus	Cabbage
Beans (green, wax, Italian)	Carrots
Bean sprouts	Cauliflower
Beets	Celery

*400 mg or more sodium per exchange serving.

Continued

APPENDIX 34 Exchange Lists for Meal Planning—cont'd

NONSTARCHY VEGETABLE LIST—cont'd
ONE NONSTARCHY VEGETABLE EXCHANGE EQUALS 5 g CARBOHYDRATE, 2 g PROTEIN, 0 g FAT, AND 25 CALORIES

Cucumber
Egg plant
Green onions or scallions
Green (collard, kale, mustard, turnip)
Kohlrabi
Leeks
Mixed vegetables (without corn, peas, or pasta)
Mushrooms
Okra
Onions
Pea pods
Peppers (all varieties)
Radishes

Salad greens (endive, escarole, lettuce, romaine, spinach)
Sauerkraut*
Spinach
Summer squash
Tomato
Tomatoes, canned
Tomato sauce*
Tomato/vegetable juice*
Turnips
Water chestnuts
Watercress
Zucchini

MEAT AND MEAT SUBSTITUTES LIST

Meat and meat substitutes that contain both protein and fat are on this list. In general, one meat exchange is:
• 1 oz meat, fish, poultry, or cheese
• ½ cup beans, peas, or lentils
Based on the amount of fat they contain, meats are divided into very lean, lean, medium-fat, and high-fat lists. This is done so you can see which ones contain the least amount of fat. One ounce (one exchange) of each of these includes:

	Carbohydrate (g)	Protein (g)	Fat (g)	Calories
Very lean	0	7	0-1	35
Lean	0	7	3	55
Medium-fat	0	7	5	75
High-fat	0	7	8	100

Nutrition Tips

1. Choose very lean and lean meat choices whenever possible. Items from the high-fat group are high in saturated fat, cholesterol, and calories and can raise blood cholesterol levels.
2. Beans, peas, and lentils are good sources of fiber, about 3 g per serving.
3. Some processed meats, seafood, and soy products may contain carbohydrate when consumed in large amounts. Check the Nutrition Facts on the label to see if the amount is close to 15 g. If so, count it as a carbohydrate choice as well as a meat choice.

Selection Tips

1. Weigh meat after cooking and removing bones and fat. Four oz of raw meat is equal to 3 oz of cooked meat. Some examples of meat portions are:
   • 1 oz cheese = meat choice and is about the size of a 1-inch cube
   • 2 oz meat = meat choices, such as
      1 small chicken leg or thigh
      ½ cup cottage cheese or tuna

*400 mg or more sodium per exchange serving.

• 3 oz meat = meat choices and is about the size of a deck of cards, such as
      1 medium pork chop
      1 small chicken leg or thigh
      ½ cup cottage cheese or tuna
      1 unbreaded fish fillet
2. Limit your choices from the high-fat group to three times per week or less.
3. Most grocery stores stock select and choice grades of meat. Select grades of meat are the leanest meats. Choice grades contain a moderate amount of fat, and prime cuts of meat have the highest amount of fat. Restaurants usually serve prime cuts of meat.
4. "Hamburger" may contain added seasoning and fat, but ground beef does not.
5. Read labels to find products that are low in fat and cholesterol (5 g or less of fat per serving).
6. Dried beans, peas, and lentils are also found on the Starch list.
7. Peanut butter, in smaller amounts, is also found on the Fats list.
8. Bacon, in smaller amounts, is also found on the Fats list.
9. A 3.5 oz hamburger patty has about half its calories from fat.
10. Meatless burgers are on the Combination Food list.

Meal Planning Tips

1. Bake, roast, broil, grill, poach, steam, or boil rather than fry these foods.
2. Place meat on a rack so the fat will drain off during cooking.
3. Use a nonstick spray and a nonstick pan to brown or fry foods.
4. Trim off visible fat before or after cooking.
5. If you add flour, bread crumbs, coating mixes, fat, or marinades when cooking, ask your dietitian how to count it in your meal plan.

APPENDIX 34 Exchange Lists for Meal Planning—cont'd

VERY LEAN MEAT AND SUBSTITUTES LIST
ONE EXCHANGE EQUALS 0 g CARBOHYDRATE, 7 g PROTEIN, 0-1 g FAT, AND 35 CALORIES

One very lean meat exchange is equal to any one of the following items

Poultry: Chicken or turkey (white meat, no skin), Cornish hen (no skin) .... 1 oz

Fish: Fresh or frozen cod, flounder, haddock, halibut, trout; lox,* tuna, fresh or canned in water .... 1 oz

Shellfish: Clams, crab, lobster, scallops, shrimp, imitation shellfish..................................... 1 oz

Game: Duck or pheasant (no skin), venison, buffalo, ostrich.. 1 oz

Cheese with 1 g or less fat per ounce:
Fat-free or low-fat cottage cheese..................... ¼ cup
Fat-free cheese....................................... 1 oz

Other: Processed sandwich meats with 1 g or less fat per ounce, such as deli thin, shaved meats, chipped beef,* turkey ham............................. 1 oz
Egg whites 2
Eggs substitutes, plain............................... ¼ cup
Hot dogs with 1 g or less fat per ounce* .... 1 oz
Kidney (high in cholesterol) .... 1 oz
Sausage with 1 g or less fat per ounce .... 1 oz

Count as one very lean meat and one starch exchange:
beans, peas, lentils (cooked) .... ½ cup

LEAN MEAT AND SUBSTITUTES LIST
ONE EXCHANGE EQUALS 0 g CARBOHYDRATE, 7 g PROTEIN, 3 g FAT, AND 55 CALORIES

One lean meat exchange is equal to any one of the following items.

Beef: USDA Select or Choice grades of lean beef trimmed of fat, such as round, sirloin, and flank steak; tenderloin; roast (rib, chuck, rump); steak (T-bone, porterhouse, cubed), ground round .... 1 oz

Pork: Lean pork, such as fresh ham; canned, cured, or boiled ham; Canadian bacon,* tenderloin, center loin chop...................................... 1 oz

Lamb: Roast, chop, leg................................ 1 oz

Veal: Lean chop, leg.................................. 1 oz

Poultry: Chicken, turkey (dark meat, no skin), chicken (white meat with skin), domestic duck or goose (well-drained of fat, no skin) .... 1 oz

Fish:
Herring (uncreamed or smoked)......................... 1 oz
Oysters .... 6 medium
Salmon (fresh or canned), catfish..................... 1 oz
Tuna (canned in oil), drained........................ 1 oz

Game: Goose (no skin), rabbit .... 1 oz

Cheese:
.5%-fat cottage cheese .... ¼ cup
Grated Parmesan .... 2 Tbsp
Cheeses with 3 g or less fat per ounce................. 1 oz

Other:
Hot dogs with 3 g or less fat per ounce*................ 1 oz
Processed sandwich meat with 3 g or less fat per ounce, such as turkey pastrami or kielbasa .... 1 oz
Liver, heart (high in cholesterol)..................... 1 oz

MEDIUM-FAT AND MEAT SUBSTITUTES LIST
ONE EXCHANGE EQUALS 0 g CARBOHYDRATE, 7 g PROTEIN, 5 g FAT, AND 75 CALORIES

One medium-fat meat exchange is equal to any one of the following items.

Beef: Most beef products fall into this category (ground beef; meatloaf, corned beef; short ribs; prime grades of meat trimmed of fat, such as prime rib)..................... 1 oz

Pork: Top loin, chop, Boston butt, cutlet .... 1 oz

Lamb: Rib roast, ground .... 1 oz

Veal: Cutlet (ground or cubed, unbreaded)............... 1 oz

Poultry: Chicken dark meat (with skin), ground turkey or ground chicken, fried chicken (with skin) .... 1 oz

Fish: Any fried fish product............................ 1 oz

Cheese: With 5 g or less fat per ounce
Feta .... 1 oz
Mozzarella.. 1 oz
Ricotta... cup (2 oz)

Other:
Egg (high in cholesterol, limit to 3 per week)............ 1
Sausage with 5 g or less fat per ounce.................. 1 oz
Tempeh .... ¼ cup
Tofu.. 4 oz or ½ cup

HIGH-FAT MEAT AND SUBSTITUTES LIST
ONE EXCHANGE EQUALS 0 g CARBOHYDRATE, 7 g PROTEIN, 8 g FAT, AND 100 CALORIES

Remember that these items are high in saturated fat, cholesterol, and calories and may raise blood cholesterol levels if eaten on a regular basis. One high-fat meat exchange is equal to any one of the following items.

Pork: Spareribs, ground pork, pork sausage .... 1 oz

Cheese: All regular cheeses, such as American,* cheddar, Monterey Jack, Swiss............................... 1 oz

Other: Processed sandwich meats with 8 g or less fat per ounce such as bologna, pimento loaf, salami .... 1 oz

Sausage such as bratwurst, Italian, knockwurst, Polish, smoked .... 1 oz
Hot dog (turkey or chicken)*........................ 1 (10/lb)
Bacon .... 3 slices (20 slices/lb)
Kidney (high in cholesterol) .... 1 oz
Peanut butter (contains unsaturated fat)................ 2 Tbsp
Count as one high-fat meat plus one fat exchange: hot dog (beef, pork, or combination)*.................... 1 (10/lb)

*400 mg or more sodium per exchange serving.

Continued

APPENDIX 34 Exchange Lists for Meal Planning—cont'd

FAT LIST

Fats are divided into three groups, based on the main type of fat they contain: monounsaturated, polyunsaturated, and saturated. Small amounts of monounsaturated and polyunsaturated fats in the foods we eat are linked with good health benefits. Saturated fats are linked with heart disease and cancer. In general, one fat exchange is
- 1 tsp of regular margarine or vegetable oil
- 1 Tbsp of regular salad dressing

Nutrition Tips

1. All fats are high in calories. Limit serving sizes for good nutrition and health.
2. Nuts and seeds contain small amounts of fiber, protein, and magnesium.
3. If blood pressure is a concern, choose fats in the unsalted form to help lower sodium intake, such as unsalted peanuts.

Selection Tips

1. Check the Nutrition Facts on food labels for serving sizes. One fat exchange is based on a serving size containing 5 g of fat.

2. Food label Nutrition Facts usually list total fat and saturated fat grams per serving. When most calories come from saturated fats, the food fits into the Saturated Fat list.
3. When selecting regular margarine, choose one with liquid vegetable oil as the first ingredient. Soft margarines are not as saturated as stick margarines and are healthier choices. Avoid those listing hydrogenated or partially hydrogenated fat as the first ingredient because they will contain more *trans*-fatty acids.
4. When selecting low-fat margarines, look for liquid vegetable oil as the second ingredient. Water is usually the first ingredient.
5. When used in smaller amounts, bacon and peanut butter are counted as fat choices, When used in larger amounts, they are counted as high-fat meat choices.
6. Fat-free salad dressings are on the Other Carbohydrates list and the Free Foods list.
7. See the Free Foods list for nondairy products such as margarines, salad dressing, mayonnaise, sour cream, cream cheese, and nonstick cooking spray.

MONOUNSATURATED FATS LIST
ONE FAT EXCHANGE EQUALS 5 g FAT AND 45 CALORIES

Avocado, medium . . . . .2 Tbsp (1 oz)	Peanut butter, smooth or crunchy. . . . . ½ Tbsp
Oil (canola, olive, peanut). . . . . .1 tsp	Sesame seeds. . . . . .1 Tbsp
Olives: ripe (black)	Tahini or sesame paste . . . . 2 tsp
green, stuffed* . . . . 10 large	
Nuts	
almonds, cashews . . . . .6 nuts	
mixed (50% peanuts) . . . . .6 nuts	
peanuts . . . . .10 nuts	
pecans . . . . 4 halves	

POLYUNSATURATED FATS LIST
ONE FAT EXCHANGE EQUALS 5 g FAT AND 45 CALORIES

Margarine: stick, tub, or squeeze . . . . .1 tsp	Salad dressing regular*. . . . . .1 Tbsp
lower-fat (30% to 50% vegetable oil. . . . . .1 Tbsp	reduced-fat. . . . . 1¼ Tbsp
Mayonnaise: regular . . . . .1 tsp	Miracle Whip Salad Dressing: regular . . . . .2 tsp
reduced-fat. . . . . .1 Tbsp	reduced-fat . . . . .1 Tbsp
Nuts, walnuts, English . . . . 4 halves	Seeds: pumpkin, sunflower. . . . . .1 Tbsp
Oil (corn, safflower, soybean) . . . . .1 tsp	

SATURATED FATS LIST*
ONE FAT EXCHANGE EQUALS 5 g FAT AND 45 CALORIES

Bacon, cooked . . . . .1 slice (20 slices/lb)	Cream, half and half. . . . . .2 Tbsp
Bacon, grease. . . . . .1 tsp	Cream cheese: regular . . . . 1¼ Tbsp (1 oz)
Butter: stick . . . . .1 tsp	reduced-fat . . . . 1 Tbsp (¼ oz)
whipped . . . . .2 tsp	Fatback or salt pork†
reduced-fat. . . . . .1 Tbsp	Shortening or lard . . . . .1 tsp
Chitterlings, boiled . . . . .2 Tbsp (¼ cup)	Sour cream: regular . . . . .2 Tbsp
Coconut, sweetened, shredded . . . . .2 Tbsp	reduced-fat . . . . .3 Tbsp
Coconut milk. . . . . .1 Tbsp	

*Saturated fats can raise blood cholesterol levels.

†Use a piece 1 in. × ¼ in. if you plan to eat the fatback cooked with vegetables. Use a piece 2 in. × 1 in. × ½ in. when eating only the vegetables with the fatback removed.

APPENDIX 34   Exchange Lists for Meal Planning—cont'd

FREE FOODS LIST

A *free food* is any food or drink that contains less than 20 calories or less than 5 g of carbohydrate per serving. Foods with a serving size listed should be limited to three servings per day. Be sure to spread them out throughout the day. If you eat all three servings at one time, it could affect your blood glucose level. Foods listed without a serving size can be eaten whenever you like.

Fat-Free or Reduced-Fat Foods

Cream cheese, fat	1 Tbsp (½ cup)
Creamers, nondairy, liquid	1 Tbsp
Creamers, nondairy, powdered	2 tsp
Mayonnaise, fat-free	1 Tbsp
Mayonnaise, reduced-fat	1 tsp
Margarine, fat-free	4 Tbsp
Margarine, reduced-fat	1 tsp
Miracle Whip, fat-free	1 Tbsp
Miracle Whip, reduced-fat	1 tsp

Nonstick cooking spray	
Salad dressing, fat-free	1 Tbsp
Salad dressing, fat-free, Italian	2 Tbsp
Salad dressing, fat-free	1 Tbsp
Sour cream, fat-free, reduced fat	1 Tbsp
Whipped topping, regular	1 Tbsp
Whipped topping, light or fat-free	2 Tbsp

Sugar-Free or Low-Sugar Foods

Candy, hard, sugar-free	1 candy
Gelatin dessert	
Gelatin, unflavored	
Gum, sugar-free	
Jam or jelly, low-sugar or light	2 tsp
Sugar substitutes*	
Syrup, sugar-free	2 Tbsp

DRINKS

Bouillon, broth, consommé†	
Bouillon or broth, low-sodium	
Carbonated or mineral water	
Club soda	
Cocoa powder, unsweetened	1 Tbsp

Coffee	
Diet soft drinks, sugar-free	
Drink mixes, sugar-free	
Tea	
Tonic water, sugar-free	

CONDIMENTS

Catsup	1 Tbsp
Horseradish	
Lemon juice	
Lime juice	
Mustard	
Pickle relish	1 Tbsp
Pickles, dill†	1½ large

Pickles, sweet (gherkin)	¾ oz
Pickles, sweet (bread and butter)	2 slices
Salsa	¼ cup
Soy sauce, regular or light†	1 Tbsp
Taco sauce	1 Tbsp
Vinegar	
Yogurt	2 Tbsp

SEASONINGS

Be careful with seasonings that contain sodium or are salts such as garlic or celery salt and lemon pepper.
Flavoring extracts
Garlic
Herbs, fresh or dried

Pimento
Spices
Tobasco or hot pepper sauce
Wine, used in cooking
Worcestershire sauce

*Sugar substitutes, alternatives, or replacement that are approved by the Food and Drug Administration (FDA) are safe to use. Common brand names include: Equal (aspartame), Splenda (sucralose), Sprinkle Sweet (saccharin), Sweet One (acesulfame K), Sweet-10 (saccharin), Sugar Twin (saccharin), Sweet 'n Low (saccharin).

†400 mg or more sodium per exchange serving.

Continued

APPENDIX 34 Exchange Lists for Meal Planning—cont'd

COMBINATION FOODS LIST

Many of the foods we eat are mixed together in various combinations. These combination foods do not fit into any one exchange list. Often it is hard to tell what is in a casserole dish or prepared food item. This is a list of exchanges for some typical combination foods. This list will help you fit these foods into your meal plan. Ask your dietitian for information about any other combination foods you would like to eat.

Food	Serving Size	Exchange per Serving
Entrees		
Tuna or chicken salad	½ cup (3½ oz)	½ carbohydrate, 2 lean meats, 1 fat
Tuna noodle casserole, lasagna, spaghetti with meatballs, chili with beans, macaroni and cheese†	1 cup (8 oz)	2 carbohydrates, 2 medium-fat meats
Chow mein (without noodles or rice)	2 cups (16 oz)	1 carbohydrate, 2 lean meats
Frozen Entrees and Meals		
Pizza, cheese, thin crust*	¼ of 12 in (6 oz)	2 carbohydrates, 2 medium-fat meats, 1 fat
Pizza, meat topping, thin crust*	¼ of 12 in (6 oz)	2 carbohydrates, 2 medium-fat meats, 1 fat
Pot pie*	1 (7 oz)	2½ carbohydrates, 1 medium-fat meat, 3 fats
Dinner type meal	14-17 oz	3 carbohydrates, 3 lean meats, 3 fats
Meatless burger, soy-based	3 oz	½ carbohydrate, 2 lean meats
Meatless burger, vegetable- and starch-based	3 oz	1 carbohydrate, 1 lean meat
Soups		
Bean*	1 cup	1 carbohydrate, 1 very lean meat
Cream (made with water)*	1 cup (8 oz)	1 carbohydrate, 1 fat
Instant*	6 oz prepared	1 carbohydrate
Instant with beans/lentils*	8 oz prepared	2½ carbohydrates, 1 very lean meat
Split pea (made with water)*	½ cup (4 oz)	1 carbohydrate
Tomato (made with water)*	1 cup (8 oz)	1 carbohydrate
Vegetable beef, chicken noodle, or other broth-type†	1 cup (8 oz)	1 carbohydrate

FAST FOODS†

Food	Serving Size	Exchanges per Serving
Burritos with beef†	2	4 carbohydrates, 2 medium-fat meats, 2 fats
Chicken nuggets†	6	1 carbohydrate, 2 medium-fat meats, 1 fat
Chicken breast and wing, breaded and fried†	1 each	1 carbohydrate, 4 medium-fat meats, 2 fats
Chicken sandwich, grilled*	1	2 carbohydrates, 3 very lean meat
Chicken wings, hot*	6 (5 oz)	1 carbohydrate, 3 medium-fat meats, 4 fats
Fish sandwich/tartar sauce†	1	3 carbohydrates, 1 medium-fat meat, 3 fats
French fries*	1 medium (5 oz)	4 carbohydrates, 4 fats
Hamburger, regular	1	2 carbohydrates, 2 medium-fat meats
Hamburger, large†	1	2 carbohydrates, 3 medium-fat meats, 1 fat
Hot dog with bun†	1	1 carbohydrate, 1 high-fat meat, 1 fat
Pizza, cheese, thin crust*	¼ of 12 in. (6 oz)	2½ carbohydrates, 2 medium-fat meats
Pizza, meat, thin crust*	¼ of 12 in. (6 oz)	2½ carbohydrates, 2 medium-fat meats, 1 fat
Soft-serve cone	1 small (5 oz)	2 carbohydrates, 1 fat
Submarine sandwich* (less than 6 g fat)	1 sub (6 in.)	2½ carbohydrates, 2 high-fat meats
Taco, soft shell* or hard shell	1 of (3 to 3½ oz)	1 carbohydrate, 1 medium-fat meat, 1 fat

*400 mg or more sodium per exchange serving.

†Ask at fast-food restaurant for nutrition information about favorite fast foods.

APPENDIX 35 National Dysphagia Diets

The following solid food texture levels have been recommended based on the food properties on the food texture scales.

Level 1: Dysphagia: Pureed

Description: This diet consists of pureed, homogenous, and cohesive foods. Food should be "puddinglike." No coarse textures, raw fruits or vegetables, nuts, and so forth are allowed. Any foods that require bolus formation, controlled manipulation, or mastication are excluded.

Rationale: This diet is designed for people who have moderate-to-severe dysphagia, with poor oral phase abilities and reduced ability to protect their airway. Close or complete supervision and alternate feeding methods may be required.

Liquid Consistency (circle one)

Thin (includes all un-thickened beverages and supplements)	Nectarlike	Honeylike	Spoon-thick

Food Textures for NDD Level 1: Dysphagia: Pureed

Food Groups	Recommended	Avoid	If Thin Liquids Are Allowed, Also May Have
Beverages	Any smooth, homogenous beverages without lumps, chunks, or pulp; beverages may need to be thickened to appropriate consistency	Any beverages with lumps, chunks, seeds, pulp, etc.	Milk, juices, coffee, tea, sodas, carbonated beverages, alcoholic beverages, nutritional supplements Ice chips
Breads	Commercially or facility-prepared pureed bread mixes, pregelled slurried breads, pancakes, sweet rolls, Danish pastries, French toast, etc., that are gelled through entire thickness of product	All other breads, rolls, crackers, biscuits, pancakes, waffles, French toast, muffins, etc.	
Cereals *(Cereals may have just enough milk to moisten.)*	Smooth, homogenous, cooked cereals such as farina-type cereals Cereals should have a "puddinglike" consistency	All dry cereals and any cooked cereals with lumps, seeds, chunks Oatmeal	Enough milk or cream with cereals to moisten; they should be blended in well
Desserts	Smooth puddings, custards, yogurt, pureed desserts, and soufflés	Ices, gelatins, frozen juice bars, cookies, cakes, pies, pastry, coarse or textured puddings, bread and rice pudding, fruited yogurt *These foods are considered thin liquids and should be avoided if thin liquids are restricted:* Frozen malts, milk shakes, frozen yogurt, eggnog, nutritional supplements, ice cream, sherbet, regular or sugar-free gelatin, or any foods that become thin liquid at either room (70° F) or body temperature (98° F)	Frozen malts, yogurt, milk shakes, eggnog, nutritional supplements, ice cream, sherbet, plain regular or sugar-free gelatin
Fats	Butter, margarine, strained gravy, sour cream, mayonnaise, cream cheese, whipped topping Smooth sauces such as white sauce, cheese sauce, or hollandaise sauce	All fats with coarse or chunky additives	
Fruits	Pureed fruits or well-mashed fresh bananas Fruit juices without pulp, seeds, or chunks (may need to be thickened to appropriate consistency if thin liquids are restricted)	Whole fruits (fresh, frozen, canned, dried)	Unthickened fruit juices

From American Dietetic Association: *National dysphagia diet: standardization for optimal care,* Chicago, 2003, ADA.

Continued

APPENDIX 35 National Dysphagia Diets—cont'd

Food Textures for NDD Level 1: Dysphagia: Pureed—cont'd

Food Groups	Recommended	Avoid	If Thin Liquids Are Allowed, Also May Have
Meats and meat substitutes	Pureed meats Braunschweiger Soufflés that are smooth and homogenous Softened tofu mixed with moisture Hummus or other pureed legume spread	Whole or ground meats, fish, or poultry Nonpureed lentils or legumes Cheese, cottage cheese Peanut butter, unless pureed into foods correctly Nonpureed, fried, scrambled, or hard-cooked eggs	
Potatoes and starches	Mashed potatoes or sauce; pureed potatoes with gravy, butter, margarine, or sour cream Well-cooked pasta, noodles, bread dressing, or rice that has been pureed in a blender to smooth, homogenous consistency	All other potatoes, rice, noodles Plain mashed potatoes, cooked grains Nonpureed bread dressing	
Soups	Soups that have been pureed in a blender or strained; may need to be thickened to appropriate viscosity	Soups that have chunks, lumps, etc.	Broth and other thin, strained soups
Vegetables	Pureed vegetables without chunks, lumps, pulp, or seeds Tomato paste or sauce without seeds Tomato or vegetables juice (may need to be thickened to appropriate consistency if juice is thinner than prescribed liquid consistency)	All other vegetables that have not been pureed Tomato sauce with seeds, thin tomato juice	Thin tomato or vegetable juices
Miscellaneous	Sugar, artificial sweetener, salt, finely ground pepper, and spices Ketchup, mustard, barbecue sauce, and other smooth sauces Honey, smooth jellies Very soft, smooth candy such as truffles	Coarsely ground pepper and herbs Chunky fruit preserves and seedy jams Seeds, nuts, sticky foods Chewy candies such as caramels or licorice	Smooth chocolate candy with no nuts, sprinkles, etc.

Level 2: Dysphagia: Mechanically Altered Characteristics

Description: This level consists of foods that are moist, soft-textured, and easily formed into a bolus. Meats are ground or are minced no larger than one quarter–inch pieces; they are still moist, with some cohesion. All foods from NDD Level 1 are acceptable at this level.

Rationale: This diet is a transition from the pureed textures to more solid textures. Chewing ability is required. The textures on this level are appropriate for individuals with mild-to-moderate oral and/or pharyngeal dysphagia. Patients should be assessed for tolerance to mixed textures. It is expected that some mixed textures are tolerated on this diet.

Liquid Consistency (circle one)

Thin (includes all unthickened beverages and supplements)	Nectarlike	Honeylike	Spoon-thick

Food Textures for NDD Level 2: Dysphagia: Mechanically Altered
(includes all foods on NDD Level 1: Dysphagia: Pureed in addition to the foods listed below)

Food Groups	Recommended	Avoid	If Thin Liquids Are Allowed, Also May Have
Beverages	All beverages with minimum amounts of texture, pulp, etc.; any texture should be suspended in the liquid and should not precipitate out; may need to be thickened, depending on liquid consistency recommended		Milk, juices, coffee, tea, sodas, carbonated beverages, alcoholic beverages If allowed, nutritional supplements Ice chips

APPENDIX 35 National Dysphagia Diets—cont'd

Food Textures for NDD Level 2: Dysphagia: Mechanically Altered—cont'd

Food Groups	Recommended	Avoid	If Thin Liquids Are Allowed, Also May Have
Breads	Soft pancakes, well moistened with syrup or sauce Pureed bread mixes, *pregelled* or *slurried* breads that are gelled through entire thickness	All others	
Cereals *(Cereals may have ¼ cup milk or just enough milk to moisten if thin liquids are restricted. The moisture should be well-blended into food.)*	Cooked cereals with little texture, including oatmeal Slightly moistened dry cereals with little texture such as corn flakes, Rice Krispies, Wheaties Unprocessed wheat bran stirred into cereals for bulk *Note:* If thin liquids are restricted, it is important that all of the liquid is absorbed into the cereal	Very coarse cooked cereals that may contain flaxseed or other seeds or nuts Whole grain dry or coarse cereals Cereals with nuts, seeds, dried fruit, and/or coconut	Milk or cream for cereals
Desserts	Pudding, custard Soft fruit pies with bottom crust only Crisps and cobblers without seeds or nuts and with soft breading or crumb mixture Canned fruit (excluding pineapple) Soft, moist cakes with icing or "slurried" cakes Pregelled cookies or soft, moist cookies that have been dunked in milk, coffee, or other liquid	Dry, coarse cakes and cookies Anything with nuts, seeds, coconut, pineapple, or dried fruit Breakfast yogurt with nuts Rice or bread pudding *These foods are considered thin liquids and should be avoided if thin liquids are restricted:* Frozen malts, milk shakes, frozen yogurt, eggnog, nutritional supplements, ice cream, sherbet, regular or sugar-free gelatin, or any foods that become thin liquid at either room (70° F) or body temperature (98° F)	Ice cream, sherbet, malts, nutritional supplements, frozen yogurt, and other ices Plain gelatin or gelatin with canned fruit, excluding pineapple
Fats	Butter, margarine, cream for cereal (depending on liquid consistency recommendations), gravy, cream sauces, mayonnaise, salad dressings, cream cheese, cream cheese spreads with soft additives, sour cream, sour cream dips with soft additives, whipped toppings	All fats with coarse or chunky additives	Cream for cereal
Fruits	Soft, drained canned or cooked fruits without seeds or skin Fresh soft/ripe banana Fruit juices with small amount of pulp. If thin liquids are restricted, fruit juices should be thickened to appropriate viscosity	Fresh or frozen fruits Cooked fruit with skin or seeds Dried fruits Fresh, canned, or cooked pineapple	Thin fruit juices Watermelon without seeds
Meats, meat substitutes, entrees *(Meat pieces should not exceed ¼-inch cube and should be tender.)*	Moistened ground or cooked meat, poultry, or fish; moist ground or tender meat may be served with gravy or sauce Casseroles without rice Moist macaroni and cheese, well-cooked pasta with meat sauce, tuna-noodle casserole, soft, moist lasagna Moist meatballs, meatloaf, or fish loaf Protein salads such as tuna or egg without large chunks, celery, or onion Cottage cheese, smooth quiche without large chunks	Dry meats, tough meats such as bacon, sausage, hot dogs, bratwurst Dry casseroles or casseroles with rice or large chunks Cheese slices and cubes Peanut butter Hard-cooked or crisp fried eggs Sandwiches Pizza	

Continued

APPENDIX 35 National Dysphagia Diets—cont'd

Food Textures for NDD Level 2: Dysphagia: Mechanically Altered—cont'd

Food Groups	Recommended	Avoid	If Thin Liquids Are Allowed, Also May Have
Meats, meat substitutes, entrees, cont'd	Poached, scrambled, or soft-cooked eggs (egg yolks should not be runny but should be moist and mashable with butter, margarine, or other moisture added to them) (cook eggs to 160° F or use pasteurized eggs for safety) Soufflés may have small soft chunks Tofu Well-cooked, slightly mashed, moist legumes such as baked beans All meats or protein substitutes should be served with sauces or moistened to help maintain cohesiveness in the oral cavity		
Potatoes and starches	Well-cooked, moistened, boiled, baked, or mashed potatoes Well-cooked shredded hash brown potatoes that are not crisp (all potatoes need to be moist and in sauces) Well-cooked noodles in sauce Spaetzel or soft dumplings that have been moistened with butter or gravy	Potato skins and chips Fried or French-fried potatoes Rice	
Soups	Soups with easy-to-chew or easy-to-swallow meats or vegetables; particle sizes in soups should be <½ inch (soups may need to be thickened to appropriate consistency, if soup is thinner than prescribed liquid consistency)	Soups with large chunks of meat and vegetables Soups with rice, corn, peas	All soups except those noted in **Avoid** list
Vegetables	All soft, well-cooked vegetables Vegetables should be <½ inch; should be easily mashed with a fork	Cooked corn and peas Broccoli, cabbage, Brussels sprouts, asparagus, or other fibrous, nontender, or rubbery cooked vegetables	
Miscellaneous	Jams and preserves without seeds, jelly Sauces, salsas, etc., that may have small tender chunks <½ inch Soft, smooth chocolate bars that are easily chewed	Seeds, nuts, coconut, sticky foods Chewy candies such as caramel and licorice	

Level 3: Dysphagia: Transition to Regular Diet

Description: This level consists of food of nearly regular textures with the exception of very hard, sticky, or crunchy foods. Foods still need to be moist and should be in bite-size pieces at the oral phase of the swallow.

Rationale: This diet is a transition to a regular diet. Adequate dentition and mastication are required. The textures of this diet are appropriate for individuals with mild oral and/or pharyngeal phase dysphagia. Patients should be assessed for tolerance of mixed textures. Mixed textures are expected to be tolerated on this diet.

Liquid Consistency (circle one)

Thin (includes all un-thickened beverages and supplements)	Nectarlike	Honeylike	Spoon-thick

Food Textures for NDD Level 3: Dysphagia: Advanced

Food Groups	Recommended	Avoid	If Thin Liquids Are Allowed, Also May Have
Beverages	Any beverages, depending on recommendations for liquid consistency		Milk, juices, coffee, tea, sodas, carbonated beverages, alcoholic beverages, nutritional supplements Ice chips

APPENDIX 35 National Dysphagia Diets—cont'd

Food Textures for NDD Level 3: Dysphagia: Advanced—cont'd

Food Groups	Recommended	Avoid	If Thin Liquids Are Allowed, Also May Have
Breads	Any well-moistened breads, biscuits, muffins, pancakes, waffles, etc.; need to add adequate syrup, jelly, margarine, butter, etc., to moisten well	Dry bread, toast, crackers, etc. Tough, crusty breads such as French bread or baguettes	
Cereals *(Cereals may have 1/4 cup milk or just enough milk to moisten if thin liquids are restricted.)*	All well-moistened cereals	Coarse or dry cereals such as shredded wheat or All Bran	
Desserts	All others except those on **Avoid** list	Dry cakes, cookies that are chewy or very dry Anything with nuts, seeds, dry fruits, coconut, pineapple *These foods are considered thin liquids and should be avoided if thin liquids are restricted:* Frozen malts, milk shakes, frozen yogurt, eggnog, nutritional supplements, ice cream, sherbet, regular or sugar-free gelatin or any foods that become thin liquid at either room (70° F) or body temperature (98° F)	Malts, milk shakes, frozen yogurts, ice cream, and other frozen desserts Nutritional supplements, gelatin, and any other desserts of thin liquid consistency when in the mouth
Fats	All other fats except those on **Avoid** list	All fats with coarse, difficult-to-chew, or chunky additives such as cream-cheese spread with nuts or pineapple	
Fruits	All canned and cooked fruits Soft, peeled fresh fruits such as peaches, nectarines, kiwi, mangos, cantaloupe, honeydew, watermelon (without seeds) Soft berries with small seeds such as strawberries	Difficult-to-chew fresh fruits such as apples or pears Stringy, high-pulp fruits such as papaya, pineapple, or mango Fresh fruits with difficult-to-chew peels such as grapes Uncooked dried fruits such as prunes and apricots Fruit leather, fruit roll-ups, fruit snacks, dried fruits	Any fruit juices
Meats, meat substitutes, entrees	Thin-sliced, tender, or ground meats and poultry Well-moistened fish Eggs prepared any way Yogurt without nuts or coconut Casseroles with small chunks of meat, ground meats, or tender meats	Tough, dry meats and poultry Dry fish or fish with bones Chunky peanut butter Yogurt with nuts or coconut	
Potatoes and starches	All, including rice, wild rice, moist bread dressing, and tender, fried potatoes	Tough, crisp-fried potatoes Potato skins Dry bread dressing	

Continued

APPENDIX 35 National Dysphagia Diets—cont'd

Food Textures for NDD Level 3: Dysphagia: Advanced—cont'd

Food Groups	Recommended	Avoid	If Thin Liquids Are Allowed, Also May Have
Soups	All soups except those in the **Avoid** list Strained corn or clam chowder (may need to be thickened to appropriate consistency if soup is thinner than prescribed liquid consistency)	Soups with tough meats Corn or clam chowders Soups that have large chunks of meat or vegetables >1 inch	All thin soups except those in **Avoid** list Broth and bouillon
Vegetables	All cooked, tender vegetables Shredded lettuce	All raw vegetables except shredded lettuce Cooked corn Nontender or rubbery cooked vegetables	
Miscellaneous	All seasonings and sweeteners All sauces Nonchewy candies without nuts, seeds, or coconut Jams, jellies, honey, preserves	Nuts, seeds, or coconut Chewy caramel or taffy-type candies Candies with nuts, seeds, or coconut	

APPENDIX 36 Renal Diet for Dialysis

Your diet depends on your kidney function. Most of the information here relates to people on dialysis. What is right for others is not always right for you. As your kidney function changes, your diet may change as well. This guide will help you do two things: plan nutritious meals you enjoy and keep your body working at its best. Your renal dietitian will work with you to make any changes needed to your usual meal plan, but this appendix contains helpful guidelines.

1. *Increase Protein*
   You will need to eat a high-protein diet. Beef, pork, lamb, fish, shellfish, chicken, eggs, and other animal foods provide most of the protein in your diet. Your protein needs are based on your weight. Most people need at least 6 to 8 oz of protein per day. A deck of cards is about the size of a 3-oz serving of protein.

2. *Limit Potassium*
   Most foods contain some potassium, but fruits and vegetables are the easiest to control. Limit fruits, vegetables, and juices to 6 servings per day. A serving is usually ½ cup.
   Do not use salt substitute or "lite" salt because they are made with potassium.

3. *Limit Salt*
   Limit the salt you eat. Don't add salt during cooking or at the table. Avoid high-salt foods such as frozen meals; canned or dried foods; "fast foods"; and salted meats such as ham, sausage and luncheon meats. Use salt-free spices or spice mixes such as Mrs. Dash instead of salt to add flavor to your food.

4. *Limit Phosphorus*
   Use only 1 serving of milk or dairy food per day. A serving is usually ½ to 1 cup. Take phosphate binders such as Tums, PhosLo, Renagel, or Fosrenol with your meals as prescribed by your doctor.

5. *Fluid*
   A safe amount of fluid to drink is different for everyone. It depends on how much urine you are making. Try not to drink more than 3 cups (24 oz) of fluid each day plus the amount equal to your urine output. If you are limiting your salt intake, you should not feel thirsty.
   Fluids include all beverages and foods that are liquid at room temperature such as Jell-O, ice cream, ice, and soup.

6. *Poor Appetite and Weight Loss*
   It is common to have a poor appetite if you are new to dialysis. If your appetite has been poor, try eating small frequent meals and extra snacks.
   Try adding high-calorie fats such as butter, margarine, and oils; sauces and gravies; and sour cream, cream cheese, or whipped cream for extra calories. Adding rice, pasta, bread, and rolls to meals also adds calories.
   Sugar and sweets such as cakes, candies, and pastries are also a good source of calories if you are *not* following a diabetic diet.
   Talk to your nutritionist about trying a nutritional supplement.

Protein

When on dialysis, you need to eat a high-protein diet. This is because you lose protein during each dialysis treatment. To stay healthy, you need to eat enough protein for your daily needs and also make up for the amount lost during dialysis. Meat, fish, poultry, eggs, and other animal foods provide most of the protein in your diet. Your body uses protein to build and repair muscles, skin, blood, and other tissues.

Albumin

Albumin is a protein found in blood. Each month a laboratory test measures your albumin. It is a good way to know how healthy you are. Your albumin level should be more than 3.4 mg/dl.

Appendix created by Katy G. Wilkens, MS, RD.

APPENDIX 36 Renal Diet for Dialysis—cont'd

Keeping a Healthy Albumin Level

Make sure that you eat enough protein every day. How much protein you need daily depends on how much you weigh.

Find your weight on the chart below to see how many protein servings you need each day.

Protein Servings for You

If you weigh:	You need:
40 kg	4-5 servings
50 kg	5-6 servings
60 kg	6-7 servings
70 kg	7-8 servings
80 kg	8-9 servings
90 kg	9-10 servings

Your weight: _____ kg

You need: _____ protein servings each day

One Serving of Protein Is:

1 egg
1 oz cooked meat, fish, poultry
¼ cup cooked/canned fish, seafood
½ cup tofu
1 cup milk
1 ounce cheese
¼ cup cottage cheese
¾ cup pudding or custard
2 Tbsp peanut butter
1 scoop protein powder
½ protein bar

Common Serving Sizes

Most people eat protein foods in portions larger than 1 serving. Here are some examples:

Average hamburger patty (3 oz) = 3 protein servings
Small beefsteak (3 in × 4 in) = 4 protein servings
Half chicken breast (3 oz) = 3 protein servings
Chicken drumstick or thigh (2 oz) = 2 protein servings
Average pork chop (3 oz) = 3 protein servings
Fish fillet (3 in × 3 in) = 3 protein servings

Estimating Serving Sizes

Here are some other easy ways to estimate protein serving sizes:

- Your whole thumb is about the size of 1 oz.
- Three stacked dice are about the size of 1 oz.
- A deck of cards is about the size of 3 oz.
- The palm of your hand is about the size of 3 to 4 oz.
- Your clenched fist is about the size of 1 cup.

Tips for Eating More Protein

Some people on dialysis dislike the taste of protein. Some people find cooking smells unpleasant. Still others are not able to eat enough protein each day.

The following tips will be helpful:

- Use gravy, sauces, seasonings, or spices to improve or hide flavors.
- Prepare meals ahead of time, or stay away from kitchen smells if they spoil your appetite.
- Eat cooked protein foods cold. Try cold fried chicken, a roast beef sandwich, or shrimp salad.
- Add cut-up meats or beans to soups or salads.
- Use more eggs. Try hardboiled eggs, egg salad sandwiches, custards, or quiches. Stir beaten eggs into casseroles and soups.
- Try other protein foods such as angel food cake, peanut butter, or bean salads.
- Eat a protein bar. Your nutritionist can help you choose one.
- Use a protein powder. Your nutritionist can help you choose one and give you ideas for using it.

Nutritional Supplements

Nutritional supplements provide extra calories and protein. In general, use one can of supplement as a snack each day. Add one extra can for each meal you miss.

Not all nutritional supplements are safe for dialysis patients. Check with your nutritionist before using any supplement. Here are some of the supplements that are used by people on dialysis:

Ensure Plus
Boost Plus
Nepro
ReNeph
Resource Diabetic
Resource Fruit Beverage
Boost Nutritional Pudding
Promod Protein Powder

Malnutrition

If you are not eating enough meat, fish, poultry, eggs, and other high-protein foods, your albumin level will drop below the recommended level.

If your albumin level is low, the cells in your body cannot hold fluid well. This leads to swelling (edema) and low blood pressure during dialysis. Low albumin increases your risk of death. Patients with albumin levels above 4.0 have the lowest death rate.

It is also important to eat enough calories. Your nutritionist can help you make sure you are getting plenty of protein and calories.

Exercise

Try to be active in some way each day (e.g., walk, swim, garden, stretch). Using your muscles helps keep them strong. Protein that is stored in your muscles helps support your albumin level.

Potassium for People on Hemodialysis

- Most foods have some potassium, but fruits and vegetables are the easiest form to control in your diet. The following list groups vegetables and fruits by the amount of potassium in one serving.
- Remember, there are no foods that you cannot eat on your diet. What is important is the amount of foods you eat and how often you eat them. Keep this list handy for shopping or eating out.
- If there are fruits and vegetables you enjoy that are not on the list, ask your nutritionist about them.

Most People on Hemodialysis May Have

- 1 serving per day from the high-potassium group
- 2 servings per day from the medium-potassium group
- 2 to 3 servings per day from the low-potassium group

This is about 2000 to 3000 mg of potassium per day with the other foods you eat. Check the serving size for each food, listed in parentheses next to the item.

Soaking Vegetables and Beans

Soaking works well for high-potassium foods such as potatoes, parsnips, sweet potatoes, winter squash, and beans. The procedure for soaking follows.

1. Peel vegetables and slice thinly (⅛ inch). Rinse well. Place them in a bowl of warm water, using four times more water than vegetable. For example, soak 1 cup of sliced vegetables in 4 cups of water. Soak at least 1 hour. Drain and rinse again.
2. Vegetables that have been soaked this way can then be fried, mashed, scalloped, put in soups or stews, or served fresh. If you are boiling the food, use four times more water than food and cook as usual.
3. Dried beans should be cooked and then chopped and soaked, using the preceding directions. Canned beans can simply be chopped, rinsed, and soaked.

Continued

APPENDIX 36 Renal Diet for Dialysis—cont'd

	Low-Potassium Foods 5-150 mg	Medium-Potassium Foods 150-250 mg	High-Potassium Foods 250-500 mg
Food Category			
Fruits	Applesauce (½ cup)	Apple (1 medium), cherries (8-10)	Apricots (3)
	Blackberries (½ cup)	Fruit cocktail (½ cup)	Avocados (¼)
	Blueberries (1 cup)	Grapes (10-15)	Banana (1 medium)
	Grapefruit (½ cup)	Mango (½ medium)	Dates (5)
	Pears, canned (½ cup)	Melons: cantaloupe, honeydew	Figs (3)
	Pineapple (½ cup)	(½ cup), papaya (½ cup)	Kiwi (1)
	Plums, canned (½ cup)	Peaches, canned (½ cup)	Nectarine (1 medium)
	Raspberries (½ cup)	Pear, fresh (1 medium)	Orange (1 medium)
	Rhubarb, cooked (½ cup	Plums (2)	Peach, fresh (1 medium)
	Strawberries (½ cup)	Watermelon (1 cup)	Prunes (5)
	Tangerine (1)		Raisins and dried fruit (¼ cup)
Vegetables	Asparagus (4 spears)	Broccoli (½ cup)	Artichoke (1 medium)
	Bean sprouts (½ cup)	Brussels sprouts (4-6)	Beans: lima, kidney, navy,
	Cabbage (½ cup)	Beets (½ cup)	pinto (½ cup)
	Cauliflower (½ cup)	Carrots (½ cup)	Greens: beet, collard, mustard,
	Corn (½ cup)	Celery (½ cup)	spinach, turnip (½ cup)
	Cucumber (½)	Eggplant (½ cup)	Lentils, split peas, chickpeas,
	Green and wax beans (½ cup)	Mixed vegetables (½ cup)	black-eyed peas (½ cup)
	Lettuce (1 cup)	Mushrooms (½ cup)	Nuts: all kinds (½ cup)
	Okra (3 pods)	Peanut butter (2 Tbsp)	Parsnips (½ cup)
	Onions (½ cup)	Pepper, green (1)	Potatoes (½ cup or 1 small)
	Peas (½ cup)	Potato chips (10)	Pumpkin (½ cup)
	Radishes (5)	Soaked potatoes (½ cup)	Spinach (½ cup)
	Rutabagas (½ cup)		Tomato (1 medium)
	Summer squash (½ cup)		Tomato sauce, tomato salsa (¼ cup)
	Turnips (½ cup)		Winter squash (½ cup)
	Water chestnuts (4)		Yams, sweet potatoes (½ cup)
Juices	Apple juice (½ cup)	Apricot nectar (½ cup)	Pomegranate juice (½ cup)
	Cranberry juices (1 cup)	Grape juice, canned (½ cup)	Prune juice (½ cup)
	Grape juice, frozen (1 cup)	Grapefruit juice (½ cup)	Tomato juice (½ cup)
	Tang, Hi-C and other fruit drinks	Pineapple juice (½ cup)	V-8 juice (½ cup)
	(1 cup), Kool-Aid (1 cup)		
	Lemonade and limeade (1 cup)		
	Peach or pear nectar (½ cup)		

Other High-Potassium Foods

- Milk is high in potassium. Limit milk to 1 cup per day unless you are told to do otherwise.
- Supplements such as Ensure Plus and Boost Plus also contain a lot of potassium. Always speak to your nutritionist before using supplements.
- Most salt substitutes and "lite" salt products are made with potassium. Do not use these products. If you are unsure, ask your nutritionist.

Shaking the Salt Habit

Salt, or "sodium chloride," is found in convenience and preserved foods. Foods that do not spoil easily are usually high in sodium. The more sodium you eat, the thirstier you will be. The following list of foods is grouped by sodium levels.

Following a low-sodium diet can be challenging. This list of sodium levels of foods is meant to help you learn what foods and how much of them you can enjoy.

Remember, there are no foods that you cannot eat on your diet. What is important is the amount of foods you eat and how often you eat them. Keep this list handy for shopping or dining.

Most People on Dialysis May Have

- 1 serving per day from the high group
- 1 serving per day from the medium group
- As many servings as desired from the low group
- 3 servings per day from the medium group
- As many servings as you want from the low group

This is 2000 to 3000 mg of sodium per day. Check the serving size for each food, listed in parentheses next to the item.

Rinsing Canned Foods to Lower Sodium (Canned Vegetables, Chunk or Flaked Fish or Shellfish, Poultry or Meats)

1. Empty can into colander or sieve.
2. Drain brine and discard.
3. Break up chunks into flakes or smaller pieces.
4. Rinse under running water for 1 min.
5. Drain food until most moisture is gone.

APPENDIX 36 Renal Diet for Dialysis—cont'd

	Low-Sodium Foods 1-150 mg	Medium-Sodium Foods 150-250 mg	High-Sodium Foods 250-700 mg
Food Category			
Breads and cereals	Breads, white, whole grain Cakes, cookies, crepes, doughnuts Cereals: cooked, granola, puffed rice, puffed wheat, Shredded Wheat, Sugar Pops, Sugar Smacks, Sugar Crisps Crackers: graham, low salt, melba toast Macaroni, noodles, spaghetti, rice	Biscuits, rolls, muffins: homemade (1) Pancakes (1) "Ready-to-eat" cereals (¾ cup) Saltine crackers (6) Sweet roll (1)	All Bran (¼ cup) Instant mixes: noodles, potatoes, rice (½ cup) Instant mixes: biscuits, breads, muffins, rolls (1 serving) Waffles (1)
Condiments	Butter, margarine, oil Horseradish, mustard, spices, herbs, sugar, syrup, Tobasco, vinegar, Worcestershire	Bacon (2 slices) Catsup, steak sauce (1 Tbsp) Commercial salad dressing (1 Tbsp) Gravy (2 Tbsp) Low-sodium soy sauce (2 tsp) Mayonnaise (2 Tbsp) Pickle relish (2 Tbsp) Sweet pickles (2 small)	Salt (¼ tsp)
Dairy products	Cheeses: cream, Monterey, Mozzarella, Ricotta, low-salt types Cream: half-and-half, sour, whipping Custard, ice cream, sherbet Milk: all kinds, yogurt Nondairy creamer	Cheeses (1-oz slice) Cottage cheese (½ cup) Pudding (¾ cup)	Buttermilk (1 cup) Processed cheeses and cheese spreads (1 slice or 2 Tbsp)
Main dishes	All unprocessed meats, fish, poultry Eggs Peanut butter Tuna: low-sodium or rinsed		Broth (½ cup) Canned fish, meat (¼ cup) Canned soups (½ cup) Hot dog (1) Luncheon meat (1 slice) Canned entrees (e.g., pork and beans, spaghetti, stew) (1 cup) Sausage (1 oz)
Fruits and vegetables	All fresh or frozen vegetables All fruits and juices Canned tomatoes, tomato paste Canned vegetables: low-sodium or rinsed	Vegetables (½ cup) Juices: tomato, vegetable (½ cup)	Canned tomato sauce or puree (¼ cup) Frozen vegetables with special sauce (½ cup) Sauerkraut (¼ cup)
Beverages and snacks	Beer, wine, coffee, tea Candy: all kinds Fruit drinks, Popsicles, soda pop, Kool-Aid, Tang Low-salt products: without potassium substitutes Unsalted nuts, unsalted popcorn	Potato and corn chips (1 cup) Snack crackers (5-10)	Commercial dips (¼ cup) Dill pickle chips (3 slices) Olives (5) Salted nuts (½ cup)

NOTE: Some foods are very high in sodium and should be used only once a week. These include Chinese, Oriental foods; corned beef, ham, pastrami; fast foods (e.g., commercial hamburgers, pizza, tacos); pickles; soy sauce; and TV dinners and frozen entrees.

Phosphorus

Why Follow a Low-Phosphorus Diet?

When phosphorus is high for too long, bones become brittle and weak. You may have joint and bone pain. Extra phosphorus may go into your soft tissue, causing hard or soft lumps. Also, you may have severe itching.

The good news is that with diet, binders, and good dialysis, you can keep your phosphorus level under control.

Phosphorus is a mineral found in most foods. Dialysis does not remove it easily. Your phosphorus level depends on the foods you eat and your medications. Keeping your phosphorus at a safe level will help keep your bones healthy.

Each month your phosphorus level will be measured. High phosphorus is a common problem for people on dialysis. A good phosphorus level in your blood is between 3 and 6 g/dl.

Continued

APPENDIX 36 Renal Diet for Dialysis—cont'd

High-Phosphorus Foods

Phosphorus is found in most foods you eat, especially protein foods. The foods that are highest in phosphorus are milk and things made from milk (dairy foods). By limiting these foods you can cut down on the phosphorus you are eating.

Most people on dialysis can have one serving daily from this list of dairy foods. The serving size is also noted.

Milk (1 cup)
Cheese (2 oz)
Cottage cheese (⅔ cup)
Yogurt (1 cup)
Ice cream (1½ cup)
Frozen yogurt (1½ cup)
Milkshake (1 cup)
Hot chocolate (1 cup)
Pudding or custard (1 cup)

You can also eat part of a serving of different foods to add up to 1 serving.

Other High-Phosphorus Foods

For some people, limiting dairy foods may not be enough. Other high-phosphorus foods are listed below. If your phosphorus level is high, you may need to limit these foods to once a week.

Bran cereals (1 oz)
Dried beans/peas (½ cup cooked)
Chili (½ cup)
Nuts (½ cup)
Frozen waffles (1)

Phosphorus and Potassium

High-phosphorus foods are often high in potassium as well. This is another reason to limit dairy foods and other high-phosphorus foods.

Phosphate Binders

Phosphate binders are pills you take when you eat. Binders help keep phosphorus in your food from going into your blood.

Your doctor will decide which binder is best for you and how many you should take each time you eat.

It is important to take all your binders planned for each day.

You can take your binders just before you start a meal, during the meal, or right after eating.

If you forget to take them or skip a meal, it may be difficult to get your full binder dose. Ask your doctor what to do if this happens.

It may take some hard work to remember to take binders each time you eat. Try these ideas:

- Each morning take out the number of binders you need that day. Put them in a small container to carry with you. It should be empty at the end of the day.
- Carry a spare container of binders for when you travel or eat out.
- Take your binders with high-protein snacks such as sandwiches or dairy foods.
- Binders may cause constipation. Talk with your nutritionist about ideas to help with bowel movements.
- There are many types of binders. If you don't like the kind you are taking, talk with your doctor, pharmacist, or nutritionist about other kinds.

Lower-Phosphorus Ideas

Below are some lower-phosphorus choices you can make in the place of milk and other creamy dairy products. Check those you will try.

- Use nondairy creamer such as Mocha Mix or Coffee Rich on cereal, for creamy sauces or soups, and in shakes.
- Try rice milk or soymilk. They are lower in potassium too.
- Try soy cheese or soy yogurt. They are available in a variety of flavors.
- Use cream cheese in the place of regular cheese or cottage cheese.
- Use sour cream or imitation sour cream on fruits or to replace yogurt in dips.
- Try a nondairy frozen ice cream made from soy, rice, or nondairy creamer such as Mocha Mix.
- Enjoy sorbet or sherbet instead of ice cream.

High Phosphorus Levels

Below are some reasons for a high phosphorus level. Check the ones that you think may apply to you:

- Eating too many high-phosphorus foods
- Forgetting to take your binders
- Not taking all the phosphate binders ordered for you
- Not taking your phosphate binders at the right times

Even if you follow your diet and take your binders, your phosphorus level may be high. When calcium and phosphorus are out of balance, your parathyroid gland becomes overactive. High levels of parathyroid hormone damage your bones. Your doctor can test for this problem and recommend treatment.

APPENDIX 37 Sodium-Restricted Diets

Sodium restriction is used in the management of essential hypertension and for cardiovascular disease, severe cardiac failure, impaired liver function, renal disease, and chronic renal failure. The goal of the sodium-restricted meal plan is to manage hypertension in sodium-sensitive persons and promote the loss of excess fluids in edema and ascites. Sodium is restricted to various degrees to meet the requirement.

Adequacy

Depending on individual food choices, sodium-restricted meal plans are adequate in all nutrients based on the Dietary Reference Intakes. When sodium is restricted to 1000 mg or less, a calcium supplement may be needed.

Special Considerations

A large volume of research has assessed the relationship of dietary sodium intake to prevention and treatment of high blood pressure. One result of this research is that sodium in combination with chloride (table salt) may aggravate hypertension is some people who are sensitive to salt. Numerous health agencies agree that sodium intake should be limited to 2.4 grams (2400 mg) or less per day for healthy people. 1 tsp salt contains 2300 mg sodium.

A therapeutic sodium-restricted meal plan should be prescribed in terms of milligrams of sodium desired on a daily basis. The following are the commonly used levels of sodium restrictions:

No Added Salt (NAS): This is the least restrictive of the sodium-restricted diets. Table salt should not be used, and salt should be limited in cooking. When high-sodium foods such as smoked, cured, or dried meats and cheeses; condiments and seasonings, salted snacks, and canned and dried soups and bouillon are also limited, the no added salt (NAS)–diet provides about 4000 mg of sodium daily.

3000 mg sodium (7.5 g NaCl or 130 mEq Na): This diet *restricts* foods and beverages that have been highly processed with sodium such as fast foods; salad dressings; soy sauce; salty snack foods; smoked, salted, and kosher meats; regular canned foods; pickled vegetables; luncheon meats; and commercially softened water. Up to ¼ tsp salt per day may be used in cooking or at the table.

From the North Carolina Dietetic Association: *Nutrition care manual*, Raleigh, NC, 2005, The Association.

APPENDIX 37 Sodium-Restricted Diets—cont'd

2000 mg sodium (5 g NaCl or 87 mEq Na): This diet *eliminates* processed and prepared foods and beverages that are high in sodium. Salt should not be used in cooking or at the table. Milk and milk products are limited to 16 oz daily. Only salt-free commercially prepared foods should be used.

1000 mg sodium (2.5 g NaCl or 45 mEq Na): Processed and prepared foods and beverages that are high in sodium are eliminated. Regular canned foods, many frozen foods, deli foods, fast foods, cheeses, margarines, and regular salad dressings are also eliminated (low-sodium or sodium-free versions should be substituted). Regular breads are limited to two servings/day. Milk and milk products are limited to 16 oz/day. Salt should not be used in cooking or at the table.

Most medical professionals no longer recommend eating patterns with less than 1000 mg sodium. In addition to being unpalatable, they are very restrictive and could result in nutritional deficiencies if followed for an extended period of time.

Guidelines for Sodium Restriction

- Obtain and evaluate a diet history before prescribing and/or instructing on a sodium restriction.
- Recommend salt substitutes containing potassium chloride only if approved by a physician. Salt-free seasoning products are readily available in most grocery stores and should be suggested instead.
- Instruct patients on reading the Nutrition Facts food label for sodium content of foods.
- Recommend potassium replacement if diuretics are used. If potassium intake from foods is not sufficient, potassium supplements may be necessary.

- Provide information on choosing low-sodium foods at restaurants.
- Recommend baked products, using sodium-free baking powder, potassium bicarbonate (instead of sodium bicarbonate or baking soda), and salt-free shortening in place of those containing sodium.
- Avoid obviously salted foods such a as bouillon, soup and gravy bases, canned soups and stews; bread and rolls with salt toppings, salted crackers; salted nuts or popcorn, potato chips, pretzels, and other salted snack foods.
- Avoid smoked or cured meats, such as bacon, bologna, cold cuts, other processed meats, chipped or corned beef, frankfurters, ham, koshered or kosher style meats, and canned meat poultry.
- Avoid salted and smoked fish such as cod, herring, and sardines.
- Avoid sauerkraut, olives, pickles, relishes, and other vegetables prepared in brine, tomato, and vegetable cocktail juices.
- Avoid seasonings such as celery salt, garlic, Worcestershire sauce and soy sauce.
- Serve cheeses (e.g., Swiss, American, and other processed cheeses) in limited amounts (approximately two times a week).
- Include sodium-containing medications, seltzer waters, toothpaste, and chewing tobacco in total sodium allotment if the restriction is below 2000 mg.
- Monitor the sodium content of various medications, including over-the-counter brands.

Sodium Content of Selected Over-the-Counter Medications

Medication	Trade Name	Sodium Content	
		Milligrams per Dose	**Milligrams per 100 ml**
Analgesic	Aspirin (various others)	49	—
Antacid analgesic	Bromo-Seltzer	717	—
Antacid laxative	Alka-Seltzer (blue box)	521	—
Antacids	Sal Hepatica	1,000	—
	Rolaids	53	—
	Soda Mint	89	—
	Alka-Seltzer (gold box)	276	—
	Brioschi	710	—
Laxatives	Metamucil Instant Mix	250	—
	Fleet's Enema	250-300	—
Sleep-aids	Miles Nervine Effervescent	544	—
Antacid suspensions	Milk of Magnesia	—	10
	Amphojel	—	14
	Basaljel	—	36
	Maalox	—	50
	Riopan	—	14
	Mylanta I	—	76
	Mylanta II	—	160
	Digel	—	170
	Titralac	—	220

Seasoning without salt: Flavorings or seasonings will make food more appetizing. For example:

- Lemon or vinegar is excellent with fish or meat and with many vegetables such as broccoli, asparagus, green beans, or salads.
- Meat may be seasoned with onion, garlic, green pepper, nutmeg, ginger, dry mustard, sage and marjoram. It may be cooked with fresh mushrooms or unsalted tomato juice.
- Cranberry sauce, applesauce, or jellies make appetizing accompaniments to meats and poultry.

- Vegetables may be flavored by the addition of onion, mint, ginger, mace, dill seed, parsley, green pepper, or fresh mushrooms.
- Unsalted cottage cheese may be flavored with minced onion, chopped chives, raw green pepper, grated carrots, chopped parsley, or crushed pineapple.
- A number of salt-free seasonings for use in cooking are available in the spice section of most supermarkets.

Continued

APPENDIX 37 Sodium-Restricted Diets—cont'd

3000-mg Sodium Diet

Food Category	Recommended	Not Recommended
Beverages	Milk, buttermilk (limit to 1 cup daily); eggnog; all fruit juices; low sodium, salt-free vegetable juices; regular vegetable or tomato juices (limit to ½ cup daily); coffee, tea, low-sodium carbonated beverages	Regular vegetable or tomato juices used in excessive amounts
Breads and cereals	Enriched white, wheat, rye, and pumpernickel bread, hard rolls, and dinner rolls; biscuits, muffins, cornbread, pancakes, and waffles; most dry and hot cereals; unsalted crackers and breadsticks	Breads, rolls, and crackers with salted tops; instant hot cereals
Desserts and sweets	All	None
Fats	Butter or margarine; vegetable oils; low-sodium salad dressing, other salad dressings in limited amounts; light, sour, and heavy cream	Salad dressings containing bacon fat, bacon bits, and salt pork; snack dips made with instant soup mixes or processed cheese
Fruits	All	None
Meats and meat substitutes	Any fresh or frozen beef, lamb, pork, poultry, fish and most shellfish; canned tuna or salmon, rinsed; eggs and egg substitutes; regular cheese, ricotta, and cream cheese (2 oz daily); low-sodium cheese as desired; cottage cheese, drained; regular yogurt; regular peanut butter (3 times weekly); dried peas and beans; frozen dinners (<600 mg sodium)	Any smoked, cured, salted, kosher, commercially prepared meat, fish, or poultry, including bacon, chipped beef, cold cuts, ham, hot dogs, sausage, sardines, anchovies, marinated herring, and pickled meats; frozen breaded meats; pickled eggs; processed cheese, cheese spreads and sauces; salted nuts
Potatoes and potato substitutes	White or sweet potatoes; winter squash; enriched rice, barley, noodles, spaghetti, macaroni, and other pastas; homemade bread stuffing	Commercially prepared potato, rice, or pasta mixes; commercial bread stuffing
Soups	Commercially prepared and dehydrated soups, broths, and bouillons (once per week); homemade broth, soups without added salt and made with allowed vegetables; reduced-sodium commercially prepared soups and broths	Commercially prepared or dehydrated regular soups (more than once per week)
Vegetables	All fresh and frozen vegetables, commercially prepared, drained vegetables	Sauerkraut, pickled vegetables, and others prepared in brine; vegetables seasoned with ham, bacon, or salt pork
Miscellaneous	Limit added salt to ¼ tsp/day used at the table or in cooking; salt substitute with physician's approval; pepper, herbs, spices; vinegar, lemon, or lime juice; hot pepper sauce; low-sodium soy sauce (1 tsp); unsalted tortilla chips, pretzels, potato chips, popcorn; salsa (2 tbsp), catsup and mustard (1 Tbsp), low-sodium baking powder	Any seasoning made with salt, including garlic salt, celery salt, onion salt, and seasoned salt; sea salt, rock salt, kosher salt; meat tenderizers; monosodium glutamate; regular soy sauce, teriyaki sauce, most flavored vinegars; regular snack chips, olives

Sample Menu for 3000-mg Sodium Diet

Breakfast	Lunch	Dinner
½ cup calcium-fortified orange juice	3-oz boneless, skinless chicken breast	1 cup spaghetti with meat sauce
¾ cup Raisin Bran	½ cup white rice	1 cup tossed salad with assorted vegetables
2 slices whole wheat toast	½ cup broccoli	1 Tbsp low-fat Italian dressing
2 tsp margarine	½ cup coleslaw	1 slice Italian bread
1 Tbsp jelly	1 whole wheat roll	½ cup apple crisp
1 cup skim milk	1 tsp margarine	2 tsp margarine
1 cup coffee	1 cup iced tea	1 cup skim milk
2 tsp sugar	½ cup chocolate pudding	1 cup coffee
	½ Tbsp whipped topping	¼ tsp pepper
	¼ tsp pepper	2 tsp sugar
	2 tsp sugar	

Nutritional Analysis

Kilocalories: 2038
Protein: 79g
Fat: 49 g
Carbohydrate: 337 g
Sodium: 3050 mg
Potassium: 3534 mg
Fiber: 21g

APPENDIX 37 Sodium-Restricted Diets—cont'd

2000-mg Sodium Diet

Food Category	Recommended	Not Recommended
Beverages	Milk (limit to 2 cup daily), buttermilk (limit to 1 cup daily), eggnog, all fruit juices, low-sodium, salt-free vegetable juices, coffee, tea, low-sodium carbonated beverages	Malted milk, milkshakes, chocolate milk, regular vegetable or tomato juices, commercially softened water used for drinking or cooking
Breads and cereals	Enriched, white, wheat, rye, and pumpernickel bread, hard rolls, and dinner rolls; muffins, cornbread, waffles; most dry cereals, cooked cereal without added salt; unsalted crackers and breadsticks; low-sodium or homemade bread crumbs	Breads, rolls, and crackers with salted tops; quick breads; instant hot cereals; commercial bread stuffing; self-rising flour and biscuit mixes; regular bread crumbs or cracker crumbs; pancakes
Desserts and sweets	All; desserts and sweets made with milk should be within allowance	Instant pudding mixes and cake mixes
Fats	Butter or margarine; vegetable oils; unsalted salad dressings; light, sour, and heavy cream; regular salad dressing limited to 1 Tbsp	Regular salad dressings containing bacon fat, bacon bits, and salt pork; snack dips made with instant soup mixes or processed cheese
Fruits	Most fresh, frozen, and canned fruits	Fruits processed with salt or sodium-containing compounds (i.e., some dried fruits)
Meats and meat substitutes	Any fresh or frozen beef, lamb, pork, poultry, fish; some shellfish; canned tuna or salmon, rinsed; eggs and egg substitutes; low-sodium cheese, including low-sodium ricotta and cream cheese; low-sodium cottage cheese; regular yogurt; low-sodium peanut butter; dried peas and beans; frozen dinners (<500 mg sodium)	Any smoked, cured, salted, kosher, commercially prepared meat, fish, or poultry, including bacon, chipped beef, cold cuts, ham, hot dogs, sausage, sardines, anchovies, marinated herring, and pickled meats; crab, lobster, frozen, breaded meats, pickled eggs, regular hard and processed cheese; cheese spreads and sauces; salted nuts
Potatoes and potato substitutes	White or sweet potatoes; winter squash; enriched rice, barley, noodles, spaghetti, macaroni, and other pastas cooked without salt; homemade bread stuffing	Commercially prepared potato, rice, or pasta mixes; commercial bread stuffing
Soups	Low-sodium commercially prepared and dehydrated soups, broth, and bouillon; homemade broth soups made without added salt and with allowed vegetables; cream soups within milk allowance	Regular commercially prepared or dehydrated soups, broth, or bouillon
Vegetables	Fresh, frozen vegetables and low-sodium commercially prepared vegetables	Regular commercially prepared vegetables, sauerkraut, pickled vegetables, and others prepared in brine; frozen vegetables in sauces; vegetables seasoned with ham, bacon, or salt pork
Miscellaneous	Salt substitute with physician's approval; pepper, herbs, spices; vinegar, lemon or lime juice; low-sodium soy sauce (1 tsp); hot pepper sauce; low-sodium condiments (catsup, chili sauce, mustard); fresh ground horseradish; unsalted tortilla chips, pretzels, potato chips, popcorn, salsa (2 Tbsp)	Any seasoning made with salt, including garlic salt, celery salt, onion salt, and seasoned salt; sea salt, rock salt, kosher salt; meat tenderizers, monosodium glutamate; regular soy sauce, barbecue sauce, teriyaki sauce, steak sauce, Worcestershire sauce, most flavored vinegars; canned gravy and mixes; regular condiments; salted snack foods, olives

Sample Menu for 2000-mg Sodium Diet

Breakfast	Lunch	Dinner
½ cup calcium-fortified orange juice	3-oz boneless, skinless chicken breast	1 cup spaghetti with low-sodium tomato/meat sauce
¾ cup raisin bran	½ cup white rice	1 cup tossed salad with assorted vegetables
2 slices whole wheat toast	½ cup broccoli	1 slice Italian bread
2 tsp margarine	½ cup coleslaw	1 tsp margarine
1 Tbsp jelly	1 whole wheat roll	½ cup apple crisp
1 cup skim milk	1 tsp margarine	1 cup coffee
1 cup coffee	½ cup homemade pudding	¼ tsp pepper
2 tsp sugar	½ Tbsp whipped cream	2 tsp sugar
	1 cup iced tea	
	¼ tsp pepper	
	2 tsp sugar	

Nutritional Analysis

Kilocalories: 1972
Protein: 78 g
Fat: 42 g
Saturated fat: 8 g
Carbohydrate: 348 g
Sodium: 2061 mg
Potassium: 3154 mg
Fiber: 26 g

Continued

APPENDIX 37 Sodium-Restricted Diets—cont'd

1000-mg Sodium Diet

Food Category	Recommended	Not Recommended
Beverages	Milk (limited to 2 cup daily); eggnog; all fruit juices; low-sodium, salt-free vegetable juices; low-sodium carbonated beverages, coffee, tea	Malted milk; milkshake, buttermilk, chocolate milk; regular vegetable or tomato juices; commercially softened water used for drinking or cooking
Breads and cereals	Enriched white, wheat, rye and pumpernickel bread, hard rolls, and dinner rolls (2 servings/day); low-sodium bread, crackers, matzo, and Melba toast; muffins, cornbread, pancakes, and waffles made with low-sodium baking powder; cooked cereal without added salt; low-sodium dry cereals, including puffed rice, puffed wheat, and shredded wheat; unsalted crackers and breadsticks; low-sodium bread crumbs and cracker crumbs	Breads, rolls, and crackers with salted tops or made with regular baking powder; quick breads; instant hot cereals; self-rising flour and biscuit mixes; regular bread crumbs and cracker crumbs, graham crackers
Desserts and sweets	Ice cream, pudding, and custard made with milk should be within allowance; fruit ice; unsalted bakery goods, homemade or commercial; sherbet and flavored gelatin (not to exceed ½ cup/day), low-salt baking powder	All candies made with sweet chocolate, nuts, or coconut; desserts made with rennin or rennin tablets; instant pudding mixes, commercial cakes, cookies, and brownie mixes
Fats	Unsalted butter or margarine; vegetable oils; unsalted salad dressings; low-sodium mayonnaise; nondairy cream (up to 1 oz daily)	Salted butter and margarine; all regular salad dressings; snack dips made with instant soup mixes or processed cheese
Fruits	Most fresh, frozen, and other commercially prepared fruits	Fruits processed with salt or sodium-containing compounds
Meat and meat substitutes	Any fresh or frozen beef, lamb, pork, poultry, fish; low-sodium canned tuna or salmon; eggs; low-sodium cheese, cottage cheese, ricotta, and cream cheese; regular yogurt; low-sodium peanut butter; dried peas and beans; frozen dinners (<150 mg sodium)	Any smoked, cured, salted, kosher, commercially prepared meat, fish, or poultry including bacon, chipped beef, cold cuts, ham, hot dogs, sausage, sardines, anchovies, marinated herring, and pickled meats; all shellfish; frozen breaded meats; pickled eggs, egg substitutes; regular hard and processed cheese; cheese spreads and sauces; salted nuts
Potatoes and potato substitutes	White or sweet potatoes; winter squash; unsalted enriched rice, barley, noodles, spaghetti, macaroni, and other pasta cooked without salt; homemade bread stuffing	Commercially prepared potato, rice, or pasta mixes; instant potatoes; commercial bread stuffing
Soups	Low-sodium commercially prepared and dehydrated soups, broths, and bouillon; homemade broth, soups without added salt and made with allowed vegetables; low-sodium cream soups within milk allowance	Regular commercially prepared or dehydrated soups, broths, or bouillon
Vegetables	Fresh, unsalted frozen vegetables, and low-sodium commercially prepared vegetables	Regular commercially prepared vegetables; sauerkraut, pickled vegetables, and others prepared in brine; frozen peas, lima beans, and mixed vegetables; all frozen vegetables in sauces; vegetables seasoned with ham, bacon, or salt pork
Miscellaneous	Salt substitute with physician's approval; pepper, herbs, spices; vinegar, lemon, or lime juice; low-sodium soy sauce; hot pepper sauce; low-sodium condiments (catsup, chili sauce, mustard); fresh ground horseradish; unsalted tortilla chips, pretzels, potato chips, popcorn	Salt and any seasoning made with salt, including garlic salt, celery salt, onion salt, and seasoned salt; sea salt, rock salt, kosher salt; meat tenderizers; monosodium glutamate; regular soy sauce, barbecue sauce, teriyaki sauce, steak sauce, Worcestershire sauce, and most flavored vinegars; canned gravy and mixes; regular condiments, including olives, horseradish, pickles, relish, catsup, and mustard, commercial salsa

APPENDIX 37 Sodium-Restricted Diets—cont'd

Sample Menu for 1000-mg Sodium Diet

Breakfast	Lunch	Dinner
½ cup calcium-fortified orange juice	3-oz boneless, skinless chicken breast	1 cup spaghetti (unsalted) with unsalted tomato and meat sauce
¾ cup shredded wheat	½ cup white rice prepared without salt	1 cup tossed salad with vegetables
2 slices low-sodium whole wheat toast	½ cup salt-free steamed broccoli	1 tbsp low-sodium salad dressing
2 tsp unsalted margarine	½ cup low-sodium coleslaw	1 slice low-sodium bread
1 Tbsp jelly	1 slice low-sodium whole wheat bread	2 tsp unsalted margarine
1 cup skim milk	1 tsp unsalted margarine	1 apple
1 cup coffee	½ cup homemade pudding	½ cup skim milk
1 tsp sugar	1 cup tea	1 cup coffee
	¼ tsp pepper	¼ tsp pepper
	2 tsp sugar	2 tsp sugar

Nutritional Analysis

Kilocalories: 1907
Protein: 78g
Fat: 45 g
Saturated fat: 10 g
Carbohydrate: 307 g
Sodium: 1070 mg
Potassium: 2956 mg
Fiber: 23 g

APPENDIX 38 Nutritional Facts on Alcoholic Beverages

Alcohol may have beneficial effects when consumed in moderation. The lowest all-cause mortality occurs at an intake of one to two drinks per day. The lowest coronary heart disease mortality also occurs at an intake of one to two drinks per day. Morbidity and mortality are highest among those drinking large amounts of alcohol. The 2005 Dietary Guidelines for Americans state:

- Alcoholic beverages should not be consumed by some individuals, including those who cannot restrict their alcohol intake, women of childbearing age who may become pregnant, pregnant and lactating women, children and adolescents, individuals taking medications that can interact with alcohol, and those with specific medical conditions.
- Those who choose to drink alcoholic beverages should do so sensibly and in moderation—defined as the consumption of up to one drink per day for women and up to two drinks per day for men.

- Alcoholic beverages should be avoided by individuals engaging in activities that require attention, skill, or coordination, such as driving or operating machinery.

Calories in Selected Alcoholic Beverages*

This table is a guide to estimate the caloric intake from various alcoholic beverages. A sample serving volume and the calories in that drink are shown for beer, wine, and distilled spirits. Higher alcohol content (higher percent alcohol or higher proof) and mixing alcohol with other beverages such as sweetened soft drinks, tonic water, fruit juice, or cream increase the amount of calories in the beverage. Alcoholic beverages supply calories but provide few essential nutrients.

Beverage	Serving (oz)	Alcohol (g)	Carbohydrate (g)	Calories	Exchanges for Calorie or Diabetes Control
Beer					
Regular	12	13	13	150	1 Starch, 2 fat
Light	12	11	5	100	2 Fat
Near beer	12	1.5	12	60	1 Starch
Distilled spirits					
80-Proof (gin, rum, vodka, whiskey, scotch)	1.5	14	Trace	100	2 Fat
Dry brandy, cognac	1	11	Trace	75	1.5 Fat
Table wines					
Dry white	4	11	Trace	80	2 Fat
Red or rose	4	12	2	85	2 Fat
Sweet wine	4	12	5	105	⅓ Starch, 2 fat
Light wine	4	6	1	50	1 Fat
Wine cooler	12	13	30	215	2 Fruit, 2 fat
Dealcoholized wines	4	Trace	6-7	25-35	0.5 Fruit
Sparkling wines					
Champagne	4	12	4	100	2 Fat
Sweet kosher wine	4	12	12	132	1 Starch, 2 fat
Appetizer/dessert wines					
Sherry	2	9	2	74	1.5 Fat
Sweet sherry, port, muscatel	2	9	7	90	0.5 Starch, 1.5 fat
Cordials, liqueurs	1	13	18	160	1 Starch, 2 fat
Vermouth					
Dry	3	13	4	105	2 Fat
Sweet	3	13	14	140	1 Starch, 2 fat
Cocktails					
Bloody Mary	5	14	5	116	1 Vegetable, 2 fat
Daiquiri	2	14	2	111	2 Fat
Manhattan	2	17	2	178	2.5 Fat
Martini	2.5	22	Trace	156	3.5 Fat
Old-fashioned	4	26	Trace	180	4 Fat
Tom Collins	7.5	16	3	120	2.5 Fat
Mixes					
Mineral water	Any	0	0	0	Free
Sugar-free tonic	Any	0	0	0	Free
Club soda	Any	0	0	0	Free
Diet soda	Any	0	0	0	Free
Tomato juice	4	0	5	25	1 Vegetable
Bloody Mary mix	4	0	5	25	1 Vegetable
Orange juice	4	0	15	60	1 Fruit
Grapefruit juice	4	0	15	60	1 Fruit
Pineapple juice	4	0	15	60	1 Fruit

From Franz MJ: Alcohol and diabetes: its metabolism and guidelines for its occasional use. Part TI, *Diabetes Spectrum* 3(4):210-216, 1990.

*The caloric contribution from alcohol of an alcoholic beverage can be estimated by multiplying the number of ounces by the proof and then again by the factor 0.8. For beers and wines, kilocalories from alcohol can be estimated by multiplying ounces by percentage of alcohol (by volume) and then by the factor 1.6.

APPENDIX 39 Nutritional Facts on Caffeine-Containing Products

Caffeine is similar in structure to adenosine, a chemical found in the brain that slows down its activity. Since the two compete, the more caffeine that is consumed, the less adenosine that is available up to a point. Caffeine temporarily heightens concentration and wards off fatigue. Within 30 to 60 minutes of drinking a cup of coffee, caffeine reaches peak concentrations in the bloodstream. It typically takes 4 to 6 hours for its effects to wear off.

The average American adult consumes about 200 mg of caffeine a day, and many may consume twice that level. Although the jury is still out on caffeine in pregnancy and lactation, it is generally safe to consume no more than the equivalent amount of caffeine in 1 to 2 cups of coffee daily. However, the mother with a fussy breast-fed baby may want to try eliminating caffeine from her diet.

Individuals with heart disease and hypertension may benefit from a reduction in caffeine consumption. To reduce caffeine and its stimulant effects, monitor intake from foods and beverages listed below.

Selected Food and Beverage Sources of Caffeine

Caffeine-Containing Products	Serving (mg)
Coffee, 6-oz Cup	
Brewed, drip method	103
Brewed, percolator method	75
Instant, 1 rounded tsp	57
Decaffeinated	2
Flavored, regular and sugar-free	26-75
Espresso, 1 oz	40
Café Latte, short (8 oz) or tall (12 oz) (Starbucks)	35
Tea	
3-minute brew, 6-oz cup	36
Instant, 1 rounded tsp in 8 oz of water	25-35
Decaffeinated, 5- minute brew, 6-oz cup	1
Tea, green (8 oz)	30
Tea, bottles (12 oz) or from instant mix (8 oz)	14
Cola Beverages, 12 oz	
Regular or diet	35-50
Decaffeinated	Trace
7-Eleven Big Gulp cola (64 oz)	190
Cherry colas, Dr. Pepper, Mr. Pibb, 12 oz	
Regular or diet	35-50
Decaffeinated	Trace
Mellow Yellow, 12 oz	
Regular or diet	52
Mountain Dew, 12 oz	
Regular or diet	54
Cocoa and Chocolate	
Cocoa beverage, 6-oz cup	4
Chocolate milk, 8 oz	8
Chocolate, sweet, semisweet, dark, milk, 1 oz	8-20
Chocolate, baking, unsweetened, 1 oz	58
Chocolate-flavored syrup, 1 oz	5
Chocolate pudding, ½ cup	4-8
Miscellaneous	
Powershot (8 oz)	800
NoDoz, Maximum Strength (1), or Vivarin (1)	200
Excedrin (2)	130
NoDoz, Regular Strength (1)	100
Red Bull (8.3 oz)	80
Water, caffeinated (Edge 2 O), (8 oz)	70
Anacin (2)	65
Jolt (8 oz)	48

APPENDIX 40 Nutritional Facts on Essential (Omega) Fatty Acids

Essential fatty acids (EFAs) are fatty acids that are required in the human diet. They must be obtained from food because human cells have no biochemical pathways capable of producing them internally. There are two closely related families of EFAs: **omega-3 (ω-3 or n-3)** and **omega-6 (ω-6 or n-6)**. Only one substance in each of these families is truly essential, since, for example, the body can convert one ω-3 to another ω-3 but cannot create an ω-3 from scratch.

In the body essential fatty acids serve multiple functions. In each of these the balance between dietary ω-3 and ω-6 strongly affects function. They are modified to make the eicosanoids (affecting inflammation and many other cellular functions); the endogenous cannabinoids (affecting mood, behavior, and inflammation); the lipoxins from ω-6 EFAs and resolvins from ω-3 (in the presence of aspirin, down-regulating inflammation); the isofurans, isoprostanes, hepoxilins, epoxyeicosatrienoic acids (EETs), and neuroprotectin D; and the lipid rafts (affecting cellular signaling). They also act on deoxyribonucleic acid (DNA) (activating or inhibiting transcription factors for NFκB, a proinflammatory cytokine).

Between 1930 and 1950 arachidonic and linolenic acids were termed essential because each was more or less able to meet the growth requirements of rats given fat-free diets. Further research has shown that **human metabolism requires both ω-3 and ω-6 fatty acids.** To some extent any ω-3 and any ω-6 can relieve the worst symptoms of fatty acid deficiency. However, in many people the ability to convert the ω-3 α-linolenic acid (ALA) to the ω-3 eicosapentaenoic (EPA) and docsahexaenoic acid (DHA) is only 5% efficient. Therefore it is important to incorporate the EPA and DHA directly into the diet usually as fish or a fish oil supplement. Particular fatty acids such as DHA are needed at critical life stages (e.g., infancy and lactation) and in some disease states.

The essential fatty acids are:

- ALA (18:3)-ω-3
- Linoleic acid (18:2)-ω-6

These two fatty acids cannot be synthesized by humans because humans lack the desaturase enzymes required for their production. They form the starting point for the creation of longer and more desaturated fatty acids, which are also referred to as long-chain polyunsaturates:

ω-3 Fatty acids:
- EPA (20:5)
- DHA (22:6)
- ALA (18:)

ω-6 Fatty acids:
- γ-Linolenic acid (GLA) (18:3)
- Dihomo-γ-linolenic acid (DGLA) (20:3)
- Arachidonic acid or AA (20:4)

ω-9 Fatty acids are not essential in humans, because humans possess all the enzymes required for their synthesis.

Adequate Intakes for ω-3 Fatty Acids for Children and Adults

Age (years)	Males and Females (g/day)	Pregnancy (g/day)	Lactation (g/day)
1-3	0.7	N/A	N/A
4-8	0.9	N/A	N/A
9-13	1.2 for males; 1.0 for females	N/A	N/A
14-18	1.6 for males; 1.1 for females	1.4	1.3
19+	1.6 for males; 1.1 for females	1.4	1.3

Adequate Intakes for ω-6 Fatty Acids for Children and Adults

Age (years)	Males and Females (g/day)	Pregnancy (g/day)	Lactation (g/day)
1-3	7	N/A	N/A
4-8	10	N/A	N/A
9-13	12 for males; 10 for females	N/A	N/A
14-18	16 for males; 11 for females	13	13
19+	17 for males; 12 for females	13	13

Dietary Sources

Some of the food sources of ω-3 and ω-6 fatty acids are fish and shellfish, flaxseed (linseed), soya oil, canola (rapeseed) oil, hemp oil, chia seeds, pumpkin seeds, sunflower seeds, leafy vegetables, and walnuts.

EFAs play a part in many metabolic processes, and there is evidence to suggest that low levels of EFAs or the wrong balance of types among the EFAs may be a factor in a number of illnesses.

Plant sources of ω-3s do not contain EPA and DHA. This is thought to be the reason that absorption of EFAs is much greater from animal rather than plant sources.

EFA content of vegetable sources varies with cultivation conditions. Animal sources vary widely, both with the animal's feed and that the EFA makeup varies markedly with fats from different body parts.

Omega-3 Fatty Acids

There is some evidence that suggests that ω-3s may:

- Help lower elevated triglyceride levels. High triglyceride levels can contribute to coronary heart disease.
- Reduce the blood's tendency to clot, which may relate to the clogging that occurs with atherosclerosis.
- Reduce the inflammation involved in conditions such as rheumatoid arthritis.
- Improve symptoms of depression and other mental health disorders in some individuals.

Dietary sources of ω-3 fatty acids include fish oil and certain plant and nut oils. Fish oil contains both DHA and EPA, whereas some nuts (English walnuts) and vegetable oils (canola, soybean, flaxseed/linseed, olive) contain only the ω-3 ALA.

There is evidence from multiple large-scale population (epidemiologic) studies and randomized controlled trials that intake of recommended amounts of DHA and EPA in the form of fish or fish oil supplements lowers triglycerides; reduces the risk of death, heart attack, dangerous abnormal heart rhythms, and strokes in people with known cardiovascular disease; slows the buildup of atherosclerotic plaques ("hardening of the arteries"); and lowers blood pressure slightly. However, high doses may have harmful effects such as an increased risk of bleeding. Some species of fish carry a higher risk of environmental contamination such as with methyl mercury.

APPENDIX 40 Nutritional Facts on Essential (Omega 3 and 6) Fatty Acids—cont'd

Common Food Sources of Omega-3 Fats

Omega-3 Fat	Food Source
ALA	Ground flaxseed and walnuts and soybeans
	Flaxseed, walnut, soybean and canola oils, and nonhydrogenated canola and soy margarines
DHA and EPA	Mackerel, salmon, herring, trout and sardines, and other fish and shellfish
	Marine algae supplements

Fish or Other Food Source	Omega-3 Content in a 4-oz Serving
English walnuts	6.8 g
Chinook salmon	3.6 g
Sockeye salmon	2.3 g
Mackerel	1.8-2.6 g
Herring	1.2-2.7 g
Rainbow trout	1.0 g
Wheat germ and oat germ	0.7-1.4 g
Halibut	0.5-1.3 g
White tuna	.97 g
Light tuna	.35 g
Whiting	0.9 g
Spinach	0.9 g
Flounder	0.6 g
King crab	0.6 g
Shrimp	0.5 g
Tofu	0.4 g (probably much less in "lite" tofu)
Clam	0.32 g
Cod	0.3 g
Scallop	0.23 g

* Exact omega-3 content varies per manufacturer. Check label.

Supplements*

Cod liver oil	800-100 mg/tsp
Fish body oil	1200-1800 mg/tsp
Omega-3 fatty acid concentrate	250 mg/capsule

Boosting Your Intake of Omega-3 Fats

- Eat fish at least two times each week.
- Include canned fish in your diet (examples: salmon, sardines, light tuna). Try sardines on toast.
- Add ground flaxseed to foods such as hot or cold cereal or yogurt. NOTE: Pregnant women should limit their intake of ground flaxseed to occasional use (not daily). Ground flaxseeds contain lignans. There is not enough information about their safety in pregnancy.
- Eat walnuts. Add walnuts to salads, cereals, baking (examples, muffins, cookies, breads) and pancakes.
- Have fresh or frozen soybeans (edamame) as a vegetable at meals.
- Use soybean oil or canola oil in salad dressings and recipes.
- Use nonhydrogenated margarine made from canola or soybean as a spread or in baking.
- Cook with ω-3 liquid eggs or eggs in the shell. Enjoy scrambled eggs or try a homemade egg sandwich.
- Use other ω-3 fortified products such as milk, yogurt, bread, and pasta.
- Substitute ¼ cup ground flaxseed for ¼ cup flour in bread, pizza dough, muffin, cookie, or meatloaf recipes.
- Replace 1 egg with 1 Tbsp ground flaxseed and 3 Tbsp water in recipes.

APPENDIX 41 Nutritional Facts on a High-Fiber Diet

This diet is a modification of the regular diet. The purpose of this diet is to decrease transit time through the intestine, promote more frequent bowel movements, and softer stools. This diet may be prescribed as a treatment for diverticulosis, irritable bowel syndrome, hemorrhoids, and/or constipation. It includes all the foods on a regular diet, with emphasis on the proper planning and selection of foods to increase the daily intake of fiber. Fluid intake should be increased.

The American Dietetic Association recommends that the average adult have a daily fiber intake of 20 to 35 g from a variety of sources. For children the child's age plus 5 g of fiber is recommended daily. In cases of severe constipation more fiber is recommended. Because of possible interactions with absorption of nutrients, regular intake of greater than 50 g of fiber per day is not recommended.

Dietary Reference Intakes for Fiber for Children and Adults

Age (years)	Males and Females (g/day)	Pregnancy (g/day)	Lactation (g/day)
1-3	19	N/A	N/A
4-8	25	N/A	N/A
9-13	31 for males; 26 for females	N/A	N/A
14-18	38 for males; 26 for females	28	29
19+	38 for males; 25 for females	28	29

Although numerous over-the-counter fiber supplements are available, food sources provide other nutrients and are the preferred method of increasing dietary fiber. Adequate liquid consumption (at least eight 8-oz glasses per day) is recommended. Fiber should be added to the diet slowly because of possible cramps, bloating, and diarrhea with a sudden fiber increase. Maximum therapeutic benefits of fiber are obtained after several months of compliance. There are two components of dietary fiber, each providing health benefits: insoluble and soluble.

Continued

Types of Dietary Fiber

Type of Fiber	Components of Cells	Food Sources	Health Benefits
Soluble fibers	Gums, mucilages, pectin, certain hemicelluloses	Vegetables, fruits, barley; legumes, oats, and oat-bran	Decrease total blood cholesterol Guard against diabetes Prevent constipation May help manage irritable bowel syndrome May protect against colon cancer and gallstones
Insoluble fibers	Cellulose, lignin, some hemicelluloses	Whole wheat products, wheat and corn bran, and many vegetables (including cauliflower, green beans, potatoes, and skins of root vegetables)	May prevent diverticular disease Prevents constipation May delay glucose absorption (probably insignificant) May increase satiety and therefore assist with weight loss Lower cholesterol May protect against colon cancer

Guidelines for High-Fiber Diet

1. Increase consumption of whole grain breads, cereals, flours, and other whole grain productions to 6 to 11 servings daily.
2. Increase consumption of vegetables, legumes and fruits, nuts, and edible seeds to 5 to 8 servings daily.
3. Consume high-fiber cereals, granolas, and legumes as needed to bring fiber intake to 25 g or more daily.
4. Increase consumption of fluids to at least 2 L (or about 2 qt) daily.
5. For a high-fiber diet of approximately 24 g of dietary fiber: use 12 or more servings of the foods from the groups below (each food contains approximately 2 g of dietary fiber). For example, ½ cup of baked beans (8 Tbsp) would count as 4 servings.

Each of these foods in this amount contains 2 g of dietary fiber:

Apple, 1 small	Strawberries, ½ cup
Orange, 1 small	Pear, ½ small
Banana, 1 small	Cherries, 10 large
Peach, 1 medium	Plums, 2 small

Whole wheat bread, 1 slice	Oatmeal, dry, 3 Tbsp
All Bran, 1 Tbsp	Shredded wheat, ½ biscuit
Rye bread, 1 slice	Wheat bran, 1 tsp
Corn flakes, ⅔ cup	Grape-nuts, 3 Tbsp
Cracked wheat bread, 1 slice	Puffed wheat, 1⅓ cup

Broccoli, ½ stalk	Potato, 2-in diameter
Lettuce, raw, 2 cups	Celery, 1 cup
Brussels sprouts, 4	Tomato, raw, 1 medium
Green beans, ½ cup	Corn on the cob, 2 in
Carrots, ⅔ cup	Baked beans, canned, 2 Tbsp

Selected Food Sources of Fiber

Food	Grams per Serving	% Daily Value*
Navy beans, cooked, ½ cup	9.5	38
Bran ready-to-eat cereal (100%), ½ cup	8.8	35
Kidney beans, canned, ½ cup	8.2	33
Split peas, cooked, ½ cup	8.1	32
Lentils, cooked, ½ cup	7.8	31
Black beans, cooked, ½ cup	7.5	30
Pinto beans, cooked, ½ cup	7.7	31
Lima beans, cooked, ½ cup	6.6	26
Artichoke, globe, cooked, 1 each	6.5	26
White beans, canned, ½ cup	6.3	25
Chickpeas, cooked, ½ cup	6.2	24
Great northern beans, cooked, ½ cup	6.2	24
Cowpeas, cooked, ½ cup	5.6	22
Soybeans, mature, cooked, ½ cup	5.2	21
Bran ready-to-eat cereals, various, 1 oz	2.6-5.0	10-20
Crackers, rye wafers, plain, 2 wafers	5.0	20
Sweet potato, baked, with peel, 1 medium (146 g)	4.8	19
Asian pear, raw, 1 small	4.4	18
Green peas, cooked, ½ cup	4.4	18
Whole-wheat English muffin, 1 each	4.4	18
Pear, raw, 1 small	4.3	17
Bulgur, cooked, ½ cup	4.1	16

*Daily values (DVs) are reference numbers based on the recommended dietary allowance. They were developed to help consumers determine if a food contains a lot or a little of a specific nutrient. The DV for fiber is 25 g. The percent DV (%DV) listed on the Nutrition Facts panel of food labels states the percentage of the DV provided in 1 serving. %DVs are based on a 2000-calorie diet.

Food Sources of Dietary Fiber ranked by grams of dietary fiber per standard amount. (All are ≥10% of adequate intake for adult women, which is 25 g/day.)

APPENDIX 41 Nutritional Facts on a High-Fiber Diet—cont'd

Selected Food Sources of Fiber—cont'd

Food	Grams per Serving	% Daily Value*
Mixed vegetables, cooked, ½ cup	4.0	16
Raspberries, raw, ½ cup	4.0	16
Sweet potato, boiled, no peel, 1 medium (156 g)	3.9	15.5
Blackberries, raw, ½ cup	3.8	15
Potato, baked, with skin, 1 medium	3.8	15
Soybeans, green, cooked, ½ cup	3.8	15
Stewed prunes, ½ cup	3.8	15
Figs, dried, ¼ cup	3.7	14.5
Dates, ¼ cup	3.6	14
Oat bran, raw, ¼ cup	3.6	14
Pumpkin, canned, ½ cup	3.6	14
Spinach, frozen, cooked, ½ cup	3.5	14
Shredded wheat ready-to-eat cereals, various, ≈1 oz	2.8-3.4	11-13
Almonds, 1 oz	3.3	13
Apple with skin, raw, 1 medium	3.3	13
Brussels sprouts, frozen, cooked, ½ cup	3.2	13
Whole-wheat spaghetti, cooked, ½ cup	3.1	12
Banana, 1 medium	3.1	12
Orange, raw, 1 medium	3.1	12
Oat bran muffin, 1 small	3.0	12
Guava, 1 medium	3.0	12
Pearled barley, cooked, ½ cup	3.0	12
Sauerkraut, canned, solids, and liquids, ½ cup	3.0	12
Tomato paste, ¼ cup	2.9	11.5
Winter squash, cooked, ½ cup	2.9	11.5
Broccoli, cooked, ½ cup	2.8	11
Parsnips, cooked, chopped, ½ cup	2.8	11
Turnip greens, cooked, ½ cup	2.5	10
Collards, cooked, ½ cup	2.7	11
Okra, frozen, cooked, ½ cup	2.6	10
Peas, edible-podded, cooked, ½ cup	2.5	10

High-Fiber Meal Plan

Breakfast	Lunch	Dinner
1 orange	3-oz boneless, skinless chicken breast	1 cup spaghetti with meat sauce
¾ cup raisin bran	½ cup broccoli	1 cup tossed salad with assorted
2 slices whole wheat toast	½ cup long grain and wild rice	vegetables and ¼ cup chickpeas*
2 tsp margarine	1 whole wheat roll	1 slice Italian bread
1 cup skim milk	½ cup chocolate pudding	½ cup apple crisp
1 cup coffee	½ Tbsp whipped topping	2 tsp margarine
2 tsp sugar	2 tsp margarine	1 cup skim milk
	1 cup iced tea	1 cup coffee
	¼ tsp salt	¼ tsp salt
	¼ tsp pepper	¼ tsp pepper
	2 tsp sugar	2 tsp sugar

Nutritional Analysis

Kilocalories: 2074
Protein: 84 g
Fat: 52 g
Carbohydrate: 313 g
Sodium: 4647 mg
Potassium: 3706 mg
Fiber: 28 g

*Fiber content may be higher, depending on vegetables selected for salad.

APPENDIX 42 Nutritional Facts on Fluid and Hydration

Adequate **hydration** is essential for life. Body water is necessary to regulate body temperature, transport nutrients, moisten body tissues, comprise body fluids, and make waste products soluble for excretion.

Principles: As the most plentiful substance in the human body, water is also the most plentiful nutrient in the diet. The amount of water recommended for an individual varies with age, activity, medical condition, and physical condition. The water in juice, tea, milk, decaffeinated coffee, and carbonated beverages contributes the majority of water in the diet. Solid foods also contribute water to the diet but usually are not counted in the amount of water provided per day.

Water deficiency, or **dehydration**, is characterized by dark urine; decreased skin turgor; dry mouth, lips, and mucous membranes; headache; a coated, wrinkled tongue; dry or sunken eyes; weight loss; a lowered body temperature; and increased serum sodium, albumin, blood urea nitrogen (BUN), and creatinine values. Dehydration may be caused by inadequate intake in relation to fluid requirements or excessive fluid losses caused by fever, increased urine output, diarrhea, draining wounds, ostomy output, fistulas, environmental temperature, or vomiting. Concentrated or high-protein tube feeding formulas may increase the water requirement.

Thirst is often the first noticed sign of the need for more water. However, athletes or workers exercising or working hard in hot climates may be significantly dehydrated before they realize they are thirsty. In these situations they should be drinking at regular intervals; they may not be able to rely on thirst to determine their need to drink.

Water excess or **overhydration** is rare and may be the result of inadequate output or excessive intake. Overhydration is characterized by increased blood pressure; decreased pulse rate; edema; and decreased serum sodium, potassium, albumin, BUN, and creatinine values. Fluid restrictions may be necessary for certain medical conditions such as kidney or cardiac disease. For those on fluid restrictions, the fluid needs should be calculated on an individual basis. The usual diet provides about 1080 ml (36 oz), a little over a quart of fluid per day.

Approximate Fluid Content of Common Foods

Food	Fluid Ounces	Household Measure	Metric Measure
Juice	2	¼ cup	60 ml
	3	⅓ cup	90 ml
	4	½ cup	120 ml
	8	1 cup	240 ml
Coffee, tea, decaffeinated coffee	6	⅔ cup	180 ml
Gelatin	4	½ cup	120 ml
Ice cream, sherbet	3	⅓ cup	90 ml
Soup	6	⅔ cup	180 ml
Liquid coffee creamer	1	2 Tbsp	30 ml

NOTE: 3 oz is approximately ⅓ cup; 6 oz is approximately ⅔ cup.

Estimating Daily Fluid Requirements for Healthy Individuals

Children	Body Weight	Daily Fluid Requirement
Infants		140 to 150 ml/kg
Children		
Method 1		50 to 60 ml/kg
Method 2	3 to 10 kg of body weight	100 ml/kg
	11 to 20 kg of body weight	1000 ml + 50 ml/kg >10
	More than 20 kg	1500 ml + 20 ml/kg >20
Adults*		
Method 1	30 to 35 ml per weight in kilograms	
Method 2	1 ml fluid per calorie consumed	
Method 3	First 10 kg of body weight	100 ml/kg
	Second 10 kg of body weight	+ 50 ml/kg
	Remaining kg of body weight (age <50)	+ 20 ml/kg
	Remaining kg of body weight (age >50)	+ 15 ml/kg
Method 4	Age in years	
	16-30 (active)	40 ml/kg
	20-55	35 ml/kg
	55-75	30 ml/kg
	>75	25 ml/kg

From the California Diet Manual, ©2003, State of California Department of Developmental Services, revised 2004.

*The 1 milliliter of fluid per calorie method should be used with caution because it will underestimate the fluid needs of those with low calorie needs. Persons who are significantly obese may best be evaluated by Method 3 because it adjusts for high body weight.

APPENDIX 43 Glycemic Index (GI) and Glycemic Load (GL) of Selected Foods*

Breakfast Cereals	GI	GL
Kellogg's All-Bran	30	4
Kellogg's Cocoa Puffs	77	20
Kellogg's Corn Flakes	92	24
Kellogg's MiniWheats	58	12
Kellogg's Nutrigrain	66	10
Old-fashioned oatmeal	42	9
Kellogg's Rice Krispies	82	22
Kellogg's Special K	69	14
Kellogg's Raisin Bran	61	12
Grains/Pastas		
Buckwheat	54	16
Bulgur	48	12
Rice		
Basmati	58	22
Brown	50	16
Instant	87	36
Uncle Ben's	39	14
Converted, white	4	
Noodles—instant	7	19
Pasta		
Egg fettuccine (avg)	40	18
Spaghetti (avg)	38	18
Vermicelli	35	16
Tortellini, Stouffer's	50	1
Bread		
Bagel	72	25
Croissant†	67	17
Crumpet	69	13
"Grainy" breads (avg)	49	6
Pita bread	57	10
Pumpernickel (avg)	50	6
Rye bread (avg)	58	8
White bread (avg)	70	10
Whole-wheat bread (avg)	77	9
Crackers/Crispbread		
Kavli	71	12
Puffed crisp bread	81	15
Ryvita	69	11
Water cracker	78	14
Cookies		
Oatmeal	55	12
Milk Arrowroot	69	12
Shortbread (commercial)†	64	10
Cake		
Chocolate, frosted, Betty Crocker	38	20
Oat bran muffin	69	24
Sponge cake	46	17
Waffles	76	10

Vegetables	GI	GL
Beets, canned	64	5
Carrots (avg)	47	3
Parsnip	97	12
Peas (green, avg)	48	3
Potato		
Baked (avg)	85	26
Boiled	88	16
French fries	75	22
Microwaved	82	27
Pumpkin	75	3
Sweet corn	60	11
Sweet potato (avg)	61	17
Rutabaga	72	7
Yam (avg)	37	13
Legumes		
Baked beans (avg)	48	7
Broad beans	79	9
Butter beans	31	6
Chickpeas (avg)	28	8
Cannellini beans (avg)	38	12
Kidney beans (avg)	28	7
Lentils (avg)	29	5
Soy beans (avg)	18	1
Fruit		
Apple (avg)	38	6
Apricot (dried)	31	9
Banana (avg)	51	13
Cherries	22	3
Grapefruit	25	3
Grapes (avg)	46	8
Kiwi fruit (avg)	53	6
Mango	51	8
Orange (avg)	48	5
Papaya	59	10
Peach (avg)		
Canned (natural juice)	38	4
Fresh (avg)	42	5
Pear (avg)	38	4
Pineapple	59	7
Plum	39	5
Raisins	64	28
Cantaloupe	65	4
Watermelon	72	4
Dairy Foods		
Milk		
Full-fat	27	3
Skim	32	4
Chocolate-flavored	42	13
Condensed	61	33

Dairy Foods—cont'd	GI	GL
Custard	43	7
Ice cream		
Regular (avg)	61	8
Low-fat	50	3
Yogurt, low-fat	33	10
Beverages		
Apple juice	40	12
Coca Cola	63	16
Lemonade	66	13
Fanta	68	23
Orange juice (avg)	52	12
Snack Foods		
Tortilla chips† (avg)	63	17
Fish sticks	38	7
Peanuts† (avg)	14	1
Popcorn	72	8
Potato chips†	57	10
Convenience Foods		
Macaroni and cheese	64	32
Soup		
Lentil	44	9
Split-pea	60	16
Tomato	38	6
Sushi (avg)	52	19
Pizza, cheese	60	16
Sweets		
Chocolate†	44	13
Jelly beans (avg)	78	22
Life Savers	70	21
Mars Bar	68	27
Kudo whole-grain chocolate-chip bar	62	20
Sugars		
Honey (avg)	55	10
Fructose (avg)	19	2
Glucose*	100	10
Lactose (avg)	46	5
Sucrose (avg)	68	7
Sports Bars		
Clif bar (cookies and cream)	101	3
PowerBar (chocolate)	83	35
METRx bar (vanilla)	74	37

From Brand Miller J et al: *The new glucose revolution*, New York, 2003, Avalon/Marlowe & Company.

*Glucose = 100.

†These foods are high in saturated fat.

APPENDIX 44 Nutritional Facts on a High-Protein Diet

The high-protein diet is designed for individuals requiring increased protein in addition to their normal diet. This diet provides additional high-quality protein, primarily from milk, eggs, cheese, soy, and meat sources. An individual's protein intake may be increased to 100 g of protein per day, or 1.25 up to 2 g/kg. Indications for use are the presence of pressure ulcers, surgery, infection, or malnutrition. Contraindications include hepatic coma and renal insufficiency. Patients on this diet may have loss of or poor appetite; therefore six feedings per day may improve patient adherence.

Adequacy: The high-protein diet is adequate in all nutrients and exceeds the dietary reference intake for protein.

Minimum Portions to Achieve 100 g of Protein

2-3 Cups or more (8 oz each) fortified milk or substitute
3-4 Servings (2-3 oz servings) meat or meat substitute
3-4 Servings fruits and vegetables (1 vitamin C–rich source daily such as 1 citrus fruit, 1 carotenoid source such as 1 dark green or yellow vegetable)
3-4 Servings or more of whole grain or enriched breads and cereals
Other foods are included to provide adequate calories.

Special Notes

1. Nonfat dry milk may be added to cooked foods to increase protein intake. One quarter cup powdered milk is equivalent to 1 cup fluid milk. Nonfat dry milk can be added to hot cereal, cream soups, and casseroles.

2. Supplemental high protein feedings may be required if the patient has a poor appetite.

3. One fluid cup (8 oz) commercial eggnog contains 15 g of protein, almost twice as much protein as 1 fluid cup (8 oz) of milk. This is a very good snack for use in a high-protein diet.

Suggested Meal Pattern: High-Protein

Breakfast	Noon Meal	Evening Meal
½ cup fruit/juice	3 oz meat/sub	3 oz meat/sub
½ cup cereal	½ cup potato/sub	½ cup potato/sub
2 eggs	½ cup veg and/or	½ cup veg and/or
1 serving bread	½ cup veg and/or	½ cup veg and/or
1 tsp margarine	½-¾ cup salad	½-¾ cup salad
1 cup (8 oz) milk	Salad dressing	Salad dressing
Coffee/tea	1 serving bread	1 serving bread
	1 tsp margarine	1 tsp margarine
	½ cup fruit/dessert	½ cup fruit/dessert
	1 cup (8 oz) milk	1 cup (8 oz) milk
AM Snack	**PM Snack**	**Bedtime Snack**
8 oz. eggnog	Cheese/crackers	Milk + sandwich

APPENDIX 45 Nutritional Facts on Vegetarian Eating

These diets are designed for those who prefer vegetarian eating for religious, ecologic, or personal reasons. Because of the variations in vegetarian diets, it is recommended that the dietitian work closely with the patient and his or her family in establishing a diet pattern. Vegetarian diets are usually classified into one of the following three types:

1. Lacto-ovo-vegetarian—a modification of the diet, which restricts all dietary sources of animal protein except dairy products and eggs. This is the most common type of vegetarian diet and is the easiest of the vegetarian diets to prepare.
2. Lacto-vegetarian—a modification of the diet, which restricts all dietary sources of animal protein except dairy products.
3. Strict vegetarian (vegan diet)—a modification of the diet, which restricts all dietary sources of animal protein.

Adequacy: the lacto-ovo and lacto-vegetarian diets require careful planning to be adequate in all nutrients to meet the dietary reference intakes. The strict vegetarian diet (vegan diet) may be deficient in protein, zinc, calcium, and vitamins D and vitamin B_{12}; therefore supplements or fortified foods are recommended.

Protein: No foods are prepared with meat-based broth. Substitute soy-based and vegetable broths.

The following foods provide approximately the same amount of protein as does 1 oz of meat (7 g of protein).

¼ cup cottage cheese	½ cup legumes, cooked
1 cup regular or soy milk	¼ cup soy beans
1 oz cheese	1 oz processed soy protein
⅓ cup mixed nuts	¼ cup tofu (soy cheese)
1 egg	¾ cup yogurt
2 Tbsp peanut butter	

Proper protein combinations combine the essential amino acids to provide high-quality proteins, but they do not have to be at the same meal. The following list provides some of the combinations:

Grains

Rice with legumes
Rice cooked in milk
Corn with legumes
Macaroni and cheese
Whole wheat bread and cheese
Whole grain breakfast cereal with milk
Whole wheat toast with poached egg

Nuts and Seeds

Peanut butter sandwich with milk
Sesame seeds with beans as in hummus

Legumes

Baked beans with whole wheat bread
Legumes with rice
Split pea soup and whole wheat bread
Soy beans with rice and wheat
Soy beans with corn and milk
Soy yogurt with granola

Vegetables

Lima beans, peas, Brussels sprouts, cauliflower or broccoli with sesame seeds, Brazil nuts, or mushrooms

Calcium: All vegetarians, especially young women, should ensure adequate calcium intake for development and maintenance of strong bones. In place of dairy products, choose abundant amounts of dark, leafy greens (i.e., kale, mustard and turnip greens, collards); bok choy; broccoli; legumes; tofu processed with calcium; dried figs; sunflower seeds; and calcium-fortified cereals and juice. The following foods provide approximately the same amount of calcium as does 1 cup of milk (about 300 mg).

1 cup calcium-fortified soy milk	3 cups cooked dried beans
1⅔ cups sunflower seeds	1 cup almonds
1 cup collards, cooked	3 pieces enriched cornbread

Data from National Center for Nutrition and Dietetics, *Food guide pyramid for vegetarian meal planning.* Chicago, Ill, 1997, American Dietetic Association Foundation; American Dietetic Association: Position of the American Dietetic Association: vegetarian diets, *J Am Diet Assoc* 103:748-765, 2003.

APPENDIX 45 Nutritional Facts on Vegetarian Eating—cont'd

Iron: Iron deficiency rates are similar between vegetarians and nonvegetarians. When consumed along with foods rich in vitamin C, plant sources of iron are better absorbed. High-iron foods include legumes, dark green vegetables (i.e., spinach and beet greens), dried fruits; prune juice, blackstrap molasses, pumpkin seeds, soy nuts, and iron-fortified breads and cereals.

Vitamin B$_{12}$: Found only in animal foods, vitamin B$_{12}$ is not a nutrient of great concern for vegetarians who regularly consume eggs or dairy products (lacto-ovo-vegetarians). Vegans should include vitamin B$_{12}$–fortified foods such as fortified soymilk and commercial breakfast cereals and/or a B$_{12}$ supplement in their diets. Vitamin B$_{12}$ is also found in Brewer's yeast.

Vitamin D: In the United States the primary source of vitamin D is dairy products, most of which are fortified with vitamin D. However, cheese and yogurt do not have to be made from vitamin D–fortified milk. The other main source results from sunlight exposure, causing vitamin D to be synthesized in the skin. If dairy products are not consumed and direct sunlight exposure is limited, supplementation is warranted. Foods containing vitamin D include fortified cow's milk, soy milk, rice milk, or nut milk. Supplementation is needed for individuals who do not consume milk products and/or spend little time in the sun.

Zinc: Because zinc is found in animal foods, the vegetarian diet may be limited. The following foods can be included in the diet to increase the needed amount of zinc:
- Wheat germ
- Nuts
- Dried beans

Minimum Portions to Be Included Daily

Food Categories	Recommended Daily Servings	Recommended Serving Sizes
Breads, cereals, rice, and pasta	6 or more	1 slice bread 1 oz ready to eat cereal, calcium fortified* ½ cup cooked cereal, rice, or pasta
Vegetables	4 or more	1 cup raw leafy vegetables, ½ cup cooked vegetables, calcium rich—1 cup cooked, 2 cups raw: bok choy,* okra,* broccoli,* collards,* kale*, Chinese cabbage*, mustard greens* ½ cup vegetable juice fortified*
Fruits	2 or more	1 medium piece of fruit ½ cup chopped, cooked, or canned fruit, figs (5)* ½ cup fruit juice, fortified*
Calcium-rich foods	8 or more	1 cup milk, yogurt, ½ cup fortified soymilk ¾ oz natural cheese 2 oz process cheese
Legumes and meat substitutes	5	½ cup cooked dry beans, soybeans* or peas, ½ cup soy nuts* 1 egg or 2 egg whites (optional) ¼ cup nuts or seeds, ¼ cup almonds* ½ cup Tempeh or calcium-set tofu* 2 Tbsp almond butter or sesame tahini,* 2 Tbsp peanut butter
Fats, sweets, and alcohol	Use sparingly	

*Calcium-rich foods.

Special Notes

Pregnancy and Lactation: Well-planned vegan and lacto-ovo-vegetarian eating patterns adequately provide for the nutritional needs of pregnant and lactating women (American Dietetic Association, 2003). Folate supplements are recommended for all pregnant women, including vegetarians. Vegans must ensure daily intake of 2 mcg of vitamin B$_{12}$ daily during pregnancy and 2.6 mcg during lactation, whether through supplements or fortified foods. Women with limited sun exposure should include vitamin D–fortified foods. Caution should be used with vitamin D supplementation because excess vitamin D can cause fetal abnormalities.

Infants, Children, and Adolescents: According to the American Dietetic Association (2003), well-planned vegan and lacto-ovo-vegetarian eating patterns adequately provide for the nutritional needs of infants, children, and adolescents. Because of the high bulk of low-fat vegetarian eating patterns, it may be difficult for children and adolescents to consume enough food to provide for their energy needs. Frequent meals and snacks with nutrient-dense foods can help meet energy and nutrient needs. If sun exposure is limited, vitamin D fortified–foods or supplements may be used. Vegan children should include a reliable source of vitamin B$_{12}$ in their diets. To provide for growth, calcium, iron, and zinc intakes deserve special attention. It is recommended that parents of vegetarian infants and youth consult a registered dietitian with expertise in the vegetarian eating pattern.

Continued

Meal Pattern: Lacto-Ovo-Vegetarian

Breakfast	Lunch	Dinner	Snack
½ cup orange juice (calcium fortified)	2-3 oz meat alt	2-3 oz meat alt	½ cup soy nuts
½ cup cereal	½ cup potato/substitute	½ cup rice/substitute	½ cup fortified tomato juice
1 egg	½ cup vegetable	½ cup vegetable	
1 serving bread	½-¾ cup salad	½-¾ cup salad	
1 tsp margarine	Salad dressing	Salad dressing	
1 cup (8 oz) milk	1 serving bread	1 serving bread	
Coffee/tea	1 tsp margarine	1 tsp margarine	
2 tsp sugar	½ cup fruit	½ cup fruit	
	½ cup (4 oz) milk	½ cup (4 oz) milk	
	Coffee/tea	Coffee/tea	
	¼ tsp salt	½ tsp salt	
	½ tsp pepper	½ tsp pepper	

Meal Pattern: Lacto-Vegeterian

Breakfast	Lunch	Dinner	Snack
½ cup orange juice (calcium fortified)	2-3 oz meat alt	2-3 oz meat alt	½ cup soy nuts
½ cup cereal	½ cup pasta/sub	½ cup brown rice/sub	½ cup fortified tomato juice
1 egg	½ cup vegetable	½ cup vegetable	
1 serving bread	½-¾ cup salad	½-¾ cup salad	
1 tsp margarine	Salad dressing	Salad dressing	
1 cup (8 oz) milk	1 serving bread	1 serving bread	
Coffee/tea	1 tsp margarine	1 tsp margarine	
2 tsp sugar	½ cup fruit	½ cup fruit	
	½ cup (4 oz) milk	½ cup (4 oz) milk	
	Coffee/tea	Coffee/tea	
	¼ tsp salt	¼ tsp salt	
	¼ tsp pepper	¼ tsp pepper	

Meal Pattern: Vegan

Breakfast	Lunch	Dinner	Snack
½ cup orange juice (calcium fortified)	6 oz lentil soup w/ ½ cup brown rice	2 burritos: 2- to 6-in soft corn tortillas	¼ cup soy nuts
½ cup oatmeal	4 sesame seed crackers	1 cup pinto beans	½ cup fortified tomato juice
2 slices whole wheat bread	Spinach salad:	¾ cup shredded lettuce	
2 Tbsp peanut butter*	1 cup raw spinach	½ cup diced tomato	
1 cup fortified soy milk	¼ cup shredded carrot	2 Tbsp diced onions	
2 Tbsp raisins	2 Tbsp chopped mushrooms	¼ cup salsa	
2 tsp sugar	2 oz tofu (calcium set)	½ cup broccoli/cauliflower mix	
	2 Tbsp low calorie Italian dressing	1 Tbsp margarine	
	1 fresh apple	½ cup fruit cocktail	
	1 cup fortified soy milk	1 cup fortified soy milk	
	¼ tsp salt	¼ tsp salt	
	¼ tsp pepper	¼ tsp pepper	

Nutritional Analysis

Kilocalories: 2395
Protein: 93 g
Total fat: 90 g
Monounsat. fat: 33.2 g
Polyunsat. fat: 30.8 g
Carbohydrates: 323 g
Sodium: 5762 mg*
Potassium: 4690 mg
Fiber: 45 g

*Use unsalted peanut butter, tomato juice, and soup to reduce sodium content.

APPENDIX 46 Nutritional Facts on Folic Acid, Vitamin B₆, and Vitamin B₁₂

Folate is a water-soluble B vitamin that occurs naturally in food. Folic acid is the synthetic form of folate that is found in supplements and added to fortified foods. Folate or folic acid helps produce and maintain new cells, which is especially important during periods of rapid cell division and growth such as infancy, adolescence, and pregnancy. Folate is needed to make deoxyribonucleic acid (DNA) and ribonucleic acid, the building blocks of cells. It also helps prevent changes to DNA that may lead to cancer. Both adults and children need folate to make normal red blood cells and prevent anemia. Folate is also essential for the metabolism of homocysteine and helps maintain normal levels of this amino acid.

Dietary Reference Intakes for Folate for Children and Adults

Age (years)	Males and Females (mcg /day)	Pregnancy (mcg/day)	Lactation (mcg/day)
1-3	150	N/A	N/A
4-8	200	N/A	N/A
9-13	300	N/A	N/A
14-18	400	600	500
19+	400	600	500

Selected Food Sources of Folate and Folic Acid

Food	Micrograms per Serving	% Daily Value*
Breakfast cereals fortified with 100% of the DV, ¾ cup†	400	100
Beef liver, cooked, braised, 3 oz	185	45
Cowpeas (blackeyes), immature, cooked, boiled, ½ cup	105	25
Breakfast cereals, fortified with 25% of the DV, ¾ cup†	100	25
Spinach, frozen, cooked, boiled, ½ cup	100	25
Great Northern beans, boiled, ½ cup	90	20
Asparagus, boiled, 4 spears	85	20
Rice, white, long-grain, parboiled, enriched, cooked, ½ cup†	65	15
Vegetarian baked beans, canned, 1 cup	60	15
Spinach, raw, 1 cup	60	15
Green peas, frozen, boiled, ½ cup	50	15
Broccoli, chopped, frozen, cooked, ½ cup	50	15
Egg noodles, cooked, enriched, ½ cup†	50	15
Broccoli, raw, 2 spears (each 5 inches long)	45	10
Avocado, raw, all varieties, sliced, ½ cup sliced	45	10
Peanuts, all types, dry roasted, 1 ounce	40	10
Lettuce, Romaine, shredded, ½ cup	40	10
Wheat germ, crude, 2 Tbsp	40	10
Tomato juice, canned, 6 oz	35	10
Orange juice, chilled, includes concentrate, ¾ cup	35	10
Turnip greens, frozen, cooked, boiled, ½ cup	30	8
Orange, all commercial varieties, fresh, 1 small	30	8
Bread, white, 1 slice†	25	6
Bread, whole wheat, 1 slice†	25	6
Egg, whole, raw, fresh, 1 large	25	6
Cantaloupe, raw, ¼ medium	25	6
Papaya, raw, ½ cup cubes	25	6
Banana, raw, 1 medium	20	6

*Daily values (DVs) are reference numbers based on the recommended dietary allowance. They were developed to help consumers determine if a food contains a lot or a little of a specific nutrient. The DV for folate is 400 mcg. The %DV listed on the Nutrition Facts panel of food labels states the percentage of the DV provided in one serving.

†Fortified with folic acid as part of the Folate Fortification Program.

Vitamin B₆

Vitamin B₆ is a water-soluble vitamin that exists in three major chemical forms: pyridoxine, pyridoxal, and pyridoxamine and performs a wide variety of functions in the body. It is needed for more than 100 enzymes involved in protein metabolism and is essential for red blood cell metabolism. The nervous and immune systems need vitamin B₆ to function efficiently, and it is also needed for the conversion of tryptophan (an amino acid) to niacin. A vitamin B₆ deficiency can result in a form of anemia that is similar to iron deficiency anemia.

Through its involvement in protein metabolism and cellular growth, vitamin B₆ is important to the immune system. It helps maintain the health of lymphoid organs (thymus, spleen, and lymph nodes) that make white blood cells. It is also important for maintaining normal blood glucose levels.

Continued

APPENDIX 46 Nutritional Facts on Folic Acid, Vitamin B_6, and Vitamin B_{12}—cont'd

Dietary Reference Intakes for Vitamin B_6 for Children and Adults

Age (years)	Males and Females (mg/day)	Pregnancy (mg/day)	Lactation (mg/day)
1-3	0.5	N/A	N/A
4-8	0.6	N/A	N/A
9-13	1.0	N/A	N/A
14-18	1.3	1.9	2.0
19+	1.3	1.9	2.0

Selected Food Sources of Vitamin B_6

Food	Milligrams per Serving	% Daily Value*
Ready-to-eat cereal, 100% fortified, ¾ cup	2.00	100%
Potato, baked, flesh and skin, 1 medium	0.70	35%
Banana, raw, 1 medium	0.68	34%
Garbanzo beans, canned, ½ cup	0.57	30%
Chicken breast, meat only, cooked, ½ breast	0.52	25%
Ready-to-eat cereal, 25% fortified, ¾ cup	0.50	25%
Oatmeal, instant, fortified, 1 packet	0.42	20%
Pork loin, lean only, cooked, 3 oz	0.42	20%
Roast beef, eye of round, lean only, cooked, 3 oz	0.32	15%
Trout, rainbow, cooked, 3 oz	0.29	15%
Sunflower seeds, kernels, dry roasted, 1 oz	0.23	10%
Spinach, frozen, cooked, ½ cup	0.14	8%
Tomato juice, canned, 6 oz	0.20	10%
Avocado, raw, sliced, ½ cup	0.20	10%
Salmon, Sockeye, cooked, 3 oz	0.19	10%
Tuna, canned in water, drained solids, 3 oz	0.18	10%
Wheat bran, crude or unprocessed, ¼ cup	0.18	10%
Peanut butter, smooth, 2 Tbsp	0.15	8%
Walnuts, English/Persian, 1 oz	0.15	8%
Soybeans, green, boiled, drained, ½ cup	0.05	2%
Lima beans, frozen, cooked, drained, ½ cup	0.10	6%

*Daily values (DVs) are reference numbers based on the recommended dietary allowance. They were developed to help consumers determine if a food contains a lot or a little of a specific nutrient. The DV for vitamin B_6 is 2 mg. The %DV listed on the Nutrition Facts panel of food labels states the percentage of the DV provided in one serving.

Vitamin B_{12}

Along with folate and vitamin B_6, vitamin B_{12} is helpful in lowering the level of the amino acid homocysteine in the blood. It has been hypothesized that at high levels homocysteine might damage coronary arteries or make it easier for blood-clotting cells to clump together and form a clot. This could increase risks for a heart attack or stroke.

Vitamin B_{12} is a member of the vitamin B complex. It contains cobalt; thus it is also known as cobalamin. It is exclusively synthesized by bacteria and is found primarily in meat, eggs, and dairy products. There has been considerable research into proposed plant sources of vitamin B_{12}. Fermented soy products, seaweeds, and algae (spirulina) have all been suggested as containing significant B_{12}. However, the present consensus is that any B_{12} present in plant foods is likely to be unavailable to humans; thus these foods should not be relied on as safe sources. Many vegan foods are supplemented with B_{12}.

Vitamin B_{12} is necessary for the synthesis of red blood cells, the maintenance of the nervous system, and growth and development in children. Deficiency can cause anemia. Vitamin B_{12} neuropathy, involving the degeneration of nerve fibers and irreversible neurologic damage, can also occur. Vitamin B_{12} can be stored in small amounts by the body. Proper vitamin B_{12} absorption requires the presence of intrinsic factor, which tends to diminish with aging. Total body store is 2 to 5 mg in adults. Approximately 80% of this is stored in the liver.

Dietary Reference Intakes for Vitamin B_{12} for Children and Adults

Age (years)	Males and Females (mcg/day)	Pregnancy (mcg/day)	Lactation (mcg/day)
1-3	0.9	N/A	N/A
4-8	1.2	N/A	N/A
9-13	1.8	N/A	N/A
14-18	2.4	2.6	2.8
19 and older	2.4	2.6	2.8

APPENDIX 46 Nutritional Facts on Folic Acid, Vitamin B₆, and Vitamin B₁₂—cont'd

Selected Food Sources of Vitamin B₁₂

Food	Micrograms per Serving	% Daily Value*
Mollusks, clam, mixed species, cooked, 3 oz	84.1	1400
Liver, beef, braised, 1 slice	47.9	780
Fortified breakfast cereals, (100% fortified), ¾ cup	6.0	100
Trout, rainbow, wild, cooked, 3 oz	5.4	90
Salmon, sockeye, cooked, 3 oz	4.9	80
Trout, rainbow, farmed, cooked, 3 oz	4.2	50
Beef, top sirloin, lean, choice, broiled, 3 oz	2.4	40
Fast food, cheeseburger, regular, double patty and bun, 1 sandwich	1.9	30
Fast food, taco, 1 large	1.6	25
Fortified breakfast cereals (25% fortified), ¾ cup	1.5	25
Yogurt, plain, skim, with 13 g of protein per cup, 1 cup	1.4	25
Haddock, cooked, 3 oz	1.2	20
Clams, breaded and fried, ¾ cup	1.1	20
Tuna, white, canned in water, drained solids, 3 oz	1.0	15
Milk, 1 cup	0.9	15
Pork, cured, ham, lean only, canned, roasted, 3 oz	0.6	10
Egg, whole, hard boiled, 1	0.6	10
American pasteurized cheese food, 1 oz	0.3	6
Chicken, breast, meat only, roasted, ½ breast	0.3	6

*Daily values (DVs) are reference numbers based on the recommended dietary allowance. They were developed to help consumers determine if a food contains a lot or a little of a specific nutrient. The DV for vitamin B₁₂ is 6 mcg. The %DV listed on the Nutrition Facts panel of food labels states the percentage of the DV provided in one serving.

APPENDIX 47 Nutritional Facts on Vitamin A and Carotenoids

Vitamin A includes a group of compounds that affect vision, bone growth, reproduction, cell division, immunity, healthy surface linings of the respiratory tract, and mucous membranes. There are two categories of vitamin A, depending on whether the food source is an animal or a plant. Vitamin A found in foods that come from animals is called preformed vitamin A and is absorbed as retinol. Sources include liver, whole milk, and some fortified food products. In the body retinol can be made into retinal and retinoic acid (other active forms of vitamin A).

Plant sources of vitamin A provide the provitamin A, called carotenoids. They can be made into retinol in the body and then to the other active forms of vitamin A. In the United States approximately 26% to 34% of vitamin A consumed is in the form of provitamin A

carotenoids. Common provitamin A carotenoids found in plants give them color and are β-carotene, α-carotene, and β-cryptoxanthin. Among these, β-carotene is most efficiently made into retinol. The darker the color of a fruit or vegetable, the greater is its carotenoid content.

Vitamin A deficiency rarely occurs in the United States, but vitamin A is needed for children with measles, infection, or eye disease in communities where vitamin A deficiency is a serious problem. Fat malabsorption can result in diarrhea and prevent normal absorption of vitamin A; this may result in vitamin A deficiency in celiac disease, Crohn's disease, and pancreatic disorders. The best absorbed form of vitamin A is in the oil form such as in cod liver oil.

Dietary Reference Intakes for Vitamin A for Children and Adults

Age (years)	Males and Females (mcg RAEs/day)	Pregnancy (mcg RAEs/day)	Lactation (mcg RAEs/day)
1-3	300	N/A	N/A
4-8	400	N/A	N/A
9-13	600	N/A	N/A
14-18	900 for males; 700 for females	1200	750
19+	900 for males; 700 for females	770	1300

RAE, Retinol activity equivalent. 1 RAE = 1 mcg of retinol = 12 mg of β-carotene = 3.33 IU of vitamin A on a label.

Food Sources of Vitamin A

Vitamin A in foods is expressed as micrograms of retinol activity equivalents (RAEs) of vitamin A per standard amount, but it is also stated as IU = 0.33 mcg RAEs. (All are ≥20% of the recommended dietary allowance for adult men, which is 900 mcg RAE/day.)

Selected Animal Sources of Vitamin A

Food	Vitamin A (IU)	% Daily Value†
Liver, beef, cooked, 3 oz	27,185	545
Liver, chicken, cooked, 3 oz	12,325	245
Milk, fortified skim, 1 cup	500	10
Cheese, cheddar, 1 oz	284	6
Milk, whole (3.25% fat), 1 cup	249	5
Egg substitute, ¼ cup	226	5

APPENDIX 47 Nutritional Facts on Vitamin A and Carotenoids—cont'd

Selected Plant Sources of Vitamin A (from β-Carotene)

Food	Vitamin A (IU)	% Daily Value*
Carrot juice, canned, ½ cup	22,567	450
Carrots, boiled, ½ cup slices	13,418	270
Spinach, frozen, boiled, ½ cup	11,458	230
Kale, frozen, boiled, ½ cup	9,558	190
Carrots, 1 raw (7½ in)	8,666	175
Vegetable soup, canned, chunky, ready-to-serve, 1 cup	5,820	115
Cantaloupe, 1 cup cubes	5,411	110
Spinach, raw, 1 cup	2,813	55
Apricots with skin, juice pack, ½ cup	2,063	40
Apricot nectar, canned, ½ cup	1,651	35
Papaya, 1 cup cubes	1,532	30
Mango, 1 cup sliced	1,262	25
Oatmeal, instant, fortified, plain, prepared with water, 1 cup	1,252	25
Peas, frozen, boiled, ½ cup	1,050	20
Tomato juice, canned, 6 oz	819	15
Peaches, canned, juice pack, ½ cup halves or slices	473	10
Peach, 1 medium	319	6
Pepper, sweet, red, raw, 1 ring (3 inches diameter by ¼ inch thick)	313	6

* Daily values (DVs) are reference numbers based on the recommended dietary allowances. They were developed to help consumers determine if a food contains a lot or a little of a nutrient. The DV for vitamin A is 5000 IU. Most food labels do not list vitamin A content. The %DV column in this table indicates the percentage of the DV provided in one serving. A food providing 5% or less of the DV is a low source, whereas a food that provides 10% to 19% of the DV is a good source. A food that provides 20% or more of the DV is high in that nutrient. It is important to remember that foods that provide lower percentages of the DV also contribute to a healthful diet.

Another way to summarize important foods is through **retinol equivalents.**

Food	Vitamin A (mcg RAEs)	Calories
Organ meats (liver, giblets), various, cooked, 3 oz†	1490-9126	134-235
Carrot juice, ¾ cup	1692	71
Sweet potato with peel, baked, 1 medium	1096	103
Pumpkin, canned, ½ cup	953	42
Carrots, cooked from fresh, ½ cup	671	27
Spinach, cooked from frozen, ½ cup	573	30
Collards, cooked from frozen, ½ cup	489	31
Kale, cooked from frozen, ½ cup	478	20
Mixed vegetables, canned, ½ cup	474	40
Turnip greens, cooked from frozen, ½ cup	441	24
Instant cooked cereals, fortified, prepared, 1 packet	285-376	75-97
Various ready-to-eat cereals, with added vitamin A, ≈1 oz	180-376	100-117
Carrot, raw, 1 small	301	20
Beet greens, cooked, ½ cup	276	19
Winter squash, cooked, ½ cup	268	38
Dandelion greens, cooked, ½ cup	260	18
Cantaloupe, raw, ¼ medium melon	233	46
Mustard greens, cooked, ½ cup	221	11
Pickled herring, 3 oz	219	222
Red sweet pepper, cooked, ½ cup	186	19
Chinese cabbage, cooked, ½ cup	180	10

*IU= International Units; RAE, Retinol activity equivalent.

†High in cholesterol.

NOTE: Mixed dishes and multiple preparations of the same food item have been omitted from this table.

Carotenoids in Fruits and Vegetables

	Neoxanthins and Violaxanthins	Lutein and Zeaxanthin	Lutein	Zeaxanthin	Cryptoxanthins	Lycopenes	β-Carotene	β-Carotene
Egg yolk	8	89	54	35	4	0	0	0
Maize (corn)	9	86	60	25	5	0	0	0
Kiwi	38	54	54	0	0	0	0	8
Red seedless grapes	23	53	43	10	4	5	3	16
Zucchini squash	19	52	47	5	24	0	0	5
Pumpkin	30	49	49	0	0	0	0	21
Spinach	14	47	47	0	19	4	0	16
Orange pepper	4	45	8	37	22	0	8	21
Yellow squash	19	44	44	0	0	0	28	9
Cucumber	16	42	38	4	38	0	0	4
Pea	33	41	41	0	21	0	0	5
Green pepper	29	39	36	3	20	0	0	12
Red grape	27	37	33	4	29	0	1	6
Butternut squash	24	37	37	0	34	0	5	0

APPENDIX 47 Nutritional Facts on Vitamin A and Carotenoids—cont'd

Carotenoids in Fruits and Vegetables—cont'd

	Neoxanthins and Violaxanthins	Lutein and Zeaxanthin	Lutein	Zeaxanthin	Cryptoxanthins	Lycopenes	β-Carotene	β-Carotene
Orange juice	28	35	15	20	25	0	3	8
Honeydew	18	35	17	18	0	0	0	48
Celery (stalks, leaves)	12	34	32	2	40	1	13	0
Green grapes	10	31	25	7	52	0	0	7
Brussels sprouts	20	29	27	2	39	0	0	11
Scallions	32	29	27	3	35	4	0	0
Green beans	27	25	22	3	42	0	1	5
Orange	36	22	7	15	12	11	8	11
Broccoli	3	22	22	0	49	0	0	27
Apple (red delicious)	22	20	19	1	23	13	5	17
Mango	52	18	2	16	4	6	0	20
Green lettuce	33	15	15	0	36	0	16	0
Tomato juice	0	13	11	2	2	57	12	16
Peach	20	13	5	8	8	0	10	50
Yellow pepper	86	12	12	0	1	0	1	0
Nectarine	18	11	6	6	23	0	0	48
Red pepper	56	7	7	0	2	8	24	3
Tomato (fruit)	0	6	6	0	0	82	0	12
Carrots	0	2	2	0	0	0	43	55
Cantaloupe	9	1	1	0	0	3	0	87
Dried apricots	2	1	1	0	9	0	0	87
Green kidney beans	72	0	0	0	28	0	0	0

Table from Sommerburg O et al: Fruits and vegetables that are sources for lutein and zeaxanthin: the macular pigment in human eyes, *Br J Ophthalmol* 82:907, 1998.

The content of the major carotenoids are given in mole%. The amounts of the carotenoids were shown in seven major groups, as neoxanthins and violaxanthins (neoxanthin, violaxanthin, and their related isomers, lutein 5, 6 epoxide), lutein, zeaxanthin, cryptoxanthins (α-cryptoxanthin, β-cryptoxanthins, and related isomers), lycopenes (lycopene and related isomers), β-carotene (all *trans* β-carotene and *cis* isomers), and β-carotene (all *trans* β-carotene and *cis* isomers). Lutein and zeaxanthin are given combined and as single amounts. The data are sorted by the combined amount of lutein and zeaxanthin.

APPENDIX 48 Nutritional Facts on Vitamin C

Vitamin C is a nutrient required in very small amounts to allow a range of essential metabolic reactions in the body. Vitamin C is principally known as a water-soluble antioxidant, and it prevents scurvy. It is also known by the chemical name of its principal form, L-ascorbic acid or simply ascorbic acid. The dietary reference intakes range from 15 to 90 mg/day as shown in the following table, with a tolerable upper intake of no more than 2 g/day (2000 mg/day).

Dietary Reference Intakes for Vitamin C for Children and Adults

Age (years)	Males and Females (mg/day)	Pregnancy (mg/day)	Lactation (mg/day)
1-3	15	N/A	N/A
4-8	25	N/A	N/A
9-13	45	N/A	N/A
14-18	75 for males; 65 for females	80	115
19+	90 for males; 75 for females	85	120

Continued

APPENDIX 48 Nutritional Facts on Vitamin C —cont'd

Selected Food Sources of Vitamin C

Food	Milligrams per Serving	% Daily Value*
Guava, raw, ½ cup	188	209
Red sweet pepper, raw, ½ cup	142	158
Red sweet pepper, cooked, ½ cup	116	129
Kiwi fruit, 1 medium	70	78
Orange, raw, 1 medium	70	78
Orange juice, ¾ cup	61-93	68-103
Green pepper, sweet, raw, ½ cup	60	67
Green pepper, sweet, cooked, ½ cup	51	56.6
Grapefruit juice, ¾ cup	50-70	55.5-78
Vegetable juice cocktail, ¾ cup	50	55.5
Strawberries, raw, ½ cup	49	54
Brussels sprouts, cooked, ½ cup	48	53
Cantaloupe, ¼ medium	47	52
Papaya, raw, ¼ medium	47	52
Kohlrabi, cooked, ½ cup	45	50
Broccoli, raw, ½ cup	39	43
Edible pod peas, cooked, ½ cup	38	42
Broccoli, cooked, ½ cup	37	41
Sweet potato, canned, ½ cup	34	38
Tomato juice, ¾ cup	33	36.5
Cauliflower, cooked, ½ cup	28	31
Pineapple, raw, ½ cup	28	31
Kale, cooked, ½ cup	27	30
Mango, ½ cup	23	25.5

*Daily values (DVs) are reference numbers based on the recommended dietary allowance. They were developed to help consumers determine if a food contains a lot or a little of a specific nutrient. The DV for vitamin C is 90 mg. The %DV listed on the Nutrition Facts panel of food labels states the percentage of the DV provided in one serving.

APPENDIX 49 Nutritional Facts on Vitamin E

Vitamin E is a fat-soluble vitamin that exists in eight different forms. Each form has its own biologic activity, which is the measure of potency or functional use in the body. α-Tocopherol is the name of the most active form; it is a powerful biologic antioxidant. Vitamin E in supplements is usually sold as α-tocopheryl acetate, a form of α-tocopherol that protects its ability to function as an antioxidant. The synthetic form is labeled *dl*, whereas the natural form is labeled *d*. The synthetic form is only half as active as the natural form. It is important to include foods high in vitamin E on a daily basis to get enough vitamin E from foods alone. Vegetable oils, nuts, green leafy vegetables, and fortified cereals are common food sources of vitamin E.

Although vitamin E deficiency is rare in humans, it is likely to occur in specific situations:

1. In persons who cannot absorb dietary fat because of an inability to secrete bile or those who have rare disorders of fat metabolism
2. In individuals with rare genetic abnormalities in the α-tocopherol transfer protein
3. In premature, very low–birth weight infants (birth weights less than 1500 g, or 3 lb, 4 oz)

Vitamin E deficiency is usually characterized by neurologic problems in the hands and feet, as well as peroxidation of cellular lipid membranes.

Most food labels do not list a vitamin E content of food. The percent daily value (% DV) listed on the table indicates the percentage of the DV provided in one serving. The DV for vitamin E is 30 IU. A food providing 5% of the DV or less is a low source, whereas a food that provides 10% to 19% of the DV is a good source. A food that provides 20% or more of the DV provides 6 units and is considered high in vitamin E.

Vitamin E content of food is stated as milligrams of α-tocopherol, milligrams of α-tocopherol equivalents (mg α-TE), or as units on supplement labels. 1 unit = 0.67 α-TE in the *d* form and about ½ of that in the *dl* or synthetic form.

Dietary Reference Intakes for Vitamin E (in milligrams) of α-TE for Children and Adults

Age (years)	Males and Females (mg/day)	Pregnancy (mg/day)	Lactation (mg/day)
1-3	6	N/A	N/A
4-8	7	N/A	N/A
9-13	11	N/A	N/A
14-18	15	15	19
19+	15	15	19

APPENDIX 49 Nutritional Facts on Vitamin E—cont'd

Selected Food Sources of Vitamin E

Food	Milligrams per Serving	% Daily Value*
Fortified ready-to-eat cereals, ≈1 oz	1.6-12.8	11-85
Sunflower seeds, dry roasted, 1 oz	7.4	49%
Almonds, 1 oz	7.3	
Sunflower oil, high linoleic, 1 Tbsp	5.6	37%
Cottonseed oil, 1 Tbsp	4.8	32
Safflower oil, high oleic, 1 Tbsp	4.6	31
Hazelnuts (filberts), 1 oz	4.3	29
Mixed nuts, dry roasted, 1 oz	3.1	21
Turnip greens, frozen, cooked, ½ cup	2.9	19
Tomato paste, ¼ cup	2.8	18
Pine nuts, 1 oz	2.6	17
Peanut butter, 2 Tbsp	2.5	16.5
Tomato puree, ½ cup	2.5	16.5
Tomato sauce, ½ cup	2.5	16.5
Canola oil, 1 Tbsp	2.4	16
Wheat germ, toasted, plain, 2 Tbsp	2.3	15
Peanuts, 1 oz	2.2	14.5
Avocado, raw, ½ avocado	2.1	14
Carrot juice, canned, ¾ cup	2.1	14
Peanut oil, 1 Tbsp	2.1	14
Corn oil, 1 Tbsp	1.9	12.5
Olive oil, 1 Tbsp	1.9	12.5
Spinach, cooked, ½ cup	1.9	12.5
Dandelion greens, cooked, ½ cup	1.8	12
Sardine, Atlantic, in oil, drained, 3 oz	1.7	11
Blue crab, cooked/canned, 3 oz	1.6	10.5
Brazil nuts, 1 oz	1.6	10.5
Herring, Atlantic, pickled, 3 oz	1.5	10

*Daily values (DVs) are reference numbers based on the recommended dietary allowance. They were developed to help consumers determine if a food contains a lot or a little of a specific nutrient. The DV for vitamin E is 15 mg α-TE. The %DV listed on the Nutrition Facts panel of food labels states the percentage of the DV provided in one serving.

Sample Meal Plan

Breakfast

¾ cup ready-to-eat cereal
½ cup low-fat/fat-free milk
1 red delicious apple
2 Tbsp peanut butter (2.5 mg vitamin E)

Lunch

1 cup mixed salad greens
3 oz tuna steak
2 slices multigrain bread
½ cup fruit salad

Dinner

3 oz grilled chicken breast
½ cup fresh steamed spinach (1.9 mg vitamin E)
½ cup whole grain rice
Side salad

Snack

1 oz sliced almonds (7.3 mg vitamin E)
1 Tbsp low-fat granola
½ cup low-fat/fat free yogurt

NOTE: Take one multivitamin/multimineral supplement daily.

APPENDIX 50 Nutritional Facts on Vitamin K

Vitamin K comes from the foods that we eat and the bacteria that normally reside in the intestines, which are able to make vitamin K. Antibiotics may interfere with this normal production. Other circumstances that may lead to vitamin K deficiency include liver disease, serious burns, health problems that can prevent the absorption of vitamin K (such as gallbladder or biliary disease, which may alter the absorption of fat), cystic fibrosis, celiac disease, Crohn's disease, and chronic antibiotic therapy. Excess vitamin E can inhibit vitamin K activity and precipitate signs of deficiency. The classic sign of a vitamin K deficiency is a prolonged prothrombin time, which increases the risk of spontaneous hemorrhage. Since vitamin K is stored in the liver, clinical deficiencies are rare.

Vitamin K is needed to make clotting factors that help the blood to clot and prevent bleeding. The amount of vitamin K in food may affect drug therapy, such as that from warfarin or other anticoagulants. When taking these medications, it is necessary to eat a normal, balanced diet, maintaining a consistent amount of vitamin K, and avoiding drastic changes in dietary habits.

In general, leafy green vegetables and certain legumes and vegetable oils contain high amounts of vitamin K. Foods that contain a significant amount of vitamin K include beef liver, green tea, turnip greens, broccoli, kale, spinach, cabbage, asparagus, and dark green lettuce. Chlorophyll, which is water soluble, is the substance in plants that gives them their green color and provides vitamin K; thus chlorophyll supplements need to be considered when assessing vitamin K intake.

Foods that appear to contain low amounts of vitamin K include roots, bulbs, tubers, the fleshy portion of fruits, fruit juices and other beverages, and cereal grains and their milled products.

Dietary Reference Intakes for Vitamin K for Children and Adults

Age (years)	Males and Females (mcg/day)	Pregnancy (mcg/day)	Lactation (mcg/day)
1-3	30	N/A	N/A
4-8	55	N/A	N/A
9-13	60	N/A	N/A
14-18	75	75	75
19+	120 for males; 90 for females	90	90

Continued

APPENDIX 50 Nutritional Facts on Vitamin K—cont'd

Selected Food Sources of Vitamin K

Food	Micrograms per Serving	Food	Micrograms per Serving
Brussels sprouts, ½ cup	460	Beef, 3.5 oz	104
Turnip greens, raw, chopped, 1 cup	364	Pork, 3.5 oz	88
Broccoli, ½ cup	248	Soybean oil, 1 Tbsp	68
Lentils, dry, ½ cup	214	Lettuce, chopped, ½ cup	63
Cauliflower, ½ cup	150	Asparagus, 1 cup, cooked	49
Kale, ½ cup cooked	150	Eggs, whole	25
Spinach, raw, chopped, ½ cup	149	Strawberries, 1 cup	23
Garbanzo beans, dry, ½ cup	132	Oats, 1 oz	18
Swiss chard, ½ cup	123	Milk, 8 oz	10

Dietary reference intake of vitamin K = 90-120 mcg.

APPENDIX 51 Nutritional Facts on Calcium and Vitamin D

Calcium

Any dietary source of calcium counts toward the daily intake, but low-fat milk or yogurt or fortified substitutes are the most efficient and readily available. Lactose-free milk and soy nut and rice drinks fortified with calcium and vitamin D are now available. In addition to milk, a variety of foods and calcium-fortified juices contain calcium and can help children, teens, and adults get sufficient levels of calcium in their diets.

If it is difficult to get the recommended amounts of calcium and vitamin D from foods, a combination of food sources and supplements is recommended.

Dietary Reference Intakes for Calcium for Children and Adults

Age (years)	Males and Females (mg/day)	Pregnancy (mg/day)	Lactation (mg/day)
1-3	500	N/A	N/A
4-8	800	N/A	N/A
9-13	1300	N/A	N/A
14-18	1300	1300	1300
19+	1000	1000	1000

Selected Food Sources of Calcium

Food	Milligrams per Serving	% Daily Value*	Food	Milligrams per Serving	% Daily Value*
Dairy Foods			**Nuts and Seeds**		
Milk, with added calcium, 1 cup	420	42	Almonds, dry roast, ¼ cup	95	9.5
Milk, whole, 2%, 1% skim, 1 cup	300	30	Whole sesame seeds (black or white), 1 Tbsp	90	9
Yogurt, low fat, plain, ¾ cup	300	30	Tahini (sesame seed butter), 1 Tbsp	63	6.3
Cheese, processed slices, 2 slices	265	26.5	Brazil, hazelnuts, ¼ cup	55	5.5
Yogurt, fruit bottom, ¾ cup	250	25	Almond butter, 1 Tbsp	43	4.3
Processed cheese spread, 3 Tbsp	250	25	**Meats, Fish, and Poultry**		
Cheese, hard, 1 oz	240	24	Sardines, canned, 3½ oz (8 med)	370	37
Milk, evaporated, ¼ cup	165	16.5	Salmon, canned with bones, 3 oz	180	18
Cottage cheese, ¾ cup	120	12	Oysters, canned, ½ cup	60	6
Frozen yogurt, soft serve, ½ cup	100	10	Shrimp, canned, ½ cup	40	4
Ice cream, ½ cup	85	8.5	**Vegetables (All Measures for Cooked Vegetables)**		
Beans and Bean Products			Turnip greens, ½ cup	95	9.5
Soy cheese substitutes, 1 oz	0-200	20	Okra, frozen, ½ cup	75	7.5
Tofu, firm, made with calcium sulfate, 3½ oz	125	12.5	Chinese cabbage/bok choy, ½ cup	75	7.5
White beans, ½ cup	100	10	Kale, ½ cup	50	5
Navy beans, ½ cup	60	6	Mustard greens, ½ cup	50	5
Black turtle beans, ½ cup	50	5	Chinese broccoli (gai lan), ½ cup	44	4.4
Pinto beans, chickpeas, ½ cup	40	4	Rutabaga, ½ cup	40	4
			Broccoli, ½ cup	35	3.5

*Daily values (DVs) are reference numbers based on the recommended dietary allowance. They were developed to help consumers determine if a food contains a lot or a little of a specific nutrient. The DV for calcium is 1000 mg. The %DV listed on the Nutrition Facts panel of food labels states the percentage of the DV provided in one serving.

APPENDIX 51 Nutritional Facts on Calcium and Vitamin D—cont'd

Selected Food Sources of Calcium—cont'd

Food	Milligrams per Serving	% Daily Value*
Fruit		
Orange, 1 med	55	5.5
Dried figs, 2 med	54	5.4
Nondairy Drinks		
Calcium enriched orange juice, 1 cup	300	30
Fortified rice beverage, 1 cup	300	30
Fortified soy beverage, 1 cup	300	30
Regular soy beverage, 1 cup	20	2
Grains		
Amaranth, raw, ½ cup	150	15
Whole wheat flour, 1 cup	40	4
Other		
Brown sugar, 1 cup	180	18
Blackstrap molasses, 1 Tbsp	170	17
Regular molasses, 1 Tbsp	40	4
Asian Foods		
Sea cucumber, fresh, 3 oz	285	28.5
Soy bean curd slab, spiced, semisoft, 3 oz	269	26.9

Food	Milligrams per Serving	% Daily Value*
Asian Foods—cont'd		
Shrimp, small, dried, 1 oz	167	16.7
Dried fish, smelt, 2 Tbsp	140	14
Seaweed, dry (hijiki),* 10 g	140	14
Seaweed, dry (agar), 10 g	76	7.6
Lily flower, dried, ¼ cup	70	7
Soy bean milk film, stick shape, 3 oz	69	6.9
Fat-choy, dried, ¼ cup	50	5
Oyster, dried, 3	45	4.5
Soy bean milk film, dried, 3 oz	43	4.3
Boiled bone soup, ½ cup	Negligible	
Laver, nori, and wakame seaweeds are low in calcium.		
Native Foods		
Oolichan, salted, cooked, 3 oz	210	21
Fish head soup, 1 cup	150	15
Indian ice cream (whipped soapberries), ½ cup	130	13

Calcium Supplements

Calcium carbonate is the most common and least expensive calcium supplement. It can be difficult to digest and causes gas in some people. Taking magnesium with it can help to prevent constipation. Calcium carbonate is 40% elemental calcium; 1000 mg will provide 400 mg of calcium. Take this supplement with food to aid in absorption.

Calcium citrate is more easily absorbed (bioavailability is 2.5 times higher than calcium carbonate), easier to digest, and less likely to cause constipation and gas than calcium carbonate. It also has a lower risk of contributing to the formation of kidney stones. Calcium citrate is about 21% elemental calcium; 1000 mg will provide 210 mg of calcium. It is more expensive than calcium carbonate, and more of it must be taken to get the same amount of calcium.

Calcium phosphate costs more than calcium carbonate but less than calcium citrate. It is easily absorbed and is less likely to cause constipation and gas.

Calcium lactate and calcium aspartate are both more easily digested but more expensive than calcium carbonate.

Vitamin D

Vitamin D is needed for the absorption of calcium from the stomach and for the functioning of calcium in the body. It also acts like a hormone in the body and has many functions throughout the body unrelated to its co-functions with calcium that are continuing to be discovered. Besides being in bone, receptors for vitamin D have been identified in the gastrointestinal tract, brain, breast, nerves, and many other tissues. The dietary reference intakes for vitamin D, as well as the content of vitamin D in foods, are stated as micrograms of calciferol. IU are used on supplement labels. 1 mcg = 40 IU of vitamin D or calciferol.

Dietary Reference Intakes for Vitamin D for Children and Adults

Age (years)	Males and Females (mcg /day)	Pregnancy (mcg /day)	Lactation (mcg /day)
1-3	5	N/A	N/A
4-8	5	N/A	N/A
9-13	5	N/A	N/A
14-18	5	5	5
19+	5	5	5

Continued

APPENDIX 51 Nutritional Facts on Calcium and Vitamin D—cont'd

There are only a few food sources of vitamin D. Good sources of vitamin D are fortified foods and beverages such as milk, fortified soy, rice and nut beverages, and margarine (check the labels on these foods). Fish, liver, and egg yolks are the only foods that naturally contain vitamin D. If you do not eat vitamin D–rich foods often, you may want to consider taking a vitamin D supplement. Most multiple vitamin supplements contain vitamin D. In addition to dietary sources, sunlight can provide the body with vitamin D because it is synthesized through the skin. Natural food sources include those listed in the following table.

Selected Food Sources of Vitamin D

Food	Micrograms per Serving	% Daily Value*
Natural Sources		
Herring, 3 oz	13.83	276.6
Herring, pickled, 3 oz	5.78	115.6
Salmon, pink, canned, 3 oz	5.30	106
Halibut, 3 oz	5.10	102
Cod liver oil,* 1 tsp	4.50	90
Catfish, 3 oz	4.25	85
Mackerel, Atlantic, 3 oz	3.06	61.2
Oyster, 3 oz	2.72	54.4
Shitake mushrooms, dried, 4	2.49	49.8
Sardines, Pacific, canned in tomato sauce	2.13 per ½ cup, 1.82 per sardine	42.6, 36.4
Sardines, Atlantic, canned in oil	2.03 per ½ cup, 0.33 per sardine	40.6, 6.6
Tuna, light meat, canned in oil, 3 oz	2	40
Shrimp, 3 oz	1.29	25.8
Egg, cooked	0.26 per whole egg, 0.25 per yolk	5.2, 5
Fortified Sources		
Tofu, fortified, ⅕ block	1.20	24
Cow's milk, all types, 8 oz	1	20
Milk, canned evaporated, 4 oz	1	20
Rice milk, fortified, 8 oz	1	20
Soy milk, fortified, 8 oz	1	20
Orange juice, fortified, 8 oz	1	20
Pudding, made with fortified milk, ½ cup	0.50	10
Cereal, fortified, ¾ cup	0.40	8
Yogurt, fortified, ½ cup	0.40	8
Supplemental Sources		
Most multivitamins for adults	Usually 10	200
Calcium with vitamin D	Amount varies	—
Vitamin D only	Amount varies	—

*Daily values (DVs) are reference numbers based on the recommended dietary allowance. They were developed to help consumers determine if a food contains a lot or a little of a specific nutrient. The DV for vitamin D = 5 mcg = 200 IU. The %DV listed on the Nutrition Facts panel of food labels states the percentage of the DV provided in one serving.

APPENDIX 52 Nutritional Facts on Chromium

Chromium is known to enhance the action of insulin; chromium was identified as the active ingredient in the "glucose tolerance factor" many years ago. Chromium also appears to be directly involved in carbohydrate, fat, and protein metabolism; but more research is needed to determine the full range of its roles in the body.

Chromium is widely distributed in the food supply, but most foods provide only small amounts (less than 2 mcg per serving). Meat and whole-grain products, as well as some fruits, vegetables, and spices, are relatively good sources, but Brewer's yeast is by far the most concentrated food source. Foods high in simple sugars (such as sucrose and fructose) are low in chromium. Dietary intakes of chromium cannot be reliably determined because the content of the mineral in foods is substantially affected by agricultural and manufacturing processes and food-composition databases are inadequate. Chromium values in foods are approximate and should only serve as a guide.

It appears that chromium picolinate and chromium nicotinate used in supplements are more bioavailable than chromic chloride.

Dietary Reference Intakes for Chromium for Children and Adults

Age (years)	Males and Females (mcg/day)	Pregnancy (mcg/day)	Lactation (mcg/day)
1-3	11	N/A	N/A
4-8	15	N/A	N/A
9-13	25 for males, 21 for females	N/A	N/A
14-18	35 for males, 24 for females	29	44
19+	35 for males, 25 for females	30	45

Selected Food Sources of Chromium

Food	Micrograms per Serving
Brewer's yeast, 1 Tbsp or 15 g	60
Broccoli, ½ cup	11
Grape juice, 1 cup	8
English muffin, whole wheat, 1	4
Potatoes, mashed, 1 cup	3
Garlic, dried, 1 tsp	3
Basil, dried, 1 Tbsp	2
Beef cubes, 3 oz	2
Orange juice, 1 cup	2
Turkey breast, 3 oz	2
Whole wheat bread, 2 slices	2
Red wine, 5 oz	1-13
Apple, unpeeled, 1 med	1
Banana, 1 med	1
Green beans, ½ cup	1

Interactions Between Chromium and Medications

Medications	Nature of Interaction
Antacids Corticosteroids H$_2$ blockers (e.g., cimetidine, famotidine, nizatidine, and ranitidine) Proton-pump inhibitors (e.g., omeprazole, lansoprazole, rabeprazole, pantoprazole, and esomeprazole)	These medications alter stomach acidity and may impair chromium absorption or enhance excretion.
β-blockers (such as atenolol or propranolol) Corticosteroids Insulin Nicotinic acid Nonsteroidal antiinflammatory drugs (NSAIDs) Prostaglandin inhibitors (e.g., ibuprofen, indomethacin, naproxen, piroxicam, and aspirin)	These medications may have their effects enhanced if taken together with chromium, or they may increase chromium absorption.

APPENDIX 53 Nutritional Facts on Iodine

Iodine is an important mineral that is found in a variety of foods, but it is most concentrated in foods from the ocean. It is mainly used to make thyroid hormones, which help to regulate metabolic rate, body temperature, growth, reproduction, blood cell production, muscle function, nerve function, and even gene expression. The most useful clinical tool for measuring thyroid function and thus iodine sufficiency is to measure thyroid-stimulating hormone (TSH), which is released from the pituitary gland and stimulates thyroid hormone production and release. If the TSH is high, thyroid function should be evaluated further.

Selenium-dependent enzymes are also required for the conversion of thyroxine (T4) to the biologically active thyroid hormone, triiodothyronine (T3); thus deficiencies of selenium, vitamin A, or iron may also affect iodine status.

Deficiency

Iodine deficiency is an important health problem throughout much of the world. Most of the earth's iodine is found in its oceans; thus parts of the world away from the oceans and exposed for millions of years longer have iodine-deficient soils, and large percentages of people living there can be iodine deficient unless public health measures are taken. Iodine deficiency can cause mental retardation, hypothyroidism, goiter, and varying degrees of other growth and developmental abnormalities. Iodine is now recognized as the most common cause of preventable brain damage in the world, with millions living in iodine-deficient areas.

The major source of dietary iodine in the United States is "iodized" salt, which has been fortified with iodine. In the United States assume that any salt in prepared foods is iodized unless the product label shows that it is *not iodized*. In the United States and Canada iodized salt contains 77 mcg of iodine per gram of salt. Iodine is also added in the diet because it is used in the feed of animals and in many processed or preserved foods as a stabilizer and a component of red food dyes.

Vegetarian and nonvegetarian diets that exclude iodized salt, fish, and seaweed have been found to contain very little iodine. Urinary iodine excretion studies suggest that iodine intakes are declining in the United States, possibly as a result of increased adherence to dietary recommendations to reduce salt intake.

Goitrogens

Substances that interfere with iodine use or thyroid hormone production are known as goitrogens and occur in some foods. Some species of millet and cruciferous vegetables (e.g., cabbage, broccoli, cauliflower, and Brussels sprouts) contain goitrogens; and the soybean isoflavones genistein and daidzein have also been found to inhibit thyroid hormone synthesis. Most of these goitrogens are not of clinical importance unless they are consumed in large amounts or there is coexisting iodine deficiency.

Dietary Reference Intakes for Iodine

Life Stage	Age	Males (mcg/day)	Females (mcg/day)
Infants	0-6 months	110 (AI)	110 (AI)
Infants	7-12 months	130 (AI)	130 (AI)
Children	1-3 years	90	90
Children	4-8 years	90	90
Children	9-13 years	120	120
Adolescents	14-18 years	150	150
Adults	19 years and older	150	150
Pregnancy	All ages	—	220
Breast-feeding	All ages	—	290

The iodine contents of some common foods containing iodine are given in the following table. The iodine content of fruits and vegetables depends on the soil in which they were grown; the iodine content of animal foods, outside of those from the ocean, depends on where they were raised and which plants they consumed. Therefore these values are average approximations.

Selected Food Sources of Iodine

Food	Serving	Micrograms per Serving	% Daily Value*
Salt (iodized)	1 g	77	51
Cod	3 oz	99	66
Shrimp	3 oz	35	23
Fish sticks	2 fish sticks	35	23
Tuna, canned in oil	3 ounces (½ can)	17	11
Milk (cow's)	1 cup (8 fluid oz)	56	37
Egg, boiled	1 large	29	19
Navy beans, cooked	½ cup	35	23
Potato with peel, baked	1 medium	63	42
Turkey breast, baked	3 ounces	34	22
Seaweed	1 oz, dried	Variable; may be greater than 18,000 mcg (18 mg)	12

*Daily values (DVs) are reference numbers based on the recommended dietary allowance. They were developed to help consumers determine if a food contains a lot or a little of a specific nutrient. The DV for iodine is 150 mcg. The %DV listed on the Nutrition Facts panel of food labels states the percentage of the DV provided in one serving.

AI, Adequate intake.

APPENDIX 54 Nutritional Facts on Iron

Iron is a nutrient found in trace amounts in every cell of the body. Iron is part of hemoglobin in red blood cells and myoglobin in muscles. The role of both of these molecules is to carry oxygen. Iron also makes up part of many proteins and enzymes in the body.

Iron deficiency anemia is common in children, adolescent girls, and women of childbearing age. It is usually treated with an iron-rich diet as well as iron supplements. Iron exists in foods in two forms: heme iron and nonheme iron. Vitamin C enhances the absorption of nonheme iron and should be consumed at the same time as an iron-rich food or meal. Substances that decrease the absorption of nonheme iron are:

Oxalic acid, found in raw spinach and chocolate
Phytic acid, found in wheat bran and beans (legumes)
Tannins, found in commercial black or pekoe teas
Polyphenols, found in coffee
Calcium carbonate supplements

Heme iron is absorbed more efficiently than nonheme iron. Heme iron enhances the absorption of nonheme iron. The richest dietary sources of iron are from:

Oysters
Liver
Lean red meat (especially beef)
Poultry, dark red meat
Tuna
Salmon
Iron-fortified cereals
Dried beans
Whole grains
Eggs (especially egg yolks)
Dried fruits
Reasonable amounts: lamb, pork, and shellfish

Iron from nonheme sources (as in vegetables, fruits, grains, and supplements) is harder for the body to absorb.

These sources include:

Whole grains	Brazil nuts
Wheat	Dried fruits
Millet	Prunes
Oats	Raisins
Brown rice	Apricots
Legumes	Vegetables/Greens
Lima beans	Broccoli
Soybeans	Spinach
Dried beans and peas	Kale
Kidney beans	Collards
Nuts	Asparagus
Almonds	Dandelion greens

Dietary Reference Intakes for Iron for Children and Adults

Age (years)	Males and Females (mg/day)	Pregnancy (mg/day)	Lactation (mg/day)
1-3	7	N/A	N/A
4-8	10	N/A	N/A
9-13	8	N/A	N/A
14-18	11 for males; 15 for females	27	10
19+	8 for males; 18 for females	27	9

Selected Food Sources of Iron

Food	Milligrams Per Serving	% Daily Value*
Clams, canned, drained, 3 oz	23.8	132
Fortified ready-to-eat cereals (various), ≈1 oz	1.8 -21.1	10-12
Oysters, eastern, wild, cooked, moist heat, 3 oz	10.2	57
Organ meats (liver, giblets), various, cooked, 3 oz†	5.2-9.9	29-55
Fortified instant cooked cereals (various), 1 packet	4.9-8.1	27-45
Soybeans, mature, cooked, ½ cup	4.4	24
Pumpkin and squash seed kernels, roasted, 1 oz	4.2	23
White beans, canned, ½ cup	3.9	22
Blackstrap molasses, 1 Tbsp	3.5	19
Lentils, cooked, ½ cup	3.3	18
Spinach, cooked from fresh, ½ cup	3.2	18
Beef, chuck, blade roast, lean, cooked, 3 oz	3.1	17
Beef, bottom round, lean, 0 in fat, all grades, cooked, 3 oz	2.8	15.5
Kidney beans, cooked, ½ cup	2.6	14
Sardines, canned in oil, drained, 3 oz	2.5	14
Beef, rib, lean, ¼ in. fat, all grades, 3 oz	2.4	13
Chickpeas, cooked, ½ cup	2.4	13
Duck, meat only, roasted, 3 oz	2.3	13
Lamb, shoulder, arm, lean, ¼ in fat, choice, cooked, 3 oz	2.3	13
Prune juice, ¾ cup	2.3	13
Shrimp, canned, 3 oz	2.3	13
Cowpeas, cooked, ½ cup	2.2	12
Ground beef, 15% fat, cooked, 3 oz	2.2	12
Tomato puree, ½ cup	2.2	12
Lima beans, cooked, ½ cup	2.2	12
Soybeans, green, cooked, ½ cup	2.2	12
Navy beans, cooked, ½ cup	2.1	11.5
Refried beans, ½ cup	2.1	11.5
Beef, top sirloin, lean, 0 in fat, all grades, cooked, 3 oz	2.0	11
Tomato paste, ¼ cup	2.0	11

*Daily values (DVs) are reference numbers based on the recommended dietary allowance. They were developed to help consumers determine if a food contains a lot or a little of a specific nutrient. The DV for iron is 18 mg. The %DV listed on the Nutrition Facts panel of food labels states the percentage of the DV provided in one serving.

†High in cholesterol.

Continued

Tips For Increasing Iron Intake

The amount of iron the body absorbs varies, depending on several factors. For example, the body will absorb more iron from foods when iron stores are low and will absorb less when stores are sufficient. In addition, certain dietary factors affect absorption:

Combine heme and nonheme sources of iron.

Eat foods rich in vitamin C with nonheme iron sources. Good sources of vitamin C include:

Bell peppers	Cantaloupe
Papayas	Tomatoes and tomato juice
Oranges and orange juice	Potatoes
Broccoli	Cabbage
Strawberries	Spinach and collard greens
Grapefruit	

If you drink coffee or tea, do so between meals rather than with a meal. Cook acidic foods in cast iron pots. This can increase iron content up to 30 times.

What About Too Much Iron?

It is unlikely that a person would take iron at toxic (too high) levels. However, children can sometimes develop iron toxicity by eating iron supplements, mistaking them for candy. Symptoms include the following: fatigue, anorexia, dizziness, nausea, vomiting, headache, weight loss, shortness of breath, and grayish color to the skin.

Hemochromatosis is a genetic disorder that affects the regulation of iron absorption. Treatment consists of a low-iron diet, no iron supplements, and phlebotomy (blood removal) on a regular basis.

Excess storage of iron in the body is known as hemosiderosis. The high iron stores come from eating excessive iron supplements or from receiving frequent blood transfusions, not from increased iron intake in the diet.

To reduce the iron from dietary sources, review the list of foods and exclude or severely limit their intake until the iron overload is alleviated. Pay particular attention to sports drinks, energy bars, and fortified cereals that have significant amounts of added iron.

Sample Meal Plan

Breakfast

½ cup low-fat/fat-free yogurt
1 whole wheat English muffin
1 Tbsp whipped cream cheese
½ cup cantaloupe

Lunch

2 grilled steak fajitas (with mixed peppers)
1 oz shredded low-fat pepper jack cheese
½ cup black refried beans
Side salad with low-fat dressing

Dinner

3 oz grilled turkey breast
½ cup mashed potatoes
½ cup fresh steamed green beans topped with almonds
1 small whole wheat dinner roll
½ cup fresh strawberries

Snack

1 med orange
¼ cup mixed nuts

The mineral magnesium is important for every organ in the body, particularly the heart, muscles, and kidneys. It also contributes to the composition of teeth and bones. Most important, it activates enzymes, contributes to energy production, and helps regulate calcium levels, as well as copper, zinc, potassium, vitamin D, and other important nutrients in the body.

Dietary Sources

Rich sources of magnesium include tofu, legumes, whole grains, green leafy vegetables, wheat bran, Brazil nuts, soybean flour, almonds, cashews, blackstrap molasses, pumpkin and squash seeds, pine nuts, and black walnuts. Other good dietary sources of this mineral include peanuts, whole wheat flour, oat flour, beet greens, spinach, pistachio nuts, shredded wheat, bran cereals, oatmeal, bananas, baked potatoes (with skin), chocolate, and cocoa powder. Many herbs, spices, and seaweeds supply magnesium, such as agar seaweed, coriander, dill weed, celery seed, sage, dried mustard, basil, cocoa powder, fennel seed, savory, cumin seed, tarragon, marjoram, and poppy seed.

Dietary Reference Intakes for Magnesium for Children and Adults

Age (years)	Males and Females (mg/day)	Pregnancy (mg/day)	Lactation (mg/day)
1-3	80	N/A	N/A
4-8	130	N/A	N/A
9-13	240	N/A	N/A
14-18	410 for males, 360 for females	400	360
19+	400 for males, 310 for females	350	310

APPENDIX 55 Nutritional Facts on Magnesium—cont'd

Selected Food Sources of Magnesium

Food	Milligram per Serving	% Daily Value*
Pumpkin and squash seed kernels, roasted, 1 oz	151	38
Brazil nuts, 1 oz	107	27
Bran ready-to-eat cereal (100%), ≈1 oz	103	25.5
Mackerel, baked, 3 oz	97	24
Halibut, cooked, 3 oz	91	23
Quinoa, dry, ¼ cup	89	22
Spinach, canned, ½ cup	81	20
Almonds, 1 oz	78	19.5
Spinach, cooked from fresh, ½ cup	78	19.5
Buckwheat flour, ¼ cup	75	19
Cashews, dry roasted, 1 oz	74	18.5
Soybeans, mature, cooked, ½ cup	74	18.5
Pine nuts, dried, 1 oz	71	17.5
Mixed nuts, oil roasted, with peanuts, 1 oz	67	17
White beans, canned, ½ cup	67	17
Pollock, walleye, cooked, 3 oz	62	15.5
Black beans, cooked, ½ cup	60	15
Bulgur, dry, ¼ cup	57	14
Oat bran, raw, ¼ cup	55	13.5
Soybeans, green, cooked, ½ cup	54	13.7
Tuna, yellowfin, cooked, 3 oz	54	13.5
Artichokes (hearts), cooked, ½ cup	50	12.5
Peanuts, dry roasted, 1 oz	50	12.5
Lima beans, baby, cooked from frozen, ½ cup	50	12.5
Beet greens, cooked, ½ cup	49	12
Navy beans, cooked, ½ cup	48	12
Tofu, firm, prepared with nigari,† ½ cup	47	11.7
Okra, cooked from frozen, ½ cup	47	11.7
Soy beverage, 1 cup	47	11.7
Cowpeas, cooked, ½ cup	46	11.5
Hazelnuts, 1 oz	46	11.5
Oat bran muffin, 1 oz	45	11.3
Great northern beans, cooked, ½ cup	44	11
Oat bran, cooked, ½ cup	44	11
Buckwheat groats, roasted, cooked, ½ cup	43	10.7
Cod, baked, 3 oz	42	10.5
Brown rice, cooked, ½ cup	42	10.5
Haddock, cooked, 3 oz	42	10.5
Chicken, cooked, 3 oz	38	9.5
T-bone steak, broiled, lean only, 3 oz	25	6.5
Turkey, roasted, white meat, 3 oz	24	6
Veal, culet, cooked, 3 oz	24	6%
Beef, ground, cooked, extra lean, 17% fat, 3 oz	17	4

*Daily values (DVs) are reference numbers based on the recommended dietary allowance. They were developed to help consumers determine if a food contains a lot or a little of a specific nutrient. The DV for magnesium is 400 mg. The %DV listed on the Nutrition Facts panel of food labels states the percentage of the DV provided in one serving.

†Calcium sulfate and magnesium chloride.

Common and Important Magnesium/Drug Interactions

Drug	Potential Interaction
Loop and thiazide diuretics (e.g., Lasix, Bumex, edecrin, and hydrochlorothiazide Antineoplastic drugs (e.g., cisplatin) Antibiotics (e.g., gentamicin and amphotericin)	These drugs may increase the loss of magnesium in urine; thus taking these medications for long periods of time may contribute to magnesium depletion.
Tetracycline antibiotics	Magnesium binds tetracycline in the gut and decreases the absorption of tetracycline.
Magnesium-containing antacids and laxatives	Many antacids and laxatives contain magnesium. When frequently taken in large doses, these drugs can inadvertently lead to excessive magnesium consumption and hypermagnesemia, which refers to elevated levels of magnesium in blood.

Sample Meal Plan

Breakfast

1 med oat bran muffin (45 mg magnesium)
1 small banana
½ cup low-fat/fat-free milk

Lunch

½ cup penne pasta with the following:
   3 oz grilled chicken breast
   ½ cup fresh cooked spinach (81 mg magnesium)
   Toasted pine nuts (71 mg magnesium)
   1 cup mixed salad greens topped with spinach leaves, tomatoes, shredded lettuce
   1 oz shredded low-fat mozzarella cheese

Dinner

2 cajun shrimp skewers
½ cup fresh steamed green beans
½ cup brown rice (42 mg magnesium)
½ cup fresh pineapple

Snack

1 cup soy fruit smoothie (47 mg magnesium)
1 oz Brazil nuts (107 mg magnesium)

NOTE: Take one multivitamin/multimineral supplement daily.

APPENDIX 56 Nutritional Facts on Potassium

A potassium-rich diet is useful for cardiac patients who are trying to lower their blood pressure using diet. If diuretics are also used, it is important to know if potassium is retained or depleted, and it should be monitored. Most patients with chronic kidney disease or on renal dialysis need to be aware of the potassium in their diets. Athletes who sweat a great deal may also need attention to the potassium in their diet.

Dietary Reference Intakes for Potassium for Children and Adults

Age (years)	Males and Females (mg/day)	Pregnancy (mg/day)	Lactation (mg/day)
1-3	3000	N/A	N/A
4-8	3800	N/A	N/A
9-13	4500	N/A	N/A
14-18	4700	4700	5100
19+	4700	4700	5100

Selected Food Sources of Potassium

Food	Milligrams per Serving	% Daily Value*
Sweet potato, baked, 1 potato (146 g)	694	19.8
Tomato paste, ¼ cup	664	18.9
Beet greens, cooked, ½ cup	655	18.7
Potato, baked, flesh, 1 potato (156 g)	610	17.4
White beans, canned, ½ cup	595	17
Yogurt, plain, non-fat, 8-oz container	579	16.5
Tomato puree, ½ cup	549	15.7
Clams, canned, 3 oz	534	15.3
Yogurt, plain, low-fat, 8-oz container	531	15.2
Prune juice, ¾ cup	530	15.1
Carrot juice, ¾ cup	517	14.8
Blackstrap molasses, 1 Tbsp	498	14.2
Halibut, cooked, 3 oz	490	14
Soybeans, green, cooked, ½ cup	485	13.9
Tuna, yellow fin, cooked, 3 oz	484	13.8
Lima beans, cooked, ½ cup	484	13.8
Winter squash, cooked, ½ cup	448	9.5
Soybeans, mature, cooked, ½ cup	443	12.8
Rockfish, Pacific, cooked, 3 oz	442	12.6
Cod, Pacific, cooked, 3 oz	439	12.5
Bananas, 1 med	422	12.1
Spinach, cooked, ½ cup	419	12
Tomato juice, ¾ cup	417	11.9
Tomato sauce, ½ cup	405	11.6
Peaches, dried, uncooked, ¼ cup	398	11.4
Prunes, stewed, ½ cup	398	11.4
Milk, nonfat, 1 cup	382	10.9
Pork chop, center loin, cooked, 3 oz	382	10.9
Apricots, dried, uncooked, ¼ cup	378	10.8
Rainbow trout, farmed, cooked, 3 oz	375	10.7
Pork loin, center rib (roasts), lean, roasted, 3 oz	371	10.6
Buttermilk, cultured, low-fat, 1 cup	370	10.5
Cantaloupe, ¼ med	368	10.5
1%-2% milk, 1 cup	366	10.4
Honeydew melon, ⅛ med	365	10.4
Lentils, cooked, ½ cup	365	10.4
Plantains, cooked, ½ cup slices	358	10.2
Kidney beans, cooked, ½ cup	358	10.2
Orange juice, ¾ cup	355	10.1
Split peas, cooked, ½ cup	355	10.1
Yogurt, plain, whole milk, 8-oz container	352	10.0

*Daily values (DVs) are reference numbers based on the recommended dietary allowance. They were developed to help consumers determine if a food contains a lot or a little of a specific nutrient. The DV for potassium is 3500 mg. The %DV listed on the Nutrition Facts panel of food labels states the percentage of the DV provided in one serving. Percent DVs are based on a 2000-calorie diet.

APPENDIX 57 Nutritional Facts on Selenium

Selenium is incorporated into proteins to make selenoproteins, which are important antioxidant enzymes. The antioxidant properties of selenoproteins prevent cellular damage from free radicals. Other selenoproteins help regulate thyroid function and play a role in the immune system. Selenium, as a nutrient that functions as an antioxidant, may be protective against some types of cancer. Its role in heart disease is not clear, but it may have a preventive role.

Plant foods are the major dietary sources of selenium. The content of selenium in food depends on the selenium content of the soil where plants are grown or animals are raised. Soil in Nebraska and the Dakotas has very high levels of selenium, and the southeast coastal areas in the United States have very low levels. Therefore selenium deficiency is often reported in these regions.

Selenium is also found in some meats and seafood. Animals that eat grains or plants that were grown in selenium-rich soil have higher levels of selenium in their muscle. In the United States meats, bread, and Brazil nuts are common sources of dietary selenium.

Most food labels do not list the selenium content of a food. The % Daily Value (DV) listed on the label indicates the percentage of the DV provided in one serving. A food providing 5% of the DV or less is a source, whereas a food that provides 10% to 19% of the DV is a good source. A food that provides 20% or more of the DV is high in that nutrient. It is important to remember that foods that provide lower percentages of the DV also contribute to a healthful diet.

Dietary Reference Intakes for Selenium for Children and Adults

Age (years)	Males and Females (mcg/day)	Pregnancy (mcg/day)	Lactation (mcg/day)
1-3	20	N/A	N/A
4-8	30	N/A	N/A
9-13	40	N/A	N/A
14-18	55	60	70
19+	55	60	70

Selected Food Sources of Selenium

Food	Micrograms per Serving
Brazil nuts, dried, unblanched, 1 oz	544
Tuna, light, canned in oil, drained, 3 oz	63
Beef, cooked, 3½ oz	35
Spaghetti w/ meat sauce, frozen entrée, 1 serving	34
Cod, cooked, 3 oz	32
Turkey, light meat, roasted, 3½ oz	32
Beef chuck roast, lean only, roasted, 3 oz	23
Chicken breast, meat only, roasted, 3½ oz	20
Noodles, enriched, boiled, ½ cup	17
Macaroni, elbow, enriched, boiled, ½ cup	15
Egg, whole, 1 med	14
Cottage cheese, low fat 2%, ½ cup	12
Oatmeal, instant, fortified, cooked, 1 cup	12
Rice, white, enriched, long grain, cooked, ½ cup	12
Rice, brown, long-grained, cooked, ½ cup	10
Bread, enriched, whole wheat, commercially prepared, 1 slice	10
Walnuts, black, dried, 1 oz	5
Bread, enriched, white, commercially prepared, 1 slice	4
Cheddar cheese, 1 oz	4

The dietary reference intakes for selenium are 20-70 mcg.

Sample Meal Plan

Breakfast

½ cup oatmeal (6 mcg selenium)
1 medium scrambled egg (14 mcg selenium)
1 small banana
½ cup low-fat/fat-free milk

Lunch

1 turkey sandwich (36 mcg selenium)
½ cup carrot sticks
1 bag baked chips

Dinner

3 oz meatloaf
½ cup macaroni and cheese (20 mcg selenium)
½ cup fresh steamed green beans

Snack

½ cup cottage cheese (12 mcg selenium)
½ cup fresh sliced peaches

NOTE: Take one multivitamin/multimineral supplement daily.

APPENDIX 58 Nutritional Facts on Zinc

Zinc is an essential mineral that is found in almost every cell. It stimulates the activity of approximately 100 enzymes, which are substances that promote biochemical reactions in the body. Zinc supports immunity; is needed for wound healing; helps maintain the sense of taste and smell; is needed for deoxyribonucleic acid synthesis; and supports normal growth and development during pregnancy, childhood, and adolescence.

Zinc is found in a wide variety of foods. Atlantic oysters contain more zinc per serving than any other food, but red meat and poultry provide the majority of zinc in the American diet. Other good food sources include beans, nuts, certain seafood, whole grains, fortified breakfast cereals, and dairy products.

Because zinc absorption is greater from a diet high in animal protein than a diet rich in plant proteins, vegetarians may become deficient if they are not monitored carefully. Phytates from whole grain breads, cereals, legumes and other products can decrease zinc absorption.

Dietary Reference Intakes for Zinc for Children and Adults

Age (years)	Males and Females (mg/day)	Pregnancy (mg/day)	Lactation (mg/day)
1-3	3	N/A	N/A
4-8	5	N/A	N/A
9-13	8	N/A	N/A
14-18	11 for males, 9 for females	12	13
19+	11 for males, 8 for females	11	12

Selected Food Sources of Zinc

Food	Milligrams per Serving	% Daily Value*
Oysters, battered and fried, 6 med	16.0	100
Ready-to-eat (RTE) breakfast cereal, fortified with 100% of the DV for zinc per serving, ¾ cup serving	15.0	100
Beef shank, lean only, cooked 3 oz	8.9	60
Beef chuck, arm pot roast, lean only, cooked, 3 oz	7.4	50
Beef tenderloin, lean only, cooked, 3 oz	4.8	30
Pork shoulder, arm picnic, lean only, cooked, 3 oz	4.2	30
Beef, eye of round, lean only, cooked, 3 oz	4.0	25
RTE breakfast cereal, fortified with 25% of the DV for zinc per serving, ¾ cup	3.8	25
RTE breakfast cereal, complete wheat bran flakes, ¾ cup serving	3.7	25
Chicken leg, meat only, roasted, 1 leg	2.7	20
Pork tenderloin, lean only, cooked, 3 oz	2.5	15
Pork loin, sirloin roast, lean only, cooked, 3 oz	2.2	15
Yogurt, plain, low fat, 1 cup	2.2	15
Baked beans, canned, with pork, ½ cup	1.8	10

Food	Milligrams per Serving	% Daily Value*
Baked beans, canned, plain or vegetarian, ½ cup	1.7	10
Cashews, dry roasted w/out salt, 1 oz	1.6	10
Yogurt, fruit, low fat, 1 cup	1.6	10
Pecans, dry roasted w/out salt, 1 oz	1.4	10
Raisin bran, ¾ cup	1.3	8
Chickpeas, mature seeds, canned, ½ cup	1.3	8
Mixed nuts, dry roasted w/peanuts, w/out salt, 1 oz	1.1	8
Cheese, Swiss, 1 oz	1.1	8
Almonds, dry roasted, w/out salt, 1 oz	1.0	6
Walnuts, black, dried, 1 oz	1.0	6
Milk, fluid, any kind, 1 cup	.9	6
Chicken breast, meat only, roasted, ½ breast with bone and skin removed	0.9	6
Cheese, cheddar, 1 oz	0.9	6
Cheese, mozzarella, part skim, low moisture, 1 oz	0.9	6
Beans, kidney, California red, cooked, ½ cup	0.8	6
Peas, green, frozen, boiled, ½ cup	0.8	6
Oatmeal, instant, low sodium, 1 packet	0.8	6
Flounder/sole, cooked, 3 oz	0.5	4

*Daily values (DVs) are reference numbers based on the recommended dietary allowance. They were developed to help consumers determine if a food contains a lot or a little of a specific nutrient. The DV for zinc is 15 mg. The %DV listed on the Nutrition Facts panel of food labels states the percentage of the DV provided in one serving.

Sample Meal Plan

Breakfast

¼ cup scrambled eggs
¾ cup ready-to-eat breakfast cereal with 25% DV (3.8 mg zinc)
½ cup sliced peaches
½ cup low-fat/fat-free milk

Lunch

1 chicken salad sandwich
½ cup carrot sticks
2 Tbsp Ranch dressing
1 bag baked chips

Snack

Yogurt, plain (2.2 mg zinc)

Dinner

3 oz grilled beef shank (8.9 mg zinc)
½ cup fresh steamed peas (0.8 mg zinc)
Side salad
1 small sweet potato
½ cup fresh pineapple

Snack

½ cup Trail mix (raisins, pecans, cashews, dried cranberries)

Index

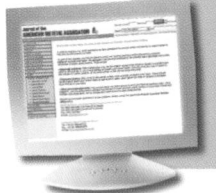

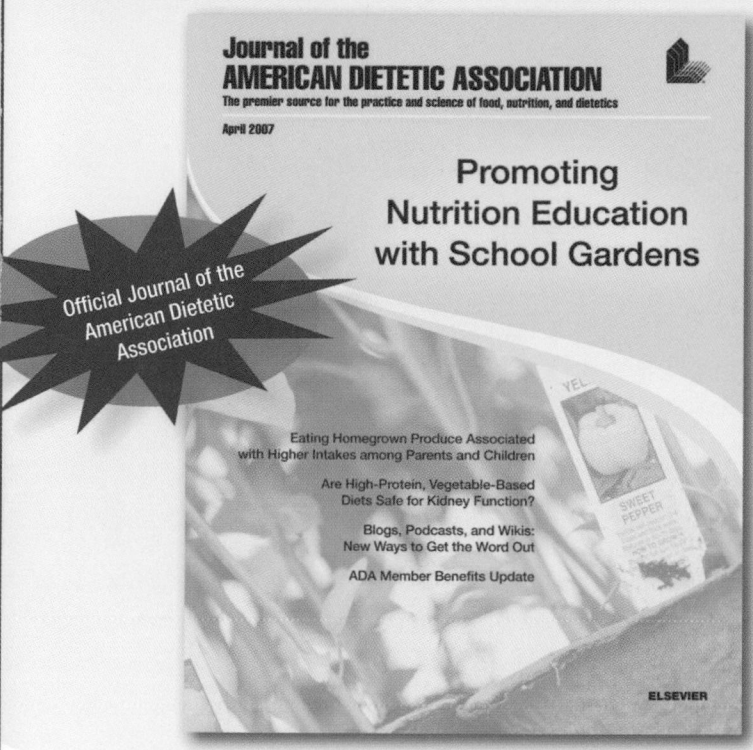
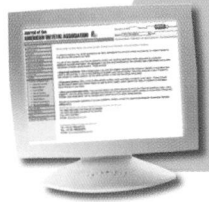